SURGERY

Principles and Practice

CONTRIBUTORS

WILLIAM E. ADAMS, M.D.

J. GARROTT ALLEN, M.D.

W. A. ALTEMEIER, M.D.

JAMES BARRETT BROWN, M.D.

LOUIS T. BYARS, M.D.

OLIVER COPE, M.D.

W. R. CULBERTSON, M.D.

ROBERT D. DRIPPS, M.D.

WILLIAM S. DYE, M.D.

WILLIAM T. FITTS, JR., M.D.

MINOT P. FRYER, M.D.

JOHN H. GIBBON, JR., M.D.

OSCAR P. HAMPTON, JR., M.D.

HENRY N. HARKINS, M.D., PH.D.

PAUL V. HARPER, M.D.

JOHN M. HOWARD, M.D.

DWIGHT J. INGLE, PH.D.

JULIAN JOHNSON, M.D.

ORMAND C. JULIAN, M.D., PH.D.

JACK LAPIDES, M.D.

H. J. McCORKLE, M.D.

K. ALVIN MERENDINO, M.D., PH.D.

FRANCIS D. MOORE, M.D.

CARL A. MOYER, M.D.

THOMAS FRANCIS NEALON, JR., M.D.

MICHAEL NEWTON, M.D.

PETER D. OLCH, M.D.

I. S. RAVDIN, M.D.

MARK M. RAVITCH, M.D.

FRED C. REYNOLDS, M.D.

JONATHAN E. RHOADS, M.D., D.SC. (MED.)

WARREN G. STAMP, M.D.

ARTHUR H. STEIN, JR., M.D.

WILLIAM H. SWEET, M.D.

SURGERY
Principles and Practice

HENRY N. HARKINS, M.D., PH.D.
Professor of Surgery, University of Washington
School of Medicine, Seattle

CARL A. MOYER, M.D.
Bixby Professor of Surgery, Washington University
School of Medicine, St. Louis

JONATHAN E. RHOADS, M.D., D.SC. (MED.)
John Rhea Barton Professor of Surgery, School of Medicine,
Professor of Surgery, Graduate School of Medicine,
University of Pennsylvania, Philadelphia

J. GARROTT ALLEN, M.D.
Professor of Surgery, Stanford University Medical School;
Attending Surgeon, Stanford–Palo Alto Hospital

SECOND EDITION

652 Illustrations

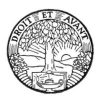

J. B. LIPPINCOTT COMPANY
Philadelphia   Montreal

DEDICATED TO

Alfred Blalock
Frederick A. Coller
Lester R. Dragstedt
Dallas B. Phemister
Isidor S. Ravdin

Contributors

WILLIAM E. ADAMS, M.D., F.A.C.S.
Raymond Professor and Chairman, Department of Surgery, University of Chicago; Attending Surgeon, Albert Merritt Billings Hospital

J. GARROTT ALLEN, M.D., F.A.C.S.
Professor of Surgery, Stanford University Medical School; Attending Surgeon, Stanford-Palo Alto Hospital

W. A. ALTEMEIER, M.D., F.A.C.S.
Christian R. Holmes Professor of Surgery and Chairman of the Department of Surgery, University of Cincinnati and the Cincinnati General Hospital

JAMES BARRETT BROWN, M.D., F.A.C.S.
Professor Clinical Surgery, Washington University School of Medicine, St. Louis; Senior Civilian Consultant in Plastic Surgery, Office of the Surgeon General, U. S. Army; Chief Consultant in Plastic Surgery, U. S. Veterans Administration, Washington, D.C.; Consultant in Plastic Surgery, Los Alamos Medical Center

LOUIS T. BYARS, M.D., F.A.C.S.
Associate Professor of Clinical Surgery, Washington University School of Medicine, St. Louis; Associate Surgeon, Barnes Hospital

OLIVER COPE, M.D., F.A.C.S.
Associate Professor of Surgery, Harvard Medical School; Visiting Surgeon, Massachusetts General Hospital

W. R. CULBERTSON, M.D.
Assistant Professor of Surgery, University of Cincinnati and the Cincinnati General Hospital

ROBERT D. DRIPPS, M.D.
Professor and Chairman of the Department of Anesthesiology, University of Pennsylvania School of Medicine; Physician-Anesthetist, Hospital of the University of Pennsylvania

WILLIAM S. DYE, M.D., F.A.C.S.
Clinical Associate Professor of Surgery, University of Illinois; Associate Attending Surgeon, St. Luke's Hospital, Chicago;

Consulting Surgeon, Veterans Administration Hospital, Hines

WILLIAM T. FITTS, JR., M.D., F.A.C.S.
Professor of Surgery, University of Pennsylvania School of Medicine; Chief of Surgical Division II, Hospital of the University of Pennsylvania

MINOT P. FRYER, M.D., F.A.C.S
Associate Professor of Surgery, Washington University School of Medicine, St. Louis; Assistant Surgeon, Barnes Hospital; Assistant Surgeon, St. Louis Children's Hospital

JOHN H. GIBBON, JR., M.D., F.A.C.S.
Samuel D. Gross Professor of Surgery and Head of the Department, Jefferson Medical College and Hospital

OSCAR P. HAMPTON, JR., M.D., F.A.C.S.
Assistant Professor of Clinical Orthopedic Surgery, Washington University School of Medicine, St. Louis

HENRY N. HARKINS, M.D., PH.D., F.A.C.S.
Professor of Surgery and Executive Officer, Department of Surgery, University of Washington School of Medicine; Surgeon-in-Chief, University Hospital; Chief Consultant in Surgery, Seattle Veterans Administration Hospital; Consultant in Surgery, Bremerton Naval Hospital, Children's Orthopedic Hospital and Madigan Army Hospital

PAUL V. HARPER, M.D., F.A.C.S.
Professor of Surgery, University of Chicago

JOHN M. HOWARD, M.D., F.A.C.S.
Professor and Chairman, Department of Surgery, Hahnemann Medical College, and Surgeon-in-Chief, Hahnemann Hospital; Consultant in Surgery, Walter Reed Army Medical Center, Washington, D.C., Fitkin Memorial Hospital, Neptune, N. J., Veterans Administration Hospital, Philadelphia; Consultant in Thoracic Surgery, Veterans Administration Hospital, Wilkes-Barre and Philadelphia, Pa.; Chief of Surgical Section (Hahnemann), Philadelphia General Hospital

DWIGHT J. INGLE, PH.D.
Professor of Physiology and Chairman of the Department, University of Chicago

JULIAN JOHNSON, M.D., D.SC. (MED.), F.A.C.S.
Professor of Surgery, University of Pennsylvania School of Medicine and Graduate School of Medicine

ORMAND C. JULIAN, M.D., PH.D., F.A.C.S.
Professor of Surgery, University of Illinois; Attending Surgeon, St. Luke's Hospital, Chicago

JACK LAPIDES, M.A., M.D., F.A.C.S.
Associate Professor, Section of Urology, Department of Surgery, University of Michigan Medical School; Chief, Section of Urology, Department of Surgery, Ann Arbor Veterans Administration Hospital; Chief, Section of Urology, Department of Surgery, Wayne County General Hospital

H. J. McCORKLE, M.D., F.A.C.S.
Professor of Surgery, University of California School of Medicine

K. ALVIN MERENDINO, M.D., PH.D., F.A.C.S.
Professor and Administrative Officer, Department of Surgery, Director of the Experimental Surgical Laboratories, University of Washington School of Medicine, Seattle

FRANCIS D. MOORE, M.D., F.A.C.S.
Surgeon-in-Chief, Peter Bent Brigham Hospital; Moseley Professor of Surgery, Harvard Medical School

CARL A. MOYER, M.D., F.A.C.S
Bixby Professor of Surgery, Washington University School of Medicine, St. Louis

THOMAS FRANCIS NEALON, JR., M.D.
Associate Professor of Surgery, Jefferson Medical College; Assistant Surgeon, Jefferson Hospital

MICHAEL NEWTON, M.D. (Penn.), M.A., M.B.B.CH. (Cambridge), F.A.C.S., F.A.C.O.G.
Professor of Obstetrics and Gynecology and Chairman of the Department, University of Mississippi School of Medicine; Chief Obstetrician and Gynecologist, University Hospital, Jackson; Consultant in Gynecology, Veterans Administration Hospital, Jackson

PETER D. OLCH, M.D.
Department of Pathologic Anatomy, National Cancer Institute, National Institutes of Health

I. S. RAVDIN, B.S., M.D., F.A.C.S., F.R.C.S. (HON.)
Professor of Surgery, Schools of Medicine, University of Pennsylvania; Vice President for Medical Affairs, University of Pennsylvania

MARK M. RAVITCH, M.D., F.A.C.S.
Associate Professor of Surgery, Johns Hopkins University School of Medicine; Surgeon-in-Chief, Baltimore City Hospitals

FRED C. REYNOLDS, M.D., F.A.C.S.
Professor of Orthopedic Surgery, Washington University School of Medicine, St. Louis

JONATHAN E. RHOADS, M.D., D.SC. (MED.), LL.D. (HON.), F.A.C.S.
John Rhea Barton Professor of Surgery, School of Medicine, Professor of Surgery, Graduate School of Medicine, University of Pennsylvania, Philadelphia; Surgeon-in-Chief, Hospital of the University of Pennsylvania; Director of the Harrison Department of Surgical Research, Schools of Medicine, University of Pennsylvania; Senior Surgeon, Children's Hospital of Philadelphia

WARREN G. STAMP, M.D.
Assistant Professor of Orthopedic Surgery, Washington University School of Medicine, St. Louis

ARTHUR H. STEIN, JR., M.D., F.A.C.S.
Associate Professor of Orthopedic Surgery, Washington University School of Medicine, St. Louis

WILLIAM H. SWEET, M.D., D.SC., F.A.C.S.
Associate Professor of Surgery of Harvard Medical School at Massachusetts General Hospital; Chief of Neurosurgical Service, Massachusetts General Hospital

Preface to the Second Edition

It is said that the child is father to the man. Similarly, with textbooks it may be true that success of a first edition patterns the development of the second. The success of the first edition of *Surgery—Principles and Practice* has exceeded our reasonable expectations. It is now up to the second edition to demonstrate its superiority over the first.

Before considering the features that are new to this edition let us summarize some of the distinctive characteristics which have proved to be useful and have been retained. Our six objectives remain as stated in the Preface to the First Edition. We have persisted in our policy of making the book basic yet practical. Again, the four editors have undertaken to write about half of the book and have assisted each other in revising their individual chapters. For the remaining chapters we have depended upon most of those individuals who worked on the first edition. The separate chapters, whether written by editors or by contributors, were gone over by two editors. Finally, all material was reviewed by the group of editors gathered round a table, discussing, analyzing and debating almost every sentence.

Features new to the second edition include Chapter 51, "History of Surgery," written by Drs. Peter D. Olch and Henry N. Harkins. It is hoped that this chapter will give a view of the background of modern surgery which will benefit student and practicing surgeon alike. The new Bibliographic Index will facilitate reference in the book to the many individual contributions to current surgical thought and technic. All of the original chapters have been brought up to date, and most of them have been drastically revised.

For this edition Dr. Henry N. Harkins assumed a major role in attending to certain logistic and production details, such as seeing that deadlines were met, but he was not in any other sense a chief editor. This is in conformity with our policy that the book be moderated in its concepts and content as a joint venture, but it is anticipated that the major responsibility will rotate with future editions, and the order of listing the editors on the title page and spine reflects this.

Dr. Henry N. Harkins is grateful to Dr. Arno G. Motulsky, Professor of Medicine and Genetics, for suggestions regarding portions of the chapter on the Spleen; to Miss Jessie Phillips, Medical Artist, and her staff who did the art work on his chapters; to his associates on the full-time staff, Drs. David Dillard, Lloyd M. Nyhus and John K. Stevenson; to members of his resident staff who helped with the proof: Drs. Earl E. Cammock, Niles D. Chapman, Robert E. Condon, Robert M. Leyse, Karl J. May, Robert A. McAlexander, Roger E. Moe, Hubert M. Radke, Lawrence E. Savage, Richard D. Sloop, L. Stanton Stavney and Loren C. Winterscheid, and especially to his editorial secretary, Mrs. Mary Stamper, and to his chief administrative secretary, Mrs. Margrette Mackey, both of whom rendered conscientious and capable assistance which was of inestimable help.

Dr. Carl A. Moyer wishes to acknowledge the constant help of his secretary, Mrs. Carol H. Wichlan.

Dr. Jonathan E. Rhoads wishes to acknowledge the aid of Drs. Lawrence C. Blair, John P. Dodds, William G. B. Graham, John Helwig, Jr., Paul G. Koontz, Jr., and Robert J. Reed, III, who as fourth-year medical students helped with the manuscripts, the references and the illustrations and gave valuable advice regarding the method of presentation on the basis of their recent and current learning experience. Miss Edna Hill is credited with the drawings in his chapters and most of those in the chapters of Drs. Hampton and Fitts, Dr. Johnson and Dr. Newton. Mr. R. L. Chapman, Mr. Robert J. Lucas and Miss Mildred M. Stelling performed most of the photographic work for these chapters. He is grateful to Dr. Eugene P. Pendergrass, Dr. Philip J. Hodes and Dr. Lawrence A. Post for radiologic illustrations, particularly in the chapters on the Biliary Tract and the Pancreas. Dr. J. Russell Elkinton was helpful with illustrative material for the chapter on

Fluid and Electrolytes; Dr. H. T. Enterline supplied illustrative material from the laboratory of surgical pathology; and Dr. John W. Thomas provided bibliographic assistance and helped prepare the section on Iron Metabolism. He is indebted to Dr. N. Henry Moss for certain data used in the chapter on the Pancreas and to Dr. James H. Robinson for bibliographic assistance for the Second Edition. He is indebted also to a former secretary, Mrs. Jane R. Lohmeyer, and to Mrs. Florence C. Fedalen for help in typing the First Edition. He is most indebted to his present secretary, Miss Jeanette B. Mager, who has carried the brunt of the preparation of his manuscripts for both editions and much of the organizational work for the book.

Finally, the Editors wish to acknowledge the helpful assistance of members of the staff of J. B. Lippincott Company, especially Mr. Stanley A. Gillet, Production Editor, Medical Department; Mr. Brooks Stewart, Medical Editor; and last, but not least, Mr. Walter Kahoe, Medical Director, whose sage counsel has been invaluable to us at all times.

THE EDITORS

Preface to the First Edition

The original reason for the writing of this textbook of Surgery was the idea that there was need for a surgical textbook that included to a greater extent the physiologic, biochemical, pathologic and anatomic bases of surgical practice. Each of the editors shared this view. A number of avenues of approach were considered, namely: the revision of an outdated text, the collection of a number of monographs covering the major surgical specialties, and the compilation of an entirely new textbook. The last approach was finally adopted because of the belief that it was the simplest way of providing the medical student with a background knowledge of anatomy, pathology, physiology and biochemistry so as to enable him to develop acumen in the diagnosis of surgical lesions; facility in the preoperative, operative and postoperative care of patients; and an understanding of the principles, aims and methods of conduct of the more important operations. More of the thought leading to the production of this book is set forth in the first chapter entitled, "Surgical Philosophy."

Our objectives, in addition to those listed above, were:

1. The provision in one volume of an introduction to general surgery and the surgical specialities (gynecology, neurosurgery, orthopedics, pediatric surgery, thoracic surgery and urology), excepting only ophthalmology and otorhinolaryngology, believing they are better presented in separate treatises.

2. The writing of the text in such a way as to lead the student to realize that surgical practice is not standardized or perfected, with the hope that by so doing research would be stimulated and open-mindedness fostered.

3. To emphasize that which is important in contemporary surgery, and more especially in the fields of cardiac, vascular and military surgery, even at the expense of omitting some of the rarer conditions and the finer points included in more compendious texts.

4. To emphasize the things that most doctors need to know about surgery rather than the more detailed points of technic that the surgeon uses. However, because we feel that one cannot understand surgery without some exposition of the central act—the operation— the text contains descriptions of several of the more important procedures with emphasis on technical principles rather than on minute details.

5. To cover the physiologic bases of surgical practice in such a way that the surgical resident, while learning technic by actual observation and experience, will find the book a useful reference in matters of nonoperative care, fluid therapy, shock, blood transfusion, nutrition and so forth.

6. To place some emphasis on what surgery has to offer, therapeutically, based on the prognosis of various conditions with and without the exercise of existent operative procedures.

Although the result of such an effort always falls short of the aspirations which lead one to undertake the task, we hope that the objectives have been realized sufficiently to justify the expenditure of time and effort.

We have concentrated responsibility for the text in the hands of as few persons as we could, without sacrifice of firsthand knowledge of the subjects covered. Thus, the four editors have undertaken about one half of the book. For the remaining half, we have called upon individuals of special competence in their respective fields, but with a broad scientific point of view, who are at the same time individuals with a gift for exposition. In an effort to obtain a cross section of surgical thought in the United States, one editor was selected from the West Coast, one from the East Coast, and two from the central part of the United States. The selection of contributors will also show a broad geographic distribution. The average age of the editors, when the book was begun in 1953, was 45 and at its completion in 1956, 48. In an effort to give the book as much cohesion and uniformity as possible, each chapter has been gone over by several of the editors, and insofar as possible this has been done at joint meetings where free discussion of differences of opinion was possible.

It should be emphasized that every effort was made to make this book a common effort of the many individuals who contributed to it. Each of the editors has contributed more than the others in some particular direction. Dr. Allen has written the largest number of chapters. Dr. Harkins has made the most exhaustive study of the proofs. Dr. Moyer had the most to do with organizing the original group and arranged for the largest number of the contributors. Dr. Rhoads kept in touch with the publisher and interrupted the active lives of the other editors to hold meeting after meeting, some for a few hours, some for as long as 12 days. Therefore, the arrangement of the names of the editors in the frontispiece is an alphabetical one. Should this text undergo subsequent editions, the editors plan a rearrangement in the order of their names, for it is hoped that the text will not come to be known by the name of a specific individual. It is desirable that such a text be moderated and maintained as a joint venture, presenting fairly and as nearly as possible the current teachings and practices in the ever-changing field of surgery.

The fact that the book has been produced without an editor-in-chief has undoubtedly increased the burdens of the publisher. To Mr. Walter Kahoe, Medical Director of the J. B. Lippincott Company, our special thanks are due. We are also grateful to Ellis Bacon, formerly Vice President of the J. B. Lippincott Company, and to Stanley A. Gillet, Production Editor of the Medical Department, who has carried so great a load in the production of the book. We also wish to express appreciation to Mr. T. A. Phillips and to Dr. Morris Fishbein for early interest and discussions.

Dr. J. Garrott Allen wishes to acknowledge the tireless efforts, in particular, of Miss Reecie Hodgson for her assistance in the preparation and the typing of his portion of this textbook of surgery, and also to Miss Wendy Kemp, Miss Lola Tucker, and Mrs. Carol Kemp for their generous secretarial services when the load became too heavy. This author is indebted to Miss Gladys McHugh for her suggestions and resourcefulness in the layout of a number of illustrations which she prepared for his portion of the text.

Dr. Henry N. Harkins is grateful to all those in his department who helped him with this work, but particularly to Miss Jessie Phillips and Mrs. Helen Halsey, who did all the new art work in his chapters; to his colleague, Dr. Lloyd M. Nyhus for much help; to members of his resident staff who helped with the proof: Drs. Paul W. Herron, John E. Jesseph, Thomas W. Jones, George I. Thomas, John K. Stevenson, and Roy R. Vetto; and especially to his administrative secretary, Mrs. Eleanore B. Ploger, whose intelligent and capable assistance was of help during all phases of the work.

Dr. Carl A. Moyer wishes to acknowledge the secretarial services of Mrs. Carmen Woelfle, Mrs. Mary Ann Sexauer and Miss Carol Hobbs.

Dr. Jonathan E. Rhoads wishes to acknowledge the aid of Drs. Lawrence C. Bair, John P. Dodds, William G. B. Graham, John Helwig, Jr., Paul G. Koontz, Jr., and Robert J. Reed, III, who as fourth-year medical students helped with the manuscript, references and illustrations and gave valuable advice regarding the method of presentation on the basis of their recent and current learning experience. Miss Edna Hill is credited with the drawings in his chapters and most of those in the chapters of Drs. Hampton and Fitts, Dr. Johnson, and Dr. Newton. Mr. R. L. Chapman, Mr. Robert J. Lucas and Miss Mildred M. Stelling performed most of the photographic work for these chapters. He is grateful to Dr. Eugene P. Pendergrass, Dr. Philip J. Hodes and Dr. Lawrence A. Post for radiologic illustrations, particularly in the chapters on the biliary tract and the pancreas. Dr. J. Russell Elkinton was helpful with illustrative material for the chapter on Fluid and Electrolytes; Dr. H. T. Enterline supplied illustrative material from the laboratory of surgical pathology; and Dr. John W. Thomas provided bibliographic assistance and helped prepare the section on iron metabolism. He is indebted to a former secretary, Mrs. Jane R. Lohmeyer, and to Miss Florence Conway for help in typing. He is most indebted to his present secretary, Miss Jeanette B. Mager, who has carried the brunt of the preparation of his manuscripts and much of the organizational work for the book.

THE EDITORS

Contents

xviii   **Contents**

Jonathan E. Rhoads, m.d., J. Garrott Allen, m.d., Henry N. Harkins, m.d., and Carl A. Moyer, m.d.

_____ CHAPTER 1 _____

Surgical Philosophy

THE FIELD OF SURGERY

Surgery is a form of service to man. It is a body of knowledge and experience developed by man to meet human needs in certain fields and has come to be entrusted to a group of individuals who have devoted themselves more or less successfully to acquiring this requisite body of knowledge and experience.

Its boundaries and those of internal medicine are more distinct in the popular mind than in practice. The practitioner of internal medicine generally abstains from performing formal operations and by doing so has more time which he can devote, at least in theory, to the study of diagnostic problems, for consideration of psychosomatic difficulties encountered by his patients, and for study of advances in the basic sciences.

A number of years ago one of our senior surgeons made the statement that internal medicine was becoming more and more surgical in its outlook, and, in all fairness, one must add that in the mid-twentieth century, general surgery has become more and more steeped in medicine and the basic medical sciences.

There is no more basic objective for the surgeon than the precept of the late John B. Deaver who said that a surgeon must be a medical man and something more—not something less.

Anyone who enters the field of surgery to escape from the rigorous mental discipline required to think straight in medicine is likely either to fail or, worse, do a great deal of harm.

HISTORICAL DEVELOPMENT OF SURGERY

The place of surgery in the whole of medicine and in our general social structure gains perspective from its historical development. The writings of Hippocrates (5th century, B.C.) reveal much valuable knowledge about the treatment of fractures, drainage of abscesses and the management of wounds. Surgery and medicine were practiced by the same people in his day. Many of the concepts in the Oath of Hippocrates are valid today, and one cannot consider the philosophy of medicine and surgery without coming back to it.

Much that the Greeks knew was transmitted to and utilized by the Romans, but medical knowledge apparently failed to grow until the Renaissance, when artists and sculptors began the study of anatomy, and Vesalius wrote *De Humani Corporis Fabrica* (1543). During the long centuries that intervened, medical care had become a function of the religious leaders, and it was not until the Church ordered the monks not to operate that they started having their barbers do it. Thus there grew up a group of barber-surgeons, the best of whom devoted themselves to surgery.

In England, there was a brief period in the early 16th century when the surgeons were associated with the physicians, but later in the 16th century Henry VIII granted a charter to the Guild of Barbers and Surgeons, and despite various attempts to break away the surgeons remained organized with the barbers until 1745. The distinction is still perpetuated in England where a surgeon is addressed as Mr. Smith while a physician is referred to as Dr. Smith.

In the United States and in other countries of the Western Hemisphere this distinction has not been made. For many years all medical men performed both medical and surgical services.

During the middle of the 19th century, the development of anesthesia, antisepsis and asepsis greatly increased the range and the effectiveness of surgery and this has been further extended by the development of roentgenology, the development of transfusion, of

1

parenteral nutrition (including water and electrolytes) and by antibiotics. Thus a great group of surgical specialties and subspecialties has developed. Today, the danger of overspecialization is often spoken of, but the probability is that the future will bring more rather than less specialization. The antidote to the danger envisioned appears to be a training period which includes a broad background in medicine and general surgery and some continued contact with these fields throughout the whole of one's professional life.

RELATION OF SURGERY TO MEDICINE

Surgery is very much a part of medicine in the broad sense. The fact that "medicine" is used to denote the whole field covered by the school of medicine in a university and also in a narrow sense to denote the department of that school which teaches internal medicine is often a source of confusion.

Certain common usages of the word "surgery" carry by implication such a slur on the profession that they cannot pass unnoticed. The British use the word as synonymous with the office of a practitioner. This usage has no place in the American language and therefore will not be commented upon. A common Americanism, however, is to say that on such and such a date the patient was taken to surgery—meaning that the patient had an operation performed. The phraseology is vaguely reminiscent of taking sheep to the slaughter, but our basic objection to it is the implication that the operation constitutes all or most of what the surgeon has to contribute. This may apply to the "ghost surgeon" but not to the more creditable representatives of the profession.

Surgery is a body of knowledge not only of operative technics but also of human anatomy, biochemistry, physiology, pharmacology, pathology, bacteriology, medicine and psychology (to mention only some of its components). This knowledge helps to determine from careful consideration of the patient's history and physical findings what laboratory aids are needed, and on the basis of these to decide the diagnosis or probable diagnosis. One must decide whether or not there is a worthwhile chance of helping the patient by operative intervention and if so when it should be done. Only on the basis of such preopera-tive study can one make proper decisions at operation about what should be done. The surgical responsibility then continues into the postoperative period for days or weeks, providing for the patient's recovery, averting and/or combating complications and endeavoring to restore the patient to complete health or to obtain for him the most in rehabilitation that his condition permits.

Obviously, the surgeon cannot do all these things alone. He must function as a member of a team helping to co-ordinate the services of clinical pathologists, radiologists, nurses, surgical house officers, social workers, rehabilitation experts and many others for the welfare of the patient.

Why, one may ask, must the surgeon concern himself with all this? Should not the job of co-ordination be left to the internist? In some cases the internist or general medical man can do a very good job of it. In other clinics, major shares of responsibility in preoperative and postoperative care are carried by anesthesiologists. Basically, however, a surgeon assumes the greatest responsibility for the patient when he operates on him. The responsibility as a rule is no less when he counsels against operation. The responsibility is of such a personal nature that it can hardly be escaped. Too often it involves life itself. A surgeon needs all the help he can get, but if things go badly when they need not go badly, the patient and the patient's family will hold him responsible, whether it be for his own acts or failure to act or for the performance of others involved in the case.

The division of responsibility between the medical man and the surgeon may be difficult. Usually agreement is reached on diagnostic probabilities and on the indications for operation. It is then generally best for the primary responsibility to shift to the surgeon during the operative and the postoperative periods. Thus, the surgeon is in the position of a consultant up to the immediate preoperative period—the internist then becomes a consultant, usually until the patient is well enough to leave the hospital. This policy is supported by a broad experience which indicates (probably without statistical proof) that the surgeon who follows his patient carefully before and after operation achieves better results than one who acts solely during the period of the operation itself.

Recently, a group of general surgeons became so alarmed by the development of sub-specialties that they proposed a special organization partially to protect the general surgeon from the inroads of men in narrower fields. Thus we have the vascular surgeon, the thoracic surgeon, the neurosurgeon, the gynecologist, the urologist, the plastic surgeon, the proctologist, etc. There is no way to predict how far this process may go. It is dependent on the size of medical units. Thus, a 100-bed hospital will do well to support men in 2 or 3 of these specialties. The 1000-bed teaching hospital probably can support most of them. What then would be possible in a 10,000-bed hospital, if such came into being? Who can say that a man who devotes 90 per cent of his time to hernia cases might not gain experience and be able to evaluate methods that would permit him to excel in this field? Another might concentrate on abdomino-perineal resections, another on gastric resections, et cetera.

It is obviously important that talent be on hand at operations to cope with unexpected findings and occurrences and especially to recognize things outside the narrowly specialized field. It is here that breadth of training appears to be an essential to safe surgery and safe medicine.

Therefore, young men entering surgery should avail themselves of broad training and education, even though they have definite plans for going into a highly specialized field.

OBLIGATIONS OF THE SURGEON BEYOND PATIENT CARE

The Oath of Hippocrates not only binds the physician to restrict his relations with patients to the care of illness or injury and to eschew social entanglements, particularly of a sexual character, but it also contains some less widely known provisions for the perpetuation of medical knowledge.

The physician is to care for his teacher as for a member of his own family and he must pass on his knowledge to the children of his teacher if they want to study medicine.

The practicing physician uses almost entirely knowledge that has been transferred to him and he often receives payment for his services without much thought of his debt to the past. If he contributes nothing either to the transfer of old knowledge to those who

must succeed him or to the discovery of new knowledge through experience or experiment, he is purely a parasite in his relations with his profession. He may still be a useful member of society as a purveyor of medical knowledge to the consumer but he adds nothing to the continuity or progress of his profession.

Particularly in surgery much depends on clinical experience. Through a proper transfer of knowledge, the experience of one surgeon may prevent others from making mistakes that cost the lives or impair the welfare of patients. When a surgeon or a physician speaks of his experience, he includes in the term knowledge which has come to him not only from his successful cases but also from his failures. It is, therefore, a serious obligation to pass on that which he has learned to the other members of his profession. This may be done by presenting case reports or analyses of series of cases to local or national medical societies and, if they prove to be of sufficient value, by publishing them in appropriate medical journals.

The further elucidation of clinical observations generally requires laboratory technics. The surgeon has certain peculiar advantages as an investigator which should be borne in mind. He is in intimate contact with patients and, if he is alert to the potentialities of modern laboratory methods, he is in a key position to see significant problems which are susceptible of solution. He may then be able to draw experts in the laboratory sciences into the study or to seek their advice in applying appropriate laboratory technics himself.

Furthermore, he has access to patients, and the decision of whether and when to try a new method or a new drug in these patients is frequently his. The moral issues raised by this situation are important ones. The obligation of the surgeon is primarily to his individual patient. He must not subject his patient to an unnecessary risk, even with the ultimate objective of benefiting thousands of other people, without full understanding by and consent of the patient. The availability of individuals clearly succumbing to disease who have more to gain than to lose by the trial of something new does much to bridge the gap which otherwise would exist between what is good for the individual and what is good for others. Here, as everywhere in surgery, the Golden Rule is the best guide to conduct.

The surgeon alone has the opportunity of

applying new operative technics. Furthermore, he has the unique opportunity of seeing and feeling internal lesions in the living patient. He also has certain opportunities to make physiologic observations at the time of operation and often to obtain biopsy material for histologic and biochemical study.

His technical skills open certain doors in animal experimentation, particularly where survival experiments are desirable. From the time of John Hunter (1728-1793) nearly all the great surgical investigators have leaned heavily on animals to try out their ideas and perfect their technics before applying them to man.

Surgery, like all of medicine, is an applied science, and the greater portion of the investigative work done by surgeons will consist in so-called applied research. However, the surgical investigator should not be blind to the opportunities he has of contributing to basic knowledge either in the clinic or the laboratory, and a number of contributions to fundamental biologic information have come from surgeons.

It should be emphasized that in clinical investigation more is generally to be learned from the careful study of a few cases than from the more casual review of long series.

Studies of great scientific contributions have shown that the years from 25 to 35 are the most productive. In medicine this means that a man's best contributions are often made during his period of study and training.

THE ART OF SURGERY

In one's pursuit of science in surgery one must not become oblivious to the fact that surgery is an art as well as a science. The art is thought of often as the manual dexterity which a surgeon must possess or acquire to do his work. This is a very important aspect but not the whole of it. It also includes much of the decision-making process which goes on constantly at the operating table. Differing degrees of skill in this field account for one man frittering away time on unimportant minutiae while another man abridges a procedure at the expense of thoroughness, and a third man strikes a proper balance by taking time to do what is important thoroughly without wasting it to achieve perfection in minutiae that are meaningless for the welfare of the particular patient.

A third and important aspect of the art of surgery lies in the field of talking to patients and their families. This is a most complicated art. What is said should depend on a host of perceptions of the patient's fears, of his doubts, of his past relationships with the surgeon and with other doctors. It is colored by the seriousness of the illness and the obstacles in the mind of the patient in the way of accepting treatment. It is necessarily colored by the surgeon's age, how well known he is in the community and how he is regarded in the patient's mind. The same surgeon at 30 may need a 10-minute exposition of facts to create the same degree of acceptance for a needed cholecystectomy that he could convey to the patient 20 years later in a sentence or two. Success in this field is again partly native ability and partly acquired skill.

One of the most important prerequisites to success in acquiring this skill is a strong enough desire for such skill to make one strive continuously to improve it. One must spend time in listening to patients and to their relatives and in trying to perceive and to understand their reactions. Considerable native modesty and a strong liking for people are most helpful. It is also extremely important to know something of one's self. When one's inner hackles rise in irritation or anger it is time to turn one's attention inward and to try to understand the why and the wherefore before giving vent to such feelings in remarks to the patient. While this brief discussion of the art of surgery is far from complete, perhaps it will convey some concept of what is involved.

Finally, if the surgeon is to do his utmost to advance his profession, he should endeavor to make opportunities for his younger colleagues to develop. This may require some self-denial on his part, some risk of being superseded in this field or that. If he is convinced that he is backing able and rightly motivated younger men, he should make some sacrifices and accept these risks.

OPPORTUNITIES FOR SURGICAL TRAINING

One purpose of setting forth our views about the obligations of surgeons in a textbook planned primarily for medical students is to provide a background for certain comments about the selection of training by those who contemplate specializing in this field.

How does one become a surgeon? How does he know a good residency opportunity from a poor one? If possible, select a medical school where the surgical department is interested in research as well as in teaching. If possible, obtain an internship in the best teaching hospital you can—be it medical, rotating or surgical in nature. Criteria which have proved useful in estimating the value of a hospital for internship are the following:

Ordinarily, the intern should have major responsibility in writing the orders for the patient's care. Rounds should be made regularly by the visiting staff with the house officers.

Do your utmost to be helpful on your hospital assignments. The unpopular assignments are often the ones where good performance will stand out most and be most appreciated.

So far as possible, steer clear of those institutions where the house is divided against itself but try to get an assistant residency in a teaching hospital. Most men are happier in a residency system which does not require progressive elimination of the fit by the more fit. The old pyramidal system which eliminates men at the end of each year may lead to competition but at the same time is apt to produce poor working relationships and bitter disappointments.

It is a good rule during one's training period, as well as in the years that follow, to participate in at least one good scientific society meeting each year.

Finally, measure your chiefs by the standards discussed above. One who takes not only an interest but an active responsibility in helping his men another step up the ladder and has been successful in doing so generally affords a much better association than a man of the "take you and leave you" type, no matter how brilliant.

Monetary advantages during the training period should not be given primary consideration. It is usually wiser to emerge from a first-class training program heavily in debt than to avoid the debt by accepting less than the best

training opportunities for which one can qualify.

THE PLACE OF THE HEALING ARTS IN SOCIETY

Today the healing arts are the subject of close scrutiny by government officials and by the rank and file of voters. There are proponents and opponents of so-called "socialized medicine." The terminology employed by its proponents has placed those who are opposed to state or corporation controlled medical care in the position of being considered antisocial. Nothing could be further from the truth. No matter how it is practiced, medicine and its branches are basically social in their attitudes. Medicine is for society—not for society as an organization but for each and every individual composing it. Thus, we would not want medical care used as a tool of the state—for instance, to be turned off or on for political minorities; but there is never any question that the job of the doctor is to help the sick and the injured and this he must do whatever the framework in which he practices.

A considerable degree of independence of thought, judgment and action must be the surgeon's if he is to perform his essential functions. This independence may be threatened in the future by economic pressures, and we shall have to depend on those in the profession who will put patient welfare ahead of financial security or so-called professional advancement to demonstrate and thereby guard against the dangers of any systems which would suppress this essential independence.

The doctors of the past often were paid little or not at all. The doctors of the present are required to perform a major tax-collecting job for the Federal Government, and the doctors of the future may be, for the most part, salaried civil servants. Despite the overtones of the last designation, the relationship of the physician to his patient can still probably be about as good as the doctor makes it, provided that he does not start "taking his profit in leisure."

Future events seldom develop in exactly the way one foresees, and it is the judgment of the editors that the possibility of changes in medical organization should not deter any rightly motivated young man from going into surgery.

HENRY N. HARKINS, M.D.

——————————— CHAPTER 2 ———————————

Wound Healing

A thorough knowledge of wound healing will lead to a more intelligent practice of our art as well as to greater perfection in it.—MONT REID.

INTRODUCTION

A knowledge of wound healing is the central core of the science of surgery; in fact, surgery is dependent upon wound healing for its very existence. In some instances the surgeon is called upon to treat patients with wounds previously inflicted; in other instances he must strategically plan the making of a wound which is to be a part of a necessary operation. In the latter instance he should not only make the wound so as to give access to the dissection which is to be required but also so that the wound itself will result in as little harm as possible and will heal in an optimum fashion.

HISTORICAL

Only a few high points can be given because the history of the study of wounds is indeed the history of surgery itself. A well-known incident is when Ambroïse Paré (1510-1590), one of the greatest army surgeons of all time, ran out of the boiling oil then used to treat battle wounds. He had to treat the wounds without it and was satisfied with the results. This was an important turning point in surgical history. Paré's appreciation of the principle of avoiding harmful interference in surgical treatment is epitomized by the inscription on his statue: *"Je le pansay, Dieu le guarit"* (I treated him, God healed him).

Many of William S. Halsted's (1852-1922) major contributions had to do with wound healing. In more recent times the contributions of Harvey (1929) and of Howes and Harvey (1935) are outstanding.

MECHANISM OF WOUND HEALING

To explain better the simultaneous catabolic and anabolic phases of wound healing, an analogy can be drawn between a bombed city and a wound. The soldiers and the repair workers on the one hand correspond to the cellular (leukocytes, etc.) and fluid elements which approach the wound both to break down and remove damaged tissue and to build up new tissue. New avenues of communication built to the damaged city correspond to the ingrowth of vascular buds to the wound which form granulation tissue. In a bombed city the work of restoration is facilitated if the workers can devote their complete attention to the job at hand. But in the presence of remnants of enemy forces (corresponding to bacteria) and unnecessary obstacles (corresponding to excessive sutures or other foreign bodies placed in the wound), they can give only a part of their time to the task of restoration, the rest being diverted to extraneous pursuits. In a wound, the digestion of large strands of catgut may seem as necessary to the leukocytes in the early inflammatory phase of wound healing as is the disposal of other dead tissue.

TYPES OF HEALING

Healing of wounds can be divided into 3 types (Fig. 2-1): (1) Healing by *first intention* (*per primam intensionum: primary union*). This involves the primary suture and healing of an aseptic, accurately closed, incised wound. An example is a healed sutured incision. In instances of primary union granulation tissue approaches the irreducible minimum. (2) Healing by *second intention* (*granulation*). This involves a defect which is first covered by granulation tissue and then closed by contraction and by secondary ingrowth of epithelium. Another way of stating this is that healing occurs by granulation in wounds where primary union fails because of excessive trauma or tissue loss, infection, or because the wound surfaces have not been brought together; an example is a neglected third-degree burn which is forced to heal without grafting. The concept of Gillman, Penn, Bronks and Roux (1955) is to be considered—that in the healing of wounds by second intention (Fig. 2-1-B), the epithelium plays a greater role in the early stages than according to the classic concept. (3) Healing by *third intention* (*secondary suture*). If a deep wound has either not been sutured primarily, or later breaks down and then is sutured or resutured several days later when granulations are present, two apposing granulating surfaces are brought together. The result is a wider and deeper scar than is the case with healing by first intention. Examples are wounds that are deliberately left open for 4 or 5 days before secondary suture (see Chap. 23, "Military Surgery") or the secondary suture of a dehisced wound.

In discussing the different types of healing, one must differentiate between flat wounds (abrasions, burns, etc.) and deep wounds (avulsion injuries, shell fragment wounds, etc.). As a corollary to this difference in type there is the difference in healing which is essentially the difference between the healing of epithelial and mesothelial tissue. Epithelium limits the growth of granulations. Even though some granulation is necessary in all wounds, this is more requisite in deep wounds. The amount of eventual scar is a direct function of the amount of granulation tissue that is formed.

PHYSIOLOGY OF WOUND HEALING

The various responses elicited by a wound present a complicated yet orderly sequence of events. The relative intensity and duration of the different phases in this sequence depend on the type of wound, the presence or the absence of infection, and whether healing is by first, second or third intention. Recent reviews of the physiology of wound healing include those of van den Brenk (1956), Gillman and Penn (1956), Jackson (1958), Cuthbertson (1959), Connell and Rousselot (1959), Hoover and Ivins (1959), Jacob and Houck (1959), McMinn (1960), and Dunphy (1960).

A new technic to study the wound fluid and its possible relationship to healing is implantation of a plastic sponge or porous metal cylinder to obtain an assay (Edwards, Pernokas and Dunphy, 1957; Schilling, Joel and Shurley, 1959).

Phase 1. Initial Productive or Substrate Phase (about 5 days). This phase is also termed the lag, autolytic, catabolic or inflammatory phase. During this phase there is an outpouring of tissue fluids, accumulation of leukocytes and mast cells, and an ingrowth of capillary buds and fibroblasts. Damaged cells are catabolized. During this phase the coapted tissues can be separated with little force; hence, there is minimal gain in tensile strength; formerly this was called the lag phase. However, as Dunphy and Udupa (1955), and Shetlar, Lacefield, White and Schilling (1959) have shown, there is a rapid increase in hexosamine content of the wound and of other positive signs of the presence of mucopolysaccharides. The relationships between adenosine 5-metaphosphate hexosamine, methionine and mucopolysaccharides has been discussed by Udupa, Woessner and Dunphy (1956), Edwards and Udupa (1957), and Reynolds, Codington and Buxton (1958). Metachromasia reaches a peak about the 5th or 6th day when the first chemical and histologic evidence of collagen fibers develops (Fig. 2-2). It would seem that the formation of collagen is dependent on a contribution of material by fibroblasts which becomes collagen only in a favorable substrate. Collagen deposition is the *sine qua non* of wound healing. The contribution of the fibroblasts may be a soluble

A. FIRST INTENTION (Primary union)

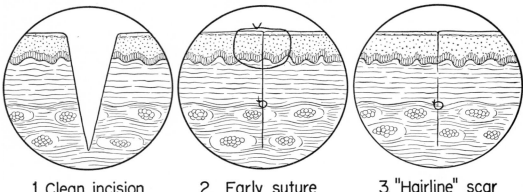

1. Clean incision   2. Early suture   3. "Hairline" scar

B. SECOND INTENTION (Granulation)

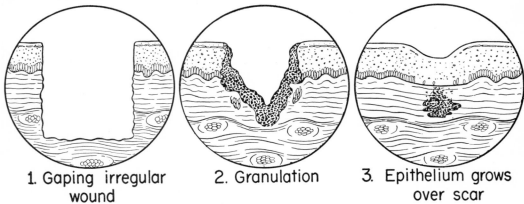

1. Gaping irregular   2. Granulation   3. Epithelium grows
      wound   over scar

C. THIRD INTENTION (Secondary suture)

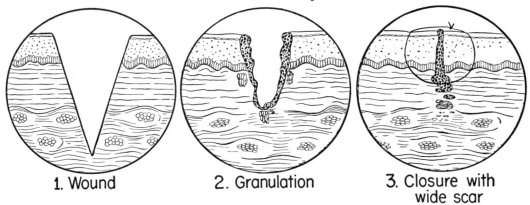

1. Wound   2. Granulation   3. Closure with
                                                wide scar

FIG. 2-1. Chronologic course of wound healing by first, second and third intention. In the final stage of second-intention healing it is to be noted that the underside of the epithelium is smooth and not serrated as normally. In the healing by second intention, the important role of contraction,

(Continued on facing page)

protein procollagenous substance essential for fiber formation. The ground substance may be related to mast cells and involves the ultimate appearance of mucopolysaccharides. Dunphy and Udupa stated:

Whatever the exact source of ground substance, it seems likely that some fraction of the mucopolysaccharides, probably a sulfated acid polysaccharide, provides a medium in which procollagen is converted to collagen. There is considerable evidence that ascorbic acid is essential to this change.

In summary, the following simplified and hypothetical equation gives a working basis for an understanding of collagen formation:

The important conclusion to be drawn from Dunphy's work is that even during the first 5 days after wounding the first 2 components of the above equation are reacting even though only in the second phase of wound healing do they culminate this reaction in the formation of collagen.

Menkin (1940, 1950) has studied the first or "inflammatory" phase of wounds from the standpoint of substances produced by injured cells. These can be *summarized* as follows:

1. Leukotaxine: A substance which increases the permeability of capillary walls and causes diapedesis of leukocytes. This substance differs from histamine in that it does not cause

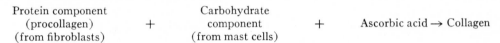

Protein component (procollagen) (from fibroblasts)	+	Carbohydrate component (from mast cells)	+	Ascorbic acid → Collagen

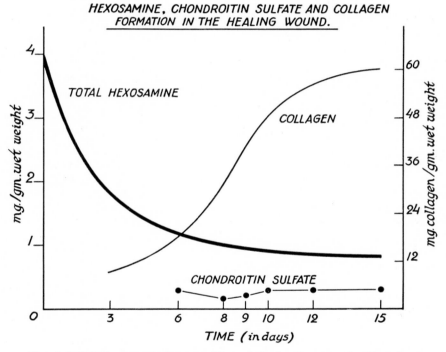

FIG. 2-2. Relative chemical composition of the healing wound with reference to (1) hexosamines; (2) the specific mucopolysaccharide, chondroitin sulfate; and (3) collagen. (Dunphy, J. E.: Ann. Roy. Coll. Surgeons England 26:82)

FIG. 2-1. (*Continued*)
which occurs in the patient in 3 dimensions and in the illustrations (B-2 and B-3) in 2, is shown. Contraction also plays a role in third-intention healing (C-2 & C-3). According to Gillman, Penn, Bronks and Roux (1955), the skin islands shown under the epithelium in B-2 and C-2 are typical of this phase of early healing. In C-3 an early phase is shown. Later the granulation tissue will be incorporated as a wide fibrous scar.

a fall in general blood pressure. (Kátó and Gözsy, 1956. Kohlson, Nilsson, Rosengren and Zederfeldt, 1960, have also reported on wound healing as dependent on the rate of histamine formation.)

2. Leukocytosis-promoting factors (thermolabile and thermostable components) (LPF)
3. Necrosin
4. Pyrexin
5. Leukopenic factors (leukopenin and the leukopenic factor)
6. Glucose
7. Possibly a growth-promoting factor

Menkin has studied these different factors and has separated them into discrete, although not chemically pure, fractions. The number of these substances indicates the complexity of the inflammatory process. This complexity is attested by the multiple symptomatology, so well expressed by Celsus (25 B.C.-A.D. 45): *"Notae vero inflammationis sunt quatuor, rubor et tumor, cum calore et dolore."*

Phase 2. Collagen or Second Phase (from about the 6th day until healing is complete). This phase is also called the proliferative or anabolic phase. As collagen forms (Fig. 2-2) there is a prompt decline in metachromasia (a histochemical test for the free sulfate groups attached to the polysaccharides) and in hexosamine content of the wound. At the same time there is a parallel rise in collagen content and in the tensile strength of the wound.

Dunphy and Udupa have also reported an alteration in these chemical changes in scorbutic guinea pigs. In such instances the productive phase is greatly extended, and there is no collagen phase. The concentration of mucopolysaccharides rises progressively, reaching levels per gram of tissue by the 12th to the 14th day far in excess of that observed in normal wounds about the 5th day. That this material is abnormal is evidenced by the fact that it does not stain metachromatically. These authors concluded:

It appears that in ascorbic acid deficiency the building blocks of wound healing are produced plentifully in the productive phase, but an important key to synthesis of collagen is lacking.

These authors summarize their work on wound healing as follows: "In this concept there is no 'lag phase' to wound healing, and normal tensile strength is a function of collagen formation not of fibroblastic multiplication as formerly postulated." (See Fig. 2-3.)

GENERAL FACTORS IN WOUND HEALING

There are both general and local influences which affect the healing of a wound. At one extreme is a clean sharp laceration of the skin of the face in a healthy young adult; at the other is a dirty ragged wound of the foot in an elderly diabetic with poor circulation and nutrition. Between these two extremes many factors determine the course of healing. These will now be considered under the separate headings of general and local factors in wound healing, realizing, of course, that to some extent these factors overlap. Also, it should be recognized that the normal rate of healing in a perfectly healthy patient is the optimum rate that can be attained. There is no known method by which healing can be forced beyond this normal rate (Zintel, 1946).

PROTEIN

Protein elements, including amino acids, are necessary as building blocks in the healing of wounds. There are several methods of diagnosing a probable protein deficiency in the tissues, most of which are, it is true, indirect methods. These include: history, as of loss of weight or of inadequate diet; physical examination, including observation of signs of recent loss of weight or of edema; blood volume estimation; and plasma protein estimation. The last listed of these, the plasma protein concentration (normal = over 6 Gm. %), may be helpful if the value is quite low, but sometimes normal plasma values do occur in the presence of tissue depletion, particularly when there is acute dehydration. Severe hypoproteinemia may not only be harmful because of a lack of "building blocks" but may also interfere indirectly with wound healing because of the local edema caused by the hypoproteinemic decrease in the colloid osmotic pressure of the plasma (Rhoads, Fliegelman, and Panzer, 1942).

Kobak, Benditt, Wissler and Steffee (1947), Williamson (1957), and Sisson, Lang, Serkes and Pareira (1958) studied the role of protein in wound healing. A special point to consider is that protein deficiency must be rather severe before it seriously interferes with wound healing. Burned rats fed on a diet containing only 0.24 per cent protein during the 60- to 90-day wound healing period healed their wounds as rapidly as control animals on a diet containing 23 per cent animal protein (Andrews, Morgan and Jurkiewicz, 1956).

The effect of endocrine factors (see below) may be indirect by improving protein synthesis (Long, 1942). Administration of 17-ethyl-19 nortestosterone (Nilevar) per os (Gouws, Silbermann and MacKenzie, 1958), and "growth hormone" (Prudden, Nishihara and Ocampo, 1958) reportedly hastened wound healing in rats.

ASCORBIC ACID

The delayed healing of wounds and even the breaking down of old healed wounds in scorbutic seamen has been described for over 200 years, the first report being by Anson (1748). More recently, Hartzell, Winfield and Irving (1941) found low vitamin C levels in the blood of patients developing evisceration following abdominal operations. Lund and Crandon (1941) showed in a human experiment that a wound can heal normally after 3 months on a vitamin-C free diet, but that after 6 months of such a diet, a typical scorbutic wound is obtained. Therefore, the element of time enters in, although in conditions of general body stress, the stores of ascorbic acid may be depleted more quickly.

Dunphy, Udupa and Edwards (1956) stated, "The basic defect of repair in ascorbic acid deficiency appears to be one of collagen synthesis . . . this defect is corrected within twenty-four hours following the intramuscular administration of ascorbic acid." Grillo and

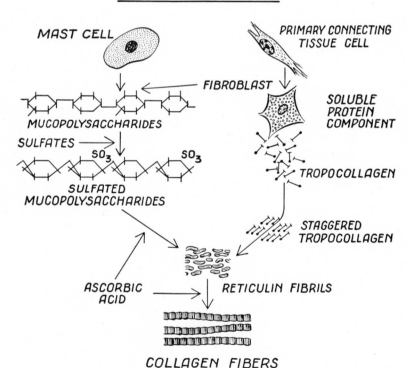

FIG. 2-3. A hypothetical model of some of the factors which contribute to the formation of collagen in the healing wound (Dunphy, J. E.: Ann. Roy. Coll. Surgeons England 26:79)

Gross (1959) reported that contraction of skin wounds in scorbutic guinea pigs shows an early delay, probably because of inadequate anchoring of the wound edges by collagen (also Grillo, Watts and Gross, 1958, and Watts, Grillo and Gross, 1958). (See also Schauble, Chen, and Postlethwait, 1960.)

Furthermore, in severe burns and after major surgical operations, vitamin C in large doses (e.g., 500-1,000 mg./day) may be advisable, even in previously well-fed individuals, to meet the general metabolic demands of the severe stress present.

Other vitamins, especially A, B and D, have been credited with beneficial action in the healing of wounds, either when applied locally or given by mouth or parenterally, but so far this action is not proved.

ANEMIA

It is commonly accepted that wounds will not heal as well as normally in an anemic patient. While this may not always be true, for practical purposes it is a good working hypothesis, and attempts to bring the red count close to normal should be made in all problems involving wound healing. The effect of "sludging" of erythrocytes is also important in wound healing (Zederfeldt, 1957).

NEUTROPENIA

A drop in neutrophils does not affect the healing of sterile wounds, but when infection is present, delay in wound healing does occur. This effect is undoubtedly secondary to the increase in the infection ("agranulocytic angina") and is especially apt to occur when the granulocytes are decreased.

EDEMA

Edema, whether of local or general causation, appears to interfere with the healing process. In some instances the edema may be secondary to hypoproteinemia as listed above.

AGE OF THE PATIENT

While there is little that can be done about this factor in any particular patient under consideration, its importance should be recognized. Du Nuoy (1916) showed that wounds heal more rapidly in young than in old animals, and that the rate of healing is inversely

proportional to a function of the age of the animal.

ENDOCRINE FACTORS

After a severe trauma (e.g., major surgical operation), there is a cyclic progression of events during part of which the survival of the organism is of pre-eminent importance and during part of which healing of the local wound gets major attention (Moore, 1953):

Phase 1. Adrenergic-Corticoid Phase (about 4 days)

Phase 2. Corticoid Withdrawal Phase (2 to 3 days)

Phase 3. Spontaneous Anabolic Phase (begins about the 7th to the 10th postoperative day and may last from 3 to 7 weeks)

Phase 4. Fat Gain Phase (may last weeks or months).

These cyclic changes are partially dependent on pituitary-adrenal alterations.

LOCAL FACTORS IN WOUND HEALING

Some of these (e.g., edema, inadequate blood supply) may be related to general abnormalities in the patient as a whole. Thus, too tight suturing or other local causes of edema may produce an exaggerated local edema in a patient with generalized hypoproteinemia. Similarly, suture of a wound with narrow or thin skin flaps which may have only a borderline blood supply will be more precarious in older patients with generalized arteriosclerosis than in children with their relatively excellent blood supply. On the other hand, others of these local factors (e.g., inadequate apposition of fascial layers) do not require the invocation of remote influences to explain their disastrous effects. A number of local factors affecting wound healing will now be considered individually under the following headings:

LOCAL TEMPERATURE

Ebeling (1922) determined that within limits for each 10° C. rise in temperature there is a twofold increase in the rate of healing of wounds in alligators. It is well known that there is a gradient in surface temperature, depending on the distance from the trunk and the head. There is a difference of about 6° C. or more in cases of peripheral arterial deficiency, between the higher temperature on the abdomen and the lower temperature on the feet. This has a practical application in that skin sutures should be left in almost twice as long for wounds of the feet (e.g., 12 days) as for wounds of the abdomen (e.g., 6 days). The wound healing delaying effects of hypothermia have been studied by Lofström and Zederfeldt (1957) and by Lundgren, Muren and Zederfeldt (1959). Similarly, Erici (1956) found that an environment of 30° C. caused quicker healing than 20° C. in rabbits. Leriche and Haour (1921) reported that wounds in sympathectomized areas heal faster than do control wounds. It is believed that the beneficial effect of higher temperatures upon wound healing, within physiologic limits, is consequent to the accelerated chemical reactions in the wound.

BLOOD SUPPLY

While blood supply is closely proportional to local temperature, it is not entirely so. The skin of the face and the neck has a better blood supply than that of the abdomen even though the local temperature is roughly comparable, the latter probably due to transmission of heat from the great body masses beneath the skin in each instance. However, with roughly equal temperature, the more adequate blood supply of the face and the neck promotes more rapid healing in these areas and permits earlier (e.g., 2 to 3 days) removal of skin sutures from the neck and the face.

Skin sutures should remain in place longer in fat persons, since their wounds tend to come apart more than in people of normal weight. As to whether this is due to mechanical factors (torsion effect of the weight of heavy fat pads) or to a less adequate blood flow through fat (not believed important by some students of wound healing) cannot be definitely stated at present. Also favoring retention of skin sutures in fat persons is the fact that disruption in an abdominal wound due to faulty apposition or healing of the fascia may not lead to the more serious evisceration if the skin sutures are still in place.

TRAUMA

A cleanly cut incised wound will heal more rapidly (healing by first intention) than an irregular ragged undébrided wound (healing by second or third intention). Similarly, an operative wound with much traumatic damage due to rough handling of tissues, prolonged pressure and tearing action of retractors, mass ligatures with large necrotic portions of tissue distal to the ligature, numerous plugs of necrotic tissue from electrocoagulation ("the tombstones of the coagulator"—Stevenson and Reid, 1947) will not "heal kindly." As in the analogy portrayed in the story of wounds given at the beginning of this chapter, this necrotic tissue must be destroyed before final wound healing is accomplished, as in a bombed city the rubble must be hauled away before rebuilding can be completed. The catabolic and destructive phase of the inflammatory process is exaggerated with prolongation of the initial "lag" period before the collagen or anabolic and proliferative phase of wound healing can take over, even though these two phases of wound healing can overlap to some extent. As a consequence, even in the absence of infection local edema and serum production and possibly a general febrile reaction are more apt to occur. Furthermore, the necrotic tissue itself, as well as the local reaction it produces, affords a highly favorable environment for the proliferation of bacteria which are present in essentially all wounds. The effect on wound healing rate of previous trauma has been studied by Sandblom (1954); Sandblom, Petersen and Muren (1953); Sandblom and Muren (1954); and Borgström and Sandblom (1956) in an excellent series of studies.

HEMATOMA FORMATION

Hematomas interfere with proper wound healing by preventing apposition of the walls of the wound ("dead space" formation), by prolonging the initial or destructive phase of wound healing, and by serving as a good culture medium for the growth of bacteria, and in some instances by interfering with the local circulation through pressure on blood vessels (Mason, 1940). In some instances respiration may be interfered with (e.g., a postoperative hematoma in the neck following thyroidectomy—usually due to slipping of a ligature on a superior thyroid artery) and in others heart action may be disrupted (e.g., pericardial tamponade). As pointed out in the discussion on drainage elsewhere in this chapter, meticulous surgical technic, including insistence on a dry field and the use of transfixion ligatures on large vessels, when there is any possibility that ordinary ligatures will slip off, is the way to control hematoma formation.

SEROMA FORMATION

A distinction must be made between postoperative bleeding and postoperative collection of serosanguineous fluid, although the two are somewhat related. Seromas contain thin fluid tinged with blood to a reddish-brown color. They may represent the degenerative state of hematomas, but more usually result from additional lymphatic leakage (as in a radical mastectomy) or from the reaction to foreign bodies as catgut or traumatized tissue. Some of the accumulation may be due to inability of the subcutaneous fat to absorb fluid as well as deep fascia and muscle. One cannot distinguish a sterile "seroma" from an infection without bacterial culture. The better the bacterial examination of "seroma" fluid, the fewer sterile seromas one will find. In this same connection, it is probable that more often the seroma precedes the infection, than the infection causes the seroma.

INFECTION

Infection may occur in an apparently cleanly incised wound but, at the same time, is favored by inadequate blood supply, trauma, and hematoma and seroma formation. Meleney (1935) estimated that from 35,000 to 60,000 bacteria fall into a sterile field during the course of a 1-hour operation with a resultant infection in 10 to 15 per cent of clean wounds. While this figure may be slightly reduced since the introduction of antibiotics (see Chap. 3, "Applied Surgical Bacteriology"), the recent prevalence of antibiotic-resistant staphylococcal infections indicates that this problem may be with us in a new form as well as in the old. Most certainly, an infection in a wound diverts some of the body forces—capillary buds, leukocytes, fibroblasts, tissue fluids, enzymes, etc. —which should go toward healing the wound, in the direction of repelling an even more dangerous trauma to the body, the secondary infection. An approximate expression of the probability of infection (I) based on controllable local factors in a given wound can be made by the following equation:

$$I = \frac{B \times P \times T}{V} \times fA$$

where B = the number of bacteria introduced into the wound; P = their pathogenicity; T = the degree of trauma; V = the blood flow; and fA = a function of the age of the patient.

The relationship of the results of the wound infection to the suture material used deserves some comment at this time. It is true that if a nonabsorbable suture such as silk is used in suturing a "clean" wound that later becomes infected (as following herniorrhaphy), that wound may continue to spew out silk sutures from troublesome sinuses for months or even years to come. This unfortunate complication, fortunately rare following careful aseptic surgery, and known as "silkosis," does not occur following the use of catgut as a suture material. On the other hand, when silk is used, even if silkosis does occur, the hernia seldom recurs, while if catgut is used, even though silkosis cannot result, once infection occurs, recurrence of the hernia is almost the rule. Furthermore, because of increased seroma formation, catgut-closed wounds may be slightly more apt to become infected in the first place.

SUTURE MATERIAL

The suture materials most commonly used include plain catgut, chromic catgut, silk, cotton, nylon and steel wire. Steel wire has the objections that it is difficult to handle and is difficult to remove if an incision has to be reopened but it has the advantage that in infected wounds it not only maintains the integrity of the wound as well as or better than silk but that it is seldom extruded. Catgut, silk and cotton, and nylon and tantalum and steel wire form a spectrum in this particular order. Plain catgut is the most rapidly absorbed, which is advantageous in some respects (if it is not accomplished before Phase 3 of the general metabolic response to injury, see above), but at the same time it produces the most reaction. Tantalum and steel are imbedded in the tissues forever but at the same time produce the least reaction. In some instances, wound healing may be progressing with difficulty either in a locally severe or infected wound or in a generally sick patient. In such cases it is not advantageous for the cellular and fluid elements of the blood to have to devote a major portion of their attention to absorbing catgut rather than to healing, according to the somewhat figurative hypothesis expressed on page 6 of this chapter. To these healing mechanisms the catgut may represent as serious an immediate menace as would staphylococci.

Localio, Casale and Hinton (1943) presented a detailed analysis of various suture materials used in surgery both from the mechanical and the bacteriologic aspects and from the standpoint of tissue reaction to the different sutures. They reported more serum collections and a higher percentage of infections following the use of catgut than after the use of nonabsorbable sutures in experimental wounds in rats. These authors reported that, "The delay in final healing of catgut sutured wounds, as noted in studies of tensile strength, and also microscopically, must be attributed to the more widespread destruction and acute inflammation of tissues in these wounds." Among the nonabsorbable sutures, silk and cotton produced more inflammatory reaction than did nylon and wire.

Dettinger and Bowers (1957) reported that Dacron was less reactive than Orlon and nylon, while the latter two were, in turn, less reactive than cotton or silk. A comprehensive study of the reaction to foreign materials, especially as used for vascular grafts, was reported by Harrison, Swanson and Lincoln (1957) and Harrison (1958).

The studies of Postlethwait, Schauble, Dillon and Morgan (1959) on plain and chromic catgut, silk, cotton, wire, nylon, Ramie, Nymo, Dacron and Teflon considered not only tissue reaction, tensile strength of the wound and tensile strength of the knot but also fraying tendency of the thread. Teflon received a high rating except from the standpoint of fraying, while Dacron's main shortcoming was the tendency of its knots to slip.

Certain suture materials may produce sensitivity reactions. This complication is most common with catgut (Kraissl, Kesten, Cimiotti, 1938).

ANTISEPTICS AND CHEMICALS

Antiseptics and chemicals may destroy bacteria but also tend to injure the body cells lining the wound. With their injudicious use, not only is wound healing impaired but also infection may be more apt to occur.

Farhat, Miller and Musselman (1959) and Rath and Enquist (1959) reported that triethylenethiophosphoramide (Thio-TEPA) does not delay wound healing in cats. On the other hand, Farhat, Amer, Weeks and Musselman (1958) found that mechlorethamine hydrochloride (nitrogen mustard) did interfere with such healing, but possibly no more than did the accompanying malnutrition induced by administration of the drug.

FOREIGN BODIES

Aside from sutures, it is now fashionable, particularly in orthopedic and vascular surgery, but to some extent in all branches of the art, to place innumerable foreign bodies in the tissues. Largely because of the pioneer work of Venable, Stuck and Beach (1937) who introduced vitallium, an alloy which is essentially nonreactive in the body, these foreign bodies (vitallium, stainless steel, nylon, Orlon, Vinyon "N," Teflon, Dacron, Ivalon, Lucite, Marlex—Usher and Wallace, 1958—etc.) do not produce much foreign body reaction, but they still are to be used with caution. Pieces of dead bone, tendon, muscle, and detached portions of intestine with mucous membrane are gross examples of *autogenous* foreign bodies that should not be purposelessly left in wounds.

One type of foreign body which caused considerable reaction in many wounds until about 1950, when its use was discontinued, is talcum (hydrous magnesium silicate). Talcum was used to facilitate putting on sterile rubber gloves. It entered into wounds not only from the outside of the gloves but also from frequent puncture of a finger of the gloves. Then the sweat-talc solution in the glove finger would leak into the wound. Talcum leads to granuloma formation, as first described by Antopol (1933). The talc, being relatively insoluble, remains in the tissues almost indefinitely and is recognized by double refractibility with polarized light.

Even though talcum is no longer used for

surgical gloves, the late results of talc granulomata are still coming to hospitals throughout the country for fistulas, chronic sinus tracts and especially intestinal obstruction associated with intestinal adhesions.

To obviate the dangers of talc granulomata, a treated powder derived from corn starch, "Biosorb" (R), was introduced. At first it was believed that this would entirely eliminate foreign-body reactions. More recent reports of starch granulomas have shown (Lee, Collins and Largen, 1952; Wise, 1955; Sneierson and Woo, 1955; McAdams, 1956; and Hyden and McClellan, 1959) that there is still a danger of foreign-body granulomata, even with the use of starch powders. Wise summarized his experiments in this regard as follows:

The starch caused less scarring and cellular reaction than talc, but more than occurred in controls in which no powder was used. In these experiments, starch was still visible in tissue sections 60 days after operation. Starch glove powder is preferable to talc, but is not entirely innocuous, and should be used as sparingly as possible. The surgeon should use as little powder as possible on his hands, and wash off all powder from rubber gloves before starting to operate.

This knowledge of the effect of foreign bodies, such as talcum or starch, on wound healing is the basis for the recommendations concerning washing of powder off surgical gloves (p. 220, Chap. 13, "Operative Surgical Care").

TECHNICAL FACTORS IN WOUND HEALING

Such factors are largely related to the local factors discussed above but are also dependent on the technical aims of the operation and on the general condition of the patient. The technic should be selected with a proper judgment as to the entire situation involved and not with a consideration of only one factor. Thus, drainage of joints must be decided upon not only from the standpoint of permitting blood to escape but also from that of the dangers of allowing infection to get in.

INCISIONS

A properly planned incision is fundamental to the performance of any surgical operation. From the practical standpoint a balance must be obtained between the desire to make a

wound which will heal as soon as possible and at the same time one which will permit as ready access to the place of operation as possible. Generally speaking, more surgical incisions are made too short than too long. The statement that a wound heals crosswise rather than lengthwise is true to a large degree. At the same time, an unnecessarily long incision involves more general trauma to the patient and more operative time is consumed in its closure.

Incisions on the surface of the body should be planned to follow certain dynamic "wrinkle lines" on the skin. As Kraissl (1951) pointed out, these lines are in many parts of the body at variance with "Langer's lines" (1861) with which they are often confused. Langer's lines are the result of a study of the static forces acting on the puncture wounds of the skin of a cadaver, whereas the wrinkle lines are produced by the dynamic forces acting on the skin of a living person. In general, the wrinkle lines run perpendicular to the action of the underlying muscles upon which they are dependent for their formation. Kraissl also pointed out that scars may become adherent

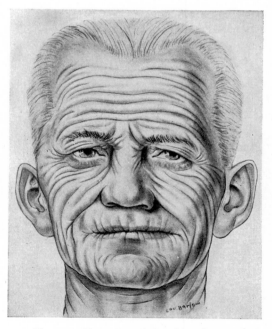

FIG. 2-4. Exaggerated drawing of normal face wrinkles. (Kraissl, C. J.: J. Plastic & Reconstruct. Surg. 8:5)

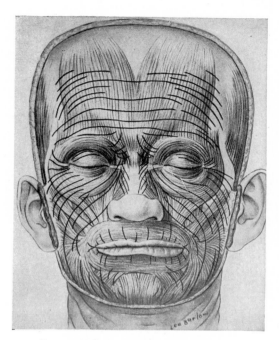

Fig. 2-5. The black lines in this Figure are tracings of the wrinkles shown in Figure 4 superimposed upon the muscles of facial expression. Note that these wrinkle lines uniformly are at right angles to the direction of contraction of the muscles. (Kraissl, C. J., and Conway, H.: Surgery 25:596)

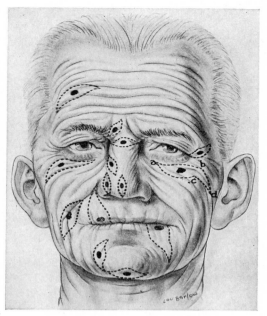

Fig. 2-6. Diagram of suggested lines of excision to allow the ultimate scar to fall in normal wrinkles. (Kraissl, C. J., and Conway, H.: Surgery 25:598)

to the underlying tissue and consequently they will least interfere with body mechanics if placed transversely across muscles and joints in the wrinkle lines. The scar then simply becomes an exaggeration of the normal physiologic perpendicular strands of connective tissue. In excising a lesion on the skin (warts, moles, tumors, etc.) incisions should be planned to have the resultant scars fall in the wrinkle lines (Metzger, 1957); whenever possible tubes, flaps and free grafts should be planned in a similar manner. Representative diagrams of the wrinkle lines according to Kraissl and Conway (1949) and Kraissl (1951) are shown in Figures 2-4 to 2-9.

Other rules concerning the placing of incisions are as follows: On the chest these should be placed parallel with the ribs. When incising an intercostal space, the incision should hug the superior border of the rib below because the neurovascular bundle is adjacent to the inferior border of the rib above. In making

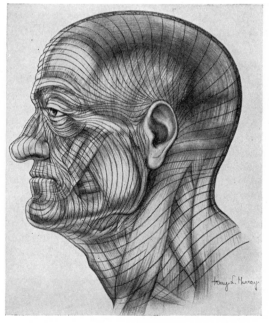

Fig. 2-7. Composite drawing of lines on the side of the head and the face superimposed on the muscles. (Kraissl, C. J.: J. Plastic & Reconstruct. Surg. 8:8)

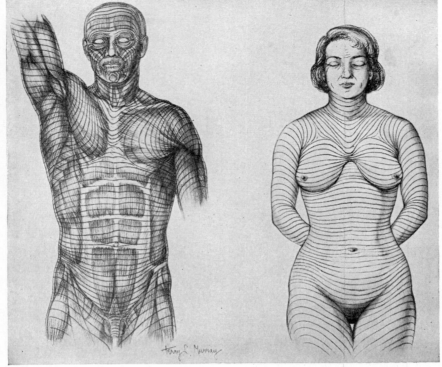

Fig. 2-8. Comparative lines on the thorax and the abdomen of the male and the female. The difference in pattern is due to the gravitational action of the mammary glands. (Kraissl, C. J.: J. Plastic & Reconstruct. Surg. *8*:11)

abdominal incisions they must be planned not only for the most probable operation but also so that if additional lesions necessitating more exposure are discovered, extension of the original incision can be accomplished most readily. For this purpose, horizontal or vertical incisions near the umbilicus can be lengthened in the desired direction with the greatest facility. In other instances, as when a McBurney (right lower quadrant muscle-splitting) incision is made for possible appendicitis and signs of perforated peptic ulcer are discovered, it may be preferable to close the McBurney incision and make a separate epigastric incision rather than to extend the original wound.

Careful consideration of underlying nerves, blood vessels, muscles and other structures is important in planning incisions. Thus, a long vertical abdominal incision will paralyze most of the muscular structure between it and the mid-line. For this reason, short transverse (or mid-line vertical of any length) abdominal

incisions are preferable since they cut the fewest important nerves in the abdominal wall.

ANATOMIC DISSECTIONS

The student of anatomy has learned to dissect out the structure he is attempting to expose, at the same time preserving important ("named") nerves, arteries, etc., in the region. The surgeon must do the same except that his dissection should be no wider than necessary and should also preserve the minute and "unnamed" blood supply. An example is the freeing of the external oblique aponeurosis in performing a herniorrhaphy: this structure should be freed no more than necessary to obtain exposure of the underlying structures and eventual apposition of fat-free edges of the aponeurosis on closure. To do more is to deprive the aponeurosis of part of its blood supply and create unnecessary open tissue spaces in which hematomas might form and infections might develop.

LIGATURES AND SUTURES

Some of the differentiating characteristics of absorbable and nonabsorbable sutures have already been considered under "Local Factors in Wound Healing." Sutures may be of various types (Fig. 2-10). In general, fine suture material inserted as atraumatically as possible and without strangulation of tissue is a desirable aim. Halsted (1913) epitomized this as follows:

I believe that the tendency will always be in the direction of exercising greater care and refinement in operating, and that the surgeon will develop increasingly a respect for tissues, a sense which recoils from inflicting unnecessary insult to structures concerned in the process of repair. . . . Healing is menaced when the circulation of the tissues to be united is impaired.

As shown in Figure 2-11, sutures which are placed too tightly cause tissues to become necrotic and tend to pull out, thus defeating their original purpose. Not only should the sutures be tied without excessive tension, but when they are inserted, the skin (or other edges to be approximated) should not be held tightly with the forceps. Stevenson and Reid (1947) go so far as to state: "Skin edges should never be picked up with hemostats or smooth forceps unless one intends to cut off the part that has been contused."

The use of "stay" sutures, either alone or to supplement a layer-by-layer closure, particularly of abdominal wounds, is advocated by many surgeons. Such sutures should also be placed without excess tension (Holman and Eckel, 1941).

CARE OF THE WOUND

During an operation, the wound edges and underlying structures should be kept moist with saline-soaked compresses applied at or slightly lower than body temperature. It is distressing to watch a surgeon who observes

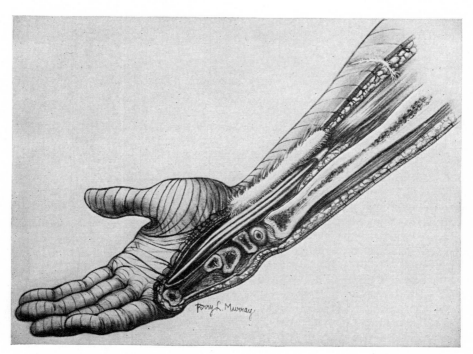

FIG. 2-9. Diagrammatic representation of transverse scar as compared with vertical scar on forearm. A transverse scar shown proximally, which is parallel with the skin lines, may become adherent to muscle without interference with function, but the vertical scar shown at the wrist, which cuts across the skin lines, splints the action of the muscle and the tendon and causes skin contraction because of muscular forces acting on it. (Kraissl, C. J.: J. Plastic & Reconstruct. Surg. 8:24)

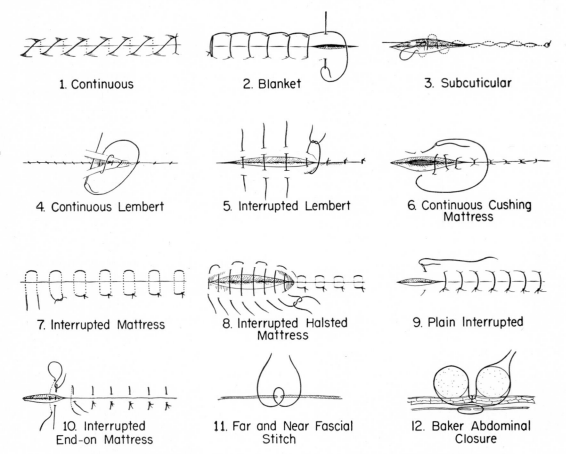

FIG. 2-10. Types of sutures commonly used. Types 4, 5 and 8 are utilized on the intestine; Types 3 and 10 on the skin; Type 11 on the fascia; and Type 12 on the entire thickness of the abdominal (or thoracic) wall. The other sutures depicted have more general applications.

all the other rules of surgical technic yet applies over-hot laparotomy pads to wounds, adding scalding to the incisional injury. At the close of most operations the author prefers that the operative field be irrigated gently with saline—again at body temperature—with the use of suction and sponging to remove all extraneous material, clots, secretions, and droplets and detached pieces of fat. As Stevenson and Reid (1947) stated:

Large strands of clot will flow into the solution like strands of water moss in a pond, but these clots will not become detached by themselves. They must be picked off with a forceps or gently rubbed loose with a gloved finger. Tissues stained with extravasated blood will become bright and fresh. Devitalized muscle will be bloody or cyanotic and should be trimmed away. All tags of tissue should be clipped loose.

Often the suction aspirator (a multiperforated Poole tip is best) will work better if it is surrounded by a gauze sponge. The sponge will catch pieces of fat and tissue that are too large to go through the perforations of the aspirator. To show the close relationship between local factors in wound healing and the general condition of the patient, one might cite the need for débridement of dead tissue, particularly devitalized muscle from extensive wounds. Not only will this permit more favorable local healing of all wounds, but if posttraumatic renal insufficiency should follow extensive injury, the lessened possibility for potassium absorption may be quite helpful.

HEMOSTASIS

This all-important element of surgical technic is too significant to be taken for granted. Hemostasis is of importance for 3 reasons: (1) it prevents blood loss and shock; (2) in a bloodless field one can dissect with greater accuracy; and (3) hemostasis helps to prevent postoperative hematomas.

DRAINAGE OF WOUNDS

Drains may be classified according to whether they are placed prophylactically, to prevent the accumulation of fluids in a fresh wound, or therapeutically, to permit the escape of fluids which have already accumulated. They may be also classified as to whether they are to drain off air (as from the pleural cavity in a patient with tension pneumothorax), pus (as from a perirectal abscess), blood (as from under a widely undermined abdominal wall flap in a fat person), or secretions (as from the region of the pancreas after

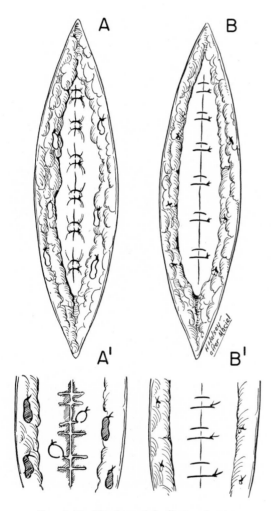

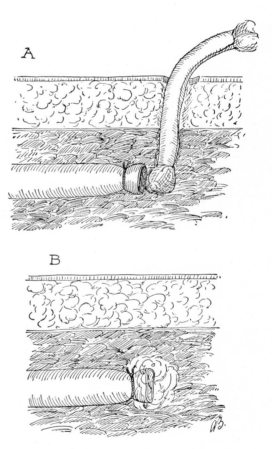

FIG. 2-11. The harmful effects of sutures that are too tight. (A) Too tight sutures and too big bites with ligatures. (A¹) Result 10 days later: necrosis of ligatured material, pulling out of sutures, necrosis and edema, etc. (B and B¹) Normal tension and result in 10 days. (Reid, M. R.: New England J. Med. *215*:756)

FIG. 2-12. A possible harmful effect of drains: (A) Showing how a drain removes the plastic exudate and invites infection by capillarity from the skin surface. (B) Showing plastic exudate about vessel when no drain is inserted. (McNealy, R. W.: Aneurysms *in* Lewis-Walters' Practice of Surgery, vol. 12, Hagerstown, Md., Prior)

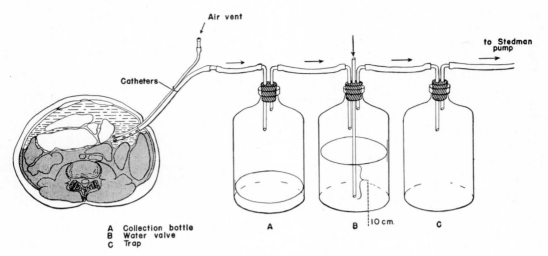

Air vent

Catheters

A   Collection bottle
B   Water valve
C   Trap

A   B   10 cm.   C

FIG. 2-13. Diagram of application of sump drain in abdominal surgery. The air vent usually has a gauze sponge loosely wrapped around the end of the catheter. (Scott, O. B., and Harkins, H. N.: West. J. Surg. *59*:619)

partial pancreatectomy). In some instances, a single drain may be placed to provide egress for more than one of these types of collections (as drainage of both blood and bile following certain biliary tract operations, or both air and pus following acute rupture of a lung abscess).

In modern surgery drains are still placed for the removal of air, pus, blood, or secretions. However, drainage for pus and for bleeding may be avoided more often than in the past and for different reasons. Most abscesses still require the placing of a temporary drain after incision. In infections of the peritoneal cavity, if operation is performed early (e.g., generalized peritonitis after perforation of a peptic ulcer), it is not considered mandatory to drain the peritoneal cavity and was not so even before the use of antibiotics. However, as advocated by Coller and Valk (1940) it is recommended that after closure of the peritoneum and the fascia in cases of peritonitis, the superficial part of the wound be drained for several days.

The harmful effects of using even soft drains must be considered. Not only will blood, etc., drain out, which is helpful, but bacteria may travel down the drains. In addition, the fibrinoplastic exudate (Fig. 2-12), which may be beneficial, is apt to be removed by drains.

Wilder (1955) stated that

A safe rule is: Use drains whenever an abnormal collection of fluid is encountered, be it contaminated, or infected material, blood, bile, or lymph, exudate or transudate; or whenever such an accumulation is anticipated. Avoid drains in joint spaces or in similar areas where excess reaction is detrimental to function.

Most drains are made of soft rubber (Penrose drains); in the neighborhood of tendons, large vessels, etc., only soft drains should be used, otherwise necrosis of these vital structures may result. Pitts (1954) showed that in rats drains made of Teflon ("dragon fur," polytetrafluorethylene) function better and produce fewer adhesions than Penrose drains. Rigid drains have an indication when suction is to be applied, particularly with an air vent producing a "sump" type of drain (Fig. 2-13) of the type popularized by Chaffin. Sump drains of rubber or stainless steel are used more widely now than formerly. *Drains should not be placed across tendon sheaths* in the foot or the hand lest the tendon become fixed and useless.

WOUND CLOSURE

Wound closure involves a final examination of the wound as to adequacy of hemostasis, a decision as to drainage, and a utilization of the type of sutures which are most applicable to the particular wound in the particular patient at hand. In all wounds inadequate or improper closure may result in wound disruption, but in the case of abdominal wounds the additional problem of evisceration is ever present. First heralded by the appearance of a *watery* blood-stained discharge on the dressings, disruption may lead to evisceration so rapidly that the first finding is that of warm coils of intestine protruding from the wound and even lying on the bed beside the patient. To prevent this catastrophe, particularly in persons with general or local factors (see above) predisposing to poor wound healing, all of the technical ability of the surgeon is called into play. Adequate bites of the fascial layers with special attention to preserving their circulation is paramount, along with a vigorous attempt to control the predisposing factors to poor healing.

DRESSINGS

As stated in Chapter 13, dressings are usually applied to wounds. All draining and discharging wounds are usually dressed. Some burns (see Chap. 17) are treated by exposure, and some surgeons do not apply dressings to sutured wounds which are not expected to drain. Dressings have 4 main functions: (1) protection, (2) absorption, as of drainage, (3) compression and (4) stabilization. Compression is still considered applicable for prevention of hematoma formation in "dead" spaces left in some wounds such as following a radical mastectomy for carcinoma of the breast. Even in such instances more aggressive means of eliminating the dead space, such as removable apposing sutures, followed by sump drainage may be preferable. On the other hand, compression may interfere with circulation, especially if considerable inflammatory swelling occurs under a compression dressing. Many surgeons no longer consider compression applicable for preventing inflammatory swelling and exudation from wounds of a type such as a thermal burn. In many instances, particularly with wounds of the extremities, a splint or plaster cast is advisable to help stabilize and immobilize the wound during the healing period.

HEALING OF SPECIAL TISSUES

Many aspects of wound healing are the same, irrespective of the special tissue involved, while others are different in each case. Some of the special features of healing are discussed below.

SKIN AND MUCOUS MEMBRANE

Epithelium shows a strong tendency to spread out and cover defects by both migration and multiplication of cells. At the same time, the farther epithelium has to travel from its original source, the thinner it is apt to become. Furthermore, the longer it takes to cover a defect, the more granulation tissue will form, and the greater will be the scar contraction. On the skin this results in deforming scars or webs; in the intestinal tract it may result in stricture formation. When scar skin spreads out to cover a granulating surface (healing by second intention, Fig. 2-1) it does not develop the wavy rete mucosum, the internal surface of the rete mucosum being more or less flat. This flatness increases the chances of separation of the rete mucosum from the cutis vera, especially from oblique blows, and explains why a large section of apparently well-healed scar epithelium may occasionally be raised up with a hematoma beneath it following a relatively trivial injury.

A rule may be stated that tissue is intended to be covered by either skin or mucous membrane which may be exposed to the air (ectodermal or entodermal layer), or by a layer of serosa which may not be exposed to the air (mesodermal layer). Examples of the former are the skin, the pharynx and the intestinal tract. Examples of the latter are the peritoneum, joint endothelium and the vascular intima. When trauma disrupts this continuity, the rule is broken, and scar tissue will result; the more scar tissue the greater the delay. Graham (1952) has expressed this as far as the skin is concerned by his alliteration: "Scab or skin." In the early stages of a flat wound when either a scab (in abrasions) or eschar (in burns) is present, skin grafting may be delayed. However, once the scab or eschar separates, usually in less than 3 weeks, skin grafting must be done promptly over any granulations that are present.

In the intestinal tract, an example of only recent observance of the rule against exposing the serosa to air is the following: Up until the past decade, practically all terminal ileostomies were fashioned by bringing the end of the loop of ileum about 2 to 3 cm. above the

ILEOSTOMY

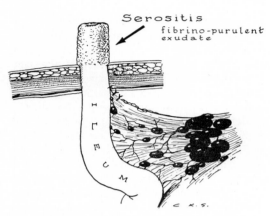

Serositis

fibrino-purulent exudate

FIG. 2-14. Serositis of an exposed ileostomy with secondary inflammatory hypertrophy of the lymph glands in the mesoileum. (Crile, G., Jr., and Turnbull, R. B., Jr.: Ann. Surg. *140*:461)

skin level, and consequently leaving a corresponding length of serosa exposed to the air. During the ensuing weeks, or months, the mucosa and the skin would tend to grow out over the serosa, finally joining so that no more serosa was exposed, and the "law" expressed in the previous paragraph was obeyed.

During this "maturation" process considerable scar tissue resulted, and certain remote effects, such as diarrhea, may have been related to the resulting serositis (Figs. 2-14 and 2-15).

Dragstedt, Dack and Kirsner (1941) attacked this problem by placing a dermatome skin graft over the exposed serosa. More recently Brooke (1952) and Crile and Turnbull (1954) devised other technics to obviate this lengthy maturation process. Brooke did this by turning down the distal half of the ileostomy stump over the proximal half and suturing the mucosal end immediately to the skin margin. Crile and Turnbull accomplished this by removing the outer seromuscular coat from the distal half of the ileostomy stump and then turning down the still attached mucosa over the proximal portion and suturing it immediately to the skin margin (Figs. 2-16 and 2-17). Peculiarly, a healed union between intestinal mucosa and skin is never attained. They merely coapt but do not unite and may be separated easily by minor trauma, producing more scar tissue each time a separation occurs.

GASTROINTESTINAL TRACT

Not only must the mucosa not have to bridge too great a gap, but for strength the

MATURATION OF ILEOSTOMY

5th DAY   8th-10th DAY   10th DAY

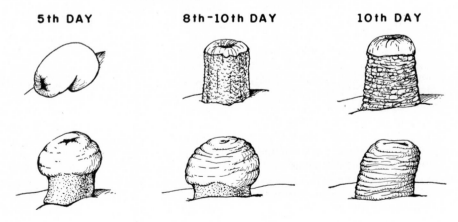

4th TO 6th WEEKS

FIG. 2-15. The usual protracted course of maturation of an ileostomy with a serosal surface exposed to the air. (Crile, G., Jr., and Turnbull, R. B., Jr.: Ann. Surg. *140*:461)

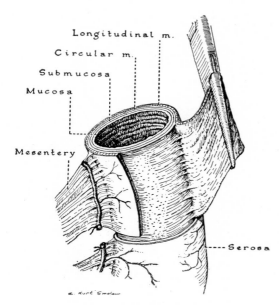

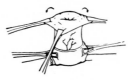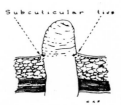

FIG. 2-17. Eversion of the submucosal-mucosal layer over the ileostomy (Crile-Turnbull technic). (Crile, G., Jr., and Turnbull, R. B., Jr.: Ann. Surg. *140*:461)

FIG. 2-16. The technic of removing the seromuscular coat from the distal half of the ileostomy. (Crile, G., Jr., and Turnbull, R. B., Jr.: Ann. Surg. *140*:461)

all-important submucosa must be approximated along with the rest of the muscular layer in intestinal suture. Approximation of the serosa, with or without inversion, is also advisable, this being done with the same row of sutures that approximates the submucosa. The importance of the submucosa in intestinal suture was first demonstrated by Halsted (1887) when he stated: "Each stitch should include a bit of the submucosa. A thread of this coat is much stronger than a shred of the entire thickness of the serosa and muscularis. . . . For us [it is] the most important coat."

NERVOUS SYSTEM

Generally speaking, nerve cells do not regenerate. Nerve fibers usually will regenerate if the cell remains intact and if they themselves are postganglionic, but not if they are preganglionic.

MUSCLE

Muscle tissue is generally considered to be so specialized that it will not regenerate after injury but will be replaced by fibrous tissue.

CARTILAGE

Since cartilage gets its nutrition, in part at least, from the joint fluid, joint wounds, even when drained, should be closed so that the cartilage is not exposed to air; furthermore, drainage is seldom advisable for other reasons. The biologic survival and growth of cartilage grafts, as opposed to the healing of cartilage in its natural locations, has been discussed by Schatten, Bergenstal, Kramer, Swarm and Siegel (1958).

BONE

Repair of bone occurs by osteoblastic growth from the periosteum and by creeping substitution of callus and of dead or transplanted bone. Thus, bone goes through a third phase of healing in addition to the productive and collagen phases, namely, a maturation or organizing differentiation (see Chap. 49, "Orthopedics").

TENDON

Since tendons are made up of parallel collagenous bundles, their repair involves a regrowth of these bundles, usually mixed with more or less connective tissue scar.

BLOOD VESSELS

When a blood vessel is injured, new tissue may arise theoretically from 3 sources: longitudinal ingrowth from the vessel walls, centripetal growth from the surrounding and supporting tissues about the vessel, and from the centrifugal deposition of platelets, fibrin and of cells from the blood stream. The first two of these sources are the most important. In the case of long pervious prosthetic vascular grafts, the second is the most important. In

CARREL

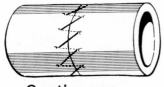

Continuous

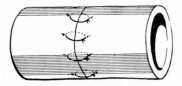

Interrupted

EVERTING MATTRESS

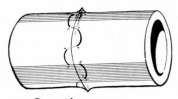

Continuous

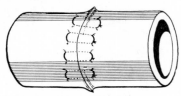

Interrupted

Fig. 2-18. Suture methods for use on blood vessels. The end-on coaptation (Carrel) method has the advantage of rapidity of performance but the disadvantage of placing considerable material in the lumen. The everting mattress, either continuous (Blalock) or interrupted (Jaboulay), method of intima-to-intima approximation has the advantage of placing little suture material in the lumen. (Sauvage, L. R., and Harkins, H. N.: Bull. Johns Hopkins Hosp. 91:279)

the case of arterial homografts, the elastic tissue layer serves as a barrier to the further ingrowth of tissue from the periarterial tissues so that the other mechanisms must play a role, the elastic tissue of the graft serving to give strength in the meantime. Sauvage and Wesolowski (1955) showed that longitudinal ingrowth of fibrous tissue seldom occurs into arterial homografts for more than 2 cm. from each anastomotic line. This implies that except near the ends, a long arterial homograft with intact elastic layer presents essentially a nonviable surface to the blood stream. These authors concluded that "the healing of arterial grafts is the same as that of other tissues that do not regenerate specialized elements." (See Chap. 40, "Peripheral Vascular Disease.")

The usual types of vascular suture are shown in Figure 2-18. The continuous over-and-over (Carrel) is the most frequently used, while the continuous everting mattress (Blalock) is used when an intima-to-intima approximation is desired, as in suturing veins, in

which the blood flow is slower and the danger of thrombosis is greater.

NEW DEVELOPMENTS IN THE STUDY OF WOUND HEALING

Progress in this field of surgical research is fundamental to all surgery. While it is impossible to compartmentalize such research, advances are being made along the following three fronts. The studies mentioned are intended to give an indication of the advances being made rather than as a comprehensive review of the subject.

HOMOGRAFTS

Autografts (from the same individual) of tissues or of organs are successfully utilized daily. Homografts (from another individual of the same species) are generally successful only if the donor is an identical twin. Apparent successes of certain homografts, as an arterial homograft implanted into the aorta to replace a thrombosed segment, are of benefit to the patient because the homograft serves as a fibrous tissue framework for ingrowth of new autogenous tissue, not because the graft survives as viable tissue. Heterografts (from another species) do not survive.

One aspect of homografting that has aroused interest is the "second-set" phenomenon. A second set of homografts taken from the same donor and transplanted to the same host sloughs more rapidly than the first set of homografts (Medawar, 1944). This observation indicates an acquired immunity and would fit in with the observations of Lehrfeld, Taylor, and Converse (1954, 1955) on the relation of survival time to implantation time of second set homografts. The cogent observation of Varco, MacLean, Aust and Good (1955) of a successful homotransplantation of skin in a patient with agammaglobulinemia offers strong support for the acquired immunity theory. When a homograft does *not* take, its rejection is accompanied by an early and uniform development of multiple thromboses in the recipient bed to which a skin homograft has been transplanted (Conway and Stark, 1954). As Dempster (1955) pointed out, one must consider not only the response of the host to the homograft but also the response of the homograft, if viable, to the host tissues.

There have been so many recent studies on the subject of homograft immunity that only a few key references can be given here (Billingham and Medawar, 1953; Andresen, Monroe, Squire, Haas and Madden, 1957; Edgerton, Peterson and Edgerton, 1957; Peer, Bernhard, Walker, Bagli and Christensen, 1957; Rapaport and Converse, 1957, 1958; Andresen and Monroe, 1958; Arguedas and Pérez-Tamayo, 1958; Braunwald and Hufnagel, 1958; Cannon, Terasaki and Longmire, 1958; Converse, Ballantyne and Woisky, 1958; Fisher, Axelrod, Fisher and Calvanese, 1958; Hubay and Holden, 1958; Kamrin, 1958, 1959; Kay, 1958; Kelly, Good and Varco, 1958; Mariani, Martinez, Smith and Good, 1958; Marino and Benaim, 1958; Markowitz and Schwartz, 1958; Martinez, Smith, Aust, Mariani and Good, 1958; Peer, Bernhard and Walker, 1958; Stark, 1958; Martinez, Smith, Shapiro and Good, 1959; Meeker,

Condie, Weiner, Varco and Good, 1959; Terasaki, Cannon and Longmire, 1959).

The grafting of organs, particularly the kidney, is also a new development. A kidney graft can be managed either by the use of an identical twin as donor (Murray, Merrill and Harrison, 1958, and Hume, 1958) or by using another type of donor and rendering the recipient able to temporarily accept the graft by preoperative sublethal whole body radiation.

RELATION OF STRESS TO WOUND HEALING

The early belief of a few that ACTH and cortisone would make all men alike as far as take of homografts is concerned was not sustained. However, such hormones and related stress do have some effect on wound healing. Howes, Plotz, Blunt and Ragan (1950) showed that very large doses of cortisone inhibit normal wound healing. Chassin, McDougall, Stahl, MacKay and Localio (1954) reported that while nonspecific stress of sufficient magnitude results in depression of the bursting pressure of standard laparotomy incisions in rats, such stress does not have this effect in adrenalectomized rats maintained on fixed doses of aqueous adrenal cortex extract. Montgomery and Green (1954) reported that tissue culture extracts applied locally will completely reverse cortisone inhibition of wound healing. Extending this into the realm of patients, Biström (1955) reported 7 patients with destructive inflammation who presented definite aggravation of symptoms after cortisone therapy. The inflammatory symptoms abated temporarily during therapy but were replaced by severe destructive changes, with increased inflammatory symptoms after cessation of cortisone therapy. This author concluded that "the examples given should serve as a warning against the uncritical use of cortisone."

Moltke (1955) studied the effects of another gland of internal secretion on wound healing, by utilizing the Sandblom-Petersen-Muren tensiometer to study healing wounds in guinea pigs. Moltke came to the following conclusions: (1) The wounds of thyroidectomized guinea pigs possess the same tensile strength as those of intact controls. (2) Thyroxine inhibits wound healing in intact as well as in thyroidectomized guinea pigs. (3) Thyrotropic hormone inhibits wound healing only in intact guinea pigs, whereas it does not appear to alter the normal course of healing in thyroidectomized guinea pigs.

Other recent work involves a study of the effect of a previous wound on the healing of a second wound. Sandblom and Muren (1954) have shown the need for careful controls in such experiments because even the change in cutaneous circulation following depilation for one wound may affect the rate of healing of the other wound. Savlov and Dunphy (1954) made observations which indicate that local factors are most important in determining the effect of preliminary local and distant incisions. Wounds of the abdomen made 15 days after wounds on the backs of rats did not show any greater tensile strength on the third day than 3-day abdominal wounds of a control group on which no previous wounding had been made. A summation of such an effect could not be demonstrated by multiple wounding on the back before an abdominal wound. On the other hand, 15-day-old abdominal wounds that were opened and resutured revealed a significant increase in tensile strength on the third day after exposure.

Raventos (1954) studied another type of stress, namely, total body exposure to ionizing radiation (500 r.). Irradiated mice showed a significant retardation of wound healing from the 6th through the 11th day after wounding, but not thereafter.

CHEMICAL CHANGES ASSOCIATED WITH WOUND HEALING

Various bits of evidence are beginning to accumulate which when fitted together will give a more precise idea of the inherent chemical changes involved in wound healing. The importance of sulfur is indicated by the work of Williamson and Fromm (1954). These authors reported a retention of sulfur after wounding in rats despite an increase in nitrogen excretion. Studies with S^{35} labeled cystine and methionine indicated that the metabolism of these amino acids is greater in wounded than in normal animals.

French and Benditt (1954) reported that, contrary to previous beliefs, alkaline phosphatase in healing wounds is not associated with connective tissue formation.

Schilling and Milch (1955) performed fractional analyses on experimental wound fluid from guinea pigs. Its crystalloidal and colloidal components were compared with those of the blood plasma of the wounded animals and of their pair-fed controls. Significant differences were observed in the protein and lipoprotein fractions.

BIBLIOGRAPHY

Andresen, R. H., Monroe, C. W., Squire, F. H., Hass, G. M., and Madden, D. A.: Types of host-graft interactions, Proc. Inst. Med. Chicago *21*:329, 1957.

Andresen, R., and Monroe, C. W.: Elimination of inflammation to homografts by transfusions of donor's blood cells, Proc. Cent. Soc. Clin. Research *31*:9, 1958.

Andrews, R. P., Morgan, H. C., and Jurkiewicz, M. J.: The relationship of dietary protein to the healing of experimental burns, S. Forum *6*:72-75, 1956.

Anson, G. (1748): Cited by Localio, Casale and Hinton (see reference below), 1943.

Antopol, W.: Lycopodium granuloma; its clinical and pathologic significance, together with a note on granuloma produced by talc, Arch. Path. *16*:326-331, 1933.

Arguedas, J. M., and Pérez-Tamayo, R.: The pattern of wound healing of skin autografts and skin homografts in the rat, Surg., Gynec. & Obst. *106*:671-678, 1958.

Billingham, R. E., and Medawar, P. B.: "Desensitization" to skin homografts by injections of donor skin extracts, Ann. Surg. *137*:444-449, 1953.

Biström, O.: The injurious effect of cortisone on destructive inflammation, Acta chir. scandinav. *109*:200-202, 1955.

Borgström, S., and Sandblom, P.: Suture technic and wound healing, Ann. Surg. *144*:982-990, 1956.

Braunwald, N. S., and Hufnagel, C. A.: Modification of homotransplantation by growth in tissue culture, Surgery *43*:501-509, 1958.

Brooke, B. N.: Management of an ileostomy including its complications, Lancet *2*:102-104, 1952.

Cannon, J. A., Terasaki, P. I., and Longmire, W. P.: Induction of tolerance to homografts by nonspecific pooled blood, A.M.A. Arch. Surg. *76*:769-773, 1958.

Celsus: Book III, cited by Menkin (see reference below), 1940.

Chassin, J. L., McDougall, H. A., Stahl, W., MacKay, M., and Localio, S. A.: Effect of adrenalectomy on wound healing in normal and in stressed rats, Proc. Soc. Exper. Biol. & Med. *86*:446-448, 1954.

Coller, F. A., and Valk, W. L.: The delayed closure of contaminated wounds: a preliminary report, Ann. Surg. *112*:256-270, 1940.

Connell, J. F., Jr., and Rousselot, L. M.: New concepts in the treatment of surgical wounds, Am. J. Surg. *97*:429-433, 1959.

Converse, J. M., Ballantyne, D. L., Jr., and Woisky, J.: The vascularization of skin homografts and transplantation immunity, Ann. New York Acad. Sc. *73*:693-697, 1958.

Conway, H., Sedar, J., and Stark, R. B.: Observations on the development of circulation in skin grafts. X. Effect of sodium salicylate on homologous skin grafts, Plast. & Reconstruc. Surg. *15*:56-60, 1955.

Crile, G., Jr., and Turnbull, R. B.: The mechanism and prevention of ileostomy dysfunction, Ann. Surg. *140*:459-466, 1954.

Cuthbertson, A. M.: Contraction of full thickness skin wounds in the rat, Surg., Gynec. & Obst. *108*:421-432, 1959.

Dempster, W. J.: Personal communication, July 20, 1955.

Dettinger, G. B., and Bowers, W. F.: Tissue response to Orlon and Dacron sutures: a comparison with Nylon, cotton, and silk, Surgery *42*:325-335, 1957.

Dragstedt, L. R., Dack, G. M., and Kirsner, J. B.: Chronic ulcerative colitis: summary of evidence implicating *bacterium necrophorum* as etiologic agent, Ann. Surg. *114*:653-662, 1941.

Du Noüy, P. le C.: Cicatrization of wounds. III. The relation between the age of the patient, the area of the wound and the index of cicatrization, J. Exper. Med. *24*:461-470, 1916.

Dunphy, J. E.: On the nature and care of wounds, Ann. Roy. Coll. Surgeons England *26*:69-86, 1960.

Dunphy, J. E., and Udupa, K. N.: Chemical and histochemical sequences in the normal healing of wounds, New England J. Med. *253*:847-851, 1955.

Dunphy, J. E., Udupa, K. N., and Edwards, L. C.: Wound healing: a new perspective with particular reference to ascorbic acid deficiency, Ann. Surg. *144*:304-317, 1956.

Ebeling, A. H.: Cicatrization of wounds. XIII. The temperature coefficient, J. Exper. Med. *35*:657-659, 1922.

Edgerton, M. T., Peterson, H. A., and Edgerton, P. J.: The homograft rejection mechanism, A.M.A. Arch. Surg. *74*:238-244, 1957.

Edwards, L. C., Pernokas, L. N., and Dunphy, J. E.: The use of a plastic sponge to sample regenerating tissue in healing wounds, Surg., Gynec. & Obst. *105*:303-309, 1957.

Edwards, L. C., and Udupa, K. N.: Autoradiographic determination of S^{35} in tissues after injection of Methionine–S^{35} and sodium sulfate–S^{35}, J. Biophys. & Biochem. Cytol. *3*:757-766, 1957.

Erici, I.: Effect of environmental temperature on the rate of wound healing, Acta chir. scandinav. *112*:346-347, 1956.

Farhat, S. M., Amer, N. S., Weeks, B. S., and Musselman, M. M.: Effect of mechlorethamine hydrochloride (nitrogen mustard) on healing of abdominal wounds, Surgery *76*:749-753, 1958.

Farhat, S. M., Miller, D. M., and Musselman, M. M.: Effect of triethylenethiophosphoramide (Thio-TEPA) upon healing of abdominal wounds, A.M.A. Arch. Surg. *78*:729-731, 1959.

Fisher, B., Axelrod, A. E., Fisher, E. R., Lee, S. H., and Calvanese, N.: The favorable effect of pyridoxine deficiency of skin homograft survival, Surgery *44*:149-167, 1958.

French, J. E., and Benditt, E. P.: Observations on the localization of alkaline phosphatase in healing wounds, A.M.A. Arch. Surg. *57*:352-356, 1954.

Gillman, T., and Penn, J.: Studies on the repair of cutaneous wounds, Mediese Bydraes *2*:121-186, 1956.

Gillman, T., Penn, J., Bronks, D., and Roux, M.: A re-examination of certain aspects of the histogenesis of the healing of cutaneous wounds: a preliminary report, Brit. J. Surg. *43*:141-153, 1955.

Gouws, F., Silbermann, O., and MacKenzie, W. D.: The effect of 17-Ethyl-19 Nortestosterone (Nilevar) on healing of experimental wounds, Canad. J. Surg. *1*:362-365, 1958.

Graham, James E.: Personal communication, 1952.

Grillo, H. C., and Gross, J.: Studies in wound healing. III. Contraction in vitamin C deficiency, Proc. Soc. Exper. Biol. & Med. *101*:268-270, 1959.

Grillo, H. C., Watts, G. T., and Gross, J.: Studies in wound healing. I. Contraction and the wound contents, Ann. Surg. *148*:145-152, 1958.

Halsted, W. S.: Circular suture of the intestine: an experimental study, Am. J. M. Sc. *94*:436-461, 1887.

———: Ligature and suture material: The employment of fine silk in preference to catgut and the advantages of transfixion of tissues and vessels in control of hemorrhage, J.A.M.A. *60*:1119-1126, 1913.

Harrison, J. H.: Synthetic materials as vascular prostheses. I. A comparative study in small vessels of Nylon, Dacron, Orlon, Ivalon sponge and Teflon; II. A comparative study of Nylon, Dacron, Orlon, Ivalon sponge and Teflon in large blood vessels with tensile strength studies, Am. J. Surg. *95*:3-15, 16-24, 1958.

Harrison, J. H., Swanson, O. S., and Lincoln, A. F.: A comparison of the tissue reactions to plastic materials, Arch. Surg. *74*:139-144, 1957.

Hartzell, J. B., Winfield, J. M., and Irvin, J. L.: Plasma vitamin C and serum protein levels in wound disruption, J.A.M.A. *116*:669-674, 1941.

Harvey, S. J.: The velocity of the growth of fibroblasts in the healing wound, Arch. Surg. *18*:1227-1240, 1929.

Holman, C. W., and Eckel, J. H.: Prevention of wound disruption with through-and-through silver wire stay sutures, Surg., Gynec. & Obst. *72*:1052-1055, 1941.

Hoover, N. W., and Ivins, J. C.: Wound debridement, A.M.A. Arch. Surg. *79*:701-710, 1959.

Howes, E. L., and Harvey, S. C.: The clinical significance of experimental studies in wound healing, Ann. Surg. *102*:941-946, 1935.

Howes, E. L., Plotz, C. M., Blunt, J. W., and Ragan, C.: Retardation of wound healing by cortisone, Surgery *28*:177-181, 1950.

Hubay, C. A., and Holden, W. D.: The effect of the properdin system upon first and second set homografts, Surg., Gynec. & Obst. *107*:311-316, 1958.

Hume, D. M.: Discussion of paper by Murray, Merrill and Harrison (see reference below), 1958.

Hyden, W. H., and McClellan, J. T.: Glove powder granuloma in peritoneal cavity, J.A.M.A. *170*:1048-1050, 1959.

Jackson, D. S.: Some biochemical aspects of fibrogenesis and wound healing, New England J. Med. *259*:814-820, 1958.

Jacob, R., and Houck, J. C.: A chemical description of inflammation and repair, Surg., Gynec. & Obst. *109*:85-88, 1959.

Kahlson, G., Nilsson, K., Rosengren, E., and Zederfeldt, B.: Wound healing as dependent on rate of histamine formation, Lancet *2*:230-233, 1960.

Kamrin, B. B.: The use of globulins as a means of inducing acquired tolerance to parabiotic union, Ann. New York Acad. Sc. *73*:848-861, 1958.

———: Successful skin homografts in mature non-littermate rats treated with fractions containing Alpha-globulins, Proc. Soc. Exper. Biol. & Med. *100*:58-61, 1959.

Kátó, L., and Gözsy, B.: Role of histamine and leucotaxin in function of cellular defense mechanism, Am. J. Physiol. *184*:296-300, 1956.

Kay, G. D.: Homologous skin grafts—factors affecting survival and a report illustrating prolonged survival, Canad. J. Surg. *2*:60-67, 1958.

Kelly, W. D., Good, R. A., and Varco, R. L.:

Anergy and skin homograft survival in Hodgkin's disease, Surg., Gynec. & Obst. *107*:565-570, 1958.

Kobak, M. W., Benditt, E. P., Wissler, R. W., and Steffee, C. H.: The relation of protein deficiency to experimental wound healing, Surg., Gynec. & Obst. *85*:751-756, 1947.

Kraissl, C. J.: The selection of appropriate lines for elective surgical incisions, J. Plast. & Reconstruct. Surg. *8*:1-28, 1951.

Kraissl, C. J., and Conway, H.: Excision of small tumors of the skin of the face with special reference to the wrinkle lines, Surgery *25*:592-600, 1949.

Kraissl, C. J., Kesten, B. M., and Cimiotti, J. G.: The relation of catgut sensitivity to wound healing, Surg., Gynec. & Obst. *66*:628-635, 1938.

Langer, K. (1861): Cited by Kraissl, C. J. (see reference above), 1951.

Lee, C. M., Jr., Collins, W. T., and Largen, T. L.: A reappraisal of absorbable glove powder, Surg., Gynec. & Obst. *95*:725-737, 1952.

Lehrfeld, J. W., Taylor, A. C., and Converse, J. M.: Relation of survival time to implantation time of second set skin homografts in the rat, Proc. Soc. Exper. Biol. & Med. *86*:849-851, 1954.

———: Observations on second and third set skin homografts in the rat, J. Plast. & Reconstruct. Surg. *15*:74-76, 1955.

Leriche, R., and Haour, J. (1921): Cited by Localio, Casale and Hinton (see reference below), 1943.

Localio, S. A., Casale, W., and Hinton, J. W.: Wound healing—experimental and statistical study, Internat. Abstr. Surg. *77*:369-375 and 457-469, 1943; Surg., Gynec. & Obst. *77*:243-249, 376-378 and 481-492, 1943.

Löfström, B., and Zederfeldt, B.: Effects of induced hypothermia on wound healing, an experimental study in the rabbit, Acta chir. scandinav. *112*:152-159, 1956.

———: Wound healing after induced hypothermia. II. An experimental investigation of the importance of intravascular aggregation of blood cells, Acta chir. scandinav. *113*:272-281, 1957.

Long, C. N. H.: A discussion of the mechanism of action of adrenal cortical hormones on carbohydrate and protein metabolism, Endocrinology *30*:870-883, 1942.

Lund, C. C., and Crandon, J. H.: Human experimental scurvy and the relation of vitamin C deficiency to postoperative pneumonia and to wound healing, J.A.M.A. *116*:663-668, 1941.

Lundgren, C., Muren, A., and Zederfeldt, B.: Effect of cold-vasoconstriction on wound healing in the rabbit, Acta chir. scandinav. *118*:1-4, 1959.

McAdams, G. B.: Granulomata caused by absorbable starch glove powder, Surgery *39*:329-336, 1956.

McMinn, R. M. H.: The cellular anatomy of experimental wound healing, Ann. Roy. Coll. Surgeons England *26*:245-260, 1960.

Mariani, T., Martinez, C., Smith, J. M., and Good, R. A.: Immunological tolerance to male skin isografts in female mice, Proc. Soc. Exper. Biol. & Med. *99*:287-289, 1958.

Marino, H., and Benaim, F.: Experimental skin homografts, Am. J. Surg. *95*:267-273, 1958.

Markowitz, A. S., and Schwartz, S. D.: Secondary rejection phenomenon elicited by primary homograft in pretreated rats, Proc. Soc. Exper. Biol. & Med. *99*:753-754, 1958.

Martinez, C., Smith, J. M., Aust, J. B., Mariani, T., and Good, R. A.: Transfer of acquired tolerance to skin homografts in mice, Proc. Soc. Exper. Biol. & Med. *98*:640-641, 1958.

Martinez, C., Smith, J. M., Shapiro, F., and Good, R. A.: Transfer of acquired immunological tolerance of skin homografts in mice joined in parabiosis, Proc. Soc. Exper. Biol. & Med. *102*:413-417, 1959.

Mason, M. L.: Wound healing, Illinois M. J. *78*:523-529, 1940.

Medawar, P. B.: The behaviour and fate of skin autografts and skin homografts in rabbits, J. Anat. *78*:176-199, 1944.

Meeker, W., Condie, R., Weiner, D., Varco, R. L., and Good, R. A.: Prolongation of skin homograft survival in rabbits by 6-mercaptopurine, Proc. Soc. Exper. Biol. & Med. *102*:459-461, 1959.

Meleney, F. L.: Infection in clean operative wounds: a nine year study, Surg., Gynec. & Obst. *60*:264-276, 1935.

Menkin, V.: Dynamics of Inflammation: An Inquiry into the Mechanism of Infectious Processes, New York, Macmillan, 1940.

————: Newer Concepts of Inflammation, Springfield, Ill., Thomas, 1950.

Metzger, J. T.: Cosmetic closure of simple lacerations, Delaware M. J. *29*:255-261, 1957.

Moltke, E.: Wound healing influence by thyroxine and thyrotrophic hormone. A tensiometric study (21665), Proc. Soc. Exper. Biol. & Med. *88*: 596-599, 1955.

Montgomery, P. O'B., and Green, C.: Reversal of cortisone inhibition of wound healing by tissue culture media, Proc. Soc. Exper. Biol. & Med. *86*:657-660, 1954.

Moore, F. D.: Bodily changes in surgical convalescence. I. The normal sequence—observations and interpretations, Ann. Surg. *137*:289-315, 1953.

Murray, J. E., Merrill, J. P., and Harrison, J. H.: Kidney transplantation between seven pairs of identical twins, Ann. Surg. *148*:343-359, 1958.

Paré, Ambroïse: Cited by Garrison, F. H.: An Introduction to the History of Medicine, ed. 4, Philadelphia, Saunders, 1929.

Peer, L. A., Bernhard, W. G., and Walker, J. C., Jr.: Full-thickness skin exchanges between parents and their children, Am. J. Surg. *95*:239-245, 1958.

Peer, L. A., Bernhard, W. G., Walker, J. C., Jr., Bagli, V. J., and Christensen, J. A.: Behavior of skin switch homografts between parents and infants, Plast. & Reconstruc. Surg. *20*:273-280, 1957.

Pitts, F. W.: Comparative study of the Penrose drain and drains of teflon, Proc. Soc. Exper. Biol. & Med. *85*:404-406, 1954.

Postlethwait, R. W., Schauble, J. F., Dillon, M. L., and Morgan, J.: Wound Healing. II. An evaluation of surgical suture material, Surg., Gynec. & Obst. *108*:555-566, 1959.

Prudden, J. F., Nishihara, G., and Ocampo, L.: Studies on growth hormone. III. The effect on wound tensile strength of marked postoperative metabolism induced with growth hormone, Surg., Gynec. & Obst. *107*:481-482, 1958.

Rapaport, F. T., and Converse, J. M.: Observations on immunological manifestations of the homograft rejection phenomenon in man: the recall flare, Ann. New York Acad. Sc. *64*:836-841, 1957.

————: The immune response to multiple-set skin homografts: an experimental study in man, Ann. Surg. *147*:273-280, 1958.

Rath, H., and Enquist, I. F.: The effect of Thio-TEPA on wound healing, A.M.A. Arch. Surg. *79*:812-814, 1959.

Raventos, A.: Wound healing and mortality after total body exposure to ionizing radiation, Proc. Soc. Exper. Biol. & Med. *87*:165-167, 1954.

Reid, Mont R.: Some considerations of the problems of wound healing, New England J. Med. *215*:753-766, 1936.

————: Introductory statement, cited by Caulfield, P. A., and Madigan, H. S.: Wound healing, Northwest Med. *54*:918-919, 1955.

Reynolds, B. L., Codington, J. B., and Buxton, R. W.: Wound healing: a study of the response of injured tissues to the coenzyme adenosine 5-monophosphate, Surgery *44*:33-42, 1958.

Rhoads, J. E., Fliegelman, M. T., and Panzer, L. M.: The mechanism of delayed wound healing in the presence of hypoproteinemia, J.A.M.A. *118*:21-25, 1942.

Sandblom, P.: The tensile strength of healing

wounds, an experimental study, Acta chir. scandinav. (Supp.) *89*:1-108, 1944.

Sandblom, P., and Muren, A.: Differences between the rate of healing of wounds inflicted with short time interval. I. Cutaneous incisions, Ann. Surg. *140*:449-458, 1954.

Sandblom, P., Petersen, P., and Muren, A.: Determination of the tensile strength of the healing wound as a clinical test, Acta chir. scandinav. *105*:252-257, 1953.

Sauvage, L. R., and Wesolowski, S. A.: The healing and fate of arterial grafts, Surgery *38*: 1090-1131, 1955.

Savlov, E. D., and Dunphy, J. E.: Mechanisms of wound healing: comparison of preliminary local and distant incisions, New England J. Med. *250*:1062-1065, 1954.

————: The healing of the disrupted and resutured wound, Surgery *36*:362-370, 1954.

Schatten, W. E., Bergenstal, D. M., Kramer, W. M., Swarm, R. L., and Siegel, S.: Biological survival and growth of cartilage grafts, Plast. & Reconstruct. Surg. *22*:11-28, 1958.

Schauble, J. F., Chen, R., and Postlethwait, R. W.: A study of the distribution of ascorbic acid in the wound healing of guinea pig tissue, Surg., Gynec. & Obst. *110*:314-318, 1960.

Schilling, J. A., Joel, W., and Shurley, H. M.: Wound healing: a comparative study of the histochemical changes in granulation tissue contained in stainless steel wire mesh and polyvinyl sponge cylinders, Surgery *46*:702-710, 1959.

Schilling, J. A., and Milch, L. E.: Fractional analysis of experimental wound fluid, Proc. Soc. Exper. Biol. & Med. *89*:189-192, 1955.

Shetlar, M. R., Lacefield, E. G., White, B. N., and Schilling, J. A.: Wound healing: glycoproteins of wound tissue. I. Studies of hexosamine, hexose, and uronic acid contents, Proc. Soc. Exper. Biol. & Med. *100*:501-503, 1959.

Sisson, R., Lang, S., Serkes, K., and Pareira, M. D.: Comparison of wound healing in various nutritional deficiency states, Surgery *44*:613-618, 1958.

Sneierson, H., and Woo, Z. P.: Starch powder granuloma: a report of two cases, Ann. Surg. *142*:1045-1050, 1955.

Stark, R. B.: Current concepts of the hemoplastic enigma, Bull. New York Acad. Med. *34*:561-577, 1958.

Stevenson, J. M., and Reid, M. R.: The fundamental principles of surgical technic *in* Bancroft, F. W., and Wade, P. A.: Surgical Treatment of the Abdomen, Philadelphia, Lippincott, 1947.

Terasaki, P. I., Cannon, J. A., and Longmire, W. P.: Antibody response to homografts. I. Technic of lymphoagglutination and detection of lymphoagglutinins upon spleen injection, Proc. Soc. Exper. Biol. & Med. *102*:280-285, 1959.

Udupa, K. N., Woessner, J. F., and Dunphy, J. E.: The effect of methionine on the production of mucopolysaccharides and collagen in healing wounds of protein-depleted animals, Surg., Gynec. & Obst. *102*:639-645, 1956.

Usher, F., and Wallace, S. A.: Tissue reaction to plastics, A.M.A. Arch. Surg. *76*:997-999, 1958.

van den Brenk, H. A. S.: Studies in restorative growth processes in mammalian wound healing, Brit. J. Surg. *43*:525-550, 1956.

Varco, R. L., MacLean, L. D., Aust, J. B., and Good, R. A.: Agammaglobulinemia: An approach to homovital transplantation, Ann. Surg. *142*:334-345, 1955.

Venable, C. S., Stuck, W. G., and Beach, A.: The effects on bone of the presence of metals; based upon electrolysis: an experimental study, Ann. Surg. *105*:917-938, 1937.

Watts, G. T., Grillo, H. C., and Gross, J.: Studies in wound healing. II. The role of granulation tissue in contraction, Ann. Surg. *148*:153-160, 1958.

Whipple, A. O., and Elliott, R. H. E., Jr.: The repair of abdominal incisions, Ann. Surg. *108*: 741-756, 1938.

Wilder, J. R.: Atlas of General Surgery, St. Louis, Mosby, 1955.

Williamson, M. B.: The Healing of Wounds, New York, McGraw-Hill, 1957.

Williamson, M. B., and Fromm, H. J.: Excretion of sulfur during healing of experimental wounds, Proc. Soc. Exper. Biol. & Med. *87*:366-368, 1954.

Wise, B. L.: The reaction of the brain, spinal cord and peripheral nerves to talc and starch glove powders, Ann. Surg. *142*:967-972, 1955.

Zederfeldt, B.: Studies on wound healing and trauma, Acta chir. scandinav. (Supp.) *224*: 1-85, 1957.

Zintel, H. A.: The healing of wounds, S. Clin. North America *26*:1404-1415, 1946.

W. A. ALTEMEIER, M.D., AND W. R. CULBERTSON, M.D.[*]

CHAPTER 3

Applied Surgical Bacteriology

Classification of Bacteria Important in
Surgery
Consideration of Effect of Pathogenic Bacteria
in Surgery
Resistance of Host to Bacterial Invasion

Applied surgical bacteriology implies the utilization of bacteriologic knowledge for the prevention, the diagnosis, or the treatment of infections seen in surgical practice. Surgery has advanced largely through contributions made by the various basic sciences—Philosophy, Anatomy, Pathology, Physiology, Bacteriology and Biochemistry—each contributing to its development. Bacteriology has given to surgery aseptic and antiseptic technics, methods of more accurate diagnosis, and effective means of preventing and treating many surgical infections. The expanding horizons of surgery have often been dependent upon the development of special methods of overcoming the hazards of postoperative infections.

Before the era of bacteriology, all wounds, both accidental and planned, became infected. The developing infections were classified as (1) benign, with "laudable pus," or (2) malignant, with "hospital gangrene" and a high mortality. With the advent of the bacteriologic era, the germ concept of infections was established, and antiseptic and aseptic technics were developed. These advances permitted the rapid expansion and the technical development of modern surgery. Without the control of bacteria and infection, this technical development would have been impossible.

During the past decade, many physicians and students had assumed that there were no longer any problems in the prevention or the control of surgical infections since a wide

selection of antibacterial agents was available. This belief was erroneous. Many of the old problems persisted, and new ones arose with the introduction of each new antibacterial agent.

Therefore, surgical bacteriology maintained its position of relative importance in clinical surgery. While it is true that we have means of controlling many infections, it is also true that bacteriologic studies and sensitivity tests are more important than ever for the successful utilization of these means. It is very questionable whether or not there are fewer infections now than 15 years ago. The number of specimens of pus submitted to clinical bacteriology laboratories for culture is much greater now than it was then. In addition, there are occurring recently an increasing number of severe and often fatal infections which are produced by bacteria that have acquired resistance to most or all of the available antibiotic agents.

CLASSIFICATION OF BACTERIA IMPORTANT IN SURGERY

A great host of micro-organisms may contaminate wounds, but the various types which produce surgical infections are fortunately more limited. Strictly speaking, the infecting agents are not all bacterial, others being spirochetal, fungal, parasitic and viral.

The more important of these may be classified as follows:

I. Aerobic bacteria
  A. Gram-positive cocci
    1. Staphylococcus
      a. aureus
      b. albus
      c. citreus
    2. Streptococcus
      a. hemolyticus

* From the Department of Surgery, University of Cincinnati College of Medicine and the Cincinnati General Hospital, Cincinnati, Ohio.

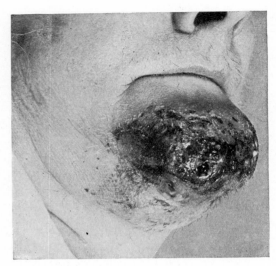

FIG. 3-1. A 65-year-old female with carbuncle of chin of 1 week's duration caused by hemolytic *Staphylococcus aureus*. No evidence of involvement of underlying mandible. Multiple draining sinuses and extensive necrosis of overlying skin are prominent.

    b. nonhemolyticus
    c. viridans
  3. Pneumococcus
B. Gram-negative cocci
  1. Neisseria gonorrhoeae
  2. Neisseria catarrhalis
C. Gram-positive bacilli
  1. Bacillus anthracis
  2. Corynebacterium diphtheriae
  3. Diphtheroid bacilli
  4. Mycobacterium tuberculosis
D. Gram-negative bacilli
  1. Escherichia coli
  2. Aerobacter aerogenes
  3. Proteus
  4. Pseudomonas aeruginosa
  5. Alcaligenes faecalis
  6. Klebsiella pneumoniae
  7. Salmonella typhosa
  8. Hemophilus influenzae
  9. Hemophilus ducreyi
II. Micro-aerophilic bacteria
  A. Gram-positive cocci
    1. Streptococcus
      a. hemolyticus
      b. nonhemolyticus

III. Anaerobic bacteria
  A. Gram-positive cocci
    1. Streptococcus
  B. Gram-positive bacilli
    1. Clostridia
      a. tetani
      b. welchii (perfringens)
      c. novyi
      d. septicum
      e. histolyticum
      f. sordellii
      g. sporogenes
  C. Gram-negative Bacteroides
    1. melaninogenicus
    2. funduliformis
IV. Spirochaeta
V. Higher micro-organisms
  A. Actinomyces
  B. Blastomyces
  C. Coccidioides
  D. Sporotrichum
  E. Candida albicans
  F. Aspergillus niger
  G. Endamoeba histolytica

The bacteria of greatest importance in acute surgical infections are the *pyogenic bacteria*. The term "pyogenic" (pus forming) is usually applied to the staphylococcus, streptococcus, pneumococcus, gonococcus and meningococcus. Sometimes it is applied to the colon bacillus and *Ps. aeruginosa* and other bacteria. The tubercle bacillus, although not considered a pyogenic bacterium, may produce typical thick creamy pus in "cold" abscesses.

The *Staphylococci* occurring in surgical infections may be classified into various subgroups on the basis of their cultural characteristics or their lysis by specific bacteriophages. As grown in culture, the *Staphylococcus* may be designated as *aureus, albus* or *citreus*, depending upon the color of its colonies. More recently it has been possible to type it by the use of approximately 32 specific bacteriophages. This organism is a normal inhabitant of the human skin and the nasopharynx, and it may be found in wounds as a pathogen or as a contaminant. In fact, it is often difficult to determine whether the organism isolated from many areas of infection represents a pathogenic or a saprophytic strain. A *Staphylococcus* which is hemolytic, coagulase positive, manitol-positive and of the *aureus* variety is usually pathogenic. In addition, the *80-81, 77* or *42B* bacteriophage types have been shown not only to be virulent varieties but also to have an unusual epidemiologic potential.

Pathogenic staphylococci usually cause rapid necrosis and suppuration, forming thick, creamy and odorless pus. Their infections display a tendency to remain localized as an abscess, which eventually heals after drainage. The favorable outcome which followed staphylococcal infection led to the old term of "laudable pus." On the other hand, strains of staphylococci may be very virulent and may produce serious or fatal invasive infections, such as septicemia and pyemia in which the organisms are circulated in the blood stream. The tendency of staphylococcic infections to remain localized is thought to be related to the production of an enzyme coagulase which produces thrombosis of vessels.

The *aerobic Streptococcus* may occur as one of several types; *hemolytic, nonhemolytic,* or *viridans.* Its strains may be normal inhabitants of the oral cavity, the upper respiratory tract, the vaginal tract, or the gastrointestinal tract. Virulent strains are prone to produce serious, invasive and rapidly developing infections which spread to involve wide areas of tissues. Necrosis may be produced, but there is much less tendency to form pus, the exudate usually being watery in character. The *Streptococcus* is regularly or frequently the etiologic agent in erysipelas, scarlet fever, acute tonsillitis, cellulitis, osteomyelitis (infrequent), septicemia, mastoiditis, lymphangitis, and many other infections. The tendency of streptococcic infection to spread has been attrib-

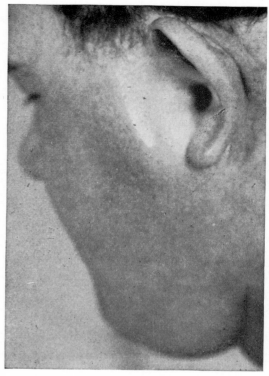

FIG. 3-2. A 24-year-old male with acute purulent parotitis and parotid abscess caused by hemolytic *Staphylococcus aureus.*

uted to the production of streptokinase which initiates fibrinolysis.

The *Pneumococcus* may be associated with infections of the lung and the pleura, septicemia, osteomyelitis, meningitis and sinusitis. Pneumococcic infections of the lung may be followed by empyema. The pus in such cases, although thin at first, rapidly becomes thick, creamy, mucoid, and contains much clotted

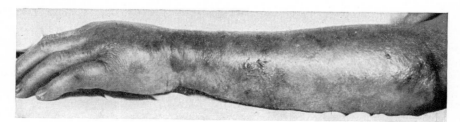

FIG. 3-3. Severe hemolytic streptococcal cellulitis of arm and hand secondary to infection of small burn. Note bronze appearance of skin and diffuseness of process with no signs of localization. Patient's temperature reached 105°. Three blood cultures were positive.

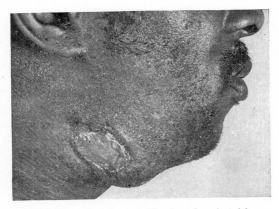

Fig. 3-4. A 25-year-old colored male with ulcerative tuberculous lymphadenopathy of 4 months' duration. Diagnosis proved by biopsy and culture.

fibrin. The *Pneumococcus* may also cause primary peritonitis in children and occasionally acute pyogenic arthritis.

The *Neisseria gonorrhoeae* or *Gonococcus* is a gram-negative coccus which does not occur as a normal inhabitant in man. In the usual infection, it grows in the urethra, the seminal vessels, the prostrate, or the epididymis in the male, and in the urethra, the cervix, or the fallopian tubes and the peritoneum in the female. However, it may occur elsewhere, as in infections of the conjunctiva. The infection produced by the gonococcus is customarily localized to the genitourinary tract, causing severe inflammation of the mucosal surface with production of a thin purulent discharge. Occasionally, the organism may become vigorously invasive and cause meningitis, arthritis (sometimes of a temporomandibular joint), septicemia, or endocarditis.

The *Neisseria catarrhalis* (*Micrococcus catarrhalis*) is also a gram-negative coccus and is frequently a normal inhabitant of the nasopharynx. It may cause disease by producing meningitis, conjunctivitis and occasionally septicemia or meningitis.

Bacillus anthracis is an aerobic gram-positive bacillus which causes anthrax. It is of historical interest because it was the first organism found to be the cause of a specific disease. Anthrax is primarily a disease of animals, but it may produce serious infection in man, either as a result of local subcutaneous invasion or as a pneumonialike infection.

Corynebacterium diphtheriae (*Bacillus diphtheriae*) is the cause of a serious toxemia in man. The organisms are gram-positive and may be present in large numbers in localized surface lesions, usually in the upper respiratory tract where a thick membrane forms which may cause respiratory obstruction and death when it becomes dislodged. However, superficial wounds of the skin may become infected with the organisms, particularly among the inhabitants of desert regions. The organism secretes a powerful exotoxin which is absorbed readily from the surface wound and produces serious systemic manifestations, especially myocardial damage.

In the *Corynebacterium* group are also included the *"diphtheroid" bacilli*. These organisms are not sufficiently virulent to produce disease by themselves but are frequently of importance as secondary contaminants in infections due to other organisms.

The gram-positive group also includes the bacillus of tuberculosis, *Mycobacterium tuberculosis*. This organism classically retains staining by the "acid-fast" technic. It produces disease of the respiratory tract, causing necrosis of lung tissue with caseation and cavitation. In addition, it may cause infection of skin, bones, lymph nodes and intestinal tract, with the formation of slowly progressive, chronic, infiltrative abscesses containing thick creamy pus and necrotic tissue in the walls of the abscesses. Characteristically, soft tissue abscesses produced by it near the body surface are devoid of the local signs of inflammation and are referred to as "cold abscesses."

The gram-negative bacillary group of bacteria includes a number of organisms of surgical import. These have become of increasing consequence since the discovery of penicillin, the use of which has often permitted secondary or superimposed infections by gram-negative bacilli during treatment, particularly by strains of *Ps. aeruginosa*, *Proteus vulgaris*, *Aerobacter aerogenes* and *E. coli*. Characteristically, they are of lesser virulence than the gram-positive pyogenic cocci, but they play an important part in the etiology of many mixed bacterial infections, such as peritonitis, putrid empyema, infected burns, urinary tract infections, postoperative cellulitis, wound infections, etc. More infrequently, they may produce monobacterial infections, such as ascending cholangitis, meningitis, urinary tract infections and septicemia.

Escherichia coli is very widespread in nature, particularly within the intestinal tracts and the excretions of man and animals. The organism appears in the intestinal tract of infants shortly after birth and remains there throughout life, usually without harmful effects. *E. coli* is of surgical interest as a partial cause of many mixed infections, including appendicitis, cholecystitis, peritonitis and infected burns, but the usual designation of the unaided activities of *E. coli* as the cause of appendiceal peritonitis is not justified or founded upon fact. The organism has little native virulence for animals when injected intraperitoneally, unless a foreign body or substance to delay its absorption is also inoculated. However, when grown and inoculated with other types of bacteria intraperitoneally, a mixed and virulent peritonitis can be produced. Frequently, it is possible to inject intravenously more than 2,500 million *E. coli* into the marginal ear vein of rabbits with no demonstrable harmful effects.

To *E. coli* has been falsely assigned also the responsibility for the putrid odor of appendiceal peritonitis. It has been shown that this organism when grown on sterile pus does not produce a foul odor, since its enzymes apparently cannot attack native protein. The principal and important causes of this foul odor are anaerobic bacteria of the *Bacteroides,* the *Clostridia,* or the anaerobic *Streptococcus* groups.

Aerobacter aerogenes is customarily a saprophyte found in the intestinal tract of man. It may become virulent and of pathologic significance in a manner similar to *E. coli. A. aerogenes* can cause urinary tract infections alone or in association with other bacteria; it can be associated with other organisms as causative agents in peritonitis and wound infections; and occasionally it may cause serious septicemia.

Proteus is usually also a nonpathogenic inhabitant of the intestinal tract, but it may cause infection alone or in synergism with other bacteria. It is seen most commonly in infections such as fecal peritonitis, urinary tract infections, infected burns, postoperative infections of abdominal or perineal wounds, or septicemia. At times, it may assume signifi-

cant virulence and invade the blood stream to produce a secondary or superimposed infection. The latter complication may develop as the result of newly assumed virulence during intensive antibiotic treatment with the various antibacterial agents.

Salmonella typhosa (the typhoid bacillus) produces disease in the human being primarily after its invasion of the gastrointestinal tract (typhoid fever). This is followed by invasion of the lymphoid tissue of the gastrointestinal tract and early dissemination in the blood stream. Hemorrhage into the intestine or perforation of the intestinal wall with secondary peritonitis may complicate the course of typhoid fever (see Chap. 35, "Peritoneum, Peritonitis and Intra-abdominal Abscesses"). As patients with typhoid fever are usually very ill, perforation must be detected early if the patient is to be saved by operation and closure of the opening. Frequent visits with a close watch for changes in abdominal rigidity are necessary. As in other ill patients, pain may not be as pronounced as in perforated peptic ulcer. Localized infection may occur later in the disease in the form of acute and chronic osteomyelitis, periostitis, pyelitis, or cholecystitis. Chronic infection may persist after subsidence of symptoms, and a carrier state may result. Wound infections may also be caused by the typhoid bacillus, particularly after cholecystectomy for the removal of the gallbladder in a carrier patient.

Klebsiella pneumoniae may produce severe pneumonia in a man and may also cause other infections such as sinusitis, empyema, pulmonary abscess, septicemia, or meningitis.

Alcaligenes faecalis is a saprophytic inhabitant of the gastrointestinal tract under normal circumstances, but it may occur in human infections as the primary etiologic agent or as a secondary invader. It has been found to be the cause of septicemia on occasions, but most frequently it is found in cases of peritonitis due to fecal contamination and occasionally is responsible for urinary tract infections.

Pseudomonas aeruginosa or *Bacillus pyocyaneus* is found frequently as a secondary infecting agent of wounds. Usually it is encountered as part of a mixed infection, particularly in large wounds containing necrotic material or consisting of large granulating defects. This bacterium is an important etiologic agent of troublesome infections of the eye, the external and the internal auditory canals, and burns. Its presence is indicated by the development of a greenish or bluish discoloration of the wound discharges and by its peculiar musty odor. Occasionally, it may assume marked virulence and produce severe invasion and life-endangering infections. Septicemia complicating burns or secondary peritonitis may be very difficult to manage and may be fatal. Meningitis caused by *Ps. aeruginosa* likewise has a high mortality. Purulent material produced by it is usually thick and blue-green in color.

Hemophilus influenzae is another gram-negative bacterium which may be found in the nose and the throat of healthy individuals. Pathogenically, it may produce sinusitis, pneumonitis, suppurative pleurisy, otitis media, or occasionally a particularly serious type of meningitis in children.

Micro-aerophilic organisms, especially the *Streptococci,* occasionally may assume importance in surgical lesions. They may be present as etiologic agents in certain chronic infections, such as chronic burrowing ulcer or chronic cutaneous progressive gangrene. At times, they may produce severe acute infections with septicemia, as in puerperal sepsis, meningitis, brain abscess, or osteomyelitis. When first isolated, they are often strictly anaerobic, but after two subcultivations they become micro-aerophilic in their oxygen requirements. They are isolated with difficulty and may be missed with ordinary methods of bacterial cultivation.

The *nonhemolytic, micro-aerophilic Streptococcus* has been found in cutaneous gangrenous lesions of the skin, peritonitis, intra-abdominal abscess and empyema.

The *hemolytic micro-aerophilic Streptococcus* has been found most frequently in chronic burrowing infections of the neck, the axillary, the perineal and the popliteal regions.

The *anaerobic Streptococcus* is also a serious invader of the human body and is encountered in various infections, such as peritonitis, lung abscess, putrid empyema, tubo-ovarian abscess, septic abortion, puerperal sepsis, or symbiotic infections. Purulent material produced by it is usually foul smelling, thick, and grayish in color. Because of its strict anaerobic requirements, frequently this organism is not isolated or identified as an etiologic agent in many surgical infections. When exposed to the air at room temperature for periods of 5 or 10 minutes or longer, the organism may die and will not grow on artificial media. In addition, if only aerobic methods of cultivation are used the organism will be overlooked. The presence of highly motile organisms in mixed culture will often obscure anaerobic *Streptococci* through their overgrowth. Although there is little or no evidence of native virulence of the anaerobic *Streptococci* for experimental animals, recent experimental work has unquestionably demonstrated their virulence and pathogenicity for man.

The pathogenic micro-organisms of the anaerobic gram-positive group which are of surgical significance include the causative agents of tetanus and gas gangrene. *Clostridium tetani* is a gram-positive sporulating anaerobe which is commonly found in the feces of animals, particularly the horse. It is also found in manured or pastured soil. As an infecting agent of wounds, *Cl. tetani* may produce the disease of tetanus through the effect of its powerful exotoxin. Absorption and distribution of this toxin affect the central nervous system and the neuromuscular end-organs to produce the typical signs and symptoms of tetanus. The local wound infected by the tetanus bacillus has no changes which are specific for this type of infection. The organism does not invade the body but remains localized in the wound. It requires very strict anaerobic environment for its growth; consequently, infection by it may occur as a complication of any deep penetrating wound. Its growth is also facilitated by the presence of necrotic material in the wound.

Cl. welchii, Cl. novyi, Cl. septicum, Cl. histolyticum and *Cl. sordellii* are anaerobic gram-positive spore-forming bacteria commonly found in the intestinal tracts of animals and man and in fertilized soil and wool clothing. Individually, or in various combinations, these organisms may cause the dreaded infectious complication of wounds known as gas gangrene. They require the presence of necrotic tissue for their growth, and the development of infection by them is aided by the presence of foreign bodies. They may cause destruc-

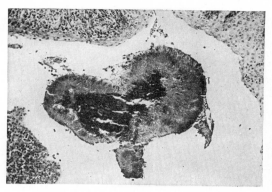

Fig. 3-5. Microscopic appearance of *Actinomyces* colony in tonsillar tissue.

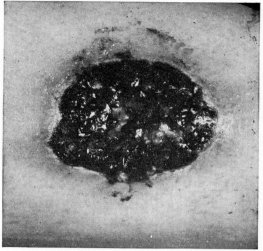

Fig. 3-6. An 81-year-old white male with blastomycotic ulcer of left leg of 5 months' duration. Diagnosis made by demonstrating *Blastomyces* in discharge at margin of wound by hanging-drop technic.

tion of adjacent and intact tissues by toxin production, thrombosis of vessels and mechanical effects of gas and edema. In military and civilian practice, gas gangrene may complicate crushing injuries, compound fractures, or fracture dislocations involving muscle masses. The infections produced by these bacteria are characteristic and serious, with severe toxemia, wet gangrene and a high mortality rate. The gas formation may be demonstrated by feeling crepitation or by roentgenogram, but it does not invariably occur.

The *Bacteroides* are pleomorphic, anaerobic, gram-negative bacilli which occasionally produce serious infections in wounds. Also, they may be of importance in such infections as fecal peritonitis, retroperitoneal cellulitis, pilonidal abscesses, or perineal abscesses. Septicemia and metastatic abscess formation can occur. The *Bacteroides melaninogenicus* may produce infections, usually in association with the anaerobic *Streptococcus*. Its growth in tissues is associated with grayish or black discoloration of the tissues, a gray exudate and a putrid odor.

The higher phylogenetic orders of microorganisms of surgical importance include the *Actinomyces*, which are the cause of actinomycosis and usually are anaerobic fungi. They may be found as nonpathogenic inhabitants of the oral cavity of man and animal. When they produce disease, they cause a chronic burrowing suppurative process which develops granulomatous lesions. Liquefaction and suppuration may occur with sinus formation and discharge of purulent material containing the characteristic sulfur granules. The usual

pathogenic strain of *Actinomyces* is the *A. bovis*. Of less importance are the *Nocardia* which are aerobic fungi assigned to this group. *N. asteroides* is occasionally the cause of disease which is clinically similar to actinomycosis. *N. madurae* is one of the causes of mycetoma or madura foot.

Blastomyces dermatitidis is a fungus pathogenic for man, which produces a very serious infection originating either as a skin surface lesion or as a pulmonary pneumonitis. The cutaneous lesion develops as a chronic, progressive, wartlike lesion composed of multiple intradermal abscesses containing the organism. It may advance to general dissemination with involvement of the lungs, bone, the kidneys and the brain. The pulmonary type is usually a fatal pneumonitis associated with cavitation.

Coccidioidal granuloma is caused by the *Coccidioides immitis*. This is usually a pulmonary infection, although there may be an involvement of the skin by nodular, ulcerative, or granulomatous lesions and, occasionally, of any parts of the body.

Sporotricha are widely distributed in nature and usually are saprophytic. However, *Sporotrichum schenckii* may cause granulomatous infections of a chronic nature with in-

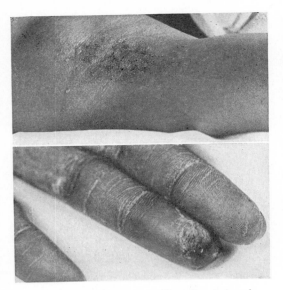

FIG. 3-7. A 30-year-old colored female with ulceration of 4th finger, lymphangitis and suppurative axillary lymphadenopathy. Diagnosis of tularemia proved by culture of ulceration and pus aspirated from abscess.

dolent ulcerations of the skin. These may progress to involve muscle, bone, or lung tissue.

Histoplasma capsulatum produces an infection in man ranging from a slight illness lasting a few days to acute and fulminating fatal disease. The organism may invade the blood stream. A pneumonia refractory to all available antibiotics is one form the disease may take. It may also produce hepatomegaly, lymphadenopathy, anemia and leukopenia.

Infections produced by *Candida albicans* are usually superficial and mild, since this organism is not vigorously invasive. The common site is the mouth where the infection is known as thrush or mycotic stomatitis. Antibiotic therapy has permitted an increased number of pulmonary and intestinal infections by this agent, many of which have become difficult to control. Meningitis and pneumonitis caused by *C. albicans* may be fatal.

Members of the *Aspergillus* group have been responsible upon rare occasions for chronic surface infections in man and occasionally for the formation of mycetoma. *Aspergillus niger* may produce cutaneous ulcerations which are chronic, mildly suppurative and covered by a black crust typical of the organism's growth.

Some *viral* infections are of surgical importance. Included are the filtrable viruses that can cause lymphopathia venereum. The initial lesion is a small ulcer of the genitalia following inoculation by sexual contact. Involvement of the lymphatics may lead to spread to the genital organs and the rectum. The resulting proctitis may cause stricture formation and obstruction requiring surgical intervention.

The *virus* causing homologous serum jaundice is transmitted from one individual to another by the injection of blood or blood products or by accidental inoculation through the medium of contaminated needles or similar objects. The incubation period is usually about 3 months but ranges from 3 weeks to 6 months. It causes a form of hepatitis of varying severity, generally associated with jaundice (see Chap. 8, "Blood Tranfusion").

Spirochetes of surgical importance include the *Treponema pallidum*, *T. macrodentium* and *T. microdentium*. The first may produce chronic ulcerations of primary syphilis or granulomatous lesions of tertiary syphilis, and these must be considered frequently in differential diagnosis of surgical lesions. The *T. macrodentium* and *microdentium* may contribute to the development of foul-smelling cervical or mouth infections or human-bite infections.

CONSIDERATION OF EFFECTS OF PATHOGENIC BACTERIA IN SURGERY

ORIGIN AND SPREAD OF INFECTIONS

Infection is the result of the entrance, the growth and the metabolic activities of microorganisms in tissues. *Surgical* infections differ from *medical* infections in 2 principal manners: (1) the infected area or primary focus is unlikely to resolve spontaneously, producing suppuration, necrosis, gangrene, prolonged morbidity, death, or other serious effects if untreated; and (2) excision, incision and/or drainage must be possible. In addition, surgical infections are often *polymicrobic* and invasive with rapid growth and spread of bacteria into the surrounding tissues or systems. In contrast, medical infections are usually *monomicrobic,* diffuse, and associated with little or no tissue reaction but a marked systemic response.

The point of bacterial entrance through the skin or the mucous membrane of the body is known as the *portal of entry*. The cutaneous surfaces and the mucous membranes of the human body are normally intact. Although often contaminated with bacteria, they are normally resistant to the invasion of micro-organisms. Bacteria cannot invade these surfaces normally except through injuries produced by trauma or some other physical, chemical, or metabolic factor which decreases the local resistance of the tissues and favors the growth of bacteria.

Obstruction to the flow of fluid excretions or secretions through tubular structures such as the ureter, the common bile duct, the intestine and the appendix usually enhances local bacterial growth and invasion of tissues by micro-organisms. In some instances, however, highly virulent bacteria may penetrate the mucous membrane without trauma, such as the typhoid, the dysentery and the tubercle bacilli, or the *T. pallidum*. In others, the bacteria will be unable to produce infection in that they will be destroyed or inhibited by the natural defenses of the body.

The period between contamination of tissues and the onset of infection is known as the *incubation period*. After invasion of the physiologic interior, bacteria may grow and produce a variety of inflammatory reactions. Their toxins may cause hyperemia, edema, increased capillary permeability, cellular infiltration, thrombosis, clot lysis and tissue liquefaction, suppuration, spontaneous bleeding or necrosis.

The reaction of the tissues locally to the growth and the products of bacterial metabolism produces the *local* signs and symptoms of infection. The reaction of tissues or organs distant to the primary focus or of the body as a whole may produce *general* signs and symptoms of the infection. *Regional* spread through adjacent tissues or neighboring lymphatics may also occur.

When infection occurs, it usually starts as a *cellulitis*, a diffuse inflammatory process without suppuration which is characterized by edema, redness, pain and interference with function. Cellular infiltration of the tissues by red blood cells, leukocytes, histiocytes and macrophages occurs. *Suppuration* often follows and is the result of local liquefaction of tissue with the formation of pus known as an *abscess*. The abscess is usually walled off by an area of inflammatory reaction which produces induration about the abscess and a softening at the center of the lesion. Cellulitis in varying degrees usually extends beyond the abscess's area of induration.

Bacterial proteolytic enzymes aid in the process of tissue liquefaction. Many bacteria produce *proteinases* which are capable of breaking down proteins. *Collagenase* is one of these which favors the liquefaction of collagen and the dissemination of infection along or even through fascial barriers. *Hyaluronidase* presumably favors the spread of bacterial toxins through alteration of the ground substances.

The hemolytic *Streptococcus* may produce a fibrinolysin, an enzyme which dissolves fibrin and makes it difficult for the body to ward off streptococcal infections.

Septic thrombosis of adjacent blood vessels frequently occurs and contributes to the local destruction and liquefaction of tissues. Small abscesses, areas of cutaneous gangrene, or infectious gangrene of entire extremities may be the result of septic thrombosis.

Thrombophlebitis of veins adjacent to infections may have additional effects. Septic emboli may be dislodged from the area of primary infection and gain their way into the circulating blood stream. The hemolytic *Staphylococcus*, in particular, produces a coagulase which clots small vessels and favors spread by septic embolization.

The dissemination of micro-organisms by a distributing focus results in either a bacteremia or a septicemia. In a *bacteremia* the primary focus distributes bacteria once or intermittently, resulting in their transient appearance in the blood. When it distributes organisms more or less constantly, their continued presence in the blood stream is known as a *septicemia*. The old concept suggested that the actual growth or reproduction of bacteria within the circulating blood stream was a septicemia in contrast with a bacteremia in which the micro-organisms found it impossible to reproduce in the circulating blood. The newer concept indicates that the difference is in the rate of dissemination from the distributing focus, it being more or less constant in a septicemia and intermittent or single in a bacteremia. Remember that any bacterium discharged into the circulation makes a complete circuit in the blood stream about every 23 seconds and, in doing so, runs the gamut of such hostile forces as circulating antibodies, polymorphonuclear leukocytes, macrophages and histiocytes of the reticuloendothelial system. It is possible to inject intravenously as many as 2,500 million bacteria in 2 cc. of culture media and to note the progressive disappearance of the bacteria from the blood stream by serial blood cultures. Usually within 2 to 6 hours the bacteria will have been completely removed, and negative blood cultures will result.

Virulent micro-organisms distributed from a *primary focus* to distant organs or tissues may set up *metastatic* infections which in turn may become *secondary* or *tertiary* distributing *foci.* Under the circumstances, the signs of invasive infection with positive blood cultures may have a cyclic sequence.

Bacteria may be carried away from the area of infection in the lymph fluid and distributed to regional areas through the *regional lymphatics or lymph nodes*. In doing so, they may cause an inflammatory reaction in the lymph vessels known as *lymphangitis,* and in the regional lymph nodes known as *lymphadenitis*. The latter may be suppurative or nonsuppurative, depending upon the resistance of the organism and the host.

Gangrene or necrosis may result in areas of infection produced by necrotizing bacterial enzymes, thrombosis of nutrient vessels, bacterial action, or ischemia resulting from the tourniquet effect caused by marked swelling of the tissues incident to infection.

Uncontrolled infections may become *chronic* and may be characterized by excessive fibrosis, sinus or fistulous tract formation, variable alterations in the local and general physiology, continued fever, anemia, sequestration of bone, fascia or tendon, contractures, limitation of function, or cosmetic disfigurement.

Thus infection may *subside spontaneously, remain localized, extend to regional or distant areas,* or *become chronic*. If the infections do extend, they do so by direct extension, lymphatic spread, venous spread or, rarely, arterial spread. Direct extension is most common, with spread by way of the subcutaneous tissues, muscles, vessel planes, or tendon sheaths. They may also spread diffusely through cavities such as the peritoneal or the thoracic cavities.

RESISTANCE OF THE HOST TO BACTERIAL INVASION

The power of resistance of a patient to bacterial infection is a complex physiologic phenomenon which is generally referred to as his *resistance* or *immunity*. The development of any infection is the result of failure of the dynamic interplay of the various factors of resistance to oppose successfully the number and the virulence of the contaminating microorganisms.

Unfortunately, resistance, immunity and their opposite, susceptibility, are *relative* and *not absolute*. Degrees of resistance exist which may be modified by a number of factors. Absolute immunity is rare, but there are isolated instances in nature in which large inoculations of micro-organisms virulent to one species will not produce significant infections in other species.

In a clinical sense, host resistance is a broad concept, representing the summation of many forces and influences in the defense mechanism which controls the relationship between the host and the parasite. An understanding of the factors which control and promote host resistance is a major responsibility of all surgeons. The basis of the treatment of infections rests essentially upon *promoting* the measures which fortify the resistance of the patient, and even the administration of antibiotic agents, which serves to control the growth of the invading parasite, cannot effect a cure without the occurrence of an adequate immune response.

Resistance or immunity of the host may be classified as *local, regional,* or *general*.

Local Resistance

Local resistance is accomplished initially by the intact barrier of the skin and the mucous membranes which is generally impermeable to bacteria. However, this barrier may be penetrated or weakened by the effects of nonbacterial disease or trauma. Occasionally, as in the case of the spirochete of syphilis, the micro-organisms may possess innate ability to penetrate the cutaneous or mucous surfaces. When the surface membranes have been broken down, permitting bacterial invasion, many other local defense mechanisms are alerted. The number, the type and the effectiveness of these depend somewhat on the tissue invaded and its vascularity. Concurrently, the phenomenon of local resistance occurs in the form of septic inflammation. This process is generally purposeful, serving to localize, destroy, or remove the invading bacteria. This inflammatory response is characterized by increased *local heat, redness, swelling* and *tenderness,* as originally noted by Celsus. Later, John Hunter added another characteristic, *interference with function.*

The increased heat and redness reflect an increase in the local blood supply to the area, with the enhancement of local defense by more oxygen and nutrition, as well as the later supply of the products which are part of general immunity.

When local pain develops in an infected area, involuntary splinting of the affected part may reduce the discomfort, decrease the dissemination of the infection and permit the tissues to localize and heal the involved area.

The swelling which develops is the result of a series of local resistance factors. One of the early changes is caused by injury to the cellular membranes which increases the vascular permeability and permits the extravasation of fluid into the intercellular spaces with the formation of an effusion. This effusion has definite antibacterial properties, and its character often varies with the type of infecting organism. Leukocytes, which have the ability to ingest and destroy many types of bacteria, migrate into the areas of edema and aid in the formation of an inflammatory exudate, the toxins and other bacterial products which may evoke different changes in areas of infection. The local lymphatics may become blocked by plugs of fibrin, venous capillaries may become thrombosed, fibrin precipitated, bacterial proteins trapped locally, and *granulation tissue* formed to create a *pyogenic membrane* or *barrier.* Either as a membrane for a surface wound or as a retaining wall about an inflammatory process, granulation tissue is a great natural protective device.

Local immunity may also be enhanced by the occurrence of a previous or recent inflammation in the same area. The effect is probably nonspecific, which in some manner potentiates a more rapid and effective mobilization of defenses to a renewed insult. It was a common observation in the preantibiotic era that the creation of a colostomy, with the associated regional soiling, protected the patient from the dangers of spreading peritonitis when a resection of the colon was performed several weeks later.

REGIONAL RESISTANCE

The second major line of defense which is elaborated by the host is a regional one. When local barriers have been overcome by the infection, spreading cellulitis or lymphangitis may occur. This extension then places the greatest burden of regional defense on the lymphatic system. With the progression of inflammation there is a great outpouring of plasma proteins, fluids and cellular elements, facilitated by bacterial spreading factors such as hyaluronidase. The rate of lymph flow, increasing greatly as extracellular pressure rises in the areas of swelling, achieves the purpose of removing waste products and cellular debris from a focus of high metabolic activity. Invading bacteria quickly appear in the regional lymph stream as though the accelerated flow washes away the organisms from the site of infection. As a consequence, the lymph vessels may become inflamed, producing the clinical picture of lymphangitis which always signifies a potentially serious process. The lymphatic pathways are filtered by the lymph nodes, which usually are located in well-defined anatomic areas along the course of major arteries and veins. When taxed beyond their capacity to react or when overwhelmed by the infection, the regional lymph nodes may become permanently damaged or permit the invasion of the blood stream with resultant *septicemia.*

The lymph nodal system serves at least two basic purposes: (1) *filtration* of infecting bacteria and cellular debris, and (2) the *production of specific antibodies* against the invading bacteria. The first of these is accomplished by the macrophages of the reticuloendothelial system which line the sinusoids of the lymph gland and there engulf the particles brought to it by the flow of lymph.

The second purpose, production of specific

antibodies, is less clearly understood. In experimental animals it has been shown that the regional nodes are an important site of the production of specific immune antibodies to a localized antigenic stimulus. The origin of the lymphoid cell which produces specific antibodies is undecided, but logically the same element which filters out the bacteria might be expected to produce these antibodies. Once formed, the specific antibodies travel from the node into the general circulation for wide distribution.

If lymphatic stasis continues and becomes chronic, its harmful effects may lower the resistance of the involved tissues. Chronic lymphedema may seriously impair resistance to bacterial infection, and a vicious cycle may develop, characterized by recurrent attacks of inflammation and increasing lymphatic damage.

GENERAL RESISTANCE

General resistance pertains to the protection afforded by antibodies which are continually circulated throughout the body in some quantity but may, upon proper stimulus, be increased significantly.

The general factors which play an important role in the over-all pattern of resistance may be natural or acquired, specific or nonspecific. *Natural immunity* refers to general resistance which is inherent, congenital, or acquired in some unknown way. Natural and nonspecific factors of general immunity include age, sex, race, individual variations, nutrition, climate and associated metabolic diseases.

Infants have inadequate resources to develop natural immunity or have not had specific stimulation for the formation of general antibodies. Therefore, they have an increased susceptibility to infection and must depend upon passive immunity acquired transplacentally from the mother. This passive immunity disappears in about 6 months and should be replaced by active general immunity.

Natural immunity may be dependent in some circumstances on nutrition, but it is not usually affected by acute processes. In long-term chronic illness associated with inadequate or unbalanced dietary replacement, there is a severe decrease in host resistance to infection.

Severe metabolic disturbances may influence a patient's resistance. In uncontrolled diabetes there is often a marked decrease in general immunity. Because of the damage to peripheral arteries in this disease, there may be a diminished local resistance to add to the over-all hazard. Other metabolic diseases which adversely influence general immunity include portal cirrhosis, vitamin deficiency states, leukopenia, multiple myeloma and Addison's or Cushing's diseases.

Specific immunity is largely dependent upon specific humeral factors which include antitoxins, bacteriolysins, agglutins and precipitins. The evidence suggests that the gamma globulin fraction of the plasma contains and stores specific bacterial antibodies. In conjunction with local measures of defense the antigen antibody response assumes great importance in controlling spreading infections.

Antibodies resulting from infection or reaction to antigens in patients confer *acquired immunity* which is lasting or permanent. *Passive immunity* follows the administration of serum containing preformed antibodies. Specific active immunity, once developed, remains more or less permanent against the particular strain of infecting parasite and confers on the host the greatest degree of serologic protection.

The specific antibodies are carried in the gamma globulin fraction of the blood stream. In recent years the fractionation of plasma proteins on a large scale has become feasible; and *gamma globulin,* made from pools of plasma representing many donors, may contain a wide spectrum of immune substances useful for the prevention or the amelioration of specific diseases.

For *in vivo* antibody-antigen reactions, *complement* is a necessary element, particularly in the lysis of bacteria. In some patients with infections it has been found that there is a complement deficiency in the blood. Recent investigations have uncovered a serum protein fraction called *properdin,* a serum protein which is essential for the proper function of complement and the antigen-antibody reaction.

An understanding of the various factors concerned with host resistance is a major responsibility of every surgeon. The physiologic process of wound healing is intimately associated with resistance, and a very valuable support to resistance lies in the intelligent care of the injured or infected area to ensure prompt and complete healing. Although much is known about the resistance of the host to the invasion of micro-organisms, there are still many gaps in our knowledge which must be filled in before the mechanisms of immunity will be clearly understood.

BIBLIOGRAPHY

Altemeier, W. A.: Bacteriology of war wounds, Internat. Abstr. Surg. *in* Surg., Gynec. & Obst. *75*: 518-533, 1942.

————: The pathogenicity of the bacteria of appendicitis peritonitis, Ann. Surg. *114*:158-159, 1941.

————: Postoperative infections, S. Clin. North American *25*:1202-1228, 1945.

Altemeier, W. A., and Wulsin, J. H.: Natural resistance to infection *in* Progress In Surgery, Karger, Basel, 1960.

Balch, H. H.: Nutrition and resistance to infection, Ann. Surg. *147*:423, 1958.

Churchill, E. D.: The American surgeon, A.U.S., Surg., Gynec. & Obst. *84*:529-539, 1947.

Editorial: The ward dressing, Lancet *2*:565, 1941.

Editorial: Surgical bacteriology, Am. Surgeon *25*:713-714, 1959.

Fleming, A.: Bacteriological examination of wounds *in* Bailey, H.: Surgery of Modern Warfare, vol. 1, chap. 16, Baltimore, Williams & Wilkins, 1941.

Hare, R.: Sources of hemolytic streptococcal infection of wounds in war and in civil life, Lancet *1*:109-112, 1940.

Meleney, F.: Bacterial synergism in disease processes, with a confirmation of the synergistic bacterial etiology of a certain type of progressive gangrene of the abdominal wall, Ann. Surg. *94*:961-981, 1931.

————: Bacteriological and surgical principles in management of surgical septicemia, Internat. Abstr. Surg. *in* Surg., Gynec. & Obst. *65*:513-521, 1938.

Meleney, F. L., and Whipple, A. O.: Statistical analysis of study of prevention of infection in soft part wounds, compound fractures and burns with special reference to sulfonamides, Surg. Gynec. & Obst. *80*:263-296, 1945.

Price, P. B.: Bacteriology of normal skin: new quantitative test applied to study of bacterial flora and disinfectant action of mechanical cleansing, J. Infect. Dis. *63*:301-318, 1938.

Reid, M. R.: Some considerations of problems of wound healing, New England J. Med. *215*:753-766, 1936.

W. A. ALTEMEIER, M.D., AND W. R. CULBERTSON, M.D.*

--- CHAPTER 4 ---

Surgical Infections

Infections of surgical significance may occur spontaneously, develop in wounds after trauma, or arise in remote areas of the body as postoperative complications. Spontaneous infections, such as acute appendicitis and acute cholecystitis, will be discussed elsewhere in the text. While many infections, such as pneumonia and pyelocystitis, may develop during the postoperative state in tissues or organs remote from the region of an operative area, most surgical infectious lesions are the result of the growth of bacteria introduced through a portal of entry caused by some type of trauma.

When infections develop in wounds resulting from accidental injury, violence, or planned operative procedures, they may have a profound effect on mortality, morbidity and the final result of the injury or the operation. Death, loss of limb, or disability which may be prolonged or permanent may result. The complication of infection, particularly in large wounds, almost certainly increases the period of morbidity after operation, since infection, the greatest enemy of wound healing, produces further destruction of tissue and suppresses the process of healing. Tissue destroyed by infection is usually replaced by scar tissue which may affect cosmetic appearance as well as function.

GENERAL CONSIDERATIONS

The primary essential for the development of infection within wounds is the growth of

* From the Department of Surgery, University of Cincinnati College of Medicine and the Cincinnati General Hospital, Cincinnati, Ohio.

bacteria. Experience and experimental work have shown that all injuries resulting in penetration of the skin or the mucous membrane are associated with contamination of the wounded tissues by micro-organisms of various types. Some may be highly virulent, others less so, and still others saprophytic. Even clean surgical wounds which heal *per primam* are contaminated by air-borne micro-organisms. Their presence in wounds may or may not be followed by infection, depending upon certain factors which influence the growth of bacteria and determine not only the development of any septic process but also its characteristics. These factors include the following:

1. The virulence, the types and the numbers of contaminating bacteria
2. Devitalized tissue within the wound
3. The presence of foreign bodies
4. The nature, the location and the duration of the wound
5. The local and general immunity response of the individual
6. The type and the thoroughness of treatment
7. The general condition of the patient

The number and the types of contaminating bacteria have long been known to increase the probability and the severity of wound infection, and the premise that infection is the unfavorable result of the equation of dose multiplied by virulence and divided by resistance still holds. However, it must be remembered that the mere presence of virulent bacteria in a wound does not make infection of that wound a certainty. The evidence indicates that the physiologic state of the tissues within the wound before and after treatment is more important than the presence of bacteria *per se*. The synergistic or cumulative activity of the bacteria present may also determine to a large extent the nature and the severity of the infection.

Unhealthy, irritated or dead tissue in wounds invites and supports the growth of virulent and nonvirulent organisms, since it has limited or little power of resistance to their growth and action. Conversely, *healthy* tissue fortunately possesses a remarkable capacity to kill bacteria or withstand their effects.

Foreign bodies, particularly those of organic composition or contamination, carry large numbers of bacteria into wounds and further the probability of infection through their local irritative action on the tissues. It must be remembered that suture material buried within a wound may act as a foreign body and therefore must be used intelligently, just enough being employed to approximate live tissues and obliterate "dead pockets" as much as possible (see Chap. 2, "Wound Healing").

The type of wound is also an important factor. Extensive wounds containing large amounts of devitalized tissues, especially muscle, fascia and bone, furnish excellent culture media for bacteria. Injuries of the thigh or the buttocks may severely damage a pound or more of muscle, and these greatly devitalized masses may become severely infected. Wounds produced by crushing and associated with heavy contamination are frequently multiple and are characterized by extensive tissue destruction, severe shock and early virulent infection.

The location of the wound is another significant consideration. Not only are the various tissues known to have different powers of local resistance to infection, but the resistance of these tissues also varies with their location in the body. For example, lacerations of the face and the neck are prone to heal kindly unless they are in communication with the mouth and the pharynx, while wounds of the perineum practically always become infected to some degree.

The multiplicity of severe wounds in one person may so compromise the treatment that adequate débridement of one or more of the wounds is not possible. Because of associated severe shock, hemorrhage, or wounds of the chest or the head, the local treatment of wounds necessarily assumes a minor role in relation to the general treatment of the patient. If the period of time required for the successful general treatment exceeds 6 to 8 hours, often infection will have occurred before local definitive treatment can be started.

The immunity response of the individual may be local, regional or general, as has been discussed previously. *Local immunity* depends somewhat on the type of tissue, especially its vascularity. The term is used mostly to describe the local resistance which an area develops after fighting off an infection so that the same organisms can no longer invade, at this point at least, though they may still get a foothold in some other part of the body. After a consideration of the available evidence, Topley concluded that "it is possible to induce an immunity which is confined to the neighborhood of the treated area, and is not shared by the body as a whole."

The resistance of the body ordinarily is largely due to a *general immunity*. The possession of such immunity is specific and resides in the body as a whole, although the protein, particularly the globulin fraction of the plasma, and the cells of the so-called reticuloendothelial system are primarily involved in the mechanisms of immunity. A third and important factor in resistance is the protective action of the lymph nodes. The development of leukocytosis during infections is also a manifestation of resistance. *Natural immunity* refers to resistance inherent or at least obtained in some unknown spontaneous way or congenitally. *Acquired immunity,* on the other hand, is the result of defenses built up in fighting a previous infection. *Artificial immunity* is a similar defense obtained, however, by passive or active immunization. Of the two, the latter is especially important in the prevention of tetanus.

Treatment influences the development of infection more than most physicians realize. Of primary importance is the surgical excision or removal of all dead or devitalized tissue and foreign bodies within the wound, preferably within 4 to 6 hours after injury in order to remove any potential pabulum for bacterial growth. Of almost equal importance, however, is the prevention of the development of devitalized tissue during the postoperative state. Impairment of the local blood supply by damage to or ligation of large vessels, by displaced fractures, by pressure of hematomas, by tourniquets or ill-applied and ill-fitting casts, or by increased subfascial tension due to edema, hemorrhage or sutures, decreases local resistance of tissues and favors the development of infection.

The physical condition of the patient is an important predisposing factor to infection, and dehydration, shock, malnutrition, exhaustion, uncontrolled diabetes and anemia may lower his resistance sufficiently to permit bacterial invasion.

PRIMARY AND SECONDARY BACTERIAL CONTAMINATION AND INFECTION

Bacterial contamination of wounds may be either primary or secondary, depending upon the time when bacteria are carried into the wound. Contamination occurring at the time of or within a few hours of injury is considered primary, while that occurring 24 hours or more after trauma is secondary. The *infection* caused by these methods is likewise designated as *primary* and *secondary*.

Primary Contamination. The sources of primary contamination include the patient's skin or hair, clothing, various foreign bodies carried into the wound, such as wood splinters, the missile, soil, pieces of glass, etc., and discharges from various tracts including the upper respiratory, the genital, or the gastrointestinal. The more common types of bacteria associated with primary contamination and infection include staphylococci, enterobacilli such as *E. coli*, *B. proteus* and the Clostridia of gas gangrene and tetanus.

Secondary contamination may be caused by contact or by airborne spread. It emanates primarily from the respiratory tract of the patient or other persons in his vicinity, particularly those treating or observing his wound. Other sources include unsterile dressings, the fingers of anyone touching the wound, dust of the operating room or the hospital ward, and contaminated dressings, instruments, or utensils. Care should be exercised in the dressing of wounds to prevent cross-contamination and secondary infection. These precautions include the wearing of the mask, the avoidance of touching the wound with the bare fingers, and the avoidance of using any instruments, material, or dressings which are not sterile.

Primary infection tends to disappear at variable rates in different wounds, depending on the type of infection, the severity of the wound and the presence of sloughs, sequestra or foreign bodies.

Secondary Infection. Primary infection is gradually replaced, often during the second week, by the stage of secondary infection caused chiefly by the pyogenic cocci, especially the hemolytic *Staphylococcus aureus* and *Streptococcus hemolyticus* and to a lesser extent by *B. pyocyaneus*, *E. coli* and *Proteus vulgaris*.

Hare and Fleming believed that the hemolytic *Streptococcus* was the most important agent in secondary infection, but it has been our experience at the Cincinnati General Hospital that the hemolytic *Staphylococcus aureus* is both more prevalent and more important.

It is interesting to recall that Lord Lister laid great stress on airborne infections, but until very recently their importance has been underestimated or overlooked. Unless strict precautions are taken, secondary or cross infections are bound to occur in a surgical ward. The longer a wound is allowed to remain open, the greater is the chance for secondary contamination and infection.

METHODS OF DIAGNOSIS OF SURGICAL INFECTIONS

Accurate and prompt methods of diagnosis of surgical infections are more important now than ever, the discovery and general use of antibiotics notwithstanding. The reasons for this continued importance of early and accurate diagnosis will be discussed in detail later.

The diagnostic methods useful in determining the location and the nature of surgical infections include the following:

1. **A careful history and physical examination,** coupled with a general knowledge of surgical infections and their etiology, may lead to the presumptive diagnosis of the lesion and the causative organism. For example, the early diagnosis of acute hematogenous osteomyelitis can be made entirely upon the history and the physical examination long before positive x-ray findings are present. In addition, we know that approximately 80 to 88 per cent of such cases are caused by the hemolytic *Staphylococcus aureus,* and that approximately 99 per cent are caused by some form of gram-positive cocci. In this manner it is pos-

sible to make a presumptive diagnosis of the lesion and the etiologic agent early in the course of the infection when antibiotic therapy will give the best results.

2. **Laboratory data,** such as red blood counts, hemoglobin, white blood counts, differential counts and urinalysis, are important sources of information which aid in differential diagnosis. Of particular importance in many patients with severe infections is the physician's recognition of the presence of diabetes by urinalysis and blood sugar determinations because of the susceptibility of diabetics to infection and the difficulty in controlling the combined diseases. Generally speaking, patients with infections exhibit varying degrees of leukocytosis, and valuable information regarding the nature and the course of the infection can be gained from serial counts. Every patient with a surgical infection of moderate or greater severity should have complete blood counts daily for 3 days and then at least twice weekly thereafter until the infection is well under control. Infections caused by hemolytic bacteria such as the *Streptococcus hemolyticus* or *Cl. welchii* may produce profound anemia.

3. **Special procedures,** such as roentgen examinations, are of considerable aid in the localization of the infection and its spread.

4. **Infectious exudates** should be obtained whenever possible from the area of infection by swab or aspiration for *examination,* 4 general procedures being possible.

Direct observation of the pus to detect its color, consistency, odor and other physical characteristics is often of great diagnostic help to the experienced surgeon.

Direct microscopic examination of a smear stained by the Gram stain, acid-fast, or other technics may yield immediate information regarding the type or general types of microorganisms present. It may also show the types of leukocytes predominant in the wound.

Culture of the pus under aerobic, microaerophilic and anaerobic conditions may indicate the specific organism or organisms causing the infection. Cultures made of infectious material should be placed *immediately* into appropriate media and then into the incubator for cultivation. Every effort should be made to do this rather than keep the material overnight in an icebox or at room temperature

which favors drying of the specimen and death of all but the hardiest organisms, which unfortunately are often not the true pathogens.

Examination of a wet preparation of the exudate, treated with 15 per cent sodium hydroxide solution, under a cover glass or by the hanging-drop technic may demonstrate the presence of yeast or fungi.

In obscure infections in which there is no purulent exudate, material aspirated by needle and syringe from cellulitic areas or areas of suspected infection may establish the diagnosis and indicate the infecting agent by examination of the smear and culture.

5. **Culture of the blood** also can provide diagnostic information. This may be the only manner of identifying the etiologic agent when pus is not available for culture or when the primary focus is hidden, obscure, or silent. Whenever possible, the blood cultures should be taken as close to the onset of a chill as possible, or when the temperature is rising rapidly.

6. **Biopsy of the lesion** in granulomatous infections, particularly tuberculous, syphilitic or mycotic, gives material for microscopic examination which may be of great value in arriving at a definite diagnosis in difficult cases.

Other special diagnostic procedures that may be used include *agglutination tests* made with the patient's serum and *skin tests* made with various antigens. The latter may be used as aids in establishing the diagnosis of lesions such as lymphopathia venereum, tuberculosis, blastomycosis, histoplasmosis and coccidioidomycosis.

TREATMENT OF SURGICAL INFECTIONS

Great advances have been made during the past 70 years in the prevention and the control of surgical infections, particularly during the last 15 years. Today it is routinely possible to prevent infection in planned operative wounds, an achievement which is one of the great milestones of surgery. In addition, considerable progress has been made in preventing or attenuating infection in accidental wounds or wounds of violence. The outlook of surgical patients with established lesions or operations performed in contaminated fields has become vastly improved. Many of the surgical infections commonly seen can now be controlled effectively in conjunction with operative intervention when indicated. However, there are still many surgical lesions of microbial etiology which are refractive to any known form of chemotherapy.

PROPHYLAXIS

In addition to directing treatment toward overcoming the various factors which predispose to the development of surgical infections, such as early excision of devitalized tissue, removal of foreign bodies, preservation of blood supply, and immobilization of injured extremities, other means of preventing infections are available.

ANTIBIOTIC AGENTS may be used to considerable advantage, but the indications for their use in civilian surgical practice are considerably more limited than those generally practiced. Their indiscriminate or blind use is to be discouraged.

1. In contaminated wounds of violence and burns, adequate débridement often cannot be accomplished, and devitalized tissue and bacteria may remain to cause infection. The systemic administration of an agent such as penicillin is indicated and usually will inhibit the growth of hemolytic streptococcal infections and prevent infection by this organism. There is no definite evidence that systemic antibiotic therapy also reduces the incidence of other invasive infections produced by the staphylococcus, *Bacillus pyocyaneus, Escherichia coli, Aerobacter aerogenes* and other gram-negative bacilli.

2. In elective procedures performed through or in contaminated areas such as the gastrointestinal, the respiratory, or the genitourinary tracts, prophylactic therapy may be useful. Here, again, unavoidable contamination of the wound by pathogenic bacteria occurs in such numbers that development of infection becomes a real probability unless the patient has the added defense of prophylactic antibiotic treatment.

3. The use of antibiotics is warranted in an effort to prevent infection in patients who have associated derangements of the urinary tract or require indwelling catheters as part of their surgical care.

4. It is also indicated in patients with pre-existing valvular heart disease who receive injuries or require elective surgical procedures in the oral or pharyngeal cavities. The well-known relationship of the initiation of subacute bacterial endocarditis under these circumstances warrants the use of penicillin or sulfadiazine as prophylaxis against this dreaded complication.

5. Prophylactic antibacterial treatment should be considered in patients requiring emergency operative surgical treatment in the presence of associated but unrelated infections, such as tonsillitis.

6. For elective preoperative preparation of the gastrointestinal tract, selected antibiotics administered orally prior to operation reduce both the numbers and the virulence of intestinal organisms which may accidentally contaminate the required operative wound.

7. In elderly people with pre-existing pulmonary disease requiring essential operative treatment antibiotics may be useful in controlling existing subclinical infection or postoperative complications. If this is done, great care should be exercised because of the danger of precipitating an antibiotic resistant infection as a complication in such patients.

The prophylactic application of antibacterial agents in circumstances other than these is usually unwarranted and potentially dangerous. The routine use of such agents in clean surgical procedures may lull the physician into a feeling of false security that infection will not occur. Such treatment may partially abort a developing infection or mask its usual and recognizable clinical signs long enough to permit serious and extensive damage to occur before its diagnosis. Some "masked infections" may even become lethal without the appearance of clinical signs diagnostic of virulent infection.

Moreover, the indiscriminate prophylactic use of antibacterial agents is causing sensitivity of an increasing percentage of the population to the various antibiotics. This may be dangerous or even fatal. It also denies the patient the benefit of that antibacterial agent in the future, should he need it. It is also possible for antibiotics used prophylactically to cause serious superimposed or secondary infections by resistant bacteria such as staphylococci or fungi which may be more serious than those to be prevented. Finally, antibiotic agents may be harmful to the patient as a result of toxicity, overdosage, or idiosyncrasy.

SEROTHERAPY may be useful to a limited degree in prophylaxis. The two surgical infections which may be considered in this regard are gas gangrene and tetanus. Experimentally and clinically, prophylactic serotherapy against gas gangrene has been found to be without benefit for practical purposes, and its use is not recommended.

IMMUNITY AGAINST TETANUS is of great value and is an essential part of the treatment of all accidental wounds.

Passive immunity can be produced by the hypodermic injection of tetanus antitoxin as soon after the injury as possible. The usual patient who is seen within 24 hours after injury should receive 1,500 units of tetanus antitoxin after proper skin-testing has shown no sensitivity to horse serum in the antitoxin. Recently it has been recommended that the prophylactic dose of tetanus antitoxin be increased to a minimum of 3,000 or even 5,000 units. In our experience at the Cincinnati General Hospital, a dose of 1,500 units is adequate, provided that it is given shortly after injury and certainly within 24 hours. If the wound is large and grossly contaminated, or if the patient has co-existing diabetes mellitus, the dose should be 3,000 or more units. If the patient is seen more than 24 hours after injury, the dose shoud be doubled for each 24 hours of elapsed time up to a maximum dose of 12,000 units. Under circumstances of delayed definitive treatment of the wound or manipulations of the injured area, passive immunity should be maintained by the injection of 1,500 units of tetanus antitoxin repeated in 7 days.

Active immunity against tetanus can be attained by 2 or 3 injections of tetanus toxoid at intervals of 3 to 6 weeks, followed by a booster injection at the time of injury. Individuals who have this active basic immunity do not require *antitoxin* in the prophylaxis of tetanus, but can be protected by reactivation of the immunity by injection of a booster dose of toxoid after injury.

THERAPY OF ESTABLISHED INFECTIONS

Factors and Principles To Be Observed. As a result of the numerous advances in the field of antibacterial therapy during the past 15 years, the outlook of surgical patients with established infections has become much improved. Experience has shown that successful treatment of surgical infections depends largely upon the physician's observance of certain factors or principles.

1. He must realize that the use of the newer antibiotic agents is adjunctive to the employment of old and established surgical principles.

2. Antibiotic agents used properly can produce profound effects in the prevention and the control of infections, but when used improperly their clinical effects may be limited, incomplete or absent.

3. He must recognize that early diagnosis is of great importance in the control of surgical infections, affecting morbidity, mortality and function. If the diagnosis is established early when infections are in the diffuse or cellulitic stage, antibacterial therapy is most apt to produce a prompt and rapid control of the invasiveness with either complete and spontaneous resolution of the infection or minimal complications. This is due to two factors. The capillary circulation is intact and can deliver adequate doses of the antibacterial agent throughout the zone of infection. There is also greater susceptibility of the bacteria to the antibiotics while they are rapidly proliferating. However, if the diagnosis is made late, the infectious process usually has become more established, and either local necrosis or abscess formation has occurred, or systemic invasion has developed. If the blood supply to an area is impaired or destroyed, insufficient concentrations of antibiotics are carried to the area of infection. In those cases in which the infection has become disseminated before a diagnosis has been made with the production of metastatic abscess or secondary infectious complications in removed areas, the control of the infection is considerably more difficult.

For the most efficient control of surgical infections, not only must the diagnosis be early, but it must be accurate and complete. The necessity of a correct clinical diagnosis as well as an evaluation of the patient's condition for intelligent treatment is obvious. This implies the recognition of the existence and the site of metastatic abscess or other complications. Failure of the elevated temperature and other general signs of infection to recede within 72 hours of the start of antibacterial therapy and other treatment generally implies the co-existence of a neighboring abscess, one or more complicating metastatic infections, resistance of the infecting bacteria to the antibiotic in use, or the development of vegetative endocarditis. This emphasizes the wisdom of re-evaluating the patient's disease and his treatment every 72 hours if a satisfactory response has not been obtained.

The importance of obtaining information regarding the infecting micro-organism is increasing. Such information can be obtained by the immediate examination of stained smears of the pus and by culture of exudate obtained by incision and drainage or aspiration with needle and syringe from the actual site of infection (see page 49). Biopsy of the lesion is often very helpful in establishing the nature of the infection, particularly in chronic infection of a specific nature, such as tuberculosis, syphilis and actinomycosis.

Errors in Diagnosis. In this regard it must be kept in mind that errors in diagnosis can be made very easily by accepting the report of the laboratory on cultures made of surface lesions. Such positive cultures may actually represent contaminants or secondary invaders, not the true pathogens which may be much more difficult to cultivate. This trend is of clinical significance, since it re-emphasizes the necessity of sound clinical diagnosis.

The selection of the proper chemotherapeutic agent is extremely important in the modern control of surgical infections. The choice of an antibiotic effective for the particular etiologic agent in any given case is obviously desirable. Whenever possible the selection should be made on the basis of data resulting from studies of the gram-stained smears, cultures of exudates obtained from the lesions and sensitivity tests. Also, whenever possible one agent should be used instead of a shotgun mixture of 3 or 4. If no infectious exudate can be obtained, or if no local lesion is demonstrable in a patient with a severe systemic infection, the selection of the antibacterial agent must be made necessarily on a presumptive diagnosis until the nature of the causative organism is determined. Such a procedure is necessarily blind.

It is important to realize that there is considerable variation in natural bacterial resistance within strains of bacteria. Consequently, the haphazard selection of an antibiotic agent which presumably should be effective for a given etiologic agent may yield an uncertain result or a failure. Many strains of bacteria in our environment, particularly in hospitals, are gradually acquiring resistance to various antibiotics. For example, only 25 to 50 per cent of the strains of hemolytic *Staphylococcus aureus* are still sensitive to penicillin, and sensitivity tests are particularly important in the management of infections caused by it.

SENSITIVITY STUDIES are of considerable value in the selection of the antibiotic agent or agents of choice for the treatment of a given infection (Fig. 4-1). Sensitivity determinations may be done in the laboratory by the serial dilution tube method or the disk method, using commercially prepared disks. The latter method is considerably less accurate than the former but is the only one that is available for general clinical use. Although not infallible, this method gives information on a qualitative basis valuable for clinical use, and it is sufficiently simple for any laboratory employing a technician trained in bacteriology. In our experience there generally has been good correlation between the results of *in vitro* sensitivity tests, as determined by the serial dilution tube method, and the clinical responses obtained.

In the treatment of serious mixed infections produced by a variety of gram-positive and gram-negative aerobic and anaerobic bacteria, it may be advisable to select two antibacterial agents for treatment of such conditions as acute septic peritonitis, intra-abdominal abscess, perinephritic abscess, urinary tract infections and various types of wound infections. Usually, aqueous penicillin G and one of the broad-spectrum group such as chloramphenicol, tetracycline, chlortetracycline, oxytetracycline, declomycin or streptomycin are selected. There is some test-tube evidence that antagonism may occur between two or more antibiotics which may decrease their effectiveness, but fortunately there is no significant evidence of this antagonism existing *in vivo*. There is also some *in vitro* evidence that synergism or increased antibacterial power occurs with the use of combinations of some of the agents such as penicillin and streptomycin.

It is advisable to *repeat cultures and sensitivity tests* at weekly intervals in severe pro-

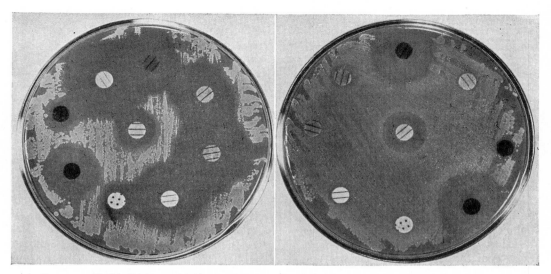

FIG. 4-1. (*Left*) Disk sensitivity studies on strain of hemolytic *Staphylococcus aureus* which is sensitive to penicillin, erythromycin, tetracycline, oxytetracycline, chlortetracycline, chloramphenicol, bacitracin and neomycin. (*Right*) Disk sensitivity studies on strain of hemolytic *Staphylococcus aureus* which is sensitive to erythromycin, bacitracin and neomycin but resistant to tetracycline, oxytetracycline, chlortetracycline, penicillin and streptomycin. It is slightly sensitive to chloramphenicol.

longed infections because of the possibility of acquired bacteria resistance or development of secondary infections. Apparently, bacteria may acquire resistance to all of the antibiotic agents in varying degrees except polymyxin B and neomycin. Occasionally, suppression of sensitive bacteria in mixed infections by antibiotics may permit other bacteria normally of lesser virulence to become invasive and to invade the blood stream, the meninges or some other tissue system. Infections produced in this manner are known as *superinfections* or *superimposed infections,* and they might be overlooked unless repeated cultures are taken.

ADEQUATE DOSAGE implies the use of the antibiotic agent in doses sufficiently large to produce antibacterial concentrations in the blood and intercellular fluids and tissues for a period of time long enough to permit the natural defense mechanism of the body to dispose of the inhibited but often still viable bacteria. The majority of the agents exert only a bacteriostatic effect which is greatest on actively growing and reproducing bacteria. In the case of some of the antibiotics, particularly penicillin, the evidence suggests that progressively large doses have an increasingly greater clinical effect and at times a bactericidal action.

TIME ELEMENT. Antibiotic treatment should be started as promptly as possible after injury. Its use may keep any infection localized, attenuated, or dormant. In established infections early antibiotic therapy gives a better chance of producing rapid and prompt control of invasiveness. Late treatment usually results in a more limited or delayed effect, and complications are more numerous, including local necrosis, abscess formation or systemic invasion (Fig. 4-2).

METHOD OF ADMINISTRATION. This is worthy of some discussion. The systemic administration of antibiotics is generally by the parenteral or oral routes, depending upon the agent used and various other factors. *Local application* of chemotherapeutic agents to wounds is seldom indicated. In traumatic shock the absorption of antibiotics from the gastrointestinal tract or muscular areas may be retarded. Consequently, the intravenous administration of aqueous penicillin G or other antibiotics is recommended during traumatic shock to guarantee rapidly an adequate blood and fluid concentration.

The timing of surgical intervention with antibiotic therapy is of special importance. Necessary operative procedures should not be delayed unless the patient's condition is too poor to withstand anesthesia and surgery. On the other hand, care should be taken to perform necessary operative procedures after the start of antibiotic treatment if possible and before the development of bacterial resistance. In general, the principles of operative treatment of surgical infection have not been changed significantly by modern chemotherapy. (See Fig. 4-3.) In serious infections such as septic peritonitis secondary to perforated appendicitis or peptic ulcer, best results have been obtained by the parenteral administration of antibiotics preoperatively and as soon as possible after the patient has been seen. This rapidly produces a bacterial-inhibiting concentration at the site of the infection, retards the progress of the infection and makes unnecessary the local application of antibiotics within the peritoneal cavity.

Supportive treatment is valuable in the management of many patients with surgical infections. Obvious local and general physiologic derangements are frequently overlooked or disregarded in present-day practice. If they are not corrected, the full therapeutic effect of the antibacterial agent will not be obtained.

Untoward reactions following the administration of antibiotic agents have been shown to be of 3 general types: toxic reactions related to the amount of the drug given, sensitivity reactions due to idiosyncrasy or sensitization of the patient, or secondary inflammations or ulcerations produced by superimposed infections. Each of the agents has been shown to be capable of producing one or more of these types of reaction. Those produced by overdosage can be readily presented or controlled. Those secondary to *sensitization* of the host are becoming more and more important, particularly in the case of penicillin. Many patients, some of whom were sensitized during the misuse of penicillin, are now deprived of its benefits and apparently will be hereafter.

IDIOSYNCRASY TO CHLORAMPHENICOL with depression of the bone marrow and leukopenia or aplastic anemia unfortunately received considerable publicity during 1951 and 1952. Many of these cases were caused by agents other than chloramphenicol, while others un-

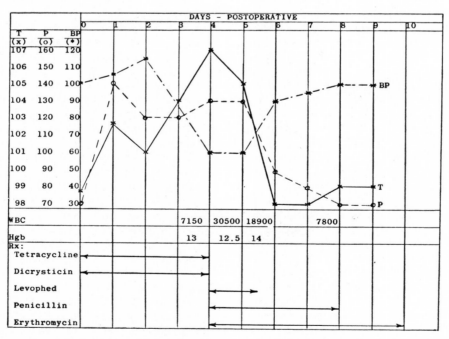

FIG. 4-2. A 14-year-old female with severe staphylococcal pseudomembranous enterocolitis developing 4 days after gastrectomy as a complication of tetracycline therapy. Note high fever, fall in blood pressure and WBC of 30,500 associated with infection. Excellent response to erythromycin and Levophed.

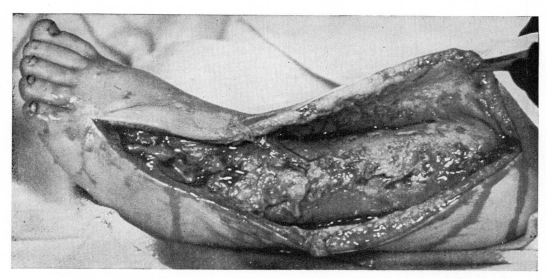

Fig. 4-3. A 2-year-old boy with extensive purulent subcutaneous cellulitis secondary to acute osteomyelitis of lower end of tibia and ruptured subperiosteal abscess caused by hemolytic *Staphylococcus aureus*. Note creamy pus. There was an associated septicemia. Although moribund when this picture was taken, the patient recovered. Without timed surgical intervention with emergency incision and drainage, the patient would have died before adequate antibiotic effect.

doubtedly were the result of its promiscuous or prolonged use in excessively large doses. A detailed study during an ensuing 4-year period revealed that there were approximately 75 proved cases of blood dyscrasia resulting from chloramphenicol which had been accumulated from the literature. In addition there was considerable evidence to indicate that the dangers of administering this agent had been greatly exaggerated. However, the wisdom of repeated and regular blood cell counts during its administration is well established. During the past 12 years chloramphenicol has been used extensively on the surgical services of the Cincinnati General Hospital, and in no instance has a blood dyscrasia developed. On only 2 cases did the white blood cell count temporarily fall below 4,000 cells per cubic millimeter, quickly returning to normal levels when the drug was discontinued.

Secondary or superimposed infections caused by the suppression of susceptible microbial agents and overgrowth of those resistant to the antibiotic administered have become of increasing importance. The most severe form has been the pseudomembranous enterocolitis which has developed in some cases,

usually after the use of chlortetracycline, oxytetracycline, or tetracycline, although it has been noted occasionally after other forms of antibacterial therapy, and even in the absence of such treatment. Fortunately, these severe and potentially fatal infections can be treated successfully by erythromycin or chloramphenicol. If they are associated with septic shock, hypotension and urinary suppression, active supportive treatment is also recommended, including the intravenous administration of Norepinephrine.

Specific serotherapy with biologic antigens or antitoxins is of limited use in surgery for the control of established infections. Vaccines or suspensions of bacteria killed by heat or chemicals occasionally are of great value in the management of infections resistant to all other forms of therapy. As the result of numerous advances in the field of antibiotic therapy during the past 10 years, the antisera have assumed lesser importance in the control of infections. Their use in established infections is probably limited to the antitoxins of tetanus and gas gangrene and will be discussed elsewhere in the text.

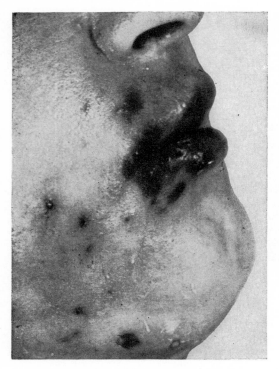

FIG. 4-4. A 33-year-old female with severe staphylococcal cellulitis of face and early carbuncle formation about lips, thrombosis of the external jugular vein, septic embolic pneumonitis and hemolytic *Staphylococcus aureus* septicemia. Recovery with penicillin therapy.

Occasionally, specific staphylococcal bacteriophage may also be used to advantage.

CLASSIFICATION OF WOUND INFECTIONS

Infections may be monomicrobic or polymicrobic, depending upon the presence of one or more varieties of infecting bacteria. Many *early infections* of wounds are pyogenic, the staphylococcus being the most frequent cause, the streptococcus the next. Mixed infections by aerobic and anaerobic, gram-negative and gram-positive bacteria may also occur, particularly in extensive wounds with retained dead tissue. Anaerobic cellulitis, clostridial myositis (gas gangrene), wound diphtheria, tetanus, anthrax and rabies are less frequent lesions.

The following is a brief classification of infections that may develop in wounds:

1. Staphylococcal
2. Streptococcal
   A. Aerobic
   B. Micro-aerophilic
   C. Anaerobic
3. Gram-negative bacillary
4. Mixed
5. Clostridial
6. Tetanus
7. Diphtheritic
8. Rabies
9. Mycotic
   A. Actinomycotic
   B. Blastomycotic
   C. Coccidioidomycotic
   D. Sporotrichotic
10. Miscellaneous
    A. Anthrax
    B. Granuloma inguinale
    C. Lymphopathia venereum

STAPHYLOCOCCAL INFECTIONS

Staphylococcal infections are usually localized and are characterized by an area of cellulitis and erythema which subsequently may undergo central necrosis or abscess formation with thick, creamy, odorless, and yellowish or reddish-yellow pus.

The hemolytic *Staphylococcus aureus,* which liquefies gelatin and produces a locally

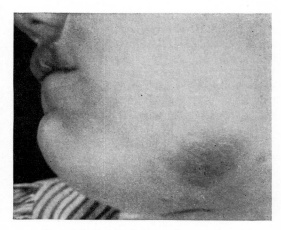

FIG. 4-5. Infected laceration of lip with purulent lymphadenopathy and cervical abscess caused by hemolytic *Staphylococcus aureus.*

necrotizing toxin, is the most important variety of staphylococcus. The coagulation of plasma by its enzyme, coagulase, favors the development of thrombosis and thrombophlebitis in the adjacent veins and is generally indicative of the pathogenicity of that particular strain. The symptoms of staphylococcal infection include swelling, erythema, and local pain which is throbbing and often synchronous with the heart beat. Fever and leukocytosis are usually present. The process may become invasive and complicated by lymphangitis, lymphadenitis, or thrombophlebitis. As a distributing focus it may produce a bacteremia and broadcast bacteria through the blood stream.

Staphylococcal infections that patients acquire during hospitalization may be particularly serious. Such infections are nearly always caused by a highly virulent staphylococcus which is resistant to most of the commonly used and available antibiotic agents. They may be characterized in some instances by a sudden onset, high fever and a fulminating course. They may have epidemic potentiality as manifested by persistent recurrences of less serious but equally refractive infections lasting for many months or years and by spread to other members of the families with whom they come in contact. Typing of the staphylococci associated with hospital-acquired infections by specific bacteriophage has revealed that the organisms responsible are one of three or four types, the most common ones being the 80-81 and the 77 strains.

The successful management of such infection may necessarily require the careful observance of established surgical principles and asepsis, meticulous selection of the proper antibiotic agent, general supportive care and active stimulation of immunity.

Folliculitis, furuncles and carbuncles are types of local staphylococcal infection of the skin and the subcutaneous tissues which usually begin spontaneously as infections of hair follicles and progress to produce small areas of induration of varying size with central necrosis. These lesions occur most frequently on the back of the neck, the face, the axillae, the groins, the buttocks and the fingers.

Treatment. The treatment of established staphylococcal infections is definitely influenced by early accurate diagnosis and consists of rest, heat, elevation of the infected area, adequate surgical drainage when pus has formed, and antibiotic therapy. Acute spreading processes should not be traumatized by incision or otherwise until the invasive characteristics have been brought under control. When pus or necrotic tissue develops in *localized* infections, its removal is extremely important for healing.

Infected wounds should be reopened with a hemostat at the point of maximum pain, swelling, or fluctuation, followed by removal of all skin sutures to enlarge the size of the cavity. In abscesses developing without reference to a wound, drainage is advocated by an adequate incision made over the area in such a manner as to avoid injury to important structures, disfiguring scars, or disabling contractures. Drainage of the wound is facilitated by fine-mesh gauze laid loosely in the cavity to keep the wound edges separated. Care should be taken not to pack the gauze tightly into the wound and thereby interfere with free drainage. The drain may be removed within 48 to 72 hours and may or may not be replaced, depending on the existing circumstances.

Antibiotic therapy should be started promptly, preferably before operation, so that a bacteriostatic concentration is produced in the blood stream to inhibit any bacteria distributed by operative manipulation. Aqueous sodium or potassium penicillin G in doses of 50,000 units intramuscularly every 4 hours or 500,000 units every 12 hours is the agent of choice. As an alternative method penicillin may also be administered effectively as a mixture of 300,000 units of procaine penicillin and 100,000 units of aqueous penicillin G every 12 to 24 hours until the infection is definitely under control. Erythromycin in doses of 100 to 200 mg. every 6 hours orally is likewise effective. The drugs of second choice include chloramphenicol, tetracycline, oxytetracycline and chlortetracycline in doses of 250 to 500 mg. every 4 to 6 hours. Declomycin and vancomycin may also be of great value in the control of these infections. In severe or fulminating cases with septicemia, aqueous crystalline penicillin G may be administered in doses of 100,000 to 200,000 units every 3 hours or 500,000 units intramuscularly every 6 to 8 hours. One of the broader-spectrum antibiotics may be used if the organism is resistant to penicillin. Bacitracin is also effective, but its administration should be controlled by daily urinalysis to detect any evidence of nephrotoxicity.

Streptococcal Infections

Streptococcal infections are produced most frequently by the aerobic *Streptococcus hemolyticus,* although some are caused by the *Streptococcus nonhemolyticus,* the *Streptococcus viridans,* the *Streptococcus anaerobicus,* or the micro-aerophilic Streptococcus.

Lesions caused by the aerobic *Streptococcus hemolyticus* characteristically are invasive and run a rapid course initially. They may develop within 12 to 48 hours after injury, or as late as 7 to 14 or more days. The incidence of infection by this organism in open wounds increases with the duration of the wound as a result of secondary contamination. In its early stages the process is usually one of diffuse inflammation with cellulitis, lymphangitis, lymphadenitis, or extension along fascial planes in deep wounds. There is little tendency to form abscesses, but gangrene of the overlying skin or thin watery pus may result. Invasion of the blood stream is frequent, and this complication should be recognized early to minimize the distribution of virulent bacteria throughout the body. Bacteremia is suggested by the development of chills, high fever, rapid thready pulse, prostration and other signs of toxemia.

Surgical scarlet fever may occur infrequently in a postoperative wound in association with the hemolytic streptococcus. The lesion is characterized by spreading cellulitis with redness, swelling, and frequently bullous formation in and about the margins of the wound. A typical scarlatiniform eruption may occur 2 to 4 days after injury or operation, starting at the wound and spreading peripherally. The local lesion may be very severe, but the general reaction may not be.

Erysipelas, also produced by the hemolytic streptococcus, may occur about small wounds, usually about the face and the neck. After an incubation period of 1 to 3 days, it is usually ushered in by chills, high fever, rapid pulse and severe toxemia. It is characterized by a spreading cellulitis with raised, irregular, indurated margins. Its appearance is characteristic, and its course is often self-limited in 4 to 8 days.

Hemolytic streptococcal gangrene (Figs. 4-6 and 4-7) occasionally follows some relatively minor injury in the extremities and is an epifascial, spreading, subcutaneous gangrene with thrombosis of the nutrient vessels and slough of the overlying skin. At the onset it is associated with pain and marked swelling at the site of wounds, chills, elevation of the temperature to 101° to 104° F., tachycardia, toxemia, marked prostration, and a rapidly spreading, painful cellulitis. The overlying skin of the diffusing cellulitis shows bullous formation and a peculiar patchy and coalescing necrosis. Hemolytic streptococci, often in pure culture, may be found in the fluid aspirated from the bullae or areas of subcutaneous slough.

Necrotizing fasciitis is an infection which involves the epifascial tissues of an operative area, laceration, abrasion, or puncture wound. It may either spread rapidly over large areas of the body or remain dormant for 6 or more days before beginning its rapid spread. In those cases which we have seen, the hemolytic staphylococcus or the hemolytic streptococcus has been found. Undermining of the skin is marked, and gangrenous changes in the skin may occur late or be absent. High fever, dehydration, anemia, marked leukocytosis and occasionally jaundice occur. The process may become chronic and may be characterized by multiple draining sinuses connected with areas of necrotic underlying fascia.

The treatment of hemolytic streptococcal infections consists of the preliminary control of their invasive characteristics by antibiotic therapy, rest and hot applications, followed by surgical drainage if abscesses or cutaneous gangrene develop. Penicillin, erythromycin, sulfadiazine, or one of the broad-spectrum antibiotics is very effective, but penicillin is usually the agent of choice in doses essentially the same as those described earlier for the treatment of staphylococcal infections. Operative treatment should be delayed until the invasive qualities of the infection have been controlled. Free drainage of collections of pus should be done along with the removal of necrotic tissue, infected hematomas, or foreign bodies. After incision, the wound is left open for further drainage and healing by granulation. The topical application of anti-biotics in such wounds is unnecessary. If suppurative thrombophlebitis exists, proximal ligation or excision of the involved vein should be considered.

In hemolytic streptococcal gangrene emergency drainage with longitudinal incision is often necessary as early as possible. It is important to make long incisions through and beyond the gangrenous area as an emergency measure without attempting to wait for control of the invasiveness by antibiotic therapy, in contrast with the usual treatment for streptococcal cellulitis. After operation the wound is treated by rest, elevation of the part if possible, and application of moist compresses. The removal of slough by sharp dissection without bleeding during subsequent dressings is possible. Before and after operation antibiotic therapy, preferably with aqueous penicillin, should be given in adequate amounts as in other aerobic streptococcal infections.

Streptococcal Fasciitis. As soon as the diagnosis of streptococcal fasciitis is established, drainage by long incisions made throughout the entire area of involvement should be made

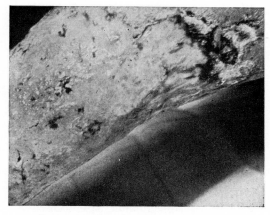

Fig. 4-7. Chronic progressive cutaneous gangrene of leg with extensive ulceration. Note gangrenous margin of ulcer where micro-aerophilic nonhemolytic *Streptococcus* and hemolytic *Staphylococcus aureus* were demonstrated.

as described for hemolytic streptococcal gangrene. The skin and the subcutaneous tissues should be separated from the deep fascia. Involved necrotic fascia should be excised completely and the wound covered with fine-

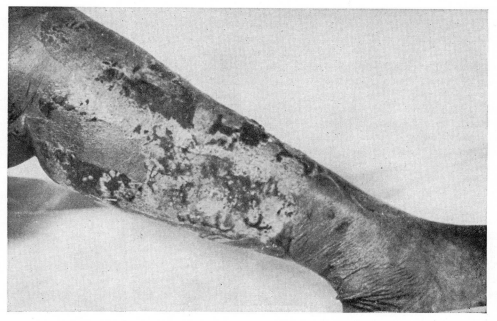

Fig. 4-6. Acute streptococcal gangrene of lower leg caused by *Streptococcus hemolyticus*. This lesion followed a slight injury to the ankle area. Note residual bullae and marked gangrene of skin.

mesh gauze. When adequate granulations have developed, skin grafting usually is necessary.

In many streptococcal infections, general supportive therapy consisting of the intelligent administration of adequate fluid and electrolytes is very important. Daily blood transfusions may be helpful, but care must be taken not to overload the heart and produce pulmonary edema. Frequent examinations for metastic infectious complications are necessary, and any that may have developed is treated according to its individual location and characteristics.

Micro-aerophilic Streptococci. Infections caused by micro-aerophilic streptococci develop and progress more slowly as a rule. Two illustrative examples are chronic burrowing ulcer and chronic progressive cutaneous gangrene. Chronic burrowing ulcer is an infrequent lesion caused by a micro-aerophilic hemolytic streptococcus and is characterized by the progressive extension of burrowing sinus tracts through the underlying tissues. Invasion and penetration of fascia, bone, muscle, peritoneum, meninges or brain have been noted. The sinus tracts usually become lined with idolent granulation tissue. General signs of infection associated with this are minimal, a low-grade fever and marked pain being likely to appear during the acute exacerbations of the lesion.

The treatment of choice consists of the radical incision and drainage of the sinus tracts throughout their entire extent, or radical excision of the sinuses in association with antibiotic therapy. Penicillin, erythromycin, bacitracin, chloramphenicol, or one of the broad-spectrum agents may be used. Antibiotic treatment without surgical treatment is inadequate.

Chronic progressive cutaneous gangrene (known also as Meleney's synergistic gangrene) may complicate operations for purulent infections of the chest or the peritoneal cavity. It is caused by the synergistic action of a micro-aerophilic nonhemolytic streptococcus and an aerobic hemolytic staphylococcus. After an incubation period of 7 to 14 days after operation for a wound involving the gastrointestinal, the genitourinary, or the respiratory tracts, the surrounding skin becomes tender, red and edematous, particularly about stay sutures. The appearance of the lesion is characteristic. A wide area of bright-red cellulitis develops about a central purplish area which widens, becomes gangrenous and finally ulcerates. The base of the ulcer is covered with dirty infected granulation tissue, and the margin is purplish black, slightly undermined and very painful.

This ulceration is slowly progressive, and ultimately it may denude larger areas and cause death unless treated adequately. Systemic manifestations at first are slight, but in neglected cases profound derangements in physiology may develop with wasting of the muscles, low-grade fever, anemia and chronic septic shock.

Local excision of gangrenous margins or other conservative methods usually fail to check this process. Radical excision of the ulcerated lesion and its gangrenous borders is indicated, along with systemic antibiotic treatment with penicillin G or erythromycin. There is some evidence that bacitracin is particularly valuable in the treatment of this condition.

During treatment of patients with chronic progressive cutaneous gangrene with penicillin the hemolytic staphylococcus may disappear and be replaced by a strain of *B. proteus*. In some instances, a synergism between *B. proteus* and nonhemolytic and micro-aerophilic streptococcus can exist primarily to cause the lesion.

Anaerobic streptococcal infections may occur as either acute or chronic lesions. In the acute type, they may occur with or without bacteremia, particularly in wounds which involve or penetrate the genital, the intestinal or the respiratory tracts. Metastatic abscesses in distant regions such as the brain may develop. These infections, which usually progress more slowly than other streptococcal infections, are characterized by the development of marked induration, foul-smelling and thick pus, extending necrosis of the involved tissues and progression along fascial planes or in muscle.

Streptococcal myositis is an infrequent type of anaerobic streptococcal infection. It is associated with massive involvement of muscle, local pain and generalized toxemia. Discoloration, edema, and crepitation of the muscle is characteristic, and a foul odor is generally apparent. Its differentiation from clostridial myositis is possible by its more pronounced cutaneous erythema, its discolored muscle which is still viable and reactive to stimuli, its different odor, and the demonstration of vast numbers of streptococci in gram-stained smears of the exudate.

The management of anaerobic streptococcal infections is dependent upon early diagnosis, operative treatment, antibiotic therapy and supportive treatment. Abscesses, areas of fasciitis, or infected groups of muscle should be incised and drained promptly, and ulcers showing phagedenic progression should be excised. Antibiotic therapy is of considerable benefit, and penicillin is the agent of choice in doses somewhat larger than those recommended for aerobic streptococcal infections. From 100,000 to 200,000 units of aqueous crystalline penicillin G every 2 to 3 hours or 500,000 units every 6 to 8 hours usually will suffice to bring the invasive qualities of the infection under control. Bacitracin or the broader-spectrum antibiotics are alternate choices.

GRAM-NEGATIVE BACILLARY INFECTIONS

Infections may be produced by gram-negative bacteria of the gastrointestinal, the urinary, or the genital tracts. *Escherichia coli, Pseudomonas aeruginosa, Proteus vulgaris* and *Salmonella typhosa* are examples capable of causing wound infections. Invasive lesions with bacteremia may occur. Often these gram-negative bacilli are relatively nonvirulent, but in the presence of such factors as necrotic tissue, general debility, or cortisone therapy, they may produce serious infections. A relatively long incubation period is also characteristic of postoperative wound infections by these bacilli.

The treatment of these lesions is dependent upon incision and drainage of abscesses, excision of necrotic tissue, and antibiotic therapy based upon *in vitro* sensitivity tests. Chloramphenicol has been particularly useful in these infections. Polymixin B. and colymycin are recommended for infections produced by *Ps. aeruginosa*.

MIXED OR SYNERGISTIC INFECTIONS

A large and miscellaneous group of infections with a polymicrobic etiology are found in surgical practice, particularly in association with injuries or operations on the gastrointestinal, the respiratory, or the genitourinary tracts. Symbiosis of aerobes and anaerobes may exist and determine the characteristics of the lesion. The bacterial toxins and enzymes usually cause a necrotizing and suppurative infection, beginning in the wound and extending along fascial and areolar tissues. Cellulitis, abscesses, necrosis and bacteremia may develop. Examples of mixed infections include deep infections of the neck, human-bite infections, putrid empyema, peritonitis and nonclostridial cellulitis.

Human-bite infections (morsus humanus) are usually severe and occur when a human being voluntarily bites another or strikes a blow with his hand which is cut by the teeth of the intended victim. The wound is usually a puncture wound through the various levels of tissue which supports the growth of the mouth organisms contaminating the tissues. A mixture of bacteria is usually found consisting of aerobic nonhemolytic streptococci, anaerobic streptococci, *Bacterium melaninogenicum,* spirochetes or staphylococci. In our experience spirochetes have never been found alone in these infections, but they are associated with the more severe lesions. If the original bite wound is treated by limited or inadequate surgical measures, evidence of inflammation appears within the first 1 to 3 days after injury and progresses steadily thereafter. Swelling, redness, pain, and limitation of motion develop and are followed by fever which is usually moderate but may be as high as 105° F. Systemic reaction is occasionally profound, and the appearance of the local infection soon becomes alarming. Granulation tissue forming within the wound becomes shaggy, gray, cyanotic and edematous and exudes a thick, foul, purulent material. Progressive necrosis extends through the tissues, particularly the areolar ones.

The prevention of infections of this type is the most effective form of treatment. Adequate excision of the wound, as soon as the patient is seen, followed by immobilization and antibiotic therapy, usually with penicillin, is the most effective means of preventing human-bite infections. When tendons are severed by human bites, primary tenorrhaphy should not be attempted. When infection has become established, radical decompression of

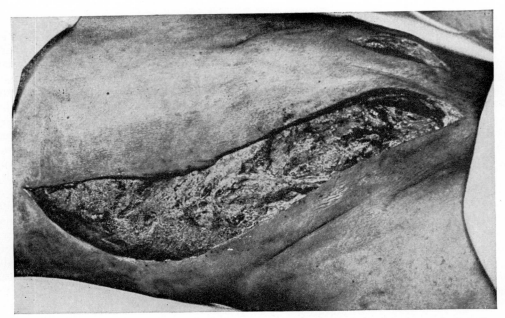

Fig. 4-8. A 50-year-old white male with acute crepitant cellulitis of abdominal wall caused by mixed infection arising in a left inguinal hernioplasty wound made for the repair of a strangulated hernia. Spread was rapid and beneath Scarpa's fascia.

the infected area and tissue planes by incision is extremely important, accompanied by antibiotic therapy.

Crepitant (nonclostridial) cellulitis is a mixed infection which is usually seen as a complication of wounds of the perineum, abdominal wall, buttocks, hip, thorax, or neck which have been contaminated by discharges from the intestinal, the genitourinary, or the respiratory tracts. When it occurs in the region of the perineum or inguinal area, its spread is often beneath Scarpa's fascia into the abdominal wall and flank. It is caused by bacteria other than the clostridia, no single type of etiologic agent being found consistently. Those associated with this process include strains of the coliform group, the anaerobic Bacteroides group such as *Bacterium melaninogenicus* and *Bacillus thetoides* and the anaerobic streptococci. The areolar and fascial tissues usually become necrotic and develop a putrid odor similar to that of an appendiceal abscess. Progressive gangrenous changes in the skin occur as a result of thrombosis of the nutrient vessels. As the process extends, toxemia usually becomes evident with dehydration, fever, a weak and thready pulse, prostration,

and elevation of W.B.C. to 20,000 or more.

Prompt surgical decompression of all involved areas by multiple incisions is imperative to control this process. Aqueous penicillin G in doses of 200,000 to 1,000,000 units every 3 to 4 hours is recommended along with one of the broad-spectrum antibiotics in doses of 500 mg. Supportive therapy may be life-saving. These infections are serious, but the prognosis is good for patients treated promptly and adequately. After the infection has been controlled and healthy granulation tissue has developed, skin-grafting is usually necessary to cover the large residual cutaneous defects.

CLOSTRIDIAL INFECTIONS

Clostridial cellulitis is a serious, crepitant, septic process of subcutaneous, retroperitoneal, or other areolar tissues which is caused by one or more of the clostridia. *Clostridium welchii* is the chief agent. However, other bacteria are usually present. It is characterized by an emphysematous cellulitis which spreads rapidly along fascial planes and is to be differentiated from clostridial myositis by the absence of invasion of living muscle.

Pain about a wound is usually the first

symptom, and it may precede any obvious swelling, erythema, or crepitation of the overlying skin by several days. A gray or reddish-brown, seropurulent or putrid discharge may develop as the infection progresses. Slough of the areolar and fascial tissues occurs, associated with thrombosis of the neighboring vessels and finally extensive gangrene of the overlying skin.

The systemic effects may be slight, moderate or severe. Compared with clostridial myositis or true gas gangrene, the fever, tachycardia, leukocytosis and anemia are more moderately altered. Clostridial cellulitis is a serious disease but does not have the high mortality of clostridial myositis if treated promptly. Prompt surgical decompression of all involved areas by extensive multiple incisions is indicated in the treatment of this condition. The incisions should be made to extend through the area of involvement into the adjacent normal tissues. The skin flaps are elevated superficial to the fascia, and any portions of necrotic fascia present should be excised. Antibiotic treatment is similar to that described for nonclostridial cellulitis, although,

in our experience, the tetracycline agents have been most efficacious, both experimentally and clinically. Antibiotic therapy should be started preoperatively and continued until all evidence of local or systemic invasiveness of the infection has disappeared. Supportive therapy is likewise important. Inspection of the involved area should be made every 24 or 48 hours and careful search made for areas of spread which are prone to develop.

Clostridial myositis is a spreading or localized gangrenous infection of muscle caused by one or more clostridia. It is usually a mixed infection which involves muscle primarily and is characterized by spreading infectious gangrene, profound toxemia and a rapidly fatal course, unless treated properly. Injuries of the extremities of the buttocks associated with devitalized, torn or contaminated muscle are prone to develop this type of infection. Interference with the main blood supply to a limb or a muscle group, the presence of foreign bodies, delay in surgical treatment, or improper surgical care are important predisposing factors. Crepitation of the tissues produced by gas occurs in most cases, par-

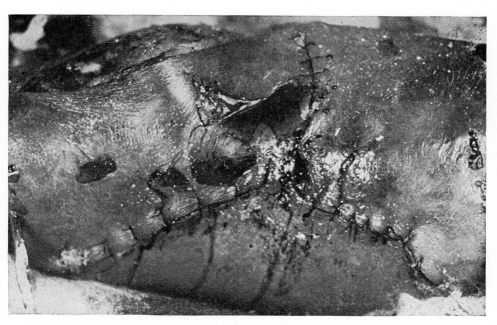

Fig. 4-9. Far-advanced gas gangrene of leg in patient 3 days after débridement and closed reduction of compound fracture of tibia and fibula. Note marked swelling, necrosis of skin, brownish watery discharge, and herniation of muscle through relaxing incision. Amputation was necessary because of irreversible gangrenous changes.

ticularly in those produced by *Clostridium welchii* and *Cl. septique*. A great variety of anaerobes have been found in this infection, chiefly *Cl. welchii, Cl. novyi, Cl. sordellii* and *Cl. septique*. The infection may be confined to a muscle or spread rapidly to involve a single group of muscles, an entire limb, or the torso. With others, edema may occur without gas, and with still others, rapid digestion and dissolution of tissue with moderate edema but no gas. The saccharolytic clostridia ferment the muscle sugar to produce acid and gas, and the proteolytic clostridia digest muscle to liquefy it. Gaseous infiltration, edema, and rapid liquefaction of the tissues may exist in the same wound. Soluble toxins diffuse into adjacent tissues, causing further destruction and thrombosis of the vessels or are absorbed into the circulation to produce marked toxemia, septic shock, damage of the liver, the heart and the kidneys, profound anemia, prostration and death.

Pain is the earliest symptom of clostridial myositis, appearing in the first 24 hours after injury and caused principally by the rapid infiltration of the tissues by fluid and gas. The patient may develop a peculiar grayish pallor, listlessness, weakness, profuse sweating, prostration and breathlessness. A striking pallor of the face develops. Anorexia is a fairly constant finding, and vomiting is not uncommon. The mental state is one of apathy and indifference to the seriousness of his condition; stupor, delirium and coma may occur later. A rapid and feeble pulse may follow the onset of pain. Circulatory collapse, which may be abrupt, progressive and severe, may develop. Fever is not a reliable index of the severity of the infectious process, varying considerably, and frequently is less than 101° F. A low temperature, a very rapid pulse and hypotension are indicative of a grave prognosis.

The skin overlying the lesion is at first white and tense, and the infected muscle visible in the wound becomes dark red, soft and swollen. It frequently herniates into the wound and discharges a brown, watery, foul-smelling exudate containing many bacteria and red blood cells but a paucity of leukocytic cells. The overlying skin becomes dusky or bronze in appearance, and vesicles filled with dark-red fluid may appear and coalesce. The distal portion of the limb involved becomes edematous, engorged, discolored, cold and finally obviously gangrenous. Laboratory data usually show a marked reduction in the number of red corpuscles with counts ranging between 1 and 2 million per cm., low hemoglobin levels of 30 to 40 per cent, and relatively low leukocytic counts not exceeding 12,000 to 15,000 cells per mm.[3] in many instances.

The early diagnosis of gas gangrene may be difficult because large dressings, casts or splints used for the treatment of the injury may mask the progress of the infection until a far-advanced process is present. Continued pain at the site of a wound containing injured muscle; a rapid and easily compressible pulse; varying degrees of fever; toxemia in association with spreading edema; a thin, brown, watery, malodorous discharge; crepitation; herniation of discolored muscle which does not bleed or contract; and typical discolorations of the skin in the regions of the wound—these are diagnostic signs. Infiltrating gas may be detected early by the experienced observer through auscultatory percussion or by serial roentgenograms.

It is important to explore surgically and without delay any wound in which the presence of clostridial myositis is suspected. Early and adequate operation is the most effective means of treating established gas gangrene; no other form of treatment, including chemotherapy and serotherapy, replaces it. Radical incision through the skin and the fascia to decompress the muscle compartments and to permit excision of all devitalized and infected muscles is imperative. If the diagnosis is made when gangrenous changes implying death of the extremity and permanent loss of function have occurred, open amputation of the guillotine type should be performed, supplemented by drainage of any infected fascial compartments and excision of any devitalized muscle remaining above the line of amputation.

Intensive antibiotic therapy is recommended in conjunction with surgery, consisting of tetracycline, oxytetracycline, or chlortetracycline in doses of 500 mg. intravenously every 6 to 8 hours. Aqueous crystalline penicillin G in large doses of 1 million units intramuscularly every 3 hours or chloramphenicol in doses of 500 mg. every 6 to 8 hours may also be used but apparently are not as effective.

Supportive therapy is of marked importance for maintaining fluid and electrolyte balance and for correcting the derangements in physiology produced by this infection. Frequent blood transfusions of whole blood are of value in correcting the severe hemolytic anemia and decreased blood volume associated with this infection, provided that prompt surgical and antibiotic therapy have also been instituted.

TETANUS

Etiology. Tetanus, also known as lockjaw or trismus, is another very serious wound infection. It is caused by the growth of *Clostridium tetani* and its generation of a potent toxin within the wound. The toxin diffuses through the adjacent skeletal muscles, acting on the neuromuscular end organs and causing a state of local tonic contraction (local tetanus). It is also distributed by the circulating blood or lymph to susceptible cells in the cord, the medulla and the motor end organs of the skeletal muscles, resulting in trismus, risus sardonicus, opisthotonos, rigidity of the abdominal muscles, spasm of the skeletal muscles of the extremities, and generalized clonic convulsions precipitated by external stimuli (generalized tetanus).

The incubation period varies from 4 to 21 or more days, the usual being 6 to 10. In general the severity of the disease decreases as the incubation period increases. A prodromal period follows the incubation period and is characterized by stiffness of jaw muscles, headache, restlessness, yawning, and twitches of pain in the region of the wound.

Pathology. In generalized tetanus, the *active stage* usually begins within 12 to 24 hours after onset of the prodromal period and is characterized by tonic spasms of the skeletal muscles. Trismus of the jaw may be extreme, and spasms of the facial musculature may produce a grimace or facial distortion. Opisthotonos with retraction of the head may be caused by tonicity of the spinal group of muscles. Extreme irritability occurs, and the slightest irritation sets up clonic spasms which may involve the musculature of the entire body, including the diaphragm. Between clonic attacks, the tonic spasm is maintained. During clonic contractions, the pain is intense, the pulse is rapid, and sweating and salivation are profuse. The leukocytic count is usually 12,000 to 15,000 with a relative polymorphonuclear leukocytosis.

During the *terminal stage,* the fever becomes greater, the pain more severe, and urinary retention may occur. There is seldom any stupor, and mental clarity persists to the end. Death is usually due to the respiratory arrest occurring during a convulsion, to asphyxia, to an exhausting toxemia, or to poisoning by barbiturates used to control the convulsive seizures.

The diagnosis of tetanus is usually not difficult, particularly when the disease is seen in the third stage or period of convulsions.

Treatment. The successful management of established tetanus depends particularly on early diagnosis and prompt adequate treatment. Severe symptoms do not necessarily indicate a fatal outcome. The main objectives of treatment are the prevention of additional toxin from reaching the central nervous system, removal of the source of toxin, adequate sedation of the patient to control convulsions, and maintenance of adequate respiration. An initial intravenous dose of 50,000 units of tetanus antitoxin is given immediately after a preliminary skin test has shown the patient not to be sensitive to horse serum. An additional injection of 40,000 units of tetanus antitoxin may also be given intramuscularly. If the skin test is positive, rapid desensitization is carried out to permit the injection of a therapeutic dose. The tissues around the site of injury may be infiltrated with 10,000 units of antitoxin. Also, a single dose of 10,000 to 20,000 units of antitoxin may be injected intrathecally by lumbar puncture. 5,000 units of antitoxin may be injected daily until the disease is obviously under control.

Whenever possible, local excision or incision of the wound should be done 1 hour later under anesthesia with intravenously administered Pentothal Sodium. Removal of any foreign bodies or infected granulation tissues should be included. Thereafter, the cleansing care of the wound is the same as that given for the average granulating wound.

The patient is placed in bed in a darkened, quiet room in order to reduce the number of external stimuli to a minimum. A nurse or a physician should be in constant attendance for the prompt recognition of respiratory arrest and the immediate institution of appropriate treatment for its correction. We have seen a patient with severe tetanus, who had been carried successfully through 11 seizures of respiratory arrest, die during his 12th seizure when the nurse left him unattended for 15 minutes.

The control of convulsive seizures is difficult. Barbiturates or paraldehyde may be administered orally, rectally or intramuscularly. Our preference is the administration of a very dilute solution of Pentothal Sodium (0.5 to 1.0 Gm. per 1,000 ml. by continuous drip in physiologic saline or glucose solution administered at the rate of 20 to 25 drops per minute. In addition, a syringe of 2.5 per cent Pentothal Sodium solution is kept in constant readiness for the emergency intravenous injection of a few ml. should convulsive respiratory arrest occur. In our experience the immediate injection of a few ml. of 2.5 per cent of Pentothal solution to a patient with a generalized convulsion and respiratory arrest is usually followed by prompt resumption of spontaneous breathing within 30 to 45 seconds. Of course, artificial respiration should be instituted.

Curarelike drugs may be given to aid in the control of the convulsive seizures. Myanesin in a 1 or 2 per cent solution may be given in amounts sufficient to meet the patient's individual requirements. The initial dose is usually 0.5 to 1.0 Gm. Thereafter, 0.2 to 1.0 Gm. per hour may be necessary. Individual requirements vary greatly. Myanesin and other curarelike drugs may be toxic or dangerous and must be used cautiously. In addition, they may not have any beneficial effect on the course of tetanus.

Tracheotomy may be considered, and oxygen therapy should be available for use if indicated. Excessive saliva should be removed by a soft rubber catheter connected to a suction pump which is kept at the bedside. Tongue blades covered with gauze may be held in place between the teeth to prevent laceration of the tongue. Adequate fluid, electrolyte and caloric intake should be maintained.

Antibiotic therapy is of no value in the treatment of established tetanus except for its control of associated wound infections or for its effect on pulmonary complications.

None of the antibiotics presently available has any influence on the tetanus toxin *per se* or its effect.

DIPHTHERITIC INFECTION

Wounds occasionally become infected by the Klebs-Löffler bacillus and develop either an acute ulceration and cellulitis, with infiltration of the skin and the subcutaneous tissues about the wound, or a chronic indolent ulceration of an open wound which fails to heal. In the acute form, the systemic symptoms may be severe. A typical diphtheritic membrane adheres to the surface of the wound, and its removal results in bleeding. If paralysis of the facial muscles, cardiac arrhythmia, or respiratory difficulty occurs in a patient with a wound covered by a gray adherent membrane, a diagnosis of surgical diphtheria should be considered until proved otherwise. The diagnosis is proved by demonstrating the organisms in stained smears and by recovering them in cultures from the wound.

The treatment consists of isolation of the patient, injection of diphtheria antitoxin, and administration of penicillin or one of the broad-spectrum antibiotics.

RABIES

Etiology. Rabies is an infection caused by a virus which is inoculated into the host by means of a bite by another animal. The disease produced is a fatal encephalitis resulting from passage of the neurotropic virus along the nerve axis cylinders to the central nervous system. Infection most frequently follows a bite by a dog but has been reported after bites by other animals, including horses, cattle, cats, squirrels and bats.

The incubation period varies almost directly with the distance of the injury from the brain and may cover from 2 weeks to several months, usually being 30 to 40 days. In the prodromal phase, the infected individual shows nonspecific malaise, but this is followed by an excitement phase in which there is the characteristic paralysis of the muscles of swallowing. Since attempts to swallow precipitate severe paroxysms of coughing, the victim becomes maniacal when he sees a glass of water. Hence the term hydrophobia.

Treatment of established rabies is unsuccessful, and prophylaxis is the only means of control for this infection. Following a bite by a suspected animal the local wound should be meticulously débrided and cleansed. The animal responsible for the injury should be carefully examined and impounded for 14 days. If the animal cannot be identified, or if it should develop rabies within the observation period, antirabies vaccine should be given immediately. Because of the very short incubation period in injuries of the face and the neck, it is probably wise to begin immunization immediately after such a bite and discontinue the treatment when the animal proves to be free from disease. It must be kept in mind that the injection of rabies vaccine is not without danger, since encephalitic paralysis may follow its use.

MYCOTIC INFECTIONS

Actinomycosis is a surgical infection caused by *Actinomyces bovis*. This fungus may also be found growing noninvasively in the pharynx of man and some mammals. It is probable that invasion is always preceded by local surface injury which may be unrecognized.

When infection develops, it is characterized by the development of nodular granulomatous areas which subsequently suppurate and discharge pus through sinus tracts. The purulent discharge characteristically contains "sulfur granules" which are masses of lightly entwined mycelial filaments. The infection is a chronic process which typically burrows through adjacent tissues and does not spread by way of the regional lymphatics.

The clinical forms of actinomycosis may be classified into 3 types:

1. The cervicofacial variety, which is seen most frequently originating near the mandible as a hard, moderately tender, inflammatory nodule. It progresses to suppuration with central necrosis and fistulous tract formation. Peripheral extension develops with similar nodules undergoing the same course.

2. The thoracic form of the infection may be well advanced before it is recognized. Its early symptoms are nonspecific and are similar to any chronic pulmonary infection. As the disease advances, its burrowing nature becomes apparent by the involvement of pleura and ribs. Far-advanced cases may develop cutaneous fistulae.

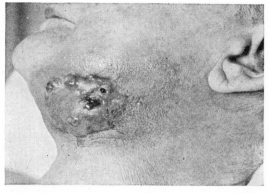

FIG. 4-10. Cervicofacial actinomycosis caused by *Actinomyces bovis*. Marked induration, discoloration of adjacent skin, and multiple sinuses apparent. Sulfur granules were identified in discharge from sinuses, and the organism was cultured anaerobically.

3. The abdominal variety may be confused with cases of appendiceal abscess or carcinoma of the cecum, even at the operating table. Persistent cutaneous abdominal fistulae may develop. The diagnosis is usually made by demonstration of the actinomycotic colonies in hanging-drop preparations, in biopsies, or in cultures.

Treatment of actinomycotic infections has become impressively more successful since the introduction of the various chemotherapeutic agents. Indicated surgical operative treatment by incision and drainage of abscesses or excision, if practical, must be accompanied and followed by a prolonged course of treatment (4 to 6 months) with chemotherapeutic agents, preferably penicillin and sulfadiazine.

Blastomycosis is another of the mycotic infections which is due to yeastlike organisms. Subsequent to local inoculation a painless papule develops and persists until it ulcerates. The ulceration has a characteristic appearance, with multiple small daughter abscesses along the advancing margin. There may occur some degree of central healing of the ulcer as it increases in diameter.

The course of blastomycosis is one of relatively slow progression while the infection remains localized. As the disease extends, distant metastases develop most often in the lungs or bone. When systemic spread has

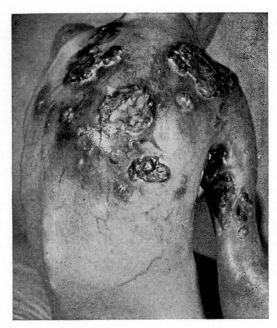

FIG. 4-11. An 11-year-old white female with far-advanced actinomycosis of thoracic type. Note characteristic discoloration of skin, granulomatous granulation tissue and marked emaciation.

occurred, the prognosis of a patient with this infection is very grave.

The treatment of blastomycosis confined to the cutaneous surface is radical excision of the involved area followed by skin grafting. Large doses of sodium or potassium iodide may be given as a systemic medication in the control of the infection. Many other forms of treatment have been used with minimal degrees of success. These include x-ray therapy, arsenicals and topical antiseptics. Recently, stilbamidine has shown some promise in the treatment of this condition.

Coccidioidomycosis is an infection caused by the fungus *Coccidioides immitis.* The most frequent type is a pulmonary infection, since the life cycle of the organism includes a sporulating stage in which it may be blown about in dust and thereby inhaled by man. The clinical picture of this infection in the chronic form resembles that of tuberculosis. An acute fulminating type is recognized in which there is an overwhelming respiratory infection which may end in death within 2 months. In the chronic form granulomatous

lesions of the lung occur and may be controlled by the patient. Progression of this form of the disease results with the occurrence of skin lesions, chronic granulomatous nodules, or spread to the bones or brain. Diagnosis is accomplished by demonstration of the organism in smears of sputum or local discharges and by examination of biopsied material. Skin sensitivity test may be useful in establishing the diagnosis.

Treatment of this infection is difficult. The principles of treatment are based on supportive measures to encourage development of body defenses and resistance against the organism. Recent experimental evidence suggests that a vaccine for this infection may be possible. Aside from drainage of abscesses, operative surgical treatment is usually of little value (see Chap. 42, "Surgery of the Lung").

Sporotrichosis. *Sporothrix schenckii* is the etiologic agent of sporotrichosis. This rare disease results from inoculation of the organisms into a small wound, usually of the hand or the foot. Ulceration with nodular lymphangitis develops along the course of the lymphatics draining the area of the wound. Secondary ulcerations of the nodules may also develop. These findings in the disease may be limited to the regional area, since systemic invasion is rare.

Treatment is usually successful with the use of large doses of potassium iodide (150 to 200 drops per day of a saturated solution).

Anthrax, formerly known as "woolsorter's disease," was the first infectious disease proved to be caused by a bacterial agent, *Bacillus anthracis,* by Robert Koch in 1877. Initially, the disease is characterized by the development of small red macules which occur in individuals who handle animals or animal products. These macules, representing the portal of entry, become vesicles. As the disease progresses, satellite vesicles occur. The primary lesion becomes necrotic, and a black eschar forms in the center. The cutaneous lesion is usually not painful, but regional lymphadenopathy, which follows, often results in localized pain and tenderness. Septicemia may occur. The general symptoms of malaise, fever and prostration develop in proportion to the stage and the severity of the infection.

A separate form of the disease may arise after infection of the victim by inhalation of these bacteria. This form is rapidly progressive and usually fatal, since the first manifestation may be septicemia with or without pneumonia.

The mortality rate in the cutaneous form of the infection in the untreated cases was approximately 25 per cent, and approximately 100 per cent in the septicemic variety.

Modern antibiotic treatment has profoundly influenced these mortality rates. Anthrax, particularly the cutaneous variety, responds rapidly to the administration of penicillin, and the tetracyclines and chloramphenicol have been reported to be similarly effective.

Granuloma inguinale is a venereal disease seen most frequently in the tropics but occasionally in all climates, particularly in the vicinity of seaports. It is caused by the bacterium, *Donovania granulomatis,* which is a gram-negative organism having a well-defined capsule and usually found intracellularly, particularly in large mononuclear cells. The incubation period, following inoculation, may vary from a few days to as long as 3 months. This is followed by the appearance of an indolent dirty ulcer on the scrotum, the penis or the groin which is slowly progressive. The associated odor is easily recognized by experienced physicians. The causative organism may be seen in smears of the exudate or in histologic section of the edge of the ulcer.

Treatment of this infection with streptomycin, the tetracyclines, or chloramphenicol is usually followed by prompt improvement.

Lymphopathia venereum is another of the venereal diseases and it is caused by a filtrable virus. Although its incidence is higher in the tropics, it is found throughout the world. The infection occurs in both males and females but is more likely to persist and cause secondary complications in the female. Colored patients are affected more frequently than white.

The infection, usually contracted by sexual intercourse, is manifested initially by a small genital ulceration which may heal slowly. Associated systemic manifestations are those of malaise, fever, which is usually low-grade, and often signs of meningeal irritation. Spread to the regional lymph nodes results in their marked enlargement and occasionally in suppuration. The disease may subside and lapse into a stage of apparent quiescence. After months or years, the process may lead to rectal stricture and associated intestinal obstruction due to fibrosis or contracture of the anogenital lymphatics, particularly in women. Diagnosis is suggested by positive skin test with Frei antigen.

In the acute infectious stage, apparent benefit in the control of the disease has been obtained by the use of chloramphenicol and the tetracyclines. In the late or cicatricial stage, these antibiotics are of no direct value, and abdominoperineal resection may become necessary.

Due to the reaction in the tissues surrounding the rectum, this operation is apt to be considerably more hazardous and difficult in this condition than in early carcinoma of the rectum. If a preliminary colostomy is done, the reaction may subside to some extent after several months, facilitating the resection at a second stage.

BIBLIOGRAPHY

Altemeier, W. A., Coith, R., Sherman, R., Logan, M. A., and Tytell, A.: Toxoid immunization of experimental gas gangrene, A.M.A. Arch. Surg. *65*:633-640, 1952.

Altemeier, W. A., and Culbertson, W. R.: Acute non-clostridial crepitant cellulitis, Surg., Gynec. & Obst. *87*:206-212, 1948.

————: The prevention and control of surgical infections, S. Clin. North America *35*:1645-1661, 1955.

————: Prophylactic antibiotic therapy, A.M.A. Arch. Surg. *71*:2-6, 1955.

Altemeier, W. A., Culbertson, W. R., and Gonzalez, L. L.: Clinical experiences in the treatment of tetanus, A.M.A. Arch. Surg. *80*:977-985, 1960.

Altemeier, W. A., Culbertson, W. R., Sherman, R., Cole, W., Elstun, W., and Fultz, C. T.: Critical re-evaluation of antibiotic therapy in surgery, J.A.M.A. *157*:305-309, 1955.

Altemeier, W. A., and Furste, W. L.: Gas gangrene, Internat. Obstr. Surg. *in* Surg., Gynec. & Obst. *84*:507-523, 1947.

Altemeier, W. A., and Garth, T.: The treatment of tetanus *in* Current Therapy, sect. 1, pp. 48-50, Philadelphia, Saunders, 1956.

Altemeier, W. A., Giuseffi, J., and Stevenson, J.: Wound infections *in* Surgery of Trauma, pp. 80-101, Philadelphia, Lippincott, 1953.

Altemeier, W. A., and Largen, T.: Antibiotic and chemotherapeutic agents in infections of the skeletal system, J.A.M.A. *150*:1462-1468, 1952.

Altemeier, W. A., and Sherman, R.: The use of antibiotics and antisera in the treatment of acute injuries, J. Kentucky M.A. *55*:428-433, 1954.

Altemeier, W. A., and Wulsin, J. H.: Antimicrobial therapy in injured patients, J.A.M.A. *173*: 527-533, 1960.

Dowling, H. F., Lepper, M. H., and Jackson, G. G.: The clinical significance of antibiotic resistant bacteria, J.A.M.A. *157*:327-331, 1955.

Edsall, G.: Active immunization tetanus, New England J. Med. *241*:18-26, 60-70, 99-107, 1949.

Hare, R., and Willits, R. E.: Bacteriology of recently inflicted wounds with special reference to hemolytic streptococci and staphylococci, Canad. M.A.J. *46*:23-30, 1942.

Hill, E. O., Altemeier, W. A., and Culbertson, W. R.: An appraisal of methods of testing bacterial sensitivity to antibiotics, Ann. Surg. *148*: 410-428, 1958.

Larrey, D. J.: Memoirs of Military Surgery, vol. I & II, Paris, Cushing, 1812-1814.

MacLennan, J. D.: Anaerobic infections of war wounds in Middle East, Lancet *2*:63-66, 94-99, 123-126, 1943.

Meleney, F.: Differential diagnosis between certain types of infectious gangrene of skin with particular reference to hemolytic streptococcus gangrene and bacterial synergistic gangrene, Surg., Gynec. & Obst. *56*:847-867, 1933.

————: Zinc peroxide in treatment of micro-aerophilic and anaerobic infections, with special reference to group of chronic, ulcerative burrowing, non-gangrenous lesions of abdominal wall apparently due to micro-aerophilic hemolytic streptococcus, Ann. Surg. *101*:997-1011, 1935.

Miles, A. A., *et al.*: Hospital infection of war wounds, Brit. M. J. *2*:855 and 895, 1940.

Pulaski, E. J.: Medical progress, New England J. Med. *249*:890-897, 932-938, 1953.

————: Surgical Infections: Prophylaxis, Treatment, Antibiotic Therapy, Springfield, Ill., Thomas, 1953.

Reid, M. R.: Infections in surgery, Internat. Abstr. Surg. *in* Surg., Gynec. & Obst. *69*:107-109, 1939.

Report of Committee: Measures to combat antibiotic-resistant infections in hospitals, Bull. Am. Coll. Surgeons *44*:73-79, 1959.

JONATHAN E. RHOADS, M.D.

—————————— CHAPTER 5 ——————————

Fluid and Electrolytes

The subject of water and electrolyte balance has been obscured by a long series of efforts to establish short cuts. It is not a simple subject but rather one that requires careful study and thought. The body ordinarily takes care of water and electrolyte requirements by impulse. Thirst and the craving for salt are familiar to most of us.

In the rat, Richter[10, 11] has demonstrated a selective thirst for calcium-containing solutions in parathyroidectomized rats and for hypertonic salt solutions in adrenalectomized rats which apparently is not as well developed in the human species. However, hunger and appetite lead to the ingestion of a varied diet, providing the usual requirements for the other electrolytes.

The body, having received sufficient water, salt and other elements by satisfying thirst and hunger, then provides an amazingly constant internal environment for its constituent cells and their enzymes. This process is known as homeostasis and is accomplished primarily by the kidney, but heart, liver, lungs, adrenals and other factors play important roles.

The great importance of this subject in surgery lies in the frequency with which normal processes of homeostasis are interfered with, (1) by certain of the diseases for which surgical treatment is required, and (2) by operation and conditions obtaining during the preoperative and the postoperative periods.

The following case is illustrative: A 43-year-old, 70-Kg. man, with a 3-year history of duodenal ulcer is admitted to the hospital because of recurrent vomiting which has been persistent for 36 hours. Study shows that he has developed pyloric obstruction. To prepare him for operation, the stomach is aspirated by tube and constant suction for 36 hours. During operation he sweats excessively and loses 600 ml. of blood. To protect the suture lines between stomach and jejunum, he is kept on gastric suction for 3 days after operation and receives only limited amounts of oral fluids during the 4th and the 5th days after operation.

Such a history is not an unusual one, and such patients could scarcely be expected to survive without replacement therapy. Consider first his water losses. He arrives dehydrated, probably having lost body fluids equal to a significant per cent of his body weight, say 6 per cent (or 4,200 ml.). This loss is accentuated by another 4½ days of suction on the

71

stomach at a rate of perhaps 500 ml. per day, by a loss of 500 ml. a day of urine if the products of body metabolism are to be excreted, by nearly 500 ml. as blood, by a daily loss by evaporation (chiefly from the respiratory tract) of 500 to 1,000 ml. and by the added loss of perspiration on the operating table of perhaps 300 ml.

The sodium loss probably would be close to 100 mEq./L. in the gastric drainage and vomitus, but in a previously healthy subject would be small in the urine and negligible in the water lost by evaporation. Perspiration would contain some additional sodium.

The daily potassium loss might run close to 10 mEq. in the gastric drainage but would also run about 15 mEq. in the urine, and this loss would persist for a time (see Table 1).

The chloride loss, like the sodium loss, would be chiefly in the gastric drainage but would be higher—relative to the normal blood concentration than the sodium loss—a part of the chloride leaving the body as hydrochloric acid, thus producing an alkalosis.

So far, then, we can anticipate the following: dehydration, sodium deficit, potassium deficit, chloride deficit and alkalosis.

To have a complete concept of what has occurred, we need to know the quantitative relationships between these losses. Thus, if the net sodium and chloride losses exceed the net

TABLE 1. SUMMARY OF APPROXIMATE
REQUIREMENTS FOR WATER, SODIUM
AND POTASSIUM IN CASE CITED

Water
Loss prior to admission		4,200 ml.
Loss by suction drainage 4½ days		2,200 ml.
Loss as urine		2,500 ml.
Loss as blood during operation		500 ml.
Loss as sweat during operation		300 ml.
Insensible loss @ 600 ml./day		3,000 ml.
Total water needed for pre-existing deficit and 5-day period		12,700 ml.

Sodium
Loss prior to admission (attributing one half the deficit to vomiting)		190 mEq.
Loss by suction drainage		220 mEq.
Loss in urine		small
Loss in perspiration		small
Loss as blood		50 mEq.

Potassium
Loss prior to admission	10 mEq./L.	20 mEq.
Loss by suction drainage	10 mEq./L.	21 mEq.
Loss in urine	15 mEq./L.	37 mEq.

water loss, that is, are larger than would be the case if extracellular fluid were lost, there probably will be a reduction in the concentration of these ions in the plasma. We need to know how the various losses are distributed between the intravascular water (plasma volume), the interstitial space (extracellular volume less the plasma volume) and the intracellular space (total body water less the extracellular volume).

From available data we can say that the water loss will be derived mainly from the extracellular water (intravascular and extravascular), normally about 20 per cent of body weight; that the sodium losses will be largely from this same area—often with some further loss of sodium from this area into the cells if the concomitant potassium loss has been rapid; and that potassium will be lost both from extracellular and intracellular sources, the larger part being derived from within the cells.

The distribution of the extracellular water between the plasma and the interstitial space will be affected by a number of factors. It is now known that the number of grams of serum albumin in the vascular system is only one of these factors. It will also be affected to some extent by sodium and chloride balance and by circulatory disorders, especially heart failure and hepatic cirrhosis.

Disturbance of the acid-base equilibrium will result not only from (1) the loss of hydrochloric acid from the stomach but also may result from (2) the loss of base in combination with keto acids which, especially in children, form during starvation when fat is catabolized in the absence of sufficient carbohydrate, or (3) from a potassium deficit which is often accompanied by an alkalosis. If factor 2 counterbalances factors 1 and 3 accurately, measurement may show normal acid base equilibrium—by a lucky chance—but at the cost of further sodium loss.

We have not considered the possibility of abnormal renal function nor have we considered other electrolytes such as magnesium, phosphate, etc., about which relatively little is known, which do not constitute such important problems in the general run of surgical patients.

Calcium and phosphorus metabolism will be considered in the section on the parathyroid gland. Bicarbonate is considered under respiratory acidosis and alkalosis.

Even after eliminating these large fields, it is clear that water and electrolyte balance is far from a simple subject, and attempts to simplify it usually have led to faulty thinking and as a result to inadequate care of those patients who most need help. These attempts at simplification have gone in 3 directions. First is the compounding of stock solutions, such as so-called physiologic saline solution, Ringer's solution, Hartmann's solution, etc., with all further thought being in terms of milliliters of this solution. Second is the measurement of concentrations of ions without regard to the volume in which such concentrations are distributed. This has led to the use of erroneous formulas for calculating electrolyte requirements from concentration figures. Third is the use of urine or whole blood as the sample for the chemical determinations needed, in place of serum or plasma.

It is proposed to review briefly the normal exchanges of water, sodium, chloride and potassium, with emphasis on normal requirements. Next, examples of abnormal losses and intakes encountered in surgical patients will be given. Third, mention will be made of the available methods of suspecting and quantitating the deficits or surpluses of these 4 substances. On the basis of these sections a method of caring for the water, sodium, potassium and chloride requirements of patients with competent kidneys will be presented. Finally, 5 special problems will be considered: (1) the patient with hyposthenuria; (2) the patient with the salt-losing kidney; (3) the patient with the lower nephron syndrome; (4) the diabetic patient undergoing surgical procedures; and (5) the effect of respiration on blood pH.

EXCHANGES OF WATER, SODIUM, POTASSIUM AND CHLORIDE OCCURRING IN NORMAL MAN BETWEEN THE INDIVIDUAL AND HIS EXTERNAL ENVIRONMENT

An adult man ingests about 1,500 ml. of water in liquid form daily and derives an additional 1,000 ml. from solid foods, partly as water and partly as a result of the oxidation of carbohydrates and fat. Of this amount, only about 200 ml. normally is excreted in the stools.

About 400 to 800 ml. is lost from the respiratory passages and the skin, without gross perspiration—the so-called insensible loss. The balance, in this example 1,500 to 1,900 ml., is lost as urine. Clearly, all of these figures are susceptible to marked variation to meet sweating, enforced fluid restriction, etc.

The average sodium chloride intake has been found to be 5 or 6 Gm., providing about 100 mEq. of each of these ions. Loss in the stool is normally small, and excretion is largely in the urine but to some extent through the skin. The sodium exchange follows a pattern similar to that of chloride. Potassium intake probably varies more widely with the diet but can be thought of as about 20 mEq. per day.

A striking difference between the body's management of sodium and potassium occurs in the kidney. Here, cessation of sodium intake is followed very soon by a marked decrease in excretion so that the sodium store in the body is conserved. However, a cessation in the intake of potassium is not followed quickly by a corresponding decrease in its excretion—the kidney continuing to excrete about 10 mEq. per day for a long period. On the other hand, in the event of an abnormally high intake of potassium, excretion of this ion by the kidneys will rise sharply.

INTERNAL EXCHANGES OF WATER, SODIUM, POTASSIUM AND CHLORIDE IN NORMAL MAN ACROSS THE WALLS OF THE ALIMENTARY TRACT

In this section, we are not considering the rapid molecular exchanges demonstrable by heavy water or isotopes but are concerned with the major moieties secreted into the alimentary tract which may be lost by fistulae or aspiration through tubes. These moieties are largely reabsorbed so that under normal conditions they do not represent an exchange with the environment. Some authors prefer to regard them as actual body tissues not in the cellular sense but as functional entities like the extracellular fluid from which these moieties are derived.

To the water ingested is added per 24 hours: as saliva, 500 ml.; as gastric juice,

1,200 ml.; as bile, 600 ml.; as pancreatic juice, 1,200 ml.; as succus entericus, 2,000 ml.* Thus, a total of 8,000 ml. of water or potential water enters the gastrointestinal tract per 24-hour period. This constitutes over 11 per cent of the body weight and over half of the extracellular water. Not all of this is in the gastrointestinal tract at any one time. Rather, there is a constant turnover of much smaller amounts. Absorption of water probably begins in the upper small bowel and assumes some importance in the distal ileum. However, it occurs especially rapidly in the right half of the colon, so that normally only about 200 ml. is excreted from the body in the feces.

Measurements of chloride concentration in gastric and small intestinal juices have averaged about 100 mEq./L. The total excretion of hydrochloric acid by the stomach is of the order of 120 mEq. in the normal adult but may be considerably higher in some individuals, especially those with duodenal ulcer. Normally, this is compensated for beyond the pylorus by the alkalinity of the juices entering the alimentary tract. Movement of chloride out of the intestine is said to proceed more rapidly than bicarbonate or sodium but not as rapidly as water.

The concentration of potassium in gastric and intestinal drainage ranges from 4 to 14 mEq./L. The higher levels may be expected in intestinal obstruction and diarrhea. Absorption is believed to parallel that of sodium and chloride, and the level in the plasma is maintained at 3.5 to 5 mEq./L. Most of the body potassium is within the cells, whereas most of the body sodium and nearly all of the chloride is outside the cells. The principal intracellular

* All of these figures are cited as representative approximations for an adult man.

TABLE 2. NORMAL RANGE OF ELECTROLYTE CONCENTRATIONS IN ADULT HUMAN PLASMA

ELECTROLYTE	CONCENTRATION (mEq./L. OF PLASMA)
Sodium	134–144
Potassium	3.5–5.3
Chloride	98–105
Calcium	4.5–5.7
	(9–11.4 mg. %)
Inorganic phosphate	2.7–4.4
(as phosphorus)	(4.6–7.6 mg. %)
Total carbon dioxide	23–29
(as bicarbonate)	(51–64 vol. %)

anion is phosphate. See Table 2 for normal serum electrolyte values and Table 3 for representative values for certain other body fluids.

EXAMPLES OF ABNORMAL LOSSES AND INTAKES OF WATER AND ELECTROLYTES IN SURGICAL PATIENTS

WATER

Vomiting is encountered in pyloric obstruction, intestinal obstruction, as a reflex phenomenon after anesthetics, after various drugs, as a response to intracranial lesions, as a psychogenic phenomenon and under innumerable other circumstances. The water losses can easily amount to 2,000 ml. in 24 hours, and often a large residual collection will remain in the stomach which, for practical purposes, is lost to the body.

Diarrhea may lead to extreme losses. The classic example comes not from surgical experience but in cholera where the "rice water" stools may carry off from 5 to 10 L. in a day. Patients with ulcerative colitis will not infre-

TABLE 3. AVERAGE ELECTROLYTE CONTENT OF ORAL AND GASTROINTESTINAL SECRETIONS[4]

SUBJECTS	SECRETION	NA (mEq./L.)	K (mEq./L.)	CA (mEq./L.)	CL (mEq./L.)
Healthy, young adults	Resting saliva	44	20.4	6.5	
Healthy, young adults	Overnight gastric	49	11.6	3.6	
Preoperative patients	Gastric	66.5	13.7		100.6
Resections	Gastric	136	5.3		98
Surgical patients	Small bowel	111.3	4.6		104.2
Surgical patients	Ileostomy (recent)	129.4	11.2		116.2
Surgical patients	Ileostomy (adapted)	46	3.0		21.4
Surgical patients	Bile	148.9	4.98		100.6
Surgical patients	Pancreas	141.1	4.6		76.6

quently lose from 2 to 4 L. of water in the stools. Pseudomembranous enteritis has been observed to produce losses as high as 11 L. in a 24-hour period.[1]

Sweating during prolonged operation may account for a loss of a liter or more, but the omission of blankets and other impediments to heat loss, such as hot humid air in the operating rooms, has tended to reduce this loss. Patients with heat exhaustion are sometimes admitted to surgical wards after probable losses of 4 or 5 L. by perspiration. Before the days of air-conditioned operating rooms, the surgeon himself not infrequently lost 2,500 ml. during a long summer operating schedule (as judged by weight changes).

Biliary fistulae and T-tube drainage may account for losses of 1,000 to 1,500 ml. per day.

Pancreatic fistulae usually drain more modest amounts, since they probably do not, as a rule, drain the whole pancreas. Potentially they could cause losses of a liter or more per day.

Salivary fistulae are seldom important as a cause of fluid loss in a patient who can swallow.

Intestinal Fistulae. A direct corollary of the finding that very large amounts of fluid enter the upper intestinal tract is that huge losses occur if a fistula opens from this area to the outside of the body. In one such case developing after failure of an anastomosis in the jejunum, Walker[15] collected up to 4 L. per day with a loss by all routes of over 40 per cent of the total chloride ion calculated to be in the extracellular space in 24 hours. Prior to the development of suitable methods for replacement therapy, such cases were invariably fatal.

Lower in the intestinal tract, however, the body may tolerate fistulae quite well. Thus, colostomy and ileostomy are established surgical procedures, and the patients do well, although some of those with ileostomy require a period of adjustment during which intravenous replacement therapy is essential.

Suction Drainge of the Alimentary Tract. This method, introduced by Wangensteen and Paine in 1933,[16] has been of inestimable value in surgery in preventing distention and many of its consequences. However, it does constitute a fistula, and occasionally as much as 5,000 ml. will drain out of the body within 24 hours. If appropriate replacement therapy is not provided, the method is capable of doing more harm than good.

Hemorrhage, whether operative or due to gastrointestinal ulceration, results in a reduction of the water content of the body. Losses of blood in the gastrointestinal tract often exceed 1,500 ml. in 24 hours.

ION LOSSES IN SURGICAL PATIENTS

Ions are almost always lost wherever water is lost from the body. Reference has already been made to the patient who lost over 40 per cent of his extracellular chloride partly through a small bowel fistula. This is calculated as the thiocyanate space times the plasma chloride concentration. Presumably, the sodium loss would have been of similar or relatively greater magnitude, since the small bowel content is alkaline, and the potassium loss can be predicted as smaller.

The loss of alkaline fluids tends to produce an acidosis, and the loss of acid gastric juice tends to produce alkalosis. Perspiration varies in its content but, when profuse, may contain from 30 to 40 mEq. of sodium chloride and 24 mEq. of potassium.

The use of irrigating fluids through tubes extending into the body can produce notable ion exchanges. When water is used for this purpose, a loss of ions always results. Thus, multiple enemas may produce hypochloremia and symptoms of water intoxication. A loss of base, most of which is sodium, occurs simultaneously.

Likewise, irrigation of tubes used for suction from the stomach and the small intestine carries away the ions found in these organs. In fact, repeated irrigation with 200 ml. of tap water every 20 minutes is a very effective method of reducing a hyperchloremia and has been used for this purpose. Unfortunately, the concentration of chloride ion after a 20-minute stay in the stomach is quite variable from one individual to another, so that fairly frequent observations of the results are necessary.

Sodium chloride, 0.9 per cent, or better yet a balanced ion solution such as that recommended by Hartmann,[6] should be used for irrigation of suction tubes, and water and ice should not be permitted by mouth in patients on Wangensteen suction, unless special provision is made to compensate for the ion losses.

Selective ion losses can be brought about by the use of ion exchange resins if the alimentary tract is functioning.

METHODS FOR SUSPECTING AND QUANTITATING THE DEFICITS OR THE SURPLUSES OF WATER, SODIUM, CHLORIDE AND POTASSIUM

Suspicion is based on history and physical examination; quantitation usually requires laboratory methods. Without the suspicion, the laboratory tests will not be done; therefore, the history and the physical examination are important.

WATER LOSS

The symptoms of water loss alone, which is rare, are thirst and dryness of the mucous membranes and at times fever. Loss of skin turgor, loss of tension of the eyeballs, and a shrunken drawn facies are characteristic of a combined loss of water and sodium.

Usually there is a concomitant loss of chloride. However, an increase in sodium and chloride concentration due to water loss alone does occur in hot areas and may result in marked rises in body temperature, causing heat stroke. Moyer[9] describes 2 patients who, in the presence of high fever and hot weather, developed evidence of increased concentration of ions in the body. If the history does not explain the water loss, it is well to look for diabetes mellitus or, rarely, insipidus. Patients with diabetes insipidus develop a rapid water loss. This may be seen following operations about the pituitary fossa.

WATER SURPLUS

A water surplus without an increase in the extracellular sodium and chloride produces water intoxication, weakness, fever and mental changes, sometimes including convulsions and coma.

A water surplus attended by normal concentrations of sodium and chloride produces no symptoms in the normal individual except diuresis until a considerable excess has been reached. Then pitting edema of the dependent portions appears about the ankles and, in bedfast patients, over the sacrum. Pulmonary edema usually comes later, but in a person with cardiac weakness it may be the first symptom. There are also increases in fluid throughout the extracellular space, for instance, in the walls of the stomach and the intestine where it may interfere with the function of gastroenterostomy stomas. There is increased excretion of fluid into the gastrointestinal tract and consequent increases in the quantities recovered by suction drainage.

If weight has been measured reliably and before the onset of symptoms, it will be found that extracellular fluid deficiency is accompanied by weight loss (6% when clinical signs become manifest, according to Coller and Maddock).[2] When extracellular fluid is present in excess, weight will be elevated.

SODIUM AND CHLORIDE LOSSES

Sodium and chloride losses, when they occur concomitantly, produce marked weakness, lethargy, often oliguria and, if severe enough, may lead to dehydration, coma and death.

If sodium is lost in excess, acidosis results, with a reduction in the serum carbon dioxide combining power. If this is marked enough, coma will supervene. If, on the other hand, chloride loss is in excess of sodium loss, alkalosis usually develops which may manifest itself by a positive Chvostek sign, a positive Trousseau sign and frank tetany due to a reduction in the concentration of ionized calcium in the plasma. Breathing may be deep and frequent in acidosis (Kussmaul) or shallow and slow in alkalosis. Imbalance may be brought about by excessive intake of one of these ions without the other as in the treatment of peptic ulcer with sodium bicarbonate.

SODIUM AND CHLORIDE EXCESS

Combined sodium and chloride excesses often are accompanied by increased water intake, producing the picture already described. They tend to produce a diuresis if kidneys are normal. However, excesses rarely develop if the kidneys are normal.

When the concentration of these ions becomes high, severe thirst is common, and dryness of the tongue and the buccal mucous membranes has been observed. In extreme situations produced by the accidental intravenous administration of highly concentrated stock solutions of sodium chloride, coma, hypotension and death have supervened rapidly.

ACIDOSIS DUE TO CHLORIDE ADMINISTRATION

If sodium ions and chloride ions are given in equivalent amounts as in 0.9 per cent sodium chloride solution, the effect is to dilute the bicarbonate which probably accounts for Van Slyke's term "dilution acidosis." Normal plasma contains approximately 140 mEq. of sodium but only 100 mEq. of chloride. If physiologic saline solution containing 150 mEq. of each is added, it increases the chloride concentration more than it does the sodium concentration and tends to lower the pH. With normal kidneys the body is able to correct for a considerable excess of chloride, but, if larger amounts are to be given or if kidney function may be impaired, sodium bicarbonate or lactate solution should be substituted for one third of the sodium chloride solution. (See Chap. 16, "Burns.")

HYPOPOTASSEMIA

Hypopotassemia is characterized by weakness and sleepiness which may merge into stupor. The electrocardiograph usually shows

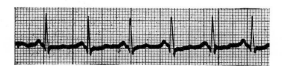

FIG. 5-1 A. Lead II—Normal.

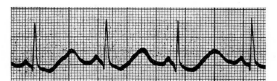

FIG. 5-1 B. Lead II—Hypokalemia. A.B. K$^+$ = 2.7 mEq./L. Note: Depression of ST segment, widening of QT interval, T-wave not lowered in this example, and U-wave superimposed on T-wave.

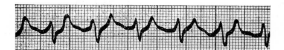

FIG. 5-1 C. Lead II—Hyperkalemia. R.S. Before dialysis K = 7.5 mEq./L. Note: Widened QRS complex, absence of P-waves, peaked T-waves, and depressed ST segments.

flattening or inversion of T-waves, prolongation of QT intervals, depression of ST segments, and appearance of U-waves (Fig. 5-1 B). It is commonly attended by an alkalosis, which will respond to the administration of ammonium chloride solution but will recur until the potassium deficit is at least partially corrected.

HYPERPOTASSEMIA

Hyperpotassemia is usually characterized by electrocardiograph changes, including spiking elevation of T-waves, depression of ST segments, and conduction defects (Fig. 5-1 C). It seldom occurs except in renal failure, and the uremic patient may lapse into coma. When the potassium concentration gets up between 8 and 12 mEq./L. it is likely to produce cardiac arrest with immediate death. This is, at times, the terminal event in uremia.

THE COMATOSE PATIENT

It will be noted that the end stage of several of the electrolyte imbalances is coma. If the patient is comatose when first seen, how does one decide whether or not this is due to electrolyte imbalance? The respirations may be deep and frequent, pointing to acidosis. The patient may have a positive Chvostek's sign, muscular twitchings or irritability, suggesting alkalosis. The breath may smell of ketone bodies, suggesting diabetic acidosis.

The possible role of metabolic aberrations in the causation of the coma can be assessed chemically by carrying out the following determinations on plasma:

Urea nitrogen
Carbon dioxide combining power
Chloride
Sodium
Potassium
Sugar

If there is any likelihood that abnormal respiration is a primary etiologic factor and not compensatory, a blood pH is important. If hypochloremia or water intoxication is present, chloride concentration will be low. If too much sodium chloride has been given, or too little excreted, the chloride will be high or it may be normal.

If coma is due to metabolic acidosis, the carbon dioxide combining power will be low, as in diabetic acidosis. If it is due to respiratory acidosis, it will be high (see below). If the coma is due to uremia, the urea nitrogen usually will be above 100 mg. per 100 ml.

If the primary abnormality is a potassium deficiency, the potassium concentration usually will be low. The author has not seen real coma from hypopotassemia alone, but deep stupor does occur. Likewise, the author has not seen unconsciousness in respiratory acidosis (CO_2 retention) or in respiratory alkalosis (blowing off CO_2 by hyperventilation) unless important metabolic changes are also present.

A low blood pH with a normal or elevated CO_2 combining capacity signifies respiratory acidosis, and a high blood pH with a normal or low CO_2 combining power signifies respiratory alkalosis.

QUANTITATIVE CONSIDERATIONS

Having suspected the abnormality and confirmed it by concentration tests of the electrolytes, what can be done to determine how large the deficit or the excess of each substance is?

Water, which is probably the most important, is one of the most difficult to quantitate. Total body water can be determined fairly accurately by D_2O, but the methods of analysis are so difficult and time-consuming as to render it impractical in most clinical laboratories. However, its relationship to body weight is inconstant, being profoundly influenced by fat which contains almost no water. Thus, body water may range from 71 per cent of body weight in the lean to 50 per cent or less in the obese subject (Moore[3, 8] and Hardy[5]).

Having determined total body water, one cannot state without knowing the figure for the same individual before he became ill, when he had about the same degree of obesity, whether or not he has a deficit.

Extracellular water is variously measured by sodium thiocyanate, inulin, chloride, etc., giving what are most safely designated as thiocyanate space, inulin space, chloride space, etc. Chloride space, which from certain standpoints would be logical, has proved to be quite unsatisfactory, probably due to binding of chloride by connective tissue (Manery and Hastings[7]).

Either inulin space or thiocyanate space provides useful information. The author has had more experience with thiocyanate space. Normally, this is about 20 per cent of body weight, but it is safer to refer it not to total weight but to total body water because of the fat factor. Thus, it should constitute about 28 per cent of total body water.

Thiocyanate space, taken as a practical measure of extracellular water, can be broken down between plasma water and interstitial water by determining the former with the blue dye, T-1824 (Evans Blue).

For accuracy, then, comparison of extracellular space with deuterium space appears to be the best laboratory method of quantitating dehydration or overhydration in an individual in whom previous observations have not been made. However, localized disease such as cirrhosis with ascites may make it unwise and unreasonable to apply the norms to a given case. Thus, if a patient had 6,000 ml. of ascitic fluid, he would be likely to have at least 6,000 ml. above the normal thiocyanate space. The attempt to dehydrate him by 6,000 ml. through fluid restriction would seriously reduce his interstitial fluid in most areas and might be dangerous. The same difficulty may arise in intestinal obstruction and other conditions characterized by a dislocation of fluid within the body. The inulin and the thiocyanate spaces provide useful information in the normal person. However, in the sick individual their use cannot be depended upon to provide accurate measurements of the *available* fluid in the various partitions.

The approximate determination of extracellular water is necessary for proper utilization of sodium, chloride and bicarbonate concentrations, as determined on plasma.

Only when one knows the amount of water in the beaker and the concentration of the solute can one calculate how much of the solute to add or subtract to bring about a desired concentration. An example will illustrate the use of this principle: A patient with anorexia nervosa is admitted in a dehydrated state. Her plasma chloride concentration is 60 mEq./L. She weighs 35 Kg. If one assumed a normal extracellular space of 20 per cent or 7,000 ml., she would require 7 L. times 40 mEq./L. of chloride to equal 280 mEq. to bring her chloride concentration to a normal value of 100 mEq./L. Actually, however, her thiocyanate space was only 4,000 ml. Had the 280 mEq. of chloride been given in concentrated form, it would have raised her chloride by 70 mEq. or to 130—a dangerously high level. Without discussing the other dangers in a situation of this kind, it is seen at once that volume as well as concentration is essential to even rough quantitation.

Since no two solutes seem to have exactly the same distribution in the body, a useful principle is to use for the test the substance needed. Thus, if chlorides are low, give a test dose of chloride (not over half the dose calculated for an extracellular space of 20 per cent body weight or one third in an obviously dehydrated or very obese individual). After administration of this amount, concentration is determined again (for accuracy, urinary loss during the interval would be required) and a rough calculation of chloride space could be made. In the case cited above, the evidence of dehydration was sufficient to suggest giving only one third of the calculated loss of 280 mEq., or 93 mEq. This should raise the chloride by only 23 mEq./L. (less if it were administered in dilute form as P.S.S.) which probably would be safe. One would know that an additional amount as a second dose would be required to bring the chloride to 100, but wisdom would suggest that this be deferred until other deficits had been partially compensated and the body, probably long adjusted to a low chloride, has time to readjust. Such estimations are chiefly useful in estimating the theoretical deficit, but it is important to remember that illness may be induced by too rapid complete correction. The experience with intravenous therapy in the chemically starved prisoners of war at the end of World War II was, in general, unsatisfactory. Some patients died unexpectedly. Apparently, under such conditions a precarious homeostasis has been established at new levels.

In the case of potassium, the chief intracellular cation, extracellular space is not of significance. Marked cellular depletion of potassium may occur with relatively small reductions in the plasma level. However, plasma levels above 5 mEq./L., probably indicate a surplus usually accumulated because of decreased urinary excretion, abnormally high intakes, or rapid tissue breakdown with release of intracellular potassium. To quantitate deficits of potassium, it has been necessary to resort to load tests. 30 mEq. of potassium is given intravenously (after one is assured that urine volume is normal), and urine is collected for a 24-hour period. When excretion equals intake, it is assumed that any intracellular deficits have been satisfied. (Note: The intercurrent administration of sodium during these tests invalidates them.)

The regulation of water between the intravascular space and the interstitial space is determined by the osmotically active colloids in the plasma (chiefly albumin), blood pressure in the various parts of the circulation, and lymph flow, as well as water and electrolyte balance. As it is essential to the discussion of shock, it is discussed in detail in Chapter 7. It is sufficient here to state that plasma volume determinations are as essential to the calculation of the plasma protein dosage needed to correct hypoproteinemia as are extracellular space estimations in calculating the dosage of chloride and sodium. Fortunately, in the management of most surgical patients with competent kidneys, one seldom requires as much laboratory work as this section describes.

PRACTICAL REGULATION OF WATER, SODIUM, CHLORIDE AND POTASSIUM BALANCE IN PATIENTS WITH COMPETENT KIDNEYS

The task of water and electrolyte regulation will be considered in 2 parts: (1) correction of existing abnormalities and (2) maintenance of equilibrium. Recognition of existing abnormalities has been discussed in the previous section. One next wants to know if the kidneys are functioning—catheterization with hourly collection is useful here, as it is in shock (see Chap. 7). While this is in process, determination of plasma chloride concentration and carbon dioxide combining power should be made. Potassium concentrations will be needed also, but in short illnesses it is usually safe to wait until the next morning to determine it, whereas the chloride and the carbon dioxide determinations are needed immediately.

The decision regarding the extent of dehydration is a difficult one. If there are clinical signs of dehydration with loss of skin turgor, dryness of the mucous membranes and the signs of diminished circulatory volume, it is reasonable to assume that a 6 per cent loss or 4,200 ml. for the 70 Kg. man has been suffered.

In general, it may be argued that if a patient is alive with his total deficit, he should be out of immediate danger when it is half corrected and probably when it is only one third corrected.

Therefore, it is seldom essential to know exactly the water deficit, but it is essential to know that the patient is suffering from a shortage rather than an excess of body fluid and to have some general idea of the magnitude of the probable change. Furthermore, if one is going to replace water, it is extremely important to know whether chloride (or sodium) concentration is low or high. If it is already low, the administration of water (5 or 10%) glucose in water) without simultaneous salt administration is dangerous but, on the other hand, if the chlorides are high and the deficit is replaced with 0.9 per cent sodium chloride, the hyperchloremia may be accentuated if chloride excretion is impaired.

If a 70-Kg. patient looks dehydrated, is very weak, has a low blood pressure, if his plasma chloride concentration is 80 mEq./L, and carbon dioxide combining power is slightly elevated, the following assumptions are made:

1. He has lost about 6 per cent of his extracellular fluid or 4,200 ml. His extracellular space is equal to 14 per cent (rather than 20%) of body weight, or 9,800 ml.

2. His calculated chloride deficit is $100 - 80 = 20$ mEq./L. in the 9,800 ml. $= 196$ mEq. plus 100 mEq./L. in the 4,200 ml. which he has lost $= 420$ mEq. or a total of 616 mEq.

3. His sodium deficit may be slightly less than the chloride deficit, since the carbon dioxide combining power is somewhat elevated.

His total water and salt deficit may be taken as 4,200 ml. of water containing about 616 mEq. of sodium chloride. However, it is dangerous to accept these assumptions as facts. It seems reasonable to doubt that they can vary from the truth by more than a factor of 2. Therefore, rather than to run a thiocyanate space determination, it seems better to give half the calculated amount fairly rap-

idly and redetermine the chloride. If the chloride has risen to about 90 mEq., one is on the right track, and the other half should be given more gradually, probably over a period of days. One may have a considerable assurance that the patient should be well out of danger of death from dehydration or hypochloremia, and it is usually wise to approach full repletion slowly if he has become adjusted to his deficiencies through a long illness.

If urinary output is above 10 ml. per hour and increases substantially with the infusion, mild aberrations in the carbon dioxide combining power may be neglected, as the normal kidneys will make the correction if they have ample water, sodium and chloride to excrete. On the other hand, if the carbon dioxide is very low, say 10 mM./L., some sodium should be given without equivalent chloride. This is usually provided as M/6 sodium lactate solution (166 mM./L.).

In the case cited, one has assumed that the extracellular space was 9,800 ml. instead of 14,000 ml. Then the amount required to raise the carbon dioxide from 10 to 25 mM./L. would be $15 \times 9.8 = 147$ mM./L. or about 885 ml. of M/6 sodium lactate solution. Here again, administration of one half the amount is prudent, and subsequent administration should be based on a repeat carbon dioxide determination.

In patients with vomiting or in those who have lost large amounts of gastric juice by suction drainage, the carbon dioxide combining power may be high, say 38 mM./L. Unless signs of tetany or impending tetany are present (Chvostek or Trousseau signs), it is probably best to see if the carbon dioxide level will return toward normal after the salt and water deficits are restored. If it does not, the plasma potassium concentration should be investigated and, if low, potassium administration should be started (see below).

In rare cases alkalosis persists after restoration of sodium, chloride and potassium concentrations and total amounts to normal. In these cases, ammonium chloride may be given intravenously, as suggested by Zintel and his associates,[17] if one is certain that the elevation of carbon dioxide is not due to respiratory acidosis. Therefore, it is wise to determine arterial pH before administering ammonium chloride, especially in aged people. Thus in the case cited, if it were desired to lower the carbon dioxide from 38 to 28, 9.800 (the e.c.s.) $\times$ 10 = 98 mEq. of NH_4Cl = about 5.2 Gm. Again, prudence suggests that one half of this be given and the carbon dioxide repeated before carrying the therapy further. Zintel found a 2 per cent concentration satisfactory for slow intravenous administration.

Surpluses of water, sodium and chloride usually have been dealt with by withholding the material or materials present in excess. Water and sodium loss often has been accelerated by the administration of one of the mercurial diuretics, such as mercuhydrin* (adult dose, 1 ml. ampule containing 39 mg. of organically combined mercury and 48 mg. of theophylline) which has the property of inhibiting reabsorption of water and sodium by the kidney tubules.

Another method is to induce sweating by external heat—a method occasionally used by jockeys and athletes to meet maximum weight criteria.

Another method is to introduce hypertonic solutions into the duodenum, preferably between 2 occluding balloons (using a 3-lumen tube). This induces a prompt outpouring of digestive juices which may be aspirated and replaced by more hypertonic glucose. While the effectiveness of the method has been demonstrated experimentally, it has not been applied generally in practice. Still another possible method is the induction of diarrhea with cathartics.

It is obvious that these methods remove ions as well as water, so that if any of them is used, the ionic loss must be taken into consideration.

Hyperchloremia and hypernatremia can be considered together. They rarely occur if the kidneys are normal and are not under the influence of excess adrenal steroids and then only in response to overdoses of salt. When a severe hyperchloremia is discovered (115 mEq./L. or more) it can be corrected by gastric lavage, 200 ml. of tap water being instilled through a tube and left in the stomach 20 minutes, then aspirated and replaced with another 200 ml. and so forth. The rate of chloride withdrawal is inconstant but probably can be as rapid as 50 mEq. per hour, so

that it is well to recheck the chloride level after 4 to 6 hours.

Potassium. Because most of the body potassium is intracellular, one cannot calculate probable deficits of potassium as for the extracellular electrolytes. If plasma potassium concentrations are normal, only maintenance doses of potassium salts are given. If plasma potassium is reduced, 50 mEq. of potassium in excess of maintenance requirements may be given daily until the potassium level is restored to normal.

In the administration of potassium it must be recalled that small absolute increments in potassium from 4 to 8 or 10 mEq./L. threaten death by cardiac standstill. Therefore, hypertonic solutions should not be used, administration should be slow (not over 20 mEq./hr.), and one should have established a satisfactory urine output (at least 30 ml./hr.) before its administration.

In the anuric patient, potassium is usually high, and in uremia it may rise to 6, 8, or 10 mEq., producing electrocardiographic changes and eventually cardiac standstill (Fig. 5-1 C). Under such circumstances one can remove potassium by *in vivo* dialysis (artificial kidney), provided that the solution against which it is dialyzed contains little or no potassium. It can be removed by the ingestion of suitable ion exchange resins prepared so as to take up potassium. Furthermore, the rate of release of intracellular potassium in the body can be reduced by feeding protein sparing foods, such as carbohydrate and fat, to minimize the breakdown of body proteins for nutritional purposes.

In formulating any such set of rules, some will be distressed at the roughness of the calculations and the breadth of the assumptions made, while others will consider the rules too cumbersome. The author has found them workable, provided that the laboratory determinations can be done promptly. In answer to those who would require less of the laboratory, one can only say that it is also possible to navigate without a compass—much of the time.

Somewhat more accurate results will be obtained if one fourth to one third of the sodium administered in salt replacement is given as the lactate rather than the chloride, but with competent kidneys this has not seemed to be essential.

* Sodium salt of meralluride with theophylline.

For a useful and ingenious bedside method of determining chloride[12] and carbon dioxide[13] the reader is referred to the paper of Stewart, Swan and Kortz from the University of Colorado[14] which provides a practical solution of the problem of the small hospital which has no laboratory staff at night.

MAINTENANCE OF WATER AND ELECTROLYTE EQUILIBRIUM

The second part of the problem is somewhat easier than the first but sometimes requires more attention because it covers a longer time period. One can keep a record of intake by mouth, by vein and by any other route which may be employed and a simultaneous record of the output of urine, vomitus, gastrointestinal drainage, etc. Such a record includes volume and description of whatever is given as 1,000 ml. of 5 per cent glucose or 600 ml. of M/6 sodium lactate solution. The output record states the volume of the urine, the vomitus, etc., in ml. and also should state the volume of the stool if it is liquid.

Furthermore, the patient can be weighed on admission and serially thereafter. A litter type scale is needed for bed patients. Short-term changes in weight are largely due to water which has entered or left the body. Thus, if the second or the third determinations of chloride, carbon dioxide and potassium reveal levels within the normal range and the urine volume is up to 1,000 ml. per day, usually the patient may be carried for 48 to 72 hours by calculating his requirements on the following assumptions:

1. That insensible loss of water will amount to 600 ml. per day plus an additional 1,000 ml. if the environmental temperature is above 90° F.

2. That a urine volume of 1,000 to 1,500 ml. will be adequate.

3. That 100 mEq. of sodium and either 100 mEq. of chloride or preferably 70 mEq. of chloride and 30 mEq. of lactate or bicarbonate will cover urinary excretion of these ions (5 Gm. of sodium chloride or 3.5 Gm. of sodium chloride and 1.5 Gm. of sodium bicarbonate).

4. That 20 mEq. of potassium will cover the urinary excretion of potassium (1.5 Gm. potassium chloride).

5. That vomitus and gastrointestinal drain-age will have an average content of about 100 mEq. of sodium and 100 mEq. of chloride and not more than 10 mEq. of potassium per liter.

The daily maintenance dose is then calculated as follows: To the abnormal losses for the preceding 24 hours (vomitus, diarrhea, gastrointestinal suction drainage) is added 2,500 ml. to determine the amount of water to be administered. For every liter of abnormal loss from the gastrointestinal tract 8.5 Gm. of sodium chloride (or 6 Gm. sodium chloride + 2.5 Gm. sodium bicarbonate) plus 6 Gm. of sodium chloride should be given. If we assume abnormal losses of 500 ml., the patient will need 3,000 ml. containing 11.5 Gm. sodium chloride or 9 Gm. sodium chloride plus 2.5 Gm. sodium lactate or bicarbonate and 22 mEq. of potassium (about 1.6 Gm. potassium chloride). It is essential that solutions to be given intravenously not be hypotonic, lest they hemolyze erythrocytes. Therefore, 50 Gm. of glucose is added to pyrogen-free distilled water and sterilized for intravenous use. Most hospitals stock certain dilute solutions of electrolytes and do not make up concentrated stock solutions because of the danger that the concentrated solutions may be administered accidentally in the dosage range needed for the dilute solutions with potentially fatal results.

The Colorado General Hospital stocks 5 per cent glucose solution (900 ml. in a flask of 1,000 ml. capacity) to which are added appropriate amounts of concentrated solutions of sodium chloride, sodium lactate, potassium chloride, etc., as needed. To prevent accidents, the concentrated solutions are stocked in flasks that will not fit the connections on the intravenous tubing. Furthermore, they are not concentrated enough to be dangerous in 100 ml. amounts—the maximum that can be added to one of the flasks containing the glucose solution.

Whatever system is used, the important point is that it should be flexible so that one is not obliged to give chloride instead of bicarbonate in order to administer a given quantity of sodium and that one can vary the potassium intake independently of either sodium or chloride.

If one has available 0.85 per cent sodium chloride (approximately 150 mEq./L.) and

5 per cent glucose, M/6 sodium lactate (166 mEq./L.) and 1.2 per cent potassium chloride (approximately 150 mEq./L.) and 5 per cent glucose in water, it becomes a typical problem in arithmetic to calculate how many milliliters of each must be used to provide, say—

3,000 cc. water
100 mEq. sodium
22 mEq. potassium
92 mEq. chloride
30 mM. lactate

Answer: approximately
200 ml. M/6 sodium lactate
500 ml. 0.85% sodium chloride
150 ml. 1.2% potassium chloride
2,150 ml. 5% glucose in water

At least every 10 liters of total water exchange it is wise to repeat the determinations of chloride, carbon dioxide and potassium in the plasma. In the average patient this is every 72 hours, but in one with large abnormal losses it will be at least every 48 hours. When the abnormal losses have stopped, and the patient has resumed normal water and food intake, the chemical determinations can be omitted, but it is still wise to chart the intake and the output until one is sure that the patient can maintain himself.

THE PATIENT WITH HYPOSTHENURIA

Especially in patients with hypertension and arteriosclerosis, the kidneys frequently lose their capacity to concentrate urine. When specific gravity becomes fixed at 1.010, 3 times as large a urine volume is required to remove a given quantity of solute as when the specific gravity is 1.030. Therefore, such patients require a larger urine output than the normal patient—possibly 2,000 ml. or more.

Recognition of this fact makes it possible to effect the improvement of many patients who appear, on the basis of rising urea levels in the blood, to be going into uremia. Formerly, many such patients were given up.

So long as the urine volume will respond to increases in water intake, there is hope that they can be salvaged. Usually additional quantities of 5 per cent glucose or 10 per cent glucose are most effective, and only basal requirements for sodium chloride are necessary. Sodium chloride and especially potassium

levels should be watched carefully in such patients, and the intake of these ions should be adjusted promptly to assist the impaired kidneys in maintaining homeostasis. Fluid intakes for such patients may be pushed up to 4,000 to 5,000 ml. unless pulmonary edema develops.

Basal rales per se are not interpreted as pulmonary edema. If one does precipitate pulmonary edema, all intravenous therapy must be stopped, and an immediate venesection should be carried out with removal of 250 to 1,000 ml. of blood.

THE PATIENT WITH SALT-LOSING KIDNEYS

A small group of patients appear to have diminished tubular resorption of sodium and chloride ions. They tend to develop hypochloremia and hyponatremia and will require larger than average amounts of sodium chloride, especially if the urine volume is high. The response in some of these patients is better if hypertonic solutions are given (e.g., 2% or 3% sodium chloride solution).

THE PATIENT WITH THE LOWER NEPHRON SYNDROME

Whether precipitated by transfusion reaction, crush, chemical poisons ($HgCl_2$, uranium salts) or other trauma, the pathologic features of this syndrome are similar. There is extensive degeneration and sloughing of tubular epithelium. This is followed after 10 to 14 days by regeneration if the patient survives. Anuria or severe oliguria is the rule during the early part of his course. If urine formation is resumed, as it is when the tubular epithelium regenerates, the urine volume increases gradually to normal amounts and then increases further so that a marked diuresis may occur. The newly regenerated organ has little power of salt retention and is, for the time being, a salt-losing kidney. Therefore, the diuresis may result in serious depletion of body sodium and chloride, and a number of patients have died because of inadequate replacement at this time.

During the period of anuria, water intake should be restricted to 700 to 1,000 ml. per day, preferably by mouth. No electrolytes should be given, and especially no potassium. Body proteins should be spared by a liberal intake of fat and carbohydrate (butter and sugar on bread or crackers). It is preferable to give no protein or protein derivatives.

The urea nitrogen and potassium concentrations should be determined at frequent intervals, usually once a day, and if the potassium level rises to 6 mEq./L. or above, electrocardiographic tracings should be made at still more frequent intervals. If characteristic changes develop (Fig. 5-1 C), strenuous efforts should be made to remove potassium. If an artificial kidney is not available, an ion exchange resin with avidity for potassium may be given by mouth, provided that the alimentary tract is functioning.

One of the wisest young surgeons the author has known was the one who transferred his anuric patient on the 3rd day of her anuria to an institution where an effective artificial kidney was available, rather than waiting until it was clear that dialysis would be necessary. If one waits until it is clear that the patient cannot recover without this aid, frequently it is too late.

THE DIABETIC PATIENT UNDERGOING SURGICAL PROCEDURES

Infection and inflammation have long been known to make diabetes mellitus more severe. Therefore, it is not surprising that diabetic patients undergoing operation often have an increase in their insulin requirement if they remain on their usual diets. However, when food intake is interrupted, they may go into insulin shock. When insufficient insulin and carbohydrate are provided, acetone, diacetic acid and β-oxybutyric acid are formed and excreted in the urine with basic ions, principally sodium. This reduces the carbon dioxide combining power and tends to lower the pH of the blood. As has been stated already, this may require sodium lactate as well as sodium chloride for correction.

At the time of operation and during the early postoperative period, it is rarely possible to regulate the diabetic surgical patient accurately (e.g., to keep his fasting blood sugar between 80 and 140 mg./100 ml. and his urine free of acetone bodies). The attempt usually fails in its objectives and is attended by bouts of insulin shock. It is far wiser to avoid insulin shock and to avoid ketosis and its attendant losses of basic ions and temporarily to abandon the third objective of keeping the blood sugar below 150. If one resolves to permit the blood sugar to remain in a high range, it is not difficult to achieve the other two objectives. About 1.5 Gm. of glucose is needed to cover one unit of insulin. The author gives 2 Gm. of glucose with each unit of insulin. Only regular insulin is used, and the insulin is actually added to each flask of glucose solution when patients are receiving parenteral solutions.

The amounts must be increased sufficiently to prevent ketosis, as shown by testing the urine for acetone and diacetic acid. A check, daily at first, is also kept on the carbon dioxide combining power of the plasma in case of losses of base with β-oxybutyric acid which is not usually analyzed in the urine.

If such infusions of glucose and insulin are given rapidly, it has been stated that the insulin effect has outlasted the glucose with resultant insulin shock. At slow rates of infusion, this has not been a problem, but if it ever should arise, additional glucose without insulin should be given.

THE RELATIONS OF RESPIRATION TO ACID-BASE BALANCE

One of the factors regulating acid-base equilibrium in the body is carbon dioxide which dissolves in water to form carbonic acid (H_2CO_3). This is an equilibrium in the body with base, chiefly sodium with which it forms (reversibly) sodium bicarbonate ($NaHCO_3$). Carbon dioxide is being formed constantly in the body by oxidation of foodstuffs and is being excreted constantly as carbon dioxide in expired air.

Anything which slows this process of excretion, be it respiratory obstruction, emphysema, pulmonary fibrosis (silicosis, pulmonary hypertension), or depressed respiratory reflexes, as during anesthesia or heavy narcosis, leads to an accumulation of carbon dioxide in the blood and plasma. This lowers the blood pH and increases the plasma carbon dioxide but not the carbon dioxide combining power (CO_2 extractable from plasma after equilibrium with a constant concentration of CO_2—usually 5.5%).

As most laboratories determine plasma carbon dioxide without equilibration, one has the confusing situation that an elevated carbon dioxide may be due to retarded respiratory excretion resulting in respiratory acidosis or it may mean that there is a relative excess of base, chiefly sodium, in the plasma which is holding the carbon dioxide as sodium bicarbonate—a situation which represents an alkalosis (metabolic alkalosis).

There are two ways of distinguishing these: The first is to do a careful carbon dioxide combining power which will be substantially unchanged from the carbon dioxide content if the patient has a metabolic alkalosis but will be lower if the patient has a respiratory acidosis; the other method is to determine the blood pH which will be below normal in respiratory acidosis and above normal in metabolic alkalosis.

There is a similar confusion between respiratory alkalosis brought about by hyperventilation and metabolic acidosis due to a relative deficiency of basic (chiefly sodium) ions in the plasma. Both give reduced serum carbon dioxide, and comparison with the carbon dioxide combining power or a pH determination must be done to distinguish between them chemically.

Clinically, however, if the respiratory tract is organically normal and if respiratory function is normal, there is little chance of serious variance between carbon dioxide and carbon dioxide combining power.

Through a series of reflex mechanisms, the body tends to use respiration to help regulate the blood pH when metabolic changes disturb it. Thus in metabolic acidosis, respirations become deep and frequent (Kussmaul breathing), which tend to blow carbon dioxide off and raise the pH. Conversely, in metabolic alkalosis, respirations tend to be shallow and slow, which result in carbon dioxide retention and lowering of pH.

REFERENCES

1. Allen, J. G.: Personal communication.
2. Coller, F. A., and Maddock, W. G.: Study of dehydration in humans, Ann. Surg. *102*: 947-960, 1935.
3. Edelman, I. S., Olney, J. M., James, A. H., Brooks, L., and Moore, F. D.: Body composition: studies in the human being by the dilution principle, Science *115*:447-454, 1952.
4. Elkinton, J. R., and Danowski, T. S.: The Body Fluids, pp. 462-463, Baltimore, Williams & Wilkins, 1955.
5. Hardy, J. D.: Fluid Therapy, Philadelphia, Lea & Febiger, 1954.
6. Hartmann, A. F., Perley, A. M., Basman, J., Nelson, M. F., and Asher, C.: Further observations on metabolism and clinical uses of sodium lactate, J. Pediat. *13*:692-723, 1938.
7. Manery, J. F., and Hastings, A. B.: The distribution of electrolysis in mammalian tissues, J. Biol. Chem. *127*:657, 1939.
8. Moore, F. D.: Determination of total body water and solids with isotopes, Science *104*: 157, 1946.
8a. Moore, F. D.: Metabolic Care of the Surgical Patient, Philadelphia, Saunders, 1959.
9. Moyer, C. A.: Fluid Balance: A Critical Manual, Chicago, Year Book Pub., 1952.
10. Richter, C. P.: Increased salt appetite in adrenalectomized rats, Am. J. Physiol. *115*: 155-161, 1936.
11. Richter, C. P., and Eckert, J. F.: Increased calcium appetite of parathyroidectomized rats, Endocrinology *21*:50-54, 1937.
12. Scribner, B. H.: Bedside determination of chloride: a method for plasma, urine and other fluids and its application to fluid balance problems, Proc. Staff Meet. Mayo Clin. *25*:209-218, 1950.
13. Scribner, B. H., Power, M. H., and Rynearson, E. H.: Bedside management of problems of fluid balance, J.A.M.A. *144*:1167-1174, 1950.
14. Stewart, B. D., Swan, H., and Kortz, A. B.: The bedside clinic and laboratory in the management of acute dehydration, Am. Surgeon *20*:93-111, 1954.
15. Walker, J., Jr.: Fluid and electrolyte replacement for the surgical patient, S. Clin. North America *29*:1849-1858, 1949.
16. Wangensteen, O. H., and Paine, J. R.: Treatment of acute intestinal obstruction by suction with a duodenal tube, J.A.M.A. *101*: 1532-1539, 1933.
17. Zintel, H. A., Rhoads, J. E., and Ravdin, I. S.: The use of intravenous ammonium chloride in the treatment of alkalosis, Surgery *14*:728, 1943.

——————————— CHAPTER 6 ———————————

Nutrition

Prior to the last two decades, nutrition was thought of chiefly in its relation to internal medicine, as in the management of diabetes and vitamin deficiencies. As other advances permitted an enlargement in the scope of surgical operations, it became increasingly evident that often nutritional factors could play a decisive role in the recovery of patients from surgical procedures. It was Ambroise Paré, who made the famous statement: "Man dresses the wound, God heals it." It is evident that wound healing involves the formation of new tissue, and new tissue requires building stones, whether they are supplied from other tissues or from currently ingested food. As the materials used in repair are basically protein in nature, it is not surprising to find that proteins occupy a central position in the nutrition of surgical patients, and that carbohydrates and fats are of value partly because of their protein-sparing qualities.

Several of the vitamins have specific roles in surgery, notably vitamin K (see Chap. 30, "Liver, Gallbladder and Bile Passages"), vitamin C, thiamine and probably others of the B group. Vitamin D has a specific usefulness in hypoparathyroidism, and vitamin E has been recommended in the treatment of Peyronie's disease and in the treatment of Dupuytren's contracture, although its effec-

tiveness in these conditions does not as yet rest on firm proof.

The subject of mineral nutrition leads us directly into the field of the electrolytes, which will be considered separately and, therefore, will be omitted from this chapter. An exception is iron metabolism, which is considered in a later section of this chapter.

PROTEIN NUTRITION

In the field of nutrition, it is a fair generalization to say that it is easier to demonstrate changes due to a deficiency of a specific food component than it is to demonstrate benefit from an amount larger than what is termed the normal requirement. In fact, it is generally doubtful whether excesses of any specific food components are definitely useful.

Hypoproteinemia

Applying this principle to the field of protein nutrition, we find that if an animal is maintained on a protein deficient regimen, a series of changes occur which have received considerable study. The animal usually will adapt himself to a moderately low protein intake, but if the intake is very low, as 1 per cent of the diet, he will go into negative nitrogen balance, putting out more nitrogen in the urine than he takes in. As this process goes forward, there will be a concomitant diminution in blood volume out of proportion to the loss in body weight and a decrease in plasma protein concentration. As a rule, the plasma albumin component will go down more rapidly than the globulin component, and this may lead to a reversal of the normal albumin-globulin ratio.

With the decline in serum protein concentration, there is of course a corresponding decline in the colloid osmotic pressure of the plasma. This permits water and electrolytes to accumulate outside the blood vessels. While this change also occurs gradually, at a serum protein level of the order of 5.0 to 5.5 Gm. per 100 ml. or at an albumin level of about 2.5 Gm. per 100 ml., edema is likely to become grossly demonstrable in dependent areas, such as the ankles. If pressure for 30 seconds or so with the finger leaves a dent, edema is spoken of as pitting, and this state usually represents an increase in the weight of the leg in the amount of 8 to 10 per cent. Similarly, a circular dent left on the abdominal wall by the examining stethoscope is suggestive of edema. The extracellular fluid increases gradually, though its appearance as detected clinically may seem rather abrupt. Therefore, it is a mistake to speak of a critical level of serum protein or serum albumin at which edema forms.

Plasma oncotic pressure is by no means the only factor in edema. Increased venous pressure produces edema by increasing the capillary pressure at the venous end of the loop so that less fluid is drawn back into the circulation at that level. Salt intake is another factor which affects edema formation, and renal function plays an important role. Jones and Eaton[26] were the first to call attention to what they called postoperative edema due to the excessive administration of sodium chloride after operation. Jones, Eaton and White[27] showed that the hypoproteinemic patient is susceptible to an excess of salt intake, and it has been shown that edema can be produced by the administration of sodium chloride solutions alone in man as well as in experimental animals.[6]

As suggested by Jones and Eaton[26] and also by Ravdin,[37] the edema is not confined to the extremities but may involve the visceral tissues also and thus be a factor in failure of gastroenterostomy stomas to function after gastric operations. Here, a local traumatic factor accentuates the edema. The picture of the nonfunctioning gastroenterostomy stoma was reproduced in the dog by Mecray, Barden and Ravdin[31] by lowering the serum protein with a low protein diet and repeated plasmapheresis and carrying out a simple gastroenterostomy. X-ray studies showed a marked delay in gastric emptying so that the gastric emptying time was almost inversely proportional to the serum protein level (Fig. 6-1). Extending their studies to dogs which had had a gastroenterostomy carried out many months earlier and finally to normal dogs, they demonstrated that hypoproteinemia retarded gastric emptying and also retarded the movement of a water barium meal from the pylorus to the cecum.

A serendipitous finding in this study was the marked frequency of wound rupture, suggesting interference with wound healing. Subsequent studies by Thompson, Ravdin and Frank[48] confirmed the observation that hypoproteinemia resulting from a low protein diet and plasmapheresis interferes with the healing of laparotomy wounds in the dog. Histologic evidence indicated that this was due to a failure or delay in fibroplasia. Whether this effect is due to the edema or to a lack of "building stones" in hypoproteinemic animals never has been completely settled. A later study by Rhoads, Fliegelman and Panzer[40] showed that in hypoproteinemia produced by the administration of acacia, this change did not occur and, furthermore, that if a dog was rendered hypoproteinemic, fibroplasia would proceed normally if acacia was given at the time the test wounds were made. This, of course, suggests that the oncotic relationships are the important thing. However, it is also possible that plasma expanders may relieve some plasma protein from the circulation for other uses.

Other studies showed that fracture healing in the dog could be interfered with by hypoproteinemia, as judged by the appearance of calcification on x-ray film after a Gigli saw transection of the ulna (Fig. 6-2).

Since a decrease in blood volume usually has been reported with hypoproteinemia, it is not surprising to find that the hypoproteinemic animal is hypersusceptible to hemorrhagic shock. This was demonstrated by Ravdin, McNamee, Kamholz and Rhoads[39] in a study in which it was found that the animal rendered hypoproteinemic by plasmapheresis could withstand only about 60 per cent as much hemorrhage per kilogram as the normal.

One of the most interesting effects of hypoproteinemia is on resistance to infection. Knowledge in this field was greatly enriched by Dr. Paul Cannon who showed in the experimental animal that certain specific antibodies form more slowly in the presence of hypoproteinemia. The response to a typhoid antigen was studied in man by Matthew Wohl,[52] who confirmed this work by finding that in hypoproteinemic patients the rise of the antibody titer is much slower.

Gell[18] studied antibody formation in undernourished men in the German Ruhr in 1946, using a group of normal subjects as controls. He used 32 cases of malnutrition from the Barmen Municipal Hospital, 25 civilian prisoners from the Siegburg jail, and 16 subjects in a good state of nutrition as controls. All were given injections of 3 antigens for which preformed immunity could not be present. The antigens used were tobacco mosaic virus, avian red blood cells, and a saprophytic vibrio, which failed to produce demonstrable agglutinins. He summarized the results for the first 2 in Table 1.

These data indicate a significant superiority of the controls over the undernourished persons at all periods and for both antigens. Gell's conclusions emphasize the following points:

(1) The extremely severe degree of undernutrition from which the test subjects were suffering

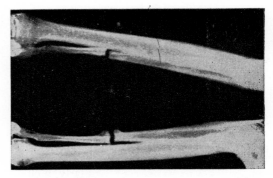

Fig. 6-2. (*Top*) Roentgenogram of Gigli saw fracture of hypoproteinemic dog after 40 days. (*Bottom*) Similar fracture of the opposite ulna of the same dog after 39 days when plasma protein levels were normal. Note increase in callus production. (Rhoads, J. E., and Kasinskas, W.: The influence of hypoproteinemia on the formation of callus in experimental fracture, Surgery *11*:38-44)

—severe enough to render active life impossible; and (2) in spite of this, the comparatively small differences between these literally famished subjects and the controls in first-class condition; (3) the significant fact that there actually has

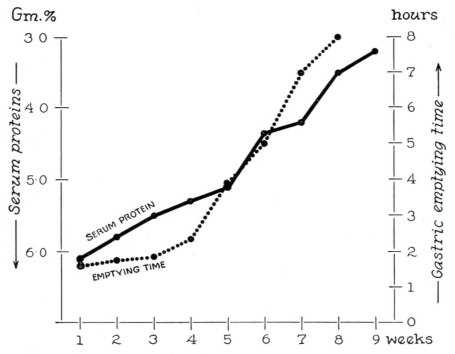

Fig. 6-1. Serum proteins and gastric emptying time. Mean values for 8 dogs.

TABLE 1. PERCENTAGES OF SERUMS GIVING AGGLUTINATION*

	WITH AVIAN CELLS			WITH TOBACCO MOSAIC		
	Before	3 Weeks	Second	Before	3 Weeks	Second
25 Prisoners	8.0	60.0	60.0	0.0	52.0	48.0
32 Patients	6.3	37.5	65.5	0.0	53.1	31.3
16 Controls	0.0	81.3	87.5	0.0	93.7	93.7

* Gell, P. G. H.: Discussion on nutrition and resistance to infection, London, Proc. Roy. Soc. Med. *41*:323, 1948.

not been any widespread epidemic disease in Germany since the war. These points taken together suggest that undernutrition does not play as large a part in widespread epidemics as is generally supposed.

Without going into further detail, it is evident that the protein deficient patient is at a great disadvantage. He is often hypovolemic. His resistance to hemorrhagic shock is decreased, and his resistance to infection may be decreased. Wound healing is likely to be delayed if hypoproteinemia is severe, and the disturbance in gastrointestinal motility may interfere with the resumption of normal nutrition, especially following a gastroenterostomy.

Unfortunately, the same group of patients who are often deprived of the use of the gastrointestinal tract for several days after operation are the ones who commonly have had digestive disturbances and consequently have developed serious nutritional deficits before operation. The extent of the deficits which individuals develop before operation is not known accurately, although it is, of course, not uncommon to find patients with gastrointestinal malignant lesions who have lost 20, 40, 60 or more pounds in weight since the onset of symptoms.

ESTIMATIONS OF PROBABLE PROTEIN DEFICITS

If hypoproteinemia has actually developed, it is safe to assume that a substantial nutritional deficit has developed unless there has been a rapid expansion of the extracellular space with solutions containing sodium. This is based on the difficulty of producing hypoproteinemia of any degree in experimental animals. A dog on a 1 per cent protein diet will require about 15 plasmaphereses in a 3-week period to carry him down to edema level. At each bleeding, hemorrhage will be

carried to or close to the point of air hunger— the blood citrated and the cells separated and returned in a saline suspension.

In some patients, weight loss may be a valuable index. In others, the dietary history may be helpful (e.g., a patient may have been put on a meat-free diet or a low protein diet by a physician who may not have been sufficiently mindful of the effects of the low protein intake). It is probable that the measurement of the total number of grams of circulating plasma protein will give a more sensitive indication of protein loss than would the serum protein concentration alone. It has been stated that the estimation of the total number of grams of circulating albumin is an even more sensitive index.

It should be emphasized that a normal serum protein concentration by no means rules out the possible existence of substantial protein deficits which may have serious significance for the patient undergoing extensive operation or a complicated postoperative course. This can be suspected in some patients if a careful dietary history is taken. Muscular wasting is an important physical sign of protein deficiency.

PREOPERATIVE PROTEIN LOSS

Some of the more acute losses of protein occurring before operation in surgical patients are shown in Table 2, and it is to be remembered that a considerable additional loss of protein is apt to occur during operation in the form of hemorrhage.[4, 8, 15, 23, 24] Unquestionably, there are additional losses as the result of tissue trauma, leakage of plasma from the circulation in the form of serum, or sequestration of plasma and possibly of cells in the local area of inflammation. The losses due to hemorrhage alone have been measured by a number of writers, and a group of such figures have been compiled in Table 3.[7, 34]

TABLE 2. NITROGEN LOSSES IN VARIOUS TYPES OF SURGICAL PATIENTS
BEFORE OPERATION*

ILLNESS	N LOSS IN GRAMS	TIME IN DAYS
Bleeding peptic ulcer—Bockus[4]	90.72	5
Thermal burn—Hirshfeld et al.[23]		
Surface oozing	7.84	1
Total nitrogen loss	30.88	1
Small bowel obstruction—Fine and Gendel[15]	11.04	1
Long bone fractures—Cuthbertson[8]	137.00	10
Long bone fractures—Howard et al.[24]	190.00	Variable number of weeks

* Rhoads, J. E.: Supranormal dietary requirements of acutely ill patients, J. Amer. Dietetic Assoc. *29*:897-903, 1953.

POSTOPERATIVE PROTEIN LOSS

After operation, the picture is a complex one. Not only is there a continuing loss of protein during a period when the intake may be quite restricted, but the loss is enhanced by a phenomenon which is known as the catabolic response to injury. The first attempt to quantitate this response in patients was made by Cuthbertson and his collaborators,[8] who studied the metabolism of patients following fractures of the long bones and reported their work in 1935. Their observations have since been confirmed by John Eager Howard[24] and others in this country. In general, it was found that there was an increase in the output of nitrogen in the urine for a period of 10 days or so following fractures. This results in a negative nitrogen balance in ordinary diets containing 3.4 Gm. nitrogen to 9.4 Gm. nitrogen, and when the dietary protein intake was increased to 11.6 Gm. nitrogen and to 14.0 Gm. nitrogen per day, the output rose also, and the patient remained in negative balance for a period in the neighborhood of 10 days. There are many ways of demonstrating this catabolic loss of nitrogen. Dr. George Whipple[50] noted it following chloroform poisoning in dogs and in a number of other conditions (see Chap. 14, "Nonoperative Surgical Care").

SIGNIFICANCE OF THE CATABOLIC RESPONSE TO INJURY AND OPERATION

The significance of this phenomenon has been the subject of much speculation among surgical physiologists. Those of one school of thought view it as a teleologic mechanism by

TABLE 3. NITROGEN LOSSES (DUE TO BLOOD LOSS) IN VARIOUS TYPES OF SURGICAL PATIENTS
DURING OPERATION (BASED ON 3 GM. OF NITROGEN PER 100 CC. OF BLOOD)*

OPERATION	NUMBER OF PATIENTS	NITROGEN LOSS IN GRAMS		
		Minimum	*Average*	*Maximum*
Radical mastectomy				
Coller et al.[7]	4	15	24	31.5
Thyroidectomy				
Coller et al.[7]	8	3	12	21
Abdominoperineal resection				
Coller et al.[7]	12	6	12	21
Gastric operations (complicated)				
Coller et al.[7]	3	9	18	24
Operations involving large body surfaces				
Coller et al.[7]	3	13.5	36	42
Pneumonectomy				
Miller, Gibbon and Allbritten[34]	16	21	57	108
First-stage thoracoplasty				
Miller, Gibbon and Allbritten[34]	10	12	22.5	60

* Rhoads, J. E.: Supranormal dietary requirements of acutely ill patients, J. Amer. Dietetic Assoc. *29*:897-903, 1953.

which the body gets rid of excess protein at a time when this may be harmful. Others view it as an attempt on the part of the body to mobilize large quantities of tissue nitrogen, possibly because of a specific need for certain moieties of the protein molecule, as for instance a particular amino acid. If one accepts the first viewpoint, one withhholds protein, or at least does not push it, and accepts a negative nitrogen balance for a period of several days following the injury. If one believes in the second hypothesis, one would be led to augment protein intake in order to provide materials to enable the body to prolong its responses for a greater period than is possible from its own stores.

While this question in the broad sense remains unanswered, experimental data are available in the case of the liver which suggest that it is the mobilization of the body's protein stores that is important. Hepatic injury produced by a standard chloroform anesthesia in the dog is better tolerated, in terms of histologic evidence of degeneration and necrosis, if the animal concomitantly receives an irritating subcutaneous injection of sodium ricinoleate capable of initiating a catabolic response. It would seem in this experimental setup that the liver injured by chloroform was actually benefited as a result of the catabolic phenomena induced by injury to subcutaneous tissue and muscle caused by the injection of sodium ricinoleate or some other irritating material.

The extent of the catabolic response in a variety of surgical conditions is presented in Table 4.[5, 24, 43] It is evident that much more protein and protein-sparing food are required to achieve nitrogen equilibrium in the patient following extensive operation than would be the case in the normal individual.

For the normal adult male of 70 Kg., the Food and Nutrition Board recommends a daily allowance of 70 Gm. of protein; and 60 Gm. for the normal adult woman of 60 Kg. (one Gm. per Kg. of body weight per day). It is considered that this provides a sufficient excess to cover ordinary variations in the character of the food protein and in the activity of the individual. It does not provide for pregnancy, for lactation or for growth of the young individual. It is based on nitrogen balance studies in more than 100 indi-

TABLE 4. NITROGEN LOSSES IN VARIOUS TYPES OF SURGICAL PATIENTS AFTER OPERATION*

ILLNESS	N LOSS IN GRAMS	TIME IN DAYS
Herniotomy[5]	18.0	10
Subtrochanteric osteotomy[24]	65.0†	14
Gastric resection[43]	54.0	5
Cholecystectomy[5]	114.0	10
Gastric resection[5]	175.0	10
Acute appendicitis (Peritonitis)[5]	49.0	10
Repair perforated peptic ulcer[5]	136.0	10
Radical mastectomy[5]	15.0	10

* Rhoads, J. E.: Supranormal dietary requirements of acutely ill patients, J. Amer. Dietetic Assoc. *29*: 897-903, 1953.

† Average of 3.

viduals carried on in some 25 laboratories and provides a 50 per cent excess over and above the average of these figures. To be compared with this is the figure of 130 Gm. of protein, arrived at by Riegel and her co-workers[43] for gastrectomy patients during the first 5 postoperative days. To obtain balance on this allowance, a relatively high caloric allowance was provided of the order of 2,100 calories or 30 calories per kilogram. These figures were average and do not provide a 50 per cent excess for individual variation. Thus it would appear that the postgastrectomy patient has nearly 3 times the protein requirement of the normal. After smaller operations, however, the change is less marked, as after herniorrhaphy there is relatively little excess nitrogen catabolism.

While the above considerations are of help in thinking of the more difficult nutritional problems, they must be mixed with much common sense when dealing with the average surgical patient. The many patients requiring minor surgical procedures and the more moderate major ones present no nutritional problem other than the provision of a normal intake, such as they might enjoy away from the hospital. Even for those patients who have a considerable accumulated nutritional deficit and who must look forward to several days after operation before food is permitted by mouth, a complicated nutritional regimen is seldom required. In most instances, if moderate support is provided, they can be expected to take sufficient food by mouth within 5 to 7 days after operation and to go into positive balance and correct any deficiencies which may have developed. However, such patients require nutritional help during the postoperative period, and it is generally advantageous to give them at least 100 Gm. of glucose and 100 Gm. of protein hydrolysates per day until a satisfactory oral intake is established. There is a real difference of opinion as to whether or not these amounts are optimal. This mixture provides only 800 calories; therefore, it is inadequate for an adult on any long-term basis. Whether or not it will be adequate on a short-term basis will depend on the manner in which the individual mobilizes his own tissues. If he mobilizes fat in sufficient quantities, it may be perfectly adequate. If, on the other hand, he does not and mobilizes more protein instead, 100 Gm. of protein and 100 Gm. of carbohydrate do not constitute a satisfactory diet.

Elman has reported that the patient receiving no protein loses no more nitrogen on 100 Gm. of glucose than when a larger amount is given. However, the studies of Zollinger and Ellison[54] indicated that with a steady nitrogen intake, increases in carbohydrate to provide higher caloric intakes are accompanied by a substantial rise in nitrogen retention.

A practical objection to providing all of these patients with a larger caloric intake during a time when they cannot take feedings by mouth lies in the concentrations which must be used intravenously to provide the intake in a reasonable quantity of water (3,000 to 3,500 ml.) and the fact that hypertonic solutions tend to thrombose veins. Therefore, it is customary to steer a middle ground in the average case, providing an intake of the order of 100 Gm. of glucose and 100 Gm. of protein hydrolysate daily until such time as the patient can eat. One then reserves the more energetic treatment for the occasional long, drawn-out case of the patient with a marked nutritional deficit in which a positive caloric and nitrogen balance seem to be urgent.

CARBOHYDRATE AND FAT

As has been stated earlier in this chapter, the surgeon's interest in carbohydrate and fat is concerned primarily with its effect in sparing proteins by supplying calories, as discussed in the section on proteins. A certain amount of carbohydrate is necessary, even if the body is able to provide ample fat from its stores for caloric requirement. If some carbohydrate is not supplied, acetone bodies will be formed and will carry off a portion of the alkali reserve, resulting in acidosis. 100 Gm. of carbohydrate a day are ordinarily more than sufficient to provide for this requirement. It should be remembered that children are probably more susceptible to the development of acidosis by this mechanism than are adults.

It is not entirely true to say that fat can be replaced in the diet by carbohydrate on an isocaloric basis. There is evidence that with extremely low fat diets the total number of calories must be increased. There is also some evidence indicating that growth can proceed at a more rapid rate if some fat is provided in the diet. Practically speaking, a fat-free diet, or even one very low in fat (less than 10% of the calories) is very unpalatable. Within a fairly wide range, however, carbohydrate and fat can be substituted for each other to provide calories and to spare proteins.

The bearing of high fat diets on the development of atherosclerosis has received much study. It has long been known that a number of disease conditions which are commonly associated with hypercholesterolemia are also associated with a high incidence of atherosclerosis and its complications. Atherosclerosis can be produced prematurely in some species by feeding a high cholesterol diet. Because of the ease with which the body produces cholesterol, it has not been sufficient to lower the cholesterol intake if one wishes to lower the blood cholesterol level. However, the blood cholesterol level generally can be reduced if the total fat intake is curtailed drastically.

Machella and his associates found that patients kept on a diet rich in protein and carbohydrate and free of fat during therapy for ulcerative colitis developed remarkably low serum cholesterol levels. Accordingly, they undertook a study[32] in which patients with a variety of gastrointestinal conditions were placed on a synthetic fat-free diet consisting of protein hydrolysate and dextrimaltose. This diet, which supplied from 2,200 to 4,000 calories a day, was supplmented with vitamins and iron and was maintained for periods up to 55 days. They found that the patients were maintained in a satisfactory stage of nutrition and health and noted an average decrease of 85 (5 to 169) milligrams of cholesterol per 100 ml. of serum in 15 days. They further noted that a significant decrease occurred within 5 days of starting this diet, and that the cholesterol level returned to the former level within 8 days of resuming a normal diet. If they added moderate amounts of fat, a significant decrease (to 96 mg. %) still occurred. They concluded that a palatable diet which is high in proteins and carbohydrate and low in fat will maintain a low serum cholesterol concentration.

The extensive studies of Keys and his associates[28] have indicated that those population groups in Western Europe whose average dietary provides about 20 per cent of the calories as fat have a far lower incidence of coronary occlusion than exists in the United States of America, where studies indicate that about 40 per cent of the calories of the diet are provided as fat. Keys's studies show further that the population groups on the lower fat intake generally have lower cholesterol levels in the blood.

The interrelationship between dietary fat, serum cholesterol and the complications of atherosclerosis with its possible effects on the incidence of vascular disease is demanding more attention. Although the evidence to date is not unequivocal, it is highly suggestive that elevated serum cholesterol levels are undesirable and should be reduced in patients with coronary artery disease, diabetes mellitus and some peripheral vascular diseases.[33] Current studies reveal that the greatest and most practical cholesterol-decreasing regimen is one in which the total fat is reduced along with a reduction in the saturated fatty acids and replaced with unsaturated fatty acids, such as those found in plant foods.[3, 33] It is emphasized that unsaturated fatty acids should not be used as a supplement but as a substitute for other dietary fatty acids.[3, 33]

ROUTES OF ALIMENTATION

Having now considered some of the unfortunate consequences and dangers of hypopro-

teinemia and the amount of protein needed under a variety of circumstances, next one must consider the means at our disposal for providing these needs. It must be emphasized again and again that the alimentary canal, if normal or only moderately impaired, is the best route for alimentation. The other routes are utilized only when the oral route is contraindicated for some particular reason, such as persistent vomiting, recent operation upon the gastrointestinal tract, severe diarrhea, etc. Generally speaking, in postoperative patients, it is wise to wait until peristaltic sounds return before using the oral route.

RECTAL ROUTE

The rectal route, although used extensively in the past (clysters), is seldom used today, but it is still a very practical route for the administration of water and isotonic sodium chloride solution. Tap water or isotonic sodium chloride solution dripped through a small catheter at a pressure of not more than 20 to 40 cm. of water ordinarily can be absorbed in amounts up to a liter or so every 12 hours. The addition of glucose to the water or saline solution retards absorption and, according to the studies of Ebeling,[13] very little glucose is absorbed. For a more detailed consideration of this subject, the reader is referred to reference numbers.[14, 42]

JEJUNOSTOMY

Allen[2] has recommended jejunostomy as a preliminary procedure in malnourished patients requiring extensive operation. The use of this method has not been uniformly successful in the hands of the author, due to the fact that instillation of food directly into the jejunum will often set up a diarrhea. A variation of the jejunostomy suggested by Ravdin and implemented by Abbott and Rawson[1] consists of placing a double lumen tube in the stomach before operation. One lumen is connected to a single tube which, during the course of a gastric operation, can be moved through the gastroenterostomy and allowed to go well down into the jejunum below the gastrojejunostomy. The tube may be passed either through the nose or the mouth, as originally suggested by the authors, or it may be brought out through the gastric wall and through the abdominal wall like the tube in a Stamm gastrostomy. The limitations of this method are influenced by the tolerance of the jejunum for food which has not been prepared in the stomach.

Studies[38] indicate that one of the functions of the stomach, in addition to storage, is to dilute hypertonic foods to or almost to isotonicity. Thus, when a large load of 50 per cent glucose was placed in the stomach of the dog, the highest glucose concentrations obtained in duodenal samples were 5.3 per cent and those in the jejunum were of the order of 2.4 per cent. In general, hypertonic materials introduced into the jejunum draw in a lot of fluid immediately. This may produce local pain, so-called "dumping Syndrome" (see Chap. 29, "Stomach and Duodenum"), or it may set up a diarrhea.[30] At times, this may be controlled with paregoric, but on other occasions the feeding mixture will have to be stopped.

PARENTERAL ROUTES

Thus we are left with the parenteral routes for the majority of patients who cannot take feedings by mouth, and of these the intravenous route is certainly the most versatile and probably the safest if one has access to pyrogen-free fluids.

Glucose is readily administered by vein in concentrations from 5 to 50 per cent. 5 per cent glucose solution is about isotonic. Weaker solutions may be given provided that the total osmotic pressure of the solution is made up with sodium chloride or some other substance suitable for intravenous injection. If this is not done, the hypotonic solution may produce hemolysis of red blood cells, with the concomitant risk of kidney injury which follows such an event.

Fructose. Intravenous fructose also has been proposed and has certain advantages. In experiments carried out by Rosenthal and his associates,[44] at a moderately rapid infusion rate about 6 per cent less sugar was spilled when using invert sugar rather than glucose. Fructose may have other advantages, although these are still being explored. Infusions at rates of 1.5 Gm./Kg. per hour resulted in the liberation of a considerable amount of lactate which may be measured in the blood stream but so far has not been shown to be defi-

nitely injurious. At times very rapid rates of infusion have produced hyperpnea.

Protein may be given either in the form of amino acid mixtures or in the form of hydrolyzed protein. Protein hydrolysates may be prepared either by acid hydrolysis which destroys tryptophane or by enzymatic hydrolysis. A common preparation results from the enzymic hydrolysis of a mixture of casein and animal pancreas. If the acid hydrolysis is used, it is essential to replace the tryptophane and tyrosine in appropriate amounts so that the resulting material will have the effect of a so-called whole or complete protein.

It is now well documented that omission of an essential amino acid from the feeding mixture results in a practically complete wasting of the rest of the material. Furthermore, all of the essential constituents must be given at approximately the same time. Thus, if an incomplete protein is fed in the morning and the moiety required to complete it is not fed until evening, most of both feedings will be lost in the form of increased nitrogen in the urine.

Ethyl alcohol is another preparation that may be administered intravenously. If there is any doubt as to whether the available ethyl alcohol is adulterated, it may be safest to use absolute alcohol, diluted to a concentration of 10 per cent or less. It is, of course, unnecessarily expensive as much of the cost of absolute alcohol is due to the expense incurred in eliminating residual water. The alcohol provides 7 calories per gram. Its pharmacologic actions are well known, although it should be emphasized that it sometimes seems to function as an excellent sedative, especially in older people who often tolerate barbiturate sedatives poorly.

Where a serious effort is being made to achieve caloric as well as nitrogen balance in the postoperative patient, a mixture of 5 per cent alcohol, 5 per cent glucose and 5 per cent protein hydrolysate can be very useful. Two liters of such a solution provide in the neighborhood of 1,500 calories and, when supplemented by an additional liter of 10 per cent glucose, often will provide a sufficient caloric intake. Such solutions are definitely hypertonic and will produce excessive thrombosis in some individuals at the site of injection. However, if the injection site is changed once every 12 to 24 hours, the majority of individuals will tolerate it.

At present, glucose, fructose, hydrolyzed protein (or amino acid mixtures) and ethyl alcohol comprise our principal repertory for parenteral alimentation.

Much-improved preparations of fat emulsions for intravenous administration have been developed during the last few years. Intravenous fat is being used as a dietary supplement in a number of institutions. One such preparation is Lipomul I.V., which is an oil-in-water emulsion containing 15 per cent w/v cottonseed oil (U.S.P.), 4 per cent w/v dextrose (U.S.P.) and the necessary dispersing agents, the dextrose being used to make the aqueous phase isotonic.

The chief deterrents to the widespread use of intravenous fats have been the immediate and late reactions after the administration of large amounts. The immediate reactions consist of one or more of the following symptoms: fever, chills, back or chest pain, dyspnea, severe flushing and urticaria. Some patients complain of nausea, vomiting and abdominal discomfort. The late reactions are of a hemorrhagic diathesis and/or jaundice. The risk of fatality appears to be extremely low if suitable precautions are taken during the administration of intravenous fat and if the infusions are stopped when a severe reaction appears.

At present it would seem that if a patient does not react unfavorably to the initial infusion of 500 ml., he can be expected to use the material to advantage up to a total of at least 10 units of 500 ml. each. The immediate reaction rate, excluding small changes in temperature (up to 2° F.), appears to be 15 per cent or less. Therefore, the material may be used advantageously in 6 out of 7 patients. The late reactions of a hemorrhagic diathesis and/or jaundice have been seen occasionally after the use of 10 to 20 or more 500 ml. units. To date (1960) the author and his associates have not experienced a clear-cut picture of this phenomenon in 34 patients receiving from 10 to 73 500 ml. units, but the average incidence may be as high as 10 per cent.[3, 41]

The advantages of the fat preparations are that they exert a negligible osmotic effect and that they carry a very high caloric value (9 calories per Gm.). Thus they may be given in concentrations up to at least 15 per cent, in which form 1 L. will supply 1,350 calories. Evidences already available indicate that several fats prepared in this way are well utilized in the body for metabolic purposes.

An interesting and probably important finding of Scott and Vars[47] is that interruption of the enterohepatic circulation of bile in an animal somewhat decreases his tolerance for intravenous fat. Some of the animals actually have died during its administration when all bile was being sidetracked from the common duct. Therefore, as intravenous fat becomes generally available, it may be wise to be cautious in the administration of these preparations to individuals with severe liver damage, obstructive jaundice, or biliary fistulas (e.g., a draining T-tube in the common bile duct).

Some authors also counsel against its use in the presence of high fever, hemorrhagic diathesis, acidosis, or persistent lipidemia of any cause.

NUTRITIONAL ROLE OF BLOOD AND PLASMA

The role of plasma proteins and whole blood in nutrition deserves consideration here. Whipple and his associates[35] showed that a dog could be maintained by giving it intravenous dog plasma as the sole source of protein (the dogs received nonprotein caloric supplements by mouth). It was believed as the result of additional studies on phlorhizinized dogs that the protein actually could be converted to various body proteins without being broken down all the way to amino acids. Allen and his associates have demonstrated recently that dog plasma permits normal growth of puppies (see Chap. 8, "Blood Transfusions"). In spite of this finding, most experts in the field of nutrition do not recommend plasma for its nutritional value, believing that its conversion to other body proteins is slow and that the plasma itself is too expensive. Blood is considered to be even less suitable as it takes a long time for protein in red cells to be converted to other proteins, if indeed this conversion takes place to any appreciable extent.

However, in spite of this, blood and plasma do provide for the blood volume deficit which is so regularly seen in hypoproteinemic patients. Certainly, they are invaluable in the preparation of a seriously malnourished anemic patient for operation. They are used extensively in such situations when the patient is confronted with an emergency operation. Furthermore, in our experience, in situations such as pyloric obstruction in which the patient has accumulated a serious nutritional deficit, usually we have found it preferable to build up his blood volume and blood protein with transfusions and carry out a definitive operation which should permit restoration of an adequate oral route after a few days rather than to attempt more complicated regimens. Attempts to build up the patient by parenteral feeding (or jejunostomy) often prove to be rather ineffective and, at times, the patient has become worse instead of better during the days when such efforts have been made. Therefore, it would seem that blood and plasma have a special role in the preoperative preparation of patients with serious nutritional deficits where these deficits cannot be definitely corrected preoperatively.

DIABETES

Any full discussion of the problems of diabetic management is, of course, beyond the scope of this book. It is of interest, however, that surgical operations, while they may accentuate diabetes and call for a temporary increase in the insulin requirement, may also have a steadying influence on the so-called "brittle" or unstable diabetic, making him easier to handle for a period. Because the insulin requirement is unpredictably affected by operation and by some of the diseases for which operation is carried out, particularly those of an inflammatory nature, it is in general unwise to attempt a precise regulation of diabetes near the time of operation. The objects of diabetic management should be: (1) to prevent ketosis and (2) to prevent insulin shock. A normal blood sugar level and freedom from glycosuria should not be objectives during the acute period. Therefore, diabetic management during such an acute period may be reduced in the opinion of the author to the administration of enough insulin to abolish ketosis and to the administration of 2 Gm. of glucose concomitantly with every unit of insulin. In the author's experience this

is accomplished most safely by administering the insulin intravenously with the glucose solution, thus starting the glucose concomitantly with the insulin, even though the initial blood sugar is exceedingly high. Plasma carbon dioxide determinations are most valuable and, if the level is low, it should be corrected. Correction may be achieved by the abolition of ketosis and the administration of isotonic sodium chloride solution in suitable amounts, but if the bicarbonate is below 20 millimols per liter, the author prefers the more direct method of giving sixth molar sodium lactate in appropriate amounts (see Chap. 5, "Fluid and Electrolytes").

Schechter and his associates[45] demonstrated marked reductions in plasma volume in 8 patients with diabetic coma. Such patients may need whole blood or plasma transfusions quite as urgently as the other elements of therapy alluded to above, and this should be considered at the time of admission.

VITAMINS

In considering the requirements of surgical patients for the various accessory food substances, attention must be focused principally on those for which storage is quite limited, as is the case with most of the water-soluble vitamins, and on those for which a conditioned deficiency may develop over a period of time in patients with surgical diseases, such as vitamin K.

THE FAT-SOLUBLE VITAMINS
Vitamin A

While a vitamin A deficiency, if fully developed, might be harmful to many surgical patients, the chance of such a deficiency developing is relatively small. The precursor of the vitamin, carotene, is fairly widely distributed in the average American diet and, as a rule, patients have an ample store of the vitamin capable of lasting them many weeks. Vitamin A has been recommended in large doses in the treatment of plantar warts. The status of this therapy is not well established, as these lesions sometimes come and go rather unpredictably without treatment. Therefore, the use of vitamin A is presented rather as something to try than as an established method of treatment.

Vitamin D

Vitamin D, another of the fat-soluble vitamins, is of course as important to infants and children who happen to be in surgical wards as it is for those in pediatric wards. This is particularly true of orthopedic patients who may be kept in a hospital for many weeks or months without exposure to sunlight. In the normal adult, however, vitamin D deficiency does not seem to be a problem of much practical importance. Considerable effort has been expended at different times to obtain faster fracture healing by the administration of additional amounts of vitamin D. However, there is no clear evidence that it effects more rapid healing of fractures. Overdosage of vitamin D can produce a complex toxic picture characterized by significant changes in renal, vascular and nervous systems.

Vitamin D does have a special role in surgery in patients suffering from hypoparathyroidism. As a rule, hypoparathyroidism comes about as a result of the removal of the parathyroid tissue during thyroidectomy, or during surgical attacks on the parathyroids themselves. The usefulness of vitamin D in this group of patients is mentioned in the chapter on the parathyroid. The usual dosage for this purpose is 50,000 to 400,000 units per day or 10 to 100 times the dosage usually employed for the correction of rickets.

Vitamin E

Vitamin E, a third fat-soluble vitamin, was identified in animal studies as being necessary for normal reproduction. While it has been administered fairly widely among patients, its field of usefulness is apparently quite limited. It has been reported to be helpful in Peyronie's disease, and some individuals have given it to patients with Dupuytren's contracture. In some of the early cases, it seems to have arrested the development of the process, but this is, of course, a clinical impression and not a well-controlled observation.

Vitamin K

Vitamin K is a nutrient of exceptional interest to surgeons. Its absence was discovered by Dam[9] when a group of chicks which he was feeding on synthetic diets developed a hemorrhagic tendency. While his original observations were made in 1929, he did not publish the discovery of the new accessory food factor until 1934, and it was not until 1938 that H. P. Smith[49] and his co-workers established the relationship of the new vitamin to hypoprothrombinemia resulting from obstructive jaundice.

It was A. J. Quick who first showed in 1934 and 1935 that the hemorrhagic tendency, so long known to develop in patients with obstructive jaundice, was due to a prothrombin deficiency. In man, the hypoprothrombinemia is due to a conditioned deficiency. Sufficient vitamin K is formed by intestinal microorganisms to supply the requirements of most individuals. It is the lack of bile salts which lowers surface tension and assists in the emulsification of fats and hence the bile salts are needed for the absorption of the naturally occurring forms of the vitamin from the bowel which leads to a relative deficiency and to hypoprothrombinemia. If the deficiency of prothrombin is to be treated orally, it is important to give either a water-soluble form of the vitamin or to give bile salts in suitable quantities to assist in its absorption. Therefore, it is not the failure of the biliary system to excrete bile but the failure of the bile (specifically, the bile salts) to reach the intestine which leads to hypoprothrombinemia. This explains the fact that patients with external biliary fistula may develop a hemorrhagic tendency even though they are not icteric. It also explains the fact that patients may develop a hemorrhagic tendency with incomplete common duct obstruction. It has long been known that the concentration of bile salts in the bile goes down as one of the earliest indications of liver damage. Therefore, it seems reasonable to explain this last group of patients on the basis that they are excreting bile pigments in adequate amounts but failing to excrete bile salts in adequate amounts.

Attention should be called to the fact that vitamin K was, perhaps, the first of the vitamins to be found in multiple forms and is still, perhaps, the only vitamin for which a synthetic substitute is more potent than the naturally occurring forms. Vitamin K_1 in the form found naturally in alfalfa and other green vegetables has the long phytyl radical found in chlorophyll and is of relatively heavy molecular weight and of low solubility in water. The central nucleus of K_1, 2-methyl-1, 4-naphthoquinone (menadione), is more effective per milligram than is K_1 itself and is slightly more soluble in water. Some of the derivatives of this proluct are considerably more soluble in water and may easily be given by parenteral injection in doses of 5, 10, or 20 mg. every 4 hours until prothrombin has returned to safe levels or risen to a maximum.

Early studies showed that not all patients with hypoprothrombinemia would respond to vitamin K, and there is now a body of evidence which indicates that prothrombin is synthesized to a large extent in the liver and that if liver damage is sufficiently pronounced, hypoprothrombinemia will develop despite large doses of vitamin K.

However, in the hypoprothrombinemia produced by Dicoumarol, there is a relatively normal level of accelerator globulin and a reduced level of prothrombin. When administered intravenously in doses of 50 to 1,000 mg., a fine emulsion of vitamin K_1 in an aqueous medium appears to have a mass action effect against Dicoumarol and can be very valuable in patients who have received excessive doses or have had excessive responses to Dicoumarol. Also, it has been given intramuscularly. The response after intravenous administration is very rapid, often being well marked within $\frac{1}{2}$ to 1 hour. The effect may be rather transient, necessitating the administration of additional doses as often as 4- or 6-hour intervals until the prothrombin concentration is stabilized at satisfactory levels. Failure to check the prothrombin at short-time intervals can easily lead to the view that no response has been obtained, as the prothrombin may have fallen back to the original level in 12 hours or so if Dicoumarol is still active in the body.

The Water-Soluble Vitamins

Thiamine. One of the most important of the water-soluble vitamins is thiamine. Its effects are tied up so much with the effects of riboflavin and nicotinic acid deficiency and possibly of other B component deficiencies that it is exceedingly difficult to be sure which of these substances is having a particular effect. In its extreme forms B_1 deficiency produces the clinical picture of beriberi with peripheral neuritis, anorexia, changes in the electrocardiogram, and eventually interference with cell metabolism. The requirement of thiamine is low, of the order of 1 to 2 mg. a day in normal adults. It may be doubled by fever or hyperthyroidism. In thyroid storm, when the temperature is high, the requirement can possibly go up as much as 4 times. Therefore, the usual custom of giving 5, 10, or 20 mg. per day should provide enormous excesses of this vitamin. So far as we know, these excesses are harmless, but their utility never has been demonstrated. It has been postulated that, when circulation to an extremity or some other local area of the body is very poor, there may be an advantage in supplying the vitamin at higher concentrations. However, this remains rather hypothetical.

At one time, it was thought that vitamin B_1 might have the property of reducing the basal metabolism in patients with Graves' disease. Under more or less controlled conditions the vitamin proved to be much less effective than iodine in reducing the basal metabolism. Still, it was noted that many more patients gained weight if they were given vitamin B_1 and brewer's yeast during the preoperative period. Frazier and Ravdin,[17] at the Hospital of the University of Pennsylvania, showed that before the use of thiamine and brewer's yeast only 28.5 per cent of the patients with Graves' disease gained weight before operation, and after treatment with small doses of these drugs, 72 per cent of the patients gained weight before operation.

Many patients other than those with hyperthyroidism also have marked improvement in appetite when thiamine is given. Anorexia and miscellaneous pains simulating peripheral neuritis are frequently treated with thiamine and other members of the B complex. Their specific usefulness remains uncertain, except where a specific deficiency exists.

Folic acid will induce a remission in patients with pernicious anemia, but unfortunately its use seems to accentuate the development of combined posterolateral sclerosis. However, this untoward result can be prevented by the use of B_{12}.

Pantothenic Acid. Another vitamin of the B group, pantothenic acid, has been shown to have an unusual influence on resistance of animals to cold stress. When given in very large doses, it significantly increased the time which rats could swim in cool or cold water and, according to Ralli,[12] in doses of 10 Gm. a day it increased, to some extent, the tolerance of young men to immersion in extremely cold water.[36] The significance of these findings remains obscure, but such experiments stand squarely in the way of the generalization that an excess of vitamins above the ordinary requirement is of no use. Inositol, pyridoxine, and the other members of the B group are commonly included in polyvitamin therapy, particularly for liver disease, although their importance in man under various conditions has not been completely studied as yet.

Vitamin C is of special interest to surgical patients because of its influence on wound healing. Early records of scurvy occurring among men on sailing ships refer to the fact that wounds long healed would sometimes break down. More recently, Wolbach[53] and others confirmed the fact that a vitamin C deficiency reduces the healing strength of wounds. While the ordinary requirement is, perhaps, 50 to 100 mg. of ascorbic acid a day, very large doses such as 1,000 mg. a day are required to evoke any excretion of the vitamin during the first 2 days after a severe thermal burn (Lund).

Recommended Daily Dietary Allowances. Obviously, the requirements of the various vitamins for health and growth are rather difficult to state. The Food and Nutrition Board in its "Recommended Daily Dietary Allowances"[16] has backed the values shown in Table 5. However, in patients who are ill, it is considered that higher vitamin intakes are safer and probably useful. A special committee of the Food and Nutrition Board on therapeutic nutrition was formed to study this problem and, as a result of its deliberations, therapeutic formulas were proposed. These were thought of as possibly advantageous in patients who may have an increased need for vitamins for short periods of time. The values given are shown in Table 6.

Undoubtedly, vitamins are being given in a very wasteful manner. Patients who are on parenteral feedings for only a day or two probably need no vitamin supplement. Those who are on parenteral feedings for 3 to 5 days or more should receive thiamine and the B

TABLE 5. RECOMMENDED DAILY DIETARY ALLOWANCES*†

	AGE YEARS	VITAMIN A I.U.	THIAMINE MG.	RIBOFLAVIN MG.	NIACIN (MG. EQUIV.‡)	ASCORBIC ACID MG.	VITAMIN D I.U.
Men	25	5,000	1.6	1.8	21	75	. .
	45	5,000	1.5	1.8	20	75	. .
	65	5,000	1.3	1.8	18	75	. .
Women	25	5,000	1.2	1.5	17	70	. .
	45	5,000	1.1	1.5	17	70	. .
	65	5,000	1.0	1.5	17	70	. .
Pregnant (2nd half)		6,000	1.3	2.0	+3	100	400
Lactating (850 ml. daily)		8,000	1.7	2.5	+2	150	400
Infants	1/12–6/12	1,500	0.4	0.5	6	30	400
	7/12–1	1,500	0.5	0.8	7	30	400
	1–3	2,000	0.7	1.0	8	35	400
Children	4–6	2,500	0.9	1.3	11	50	400
	7–9	3,500	1.1	1.5	14	60	400
	10–12	4,500	1.3	1.8	17	75	400
Boys	13–15	5,000	1.6	2.1	21	90	400
	16–19	5,000	1.8	2.5	25	100	400
Girls	13–15	5,000	1.3	2.0	17	80	400
	16–19	5,000	1.2	1.9	16	80	400

* The allowance levels are intended to cover individual variations among most normal persons as they live in the United States under usual environmental stresses. (Adapted from Cooper, L. F., Barber, E. M., Mitchell, H. S., and Rynbergen, H. J.: Nutrition in Health and Disease, Philadelphia, Lippincott, 1958.)

† Food and Nutrition Board, National Research Council Recommended Daily Dietary Allowances, Revised 1958 (Publication No. 589).

‡ Niacin equivalents include dietary sources of the preformed vitamin and the precursor tryptophan. Sixty mg. tryptophan equals 1 mg. niacin.

TABLE 6. VITAMIN REQUIREMENTS DURING
ILLNESS OR INJURY*

	MODERATE ILLNESS OR INJURY	SEVERE ILLNESS OR INJURY
Thiamine (mg.)	2	10
Riboflavin (mg.)	2	10
Nicotinic Acid (mg.)	20	100
Pantothenic Acid (mg.)	18	40
Pyridoxine Hydrochloric Acid (mg.)	2	40
Folic Acid (mg.)	1.5	2.5
Vitamin B_{12} (mcg.)	2	4
Ascorbic Acid (mg.)	75	300†
Vitamin A, I.U.	5000	5000‡
Vitamin D, I.U.	400	400‡
Vitamin K (mg.)	2	20‡§

* Adapted from "Therapeutic Nutrition With Special Reference to Military Situations," National Academy of Sciences, National Research Council, Jan., 1951.

† Up to 1,000 mg./day may be needed to cause excretion of the vitamin in a severely burned patient.

‡ Not needed in short-term therapy unless specific deficiency exists.

§ Dose for severe and resistant hypoprothrombinemia may be as high as 500 mg. of emulsified K_1 prepared for intravenous administration.

complex vitamins and vitamin C. The indications for vitamin K are special ones, and vitamins A, D and E are not required in surgical patients as a general rule.

IRON

One is often faced with problems in disturbed iron metabolism in surgery in conditions such as malnutrition, hemorrhage, malignant disease, chronic infection, hemolytic anemia, hemosiderosis from repeated transfusions, and diseases of the upper gastrointestinal tract and the liver. In recent years our knowledge of the essential role of iron in cellular function has been increased by a number of extensive studies, and the reader is referred to these for a more detailed discussion of the subject.[10, 19, 20, 21, 25, 46, 51]

Iron plays an essential role because of its widespread distribution in hemoglobin, myoglobin and in fundamental enzyme systems such as cytochrome, catalase and peroxidase. In this way, it is indispensable for the transport and the utilization of oxygen.

The average adult contains approximately 4.5 Gm. of iron, of which 60 to 70 per cent is in hemoglobin, 3 to 5 per cent in myoglobin, 0.1 per cent in essential enzyme systems, 0.1 per cent in transport in the serum, and the remainder in storage mainly in the liver, bone marrow and the spleen.

Iron metabolism differs from that of the other electrolytes and elements in the manner in which it is absorbed and excreted. Reutilization of iron liberated by normal disintegration of red blood cells supplies most of the iron needed for hemoglobin synthesis. The remainder is derived from storage iron, and a small fraction from recently absorbed iron, 27 to 28 mg., is released daily, and most of this is utilized over and over again. As a result, only 0.6 to 1.5 mg. need be absorbed from the diet each day. 0.5 to 1.5 mg. is excreted daily in urine, bile, sweat and feces, which is derived entirely from the desquamation and the disintegration of cells.

McCance and Widdowson[29] first noted that the intestines regulate the amount of iron absorbed. According to this hypothesis, called the "mucosal block theory," and given considerable experimental support by the work of Granick[19] and Hahn,[21] the mucosal cells of the duodenum and the jejunum absorb iron in the ferrous ionic form. It is oxidized to the ferric state and combines with a protein acceptor, apoferritin, to yield ferritin, one of the storage forms of iron. When the mucosal cells become saturated, they form a barrier to further absorption until this supply is utilized. This mechanism maintains iron absorption at the fairly constant rate of 0.6 to 1.5 mg. a day when the individual is in a healthy state. However, if the need for iron is increased, the degree of absorption is increased 5 to 15 times. Following an acute massive hemorrhage in a previously healthy person, this response does not occur for 6 or 7 days. This suggests that the body stores must first be utilized by accelerated hemopoiesis before the intestinal mucosa will respond to a reduced hemoglobin level.[20, 22] In chronic states of iron deficiency, the degree of iron absorption is increased in spite of an adequate or even excessive iron store.[11] In response to whatever the body needs may be, the ferritin in the mucosal cell releases iron in the ferrous form. It enters the blood stream, is oxidized again to the ferric state and combines with a specific B_1-globulin called siderophilin. By this means it is transported by the blood to the tissues for storage and utilization.

0.1 per cent of the total iron circulating in the blood is contained in plasma, and 99.9 per cent is in the hemoglobin of red cells. The normal whole blood content of iron is 40 to 50 mg./100 ml., and the normal serum iron level is 100 to 110 mcg./100 ml. The total iron-binding capacity (TIBC) of the serum is 300 to 350 mcg./100 ml. when siderophilin is completely saturated, and normally it is about one third saturated.

The serum iron level is lowered in iron deficiency anemia and raised in certain other types of anemia and in conditions of iron overload. Therefore, the measurement of serum iron levels and the total and unsaturated iron binding capacity (UIBC) are of importance. In cases of iron need, as in iron deficiency and chronic hemorrhage, the total capacity to bind iron increases, and the degree of saturation decreases markedly. On the other hand, an excess of iron in the storage depots, as in transfusional hemosiderosis, is associated with a decrease in the total iron-binding capacity and a marked increase in the degree of saturation. In infection and malignant disease the total iron-binding capacity and the serum iron are decreased, which results in a slightly decreased degree of saturation.

Iron is stored in the tissues as ferritin, mainly in the liver, bone marrow and the spleen. Some of it is released for synthesis of heme compounds as the need arises. When the

capacity to store iron as ferritin is exceeded in conditions of iron overloading, it is stored as hemosiderin and can be detected microscopically with appropriate iron stains.

Due to the re-utilization of iron released from hemoglobin breakdown and the very small amount excreted, the daily requirement for a normal male is 0.8 to 1.0 mg. a day, and about twice that amount for a female. Since only 2 to 10 per cent of the oral iron intake is absorbed, the minimal daily requirement must be increased as shown in Table 7.

TABLE 7. RECOMMENDED DAILY DIETARY ALLOWANCE OF IRON*

	IRON (MG.)
Man (70 Kg.) or 154 lbs.	10
Woman (58 Kg.) or 128 lbs.	12
Pregnancy (latter half)	15
Lactation	15
Children	
1–6 months	5
7–12 months	7
1–3 years	7
4–6 years	8
7–9 years	10
10–12 years	12
Over 12 years	15

* Food and Nutrition Board, National Research Council Recommended Daily Dietary Allowances, Revised 1958 (Publication No. 589).

REFERENCES

1. Abbott, W. O., and Rawson, A. J.: A tube for use in the postoperative care of gastroenterostomy cases, J.A.M.A. 108:1873, 1937.
2. Allen, A. W., and Welch, C. E.: Jejunostomy for relief of malfunctioning gastroenterostomy, Surgery 9:163, 1941.
3. Beeson, P. B., Muschenheim, C., Castle, W. B., Harrison, T. R., Ingelfinger, F. J., and Bondy, P. K.: Year Book of Medicine, 1959-1960 Series, p. 687, Chicago, 1959.
4. Bockus, H. L.: Gastro-Enterology, Philadelphia, Saunders, 1949.
5. Brunschwig, A. D., Clark, D. E., and Corbin, N.: Symposium on abdominal surgery: postoperative nitrogen loss and studies on parenteral nitrogen nutrition by means of casein digest, Ann. Surg. 115:1091, 1942.
6. Coller, F. A., Campbell, K. N., Vaughn, H. H., Iob, V., and Moyer, C. A.: Postoperative salt intolerance, Ann. Surg. 119:533-541, 1944.
7. Coller, F. A., Crook, C. E., and Iob, V.: Blood loss in surgical operations, J.A.M.A. 126:1, 1944.
8. Cuthbertson, D. P.: Further observations on the disturbance of metabolism caused by injury, with particular reference to the dietary requirements of fracture cases, Brit. J. Surg. 23:505, 1936.
9. Dam, H.: Hemorrhages in chicks reared on artificial diets; new deficiency disease, Nature 133:909, 1934.
10. Drabkin, D. L.: Metabolism of the hemin chromoproteins, Physiol. Rev. 31:345, 1951.
11. Dubach, R., Callender, S. T. E., and Moore, C. V.: Studies in iron transportation and metabolism; absorption of radioactive iron in patients with fever and anemias of varied etiology, Blood 3:526-540, 1948.
12. Dumm, M. E., and Ralli, E. P.: The critical requirements for pantothenic acid by the

adrenalectomized rat, Endocrinology *43*:283, 1948.

13. Ebeling, W. W.: Absorption of detxrose from the colon, Arch. Surg. *26*:134, 1933.

14. Edsall, D. L., and Miller, C. W.: Study of two cases nourished exclusively per rectum; with a determination of absorption nitrogen metabolism and intestinal putrefaction, Tr. Coll. Physicians, Philadelphia *24*:225, 1902.

15. Fine, J., and Gendel, S.: Plasma transfusion in experimental intestinal obstruction, Ann. Surg. *112*:976, 1940.

16. Food and Nutrition Board, National Research Council: Recommended Daily Dietary Allowances, revised 1958. Publication No. 589.

17. Frazier, W. D., and Ravdin, I. S.: The use of vitamin B_1 in the preoperative preparation of the hyperthyroid patient, Surgery *4*:680, 1938.

18. Gell, P. G. H.: Discussion on nutrition and resistance to infection, Proc. Roy. Soc. Med. *41*:323, 1948.

19. Granick, S.: Iron and porphyrin metabolism in relation to red blood cells, Ann. New York Acad. Sc. *48*:657, 1947.

20. Gubler, C. J.: Absorption and metabolism of iron, Science *123*:87, 1956.

21. Hahn, P. F.: Metabolism of iron, Fed. Proc. *7*:493, 1948.

22. Hahn, P. F., *et al.*: Radioactive iron absorption by gastrointestinal tract; influence of anemia, anoxia, and antecedent feeding distribution in growing dogs, J. Exper. Med. *78*:169, 1943.

23. Hirshfeld, J. W., Williams, H. H., Abbott, W. E., Heller, C. G., and Pilling, M. A.: Significance of nitrogen loss in exudate from surface burns, Surgery *15*:766, 1944.

24. Howard, J. E., Parson, W., Stein, K. E., Eisenberg, H., and Reidt, V.: Studies on fracture convalescence: I. Nitrogen metabolism after fracture and skeletal operations in healthy males, Bull. Johns Hopkins Hosp. *75*:156, 1944.

25. Hynes, M. J.: Distribution of leukocytes on counting chamber, J. Clin. Path. *1*:57, 1948.

26. Jones, C. M., and Eaton, F. B.: Postoperative nutritional edema, Arch. Surg. *27*:159, 1933.

27. Jones, C. M., Eaton, F. B., and White, J. C.: Experimental postoperative edema, Arch. Int. Med. *53*:649-674, 1934.

28. Keys, A. B., Brozek, J., Henschel, A., Mickelson, O., and Raylor, H. L.: The Biology of Human Starvation, vol. 2, p. 1006, Minneapolis, Univ. Minnesota Press, 1950.

29. McCance, R. A., and Widdowson, E. M.: Absorption and secretion of iron, Lancet *2*:680, 1937.

30. Machella, T. E.: The mechanism of the postgastrectomy "dumping" syndrome, Tr. Am. Clin. & Climatol. A. *60* (1948), 206-231 (1949).

31. Mecray, P. M., Barden, R. P., and Ravdin, I. S.: Nutritional edema; its effect on gastric emptying time before and after gastric operations, Surgery *1*:53, 1937.

32. Mellinkoff, S. M., Machella, T. E., and Reinhold, J. G.: The effect of a fat-free diet in causing low serum cholesterol, Am. J. M. Sc. *220*:203, 1950.

33. Meltzer, L. E., Bockman, A. A., and Berryman, G. H.: A means of lowering elevated blood cholesterol levels in patients with previous myocardial infarction, Am. J. Med. Sc. *236*:595, 1958.

34. Miller, B. J., Gibbon, J. H., Jr., and Allbritten, F. F., Jr.: Blood volume and extracellular fluid changes during thoracic operations, J. Thoracic Surg. *18*:605, 1949.

35. Pommerenke, W. T., Slavin, H. B., Kariher, D. N., and Whipple, G. H.: Dog plasma protein by vein utilized in body metabolism of dog, J. Exper. Med. *61*:261, 283, 1935.

36. Ralli, E. P.: The effect of certain nutritional factors on the reactions produced by acute stress in human subjects, Recent Advances in Nutrition Research, Nutrition Symposium Series 5, 78, Aug., 1952.

37. Ravdin, I. S.: Factors involved in the retardation of gastric emptying after gastric operations, Pennsylvania M. J. *41*:695, 1938.

38. Ravdin, I. S., Johnston, C. G., and Morrison, P. J.: Comparison of concentration of glucose in the stomach and intestines after intragastric administration, Proc. Soc. Exper. Biol. & Med. *30*:955, 1933.

39. Ravdin, I. S., McNamee, H. G., Kamholz, J. H., and Rhoads, J. E.: Effect of hypoproteinemia on susceptibility to shock resulting from hemorrhage, Arch. Surg. *48*:491, 1944.

40. Rhoads, J. E., Fliegelman, M. T., and Panzer, L. M.: The mechanism of delayed wound healing in the presence of hypoproteinemia, J.A.M.A. *118*:21-25, 1942.

41. Rhoads, J. E., and Lehr, H. B.: Intravenous nutrition with fat emulsions (Presented before Fifth International Congress on Nutrition, Session on Lipids: Man II, 9/3/60, Washington, D. C.).

42. Rhoads, J. E., Stengel, A., Riegel, C., Cajori, F. A., and Frazier, W. D.: Absorption of protein split products from chronic isolated colon loops, Am. J. Physiol. *125*:707, 1939.

43. Riegel, C., Koop, C. E., Drew, J., Stevens, L. W., and Rhoads, J. E.: The nutritional requirements for nitrogen balance in surgical patients in the early postoperative period, J. Clin. Invest. *26*:18, 1947.

44. Rosenthal, O., Stainback, W. C., Rhoads, J. E., and Engelberg, J.: The utilization of invert sugar and glucose following intravenous administration to postoperative patients, S. Forum *3*:585-589, 1953.

45. Schecter, A. E., Wiesel, B. H., and Cohn, C.: Peripheral circulatory failure in diabetic acidosis and its relationship to treatment, Am. J. M. Sc. *202*:364, 1941.

46. Schultz, M. O.: Metallic elements and blood formation, Physiol. Rev. *20*:37, 1940.

47. Scott, S. M., and Vars, H. M.: Response of animals with biliary fistula, bile duct occlusion, or chloroform intoxication to parenteral fat feeding, S. Forum *5*:350-354, 1955.

48. Thompson, W. D., Ravdin, I. S., and Frank, I. L.: Effect of hypoproteinemia on wound disruption, Arch. Surg. *36*:500, 1938.

49. Warner, E. D., Brinkhous, K. M., and Smith, H. P.: Bleeding tendency of obstructive jaundice, Proc. Soc. Exper. Biol. & Med. *37*:628, 1938.

50. Whipple, G. H.: Protein production and exchange in the body, including hemoglobin, plasma protein, and cell protein, Am. J. M. Sc. *196*:609, 1938.

51. Wintrobe, M. M.: Clinical Hematology, Philadelphia, Lea & Febiger, 1952.

52. Wohl, M. G., Reinhold, J. G., and Rose, S. B.: Antibody response in patients with hypoproteinemia, Arch. Int. Med. *83*:402, 1949.

53. Wolbach, S. B., and Howe, P. R.: Intercellular substances in experimental scorbutus, Arch. Path. & Lab. Med. *1*:1-24, 1936.

54. Zollinger, R. M., and Ellison, E. H.: Nutrition in surgical patients, GP *2*:37, 1950.

──────────CHAPTER 7──────────

Shock

Included under the designation of "shock" are many conditions, medical and surgical. In this chapter the term will be considered to cover only the condition of *hypovolemic shock,* in which an acute reduction in the circulating blood volume occurs. In this chapter "shock" due to carotid sinus reflexes, to spinal anesthesia, to coronary thrombosis, to diarrhea, to anaphylactic reactions, or to similar causes will *not* be considered.

Classifications of the broad subject of "shock" are many. A few of these are pertinent at this time to show the exact place which hypovolemic, or as we consider it, true shock plays in the over-all "shock" picture. One classification is that of Blalock (1934) as follows:

1. Hematogenic shock (hypovolemic, or true shock)

2. Neurogenic "shock" (spinal "shock," syncope or fainting, carotid sinus reflex "shock," etc.)

3. Vasogenic "shock" (histamine "shock," etc.)

4. Cardiogenic "shock" (due to myocardial infarction or pericardial tamponade)

Another classification is based upon the blood volume, as follows:

1. Hypovolemic shock

2. Normovolemic "shock" (spinal "shock," etc.)

3. Hypervolemic "shock" (some instances of myocardial infarction)

Still another classification is by origin; i.e., hemorrhagic shock, traumatic shock, surgical or operative shock, burn shock, etc. These and other similar conditions representing hypovolemic shock are considered on pages 107 to 110. The final classification to be mentioned here is into primary (syncope or fainting) or other conditions in which the blood pressure fall is independent of any hypovolemia and secondary (hypovolemic) shock.

The rest of the discussion in this chapter will deal with hypovolemic shock.

DEFINITION

Shock comprises a group of conditions of various etiologies, usually acute, which mainly occur in surgical patients and are associated with a lowered blood volume due to loss of fluid from the blood stream. Definitions which show the evolution of ideas concerning it are as follows:

"Shock is a species of functional concussion by which the influence of the brain over the organ of circulation is deranged or suspended."—Travers (1826).

"A manifestation of a rude unhinging of the machinery of life."—Gross (1850).

"Peripheral circulatory failure resulting from a discrepancy in the size of the vascular bed and the volume of intravascular fluid."—Minot and Blalock (1940).

"A progressive vasoconstrictive oligemic anoxia."—Harkins (1940).

"Wound shock may be defined broadly as the clinical manifestations of an inadequate volume of circulating blood accompanied by physiologic adjustments of the organism to a progressive discrepancy between the capacity of the arterial tree and the volume of blood available to fill it."—Simeone (1953).

"Hypovolemic shock is an acute reaction to a rapidly reduced volume of circulating blood."—J. Garrott Allen (1955).

"A state of profound depression of the vital processes of the body. . . . The total blood volume is reduced. . . . Shock occurs as a result of extensive wounds, hemorrhage, crush-injuries . . . etc."—Webster's New International Dictionary of the English Language, ed. 2. Unabridged (1959).

Because of the rapid nature of the development of the hypovolemic shock syndrome, it is less often encountered in nonsurgical patients. An exception to this may be the sudden loss of large amounts of plasma-like fluid into the lungs in certain instances of pneumonia (Andrews and Harkins, 1937).

Definition by example may be helpful. The following patient seen over 25 years ago before the use of adequate blood replacement was recognized is illustrative:

J. J., a college student aged 21 years, was run over one morning by a truck, and both legs were severely crushed. He became temporarily unconscious but was able to talk on the way to the hospital. Three broken bones were easily set; there was no visible bleeding, and after taking a sedative he felt well enough to smile and appeared to be on the road to recovery. In the afternoon, however, he became restless; his face showed an anxious expression, with pallor; his pulse became weak and rapid, his skin cold and clammy and his breathing labored and shallow; he sank into coma despite a 500 ml. blood transfusion and, toward evening, died.

This boy died of shock. Such injuries may be accompanied by large concealed hemorrhages which may correspond to the loss of over 2 or 3 liters of blood. It is generally said that it takes a 10 to 25 per cent reduction in the blood volume to cause a reduction in blood pressure. The same applies to loss of whole blood or plasma or both during surgical operations, as a result of burns, and following other types of trauma.

HISTORICAL BACKGROUND

The history of shock can be divided into 3 periods. Unfortunately, at present we are in only the second of these periods. The first, or qualitative period, includes the years up to about 1930, during which the physiologic and pathologic changes accompanying shock were demonstrated and correlated. During this first period there was a beginning awareness of the advisability of blood transfusions, but this awareness was more qualitative than quantitative and usually was satisfied by giving one pint.

The publications of Blalock (1930) and of Phemister (Parsons and Phemister, 1930), working independently, can be selected arbitrarily as ushering in the second or quantitative period in the history of shock. These authors applied mechanical trauma to one hind limb of anesthetized dogs so that shock and death resulted. At necropsy there was extensive swelling of the traumatized limb, and the amount of swelling as measured by hindquarter amputation and comparison of the weight of the traumatized and opposite untraumatized limbs was essentially enough to account for death of the animal (Fig. 7-1). This quantitative assumption was based on a further comparison of this weight difference with the amount of bleeding necessary to cause death in dogs of similar size. Finally, the excess fluid which was present in the swollen limb was found to be a mixture of extracellular fluid, blood and plasma and was *not* just water.

The whole modern blood and plasma bank program is based on the quantitative concept brought out by these papers. Next to the conquest of pain (by anesthesia) and of infection (by antisepsis, asepsis and possibly by antibiotics) one of the greatest advances in surgery has been the control, in large part at least, of surgical and traumatic shock. It is of great historical interest that this same experiment later performed by Blalock and by Phemister was reported by Cannon and Bayliss in 1919. Because of the terrific number of casualties occurring in the Allied Troops in World War I, a Joint Commission headed by two of the leading physiologists of the world, Walter B. Cannon of Harvard, representing the United States, and William M. Bayliss of London, representing Great Britain, performed a simple experiment. On the basis of their interpretation of this jointly performed experiment they concluded that local fluid loss could not be the major factor in the production of shock. Because of the authority of these two great men, this view held sway until 1930 when Blalock and Phemister showed that a simple error had been made in setting up the terms of the experiment and that, when correctly performed, the logical conclusion follows that fluid loss *is* a major factor in the production of shock. This incident is recited, not to cast doubt on the experimental abilities of these two workers in the 1917-1919 Joint Commission on Shock (the writer of these pages still believes them to be two of the greatest physiologists of all time), but rather to point out the hazard of blindly accepting an authoritarian statement which held back progress in the understanding of shock for over half of the period between the two wars.

The third period in the history of shock began recently. At some future date we may understand not only what causes shock in the beginning, which we now understand fairly well, but also why it is irreversible when it has progressed beyond a certain point. This aspect of the subject is considered further on pages 114 and 115 of this chapter.

ETIOLOGY

Predisposing Factors

Predisposing factors in shock may be of various types. Certain patients, when operated upon, are more susceptible to shock than others, even though the degree of trauma and blood loss during the operation may be equal in each instance. The condition of heart, lungs, liver and kidneys is important (see Chap. 14, "Nonoperative Surgical Care"). Fluid and salt balance irregularities may be a predisposing factor. Certain anesthetic agents may predispose toward shock. Many patients, particularly those with chronic debilitating or wasting diseases such as carcinoma, may have a diminished blood volume which has been at subnormal levels for some time, as shown by Lyons and associates (1947) (see Clark, Nelson, Lyons, Mayerson, and De Camp, 1947). Such patients cannot be said to be suffering from true shock because they are more or less compensated to this low level, and there is no inherent tendency for the hypovolemia to progress rapidly. In true hypovolemic shock,

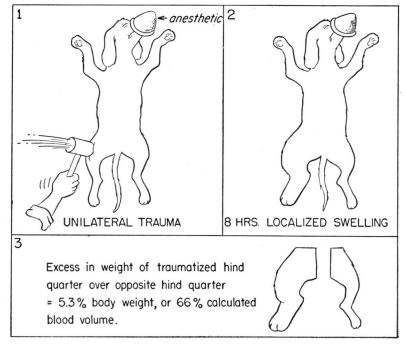

Fig. 7-1. Diagrammatic representation of classical hindquarter weight comparison experiment of Blalock and of Phemister following unilateral traumatic shock.

on the other hand, the diminished blood volume is essentially of rapid onset and usually tends to progress unless treatment is instituted promptly. Therefore, such patients with a chronic reduction in blood volume are susceptible to shock; they do not by definition have shock.

INITIATING FACTORS

Initiating factors in shock may be discussed under 2 headings: (1) basic factors leading to shock, and (2) clinical conditions in which such basic factors may operate and, hence, in which shock may result.

Basic Factors Leading to Shock. These may be listed briefly as follows:

1. Fluid loss (whole blood, plasma, or extracellular fluid, alone or together)
2. Toxic factors (see pp. 114 and 115 and 120)
3. Bacterial factors (see pp. 114 and 115 and 118 and 119)
4. Adrenal factors (See Hammond, Vandam, Davis, Carter, Ball and Moore, 1958; Egdahl, 1959, and Moore, 1959).
   A. Medullary overaction
   B. Cortical insufficiency
5. Nervous factors

The "fluid loss" factor is now regarded as being the most important. Furthermore, it is a factor about which something can be done (blood or plasma transfusion). Finally, many, if not most, of the accompanying signs and symptoms of shock (see pp. 110 to 113), regardless of the exact etiology (loss of blood, plasma, or extracellular fluid), are explainable by, or are directly related to, the hypovolemia which results from the loss of fluid from the blood stream. It is important to note that this loss is of red blood cells, protein, or sodium-containing fluid and not just water. A patient may lose several liters of urine or perspiration a day without difficulty but cannot lose nearly that amount of blood in the same period of time without serious trouble.

As discussed in the following sections, "Perpetuating Factors in Shock" and "Present-Day Problems in Shock," many of the other possible etiologic factors listed above may be more important as perpetuating factors than as initial etiologic factors. At the same time, shock tends to be a progressive syndrome, and it is

possible that the perpetuating factors start their insidious effect from the very moment that shock begins. For a further discussion of the adrenal factors, see Chapter 15, "The Endocrine and Metabolic Basis of Surgical Care."

Clinical Conditions in Which Shock May Occur. These conditions are primarily surgical but may include certain medical conditions. Essentially, they include situations in which the blood volume may be lowered rapidly, particularly by loss of whole blood, plasma, or both (Table 1).

1. "HEMORRHAGIC SHOCK"—e.g., externally from a lacerated vessel, or internally into a free cavity, as from a ruptured spleen or ectopic pregnancy. An example of fatal postoperative intraperitoneal hemorrhage treated 20 years ago is shown in Figure 7-2. (See also the review of shock by Harkins, 1941). Extensive retroperitoneal hemorrhage is another condition which, when encountered at operation or necropsy, has, according to Cushman (1953), "usually been reported as an uncommon and puzzling condition in which loss of blood has not been suspected."

It has been stated that hemorrhage and shock are separate entities because the former is not accompanied by hemoconcentration, while the latter is. As shown in Figure 7-3, this is not a differentiating factor, and the extent of hemoconcentration merely depends

TABLE 1. PATHOGENESIS OF HYPOVOLEMIC HYPOTENSION
(From Allen, J. G., 1955)

A. *Blood loss*
1. External, as in lacerations, bleeding ulcer, etc.
2. Internal, as in femoral fracture, crushing injury, ruptured spleen, etc.
B. *Plasma loss*
1. External, as in burns (where blood also may be lost and some loss of plasma occurs into the tissues)
2. Internal, as in peritonitis
3. Crushing injury (where generally more blood is lost than plasma)
C. *Water loss* (not under discussion here)
1. Water deprivation: electrolytes are concentrated and not lost. (The therapy indicated is water without salt.)
2. Water loss: as from vomiting, high intestinal pancreatic or biliary fistula, or diarrhea. (Since electrolytes are also usually lost, the therapy indicated is water with electrolytes.)

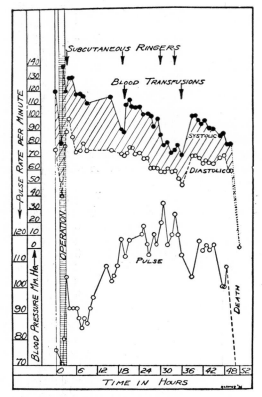

FIG. 7-2. Inadequacy of observation of fall in blood pressure in diagnosis of shock due to hemorrhage. In this patient with malignancy of the head of the pancreas, marked jaundice, and postoperative bleeding into the peritoneal cavity, treated before the days of vitamin K, it is seen that the fall in blood pressure was not a perfect guide as to the seriousness of the condition until shortly before death. The increase in pulse rate was a much better guide early, but its late improvement was deceiving. (Harkins, H. N.: Surgery 9:268)

on the proportions of blood cells and plasma lost and upon the adjustments that the body is able to make after the loss. To show how at one time it was erroneously believed that hemorrhage and shock are completely discrete, the following quotation is taken from Gross (1882):

In shock [in contradistinction to hemorrhage], the same effect [death] may happen, and yet the body be literally surcharged with blood, not a single drop, perhaps, having been spilled in the accident causing the fatal result.

2. "TRAUMATIC SHOCK"—e.g., crushed thigh after automobile accident (see case history, p. 105). In such instances the loss is primarily of whole blood, but also of some plasma. In 1937, Harkins and Roome presented 10 clinical traumatic cases with quantitative measurements of the injured parts indicating that the "concealed hemorrhage" present was (1) far greater than casual inspection would indicate and (2) large enough to be of definite significance as a causative factor in the resultant shock.

3. "SURGICAL OR OPERATIVE SHOCK." Such cases are in the main a variety of hemorrhagic shock. Formerly, surgical shock was chiefly attributed by many authors to the reflex phenomena which follow handling of intestines. Now it is generally recognized that underestimated blood loss at the time of operation is the usual causative factor. Gatch and Little (1924) determined the blood loss during surgical operations by testing the sheets, sponges, etc., and found it greater than was anticipated (mastectomy, 710 ml.; nephrectomy, 816 ml.; laminectomy, 672 ml., etc.). They advised the transfusion of as much as 3 liters of blood to counteract the blood loss attending operation.

Coller and Maddock (1932) confirmed Gatch's observations and concluded:

In general, the operator is surprised to find the blood loss as high as calculated, since he does not think of the gauze sponge as absorbing much blood. . . . It is probable that most surgeons underestimate the amount of blood lost, especially in operations . . . in which wide areas of the body are uncovered with many small points of hemorrhage, control of which is attempted by gauze packing.

One patient upon whom radical mastectomy was performed under nitrous oxide-oxygen anesthesia lost 1,272 ml. of blood.

In patients with tuberculosis subjected to thoracoplasty, Allbritten, Lipshutz, Miller, and Gibbon (1950) not only found that such individuals were admitted with a low blood volume to begin with (hence, a "predisposing factor" to shock was present), but they lost considerable blood with each stage of the thoracoplasty. The blood loss from a single stage of the procedure was as much as 1,407 ml. (as determined by weighing the sponges) or 1,558 ml. (as determined in the patient by the dye method). This important subject has also been analyzed with exactly the same conclusions by Coller, Crook, and Iob (1944), Bonica and Lyter (1951), Engberg (1956), Borden (1957), Williams and Parsons (1958), and Cáceres and Whittembury (1959).

Rains (1955) studied 4 methods of measuring blood and fluid loss at operation: (1) sponge weighing, (2) sponge washing and hemoglobin determination, (3) weighing the patient, and (4) blood volume estimation (Evans blue). All of these methods have advantages and disadvantages. This author also pointed out that one third of each unit of blood to be administered represents citrate solution. Furthermore, since some of the blood is left in the bottle or tubing "one finds that just over half a pint of blood is given when one thinks one has given a patient a pint of blood."

LeVeen and Rubricius (1958) reported the use of a continuous, automatic, electronic method for determining operative blood loss.

At the hospital of the writer of this chapter it is routine to measure the blood loss at major operations by weighing the sponges and laparotomy pads and comparing such weight with a control dry weight. The amount of blood in the suction bottle, etc., is added, and a running total figure is written in large letters on a large sheet of wrapping paper on the wall within view of the surgeon. In another column the amount of blood administered is similarly totaled, and an attempt is made to keep the total of the second column at least equal to that of the first column. Further details of technic are given in the papers by Baronofsky, Treloar, and Wangensteen (1946), Gross (1949), and by Saltzstein and Linkner (1952), and in Chapter 8, "Blood Transfusion." A useful scale for measuring the blood in sponges is shown in Figure 7-4. Ditzler and Eckenhoff (1956) reported that controlled hypotension definitely reduces blood loss in standard surgical procedures. Thus the average total blood loss in the controlled hypotension cases as opposed to control patients was as follows: radical dissections of the neck, 910 and 1,415 ml.,

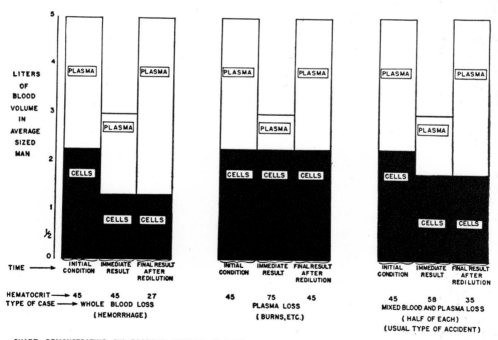

CHART DEMONSTRATING SIX POSSIBLE RESULTS IN SHOCK CASES AND THE FALLACY OF USING HEMOCONCENTRATION AS THE ONLY GUIDE TO TREATMENT

Fig. 7-3. Hemoconcentration and shock. The variability in blood concentration in various types of shock is shown graphically. The chart demonstrates the fallacy of using hemoconcentration as the only guide to treatment. (Harkins, H. N.: Surgery 9:258)

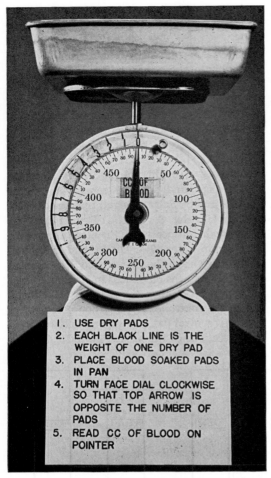

FIG. 7-4. Diabetic scale adjusted for weighing dry sponges, with a metal instrument pan (8 by 8 by 2 in.) fastened to the weighing platform. (Dr. H. C. Saltzstein, Detroit)

and for radical dissection within the pelvis was 1,870 and 2,805 ml., respectively.

4. "BURN SHOCK." In this instance (see Chap. 16, "Burns," and Chap. 8, "Blood Transfusion"), the loss of fluid from the blood stream is primarily of plasma, but some early destruction and loss of red cells occurs at the same time. In general, the loss of plasma is earlier and greater; the loss of cells later and less, but the latter is appreciable in severe burns. The greater plasma loss results in hemoconcentration, as evidence for which the hematocrit may exceed 70 per cent in some severe untreated burns.

5. MISCELLANEOUS CAUSES OF SHOCK. These include intestinal strangulation, release of a tourniquet which has been in place for several hours, mesenteric vascular occlusion, bile peritonitis, freezing, acute pancreatitis, certain acute pneumonias, irritant war gas (e.g., phosgene [carbonyl chloride, $(COCl_2)$]) poisoning, etc. Concomitant water and salt loss is commonly considered to be a cause of shock but must be severe to produce it in the absence of other factors (see Chap. 5, "Fluid and Electrolytes").

ACCOMPANYING FACTORS

If one accepts hypovolemia as the primary disturbance in the surgical types of shock, one may list other changes as secondary to the reduced blood volume. Table 2 lists a series of pathologic physiologic changes which are dependent upon the hypovolemia and may disappear once the hypovolemia is corrected. In the early phases of shock, while the cardiac output is still only moderately reduced, the heart rate is usually normal, at least if the patient is lying down. Later, when the hypovolemia has advanced to such a degree that the cardiac output is much decreased, tachycardia or even bradycardia may ensue. Shenkin and associates (1944) studied human volunteers following bleeding of 1 liter or more. They observed that in the recumbent position, the pulse rate and blood pressure tended to remain normal, while if the patient became erect, the blood pressure fell, and the pulse became rapid in early cases and slow in patients with severe symptoms. On the other hand, even when recumbent, almost all the subjects demonstrated a significant fall in cardiac output as determined by ballistocardiographic tracings. These authors concluded:

that the slowing of the pulse was more common than acceleration greatly surprised us. In subjects first seen after the event, the hemorrhage could never have been diagnosed from the pulse rate. . . . The old concept that acute hemorrhage can be readily diagnosed by a rapid pulse and a low blood pressure is erroneous.

As stated above, bradycardia may occur early. However, tachycardia is generally considered to be characteristic of shock and when it occurs results from a reflex cardiac mechanism according to Marey's law, whereby it is

TABLE 2. ACCOMPANYING PATHOLOGIC
PHYSIOLOGIC FACTORS IN HYPOVOLEMIC SHOCK

1. Decreased cardiac output
2. Decreased peripheral blood flow
3. Blood pressure fall
4. Sympathetic overactivity
5. Vasoconstriction
6. Hypocapnia
7. Hypoxia
8. Decreased metabolism
9. Lactacidemia
10. Parenchymatous tissue damage

activated by the lowered arterial pressure.

Additional factors include the increased sympathico-adrenal activity brought on reflexly by the carotid sinus and aortic reflexes and by direct action of the excitement associated with the injury. The heart rate may not be as closely associated with the degree of shock as is the blood pressure and, furthermore, bradycardia may occur in the terminal stages of fatal shock. The relationship of some of these factors, as correlated by Zweifach, Lee, Hyman, and Chambers (1944) is shown in Figure 7-5.

Reasons for not depending too much on a blood pressure fall alone in the diagnosis of shock, particularly at the operating table, are as follows: (1) It is generally a late sign, especially in the horizontal position. (2) A compensatory hypertension may result, especially in the young patient (Howard, 1953). (3) Anesthesia hypercapnea may induce such vasoconstriction as to mask the shock hypotension. (4) The anesthetist may have given vasospastic drugs which also may mask the shock hypotension.

The spleen contracts when shock due to hemorrhage occurs. This contraction represents a protective mechanism, the spleen serving as a blood reservoir in case of accident. In dogs (Lewis, Werle and Wiggers, 1942) the amount of contraction may be over 50 per cent of the control volume, but in human beings it is unlikely that it often exceeds 100 ml., the spleen being relatively smaller in the human patient.

The lack of blood in the vascular bed is contributory to the decreased cardiac output. As the cardiac output decreases, the peripheral blood flow tends to decrease also, and this tendency is accentuated by peripheral vasoconstriction. A fall in blood pressure, particu-larly in young patients, may be a late occurrence and hence is a relatively poor early diagnostic sign of shock. So long as the blood pressure is maintained at reasonable levels despite the decreased cardiac output, the vasopressor activity must not only be intact but possibly exaggerated. The vasoconstriction that exists in hypovolemic shock may be considered as practically maximal. Therefore, vasoconstrictor agents such as ephedrine, Neosynephrine, epinephrine, and even levorotatory norepinephrine should not be depended upon for definitive treatment, and reliance upon them may delay the introduction of appropriate fluid replacement. Watts (1956) found a significant rise in blood epinephrine levels (up to 37 μg/1) during hemorrhagic shock in dogs.

Associated with the early decrease in cardiac output coupled with vasoconstriction during this period, the volume flow of blood shows a marked early decrease. Gesell (1919) studied the effects of hemorrhage and of intestinal trauma on the volume flow of blood through the submaxillary gland of the dog. He found that a decrease in blood volume of less than 10 per cent produced by hemorrhage may elicit a decreased flow of blood through the submaxillary gland of more than 60 per cent even though accompanied by a rise in blood pressure. Changes of similar nature and degree were produced by intestinal manipulation. Gesell and Moyle (1922) found that hemorrhage produces a similar decrease in blood flow through the striated muscle of the dog. Sometimes the early decrease in minute volume flow can be detected by determining how long it takes finger pressure pallor on the skin of the patient to return to the color of the surrounding skin. The decrease in minute volume flow also applies to the coronary arteries (Edwards, Siegel and Bing, 1954).

The hypocapnia present in shock is a result of reflexly stimulated overbreathing. The hypoxia, decreased metabolism and accompanying lactacidemia together are results of the decreased circulation. One of the effects of anoxia is to increase capillary permeability. Landis (1928) showed by quantitative experiments on single capillaries of the frog mesentery that immediately after a 3-minute period of oxygen lack, fluid filters through the capil-

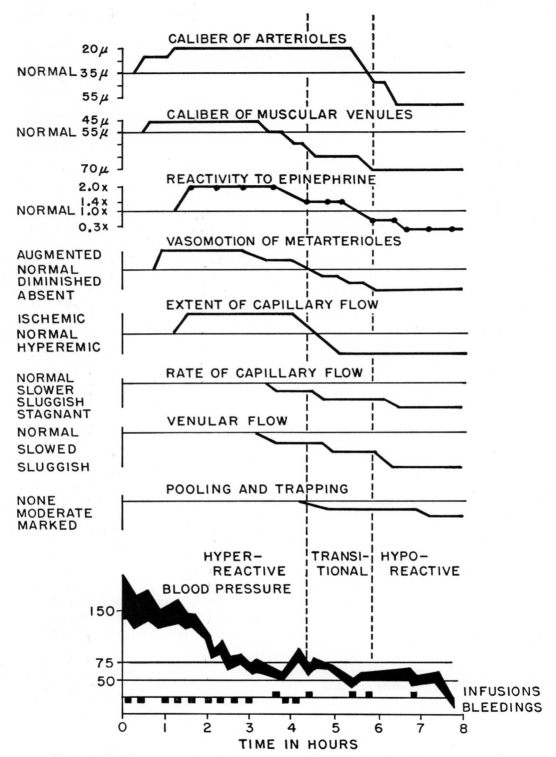

FIG. 7-5. Graphic presentation of observations made during shock on the terminal vascular

(*Continued on facing page*)

lary wall at approximately 4 times the normal rate. The increased permeability of the wall permitted also the passage of protein, thus reducing the effective osmotic pressure of the plasma proteins in these particular experiments to almost one half their normal value.

McClure, Hartman, Schnedorf and Schelling (1939) pointed out that anoxic anoxia occurring during general anesthesia, particularly with nitrous oxide, is apt to produce tissue damage. Not only will this increase the tendency to shock but also it may give permanent cerebral damage. These authors cited the instance of a girl who previously had done well in school but after having a tooth pulled under some difficulty with nitrous oxide alone did very poorly in school. Instances of prolonged cardiac arrest in which the patient lives but his mind remains cloudy are also examples of the same effects of anoxia, in this case both anoxic and stagnant anoxia (see list below). An increased body temperature also disturbs the balance between the body's demand for oxygen and the supply thereof, and in cases of marked hyperthermia with the increased demand involved, additional oxygen may have to be given to the patient. The importance of an adequate airway is always paramount. These authors classified anoxia into 4 types as follows:

1. *Anoxic anoxia*—due to inadequate oxygen reaching the lungs

2. *Anemic anoxia*—due to lack of, or inactivation of, hemoglobin, decreasing its capacity to take up oxygen

3. *Stagnant anoxia*—due to retardation of the circulation and transportation of oxygen

4. *Histotoxic anoxia*—due to drugging of the tissue cells so that they cannot utilize the available oxygen

Finally, parenchymatous tissue damage, which is the cumulative consequence of all the above-mentioned changes, is the harbinger of irreversibility. All treatment of shock should be aimed at preventing such parenchymatous tissue damage by increasing the blood volume and, hence, improving the circulation before irreversibility occurs.

Chemical changes are numerous (many of these are discussed in Chapter 16, "Burns," and Chapter 5, "Fluid and Electrolytes"). The cellular destruction accompanying shock results in a liberation of potassium with resultant high serum levels of this cation. In tourniquet shock in rats, the potassium content of muscle was reported to drop to 10 per cent of the normal value (Ravin, Denson and Jensen, 1954). At the same time the serum concentration rose from 5.7 to 11.5 mEq./1. The serum sodium fell only slightly, while the calcium and magnesium values rose. The alterations in the adrenal cortex are appreciable; Harkins and Long (1945) found a decrease in adrenal total cholesterol to only 30 per cent of the control value in 6 hours following burn shock in rats. It is significant that previous hypophysectomy entirely abolished this response. At the same time, the plasma amino nitrogen level became 4 times the control value. Changes in the blood hormonal concentrations are considered in Chapter 15, "The Endocrine and Metabolic Basis of Surgical Care."

Secondary effects of shock include a predisposition to other conditions such as acute peptic ulcer of the Curling's type (see Chap. 16, "Burns"), lower nephron anuria, pulmonary embolism, possibly acute enterocolitis, and possibly infections in general (see pp. 118 to 119). Some of the aspects of the "crush syndrome" appear to be related to shock and to immunologic hemolytic transfusion reactions. These 3 syndromes are also related to postoperative renal shutdown. Crush syndrome was described by Bywaters and Beall (1941) and was studied especially in Great Britain during World War II as a result of the bombing catastrophes in London. Patients with crush syndrome usually have been buried or pinned down for several hours by beams or debris impinging on a limb. In the same year, Bywaters and Delory attributed the condition, with its accompanying oliguria, to deposits of myohemoglobin from the damaged muscle in the kidneys. While a true crush syndrome may exist, in many instances the supposed syndrome is merely hypovolemic shock with in-

---

Fig. 7-5 (*Continued*).

bed, contrasting the findings in the hyperreactive or reversible phase and the hyporeactive or irreversible phase of shock. Note the beneficial results on blood pressure from a reinfusion of blood during the reversible state and the failure to improve the hypotension by repeated transfusions in the irreversible state. (Redrawn from Zweifach, Lee, Hyman, and Chambers: Ann. Surg. *120*:241)

adequate fluid replacement because of under-estimated blood loss into the crushed tissues or is an instance of reaction to mismatched blood.

DIAGNOSIS

The diagnosis of shock is chiefly based on (1) recognition of the possibility of shock when etiologic factors are present, such as crushed limb, burns, intestinal strangulation, etc.; (2) observation of the symptoms and signs of shock—pallor, cold sweat, anxious expression, weak pulse, thirst, etc.—and (3) special tests. Among the last is the "tilt test," first suggested by Duncan (1944) and later developed as a practical test by Green and Metheny (1947). This test brings out the *latent* arterial hypotension which does not demonstrate itself early in shock patients—probably because most patients with injuries or conditions severe enough to produce shock are examined when they are lying down—by tilting the head of the patient up. Tachycardia of varying degrees at certain angles of tilt is roughly proportional to the amount of blood lost.

In the differential diagnosis, syncope (for-merly called "primary shock") must be con-sidered. A knowledge of the basic mechanisms underlying syncope is useful, not only because of the direct practical importance of its pre-vention and therapy, but also because of the need for arriving at a basic understanding of the more complicated and more serious "sec-ondary" or hypovolemic shock. In shock the *blood volume is too small for the vascular bed* under normal tone. In syncope the disparity exists because the blood vessels are relaxed even though there has been no blood loss and the volume of blood is normal. In shock the disparity exists because there has been whole blood (e.g., hemorrhage) or plasma (e.g., ex-tensive thermal burns) loss; the blood vessels, instead of being relaxed, are actually more contracted than normal in an attempt to com-pensate for the decreased blood volume. For this reason the blood pressure falls at once in syncope but is a late warning sign in secondary shock. The cardiac output may be normal in syncope; in shock it is lowered.

In syncope, due to a nervous imbalance or too-long maintained erect posture, the blood tends to go to the legs and leave the brain. The important thing is that the cerebral cir-culation is not adequate. Soffer (1954) has shown that the most effective therapy "is not the head-between-knees position but rather the Trendelenburg or supine or prone posi-tion with the legs raised. Recent evidence of the primary importance of the lower extremi-ties in the production of syncope secondary to postural hypotension explains why leg binding (extending to the hips) may be more effective in prophylaxis than sympathomimetic drugs or abdominal binders."

Several practical points concerning syncope should be borne in mind:

1. Whereas in normal individuals a large amount of blood may pool in the lower ex-tremities, this amount may be abnormally large in patients with varicose veins.

2. Fainting is also more common in taller men, probably due to the gravity factor.

3. Persons who have been ill recently have often lost their ability to adjust to the erect posture and are more apt to faint.

4. A warm office relaxes the patient's blood vessels and makes fainting more likely. With susceptible patients keep the room cool.

PERPETUATING FACTORS

After the recognition of the importance of the work of Blalock and of Phemister, the pendulum swung too far the other way, and for a while some students of shock recognized no other cause than fluid loss. Gradually, it was realized that other factors do exist and that shock is not a simple mechanism but is extremely complex in its etiology. Quite often in experimental studies, the total fluid loss de-termined (as in bile peritonitis) was almost enough, yet not quite enough, to explain by itself the death of the animal. Certain other causative factors, it is true, probably act pri-marily as *perpetuating* factors rather than as *initiating* factors, but now it is recognized that certain of them may play a role in the initia-tion of shock. These include especially the toxic, bacterial, adrenal and nervous factors. In some cases of shock when the hypovolemia is corrected, certain of the accompanying fac-tors may not return to normal and may in themselves act as perpetuating factors. Cohn (1956) raises the possibility that overgrowth of intestinal bacteria may be the cause of irreversibility.

The study of simple hemorrhagic shock is revealing in this regard. If an experimental animal is bled an amount sufficient to produce definite shock, immediate restoration of the amount of blood removed—or even a little less—will result in rapid and permanent improvement of the animal. If blood restoration is delayed somewhat, it usually requires a restoration of more than the amount of blood originally removed to result in recovery of the animal. If blood restoration is delayed several hours, restoration of not only the amount of blood originally removed but even several times that volume may not result in recovery of the animal. This is the basis for the concept of irreversibility of shock.

In some of the more complicated types of shock, such as that following burns or intestinal strangulation in which many more factors than simple blood loss exist, irreversibility may occur earlier or be otherwise a more important factor.

Any or all of the factors listed on pages 106 to 110 may act as perpetuating factors as well as initiating factors, even fluid loss. In burns, on the one hand, it was shown experimentally (Harkins, 1935) that half of the eventual fluid loss will occur during the first hour after the burn, but, on the other hand, it is known that severe fluid loss will continue in burns for at least 24 hours. The therapeutic implications of this double concept are clear: a necessity for speed in instituting treatment, on the one hand, and persistence coupled with repeated and continued observation of the patient on the other.

It is always important to be sure that the particular case with supposedly "irreversible" shock is not a mere instance of incorrect diagnosis or inadequate therapy. A summary of such possibilities is given in Table 3.

TREATMENT OF SHOCK

The treatment of shock is urgent and should be accomplished before irreversible changes intervene. At the same time, even more urgent than shock are the important trio of preservation of an adequate airway, control of sucking wounds of the chest, and the control of hemorrhage.

TABLE 3. SOME CAUSES FOR FAILURE OF RESUSCITATION IN WOUND SHOCK
(From Simeone, 1953)

A. Inadequate volume or rate of replacement
B. Error in diagnosis of mechanism of shock
  1. Interference with cardiopulmonary function
    a. Atelectasis
    b. Tension pneumothorax
    c. Cardiac tamponade
    d. Fat embolism
  2. Infections
    a. Peritonitis and retroperitoneal cellulitis
    b. Clostridial myositis
    c. Cerebral infection
  3. Head injury
C. Continuing bleeding
  1. From primary wound
  2. From other wounds
  3. Concealed
    a. Pleural cavity
    b. Peritoneal cavity
    c. Injured soft parts

The treatment of shock itself involves six standard items, as follows:

1. **Fluid Replacement.** This should include the early and quantitative replacement into the blood stream of fluid similar to that which was lost. If whole blood was lost (e.g., hemorrhage), whole blood should be restored. If plasma was lost, plasma should be restored. In many conditions both of these are lost. The hematocrit reading may serve as a rough guide for quantitative treatment in cases in which the principal loss is plasma. In the operating room, weighing of the sponges (see p. 110) helps determine the amount of blood lost. It goes without saying that hemostasis is essential in treating shock; in fact, it is an important preliminary to all other treatment.

So-called "plasma-expanders" or "blood substitutes," such as dextran, polyvinylpyrrolidone (PVP) and gelatin, are inferior to whole blood when the latter is indicated but may have some usefulness under emergency conditions. Under these circumstances, dextran is generally advised in doses up to 1,000 ml. Under urgent circumstances the dose can be increased to 2,000 ml. if a slight risk of introducing a hemorrhagic tendency is acceptable. Saline solution may be useful because of the contained sodium but is not a substitute for blood (see pp. 119-120). Potassium is dangerous in the early stages (first 48 hours) because the plasma potassium is often already elevated due to breakdown of cellular elements of the body. Dried pooled plasma, whether irradiated or not, should be given with caution because of the danger of serum hepatitis, unless storage in the liquid state at room temperature has been carried out (see Chap. 8, "Blood Transfusion"). The efficacy of the prolonged room temperature storage method of rendering plasma serum hepatitis virus free has been rather well established (Sayman, Gauld, Star and Allen, 1958, and Hoxworth, Haesler and Smith, 1959).

The experiments of Millican (1954) indicate certain advantages of whole blood over plasma. Tracer doses of S^{35}-plasma protein and S^{35}-erythrocytes were administered intravenously after the release of lower extremity tourniquets in mice. When tourniquet shock was present, over 90 per cent of the tagged plasma protein leaked out of the blood vessels into the injured lower portion of the body, while under comparable conditions only 9 per cent of the erythrocytes were similarly lost. The relative advantages of plasma, dextran and whole blood in the treatment of shock have been analyzed by Sayman and Allen (1959), by Serkes, Lang and Pareira (1959), and by Howard, Ebert, Bloom and Sloan (1959).

2. **Drugs.** In some instances, antibiotics may help control the uncertain bacterial factors (see pp. 118 to 119) which may be present in shock. Generally speaking, the administration of adrenal cortical substances may produce other effects more certainly than the control of shock. Frank, Frank, Korman, Macchi and Hechter (1955) reported that in dogs suffering from hemorrhagic shock, while the output of corticosteroids in the adrenal veins tended to be reduced as compared with the levels before the induction of shock, there was no correlation between the extent of reduction and the fate of the animal. ACTH is usually not helpful because the patient's own stress reaction is already stimulating the adrenal cortex to its full capacity so that adding more ACTH would be like "whipping a tired horse." In fact, Hechter, Macchi, Korman, Frank and Frank (1955) studied the corticosteroid output in adrenal veins of "normal" dogs before and after exogenous ACTH administration and found no significant increase. They concluded that "the conditions of the

experiments provided maximum endogenous stimulation." Hume and Nelson (1955) reported that the increase in adrenal venous blood corticosteroid secretion following hemorrhage did not occur in hypophysectomized dogs.

Steenburg, Lennihan and Moore (1956) observed an early and extensive (4-fold in 4 hours) increase in the free serum 17-hydroxycorticoids after major operation in man. This use was greater than that produced by maximal doses of ACTH over similar periods of time. The level of 17-hydroxycorticoids seemed to be an index of the timing and the intensity of adrenal response to injury while the urinary excretion of total steroid provided a more suitable index of the duration of this response. The excretion of 17-hydroxycorticoids was proportionate to the extent of trauma, while that of 17-ketosteroids was not a suitable index in this regard.

L-norepinephrine may be helpful in nonhypovolemic types of shock, but in true hypovolemic shock it is of chiefly symptomatic value and does not get at the source of the difficulty. Catchpole, Hackel and Simeone (1955) reported that in controlled experiments using dogs with hemorrhagic hypotension, the use of l-norepinephrine in doses sufficient to correct the hypotension did not result in a higher rate of survival for the dog so treated. Howard (1955) succinctly summarized his opinion as follows: "Prior to anesthesia vasoconstrictors have no place" in the treatment of shock. "If you use blood pressure as your assay, vasoconstrictors have a place, but if you use mortality, they do not." The danger from tissue necrosis if the l-norepinephrine leaks out of a vein is well known (deAlvarez, Nyhus, Merendino, Harkins and Zech, 1957). On the other hand, if the surgeon is *absolutely* sure that fluid replacement has been adequate and the blood pressure *still* is low for that particular patient, l-norepinephrine may be useful.

3. **Heat.** The application of external heat is usually harmful, but conservation of normal body heat is helpful. The recovery rate from experimental shock in mice was found by Bergman and Prinzmetal (1945) to be greatest at a room temperature of 68° F. and to be progressively less at temperatures higher or lower than this figure (Fig. 7-6).

4. Analgesics and Sedatives. Analgesic drugs should be given only for actual pain, not for restlessness, and should be administered intravenously, the initial dosage being from one half to two thirds that usually employed hypodermically. Sedatives, such as the barbiturates, are of little value and may be harmful in large amounts or even in normal therapeutic doses.

The danger of giving repeated doses of subcutaneous morphine to men with shock from war wounds was emphasized by Beecher (1944) in the African Theater of World War II. When shock is severe enough to prevent ready absorption of the morphine it becomes pooled in the subcutaneous tissues, and morphine poisoning follows the absorption of the several doses when the patient receives blood replacement therapy. For these reasons, morphine given to patients in shock should be by the intravenous route and should not exceed gr. ⅙ (10 mg.) as an initial dose.

In addition to the dangers of overdosage of analgesics and sedatives, there is a definite possibility of overdosage of anesthetic agents in the shock patient (see Chap. 12, "Anesthesia," and Chap. 23, "Military Surgery").

Reports continue to appear concerning the benefits of certain sedative agents in shock. These should be approached with caution. A recent study is that of Hershey, Gucciune and Zweifach (1955) who reported a beneficial action of pretreatment with chlorpromazine following graded hemorrhage in the rat; Overton and DeBakey (1955) used the dog for their studies. The application of this preliminary work to human patients awaits further studies. Sensitivity to these drugs must also be considered.

5. Oxygen. Maintenance of an adequate airway for ready inhalation of air is mandatory. As Fitts (1955) listed them, the priority of treatment in injury is as follows: (1) airway, (2) sucking wound of the thorax, (3) stop hemorrhage, (4) shock.

Supplemental oxygen may be tried and

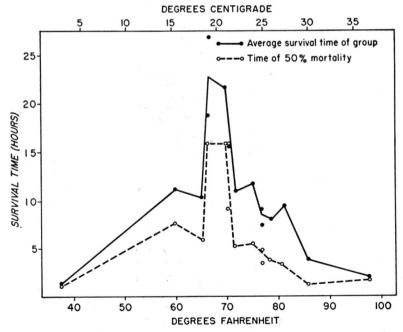

FIG. 7-6. Effect of environmental temperature on mortality in burn shock. Each point represents 20 to 26 mice, etherized and scalded up to the head at 65° C. for 10 seconds, kept in rooms at various constant temperatures. The range of environmental temperatures for optimal survival is 65° to 71° F. (Redrawn from Bergman and Prinzmetal: Arch. Surg. 50:202)

should be continued if it improves the color, lowers the pulse rate, or otherwise benefits the patient.

6. **Position of the Patient.** Elevation of the foot of the bed to relieve shock—the opposite of the tilt test which is used to test for shock—is a useful temporary measure. Caution must be employed in using this maneuver in fat people (because of interference with movement of the diaphragm), or in patients with peripheral arterial disease (because of danger of permanent ischemic changes in the feet due to reduction in local arterial blood flow).

The prime factor in the treatment of oligemic shock is to restore the blood volume to normal levels, starting at the earliest possible moment. As Howard (1955) stated, "Never give up." Other measures, while useful, should not be utilized as an excuse to avoid this main element in the treatment.

PRESENT-DAY PROBLEMS IN SHOCK

There are a number of unsettled problems concerning shock, and much remains to be done in this field. Research work on shock usually goes through a lull after each major war. Only by further elucidation of some of the biochemical factors in shock can our knowledge of the syndrome evolve from the second period of understanding of the subject (wherein we have demonstrated that fluid loss is the prime factor in early shock and that early restoration of that fluid loss is the most efficacious early treatment) into the third period of understanding of shock (wherein it will be demonstrated why late shock may be irreversible and how it may be controlled). In other words, while we may now understand something about early shock we do not at all understand late shock, either from the standpoint of etiology or treatment.

At present, interesting work is going on in an attempt to answer the following important questions:

1. *Is there an important bacterial factor in shock?* During World War II one group of investigators reported that in experimental shock in dogs, bacteria were regularly recovered on blood culture. Later these observers had to state that all the previously reported

dogs were connected with a nonsterile citrate bottle for recording the blood pressure. When other experiments were done without such a nonsterile hookup, only occasional blood cultures were reported as positive. Aub (1944) reported that muscle extracts from anoxic extremities of dogs were toxic, but at the same time they were routinely infected, usually with clostridial organisms. This work, indicating a bacterial origin for a possible toxic factor in shock, is not completely applicable to shock in human beings because dog muscle regularly contains Clostridia while human muscle rarely does. More recently, Fine (1954, 1955) has studied the possible role of bacterial invasion in the causation of the irreversibility of shock, even though apparent infection may seem to be absent or of little consequence. *Escherichia coli*, which in the healthy dog is relatively nonvirulent, was found to possess lethal power in a dog subjected to hemorrhagic shock of only 2 hours' duration. It was postulated that these organisms, as well as others, normally invade the blood stream and the tissues from the intestine but are inactive in the absence of shock. Antibiotic therapy seemed to be effective in many instances. Still more recently, Frank, Kaufman, Korman, Schweinburg, Frank, and Fine (1955) treated shock in dogs produced by injecting feces into the peritoneal cavity. Such peritonitis was accompanied by hypovolemia, but treatment of the hypovolemia did not result in recovery of the animals. On the other hand, antibiotic therapy did not result in immediate relief of the hypovolemia but did spare the lives of some of the animals. The application of this particular experiment to the treatment of other types of shock is uncertain.

This work by Fine offers great potentialities, but other recent work (Hardy, *et al.*, 1954) indicates no difference in the recovery rate of dogs suffering from shock either with or without antibiotic therapy.

In an extension of this work, Schweinburg, Yashar, Aprahamian, Davidoff, and Fine (1955) reported that an important factor in the decreased resistance of dogs suffering from hemorrhagic shock to intravenously injected bacteria may be a considerable reduction in the phagocytosis-promoting activity of the serum in hemorrhagic shock. Balch (1955), in studying severely wounded soldiers in

Korea, also found a reduction of the phagocytic capacity of neutrophilic polymorphonuclear leukocytes during the first day. However, he was unable to relate this temporary change to the development of clinical infection and concluded: "No evidence was found that battle casualties with or without complicating acute renal failure are more prone to develop infection because of a possible deficiency in the antibacterial defense mechansims studied."

Schweinburg and Fine (1955) reported still another possibility, namely, that in rabbits, during the immediate post-transfusion recovery phase of hemorrhagic shock, the sensitivity to a purified *E. coli* toxin is increased 100,000 times normal. Return to normal tolerance to the endotoxin was stated to require about 48 hours. Recent studies on bacterial factors in shock include those of Altemeier and Cole (1956, 1958); Culbertson, Elstun, Cole and Altemeier (1959); Egdahl (1959); Egdahl, Melby and Spink (1959); and Fine, Frank, Ravin, Rutenberg and Schweinburg (1959).

Properdin, a serum globulin, which acts in association with complement and magnesium ions as a natural bactericidal system, is a factor of importance in resistance to infection. Frank, Fine and Pillemer (1955) reported that properdin levels in the serum of dogs with hemorrhagic shock fall early and progressively. These authors stated that this decrease may be a factor in the decreased bacterial resistance in shock which they have reported in their other papers. The observation that properdin falls in hemorrhagic shock has been confirmed by Blattberg and Levy (1960).

2. *Is the agglutination and "sludging" of red cells important in shock?* The importance of this factor, emphasized by Knisely (1951), has been elaborated upon recently by Gelin and Löfström (1955) and Gelin (1955, 1956). In the first report Gelin stated that in hypothermia severe agglutination occurs. In the second he presented data showing that this condition is accentuated by the administration of dextran of high molecular weight but is prevented by the administration of dextran (Macrodex) of low molecular weight. Since he found whole blood to accentuate the condition somewhat, he concluded that in this respect dextran of low molecular weight may be superior to whole blood. Recently, Drawhorn and Howard (1955) have advocated Dextra-

ven, a British dextran of high (230,000) molecular weight, because it remains in the blood stream longer than low-weight dextran. Howard, Teng and Loeffler (1956) reported that high-molecular-weight dextran is more apt to lead to hemorrhagic tendencies. This work on dextran has been extended by Thorsén (1959).

The effect of trauma on the agglutination of red cells may also be related to the changes in the patient's own plasma. Wadström (1958) found that trauma affects the plasma lipids, causing particularly an increase in the unesterified fatty acid level.

3. *Is normal saline solution alone efficacious in the therapy of shock?* The general applications of the work of Moyer, Coller, Iob, Vaughan and Marty (1944) and of Fox (1944), showing the efficacy of sodium salts in burns, is considered in Chapter 17, "Burns." In traumatic shock, such solutions were first advocated on a comparative basis as related to whole blood or plasma by Hoitink (1935) and by Allen (1939). Experimental observations by Rosenthal (1943) on mice and by Harkins (1947) on rats indicated that normal saline solution by mouth greatly lowered the mortality rate in a standard tourniquet shock preparation.

More recently, Koletsky and Gustafson (1954) also worked with a standard tourniquet shock preparation which produced 100 per cent mortality and studied the effects of (1) no treatment, (2) treatment with intravenous saline and (3) treatment by reapplication of the tourniquet. They found that a combination of the last two-named procedures reduced the mortality to 10 per cent. It was concluded that this indicates that with the injured part still in contact with the circulation, saline was of no value (in this particular preparation), but that if the injured part were isolated by reapplication of the tourniquet, saline would restore 9 of 10 rats which otherwise would die. Still more recently, Koletsky and Klein (1955) reported that massive doses of saline, equal to 15 per cent of body weight, given by combined intravenous and intraperitoneal routes to rats in terminal shock, caused reversibility in 75 per cent of animals. From this they concluded that the irreversible phase is in large part quantitative rather than qualitative. Hall and Hall (1955) reported that tourniquet shock which was 92 per cent fatal in single rats was not fatal in any of 10 pairs of parabiotic rats when the tourniquets were applied to one of each of the pairs. This work fits in well with the observations of Millican, Tabor, Stohlman and Rosenthal (1952) who reported that within an hour of the administration of either saline or plasma to mice suffering from burn or tourniquet shock, all the fluid was recovered in the injured areas, except for that part which corrected dehydration in the uninjured tissues. This work would also tie in with the observations of Baratz and Ingraham (1955) who reported that in rats, in a study of the disappearance curves of fluorescein-labeled albumin conjugate, there is no difference between control animals and those surviving or succumbing to hemorrhagic procedures. On the basis of this observation they concluded that in the rat an increase in capillary permeability is not a major factor in the transition from reversible to irreversible hemorrhagic shock. Millican (1955) reported that when administered immediately after tourniquet release, intravenous saline or serum was equally effective in preventing death from tourniquet shock in mice. However, when given 5 hours later, serum was definitely more effective.

The present status of the entire problem as to the efficacy of normal saline solution in shock is as follows: It would seem that such therapy may be of some value in mild shock, or in severe shock of short duration in which the damaged part has been isolated or controlled. However, such an effect is not definite enough to forego the use of more definitive means of treatment such as whole blood, plasma, or dextran, if these are available.

4. Is intra-arterial transfusion superior to intravenous transfusion? The special advantages of intra-arterial transfusion have been promulgated for 80 years. Particular recent advocates of this technic have been Seeley and Nelson (1952) and Veal, Russell, and Stubbs (1952). More recently, Maloney, Smythe, Gilmore, and Handford (1953) reported that the hydraulic effect of intra-arterial transfusion in elevating arterial pressure is insignificant at the rates of transfusion employed clinically. The weight of evidence against the special merits of the arterial route is summarized by Hampson, Scott and Gurd (1954) (Fig. 7-7) and by Gurd and Gardner (1955).

These latter authors concluded that "The side of the circulation into which the blood is transfused is of no importance provided that a rapid rate can be assured." It should also be pointed out that instances of gangrene, e.g., of the hand after use of the radial artery for transfusion, have been reported. For all these reasons the present situation is that the intravenous route is generally preferable for blood or fluid infusion. In certain instances when a surgeon is operating within the abdomen or the chest and a sudden large loss of blood occurs, rapid introduction of equivalent amounts into the aorta may offer certain practical advantages. Howard (1955) epitomized these studies by stating that intra-arterial transfusions have "no place provided intravenous transfusion is possible."

5. Are certain autogenous vasotropic substances (VEM and VDM) an important factor in shock? Shorr (1953) has postulated that these two factors are important. VEM is a product of hypoxic or anaerobic metabolism of the kidney which is rendered vasoinert by the aerobic kidney. This substance potentiates the response to topical epinephrine of the muscular vessels of the capillary bed. It assists in the compensation of the vascular system to reduction in blood volume. It appears early and is said to be a factor in the first, or reversible, stage of shock. Lack of its production is stated to be the explanation for increased susceptibility to shock of arenal animals.

The other important substance, liver VDM (SH-ferritin), on the other hand, is a product of anaerobic or hypoxic metabolism of the liver. Under normal oxidative conditions it is acted upon by the liver to render it vasoinert. VDM depresses the capacity of the terminal capillary bed of the mesentery of the rat to react to epinephrine. It is said to be the cause of breakdown of the compensatory stage and of transition into the irreversible stage of shock. Shorr also postulates the production of vasodepressor material in the muscles.

This hypothesis is not universally accepted but indicates one of the directions in which present research on shock is going. Nickerson (1953) summarized his skepticism by stating: "We are still faced with the question of whether it (SH-ferritin) is actually part of the chain of cause and effect which ultimately kills an animal, or is simply a manifestation of the fact that the animal is going to die." This confusion of cause and effect has occurred before in the history of shock and undoubtedly will occur again. Rothstein, Rosen, Markowitz and Fuller (1960) performed experiments on dogs which failed to indicate that circulating ferritin is a major factor in the genesis of irreversible traumatic shock.

In a recent study of 20 Korean battle casualties, Scott, Howard, Shorr, Lawson and Davis (1955) found that VDM is often present in the plasma in high concentration fol-

lowing major injury. However, within the limitations of the study no positive correlation could be made between the VDM-VEM titers and the blood pressure, the development of refractory shock, the transfusion requirements, the development of post-traumatic renal insufficiency, or the ultimate prognosis of the patient.

SUMMARY

Shock is an important and frequent condition which occurs in a variety of traumatic, surgical and medical conditions. The major

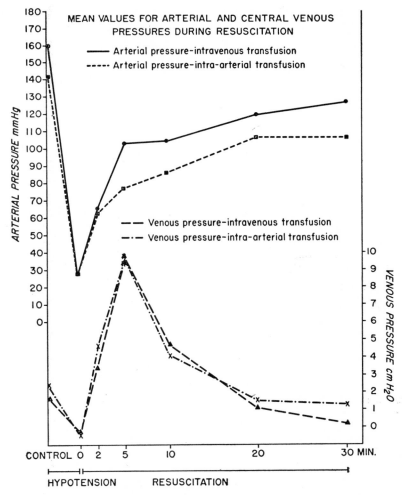

FIG. 7-7. Graphic presentation of mean values for arterial and central venous pressures during resuscitation in control animals with normal hearts. (Redrawn from Hampson, Scott and Gurd: Ann. Surg. *140*:57)

factor is a decreased blood volume (hypovolemia, oligemia) caused by a rapid and primarily local loss of blood, plasma, or both, but other factors play an accessory causative role. Treatment should be prompt before irreversibility occurs and should include quantitative restoration of blood volume with blood or plasma, depending on the type of fluid originally lost.

BIBLIOGRAPHY

Allbritten, F. F., Jr., Lipshutz, H., Miller, B. J., and Gibbon, J. H., Jr.: Blood volume changes in tuberculous patients treated by thoracoplasty, J. Thoracic Surg. *19*:71-79, 1950.

Allen, F. M.: Physical and toxic factors in shock, Arch. Surg. *38*:155-180, 1939.

Allen, J. Garrott: Personal communication, June, 1955.

Altemeier, W. A., and Cole, W.: Septic shock, Ann. Surg. *143*:600-607, 1956.

Altemeier, W. A., and Cole, W. R.: Nature and treatment of septic shock, A.M.A. Arch. Surg. *77*:498-507, 1958.

Andrews, E., and Harkins, H. N.: "Surgical shock" factors in pneumonia, Ann. Int. Med. *10*:1503-1507, 1937.

Aub, J. C.: Toxic factor in experimental traumatic shock, New England J. Med. *231*:71-75, 1944.

Balch, H. H.: The effect of severe battle injury and of posttraumatic renal failure on resistance to infection, Ann. Surg. *142*:145-163, 1955.

Baratz, R. A., and Ingraham, R. C.: Capillary permeability during hemorrhagic shock in the rat, Proc. Soc. Exper. Biol. & Med. *89*:642-644, 1955.

Baronofsky, I. D., Treloar, A. E., and Wangensteen, O. H.: Blood loss in operations: a statistical comparison of losses as determined by the gravimetric and colorimetric methods, Surgery *20*:761-769, 1946.

Beecher, H. K.: Delayed morphine poisoning in battle casualties, J.A.M.A. *124*:1193-1194, 1944.

Bergman, H. C., and Prinzmetal, M.: Influence of environmental temperature on shock, Arch. Surg. *50*:201-206, 1945.

Blalock, A.: Acute circulatory failure as exemplified by shock and hemorrhage, Surg., Gynec. & Obst. *58*:551-566, 1934.

———: Experimental shock: the cause of the low blood pressure produced by muscle injury, Arch. Surg. *20*:959-996, 1930.

Blattberg, B., and Levy, M. N.: Properdin titers of dogs surviving hemorrhagic hypotension, Proc. Soc. Exper. Biol. & Med. *104*:155-158, 1960.

Bonica, J. J., and Lyter, C. S.: Measurement of blood loss during surgical operations, Am. J. Surg. *81*:496-502, 1951.

Borden, F. W.: Loss of blood at operation, California Med. *87*:91-97, 1957.

Bywaters, E. G. L., and Beall, D.: Crush injuries with impairment of renal function, Brit. M. J. *1*:427-432, 1941.

Bywaters, E. G. L., and Delory, G. E.: Myohaemoglobinuria, Lancet *1*:648, 1941.

Cáceres, E., and Whittembury, G.: Evaluation of blood losses during surgical operations, Surgery *45*:681-687, 1959.

Cannon, W. B., and Bayliss, W. M.: Note on muscle injury in relation to shock, Report of Shock Committee, Medical Research Committee, No. 26, 19-23, March, 1919, cited by Blalock, (1930).

Catchpole, B. N., Hackel, D. B., and Simeone, F. A.: Coronary and peripheral blood flow in experimental hemorrhagic hypotension treated with *l*-norepinephrine, Ann. Surg. *142*:372-381, 1955.

Clark, J. H., Nelson, W., Lyons, C., Mayerson, H. S., and De Camp, P.: Chronic shock: The problem of reduced blood volume in the chronically ill patient, Ann. Surg. *125*:618-646, 1947.

Cohn, Isidore, Jr.: Strangulation obstruction—Thirty fistula studies, S. Forum *6*:344-347, 1956.

Coller, F. A., Crook, C. E., and Iob, V.: Blood loss in surgical operations, J.A.M.A. *126*:1-5, 1944.

Coller, F. A., and Maddock, W. G.: Dehydration attendant on surgical operations, J.A.M.A. *99*:875-880, 1932.

Culbertson, W R., Elstun, W., Cole, W., and Altemeier, W. A.: Bacterial studies in irreversible hemorrhagic shock, A.M.A. Arch. Surg. *79*:185-189, 1959.

Cushman, G. F.: Subperitoneal hemorrhage, California Med. *78*:11-16, 1953.

deAlvarez, R. R., Nyhus, L. M., Merendino, K. A., Harkins, H. N., and Zech, R. K.: Tissue necrosis associated with intravenous norepinephrine administration, Am. Surgeon *23*:619-635, 1957; J.A.M.A. *165*:1878, 1957.

Ditzler, J. W., and Eckenhoff, J. E.: A comparison of blood loss and operative time in certain surgical procedures completed with and without controlled hypotension, Ann. Surg. *143*:289-293, 1956.

Drawhorn, C. W., and Howard, J. M.: Clinical evaluation of "Dextraven," a dextran of high molecular weight, U. S. Armed Forces M. J. *6*:1576-1580, 1955.

Duncan, G. W., Sarnoff, S. J., and Rhode, C. M.: Studies on effects of posture in shock and injury, Ann. Surg. *120*:24-33, 1944.

Edwards, W. S., Siegel, A., and Bing, R. J.: Studies on myocardial metabolism. III. Coronary blood flow, myocardial oxygen consumption and carbohydrate metabolism in experimental hemorrhagic shock, J. Clin. Invest. *33*: 1646-1661, 1954.

Egdahl, R. H.: Pituitary-adrenal response following trauma to the isolated leg, Surgery *46*:9-21, 1959.

————: The differential response of the adrenal cortex and medulla to bacterial endotoxin, J. Clin. Invest. *38*:1120-1125, 1959.

Egdahl, R. H., Melby, J. C., and Spink, W. W.: Adrenal cortical and body temperature responses to repeated endotoxin administration (24944), Proc. Soc. Exper. Biol. & Med. *101*: 369-372, 1959.

Engberg, H.: Blood loss in operations: A practical colorimetric method, Acta chir. scandinav. *111*: 235, 1956.

Fine, J.: The Bacterial Factor in Traumatic Shock, Springfield, Ill., Thomas, 1954.

————: Host resistance to bacteria and to bacterial toxins in traumatic shock, Ann. Surg. *142*:361-371, 1955.

————: Relation of bacteria to the failure of blood volume therapy in traumatic shock, New England J. Med. *250*:889-895, 1954.

Fine, J., Frank, E. D., Ravin, H. A., Rutenberg, S. H., and Schweinburg, F. B.: The bacterial factor in traumatic shock, New England J. Med. *260*:214-220, 1959.

Fitts, W. T., Jr.: Postgraduate Course on Preoperative and Postoperative Care, 41st Annual Clinical Congress, American College of Surgeons, Chicago, November 2, 1955.

Fox, C. L., Jr.: Oral sodium lactate in the treatment of burn shock, J.A.M.A. *124*:207-212, 1944.

Frank, E. D., Kaufman, D., Korman, H., Schweinburg, F., Frank, H. A., and Fine, J.: Effect of antibiotics on hemodynamics of hypovolemic septic shock, Am. J. Physiol, *182*:166-176, 1955.

Frank, E., Fine, J., and Pillemer, L.: Serum properdin levels in hemorrhagic shock, Proc. Soc. Exper. Biol. & Med. *89*:223-225, 1955.

Frank, H. A., Frank, E. D., Korman, H., Macchi, I. A., and Hechter, O.: Corticosteroid output and adrenal blood flow during hemorrhagic shock in the dog, Am. J. Physiol. *182*:24-28, 1955.

Gatch, W. D., and Little, W. D.: Amount of blood lost during some of the more common operations, J.A.M.A. *83*:1075-1076, 1924.

Gelin, L.-E.: Macrodex in burns, International Surgical Society Travel Club Meeting, Lund, Sweden, August 4, 1955.

————: Studies in anemia of injury, Acta chir, scandinav., Supp. *210*:130, 1956.

Gelin, L.-E., and Löfström, B.: A preliminary study on peripheral circulation during deep hypothermia: Observations on decreased suspension stability of the blood and its prevention, Acta chir. scandinav. *108*:402-404, 1955.

Gesell, R.: Studies on the submaxillary gland. III. Some factors controlling the volume-flow of blood, Am. J. Physiol. *47*:438-467, 1919.

————: Studies on the submaxillary gland. IV. A comparison of the effects of hemorrhage and of tissue-abuse in relation to secondary shock, Am. J. Physiol. *47*:468-506, 1919.

Gesell, R., and Moyle, C. A.: On the relation of blood-volume to tissue nutrition. II. The effects of graded hemorrhage on the volume-flow of blood through the striated muscle of the dog, Am. J. Physiol. *61*:412-419, 1922.

Green, D. M., and Metheny, D.: The estimation of acute blood loss by the tilt test, Surg., Gynec. & Obst. *84*:1045-1050, 1947.

Gross, R. E.: A scale for rapid measurement of blood which is lost in surgical sponges, J. Thoracic Surg. *18*:543-545, 1949.

Gross, Samuel D.: System of Surgery, 1850, cited by Mann, F. C.: Bull. Johns Hopkins Hosp. *25*:205-212, 1914.

————: System of Surgery, ed. 6, vol. 1, p. 412, Philadelphia, H. C. Lea's Son & Co., 1882.

Gurd, F. N., and Gardner, C. McG.: Reappraisal of the treatment of hemorrhagic shock, Am. J. Surg. *89*:725-729, 1955.

Hall, C. E., and Hall, O.: Protection against tourniquet shock afforded by parabiosis, Proc. Soc. Exper. Biol. & Med. *90*:230-232, 1955.

Hammond, W. G., Vandam, L. D., Davis, J. M., Carter, R. D., Ball, M. R., and Moore, F. D.: Studies in surgical endocrinology. IV. Anesthetic agents as stimuli to change in corticostereroids and metabolism, Ann. Surg. *148*:199-211, 1958.

Hampson, L. G., Scott, H. J., and Gurd, F. N.: A comparison of intra-arterial and intravenous transfusion in normal dogs and in dogs with experimental myocardial infarction, Ann. Surg. *140*:56-66, 1954.

Hardy, E. G., Morris, G. C., Jr., Yow, E. M., Haynes, B. W., Jr., and DeBakey, M. E.: Studies on the role of bacteria in irreversible hemorrhagic shock in dogs, Ann. Surg. *139*: 282-286, 1954.

Harkins, H. N.: Experimental burns. I. The rate of fluid shift and its relation to the onset of shock in severe burns, Arch. Surg. *31*:71-85, 1935.

————: Physical factors in surgical shock, Nord. med. *6*:1112-1115, 1940.

————: Recent advances in the study and management of traumatic shock, Surgery *9*:231-294, 447-482, 607-655, 1941.

————: Sodium therapy of experimental tourniquet shock, Am. J. Physiol, *148*:538-545, 1947.

Harkins, H. N., and Long, C. N. H.: Metabolic changes in shock after burns, Am. J. Physiol. *144*:661-668, 1945.

Harkins, H. N., and Roome, N. W.: Concealed hemorrhage into tissues and its relation to traumatic shock, Arch. Surg. *35*:130-139, 1937.

Hechter, O., Macchi, I. A., Korman, H., Frank, E. D., and Frank, H. A.: Quantitative variations in the adrenocortical secretion of dogs, Am. J. Physiol, *182*:29-34, 1955.

Hershey, S. G., Guccione, I., and Zweifach, B. W.: Beneficial action of pretreatment with chlorpromazine on survival following graded hemorrhage in the rat, Surg., Gynec. & Obst. *101*: 431-436, 1955.

Hoitink, A. W. J. H.: Treatment of acute fatal hemorrhage by injection of artificial blood substitutes, Surg., Gynec. & Obst. *61*:613-622, 1935.

Howard, John: Experiences with shock in the Korean Theater *in* Tr. Third Conf. on Shock and Circulatory Homeostasis, 1953, New York, Macy, 1954.

————: Postgraduate Course on Preoperative and Postoperative Care, 41st Annual Clinical Congress, American College of Surgeons, Chicago, November 1, 1955.

Howard, J. M., Ebert, R. V., Bloom, W. L., and Sloan, M. H.: The present status of dextran as a plasma expander, Am. J. Surg. *97*:593-596, 1959.

Howard, J. M., Teng, C. T., and Loeffler, R. K.: Studies of dextrans of various molecular sizes, Ann. Surg. *143*:369-372, 1956.

Hoxworth, P. I., Haesler, W. E., Jr., and Smith, H., Jr.: The risk of hepatitis from whole blood and stored plasma, Surg., Gynec. & Obst. *109*: 38-42, 1959.

Hume, D. M., and Nelson, D. H.: Adrenal cortical function in experimental shock, measured by adrenal venous blood corticosteroid secretion, Nav. M. Res. Inst. Res. Rep. *13*:167-176, 1955.

Koletsky, S., and Gustafson, G. E.: Tourniquet shock in rats; reversibility in the terminal phase, Am. J. Physiol. *178*:229-232, 1954.

Koletsky, S., and Klein, D. E.: Reversibility of tourniquet shock with massive saline therapy, Am. J. Physiol, *182*:439-442, 1955.

Knisely, M. H.: An annotated bibliography on sludged blood, Postgrad. Med. *10*:15-24, 80-93, 1951.

Landis, E. M.: Micro-injection studies of capillary permeability. III. The effect of lack of oxygen on the permeability on the capillary wall to fluid and to the plasma proteins, Am. J. Physiol, *83*:528-542, 1928.

LaVeen, H. H., and Rubricius, J. L.: Continuous, automatic, electronic determinations of operative blood loss, Surg., Gynec. & Obst. *106*:368-374, 1958.

Lewis, R. N., Werle, J. M., and Wiggers, C. J.: The behavior of the spleen in hemorrhagic hypotension and shock, Am. J. Physiol. *138*: 205-211, 1942.

Maloney, J. V., Smythe, C. M., Gilmore, J. P., and Handford, S. W.: Intra-arterial and intravenous transfusion: a controlled study of their effectiveness in the treatment of experimental hemorrhagic shock, Surg., Gynec. & Obst. *97*: 529-539, 1953.

McClure, R. D., Hartman, F. W., Schnedorf, J. G., and Schelling, V.: Anoxia: a source of possible complications in surgical anesthesia, Ann. Surg. *110*:835-850, 1939.

Millican, R. C.: S^{35}-plasma and erythrocyte distribution in tourniquet-shocked mice, Am. J. Physiol. *179*:513-519, 1954.

————: Tourniquet shock in mice: comparison of serum and saline therapy administered early and late after injury, Am. J. Physiol, *183*: 187-192, 1955.

Millican, R. C., Tabor, H., Stohlman, E. F., and Rosenthal, S. M.: Traumatic shock in mice: acute hemodynamic effects of therapy, Am. J. Physiol. *170*:187-195, 1952.

Minot, A. S., and Blalock, A.: Plasma loss in severe dehydration, shock and other conditions as affected by therapy, Ann. Surg. *112*:557-567, 1940.

Moore, F. D.: Metabolic Care of the Surgical Patient, Philadelphia, Saunders, 1959.

Moyer, C. A., Coller, F. A., Iob, L. V., Vaughan, H. H., and Marty, D.: A study of the interrelationship of salt solutions, serum and defibrinated blood in the treatment of severely scalded, anesthetized dogs, Ann. Surg. *120*:367-376, 1944.

Nickerson, M.: Epinephrine and norepinephrine, Tr. Second Conf. on Shock and Circulatory Homeostasis, 1952, New York, Macy, 1953.

Overton, R. C., and DeBakey, M. E.: Experimental observations on the influence of hypothermia and autonomolytic drugs in hemorrhagic shock. Paper given before Annual Congress, American College of Surgeons, November 2, 1955.

Parsons, E., and Phemister, D. B.: Haemorrhage

and "shock" in traumatized limbs: an experimental study, Surg., Gynec. & Obst. *51*:196-207, 1930.

Rains, A. J. H.: Experience in the measurement of blood- and fluid-loss at operation, Brit. J. Surg. *43*:191-196, 1955.

Raker, J. W., and Rovit, R. L.: The acute red blood cell destruction following severe thermal trauma in dogs, Surg., Gynec. & Obst. *98*:169-176, 1954.

Ravin, H. A., Denson, J. R., and Jensen, H.: Electrolyte shifts and electrocardiographic changes during tourniquet shock in rats, Am. J. Physiol. *178*:419-426, 1954.

Rosenthal, S. M.: Experimental chemotherapy of burns and shock. IV. Production of traumatic shock in mice; V. Therapy with mouse serum and sodium salts, Pub. Health Rep. *58*:1429-1436, 1943.

Rothstein, D. A., Rosen, S., Markowitz, A., and Fuller, J. B.: Ferritin and antiferritin serum treatment of dogs in irreversible hemorrhagic shock, Am. J. Physiol. *198*:844-846, 1960.

Saltzstein, H. C., and Linkner, L. M.: Blood loss during operations, J.A.M.A. *149*:722-725, 1952.

Salzberg, A. M., and Evans, E. I.: Blood volumes in normal and in burned dogs: a comparative study with radioactive phosphorus tagged red cells and T-1824 dye, Ann. Surg. *132*:746-759, 1950.

Sayman, W. A., and Allen, J. G.: Blood, plasma and expanders of plasma volume in the treatment of hemorrhagic shock, S. Clin. North America *39*:133-143, 1959.

Sayman, W. A., Gauld, R. L., Star, S. A., and Allen, J. G.: Safety of liquid plasma—A statistical appraisal, J.A.M.A. *168*:1735-1739, 1958.

Schweinburg, F. B., Yashar, Y., Aprahamian, H. A., Davidoff, D., and Fine, J.: Resistance to bacteria in hemorrhagic shock. I. Decline in phagocytosis-promoting capacity of serum in shock, Proc. Soc. Exper. Biol. & Med. *88*:587-589, 1955.

Schweinburg, F. B., and Fine, J.: Resistance to bacteria in hemorrhagic shock. II. Effect of transient vascular collapse on sensitivity to endotoxin, Proc. Soc. Exper. Biol. & Med. *88*:589-591, 1955.

Scott, R., Jr., Howard, J. M., Shorr, E., Lawson, N., and Davis, J. H.: Circulatory homeostasis following massive injury, studies of vaso-

depressor and vasoexcitatory substances in the circulating blood, Ann. Surg. *141*:504-509, 1955.

Seeley, S. F., and Nelson, R. M.: Intra-arterial transfusion, Internat. Abstr. Surg. *94*:209-214, 1952.

Serkes, K. D., Lang, S., and Pareira, M. D.: Efficacy of plasma and dextran compared to saline for fluid replacement following tourniquet shock, Surgery *45*:623-633, 1959.

Shenkin, H. A., Cheney, R. H., Govons, S. R., Hardy, J. D., Fletcher, A. G., Jr., and Starr, I.: On the diagnosis of hemorrhage in man: a study of volunteers bled large amounts, Am. J. M. Sc. *208*:421-436, 1944.

Shorr, E.: Tr. Second Conf. on Shock and Circulatory Homeostasis, 1952, New York, Macy, 1953.

Simeone, F. A.: Wound shock *in* Bowers, W. F., ed.: Surgery of Trauma, Philadelphia, Lippincott, 1953.

Soffer, A.: Therapy of syncope, J.A.M.A. *154*:1177-1179, 1954.

Steenburg, R. W., Lennihan, R., and Moore, F. D.: Studies in surgical endocrinology; II. The free blood 17-hydroxycorticoids in surgical patients; their relation to urine steroids, metabolism and convalescence, Ann. Surg. *143*:180-209, 1956.

Thorsén, G.: The use of dextrans as infusion fluids, Surg., Gynec. & Obst. *109*:43-52, 1959.

Travers, B.: An inquiry concerning irritation, London, 1826, cited by Mann, F. C.: Bull. Johns Hopkins Hosp. *25*:205-212, 1914.

Veal, J. R., Russell, A. S., and Stubbs, D.: Intra-arterial transfusions: indications and technic, Am. Surgeon *18*:1150-1159, 1952.

Wadström, L. B.: Effect of trauma on plasma lipids; an experimental study on the rat, Acta chir. scandinav. *115*:409-416, 1958.

Watts, D. T.: Arterial blood epinephrine levels during hemorrhagic hypotension in dogs, Am. J. Physiol. *184*:271-274, 1956.

Williams, W. T., and Parsons, W. H.: The indications for blood volume determinations in major surgical procedures, Surg., Gynec. & Obst. *106*:435-440, 1958.

Zweifach, B. W., Lee, R. E., Hyman, C., and Chambers, R.: Omental circulation in morphinized dogs subjected to graded hemorrhage, Ann. Surg. *120*:232-250, 1944.

J. GARROTT ALLEN, M.D.

CHAPTER 8

Blood Transfusions and Allied Problems

The development of blood transfusion is one of the most fascinating stories in the history of medicine. It is of special significance to surgery, for the evolution of the circulation, transfusion, hemostasis and shock are much of the warp and the woof of the fabric of modern surgery. In essence, present-day blood and plasma replacement is the inevitable result of the scientific studies in many fields.

DEVELOPMENTAL INTERRELATIONS OF SURGERY AND THE DISCOVERY OF THE CIRCULATION, TRANSFUSION, HEMOSTASIS AND SHOCK*

The story of transfusion is that of the scientific method itself. While the discovery of the circulation was prerequisite to its experimental and clinical trial, the developments in immunology and coagulation 250 years later were essential to its success and general usage. The interval between the first transfusion and its mature development demanded careful attention to hemostasis if operative surgery was to take advantage of the advances which anesthesia and bacteriology made possible after the mid-portion of the 19th century.

To recount, as often done, the fables and the folklore of transfusion history is to ignore

* The author wishes to express his appreciation to Dr. Ilza Veith of the Departments of Medicine and History of the University of Chicago for checking historical accuracy and for her helpful suggestions in the first part of this chapter.

or to relegate to an inferior position the wealth of historical facts which have accrued through nearly 2000 years.

THE DISCOVERY OF THE CIRCULATION

The concepts of the circulation required no less than 1200 years of recorded history to emerge from its Galenic shackles before it could assume a sound scientific footing. The writings of Aristotle (384-322 B.C.) are among the first to be cited in this epic. He studied the movement of blood in the chick embryo and believed that the arteries connected with the veins through pores in the septum of the heart. He believed that the heart was the source of body heat and the seat of the soul, that expansion of the heart was the result of boiling blood heated within the heart, and that the heart was the all-important organ to the body, as well as to the vessels.

Erasistratus (330-245 B.C.), an early Greek physiologist, described the auriculo-ventricular valves, but unfortunately assigned to the liver the role that Aristotle accredited the heart. He introduced a second misconception to be long perpetuated, that of believing that the arteries carried air rather than blood. Both Aristotle and Erasistratus believed that the arteries communicated with the veins through pores in the intraventricular septum. Their views might well seem to be reaffirmed were Aristotle and Erasistratus to witness today an operation for the closure of a septal defect in the heart. It is possible that in their limited dissections they encountered a septal defect and, failing to find such obvious communications between the right and the left chambers of the heart in the vast majority, postulated the invisible pores to account for the passage of blood from the right ventricle to the left.

Some of the views credited to each of these

men may have been in some measure those of Galen (A.D. 130-200) because of the difficulties often entailed in the course of translations. Therefore, there is a moderate degree of uncertainty expressed among scholars as to some of the interpretations attributed to the ancient Greeks. Harvey[21] quotes Aristotle as writing

. . . the blood of animals pulsates within their veins (meaning the arteries) and by the pulse is sent everywhere simultaneously . . . thus do all the veins pulsate together and by successive strokes, because they all depend upon the heart; and, as it is always in motion, so are they likewise always moving together, but by successive movements.

A similar but not identical view also was expressed by Erasistratus, but it was the Galenic view that the pulse was a function of respiratory motion which was to prevail for more than 1200 years.

Galen was forced to limit his prodigious dissections to animals, especially to apes. He taught Erasistratus' belief "that the blood is prepared in the liver and is thence transferred to the heart to receive its proper form and last perfection."[47] To him, blood ebbed to and fro in the veins and the arteries, passing from side to side through the porous intraventricular septum as suggested by Aristotle. Galen believed that arteries distributed both air and blood through the body and that in some manner air was derived from the lungs, whereas Erasistratus conceived the arteries to contain "nothing but spirits" (air); hence, they were named "arteria" from the Latin. Born in Athens, Galen later migrated to Rome.

Harvey and De Motu Cordis. History often discloses serious injustice in science— perhaps Galen was such a victim. But errors need not always be stumbling blocks; they may also be steppingstones. It is easy to see that a discoverer profits by the discoveries of his predecessors, but it may not be so evident that their errors also may serve him equally well—and sometimes better. There can be no doubt that the misfortunes of Galen, especially his endorsement of the Erasistratic concept, namely, that it was the liver and not the heart which was the all-important circulatory organ, provided a most important stimulus to Harvey. His logic had to be made absolutely clear if he was to refute the ancients successfully. Because of the importance of Harvey's

discovery and that mention of his debate in *De Motu Cordis et Sanguinis* directly cited Galen so prominently, the latter's contributions made 1400 years earlier may have suffered somewhat unfairly. On the other hand, the argument can be advanced that Galen's position today would be of much less consequence had he not been so important a target in Harvey's immortal contribution. Galen and his work were perpetuated primarily because the spirit of the Middle Ages was essentially that of the acceptance of ancient beliefs and suppression of new thought. Moreover, Galen must have appeared to Harvey as an unusually strong opponent, for Galen's work had been brought to England less than a century in advance of Harvey's times and hence likely was under critical review at that time. Linacre translated Galen from Greek into Latin in England; Linacre was the first president of the Royal College of Physicians of London. Harvey's attack upon Galenic doctrines and Galens' students and admirers was relentless, dissecting as it were, truth from fantasy, logic from confusion, and candor from "divine expression." However mild Harvey is depicted by some, there is little evidence of fear as to the correctness of his own scientific conclusions or of any reservation or concern for reprisal to be found in his vigorous writings:

Good God! how should the mitral valves prevent the regurgitation of air and not of blood? I do not see how he (Galen) can deny that the great artery is the very vessel to carry the blood, when it has attained its highest term of perfection for distribution to all parts of the body. Or would he perchance still hesitate, like all who come after him, even to the present hour, because he did not perceive the route by which the blood was transferred from the veins to the arteries, as I have already said, of the intimate connection between the heart and the lungs? And it plainly appears that this has puzzled the anatomists no little when, in their dissections, they found the pulmonary artery and left ventricle full of thick, black, and clotted blood, and felt themselves compelled to affirm that the blood made its way from the right to the left ventricle by transudating through the septum of the heart. But this fancy I have already refuted. A pathway for the blood must therefore be prepared and thrown open, and being once exposed, no further difficulty will, I believe, be experienced by anyone in what I have already proposed in regard to the pulse of the heart and the arteries, viz., the passage of the blood from the veins to the arteries and its distribution to the whole of the body by means of these vessels.

In *De Motu Cordis,* Harvey clearly postulated a peripheral communication between the small arteries and the veins based on observations made upon the comb of the young cock, the ears of white rabbits, the wings of the bat, the tails of tadpoles, the fins of fish, and other more primitive forms of animal life. He assumed that the arteries delivered blood to the tissues, flowing through a structureless parenchyma to enter the venous side of the circulation. However, Harvey, an Aristotlean devotee, could not bring himself to refute the latter's concept that the heart was the source of body heat.

Capillaries. The anatomic demonstration of the capillary circulation was to come from the microscopic observations of Marcello Malpighi (1628-94)[41] in 1661. This practicing clinician and professor of medicine is said by some to have used a compound microscope, whether the one invented by Zacharias and Hans Janssen about 1590 or the much improved Drebbel version made about the same time is unknown to me. Others say that he used the simple microscope of von Leeuwenhoek (1632-1723) invented before 1673. In any case, the microscope allowed Malpighi to describe the capillaries, though he misinterpreted blood corpuscles as fat cells. In letters to his mathematician friend, Borelli, is contained his first description of the capillary circulation. Malpighi wrote:

Hence, it was clear to the senses that blood flowed away along tortuous vessels and was not poured into spaces, but was always contained within tubules, and that its dispersion is due to the multiple winding of these vessels.

His studies were greatly extended by Leeuwenhoek, beginning in 1668.

The Pulmonary Circulation. Recognition of the pulmonary circulation in 1553 is to be found in the writings of Michael Servetus (1509-53),[57] as student prosector and contemporary of Vesalius. By nature, Servetus was a dissenter and nonconformist, if not a heretic. He decried with contempt the formalities of religion of his day, advocating simplicity and an ungarnished Christianity. This same spirit prevailed upon Servetus in his scientific attitudes, especially as applied to Galen; interestingly, his friend and colleague, Vesalius, the father of gross anatomy, discredited much of Galen's anatomy, though perhaps with less malice.

Servetus recognized the pulmonary circuit and emphatically denied Galen's concept of septal pores as the means of transit for blood from the right ventricle to the left. This unfortunate soul, like Vesalius, was to come to an untimely end, the result of his religious fervor and fanaticism. A copy of Servetus' *Christianismi Restituto,* which also contained his views on the pulmonary circulation, fell into the hands of his one-time friend, Calvin, in Geneva. Through the latter's influence, Servetus was condemned. Calvin seems to have cunningly mobilized the opposing forces of the Reform movement and of the Catholic Church against Servetus. Brought to trial in Geneva, imprisoned but escaped, he was burned in effigy with his 5 bales of books, April 17, 1553. Subsequently recaptured and tried, he was sentenced to death by slow burning at the stake carried out at noon, October 27, 1553. With all but 2 copies of *Christianismi Restituto* devoured in the flames of April 17, there is little reason to believe that Harvey was aware of the contributions of Servetus. His failure to acknowledge Servetus is no surprise.

In *Christianismi Restituto* were Servetus' comments on the pulmonary circuit:

The vital spirit has its source in the left ventricle of the heart, the lungs aiding most essentially in its production. . . . The right ventricle of the heart communicates to the left. This communication, however, does not take place through the septum, partition, or midwall of the heart, as is commonly believed, but by another admirable contrivance, the blood being transmitted from the pulmonary artery to the pulmonary vein by a lengthened passage through the lungs, in the course of which it is elaborated and becomes a crimson color. It is finally attracted by diastole and reaches the left ventricle of the heart. Moreover, it is not simply air, but air mingled with blood that is returned from the lungs to the heart through the pulmonary vein. . . . It is in the lungs that the mixture of blood with inspired air takes place, and it is in the lungs, not in the heart, that the crimson color of the blood is acquired. To conclude, the septum or middle portion of the heart, seeing that it is without vessels or special properties, is not competent to permit and accomplish the communication and elaboration in question, although it may be that some transudation occurs through it.

TRANSFUSION DEVELOPMENTS

One of the natural outgrowths of Harvey's discovery was to be the first documentation of blood transfusion by Richard Lower (1631-91)[37] carried out at Gresham College in Oxford late in February of 1665 in dogs. Sir Christopher Wren (1632-1723) experimented earlier with the intravenous infusion of ales, wines and drugs as a method of administration of drugs while at Oxford and is credited by many as having also infused blood. This latter activity seems to be unconfirmed. Lower, in publishing his observations in the *Transactions of the Philosophical Society*, December 17, 1666, recognized transfusion to have its greatest potential value in the replacement of blood lost in hemorrhage. His successful demonstration of transfusion in dogs on November 14, 1666, before the Royal Society (newly formed at Oxford in 1662) proved the feasibility of transfusion and its value in hemorrhage. About this event, Dr. Samuel Pepys recorded in his Diary of that date: "This did give occasion to many pretty wishes, as the blood of a Quaker to be let into an Archbishop, and such like." Lower, himself, did not deny the importance of his observation, writing,

At least it is a comfort to our Nation and credit to our fame that Harvey became pre-eminent by first demonstrating that blood circulated inside the body. That this circulation could be extended outside the body was first discovered by me.

Unfortunately, the freedom with which dogs may be transfused without resort to crossmatch or typing, in sharp contrast with man, was not to be recognized until 250 years later. Thus, the excellent results of Lower obtained on dogs were doomed from the start so far as human transfusion was concerned. Denis (1630-1695) administered 2 human transfusions in 1667, but his 3rd patient died with all the symptoms of an acute transfusion reaction and its attendant shock.[14] Charged by the patient's wife of murdering her husband, Denis was tried but eventually exonerated in the French courts, but not without the wise decree prohibiting further trial of human transfusions

unless sanctioned by the Faculty of Medicine of Paris. A decade later, similar action was taken by Parliament and soon thereafter by papal and governmental decree in Italy.

More than 125 years elapsed until John Blundell (1790-1877), a London obstetrician, once again gave human transfusions and once again with disastrous result in 1818.[26] Five of his 10 patients died; his work is said by some to have served to reawaken interest and to reopen the subject of transfusion, but certainly there was no great tendency to resume its use.

Blood Typing. As William Harvey set in order the knowledge of the circulation, so Karl Landsteiner (1868-1943) accomplished the same for the field of blood transfusion immunology. Examining bloods of various members of his laboratory, he was able from this limited experience to recognize 3 blood types (A, B and O) in 1900. In this publication[27] he emphasized the importance of blood typing preliminary to transfusion. Decastello and Sturli[13] described the 4th and rarest type, AB, in 1902. Landsteiner provided the classification which is the international nomenclature used today. Within the intervening 40 years of his study, Landsteiner described cold agglutinins, the M and the N factors, the Rh factors and their significance, as well as certain other minor types and agglutination irregularities. His subject matter and accomplishments deserve hardly less recognition than those of Harvey.

Crossmatching. Ludwig Hektoen[23] reemphasized in 1907 the need for selecting donors according to blood type, and in 1908 Epstein and Ottenberg devised the slide method for the detection of incompatible mixtures of blood. To Ottenberg must also go the credit for the first large-scale use of blood typing in the selection of donors for patients to be transfused, reporting with Kaliski in 1913[45] the transfusion of blood to 128 patients with only 3 deaths, and these he proved to be fatalities from mismatched blood. They observed agglutination of the donors' cells by the patients' serum to be more important "to avoid than the reverse." Thus developed the concept of "major" and "minor" fields of agglutination in transfusion crossmatchings, as well as the concept of the "universal donor" (Type O) and the "universal recipient" (Type AB).

Anticoagulants in Transfusion. Lower described the use of defibrinated blood and his transfusions among dogs in 1669 and pointed out that coagulation presented one of the most serious problems in blood transfusion. Braxton-Hicks,[9] encountering hemorrhage in his obstetric practice, introduced sodium phosphate as an anticoagulant to facilitate blood transfusion, but its toxicity prevented its general acceptance.

The role of the calcium ion in blood coagulation needed to be elucidated before transfusions were to become practical, even though typing and crossmatching procedures would eliminate most incompatibilities. By precipitating blood calcium with sodium oxalate, Arthrus and Pages in 1890 were able to prevent coagulation *in vitro*. Schmidt in 1895[54] was unable to accept the Arthrus and Pages explanation for the anticoagulant action of oxalate, because he noted that sodium citrate added to blood had the same anticoagulant effect without altering the concentration of calcium in blood. Sabbatani in 1903[51] explained this seeming discrepancy, demonstrating the action of citrate as one in which the calcium ion is firmly bound but not precipitated. In this bound state, calcium was incapable of participating in blood coagulation.

Lewisohn, Agote, Dustin, and Weil all independently suggested the use of sodium citrate as an anticoagulant adequate to prevent coagulation of blood drawn for transfusion purposes. Lewisohn's[35] contributions continued for more than 10 years, logically answering each of the many objections raised, and finally established sodium citrate as an anticoagulant useful and safe in the preparation for blood transfusion. Citrate remains the basic anticoagulant of choice today and has eliminated the need for haste in transference of blood from donor to recipient. To Lewisohn belongs the credit.

Hemostasis. One of the benevolent influences of the "transfusion failures" after Lower's 17th-century experiments was the continuing emphasis for improvements in technics for operative hemostasis. If surgery was to take advantage of the opportunities to be afforded by the mastery of anesthesia and operative sepsis 200 years later, careful hemostasis was essential. Recognizing the importance of hemostasis was not new. For centuries it was proposed that amputation be carried out in the gangrenous or necrotic portions of limbs where bleeding would not occur, or that *en masse* ligation of the vessels be employed at the time of amputation.

Archigenes and Celsus recommended the use of the ligature as early as A.D. 100, and compression bandages were applied by the early Greeks. However, as a technic for hemostasis, compression bandages were of little value until the tourniquet or garrot technic was introduced in 1674 by Morel. Both linen and catgut were employed as ligature material by the ancients and were mentioned so frequently in the early writings as to mask the exact identity of their origins.

Cautery, too, was used at an early date in the control of hemorrhage and certainly was in general use at the time of Hippocrates and Galen and later was advocated in the writings of John de Vigo (1460-1520) to whom Paré referred.[46]

At Tourin in 1537, Ambroise Paré (1510-1590) exhausted his supply of boiling oil used for hemostasis and the general wound care before he could treat the large numbers of wounded soldiers assigned to him. Thus he was forced to treat the remaining casualties with a medicament comprised of egg yolk, oil of roses and turpentine. Fearing that all the latter group might die before morning for the want of boiling oil, he arose early to visit them

where beyond my expectation, I found that those to whom I had applied my digestive medicament had but little pain, and their wounds were without inflammation or swelling, having rested fairly well that night; the others, to whom the boiling oil was used, I found feverish, with great pain and swelling about the edges of their wounds. Then I resolved never more to burn cruelly poor men with gunshot wounds.

To Paré belongs the credit for recognizing that the treatment of wounds with cautery was harmful. But it was not until 15 years later that he abandoned the searing cautery as a means of hemostasis in amputation. The occasion was his military journey to Danvilliers in 1552, where he reports that he drew forth the vessels with bullet forceps, ligated them *en masse* and amputated above the line of demarcation. Thereby the surgical use of ligature was rediscovered.

Through the ages, materials for ligature have included many items: among them were linen, catgut, "animal sinews," strips of doeskin, silk and cotton. Joseph, Baron Lister (1827-1912), originally a student of colloidal chemistry under Sir Thomas Graham and later entering surgery, revived the use of catgut. He invented the chromasizing process in 1876[36] and was the first to use it. By chromasizing catgut, he hoped to prolong its effectiveness in tissue on one hand and, at the same time, to avoid its unnecessary persistence when ligatures no longer served as useful purpose.

William Stewart Halsted (1852-1923), a great admirer of German aseptic technic and of the operative meticulousness of the Swiss surgeon, Theodor Kocher (1841-1917), was among the first to emphasize the principles of hemostasis in this country. Halsted, like Kocher, favored the use of silk ligatures and despaired of catgut.[17] Doubtless, catgut was a troublesome product in that day, but in his condemnation of it, Halsted overlooked or failed to appreciate the biologic principles which were always so much a part of Lister's investigations. Perhaps more to the point are the principles of careful hemostasis and the gentle handling of tissues, for these have not changed—suture material has.

Hemostatic instruments, beginning with the bullet forceps, developed shortly after the invention of firearms, were otherwise very slow to develop and to come into extensive use. Centuries later, Physick, Liston, Péan, Kocher, Halsted and many others designed or made contributions to the various types of hemostats, some of which bear their names and are still in use today. Samuel Harvey's[20] account of the story of hemostasis and Halsted's excellent review of surgery in general, related in his 1920 *The Operative Story of Goitre*,[18] afford a pleasant evening's reading for the student of surgery who is searching for or seeking out the "genetics and mutations" of his professional heritage. In these two tracts are told the stories of many of the men and their accomplishments in the long search to overcome the hazards and the fears of operative hemorrhage.

Historical developments of shock and its relationship to hemorrhage, hemostasis and transfusions are not easily explained, for one of the curious failures in the historical trails left by the surgeon and the physician alike was their inability to understand that hemorrhage was the chief cause of operative or hemorrhagic shock. For 500 years can be found written evidences of many shots striking the target circle but never once quite hitting the "bull's-eye." While all recognized the important association of shock and hemorrhage, the concepts of hidden, internal or sequestered hemorrhages and/or of plasma loss did not receive serious consideration until the 1930's. In such patients, shock seemed to have occurred without hemorrhage or at least with less bleeding than was realized. This reason, more than any other, clouded the issue and delayed its understanding. The choice and the derivation of the word "shock" (Fr. *choquer:* the phenomenon following a blow, impact, or collision, especially as applied to combat injuries) to define the patient's condition connotes to a certain extent the misinterpretation of its nature and of the patient's response. Much of its earlier meaning yet remains and is a term all too frequently abused by the medical profession and the laity alike even today.

As recently as 1923, Walter Cannon (1871-1945), in a monograph entitled *Traumatic Shock*, presented data of his own as well as referring extensively to those of others, especially to Keith and to Gasser. By 1923 all of these reports had demonstrated conclusively a diminished circulating blood volume as a constant finding in traumatic shock and that frequently this was also accompanied by a rise in the hematocrit reading; nonetheless, the cardinal point, while acknowledged and extensively discussed, failed to impress Cannon and others of its all-important role in the genesis of hemorrhagic, burn, or traumatic shock.

Cannon agreed with O. H. Robertson that the transfusion of compatible blood was the most effective treatment of shock but did not emphasize the singular importance of hypovolemia as its cause. He wrote in his preface, "because of its mysterious onset and nature, traumatic shock has long suggested problems of unusual clinical and scientific interest . . . it has remained an enigma." Toxemias and neural reactions continued to cloud the ultimate and basic disturbance for another 2 decades.

Out of the experimental studies of Phemister and of Blalock in the late 1920's and the early 30's was to emerge the full significance of the role of hypovolemia in shock of traumatic, hemorrhagic or burn origin. The experimental observations of these 2 men were soon to be confirmed and the soundness of treatment with blood and/or plasma to be documented thoroughly by the military experiences of World War II.

Thus from the cumulative observations, beginning 400 years ago with Paré, Servetus, Harvey, Lower, and revived 300 years later by the works of Landsteiner, Lewisohn, Robertson, Cannon, Blalock, Phemister and many others evolved the knowledge and the background which were to provide the present-day indications and status of one of our greatest therapeutic pillars: the proper use of blood transfusion and allied substances. If one man's contributions in this field are to be singled out above all others, they would seem to be that of Karl Landsteiner. Because of his brilliance and keenness of insight, his contributions must stand abreast of those of all time.

Glycerolized Frozen Blood. One important new development in blood preservation is the use of glycerolized frozen blood (Tullis, Ketchel, Pyle, Pennell, Gibson, Tinch and Driscoll, 1958; Haynes, Tullis, Pyle, Sproul, Wallach and Turville, 1960; and O'Brien and Watkins, 1960). Such blood collected in acid-citrate-dextrose solution and stored at −80° C. for up to 31 months, showed less deviation of the oxyhemoglobin saturation curve than blood stored by conventional methods at 4° C. beyond 7 days. Frozen blood also can be used for pump priming and transfusion in cardiovascular surgery (see Chap. 41, "Cardiac Surgery").

Cadaver Blood. Used in Russia for at least 25 years, transfusion of cadaver blood has recently been redescribed in the American literature by Petrov (1959) of Moscow. Chief credit for originating this method should go to the late Serge S. Yudin (1936), also of Moscow. The obtaining of cadaver blood is in turn based on the principle of postmortem fibrinolysis discovered by Skundina and Rusakov (1934). One of the editors (H.N.H.) has visited the laboratories of both Yudin and of Skundina.

PRACTICAL ASPECTS AND PRECAUTIONS IN BLOOD TRANSFUSIONS

Although blood transfusion became a practical possibility with Landsteiner's initial discovery, nearly 15 years were to elapse before the general use of transfusions was to receive serious consideration. Even then, its development was to be slow; each point of theory or practice was to be debated extensively but to the ultimate advantage and safety of the patient. From this sound approach was to emerge one of the important improvements in the general care of the patient, especially the surgical patient. It was well after 1930 before transfusions were to be employed as procedures other than those of last resort or desperation.

For 40 years (1900-1940), only 4 blood types or groups were considered as groups of consequence. In the last year, Landsteiner and colleagues,[29, 33] particularly Levine, introduced a secondary series of blood groups, the Rh groups. The Rh groups were destined to explain many of the hemolytic transfusion reactions not accountable on the basis of Landsteiner's initial discoveries of 1900. To distinguish between the groups, AB, A, B and O and those of the Rh family, the terms "Standard or Major" blood groups, or iso-agglutinogens, have been employed in the identification of the former, and the latter is referred to as the "Rh Group or Type."

BLOOD GROUPS

Major or Standard Blood Groups (AB, A, B and O). The standard nomenclature identifying major blood groups is that of Landsteiner, which is now employed internationally. Its advantage over the Moss or Jansky numerical classification is that the International nomenclature is descriptive of the iso-agglutinogen and iso-agglutinin content of each blood group (Table 1).

It is clearly evident from this Table that 4 factors are concerned in establishing any blood group. Two of these, Factors A and B, may be present in the red cells and are referred to as *iso-agglutinogens*. Two may be present in the serum *a* and *b* and are termed

TABLE 1. ISO-AGGLUTINOGENS AND ISO-HEMAGGLUTININS OF THE MAJOR BLOOD GROUPS

BLOOD GROUP INTERNATIONAL	CELLS CONTAIN ISO-AGGLUTINOGENS	SERUM OR PLASMA CONTAINS ISO-HEMAGGLUTININS	APPROX. % OF POPULATION (U.S. WHITE)
O	None	ab (Anti-A and Anti-B)	40–45
A	A	b (Anti-B)	40
B	B	a (Anti-A)	10–15
AB	A & B	o (Neither Anti-A nor Anti-B)	5

agglutinins. Blood groups are known by the cellular agglutinogens they contain and not by their serum iso-agglutinin. Thus, blood whose cells bear only iso-agglutinogen A is known as Group A, and blood cells whose iso-agglutinogens contain only B are known as Group B blood. Cells containing both iso-agglutinogens A and B belong to Group AB, and those containing neither iso agglutinogens A or B are referred to as Group O (meaning zero).

Serum iso-agglutinin *a* will coat or be absorbed upon erythrocytes containing iso-agglutinogen A, causing them to clump and/or hemolyze. For this reason, serum containing only the iso-agglutinin *a* is antagonistic to cellular agglutinogen A; therefore, this serum is known as *Anti-A.* The same holds for serum containing only iso-agglutinin *b,* which agglutinates the cellular iso-agglutinogen B. This serum is known as *Anti-B* serum. Serum containing both iso-agglutinogens A and B is known as Anti-A and Anti-B. Sera containing neither iso-agglutinins *a* or *b,* of course, are not antagonistic to erythrocytes of any of the 4 major blood groups. Thus, Group A blood is incompatible with Group B blood because the serum of Group B contains iso-agglutinogen Anti-A, and vice versa; whereas, Group AB erythrocytes are compatible with the sera of all 4 blood types, as its serum contains neither the Anti-A nor the Anti-B agglutinins.

Blood Groups or Types. These are estab-lished by determining the presence or the absence of agglutination when whole blood of the unknown group is mixed separately with Anti-A serum and Anti-B serum (Table 2).

The Rh Factors or Groups. Six different cell characteristics are identifiable in the Rh system. These are designated as Rh_0, rh′, rh″, Hr_0, hr′, and hr″, respectively; or by the British corresponding nomenclature of D, C and E, and *d, c* and *e.* However, these do not refer to the potential number or combinations of Rh groupings which total 27 possibilities.

The erythrocytes of every person must contain at least one member of each of these 3 pairs of antigens. The red cells of some individuals may contain 4, 5 or even 6, so that the combinations possible are rather large.

In testing erythrocytes for the Rh antigens that they may contain, it is practical at the present time to examine cells for the presence of Rh_0, rh′ and rh″, using the corresponding antisera—Anti-Rh_0 (Anti-D), Anti-rh′ (Anti-C) and Anti-rh″ (Anti-E). Of these 3, the most important is D or Rh_0, as it is most frequently antigenic and is encountered most commonly. However, it is advisable to examine for the presence of C and E as well (Table 3 A and B).

Testing for the presence of *c, d* and *e* antigens (Hr_0, hr′ and hr″) with each respective antisera is not performed by all blood banks, although within the past year or two these

TABLE 2

ANTI-A SERUM	ANTI-B SERUM	UNKNOWN BLOOD UNDER TEST
Serum containing only Iso-agglutinin *a*	Serum containing only Iso-agglutinin *b*	Blood Group or Cell Type Indicated (International)
Agglutination	Agglutination	AB
Agglutination	No agglutination	A
No agglutination	Agglutination	B
No agglutination	No agglutination	O

TABLE 3 A. COMPARATIVE NOMENCLATURES

RH SYSTEM	CDE SYSTEM
Rh$_o$	D*
rh'	C
rh"	E
Hr$_o$	d
hr'	c
hr"	e

* It is unfortunate that in the CDE designation Rh$_o$ does not correspond to C rather than to D.

procedures have been introduced as a routine procedure by many.

The production of Rh antibodies is stimulated in the patients receiving an Rh antigen which their blood does not contain. Sensitization generally occurs by one of two mechanisms or both. Either the Rh negative patient receives an Rh positive blood transfusion and thereby is stimulated to produce antibodies to the Rh antigen given, or the patient is an Rh negative mother bearing an Rh positive fetus whose red cells manage to enter the maternal circulation and stimulate the production of maternal Rh antibodies. The initial transfusion of Rh positive blood in an unsensitized Rh negative patient causes no reaction. However, Rh positive blood administered again several weeks later can induce serious or fatal hemolytic transfusion reactions. The following case report and the data presented in Figure 8-1 illustrate this point:

A 43-year-old married female was admitted in January, 1944, with bleeding from ulcerative colitis. Four daily transfusions were administered for anemia. Under medical management, her colitis symptoms subsided, and she improved. 43 days after this series of transfusions, she was given a single transfusion of blood for mild persistent anemia with the expectation of discharge to home the following day. Severe chill and symptoms of an acute hemolytic reaction near the termination of her transfusion developed. Jaundice and anemia followed the next day. Slowly, she recovered. Finally, she was discharged 6 weeks later (Fig. 8-1).

Rechecking of the last donor disclosed his blood to be Rh positive and the blood of the patient to be Rh negative. The 4 preceding donors were recalled and proved to be Rh positive also. Further encouragement to adapt Rh determinations as routine for the bloods of all donors and recipients was not necessary thereafter.

Hence, a female patient always should receive blood from a donor of the corresponding group and of the corresponding Rh type if she has been pregnant or is or will be of the childbearing age.

However, in the male, under emergency situations only, the administration of an Rh positive blood to an Rh negative recipient may be condoned when appropriate Rh negative blood is not available or when suitable typing facilities are not at hand. Rh negative women who never have been pregnant and are beyond the childbearing age fall into this same category. However, it should be remembered that subsequent transfusion of Rh positive blood a few weeks later may lead to serious hemolytic reactions.

The Coombs' Test (Antihuman Serum) has been most helpful in the recognition of Rh antibodies in Rh negative patients, thereby alerting the physician to potential trouble. The Coombs' serum reacts *only with coated* cells. Coated or sensitized red cells occur at times from autosensitization and are found in certain hemolytic diseases. The Coombs' serum is believed to react under these *in vitro* conditions because this Antihuman Serum adds a second coat to the already *in vivo* coated red cells, making them more susceptible to agglu-

TABLE 3 B. TEST SERUM AND USUAL RH TYPING

CELL TYPE	(ANTI-D) ANTI-RH$_o$	(ANTI-C) ANTI-RH'	(ANTI-E) ANTI-RH"	APPROXIMATE % WHITE
rh (cde)	—	—	—	15.0
rh' (Cde)	—	+	—	1.0
rh" (cdE)	—	—	+	0.7
rh'rh" (CdE)	—	+	+	0.02
Rh$_o$ (cDe)	+	—	—	1.5
Rh$_o$' (CDe)	+	+	—	54.0
Rh$_o$" (cDE)	+	—	+	14.5
Rh$_o$' Rh$_o$" (CDE)	+	+	+	13.2

tination. This coating or sensitivity occurs *in vivo* generally but is not sufficient to induce agglutination when tested *in vitro* against ordinary sera. The Coombs' serum, which will not react with erythrocytes unless they are already coated *in vivo,* thus acts as a booster in such reactions and makes possible the detection of sensitized or coated erythrocytes not otherwise found by laboratory methods.

Two kinds of Coombs' tests have been devised. They are known as the Direct and the Indirect Tests.

The Direct Coombs' Test is a diagnostic procedure, designed to pick up coated red cells which have been coated or sensitized by the patient's own serum when it possesses some antibody for an antigen contained on his erythrocytes. Therefore, it is a diagnostic test for unusual autohemolytic diseases and is especially useful in the recognition of erythroblastosis, certain of the hemolytic anemias,

especially "splenic" anemia, and to assist in the avoidance or the explanation of hemolytic transfusion reactions. It should be requested when these conditions are suspected.

The Indirect Coombs' Test is essentially a crossmatch, wherein an attempt is made to determine whether the donor's red cells when given to the recipient are coated or sensitized by an unusual antibody contained in the donor's serum which is not otherwise recognizable and will react with an antibody in the patient's serum. Therefore, one orders a direct Coombs' test when one wishes diagnostic assistance as to the nature of the hemolytic reaction within his patient. An indirect Coombs' test is requested when one suspects that the patient's plasma may contain some unusual antibody which may antagonize the erythrocytes of a prospective donor.

The indirect Coombs' test is particularly valuable when the patient's serum is Rh nega-

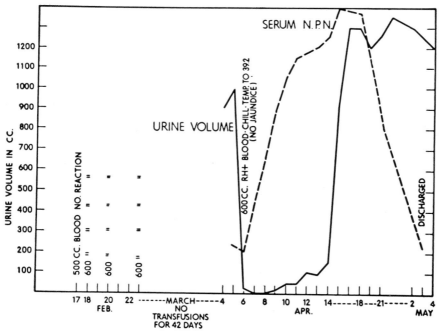

FIG. 8-1. Hazards of giving RH+ blood to an RH— patient. (A.C., aged 35, 321275 ulcerative colitis RH— Type O, one child L and W, no miscarriages.) The oliguric state with renal azotemia with near fatality in an RH negative patient sensitized to RH positive blood in 1944, as demonstrated by chart. The 4 transfusions administered over a 7-day period in February of that year were examined subsequently and proved to be RH positive. Accidents such as this one occurred in many institutions and forced the inclusion of RH typing as a part of the standard routine in the preparation of blood for any and all recipients.

tive to *d* but not to *c* or *e*. An Rh negative D donor whose C and E antigens have not been established may be recognized by the Indirect Coombs' test, and then further subtyping is carried out. The indirect Coombs' is also indicated in patients receiving repeated transfusions which may have sensitized the patient to erythrocytic antigens of potential donors. The indirect test is also indicated in patients with so-called "splenic" anemia. Indeed, to provide the patient with the greatest safety in his transfusions, an indirect Coombs' test always should be performed, but often the amount of work and time consumed does not make so broad a usage possible in many blood banks.

Undoubtedly, more blood antigens will be identified and found to play an important etiologic role in some transfusion reactions. Four of the more common ones are discussed below.

Other Blood Antigens.

COLD AGGLUTININS. These were first described by Landsteiner and Levine in 1926[28] and represent the phenomenon of autoagglutinins. The erythrocytes of an individual become agglutinatible by his own plasma or serum at temperatures less than that of body heat. Landsteiner demonstrated that after thorough washing of erythrocytes when cold agglutinins existed, the cells could be resuspended in the plasma of an individual free of cold agglutinins without agglutinations taking place upon lowering the ambient temperature. Thus he proved that cold agglutinins were real and not an artifact.

Cold agglutinins are said to be present in a higher percentage among Negro donors than among Caucasians. They are also frequently present in Raynaud's disease, paroxysmal hemoglobinuria, cirrhosis, in severe anemia, hemolytic anemias, and in fact in an almost unending list of chronic diseases.

Two clinical facts are important and practical with reference to cold agglutinins. First, if blood typing is carried out in a cool room, the blood being typed can show agglutination against both Anti-A and Anti-B sera from the presence of cold agglutinins rather than from an incompatibility with the specific typing serum. Thus, a Group O, a Group A, or a Group B donor could be identified erroneously as Group AB. The blood of all individuals, when agglutinated by both Anti-A and Anti-B serum, may be reexamined at 37° C. for the presence of cold agglutinins, thereby eliminating this source of typing error. This procedure is a relatively simple one. It is readily feasible, also, as only about 5 per cent of the Caucasian population normally have Group AB blood.

The second malevolent influence of cold agglutinins is the ability of the chilled blood of a donor with erythrocytic cold agglutinogens to be agglutinated in the course of transfusion by a patient whose plasma contains cold agglutinins, causing a hemolytic reaction. Cold agglutinins were seldom a factor of concern prior to the introduction of blood banking wherein blood is refrigerated before use. Most blood was administered 20 years ago very shortly after its withdrawal from the donor and without cooling. Its temperature was more nearly that of body heat. In a normal individual whose serum possesses cold agglutinins, the administration of chilled blood may result in a transient rise in temperature, a chill and mild to moderate hemolysis of little consequence. However, in the critically ill individual, a similar reaction is less well tolerated and may cause a severe enough reaction in some patients to be disastrous. At the University of Chicago, the practice of administering cold blood is generally employed, excepting where the patient is known to possess cold agglutinins. Under these conditions, it is advised that the donor's blood be brought slowly to 37° C. and administered, maintaining heat by placing warm water bottles about the tubing.

Other blood antigens also are recognized as capable of producing antibodies in the plasma of patients whose blood cells do not contain them. Three of these appear to be of clinical importance. They are the Kell, the Luther and the Duffy factors, so termed because they were first described in patients bearing these respective names. The Kell antigen may be demonstrated by anti-Kell serum; those cells not reacting with Anti-K serum are labeled *k* cells. Those reacting with Anti-K serum are called K. The Duffy and the Luther factors are less well defined, but similar anti-Duffy or anti-Luther serum antibodies can be developed.

Transfusion Safeguards and the Common Sources of Transfusion Accidents and Their Prevention. The central and practical point relative to the safety of blood transfusions depended upon the development and the general availability of highly reactive and reliable typing serum. Excellent typing sera did not become generally available until after 1940. Consequently, in spite of the contributions of Landsteiner,[27] the introduction of crossmatching by Ottenberg[45] and the development of citrate as an anticoagulant by Lewisohn,[35] reliable typing sera was still a quarter of a century away. Fatal transfusion reactions continued to occur for many years at a rate too high to encourage the use of blood as a replacement therapy in surgery or trauma other than as an emergency fluid, and then its use generally was one of desperation. In the years from 1936 to 1940, at the University of Chicago Clinics, death attributed to transfusion reactions occurred in 1 out of every 366 patients transfused; this example represents the results usually obtained as recently as 20 years ago. However, since 1940, when highly potent Anti-A and Anti-B typing serum became available, no deaths have occurred from 1942 to 1956 in this hospital from mistaken blood groups where high titer agglutinogens were employed. During the 16-year period, more than 15,000 patients have received more than 60,000 units of blood. Although some mismatched transfusions of low titer have been given with serious consequences, none has been fatal.

Mistakes in blood group identification can now be reduced to those related to or caused by human error. To a lesser or greater extent, probably these limitations always will impose a slight degree of hazard in blood transfusion, regardless of what checks and counterchecks are employed. The most important of these errors or hazards appears to arise from fatigue and vexation of blood bank personnel, assuming that excellent personnel and technics are employed. The physician, concerned with the safety of his own patient, must recognize that an unreasonable attitude on his part toward the blood bank trying to serve the needs of his patients will almost certainly increase unwittingly the frequency of human error. This result is exactly what he wishes to avoid; the safety of all patients is jeopardized

—not merely those of the dominant complainer. The blood bank should be able to function with the element of human error usually less than 0.05 per cent. Unfortunately, errors in the range of 1 per cent, or greater, still persist in many blood banks throughout the country.

The dictum of *primum non nocere*, yes—always! but this ideal when applied to the use of blood transfusions involves not only the risk entailed in the preparation of the transfusion itself but also the recognition on the part of the physician or the surgeon that unwillingness to employ blood when needed often subjects his patient to a much greater hazard. All things considered, many physicians continue in the practice of "too little and too late," failing to appreciate fully the patient's blood requirements, particularly in the field of trauma and in the course of extensive operations.

Errors can arise in the blood bank. But the house staff, the attending physician and the nursing staff also contribute to the total hazard involved. Insofar as errors attributable to the blood bank are concerned, the most important is faulty identification of the blood group—of either the donor, the recipient, or both. When blood groups are identified properly, the occurrence of serious or fatal reactions attributable to the blood bank are essentially abolished. The all-important concern of the blood bank is to be certain that the blood groups of the donor and the recipient correspond or at least the combination of the donor's is not affected adversely by the patient's serum or plasma, and that the blood issued for the patient is actually the one which has been typed and crossmatched for the particular patient.

At present the crossmatching of the donor cells with those of the patient is of secondary importance, provided that a high titer and active typing sera are employed. Nonetheless, the crossmatch has not lost its usefulness and always should be carried out. It serves as a check on blood typing and assures one that labeling errors have not occurred.

There are two important sources of typing errors. Foremost is the use of low-potency typing sera or sera which has lost its initial potency either from bacterial contamination or age. This is prevented by checking at least once a week the potency of typing sera on hand. Typing sera should be maintained under refrigeration. The second error is of human origin and relates to the faulty recording of properly typed bloods, improper identification of Anti-A or Anti-B typing sera, or the accidental placing of the donor cells in his own serum in crossmatching rather than in that of the recipient. These errors may be prevented by typing twice the bloods of the recipient and the donor—performed independently by 2 different persons—and the independent recording of the identification of the blood groups concerned. No precautions should be overlooked.

The house staff or physician administering the blood may introduce errors of another nature. Unwittingly, he may administer to the wrong patient the blood that he takes from the blood bank. This error may be avoided by limiting to one unit of blood that which the physician may take from the blood bank at any one time and by writing in bold lettering on its label the name of the patient for whom it is intended and his blood group, as well as that of the donor. The physician's second error is the inadequate identification of the recipient's blood sample which he brings to the blood bank in requesting his transfusion. At the University of Chicago, where some 9,000 transfusions are given per year, we have been both surprised and terrified by the frequency with which the full name of the recipient and, indeed his diagnosis, will correspond exactly to that of another patient hospitalized at the same time. Therefore, in requesting the transfusion, recording the patient's name on the transfusion requisition is not enough; the requisition should bear his hospital unit number as well. Third, if irregular antibodies or sensitization are suspected, it is up to the physician to communicate his suspicions to the blood bank. Direct Coombs' testing should be the physician's responsibility to request; indirect Coombs' crossmatch is the joint responsibility of the blood bank and the physician. There remains a fourth source of potential error on the part of the physician in that he may draw from several patients samples of blood to be typed and crossmatched, unwittingly mixing his requisition slips with the sample submitted to the blood bank. In our experience, this has proved the

smallest source of transfusion error and may be avoided if the person drawing the blood sample fills out each requisition individually at the patient's bedside at that time.

The National Institutes of Health established certain minimum standards for the safe preparation and preservation of blood for transfusion purposes.[62] These have been adopted by the American Association of Blood Banks and endorsed by the American College of Surgeons.[43] This is no guarantee of safety, for no body of authority is charged with the responsibility of seeing to it that such precautions will be carried out. Therefore, in the final analysis the safety of transfusion is a summation of the joint efforts of the attending physician, all hospital personnel concerned with patient care, as well as those in the blood bank.

The medical staff should see to it that the best practices possible are employed by blood banks. At the same time, they must realize the limitations in blood banking procedures in general and of their personnel in particular. As the efficiency of personnel and blood banks is subject to variation, these variations affect, to some extent, the "ground rules" concerning the indications and the contraindications for transfusion from one hospital to another. Thus, among the indications for transfusion is the past experience with the particular blood bank concerned. Yet, the physician must also realize, as with his own operative procedures, that however much care is exercised, some errors creep in and often when least expected —a situation not foreign to the surgeon's own operative experience. He never will be able to employ transfusion with complete safety; he can only hope that the accidents will be few and far between.

Crossmatching Principles. The matching of the donor's red cells with the patient's serum and the patient's cells with the donor's serum serves as a final check upon the correctness of the typing of both the blood donor and the patient, as well as the identity of both donor and recipient. As mentioned above, this procedure was more important in the days prior to the development of reliable high-titer Anti-A and Anti-B typing sera. Nonetheless, crossmatching should be carried out if at all possible. These procedures continue in our hands to detect an occasional error in labeling of a blood type or indicate a blood of mistaken identity. However, it seldom discloses any abnormalities other than those resulting from the mixing of major groups of incompatible bloods. It will not identify incompatibilities of the Rh type, the Kell, the Duffy, or Luther type or the Du factor. Specific antisera are needed for each of the latter.

In general, 3 types of crossmatching procedures are employed. The first and most generally used is the *saline* crossmatch, wherein a saline suspension of donor and recipient cells is mixed respectively with recipient and donor sera. The second technic, and considered by many to be more nearly accurate than the saline crossmatch, is the *gross* crossmatch. It tests only the compatibility of the donor's cells with the recipient's serum; but this is the all-important aspect of compatibility. A 4 per cent saline suspension of red cells is mixed directly with an equal volume of the recipient's serum. The final mixture, generally about 1 ml., is centrifuged at 1,000 r.p.m. for a period of 3 minutes and then agitated gently. An incompatibility is revealed by the presence of agglutinated clumped cells; the compatible reaction is revealed by the uniform suspension of all cells throughout the serum.

The High-Protein Crossmatch is the third and was introduced to overcome the problem of "blocking" antibodies. These are incomplete antibodies affecting the Rh system and they are not detected in saline suspensions. However, clumping of incompatible Rh bloods does occur when serum, plasma or albumin are present in sufficient concentrations. The high-protein crossmatch, wherein 30 per cent bovine albumin is used as the fluid for suspension of the red cells being tested, has been recommended and adopted for general use. However, with passage of time, the high-protein crossmatch has not proved its ability to replace entirely saline crossmatch. At the University of Chicago, both crossmatching procedures are used for each patient.

The all-important aspect of crossmatching by any procedure is that the donor cells be compatible with the patient's serum. This is known as major field crossmatch.

The Universal Donor. Since the days of Ottenberg, the fact has been known that the Group O donor may give blood to recipients of any of the 4 major blood groups; he is known as the "universal" donor. His erythrocytes, containing neither agglutinogens A nor B, obviously cannot be attacked by the patient's agglutinins *a* and/or *b*. However, it will be recalled that the Group O donor's plasma contains both agglutinins *a* and *b*. Generally, this is of little consequence, for as his blood is administered to the recipient, his iso-agglutinins *a* and *b* are rapidly diluted throughout the patient's circulation and cause no important hemolysis. Occasionally, however, the iso-agglutinin titers of *a* and *b* in a Group O donor's blood are very high and can induce severe hemolysis of the patient's cells should he be of another blood group. A case in point is that which follows:

A 76-year-old man was operated upon in July, 1946, for a carcinoma of the rectum. A Miles procedure was performed by the author without difficulty. Because of an uncorrected anemia, 3 blood transfusions were administered during the day of operation. Certainly 2 were all he needed. The first 2 transfusions were AB Rh positive and compatible with the patient's own type. The 3rd blood was administered late in the day and was given in the hope that an improved blood count, over that of the preoperative one, would result. As no other AB bloods were available, a Type O Rh positive blood was administered without incidence until it was noted a few hours later that the urine contained an abundance of hemoglobin. The following day the patient's color was deeply icteric and for 48 hours no urine was secreted (Fig. 8-2).

Beginning with the 4th day, urine flow returned, and the high bilirubin levels (28 mg.%) receded. Slowly his general course began to improve, but his erythrocyte count was now 1,800,000 per cm. ml., and his hemoglobin determination was 5.6 Gm. per cent. On the 8th day, without previous warning, he suddenly expired from acute left heart failure.

Rechecking of the blood types of the 3 donors and the patient assured their correctness. Then the Type O donor sample was titered and found to be in excess of 1:2096 or of a titer 10 to 20 times that of the maximum allowed. That this transfusion was not immediately fatal is in itself surprising, but it must also be admitted that this hemolytic reaction posed a threat to this 76-year-old man which might have been much less harmful to a younger and more vigorous patient. Autopsy disclosed no special cause for his acute heart failure.

As the Group O donor constitutes 40 to 45 per cent of the Caucasian population, his usefulness is an invaluable asset in times of catastrophe and emergency, especially if his titer is known. Crosby and Akeroyd[12] employed Group O Rh positive blood of low titer in the Korean War, administering as much as 10 to 30 units of blood without regard to the recipient's blood group. All Group O blood used in their casualty work had an agglutinin titer of less than 1:200. The results they achieved were remarkable indeed, for it made possible the administration of blood to the wounded as soon as they could be reached and undoubtedly saved many lives. This practice should be used in civilian emergencies with the same precautions when blood is needed before typing procedures can be carried out. It should be remembered that in Rh negative recipients, the use of Rh positive Group O blood as emergency fluid may induce the production of Anti-Rh antibodies within the recipient or that its use can present a serious hazard in Rh negative women whose anti-Rh titer has already been developed by pregnancy. Subsequent transfusions administered a week or two later should be group specific Rh negative blood (see p. 134). Thus, the administration of Rh positive Group O blood should not be employed electively other than in Rh positive patients, for it may cause trouble at a later date should it be necessary to administer

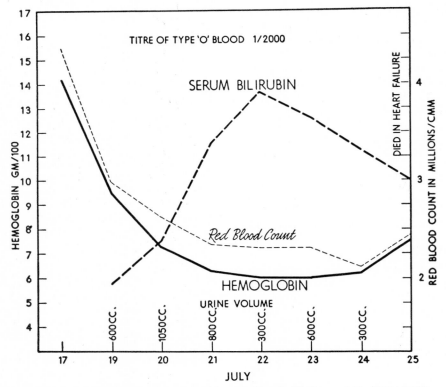

Fig. 8-2. Hazards of using universal type O blood. (D.C., aged 73, 385410, Wt. 77.4 Kg. Type A RH+.) The rare but distinct risk of group O blood administered to a patient of another blood group when the iso-agglutinin titer of Group O is excessive, as illustrated graphically by the acute decline in the red cell count and hemoglobin concentration with concurrent development of icterus. This is the so-called "minor" field or crossmatch wherein the incompatibility is that of the donor's serum for the patient's cells. Note that in spite of the severe degree of hemolysis, the daily urine volume was moderately good. This is in contrast with the oliguric or anuric states which follow reactions wherein the cells of the donor are incompatible with the serum of the recipient (compare with data in Fig. 8-1).

Group O Rh positive blood under emergency circumstances.

The universal recipient is a Group AB patient whose cells contain iso-agglutinogens A and B. His plasma contains neither iso-agglutinins *a* nor *b*. He may receive blood from donors of any blood group, as his plasma will not agglutinate the cells of any donor with major agglutinogens A and/or B. Therefore, this recipient is designated as the "universal" recipient. Although this knowledge is useful in some instances, its greatest limitation is the fact that only about 5 per cent of the recipients have blood of the AB variety.

Witebsky[66] has shown that the addition of a blood group specific substance to human blood neutralizes about 50 per cent of the iso-agglutinins contained in many such bloods. This material is obtained from animal tissues and is by nature polysaccharide. It can be highly purified and is essentially nonantigenic. When added to Group O blood, it tends to neutralize the Group A and B antibodies in plasma and should be used whenever it is necessary under emergency conditions to give blood to a recipient whose type is not yet established. It is not always successful and cannot be fully relied upon to accomplish its purpose.

THE NATURE OF BLOOD TRANSFUSION REACTIONS

Until 15 years ago only 3 types of transfusion reactions were recognized. They were classified as hemolytic, pyrogenic and allergic. As further experience has accumulated, additional untoward manifestations have been recognized as resulting from certain reactions from the transfusions of blood. Most of these relate directly or indirectly to the larger volumes of blood replacement employed in the extensive operative surgery in the fields of cancer, heart surgery and that of trauma; or they are related to the prolonged storage of blood. They include homologous serum jaundice, circulatory overload, potential citrate intoxication and the growth of bacteria under prolonged periods of refrigeration, as well as the increases in serum potassium as blood ages or hemolyzes. The importance of a normal pH in bank blood has been emphasized recently by McLaughlin, Nealon and Gibbon (1960).

Excess acidity of stored bank blood may lead to cardiac arrest. The extent and the seriousness of such acidity has not been recognized sufficiently in the past.

HEMOLYTIC REACTIONS

Hemolytic transfusion reactions may or may not be of importance. Stated otherwise: some hemolytic reactions are serious; some are not. Hemolytic reactions are always a source of concern to the clinician, and their origin always must be determined as soon as possible. Only when the cause is known can proper treatment be implemented and the importance of the reaction be assessed.

Common to all hemolytic reactions usually is the early but transient occurrence of hemoglobinemia and hemoglobinuria and a few hours later an increase in serum bilirubin and usually clinical icterus. Generally, hemoglobinuria can be detected only within the first urine sample after the reaction has occurred, as free circulatory hemoglobin is soon converted to bilirubin. Hemoglobinemia will be detected only if the serum is examined early and for the same reason. Whether or not acute and pronounced anemia occurs depends upon the extent of hemolysis; in extensive hemolytic reactions, severe anemia may develop (see case report on p. 134). The effect of the hemolytic reaction upon renal function, particularly urine secretion, depends upon its cause and kind. In general, hemolytic reactions are one of two varieties: rapid hemolysis of aged (14 to 28 days) donor blood, or the hemolysis of mismatched blood. The latter is the serious threat to the life of the patient and his renal function.

Causes of Less Serious Types of Hemolytic Reactions.

AGED BLOOD, 14 to 28 days or older: The "life" span of the normal erythrocyte, freshly drawn and transfused without delay to the normal recipient of the same blood groups, is approximately 120 days. However, the length of life span rapidly falls off as blood ages *in vitro* under blood-banking conditions. The residual life span of erythrocytes of a 2-week unit of blood may be less than 1 week, even when transfused into a recipient of the same blood groupings, including subtypes. If several units of aged blood are transfused within a day or two, physiologic hemolysis of the donors' erythrocytes may proceed at a rate sufficiently rapid to produce hemoglobinuria, to elevate materially the serum bilirubin levels and cause extensive clinical icterus. Transfusion icterus of this origin is generally unimportant except that the beneficial effects of such transfusions upon the patient's anemia is short-lived. Urine flow generally is not affected appreciably. However, the diagnosis as to the origin of the hemolytic reaction is one made by exclusion. All typing and cross-matchings must be rechecked and found satisfactory before the conclusion can be justified that hemolysis is due to outdated erythrocytes.

IMPAIRED HEPATIC BILIRUBIN EXCRETION. As the liver is the prime organ of bilirubin clearance, impaired hepatic excretion of bilirubin of any origin may result in an increased retention of serum bilirubin. If icterus is already present, it is obvious that the patient cannot clear his plasma of his own erythrocytic breakdown products. Thus, after the transfusion of relatively aged blood, an increase in clinical icterus and of the serum bilirubin level is observed so frequently as to be the rule rather than the exception. The larger the number of transfusions of properly matched bloods the icteric patient receives, the greater the post-transfusion icterus is likely to be. The extent of the increase in icterus is likely to be greater when aged bloods are given to patients with normal liver function and when Group O bloods are administered when the recipient is of another blood group. While the hemolysis from the transfusion of aged blood often results in an increase in icterus and bilirubinemia, it is seldom of great clinical importance.

THE HIGH AGGLUTININ TITER UNIVERSAL DONOR. The results of hemolysis, this time the destruction of the patient's cells, can be more serious (see p. 139 and Fig. 8-2). The use of Group O Rh positive blood whose titer is low, as Crosby and Akeroyd[12] found, rarely causes icterus when the recipient is of another blood group, even when administered in large quantities, unless the recipient suffers from a high degree of impairment in his bilirubin clearance or the blood was old.

COLD AGGLUTININS. When the patient's serum has a high titer of cold agglutinins, the administration of chilled blood usually incites hemolysis of donor cells containing this antigen. As pointed out on page 136, this is an agglutinative and/or hemolytic reaction which may be prevented by warming the donor's blood slowly (several hours) to 37° C. before administering to patients and by the selection of a donor free of cold agglutinins. Hemolytic reactions from cold agglutinins are not generally as severe as those following the transfusion of the incompatibility of the major AB, A, B and O groups or of an Rh positive blood given to a sensitized Rh negative patient. On the other hand, the patient with cold agglutinins appears to acquire this antigen-antibody phenomenon in many instances in association with serious disease, if he does not possess it by inheritance. In the critically ill patient, any reaction is likely to be tolerated poorly and can contribute to, if not occasionally cause, his death.

Hemolytic Reactions from Mismatched Blood. The administration of mismatched blood was undoubtedly one of the most commonly encountered causes of acute hemolysis following blood transfusion prior to about 1940. It should be encountered rarely today. Certainly this accident should occur with a frequency less than 1 in 5,000 to 10,000 transfusions if proper precautions are observed assiduously. In the carefully controlled blood bank, errors of this origin are those of the "irreducibility of human error" (p. 137). Unfortunately, most blood banks do not function this well.

To many physicians, any hemolytic transfusion implies only that a mismatched blood was given. This belief is invalid and is encountered more often among doctors whose clinical experience antedates 1940, prior to the advent of excellent typing sera and our knowledge of the Rh factors. At the same time, the doctor's alarm reaction in this regard is good for all concerned, for the early diagnosis of hemolytic reactions of mismatched bloods is of the greatest importance. It is incumbent upon the attending physician, the house officers and the nursing staff to report such reactions to the blood bank at once so that their nature can be established and the most effective method of treatment implemented immediately. When any transfusion reaction occurs, the transfusion should be discontinued immediately. *Any residual blood in the transfusion equipment should be returned immediately with the transfusion set to the blood bank for analysis.* Too often, the residual blood is discarded or allowed to stand for many hours before returning; not only is valuable time lost but the trail becomes too cold to track down the cause.

Certain clinical features of a hemolytic transfusion reaction are very suggestive that it does or does not arise from the transfusion of mismatched blood. However, these symptoms are not to be considered as diagnostic, as some of them may also occur from a hemolytic reaction of other cause, in the so-called pyrogenic reactions and from blood which is either hemolyzed or bacteriologically contaminated. These symptoms and signs which are suggestive of mismatched blood may be classified as immediate, intermediate and delayed.

The earlier and the more serious the reaction, the more disastrous the consequences are likely to be (Table 4).

Treatment procedures employed in serious incompatible blood transfusion reactions should have some degree of priority. But no form of treatment is as effective as the prevention of the transfusion of mismatched bloods.

1. Discontinue transfusion at once but do not remove the needle in the patient's vein, as peripheral vascular collapse usually makes impossible the reintroduction of a needle into a vein. This creates unnecessary delay in treatment and may necessitate a venous cut-down in order to institute intravenous fluids.

2. Institute immediately an intravenous infusion of 10 per cent glucose in water to induce diuresis. To this should be added, as soon as obtainable, an ampule of sodium lactate containing 4.48 Gm. or 40 mEq. to ensure immediate alkalinization of urine. An acid urine favors the precipitation of an acid hematin and possibly hemoglobin in the renal tubules. If peripheral collapse is present, a second intravenous infusion of glucose is started to which has been added the contents of an ampule containing 4 mg. of norepinephrine. Sufficient volumes of 10 per cent glucose in water to induce a diuresis cannot be administered as rapidly as necessary if the glucose solution also contains norepinephrine. The quantity of norepinephrine given needs to be regulated carefully and therefore to be administered separately (see Chap. 27, Sect. 2).

3. If respiratory difficulty occurs, particularly a severe asthmatic attack, 25 mg. of ephedrine sulfate should be administered intravenously if peripheral collapse is present. Should the blood pressure be normal, 50 mg. of this drug may be administered intramuscularly unless the attack is abating.

Nasal oxygen should be instituted promptly if cyanosis is present.

5. Analgesia and occasionally sedation may be required. Generally, 7.5 mg. of intravenously administered morphine sulfate for the 70 Kg. patient produces an effective analgesia and is the agent preferred by this author.

6. A 30 ml. sample of the patient's blood is withdrawn as soon as practical and centrifuged to check for the presence of hemoglobinemia. Sufficient blood is obtained to resubmit the patient's blood to the blood bank for checking and identity of blood groups. Also a portion is sent to the clinical laboratory for analysis of the nitrogen as well as urea nitrogen determinations; these 2 chemical determinations provide baseline data for subsequent comparisons should renal function be seriously impaired within the days to follow.

7. The donor's blood should also be rechecked and cultured for bacterial growth.

TABLE 4. SIGNS AND SYMPTOMS SUGGESTING INCOMPATIBLE BLOOD TRANSFUSION REACTION

IMMEDIATE (FIRST FEW MINUTES)	INTERMEDIATE (20 MINUTES TO 2 HOURS)	DELAYED (2 HOURS TO 24 HOURS)
1. Acute anaphylaxis	1. Pain in lumbar area	1. Chills and fever
2. Acute dyspnea and/or asthma, usually with cyanosis	2. Chills and fever	2. Hemoglobinemia and hemoglobinuria are likely overlooked unless checked for within the first 2 to 4 hours
3. Peripheral vascular collapse	3. Restlessness and hypotension	3. Oliguria, often followed by anuria in less than 24 hours
4. Hemoglobinemia	4. Hemoglobinemia	4. Anemia and icterus
5. Hemoglobinuria	5. Hemoglobinuria	

8. An indwelling catheter is placed in the urinary bladder to provide a means for the hourly measurement of urine flow and the early detection of hemoglobinuria. The importance of the hourly record of the urinary output cannot be overemphasized. A patient may secrete as much as 1,000 ml. of urine within the first 6 hours after his transfusion reaction, only to develop complete renal shutdown thereafter. Consequently, if urine volume is measured on the 24-hour schedule, 18 hours or more may elapse before renal shutdown is detected. This information bears directly upon the subsequent volumes and characteristics of the fluids to be administered intravenously or by mouth. (See Chap. 48, "Urology," the section on Acute Renal Failure.) Hourly records are essential.

9. Avoid the infusion of electrolytes, except when their need is demonstrated by reliable chemical data.

PYROGENIC REACTIONS

Febrile reactions occur in association with the administration of any intravenous fluids, including blood and plasma. They have been recognized as long as transfusions have been employed. Halsted, in 1883, describing a transfusion given in the treatment of monoxide poisoning, remarked: "the usual post-transfusion recurrence lasted for half an hour."[19] Jean Baptiste Denis was nearly beheaded for the same reason 200 years earlier!

Seiver[56] demonstrated that certain nonpathogenic bacteria often multiply in distilled water and cause fever when injected into animals. For many years in the preparation of intravenous fluids it was assumed that bacterial cultivation in distilled water was unlikely. This proved to be an error. All fluids for parenteral use should be prepared from freshly distilled water only and autoclaved promptly prior to storage.

A second common source of pyrogens are the chemical contaminants in intravenous tubing, glassware or unclean needles. Now that most blood banks employ disposable administration sets, pyrogenic reactions have largely disappeared.

Pyrogenic reactions are characterized by fever and/or chills, occasionally by lumbar pain and rarely by peripheral collapse. If blood is refrigerated promptly when drawn, and if disposable sets are employed for administration, pyrogenic reactions should not exceed an incidence of 2 per cent of transfusions given— preferably less. Generally, pyrogenic reactions are mild and not serious, but, as stated above, any reaction in the debilitated or critically ill patients can be disastrous.

If the reaction occurs while blood or plasma is still in the process of administration, the infusion fluid should be discontinued. The chill may be partially controlled by the intravenous injection of 1 Gm. of calcium gluconate combined with 7.5 mg. of morphine sulfate by vein. Some have reported benefit from the administration of certain of the antihistaminic drugs.

ALLERGIC REACTIONS

Urticarial or allergic reactions are characterized by the appearance of hives and occasionally by attacks of angioneurotic edema and asthma. The exact mechanism of this phenomenon is not clearly understood. Occasionally, a patient, sensitive to a particular food or drug, will display urticarial or allergic reactions when the donor has eaten a food recently or is under a drug therapy to which the patient is sensitive. For example, the donor may have eaten tomatoes or shrimp recently, or he may be under sulfonamide therapy to which the patient is sensitive. Then the recipient may develop urticaria, angioneurotic edema or an acute asthmatic attack.

Reactions of this type generally occur in less than 1 per cent of the patients transfused with either blood or plasma. The administration of calcium gluconate is often beneficial if given promptly. In more severe reactions, especially asthmatic attacks, antihistaminics and/or ephedrine sulfate may be administered. In general, reactions of this type are not serious.

CIRCULATORY OVERLOAD

Circulatory overload from excessive transfusion is seldom seen in surgical patients undergoing an operation. This does not imply that the circulation cannot be overloaded, for it can be. The volume of blood lost at operation or in trauma is underestimated much more often than it is overestimated; therefore, overload is seldom encountered under these conditions. Circulatory overload is observed more commonly in the course of preoperative transfusions where an attempt is made to correct anemia or hypoproteinemia with blood and/or plasma being administered either too rapidly or in too large a volume at one time. However, it is remarkable that even under these circumstances this complication seldom occurs. Its failure to do so is excellent testimony to the ability of the vascular system to compensate for the increase in blood volume if fluids are not administered too rapidly and if cardiopulmonary reserve is reasonable. Generally, little if any increase in plasma volume can be detected 6 hours after the administration of a liter of plasma. The water in transfused blood or plasma is lost from the circulation fairly rapidly, either by diffusion into the extravascular spaces or via the kidneys as urine. Overload from plasma transfusions is less likely to be encountered than from blood, where the transfused red cells remain within the circulation. The transfusion of blood is tolerated best in patients with anemia, provided that they are without marginal cardiovascular reserve; the increase in total blood volume probably is compensated in part by the rapid disappearance from the circulation of plasma and water contained in whole blood transfusions.

The symptoms of circulatory overload are those of left-sided heart failure and pulmonary congestion and/or edema. This complication can be rapidly fatal if not recognized promptly and treated appropriately. Its treatment may consist of the intravenous administration of digitalis preparations in patients with marginal cardiovascular function. It may be necessary also to perform phlebotomy promptly. But first one should apply the usual blood pressure tourniquets to 3 of the 4 extremities, elevating the constricting pressure above that of the systolic blood pressure. By rotating one tourniquet to the unconstricted extremity once every 20 minutes, no extremity remains occluded for more than 1 hour at a time.

ABNORMAL BLEEDING

Abnormal bleeding is occasionally a disastrous complication of blood transfusions. Its pathogenesis is by no means clearly understood, although certain disorders in coagulation can be detected in some patients. The importance of such a defect probably varies from patient to patient. This is principally a complication of transfusions administered during operation and is seen more frequently under hypothermic than under normothermic conditions.

The clinical pattern is frightening indeed. The exposed surfaces suddenly begin to ooze blood from even the minutest of vessels. Death may occur in a few hours in spite of any treatment.

Although abnormal bleeding of this type generally is encountered more frequently in patients receiving massive transfusions in the course of an operative procedure, occasionally it is observed when only 1 or 2 transfusions have been administered. Characteristically, the blood is unusually dark in spite of the administration of oxygen in seemingly adequate quantities or of the type of anesthesia employed. Its appearance is also unusual in that clotting appears to be delayed; the blood appears less viscid than usual. As puddles of blood accumulate in the tissues or on drapes, coagulation generally takes place. Coagulation will not take place at all if the fibrogen also has been destroyed. Once this condition occurs, the continued administration of blood seems to be more harmful than beneficial; the author prefers to change to plasma but for no well-documented reason. Continued effort at hemostasis appears to be essentially hopeless, for the bleeding points are so numerous as to preclude satisfactory hemostasis by the ligature technic.

Blood samples examined under these conditions generally disclose more than one type of clotting disorder. The platelet count is usually at near thrombocytopenic levels (10,000 to 50,000 per cu. mm.). Prothrombin activity also may be depressed sharply, and in some patients the circulating heparinlike anticoagulant may be found.[49]

Another of the more important disorders is that of an increased tendency of the fibrin clots to undergo lysis. The enzyme responsible for lysis appears to be similar to, if not identical with, that normally present in the activate fibrinolytic (plasmin) system. Fibrinolysin normally exists as a relatively inactive substance; its precursor is abundantly present in plasma and is known as profibrinolysin. Although it is normally activated at all times, its rate of activation in the course of thrombin generation or fibrin formation is accelerated. In the highly active fibrinolytic state, fibrinogen and, to some extent, prothrombin are attacked as well as fibrin. Therefore, fibrinogen and prothrombin deficiencies also may exist along with thrombocytopenia.

There is also normally present an inhibitor of fibrinolysin known as antifibrinolysin (antiplasmin). An increasing fibrinolytic activity may result then from two mechanisms. There may be an actual increase in the rate at which fibrinolysin is activated, or fibrinolysin may accumulate because it is not destroyed by its inhibitor—antifibrinolysin or both.

The inhibitor apparently is produced by the liver. In far-advanced liver disease, the loss of the inhibitor appears to account for some of the fibrinolytic states described. The prostatic secretions contain the fibrinolytic enzyme or a similar enzyme whose properties affect fibrin, fibrinogen and prothrombin in a manner indistinguishable from that of fibrinolysin. Abnormal bleeding from the prostatic bed is often from the fibrinolysin of prostatic origin but is mistaken for poor mechanical hemostasis. General hemorrhagic states characterized by lysis of both fibrinogen and fibrin were first observed by the author in 1949 in patients with metastatic prostatic carcinoma irrespective of surgical operations. A number of others have reported similar cases. In general, such patients are encountered infrequently.

The hemorrhagic complication of abruptio placenta is one illustration of a highly activated fibrinolytic system.[55] Fibrinogen also may disappear completely from the circulation. It is believed that fibrinogen is exhausted by the formation of multiple small thrombi throughout the circulation, caused by the introduction of thromboplastic juices of placental origin entering the circulation spontaneously under these conditions. It is possible to coagulate experimentally all of the fibrinogen within the circulation over a period of 15 minutes or less without fatal embolism. Minute quantities of fibrin can be demonstrated in the capillary bed of the liver, the lungs and the kidneys. Platelets are trapped in these thrombi and probably account for the acute thrombopenia. The plasma remaining is essentially circulating serum and has considerable increase in fibrinolytic activity.

Although the exact mechanism which excites the state of fibrinolytic activity in transfusions at operation is not known, it may be due to the entrance of thromboplastic substances into the circulation, either from the operative bed or from an unrecognized transfusion reaction with release of thromboplastic materials.

To establish an accurate diagnosis when abnormal bleeding is occurring so extensively in the course of an operation is essentially impossible. Consequently, the surgeon is driven to the use of certain antihemorrhagic agents empirically, hoping that at least one or more of the compounds employed will control the bleeding diathesis. The author prefers to administer at least 5 to 7 Gm. of fibrinogen intravenously, given in less than 30 minutes' time. Concurrently, 100 mg. of protamine sulfate is administered into another vein over a 10-minute period to combat a possible concurrent heparinoid effect. Protamine sulfate and fibrinogen should not be given in the same flask or through the same tubing. Then fibrinogen administration is continued at the rate of 2 to 4 Gm. an hour for several hours if required. Platelet transfusions are very helpful but seldom available.

The all-important feature of this type of abnormal bleeding in the surgical patient receiving blood is its self-limiting nature. Consequently, prompt and heroic measures with reference to the administration of these three agents are imperative. If they prove to be effective, the patient will recover, and further hemorrhage is unlikely to recur. The surgeon should check with the anesthesiologist to make certain that adequate calcium gluconate has been administered in the course of transfusions to obviate the possibility of citrate intoxication.

CITRATE INTOXICATION

On repeated occasions during the past 40 years, warnings have been issued that toxic concentrations of citrate occasionally occur following the use of citrated blood or plasma transfusion. Abnormal bleeding, hypotension and other difficulties relative to the depletion of the calcium ion have been suggested. The earlier advocates of this view were answered readily by the studies of Lewisohn from 30 to 40 years ago. Within the past 15 years, however, when more extensive elective or traumatic surgery has been made possible by the liberal use of citrated blood and plasma, it has not been so easy to deny that citrate intoxication might not occur in the occasional patient.

In 1944, a study of all patients receiving transfusions where the amount of citrate ranged from 7.6 to 40.0 Gm. disclosed no evidence at the University of Chicago that bleeding attributable to citrate had occurred.[3] This study was followed by an experimental study by Adams, Thornton, Allen and Gonzalez[2] on dogs. They demonstrated that dogs given large doses of sodium citrate would develop tetany very rapidly and die unless extra sources of calcium ion were made available, but hemorrhage was not noted except during the agonal state. Tetany appeared before coagulation was retarded and proved to be an excellent indication as to when calcium gluconate therapy should be instituted in their studies, but only when the animals were under light or no general anesthesia. With deep anesthesia tetany was absent.

Practically, these observations led to routine administration of 1 Gm. of calcium gluconate after the 2nd or the 3rd transfusion during surgery involving rapid blood loss and entailing rapid infusion of citrated blood as replacement therapy. One precaution is necessary; the calcium gluconate must be administered through a separate venous infusion set; if added to the blood transfusion, coagulation of the blood in the transfusion container occurs. No evidence of calcium intoxication has been observed with this regimen.

Although it is doubtful that calcium gluconate so administered prevents the occasional hemorrhage associated with blood transfusion, it may be useful in reducing toxic effects of excessive citrate, and we have continued its use for 12 years. As late as 1955, reports continue to indict citrate intoxication,[10] but a review of the data published disclosed that only infrequent attempts were made at calcium replacement in patients receiving massive transfusions in brief periods of time. Better results can be achieved if severe calcium depletion is prevented by the intermittent administration of calcium gluconate to prevent citrate intoxication and if reasonable attempts at surgical hemostasis are carried out so that less blood is needed.

It is possible that patients under hypo-thermic anesthesia or with severe liver disease may detoxify citrate at a much slower rate than normal. However, in the author's experience, the administration of 1 Gm. of calcium gluconate for each 2 transfusions administered in the operating room has given rise to no suspicion that citrate intoxication has occurred in any of our patients during the past 12 years. This may not apply to hypothermic anesthesia.

BACTERIAL CONTAMINATION

Borden and Hall[7] describe 2 fatal reactions from blood transfusion containing massive numbers of bacteria. Other reports have described similar accidents. The principal feature in these circumstances is peripheral vascular collapse. The organisms generally cultured have been of the coliform or Pseudomonas families, although other organisms also have been involved.

It is inevitable that an occasional unit of blood will be contaminated with some bacteria. When blood is stored under conditions of refrigeration, bacterial growth is slow, but when storage is prolonged, the problem of contamination can be a serious but infrequently encountered one.

Braude and collaborators[8] studied the problem of bacterial contamination in donor blood and the rates of growth of various organisms in citrated blood under refrigerated conditions. Although they encountered in approximately 2 per cent of their bloods bacterial contamination, growth of bacteria under conditions of refrigeration was infrequent. Nonetheless, a number of organisms were found to grow slowly but continuously in refrigerated citrated blood. Some of their contaminated bloods exhibited coagulation, and they suggest that the presence of a clot in *aged* blood serves as a useful indication that the unit may be contaminated. Bacterial contamination is seldom a hazard, if blood is less than 2 weeks in age and has been stored properly under refrigerated conditions. However, it is one that will arise with increasing frequency as it becomes possible to store liquid blood for longer periods of time. This occurrence can be minimized by the employment of adequate aseptic precautions and, if necessary, culture technics.

Hyperkalemia. One of the features of aging blood is the diffusion of potassium into plasma from the erythrocytes. Diffusion of this ion continues at a fairly steady rate from the moment the cells of citrated blood are withdrawn until they are given. As potassium in blood is largely an intracellular erythrocyte cation, plasma potassium levels are higher in hemolyzed blood but may increase by diffusion to as much as 10 times the normal level by diffusion alone, with little or no evidence of concurrent hemolysis. It is a safe assumption that the greater the degree of hemolysis of refrigerated blood, the greater the concentration of potassium in its plasma. Concentration of potassium in citrated blood stored under refrigeration with little or no evidence of hemolysis may reach levels as high as 35 to 40 mg. per cent (9 to 10 mEq. per liter).[42]

The diffusion of potassium into the plasma of aging blood occurs at a slower rate when glucose is added to the citrate solution into which blood is drawn. There is some evidence that the addition of glucose to the hyperkalemic plasma of aged blood can drive potassium back into the cells, but thus far the addition of glucose to outdated blood has not proved to be a practical technic in blood banking practices. More useful to this end is the decanting of plasma in aged blood (2 to 3 weeks of age) and administration of packed red cells or their resuspension in dextran or isotonic saline solution, should one be concerned with this type of hyperkalemia.

The possibility that potassium intoxication will result from the transfusion of large volumes of aged blood is difficult to assess. Melrose and Wilson[42] were unable to detect any significant changes in electrocardiographic tracings attributable to potassium intoxication when aged blood with elevated potassium concentration in the plasma was administered. It should be remembered that the increased serum potassium levels of the patient under abnormal conditions is largely at the expense of his intracellular potassium and often is associated with a depletion of intracellular protein. It may be that hyperkalemia from blood transfusion in the nondepleted patient is tolerated better in man than is generally believed. Much of the evidence of potassium intoxication or depletion has been obtained in the burned or traumatized patient or in the patient under corticoid therapy or with adrenal insufficiency.

Although many deaths, including those of cardiac arrest, occur in the course of the use of massive transfusions, there is insufficient evidence at the present time to warrant withholding blood that is 2 to 3 weeks old in the fear that the increase in potassium concentration within the plasma of aged blood is often, if ever, a cause. Once again, the excellent results obtained by Crosby and Akeroyd[12] are to be cited, for in their use of 10 to 30 pints of blood in the Korean war, the chief source of their Rh positive Group O blood was that drawn in this country, flown to Korea, in which the agitation of the blood in flight should be expected to favor an accelerated hemolysis and hyperkalemia. No suggestion of potassium intoxication was reported among the recipients.

Schechter, Nealon and Gibbon (1959) and McLaughlin, Nealon and Gibbon (1960) presented an ingenious technic to remove excessive potassium and ammonium from bank blood prior to transfusion. This method may help in solving the problem of such excess in instances of blood subjected to prolonged storage.

Intra-arterial Transfusion. Some have advocated the intra-arterial route for the rapid administration of banked blood as a means for minimizing the potential potassium intoxication of this origin.[42] Originally this technic was suggested as a means for achieving an increase in the arterial blood, increasing more rapidly the volume of blood constrained by the aortic valve at one end and the arteriolar peripheral resistance at the other. This benefit is largely a theoretical one if the intravenous infusion is given at the same rate as the intra-arterial transfusion.[40]

Aged blood administered intra-arterially has the benefit of greater dilution by its passage through the peripheral circulation before reaching the heart and the coronary circulation than when administered by the intravenous route. This suggestion in principle is doubtlessly correct, but until it can be shown that the elevated serum potassium concentration of this origin in the nondepleted recipient is definitely harmful, this consideration is not sufficient to advocate use of the intra-arterial route of transfusion. Arterial transfusions carry certain special hazards which seemingly are not compensated for by any demonstrated superiority over that of blood administered at the same rate by vein.[40] Among the reported hazards by intra-arterial blood is arterial damage with gangrene of the extremity peripheral to the arterial puncture, as well as the need for greater technical skill in the introduction of the intra-arterial needle; the latter introduces the hazard of delay as well as that of arterial injury. Although certain other theoretical considerations have been advocated for the intra-arterial route of administration of blood in the patient in peripheral collapse, such as reducing the hazard from air ambolus, should this occur, and the reported greater ease with which the artery may be entered in shock, the author does not recommend or employ this route for blood administration.

THE SINGLE TRANSFUSION AND ITS MULTIPLE HAZARDS

The adult surgical patient (70 Kg.) receiving one unit of blood represents one of the most frequent abuses of blood transfusions currently encountered. If acute blood loss from any cause has been excessive, the treatment of the hypovolemic shock incurred usually requires administration of several to many blood transfusions if shock is to be treated successfully. On the other hand, if one transfusion is sufficient to restore and maintain the normal blood pressure, it is probable that liquid plasma, heated albumin, or dextran would have served equally well. These fluids do not carry the risks entailed in crossmatching, the identification of the patient, or the transmission of homologous serum jaundice. The case reports on pages 134 and 139 illustrated 2 of the hazards in blood transfusion. In both instances, these occurred from the elective or nonessential use of a transfusion; one terminated fatally. Another hazard which ended in death is also illustrated by the following case report in a patient receiving *one* transfusion. In retrospect, this transfusion may not have been essential.[25]

A 61-year-old man was admitted to the University of Chicago Clinics on January 26, 1953,

having been in coma for 1 day. 80 days previously, in his community hospital, he was operated upon for ruptured appendicitis. During the operation, one transfusion of whole blood was administered. His postoperative course was a stormy one, as he was a severe diabetic.

At the time of admission to the University of Chicago Clinics, he was deeply icteric. The abdomen was soft, normal peristaltic sounds were heard, and the blood pressure was 70/58 mm. of mercury. Laboratory studies disclosed a leukocyte count of 16,750 with a hemoglobin level at 10.5 Gm.100 cc. of blood. Emergency treatment was instituted immediately; it consisted of plasma, glucose and saline administration, as well as norepinephrine. The patient did not respond and succumbed a few hours later.

From the autopsy examination it was concluded that the cause of death was acute necrosis of the liver, presumably from homologous serum jaundice. Histologic examination showed that only a few scattered islands of parenchymal cells remained. There was no evidence of bile duct obstruction.

The circumstances of the patient responsible for the decision to employ a blood transfusion in the course of appendectomy can be assessed only by the surgeon in the course of his operation. However, the decision to use the transfusion was also the decision eventually to be responsible for the patient's death. At the University of Chicago Clinics, where 84 patients have developed homologous serum jaundice from whole blood transfusions, 38 received but *one* unit of blood! The circumstances under which these 38 transfusions were given suggest that some other fluid or medication with less hazard probably would have served the patient's needs equally well in many, if not in most, instances better. When transfusion accidents occur under these circumstances, it is often difficult in retrospect to satisfy all concerned that the use of one transfusion was actually justified. The benefits expected from the single transfusion seldom outweigh the risk entailed when administered to adult patients.

These remarks are not intended as an indictment of blood transfusion when blood is needed, for if this is the surgeon's response, he immediately becomes the victim and the source of another important abuse of blood transfusion—that of administering too little and too late. The risk entailed in multiple transfusions in the treatment of hypovolemic shock, while increasing at an arithmetic rate, is accepted much more readily, provided that every reasonable precaution in the administration of blood has been observed.

The adult patient receiving the isolated 500 ml. transfusion is by no means restricted to surgical patients alone. Many patients with iron deficiency anemia are given the single transfusion on medical services when suitable preparations of iron in conjunction with a diet adequate in proteins, vitamins and calories would serve equally well. Although there always will remain a small risk in blood transfusion which is beyond the pale of human endeavor to prevent, the physician is in a much more defensible position when such accidents occur in patients in whom the question of need for blood cannot be challenged.

SPECIAL TRANSFUSIONS

Under certain circumstances it may be desirable to administer "washed" red cell concentrates, platelet transfusions, freshly prepared citrate transfusions and in some instances "direct" transfusions wherein no anticoagulant is employed as well as to employ exchange transfusions.

EXCHANGE TRANSFUSIONS

Such transfusions are limited principally to 3 general types of disorders: (1) those wherein the patient's hemoglobin has been rendered incapable of carrying oxygen; (2) that of eliminating or reducing insofar as possible the abnormally sensitized blood cells of the infant suffering from erythroblastosis foetalis; and (3) the surgical patient whose volume of operative blood loss is excessive and the replacement volume assumes exchange proportions in an attempt to sustain life by supporting the blood volume until hemorrhage is under control and the vital signs become stabilized.

Erythroblastosis foetalis was first explained on a rational basis by Landsteiner[29] and developed by Levine, his pupil, in a series of papers.[32] They attributed this disease to Rh positive cells which enter the mother's circulation from the fetus, she having Rh negative blood and being vulnerable. It has been presumed with good evidence that the blood antigen is the Rh positive red cell of the infant

in most instances and that in the course of pregnancy, small quantities of the infant's blood enter the maternal circulation by one means or another. The production of Rh antibodies is thereby stimulated in the Rh negative mother. These maternal antibodies then pass freely across the placental barrier, inducing hemolysis of the infant's red cells and other serious disorders.

Erythroblastosis foetalis is treated by means of exchange transfusions as soon after birth as the diagnosis is made. The purpose of blood exchange in this disease is to remove the infant's own red cells which are sensitized to the maternal anti-Rh antibodies which have been transmitted across the placental barrier. The use of exchange transfusions in this disease has reduced effectively the incidence of kernicterus, although jaundice alone probably is not responsible for the damaged basal nuclei often associated with this disease. Exchange transfusions where severe hydroptic changes have occurred prenatally have little to offer. The diagnosis of impending erythroblastosis is anticipated by a detection of a rise in anti-Rh titer within the maternal blood. Other antigens are also believed to be responsible occasionally for this disease in some patients.

If treatment is to succeed, exchange transfusions should be commenced within the first hours of infant life. Into the umbilical vein is threaded a polyethylene catheter, and the exchange is carried out by repeatedly withdrawing 20 ml. of the infant's blood and replacing this with 20 ml. of donor blood until from 300 to 500 ml. have been transferred. The donor considered best suited is an Rh negative individual of the same blood group who has no Rh antibodies. Intermittently, calcium gluconate is administered to prevent possible citrate intoxication (p. 147). In some instances, repetition of the exchange may be necessary on several occasions during the first day or two. Generally, the umbilical vein can be re-entered, but should it be thrombosed by that time, a femoral vein may be used.

Monoxide poisoning is the other usual reason for the use of exchange tranfusions. In this instance, as in other types of hemoglobin poisoning affecting its oxygen-carrying capacity of red cells, the immediate problem is to provide compatible donor cells in sufficient quantity to meet oxygen transport needs. No problem of isosensitization exists in these patients. In many instances, 2 or 3 units of blood promptly given in monoxide poisoning is all that is necessary. In the course of their administration, bloodletting can be instituted to avoid circulatory overload. Because of the extreme urgency, the use of Group O Rh negative blood without resorting to typing may be necessary in many instances. Generally, if the transfer of 40 to 50 per cent of the patient's estimated blood volume in monoxide or similar types of poisoning does not prove to be beneficial, further exchange is likely to be fruitless.

DIRECT TRANSFUSIONS

A "direct" transfusion, as opposed to "indirect" one, refers to the rapid intravascular transfer of blood from the donor to the recipient without the use of an anticoagulant. This, of course, is the type of transfusion used early and was one of the reasons why blood transfusion was such a formidable procedure prior to the citrate era. Any specific merit that this procedure has over the more deliberate and carefully planned citrated transfusion is sharply limited, if indeed a benefit actually does exist other than in the hemophiliac patient.

Many clinicians believe that direct transfusion has certain beneficial properties in the treatment of patients with abnormal bleeding that are not possible with freshly prepared citrated blood or plasma. The available facts do not support this contention, except for the treatment of hemophilia, assuming that the citrated blood is less than a day or two in age. Of greater importance is the fact that the *in vivo* turnover times are so rapid that their beneficial effect is evanescent (Figs. 8-3 and 8-4) in many of the clotting disorders.

The *in vitro* stability of the more important clotting factors in citrated blood under refrigeration is about as follows:

Fibrinogen and prothrombin are comparatively stable for several days.

Prothrombin is active for less than a week.

Factor V or Accelerator Globulin are more labile, generally less stable, but continue to be active for a few days.

Platelets adhere to the sides of glassware ordinarily used in transfusions, and blood transfusions of this type are useless in attempting the correction of thrombocytopenia (p. 153). The antihemophiliac factor is highly labile, but apparently no more so in citrated blood freshly drawn than in blood without anticoagulants. The myriads of other reported clotting factors need not be considered now. They offer little opportunity for clinical trial at this time, as their identity is not established, and the cause and the consequence of their deficiencies has not been determined.

PACKED AND/OR WASHED RED CELLS

Under certain circumstances, it may be advisable to administer "packed" red cells. The unit of blood is centrifuged, its plasma withdrawn, and only the red cell mass is transferred. Several units of transfused packed red cells will permit the rapid correction of anemia with only about half of the volume entailed when whole blood is given. However, the use of packed cells in this connection overlooks the fact that transfused plasma diffuses rapidly from the circulation of the recipient when whole blood is given. Plasma is of considerable nutritive value, whereas red cells are metabolized very slowly (see below). In essence, the patient retains the transfused red cells for days to weeks, whereas plasma in transfusions leaves the circulation in a matter of hours. Thus the patient performs his own plasmapheresis and thereby packs the transfused red cells himself. One should remember that packed red cell transfusions are nearly twice as effective in blood volume expansion as compared with whole blood. Therefore, if the circulation is not to be overloaded, only half the volume of packed cells should be transfused when compared with whole blood. The use of red cell concentrates in the patients with cardiac disease suffering from severe anemia does have definite advantages over that of whole blood. Undoubtedly, anemia under these conditions is corrected more safely by the administration of red cell transfusions. Not only are smaller volumes required but red cell concentrates carry a minimum of sodium chloride. Some maintain that fewer pyrogenic reactions occur following transfusions of red cells than when whole blood is given; at best, these data show only a minor difference in rates of reactions and are not observed consistently or generally in most patients.

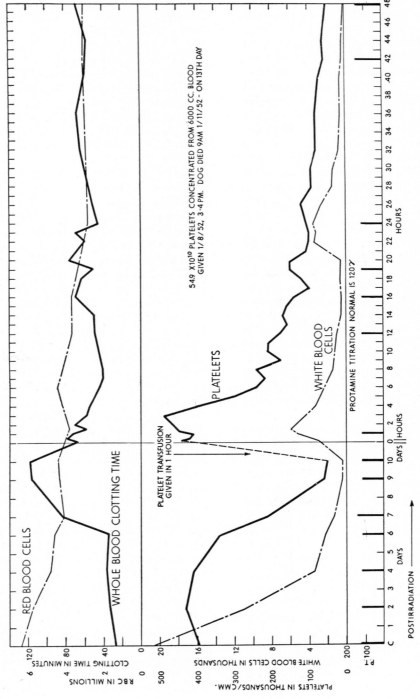

Fig. 8-3. Platelet transfusion. Illustrating the rapid declines in platelet count after platelet transfusions. Animals were rendered thrombocytopenic by total body radiation.

Most advocates of transfusion of red cell suspensions believe it to be the treatment of choice for anemia when the blood volume is normal. However, unless the anemia cannot be treated otherwise by appropriate medication, or its rapid correction is essential before surgery can be undertaken safely; the use of transfusions under these conditions carries in addition to the risk of errors incurred in typing and crossmatching the unpreventable hazard of transmission of homologous serum jaundice. Hence, in the decision to employ blood transfusions for the correction of anemia alone, whether as packed red cells or whole blood, the risk of transfusion hazards must be weighed carefully against the benefits expected, the needs of the patient, and the possibility that these needs can or cannot be met satisfactorily by alternative procedures (iron, liver, vitamin B_{12} and a sound diet). Of the 3 case reports included in this chapter (pp. 134, 139 and 149) illustrating the hazards of blood transfusion, 2 were employed for the correction of anemia alone. In retrospect, both patients could have been treated conservatively with greater safety.

If the anemia can be treated only by transfusion or with greater safety—for many patients this is the case—blood transfusion as packed red cells or whole blood should be used without hesitation. On the other hand, the use of the "cosmetic" transfusion carries too great a risk to warrant its use. This risk does not exist when conservative therapy and a little patience will do equally well or better. The cosmetic transfusion constitutes one of the major abuses of blood transfusion in many hospitals.

Platelet Transfusions

Platelet transfusions can be prepared which permit the transfusion of platelet concentrates. Many units of fresh blood are needed to accumulate sufficient platelets for transfusion purposes if the resulting platelet concentrates are to elevate the platelet count in thrombocytopenic patients.[15] Unfortunately, the increased thrombocyte level achieved is transient, lasting for only a day or two (Fig. 8-3). In the author's opinion, platelet transfusions present interesting opportunities for physiologic studies, but there is little current evidence that they offer essential therapeutic

assistance in the preparation of the thrombocytopenic patient for splenectomy necessitated by hyperplenism. In fact, once the diagnosis of idiopathic thrombocytopenia is made, usually there is greater safety to the patient in prompt splenectomy than in delaying until platelet concentrates can be prepared. Platelet concentrates are better delayed until after splenectomy and transfused then only if the platelet count does not rise promptly and bleeding continues.

Platelet transfusions in the bleeding patient who suffers from thrombocytopenic purpura of other origin, i.e., leukemia, aplasia of marrow, etc., is also a measure of temporary therapeutic value. To continue such transfusions for more than a few days soon presents problems in blood procurement that are not likely to be surmounted (Fig. 8-3).

Fibrinogen Transfusion

In afibrinogenemia, whether congenital or acquired, or from acute fibrinolysis, the transfusion of the fibrinogen (Cohn Fraction I) offers an immediate means for the restoration of the plasma fibrinogen concentration and effectively controls hemorrhage of this origin for short periods of time (see p. 145, Abnormal Bleeding and Transfusion). Because of the high incidence of serum hepatitis, fibrinogen transfusions should be used only when in the clinical judgment of the surgeon the potential advantages outweigh the risk.

Plasma Transfusion

Its Development, Use and Problems in the Treatment of Hypovolemic Shock. Although serum transfusions in the treatment of hypovolemic shock had been employed prior to the turn of the century, the need for serum or plasma as a substitute for blood transfusion did not receive serious attention prior to World War I. Abel, Rowntree and Turner[1] demonstrated that healthy dogs withstood great losses of blood when they were infused quickly with plasma. Rous and Wilson[50] reported that rabbits could be bled down to a hemoglobin concentration of 20 per cent of the initial level when plasma infusions were given as replacement. They pointed out that at slightly lower hemoglobin concentrations, death occurred with regularity. They did not believe that death was due to lack of oxygen-carrying power but rather to the inability to maintain "blood bulk," which we now call blood volume. Today these conclusions may appear as an oversimplification. Most agree that a blood loss of more than 15 per cent of the calculated total from acute hemorrhage in man requires that a major portion of the replacement therapy be in the form of whole blood transfusion rather than as plasma therapy. Nonetheless, all agree that in the absence of available blood for transfusion, pooled plasma or intravenous 6 per cent albumin therapy are the safest and most effective blood substitutes currently available (see Chap. 7, "Shock").

Plasma Preparation. Ward[65] urged the use of plasma as a substitute for blood transfusion in the treatment of shock late in World War I. He believed that the risk of blood transfusion remained too high and that suitable donors and typing facilities were seldom available when such emergencies developed. He believed that plasma always should be on hand and would serve as a substitute until blood transfusion could be prepared and carried out safely.

Rous and Wilson[50] maintained that the loss of fluid from the tissues and the organs was as important as the loss of blood per se, "a fact long known to the physiologist." However, it was recognized by these investigators that replacement of intravascular fluid had little to offer unless the fluid was one bearing colloids. The failure of replacement therapy when it consisted of glucose, saline and/or of Ringer's solution, was correctly attributed to its rapid departure from the vascular bed to the tissues or to its rapid loss in the urine, the latter escape of such fluids being of much less consequence than that lost into the tissues.

The basic discoveries relating to the important distinction between colloid-bearing fluids as opposed to crystalloids were those made by Starling in 1896[59] and by Claude Bernard as early as 1859. To Starling belongs the credit for first having demonstrated that the crystalloids of blood (plasma) and water pass very rapidly into the extravascular spaces and tissues in contrast with the colloids of plasma. The latter were shown to escape much more slowly. In consequence, Starling concluded that there exists normally a protein gradient across the vascular walls, often referred to as "oncotic pressure." He believed that this phenomenon tended to draw water into vessels from the tissues. At the arteriolar end of the capillaries, the blood pressure being higher than the oncotic pressure, water and crystalloids tend to enter the extravascular spaces. On the venous side, the oncotic pressure exceeds that of blood pressure so that reversal of flow occurs; thus, fluid normally enters and leaves the circulation at a homeostatic rate.

Although more recent developments indicate the diffusion or fluid exchange to be more complex, Starling's observations have lost none of their original importance. With his observations available as common knowledge at the time of World War I, it should come as no surprise that artificial colloid-bearing fluids should have been employed more extensively in the clinical treatment of shock among the wounded soldiers than plasma, whose properties, availability and large scale preparation were yet to be developed.

Strumia, Wagner, and Monaghan[61] revived the interest in plasma as a blood substitute in 1940, but its usefulness was hampered to some extent because of the iso-agglutinin titer of unpooled plasma. Type-to-type plasma was originally used by many. The delay in plasma administration incurred by the time required for typing aborted any benefits that plasma might have. All acknowledged that a transfusion of properly typed blood could be prepared within the same period of time and had the advantage that it accomplished complete replacement.

With the advent of World War II, once again interest in plasma as a blood substitute came into the foreground. Its stability was well recognized, and this afforded the great advantage of indefinite storage, particularly if lyophilized.[16] Drying of plasma lent itself well to large-scale plasma production for several reasons. If bacterial contamination of the donors' blood occurred, this was of little consequence, for if the lyophile process was carried out promptly, bacterial growth could not occur. Plasma dried by this process could be reconstituted readily and was available for instant use. The goal of stock-piling of emergencies was now a reality. Further encouragement came with the demonstration by Levinson and Cronheim[34] that, by pooling the plasma from many donors, the risk of encountering a high iso-agglutinin from any one donor was minimized by virtue of dilution in the sum total of the pool. Pooling had the additional advantage in that it greatly facilitated the commercial production of plasma. The result was the preparation of some 15 million units of lyophilized pooled plasma in this country for military use during World War II. Pools consisted generally of the plasma from 300 to 400 donors. The liberal use of this product undoubtedly played an important part in the reduction of mortality among soldiers surviving long enough to be reached, transfused and evacuated for more definitive care (see Chap. 23, "Military Surgery"). However, the plasma story was not to end here, for already the serious complication of homologous serum jaundice was becoming evident.

Homologous Serum Jaundice. This complication, previously mentioned for blood transfusion, is of much more serious consequence for pooled plasma. The presence of this virus in the carrier donor cannot be detected by any method at present. Because the blood of one carrier goes to only one recipient when the donor's blood is transfused as such, only one recipient is exposed. The hazard for pooled plasma proved to be of much more serious consequence because the plasma from one donor carrying the virus contaminates the entire plasma pool and exposes all of its recipients to the disease. The virus carrier rate among healthy donors appears to be about 1 donor among every 150 to 200, and the attack rate among recipients of blood or plasma containing virus appears to be approximately on the order of 25 per cent. It is obvious that many of the recipients of an infected pool of plasma will come down with serum hepatitis; the larger the number of recipients, the greater will be the number coming down with the disease. Actual attack rates among the recipients of a single pool of virus-infected plasma will be about 25 per cent, whereas that for blood alone ranges between 0.2 to 0.5 per cent.[5]

After the war, it became increasingly evident that hepatitis of this origin often carries a morbidity of weeks to months and in a few instances of years' duration and is accompanied by a mortality rate ranging between 5 and 10 per cent. There was nothing else to do but abandon the use of plasma save as an emergency fluid to be used where no other fluid was available, until some method to eradicate this hazard could be developed.

The serum hepatitis problem is made even more difficult because of the prolonged incubation period. Generally 2 to 4 and even 5 months elapse from the time of exposure to the time of onset of symptoms. Moreover, about 1 in 5 patients developing hepatitis of this origin display some degree of impairment in liver function but fail to develop icterus. Usually, the shorter the period of incubation, the more severe the attack, but exceptions to this generalization are numerous.

Homologous serum jaundice was first described by Lürmann in 1883.[38] A vaccine for smallpox was prepared by pooling human lymph obtained from vesicles; this was pooled and stored in glycerine. 191 of 1,293 persons vaccinated developed the disease. Several other outbreaks of the hepatitis of this origin were reported prior to World War II, particularly during the 1930's when pooled immune serum was employed in the treatment of various infectious and contagious diseases. In the early stages of World War II, yellow fever vaccine was prepared, using pooled plasma or serum as a stabilizing agent. Over 32,000 of those vaccinated were reported to have developed serum hepatitis believed due to the yellow fever vaccine prepared by this method. This complication immediately disappeared as soon as plasma was removed from the vaccine.

The emergency conditions of World War II undeniably made necessary the continued use of pooled plasma. The numbers of cases of hepatitis arising from the virus in pooled plasma in World War II never will be known, for one of the other common diseases of wartime conditions is that of infectious hepatitis. No means of distinguishing between these two diseases exists, although generally in infectious hepatitis, the incubation period is about 3 weeks. Whether they represent two separate diseases or the same disease acquired by different portals of entry is still debated.

However, the value of plasma was not lost sight of, and every reasonable effort to kill the virus without injuring the plasma has been tried. Among the more common procedures employed has been the use of ultraviolet light exposure introduced by Lehane and associates in 1949.[30] Several encouraging reports followed immediately, suggesting that this method was effective. However, within 2 years, it was clearly evident that ultraviolet light, while effective in killing many viruses and bacteria, had little, if any, influence upon the attack rates of homologous serum jaundice and pooled plasma.[11] Admittedly, radiation was not beneficial to virus survival.

At the University of Chicago Clinics, where pooled liquid plasma stored for 6 months at room temperature, 26° C. to 36° C., has been employed for many years for the correction of hypoproteinemia in depleted surgical patients, no hepatitis attributable to plasma has yet been observed. The pooled plasma administered at this institution has been citrated without glucose. Its storage for 6 months at warm room temperature in the liquid state prior to administration was an unusual but fortunate precaution. Initially, this method of storage was introduced at Chicago as a means for allowing deterioration of plasma iso-agglutinins; the benefits derived in this connection, while excellent, were of much less consequence than the observation that this method proved to be an effective means for reducing, if not essentially eliminating, the hazard of homologous serum jaundice in pooled plasma. The basic principle involved in the viricidal action of this procedure is well stated by Topley and Wilson.[63]

Most viruses appear to be very resistant to cold. Frozen and dried, they may live for many months. Survival in distilled water, saline or Ringer's solution varies considerably. In the icebox, many viruses will survive a long time, but most of them perish rapidly if kept at room temperature or 37° C.

On the other hand, among the best ways to preserve a virus is by freezing, refrigerating, or lyophilizing the product. The virologist interested in preserving his virus for further study day after day generally uses one of these procedures to accomplish his purpose. He assiduously avoids storing his virus in liquid cell-free medium at room temperature for prolonged periods of time. In lyophilizing, freezing, or refrigerating of pooled plasma, the preservation of the hepatitis virus, should it be present, is clearly augmented.

Contrariwise, storing plasma in the liquid state at room temperature inevitably leads to its deterioration.

Storage Time and Temperature in Relation to Plasma Safety. The rate at which virus activity deteriorates upon standing in a liquid cell-free medium increases exponentially as the ambient temperature is elevated. In general, for each 10° C. increase in temperature, the time required to achieve the same extent of virus inactivation is reduced by 50 per cent or more. Contrariwise, for each 10° the temperature is reduced, the storage time required to achieve comparable virus inactivation by the storage technic should be doubled. These are very conservative estimates.

Thus, it becomes strikingly evident, when "room temperature" storage is employed to inactivate the virus of serum hepatitis in pooled plasma, that it is highly important to establish with reasonable accuracy the mean room temperature employed, as its ranges are essential considerations to the preparation of a safe plasma. The term "room temperature storage" as a concept relating to the safety of plasma must be defined not only in terms of storage duration but also in terms of ambient temperature. *It should be in excess of 31° C.*

Fortunately, data are now available from several sources relating to time and temperature storage of liquid pooled plasma and its safety. These can be applied in general to this important problem, thereby materially assisting in the achievement of safety (Table 5).

All evidence currently available suggests that 6-month storage at a mean temperature of 31.6° C. produces a pooled plasma essentially free from the risk of transmitting serum hepatitis. No cases of hepatitis have been known to occur at these temperatures. Should room temperature of 25° C. be employed, the storage duration to achieve a comparable degree of inactivation of the virus should be increased to approximately 9 months. Using this lower temperature range of 26° C. for 6 months, Murray *et al.*[5] were able to reduce the attack rate for their highly virulent plasma from 52.6 per cent to 5 per cent. Should the room temperature average 20° C., the duration of storage should be approximately 12 months, and so on. Stated otherwise, the mean temperature at which seemingly complete safety of pooled plasma was achieved

TABLE 5. APPROXIMATE RELATIONSHIPS BETWEEN THE DURATION OF STORAGE TIME FOR
VIRUS INACTIVATION AND VARIOUS TEMPERATURES EMPLOYED

VIRUS AGENT	AMBIENT STORAGE TEMPERATURE DEGREES CENTIGRADE	APPROXIMATE TIME REQUIRED FOR INACTIVATION	EXTENT OF INACTIVATION
		Minutes	
Bacteriophage (Virus T5)	63.4	480	Complete
	69.5	50	Complete
	73.0	15	Complete
Serum Hepatitis	60.0	600	Complete
	60.0	240	Incomplete
		Days	
	31.6	180	Complete
	26.0	180	Nearly complete
	20.0	180	Incomplete

COMMENTS. At the 31.6° C. employed here, the average temperature stability of plasma proteins in sodium citrate is remarkably good with reference to the use of plasma as a substitute for blood or as an intravenous source for protein administered for nutrition. However, this plasma is not useful in providing the proteins concerned with coagulation; only freshly prepared plasma or blood should be used in these latter and unusual circumstances (see p. 153).

at the University of Chicago and at the University of Cincinnati was in excess of 30° C. when stored for 6 months. By extrapolating for each 1° C. below the mean temperature of 31.6° C., the duration of storage time should be increased approximately 3 weeks beyond the 6-month storage time.

As the stability of plasma prepared from citrated blood is remarkably good, plasma can be stored under these conditions for several years without concern of deterioration (Fig. 8-4). However, plasma collected in A.C.D. (glucose) solution is much less stable but still serviceable if administered between 6 and 24 months of age. In both instances, however, the proteins concerned with blood coagulation lose their activity sufficiently rapidly so that plasma is not suited for the correction of coagulation defects.

As plasma is generally employed in conjunction with blood transfusion, it is of interest that the attack rate of hepatitis is no greater than when blood is used alone, provided that the warm room temperature procedure has been used in plasma preparation. Undoubtedly, other methods for sterilization of plasma or combinations of methods will be developed in the future which will eliminate the need for its storage at room temperature for long periods of time. Until such time, it appears that the room temperature storage

technic offers a means whereby pooled plasma can be safely resumed as a substitute for blood, as well as providing an excellent means for rehabilitating the depleted surgical patient unable to eat. The combination of warm room temperature plus exposure of plasma to ultraviolet light has the advantage of potentially greater lethal rates to viruses and is used by some.

Sayman, Gould, Star and Allen (1958) did follow-up studies in 3 categories of patients: (1) those receiving pooled plasma but no blood; (2) those receiving plasma and blood; and (3) those receiving blood alone. All the plasma had been prepared with 6 months' storage at slightly above room temperature. In category 1 (305 patients) no case of hepatitis occurred; whereas with ordinary pooled plasma, 48 cases would have been expected. The incidence in category 2 was what could be accounted for by the administration of the whole blood given. In category 3 (1,894 patients) there were 44 who developed hepatitis (2.3%). These figures indicate the value of the slightly above-room-temperature storage of pooled plasma in inactivating the serum hepatitis virus. Hoxworth, Haesler and Smith (1959) have confirmed Allen's work on the elimination of danger of hepatitis from plasma transfusions by 6 months' storage.

That pasteurization (60° C. for 10 hours)

of pooled plasma may also be effective is suggested by the report of Levin, Blocker, Dunton and Casberg (1958).

Intravenous Plasma for the Correction of Hypoproteinemia and Protein Depletions. Surgical patients in whom their pathology prevents or seriously interferes with the oral intake or absorption of food, often present important systemic disorders in nutrition which increase the surgical risk over and above that presented by the local pathology. These nutritive disorders are likely to involve depletion of body fat, carbohydrate and protein reserves as well as those of minerals, vitamins and body water (see Chap. 6, "Nutrition"). Mineral, water and vitamin deficiencies are easy to correct by the parenteral administration of each according to estimated needs. However, if the patient cannot eat or assimilate enough food to meet the total ca-

loric and protein requirements, operative mortality as well as morbidity are likely to be increased.

For many years the surgeon has sought ways and means for improving the caloric and protein intake of depleted surgical patients prior to operation, as well as in the postoperative period. All are agreed that whenever possible the oral route of feeding of natural foods is preferable. Unfortunately, this is not always possible, even when the patient suffers from benign diseases such as stricture of the esophagus, a stenosing duodenal ulcer, a gastroenterocolic fistula or from ulcerative colitis. Parenteral alimentation, gastrostomy or enterostomy feedings have been employed, but none of these procedures is totally satisfactory in all patients. At present, the greatest problem appears to be the inability to meet the total caloric needs. Intravenous fat emul-

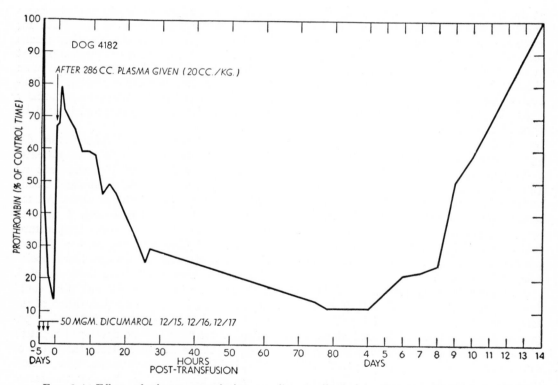

Fig. 8-4. Effect of plasma transfusion on dicumarolized dog. Shows rapid rate at which transfused prothrombin concentrates are consumed. Similar turnover rates for transfused platelets are shown in Figure 8-3 and are found for fibrinogen (actually for fibrinogen the rate is even more rapid). To keep pace with the demands of the clotting constituents by transfusions of concentrates is difficult and soon becomes impossible if the normal mechanisms do not take over soon.

sions hold promise but are not yet fully developed for general use.

It should be acknowledged also that in the catabolic state of serious malnutrition there are many associated disorders which are poorly understood. This is particularly true in the protein-depleted patient whose enzymatic systems may be disordered and consequently he responds slowly to protein administration. The crux of this problem probably is related to the fact that all enzymes are proteins; therefore, in a sense the protein-depleted patient is also one depleted of some or many enzyme systems. Thus, the very mechanisms responsible for the activation of some of the fundamental metabolic reactions can be seriously disordered or retarded and the body be incapacitated to this extent in its early response to feeding.

Correction of hypoproteinemia can be accomplished fairly rapidly by the infusion of plasma daily.[4] Generally, 3 to 7 days of a liter to 1,500 ml. of plasma, given in divided doses, will restore safely the normal concentration of plasma proteins in most patients (Figs. 8-5, 8-6).

If the benefits of plasma transfusion were limited only to those of improving the oncotic relationships of the circulation in depleted patients, its administration on this basis alone could be justified. Fortunately, plasma serves as an excellent source of protein nutrition as well as a substitute for blood.[60] A state of strongly positive nitrogen exists under plasma therapy, and the patient's general condition likewise generally improves. Admittedly, plasma and glucose alone do not supply the desired daily caloric intake, but in many cases the correction of hypoproteinemia by plasma transfusion and the restoration of the normal hemoglobin values with blood assists materially in the preparation and in the tolerance of the patient for operation. This regimen is not the final answer to the correction of malnutrition, but it does serve as well if not better than any other parenteral feeding currently available. Plasma is used more rapidly than originally believed possible.

It has been demonstrated recently that litter-mate pups grow at least as well with intravenous plasma as their only source of protein over a 3-month period as do their sisters and brothers fed the same amount of protein by mouth (horse meat and liver).[60] These results are illustrated in Figure 8-7.

The concentration of the calcium and potassium ions in plasma is governed partly by their being bound to some extent to plasma proteins. In the protein-depleted patient, occasionally the serum levels of these ions may

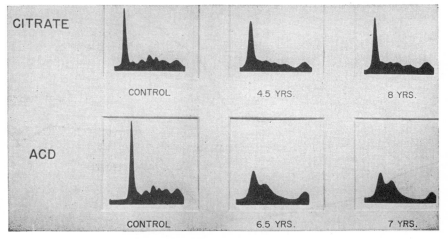

FIG. 8-5. Comparison of electrophoretic patterns. Reveals greater stability of plasma proteins when plasma is drawn in sodium citrate than in acid citrate dextrose (ACD). Note that there is a distinct difference in electrophoretic patterns. Plasma proteins are less stable in pooled plasma anticoagulated with acid-citrate-dextrose (ACD) than when anticoagulated with sodium citrate alone. (From Chanutin)

be reduced simply because the extent of hypoproteinemia is so severe as to reduce the quantity of these ions that can be bound. In a few such patients, the administration of calcium or potassium salts will not correct existing deficiencies, presumably because there is insufficient plasma protein to hold these ions within the circulation. If the protein deficits can be corrected by any means, calcium and potassium are retained more easily. The reverse also appears to be true: namely, that protein depletion is difficult if not impossible to correct in the absence of the potassium ion and possible in others (calcium, phosphorus, magnesium, iron, etc.). Proteins fed orally or given by vein as plasma contain both calcium and potassium. Generally, the correction of hypoproteinemia automatically corrects any existing potassium or calcium deficiency unless there are other continuing losses of these minerals.

PLASMA SUBSTITUTES have been employed longer than plasma itself in the treatment of hypovolemic shock. They are "standby fluids" until blood transfusions can be prepared. Among the first was gum acacia, introduced by

Bayliss[6] and used extensively in World War I. Later its use was abandoned because of its retention within the body, where it appeared to concentrate within the reticuloendothelial system and the liver. Much of it appeared to remain permanently.

Oxypolygelatin also has been extensively used and is a valuable plasma volume expander. Unlike some of the heterologous sera or plasma tried earlier, gelatin as now prepared is nonantigenic and appears to display no harmful effects. It is stable in liquid form but does tend to gel at cooler temperatures. This feature has presented a difficult problem in the military services. Gelatin is largely excreted in the urine over a period of several days and may be metabolized slowly, but to an extent unimportant to nutrition. Gelatin sustains the colloidal properties of the circulation for about the same period of time as plasma or serum albumin when given in equivalent amounts.

Dextran was developed and used extensively as a substitute for plasma by the Germans during World War II. The dextrans are a series of polysaccharides with a broad

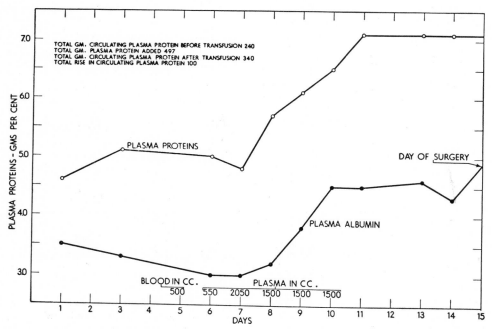

FIG. 8-6. Illustrates response of hypoproteinemia when plasma is given in volumes of 1,000 to 1,500 ml. in divided daily dosages. RA. 398635. Gastro-entero-colic fistula. Weight loss 13.5 Kg.

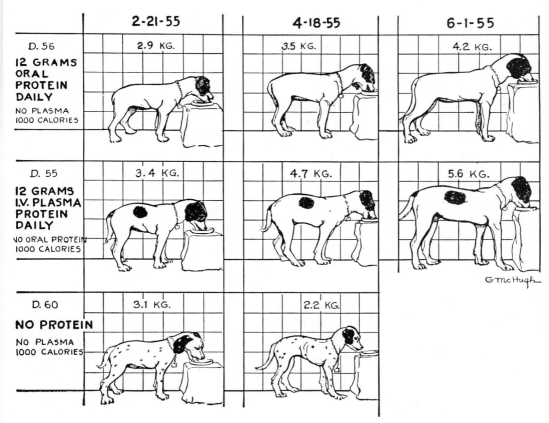

	2-21-55	4-18-55	6-1-55
D. 56 12 GRAMS ORAL PROTEIN DAILY NO PLASMA 1000 CALORIES	2.9 KG.	3.5 KG.	4.2 KG.
D. 55 12 GRAMS I.V. PLASMA PROTEIN DAILY NO ORAL PROTEIN 1000 CALORIES	3.4 KG.	4.7 KG.	5.6 KG.
D. 60 NO PROTEIN NO PLASMA 1000 CALORIES	3.1 KG.	2.2 KG.	

Fig. 8-7. These are exact tracings of litter-mate animals receiving the same amount of daily protein for a 99-day study period. In one case, 12 Gm. as horsemeat and liver was administered by mouth. The pup receiving its daily 12 Gm. of protein as intravenously administered plasma with no oral protein grew in height and gained equally well in weight with its litter-mate on oral protein. Total daily calories were the same. (Tracings were made directly from the photographic negatives; all photographs were made at 114 cm. distance between camera lens and pup.) (Ann. Surg. *144*:349-355)

spectrum of molecular weights, ranging from a few thousand to a half million. Those most useful for plasma volume expansion are selected from that portion of the spectrum corresponding to that of the plasma proteins in molecular weight. The wide range of molecular weights lends certain theoretical advantages to dextran in that it is possible to select the range which best suits the needs envisioned.

About 80 per cent of infused dextran is excreted in the urine over a period of 3 to 4 days. The remainder is metabolized and exhaled as CO_2 over a period of 3 to 4 weeks. None remains permanently within the body.

Polyvinylpyrrolidone or PVP is a polymer of formaldehyde. This agent was also devel-oped by the Germans and used extensively during World War II as a plasma substitute. Much of the infused PVP is excreted in the urine. That which remains within the body seems to remain indefinitely. Eosinophilic amorphous deposits have been described as appearing in a number of the tissues of the body many months after the infusion. These deposits provoke little if any reaction, and their significance is not known. For these reasons, PVP is looked upon by most with less favor than gelatin or dextran as substitutes for plasma at this time.

A state of abnormal bleeding has been observed in a few patients when large volumes of dextran, PVP, or gelatin have been administered. It is rarely observed when volumes less than a liter have been given: for this reason it is currently recommended that not more than a liter of these substitutes be administered to any one adult patient. The nature of the clotting abnormality responsible for the bleeding state is not understood. It is characterized principally by a prolonged bleeding time. As experience accumulates, it may be that this bleeding state will prove to be of little consequence.

SERUM ALBUMIN is the most valuable of all plasma substitutes. It serves not only the needs of oncotic pressure supplied by plasma equally well or better, but it is also metabolized in a similar manner.

Fortunately, serum albumin will withstand 10 hours of heating at 60° C. which kills the hepatitis virus. Its great drawback is cost; only about 40 per cent of serum albumin present in plasma is recoverable by commercial processing at this time. The remainder of the protein fractions of plasma are not suited to transfusion purposes.

Serum albumin can be prepared salt-poor and administered intravenously as 6 per cent solution if desired. Because of its smaller molecular weight, serum albumin should be diluted adequately with normal saline in the treatment of hypovolemic shock lest it cause the circulation to imbibe water at the expense of extravascular water. It may be given as a 25 per cent solution as a dehydrating agent when this function is desirable to accomplish; in this capacity circulatory overload must be guarded against.

In general, the field of blood and allied problems is one of continuing change and advancement. The student and the practitioner of surgery will find it to his own advantage as well as to that of his patient to keep himself informed of these developments, to pursue them with an open mind and to employ them in his practice with caution and restrained judgment.

REFERENCES

1. Abel, J. J., Rowntree, L. G., and Turner, B. B.: Plasma removal with return of corpuscles (plasmapheresis), J. Pharmacol. & Exper. Therap. *5*:625, 1914.
2. Adams, W. E., Thornton, T. F., Jr., Allen, J. G., and Gonzalez, D. E.: The danger and prevention of citrate intoxication in massive transfusions of whole blood, Ann. Surg. *120*: 656, 1944.
3. Allen, J. G., Clark, D. E., Thornton, T. F., Jr., and Adams, W. E.: The transfusion of massive volumes of citrated whole blood in man: clinical evidence of its safety, Surgery *15*:824, 1944.
4. Allen, J. G., Egner, W., Brandt, M. B., and Phemister, D. B.: Use of blood and plasma in correction of protein deficiencies in surgical patients, Ann. Surg. *131*:1, 1950.
5. Allen, J. G., Inouye, H. S., and Sykes, C.: Homologous serum jaundice and pooled plasma—attenuating effect of room temperature storage on its virus agent, Ann. Surg. *138*:476, 1953.
6. Bayliss, W. H.: Arch. med. belg. *70*:793, 1917 (Quoted by Rous and Wilson[50]).
7. Borden, C. W., and Hall, W. H.: Fatal transfusion reactions from massive bacterial contamination of blood, New England J. Med. *245*:760, 1951.
8. Braude, A. I., Sanford, J. P., Bartlett, J. E., and Mallery, O. T., Jr.: Effects and clinical significance of bacterial contaminants in transfused blood, J. Lab. & Clin. Med. *39*: 902, 1952.
9. Braxton-Hicks, J.: On transfusion and new mode of management, Brit. M.J. *2*:151, 1868.
10. Bunker, J. P., Stetson, J. B., Coe, R. C., Grillo, H. C., and Murphy, A. J.: Citric acid intoxication, J.A.M.A. *157*:1361, 1955.
11. Cannan, K.: Some problems in the National Blood Program, Nat. Acad. Sc. News Rep. *2*:81, 1952.
12. Crosby, W. H., and Akeroyd, J.: Some immunologic results of large transfusions of Group O blood in recipients of other blood groups, Blood *9*:103, 1954.
13. Decastello, A., and Sturli, A.: Ueber die Isoagglutinine im Serum gesunder und kranker Menschen, München med. Wchnschr. *49*:1090, 1902.
14. Denis, Jean Baptiste: Extrait d'une lettre de M. Denis (professeur de philosophie et de mathématiques) touchant la transfusion du sang, J. des Scanvans, 86 (Mar. 9), 1667; 123, 178 (April 2), 1667. (See Roussel, J.: Transfusion of Human Blood by the Method of Roussel, translated by Guiness, C. H. C., London, 1877.)
15. Dillard, G. H. L., Brecher, G., and Cronkite, E. P.: Separation, concentration, and transfusion of platelets, Proc. Soc. Exper. Biol. & Med. *78*:796, 1951.

16. Flosdorf, E. W., and Mudd, S.: An improved procedure and apparatus for preservation in lyophile form of serum and other biologic substances, J. Immunol. *29*:389, 1935.

17. Halsted, W. S.: Ligature and suture material, J.A.M.A. *60*:1119, 1913.

18. ———: The operative story of goitre, Johns Hopkins Hosp. Rep. *19*:71, 1920; Surgical Papers by William Stewart Halsted, vol. 2, second printing, Baltimore, Johns Hopkins Press, 1952.

19. ———: Surgical Papers, vol. 1, second printing, p. 4, Baltimore, Johns Hopkins Press, 1952.

20. Harvey, S. C.: The History of Hemostasis, New York, Hoeber, 1929.

21. Harvey, William: Exerciata Anatomica De Motu Cordes et Sanguinis, 1628.

22. Haynes, L. L., Tullis, J. L., Pyle, H. M., Sproul, M. T., Wallach, S., and Turville, W. C.: Clinical experiences with the use of glycerolized frozen blood, J.A.M.A. *173*: 1657, 1960.

23. Hektoen, L.: Iso-agglutination of human corpuscles, J.A.M.A. *48*:1739, 1907.

24. Hoxworth, P. T., Haesler, W. E., Jr., and Smith, H., Jr.: The risk of hepatitis from whole blood and stored plasma, Surg., Gynec. & Obst. *109*:38, 1959.

25. Jennings, F. L., and Allen, J. G.: Diagnostic problems; presentation of a case, J.A.M.A. *156*:1498, 1954.

26. Jones, H. W., and Mackmull, G.: The influence of James Blundell on the development of blood transfusion, Ann. M. Hist. *10*:242, 1928.

27. Landsteiner, K.: Zur Kenntniss der Anti-fermentativen, Lytischen and Agglutinieren-den Wirkungen des Blutserums und der Lymphe, Zentralbl. Bakt. *27*:357, 1900.

28. Landsteiner, K., and Levine, P.: On the Cole agglutinins of human serum, J. Immunol. *12*:441, 1926.

29. Landsteiner, K., and Wiener, A. S.: An agglutinable factor in human blood recognized by immune sera for Rhesus blood, Proc. Soc. Exper. Biol. & Med. *43*:223, 1940.

30. Lehane, D., Kwantes, C., Upward, M. G., and Thomson, D. R.: Homologous serum jaundice, Brit. M.J. *2*:573, 1949.

31. Levin, W. C., Blocker, T. G., Jr., Dunton, E. F., and Casberg, M. A.: Clinical trial of pasteurized pooled human plasma, U. S. Armed Forces M.J. *9*:1249, 1958.

32. Levine, P.: The pathogenesis of erythroblastosis fetalis; a review, J. Pediat. *23*:656, 1943.

33. Levine, P., and Katzin, E. M.: Iso-immuni-zation in pregnancy and the varieties of isoagglutinins observed, Proc. Soc. Exper. Biol. & Med. *45*:343, 1940.

34. Levinson, S. O., and Cronheim, A.: Suppression of iso-agglutinins and the significance of this phenomenon in serum transfusions, J.A.M.A. *114*:2097, 1940.

35. Lewisohn, Richard: Blood transfusion—50 years ago and today, Surg., Gynec. & Obst. *101*:362, 1955.

36. Lister, J.: On the catgut ligature *in* The Collected Papers of Joseph, Lord Lister, vol. 2, Oxford, London, 1909.

37. Lower, Richard: De Transfusione Sanguinis, 1665-66, and Tractus de Corde, 1669, tr. by Hollingsworth, M. W.: Ann. M. Hist. *10*: 213, 1928.

38. Lürmann of Bremen: Eine Icterusepidemie, Berl. klin. Wchnschr. *22*:20, 1885 (Quoted by Hirsch, A.: Handbook of Geographical and Historical Pathology, tr. by C. Creighton, London, New Sydenham Soc. *3*:420, 1886.

39. McLaughlin, E. D., Nealon, T. F., Jr., and Gibbon, J. H., Jr.: Treatment of bank blood by resins, J. Thor. & Cardiovasc. Surg. *40*: 602, 1960.

40. Maloney, J. V., Jr., Smythe, C. McC., Gilmore, J. P., and Handford, S. W.: Intra-arterial and intravenous transfusion: a controlled study of their effectiveness in the treatment of experimental hemorrhagic shock, Surg., Gynec. & Obst. *97*:529-539, 1953.

41. Malpighi, Marcello: De Pulmonibus Observationes Anatomicae *in* a letter to Borelli, tr. Foster, Lane Lectures on the History of Physiology, London, Cambridge, 1901.

42. Melrose, D. G., and Wilson, A. O.: Intra-arterial transfusion: the potassium hazard, Lancet *1*:1266, 1953.

43. Minimum Standards for Blood Transfusions Outlined: Bull. Am. Coll. Surgeons, March-April, 1956.

44. O'Brien, T. G., and Watkins, E., Jr.: Gas-exchange dynamics of glycerolized frozen blood, J. Thor. & Cardiovasc. Surg. *40*:611, 1960.

45. Ottenberg, R., and Kaliski, D. J.: Accidents in transfusion, their prevention by preliminary blood examination, J.A.M.A. *61*:2138, 1913.

46. Paget, Stephen: Ambroise Paré and His Times: 1510-1590, New York, Putnam, 1899.

47. Payne, J. H.: Harvey and Galen, Lancet *2*:1133, 1896.

48. Petrov, B. A.: Transfusion of cadaver blood, Surgery *46*:651, 1959.

49. Pifer, P. W., Block, M. A., and Hodgkinson, C. P.: Thrombocytopenia and hemorrhage in hemolytic blood transfusion reactions, Surg., Gynec. & Obst. *103*:129, 1956.

50. Rous, P., and Wilson, G. W.: Fluid substitutes for transfusion after hemorrhage, J.A.M.A. *70*:219, 1918.

51. Sabbatani, L.: Action antagoniste entre le citrate trisodique et le calcium, Mosso's Arch, ital. biol. *36*:416, 1901.

52. Sayman, W. A., Gould, R. L., Star, S. A., and Allen, J. G: Safety of liquid plasma—a statistical appraisal, J.A.M.A. *168*:1735, 1958.

53. Schecter, C., Nealon, T. F., Jr., and Gibbon, J. H., Jr.: The removal of excessive potassium and ammonium from bank blood prior to transfusion, Surg, Gynec. & Obst. *108*:1, 1959.

54. Schmidt, A.: Weitere Beitrage zur Blutlehre, Weisbaden, Bergmann, 1895.

55. Schneider, C. L.: Rapid estimation of plasma fibrinogen concentration and its use as a guide to therapy of intravascular defibrination, Am. J. Obst. & Gynec. *64*:141, 1952.

56. Seiver, F. B.: Fever-producing substances found in some distilled waters, Am. J. Physiol. *67*:90, 1923, and *71*:621, 1925.

57. Servetus, Michael: Christianismi Restituto, Vienna, 1553, Tr. in part by Williams, G. A.: Ann. Med. Hist. *10*:287, 1928.

58. Skundina, M. G., and Rusakov, A. V. (1934): Cited by Petrov (1959).

59. Starling, E. H.: On the absorption of fluids from the connective tissue spaces, J. Physiol. *19*:312, 1896.

60. Stemmer, E. A., Head, L. R., and Allen, J. G.: Comparative growth rates of litter mate puppies maintained on oral protein with those on the same quantity of protein as daily intravenous plasma for 99 days as only protein source, Ann. Surg. *144*:349-355, 1956.

61. Strumia, M. M., and McGraw, J. J.: Blood and Plasma Transfusion, Philadelphia, Davis, 1949.

62. Technical Methods and Procedures of the American Association of Blood Banks: Minneapolis, Burgess Printing Co., 1953.

63. Topley, W. W. C., and Wilson, G. S.: Topley and Wilson's Principles of Bacteriology and Immunology, rev. by Wilson, G. S., and Miles, A. A., ed. 3, London, Arnold, 1946.

64. Tullis, J. L., Ketchell, M. M., Lyle, H. M., Pennell, R. B., Gibson, J. G., II, Tinch, R. J., and Driscoll, S. G.: Studies on the in vivo survival of glycerolized and frozen human red blood cells, J.A.M.A. *168*:399, 1958.

65. Ward, G. R.: Transfusion of plasma, Brit. M.J. *1*:301, 1918.

66. Witebsky, E., and Klendshoj, N. C.: The isolation of an O specific substance from gastric juice of secretors and carbohydrate-like substances from gastric juice of nonsecretors, J. Exper. Med. *73*:655, 1941.

67. Yudin, S. S.: Transfusion of cadaver blood, J.A.M.A. *106*:997, 1936.

PAUL V. HARPER, M.D., F.A.C.S.*

——————————— CHAPTER 9 ———————————

The Principles of
Isotope Technics in Surgery

Physical Properties
Istotopic Radiation Measurements
Practical Considerations
Applications

The contribution made to surgery by isotopic methods is difficult to separate from that made to biology and medicine as a whole, and no effert to do so will be made in the present discussion. Rather, certain of the physical properties of the radioactive isotopes and their radiations will be presented, together with the general methods by which these properties may be utilized in the study and the treatment of surgical disease.

PHYSICAL PROPERTIES

An istotope may be defined as a unique nuclear species with a definite mass, charge and energy content. For the most part, the artificial radioactive isotopes with which we are largely concerned are indistinguishable chemically from the naturally occurring stable isotopes, and in biologic systems they behave in a manner identical to the corresponding stable element. This property is the basis of the tracer method, in which the isotopic label may be detected and measured by virtue of its radioactivity.

By definition, radioactive isotopes disintegrate eventually, emitting a variety of radiations and usually giving rise to elements differing from the original ones. This process occurs at random at faster or slower rates for different isotopes. The average time required for

* Professor, Department of Surgery, University of Chicago, and the Argonne Cancer Research Hospital Operated by the University of Chicago for the Atomic Energy Commission).

half of a given number of atoms to disintegrate is characteristic of the isotope and is called the half life. This may vary with different isotopes from a fraction of a microsecond to many billion years. For practical purposes, in biologic work a half life of at least 12 hours is desirable, although some studies have been done with 20-minute carbon 11.

The unstable radioactive nuclei may be divided into two principal classes: (1) those containing an excess of neutrons (formed by neutron bombardment or fission) and (2) those deficient in neutrons (formed by cyclotron bombardment). Most of the elements have isotopes in both classes. The number of protons in the nucleus is, of course, fixed by the atomic number of the element. Isotopes containing a neutron surplus disintegrate by beta decay, converting one of the excess neutrons to a proton, emitting in the process an ordinary negative electron or beta particle. Often this is accompanied by one or more gamma rays. The gamma rays are rather energetic monochromatic photons, representing transitions between energy levels inside the nucleus. On the other hand, the beta particles have a continuous energy distribution from zero to a maximum value and an average value of about one third of the maximum. Some of the gamma radiation is absorbed by orbital electrons, which then appear as ejected monoenergetic photoelectrons along with the beta particles.

Neutron-deficient isotopes decay in an exactly analogous manner, except that they emit positrons, or positive electrons, instead of beta particles. The positrons, after losing their energy by collision, combine with ambient electrons and are annihilated, giving rise to two photons of 512,000 electron volts energy each, traveling in exactly opposite directions. This process is used in positron scanning, in which detectors placed on opposite sides of a source can detect specifically these simultaneous annihilation photons. This method of detection eliminates all but those disintegrations which can be viewed by both detectors along the line, joining them and thus producing what is essentially electronic collimation for the radiation to be detected.

An alternative mode of decay in this class of isotope is called electron capture, which occurs when the neutron-deficient nucleus captures an orbital electron from the inner, or K, shell (thus the term "K-capture"), converting one of the nuclear protons to a neutron. This leaves the resulting atom in an ionized state, in which it emits the characteristic fluorescent roentgen rays.

The various alternative modes of decay which may be possible for an isotope are usually not observed, as one mode is overwhelmingly more probable than the others. However, in a few isotopes, in particular Cu^{64}, the relative probabilities are of the same order of magnitude, and this isotope decays by electron capture 42 per cent, beta decay 39 per cent and positron decay 19 per cent.

A number of the heavier isotopes, which are intrinsically less stable, decay by emission of monoenergetic alpha particles (helium nuclei).

In using an isotope for tracer work, it is usually necessary to use chemical quantities which are negligibly small compared with those in the system under study. In this application it is often desirable to use isotopic preparations, which are referred to as "carrier free"; that is, the only atoms of the element present are those of the radioactive isotope. Radioactive phosphorus, for instance, may be prepared from normal phosphorus by neutron bombardment by the reaction P^{31} (n,γ) P^{32}, in which the radioactive isotope is obtained mixed with a rather large quantity of inert or carrier P^{31}. It also may be prepared by neutron bombardment of sulfur (S^{32} [n,p] P^{32}). The resulting phosphorus in this case may then be separated from the sulfur chemically, uncontaminated with stable P^{31}.

For detailed information concerning any particular isotope, the student is referred to the standard compilations of nuclear data, which are extremely useful, although not always entirely up to date.[1-3]

ISOTOPIC RADIATION MEASUREMENTS

The detection of isotopic radiation is easily accomplished with relatively simple, inexpensive and reliable electronic equipment. The classic Geiger-Mueller counter tube consists of a cylindrical cathode surrounding a fine wire anode in a gaseous atmosphere. When ionizing radiation enters the sensitive volume of such a tube, the resulting electrons are strongly accelerated toward the anodes, producing by collision an increasing cascade of similar electrons that finally reach the anode and cause a large voltage pulse, which is recorded. The larger positive ions move more slowly toward the cathode, and for a significant length of time following a pulse they act as a shield between the anode and the cathode, during which times the tube is dead. The Geiger counter thus detects individual ionizing events so long as they do not occur too rapidly. The counting efficiency for various types of isotopic radiation is variable. Any beta particle that enters the sensitive volume gives rise to a count, while a gamma ray has to be absorbed in the gas of the tube or in the wall with ejection of a secondary electron before it triggers the counter. Thus, the gamma counting efficiency of a Geiger tube is quite low, of the order of 1 per cent. A great variety of such tubes are available for different applications, with thick walls, thin walls, thin windows for counting weak beta radiation and flow counters in which the sample is placed within the tube itself, or where the sample in gaseous form is actually mixed with the counting gas.

When a Geiger tube is operated at a lower voltage, the electrons formed are collected as before on the anode but do not form cascades. Thus, while the recorded pulses are smaller, about one tenth of 1 per cent of the Geiger pulses, there is no dead time limitation on the tube. The size of the pulse is proportional to the amount of ionization caused by the incident radiation, and for this reason such a device is called a proportional counter. An alpha particle pulse in a proportional counter is much greater than a beta or gamma pulse because of the much greater ionization produced and may be distinguished easily by this means.

Instead of counting individual pulses, the total ionization current created in the gas of the tube by the incident radiation may be measured. Such a device is called an ionization chamber. These have been designed for a variety of different applications, and the fundamental unit of radiation dosage, the roentgen, is based on such measurements. Ionization chambers usually are used in connections with intense radiation fields in therapeutic work, while counters are used in analytic and tracer work.

A very sensitive and efficient method of counting ionizing events is based on the properties of certain crystalline materials or phosphors to emit light quanta when exposed to ionizing radiation. These light quanta or scintillations are counted by a photomultiplier tube. The principal advantage of this method in gamma counting is a counting efficiency of 20 per cent to 50 per cent, which reduces the amount of isotope necessary to produce the detectible counting levels, especially in external survey in localization work. In beta counting, the liquid scintillation method, in which the sample and the phosphor are dissolved in a common solvent that then is viewed by photomultiplier tube, greatly increases the efficiency of counting soft beta rays such as of C^{14} and H^3, which are both extremely valuable tracer elements in biologic work. This method is nondestructive, so that after counting, the sample is still available for chemical or biologic analysis.

PRACTICAL CONSIDERATIONS

Production, sale, possession and disposal of all reactor-produced isotopes is under control of Federal statutes, which define the conditions of safety under which isotopes may be used. Most institutions using isotopes have committees that are responsible for radiation hazards, approval of isotope projects, etc., and a health physics department responsible for enforcing decisions of these committees.

Dangers

The dangers of using isotopes fall into several categories. The accidental ingestion of long-lived isotopes which are not excreted rapidly is probably the most serious hazard. This is particularly well exemplified in the case of the radium dial painters. Alpha emitters or high energy beta emitters are particularly dangerous in this connection, especially in bone-seeking isotopes such as Sr^{90} and plutonium. The permissible body load for various isotopes may be found in the Bureau of Standards Hand Book 52.

Radiation exposure from handling beta and gamma emitters must be limited to tolerable levels—by adequate shielding, by reducing exposure time or by using long instruments and relying on inverse square attenuation of the radiation. Low level contamination with radioactive isotopes, although often not a health hazard, can distort counting and survey measurements and must be strictly avoided.

In general, the clinical use of isotopes in children and in pregnant women should be avoided. This is particularly true of radio iodine. It has been definitely shown that modest doses of radiation to the thyroid gland in children (200r-700r) give rise to a substantial incidence of thyroid carcinoma. This dose level could easily be achieved by careless use of I^{131} "tracer" studies.

A brief table is appended, giving pertinent physical constants of some representative isotopes, to illustrate the characteristics of the various types of isotopic radiation, nuclear reactions, shielding requirements, etc.

Quantitative Considerations

Tracer Level. The quantity of isotope required for any given application depends both on the isotope and the application. In tracer work, it is desirable to use a counting rate that is large compared with the cosmic ray background, and for statistical accuracy at least 1,000 counts should be recorded which gives a standard deviation of $\pm$ 3 per cent. Thus, with a background of 20 counts/min., the sample should count 200 counts/min., and sufficient counts will be recorded in 5 to 10 minutes. Assuming a counting efficiency of 20 per cent, which is reasonable for a thin-window beta counter or scintillating gamma counter, this means that the sample for counting should contain at least 5×10^{-4} microcuries (1 microcurie = 3.7×10^4 disintegrations per second). If a sample contains too much activity for counting, it may be placed at a distance from the counter, or absorbing material (usually aluminum) may be interposed between the sample and the counter. Occasionally, other agents are preferable.

A standard sample of uranium, radium or some other long-life isotope should be counted with each series of experimental samples to control changes in sensitivity of the counter; or, alternatively, a standard may be made using the isotope in question, and the counts expressed as per cent of the standard, thus automatically correcting for decay.

Therapeutic Level. In considering the quantity of isotope for use as a diffuse radiation source in tissue, it is necessary to calculate the amount of energy absorbed by the tissue from the radiation traversing it, since this is the basis for radiation dosage measurements. (The unit of absorbed dose of radiation, the rad, is 100 ergs absorbed per gram of tissue, equivalent roughly to an exposure of 1 roentgen). This is easily done for beta ray emitters, since practically all the emitted energy is absorbed within a few millimeters of its point of origin. The radiation dosage produced in tissue by the complete disintegration of 1 microcurie/Gm. depends on the energy of the radiation and the average life of the isotope. For P^{32} the value is 730 rad; for I^{131}, 120 rad. These calculations represent ideal distributions. For irregular distributions such as those obtained by the infiltration of radioactive colloidal material into tumors, the effective radiation dosage is much less, and to accomplish the same result the amount of isotope must be increased many times.

Energy absorbed from gamma radiation and from beta radiation is essentially the same in its biologic effects. On the other hand, the relative biologic efficiency (RBE) of alpha particles in tissue is many times greater in terms of energy absorbed.

The use of a gamma emitter in tissue in diffuse or discrete sources requires much more isotope than a beta emitter to produce the same radiation dosage, as most of the energy released leaves the neighborhood of the source. The radiation dosage calculations here depend on the average life of the isotope, the energy of the radiation and the absorption constants in tissue for the radiation. While straightforward, the dosage calculations are somewhat

involved. The available data on radium and radon can serve as a model for many of these calculations. In general, from 10 to 100 millicurie quantities of isotope are required in this type of use.

When gamma emitters are substituted for radium teletherapy units, the quantity required is immensely greater, being measured in kilocuries.

APPLICATIONS

Tracer Level. The application of isotope methods in surgical diagnosis is principally in the fields of selective localization and measurements of physiologic and chemical compartments.

For practical purposes, specific localization is limited to thyroid tissue. Here injected or ingested, I^{131} in a carrier-free state will localize to a considerable extent in the thyroid gland or in functioning thyroid metastases. Very sensitive survey methods using scintillation crystal gamma detectors and focused lead collimators have been devised in connection with mechanical scanning and recording equipment, so that the size and the shape of the thyroid gland, for instance, may be delineated quite accurately and distant metastases located accurately. Astatine, the higher homologue of iodine, will give somewhat similar localization.

Specific localization of isotopes in tumors has also been produced experimentally by injecting antibodies to the tumor iodinated with I^{131}.

In nonspecific localization, where differences in vascularity between tumor and surrounding tissue are detected, brain tumor and liver metastases have been demonstrated, and the methods of positronic scanning (see above) have proved to be useful. This approach also has been used in the eye for ocular tumors that have been distinguished from retinal detachment on the basis of vascularity, using a small probe counter.

In the brain, localization studies are aided by the fact that the blood-brain barrier, which is impervious to many substances, may be absent in a brain tumor, allowing radioactive material to enter the tumor tissue from the blood stream. This may then be detected by external scanning or with a small probe counter inserted into the brain tissue.

The use of isotopic methods for studying fluid spaces differs little from similar chemical methods. A quantity of tagged material is injected intravenously, and, after mixing has been completed in the compartment in question, determination of the dilution of the isotope is made, and the size of the compartment may be calculated by knowing the quantity of isotope given. Serum albumin tagged with I^{131}, red cells tagged with P^{32} or Cr^{51}, give blood-volume values more or less identical with those obtained by tagging the albumin with Evans blue or the red cells with carbon monoxide. In some cases the differences in analytic methods result in a more expeditious determination.

However, the isotope methods go beyond the chemical methods by permitting chemical spaces or pools, as well as volumes, to be determined. For instance, after injecting intravenously a millimol of sodium with a "specific activity" of 100,000 counts/sec. per millimol, the serum, after mixing, is found to contain 25 counts/sec. per millimol of sodium. It then is said that the injected sodium has been diluted by the sodium pool, which consists consequently of 4,000 millimol. Other body fluid elements may be studied in this way. Potassium, carbonate and water have suitable isotopes for use of this type in human patients. Chlorine does not have a suitable isotope, but bromine has been substituted in these circumstances. A recent development in this line is the determination of the total body potassium. Naturally occurring potassium is slightly radioactive, so that with special shielding and using large scintillation crystals, the total potassium in the body may be measured with about 5 per cent accuracy in 15 minutes.

When pursued in detail, studies of this sort become very complex, since, in fact, they involve transient, rather than steady state measurements. In most cases, correction for excretion must be made, and the ions under study exist in several physical compartments rather than one, with varying exchange rates between the compartments. The mathematical analysis of such systems rapidly becomes impracticable, and often they are best studied by using hydrodynamic or electronic models. In general, this is true of many biochemical systems, such as the plasma phosphate, urine phosphate, organic phosphate, bone phosphate, phosphoplipid system, or the plasma iodine, urine iodine, thyroid iodine, plasma protein bound iodine system.

A number of transient phenomena of medical and surgical interest may be studied using isotopes. Curves showing the rate of uptake of radioiodine by the thyroid may be made by external survey of the gland. The life of the red cell may be determined by tagging it with radioactive iron or chromium. The circulation in the extremities, for instance, may be studied by watching the change in counting rate over the leg following injection of radioactive sodium intravenously. Radioisotopes have been used extensively for cardiac output studies in a manner similar to the method using dye curves, and various cardiac shunts may be demonstrated using isotopic methods.

Therapeutic Level. Isotopes have been used in a variety of ways in radiotherapy. These may be classified as (1) *teletherapy,* in which long-lived gamma emitters such as Co^{60} or Cs^{137} are substituted for radium to produce an intense gamma ray beam; (2) *brachytherapy,* in which small sources are implanted in tissue to produce the desired radiation fields; and (3) in the use of *diffuse sources* such as P^{32}, I^{131} and Y^{90} spread evenly through the tissues or injected into cavities. Surgical applications are limited to the use of brachytherapeutic devices and the attempts to produce diffuse sources by the injection of radioactive colloidal material.

Radium needles and radon seeds, which have been used for many years, are gradually being supplanted by the various isotopes with their more flexible radiation characteristics and more general availability. Much attention has been directed toward reducing the exposure hazard to the operator, since it is clear that, in addition to causing local damage, exposure to radiation induces leukemia. This has been accomplished by using isotopes emitting softer gamma radiation than radium and radon. This softer gamma radiation behaves in tissues in a manner similar to that of the familiar radium gamma radiation, but it is much more easily shielded by lead (see Table 1). Additional efforts along these lines include fixing sources in threads or tapes and drawing

TABLE 1. PRINCIPAL PHYSICAL CONSTANTS OF SOME REPRESENTATIVE ISOTOPES

K indicates K-Capture. Energies of particles and photons are given in MEV (million electron volts). E_{max} indicates maximum energy, $\bar{E}$ indicates average energy. HVL (half value layer) figures are approximate. Abbreviations for nuclear reactions: Na^{23} (n,γ) Na^{24} means sodium[23] absorbs 1 thermal neutron, emits 1 gamma ray and becomes sodium[24].

			RADIATION CHARACTERISTICS								
			PARTICLES				PHOTONS				
					TISSUE			HVL CM.			
ISO-TOPE	MODE OF DECAY	HALF LIFE	E_{max}	$\bar{E}$	Range mm.	HVL mm.	MEV	Tissue	Lead	PRODUCTION	USE
C^{14}	$\beta-$	5720 y	.155	.050	.2	—	—	—	—	$n^{14}(n,p)C^{14}$	Tracer studies
Na^{24}	$\beta-,\gamma$	14.9 h	1.39	.54	6.4	.85	2.76 1.38	14	1.3	$Na^{23}(n,\gamma)Na^{24}$	Tracer studies
P^{32}	$\beta-$	14.3 d	1.71	.695	8.1	1.3	—	—	—	$S^{32}(n,p)P^{32}$ $P^{31}(n,\gamma)P^{32}$	Tracer studies Bone-marrow irradiation
Fe^{55}	K	2.91y	—	—	—	—	.0065	.032	—	$Fe^{54}(n,\gamma)Fe^{55}$	Tracer studies
Co^{60}	$\beta-,\gamma$	5.3 y	.31	.10	.8	.09	1.17 1.33	11	1.0	$Co^{59}(n,\gamma)Co^{60}$	Tracer studies Brachytherapy Teletherapy
As^{74}	K $\beta-,\gamma$ $\beta+$	17.5 d	1.4 $\beta-$ .95$\beta+$	—	—	—	.596 .635 .51*	7.8	.42	$Ge^{74}(d,n)As^{74}$	Positron Scanning
Y^{90}	$\beta-$	2.54d	2.18	.89	11	1.48	—	—	—	$Y^{89}(n,\gamma)Y^{90}$ Daughter of Sr^{90}	Brachytherapy Interstitial therapy
I^{131}	$\beta-,\gamma$	8.0 d	.61	.205	2.1	.25	.365	7.0	.25	Fission of uranium	Tracer studies Diffuse source Brachytherapy
I^{125}	K, γ	60 d	—	—	—	—	.027	2	.002	Daughter of Xe^{125}	Tracer studies
Au^{198}	$\beta-,\gamma$	2.69d	.97	.32	3.9	.36	.411	7.2	.32	$Au^{197}(n,\gamma)Au^{198}$	Brachytherapy Diffuse source
Rn^{222}	α	3.85d	5.48	5.48	41.1μ	—	—	—	—	Daughter of natural Ra	Brachytherapy (with decay products)

them rapidly into the tumor from a shielded container, thus avoiding prolonged exposure to the operator. Fine polyethylene tubing has also been used to form implants, which are later filled with appropriate isotopes in solution. These brachytherapeutic methods are extremely flexible, and by using them it is possible to produce many types of extremely well-localized radiation fields of any desired intensity.

The efficacy of diffuse beta ray sources in tissue has been amply demonstrated by the experience with radioactive iodine in the treatment of diseases of the thyroid gland. The thyroid tissue may be essentially destroyed with a relatively small dose of isotope without resultant damage to the surrounding tissue. Attempts have been made to reproduce in tumors the even distribution of isotope responsible for these effects by the injection

of radioactive colloidal materials such as Au^{198}, $CrP^{32}O_4$, $Y^{90}(OH)_3$ and $Y^{90}F_3$. These materials have been used clinically by injection into the prostate and the parametrium, where they move about in the lymphatics much as any other colloidal material. It has been found impossible to achieve more than a patchy distribution of isotope in a given volume of tissue by such local infiltration technics, and the high hopes first held out for this application have not been achieved.

The treatment of pleural effusion and ascites due to tumor by the injection of the above materials into the affected cavity has met with some success, but again the isotope is deposited in irregular patches on the cavity walls and does not produce an even radiation dosage to the cavity wall.

Certain special applications have been made of strong radioactive sources to destroy local areas of tissue. The implantation of strong (10-15 millicurie) radon seeds or the use of a number of Y^{90} sources implanted into the hypophysis has accomplished destruction of this gland without serious damage to surrounding structures.

A completely different approach has been devised in connection with brain tumors, in which a nonradioactive compound containing boron is made to localize in the tumor. The patient is then exposed to a beam of thermal neutrons that react with the boron-producing alpha particles, thus subjecting the tissue where the boron is located to a greatly increased radiation dosage compared with the other tissues in the neutron beam. This method could also be applied using lithium, or in the case of uranium the fission reaction could be utilized.

It is our feeling at the present time that the place of isotopes in the diagnosis and the study of disease is quite secure. However, many of the therapeutic methods presently available will have to undergo considerable evolution before their value is established. The student can expect to encounter many advances and changes within the next few years.

REFERENCES

1. Nuclear Data Sheets, National Academy of Sciences, National Research Council, Washington, D.C. (Published bi-monthly).
2. Strominger, D., Hollander, J. M., and Seaborg, G. T.: Table of isotopes, Rev. Modern Physics 30:585-904, 1958.
3. Sullivan, W. H.: Trilinear chart of Nuclides (Atomic Energy Commission), U.S. Government Printing Office, Washington 25, D.C.

CARL A. MOYER AND JONATHAN E. RHOADS

CHAPTER 10

Neoplastic Disease—General Considerations

Neoplasms
Certain Practical Considerations in Cancer
  Surgery

NEOPLASMS

DEFINITIONS

Neoplasms are nonconformist cellular populations no longer dedicated to the purposes of the organism as a whole. In contrast with normal cellular populations, ontogenetically grouped to form organs that remain fixedly related to one another and are integratively functional, neoplastic cells do not form organs, are not fixedly related to other cells, and function physiologically as relatively independent uncontrolled elements. They are separated behavioristically into the benign and the malignant types.

Benignity implies local noninvasive growth; and malignancy, invasive growth and metastasis (transplantation of cells with secondary growth at other sites in the body). The assignation of benignity or malignancy to particular neoplasms rests upon knowledge gained by the observation of the growth and the functional characteristics of other neoplasms of similar appearance in comparable locations in other individuals. The designation of benignancy or malignancy to some tumors can be made with certainty, e.g., xanthomas and keloids are benign, while Ewing's tumor, adenocarcinoma of the stomach and squamous carcinoma of the lung are malignant. However, the classification of some tumors is often impossible without knowledge of that tumor's behavior in the individual harboring it. Carcinoids of the appendix and the colon, leiomyomas, chondromas and juvenile melanomas fall into this category.

Malignancy does not always connote meta-static propensity in the individual tumor, but a tumor type that never metastasizes is regarded as benign. Medulloblastomas and glioblastomas of the brain are considered as malignant, although they metastasize with extreme rarity; they are malignant because of their local invasiveness and because metastasis has been known to occur. One of the important basic characteristics of malignant cells is a decrease in the adhesiveness of one cell to the next. This was originally demonstrated by Coman (1944) and in general differentiates malignant tumors from benign tumors as well as from normal tissue. It may be demonstrated in tissue cultures and by appropriate methods in tissues as they come from the body.

ETIOLOGY

The primary etiologic factors involved in the inception of neoplasms in man are still unknown. Presumtively, something happens to the constitution of nuclear material of a cell, rendering it no longer obeisant to regulation of its growth. Although the primary cellular genesis of neoplasia is unknown, it can be induced by a variety of agents. These may be classified as mechanical, infectious, chemical and physical (chiefly, ionizing radiation). The long exposure of skin to ultraviolet light induces cutaneous carcinomata, as does the repeated exposure to x-rays. Long exposure to x-radiation leads to leukemia in some individuals, radium ingestion to osteogenic sarcomas and, in rats, radioiodine to carcinomas of the thyroid. Long exposure to certain aniline dyes promotes carcinomas of the bladder. Butter yellow (a dye) induces hepatic carcinomas in animals, while arsenic, chromates and pitchblende promote the development of carcinomas of the lung in man. Viruses are known to incite many types of tumors, benign

and malignant, in many animals, and neoplasms in plants; coal tars, human scrotal
cancer; heat and infrared rays, kangri cancer;
and cigarette tars, cutaneous carcinomas of
mice and rabbits and probably carcinomas of
the lung in man.

GROWTH FACTORS

The growth of neoplasms, both benign and
malignant, often appears to be unsteady in
rate and occasionally even retrogresses. The
growth rate of visible or palpable tumors
rarely approaches the theoretical maximal
growth rate, which may be expressed as:
$X = 2^{(y-1)}$. In this formula, X represents the
number of cells, and y the number of division
time intervals. Should there be no biologic
restrictions upon neoplastic growth, a cancer
cell of 1,000 cu. micron size (10 × 10 × 10
microns) with a division time interval of 1
month would grow into a mass of about 4 cu.
cm. in 31 months, 268 cu. cm. in 37 months,
and 9,400 cu. cm. in 42 months! Peritoneal
metastases of anaplastic carcinomas of the
stomach may almost attain such a rate of
growth. At celiotomy, nodules varying in size
from the barely visible to 0.5 cm., tagged with
silk sutures, become masses from 2 to 10 times
larger in 1 or 2 months. The principle of

exponential growth as applied to neoplasms is
illustrated in Figure 10-1. Obviously, whatever the rate of growth of a tumor may be, at
least two thirds of the life span of a tumor
has transpired before it attains to a visible
size, assuming that the minimal visible diameter is 4 mm. and the diameter attainable
before it kills the host is 12 to 20 cm.

The rate of growth of an adenocarcinoma
in a human colon is shown in Figure 10-2. The
observed rate of growth of this one colonic
cancer during 7 years, in a person judged to
be an "impossible" surgical risk because of
pulmonary and myocardial infarcts, hypertension, diabetes, advanced arteriosclerosis and
obesity, indicates that it doubled in size about
every 636 days. The time required by a neoplasm to double its size has been termed the

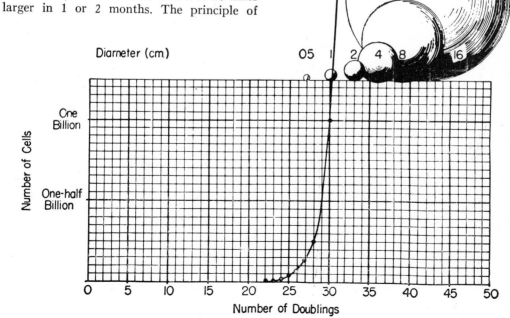

FIG. 10-1. Diagrammatic illustration of the theoretical exponential growth rate of
neoplasms demonstrates the relationship of the size of the neoplasm relative to its
age. (Collins, V. P., *et al.:* Am. J. Roentgenol. *76*:988)

doubling time. So far few measurements of the doubling times of human tumors have been made. Some of them made so far of pulmonary metastases, the sizes of which may be determined roentgenographically, are from embryonal carcinomas of the testis, 11 to 40 days; from carcinomas of the breast, 28 to 184 days; from carcinomas of the rectum, 49 to 123 days; and from one carcinoma of the esophagus, 164 days (Collins, et al.).

There are local and general factors which tend to limit the growth rate of neoplasms. The generally accepted local factors are: vascularity, fibroplasia, and lymphatic and vascular resistance to invasion. Many tumors are said to grow away from their blood supply. Such tumors are prone to undergo avascular necrosis. Hodgkin's sarcoma, leiomyosarcoma and astrocytomas often demonstrate this phenomenon.

Within many neoplasms a relatively avascular fibroplasia encases the neoplastic cells into small nests. Presumtively, such encasements interfere with the growth of neoplasms as a whole.

The propensity for entry into lymphatics and veins varies a great deal from neoplasm to neoplasm. Arteries are peculiarly resistant to invasion. Malignant brain tumors have little tendency to invade the blood vessels of the brain or the lymphatics in the meninges (the brain itself contains no lymphatics), while the chorio-epithelioma and primary renal parenchymal carcinomas invade veins readily. The carcinomas of the intestinal tract invade both the lymphatics and the veins, and squamous cell carcinomas of the lip invade lymphatics regularly but veins rarely. The reasons for these differences in propensity of invasion of lymphatics and blood vessels are not adequately explained.

The known general factors limiting neoplastic growth are hormonal and nutritional. Reduction of the rate of growth and even retrogression of carcinomas of the breast may attend the administration of estrogenic or androgenic substances, the ablation of ovarian hormones by oophorectomy, and the removal of the adrenal or pituitary glands. The growth of prostatic carcinoma may be stayed for a time by castration, the administration of estrogen and hypophysectomy.

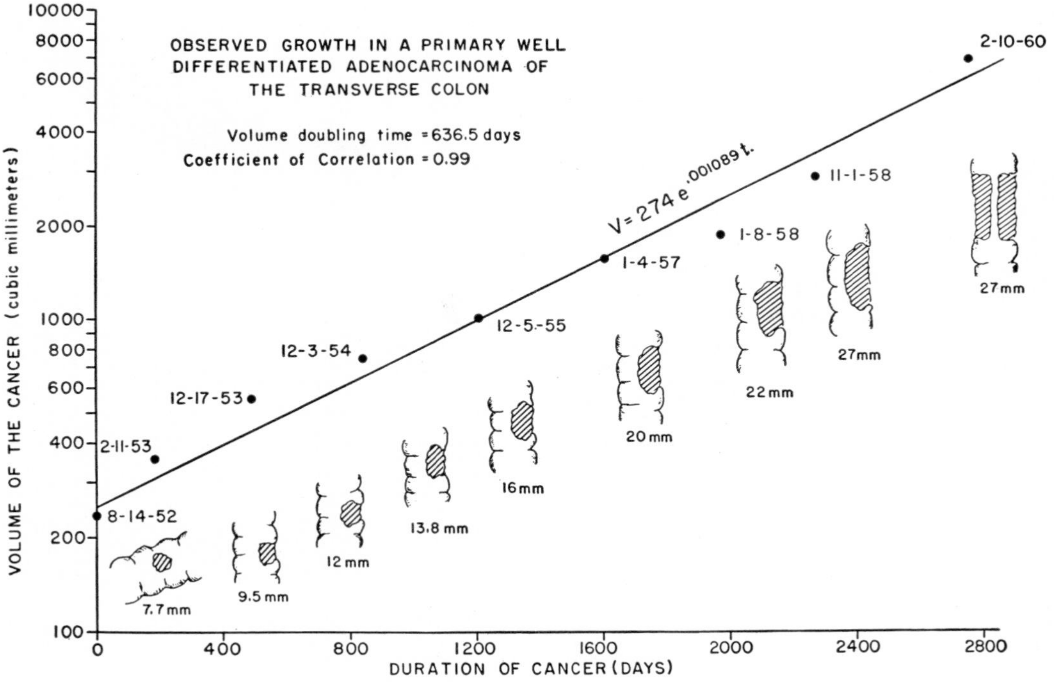

OBSERVED GROWTH IN A PRIMARY WELL DIFFERENTIATED ADENOCARCINOMA OF THE TRANSVERSE COLON

Volume doubling time = 636.5 days
Coefficient of Correlation = 0.99

$V = 274 e^{.001089 t}$

FIGURE 10-2.

Although protein, carbohydrate or fat starvation has practically no detectable effect upon the growth of neoplasms in man, functional deficits of accessory foodstuffs do. The folic acid antagonists, such as Aminopterin, reduce the growth rates of a number of neoplasms such as lymphosarcoma, Hodgkin's sarcoma and leukemia but do not destroy them.

The growth of some malignant neoplasms may be reduced significantly by such diverse substances as arsenic (Fowler's solution), urethane (ethyl carbamate), toxins of streptococci and *Bacillus prodigiosus* (Coley's toxin or fluid), viruses and nitrogen mustard. Some individual tumors among the seminomas, the lymphomas and the basal cell carcinomas can be destroyed completely by x-radiation, while the irradiated contiguous normal tissue cells about the neoplastic ones remain viable. However, there are other neoplasms that are so tough that normal cells about them are killed before the majority of the neoplastic cells are affected by the irradiation. Leiomyosarcomas, adenocarcinomas of the stomach and the rectum, chondrosarcomas and melanocarcinomas are examples of this type of radiation-resistant tumor. In addition, many neoplasms are made

up of cellular populations having remarkably different individual capacities to withstand radiation. Some cells of these neoplasms die while their normal neighbors live on, and others still live after such heavy radiation that their normal companions are destroyed. Carcinomas of the breast, some ovarian cancers, squamous cell cancers of the esophagus and the buccal mucosa, papillary cancers of the thyroid, and astrocytomas often exemplify this type of behavior after radiation.

SYMPTOMS AND SIGNS

The symptoms and signs of neoplasms are extremely variable. However, the formulation of some generalizations regarding them can be made. In general the signs and symptoms of cancer may be divided into 5 categories that are related to the biologic behavior of the neoplasm: (1) those related to expansive growth, (2) those related to infiltrative growth and metastasis, (3) those relatable to avascular necrosis and/or ulceration, (4) those attributable to the peculiar physiologic activities of neoplasms, and (5) those related to destruction of the tissue in which the neoplasm grows. There are only a relatively few neoplasms that give rise to symptoms and signs

TABLE 1. PHYSIOLOGICALLY FUNCTIONAL NEOPLASMS

LOCUS	TYPE	SIGNS
Hypophysis	Adenoma, basophilic	Cushing's syndrome "pituitary basophilism"
	Adenoma, eosinophilic* or mixed (rarely carcinoma in adults)	Gigantism (prepubertal) Acromegaly (postpubertal)
Thyroid	Adenoma*	Hyperthyroidism
Parathyroid	Adenomas and carcinomas of all types excepting oxyphil*	Hyperparathyroidism
Pancreas	Islet cell adenoma*	Hyperinsulinism
	Islet cell carcinoma	
Adrenal medulla	Pheochromocytoma*	Episodic hyperadrenalism and hypertension
Adrenal cortex	Cortical adenoma and cortical carcinoma	Cushing's syndrome
	Cortical carcinoma* in women and children	Adrenal virilism and adrenogenital syndrome
Testis	Chorio-epithelioma*	Gynecomastia
	Leydig cell tumors* (interstitial cell)	Precocious puberty, the "infant Hercules"
	Sertoli cell (very rare)	Feminization
Ovary	Arrhenoblastoma	Masculinization
	Fibroma	Meigs' syndrome
	Granulosa and theca cell*	Precocious puberty, postmenopausal bleeding, menstrual irregularities
Intestine(mainly)	Malignant carcinoid	Flushing spells, pulmonic stenosis, tricuspid insufficiency, cyanosis
Thorax and abdomen (mainly)	Sarcoma	Hypoglycemia and signs thereof
	Choriocarcinomatous* teratoma (very rare)	Prepubertal uterine bleeding

* These neoplasms are very frequently associated with the signs indicated.

attributable to the physiologic or biochemical activities of the neoplasm. In man most of these appear to originate in the endocrine glands or gonads (see Table 1).

The frequency of the association of the signs with these specific neoplasms in Table 1 varies much. With the starred entities, the neoplasm and the signs are associated very frequently, while in the case of the others they are not. In other words, the unstarred entities often exist without signs of physiologic overactivity. Peculairly, carcinomas of the thyroid are accompanied only very rarely by signs of hyperthyroidism.

Expansive Growth. The signs of neoplastic growth associated with expansiveness are the most protean (see Table 2). However, they may be sorted out into a fairly orderly array because they are peculiar to the function and the location of the organ wherein the tumor is located. Clearly, expansive growth of tumors within or near the skin, or in the mouth and the anus will produce visible and palpable lumps. In the respiratory, the gastro-intestinal, the biliary, the urinary and the cerebral spinal conductive tracts expansive tumor growth may lead to obstruction of the tract. In fact, the signs of neoplasms in these places are frequently related to obstruction. The expansive growth of tumors within rigid cavities, such as the skull and the spinal canal, blocks conduction over nerve fibers and may lead to a multiplicity of paralyses as well as pain. In brief, the expansive growth of tumors leads in man to palpable and visible lumps, the signs and symptoms of the obstruction of tubed structures, and disturbances of the nerve supply of parts of the body.

Necrosis of the tumor is especially prone to provide some of the early signs of cancer when it originates within the skin or the epithelium of the respiratory tract, the wall of the intestine, the cervix uteri, or the genitourinary tract (see Table 3). In other words, cancers arising in parts of the body that lead to the external environment will often first make themselves known by signs and symptoms of inflammation secondary to necrosis or ulceration of the tumor. With partial death of cancers of skin, lips, tongue, pharynx, larynx, penis and anus, ulceration often occurs. The ulcer supports bacterial growth, and inflammation is thereby stimulated, leading to redness, heat, pain, swelling, and impairment of function. Necrotic tumors of the bronchi also ulcerate, and the peritumorous inflammation mimics pneumonia, tuberculosis or pulmonary abscess. By virtue of this secondary bacterial inflammatory component of partially necrotic cutaneous, visible mucosal and pulmonary cancers, frequently the antibiotics will relieve the infection, and often the lesion will subside remarkably, and occasionally the ulcer will even heal. For this reason any ulcer within

TABLE 2. SIGNS ATTRIBUTABLE TO EXPANSIVE GROWTH

LOCUS	SIGNS
Skin and subcutaneous tissues, including mouth, breast, testes, penis and anus	Visible and palpable mass
Superior mediastinal, extratracheal	Occlusion of trachea—dyspnea and wheezing; occlusion of esophagus —dysphagia; occlusion of great cephalad veins—cyanosis and swelling of head and arms
Trachea and bronchi	Cough, dyspnea and obstructive atelectasis
Gastrointestinal tract	Signs of obstruction: esophagus—dysphagia stomach—vomiting intestine—abdominal distention, intestinal colic, obstipation
Common hepatic and common bile ducts	Jaundice and elevated serum alkaline-phosphate
Urinary tract, ureter, prostate	Ureteral colic (rare) and hydronephrosis, prostatism
Eustachian tube	Impaired hearing ("plugged-up ear")
Bone	Pain and directly or roentgenographically visible masses and defects
Intracranial	Headache; nerve and tract conduction deficits or palsies; signs of increased intracranial pressure
Spinal cord and cauda equina	Pain and paralyses
Liver	Hepatomegaly
Spleen	Splenomegaly

TABLE 3. CLINICAL SIGNS ATTRIBUTABLE TO NECROSIS OF THE TUMOR

LOCUS	SIGNS
All loci	Signs of tissue death: 1. Fever 2. Leukocytosis 3. Elevation of sedimentation rate 4. Anorexia, malaise
Visible loci	Ulceration
Intestinal tract, including biliary	1. Micro- and macro-intestinal hemorrhage, leading to anemia with its signs such as weakness, dyspnea on exertion, etc. 2. Signs of inflammation, especially with esophageal and colonic neoplasms manifest by intra-abdominal inflammatory pain often mimicking cholecystitis, appendicitis and pancreatitis
Lung	Signs of cavitation and inflammation imitating bronchopneumonia and viral pneumonias, pulmonary abscesses, and pulmonary tuberculosis
Urinary tract: renal pelvis, ureter, bladder	Hematuria and pyuria
Uterus, corpus and cervix	Intermenstrual and postmenstrual bleeding and vaginal discharges

the above structures requires a biopsy before the possibility of cancer can be reasonably dismissed. A favorable response to antibiotics is not a sign that the lesion is not neoplastic.

Necrosis of tumors within the gastrointestinal tract accounts in part for carcinomas of the stomach masquerading as peptic ulcers and carcinomas of the right colon mimicking appendicitis and cholecystitis. Many a gallbladder and appendix have been removed because of symptoms and signs arising from an ulcerated carcinoma of the right colon, while at the same time the cancer has been missed. Similarly, many a cancer of the stomach has been left to grow for months before a surgeon is consulted because the gastric ulcer healed symptomatically and even roentgenographically when the patient was placed on an ulcer regimen.

Partially necrotic tumors within parenchymatous organs, such as the liver, the spleen, the kidney, the bone marrow and the retroperitoneal region constitute one of the causes of the so-called "fever of undetermined origin." Tumors encased within the body may give rise to fever, leukocytosis and an elevated sedimentation rate even as the dead cardiac muscle cells within a cardiac infarct do. Actually these signs of localized tissue death may be the sole early signs of tumor within the liver, the spleen or the kidney.

Bleeding and Anemia. Necrosis of the tumor also leads to bleeding and consequently, at times, to anemia. Slowly bleeding carcinomas of the stomach and the right colon are especially prone to produce a secondary anemia; and this secondary anemia, together with its attendant exertional dyspnea, ease of fatigue, and weakness, may constitute the sole signs of these cancers. Unfortunately, this anemia, together with its signs, usually responds favorably to the administration of salts of iron. Consequently, some cancers of the stomach and the colon are permitted to grow until signs other than those of anemia appear, because the patient takes iron-containing nostrums or, what is worse, the physician prescribes iron for the secondary anemia without examining the gastrointestinal tract with the proper " 'scopes" and appropriate roentgenologic methods.

Occasionally, neoplasms give rise to massive gastrointestinal bleeding. Necrotic leiomyosarcomas of the stomach and the duodenum, ulcerating carcinomas on the lesser curvature of the stomach, and the rare carcinomas of the duodenum and the jejunum may bleed profusely. Cancers of the renal pelvis, the bladder, the uterus and the cervix are also prone to bleed. Hematuria and bloody intermenstrual vaginal discharges must be considered as of neoplastic origin unless specific diagnostic procedures contradict this view.

TABLE 4. CLINICAL SIGNS OF INFILTRATIVE GROWTH

LOCUS	SIGNS
Nerves in region:	
1. Parotid	Paralysis of the facial nerve
2. Thyroid (carcinoma)	Recurrent laryngeal nerve palsy and fixation of thyroid to contiguous structures
3. Apex of thoracic cavity and axilla (Pancoast's tumor and metastatic axillary carcinomas)	"Brachial plexus" pain and palsies and fixation of palpable tumors
4. Pancreas (carcinoma of body of pancreas and retroperitoneal malignant neoplasms)	Pain over lower dorsal and upper lumbar spine
5. Pelvis (carcinoma of cervix and rectum)	Lumbosacral plexus pain
Lymphatics	Lymphedema, chylous ascites or chylothorax and hydrothorax
Veins	Venous occlusive edema and nonchylous ascites or pleural effusion
Breast	Fixity of the skin to the tumor
Cervix	Thickening of palpable ligamentous support

In summary, the tendency of tumors to die in part and to ulcerate may lead to a number of signs such as fever and leukocytosis, anemia secondary to the seepage of blood, massive gastrointestinal hemorrhage and localized signs of inflammation mimicking benign gastric ulcer, appendicitis, cholecystitis, sinusitis, and so forth.

Infiltrative Growth. The infiltrative growth of malignant tumors gives rise to signs that in the main are related to the invasion of nerves (pain), the blocking of the low pressure fluid conduits, the veins and the lymphatics and the bronchi (edema, ascites and hydrothorax, and atelectasis), and the fixation of normally mobile structures, such as the cervix and the skin (see Table 4). Nerve invasion with its unremitting, demoralizing pain is especially prone to attend neoplasms growing in organs located near the major nerve plexi: for example, the invasion of the brachial plexus by cancers in the apex of the lung and in the axillary lmph nodes, and the infiltration of the lumbosacral plexus by carcinomas in the rectum, the cervix and the iliac lymph nodes.

Generally, the signs of infiltrative growth are signs of incurability, some mammary cancers excepted.

The neoplastic signs attributable to destruction of the host tissues, excepting panhypopituitarism, are frequently signs of incurability (see Table 5). Table 6 provides a cursory summary of this brief discussion of the clinical manifestations of neoplasia.

CERTAIN PRACTICAL CONSIDERATIONS IN CANCER SURGERY

A number of problems confronting the surgeon who cares for patients with cancer or suspected cancer are common to many types of the disease. Some of these will be considered here. Breast cancer (see Chap. 25) will serve to illustrate these points.

One is confronted first with the case only suspected of having cancer. What are the minimal criteria for doing a biopsy? Should this be a wedge or a chip biopsy, or should it always be an excision biopsy? Is a needle biopsy ever justified? If so, when?

What are the chances of spreading cancer by doing an incomplete biopsy? What are the chances of a sampling error (i.e., missing the cancer) by doing a limited biopsy, a needle biopsy, or a biopsy before a dominant lump is found? How reliable is the gross appearance of the lesion as a basis for diagnosis? How reliable is frozen section? Will waiting for a paraffin section reduce the chances of cure if malignancy is present?

These are questions which arise in connec-

TABLE 5. CLINICAL SIGNS OF DESTRUCTION OF HOST TISSUE

LOCUS	SIGNS
Bone	Pathologic fractures
Liver	Hepatic insufficiency
Bone marrow	Aplastic anemia, neutropenia and thrombocytopenia
Pituitary	Panhypopituitarism
Brain and spinal cord	Palsies and anesthesia

TABLE 6. SIGNS OF NEOPLASIA

Neoplastic Location	Physiologic Function	Expansive	Necrotic Inflammatory	Infiltrative	Destruction of Host Tissue
Brain		+++ Headache and palsies		+ Pain	+ Palsies, etc.
Endocrine glands	+++ Hyperfunction	+ Tumor		+ Recurrent nerve palsy ca. thyroid	
Lung		+++ Cough and atelectasis	++ Pneumonia, hemoptysis	+ Brachial plexus pain, pleural effusion	
Gastrointestinal tract		+++ Intestinal and gastric obstruction	++ Inflammation, anemia, hemorrhage	+ Ascites	
Biliary tract		+++ Jaundice			
Urinary tract		++ Prostatism	+++ Hematuria, pyuria		
Female genital tract		+ Tumor	+++ Intermenstrual bleeding, vaginal discharge, ulceration	+ Lumbosacral plexus pain	
Bone		+ Pain	++ Inflammation mimicking osteomyelitis		+++ Pathologic fracture
Bone marrow					+ Panhematopenia
Liver		+++ Tumor			+ Hepatic insufficiency
Spleen		+++ Tumor			
Skin and breast		+++ Tumor	++ Late ulceration	+ Fixation to skin or chest	

+ Present
++ Marked
+++ Very marked

tion with establishing a diagnosis of malignancy in many areas in which cancer may be suspected.

In more advanced cancer one must answer other questions. Is the patient operable in the sense that he can stand an exploratory operation and biopsy? Is the tumor resectable in the sense that all gross tumor can be removed completely? There follow many additional questions about the absolute efficacy of alternative methods of treatment, such as roentgen therapy; the relative efficacy of radiation as compared with attempted surgical excision as compared with no treatment at all, in various stages of advancement of the tumor.

In the cancers that are incurable by present methods, one must evaluate the results of therapy in terms of symptomatic relief, as well as in terms of life expectancy.

Such considerations bring one face to face with the philosophical problem of whether a physician has an obligation to prolong life into a period of uselessness, pain and slow dissolution in the face of a prognosis which appears on the best evidence to be hopeless.

What answers can be provided to these

questions? In many instances, rather little factual material has been assembled on which answers can be based. Therefore, the following are based in part on clinical experience and opinion.

In the realm of diagnosis, a definite basis should exist for doing a biopsy for malignancy. Occasionally, this is based on suspicion of a generalized or widespread disease, such as a bone marrow biopsy in leukemia, but generally it is based on palpation of an abnormal lump or of abnormal consistency in otherwise normal tissues. In the absence of such findings, random biopsies are valueless unless they turn out to be positive, and this occurs but seldom. Furthermore, the healing of such biopsy wounds leaves areas of induration and scarring which may interfere with accurate palpation of the area for months and sometimes for years, thus diminishing the chance of discerning significant changes at subsequent examination.

In all breast lesions, except very advanced ones, and where possible in most other lesions suspected of malignancy, excision biopsy should be practiced rather than incision or chip biopsy. Wedge or chip biopsies are of limited value when negative, and needle biopsies in general cannot be relied upon at all if they are negative. It is essential in doing a biopsy to avoid an error in sampling. With all hard-to-feel lumps near the surface of the body, local infiltration anesthesia should be avoided, if possible, as it often makes it impossible to identify the lesion by touch during the operation. Of course, regional nerve blocks at a distance from the lesion do not have this drawback.

Tumors of hollow viscera usually cannot be subjected to excision biopsy without undertaking a major resection (see Chap. 29, "Stomach and Duodenum"). Even when an intraluminal approach is used (e.g., proctoscopic examination of rectum), only a chip or partial biopsy is possible in many instances, but many a polyp which appeared to be benign in the portions removed by the biopsy forceps has revealed carcinoma when the entire specimen reached the pathologist. (See Chap. 31, "Pancreas," regarding the problems of pancreatic biopsy).

The reliability of frozen section diagnosis can be high in the breast (90 to 95% correct), though it is closely approached by the examination of the gross appearance of the cut surface of the lesion. However, it is not as good as the histologic diagnosis of the paraffin section. What evidence is available would indicate that when the pathologist is in doubt after examination of the frozen section, a delay of 2 to 5 days in carrying out a definitive cancer operation should be permitted so that examination of the paraffin section can be done. Such a delay does not result in a demonstrably worse prognosis. Such cases are usually early cases, however, and it has been argued that the 5-year cure rate should be better than average rather than about the same. Furthermore, the increased psychic trauma to the patient caused by staging the operation is an important consideration.

In certain other areas the value of the frozen section is less, e.g., polyps of the colon, and in still other areas its value is nil unless certain positive findings happen to exist. This is especially true in the examination of lymph nodes where little is certain on frozen section, unless the node is invaded by evident metastatic carcinoma.

It is not too much to hope that eventually means will be developed for producing sections of tissue suitable for definitive microscopic examination within a few minutes, but with present methods one must know when to rely on frozen section diagnosis and when not to.

Turning toward the other end of the spectrum in carcinoma, when is a cancer so advanced as to make a radical attempt to remove it not worth while? In breast carcinoma, this problem was studied carefully by Haagensen and Stout (1943), who set up criteria of nonoperability by correlating preoperative findings with 5-year postoperative survival. Even though the series included about 700 cases, the subgroups were in some instances small, and some of the conclusions reached have had to be modified (1951). No comparable study has been achieved for cancer in any other site with the possible exception of the cervix uteri.

How serious a mistake is it to do a radical mastectomy even though it violates a criterion of nonoperability as evidenced by the study of Haagensen and Stout? Mortality, morbidity and the chances of increasing the spread or the rate of growth of unremoved tumor are all factors to be considered.

In a recent review of clinical experience, Boyd, Enterline and Donald (1954) report an operative mortality of 0.2 per cent for radical mastectomy. The risk to life, then, is small if available safeguards are employed during operation and the postoperative period. Disability is marked for 1 to 4 months. Residual disability is slight for the activities in which most women engage. There are also the economic factors, but it is doubtful that irradiation therapy is much less expensive than operative treatment, and there remain psychological factors. The removal of a breast for a tumor is a heavy blow to face, but is it worse than living with the tumor visibly and palpably growing and ultimately often ulcerating? And, is it worse than prolonged x-ray therapy with its attendant "radiation" illness and local radiation reactions?

The late Dr. Eldridge L. Eliason frequently said, "In this country a person cannot be condemned to death without a fair trial." Certainly, in all borderline cases, it is better to attempt radical treatment when the operative mortality is low. However, there are cases which are clearly beyond help, and the surgeon should avoid embarking on an operation if it is a useless gesture.

The degree of palliation offered by operation in incurable cancer is a moot point. In breast cancer, it is doubtful if it offers any more for the patient with distant metastases than x-ray therapy. In colon cancer, it has been thought that liver metastases grew more slowly after surgical eradication of the primary tumor. The above is a clinical impression neither supported nor contradicted to the author's knowledge by statistically significant data. It seems improbable that removal of a primary in the colon actually decreases the growth rate of established liver metastases. However, its removal should halt the seeding of the liver with fresh metastases. Many of the liver metastases appear to be well localized or somewhat encapsulated and may grow very slowly. At least, metastases in the liver are essentially sterile, while the original colon growth is always infected.

Bruschwig (1947, 1954), who has been a strong advocate of radical surgery in advanced cancer, has been able to report significant numbers of 5-year survivors among persons who have what are generally considered "hopeless" cancers, especially of the cervix uteri and the rectum. An interesting discussion of the problems and various types of procedures of the "supraradical" nature is presented by Fisher (1954).

MISCELLANEOUS PALLIATIVE CANCER OPERATIONS

In addition to attempts at resection, there are many other palliative operations carried out in cancer patients. Many of these are side-tracking procedures for relief of obstructions in hollow viscera. Examples are tracheostomy for carcinoma of the larynx, gastrostomy for carcinoma of the esophagus, gastro-enterostomy for carcinomas obstructing the pyloric area, entero-enterostomy, ileocolostomy, et cetera. Cholecystojejunostomy or choledochojejunostomy may relieve jaundice due to neoplastic obstructions low in the common bile duct. Similar shunting procedures are used in the urinary tract. It is hard to evaluate these methods of treatment fairly. Gastrostomy, for relief of obstruction of the esophagus by carcinoma, has been followed by an average survival of only 3 months in some series. Unfortunately, some of these patients develop pain from the advance of the malignancy, whereas they probably would have died painlessly from inanition if left alone. In arriving at final decisions in such situations, it is generally wise to have the appropriate members of the patient's family and a consultant share the responsibility for the decision.

Neurosurgery has made a great contribution to the palliative treatment of cancer by developing methods of interrupting the sensory pathways for pain with minimal interference with other modalities of sensation, or by destroying so-called association pathways. These procedures are discussed in Chapter 51, "Neurosurgery."

CANCER STATISTICS

To evaluate the published experience of other physicians is nowhere more important than in the field of malignant disease. The pitfalls are numerous. To illustrate, a report may state that the 5-year cure rate after subtotal gastric resection for gastric cancer is 30 per cent. This statement does not tell one the following things:

How was cure judged at 5 years: by survival, by letter follow-up, by physical examination, or by physical examination plus x-ray studies of the gastrointestinal tract and the chest? Most careful authors now use the terms

"5-year survival" or "5-year survival without clinical evidence of recurrence."

Does the 30 per cent relate to all of the hospital's admissions with carcinoma of the stomach, to all admissions on the entire surgical service of the hospital, to all admissions to a particular surgeon's service, to all operable cases in one of the above categories, to all such cases that were resectable, to all that were resected without leaving gross tumor behind, or to all that were resected and found to have no lymph node mastases?

One can think of other variables that might be important. For instance, with breast cancer, the incidence of axillary metastases at the time patients seek treatment has been much higher among indigent patients than among private patients.

In order to compare or combine different series, it is necessary to know how the statistics were compiled. Usually, it is best to report the 5-year survivals as a percentage of all patients in which the diagnosis was well established, admitted to an institution or, at least, to a service. The criteria for including or excluding cases should be stated in some detail. The 5-year survivals may then also be related to the total number operated upon, the total number resected with the hope of cure, the total number without lymph node metastases, etc. A good reference on the subject is Johnson (1955).

PROPHYLACTIC SURGERY IN THE FIELD OF CANCER

It is now reasonably well established that certain lesions are potentially malignant. In some cases, the lesion is a benign tumor or ulcer, which it is believed may undergo malignant transformation. In other situations, some pathologists oppose the concept of transformation and maintain that those lesions which are malignant in their late stages were always malignant, even though at the earlier stage they were grossly indistinguishable from a benign lesion. In both groups of patients having potentially malignant though probably benign tumors, it is desirable to remove the lesions if the price in terms of operative mortality, disability (both temporary and permanent) and psychological factors is not too high.

Examples in which such removal is generally considered worthwhile, except where special contraindications exist, are nodules in the thyroid gland, especially if they appear to be solitary, polyps of the rectum and the colon, and chronic sores on the lip, the tongue, or the buccal mucous membrane. An example in which the price is generally considered too high is the following:

Morbidity statistics would seem to indicate that 50 per cent of cancer in women would be eliminated if the uterus and the breasts were removed after the woman had her family and had attained the age of 38 to 40 years. The mortality of the two simple mastectomies would be very low—about 0.1 to 1.0 per cent; the mortality of the total hysterectomy in healthy individuals at that age should be under 1.0 per cent—so that the total risk would be of the order of 1.2 per cent if proper safeguards were observed carefully. It is estimated that 20 to 25 per cent of women die of cancer, and 10 to 12 per cent die of cancer in one of these loci. There should be little permanent disability as pectoral muscles could be left intact, and the axillary lymphatics would be left intact or nearly intact. Why then is it not done? There are several reasons:

(1) The individuals who would die of the procedure would lose 35 to 40 years of expected life, including 10 to 20 years when they were of especial importance as mothers, whereas deaths due to cancer would be distributed at all ages. (2) Some of those who waited until cancer developed could still be saved by operation at that time (though this factor has already been taken into consideration in the mortality figures). (3) Such treatment involves considerable expenditure of both time and money, especially if one considers the several months of feeling below par after discharge from the hospital. (4) Probably the real reasons are the psychological ones. Breasts are too much a part of a woman's total being to be dispensed with lightly. It is possible that, in a different psychological climate, this factor might change (remember the Amazons), but this does not appear probable here and now. Practically, since current surgical practice does not include these procedures on a purely prophylactic basis, the surgeon who began them might have difficulty in defending himself legally, even though he had acted in accordance with his best judgment.

Preventive surgery presents its own special problems. Superficially, at least, it is in contradiction of Sydenham's famous adage, *"Primum non nocere"* (First, do no harm). In preventive surgery, the harm is done first, and the benefits accrue to the survivors later. The same is true of some phases of preventive medicine as in the early poliomyelitis vaccine experiences of 1955.

The advisability of preventive surgery must be determined by mathematical analysis of experience—in other words, by statistics. In many fields, we do not have experience recorded in ways which permit analysis. What does one need, for instance, to determine whether or not one should advise a patient with a questionable gastric ulcer to have an immediate gastric resection rather than to wait 3 to 4 weeks for a trial of medical treatment? One needs a long series of such patients treated by the alternate case method in which all patients in each half of the series are followed to the time of death and the average months of life for patients in the 2 groups is compared.

Because of the lack of such data and the long time required to obtain them, one looks for more expedient methods. One interesting method depends on only 5 factors: (1) operative mortality when the lesion is benign; (2) the proportion who have or would develop malignancy in the ulcer; (3) the proportion of those who would not come to gastric resection eventually, either for carcinoma or intractability; (4) the 5-year survival rate of those with carcinoma who were operated upon without delay; and (5) the 5-year survival rate for those with carcinoma who are not operated on until lack of response to a trial of medical treatment or other evidence suggested carcinoma.

Let us pick some statistics from the literature and see how far we can get in a concrete example. The mortality of gastric resection for benign lesions as obtained by combining the statistics of Walters *et al.* (1952), Lahey and Marshall (1952), Druckerman *et al.* (1953), Priestley *et al.* (1954), and Wallensten and Gothman (1953) was about 2 per cent.

The incidence of gastric ulcers which proved to be malignant is at least 10 per cent, according to Ransom (1947) and Ravdin and Horn (1953). The percentage of those responding to medical treatment who eventually come to gastric resection is estimated by Smith and Jordan (1948) and by Marshall (1953) at 20 per cent.

The 5-year survival rate for patients with gastric carcinoma has long been given as 5 per cent and will be taken at 8 per cent on the basis of Ransom (1953). In 2 series, Lampert, Waugh and Dockerty (1950) and Ransom (1947), the 5-year survival rate for patients with gastric carcinoma after resection for "undiagnosed" gastric ulcer was over 40 per cent.

The cost in lives lost unnecessarily is the mortality which was 2 per cent multiplied by the patients who would escape operation entirely if not operated upon prophylactically. Of 100 patients with doubtful ulceration of the stomach, experience indicates that 10 will have cancer and 20 will have intractable ulcers. This leaves 70 who would escape operation if it were delayed. Thus, the cost of a policy of prophylactic resection would be seen to be $.02 \times 70 = 1.4$ per cent or 14 per thousand.

Offsetting this is the difference between the 5-year survival rate for carcinomas operated on prophylactically (S_1) and the 5-year survival rate for carcinomas operated on after the diagnosis had become apparent (S_2) multiplied by the number who have carcinoma (C). Expressed mathematically, this is ($S_1 - S_2$)C, or $(40 - 8) .10 = 3.2$ or 32 per thousand. Thus, in the example given, preventive surgery would appear to save over twice as many lives as it cost.

When one considers the many other variables, such as the number dying of the cancer after 5 years, the tendency of patients who have had one cancer to develop another, the fact that the months the patient with cancer would live before diagnosis became definite are lost by the unfortunate person without cancer who dies of operation and other factors that the thoughtful student will consider, this is not a very wide margin. However, if the operative mortality could be reduced to 0.5 of 1.0 per cent, the advantage becomes about 9 to 1. This shows that preventive surgery is for the good-risk patient rather than the poor -risk one, and that greater reduction in operative mortality rates could ex-

TABLE 7. ESTIMATED 5-YEAR SURVIVAL RATES
OF COMMON CANCERS

Locus	FIVE-YEAR SURVIVAL (All patients receiving definitive treatment) PER CENT
Breast	
Without axillary metastases	70
With axillary metastases	30
Lip	80
Tongue	25
Stomach	
Resectable without gross residual tumor	25
Resectable without node metastases	50
Rectum (and rectosigmoid)	40
Cervix—over-all	45
Stage 0	95
Stage I	80
Stage II	50
Stage III	25
Stage IV	10
Uterus	
Limited to uterus	70
Spread beyond uterus	20
Thyroid	65
Lung (resectable)	10
Skin	95

tend the indications for prophylactic surgery further. This example is cited partly to point up how complicated these issues are and partly to indicate a more quantitative approach to the answers.

The surgery of cancer has become a major preoccupation of many surgeons. However, it is not expected that the ultimate solutions will be found by surgical means. Pending the development of what might be called a satisfactory molecular attack on cancer, surgery is the most effective means of treating most early forms of malignancy. Some estimates of the 5-year survival rates for cancer originating in some of the common loci are presented in Table 7.

In addition to the survivors at the 5-year level, much is accomplished in prolongation of life and alleviation of symptoms by palliative procedures.

BIBLIOGRAPHY

Boyd, A. K., Enterline, H. T., and Donald, J. G.: Carcinoma of the breast: a surgical follow-up study, Surg., Gynec & Obst. 99:9-21, 1954.

Brunschwig, A.: Radical Surgery in Advanced Abdominal Cancer, Chicago, Univ. Chicago Press, 1947.

———: Total and anterior pelvic exenteration: report of results based upon 315 operations, Surg., Gynec. & Obst. 99:324-330, 1954.

Collins, V. P., Loeffler, R. K., and Tivey, H.: Am. J. Roentgenol. 76:988, 1956.

Coman, D. R.: Decreased mutual adhesiveness, a property of cells from squamous cell carcinomas, Cancer Res. 10:625-629, 1944.

Druckerman, L. J., Weinstein, V. A., Klingenstein, P., and Colp, R.: Duodenal ulcer treated by subtotal gastrectomy with and without vagotomy, J.A.M.A. 151:1266, 1953.

Fisher, B.: Editorial: supraradical cancer surgery, Am. J. Surg. 87:155-159, 1954.

Haagensen, C. D., and Stout, A. P.: Carcinoma of the breast; criteria of operability, Ann. Surg. 118:859, 1943.

———: Carcinoma of the breast; results of treatment, Ann. Surg. 134:151-172, 1951.

Johnson, R. E.: Editorial: deceptive associations in clinical data, Ann. Surg. 141:567-571, 1955.

Lahey, F. H., and Marshall, S. F.: The surgical treatment of peptic ulcer, New England J. Med. 246:115, 1952.

Lampert, E. G., Waugh, J. M., and Dockerty, M. B.: Incidence of malignancy in gastric ulcer believed preoperatively to be benign, Surg., Gynec. & Obst. 91:673, 1950.

Marshall, S. F.: The relation of gastric ulcer to carcinoma of the stomach, Ann. Surg. 137:891, 1953.

Priestley, J. T., Walters, W., Gray, H. K., and Waugh, J. M.: Annual report on surgery of stomach and duodenum for 1953, Proc. Staff Meet. Mayo Clin. 29:638, 1954.

Ransom, H. K.: Cancer of the stomach, Surg., Gynec & Obst. 96:275, 1953.

———: Subtotal gastrectomy for gastric ulcer: a study of end results, Ann. Surg. 126:633, 1947.

Ravdin, I. S., and Horn, R. C.: Gastric ulcer and gastric cancer, Ann. Surg. 137:904, 1953.

Smith, F. H., and Jordan, S. M.: Gastric ulcer: a study of 600 cases, Gastroenterology 11:575, 1948.

Wallensten, S., and Gothman, L.: An evaluation of the Billroth I operation for peptic ulcer, Surgery 33:1, 1953.

Walters, W., Gray, H. K., Priestley, J. T., and Waugh, J. M.: Report on surgery of the stomach and duodenum for 1950, Proc. Staff Meet. Mayo Clin. 27:39, 1952.

Carl A. Moyer, m.d.

CHAPTER 11

The Assessment of Operative Risk

Intuition based upon personal experience and the observation of a patient's total reaction are important for judging operative risk.

Ideally, the assessment of operative risk should be approached as a statistical problem, and the risk expressed as the probability of dying during an operation and convalescence. However, the statistical approach demands accurate data pertaining to the effects of many factors such as age, starvation, heart disease, etc., upon the operative risk. These are practically nonexistent. Furthermore, the risk attending practically all operations performed upon a random population has undergone remarkable reduction during the past half-century (Table 1). Obviously, because of these factors the accurate assessment of the operative risk for an individual case is impossible today. All we can do is guess. Therefore, the sole purpose of the discussion to follow is to enable the reader to make a better guess than he could before reading it as to the risk that an individual takes when submitting to an operative procedure.

The factors ostensibly affecting the operative risk are: the anatomic site, the magnitude of the procedure, the age of the person, the character of the disease, the duration of the illness, the metabolic state of the individual, the technic employed to perform an operation, the quality of ancillary medical care and anesthesia.

To be sure, there are others such as emotional state, insanity, the duration of anesthesia and soporific and analgesic drugs. However, they will not be discussed because their influence cannot be assessed.

The locus of an operative procedure plays an important role in the risk attending an operation. Operations performed upon the heart, the thoracic esophagus and the brain are more risky than those performed upon the gallbladder, the stomach, the appendix, the lung or the breast. Even the location of the disease within a single organ affects risk; the operative death rate is higher with resections of upper esophageal carcinoma than it is with resection of lower lesions (Table 2).

TABLE 1. CHANGE IN OPERATIVE RISK
(Between 1916 to 1938 and 1948 to 1953)

	1916–1945		1948–1953	
OPERATION	TIME PERIOD	OPERATIVE MORTALITY PER CENT	TIME PERIOD	OPERATIVE MORTALITY PER CENT
Choledochostomy	1916–1938	16	1948–1952	2
Thyroidectomy for toxic goiter	1920	5–8	1953	1
Closure of perforated peptic ulcer	1935	41	1949	7
Correction obstructions of small intestine	1928	37	1950–1953	8
Esophagectomy for cancer	1933	55	1952	16
Partial gastric resection for duodenal ulcer	1936–1945	4	1952	2
Surgical therapy of hepatic wounds	1934	62	1953	10
Surgical therapy of colonic wounds	1941	62	1953	14
Radical mastectomy	1925	1	1952	0.2

The combined unit surgical mortality rate of the above procedures between 1916–1945 was 34.1%, while it was 7.6% between 1948–1953. The 1948–1953 rate was only 22% of the 1916–1948 rate.

TABLE 2. OPERATIVE MORTALITY RELATIVE TO THE ANATOMIC SITE

	OPERATION	MORTALITY RANGE PER CENT	MORTALITY MEAN PER CENT	TIME PERIOD
Group I				
Heart	Mitral commissurotomy	6–11.5	..	1949–1953
Esophagus	Thoracic esophagectomy	13–37.5	..	1948–1953
	Repair of congenital atresia and fistulae	42–68	..	1944–1953
Brain	Resection of infiltrating tumors of brain (astroblastoma, glioblastoma, and medulloblastomas)	25–45	..	1946–1953
Group II				
Gallbladder	Cholecystectomy	0.0– 1:8	0.4	1948–1952
Stomach	Partial gastrectomy for duodenal ulcer	0.8– 1.9	..	1945–1952
Breast	Radical mastectomy	0.0– 1.8	..	1935–1952
Colon	Colectomy	4.6– 7.7	5.7	1948–1952
	Radical resection of the rectum	0.0–11.7	6.9	1948–1952
Group III				
Esophagus	Resections of upper esophagus for carcinoma	24	..	1943–1954
	Resections of lower esophagus for carcinoma	7	..	1943–1954
Group IV				
Stomach	Closure of perforation of peptic ulcer	16.6 (gastric)	..	1948–1952
Duodenum	As above	2.7 (duodenal)	..	1948–1952

The risk attending a surgical procedure upon an organ or within an anatomic cavity tends to be directly related to the magnitude of the procedure: a higher mortality rate obtains with a resection of the entire stomach than it does with a resection of a part of it. This and other examples of the influence of the magnitude of the operation upon operative risk are tabulated in Table 3.

The comparison of gross operative mortality rates among the aged and the young leads to this generalization: aging increases the operative risk. J. and J. C. Mithoefer[10] found during 1952 and 1953 a gross operative mortality rate of 8.3 per cent among 240 individuals aged over 70 years and a rate of 1.9 per cent among 1,073 persons less than 70 years old. Between 1948 and 1952 Cole[3] noted gross operative mortality rates of 2.07 per cent and 5.1 per cent among 2,577 per-

TABLE 3. OPERATIVE MORTALITY RELATIVE TO MAGNITUDE OF THE PROCEDURE

	OPERATION	MORTALITY RANGE PER CENT	MORTALITY MEAN PER CENT	TIME PERIOD
Stomach	Partial gastrectomy for carcinoma	6.7–13.6	..	1940–1952
	Total gastrectomy for carcinoma	20 –35.7	..	1947–1952
Colon	Appendectomy	0.1– 0.45	..	1943–1953
	Colectomy (exclusive of rectum)	4.6– 7.7	5.7	1948–1952
	Radical resection of rectum	0.0–11.7	6.9	1948–1952
Lung	Lobectomy	0.0– 2.3	2.1	1948–1952
	Pneumonectomy	12.2–27.7	16.5	1948–1952
Biliary Ducts	Cholecystectomy	0.0– 1.8	0.4	1948–1952
	Cholecystectomy and choledochostomy	0.0–10	2.0	1948–1952
	Choledochoplasty	2.3– 8.3	3.7	1948–1952

TABLE 4 A. OPERATIVE RISK AND AGE

OPERATION	AGE	MORTALITY PER CENT	NUMBER IN SERIES	TIME PERIOD	P OLD = YOUNG
Closure of perforated peptic ulcer	20–39	5	41		
	40–59	15.6	64	1935–1941	0.01
	60–79	40.0	28		
Radical surgery for cancer of mouth and neck	Under 60	1.0	105		
	Over 60	11.5	121	1948–1952	0.001
*Cholecystectomy with and without choledochostomy	Under 70	1.18	513		
	Over 70	5.7	70	1944–1951	0.01
Radical resection of rectum for cancer	Under 60	0.0	53		
	Over 60	11.7	62	1948–1952	0.01
†Gastrectomy for duodenal ulcer	Under 40	1.3	77		
	Over 40	7.9	240	1940–1950	0.05
Pneumonectomy	Under 60	12.2	49		
	Over 60	27.2	18	1948–1952	0.01

* Between 1948 and 1952 Cole found no significant difference between individuals less than and over 60 years (see Table 30 B, Cholecystectomy).

† At variance with Cole's later finding (see Table 30 B, Gastrectomy).

sons under 60 and 1,099 over 60 years of age, respectively. However, after comparing the operative mortalities pertinent to the old and the young obtaining during and after specific operations one is led to conclude that the effect of aging upon the operative risk is variable. The risk attending some operations is the same for the aged and the younger persons (Table 4 B), while it is distinctly lower for the younger in others (Table 4 A).

The probabilities that the death rates attending the operations in Table 4 A are the same among the older and the younger are so small as to permit the assumption that there is very small likelihood of chance accounting for the observed variances in mortality between the young and the old. Therefore, one may conclude that the operative risk attending the operations listed in Table 4 A is greater for the aged than for the

TABLE 4 B. OPERATIVE RISK AND AGE
(From Cole—Operability in young and aged)

OPERATION	AGE	MORTALITY PER CENT	NUMBER IN SERIES	TIME PERIOD	P OLD = YOUNG
Esophagectomy for cancer	Under 60	29.4	17		
	Over 60	41.9	31	1948–1952	0.4
Colectomy	Under 60	4.6	43		
	Over 60	7.7	26	1948–1952	0.6
Radical mastectomy	Under 60	0	122		
	Over 60	0	67	1948–1952	..
Cholecystectomy	Under 60	0	169		
	Over 60	1.8	54	1948–1952	> 0.1
Thyroidectomy	Under 60	0	287		
	Over 60	0	44	1948–1952	..
Herniorrhaphy	Under 60	0.3	313		
	Over 60	1.5	68	1948–1952	0.3
Partial gastrectomy for cancer	Under 60	5.8	34		
	Over 60	2.8	36	1948–1952	0.5
	Under 40	17.7	17		
	Over 40	13.2	59	1940–1950	0.7
Partial gastrectomy for peptic ulcer	Under 60	1.5	67		
	Over 60	0.0	24	1948–1952	0.6

TABLE 5. CHANGING RELATIONSHIP OF OPERATIVE RISK TO AGE

OPERATION	AGE		MORTALITY PER CENT	
			1941	1951
Cholecystectomy	10–60		4.0	1.1
	61 and older		16.6	5.7
	Difference		12.6	4.6
		1928	1927–1931	1940–1949 5th decade only
Appendectomy for simple and complicated appendicitis	0–60	0.4	4.1	0.7 (274)
	61 and older	54	24.0	4.5 (88)
	Difference	53.6	19.9	3.8
		(Fitch)	(Boland)	(Wolff)

young. However, such is not the case for the operations listed in Table 4 B; the probabilities that the operative mortalities are the same among the old and the young are so large as to permit the conclusion that the risk attending the operations in Table 4 B is the same for the old and the young.

Obviously, one cannot formulate a generalization pertinent to the influence of aging upon operative mortality. The rapidity with which the operative mortality rates attending certain operations upon the elderly and the young have approached or are approaching one another (Table 5) indicates that aging likely has little inherent effect upon one's capacity to live during an operation and the convalescence after it, provided that the time requisite for physiologic recovery postoperatively is not prolonged. A cursory search for possible reasons for the lack of difference between the operative mortalities among the young and the old attending such major physically deforming operations as colectomy, radical mastectomy and partial gastrectomy (1948-1952), while a difference exists between the mortalities of the 2 age groups following lesser physically deforming operations such as closure of perforated peptic ulcers and radical surgery of the mouth and the neck, is highly suggestive that the time requisite for physiologic recovery is more important than the anatomic magnitude of the procedure in determining the relative capacity of an aged individual to live after an operation. In other words, of 2 operations effecting equal physical and physiologic deformations, that one producing the physiologic deformation of shortest duration will be the one least likely to be attended by a higher operative mortality among the aged.

This thesis is supported by the following observations: (1) A higher mortality exists among the aged after those operations which are especially prone to be followed by suppuration and other complications (closure of perforated peptic ulcer, radical resection of the rectum, and radical surgery of the mouth and the neck). (2) The same operative mortality exists among young and old after operations seldom attended by complications (mastectomy, thyroidectomy, herniotomy and partial gastrectomy). (3) Burns which usually are followed by a longer period of physiologic deformation than any operative procedure listed in Tables 4 A and B are associated with a discrepancy between the mortality rates among old and young greater than that attending any operation (Table 6).

In other words, the old person is as capable as the young one of withstanding an operation having a short period of physiologic upset, but he is less capable of taking in stride one with a prolonged period of physiologic derangement. A way to say the same thing is a paraphrase of one of Mithoefers' conclusions: An increased operative fatality rate among the aged when it exists is not dependent upon old age itself but is relatable to the lack of tolerance of the aged to complications and misdirected therapy.

These observations and surmises concerning the relationship of operative risk to age provide a basis for the expectation that surgeons may well abolish the influence of age upon operative risk by learning how to shorten the postoperative period of physiologic deformation, how to reduce further the frequency

TABLE 6. AGE AND MORTALITY

Area injured % body surface	BURNS			OTHER OPERATIONS*			
	Mortality %†				Mortality %		
	Age 0–60	Age 60 +	Difference	Operations‡	Age 0–60	Age 60 +	Difference
5	0.005	2	..				
10	0.1	10	..				
15	1	35	34	2	1	11.5	10.5
20	2	60	58	4	5.8	2.8	
25	4	88	84				
30	8	95	87	1	10	40	30
35	16	98	82	3	12	27	15

* Arranged in order of mortality comparable with burns of persons 0–60 years old.

† Minimal death expectancies derived from probit analysis of thermal injuries in Dallas, Texas, between 1945 and 1952.

‡ Operation: (1) closure perforated peptic ulcer, (2) radical surgery for cancer of mouth and neck, (3) pneumonectomy, (4) partial gastrectomy for cancer.

of complications, and how to avoid the use of misdirected therapy.

Operative risk and disease are related. Partial gastrectomy, esophagectomy, and thyroidectomy performed for cancer are more risky than partial gastroectomy for duodenal and gastric ulcers, esophagectomy for benign esophageal stricture, and thyroidectomy for thyrotoxicosis. The comparative mortalities are listed in Table 7.

It might well be argued that the disease, cancer, is not the direct cause of this phenomenon, but rather that the greater age of the cancerous person, his poorer nutrition,

TABLE 7. OPERATIVE MORTALITY RELATIVE TO THE DISEASE OF THE ORGAN

OPERATION	MORTALITY PER CENT	NUMBER OF CASES
Partial gastrectomy (Kurzweg) 1940–50		
for: carcinoma of stomach	13.64	176
gastric ulcer	5.26	152
duodenal ulcer	6.25	320
Partial gastrectomy (Cole) 1948–52		
for: carcinoma of stomach	4.3	70
duodenal and gastric ulcers	1.1	91
Thyroidectomy		
for: carcinoma (1924–52)	8.5	64
toxic goiter (1928–29)	0.5 to 2	over 100
Esophagectomy and primary anastomosis (Burford) 1948–53		
for: chemical strictures	0.0	30
peptic esophagitis	2.4	41
carcinoma	20.0	98

and the wider extent of the operation for cancer are. These may be the real causes, but there is no objective evidence that they are. So until data are collected to prove or disprove this argument it needs be said that a particular operation performed for cancer carries a higher risk than it does when performed for another disease.

There is much to the saying that the longer the lapse of time between the onset of illness and the operation to correct it, the greater the surgical risk. The direct relationship between operative risk and procrastination is especially apparent in a number of diseases with inflammatory components. The association of risk with time in a number of such disease entities is shown in Table 8. By virtue of the direct relationship of time-lapse to perforation of the gallbladder with cholecystitis and gangrene of the intestine with intestinal obstructions Parts 2 and 3 of Table 9 are also illustrative of the increase in operative risk with increase in time between the onset of the disease and the operation.

Although for some time great emphasis has been placed upon the influence of the metabolic state of the individual upon his capacity to withstand surgical therapeusis, remarkably little human data is available for the quantitative assessment thereof. Although everyone agrees that individuals ill with adrenal cortical insufficiency, uncontrolled diabetes or myxedema are "poor operative risks," one cannot find data that might permit the formulation of an idea of how much these metabolic

TABLE 8. INFLUENCE OF DURATION OF ILLNESS UPON OPERATIVE MORTALITY

OPERATION	DURATION OF ILLNESS	MORTALITY	
		1940–1944	*1945–1949*
Closure of perforated peptic ulcer	0–12 hours	21.6%	3.8%
	12 or more	45.5%	18.7%
		1934–1951	
Reduction of intussusception, or resection for	0–24 hours	1.5% (66)	
	0–48	3.4% (89)	
	Longer than 48	25.6% (27)	
		1930–1935	
Appendectomy (all types of appendicitis— simple and complicated)	0–6 hours	0.0% (219)	
	6–12	1.0% (578)	
	13–18	1.0% (204)	
	19–36	4.4% (1,004)	
	37–72	5.4% (930)	
	72 plus	8.0% (578)	
		1936	
Appendicitis, complicated by rupture, peritonitis, etc. (appendectomy and drainage of abscesses)	0–12 hours	1.8% (212)	
	12–24	2.4% (411)	
	24–36	3.0% (134)	
	36–48	8.1% (296)	
	48–72	8.6% (221)	
	72–96	10.5% (86)	
	5 days plus	14.2% (225)	

diseases increase risk. A rough idea of the influence exerted by two metabolic dyscrasias—myasthenia gravis and thyrotoxicosis—may be drawn from the figures presented in Table 10.

Because suppuration induces appreciable metabolic alterations, the relationship of operative risk to suppuration may well be considered as an example of the relationship of

metabolic state to operative risk. The development of local or general peritonitis increases the postoperative mortality rate significantly, although the influence it bears is less today than it was 30 years ago. Compare parts (A) and (B) of Section 1, Table 9.

Malnutrition in general and more especially "protein depletion" and vitamin deficiencies

TABLE 9. INFLUENCE OF SUPPURATION UPON OPERATIVE RISK

OPERATION	MORTALITY PER CENT	NUMBER IN SERIES	SOURCE AND TIME
1. Appendectomy			
A. For: acute local appendicitis	1.7	1340	St. Thomas Hospital
appendicitis with local abscess	8.0	189	London
appendicitis with generalized peritonitis	21.1	226	1920–1929
B. For: appendicitis without peritonitis	0.45	2160	Seneque
appendicitis with generalized peritonitis	4.4	253	1934–1953
2. Cholecystectomy			
For: uncomplicated acute cholecystitis	6.5	. .	Pines
acute cholecystitis with walled-off perforation	15.0	90	1942–1952
acute cholecystitis with free perforation	23.3		
3. Resection of small intestine			
For: nongangrenous bowel	7	14	Bollinger
gangrenous nonperforated	31	32	1953
gangrenous perforated	40	15	
4. Pneumonectomy			
For: tuberculosis			
A. Before streptomycin	66	6	Efskind
B. With streptomycin	6	90	1946–1953

TABLE 10. INFLUENCE OF METABOLIC STATE UPON OPERATIVE MORTALITY

OPERATION	MORTALITY PER CENT	NUMBER IN SERIES	TIME PERIOD
Superior Mediastinal Exploration			
Removal of benign			
(A) mediastinal tumors	1–3		1945–1950
Removal of thymus			
(B) or thymic tumors from persons	16.6	12	1946–1953
having myasthenia gravis	33.0	12	1953
Subtotal Thyroidectomy			
For: (A) nontoxic goiter	1	900	1895
(B) toxic goiter	3–12	+1000	1920

are imputed to exert relatively enormous effects on operative risk. To be sure, animals are poor operative risks when so starved as to be barely alive, or so subjected to repeated plasmaphoresis as to be so ill that some die without being operated upon, but extreme states such as these are rarely seen among men, women, or children in the United States.

Without a doubt, the administration of vitamin K to jaundiced persons has reduced materially the operative hazard of choledo-chostomy. A statement such as this and applicable to all operations cannot be made with equal surety for the administration of vitamins A, B, C, D, or E to the malnourished person.

Although the imputation to starvation and more especially to protein-starvation of a major detrimental influence upon operative risk is logical and is supported by some experimental work performed upon animals other than man, the human evidence in support of this belief is practically nonexistent. However, human starvation effecting a loss of weight so as to reduce the individual to below 80 per cent of normal is attended by diarrhea in 20 to 50 per cent of men and a mortality up to 10 per cent among those having the flux. Obviously, the performance of surgery upon starved individuals should carry a greater risk for that reason alone. However, the experiences of American and European military physicians in Japanese prisoner-of-war camps during the last conflict were such as to indicate that even severe starvation has relatively little influence upon operative risk. In Gottlieb's words:[6]

An interesting observation is that men who in ordinary times would be considered very poor surgical risks because of their emaciation, amebia-sis, and vitamin deficencies responded very well under surgery. In fact, most of them sat up and asked for rice in about 36 hours. There were no cases of pulmonary embolism. Excellent results were obtained in abdominal surgery even though there was very little asepsis. There was no post-operative peritonitis, very little abdominal distention, and no stitch abscesses appeared.

Apparently, the deleterious effects of caloric and protein starvation and vitamin deficiencies upon one's capacity to live during and after an operation are not as remarkable or as general as many supposed them to be. For this reason delay of indicated operations should not be based upon need to improve nutrition and especially when the malnutrition has a surgically remedial intestinal lesion at the bottom of it.

This statement must not be construed as an argument for the reduction of attention to improving a starved individual's nutritional status before and after operating upon him. Nonetheless, it may well be used as an argument for an immediate attack upon such lesions as pyloric and intestinal obstructions, enteral fistulas and the placement of grafts on burns.

That severe anemia increases operative hazard is well established through animal experimentation and clinical observations. Such a dogmatic statement cannot be made in regard to the effect of hypoproteinemia alone, notwithstanding many positive statements to the contrary.

The operative risk attending an operation is in part dependent upon the technical manner with which the operation is performed. Table 11 illustrates this point.

Much attention has been placed upon the so-called pulmonary-cardiac status as an im-

TABLE 11. OPERATIVE MORTALITY RELATIVE TO TECHNIC EMPLOYED TO PERFORM A PROCEDURE

OPERATION	MORTALITY PER CENT	NUMBER IN SERIES
Partial gastrectomy (Kurzweg)* 1940–50		
with an antecolic gastro-jejunostomy	10.5	210
with a retrocolic gastro-jejunostomy	5.8	398
Polya	9.8	275
Hofmeister	4.6	326
Drainage of Subphrenic Abscess (Ochsner and DeBakey) 1938		
Extraperitoneal	10.8	67
Transpleural	36.2	394
Transperitoneal	35.1	327
Prefrontal Lobotomy (W. Freeman) 1936–52		
Transcranial	3.6	624
Transorbital	1.7	1239
Closure of Perforated Peptic Ulcer (Donhauser) 1935–51		
Closure without drainage of peritoneal cavity	3.2	61
Closure with drainage (non-suction) of peritoneal cavity	20.3	54

* Partial gastrectomy for carcinoma, and peptic ulcers of stomach and duodenum. The use of the various technics, so far as can be determined, was applied randomly in the treatment of carcinoma and ulcer.

TABLE 12. ANESTHESIA AND OPERATIVE RISK*

AGENT	ANESTHESIA DEATH RATE PER CENT	NUMBER IN SERIES
Nitrous oxide	0.0190	26,200
Thiopental	0.0430	14,000
Thiopental and nitrous oxide	0.0400	43,000
Thiopental and/or nitrous oxide with "curare"	0.1280	38,100
Cyclopropane	0.0188	37,100
Cyclopropane—"curare"	0.0833	2,400
Ether	0.0390	171,300
Ether—"curare"	0.4000	2,000
Ethylene	0.0068	29,200

* Beecher and Todd, Ann. Surg. *140*:2, 1954.

portant determinant of risk. However, as more surgical experience is gained upon persons suffering from pulmonary and cardiac ills, the less important as a risk factor does pulmonary-cardiac disease become. In fact, excepting the existence of angina pectoris, malignant hypertension, repeated or recent myocardial infarction, physically disabling pulmonary emphysema and uncontrolled cardiac failure, the pulmonary-cardiac status changes operative risk very little. The Mithoefers[10] studied 240 aged individuals who were classified as poor or good cardiopulmonary risks preoperatively and found no significant difference in operative mortality between the 2 groups. This led them to the conclusion that cardiopulmonary disease, when unaccompanied by angina pectoris, has no apparent influence upon the surgical mortality among the aged.

Advanced renal and hepatic insufficiency reduces the chance of living after an operation. The postoperative mortality rate attend-

ing portocaval shunting for bleeding esophageal varices was 3 to 5 times higher for those individuals having serum albumin concentrations less than 3 Gm. per cent or cephalin flocculations of 3+ to 4+, or B.S.P. retentions greater than 10 per cent, or ascites that did not disappear with medical treatment, than it was for those persons having serum albumin above 3 Gm. per cent, cephalin flocculations of 1+ to 2+, B.S.P. retention less than 10 per cent, and ascites that disappeared with medical therapy.[9] Blakemore's[2] experience was similar to Linton's. Both Linton and Blakemore found that the mere existence of ascites, the level of serum bilirubin and the prothrombin time were no indicators of the operative risk attending portocaval shunting for bleeding esophageal varices or portal hypertension.

The anesthetic agent employed to perform an operative procedure often has been incriminated as a very important risk factor. The anesthetic risks associated with the administration of 9 agents or combinations thereof are listed in Table 12.[1] More than 60 per cent of anesthesias were performed by nurse anesthetists and residents. Clearly, today anesthesia carries relatively little of the burden of the total operative risk. Only with operations bearing little risk, such as herniorraphy, appendectomy, thyroidectomy and the like, is the anesthetic risk a highly important factor.

A gross idea of the relative importance of anesthetic risk in the total picture of operative risk can be gained from Beecher and Todd's[1] figures listed below:

CAUSE OF DEATH (PRIMARY)	NUMBER	MORTALITY RATE	
Patient's disease	6325	1:95	1%
Surgical error	1428	1:420	0.23%
Anesthesia, primary and contributory	384	1:1560	0.06%

Clearly, surgical errors in diagnosis, judgment and technic contribute 4 times as much as anesthesia to operative risk. This statement is in part unfair to anesthesia because when the calculation of the relative contributions of surgical error and anesthesia is based upon

TABLE 13. INFLUENCE OF QUALITY OF NURSING UPON OPERATIVE RISK*

OPERATION	MORTALITY PER CENT	NUMBER	P
Pneumonectomy			
Poor nursing	29.6	91	P:G
Good nursing	11.8	68	0.1
Lobectomy			
Poor nursing	7.5	13	P:G
Good nursing	3.5	28	0.5

* Brea, Buenos Aires, 1944–52.

TABLE 14.

Formula for Adjusted X^2 (chi square)

$$X^2 = \frac{[(ad - bc) - N/2]^2 N}{(a + b)(c + d)(a + c)(b + d)}$$

Treatment Series	Living	Dead	
I	a	b	a + b
II	c	d	c + d
	a + c	b + d	a + b + c × d = N

a—number patients living } of Treatment
b—number patients dead } Series I
c—number patients living } of Treatment
d—number patients dead } Series II

Table of Values of Probabilities for Adjusted Chi Square (X^2)
One Degree of Freedom from Table IV[4]

If X^2 =	.000157	.000628	.00393	.0158	.0642	.148	.455	1.074
Then P =	.99	.98	.95	.90	.80	.70	.50	.30

If X^2 =	1.642	2.706	3.841	5.412	6.635	10.827
Then P =	.20	.10	.05	.02	.01	.001

Example:

Treatment Series		Living	Dead	
I	Albumin: <3.0 gm.	a 1	b 5	6
II	>3.0 gm.	c 63	d 6	69
		64	11	75

$$\text{Adj. } X^2 = \frac{[(1 \times 6) - (5 \times 63) - 75/2]^2\, 75}{(1 + 5)(63 + 6)(1 + 63)(5 + 6)} =$$

Calculation of example: $\text{Adj. } X^2 = \dfrac{[(6 - 315) - 38^2]\, 75}{6 \times 69 \times 64 \times 11} = 18.9, \therefore P = <.001$

Conclusion: Individuals having portacaval shunts for bleeding esophageal varices who have serum albumin concentrations above 3 grams percent do not die postoperatively with the same frequency that persons having serum albumin concentrations below 3 grams percent do.

death attributable to anesthesia alone, surgical error is found to contribute 4 times as much as anesthesia to the operative risk.

The quality of nursing and general hospital services, and the capacity of the surgeon are very important risk factors, though data supporting this statement is remarkably scarce. Table 13 shows presumably the effect of quality of nursing upon operative risk. The mortality rate attending pneumonectomy is considerably higher with "poor" nursing than it is with "good" nursing, but the mortality associated with lobectomy is not significantly higher. Data should be gathered to permit an assessment of the parts played by the surgeon and the hospital in operative risk. It may well be that the surgeon, or he who calls himself one, may be in some hospitals the major factor in the total picture of surgical risk.

Although this discussion of operative risk is sketchy and brief, it should be adequate to permit this statement: the accurate assessment of operative risk is impossible today and can be no more than a guess at best.

In a number of tables in this chapter there is a column designated "P." "P" represents the probability or the chance that if one condition exists, a "given" result will occur. Thus, a "P" value of 0.05 means that if 100 tests were run, one could expect the "given" result 95 times. The numbers in these columns were derived from calculations of chi squares (X^2) using the formula of Table 14 and the Fisher and Yates table which is also included in Table 14 for the conversion of the X^2's to probabilities (P's).

The sample calculation of a chi square in Table 14 uses figures taken from Linton's article.[9]

The hypothesis tested in this way may be simply stated: "The outcome of the operation is the same regardless of the value of the variable"—the variable being such things as age of patient, sex, type of operation, etc. The derivation of a probability (P) larger than 0.05 indicates that under the conditions of the test the hypothesis stated above is conventionally acceptable and the more especially should the P be greater than 0.1.

The utility of statistical methods in evaluating the merits and the demerits of various forms of treatment, and the influence of varied factors upon the outcome of different ills and operations is now unquestioned. The medical student should look upon his mastery of the elements of statistics as an invaluable part of his education for the actual practice of medicine. He must be able to evaluate critically the claims made for the effectiveness of drugs and operations, and to do this he needs a working knowledge of statistical methods and of experimental design.

REFERENCES*

1. Beecher, H. K., and Todd, D. P.: A study of the deaths associated with anesthesia and surgery, Ann. Surg. 140:2-34, 1954.
2. Blakemore, A. H.: Portocaval shunting for portal hypertension, Surg., Gynec. & Obst. 94:443-454, 1952.
3. Cole, W. H.: Operability in the young and aged, Ann. Surg. 138:145-157, 1953.
4. Fisher, R. A., and Yates, F.: Statistical Tables for Biological, Medical and Agricultural Research, London, Oliver, 1939.
5. Gibbon, J. H., et al.: Cancer of the lung; an analysis of 532 consecutive cases, Ann. Surg. 138:489-501, 1953.
6. Gottlieb, M. L.: Impressions of a P.O.W. medical officer in Japanese concentration camps, U.S. Naval Med. Bull. 46:663-675, 1946.
7. Hill, A. B.: Principles of Medical Statistics, ed. 5, New York, Oxford, 1950.
8. Johnson, P. O.: Statistical Methods in Research, New York, Prentice-Hall, 1949.
9. Linton, R. L.: Selection of patients for portocaval shunts, Ann. Surg. 134:433-443, 1957.
10. Mithoefer, J., and Mithoefer, J. C.: Studies of the aged; surgical mortality, A.M.A. Arch. Surg. 69:58-65, 1954.
11. Nemir, P., Jr.: Intestinal obstruction, Ann. Surg. 135:367-375, 1952.
12. Sparkman, R. S., and Fogelman, M. J.: Wounds of the liver, Ann. Surg. 139:690-719, 1954.
13. Sweet, R. H.: Total gastrectomy by the transthoracic approach, Ann. Surg. 138:297-310, 1953.
14. Young, M., and Russell, W. T.: Appendicitis: A Statistical Study, Spec. Rep. Ser. 233, Med. Res. Council, Great Britain, 1939.

* The items listed here (but not referred to in the text) have been selected for their excellent bibliographies and comparative statistics concerning the entities named in the titles.

ROBERT D. DRIPPS, M.D.

Anesthesia

Among his professional achievements a physician should have the ability to administer an anesthetic and to supervise intelligently a patient under the influence of that anesthetic. Practical skill in anesthesia can be acquired only in the operating room through personal experience, but certain principles can be set down as guides toward that experience. Some of these will be presented in this chapter. Others can be found in a monograph recently published by the author and his associates.[5]

The signs and the stages of general anesthesia are described in current pharmacologic texts and should be reviewed by the student. These guides to progressive degrees of narcosis are most accurate for ether. However, familiarity with the basic pharmacologic properties of the other general anesthetic agents permits a reasonable estimate of the depth of anesthesia with these substances. Technical aspects of anesthesia will not be considered.

INHALATIONAL ANESTHESIA

Nitrous oxide, cyclopropane and ethylene are the gaseous agents used most commonly, while diethyl ether, fluothane, trichlorethylene, divinyl ether and, to a lesser extent, ethyl chloride and chloroform are the volatile liquids administered for inhalational anesthesia.

GASEOUS AGENTS

Nitrous Oxide. Of the inhalational agents this drug causes the least disturbance to normal bodily function if it is given with a concentration of oxygen equal to or exceeding that in room air (21%). The onset of and the emergence from anesthesia is rapid. Nitrous oxide is a weak anesthetic, but its lack of potency can be overcome in several ways. Preoperative medication with narcotics can be provided in doses larger than are used for the more powerful inhalational anesthetics. An increase in the partial pressure of nitrous oxide in arterial blood, with a consequent intensification of its effect, can be produced by denitrogenation, i.e., displacement of the nitrogen in the lungs, and to a lesser extent in the blood stream and the tissues. This can be accomplished by repeated emptying of the breathing bag of the anesthesia machine, or by use of large flows of gases and minimal or no rebreathing. Nitrous oxide is also frequently combined with the intravenous injection of a short-acting barbiturate. The inability of the latter to provide analgesia is overcome by the ability of nitrous oxide to interrupt afferent impulses, and the two drugs supplement one another. Another combination includes nitrous oxide, thiopental and a "curare" drug, the last being added to provide muscular relaxation. For the patient in profound shock, nitrous oxide alone in concentrations of as low as 50 per cent has proved to be capable of providing an adequate depth of anesthesia for many surgical procedures. This susceptibility to narcosis of the patient in shock is discussed in the section on the anesthetic management of battle casualties.

Cyanosis may occur during recovery from nitrous oxide anesthesia despite ample ventilation with regular, unobstructed respiratory movements in patients who are awake shortly after removing the mask. The duration of this hypoxia may be as long as 10 minutes and may cause an unwanted stress to patients with cardiopulmonary disease. This phenomenon has been termed diffusion anoxia.[6] It is related to the large amount of nitrous oxide which is dissolved in the blood of a patient during anesthesia with this substance. When anesthesia is stopped, nitrous oxide pours out from the blood into the alveoli. The volume of expiration exceeds that of inspiration by as much as 10 per cent at this time. The outflowing nitrous oxide dilutes the alveolar oxygen, and decreased saturation of hemoglobin results. This sequence of events should be prevented by providing at the end of anesthesia with nitrous oxide an inspired concentration of oxygen greater than that of room air.

Ethylene. This unsaturated hydrocarbon is the only inhalational anesthetic agent lighter than air. It is relatively insoluble in blood and is administered, because of its lack of potency, in high concentrations, e.g., 70 per cent in the inspired atmosphere. Onset of anesthesia and emergence from anesthesia are prompt. Except in one or two centers, the drug has not achieved great popularity in this country, perhaps because its odor is unpleasant, and it is explosive. Its only advantage over nitrous oxide is a somewhat greater degree of potency with a lesser likelihood of the development of hypoxia.

Cyclopropane. This drug offers a rapid, smooth induction and emergence from anesthesia, easy controllability and, since it is potent, it can be given with a high concentration (60-80%) of inspired oxygen. Arguments over its value center about certain circulatory reactions. The drug causes a rise in central venous and right auricular pressures. The cause of this is unknown, but the rise may contribute to bleeding in skin and muscle which some believe occurs to a greater degree with cyclopropane than with other general anesthetics.

A decline in blood pressure below preoperative levels may occur at the conclusion of anesthesia. When marked, this response has been termed "cycloyropane shock."[2] One factor possibly responsible for this postanes-thetic decline in blood pressure is the acidosis incident to the retention of carbon dioxide, which may accompany underventilation with any agent, e.g., cyclopropane, thiopental, curare or other respiratory depressants. A second and probably more important factor relates to the mobilization by cyclopropane of norepinephrine, and to a lesser extent of epinephrine. When a norepiniphrine infusion is stopped in a conscious individual, blood pressure not infrequently declines below normal values. Cessation of a cyclopropane anesthesia is tantamount to interrupting a norepinephrine infusion, and the hypotension resulting appears to be analagous.

Abnormalities of cardiac rate and rhythm may follow the administration of cyclopropane. These are of 2 types. The first consists of slow rhythms caused by a downward displacement of the pacemaker, probably reflecting the parasympathetic stimulant property of cyclopropane. These slow rhythms have little clinical significance. The second type consists of more rapid rhythms caused by an increased irritability of the myocardium. There may be ventricular extrasystoles, ventricular tachycardia or infrequently ventricular fibrillation.

Increased production of norepinephrine and epinephrine unquestionably contribute to the cardiac irritability which is further increased if respiratory acidosis is permitted to develop. Therefore, efforts should be made to maintain adequate alveolar ventilation.

If, as is done by some clinicians, ethyl ether is added in small amounts, the incidence of ventricular tachycardia occurring during cyclopropane anesthesia appears to be reduced. The mechanism for such protection is not clear, although interruption of sympathetic impulses arising in the hypothalamus and passing to the heart has been suggested. Indeed, the role of the hypothalamus in the production of cardiac arrhythmias occurring during inhalational anesthesia deserves considerable further study. Clinical experience indicates that ventricular tachycardia is rarely followed by ventricular fibrillation. Many instances of ventricular tachycardia are reported in the literature. Authentic reports of ventricular fibrillation occurring during cyclopropane anesthesia are rare. Sudden circulatory collapse may occur during cyclopropane anesthesia as with any other powerful anesthetic. Such a catastrophe cannot properly be assumed to be due to ventricular fibrillation unless an electrocardiogram was being taken at the time or unless the heart was visualized directly and seen to be in fibrillation. The most common cause for such a calamity is overdose of the agent.

We have anesthetized with cyclopropane many patients with serious cardiac disease. It is our belief that the opponents of this agent have exaggerated the possibilities of harm following its use and have overlooked the advantages of smooth induction, relatively prompt recovery and controllability. Since other technics are available to the modern anesthesiologist, some avoid this agent in the presence of thyrotoxicosis or other instances in which myocardial irritability is known to be increased.

VOLATILE LIQUIDS

Diethyl Ether. This volatile liquid was apparently first prepared in 1540 by Aureolus Phillipus Theophrastus Bombastas von Hohenheim, self-named Paracelsus! Primarily because there is a rather wide margin between the concentration of the drug required to produce respiratory arrest and that required to cause cessation of the heart beat, ether has achieved almost universal use.

Ether is irritating to the respiratory tract. Its unskilled administration may be followed by increased secretions in the respiratory tract, swallowing of ether-laden mucus, and by nausea and emesis in the postoperative period. During its administration by the open-drop technic, anoxia and carbon dioxide retention are likely to occur, particularly if thick layers of gauze are used on the mask, if the gauze becomes saturated with expired water vapor or if a flow of 300 to 400 ml. per minute of oxygen is not added under the mask. A prolonged period of induction is often observed. Attempts to hurry the induction may be accompanied by cough, excessive secretions, laryngospasm and excitement. These sequelae are not inevitable and occur less commonly as experience with the drug increases.

Ether stimulates the sympathetic nervous system. Blood sugar increases through mobilization of liver glycogen. Cardiac rate and output tend to rise, in part, at least, as the result

of mobilization of norepinephrine and to a lesser extent in man, epinephrine.[8, 9] In patients with extensive resection of the sympathetic chain, ether may produce circulatory depression, even in relatively light planes of anesthesia, since the protective or buffering mechanism against the direct cardiac and vascular depression of ether has been reduced. Smooth muscle is relaxed, and for this reason ether is preferred to such parasympathetic stimulants as cyclopropane or thiopental for patients with bronchial asthma and allergic phenomena.

Ether blocks transmission across the nerve-skeletal muscle junction more than do most anesthetics. For this reason it acts synergistically with the antidepolarizing or competitive blocking muscle relaxants such as d-tubocurarine, Flaxedil or Metubine. Therefore, smaller doses of these relaxants are indicated during ether anesthesia. Through a variety of mechanisms ether tends to stimulate respiration, and respiratory acidosis is less common following its administration than when thiopental or cyclopropane has been given. This is particularly true if opiates are omitted from preanesthetic medication. If hypoxia is avoided there is little evidence that ether damages the liver. The drug has a wide field of usefulness, particularly for the occasional anesthetist; it is cheap and can be administered with minimal equipment.

Fluothane. It was considered dangerous to use drugs with fluorine in them until it was realized that some hydrocarbons containing fluorine were among the most stable in organic chemistry. Therefore, fluorinated compounds were studied as anesthetics, primarily because some of them could be made nonflammable. Fluothane—CF_3-$CHClBr$—although expensive, has created considerable interest during the last few years. Because it fails to mobilize norepinephrine in man to the degree characteristic of cyclopropane or ether, fluothane can cause profound hypotension unless the inspired concentration is controlled within fairly narrow limits. Current practice suggests that induction concentrations rarely should exceed 3 to 4 per cent, with maintenance at the 0.5 to 1.5 per cent level. As a rule, these concentrations are attained with special apparatus or with such vaporizers as a copper kettle.

Despite hypotension, some observers regard

the patient's condition as excellent, pointing to a full pulse and warm dry skin which is often of good color. Certainly, within reason, a given level of low arterial blood pressure is less important than is the mechanism underlying the reduction. The prognosis, for example, is more grave with hypotension produced by histamine than at the same level of pressure resulting from the injection of acetylcholine. Capillary circulation is better preserved in vital areas in the latter set of circumstances. Perhaps this same situation will obtain with fluothane. In the absence of respiratory acidosis, cardiac arrhythmias are rare during anesthesia.

The drug is extraordinarily soluble in fat, a fact which may explain the slow awakening sometimes seen after its administration. Postoperative nausea and vomiting appear to be diminished, but this may be due to the fact that fluothane is not commonly given for intraabdominal operations. Originally regarded as valuable because of its nonexplosibility, this volatile liquid currently is being explored in a variety of circumstances by many enthusiastic individuals. Its ultimate place remains to be determined, but it does appear to have many desirable features.

Divinyl Ether (Vinethene). This potent drug is usually administered in an open system for brief operative procedures, or as an induction agent to ether. Prolonged administration to man and animals has been followed by renal and hepatic cellular damage, particularly if hypoxia was present during anesthesia. The incidence of muscular twitching and convulsions is higher after Vinethene than with other volatile liquids, reaching 3 per cent in some series. Its relatively greater capacity to induce convulsions makes its use somewhat hazardous in the face of high fever, dehydration and electrolyte imbalance, especially in infants and children. Because of its potency Vinethene has been used to supplement nitrous oxide during dental operations. Emergence is rapid, and recovery is usually free of nausea and vomiting.

Trichlorethylene (Trilene, Trimar). This agent is used to produce analgesia for vaginal delivery, cystoscopy and other minor procedures. Because it is nonexplosive, it is also useful for major operations that do not require muscular relaxation or profound depth of anesthesia. The drug has several interesting properties. If administered in too high a concentration, it causes an increase in respiratory rate up to 50 to 60 per minute. It is the only inhalational anesthetic which is partially metabolized in the body. Nausea and vomiting are not common following its administration. Because of its low volatility, opendrop administration is difficult. Therefore, the drug is given by means of a specially constructed inhaler or via a standard gas machine. Volatilization with nitrous oxide and oxygen is currently popular. A closed system with soda lime absorption of expired carbon dioxide cannot be used, since the drug decomposes in the presence of heat to form toxic or irritant products.

Ethyl Chloride. Halogenation of a hydrocarbon increases the potency of a compound but also makes it more of a cellular toxin. Examples of this chemical fact include chloroform, Avertin and ethyl chloride. Ethyl chloride is highly volatile, boiling at 12° C. Induction is rapid, but circulatory depression may be profound. In skilled hands the drug has been used for an induction agent to ether. As a surface spray the resulting local analgesia, related to cooling of the tissues sprayed, is often inadequate for the performance of operations.

Chloroform. The anesthetic properties of this liquid were discovered by Flourens in 1847, and Simpson the great British obstetrician, administered it to patients that same year. Simpson attended Queen Victoria during several of her deliveries, using chloroform as an analgesic. From this has come the term *anesthesia à la reine*. An amusing story is told about Simpson, who was a rather pompous individual. On one occasion he placed a note on the door of his consulting room, which read, "Have gone to London to deliver the Queen." Beneath this impressive statement, an irreverent is said to have scrawled, "God Save the Queen."

Early experiences with chloroform in patients poorly prepared for operation and in whom hypoxia was not prevented tended to discredit the drug in the minds of many. It is not used often by physician-specialists in anesthesia. Chloroform is a potent nonexplosive anesthetic agent. When means were provided for controlling the inspired concentration within narrow limits, e.g., 0.1 per cent, and when unevenness in depth of anesthesia was avoided, studies at the University of Wisconsin indicated that the safety of chloroform could be increased considerably.[10]

INTRAVENOUS ANESTHESIA

Thiopental is the drug most frequently given intravenously to produce unconsciousness for surgical operations. The outstanding advantage of this substance for the patient is the smooth induction afforded. Excitement is absent, as are the unpleasant buzzing, roaring, and sinking feelings experienced during induction with inhalational agents. Its chief usefulness is for induction of anesthesia, for brief operations, or in combination with nitrous oxide for procedures not requiring muscular relaxation. Should relaxation be necessary a "curare"-like drug must be added. If large doses of thiopental are used and if the anesthetist attempts to obtain deep planes of anesthesia, hypotension and tachycardia may develop.

The barbituric acid derivatives do not block sensory pathways as readily as do most anesthetics. Afferent impulses from the operative site can reach the brain more readily than when inhalational anesthetics are used. Therefore, in response to surgical manipulations, reflex spasm of the vocal cords or the abdominal muscles may occur. In attempting to treat or prevent these reactions the anesthetist may add more and more drug until dangerous degrees of respiratory and cardiovascular depression result. Therefore, there are certain disadvantages to thiopental for operations in which reflex stimulation is undesirable. To combat this pharmacologic weakness, the analgesic action of nitrous oxide is combined with the sedative quality of thiopental as has been described. However, this is only a partial solution.

CONDUCTION ANESTHESIA

REGIONAL OR LOCAL ANESTHESIA

Isolation of a discrete area of the body by infiltration or block of individual nerves with a local anesthetic agent should theoretically disturb vital functions least of all of the anesthetic methods. In practice this is true for many patients, and often pain relief for operations on seriously ill individuals can be obtained with little added strain. However, this statement must be qualified. Intra-abdominal manipulations, when only block of the abdominal wall has been performed, may be attended by a reflex decrease in blood pressure and unpleasant subjective reactions such as pain, nausea and vomiting (Fig. 12-1). The pathways of this reflex are ill-defined. Occasionally, atropine will reverse the untoward signs and symptoms, suggesting that at least part of the response is parasympathetic in origin. Injection of large amounts of a local anesthetic or unusual sensitivity to the drug may be followed by serious hypotension, convulsions, loss of consciousness, or disturbance in cardiac conduction. The absorption of epinephrine, used to prolong the action of the anesthetic solution, may increase cardiac work beyond the capacity of the coronary arteries to supply blood, and evidences of coronary arterial insufficiency may occur.

Despite these objections, local anesthesia remains of great value for operations on the head, the neck, the extremities, the trunk surface and certain mucosal areas. The cardinal principle in the safety of this method lies in the use of the smallest volume of the lowest concentration of drug which permits satisfactory pain relief. Too frequently, perhaps because of lack of skill or unfamiliarity with the properties of the local anesthetics, surgeons and anesthetists inject large volumes of highly concentrated solutions. Signs of overdosage often result. A 0.25 or 0.5 per cent concentration of procaine provides adequate pain relief during infiltration anesthesia, and the custom of using a 2 per cent solution subjects the patient to an unnecessary hazard of overdosage. For block of individual nerve roots such as the brachial plexus a stronger solution is needed.

A rough guide to the relationship of the safe volume of procaine and its concentration is as follows:

CONCENTRATION (%)	TOTAL VOLUME (CC.)
0.5	200
1	100
2	30

Lidocaine (Xylocaine) is currently popular for local anesthesia, primarily because it spreads more readily through tissues.

Spinal Anesthesia

Spinal anesthesia produces excellent muscular relaxation and affords ideal working conditions for the surgeon during intra-abdominal operations. Two *immediate sequelae* of subarachnoid nerve block must be anticipated: (1) a decrease in mean arterial blood pressure from block of vasomotor nerves and reduction in the thoracic pump effect; and (2) respiratory inadequacy from block of intercostal nerves. If these possibilities are kept in mind and prevented or treated intelligently, as they can be, the safety of spinal anesthesia is greatly increased even for substandard patients. The method is probably contraindicated in the presence of low blood volume because the resulting vasodilation may be followed by marked hypotension.

Many patients and physicians fear that spinal anesthesia will be followed by serious neurologic disturbances. Foster Kennedy[7] has stated:

From a neurological point of view we give the opinion that spinal anesthesia should be rigidly reserved for those patients unable to accept a local or general anesthetic. Paralysis below the waist is too large a price for a patient to pay in order that the surgeon should have a relaxed field of operation.

If spinal anesthesia is given to patients with pre-existing neurologic disease, sequelae are more apt to occur. If faulty sterilization of

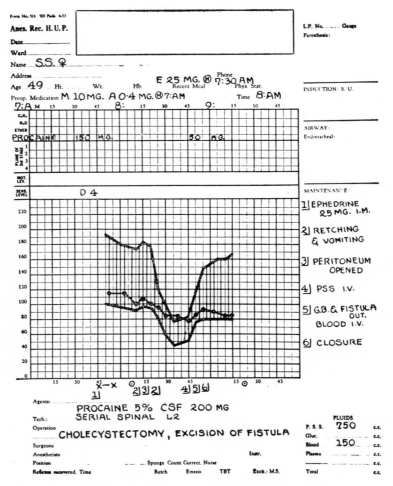

FIG. 12-1. Hypotension occurring during local anesthesia and caused by intra-abdominal manipulations.

the drugs, needles and syringes used for this method is permitted, an increased number of complications will be noted. *But if the technic of lumbar puncture is refined, if foreign materials such as talcum powder applied to gloves or skin antiseptics do not contaminate the subarachnoid space, and if all drugs are autoclaved,* spinal anesthesia is an exceptionally safe and useful method. The author and his associates have followed patients to whom spinal anesthesia was given, not only during the immediate postoperative period but for 6 to 60 months after operation. Of approximately 9,300 patients, 89 per cent have been followed in this fashion. Not a single instance of adhesive arachnoiditis has been found during this study. Indeed, no patient appears to have suffered permanent neurologic damage of any consequence.[4] Instances of persistent numbness, backache, pain, or weakness were reported, but on examination these proved to be trivial or minor in nature. We believe that spinal anesthesia is a particularly useful method, and one which has suffered unjustly because of fear of medicolegal consequences. However, consciousness during an operation is frequently unpleasant, with fear, nausea, vomiting and pain among the undesirable aspects. The management of spinal anesthesia must be carried out with skill and understanding. Supplementation of the block with intravenous barbiturates and nitrous oxide is often essential. If no additional general anesthesia is provided the patient must be reassured constantly and given adequate psychological support.

MUSCLE RELAXANTS

Prior to 1940 curare was a medical curiosity. Injection of crude solutions of the drug into animals resulted in such depression of blood pressure that the possibility of use in man seemed to be remote. However, the development of the field was rapid as soon as acceptable products became available. A vast clinical experience has now been accumulated. Overenthusiasm marks the reaction of some. Skepticism is equally apparent. We must view the "curare" drugs in a proper perspective which time alone can provide.

The "curare" drugs are administered to anesthetized patients primarily with the view

of reducing the amount of other drugs required to produce muscular relaxation and reduction in reflex activity. Without a curarizing agent profound muscular relaxation *during general anesthesia* can be achieved only by relatively deep narcosis. This greater depth of anesthesia is accompanied by greater interference with function (e.g., heart, liver and kidney) during operation and by a more disturbed postoperative course. One must attempt to discover whether the hazards of the "curare" drugs outweigh the disadvantages of deeper general anesthesia.

In a study by the author of 2,800 patients receiving various muscle relaxants, 0.5 per cent exhibited profound respiratory depression or apnea. These lasted from 1 to 3 hours after completion of the operation, even though acceptable or safe amounts of drugs had been given.[3] To have a patient not breathing or requiring constant assistance to respiration when the operative procedure has been finished is indeed disturbing. In inexperienced hands one can anticipate fatalities under such circumstances. Although the causes of these abnormal respiratory responses to the "curare" drugs remain unknown, the available evidence suggests that interference with central nervous system activity is involved in addition to block at the peripheral neuromyal junction. It has been shown, for example, that stimulation of the phrenic or intercostal nerves in the apneic patients will result in contraction of the diaphragm or intercostal muscles, indicating that the junctional pathways are intact. Similarly, movements of the arms, the legs and the head have been observed in such patients despite the absence of respiration. This bizarre situation emphasizes the complexity of the "curare" action and indicates that neuromyal block alone is insufficient to explain some of the untoward sequelae of the drugs. The therapy of prolonged respiratory depression is artificial ventilation until tidal volume has returned to normal. Pharmacologic antidotes such as prostigmine, preceded by atropine, may be useful against *d*-tubocurarine and drugs resembling it. These antidotes affect conduction through the nerve-muscle junction and are of no value if the abnormality responsible for apnea lies within the central nervous system.

Depression of blood pressure may follow

administration of the muscle relaxants. The mechanisms responsible for this include autonomic ganglionic blockade, liberation of histamine, diminished muscular tone, the use of positive pressure respiration, or the simultaneous injection of thiopental.

Succinyldicholine Chloride (Anectine). Of the newer substances succinyldicholine chloride (Anectine) is the most interesting. Its duration of action following a single intravenous dose is brief, ranging from 2 to 5 minutes. Short periods of relaxation can thus be afforded by single injections of 20 to 40 mg. for such procedures as endoscopy, reduction of fractures and electroshock. If more prolonged relaxation is required, the drug may be administered as a continuous intravenous drip in doses of 2 to 8 mg. per minute. Regulation of the rate of flow affords relaxation of varying degree. Cessation of flow is usually followed by a prompt return of muscle tone. This is not inevitable, however, since the rate of destruction depends in part upon the availability of pseudocholinesterase, an enzyme which may be reduced in concentration under certain circumstances, e.g., liver disease. Administration of large amounts of the drug may saturate body depots, and prolonged action results.

Summary. The author's attitude toward the curare group of drugs can be summarized as follows. The balance sheet is in favor of these substances. In the United States the doses used are more conservative than abroad, where amounts administered are double or triple those used in this country. With this more cautious approach it is our belief that these drugs carry little if any hazard to the patient whose preoperative physical condition is within normal limits. Indeed, the sparing of deeper planes of anesthesia for such patients may result in a smoother, safer convalescence. There are data to suggest that the incidence of untoward reactions to the curare group rises as the physical condition of the patient deteriorates.[3] But the hazard of any anesthetic procedure increases under these conditions. Suggestions of individual susceptibility to various of the curare group have been made by some. Preliminary injection of a small amount of the agent to the conscious patient may reveal such a sensitivity. In the absence of this type of response and in the hands of

an intelligent anesthetist the muscle relaxants have much to offer.

RESPIRATORY PROBLEMS ASSOCIATED WITH UNCONSCIOUSNESS

Unconsciousness carries with it the threat of certain respiratory difficulties which must be anticipated constantly and treated promptly. These potential hazards exist in every unconscious individual whatever the cause of the unconsciousness. Thus the problem may complicate any type of general anesthesia, as well as such medical ills as narcotic poisoning, diabetic coma, uremia, or cranial injuries. It is unfortunate that so many physicians are unfamiliar with the management of these respiratory abnormalities and permit inadequate breathing to persist when often simple measures would suffice to correct them. Therefore, it is stressed that the following discussion is not limited solely to the management of the anesthetized patient but applies equally to any comatose person.

Air must be allowed to move in and out of the lungs freely with movement of the thoracic cage and the diaphragm. Obstruction to this movement of air causes increased work on the part of the respiratory muscles, asphyxia of a degree dependent upon the degree of obstruction, and carries with it the threat of sudden death due to exhaustion, medullary damage or if obstruction becomes complete.

RECOGNITION OF RESPIRATORY OBSTRUCTION

A disparity between the activity of the thorax, the muscles of respiration and the volume of air moved suggests obstruction of the air passages. This may be noted by watching or feeling the chest, the abdomen and the neck and holding the palm of the hand in front of the nose and the mouth. If the air current perceived by the palm is less than the activity of the respiratory muscles indicate that it should be, a diagnosis of obstruction is reasonable. The sounds of breathing also have diagnostic import. "Noisy" breathing is "obstructed breathing." The nature of the sound may localize the site of obstruction, with stertor or snoring indicating soft tissue block (e.g., tongue, epiglottis) and stridor or crowing implicating glottic spasm. If the degree of obstruction is sufficient, cyanosis will occur.

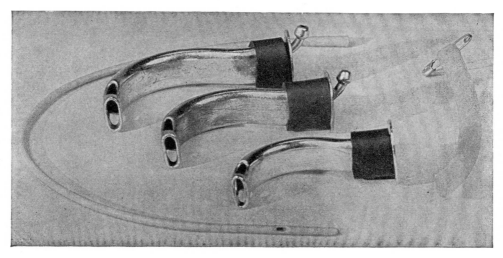

FIG. 12-2. Artificial airways.

TREATMENT OF RESPIRATORY OBSTRUCTION

If obstruction of the soft tissues exists, a number of maneuvers may be of value. The patient should be placed prone or in the lateral position, since the tongue tends to fall back and block the passage of air when an individual lies on his back. The mandible can be moved up and out by fingers placed behind the angles of the jaw. This movement carries the tongue forward and tends to reduce soft tissue block in the mouth and the pharynx. If the mouth can be opened, the tongue can be grasped with gauze or a forceps, or a suture can be placed through the tongue and mild traction exerted. By pulling the tongue forward toward the lips the pharynx may be freed of obstruction. Artificial metal or rubber airways may be inserted in the mouth to hold the tongue forward (Fig. 12-2); rubber tubes may be passed through the nose into the posterior pharynx. Finally, an endotracheal tube may be placed or a tracheostomy performed.

INADEQUATE VENTILATION

The unconscious patient may have such depression of the respiratory center or poor tone of the respiratory muscles that the volume of air moved is not sufficient for alveolar ventilation. Then artificial respiration must be provided. This can be accomplished manually by the Holger Nielsen technic if the patient is prone, or by compression of the chest anteriorly if he is supine. Mouth-to-mouth, or mouth-to-nose breathing can be used. If as a result of artificial respiration the patient's color remains good, room air will suffice. If cyanosis is noted, 100 per cent oxygen should be used. Should support of respiration be required for hours or days, a concentration of 50 per cent oxygen may avoid signs and symptoms of oxygen toxicity.[1] Mechanical resuscitators may be applied when they become available, but valuable time must not be lost in searching for them (a simple device is a hand bellows resuscitator illustrated in Fig. 12-3).

SELECTION OF ANESTHETIC AGENTS AND TECHNICS

An anesthetist skilled in the administration of a variety of agents can so apply these that a specific problem usually may be solved in one of several ways. Gastric resections, for example, have been performed satisfactorily on patients during continuous spinal anesthesia or single dose spinal anesthesia supplemented with inhalational or intravenous anesthesia; during closed system ether, open-drop ether with or without tracheal intubation; or during field or splanchnic block. Skillfully managed, any one of a number of agents and technics can be applied in a given instance, with the final selection being often a matter of individual preference and experience.

The former examination question was unjust when it described a patient with several complicating ailments facing an operation, and required a student to select from a prescribed list the one and only procedure which fitted the conditions outlined. One should be more concerned with *why* a particular method is selected. The student should define his choice of method fortified by reasons for so doing.

The rational point of view recognizes that choice of anesthesia is not a matter of matching a drug or a technic to a disease and of stating dogmatically that such a mating is inevitable and final. Rather, it concerns itself with a broader approach in which the training of the anesthetist, his acquaintance with the surgeon's methods, the accepted procedures in the community, the specific request of the patient, and the former experiences of the patient, must all be considered. We do not believe that an internist called as a consultant to evaluate the physical status of a patient scheduled for operation should dictate the type or method of anesthesia to be used, particularly if a physician specializing in anesthesia is available. Few internists accompany their patients to the operating room, watch the problems of induction and maintenance, realize the difficulties posed by the body habitus of the patient, or appreciate the requirements of individual surgeons. Until they have practical, first-hand experience with the conduct of anesthesia it is unwise for them to insist upon a particular course of anesthesia. If an internist is asked to evaluate a patient for operation in a hospital where technician-anesthetists are employed, it is equally unwise for him to do more than suggest a plan of management. *It is undoubtedly safer for the patient to receive that anesthetic agent with which the technician is most familiar than to attempt a theoretically safer procedure in which he is less skilled.*

ANESTHETIC MANAGEMENT OF THE "POOR RISK" PATIENT

The term "risk" involves an estimate of prognosis. A consideration of the factors which influence the final outcome of a given case suggests that "estimating the risk" is frequently approached improperly. To designate the "risk" accurately would necessitate foreknowledge of such variables as the reliability of the suture material, the fallibility of asepsis, the availability of drugs, the responsibility of those in charge of postoperative nursing care, and a host of other aspects which cannot always be assessed for each patient by the anesthetist or the surgeon. A patient anesthetized by a medical student and operated upon by a junior surgeon has less of a chance than would the same patient in the hands of an experienced anesthesiologist and a senior

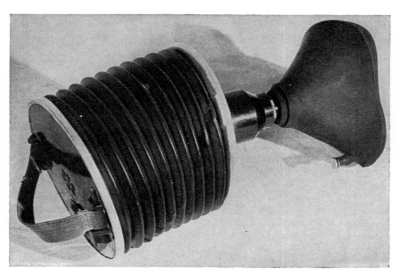

Fig. 12-3. Hand bellows resuscitator. (Kreiselman)

surgeon. In the latter case the patient's condition has not changed, but the likelihood of survival has been increased materially. Likewise, the patient's prognosis is more favorable if the personnel responsible for his care are not tense and overworked. Again, the patient's condition remains the same, but the risk is less. The success or failure of a given procedure often depends upon many things which have little to do with the patient's physical condition.

The above is perhaps an academic discussion. Obviously, there are patients who, for a variety of reasons, are less likely to survive anesthesia and operation than others. Such patients are encountered among candidates for emergency, as well as for less urgent operations. Their anesthetic management will be considered first, in general terms.

Many an anesthetic or surgical accident could have been avoided had a careful appraisal of a patient's problems been made and appropriate corrective measures instituted prior to operation. Too often, for example, the medical work-up of a seriously ill patient or one deemed an "emergency" is inadequate. The very seriousness of the patient's condition creates an atmosphere of tension in which logical analysis is replaced by hurried decision, and attention to detail is subordinated to a cursory survey. The history is glossed over, physical examination is limited, and laboratory data are minimal. The operating room is prepared in haste, the patient is anesthetized hurriedly, and troubles which could have been avoided present themselves in rapid succession.

If the above be true for emergency situations it is at least as pertinent when time is of less concern. Thoroughness of work-up, careful appraisal of systems other than those involved by the primary surgical condition and efforts designed to correct abnormalities of these systems form the backbone of an intelligent preoperative regimen. Such measures ease the anesthetist's burden significantly. Often the patient is classified as "poor risk" from the anesthetic standpoint solely because of inadequate preparation for the operation. The more seriously ill the patient is to begin with, the more important these principles become. Certain examples may be illustrative.

The patient with intestinal obstruction poses problems of anesthesia, many of which can be minimized by preoperative preparation. Aspiration of intestinal contents into the respiratory tract is prone to occur during induction of anesthesia or during surgical manipulation of the distended bowel. The higher the point of obstruction, the greater is the hazard. In the presence of gastric dilation and atony stomach contents may pour into the pharynx at any time and be aspirated into fhe lungs. The best solution to this problem is preoperative decompression and drainage of the stomach and the distended bowel. The time spent in preparing the patient with bowel obstruction for operation is obviously important to the patient's safety and reduces considerably the problems presented to the anesthetist and the surgeon. Since suction-drainage cannot empty the entire intestinal tract, the anesthetist must continue to be aware of this problem. If general anesthesia is selected, there is much to be said in favor of rapid intubation of the trachea with a cuffed tube. Intubation can also be accomplished under topical anesthesia of the mucous membrane of the upper respiratory tract while the patient is still conscious. Spinal anesthesia has been recommended because, among other virtues, it does not impair laryngeal and tracheal reflexes. However, it must be realized that many patients with intestinal obstruction have depression of all reflexes. They may be semistuporous because of dehydration and loss of electrolytes among other reasons, and aspiration of intestinal contents into the lungs is not unlikely even if the operation be conducted during local anesthesia. In addition, these patients have difficulty maintaining an adequate circulation. Spinal anesthesia may precipitate severe hypotension unless blood volume and electrolyte balance have been restored toward normal.

A second example is the patient with chronic suppuration in the respiratory tract. Administration of inhalational anesthesia to an individual with a considerable amount of purulent material in the tracheobronchial tree is difficult because of the following:

1. The exudate in the bronchioles or bronchi tends to block access of the anesthetic to the alveoli.

2. For the same reason adequate oxygena-

tion and elimination of carbon dioxide may be less likely.

3. A smooth plane of anesthesia is difficult to maintain, since frequent aspiration of the respiratory passages is required.

4. Spread of contaminated material throughout the lung fields may occur with change of position, compression of the lung by the surgeon, and because of loss of the cough reflex.

5. There tends to be greater irritability of reflexes in the respiratory passages with more secretions, coughing and cyanosis likely.

These problems are reduced in degree by such preoperative measures as postural or bronchoscopic drainage, inhalation of aerosols, use of antibiotics, use of positive-pressure breathing and elimination of smoking. Many days may be required before the patient with advanced bronchiectasis becomes "relatively dry," but the chances of a fatal outcome or of undesirable postoperative sequelae are reduced for each day that such prophylaxis is carried out. The anesthetist can contribute further to safety by frequent aspiration of the trachea and the bronchi during anesthesia; by having the patient awake at the conclusion of the operation so that he can rid himself of secretions by coughing; and by having injected the intercostal nerves with a local anesthetic agent so that coughing produces less incisional pain. However, the chief contribution that can be made toward the successful surgical and anesthetic management of the patient with copious pulmonary secretions is the preparatory regimen referred to above. The actual anesthetic agent is not of as great importance. Cyclopropane or ether may be given if the cautery is not to be used; a combination of thiopental and nitrous oxide and a muscle relaxant also is popular. Regional anesthesia may be used.

In the cases just discussed it has been pointed out that a lowered mortality and morbidity rate may be achieved by adequate preoperative care. However, there are some patients whose condition is such that they cannot be greatly improved before operation. Under these circumstances the anesthesiologist must select that method which will interfere least with the abnormalities already present. The individual with coronary arterial disease falls into this group. In this type of patient the essential problems are to prevent an increase in cardiac work, or a decrease in coronary arterial flow with a consequent disparity between the metabolic requirements of the cardiac muscle and the available supply of oxygen.

There is no single satisfactory approach to the anesthetic management of these patients, particularly if an intra-abdominal operation is planned. The following suggestions are recommended:

1. Assurance through personal contact that the anesthetist is aware of the patient's particular problem. This relieves a great source of anxiety on the part of the patient who frequently worries lest those concerned with his care be not completely familiar with his cardiac disability.

2. Adequate sedation prior to operation. The mental stress of a trip to the operating room is understandable, and attacks of angina pectoris or coronary insufficiency may be precipitated by such an emotional crisis if proper sedation has not been achieved.

3. Smooth induction of anesthesia. A stormy induction with the likelihood of struggling, respiratory obstruction, anoxia, and retention of carbon dioxide is hazardous for a heart whose blood supply is marginal. Since this blood supply in all probability cannot be increased in the normal fashion by coronary artery dilation, further demand for blood secondary to increased cardiac work should be avoided.

4. Maintenance of blood pressure. A reduction in mean arterial blood pressure will reduce the amount of blood flowing through the coronary arteries if there cannot be compensatory dilatation. Although during hypotension work of the heart against peripheral resistance may be reduced, one cannot be certain that the demand for oxygen will be lowered sufficiently to be met by the decreased supply.

5. Administration of oxygen. The value of this procedure is self-evident.

Regional anesthesia is thought by some to be the safest form of pain relief for patients with coronary arterial disease. We prefer inhalational anesthesia with ether or cyclopropane to unsupplemented regional anesthesia for the following reasons: Under local anesthesia the patient is conscious and aware of the sight, the sounds and the odors of the operating room. This is not calculated to provide mental calm unless large amounts of sedatives are provided. Furthermore, despite satisfactory anesthesia of the abdominal wall, intra-abdominal manipulations are often accompanied by severe pain, nausea, vomiting, dyspnea and a lowered blood pressure. The decrease in blood pressure has been ascribed by some to a reflex constriction of the portal venous system with diminished venous return to the heart and a lowered cardiac output. The pain, frequently substernal, and the subjective feeling of shortness of breath, have been attributed to a reflex reduction in coronary arterial blood flow, although evidence on this point is not conclusive.

If there is virtue in urging the patient with coronary arterial disease to live quietly, avoid stress and strain and adjust his way to a calmer existence, it seems unwise to subject this same individual to the mental and physical upset occasioned by an operation performed under local anesthesia, when a *properly administered* general anesthetic can abolish the mental disquiet and minimize the untoward effects of intra-abdominal traction.

Despite these beliefs, it must be admitted that such procedures as cholecystostomy, colostomy, gastrostomy or suprapubic cystotomy have been carried out successfully during local anesthesia.

A second type of patient whose problems must be solved during the anesthesia is the individual with mitral stenosis, a history of heart failure, who has a complicating surgical illness or is ready for obstetric delivery. Where the location of operation permits their use, spinal or epidural anesthesia has much to recommend it for these patients. Both methods produce a circulatory response which might be termed a bloodless phlebotomy. Vasomotor fibers to arterioles and venules are blocked in varying numbers according to the level of anesthesia. Venous pressure decreases, and blood is pooled in the peripheral circulation, largely in the legs. This is obviously of advantage to the patient with incipient pulmonary edema. However, for mitral commissurotomy, general anesthesia is used. Here the selection of drug seems to be unimportant. Of greatest concern is maintenance of an extraordinarily light plane of anesthesia, lest major depression of blood pressure result.

Positioning of the cardiac patient on the operating table is important. It is wise to test preoperatively the effects of the position required. Should the patient complain of additional dyspnea or should blood pressure be reduced as the unanesthetized individual is placed in the surgical position it may become necessary to modify the operative approach. The head-down jackknife and lateral positions are difficult for the cardiac patient to tolerate. In some of these individuals pulmonary edema can be precipitated by assumption of even the horizontal supine position. These people can be operated upon in the semi-Fowler position. This is of great importance when the myocardial weakness is combined with the elevated diaphragm and respiratory embarassment of a full-term pregnancy. Under no circumstances should the orthopneic patient be placed flat after induction of general anesthesia merely because he is asleep and cannot complain of dyspnea.

Anesthesia for Battle Casualties

Until shock is corrected the severely wounded soldier is inordinately susceptible to narcosis, regardless of the agent or the technic selected. Prior to anesthesia he presents a picture of apathy and depression. He appears to be already partially narcotized. In such a patient even small amounts of central nervous depressant drugs evoke a response out of proportion to the size of the dose administered. Each war has accented this fact. The prolonged postoperative sleep of these patients tends to support this contention.

The physiologic basis for this susceptibility is not completely understood. It is undoubtedly bound up with the numerous factors responsible for shock; hence, it has humoral, endocrine, hemodynamic and psychic aspects, to mention only a few. Exhaustion of adrenal cortical and medullary hormone output is receiving increasing attention.

The guiding principle in the administration of anesthesia to any patient is use of the least amount of narcotic compatible with the surgical requirements. As already stated this is of paramount importance in the severely wounded. The susceptibility of the serious battle casualty to anesthesia enables one to provide satisfactory working conditions with 50 to 60 per cent nitrous oxide in oxygen in many such patients. This concentration may not produce even minimal surgical anesthesia in normal individuals; but if satisfactory results can be obtained, the shocked patient has been spared the consequences of a more potent depressant. In the severely wounded marked hypotension may even follow first plane anesthesia with ether. It must be administered with caution. An intravenous injection of 25 to 50 mg. thiopental may reduce blood pressure profoundly. This drug must be given slowly and in small amounts until the patient's tolerance is established. Cyclopropane would appear to have certain advantages, but experience with it is limited. Spinal anesthesia probably has little or no place in the management of the seriously wounded. Regional and local anesthesia are of value.

Regardless of the method finally selected, certain problems of the seriously wounded will affect the casualty's response to the stress of anesthesia and operation. These reactions must be anticipated and treatment begun promptly. As the patient is moved from the resuscitation unit to the operating room his blood pressure may fall markedly. Motion appears to have an adverse effect on the circulation of these patients as though compensation had been maintained by a delicate balance, almost any alteration of which proves to be upsetting. If hypotension does not follow this degree of activity, it may occur as the patient is placed in position on the operating table. Constant awareness of this possibility and treatment with parenteral fluids or pressor drugs may prevent disasters.

SPECIAL ANESTHETIC TECHNICS

CONTROLLED OR DELIBERATE HYPOTENSION

The deliberate reduction of arterial blood in an effort to produce a relatively bloodless field for operation is being re-explored. This is a challenging concept and one worthy of careful study, since its successful application might minimize the need for blood transfusions, reduce the incidence of transfusion reactions, improve the results of certain operative procedures by minimizing bleeding and decrease operating time.

The alleged improvement in surgical working conditions attributed to the lowered blood pressure is open to question. There can be little doubt but that capillary oozing can pro-

long an operation, if not actually prevent its successful conclusion. However, bleeding from larger vessels can be severe, even during deliberate hypotension, and unless this blood is replaced as it is lost the result may lead to irreversible hypotension. Data are needed to compare the extent of blood loss during operations of comparable extent and in comparable groups of patients with and without hypotension. Proof of the sparing action of deliberate hypotension on blood loss is sketchy at the moment. Likewise, there is little convincing evidence of the decreased operating time and the facilitation of surgery which has been attributed to the lowered arterial pressure. Postoperative hemorrhage, although not reported frequently, is always a possibility as the pressure-head returns toward normal following operation. There is danger lest this procedure be attempted in instances in which perfectly satisfactory results can be obtained otherwise. Neurosurgical, plastic and radical procedures for eradication of malignancy are the most likely operations for trial of this method.

A number of methods are available for the intentional reduction of blood pressure. The primary principle is dilatation of the vascular bed with pooling of blood probably in the venous reservoirs. This may be achieved by block of the vasomotor outflow with epidural or spinal anesthesia, by ganglionic blocking agents such as hexamethonium salts or by Arfonad, a drug which dilates blood vessels peripherally, blocks ganglia and may liberate histamine. Further pooling of blood can be achieved by lowering the legs or by applying suction to a box enclosing the legs.

The successful use of deliberately produced arterial hypotension will depend on whether nutrition for the heart, the brain and the liver can be maintained during the period of low blood pressure. The kidney apparently will survive reasonable insults. Therefore, the clinician electing to employ this procedure must be able to predict which patient will tolerate it. Most observers will agree that young, healthy subjects can withstand reduced blood pressure satisfactorily. Most will agree that older subjects with sclerotic vessels and previous histories of coronary, cerebral or renal insufficiency are poor candidates.

INDUCED HYPOTHERMIA

Deliberate reduction of both temperature during anesthesia and operation offers advantages to certain types of patients. Such patients include those scheduled for open heart operations, grafting of aortic aneurysms or other procedures which involve prolonged interruption of blood supply to tissues, and patients with uncontrolled hyperthyroidism, marked degrees of fever or anoxia. The purpose of hypothermia is to reduce metabolism so that tissues may better tolerate reduction in blood supply or may no longer require excessive oxygenation. Oxygen consumption is reduced by about 50 per cent when a body temperature of 78° F. is reached.

Cooling is unpleasant for a conscious subject, and the majority of patients are anesthetized lightly prior to reduction of their temperature. The anesthetic agents or technics do not appear to be of great importance so long as adequate pulmonary ventilation is provided. Since the heat production associated with shivering makes hypothermia more difficult to achieve, muscle relaxants may be used. The technics of cooling vary from surface application of cold to the direct cooling of blood as it passes from an arterial cannula through coils immersed in ice water back to a vein. Specially constructed blankets are also available which contain coils through which circulates a refrigerant. The patient lies between two layers of coils. Immersion of the trunk and the extremities in cold water is also used. The rate of cooling is relatively slow for adults—several hours being required to decrease rectal temperature from normal to 30° C. with surface cooling. Children may be cooled more rapidly.

Many physiologic alterations accompany hypothermia. Cardiac output is reduced, blood pressure declines, and pulse rate falls. As part of the general depression of tissue activity and reactivity respirations become inadequate. If this is not treated, respiratory acidosis may develop. Cardiac irritability increases, and ventricular fibrillation may occur. The cause of this apparent increase in myocardial irritability is unknown. Conduction of impulses in the nervous system is reduced by cooling. Blood viscosity increases. Hemoglobin tends to hold on to oxygen more tenaciously at low temperatures. The solubility of all gases increases so that much more oxygen and carbon dioxide, for example, are dissolved than at normal body temperature. The same holds true for anesthetic gases and vapors.

The length of time which tissues can survive absence of all blood supply has not yet been determined for man at varying body temperatures. However, it is known in dogs, that the liver will tolerate only 20 minutes of complete ischemia at normal temperatures, while 60 minutes is permissible at a temperature of 27° C. Similar data are being obtained for the brain, the heart, the gastrointestinal tract and the kidney.

It is unlikely that deliberate reduction of body temperature will prove to be the answer to the problems posed when a surgeon attempts "open heart" operations. However, the technic may be useful in neurosurgery and in operations which can be performed only when the blood supply to tissues must be interrupted for relatively prolonged periods of time, e.g., thoracic aortic grafting, or resection of the liver. Hypothermia also deserves study as a method of anesthesia for substandard patients.

HYPNOSIS

Hypnosis as an adjuvant to anesthesia has been re-explored recently. Even enthusiasts agree that its role is limited, but with proper training in technic, an anesthetist can either induce anesthesia or provide total anesthesia in certain selected patients.

Hypnosis involves the uncritical acceptance of ideas by the subject from the operator and requires an exaggerated state of suggestibility. About 10 to 20 per cent of the population can respond sufficiently so that total anesthesia is possible. Children above the age of 5 or 6, anxious to explore new things, and with an ability to create a fantasy, are often good subjects. The procedure is time-consuming and, if a deep trance is to be provided for an operation, rehearsal of each step of the procedure is believed to be desirable. Constant reinforcement during operation is usually required.

Hypnosis has certain potential dangers. It may uncover critical problems or internal repressions in a patient's background which, when brought to the surface, cause a serious threat to the individual's mental balance. An anesthetist should not use the technic for psychotherapy lest lack of knowledge of psychodynamics result in tragic consequences.

UNUSUAL COMPLICATIONS OF ANESTHESIA

The administration of anesthesia involves the avoidance and the treatment of all types of complications which may be inherent in the patient, the agents employed, the technic of application, or the supportive measures used. A number of these complications have been discussed in other sections of this chapter. Those listed here have occurred with sufficient frequency or have sufficient potential to warrant mention.

INJURIES TO THE EYES

Careless application of a face mask, certain positions of the patient on the operating table (e.g., face down), the anesthetic agent employed and the activities of the surgeon in cleansing the skin about the face may predispose the patient to ocular injury. Open technics with liquid anesthetics are particularly liable to result in conjunctivitis or corneal abrasions, while large masks pressing on the orbits have been known to produce intraocular injuries and to give rise to reflex vagal activity.

In general, the best precaution against injury is to keep the eyelids closed. The procedure of eliciting a corneal reflex to determine depth of anesthesia is not a good one because of the possibility of abrading the cornea. It may be necessary to approximate the lids with Scotch tape or adhesive, particularly during long operations, to keep the eyes closed. Instillation of a 5 per cent boric acid ophthalmic ointment will prevent drying of the corneas in the deeper planes of anesthesia. The eyes should be inspected at the conclusion of anesthesia. Should injury have occurred, ophthalmologic consultation is indicated. Simple conjunctivitis is treated best by irrigations with saturated solutions of boric acid. Corneal abrasions are not only painful but may progress to inflammation of the uveal tract if untreated. If treated early with antibiotics locally, abrasions often begin to reepithelialize within 24 hours.

RESPIRATORY TRACT INJURIES DUE TO EXCESSIVE GAS PRESSURE

Since oxygen and the commonly employed gaseous anesthetic agents are supplied for clinical use at greater than atmospheric pressure, the possibility of high pressure injuries to the lungs is ever present. The exact limits of pressure which can be supplied safely to the lungs of man have not been defined clearly. If a gas reaches the alveoli under increased pressure, rupture of alveoli may ensue with the subsequent hemorrhage, capillary air embolization, or dissection of gas into the interstitial tissues of the lung. Gas that collects in the interstitial tissues of the lungs under pressure may rupture through subpleural blebs to produce unilateral or bilateral pneumothorax or dissect back through the hilum into the mediastinum to give rise to pneumomediastinum. The lungs may remain partly inflated and "stiffened" with gas (pulmonary interstitial emphysema), and venous return to the heart may be impeded in the mediastinum (air block). Further dissection from the mediastinum explains the appearance of subcutaneous emphysema about the neck, the face and the chest.

Fatalities may occur with any of the aforementioned events. They are especially apt to occur during endotracheal anesthesia when the protective closing action of the larynx in response to stimulation has been prevented. Maximum protection is afforded by the placement of safety valves between the source of pressure and the patient's airway. Gas tanks should be turned on and flows adjusted before connections to the patient are made. As a life-saving measure bilateral tension pneumothorax must be diagnosed almost at once. Insertion of large-bore needles and rapid withdrawal of air from chest will allow re-expansion of the lungs under simultaneous positive pressure.

INSUFFLATION OF LIQUID ETHER INTO THE LUNGS

The design of some anesthetic apparatus with respect to vaporization of volatile liquids with gases under pressure creates the possibility of blowing liquid ether into the lungs. Again, the likelihood for this accident is greater during endotracheal anesthesia when the glottis cannot close. Liquid ether may produce bronchoconstriction, pulmonary edema and, should the victim survive, an inflammatory reaction and bronchopneumonia. The precautions which we have used to avoid this catastrophe include placement of a trap between the vaporizer and the patient's airway, adjustment of proper gas flows before the vaporization of liquids is started, and making all of these adjustments before connecting the vaporizing apparatus to the patient.

Injuries to Nerves

Peripheral nerves can be damaged during anesthesia by overstretching between two points of fixation, pinching between unyielding structures, or direct pressure, mainly because the patient is unable to complain, and the protective action of muscle tone is lacking. The nerves most commonly injured are those which are placed superficially: the brachial plexus, the ulnar nerve, the common peroneal and the radial.

The nerves forming the brachial plexus have two points of fixation: one centrally at the transverse processes of the cervical vertebrae, and the other peripherally at the point of attachment to the tissues of the arm. Excessive separation of these two points may stretch the nerves, and nerve palsies may ensue. The presence of several natural anatomic fulcrums, such as the scaleni muscles which can compress the plexuses against the first rib, the attachment of the pectoralis minor muscle to the coracoid process of the scapula around which the plexus is stretched in hyperabduction of the arm, and the rounded head of the humerus provide additional possibilities for stretch. The use of a shoulder brace improperly applied to the soft tissues of the cervical triangles may not only act as an artificial fulcrum but also compress the brachial plexus against the underlying structures. Lastly, the plexus may be pinched between the scalene muscles and the first rib or between the clavicle and the first rib with downward displacement of the shoulder.

To avoid these brachial plexus injuries one must bear the possibility in mind constantly and avoid extremes of position of the head and the arm. Should a palsy result after operation, a careful neurologic examination must be made as a base line for future improvement, and measures for restoration of function must

be begun. The latter include proper support of the weakened muscles and physiotherapy. In the case of severe injuries, restitution of normal function may not take place until 6 months or a year have elapsed.

The ulnar and the common peroneal nerves and to lesser degree the radial nerves are superficial structures liable to be compressed against bone by outer pressure or stretched around bony eminences. Again, certain operating positions will predispose these nerves to injury, and they are more apt to occur in debilitated patients where the subcutaneous protective layer of fat is absent. If the latter occur, treatment is the same as that described for brachial plexus palsies.

Injuries Associated with Intravenous Anesthesia

The extravasation of thiopental may produce necrosis of tissue and indolent sloughing types of ulceration. Hence, every precaution must be taken to avoid extravasation and to recognize this incident if it occurs. It is said that the immediate infiltration of the area with procaine solution may be useful, probably through dilution, pain relief and vasodilation.

A rare accident is the inadvertent injection of thiopental into an artery rather than a vein. Intense pain results in most instances and, if present, suggests the diagnosis. Such accidents have been reported following attempts to seek a vein in the antecubital space, the forearm and the back of the hand. If a syringe and needle technic is used, it is not always easy to recognize that one is in an artery prior to injection, for blood may not pulse into the syringe, nor can one be certain of the color of the blood. Injection of thiopental into the running stream of an intravenous set would appear to be a prophylactic measure.

The pathologic lesion produced is that of intimal destruction with thrombi forming at the sites of destruction. In experimental animals, arterial injection of solutions buffered to the pH of thiopental solutions (about pH 10.5) cause little damage. This suggests that the thiopental molecule is at fault, rather than alkalinity per se. There are also observations indicating that some patients react more intensely than others to the local chemical irritation.

Treatment is discouraging, irreversible damage apparently occurring at the instant of injection in some instances. Efforts aimed at active vasodilation have been recommended, including the administration of light general anesthesia with cyclopropane or ether, the application of heat to uninvolved portions of the body, stellate ganglion or brachial plexus block and the use of dilator drugs such as Priscoline. Attempts to treat the damage locally by intra-arterial approach have included injection of procaine and heparin. Apparently, large doses of the latter are required. Surgical exploration has been advocated. Amputation may be required ultimately, despite prompt treatment. The recent demonstration that norepinephrine may be liberated from the arterial wall as the result of the injection of thiopental, if confirmed, suggests the use of a substance such as regitine.

FIRE AND EXPLOSION HAZARDS

In comparison with the other hazards of anesthesia, explosions occur so infrequently as to be almost insignificant. However, the emotional factors involved in an anesthetic explosion make it a dreaded disaster.

Fires and explosions are combustive processes differing merely in the speed of the reaction and the magnitude of the forces released. Three elements are necessary for the production of combustion: (1) a combustible substance; (2) a supporter of combustion, oxygen, from whatever source; and (3) a source of ignition.

All hydrocarbons are subject to decomposition by heat. Several burn readily or explode when in proper mixture with air, oxygen or nitrous oxide. The volatile liquids and gases used in anesthesia may be classified as follows:

1. The vapors of divinyl ether, diethyl ether, ethyl chloride, ethylene and cyclopropane will explode violently under suitable conditions. Trichlorethylene vapor is not flammable either in oxygen or air at ordinary temperatures; however, phosgene and dichloracetylene may be liberated if the trichlorethylene vapor is heated. Chloroform vapor will not ignite but will liberate phosgene if heated. Fluothane vapor is not flammable.

2. Oxygen and nitrous oxide are not explosible but support combustion. Explosions have occurred with nitrous oxide alone, presumably because of the presence of explosive contaminants derived from the anesthetic machine.

It is impractical to memorize the flammable ranges for the various anesthetics in air, nitrous oxide and oxygen. The general order of magnitude of the flammable ranges for anesthetics is: 1.7 per cent to 37 per cent in air; 1.4 per cent to 40 per cent in nitrous oxide; and 1.8 per cent to 85 per cent in oxygen. The anesthetic concentrations of flammable gases lie within these ranges.

Prevention

Measures for the prevention of explosions will be discussed under the heading of the 3 conditions necessary for combustion.

The Combustible Substances

1. **Avoidance.** Agents or methods which do not carry the hazard of explosibility should be used whenever possible in situations involving the use of x-rays, the cautery, flame, etc. However, it must be recognized that under no circumstances must a greater hazard be substituted for a lesser one. For example, if a 4-year-old child were scheduled for the closed reduction of a fracture under general anesthesia and the fluoroscope were to be used in a darkened room, the possibility of circulatory depression from chloroform which is nonexplosive would be a greater danger than the possibility of an explosion from ether, which is flammable.

2. **Storage of Agents and Care of Equipment.** Cylinders and containers of volatile liquids should be stored in well-ventilated places at a safe distance from radiators, steam pipes and other sources of heat. Oxidizing substances (oxygen, nitrous oxide) should be separated from the reducing substances (the hydrocarbons).

The Presence of Substances That Support Combustion

1. **Dilution with Air or Inert Gases.** Since the explosive range of the flammable agents is narrower in air than with oxygen or nitrous oxide, the explosion hazard may be reduced by administering anesthetics with the minimal effective or safe concentrations of oxygen or nitrous oxide. This increased safety from fire must be weighed against the physiologic advantages of the higher tensions of oxygen in

inspired mixtures. "Open" ether may be administered with relative safety in the presence of the cautery or x-ray equipment provided that the container, the mask and the material saturated with the agent are removed at a time when sparking or heating is apt to occur. Further protection is offered by molding a water-soaked cloth about the patient's face.

2. **Closed System Technic.** The closed system of administering anesthetics confines the explosive mixture to the apparatus and the patient's respiratory tract save when leaks occur or the reservoir bag is emptied. Thus the hazard of ignition from exogenous sources such as sparks is lessened, but there remains a greater likelihood of injury to the patient in the event of an explosion.

Sources of Ignition

1. **Obvious sources** of ignition such as flames, cigarettes and matches should be banned from anesthetizing locations (anesthesia rooms, operating room, corridors and storage places).

2. **Electrical wiring and equipment** when installed in anesthetizing locations should conform to the specifications advised by the National Electrical Codes and National Board of Fire Underwriters, although the Underwriters occasionally appear unreasonable to the author.

3. **Static sparks** probably constitute the greatest danger as sources of ignition. Since they may be generated in so many different ways, they are most difficult to control. There can be no accumulation of static electricity if all objects present are isoelectric, i.e., at the same electrical potential. The chief means of achieving isoelectric conditions is the grounding of all objects and persons within the "hazardous area." A list of preventive measures is appended.

A. Equipment

a. Floors in anesthetizing locations should provide a path of moderate electrical conductivity for grounding purposes. Too low a resistance may permit electrocution if faulty wiring is present. Too high a resistance may prevent run-off of static charge and, hence, an increased likelihood of sparking.

b. Furniture, equipment and operating tables should make contact with the ground via metal or conductive rubber contacts.

c. Woolen blankets are prohibited in anesthetizing locations, and mattresses and cushions should be conductive.

B. Activity of Personnel

a. Breaking connections on anesthetic apparatus should be carried out with both parts held by the anesthetist to maintain isoelectric conditions.

b. Persons other than the anesthetist should keep away from maximal and dangerous accumulation points of combustible substances. These are (1) the patient's respiratory tract and (2) the anesthetic machine.

c. Personnel should wear shoes with conductive soles or with conductive strips. Silk, wool, rayon or sharkskin may be worn if in contact with the skin.

C. Other Measures

a. Cautery and high-frequency equipment. If the cautery is used during operations, it should be beyond a 2-foot radius from the head of the patient, provided that there is a suitable intervening barrier and ventilation about the head.

b. Humidification. A film of moisture may serve as a means of dissipating electrical charges. This is especially important in dry climates or in winter.

POSTANESTHETIC OBSERVATION ROOM (RECOVERY ROOM)

From the standpoint of anesthesia the most critical period in a patient's postoperative course is that of the first few hours after operation. During this time the unconscious or semiconscious patient is dependent upon others for his well-being. Even the individual who has received regional anesthesia and is in control of his faculties may require prompt attention for circulatory or other abnormalities. A specially staffed and specially equipped room should be available for the care of these patients. This room should be immediately adjacent to the operating suite, for if a patient has to be transported for any distance the purpose of the room is defeated in the interim. The facilities in such an area should include oxygen and suction outlets, solutions for parenteral administration, laryngoscopic and bronchoscopic equipment, and an assortment of drugs which might be required for the treatment of various respiratory or circulatory emergencies.

If space is limited the following patients, at least, should be admitted to the recovery room: (1) any patient who has spinal anesthesia and has had significant circulatory or respiratory insufficiency; (2) any patient who has been given general anesthesia and is not oriented as to time and place; (3) any patient whose immediate postanesthetic condition concerns the anesthetist; (4) an outpatient who has received general anesthesia and needs to recover prior to departing from the hospital.

During the recovery room stay blood pressure, pulse and respiratory rate should be recorded at regular intervals. Bodily temperature should be determined in infants, and if changes in temperature are suspected. A careful physical examination of the chest should be made on patients who have a rapid respiratory rate, who have respiratory obstruction and are cyanotic, orthopneic or dyspneic. For example, pneumothorax may be found after thoracolumbar sympathetic resections, renal, thyroid, or intrathoracic operations. Atelectasis may occur at any time during or after anesthesia. Pulmonary edema may occur in patients with myocardial disease, respiratory obstruction, or after pneumonectomy. Appropriate therapeutic measuers for these sequelae should be instituted promptly.

The average patient who has had general anesthesia may be dismissed from the postanesthetic observation room if he can obey simple commands (i.e., "open your eyes," "stick out your tongue"). The discharge of other patients will depend upon improvement in the primary reason for their admission. Frequently, the chief criterion for dismissing a patient from the recovery room will be the clinical judgment of the attending anesthetist and surgeon.

REFERENCES

1. Comroe, J. H., Jr., and Dripps, R. D.: The Physiological Basis for Oxygen Therapy, Springfield, Ill., Thomas, 1950.
2. Dripps, R. D.: The immediate decrease of blood pressure seen in the conclusion of cyclopropane anesthesia: "cyclopropane shock," Anesthesiology 8:15-25, 1947.
3. ———: Abnormal respiratory responses to various "curare" drugs during surgical anesthesia, Ann. Surg. 137:145-153, 1953.
4. Dripps, R. D., and Vandam, L. D.: Long-term follow-up of patients who received 10,098 spinal anesthetics, J.A.M.A. 156:1486-1491, 1954.
5. Dripps, R. D., Eckenhoff, J. E., and Vandam, L. D.: Introduction to Anesthesia, Philadelphia, Saunders, 1957.
6. Fink, B. R.: Diffusion anoxia, Anesthesiology 16:511-519, 1955.
7. Kennedy, F., Effron, A. S., and Perry, G.: The grave spinal cord paralysis caused by spinal anesthesia, Surg., Gynec. & Obst. 91:385-392, 1950.
8. Orth, O. S., Stutzman, J. W., and Meek, W. F.: Relationship of chemical structure of sympathomimetic amines to ventricular tachycardia during cyclopropane anesthesia, J. Pharmacol. & Exper. Therap. 81:197-202, 1944.
9. Price, H. L., Linde, H. W., Jones, R. E., Black, G. W., and Price, M. L.: Sympatho-adrenal responses to general anesthesia in man and their relation to hemodynamics, Anesthesiology 20:563-573, 1959.
10. Waters, R. M.: Chloroform, Madison, Wisc., Univ. Wisconsin Press, 1951.

HORACE J. McCORKLE, M.D.

—————————————— CHAPTER 13 ——————————————

Operative Surgical Care

INTRODUCTION

Good manners and correct conduct in the surgical operating rooms as well as elsewhere reflect the traditional education and training of the physician. Furthermore, they help to ensure the strict maintenance of asepsis. Modern methods of anesthesia make it possible for most surgical procedures to be done without haste. Enough operating time should be taken by the surgeon to assure the maintenance of aseptic procedure, ensure that a minimum of trauma is inflicted, secure hemostasis and ascertain that each detail of the operation is completed accurately and securely.

It is the duty of the surgeon to inquire frequently into the methods used for the preparation of materials and supplies used in the operating room and to observe the care with which these important things are handled. Also, observation by the surgeon of the activities of all persons in the operating room during the surgical procedure is essential to protect the patient from bacterial contamination from external sources. The use of antibacterial substances does not minimize in any way the need for the strictest possible regimen to maintain aseptic technic.

Usually medical students who have been assigned to study a surgical case will introduce themselves to the operating surgeon several minutes before his preparations for the operation are begun. Often there follows a brief discussion of the diagnosis and the management of the case, following which the surgeon will ask the student to observe or to participate in the operation as a member of the surgical team, depending on the nature and the circumstances of the operation. Otherwise, visitors to operating rooms usually introduce themselves to the chief operating room nurse who will obtain the permission of the surgeon and then instruct the visitor regarding the changing of clothing; she will supply caps, smocks and masks, which should be donned (the mask covering the nose as well as the mouth) and fastened in place before the visitor is conducted into the operating room. It is well for the student or visitor to enter the operating room deliberately and to survey the location of sterile tables, basins and other equipment, and the areas of activity of the operating room personnel before moving quietly into an unused corner or other part of the theater. After the operating team has assembled about the table the visitor may carefully approach to a place where he may observe, or will assume a place designated by the surgeon or one of his assistants. All movements in the operating room should be made slowly and deliberately and the visitor or student must be constantly aware of all sterile things in the operating room and he must avoid contaminating them.

The operating room personnel must be vigilant at all times to detect any possible break in aseptic technic. If such a fault in technic is detected or even suspected the head nurse and the surgeon must be notified and the situation corrected immediately and without any question or discussion, regardless of its cause. These rules apply to all persons in the operating room—visitors, students, orderlies, nurses, assistants and the chief surgeon.

The development of antibiotics in recent years cannot be considered to have altered in any way the duties of operating room personnel to carry out in the most precise way the methods of aseptic operating room technic.

STERILIZATION IN THE OPERATING ROOM

Much time and great care are required for preparation of the sterile linen, instruments and other materials used in aseptic procedures.

All cloth materials must be freshly laundered, folded and packaged loosely enough to permit sterilizing steam heat to penetrate into the deepest part of each package. The packaging also should be designed to protect the linens from contamination after sterilization and, to allow their easy removal and transfer from packages to the sterile tables. Packages of linen, including sheets, gowns and sponges should be 25 x 12 x 12 inches in size, or smaller. They should be fixed in double-layered cloth (muslin) wrappers and autoclaved at 250° F. for 30 minutes. Blue-gray colored cloth material appears to subdue glare in the field of operation. Rubber gloves must be cleaned carefully and placed in double-layered cloth (muslin) envelopes containing cloth flaps that fit loosely into the cuffs of the gloves and hold the gloves slightly open, then packaged in double-layered cloth (muslin) and autoclaved at 250° F. for 15 minutes. The sterilized gloves should be kept overnight before being used. Water, normal saline solution and other solutions used in the operating room should be autoclaved in flasks (with gauze-covered openings or loosely applied caps) at 250° F. for 20 minutes. Needles, scalpel blades and scissors also may be "cold-sterilized" in a formaldehyde-alcohol preparation (such as Bard-Parker antiseptic) or autoclaved. All metal instruments must be scrupulously clean, free of corrosion, oiled (and all excess of oil wiped away) and tested for ease of operation before being sterilized in open metal trays or pans bundled in suitable cloth wrappings. Glove powder is prepared in small individual paper packages containing just enough powder ("Biosorb") for one person's hands, enclosed in the glove package, and autoclaved with them at 250° F. for 15 minutes. (Talc should *never* be used. See Chap. 2, "Wound Healing," and Chap. 35, "Peritoneum, Peritonitis and Intra-abdominal Abscesses.")

Caps and masks are laundered and sterilized by autoclaving in muslin bags that may be fitted into suitable covered metal containers and kept ready for use. The scrubbing brushes and fingernail cleaners are cleaned thoroughly, packed in cans and autoclaved at 250° F. for 30 minutes. These items are kept in convenient shelves or tables in the scrub-up room.

It should be emphasized that all materials and instruments must be packed loosely enough and in packages that are small and porous enough to admit live steam to all parts of the packages during autoclaving. All solid containers should be placed on their sides for sterilizing in the autoclave. Tops of cans should be left off or loosely applied since otherwise the inner parts of tightly closed metal containers may not be sterile after autoclaving.

THE PLAN FOR OPERATION. PREPARATION OF THE OPERATING ROOM PERSONNEL, THE PATIENT AND THE FIELD OF OPERATION

Emergency situations can arise where there is little time to plan the surgical procedure; but most often a careful study of the patient, including a review of the history of the case, the physical, x-ray and laboratory findings, may be done before going into the operating room. A plan for the operative procedure and possible alternative courses of procedure should be made before the surgeon begins the operation. As the operation proceeds it may be necessary to alter the plans according to the pathologic findings or the changing condition of the patient. The careful planning of surgical procedures before they begin aids considerably in reducing conversation, discussion, consultation of the records and waste of time in the operating room.

Usually an operating room that is kept in service daily can be readily maintained in suitable condition for major aseptic surgery, but rooms seldom used may be more difficult to keep in operating condition. The operating rooms should be designed so that they can be cleaned easily and quickly. As far as possible they should be kept free of dirt by minimizing traffic in the room, by filtering the air intake, and by cleaning floors, walls, ceilings and fixtures several hours before the rooms are to be used. If contamination with pathogenic bacteria occurs during a surgical procedure, the operating room must be decontaminated before another operation is done in it. This is accomplished by isolating and removing all contaminated materials, including instruments, drapes, caps, gowns, masks, gloves, etc., and cleaning floors, walls and fixtures with an antiseptic detergent solution.

Persons with acute respiratory infections should not enter the operating rooms.

Street clothing and shoes should not be worn into the operating room; instead, clean freshly laundered garments and clean shoes kept especially for operating room use should be donned, and the street clothing left in an adjacent locker room. All persons must apply caps and masks before entering the operating room, and must wear caps and be masked over both mouth and nose while in the operating room (Fig. 13-1).

All sterile packs and trays should be kept closed or covered until a few minutes before they are to be used. When the patient is anesthetized the first assistant proceeds with the preparation of the skin of the patient in the proposed field of operation, according to the author's method, in the preparation room adjoining the operating room. During this period the surgeon and other assistants proceed with the hand-scrubbing technic (see pp. 219-220). First, the skin of the patient is lathered and shaved over an area somewhat larger than the area later to be bordered by sterile drapes. The skin is shaved with great care in order to remove all hair cleanly, yet avoid scratching or cutting the skin. In many hospitals this part of the preparation is carried out before the patient comes to the operating suite. Following this the skin is washed with water and soap or one of the more recently developed antiseptic detergents. Usually this is done with clean sponges of gauze, while brushes are used also if the nails of an extremity are in the field of preparation. The scrubbing should be done with light pressure in order to avoid abrading the skin. The length of time required for shaving and cleaning the skin of the patient varies with the size and the

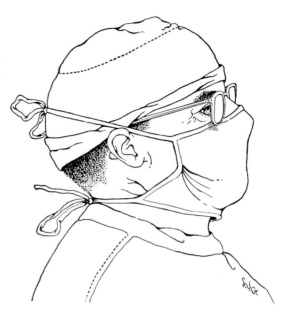

FIG. 13-1. The surgeon's cap should cover as much of the head as is possible. The gauze mask covers nose, mouth and chin.

configuration of the area to be cleaned and thus may vary from 3 to 20 minutes. Some care must be used to select the detergent in order to avoid skin reactions and eliminate chemical incompatibility that may interfere with the bactericidal properties of the antiseptic agents to be used in the sterile preparation. An antiseptic detergent that contains an antiseptic with an organic iodine-complex together with agents that cause a satisfactory lathering for scrubbing purposes, is suitable for this purpose. This antiseptic detergent can be used prior to, and does not interfere with the bactericidal properties of, the organic iodine-complex used in the sterile skin preparation. (70% ethyl alcohol is also a widely used skin antiseptic.) A sterile towel should be used to cover the clean field if the sterile preparation is delayed for a few minutes, otherwise the sterile preparation immediately follows the shaving and cleaning preparations (Fig. 13-2).

While the anesthetist and the first assistant are proceeding with the anesthetization and the preparation of the patient's skin in the proposed field of operation, the surgeon and other assistants carry out their sterile hand-scrubbing technic. The object of this proce-

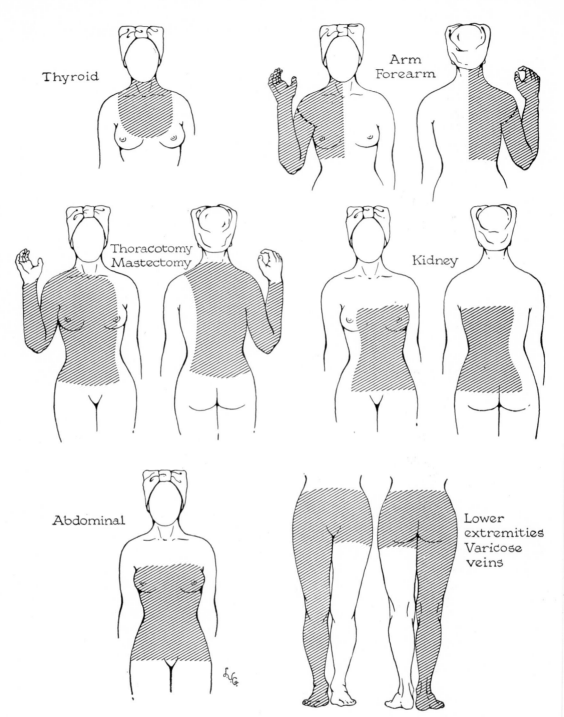

Fig. 13-2. Diagrams indicating the fields of preparation for common aseptic operations. (Redrawn from similar diagrams in Moseley's Textbook of Surgery, ed. 2, St. Louis, Mosby, 1955)

dure is to eliminate as far as is possible the bacteria from the skin of their hands and arms. The hands of all operating room personnel should be kept as clean as possible at all times. Surgical wound dressings should not be done on the morning prior to operations, and septic dressings always should be handled with rubber gloves and with instruments. The fingernails should be neither too long nor clipped too short, but of such a length and shape that conforms to the configuration of the fingertip. Nail polish must be removed with acetone or other nail polish remover. All rings, bracelets and wrist watches must be removed. A sterile cloth cap is removed carefully from the sterile container and held by each side of the rim while it is fitted over the head. This care is necessary because of the possibility of tiny bits of lint dropping from the cap into the sterile field during the operative procedure. The cap should fit as far as possible over all of the hair (front, back and sides) and should be drawn down to the level of the brows in front (so as to absorb perspiration), to the ears on both sides and as far as is possible down the back of the head to prevent loose hairs or dandruff from falling into the wound. [All participants in surgical operations should wash their hair after getting a haircut to remove the numerous segments of hair that result from such a procedure: H. N. H.; Editor.] Then a sterile gauze mask is removed from its container; it too should be handled as little as possible and preferably by touching only the tying strings. The mask should consist of several layers of gauze, and it must fit as comfortably as possible completely over the nose, the mouth and the chin. If eyeglasses are to be worn the upper margin of the mask may be molded to fit tightly against the nose and the cheeks, either with a malleable metal (aluminum strip that is inserted into a slot in the mask, or with a strip of adhesive tape, in order to prevent fogging of the glasses. It is essential that the operating room cap and mask be applied correctly and comfortably before beginning to scrub hands and arms.

The sterile containers of brushes and fingernail cleaners are opened before starting the scrubbing procedure. The running water in the scrubbing sink is regulated to a comfortably warm temperature. At this time it is preferable to use one of the available antiseptic detergent preparations containing hexachlorophene ("pHisohex") or one of the organic iodine complex antiseptic detergent combinations for hand and arm scrubbing purposes. The time of beginning the scrubbing procedure is observed on a clock, so placed as to be viewed easily during the procedure. The surgeon's and the assistants' hands and arms are washed thoroughly with running water and the antiseptic detergent up to a level of about $2\frac{1}{2}$ in. above the elbows. After rinsing hands and arms in the running water a sterile brush is removed from the container; after wetting it thoroughly with water, antiseptic detergent is applied to the wet brush and, beginning with the hands and the fingers, both hands and arms are scrubbed up to a level of 2 in. above the elbows for 5 minutes by the clock. A system for accomplishing this in a routine manner should be established so that it becomes a method whereby the entire skin surface of the hands and the arms is scrubbed completely each time. More time is spent scrubbing the fingernails and the creased areas of the hands and the wrists than on the forearms and the elbows. After the first 5 minutes of scrubbing the brush is discarded, a fingernail cleaner (orangewood stick or file) is removed from the sterile container, and each fingernail is cleaned under the running water. The fingernail cleaner should be rinsed after each fingernail is cleaned; when all nails have been cleaned it is discarded. Then a second scrubbing brush is removed from the sterile container, and the systematic scrubbing of the hands and the arms from the fingertips to a level 1 in. above the elbows is carried out for a second period of 5 minutes by the clock. Thus, a routine hand scrubbing is established for a 10-minute period for all operating room personnel—surgeons, assistants, nurses and students. (The first assistant carries out his hand-scrubbing technic after he has finished the unsterile preparation of the skin of the patient.) If the hands or the arms touch unsterile things at any time after the scrubbing has been started, the entire 10-minute period of scrubbing must be repeated. Even with the excellent antiseptic detergents available for hand-scrubbing purposes in surgical operating rooms, it is unwise and unsafe to designate a total period for hand-scrubbing routine of less than 10 minutes.

When antiseptic detergents are used it is unnecessary and undesirable to rinse off completely the antiseptic detergent after finishing the 10-minute period of scrubbing. Instead, a film of the antiseptic detergent is left on the hands and the arms, which are carefully blotted dry with sterile towels.

Next, a sterile gown is put on. The gown must be unfolded completely before putting it on, and it must be donned with great care to avoid contaminating its outside surface. Usually the gown is tied at the surgeon's back by the unsterile circulating operating room nurse. Sterile vests which tie in front and keep the back as well as the front of the operator relatively sterile are used in some hospitals over the gown. It is important to be aware of the fact that the backs of such vests may become contaminated without the wearers' being aware of it. The hands are powdered from a small sterile individual packet of glove powder ("Biosorb," an especially prepared starch powder containing a minute amount of magnesium oxide), following which sterile gloves are applied. The glove powder in the individual packet should be exactly enough to powder the hands of one person, and the excess of powder should be kept away from the sterile operating room supplies. The sterile rubber gloves are inspected carefully to be certain that they are free from perforations or patches. Excess powder, "Biosorb" should be washed from the gloves (see Chap. 2, "Wound Healing"). The gloved hands are folded in a sterile towel until the operation begins.

The sterile preparation of the patient's skin is done by the surgeon from a sterile tray that holds a sponge forceps, gauze sponges and a small basin containing an organic iodine-complex solution. The surgeon touches only the handle of the sponge forceps with which he picks up one of the sterile sponges, soaks it with the organic iodine-complex solution and gently and methodically scrubs the skin over an area several square inches larger than the area of sterilized skin proposed for the field of operation. This sterile preparation requires several minutes, and a number of sponges are used to make several applications of the antiseptic to the skin in the area of sterile preparation, following which the sponge stick and the preparation solution basin are discarded. Larger or more complicated fields of operation require a proportionally longer period of time for the preparation of the skin. In certain cases it may be desirable to apply a sterile adherent transparent plastic film over the prepared sterile field of operation.

When the proposed field of operation has been prepared (i.e., shaved, cleaned and painted with antiseptic solution) the surgeon applies sterile drapes (from the sterile supply table) about the proposed field of operation. The size of the patient's skin surface exposed in the draped field should not be larger than necessary for the proposed operation, but it should include enough skin surface for possible extension of the initial incision or for additional incisions if they should become necessary during the course of the procedure. Several sterile towels folded once longitudinally are carefully placed so as to border the proposed field of operation. Once placed, these towels should not be shifted. They are fixed to the skin in proper position with towel clips or sutures or both. Then suitable large sterile drapes are placed so as to provide a wide sterile area around the zone of operation, leaving only an aperture for the exposure of sufficient sterilized skin for the proposed site of operation. The sterile instrument tray is moved into the draped sterile field. Suitable operating room lights are directed on the proposed site of operation. For most major procedures the light should come into the surgical incision from at least 2 separate sources—the light beams must be focused to give a uniform lighting over the field of operation. An auxiliary source of electric power should be available for the operating room illumination in case of failure of the main electrical power service.

The surgeon and the assistants (capped, masked, scrubbed, gowned and gloved) assume their positions at the sterilely draped table. It is time for the incision to be made.

PRINCIPLES OF OPERATIVE PROCEDURE

It is preferable that the patient be brought to the operating room in his own bed, but he should have been ambulated on the day of his operation before receiving his preoperative medication and other final preparations for operation, unless he is in a state of shock, has severe peritonitis, cardiac failure, or has fractures or other disabilities that make ambulation undesirable or impossible. It is also desirable that the patient be moved from his bed to the operating table, the anesthetic induced (unless it is an explosive one) and the proposed site of operation be prepared in a special room that is adjacent to the operating room.

The present-day polypharmaceutic approach to anesthesia makes it almost essential that an intravenous solution be administered to patients throughout the period of anesthesia and operation. Usually this intravenous infusion consists of a solution of 5 per cent dextrose in water given at a slow rate, so that during an operative procedure of 1 to 3 hours the patient receives from 500 to 1,000 ml. of the solution. It is preferable that the infusion be injected into an arm vein rather than a vein in the foot or the leg, but on some procedures the arm is not accessible for this purpose, and a vein in the lower extremity is used. Every effort should be made to conserve the patient's own blood rather than transfuse to replace blood lost at the operation. However, when the estimated blood loss exceeds 500 ml. in adults or even smaller amounts in debilitated patients, children or infants, or if the

procedure is unusually shocking for any other reason, then transfusions of whole blood to replace losses or to correct shock are indicated.

Several considerations are involved in minimizing trauma to the patient during an operation. The first of these is the gentle and skillful handling of all phases of the operative procedure by the surgeon and his assistants. All movements and manipulations should be deliberate, purposeful and with the softest possible touch. Whenever possible, incisions and dissections should be done with sharp instruments—preferably with the scalpel (Fig. 13-3), or in certain situations by cutting with dissecting scissors. Only in dissecting near certain structures, such as essential nerves or blood vessels, is some gentle spreading of the tissues with a small pointed hemostat or with the blunt end of a scalpel justified. If an incision of adequate size is employed, if lighting is satisfactory, and anesthesia sufficient, then the need for the retraction of tissues is minimized. Strong and prolonged retraction traumatizes tissues and should be avoided. Sponging is done by blotting accurately once or twice to remove the blood from the wound before the bleeding point is caught with a fine-pointed hemostat and then ligated. Repeated sponging or firm rubbing with gauze sponges should not be done, because these practices inflict some

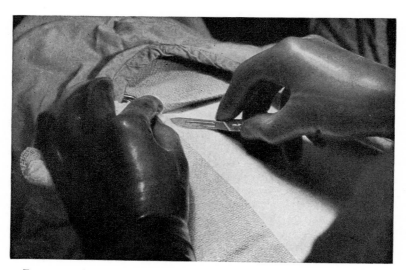

Fig. 13-3. Sharp dissection. The skin incision and most other dissections are made with the curved part of the scalpel blade. Only the lightest pressure is required for dividing tissues with sharp dissection.

trauma to the tissues (see Chap. 2, "Wound Healing").

It is much better to conserve the patient's own blood by careful control of all blood vessels and bleeding areas before significant amounts of blood are lost than to transfuse to replace lost blood. In order to accomplish this the surgeon must take much of the operating time to clamp each bleeding point with a fine-pointed hemostat as it is encountered; or, when blood vessels can be seen before they are cut, to clamp and divide them between small pointed hemostats; then replacing hemostats with ligatures of fine cotton (Fig. 13-4). Packing with gauze or suturing large areas in wounds to control bleeding should be avoided unless the usual methods of clamping and ligation are not applicable or are regarded as inadequate.

Perhaps the most important of all factors that have to do with minimizing the operative risk for patients are the care and the skill employed by the surgeon in removing the diseased parts and in repairing vitally important viscera, as well as the incisions used to gain access to them. It is obvious that blood vessels must be repaired with a suture line that does not leak at the time of repair or later. Each ligature must be secure. The hollow viscera should be arranged and repaired so that their comfortable functioning is assured as well as their security against the leakage of fluids or gas. All sutures that maintain the essential strength of the repaired tissues, whether they secure the fascia of the abdominal wall, the submucosa of the intestine or some other equally important structure, preferably should be interrupted sutures of nonabsorbable material such as cotton. The size of the suture material should be the smallest that will give the repaired tissue its normal (or usual) tensile strength. It is desirable that such sutures be interrupted, not continuous. They must be placed with absolute accuracy and spaced correctly. They should be tied just tightly enough to approximate the tissues correctly but not to cut them or impair their vascular supply. These principles apply also to the securing of ligatures and sutures in ducts and pedicles, so that they will hold securely enough to avoid slipping but will not cut through the wall into the lumen.

Following most cleanly and properly performed operations, drainage is seldom indicated. However, when an uncontrollable oozing of blood, bile or other secretion is expected to continue for some time after closure of the incision, a small soft rubber dam drain may be inserted to the oozing area and brought out through a small slit in the main incision or, preferably, through a nearby separate small incision. The soft rubber dam drain should be fixed in place with a nonabsorbable suture in the skin or transfixed with a closed safety pin to prevent the drain from retracting into the incision.

Tiny plastic tubes, containing several openings near the submerged tip, may be placed into wounds that are likely to accumulate serum and air (e.g., axillary, groin, and cervical dissections) and connected to a continuous aspiration device postoperatively.

Practices regarding the application of dressings to incisions vary. In some climates and in certain incisions (e.g., on the face) surgeons may not apply any dressing to the wound, and a few surgeons have extended this practice to leave all closed clean incisions uncovered by dressings. Some coat clean incisions with a film of plastic material (e.g., collodion or Aeroplast) which is painted or sprayed on the incision just after the completion of the operation. It is the practice of most surgeons, however, to cover cleanly made incisions with a dressing. This may consist of a single layer of petroleum jelly or plastic (Telfa) gauze next to the wound, followed with several layers of surgical gauze held in place with adhesive tape applied to the skin over a protective coating of compound tincture of benzoin. Elastoplast is preferable to adhesive tape for holding gauze dressings in place over mobile areas such as the extremities or the neck. Stockinette cut on the bias makes a suitable wrapping for dressings over incisions in the thoracic region and on the lower extremities. Wounds that may drain usually require very much more gauze dressing than clean wounds without appreciable drainage. Severely contaminated wounds may have to be unsutured, partially or completely, and covered with sterile petrolatum gauze and many layers of sterile surgical gauze dressings (delayed closure of the wound may be accomplished later).

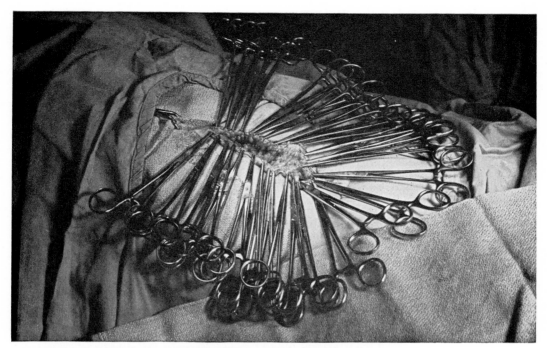

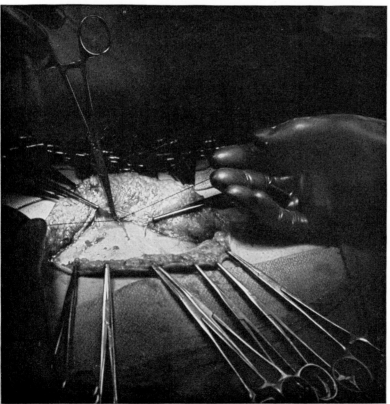

Fig. 13-4. Hemostasis is accomplished by clamping vessels with sharply pointed small hemostats, then removing the hemostats as the vessels are tied with fine cotton ligatures (or other suitable material). It is preferable to conserve the patient's own blood with the application of many hemostats rather than replace lost blood by transfusion.

GENERAL CARE

Cardiac arrest is a rare complication of surgical procedures (the incidence may be approximately one cardiac arrest in 5,000 operations), but it is a situation that must be recognized and treated immediately by the surgeon and the anesthesiologist if the patient is to be helped. Any circumstances that result in a deficiency of oxygen disturbance in pH or other chemical abnormality in the myocardium may cause cardiac arrest (see Chap. 41, "Cardiac Surgery").

Temperature Control. Hyperthermia is dangerous, and in indicated cases induced hypothermia may be indicated. In such cases a recording rectal termometer is advisable. A refrigeration mattress should be placed under the patient in all instances in which the rectal temperature is above 40° C. when the patient comes to the operating room.

Shock. The prevention and the treatment of shock is important (see Chap. 7). A current recording of blood loss with associated quantitative replacement is mandatory. In major operations, even if blood is not to be used immediately, a vein should be kept open with 5 per cent dextrose in water solution at the rate of 500 ml./hour in adults, and in children on the low side of an amount less than this in proportion to body weight.

RETURN OF PATIENT TO THE WARD OR POSTANESTHETIC RECOVERY ROOM

A professional member of the surgical team must accompany the patient to the ward or, preferably, to a postanesthetic recovery room. During this early postoperative period before the patient is fully awake two precautions are important: (1) the maintenance of an adequate respiratory airway and (2) the prevention of the aspiration of vomitus. It is the assistant's duty to see that these precautions are observed and to institute controls against any other postoperative complications, as well as to write the postoperative orders. The responsibility of the operating team is not fulfilled until the patient is completely awake.

BIBLIOGRAPHY

McCorkle, H. J.: The role of technical factors in reducing the operative risk, 16th Congrès de la Société Internationale de Chirurgie, Copenhagen, Bull. Soc. Internat. Chir. *14*:992-994, 1955.

CHAPTER 14

Nonoperative Surgical Care

General
Fever
Postoperative Pain
Gas Therapy
Postoperative Urinary Retention

Edema
Nausea and Vomiting
Headache
Symptomatic Psychoses

Section 1. General

PATIENT REACTION

An operation performed today is often preceded and followed by many discomfiting maneuvers not employed a half century ago. To the laymen, for instance, ignorant of the nature of modern medical diagnostic methods, the placing of the electrodes and the taking of the record for an electrocardiogram is often a harrowing experience. "My God! I thought they were going to electrocute me" was once thrown at me by an ill man whom I in haste had not apprised of his coming medical nightmare.

The taking of blood for the hemogram requires "only a little stick"! But who is there who takes pleasure from a stick, no matter how small, unless he be psychopathic? The drawing of larger samples of blood for "blood chemistries" requires larger sticks, and the sight of one's own life-blood being drained from him is unnerving.

A measure of the psychological trauma of the procedures entering into the care of a person while undergoing a gastrectomy is illustrated by the story told me by a farmer. What follows is his tale—not told as well as he did—after he learned that I was a doctor.

I had gone to the clinic to see about my stomach hurtin' two to three times. They'd taken some exer rays which didn't hurt none but were some scary! They darkened up the room as dark as a moonless night and told me to drink some stuff

I couldn't see or taste from a beer-mug. While I was drinking this stuff that felt like some slaked lime I drank once, a fella was a punchin' on my stomach and running a board up and down in front of me. So he finds a right sore spot and says, "There it is." So I thinks, "I got a cancer!" They have me lie on a shiny table that's as hard as cement and cold—them city boys must have air conditionin'! After a while they let me go. I go back to the clinic frettin' about cancer! I wait about three hours when a doc tells me I have one of those stomach ulcers and not to worry. He'd give me medicine to heal it. That's what they told Jim Dyer when he took sick, and he died in three months. When he was embalmed twern't a free piece of innard in him and his belly almost a-busting with water. I know! I was there! So I goes home and takes the medicine like Doc says to, only it don't do me no good! I began puking. It took me two weeks to get up enough gumption to go back—and then I really didn't all by myself because Harry, my boy, carries me and I so weak I couldn't help myself, I just let him.

They take me into the hospital right off and in ten minutes they took my clothes. I hoped they wouldn't lose them because they were the only clothes I had fittin' to bury me in and I didn't want Ma spendin' the milk money just to buy clothes to cover a good-for-nothin' corpse.

Well, they shooed Harry and Ma out and went to work. First, a fresh lookin' little thing a-comes and without sayin' nothing grabs my ear and—wham!—I'd thought the dangdest biggest horse fly that ever growed had a-bit my ear! I found out next day she was taken' my blood to count.

Then a young studying doctor comes in and asks me a whole lot of questions that weren't especially fittin'. 'Twas in a way a-pesterin' of a sick man. All I wanted was to be alone a while to get used to the smells and the strange quarters. You know not even dumb chickens like new places! They really don't! They'll a-quit layin' for a week when you move 'em off'n the roost they're used to.

So I answered his questions mostly "No" cause I found that's easiest 'cause if you say "Yes" to anything then it's "When?" and "Where?" and "What did you do for it?" He leaves and comes back shortly with a small syringe like the one I use to give the shoats the cholery vaccine. He wraps a rubber tube around my arm, a-pullin' the hair, and wipes it with cold alcyhol and then jabs a needle in! All the while tellin' me nothin' he's about. That needle must have been used to puncture a tin can! It felt like a scorpion sting. Even though I have blood-veins like a fresh cow's udder —it was plain he was tryin' to stick one of them— he couldn't stick the needle in. So he draws that needle out and it's plain why it wouldn't stick into the vein, it caught in the skin-hole like it had a fish hook on the end. The next needle he tried must have been new—it went right in. Then he drawed out four of them syringes full of blood and I knew I didn't have much more of that stuff to give to anybody!

After that I was let rest for about two hours and in comes an older young doctor who asks me the same questions and looks me all over. He goes, and in comes another with a nurse and a panful of ice and a little rubber hose in it. Though that hose looked little it felt as big as an irrigation pipe going through my nose. The nose wasn't made to push tubes through. Anyway he carefully pushes this tube through my nose and I felt like my head was a-bustin', till it got in back of my throat and I suddenly feel like throwin' up which I do easy (and I do!) and out my mouth comes the tube and I feel like a bull bein' led around by his nose! Back he pulls the tube and down he tries to push it quicklike. Oh! It goes down the wrong way and I can't stop coughin' and chokin'. After what seems like an hour I play out and he gets it into my stomach. They hook it up to some bottles after fastening it to my nose. I rest for a while; then that little hose evidently kicks a little because I feel like vomitin' again.

Then this doctor comes back with a nurse and bottles. They hang these on a stand that leans over so I'm sure it'll fall. I've never liked leaning things since Pa's leaning haystack fell over on me as a kid and I near died before they dug me out. Well, Doc sticks my vein easy, he tested the needle for hooks, and they hook the bottle-tube to it and tie my arm to a board and the board to the bed. I never thought that stuff would ever get in. I was a-feared to move because the nurse told me as she left, "Don't move or the needle will come out." I wasn't goin' to move a whisker. I'd been stuck enough for one day.

Well, my elbow ached, my shoulder ached, and my rump ached before that fluid got in; in fact, they didn't ache all at once but took turns achin'.

I wear this tube in my stomach and drink and eat, so they told me, through my veins for two days then more exer rays. And after they was took the older young doctor came with an older one I'd never seen and he says to me, "Mr. Beiner, you need a part of your stomach taken out so you can eat. You have a gastric ulcer blocking off your stomach." "Thank you," I says very polite like; feelin' like I'd like to crawl in a hole under the barn like Shep did when he was a-dyin'. I knew now—I just knew! I had a cancer like Jim Dyer—and I sees him again—open at the undertaker's.

Well, I signs so's they can cut as they like and the next mornin' they takes me to the surgery, they calls it. Before I go the nurse gives me a shot that feels cool like ice in hot weather and before I know it I feel sleepy and don't give a dangish, and I don't recall none until somebody covers my mouth and nose with a little rubber feed bag and in no time at all I see flashes that look like lightnin' and there comes a-roaring sound like those jet planes flyin' low and then I just floats off—

When I wake up my belly hurts like it was a-fire, my mouth feels like I been drunk for a week, and I can't hardly talk for my throat being sore. I knew the stomach wasn't in the throat but until the studyin' doctor told me that the throat was sore from a tube to get wind into me while I was being cut, I thought they'd maybe taken all my eating machinery out.

The next day in comes the old doctor with the young ones and he asks a few questions and says, "Dave," he says, "we're going to get you up!" "When, next month?" says I. "No, Mr. Beiner— right now." "Is he crazy?" I thought! I hadn't heard of this early perambulatin' they expect of you these days. My father had his breach fixed about forty years back and he laid in bed in the hospital for two straight weeks. Finest rest he ever had with everybody waitin' on him hand and foot. Better than stayin' in the Jefferson Hotel. I expected that too but, though I had a goodly portion of my stomach cut out yesterday, up I go! No rest! They pry me from my bed, my head swims and I almost black-out. I suppose that's good because when I fully come to, my belly is hurtin' like everything where it was cut, but up I get! I've always liked gettin' out of bed,

I almost always feel so good I pound my chest a little. This was one time that I got up and wanted to pound Doc, not my chest. I didn't because I was sure if I tried it the stitchin'd tear loose. I am sure being able to contain my feelin's saved me from bustin' my stitches trying to lick those doctors. I'm sorry I felt that way! 'Twasn't really a fittin' feeling to have, but who wouldn't feel that way after expectin' a rest but getting only a real passle of sufferin' and being hauled out of the bed a-hurtin' like I'd never hurt before. It's not that I' never suffered because I've had two felons and real bad piles that had to be lanced.

In fact, that there penicillin they'd shot into my rump for ten days was worse'n the piles. I never knew a man's rump could look like a worn-out pin cushion until I looked at it with the shavin' mirror Harry brought me after he saw me all a-whiskered-up like a mangy old he-goat.

Well, the next few days go all right. I knew now what to expect! Bein' stuck! A-lyin' still like a stove-poker! Gettin' up a-hurtin' and wearin' the little hose that wasn't botherin' much until my ear began to ache and my throat felt scratchy at the back. Finally they pull it out! On it was stuck the worst lookin' stuff you'd ever want to see. I'd never seen nothin' like it and I've seen a heap of sights.

They give me a little water to drink, and I never knew water'd taste so good. It even tasted better'n than that I remember drinkin' while puttin' up hay in August. Next day I get a little mush to eat. It tasted good but I got filled up so quick I couldn't eat half of it. Oh! I thought—"did they take out so much stomach I can never eat a square meal again?" I worry all day about that and finally ask the resident, as they call one of them young doctors, about it. He tells me the stomach needs a little stretchin' and then I can eat a *small* meal again. I didn't like that "small-meal" sayin' but I felt better and almost quit worrying.

About ten days after they cut me I hear a rattling and in comes a young doc pushing a table on rollers that were almost square—that's what made it rattle so. A nurse seemed to be riding on the front of it. My, how these young ones make light of things! Playing around sick people like they were kids! No, they were not playing, it only looked that way with my imaginin'.

They come to my bed; off come the bed clothes I was lying under right proper, because the night shirt they give me that mornin' had been shrunk so, exposin' my privates in plain view of that young nurse who had no weddin' ring on! Then off came the sticky-tape. It had been taken off before but didn't bother much the first time

because the hair they'd shaved off my belly had not growed yet, but this time it seemed like the hair had growed into the tape because when he pulled it off I almost went off the bed!

Then out came a scissors and Doc told me he was going to take the stitches out. I bet that'll hurt—everything else they've did to me had! So I grit my teeth, begin to sweat, my heart pounds away—and out comes the first stitch. Well! that was the first thing that didn't hurt! I thought that was only luck and bet to myself that the next one would make up for it! No, it didn't either. Well, at least there were two things that didn't need sufferin'—the taking of the stitches and the urine analysis, they call it! Giving them the water for that was the only simple pleasure I had in two weeks in the hospital!

But after all, these doctors are wonderful! Here I am now, feelin' fit as a tom-cat! Eatin' greens and all and even takin' a little nip now and then when Ma's away visiting her kinfolk in St. Lewi. I hadn't been able to take one for three years because it burned so after. I can work or walk all day now and I feel like 40 'stead of the 66 I am!

This tale embraces some of the mental trials imposed upon a person by a major operative procedure. Although our capacity to save the lives of persons having surgically remediable ills is remarkably greater today than it was a half century ago, the mental trial of surgery is no less for the individual today than it was and, in fact, it may even be somewhat greater.

PREOPERATIVE PATIENT CARE

What can be done to minimize the psychological upsets connected with an operation?

Obviously, a high regard for the feelings of the sick person is of first importance. He is usually apprehensive of surgery itself and is ignorant of the many protective and therapeutic details accompanying it. Therefore, no painful act should be performed on his body without telling him of the necessity for it. Not to do so serves to raise his fear and may at times lead him to believe that he is being used for experiment without his knowledge. Only the very young, the very old, and the mortally ill are insensitive to the sanctity of the body, and a sick person clings to the primary biologic urge not to be hurt or exposed without knowing why.

His capacity, too, to stand mental trial

and physical suffering without losing the will to live is remarkably enhanced by the presence of kind, truthful, conscientious and knowledgeable men and women, whether they be orderlies, nurses, or physicians.

His questions should be answered without evasiveness. Occasionally, the only truthful answer must be given in the form, "I really don't know until we have examined the tissues," and questions about the character of a tumor or the cause of many ailments must be answered in this way. After the operation fewer questions will be asked, seemingly because the sick person senses what is really wrong.

Sometimes a moribund patient seems to be dimly aware of the approaching end but prefers to know it, as it were, obliquely. The physician usually can follow suit and need not state directly what the patient prefers to know indirectly.

The signs of approaching death become familiar to the medical man all too soon in his career. Fear is not commonly one of these signs. In fact, the energy required to give vigorous expression to fear is rarely found in the dying. More often the picture is like that which Shakespeare gives of the dying Falstaff:

He parted even just between twelve and one, even at the turning of the tide: for after I saw him fumble with the sheets, and play with flowers, and smile upon his finger's end, I knew there was but one way; for his nose was as sharp as a pen and 'a babbled of green fields. . . . 'A bade me lay more clothes on his feet: I put my hand into the bed, and felt them, and they were as cold as any stone; then I felt to his knees, and so upward, and upward, and all was as cold as any stone.

When we ask their help, the priest, the rabbi and the minister serve the religious well in time of trial. Often the man of religion quiets the fears of the one to be operated upon more rapidly and surely than drugs, reassurance or the psychiatric consultant. The soporific drugs help in allaying fears. Amytal Sodium, 0.06 to 0.3 Gm.; pentobarbital Sodium, 0.1 to 0.2 Gm.; Seconal, 0.1 Gm. (sodium propyl methyl carbinyl allyl barbiturate); and chloral hydrate, 1 to 2 Gm., are effective and widely used for this purpose. Scopolamine, 0.25 to 1 mg., also has the capacity to render most individuals less sensitive to their surroundings and much less apprehensive of danger and pain. The need for these drugs is especially acute on the night preceding and on the day of the operation.

The dictates of humanity require that the person having physical pain before an operation be relieved of the consciousness of his pain. For this purpose the analgesics, morphine (0.014 Gm.) and Demerol (0.050-0.150 Gm.) are remarkably effective. The patient who has peripheral circulatory failure, whatever be its cause, and pain should be given the analgesic intravenously. The intravenous dosage of most drugs usually given subcutaneously, such as morphine and Demerol, is one half to two thirds of the subcutaneous dosage with at least 5 ml. of liquid vehicle.

Although the soporifics and the analgesics are very beneficent drugs, their use at times poses unexpected and disturbing problems. Few situations are more discomfiting than to have everything and everyone prepared to begin an operation and then to have the anesthetist say: "I am afraid to start the anesthesia because the blood pressure is 60/20." The surgical resident says, "It wasn't low when I took it this morning; it was 160/90." Has the patient suffered a myocardial infarct? Is he bleeding internally? Is he dehydrated? Has he suffered an acute massive collapse of the lung? Is he about to die? These are some of the questions raised immediately. Whereas 5 minutes ago there was certainty, now there is only uncertainty and consternation.

The commonest cause of acute preoperative preanesthesia hypotension, especially among the elderly and the starved, is preoperative soporific-analgesic idiosyncrasy or overdosage. The combination of morphine and barbiturate is somewhat more prone to induce hypotension than is the combination of Demerol and barbiturate.

Should acute preoperative hypotension occur, the operation should be delayed whenever possible. When a delay of the operation jeopardizes the life of the patient, a vasopressor agent may be employed. Ephedrine hydrochloride, 0.03 to 0.12 Gm., or neosynephrine, 0.005 to 0.01 Gm., are effective and safe. The physiologic action of norepinephrine (Arterenol) does not differ significantly from that of ephedrine. Ephedrine's vasopressor action is effected largely by its inhibition of the enzyme which normally destroys norepinephrine. In effect, the giving of ephedrine provides the person a higher titer of his own norepinephrine.

Besides hypotension, unwanted actions of morphine and the barbiturates are respiratory depression and hypothermia.

Demerol, atropine and to a lesser degree scopolamine inhibit sweating. This action favors hyperthermia especially during hot weather and febrile illness. This complication is occasionally lethal, especially in hot operating and recovery rooms and especially among children having suppurative processes (see Heat Stroke in this chapter).

The preoperative general care of the surgical patient other than that directed toward the amelioration of psychological stimuli and pain is directed toward providing him with optimum conditions for recovery, but these procedures are tolerated better if he is completely apprised of their nature. In other words, it is aimed at the prevention of complications and therefore constitutes a major part of the preventive medical aspect of surgery.

ASPIRATIONAL PNEUMONITIS

One of the gravest dangers attendant upon anesthesia is the aspiration of vomitus into the lungs. The pulmonary aspiration of gastric juice with or without food particles in it induces a fulminant, necrotizing chemical pneumonitis. In effect, the living lung becomes acutely inflamed and edematous, and the bronchial secretions are increased, adding further to the hypoxia and promoting atelectasis. Aspiration of intestinal juice into large segments of lung is often lethal in 36 hours and sometimes within 30 minutes. The aspiration into small segments may be followed by bronchopneumonia and pulmonary abscesses, especially when food particles are inhaled with the juice.

Ensuring an empty stomach before an anesthetic is given and keeping it empty during the operation obviate the danger of aspirational pneumonitis. In the absence of esophageal, pyloric or intestinal obstruction or ileus, an empty stomach *usually* is attained by merely withholding all but liquid foods for 12 hours, all liquid foods for 6 to 8 hours,

and water for 4 hours preoperatively. Occasionally, the application of this rule will not secure an empty stomach. Actually, the only way to be reasonably sure of an empty stomach before an operation is to aspirate it through a tube.

The placement of an inlying gastric tube before anesthesia is begun should be mandatory for all major intra-abdominal operations excepting pelvic. However, even with pelvic operations, nephrectomy and appendectomy, trouble with postoperative ileus and gas pains is reduced remarkably by ensuring an empty stomach with the use of an inlying gastric tube before and during the operation.

The placement of a tube into the stomach should precede gastrectomy by at least 8 hours, and in cases of pyloric obstruction by 24 or more hours. The use of the long and the short intestinal tubes for intestinal obstructions and ileus is discussed in Chapter 36, "Intestinal Obstruction."

COMPLICATIONS OF GASTRIC INTUBATION

The indwelling gastric and intestinal tubes are mixed blessings. Occasionally, their use is attended by two complications rarely lethal but often crippling, namely, cicatricial laryngeal and esophageal stenosis. Pain in the throat radiating up behind the ear, earache and dysphonia (indications of laryngeal inflammation) and heart burn or low substernal and epigastric discomforts (indicative of lower esophageal inflammation) appearing while the intestinal tube is being worn are indications for its immediate removal and inspection. Should *bloody mucus* be found upon the tube, a tube should not be reinserted. If the illness requires further use of gastric or intestinal decompression it should be effected through a gastrostomy or a jejunostomy; fortunately, this is rarely needed.

Necrosis of the ala nasae may attend the wearing of an indwelling gastric tube. This complication is attributable to the ignorance of the person securing the tube to the face. The tube never should be secured while lying in the nasolabial groove or over the lateral aspect of the nose and being directed upward toward the eye, since the acute bend of the tube about the ala nasae compresses it.

The irrigation of gastric and intestinal tubes

with water to maintain their patency may induce fluid balance disturbances. Water introduced into the stomach or the intestine, if not removed immediately, will be attended by the rapid movement of salts from the plasma into the water in the lumen of the intestine (see Chap. 36, "Intestinal Obstruction"). As the fluid is removed subsequently through the tube, it withdraws with it salts that would not have been lost from the body if water had not been instilled into the gut. In the process the water in the plasma previously holding the withdrawn salts is redistributed throughout the body, and the osmolar concentration of the body's fluids is reduced. The physiologic consequences of fluid changes attending the repeated instillation of water into the gastro-intestinal tract and its subsequent withdrawal through tubes are a decreasing plasma volume, a decreasing interstitial fluid volume, an increasing intercellular water volume and a decreasing osmolar concentration. These changes may lead ultimately to peripheral circulatory failure coupled with water intoxication.

The rate of loss of potassium from the body of a person wearing an indwelling gastric or intestinal tube also is increased by irrigating the tubes with water or a solution containing no potassium.

If a tube must be irrigated, the use of Ringer's solution will prevent the development of the above disturbances of fluid balance associated with irrigating indwelling intestinal tubes with water.

Section 2. Fever

ETIOLOGY

The predominant causes of the postoperative fever are: (1) infection within the wound, (2) infection within the urinary tract, (3) pulmonary complications, (4) thrombophlebitis and (5) increased osmolar concentration secondary to a lack of water or a salt-excess (see Chap. 5, "Fluid and Electrolytes"). Less common causes are: (1) drug reactions (e.g., allergic-penicillin, etc.; specific-atropine), (2) malarial relapse, (3) central neurologic disturbances, (4) bacterial enterocolitis and (5) factitial factors such as the heating of the thermometer with hot liquids, radiators, matches, lighters or friction *et alia*.

WOUND INFECTION

Diagnosis. With such a variety of factors to consider, the search for the cause of any postoperative fever must be orderly. The wound must be examined first. Yet it is often difficult and sometimes impossible after a single examination to be sure of infection in a wound. To some degree, all the classic signs of infection—redness, heat, tenderness, swelling—are present in the primary stage of healing of a thoroughly healthy and uninfected wound. Even the systemic signs of an infection—leukocytes and fever—may be stimulated by the very small amounts of sterile dead tissues inescapably left within the wound. A single examination, therefore, is seldom enough, and repeated examinations are required to disprove the existence of a wound infection.

Clearly, repetitive examination of the wound is often required to determine the existence of an infection within it unless pathognomonic signs of a wound infection exist. These pathognomonic signs are: drainage of fluid containing numerous bacteria from the wound, fluctuation, erysipelas, necrosis of skin (phlegmonous erysipelas), vesiculation, and with clostridial infections rapidly expanding crepitus or crepitus associated with physical prostration and a tachycardia greater than that compatible with the height of the fever (see Chap. 4, "Surgical Infections").

The aim of the repetitive examination of a wound in which infection is suspected is to determine whether the heat, the redness, the swelling and the tenderness are increasing or decreasing. Increasing or spreading heat, redness, swelling and tenderness indicate the probable existence of infection, and diminishing heat, redness, swelling, or tenderness indicate its nonexistence or biologic control.

Treatment. As soon as the diagnosis of a wound infection can be made with reasonable certainty the wound is opened at the point of maximum tenderness and swelling down to the subcutaneous fascia. Of course, aseptic precautions must be exercised. A sample is collected immediately for smearing and bacterial culturing (see Chap. 3, "Applied Surgical Bacteriology"). The depth of the wound is then inspected and probed gently. Free drainage should be maintained by introducing one end of a suitable drain. Wet dressings such as gauze saturated with sterile 0.9 per cent sodium chloride solution often are helpful in preventing the secretions from the wound from forming a dry coagulum which may interfere with free drainage. If the probe passes freely beneath the wound or if the tissue in its depths is shaggy, avascular and gray, suggesting one of the more serious types of infection, the entire wound should be laid open and packed loosely with fine meshed cotton or linen gauze. Failure to open an infected wound completely may lead to loss of the patient's life. In the case of laparotomy wounds, the peritoneum and the deep fascia are left intact except for the purpose of draining a subjacent intra-abdominal abscess.

The use of antibiotics has complicated the picture of wound infections. The local and systemic signs of a wound infection arising while these drugs are being administered often are remarkably delayed in their appearance and are attenuated. At times a near-fatal wound infection is attended by so few local signs that it is overlooked until the wound opens and drains spontaneously.

ACTH and the corticoids also may inhibit the development of the local and general signs of a wound infection and render the detection of suppuration difficult. Rapid physiologic deterioration occurring in a postoperative patient receiving corticoids or ACTH in whom no signs of a pulmonary, otitic, or urinary infection can be found, is sufficient indication for opening of the wound. It may be closed should no infection be found.

Diabetics and especially those who have peripheral neuropathy often respond peculiarly to a wound infection. They may manifest little fever, slight leukocytosis, little pain, tenderness, redness or warmth of the wound even though much pus be contained in it: swelling there is and little else. However, the diabetes "goes out of control" regularly with infection, the glycosuria increases, and acetone bodies appear in the urine, though the amount of insulin given previously was adequate to prevent both. In other words, a diabetic who

has been stabilized postoperatively and then goes out of control probably has developed an infection somewhere in the wound, the lung or the urinary tract, and the possible location of it in the wound cannot be excluded because of lack of the classic signs of an infection about the incision.

After the wound has been examined a search always is made for the other possible causes of postoperative fever. The chest is percussed, the character of the breath sounds carefully auscultated in order to determine their qualities and the presence of concomitant adventitious sounds such as rales, rhonchi or rubs. The type of breathing is observed, and the position of the trachea is determined. In addition, the relative intensity and quality of the aortic and the pulmonary second sounds are to be noted. Gallop rhythm, especially along the left border of the sternum, and cardiac irregularities are to be looked for. The quality of the apex beat and the size of the heart also are important.

PULMONOCARDIAC DISTURBANCES

The pulmonocardiac disturbances commonly associated with fever are: atelectasis (collapse of the lung) due either to bronchial obstruction, which is common, or less often to compression, congestive atelectasis (acute nonobstructive massive collapse of lung), pneumonitis (bacterial or from aspiration of gastrointestinal contents), pleuritis, acute cardiac failure, pulmonary embolism and myocardial infarction. Obviously, *roentgenograms of the chest and electrocardiographs* are invaluable for the detection and the analysis of a postoperative pulmonocardiac complication.

Brief descriptions of the characteristics of some of the above-named possible causes of postoperative fever follow:

Bronchial Obstructive Atelectasis. USUAL ORIGIN. Inspissated mucus: foreign bodies (teeth, dentures and food particles) are less frequent causes.

GENERAL COURSE OF THE ILLNESS. Tachycardia, tachypnea and fever often occur practically simultaneously. Cyanosis is an inconstant sign, but when present it indicates that a rather large segment of lung is unaerated and that a significant quantity of blood is flowing through its pulmonary arteriovenous circuit, having much the effect of a right-to-left cardiac shunt. The administration of oxygen does not abolish the cyanosis, though it may reduce it somewhat. Dyspnea is experienced only when a large segment of the lung is airless.

The trachea and the mediastinum tend to shift toward the atelectatic lung. Obviously, tracheal and mediastinal shift will be slight or undetectable with a unilateral slight or a bilateral atelectasis of equal extent. The respiratory excursion of the chest is limited and lags on the involved side. Breath sounds are diminished in intensity (distant) and tend to be bronchial in character over atelectatic segments in contact with the chest wall. Obviously, should the atelectasis occur solely within the hilar segments, the upper lobes, the lingular segment of the left upper lobe, or only in small portions of lung in contact with the chest wall, abnormalities of quality and character of breath sounds may not be detectable. For this reason atelectasis cannot be excluded as a cause of postoperative fever on the basis of absence of auscultatory or percussional signs, and roentgenographic studies are necessary. The roentgen signs of atelectasis are opacification of lung, homolateral shift of mediastinum and trachea, accentuation of bronchovascular markings, and limitation of motion of the diaphragm.

Rales, rhonchi and wheezes almost always accompany obstructive atelectasis.

TREATMENT OF OBSTRUCTIVE ATELECTASIS. This is directed toward the removal of the obstruction, permitting air to enter the lung again. The methods used consist of increasing the activity of the patient, deep breathing exercises, coughing, tracheal aspiration and bronchoscopy.

Increased activity of the patient may be obtained by having him roll from side to side in bed or getting him out of bed to walk. With the assumption of physical activity, coughing is often stimulated, and the atelectasis may disappear with great rapidity. However, this method of treating atelectasis is rarely effective when the atelectasis is extensive or accompanied by numerous rhonchi.

Coughing can be rendered more effective by supporting the thoracic or abdominal wound. A pillow held tightly over the would by grasping it at the ends and pressing it about the body provides an effective external splint, permitting a much more effective cough.

If neither activity nor coughing will clear the bronchial tree, *aspiration of the trachea* is required. This may be done blindly by use of a suction apparatus.

A lubricated catheter is passed through a nostril, and the tip is advanced to the epiglottic region. The passage of the length of catheter spanning the distance between the tip of the nose and a mastoid process will place the tip near the epiglottis. Then while the patient's head is tipped backward with the chin held forward, the catheter is advanced quickly *while the patient inspires deeply*. The entry of the catheter into the trachea will be attended by a fit of coughing. Then the top of the trap connected to suction is stoppered rapidly and intermittently with the thumb or the forefinger. Next, the catheter is advanced, while the trap is being alternately opened and closed. The intermittent aspiration is kept up until secretions are not obtainable. Then the examination of the chest is repeated Should remarkable improvement be found, bronchoscopy may not be necessary. However, should little or no improvement be found, bronchoscopy should be done.

Often *bronchoscopic aspiration* is indicated without antecedent attempts to clear the atelectasis with increased activity, coughing and tracheal aspiration. It is indicated as the primary therapeutic step in cases of massive collapse of one lung or bilateral extensive atelectasis, atelectasis secondary to aspiration of a foreign body, and atelectasis associated with hypotension, disorientation, stupor, or coma, paralysis of intercostal and abdominal musculature, or profound weakness. Skillful bronchoscopy is safe and without much discomfort and has so much potential benefit that one should not hesitate to employ it as a therapeutic measure for atelectasis. At times a tracheostomy is required to permit the repeated aspiration of mucus in order to keep the airway unobstructed. This is especially applicable to the treatment of atelectasis occurring after crushing injuries of the chest, severe facial-cervical burns, pulmonary aspiration, and among those persons who have obstructive atelectasis and are very weak or have far-advanced chronic pulmonary diseases such as pulmonary fibrosis and emphysema.

Associated measures to be taken in conjunction with and subsequent to the above methods of treating obstructive atelectasis are: (1) the giving of a wide-spectrum antibiotic; (2) the discontinuance of use of any drug having an atropinelike action, such as scopolamine, atropine, tincture of belladonna, and Demerol as these drugs increase the viscidity of the bronchial secretions, making them more difficult to expel; (3) the avoidance of drugs which depress the cough reflex, such as opium, codeine, morphine, Dilaudid, Pantopon, etc.; (4) the use of a route other than the intravenous for the administration of needed water and electrolytes. When fluids are given intravenously while atelectasis exists they tend to increase it or at least delay its resolution. For unknown reasons, fluids given orally, subcutaneously, or rectally apparently are less prone to do so; (5) agents which increase the fluidity of the bronchial secretions may be given. Potassium iodide does so. Recently, certain surface-tension-reducing agents have been shown to effect dissipation of mucus within the respiratory tract. Their effectiveness in the prevention and the after-treatment of atelectasis has not been established. However, they appear to do no harm so far as is known and consequently may be tried. These are usually given in a solution which is volatilized as a mist and inhaled.

Oxygen therapy has a limited usefulness in the treatment of bronchial obstructive atelectasis as a supportive measure before and during bronchial aspiration. A lung filled with oxygen becomes atelectatic far more rapidly than one filled with air. Consequently, the giving of oxygen after tracheobronchial aspiration may retard recovery, especially when the secretions are copious. However, it should be given with air-hunger or cyanosis.

Compressional atelectasis attends internal encroachment upon the lung space by fluid or air within the thoracic cavity or by fluid, air or distended viscera within the peritoneal cavity. It is attended by the same physical signs as obstructive atelectasis, except that the breath sounds may be accentuated occasionally and bronchial in character since the bronchus to the atelectatic lung is open. Deviation of the mediastinum and the treachea either does not occur or is in the direction away from the disease. Circumferential bind-ing of the abdomen with tape or a Scultetus binder is a frequent cause of compressional atelectasis. Fatal compressional atelectasis with pulmonocardiac failure is easily produced by circumferentially binding the abdomen of an anesthetized dog. The application of a circumferential abdominal dressing to an anesthetized person may be a grave surgical error.

Treatment of Compressional Atelectasis. This consists of the removal of the cause, e.g., thoracentesis, drainage of empyema, drainage of subphrenic abscess, the relief of meteorism, paracentesis, and removal of abdominal binders and circumferentially bound dressings.

For many years the administration of 7 to 20 per cent carbon dioxide in oxygen was recommended for the treatment of bronchial obstructive and compressional atelectasis. It is no longer recommended.

The *antibiotics* are valuable adjuncts in the therapy of all forms of atelectasis and postoperative pneumonitis. Purulent tracheobronchitis and bronchopneumonia frequently attend or follow atelectasis. The organisms vary, with pneumococci, streptococci and staphylococci predominating. Consequently, a broad-spectrum antibiotic is best (see Chap. 4, "Surgical Infections").

Postoperative Pneumonia. Before the nature of bronchial obstructive atelectasis was known "ether pneumonia" was presumed to be the cause of postoperative pulmonary troubles. However, it is now known that ether does not produce pneumonia. Today primary lobular and lobar pneumonias occur rarely after operations, and the appearance of lobular pneumonia postoperatively now indicates most likely that the aspiration of gastrointestinal fluid has taken place or that bronchial obstructive atelectasis has occurred, is developing or clearing.

Treatment of postoperative lobular pneumonia depends somewhat upon the nature and the quantity of the bronchial secretions and upon the organisms found in the sputum. Copious tenacious secretions require the use of bronchial aspiration in addition to the giving of a wide-spectrum antibiotic. Since incomplete saturation of the pulmonary venous blood is characteristic of lobular pneumonia, the giving of oxygen is an important part of its therapy.

Congestive Atelectasis. The air-containing space of lung may be encroached upon by blood contained within the pulmonary capillaries. Occasionally, the encroachment is so great as to render large parts of the lung essentially airless. The condition is called congestive atelectasis. It follows rapid decompression (extrusion from a pressurized airplane at very high altitudes), and occurs spontaneously among persons suffering from severe kyphosis and is then usually called pulmonocardiac failure. Congestive atelectasis occasionally occurs during or after an operation when it may be called acute postoperative nonobstructive massive collapse of the lung.

The signs of congestive atelectasis are a fulminant fever, hypotension, a cyanosis that cannot be cleared by administering pure oxygen, forceful expiratory abdominal breathing, limitation of costal breathing, tachycardia, and severe oliguria or anuria. Viewed through a bronchoscope, the bronchi are seen to be wide open during inspiration and partially or completely collapsed during expiration. Pulmonary roentgenograms may show nothing amiss, and often thoracic auscultation and percussion are not particularly abnormal until shortly before death.

No effective treatment is known. Digitalis, transfusions, phlebotomy, bronchoscopic aspiration, assisted forced breathing are all ineffective. A compression chamber should be tried; practically everything else has been tried and has failed.

Other postoperative intrathoracic complications attended by fever are pulmonary embolism (see Section on Thrombophlebitis), fat embolism, mediastinitis and pleuritis (see Section on Pain).

Fat Embolism

Fat embolism most often follows fractures and contusional trauma; however, it occurs rarely after mastectomy, the removal of arterial emboli, spinal and other osseous fusions, and celiotomy. The clinical picture, though often confusing, may be very clear-cut. Characteristically, a person who is recovering from an accident or an operation in fine fashion becomes short of breath, then febrile and disoriented, hypotensive with a fast small pulse, oliguric and finally comatose. The discovery of petechiae over the neck and the anterior

axillary folds, the anterior chest and the inner aspect of the thighs when coupled with the above clinical picture practically clinches the diagnosis. The demonstration of globules of fat in urine and saliva and seeing them in the retinal vessels add much to the credibility of the diagnosis.

The treatment of fat embolism is poorly developed. It consists of the cessation of oral feeding, the control of the pyrexia with aspirin and tepid sponge baths, the treatment of peripheral circulatory failure with transfusions of blood, and the maintenance of fluid balance.

Air Embolism

Air embolism, though not attended by fever and a very rare surgical complication, is one of the most feared complications of intracranial and intracardiac surgery, hepatectomy, thyroidectomy and pulmonary operations. It may account for more of the unsolved operative deaths than was suspected heretofore. The syndrome varies from one of fulminating circulatory failure to that of coma and death after a completely lucid interval. The rapid entry of 200 to 600 ml. of air through the systemic veins into the right heart may kill by turning the blood in the right heart to a bloody froth which cannot be pumped effectively. The opening of sigmoid venous sinuses in the skull and the transection of thyroid veins while the patient is in the head-up position, and transection of the hepatic veins while the patient is in the head-down position occasionally lead to the massive right heart type of air embolism. However, it may occur through these same vessels without regard to the position of the patient. Tachycardia, acute hypotension, cyanosis and crunchy heart sounds are its signs. The most direct form of treatment is aspiration of the right ventricle; it has been tried with some reports of success.

Air entering the pulmonary veins with thoracentesis or pulmonary operations or from the previously opened isolated left ventricle kills without foaming the blood in the heart. A small volume of air, 4 to 10 ml., entering the coronary and the cerebral circulations may kill. Acute, irreversible respiratory arrest, acute cardiac standstill and failure to recover from anesthesia are variants of left-side cardiac or pulmonary venous air embolization in anesthetized animals. No effective therapy is known. The emphasis must be on prevention.

THYROID STORM OR CRISIS

Fever may have peculiar connotations when it follows thyroidectomy and craniotomy. Before the discovery that the thioureas and iodine could effect the complete remission of Graves's disease, the performance of thyroidectomy for thyrotoxicosis was followed regularly by fever, and in some cases the fever was fulminant and, together with other metabolic disturbances, killed. The whole train of events was called a thyroid storm or crisis. Storm it was and still is: fulminant fever, mania, tachycardia up to 200, vomiting, diarrhea, coma and death. Among the aged occasionally it is relatively quiet, the fever being relatively small, and the mania absent. It is exceedingly rare after thyroidectomy today but it is still to be seen. It occasionally follows the administration of I^{131} in therapeutic doses to thyrotoxicotics, the performance of any operative procedure upon them before they have been given the thioureas, and the delivery of a child or the sufferance of an accident by untreated thyrotoxic persons.

Treatment. The treatment consists of: (1) the control of the fever by sponging the torso and the legs with tepid alcohol, placing ice bags and packs to head, axillae and chest, and the giving of aspirin (0.6 to 1.0 Gm.) every 2 hours until the rectal temperature taken at intervals of 15 to 30 minutes is 100° F. or less; (2) the provision of carbohydrate and water by intravenously infusing a cooled solution of 10 or 15 per cent dextrose in water (2,500 to 4,000 ml.); (3) raising the oxygen tension of the air breathed with a good oxygen tent; (4) quieting the mania with Seconal (0.1 to 0.2 Gm.) or Pentothal Sodium intravenously; (5) digitalizing if signs of cardiac failure appear with lanatoside C (Cedilanid) 1.0 to 1.6 mg. intravenously; and (6) providing adrenal cortical support, especially if the eosinophile numbers exceed 30 to 50 per/c.mm., with cortisone 100 mg. every 6 hours.

POSTCRANIOTOMY FEVER

Hyperpyrexia occasionally attends or follows craniotomy. Hypophysectomy and the resection of craniopharyngiomas are frequently followed by it. Formerly, disruption of the function of the temperature-regulating center was implicated as the cause. However, increased osmolar concentration is recognized now as one of the causes of postcraniotomy hyperpyrexia. When it is the cause the serum sodium concentration is found to be remarkably elevated, occasionally reaching 180 mEq./liter. Presumptively, an acute insufficiency of secretion of antidiuretic hormone permits the reduction of the renal tubular facultative absorption of water while the renal tubular absorption of electrolytes is enhanced by the operative stimulation of the adrenal cortex. The result is retention of solutes and loss of large amounts of water and an elevation of the osmolar concentration of body fluids. This is sufficient to induce fever.

Treatment. The treatment of fever attributable to hyperosmolarity by the discovery of a serum sodium concentration above 155 mEq. when it was normal preoperatively is easily effected by giving water rectally and orally, 5 per cent dextrose in water subcutaneously and intravenously. Care must be exercised lest too much water be given. For this reason the serum concentrations of sodium should be performed at hourly intervals while the water is being administered.

Some postcraniotomy fevers are not attributable to hyperosmolarity, infection, or other febrile general postoperative complications. Such need not be treated unless they exceed 104° F. (40° C.) or persist for longer than a day. Giving aspirin (acetylsalicylic acid) 0.65 to 1.0 Gm. every 4 hours and/or sponging the body with tepid water or 70 per cent alcohol usually will control nonspecific neurogenic fevers.

HEAT STROKE

Heat stroke is an occasional cause of a very high fever postoperatively. Thyroid storm, intracranial disturbances and extreme elevations of osmolar concentration (serum sodium of 170 mEq./1. or above) and heat stroke are the main causes of fever above 108° F. (42° C.).

Heat stroke is attributable to an environmental heat overload and is especially likely to occur during the first days of a hot spell.

A febrile illness, lack of water, physical exertion, alcoholism, anesthesia, debility, and nonfunctioning sweat glands secondary to diabetic neuropathy and drugs such as atropine predispose one to it. Unless treated vigorously, it soon kills.

Classically, heat pyrexia or stroke consists of a rapidly mounting fever in a person having dry hot skin. He is first apathetic, then stuporous, and then comatose. Early, he is flushed, has visibly full pulses with a wide pulse pressure and exaggerated heart sounds. Later, he becomes ashen gray, has small pulses, low blood pressure and becomes anuric. Occasionally, signs of acute cardiac collapse may be found late in the illness.

Treatment. Although the pathogenesis of heat stroke is unknown, it can be treated successfully if the treatment is begun early and conducted vigorously. Reduction of the fever by immersing the person in a bathtub filled with water and ice is the basic step. After the rectal temperature falls to 100° F. (38° C.) the patient is placed upon a bed, and the rectal temperature is determined continuously with a thermistor or thermocouple or frequently with a thermometer. If the temperature begins to rise he is covered with wet sheets and fanned. Should the temperature fall below 96° F. (36° C.) he is covered with a blanket. Sponge bathing and fanning are inferior to immersion in ice water for the primary control of heat stroke. Speed is of utmost importance.

When peripheral circulatory failure persists after reducing the temperature to normal, appropriate intravenous fluids are given. Lactated Ringer's solution is suitable until a specific choice of fluids can be made upon receiving the necessary laboratory reports. While the fluid is being given careful watch for signs of acute heart failure must be exercised. Should signs of heart failure appear, digitalization with Cedilanid is indicated.

Occasionally, heat stroke may develop during an operation. F. L., aged 6, on a day with a maximum temperature of 96° F. developed appendicitis and a preoperative temperature of 38.6° C. She was given 1/300 gr. of atropine a half hour before being anesthetized with ether and heavily covered with drapes in a hot operating room (31° C.). The surgeon, upon placing his fingers within the abdomen, noted great warmth and asked that the rectal temperature be taken—it was 41.6° C. The appendix was removed quickly, the wound closed, and the temperature was reduced by immersion in ice water. However, 6 hours later the child died. Necropsy demonstrated only widespread petechial hemorrhages. Extreme hyperpyrexia may be quickly lethal. One must be particularly aware of the great hazard an operation holds for a dehydrated, atropinized person subjected to high environmental temperatures.

Such cases often are complicated by convulsive movements or twitchings, the so-called ether convulsions (see Chap. 12, "Anesthesia").

HYPOTHERMIA

At ordinary hospital temperatures (20 to 30° C.) noniatrogenic hypothermia is not dangerous per se. It is a rather frequent complication of morphine and barbiturate overdosage, ileostomy and colostomy diarrhea, profuse fistulous drainage, enteral aspiration and pyloric obstruction with vomiting. Of course, simple exposure to cold is a likely cause. Briefly, exposure to cold, extracellular fluid volume deficit with hyponatremia, and overdosage with morphine and barbiturates are the main causes. Treatment is simple: warm surroundings for exposure hypothermia; saline solutions for dehydrational hypothermia; and withholding the drugs and warming for drug hypothermia.

Section 3. Postoperative Pain

Pain is a fearsome sensation, indicating environmental abnormality. Adequacy of stimulus varies in different tissues. The application of a hot rod to the skin, a tooth, the cornea, or the parietal peritoneum is painful, while its application to muscle, fat, mucosa of the stomach or the intestine and the visceral peritoneum is not painful. An incision is exquisitely painful in skin, barely discernible in fat, nondiscernible in muscle, moderately painful in tendon or fascia, exquisitely painful in periosteum, and not felt in intestine. Incision into a mixed nerve is agonizing.

ETIOLOGY

The possible causes of postoperative pain are relatively few: namely, inflammation, pressure, tension and ischemia. Pains stimulated by pressure, tension, ischemia and inflammation have somewhat similar characters: they are steady, aggravated by motion and may be throbbing. Only that pain associated with intermittent increases in tension is truly and regularly intermittent. The pains of ureteral and intestinal colics are of this type; they come and go as the peristalses in these structures come and go.

SITE

The commonest site of postoperative pain is the wound. All wounds are somewhat painful for 48 to 72 hours; however, normal incisional pain is not severe. Therefore, severe pain in a wound at any time signifies infection, undue pressure and tension, ischemia about the wound or of the wounded member; or the reference of pain to the wound. The phenomenon of reference of pain to the wound is especially important during the immediate postoperative period. The pain of myocardial infarction, pulmonary infarction, gastric dilatation, and vesical dilatation are frequently referred to a healing abdominal incision. Consequently, the search for the cause of unusual pain ostensibly located in an abdominal wound needs to be thorough and ofttimes extensive.

PAIN OF ISCHEMIA

Pain in a hand, a foot, an arm, a leg, or the head contained within a cast or an enveloping dressing is often ischemic in origin and demands immediate attention. Testing the painful part distal to the cast or the bandage for arterial pulses, speed of capillary flow and sensation is mandatory before an analgesic is prescribed. The speed of capillary flow can be gauged roughly by pressing upon the skin or the base of fingernail or toenail, and noting the rate of return of blood-color after the removal of pressure. A slow return of color in-

dicates impairment of blood flow through the arteries to the part. Pressure upon nerves quickly blocks conduction in them so that parts distal to the point of pressure become hypesthetic or anesthetic. Consequently, testing the finger or toe pads with a pin is also an important part of the examination of all and more especially of the painful extremities contained in casts or encircling bandages. A slow capillary flow or a change in the sensation of a part are sufficient indications for splitting, spreading or otherwise loosening the cast and if necessary its removal. They are always indications for the removal of the encircling dressing, including materials used to line the cast. Gangrene, Volkmann's ischemic contracture, neural palsies and pressure sores are dire consequences of failure to remove or at least to loosen tight casts and bandages.

Although capillary flow and sensibility of the distal parts of an extremity may be normal, the pain in a leg or an arm still may be ischemic in origin. The cast or the bandage may be pressing upon bony prominences. Should this be the case and the cast or the bandage is not loosened or fixed, a pressure sore will form. The pain of the localized ischemia preceding a pressure sore usually is sharply localized to the part bearing the pressure.

Incisional pain is stimulated most frequently by wound infections and faulty technic of wound closure and dressing, and adherence of the dressing to the wound. The signs of wound infections have been discussed. Tying cutaneous sutures tightly is followed by a painful wound wherever it is located. However, wounds of the chest wall and the upper abdomen are especially painful when closed with tightly tied sutures; every breath hurts.

The aim of wound closure is coaption without tension. Tight sutures about muscle fibers kill them; they turn fascia and tendon into a gluey liquid and widen the holes through the skin, leaving unsightly scars.

Meticulous adherence to the principles of wound closure and dressing, namely, coapt but do not strangulate and bind it not so tightly as to impair the venous or arterial flow of blood, ensure minimally painful wounds. Tightly sutured wounds must be suffered, but the error need not be repeated (see Chap. 2, "Wound Healing").

WOUND DISRUPTION

A sudden short-lived pain in an abdominal wound brought on by coughing, sneezing, or movement never should be passed over lightly. It is indicative of disruption of the incision. Should such a pain occur, the dressing must be removed and the wound inspected. The seepage of a serosanguineous fluid from an abdominal wound at any time is indicative of disruption or infection and the more especially disruption after a sudden sharp short-lived effort pain. Some of this fluid should be collected for culture and some smeared and stained. Should the fluid contain very few or no organisms, it may be inferred that disruption of the wound has most likely taken place and that it should be opened further in an operating room, and the disrupted layers reapproximated. Should this not be done, spontaneous evisceration may follow the next cough, hiccough or movement. Bowel, especially small intestine, may catch in an incomplete disruption and become obstructed. The least life-endangering consequence of nonclosure of a deep fascial disruption of an abdominal wound is an incisional hernia. All of these consequences of disruption may be prevented by reclosure of the wound in layers, or en masse with strong through-and-through heavy malleable wire or monofilic nylon sutures (see Chap. 2, "Wound Healing").

THE PROBLEM OF NONINCISIONAL ABDOMINAL PAIN

Postoperative abdominal pain not restricted to the wound confronts the surgeon with two very perplexing problems, namely, what is the cause of the pain and what is its significance? For example, 36 hours after the performance of a resection of the ascending colon and an ileotransverse colostomy, the patient complains of intermittent epigastric pains. Are these pains merely a phase in the restitution of functional peristalsis, the so-called normal postoperative gas pains or do they signify the existence of a mechanical intestinal obstruction? Or 15 hours after a splenectomy for idiopathic thrombocytopenic purpura we are presented with a febrile person having a distended silent abdomen, complaining of constant deep upper abdominal pain and pain in the left supraclavicular region and the midback. Do these pains have as their cause: a traumatic necrosis of the tail of the pancreas, an infection beneath the left hemidiaphragm, a normal abacterial nonchemical inflammatory reaction secondary to the physical trauma of the operation, a thrombosis of the portal vein, an embolus lodged in the lower lobe of the left lung, or a myocardial infarct?

Clearly, the picture is often so confusing as to prevent the formulation of a specific diagnosis. Consequently, the questions that the surgeon needs to answer soon are: shall I operate again now? Shall I wait and watch? What laboratory and roentgen examinations should be performed to permit me the maximum exercise of judgment?

In general, painful intra-abdominal postoperative complications which can be corrected by surgical intervention fall into 3 categories: (1) peritonitis with the leakage of the contents of hollow organs into the peritoneal cavities or fascial planes, (2) the obstruction of hollow viscera, (3) the impedance of the flow of blood to abdominal organs.

Postoperative abdominal pains not amenable to correction by surgical procedures may have as their origin: myocardial infarction, pulmonary infarction, pneumonia, post-traumatic sterile inflammation, and infections within the genitourinary tract.

Surgical intervention is indicated should the complication be amenable to correction by an operation and is not indicated should the illness fall into the second category. Would the postoperative patient respond to the above-named troubles as the patient who has not been operated upon does, the differentiation of the surgical significant pain from the nonsurgically significant would be relatively easy. However, the postoperative patient often does not respond to any of the above jeopardies to his life in the manner that a person who has not been operated upon does. The pain of a myocardial infarct after a celiotomy tends not to have an upward and left arm radiation but tends to be strictly abdominal. Free leakage of the contents of the stomach, the duodenum and the jejunum into the peritoneal cavity postoperatively is often unattended by abdominal muscle spasm greater than that associated with an abdominal wound without complications; likewise, the tenderness is often relatively slight. The same insult to the peritoneum of a person who has not been operated upon is attended almost immediately by a spastically rigid abdominal musculature and great tenderness. The reason for the paucity of local response to peritonitis postoperatively is unknown. However, the person receiving cortisone or ACTH may react to a peritoneal inflammation just as a person often does during the immediate postoperative period, the response being abnormally small. It is known that the secretion of corticoids during and for a short time after an operation is remarkably enhanced. Perhaps this increase is sufficient to produce the inhibition of response to peritonitis postoperatively. Many a physician arguing that the patient he had operated upon could not have peritonitis because little tenderness and muscle spasm existed has had his argument refuted and his pride punctured by the pathologist's irrefutable revelations in the autopsy room.

Similarly, complete mechanical intestinal obstruction during the immediate postoperative period often lacks the gurgles, the tinkles and the rushes coincident with cramps characteristic of the intestinal obstructions occurring at other times.

The excruciating pain so frequently experienced with interference with blood flow to abdominal viscera may be lacking postoperatively even though the arterial and venous blood flow to the entire small intestine be occluded by volvulus, thrombi or emboli. How then does one go about the process of differentiating the surgically correctable from the nonsurgically correctable origin of abdominal pain postoperatively?

Shock rarely supervenes quickly in the case of complications that cannot be corrected by operations except with myocardial and pulmonary infarction. Consequently, in instances in which pain and shock are joined, an electrocardiogram and a roentgenogram of the chest and the abdomen become very important parts of the examination of a patient who suffers from abdominal pain postoperatively.

The determination of the concentration of red cells with an hematocrit, a red blood cell count or a hemoglobin determination is very important. Progressive hemoconcentration means a rapid plasma loss and in a previously stable patient is indicative of peritonitis or intestinal obstruction. Therefore, it is usually an indication for reoperation. In addition, volvulus, venous vascular occlusions and pancreatitis are often attended by hemoconcentration, while myocardial and pulmonary infarction, bronchopneumonia and genitourinary infections and obstructions rarely are.

The white blood count is of relatively little differential diagnostic importance. Leukocytosis and a shift to the left occur regularly during the immediate postoperative period—complications or not.

The search of a clean voided or better a catheterized specimen of urine for white blood cells, bacteria and albumin is the only relatively certain means of detecting an infection within the urinary tract.

Should the operation antecedent to the pain have been performed upon the biliary tract or near it, for instance, gastrectomy, the urine should be tested for the presence of bilirubin. Occlusion of the common or the hepatic ducts by ligature is soon followed by the excretion of bile in the urine. The Gmelin and the fuming nitric acid tests are satisfactory screening tests for bile in urine.

Abdominal pain coupled with tenderness or pain in the costovertebral angle or flank following an operation within the pelvis or in proximity to the abdominal ureter such as resections of the ascending, the descending and the sigmoid colons, resections of the aorta and the iliac arteries, ligation of the vena cava, and lumbar sympathectomy are sufficient indication for a pyelographic examination. One or both ureters may have been ligated.

The determination of serum amylase or diastase concentrations do not always have the customary significance. Moderate elevations are not infrequent following a variety of upper abdominal operations. They may indicate postoperative pancreatitis but they may not! The author knows of 3 cases of intestinal gangrene in which the serum amylase concentration was very high, in one case being 3,600 Somogyi units.

All the while the aforementioned examinations are being conducted the person is to be examined and observed repeatedly. Pulse rate, blood pressure, rectal temperatures, the amount of abdominal tenderness and spasm are to be determined and recorded repeatedly. Postoperative abdominal pain with increasing tachycardia, a narrowing pulse pressure, or falling systolic and diastolic pressures with progressive hyperpyrexia and deterioration of general physiologic state coupled with absence of electrocardiographic signs of myocardial infarction and lack of electrocardiographic and roentgen signs of pulmonary infarction usually constitute sufficient reason for surgical re-entry of the abdominal cavity; almost certainly a postoperative surgical catastrophe has taken place, and the surgeon must make an attempt to correct it. Many an untimely death is attributable to postoperative procrastination.

However, few situations tax the judgment of the surgeon more severely than such a crisis in a postoperative patient. He must weigh all the risks and the probabilities as accurately as possible. Paracentesis may be indicated. In general, he will do well not to re-enter a closed abdomen without objective evidence of an intra-abdominal catastrophe. However, on the other hand, he must guard against any unwillingness to face the possibility that he has made a technical error. The treatment of postoperative complications productive of abdominal pain needs to fit the cause.

PAIN OF POSTOPERATIVE ILEUS

Ileus is a common cause of abdominal pain postoperatively, and the determination of cause is especially difficult because mechanical intestinal obstruction arising during the immediate postoperative period is often unattended by intestinal colic (see Chap. 37, "Intestine").

The causes of postoperative ileus fall into two groups: mechanical and adynamic, and the adynamic is divisible into 3 categories: vascular, chemical, of which hypokalemia is most common, and reflex.

The treatment of the ordinary mild postoperative adynamic ileus varies with its cause, e.g., for that associated with vesical distention —catheterization; for that after manual handling of the intestine—gastroduodenal suction. Prostigmine and the acetylated cholines occasionally work and are the safest of the drugs employed to stimulate peristalsis, although at times their flatal actions may serve more to allay the disquietude of the physician than to better the patient.

Enemas are relatively ineffectual treatments of adynamic ileus. They often are largely retained and when they are, their least objectionable action is supplementation of the meteorism. Should the retained enema be water and not saline, it will abstract salts from the plasma and the interstitial fluid into the lumen of the bowel, producing a decrease in plasma volume before the water is absorbed. In moderately dehydrated patients, as many with ileus are, the acute drop in plasma volume induced by the retained water enema may be sufficient to induce shock. The use of isotonic saline for enemata removes this danger of retention.

PLEURISY

After operations on parts of the body other than the thorax, pleuritis and myocardial infarction are common causes of postoperative chest pain. Pleuritic pain is rhythmic and synchronous with breathing. Deep breathing and coughing accentuate it. A rub is almost always audible in the region of the pain. Generally, pleuritis is a manifestation of an inflammatory lesion of the lung in contact with parietal pleura such as a localized aspirational pneumonitis, pulmonary infarction or lobar pneumonia. Consequently, roentgenograms of the chest and meticulous examination of the extremities for signs of thrombophlebitis, and of the sputum for pneumococci are necessary in attempting the discovery of the cause of the pleurisy. Pleuritic pain is usually short-lived, and analgesics readily control it, while appropriate specific medications such as antibiotics and anticoagulants are given to treat the cause of the pulmonary lesion.

POSTOPERATIVE MYOCARDIAL INFARCTION

Postoperative myocardial infarction is especially prone to follow amputations for ischemic gangrene of the foot and the leg. Peripheral circulatory failure attending or following an amputation is often traceable to myocardial infarction. Should the infarction take place while the person is anesthetized it is painless, and when it occurs while the patient is under the influence of analgesics and soporifics the retrosternal pain and oppression may be lacking or so slight as to be readily disregarded by patient and physician. Consequently, obscure weakness, fever, anterior chest pains, tachycardia, cardiac irregularities and shock postoperatively are indications for electrocardiograph.

MEDIASTINITIS

Retrosternal pain may be indicative of mediastinitis when associated with fever and dyspnea after esophageal diverticulectomy, esophagectomy, pneumonectomy, gastroscopy, esophagoscopy, the removal of foreign bodies from the main stem bronchi or the trachea and the esophagus, and rarely after thyroidectomy. Mediastinitis was a highly fatal complication before the sulfonamides and the antibiotics were discovered. Today it is not, if its existence is detected and if appropriate operative measures are taken to control it.

POSTOPERATIVE DYSPNEA

Dyspnea, the consciousness of needing to breathe, has a number of important connotations postoperatively: (1) partial obstruction of the trachea or the bronchus; (2) stiffening of the lung with edema (pulmonary edema) or blood (congestive atelectasis) or obstruction of a bronchus (obstructive atelectasis); (3) the reduction of pulmonic volume by extrapulmonic intrathoracic air (pneumothorax), similarly located fluid (pleural effusion and empyema), or elevation of the diaphragm by ascites, meteorism, abdominal obesity, or tight abdominal binders; (4) muscular weakness (shock, myasthenia gravis and adrenal insufficiency); and (5) acidosis.

AIRWAY OBSTRUCTION

Often after operations upon the tongue and the neck dyspnea is attributable to obstruction of the airway. In particular after thyroidectomy dyspnea may be caused by partial obstruction of the airway within the larynx by paralysis of the vocal cords or laryngeal edema, tracheal obstruction from tracheal ring collapse or pressure from a hematoma (hemorrhage); or by acute cardiac failure or acute hypoparathyroidism. All but hypoparathyroidism pose an immediate threat to life. Consequently, post-thyroidectomy dyspnea is a real danger signal and dictates immediate

steps to determine its genesis. Inspection of the wound is first. A tense swollen neck is indicative of *hemorrhage* with tracheal or pharyngeal compression and requires *immediate opening* of the wound because arterial bleeding is the predominant cause of strangulating peritracheal and retropharyngeal hemorrhage and it leaves little time between the onset of dyspnea and death.

The breathing with tracheal obstruction is characteristic. It is audibly labored with retraction of the supraclavicular and the intercostal spaces. Finding the pharyngeal airway obstructed or the vocal cords edematous or in the cadaveric position indicates the need for tracheostomy. It is to be performed at the bedside should the patient be severely dyspneic or unconscious. In the meantime, should the dyspnea be severe, the insertion of a pharyngeal airway and the administration of helium and oxygen usually will relieve the dyspnea *but not the necessity for tracheostomy*. Attempting to ride out partial laryngeal obstruction from paralyzed vocal cords invites disaster. Acute fulminant pulmonary edema is prone to occur, and before tracheostomy can be done the patient may be dead. Tracheostomy bears little risk to life, while asphyxia and pulmonary edema attendant upon laryngeal obstruction do.

Bronchoscopy is requisite for viewing the size of the tracheal lumen and is the only means of ascertaining the existence of tracheal ring collapse. Immediate tracheostomy is the treatment for tracheal collapse. The tracheal rings will soon stiffen, and the tracheostomy tube may be removed and the wound permitted to close, often within a week.

Dyspnea is rarely the first sign of parathyreoprivia to be appreciated. Failure to find an organic cause of post-thyroidectomy dyspnea raises the probability that hypoparathyroidism is its cause and dictates the ascertainment of the serum calcium level and search for Chvostek's and Trousseau's signs. The treatment of parathyreoprivia is discussed in Chapter 26.

CARDIAC FAILURE

SIGNS AND SYMPTOMS

Dyspnea may be the first sign of acute cardiac failure. Cardiac failure is a relatively infrequent postoperative complication. When it occurs it usually presents the picture of "acute cardiac collapse" rather than that of "congestive failure." Consequently, it resembles hemorrhagic shock or peripheral circulatory failure of the hypovolemic type. However, its differentiation from hematogenic shock, though usually easy, is occasionally very difficult.

The differentiation of postoperative acute cardiac failure or collapse from surgical shock depends largely upon the detection of signs of pulmonary congestion and cardiac dilatation. They appear with or soon after the beginning of acute cardiac failure, while with hemorrhagic shock they are absent or appear very late, and then in lesser degree. The measurement of venous pressure is also helpful. It is high with cardiac failure and low or normal with shock.

The signs of pulmonary congestion are dyspnea, labored breathing, rales and venous distention, most easily observed in the cervical veins although inconstant and late in appearance. The detection of left ventricular cardiac dilatation is more difficult, especially in the obese and emphysematous patient. When the physical signs of dilatation can be elicited they are diffuseness of the apical beat, shift of the point of maximum impulse to the left of the midclavicular line, and gallop rhythm.

The point of maximal impulse may be shifted toward the left by dorsal scoliosis, right pleural effusion or pneumothorax or left bronchial obstructive atelectasis. Consequently, the careful examination of the spine and the pulmonary fields is requisite to the interpretation of finding the cardiac impulse to the left of its normal position.

Gallop rhythm or three-sound rhythm has varied significance. A distinct three-sound rhythm, LUBB-dup-da, may be heard in normal persons with slow pulse rates. The third sound, the -da, disappears with a little exercise. It has no pathologic significance. True gallop rhythms do not disappear with exercise and they exist with tachycardia. They have the varied cadences of a galloping horse: da-LUBB-dup, da-LUBB-dup (presystolic gallop); LUBB-dup-da, LUBB-dup-da (protodiastolic gallop); or lupp-dup-DA, lupp-dup-DA (summation gallop). The discovery

of any of the true gallop rhythms is very helpful; it means that the heart is dilated, and heart failure is imminent or exists.

Left ventricular dilatation is best determined by roentgenogram. Frontal and left anterior thoracic oblique projections are the most useful. A rounding of the apex and a widening of the transverse cardiac diameter relative to the transverse diameter of the chest, and backward displacement of the cardiac shadow are the frontal and left anterior oblique signs of left ventricular dilatation. Cardiac hypertrophy without significant dilatation is not readily apparent roentgenographically. Acute postoperative cardiac collapse or failure is often associated with abnormal cardiac rhythms, such as the ectopic tachycardias of auricular fibrillation and flutter, and extreme sinus tachycardia. Peripheral circulatory failure is rarely associated with disturbances of rhythm other than simple sinus tachycardia. The definitive termination of type of disturbance in cardiac rhythm existing in a patient requires electrocardiography. The differential signs of acute heart failure and shock are listed in Table 1.

Such signs as mottled cyanosis of the trunk, cold extremities, small peripheral pulses, sweating, slight fever and psychic disturbances are common to acute cardiac failure and shock alike and consequently have no differential diagnostic significance.

TREATMENT

The treatment of acute postoperative cardiac failure varies somewhat with the stage and the rate of development. Venesection has a place in the treatment of the acute fulminant form and the late stage of the nonfulminant type with pulmonary edema, e.g., F.H., male aged 67 years, and hypertensive was catheterized at 2:30 P.M. to measure residual urine. About 5 minutes after the catheterization he was found struggling for breath, cyanotic, losing consciousness, and with gurgling breathing. Within 3 minutes venous occlusive tourniquets were placed on arms and thighs, and the antecubital veins were opened through incisions which he did not feel even though no anesthetic was used. At first blood dripped slowly from the transected veins, then the flow gradually quickened, and as it did breathing became less laborious, cyanosis

TABLE 1

Symptom or Sign	Acute Heart Failure or Acute Cardiac Collapse	Hypovolemic Shock
Dyspnea	Prominent	Slight or absent
Orthopnea	Prominent	Absent
Circulation time	Slow	Within normal limits
Rales	Prominent feature	Rare excepting preterminally
Heart size	Large	Normal
Maximum impulse	Outside midclavicular line	Within midclavicular line
Apical impulse	Diffuse	Sharply localized
Apical gallop	Often present	Absent
Cardiac arrhythmias	Frequent	Rare excepting sinus tachycardia
Venous pressure	Often elevated	Infrequently elevated, is often low
Roentgenogram Frontal	Rounded apex	
	Increased transverse diameter	Normal apical contour
	Prominent hilar Vascular shadows	Normal or faint hilar vascular shadows
Left ant. oblique	Filling of retro-cardiac space	Retrocardiac space normal
ECG	Left axis deviation	Normal axis
	Ectopic rhythms	Sinus tachycardia

began to clear, and when the blood flowed a stream, consciousness returned. Then the tourniquets were removed, pressure dressings were placed over the antecubital incisions, and a digitalis glucoside was given. That evening he walked about the ward unmindful of his proximity to death 4 hours earlier. Admittedly, such a dramatic response is seldom seen.

Venesection is rarely required for less fulminant and lesser degrees of cardiac collapse without extensive pulmonary edema. Venous occlusive tourniquets, the pressure breathing of oxygen, and cardiac glucosides usually control them rapidly.

Because the nature of the cardiac abnormality that underlies acute postoperative cardiac failure is rarely ascertainable before digitalization, lanatoside C ("Cedilanid") is most satisfactory. It acts quickly and disappears rapidly from the body, thereby minimizing the danger of overdosage. For adults the initial digitalizing dose of lanatoside C is 1.0 to 1.6 mg. parenterally. The intravenous route is used whenever there is pulmonary edema and one is reasonably certain that myocardial infarction is absent. The intramuscular route is used for acute cardiac failure without pulmonary edema.

The treatment of cardiac collapse with post-operative myocardial infarction almost defies description. Oxygen by mask, anticoagulants, heparin and Dicoumarol, papaverine 0.1 to 0.2 G. every 4 to 6 hrs. and atropine 0.3 to 0.4 mg. every 6 hrs. subcutaneously are recommended. With pronounced or progressive pulmonary edema venous occlusive tourniquets or cautions venesection may be used. With pronounced signs of peripheral circulatory failure and severe oliguria or anuria and few signs of pulmonary edema the careful transfusion of blood may help. According to some internists digitalization is indicated only rarely. Because myocardial infarction is often painless postoperatively, an electrocardiogram should be performed before digitalizing a person showing signs of cardiac collapse during or after an operation. As with diabetic coma, the treatment of postinfarctional cardiac collapse demands the artistry and the experience that an internist is best able to provide.

Dyspnea of Weakness

Persistent dyspnea and weakness after thyroidectomy is occasionally ascribable to myasthenia gravis which is occasionally associated with thyrotoxicosis. When persistent dyspnea and weakness are accompanied by difficulty in swallowing and speaking, and the rapid fatigue of used muscles, including a drooping of the upper eyelids, myasthenia gravis should be considered as a possible cause. Rapid fatigue of muscles upon repetitive motion of an extremity and progressive weakness and slurring of speech with sustained speaking are rather peculiar to this disease. Should these signs be demonstrable, neostigmine (1 mg.) intramuscularly may be given. Any improvement tends to confirm the diagnosis.

Section 4. Gas Therapy

OXYGEN

Increasing the partial pressure of oxygen in the inspired air increases the rate with which pulmonary arterial blood is oxygenated and reduces the mass of gaseous nitrogen in solution within the body.

The primary action of oxygen therapy is the augmentation of the rate of oxygenation of pulmonary arterial blood. This action is of clinical significance for patients with abnormally incomplete oxygenation of the peripheral arterial blood. The main causes of incomplete oxygenation of the peripheral arterial blood are: patchy atelectasis, bronchopneumonia, pulmonary fibrosis, hypopnea, pulmonary edema, incomplete obstructions of the trachea or the major bronchi and severe reductions of the residual air such as attend removal of lungs. Oxygen therapy for these conditions usually will serve to improve the saturation of the systemic arterial blood if it is below normal. Oxygen therapy should be tried whenever the signs of anoxic hypoxia appear. The signs of hypoxia are: exertional dyspnea, tachycardia, fever, changes in psyche, such as euphoria, disorientation, delirium, convulsions and coma. These are more important signs of indication for the institution of oxygen therapy than is peripheral cyanosis. Often peripheral cyanosis may be lacking, even though the individual is suffering from a severe hypoxic hypoxia. Indications that oxygen therapy is effective in a particular patient are: the reduction of the pulse rate, improvement in sensorium, and the relief of breathlessness and restlessness when it is given.

Oxygen therapy has often been recommended for the treatment of peripheral circulatory failure. It is doubtful that it is particularly valuable in the treatment of the circulatory anoxia that attends shock, excepting when anoxic anoxia exists with it. When in doubt, oxygen may be given, but its use never should be accepted as a substitute for specific therapy such as transfusions of blood or other fluids.

The giving of oxygen in high concentrations may be accomplished with the use of oxygen tents, nasal catheters and the oronasal Boothby mask. The administration of oxygen with a tent or through a nasal catheter will effect increases in the oxygen tension of alveolar air to about 300 mm. Hg pressure. Alveolar partial pressures of oxygen above 400 mm. Hg can be obtained with the use of the oronasal Boothby mask or the administration of oxygen through an endotracheal tube attached to a special respiratory apparatus or anesthesia machine. The choice of the way the oxygen is given depends upon what needs to be accomplished. The nasal catheter route is usually adequate for the administration of oxygen to individuals who are not comatose and do not have high body temperatures. The oxygen tent is superior to the nasal catheter for patients who have hypoxic hypoxia and hyperpyrexia. The oxygen tent, besides increasing the oxygen in the inspired air, serves as an air-conditioning mechanism. The oronasal mask route of administration is especially applicable whenever the anoxia is particularly severe and ileus with meteorism exists.

The breathing of tensions of oxygen above 500 mm. Hg pressure is at times beneficial to individuals suffering from ileus and meteorism, partially by virtue of the denitrogenating action of breathing high concentrations of oxygen. Breathing oxygen for an hour or two denitrogenates the body because though only oxygen is breathed in, nitrogen, oxygen and carbon dioxide are breathed out. Since more than two thirds of the gas in the intestines of an individual suffering from meteorism is made up of nitrogen, the denitrogenation of the body attendant upon the breathing of pure oxygen serves to reduce the meteorism (see Chap. 36, "Intestinal Obstruction"). This action of high oxygen therapy has been well substantiated by Fine.

There is some danger attendant upon the administration of pure oxygen through tight-fitting masks or through endotracheal tubes for periods of time longer than 4 to 6 hours. The breathing of pure oxygen for long periods promotes a hemorrhagic pneumonia. This has been termed oxygen poisoning. It can be prevented by breaking the administration of pure oxygen every 3 to 4 hours for 5 minutes.

The danger of oxygen poisoning is not the only one attendant upon the administration of pure oxygen. The giving of pure oxygen to individuals is capable of inciting respiratory arrest in persons who by reason of their illness or drugs given to them have lost their respiratory sensitivity to carbon dioxide and whose breathing, therefore, is being maintained in part by the anoxic drive of breathing. Patients who have been given morphine and short-acting barbiturates, emphysematous asthmatics and comatose persons tend to have respiratory centers that are insensitive to carbon dioxide and are prone to reduce their rate and depth of breathing when given oxygen to breathe. With the decline in pulmonary ventilation attendant upon the receipt of oxygen, carbon dioxide is retained in their bodies, and the pH of their blood falls. As the carbon dioxide tension builds up their respiration slows and ultimately stops. Carbon dioxide is a respiratory depressant in individuals whose respiratory mechanisms have lost their sensitivity to it.

Because of the danger of respiratory depression attendant upon the administration of oxygen the institution of oxygen therapy to all comatose, emphysematous, asthmatic and drugged patients should be conducted under the cognizance of a physician for at least 30 minutes to 1 hour, and the respiratory rate and pulse rate should be determined and charted every 15 minutes for at least 3 hours.

The administration of high oxygen tensions to individuals who have large amounts of tenacious secretions in their tracheal-bronchial tree predisposes them to the development of obstructive atelectasis. The occlusion of a major bronchus of an animal breathing air is not attended by collapse of the lung for 24 to 72 hours. However, the obstruction of the bronchus of an animal breathing oxygen is followed by collapse of the obstructed segment of lung within 3 or more hours. Because of the enhancement of atelectasis by oxygen breathing in the presence of bronchial obstruction, the clearance of the airway of secretions becomes a very important part of oxygen therapy.

CARBON DIOXIDE THERAPY

For many years from 5 to 10 per cent carbon dioxide in oxygen was administered for 3 to 5 minutes every hour or two of the operative day to stimulate breathing. Today it is used very infrequently for this purpose. The administration of 5 per cent carbon dioxide in oxygen is valuable as a temporary therapeutic measure for the control of carpopedal spasms, due to tetany resulting from respiratory alkalosis, and hiccoughs. It is also valuable occasionally for the treatment of the acute nonoligemic hypotension which sometimes follows a prolonged anesthesia with cyclopropane. Seemingly, some of the acute hypotensions which attend the recovery from cyclopropane anesthesia are attributable to hypocarbia. Sometimes children who have been relieved of severe partial obstructions of the upper airways by tracheostomy or intubation stop breathing soon after the obstruction is relieved while breathing air or oxygen. Sometimes 5 per cent carbon dioxide in oxygen will maintain the breathing of such children.

HELIUM

From 30 to 50 per cent helium in oxygen is a valuable gas mixture for the temporary relief of local partial obstructions of the major air passages. The effort required to move air through a narrowed larynx, trachea or bronchus is reduced significantly by the helium. The administration of helium in oxygen must be considered only as a temporary expedient before the correction or the removal of the obstruction of the trachea or the bronchi. It is without value in the treatment of obstructions of the minor air passages.

Section 5. Postoperative Urinary Retention and Oliguria

URINARY RETENTION

Overfilling of the bladder, the incapacity to urinate in the horizontal position, obstructive uropathy, and operative disturbances of the nerves or the position of the bladder are the prominent causes of postoperative urinary retention. A distention of the bladder with urine while the patient is anesthetized or deeply depressed with opiates or barbiturates, or unconscious for other reasons renders the smooth muscle of the bladder practically incapable of contracting. This might well be termed "acute decompensation of the bladder." Peculiarly, many normal young men are unable to void while lying in bed. Many postoperative urinary retentions that occur among middle-aged and elderly men can be traced to an incomplete obstruction of the bladder neck or the urethra by prostatic hypertrophy or stricture.

After combined abdominoperineal resections of the sigmoid colon and the rectum, difficulty with the passage of urine is commonplace. At one time these difficulties were ascribed to the interference with the nervous outflow to the bladder. However, some authors believe that retroposition of the bladder and descent of the base of the bladder are partly responsible for the difficulty in the passage of urine following combined abdominoperineal resections of the sigmoid colon and the rectum.

Treatment of postoperative urinary retention consists of first having the individual stand or sit upon the toilet and attempt to urinate. Should he be unable to do so, a small catheter is passed, and the urine is withdrawn. If the volume of urine exceeds 700 to 800 ml. the catheter should be left in place for 24 to 36 hours and connected to a continuous drainage system to permit the bladder musculature to recover from the stretching. Should smaller amounts of urine be obtained, the catheter is withdrawn, and from 4 to 6 hours later the individual is encouraged to empty the bladder.

If the catheter is left indwelling for more than 24 hours the urinary tract shoud be protected from infection to the extent afforded by an antibacterial drug (see Chap. 48, "Urology").

OLIGURIA

Mechanical obstruction of the urinary tract, neurogenic disturbances of micturition, changes in renal function attendant upon endocrine, hemodynamic and fluid balance alterations singly or in combination may give rise to postoperative oliguria.

Because obstruction of the flow of urine by ureteral ligation and vesical obstruction from prostatic hypertrophy and sphincteric dysfunction may be the cause of oliguria or anuria postoperatively, catheterization is the first diagnostic step. (See Chap. 48, "Urology," for a full discussion of obstructive uropathy.)

Actually, even though obstructive uropathy be lacking, slight oliguria is to be expected after major operative procedures. Some of the changes in the rates of renal excretion of water and urea during the induction of anesthesia, the operation and the postoperative period are shown in Figure 14-1. These observations are a half century old. Notice the remarkable slowing of the rates of excreting water and urea during the operation and the time taken for recovery. Stewart and Rourke were the first to study the alterations in the rates of renal excretion of water and salts associated with anesthesia and surgery. Many others have corroborated their discoveries. An operation greatly reduces the capacity of man to excrete water for 1 to 5 days (Fig. 14-2).

The degree of reduction in the rate of excreting a load of water attendant upon a major operation is readily secured in normal persons by injecting pitressin while infusing dextrose in water.

Such observations lend credence to the theory that operative pituitary stimulation is responsible for at least a portion of the postoperative oliguria. This theory is better supported by the observations of Theobald that traumatic inhibition of water diuresis does not occur in a dog after removal of the hypophysis. The inhibition of water diuresis attributable to the antidiuretic effect of an operation will not induce anuria or rates of urine flow less than 400 ml. per day. Slower rates of excretion of urine postoperatively must have additional cause. However, inhibition of water diuresis is an important cause of minor postoperative oligurias and is often so pronounced as to fix the flow of urine at rates of 450 to 800 ml. daily for hours and even days postoperatively.

During the time that the operative inhibition of water diuresis exists attempts to break it by infusing glucose in water intravenously are

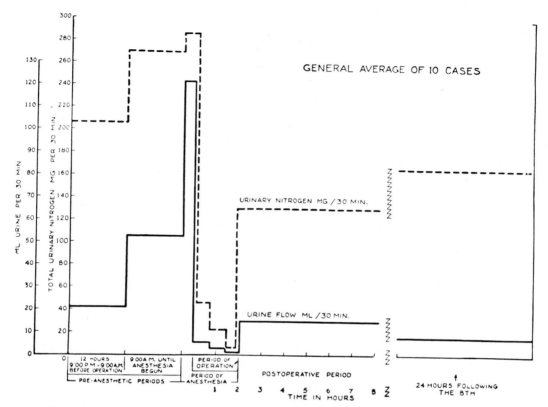

Fig. 14-1. Rates of excretion of urine and urinary nitrogen by man before, during and after ether anesthesia and various operations. Graphic representation of data of Pringle, Maunsell and Pringle (published in the British Medical Journal, September 9, 1902), showing the remarkable reduction of urea excretion and urinary flow during the operation and the immediate postoperative period. (Moyer, C. A.: Surgery 27:199)

It must not be inferred that the anesthetic agent is the only factor influencing the changes in renal function during and immediately after an operation. Practically all of the soporific and analgesic drugs used preoperatively and postoperatively exert an antidiuretic influence. (Bibliographical references pertaining to the above statement are to be found in "The Kidney" by H. W. Smith, Oxford University Press, New York, 1951, pages 283, 444, 445, and 446)

In addition to the antidiuretic influences exerted by the soporific, analgesic and anesthetic agent employed to permit the operation, the painful sensory stimuli, attendant upon the operation and bodily movements, such as breathing and rolling about before the wound is well along the road to healing, lead to antidiuresis (Theobald, G. W., and Verney, E. B.: J. Physiol. 83:341, 1935). The nature of the surgical illness is important also; obstructive jaundice in man is attended by a remarkable inhibition of water-diuresis. (Abe, S.: Tohoku J. Exper. Med. 17:174, 1931)

Of course, oligemia incident to the loss of blood and the sequestration of extracellular fluid in the tissues injured during the operation are determinants of the degree of functional renal incapacity attendant upon an operation. However, though oligemia be prevented by the transfusion of blood and a balanced saline solution, renal function is disturbed during and for a time after major operations by nervous stimuli, drugs and the anesthetic agent.

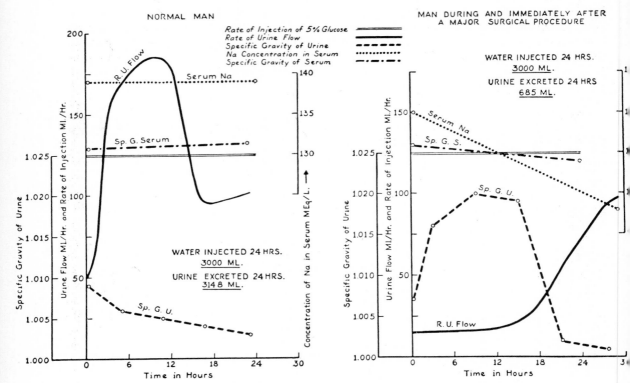

FIG. 14-2. Responses to intravenous 5 per cent glucose in distilled water. Graphic representation of data of Coller, *et al.* The left half of the figure shows the response of a normal adult to the intravenous injection of 125 ml. of 5 per cent dextrose in water per hour for 24 hours. The urine flow accelerates rapidly and for a time exceeds the rate of injection, the urinary specific gravity falls, while the serum specific gravity and sodium change little, and at the end of the injection the urine excreted exceeded the volume of water given.

The right half shows a typical response of man to the intravenous injection of 125 ml. of 5 per cent dextrose in water per hour for 24 hours after a major operative procedure such as a combined abdominoperineal resection of the rectum, choledochostomy and gastrectomy. The urine flow accelerates slowly and does not exceed the rate of injection; the serum sodium concentration and the specific gravity of serum fall; while the specific gravity of the urine rises for a time and then belatedly falls, and only 685 ml. of urine is excreted, while 3,000 ml. of dextrose solution was given. (Moyer, C. A.: Surgery 27:201)

prone to fail and are dangerous because the retained water reduces the osmolar concentration of the body's fluids and may precipitate water intoxication.

As stated above, urine flows of less than 400 ml. a day cannot be ascribed to operative inhibition of water excretion alone, because 400 ml. daily is the slowest urine flow attainable by the maximal enhancement of the facultative absorption of water by the distal renal tubular cells in normally hydrated adults. Consequently, the excretion of less than 400 ml. of urine per day at any time

during a postoperative or post-traumatic period should immediately prompt a search for other causes of oliguria such as oligemia, obstructive uropathy, extracellular fluid volume deficit, osmolar dilution (water intoxication) and organic renal disease. Oligemia is the most frequent cause of the postoperative excretion of less than 400 ml. daily. A large incompletely replaced operative loss of blood is the main cause of postoperative oligemia. The signs and symptoms of hemorrhagic shock and dehydration are covered in Chapters 7 and 5, respectively. Clearly, whenever signs of oligemia are found in an oliguric patient the oliguria is properly treated by correcting the oliguria by appropriate measures—blood transfusion for whole blood lack and lactated Ringer's solution for interstitial fluid volume translocation or external loss.

Postoperative anuria—the absence of urine flow—is a manifestation of shock, complete ureteral occlusion, a transfusion reaction, organic occlusion of the blood flow through the kidneys by emboli or thrombi, acute cardiac failure or the removal of the only functioning kidney.

No definitive treatment exists for the nephrectomy type of anuria. Ureteral catheterization and ureteral lavage have effected remarkably rapid corrections of anuria attributable to ureteral obstruction by crystals of sulfonamides or creatine. Ureteral catheterization alone has done the same thing for ureterolithiac obstructive anuria. The transfusion of blood has corrected many an anuria associated with hemorrhagic peripheral circulatory failure, and the infusion of sodium salt solutions has done the same for anurias attendant upon extracellular fluid volume deficit (dehydrational) shock.

The treatment of an anuria persisting after the correction of oligemic shock, after transfusion reactions, and after the removal of obstructions is discussed in Chapter 48, "Urology."

Section 6. Postoperative Jaundice

Jaundice that develops during the immediate postoperative period is mainly related to one of two causes—obstruction of the extrahepatic biliary ducts or a porphyrin overload. A steadily increasing jaundice appearing after cholecystectomy and difficult gastric resections usually means that the common hepatic or the common duct has been encircled by a ligature or cut off and tied. Acholic feces and the absence of bile in duodenal drainage are characteristic of it. The jaundice of porphyrin overload accompanies fulminant wound infections and the more especially those caused by certain anaerobes such as *Cl. histolyticum,* the hemolytic streptococci and staphylococci and the transfusion of much stored blood during the operation. The differentiation of jaundice appearing during the first postoperative week is relatively easy. Duodenal drainage will serve to differentiate the obstructive from the porphyrin-overload type. The lack of or the existence of signs of a fulminant infection distinguishes the transfusional from the infectional porphyrin overload variety.

The treatments are obvious: For the obstructive jaundice the obstruction must be removed. This requires that an operation be done as soon as the condition of the patient permits it. For that associated with infection, drain and débride and give antibiotics. For the transfusional no treatment is needed; it will disappear in a few days.

Section 7. Edema

Edema, the swelling of a part of the body with fluid, has many causes: increased venous pressure, decreased arterial blood flow, decreased intravascular oncotic pressure (serum albumin deficiency), decreased lymph flow, dependency, immobility, physical trauma, infection, excessive sodium intake and cardiac failure.

VENOUS OCCLUSIVE EDEMA

Edematous swelling associated with increased venous pressure attends venous thrombosis, the application of tight encircling bandages and casts, the ligation of major veins and the obstruction of veins by neoplastic invasion or encirclement.

During the development phase venous occlusive edema is accompanied by some blueness of the swollen member; it is tender and painful and is firm and relatively nonpitting. Just prior to measurable subsidence, the swelling softens and pits deeply.

THROMBOPHLEBITIS

Edema is often the first sign of thrombophlebitis. Acute thrombophlebitis is an inflammatory disease of veins: the intima swells and in places disappears, the media swells and is infiltrated with wandering cells and lymphocytes, the adventitia becomes edematous, and the perivenous lymphatics are irregularly occluded. Blood clots within the lumen, and the thrombus is attached with more or less fixity to the intimally denuded vein wall. Thrombophlebitic edema varies remarkably in degree: usually it is slight when the superficial veins such as the saphenous and the cephalic are afflicted alone. It also may be slight and attended with little pain or tenderness even when the deep veins are extensively thrombosed (phlebothrombosis). However, thrombophlebitic edema may develop with remarkable rapidity and to an alarming extent. The collection of about 8 L. of edema fluid in the thighs and the legs has been observed to take place in 24 hours in a case of bilateral phlegmasia cerulea dolens.

The other signs and symptoms of thrombophlebitis also vary greatly in degree and character. The extremity may become very painful, tender and diffusely violaceous and develop bloody blebs on the digits and the dorsums of hand or foot (phlegmasia cerulea dolens), indicating a grave prognosis because few cases of phlegmasia cerulea dolens recover. It may be painful, tender and gray-white (phlegmasia alba dolens), or be practically painless, slightly tender and be normally colored (phlebothrombosis). Movement of the part may be impossible because of pain (phlegmasia dolens) or practically unrestricted (phlebothrombosis). The systemic manifestations vary from a very transient mild fever and tachycardia and slight illness to chills and very high fever, oligemic shock from sequestration of extracellular fluid within the zone of thrombosis, and the severe respiratory and circulatory disturbances of pulmonary embolization.

Chills and high fever with thrombophlebitis are indicative of thrombophlebitis purulenta, a thrombophlebitis complicated with bacterial invasion and break-up of the clot. These bacterially laden clot-fragments enter the circulation and are disseminated especially to the lungs where they are prone to produce septic pulmonary infarcts.

Tenderness is practically always elicitable in the afflicted part. Gentle dorsiflexion of the foot (Homan's sign), pressure upon the gastrocnemius-soleus and the anterior tibial muscles, and the application of a blood pressure cuff about the thigh with a pressure of 60 mm. Hg generates pain in cases of thrombophlebitis of the leg.

The arterial pulses are reduced and may even be practically obliterated during the early stages of phlegmasia cerulea and alba dolens. Presumably this is initiated by reflex arterial spasm, because blocking of the sympathetic nerves to the part restores the pulses.

Thrombophlebitis is not the only peripheral affliction attended by swelling, color changes, pain and tenderness in the leg. Consequently, the differential diagnosis is often difficult. Rupture of the tendon of the plantaris muscle, myositis, acute lymphadenitis and angiitis, and acute arterial thromboses produce many of the physical signs that thrombophlebitis does.

The treatment of thrombophlebitis is empirical. The therapeutic measures now in use are: rest and elevation, elastic bandaging, hot fomentations, blocking the sympathetic nerves, ligation and transection of veins and the administration of the anticoagulants (heparin and Dicumarol).

Rest is universally applicable. Lumbar sympathetic nerve block is especially useful in the treatment of phlegmasia alba and cerulea dolens; it frequently relieves the pain, often restores arterial pulses and seemingly hastens the disappearance of the edema.

Venous ligation and transection proximal to the thrombosis is indicated for all cases of thrombophlebitis purulenta. Vena-caval ligation is preferable to ligation of the iliac or the common femoral veins whenever the thrombosis purulenta involves the common femoral, the external iliac or the hypogastric veins, because the disabling sequelae of vena-caval ligation apparently are fewer than those which follow interruption of the common femoral or the iliac veins. In women the ovarian veins should be ligated as well as the vena cava in treating pelvic thrombophlebitis purulenta. Ligation and transection of the saphena magna at its point of entry into the femoral is a very effective way of treating thrombophlebitis limited to the saphenous vein. Persons having varicose veins frequently develop thrombophlebitis within the saphena magna postoperatively.

The anticoagulants are being given now for

all forms of thrombophlebitis excepting the purulenta variant. Although their effectiveness is variable and still cannot be defined accurately for a given case, there is equivocal evidence that the use of these drugs has reduced the frequency of massive pulmonary embolization and has shortened the period of swelling and pain.

Before giving Dicumarol, the prothrombin time or concentration must be performed because a prothrombin deficiency may be present before the drug is given, and should the recommended initial dose of Dicumarol be given to a prothrombin-deficient patient a lethal intracranial or other hemorrhage may occur.

For the treatment of thrombophlebitis in a person with a normal prothrombin concentration the dosage of Dicumarol is 300 mg. during the first day, 200 mg. the second, and 100 mg. the third, provided that the prothrombin time does not exceed 2 to 3 times normal. Should the prothrombin time be close to 2 to 3 times normal, the dose for that day is reduced or interrupted. The therapeutic aim is the maintenance of the prothrombin time at 2 to 3 times normal until signs and symptoms of the thrombophlebitis have been absent for a week or more.

The antidote for Dicumarol is K_1 oxide, 50 mg. i.v. This dose often will restore the prothrombin time to normal within 1 or 2 hours. The anticoagulant effect of Dicumarol is not exerted fully for 24 to 36 hours after the first dose has been given. Whenever an immediate anticoagulant action is wanted, heparin will fill the need. Heparin should be given in the aqueous form in doses of about 50 mg. i.v. every 4 hours. Controlled clotting times serve as the basis for dosage regulation; the clotting time of the patient's blood should be kept about twice as long as that of the control 4 hours after the preceding dose was given. After one is assured that the dosage of 50 mg. every 4 hours keeps the clotting time about twice normal, 50 mg. is given every 4 hours, and the clotting time is determined only once a day.

The antidotes for heparin are: protamine sulfate 50 mg. i.v. and toluidine blue 100 mg. A single dose of either drug counteracts the effects of heparin.

Elastic bandaging of the leg alone is a very important part of the treatment of thrombophlebitis. Bandages should be worn for 2 to 3 months after all signs of the disease disappear. Elastic bandages or stockings should not be placed or worn above the knee because they become constricting bands about the knee when the leg is flexed, tending to promote rather than ameliorate swelling of the foot and the leg.

The frequency of postoperative thrombophlebitis in the veins of the leg may be reduced somewhat by avoiding saphenous venoclysis during an operation and the preambulant postoperative period, by taking care that the straps binding the patient to the operating table are applied carefully and not too tightly, by binding the legs of persons having varices with elastic banages before, during and after the operation, and by early active motion of the legs and the feet.

EDEMA FOLLOWING PLANTARIS TENDON RUPTURE

Plantaris tendon rupture occurs suddenly, usually as the person quickly places his weight upon an extended leg while the foot is held in an extreme equinus position, as when getting out of a high hospital bed. With the rupture the person usually falls to the floor. Synchronously, a sharp stabbing pain is felt in the calf of the leg. The leg swells, and great tenderness is immediately elicitable over the upper part of the body of the gastrocnemius muscle. Dorsiflexion of the foot is painful. Within 4 to 24 hours, ecchymosis usually appears along the Achilles tendon. Elastic bandaging of the foot and the leg so as to limit dorsiflexion of the foot while walking constitutes adequate treatment.

TRAUMATIC MYOSITIS

Postoperative myositis is not rare. It occurs as the convalescent patient begins to walk freely in footwear having heels lower than those customarily worn. It might be called the carpet-slipper syndrome. Women who have long worn only high-heeled shoes are especially prone to suffer from carpet-slipper myositis. Homan's sign is positive; the leg and the foot are often visibly edematous; and the calf muscles are tender. All these signs subside with a day of rest and the use of their high-heeled shoes when walking is resumed.

EDEMA OF LYMPHADENITIS

Acute lymphadenitis without visible superficial lymphangitis occasionally gives rise to a tender edema of the arm or the leg. Exploration of the femoral veins of 39 people presumed to have thrombophlebitis, because all of the signs of thrombophlebitis existed, turned up 8 cases in which blood flowed freely in the superficial femoral and saphenous veins, and no clots could be aspirated from them. In every such case the inguinal lymph nodes were much enlarged, and the periglandular and the perifemoral venous tissues were edematous. No sign of superficial lymphangitis existed preoperatively. Acute lymphangitis should be suspected as the cause of swelling of an extremity whenever the lymph nodes of the groin or the axilla are *enlarged, matted together* and *tender*. In the author's experience acute postoperative inguinal lymphadenitis without signs of superficial lymphadenitis is especially prone to follow vaginoperineal repair, hemorrhoidectomy and herniotomy.

ARTERIAL OCCLUSIVE EDEMA

The swelling of a leg or an arm that follows the interruption of blood flow through its major arteries is very hard and painful. The muscles within the zone of deficient blood flow are tense and do not contract. Consequently, free active or passive motion of the parts moved by these muscles cannot be effected. Passive motion is very painful. The differentiation of thrombophlebitis from acute incomplete arterial occlusion is often extremely difficult and occasionally is impossible without repeated examination and the ascertainment of the course of events: the loss of sense perception practically clinches the diagnosis of arterial occlusion. Restoration of arterial flow by the methods discussed in Chapter 40 constitutes the only means of preventing loss of the part. Arteriography is often necessary to differentiate arterial occlusive edema from the others.

HYPO-OSMOTIC EDEMA

Hypo-osmotic or hypoalbuminemic edema is readily pitable and with changes of position shifts rapidly from one part of the body to another, collecting about the eyes and in the hollow of the back when the person is dorsally recumbent, and flowing into the legs and the feet when he sits or stands. It is especially prone to occur in the aged, the starved, the cirrhotics and the nephritics. It may be increased by giving sodium salts. The administration of plasma or salt-free albumin temporarily reduces it. Prolonged control can be effected only by dietary measures, the feeding of sufficient protein and other foods to meet the caloric needs and to repay the deficits, and the giving of only that amount of sodium chloride necessary to prevent the low-salt syndrome. In the absence of enteral losses of salt from 500 to 1,000 mg. daily is usually enough.

LYMPHATIC OBSTRUCTIVE EDEMA

The painless swelling of the hand and the arm after radical mastectomy and of the leg after inguinal node resections has often been attributed to lymphatic obstruction. Injection of sky-blue dye into the superficial cutaneous lymphatic network of the swollen member readily differentiates lymphatic block swelling from other types. Lymphatic obstructive edema is attended by superficial lymphangiectasis while the others, excepting that associated with erysipelas, are not. Elevation of the arm, massage and active motion while the arm and the hand are encased in elastic bandages constitute its treatment.

POSTFIXATION EDEMA

The resumption of walking or sitting after long confinement to bed or after having a part encased in a cast is regularly followed by swelling of the legs or the casted arm. It is practically painless, is readily pitted and subsides rapidly upon elevating the part above the trunk. It is easily treated by the application of elastic bandages until full restoration of function is attained.

SALT-OVERLOAD EDEMA

The administration of more sodium salts than are needed to make up for fistulous, transpiratory, diarrheal, gastric and renal losses frequently leads to generalized postoperative edema. Salt-overload edema is frequently mistaken for hypoalbuminemic edema, because the serum albumin concentration falls as the edema grows. The following case illustrates this.

does not so occlude a pulmonary arterial branch as to kill a piece of lung. Pulmonary infarction signifies pulmonary parenchymal arterial obstructive necrosis. The signs of pulmonary embolus and infarction differ appre-

CASE: B. G. W., male, aged 56 years

	WEIGHT	HB.	SERUM ALBUMIN
Preoperative	67.5 K	13.1	4.7
Postoperative (partial gastrectomy)			
Day 1 } 27 Gm. NaCl daily	66.9	12.3	4.9
Day 3 } 3 liters of 0.9% NaCl i.v. daily	71.4	11.1	2.7
Day 4 }	68.0	. . .	3.5
Day 5 } 3 liters of 5% dextrose i.v. daily	66.3	12.8	4.4

Postoperative Day, 3 edema + to + + of hands, feet, legs, eyelids and back.
By the 5th postoperative day the edema was gone.

Salt-overload edema is readily differentiated from hypoalbuminemic edema by withholding all sodium salts for 48 to 72 hours; the serum protein deficiency edema does not subside remarkably within this short time when salt is withheld, while salt-overload edema does, and as it does the serum albumin level rises rapidly. Withholding salt generally constitutes adequate therapy. The mercurial diuretics may be used to hasten resolution in cases of massive saline overloads.

Edema attributable to cardiac failure is a rarity postoperatively. When it does occur, the associated dyspnea, orthopnea, and signs of pulmonary and hepatic congestion serve to differentiate it readily from other types of edema.

PULMONARY EMBOLUS AND PULMONARY INFARCTION

Pulmonary embolus and pulmonary infarction are major postoperative worries; the gastrectomy was well done, the wound has healed per primam, the man is eating well and has high spirits, he strains at stool—and dies before he can be moved from the bathroom floor. Fortunately, most pulmonary emboli are not so deadly. Pulmonary emboli usually are blood clots detached from the veins of the leg or the pelvis. They rarely arise from clots within the veins of the arm or the right auricle or ventricle. Pulmonary infarction does not attend the lodgment of all pulmonary emboli; many a pulmonary embolus

ciably. The signs and symptoms of pulmonary embolus vary from extreme dyspnea, shock, retrosternal oppression and quick death to a mild transient dyspnea and apprehension. The lungs are usually clear to auscultation and roentgenogram. The pulmonary second sound may be accentuated.

Pulmonary infarction adds to the above signs and symptoms of embolus: leukocytosis, fever, pleurisy, dark blood-stained sputum, and ausculatory and roentgen signs of pulmonary consolidation.

The treatment of pulmonary embolus and infarction is changing. Today the giving of the anticoagulants as described in the section on thrombophlebitis and the ligation of veins either alone or combined are recommended. If venous ligational therapy is selected, both superficial femoral veins or the vena cava should be tied, because the source of the embolus cannot be determined with any degree of certainty, and the thrombi are so often bilateral. Interruption of the common femoral veins should not be performed, because persistent edema, varicosities and stasis ulcers follow interruption of the common femoral veins with remarkable regularity while they very seldom follow interruption of the superficial femoral vein.

After ligation of veins the anticoagulants should be given, excepting when there are specific contraindications to their use, e.g., prolonged clotting time, low prothrombin concentration, hemorrhage, hepatitis, or cirrhosis.

Section 8. Nausea and Vomiting

Nausea is the sensation of needing to empty the stomach. Its causes are many: emotions, overdosage or idiosyncrasy to drugs, cardiac failure, uremia, obstructions of the cystic duct, the common duct, the ureters and the digestive tract, enteritis, pneumonia, pain, great fatigue, acidosis, adrenal cortical insufficiency, etc. Vomiting supposedly initiated by the "vomiting center" usually follows nausea. Obviously, nausea and vomiting alone cannot serve as important differential signs of illness. However, they have more limited connotations postoperatively.

Some nausea and vomiting may be considered as temporary accompaniments of the process of normal recovery from anesthesia. However, protracted postoperative nausea and vomiting indicate that something is seriously amiss.

GASTRIC DILATATION

Acute gastric dilatation or atony is one of the serious postoperative causes of protracted nausea and vomiting; unrelieved, it may be lethal in only an hour or two. Often the vomiting attending acute gastric atony or dilatation is effortless; the vomiting simply pours out of the mouth without retching. The vomit is foul, dark, and contains altered blood. Tachycardia, prostration and hypotension often accompany it. Remarkably, little pain is usually suffered. Thirst may be insatiable. The epigastrium bulges and tympanites extends far up into the left thoracic cavity. Erect scout films of the abdomen show a very large gastric gas bubble and elevation of the left leaf of the diaphragm. Roentgen examination is not requisite to diagnosis. In any case of protracted nausea and vomiting gastric suction should be instituted: the rapid aspiration of 2 or more liters of gas and dark, foul fluid from the stomach is sufficient to establish the diagnosis of acute gastric atony.

In most cases acute gastric dilatation has no demonstrable organic obstructive lesion of the stomach or intestine for its genesis. It frequently complicates operations within the chest and upon the spine as well as central nervous troubles such as strokes and acute psychosis. However, in some instances its cause may be unsuspected cicatricial pyloric or duodenal stenoses; pyloric tumors; intestinal obstruction from bands, herniae and congenital anomalies; and obstruction of the efferent stoma of a gastrojejunostomy. Hypokalemia alone at times is capable of inciting and maintaining gastric atony, as are diabetic acidosis, acute adrenal insufficiency and uremia. Hyperextension of the spine in a cast or on a frame, retroperitoneal hemorrhage, and ureterolithotomy or catheterization may be followed by gastric atony.

Regardless of etiology, the initial treatment of gastric dilatation is: (1) the immediate emptying of the stomach (proved by irrigation with clear return) and institution of continuous gastric suction and its maintenance for 36 to 48 hours (the appropriate period of time required for the regaining of functionality by the stretched stomach) and (2) the restoration of fluid balance with the administration of requisite salts, e.g., potassium salts for hypokalemia, and sodium salts for deficit of extracellular fluid. These are lifesaving measures (see Chap. 5, "Fluid and Electrolytes").

While the gastric aspiration and fluid therapy are being conducted search must be made for signs of intestinal obstruction while constantly bearing in mind the relative paucity of symptoms of intestinal obstruction during the early postoperative period.

EMETIC DRUGS

Other associates of postoperative nausea and vomiting, namely, ileus, cardiac failure and infections, have been discussed. Drug overdosage or idiosyncrasy is a more prominent cause of postoperative nausea now than it was 30 years ago; then digitalis, morphine, belladonna, hyoscine, barbiturates and potassium iodide constituted practically the entire gamut of the occasionally nauseating and emetic medicaments given postoperatively. Today the list is much longer and includes vitamins, sulfonamides, antibiotics, Demerol, spasmolytics such as Banthine and dicyclamine hydrochloride, and the protein hydrolysates. Iatrogenic nausea and emesis are often coupled with cutaneous signs of a drug-reaction. Except in the case of such drugs as provide specific signs of toxicity, e.g., digitalis, morphine, atropine and scopolamine, ascribing postoperative nausea and vomiting to drugs is justified largely by the exclusion of possible organic and metabolic causes, by the time relationships of the nausea to the dosage schedule and to subsidence of the nausea when the drugs are stopped. The withdrawal of drugs or the giving of chlorpromazine (Thorazine) or barbiturates without ruling out gastric atony, ileus, uremia, hypokalemia, etc., as possible causes of the nausea and vomiting is ill-conceived and dangerous practice. However, whenever mechanical and biochemical causes for nausea and vomiting can be excluded, the discontinuance of drugs and the giving of tranquilizers may be warranted.

PROJECTILE VOMITING

Projectile vomiting is a phenomenon peculiar to increased intracranial pressure and is associated with such abnormalities as intracranial tumors, encephalitis, meningitis, head injuries and water intoxication. Characteristically, it is neither preceded by nor attended with nausea. It occurs suddenly, and the ejection of the vomitus may be so forceful as to propel it many feet. Obviously, the occurrence of projectile vomiting at any time dictates the need for a neurologic and an ophthalmoscopic examination and the determination of the serum sodium concentration. See Chapter 50, "Surgery of the Nervous System," for the treatment of increased intracranial pressure and meningitis and Chapter 5, "Fluid and Electrolytes" for the treatment of water intoxication.

HICCOUGH

Hiccough (singultus) was a rather frequent postoperative trouble 20 years ago. Today it is rare. Hiccoughs occur in conjunction with peritonitis, subphrenic abscesses, empyema, uremia, gastric dilatation, ileus, anxiety and other illnesses. It tends to occur periodically and consequently is not dangerous ordinarily. However, occasionally it may last for days and exhaust the patient physically. Ordinarily, some measure of control may be effected with gastric emptying and lavage of the stomach with an alkaline saline solution, sedation, and changing the position of the patient. Occasionally, conduction over the phrenic nerve or nerves needs to be blocked with a long-acting local anesthetic such as lidocaine in order to provide the patient with some relief from them. However, even this may not do so; the person hics with the intercostal musculature after the phrenic nerves are blocked.

Obviously, the surest treatment is that which corrects the associated disease. The primary surgical significance of hiccough is the implication that something that does or may soon endanger life exists, prompting the surgeon to search for the signs of such entities as subphrenic abscess, empyema, uremia, gastric atony, ileus and acidosis. Hiccoughs occasionally are the earliest sign of their presence.

Vagal pressure, breathing 5 per cent carbon dioxide, breathing into a bag, tickling the nose with a feather and the feet with a pin will often stop them, but after these and other maneuvers they are prone to return.

Section 9. Headache; Care of Mouth and Skin

Headache is a frequent complaint following spinal anesthesia. The leakage of spinal fluid through the site of puncture of the dura is presumed to be its cause. It is aggravated by sitting, standing, coughing or sneezing. The avoidance of the upright position for 3 to 5 days usually controls it.

Some severe postoperative headaches are merely the signs of caffeine withdrawal. Patients who were in the habit of drinking 3 to 10 cups or more of coffee a day before they were operated upon frequently complain of severe, throbbing frontal headaches during the postoperative period of fasting. These are quickly relieved by giving caffeine sodium benzoate or a cup of coffee.

Headache and blurring of vision may be the first sign of water intoxication. However, most of the postoperative headaches other than those which follow spinal anesthesia cannot be attributed to any specific biochemical disturbance. Aspirin, codeine, or other weak analgesics control them readily.

CARE OF THE MOUTH

Preoperative and postoperative oral cleanliness is important. The mouth should be looked upon as a part of the operative field during esophagectomy and gastrectomy. Consequently, meticulous cleanliness of the oral cavity should be attained before these operations are undertaken. Whenever possible badly decayed teeth should be removed before the operation is performed; however, this is often impossible. Nevertheless, even in the worst cases of dental caries a fair degree of oral cleanliness can be obtained with a dental prophylaxis or the extensive use of toothbrush and a foaming toothpaste for 3 or 5 days before the operation is performed.

Postoperatively, the maintenance of oral cleanliness is a very important part of nursing. A dry, dirty mouth may lead to surgical parotitis, and the pulmonary aspiration of bits of filth is prone to lead to lung abscesses.

CARE OF THE SKIN

The care of the skin consists of keeping it clean and dry and preventing localized ischemia. A bedsore or decubitus ulcer is evidence for poor care of the skin. Constant dryness is often very difficult to obtain. The febrile individual may sweat a great deal. Copious sweating requires frequent bathing, massaging and powdering of the skin, especially of the back. Any patient who is incontinent of urine requires the insertion of an indwelling catheter in order to keep the skin of the buttocks, the back and the legs dry. The unconscious patient and paraplegic, and the weak and the aged need to be turned in bed every 1 to 2 hours to prevent ischemic necrosis of the skin overlying the sacrum and the bony prominences such as the ischial tuberosity, the greater trochanters of the femurs, the shoulders and the elbows.

Herpes simplex, or fever blisters, occasionally are a complication of surgery. Their resolution can be hastened materially by coating them with a clear nail polish or tincture of benzoin.

The pruritic rashes that appear following operative procedures are usually attributable to the antiseptic applied to the skin preoperatively, or to medicaments given internally. The determination of the cause of the postoperative rash is usually relatively simple; the antiseptic rashes are limited to the area to which the material was applied while the drug sensitivity rashes are more generalized. Usually the removal of the cause terminates the rash. Washing the skin with alcohol and soap and water will serve to remove the antiseptic. Discontinuance of the antibiotics or such medications as iodides, bromides and penicillin and the giving of pyribenzamine and codeine is usually all that is required to control the symptoms and the rash. However, occasionally the sensitivity reaction is so severe as to require the administration of ACTH, cortisone and epinephrine to obtain relief.

If exfoliative dermatitis is threatened, corticoids should be begun early, as this complication was formerly often fatal and still is in some instances.

Section 10. Symptomatic Psychoses

Today surgeons and internists alike largely disregard the psychological abnormalities associated with the ills they meet and the treatments they apply, in spite of the emphasis placed upon the symptomatic psychoses during the 19th century. Evidently, we look upon the symptomatic psychoses as "normal" behavior among the ill and consequently disregard them just as we are prone to disregard the normal leg, tooth, or heart.

However, the symptomatic psychoses (Bonhoeffer's terminology) are important signs of organic illness, especially during the postoperative period, because they often constitute the earliest manifestations of trouble. Although an operation or its complications may be the factor that relights or precipitates a functional psychosis such as a manic depression or schizophrenia, this discussion of psychoses will be limited to the symptomatic group.

CLASSIFICATION

I. NUTRITIONAL
   Origin
   1. Elemental
      Potassium deficiency
      Sodium deficiency
      Hypocalcemia
      Bromide excess
      Lead excess
   2. Water
      Water deficit with hyperosmolarity
      Water excess with hyposmolarity
   3. Organic foodstuffs
      Vitamine deficiency
         Nictonic acid
         Thiamine
      Protein intoxication
      Hypoglycemia
   4. Gases
      Hypoxia
         Circulatory
         Respiratory
II. COMPLEX METABOLIC
   1. Uremia without hypertension
   2. Uremia with hypertension
III. THE PHARMACOPSYCHOSES
   1. Anesthetics
   2. Ethyl alcohol
      Delirium tremens
      Korsakoff's syndrome
      Wernicke's syndrome
   3. Barbiturates
   4. Lysergic acid and its derivatives
IV. ENDOCRINOPATHIC
   1. Hyperthyroidism
   2. Hypothyroidism
   3. Hypoparathyroidism (calcium deficiency)
   4. ACTH and cortisone
   5. Acute adrenal cortical insufficiency
V. SEPTIC TRAUMATIC
   1. Acute septic
   2. Chronic septic
   3. Cranial traumatic
   4. Burn psychosis

DELIRIUM

Delirium is the term usually used to describe some of the psychotic manifestations of the symptomatic psychoses. It connotes much more than mental confusion and is distinct from the dementias, the affective disorders and stupor. Essentially, delirium consists of: (1) disorders of perception manifested as visual, auditory and tactile hallucinations; (2) disturbances of interpretation: namely, illusions and delusions; (3) psychomotor abnormalities, predominantly of the overactive type; (4) and evidence of stimulation of the sympathetic nervous system.

The clinical signs of delirium are:

1. Signs of stimulation of the sympathetic system: tachycardia, mild fever and sweating

2. Disturbances of perception: hallucinations

3. Disturbances of interpretation: delusions and illusions

4. Abnormalities of somatic motor activity: perseveration, iteration, overtalkativeness, tremors, restlessness, picking at bedclothes, convulsions

5. Disturbances of affect such as uncontrolled laughter, weeping, or moaning

6. Alterations of mood from euphoria to abject fear and violent temper

7. Disturbances in sensorium varying between coma and transient disorientation in place and time

The signs of sympathetic overactivity may be the earliest signs of delirium, especially among thyrotoxicotics. The sweating of delirium predominantly occurs on the face, the hands and the feet, though at times the whole body is drenched with sweat. The fever is usually mild, rarely above 101° F., excepting in those deliria attending infections, head injuries, hyperosmolarity, and thyroid storm when it may reach lethal heights of 108° to 112° F.

The disturbances of perception are hallucinations (*the perception of animate and inanimate objects or their relationships which have no realistic basis*). The visual and auditory forms predominate. Their characters often change frequently: one minute the delirious one is being trampled by a herd of giant mice, the next he is being eaten by a single pigmy ant, the next he is being scolded and whipped by a 10-headed grandfather, and 20 minutes later is cowering beneath the bedclothes, holding his ears because jet bombers are buzzing him. Unpleasant or horrifying hallucinations stimulate motor reactions which may be violently combative or evasive or loudly vocal. Some of the illusions of delirium are pleasant and are accompanied by tranquility: God speaks as a father to a favorite son, or the bed floats among vividly colored hanging gardens to the accompaniment of a well-ordered mélange of the music of Strauss, Beethoven, Debussy, Gershwin, and Handel. Ofttimes some components of hallucinations are remembered with remarkable tenacity.

The disturbances of interpretation are practically indistinguishable from those of perception. The difference between a hallucination and an illusion or delusion is lack of an external environment stimulus: the hallucination has no apparent real stimulus, while the illusion and the delusion have.

A delirious person looking out of a window in Kansas at the sky and saying "We're sailing on a beautifully calm sea" is suffering an illusion, and if after being told that he is not at sea and nowhere near a ship or water he persists in the belief that he is at sea he is *deluded*. However, the same statements made by a man in a completely darkened, windowless room would indicate that he is suffering hallucinations. However, this man may have heard the Sisters' raiments as they passed his doors rustling as does the quiet sea. The hallucination then becomes an illusion.

The relationship of delirium to the illness varies; at times it appears before the other signs of illness, at others with them, and occasionally after the crisis. Peculiarly, the sick person is often delirious at night and soporous during the day. The passage of delirium usually is heralded by profound sleep and leaves a weak, easily fatigued, emotionally unstable, despondent or complaining, whining patient who may be hypersensitive to odors, light and noise and he may be unco-operative.

During the delirium the patient is apt to injure and occasionally to destroy himself by jumping from a window or throttling himself with the bedclothes or venetian blind cords. Constant physical restraint often aggravates the motor activity of delirium.

At one time physicians believed that characteristic forms of deliria were associated with specific disease entities. We do not. However, there are certain differences between the compositions of the total pictures of the symptomatic psychoses that permit an initial presumptive determination of the possible causes of an observed postoperative symptomatic psychosis.

A careful history of the person's illness, a meticulous examination of the patient's hospital record, including the nurses' notes, and intelligent examinations of the patient will serve to determine the cause of most symptomatic psychoses among surgical patients.

The major categories of postoperative symptomatic psychoses are the septic, the traumatic and the nutritional. Within these categories, the acute septic, the cranial traumatic, elemental deficiencies and circulatory hypoxia (shock) are the most frequent. Space does not permit more than a cursory description of the clinical aspects of the postoperative symptomatic psychoses.

NUTRITIONAL PSYCHOSES

POTASSIUM DEFICIT

The onset of the psychoses associated with potassium deficit is preceded by the history of or the actual observation of the loss of body fluids through diarrhea, vomiting and fistulous drainage, or the administration of ACTH or cortisone without the administration of supplemental potassium.

The physical signs associated with it are: weakness, atonic musculature, ileus, and flattening and inversion of T-waves on the electrocardiogram.

The neurologic signs are: hyperactive tendon reflexes with mild deficits, and hypoactive to absent tendon reflexes and motor paralysis with the severe deficits.

The psychotic behavior is characterized by a mild delirium with overtalkativeness, iteration, confabulation and wakefulness. Vacillating disorientation in time and space is seen often.

Sodium Deficits (Extracellular Fluid Volume Deficits)

The abnormal psychotic behavior associated with sodium deficit is also preceded by a story of evidence of loss of body fluids through diarrhea, vomiting, fistulous drainage, profuse sweating, and trauma such as fractures of the femur, burns and peritonitis.

The physical signs associated with it are: weakness, tachycardia, softening of the pulse, varying degrees of hypotension, shrunken tissues, soft muscles, and subnormal temperatures in the absence of infection. The tendon reflexes tend to be hypoactive. Apathy and somnolence progressing to coma are the major psychic manifestations. Disorientation, hallucinations, illusions, or delusions are extremely infrequent.

Hypocalcemia

This is generally preceded by a recently performed thyroidectomy, removal of a parathyroid adenoma, or associated with severe, acute pancreatitis or prolonged diarrhea. Tachycardia, muscle spasms brought on by exercise or occlusion of the arterial blood flow, and hyperactive reflexes manifested by such signs as Chvostek's, are the predominant physical signs.

Psychic manifestations are paresthesia, circumoral numbness, itching of the nose, apprehension, and increased sensitivity to noise and bright lights. There is no delirium, although often the individual may manifest hysterical behavior.

Bromide Excess

Persons suffering from brominism are occasionally to be seen on the surgical services, especially for the treatment of injuries and chronic ulcers of the lower extremities. There is usually a history of taking a "nerve medicine" and of headache.

The physical signs are an acniform eruption upon the face and the body, occasional ulcers of the extremities, coldness of the extremities and fetid breath. There are no neurologic signs. Sleepiness, slowness of speech and mental detachment are the main psychic manifestations.

Lead Poisoning

Persons suffering from acute plumbism are occasionally subjected to celiotomy because of the severe colicky abdominal pain that may attend acute lead poisoning. Plumbism has been mistaken for acute mechanical intestinal obstruction, intussusception, appendicitis, cholecystitis and ruptured peptic ulcer.

A history of chewing painted furniture and woodwork usually can be obtained from parents of children having lead colic, and a story of working with lead paints or lead-containing insect poisons, battery salvaging or battery casing burning is sometimes obtained from adults. There may be abdominal signs of acute intestinal obstruction. Anemia, basophilic stippling of the red cells, constipation, lead line, and motor nerve paralysis predominating in the muscles used most, such as the antebrachial and the leg muscles (wrist drop and foot drop, respectively), are signs of plumbism. Kernig's sign and convulsions often develop in children.

The mental picture varies from depression to violent mania. Delirium occurs, especially among children.

Water Deficit with Hyperosmolarity

This occasionally follows cranial injury and intercranial operative procedures, especially resections of craniopharyngiomas and pituitary tumors.

Under other circumstances an incapacity to drink water usually precedes the onset of the syndrome. Thirst is a prominent symptom until consciousness is lost. Fever, dry mucous membranes, high urinary specific gravity and a serum sodium above 155 mEq./L. constitute the main physical aspects. Disorientation and hyperactivity are the early psychic signs and violent delirium a late accompaniment.

Water Excess with Hyposmolarity

A story can usually be obtained of vomiting, diarrhea or injury, coupled with the avid drinking of water. Muscle cramps, blurring of vision, and headache are the main symptoms. Physical signs are: practically no sodium salts in the urine, increased cerebral spinal fluid pressure, and a serum sodium concentration below 130 mEq./L. Apprehension, restlessness, mild delirium and epileptiform convulsions among the young are the psychic manifestations.

Nicotinic Acid Deficit (Pellagra)

This occurs mainly in individuals who have been unable to eat or have followed a very poor diet, such as cornbread, fat pork and molasses. The early physical signs are a fiery red erythema of skin exposed to sunlight, diarrhea and anorexia. Later, sharkskin and beefy redness and soreness of the tongue appear. The neurologic signs of acute deficits, such as those precipitated by an operation, are cogwheel rigidity, and grasping and sucking reflexes. Irritability, insomnia, slow reactions, poor memory and delirium constitute the psychosis. This is part of the syndrome of pellagra (dermatitis, diarrhea, dementia and death).

Thiamine Deficit (Dry Beriberi)

Alcoholism, a polished rice diet, or inability to eat are its main causes. The predominant sign is generalized muscular tenderness, which in the leg is especially prominent upon squatting. Signs of congestive heart failure may appear. The neurologic picture is made up of paresthesia, hyperesthesia, loss of superficial cutaneous senses, diminution of tendon reflexes and very rarely flaccid paralysis such as foot drop. Neurasthenias, irritability, failure of memory and confusion of thought, sleeplessness, increased sensitivity to noise and pain are the predominant psychic features.

Protein Intoxication

One type of protein intoxication has all of the features of water deficit with hyperosmolarity. It attends the forced feeding of protein to individuals who by reason of weakness or physical or mental incapacity are unable to drink enough water to counter the increased need for water imposed by the large protein loads. The physical and psychic signs are those of water deficit.

The other form of protein intoxication appears among cirrhotics and individuals who have had portacaval or rarely splenorenal venous shunts performed upon them. There is usually physical evidence of cirrhosis such as esophageal varices and splenohepatomegaly and laboratory evidence of hepatic insufficiency. Failure of memory, lack of care of person, loss of inhibitions, and depression are

early signs, and delirium and coma the late ones. A decreased rate of ammonia catabolism is held to account for some cases.

Hypoglycemia

Of course, this occurs most frequently among individuals taking insulin. However, surgically it may follow gastrectomy, the more especially total gastrectomy. Also, it is occasionally seen following the termination of a prolonged period of intravenous alimentation with concentrated glucose solutions. Hypoglycemia may also occur in cases of pancreatic islet cell tumors (see Chap. 32, "Pancreas"). Profuse sweating, tremors, in-co-ordination, slurring of speech, apprehension, and inability to communicate with others precede convulsions or coma. For a brief time interval between incapacity to speak and coma, the person gives evidence with eye movements that he is conscious of his trouble and of what is going on about him.

Hypoxia

Oligemic shock, injuries to the chest, and the removal of lungs are the predominant causes of circulatory and anoxic hypoxia in surgery (see Chap. 7, "Shock"). The main physical signs are breathlessness, Cheyne-Stokes type breathing, and signs of shock. Cyanosis is rare excepting in the presence of anoxic anoxia. Psychic variances with mild anoxia are euphoria, deterioration of judgment and in-co-ordination (a picture of moderate drunkenness). Delirium is common with severe hypoxia. Surgically, one of the important signs of hypoxia is delay or failure to recover from anesthesia. If fever is present with the hypoxia, the danger from it is enhanced. In such cases the reduction of the fever becomes a very important part of the treatment of the hypoxia.

COMPLEX METABOLIC PSYCHOSES

Uremia

The symptomatic psychosis associated with uremia is extremely variable. However, the variability of the picture may be reduced by separating the uremias without hypertension from those with hypertension. The psychologic manifestations differ: with uremia without hypertension the picture is one of apathy, sleeplessness, reduction of spontaneous movement, and coma without delirium; with uremia with hypertension there are restlessness, twilight states, fits and delirium. The picture of uremia with hypertension is often that of a major psychosis.

PHARMACOPSYCHOSES

ANESTHESIA

(See Chap. 12, "Anesthesia")

ALCOHOL

The alcoholic psychoses are especially troublesome in surgery because they are prone to appear after injuries or operations. There are 3 types of alcoholic psychoses that the surgeon may see: (1) delirium tremens, (2) alcoholic hallucinations and (3) Korsakoff's psychosis.

Delirium tremens appears after the cessation of the imbibition of alcohol. It is one of the commonest, if not the commonest, symptomatic psychosis seen on the surgical wards of charity hospitals. In-co-ordination, coarse tremors of all extremities, sleeplessness, agitation, and a highly active delirium with remarkably vivid visual and auditory hallucinations make up the picture.

Alcoholic hallucinations are a complication of chronic active alcoholism. Although the person is well oriented and has clear senses, his actions speak for distrust, suspicion and jealousy. These overt reactions are attributable to auditory hallucinations. Persons suffering from alcoholic hallucinations are especially troublesome on large wards because of their tendency to seemingly unprovoked combativeness.

The signs of **Korsakoff's psychosis** are the loss of memory for recent events and remarkable confabulation. The loss of memory for recent events is often striking in that one may be greeted by such a person upon seeing him for the second time within a matter of minutes by, "Hi, Doc. I have been looking for you all day. Why don't you come and see me more often?" While the condition is usually chronic, it occasionally begins with a delirious episode after an operation or injury.

BARBITURATES

The barbiturate symptomatic psychosis **is** divisible into two types: the chronic and the acute.

The chronic type is associated with muscle tremors, ataxia, nystagmus, vertigo, poor memory, thick speech and episodic hallucinations. All of these signs may be aggravated upon withdrawing the drug.

The acute intoxication is associated with hypotension, hypothermia, and stupor progressing to coma. The stupor may be preceded by a short phase of delirium. In brief, the acute intoxication has many of the aspects of general anesthesia.

ENDOCRINOPATHIC PSYCHOSES

HYPERTHYROIDISM AND HYPOTHYROIDISM

(See Chap. 26, "Thyroid, Thymus and Parathyroids")

HYPERPARATHYROIDISM

(See Hypocalcemia, Calcium Deficits, this chapter)

ACTH AND CORTISONE

The psychotic picture varies from euphoria to severe depression. Delirium is rare.

ACUTE ADRENOCORTICAL INSUFFICIENCY

Anorexia, vertigo, vomiting and weakness are the main objective complaints. Hypotension is often detectable. Disorientation in time and place, especially during the night, with remembrance of the abnormal behavior during lucid intervals, may take place.

SEPTIC PSYCHOSES

The septic symptomatic psychoses are very interesting because a number of psychic manifestations often appear before the systemic signs of illness do. Restlessness, oversensitivity to noise and light, decreased emotional control, inability to concentrate, talkativeness, euphoria and vivid dreams often precede the systemic signs of illness. At times the psychic behavior disturbance does not appear until after the crisis or subsidence of the fever or infection. In general, though, the symptomatic psychoses and the illness are associated temporally. During the febrile illness the septic psychoses may assume all of the aspects of a violent delirium. Among children the delirium may be interrupted by epileptic seizures. With the subsidence of the delirium, a period of postinfection neurasthenia or depression occasionally occurs. Frequently, the postinfection depression is not preceded by delirium. Malaise, headache, weakness, fatigue, emotional instability, episodic frightening hallucinations, and despondency with depression, or un-co-operativeness with complaining and whining are the main signs of postinfection depression.

CRANIAL TRAUMATIC PSYCHOSIS

The cranial traumatic symptomatic psychoses are increasing in number. Automobile accidents constitute the main cause. Occasionally, hyperosmolarity is the precipitating factor, and at other times it is alcoholism. However, contusional injury to the brain itself is presumed to be the predominant underlying organic disturbance. Besides the alcoholic psychosis, the cranial traumatic seems to have the longest duration of the symptomatic psychoses.

The signs and symptoms run the gamut from facetiousness to delirium and coma.

SITUATIONAL, CONTINUOUS PAIN

Penetrating peptic ulcers, chronic active pancreatitis and burns are especially prone to be attended by situational symptomatic psychoses, although with burns the septic factor may be predominant. Persons suffering from penetrating peptic ulcers and chronic active pancreatitis occasionally go beserk, throwing chairs and the like through windows, and injuring themselves by running head-on into walls. During the psychotic episodes they may attempt self-destruction. The psychotic behavior of a person during the first day following a severe burn is seemingly primarily attributable to hypoxia (shock) because it usually disappears as the signs of shock do. Later, the abnormal psychic behavior ascribable to various nutritional disturbances may make their appearances, and later after a dressing change or two has been performed, the burned person becomes a detached, despondent, crying, un-co-operative physical wreck. Delirium is rare after the first week unless uncontrolled sepsis occurs.

TREATMENT OF PSYCHOSES

The treatment of the symptomatic psychoses needs to be varied according to the biochemical and nutritional disturbance attending it.

The delirium of many patients quickly subsides with the institution of specific treatment of the underlying biochemical or bacterial cause (see Table 2). However, many such as the cranial traumatic, the alcoholic and the situational cannot be treated specifically and require symptomatic care, according to the following rules of general treatment:

1. Continuous attendance upon a delirious patient by physicians, nurses, trained attendants, or intelligent relatives is mandatory.

2. All drugs that may even remotely abet or promote the delirium, such as barbiturates, analgesics (excepting in the case of pain), atropine, hyoscine, salicylates, bromides, ACTH and cortisone (excepting in the case of adrenocortical insufficiency and delirium tremens), are to be avoided.

3. *Fresh* paraldehyde (10 to 15 ml. in fruit juice orally or in 50 to 100 ml. of water rectally) is a satisfactory sedative, as is also chloral hydrate. The amount of sedative given should not be so great as to abolish all signs of delirium or excitement, because to do so requires so much drug as to endanger life.

4. Place the patient in quiet and well-lighted surroundings so as to reduce the intensity of hallucinatory reactions.

5. All the while, strict attention must be paid to the pulse rate, temperature and blood pressure as well as the intake of fluid and the output of urine. An indwelling catheter is necessary for the latter.

6. Circulatory collapse may appear suddenly and requires alert and energetic treatment such as transfusions of blood and plasma, or saline solutions and vasopressor agents for shock, and digitalization for acute heart failure.

7. The delirious patient should be permitted to be up and about unless he is physically incapable of safe walking. Restraints often excite the delirium; therefore, they should be used with care.

8. Whenever coma occurs meticulous attention must be paid to the maintenance of the full patency of the airway. When neces-

TABLE 2. TREATMENT OF SYMPTOMATIC PSYCHOSES

TYPE	TREATMENT
Potassium Deficiency	KCl or K_2HPO_4 (0.2 to 0.4%), 2–4 Gm./L. of 10% dextrose intravenously, provided that the patient is not anuric
Sodium Deficiency (with normal osmolarity)	Hartmann's solution (Ringer's lactate) when pH of serum is normal or below normal. NaCl 0.9% with or without NH_4Cl 0.6 to 1.1% for Na+ deficit with alkalosis
Hypocalcemia	Calcium gluconate 10% solution, 20–120 ml. intravenously Calcium lactate 10–40 Gm. daily orally Vitamin D, but no milk or cheese in diet Occasionally, dihydrotachysterol or parathormone may be required for a short time
Bromide Excess	Sodium chloride 10–20 Gm. daily
Delirium Tremens	Cortisone or metacorten as for adrenal insufficiency I.V. fluids containing glucose and sodium chloride
Lead Excess	For colic: calcium gluconate i.v., atropin For psychosis: sodium citrate 12 Gm. orally daily (Consult toxicologic text for use of B.A.L., etc.)
Water Deficit (with hyper-osmolarity)	Water orally or rectally, 5% dextrose in water i.v. and subcutaneously Also, give pitressin, aqueous 2–10 I.U. (0.1 to 0.2 ml.) every 4 hours i.m. *if hyperosmolarity is associated with acute postoperative diabetes insipidus*
Water Excess (with hyp-osmolarity)	Withhold water if extracellular fluid volume is normal or above normal Administer i.v. 3.0 to 5.0% NaCl if extracellular fluid volume is subnormal and the person is alkalotic or M/2 or molar sodium lactate should there be an extracellular fluid volume deficit and acidosis Reduce the dosage or discontinue pitressin if it is being used

Vitamin Deficiency
  Nicotinic Acid
  Thiamine
	
	Niacin 50 mg. orally t.i.d. or nicotinamide 100 mg. daily parenterally
	Thiamine 2–6 mg. t.i.d. orally or 15–25 mg. daily parenterally
	Watch especially for signs of acute heart failure and digitalize should its signs appear

Protein Intoxication
  With Hyperosmolarity
  With Normal Osmolarity
	
	As for water deficit (see above)
	Reduce dietary protein to 40–60 Gm. daily

Hypoglycemia	25% glucose i.v. for hypoglycemic shock, convulsions or coma For postgastrectomy hypoglycemia remove free sugar from the diet and raise the protein in it to 120–150 Gm. daily taken in 5 to 6 meals

Hypoxia
  Circulatory
    Oligemic Shock
    Vasoparalytic
    Acute Cardiac Failure
	Reduce accompanying fever if present
	
	Blood, plasma and saline solutions (see Chap. 7, "Shock")
	Vasopressor agents (see Chap. 7, "Shock")
	(See page 241, this chapter)

Respiratory	Oxygen
Uremia	(See Chap. 48, "Urology")
Hyperthyroidism	(See Thyroid Storm, this chapter)
Hypothyroidism	(See Chap. 26)
Hypoparathyroidism	(See above, Hypocalcemia)
ACTH and Cortisone	Reduce dosage or discontinue
Acute Adrenal Insufficiency	Cortisone 20–100 mg. daily or metacorten 5–10 mg. with sodium and potassium salts
Septic	Appropriate antibiotics and surgery and control of hyperpyrexia and hypoxia if present
Situational	Morphine i.v. for severe pain Gentleness in care of the injured

sary, an intratracheal tube may be inserted. Usually this may be done without difficulty. Rarely, a tracheostomy may be needed. Secretions must be removed from the airway regularly by suction. Aminophylline will often serve to abolish Cheyne-Stokes breathing. Artificial control of body temperature with sponge bathing and ice packs may be necessary. Atropine should not be given, because it thickens secretions and disturbs temperature regulation by inhibiting sweating. The maintenance of fluid and electrolyte balance and parenteral feeding are very difficult problems in the comatose patient.

FRANCIS D. MOORE, M.D.

—————————————————— CHAPTER 15 ——————————————————

The Endocrine and Metabolic Basis
of Surgical Care

INTRODUCTION

That there is a systemic reaction to bodily injury has been an observation made by physicians and surgeons over the centuries. Until the advent of asepsis and more recently antibacterial therapy, many of the systemic effects observed were those of bacterial invasion and host resistance. Tissue trauma as a physiologic stimulus could not be distinguished from the subsequent inevitable infection.

In the past decade there has emerged a much clearer understanding of this systemic response to tissue trauma. This understanding traces its origin to the work of Walter Cannon (1871-1945), who studied the effects of nonspecific stress and trauma on the activity of the adrenal medulla. This systemic response to disease, operations and injury determines the adaptation of supportive treatment to the needs of the surgical patient. We must understand what the patient is doing for himself if we are to help him effectively. It is the purpose of the author in this chapter to review the known evidences of an endocrine response to trauma and its metabolic counterpart. Then the significance of this metabolism in daily surgical care is discussed in some detail.

Because the response of the adrenal cortex is better known than others, it is documented in greatest detail. But this should not be construed as indicating that the postoperative endocrine adjustment involves only one gland; other endocrine changes are of great importance. Beyond the endocrine changes are many metabolic facts (such as the replacement of extrarenal losses or treatment of renal acidosis), wherein the biochemical alteration determines therapy, and endocrine responses are unknown, poorly understood or of little importance.

EVIDENCES OF ENDOCRINE ACTIVATION AFTER TRAUMA

ADRENALS

Eosinophils. In the presence of normally functioning adrenal glands, the predominant influence bearing on the concentration of eosinophils in the peripheral blood is change in serum concentration of the glucocorticoids of the adrenal cortex. A rise in corticoid concentration produces a fall in eosinophils, and conversely a drop in steroid concentration is followed by a rise in eosinophils. A maintained high steroid level will not necessarily maintain a continuously low count of eosinophils. Factors of allergy and adrenomedullary effects also influence the circulating eosinophil count. Despite this variety of influences, the normal eosinophil course after surgery is quite constant, and, therefore, departures are of significance.

The normal eosinophil count in the adult averages between 150 and 300 per cu. mm., with extremes well beyond these limits. The counting technic is inaccurate, and counts are variable. Changes in the count must be checked by subsequent observation, and must be of the order of magnitude of 50 per cent to be of significance.

Major surgical operations of minor extent such as herniorrhaphy lower this count to 10 to 30 per cent of the starting level, observed values being in the general range of 40 to 80 per cu. mm. Operations of greater extent lower the count substantially to zero, and beyond this the lowering obviously cannot go. For this reason, there is no further effect on the eosinophil lowering by further increasing the amount of trauma; the effect can only be manifested by the subsequent course of the count.

The post-traumatic fall is rapid and is often complete before the end of surgery, and usually so on the day of the trauma. In some instances there is a transient rise in eosinophil count during the induction of anesthesia or during the early phases of surgery. This is a normal change, and does not denote adrenal insufficiency. Spinal anesthesia delays the fall in count for a few hours, and ether anesthesia accelerates it. Indeed, ether anesthesia alone will produce a significant eosinopenia. Apprehension and other psychological factors present prior to surgery are occasionally associated with a lowering of the eosinophil count.

The course of the count after its initial lowering depends upon the nature of the trauma and the subsequent course of the patient. After a lesser trauma the eosinophils quickly return to normal, often within 24 hours. After more major injury or trauma the count remains low, near zero, for from 2 to 5 days. When a continuing open wound is present, as in a burn, open fracture or crush injury, the eosinophil count remains low much longer, returning upward after 7 to 14 days have passed.

The course of the eosinophil count, after starting its upward trend, may take one of two rather characteristic courses. The curve may return to normal values and stay there. Or, in some instances, the count rises to a value well above the starting normal, remaining there for from 1 to 10 days before returning to normal. This "backswing overshoot" is especially noticeable in those instances in which the trauma has been massive, sudden and intense but has totally passed after definitive surgery. A characteristic example is to be found in moderately severe war wounds after definitive surgery; occasionally in burns. A high prolonged count is observed during the phase when the wound closure is becoming complete and immediately thereafter. Pathologic variations in the eosinophil count are described in a later section.

The fall in lymphocytes and the rise of neutrophilic granulocytes which occur after trauma are also characteristic and probably endocrine mediated. Details and interpretation are too meager to merit further discussion as manifestations of a systemic endocrine adjustment. The leukocytosis of infection far outweighs in importance that seen from tissue trauma alone.

Urinary Steroids. The 17-ketosteroids are urinary end-products of steroids arising from both the adrenal and the testicles. The 17-ketosteroids are derived from their precursors by configurational changes which occur in the liver. Although there is measurable increase after extensive surgery or trauma, the urinary excretion of 17-ketosteroids is insensitive and unreliable as an index of the systemic endocrine adjustment which follows surgery. It is of greater value in the study and the treatment of such disorders as adrenal virilism and Cushing's disease.

Glucocorticoids of the adrenal cortex include a large number of steroid compounds, of which compounds E and F (cortisone and hydrocortisone) are physiologically the most important and compound F the predominant secretory product in man. Measurement of these substances in the urine has often been done by bio-assay, a laborious and nonspecific (but biologically very significant) method. These substances may also be measured by their "formaldehydogenic" property, both before and after hydrolysis. The latter serves to free the conjugated steroids so that they may be detected analytically. Recently, chromatographic and spectrophotometric separation has become available as means not only of measuring but of positively identifying urinary steroids. Of these various methods, the Porter-Silber color reaction is one of the most simple and useful, and, as developed for urinary steroids, it measures the total urinary 17-hydroxycorticoids quite effectively. It is not entirely free of fault, as positive results in the low range of values may be produced by the administration of certain drugs such as iodides and paraldehyde, which interfere with the final color reaction. By all these methods, both chemical and biologic, a rise in urinary excretion of glucocorticoids is readily demonstrable after trauma or surgery.

The normal excretion of total urinary 17-hydroxycorticoids in the adult is from 5 to 10 mg. in 24 hours. Lesser traumata (herniorrhaphy, appendectomy) produce significant increases (up to 25 mg.) usually lasting only 1 day. More major injury (long bone fracture) may produce increases up to 50 mg. in 24 hours, lasting a day or two. Intraperitoneal surgery of an extensive sort produces increases in the 30 to 60 mg. range, lasting from 1 to 5 days. Burns produce increases persisting for as long as 2 weeks.

Ordinarily, the course of urinary steroid excretion after the operative rise is a fall to normal levels. Occasionally, there is a period of subnormal excretion prior to the resumption of normal levels.

Since the urinary excretion of total 17-hydroxycorticoids is in a sense an integrated total of the entire secretory pattern, it may serve as a better index of the total magnitude of the adrenal discharge than the serum peak in free 17-hydroxycorticoids. However, the latter serves as a better index of the timing and the mechanism of the steroidal change.

The adrenal cortex also secretes a very potent "electrolyte-active" hormone known as aldosterone ("electrocortin"). Scanty evidence to date suggests that this material is present in the urine in increased quantities in a variety of situations, including the postoperative period. The secretion of this hormone is evidently under pituitary control to a considerably lesser extent than is the case with the glucocorticoids.

The physiology by which these secretory patterns emerge after injury is beyond the scope of this chapter. For the sake of completeness, it should be mentioned that many of these endocrine alterations are abolished or altered by experimental procedures which destroy tracts or centers in the peripheral nerves, the spinal cord, the hypothalamus and the pituitary. Increased amounts of ACTH have been demonstrated in the blood following injury, and this increased ACTH secretion is doubtless responsible, at least in part, for the changes observed in serum and urine steroids.

Blood Steroids. The free serum 17-hydroxycorticoids may be measured also by the Porter-Silber color reaction and the total corticoids similarly after hydrolysis. The method is accurate and reproducible with normal values for the free hormone in the range of 5 to 15 gamma per cent.

The alteration in blood corticoids produced by surgical operation is a very spectacular one. After surgery of moderate magnitude, the free serum 17-hydroxycorticoid level rises to 30 to 50 gamma per cent within an hour or two of making the incision. The peak is usually passed and normal values are rapidly resumed within 24 hours of surgery. Ether anesthesia alone produces a rapid rise to a level in the 20 to 40 gamma per cent range.

As evidence of increased adrenal activity after operation, this change in blood corticoids is of great significance. The rise at the time of surgery is the chemical reflection of a very rapid and drastic alteration in endocrine balance produced by the surgical experience. Yet, there are many other factors besides adrenal secretory change which determine the absolute blood level attained and the rate of fall in concentration of the free steroid; alterations in liver and kidney function affect both.

OTHER ENDOCRINE FACTORS

Adrenal Medulla. The classic evidences for activation of the adrenal medulla have been the increase in rate of the denervated heart in the cat, when the cat was angry, excited or injured. This work, carried out by Dr. Cannon, has not been extensively corroborated or confirmed in any type of study in the human being. The clinical finding of tachycardia in the injured patient is usually thought to be adrenal medullary in origin, and the occurrence of increased circulating epinephrine is considered to be responsible for this tachycardia. Peripheral blanching and narrowing of the pulse pressure by a rise in the diastolic pressure are also regarded as peripheral effects of vasoconstriction due to the action of adrenal medullary substances, probably norepinephrine. Although increased sweating in the periphery is cholinergic in its end-organ mediation, it is a sympathetic effect in terms of nervous pathways. The total combination, then, of tachycardia, vasoconstriction and sweating has long been considered to be evidence of sympathetic and adrenomedullary activity.

This adrenomedullary triad (tachycardia, vasoconstriction and sweating) is readily produced by psychological stimuli, particularly apprehension. Its most marked evidences occur in traumatic shock. The entire triad may often be missing during surgery carried out in an anesthetized patient who is not frightened, who has confidence in his surgical care, who has little pain and in whom blood volume is normal. Therefore, the adrenal medullary effects fall into a special group, being activated most particularly by psychological stimuli (as indeed they were in much of Dr. Cannon's early work) and by traumatic shock.

Posterior Pituitarylike Effects. There is an alteration in water metabolism after trauma which is quite similar to that produced by injections of posterior pituitary hormone. This alteration in water metabolism might be called a decreased "water tolerance," by which is meant that administered water loads are cleared through the kidney much less rapidly, the urine has a high specific gravity (and high osmolarity), regardless of the need of the organism to excrete water and quite independent of any alterations in electrolyte metabolism.

Recently, it has been demonstrated that there is a substance in the urine of postoperative patients which resembles the antidiuretic hormone of the posterior pituitary. Positive identification of this material in the blood in increased amounts after surgery is still wanting. Demonstration that the antidiuretic substance present in the urine is in point of fact posterior pituitary in origin is also lacking. However, the physiologic effects remain, and there is strong presumptive evidence that the antidiuresis which follows surgery is posterior pituitary in origin.

Gonads. After massive injury or burns there is a period of amenorrhea in the female and a period of loss of libido in the male. In the female there may also be marked growth of body hair, often a male distribution, which is lost when the trauma is past and healing is complete. Menstruation then returns. In terms of clinical endocrinology, these observed changes are evidence of decreased gonadal function. Specific demonstration that there is a decrease in gonadal function must await further work on urinary androgens and estrogens after surgery. It is not unusual for the female to miss one menstrual period after moderately extensive surgery. It is also not unusual for the female to have a period of uterine bleeding while still in the hospital after surgery. This would suggest that a secretory endometrium had been built up under preoperative estrogenic influences, and that their sudden withdrawal as a result of surgical inhibition of gonadal function results in uterine bleeding rather than true menstruation. The few quantitative measurements available to date are based on sporadic studies of gonadal hormones after surgery and fail to show a consistent pattern, although changes may be marked.

Thyroid. That there is an increased demand for oxygen after injury has been demonstrated by several workers. The patient immediately after surgery or with a continuing open wound and infection has a high oxygen consumption, indicating an increased conversion of endogenous or exogenous substrates to heat or kinetic energy. In considering this fact, it is important to remember that the thyroid is not the only mechanism in the body by which oxygen consumption may be increased. Increased oxygen consumption is found in widespread malignancy, in lymphoma and in infection, in which there is no evidence of increased thyroid activity. Although there is good evidence of a reciprocal thyroidadrenal relation, the evidence that the thyroid increases its activity after surgery is inconclusive at the present time: some studies carried out in animals indicate that the thyroid undergoes no particular change in function after trauma. Other work would imply that there is an increase in thyroidal function after surgery, although the evidence for this is scanty. Thus we are left with the fact that in the early post-trauma period there is increased oxidation of fat and sugar, and that such may persist for many weeks should infection or an open wound persist. The role of the thyroid in this change is not clear at present.

Pancreas. After surgery there is an increase in blood sugar. This is regarded as adrenomedullary in origin, and as occurring at the expense of liver glycogen, since the same change is produced by the injection of epinephrine. The possibility that surgery may inhibit the peripheral utilization of glucose by alteration in the function of the pancreatic islets is also a possibility, and the increased amounts of adrenal steroids present in the blood after surgery would in themselves tend to counteract some of the peripheral effects of insulin. Suffice it to say that at the present time there is no clear-cut evidence that the pancreatic islets change their function after trauma, although there is a clear tendency to hyperglycemia and glycosuria.

POSTOPERATIVE METABOLISM, RELATION TO ENDOCRINE ACTIVITY

Tissue trauma excites a number of changes in the metabolic functions of the organism, many of which appear coincident with the endocrine changes just described. These metabolic changes will be described in relation to the elements involved.

NITROGEN

Trauma is followed by a period of starvation. This varies in duration from the loss of a single meal to protracted periods of lack of dietary intake due to direct injury to the gastrointestinal tract and its glands, to alterations in gastrointestinal motility or to loss of appetite from other sources. This starvation tends to produce a negative nitrogen balance which in the adult male would be expected to amount to urinary nitrogen excretion rates (on zero intake) in the neighborhood of 7 to 10 Gm. a day.

Superimposed on this period of starvation is an additional loss of nitrogen which is rightly termed catabolic in nature, since it occurs with or without intake. It may continue to occur (unlike starvation losses) as intake and caloric supply are gradually increased. In surgery of minor extent, such as inguinal herniorrhaphy or appendectomy or a fractured ankle, the nitrogen loss on the first day or two after surgery is not greatly in excess of that observed in starvation alone. With more extensive surgery, the nitrogen loss is increased to the neighborhood of 12 to 15 Gm. of nitrogen per day on zero intake; and after major fractures, burns and extensive soft tissue injury, this nitrogen loss may exceed 25 Gm. per day per 70 Kg. of body weight.

If, as intake is resumed a few days after trauma, nitrogen-excretion rates remain high, the extent of negative nitrogen balance is determined to some extent by the intake. After major trauma, negative nitrogen balances may persist in the face of normal intakes for periods up to a week or two at rates of 7 to 12 Gm. per day. Such negative nitrogen balances may involve urinary nitrogen-excretion rates as high as 20 to 30 Gm. per day. At the cessation of this catabolic phase, one often observes a very sudden decrease in urinary nitrogen-excretion rate (termed the "corticoid withdrawal phase"), in which the nitrogen-excretion rate is sharply reduced. This reduction in urinary nitrogen-excretion rate may occur even if intake is zero.

If the reduction in urinary nitrogen-excretion rate occurs on an ascending intake of nitrogen and calories, positive nitrogen balance quickly results, and a long period of positive nitrogen balance then ensues. After operations of moderate magnitude, this positive nitrogen balance (the "spontaneous anabolic phase") begins about the 6th day and lasts until about the 20th day. After more extensive soft tissue injury, fractures or burns the positive nitrogen phase may not begin for several weeks, and, when it does occur, it may last for several months. In either case the tendency is for the body to reload the amount of nitrogen previously lost, synthesizing body protein from the absorbed amino acids and polypeptides. Exceptions to this are found after operations involving the gastrointestinal tract itself, if the disease or the procedure makes adequate dietary intake impossible. In such instances the patient does not regain his preoperative weight and remains for many months, or even years, below normal weight and muscular vigor.

Most of the nitrogen lost after trauma is excreted in the urine as urea. The amounts of nitrogen lost are so great as to suggest that they come from some very large mass of protein in the body. There are marked weakness and loss of muscle mass during the catabolic phase, and every evidence points to skeletal muscle as being the predominant site of postoperative nitrogen loss.

Where a large amount of blood is lost into the tissues, the products of degradation of this blood are excreted in the urine and the feces.

Nitrogen appears in the urine in increased quantities, and urobilinogen appears in the feces. In compound fractures of the femur and in crushing injuries of the pelvis, the amount of blood so trapped and subsequently excreted adds significantly to the negative nitrogen balance observed.

The sequential change in nature of this negative nitrogen balance is of great importance. At first the nitrogen negativity appears to be "obligatory," in the sense that it is very difficult to abolish it by high nitrogen and caloric intakes, although these may mitigate or reduce the loss. After this, following the corticoid withdrawal phase, urinary nitrogen excretion is much less, and it is at this stage that the intake of nitrogen and calories becomes of critical importance in recovery. Positive nitrogen balance during postoperative anabolism cannot be attained without an adequate caloric intake and a liberal supply of vitamins. In the vast majority of instances, oral intake is an essential for this muscle-rebuilding phase.

POTASSIUM

Potassium is the predominant intracellular base. It is lost after trauma in amounts in the range of 70 mEq. the first day after surgery of moderate to major magnitude, and thereafter in lesser amounts in the range of 20 to 30 mEq./day. In most instances, potassium losses are predominantly in the urine. Over the first few days, more potassium is lost than would be predicted from the nitrogen loss. The K:N ratio of the negative balance, instead of being the "starvation ratio" (about 3 mEq./Gm.) will be higher, in the range of from 5 to 10 mEq./Gm. Potassium balance tends to become weakly negative, zero or slightly positive prior to the achievement of positive nitrogen balance. And after loading begins, the K:N ratio of the positive balance is also high. Therefore, the implication of these changes is that the body cells lose electrolyte and water before they lose matrix (as indicated by nitrogen) and in large relative proportion to matrix. By the same token, cells appear to load electrolyte and water a little sooner and a little faster than they reconstruct matrix.

The course of serum-potassium concentration undergoes changes which bear little relation to the balance changes. Any one of the three possible courses may be seen, depending on circumstances.

1. In major injury with no evident metabolic acid-base change (although respiratory acidosis may play a role here), there is characteristically a minor rise in serum potassium to the range of 4.7 to 5.5 mEq./L.

2. In lesser trauma there is no change.

3. When trauma has occurred in the presence of metabolic alkalosis, the alkalosis is worsened and the serum potassium falls (*vide infra*). Levels in the range of 2.5 to 3.0 mEq./L. are common.

SODIUM AND CHLORIDE

The extracellular ions, sodium and chloride, are conserved after surgery. This takes the form of a reduced excretion rate in the urine. Sodium excretion is reduced to a greater extent than chloride. The onset of this sodium conservation may occur immediately with operation, or it may be delayed a day or two. If it occurs immediately, it is often of short duration but intense, with urinary sodium-excretion rate reduced from 100 to 150 to the range of 1 to 5 mEq./day. This is to be compared with the starvation urinary sodium-excretion rate of 80 to 100 mEq./day. This conservation is often followed by a "sodium-release phenomenon" with a sudden increase in sodium excretion and considerable diuresis. If, on the other hand, sodium conservation is slow to begin, commencing on the 2nd and the 3rd days after trauma, the sodium conservation may persist for many days or even weeks. We have not been able to predict which type of pattern will occur, although sudden massive trauma in the healthy male tends to produce the early type of sodium conservation, whereas in depleted individuals a more gradual but very prolonged sodium conservation is rather characteristic. This trend is not always reliable.

If sodium is administered in any quantity during this period of sodium conservation, two important results obtain. First, the absolute urinary sodium-excretion rate is considerably increased. It may be as high as 30 to 50 mEq./day on intakes of 150 mEq./day. But, so long as sodium conservation persists, a positive sodium balance ensues, the magnitude of which is a function primarily of the intake.

For this reason, it is erroneous to speak of a patient as being in "postoperative positive sodium balance" if no sodium is being given, even if excretion is reduced. Clearly, sodium must be administered during a phase of conservation for positive balance to be attained. If no intake is provided and urinary sodium conservation is marked, the situation is produced of an essentially zero balance on zero intake. This is seen occasionally in patients with heart disease in whom sodium conservation is extremely marked when they are managed postoperatively without sodium administration. As a general rule, the clinical objective of management should be zero balance, except in those instances in which there is an obligatory accumulation of traumatic edema.

The tendency to retain chloride after surgery is not as marked as is the case with sodium. This results in a tendency to gain sodium in greater quantities than chloride, and is in part responsible for the tendency of postoperative patients to become slightly alkalotic with an acid urine.

Coincident with these changes in sodium excretion there is a very distinct tendency after surgery for the serum sodium to be lowered to the range of 130 to 135 mEq./L. One might predict that retention of sodium would raise the serum-sodium concentration. Quite the reverse is the case. Those patients who show the most marked restriction of urinary sodium excretion will often be those in whom the serum sodium is most markedly lowered. Water retention may play some role in its lowering, and there is evidence that after injury an unusual amount of sodium appears in muscle cells.

WATER

There is a tendency to retain water after surgery. As mentioned above, this takes the form of diminished urine volume, which in the early post-traumatic phase may be of rather high specific gravity. This also manifests itself by decreased excretion of a given water load: there is an inability of the kidney to respond by diuresis to large water infusions. If too much water is given, there is a tendency to dilute all serum constituents, producing a fall, particlarly of red blood cells, protein and sodium.

Certain crystalloids such as glucose, urea and mannitol increase total postoperative water excretion when antidiuresis is evident and osmolarity fixed.

Changes in the total body water are not marked after closed soft tissue trauma. The normal male total body water is about 60 per cent of body weight; the female, 50 per cent. In burns or massive tissue injury, body water changes are great, and commence with a rapid rise under treatment. Although total body water does not change markedly in ordinary circumstances, there is a consistent tendency for the extracellular fraction (normally 20-25% of body weight) to enlarge; this is due in part to water retention, new water production by fat oxidation and, in some instances, a demonstrable change in cell permeability.

SERUM PROTEIN

The postoperative conservation of water and salt produces no consistent protein dilution if excessive administration is avoided. If large amounts of water are given, there is a significant post-traumatic fall in the concentration of sodium and protein. If large amounts of sodium are given, the sodium-concentration fall is not so great but the drop in serum-protein concentration is greater. Hypoproteinemia on a hepatic basis is a rarity in those without overt liver disease; functional reserve is great. The role of starvation and the syndrome of depletion are discussed below.

GLUCOSE

There is a rise in blood sugar after trauma. This persists for from 1 to 2 days, depending on the magnitude of the trauma. It is associated with the complete exhaustion of liver glycogen and, in some instances, by the spilling of sugar in the urine.

Gluconeogenesis from protein and the production of short chain carbon compounds from fat thereafter provide the oxidative substrates for energy metabolism after trauma until intake is resumed.

BODY FAT

There is rapid oxidation of body fat after major trauma. In starvation the fat-loss rate is about 75 Gm. per day. After moderately extensive surgery this is from 150 to 200 Gm./day, and after massive trauma the fat-oxidation rate runs as high as 500 Gm. a day. This rapid fat oxidation persists only a few days after closed soft tissue trauma, and then, as oral intake is resumed and endogenous substrates form a lesser fraction of the energy supply, the patient remains for many days or weeks in "zero fat balance," neither gaining nor losing fat. Then, late in convalescence, and often long after protein resynthesis has begun in the anabolic phase, restoration of body fat slowly occurs.

RELATION OF THESE METABOLIC CHANGES TO ENDOCRINE MECHANISMS

The changes in nitrogen, sodium, chloride, potassium and carbohydrate metabolism are all similar to those produced by short-term adrenal stimulation in a starving individual. There are many interesting differences between the post-traumatic metabolism and that produced by ACTH, but the resemblances far outnumber the differences. The injection of cortisone will produce similar changes, though less marked, in sodium and chloride metabolism. The injection of aldosterone produces marked restriction in sodium and chloride excretion. These facts, that the adrenal glands are markedly activated by trauma, and that certain of the metabolic changes are steroidal in character, have led to the assumption that the metabolic changes are themselves produced by adrenal secretory alterations. Doubt has been cast on this hypothesis by the demonstration in adrenalectomized animals (maintained on constant doses of cortisone) that the same changes occur. However, such evidence is diminished in importance upon the demonstration that injury alters the metabolism, inactivation or excretion of steroids in a way that increases their concentration in body fluids in addition to causing marked secretory changes. Whether or not the steroid increase per se causes these metabolic alterations, the two occur together, and survival is threatened without both of them. The exhaustion of liver glycogen and the sudden shift over to fat oxidation may also be related etiologically to alterations in the blood level of hormones which diffusely affect oxidative energy metabolism throughout the body.

As mentioned previously, the changes in water and glucose metabolism appear to be due to alterations in the function of the posterior pituitary and the adrenal medulla, respectively, although here the evidence is much less conclusive.

The endocrinology of that most important phase—spontaneous anabolism—is unknown at present.

Before leaving these metabolic changes and their relation to post-traumatic endocrinology, it should be re-emphasized that the postoperative patient is in a dynamic metabolic state. Each day he changes. For instance, after a subtotal gastrectomy there is a period of 1 or 2 days of water-excretion restriction, with increased nitrogen and potassium excretion, and a tendency to sodium retention. Then there follows a period of 2 or 3 days in which water is diuresed and the nitrogen-excretion rate is markedly reduced. Potassium balance may become positive before nitrogen. Then the patient passes into a long phase of spontaneous anabolism of nitrogen and potassium, at some time during the course of which he usually diureses sodium and water. This, then, passes along to a period of zero nitrogen balance with continued weight gain due to fat accumulation. A description of these sequential changes viewed as periods in convalescence may be found in the bibliography. The reader is referred to these accounts for fuller detail. It is this dynamic nature of surgical convalescence which renders its understanding of such importance in surgical care should complications arise or should there be complex disease involving loss of gastrointestinal function, extrarenal losses of body fluid, visceral damage or severe infections. It is this dynamic and often fast-changing state which renders ineffective any therapeutic plan based only on a static situation as observed on a certain day and considered as discrete from the unfolding pattern of which it forms a part.

WOUND HEALING IN RELATION TO NITROGEN AND CALORIC BALANCE

Because of the enthusiasm of most surgeons to improve the nutrition of their patients, an enthusiasm which has resulted in much good, the assumption has become current that wounds will not heal unless patients are in positive nitrogen balance. Nothing could be farther from the case.

The normal healing of the postoperative wound occurs almost completely during the nitrogen-negative phase. After an operation such as gastrectomy, intestinal resection, pneumonectomy, etc., the most important period of wound healing—that period during which tensile strength is gained and failure of wound healing is associated with wound dehiscence—occurs in the nitrogen-negative phase. The mobilization of low molecular weight nitrogen compounds from body protein may indeed be devoted to wound healing. Those injuries which are characterized by prolonged wound healing (major long bone fractures and burns) are the metabolic situations associated with the most prolonged negative nitrogen balance. Whatever the explanation is, the fact remains that while early resumption of anabolism is desirable, a negative nitrogen balance is not unfriendly to normal wound healing. Therefore, it is a mistake to treat an elderly patient or a feeble individual, a sick child or a burned person by forced feeding immediately after surgery in the hope that this is somehow going to help the wound. So far as we know, it will have no effect whatsoever on the wound, and it may be extremely deleterious to the patient by the production of distention and aspiration pneumonitis.

Primary failure of wound healing is manifested in abdominal surgery by wound dehiscence. The factors responsible for this failure of wound healing are unknown. Starvation may have been absent. Sepsis is unimportant. Vitamin C levels are indubitably important. Serum-protein concentrations may be normal. When the wound is resutured promptly, immediate and excellent healing usually occurs.

It is known that very large doses of compound E or F, given to experimental animals, will inhibit wound healing. It has not been demonstrated in man that wound dehiscence is due to excessive stimulation of the adrenal glands, or altered metabolism of steroids.

In contrast with the mystery of dehiscence, the late unhealed surface wound, as in a burn, seems to us to have a definite metabolic significance. It is a late occurrence and is often present in the face of a positive nitrogen balance. The early post-traumatic phase of metabolism is apparently that phase most favorable to wound healing. The organism places the wound at the top priority of substrate competition in the early post-traumatic phase: the wound has precedence, and the rest of the body must devote substances to the wound, after which tensile strength is readily gained. Later on, when the patient passes into positive nitrogen balance, the tissues that are being rebuilt are chiefly skeletal muscle and later storage fat. The wound has fallen from its favored position. The positive nitrogen balance of late convalescence represents reaccumulation of striated muscle, as can be readily demonstrated by limb measurements or measurements in body strength, as well as by the simple arithmetic calculation that there is no place else in the body where so much protein can be stored so rapidly. If, during this period of late body rebuilding, the wound is not already healed, it is very difficult to make it heal except by reoperation or administration of ACTH. It is our interpretation of these events —if chronic anemia or invasive infection is not a part of the picture—that the trauma has restored the wound again to top priority in the body's economy.

The statement made above, that wounds normally heal in the presence of a negative nitrogen balance, should not be taken to mean that it is unimportant for the surgical patient to pass into positive nitrogen balance. When the time comes for anabolism to ensue, adequate intake must be given the patient. If he does not go into nitrogen positivity at this time, convalescence will not progress. It is his muscular mass, not the wound, which gains protein during anabolism.

CLINICAL METABOLIC MANAGEMENT

It is not the purpose of this chapter to describe in detail all of surgical care as regards the treatment of water and electrolyte abnormalities, nutritional deficiency, burns, heart failure or renal failure. These are detailed elsewhere in this book. Instead, it is our purpose to outline those endocrine and metabolic processes which form the basis of surgical care. In this section will be described briefly a few of the most important aspects of convalescence the daily clinical management of which rests on these metabolic principles.

NORMAL CONVALESCENCE AFTER MODERATELY SEVERE SURGERY WITH TEMPORARY INTERRUPTION OF GASTRO-INTESTINAL FUNCTION

The endocrine and metabolic response to surgery does most of our job for us here. This is the traumatic situation for which nature has "designed" the trauma response. Only a few therapeutic details need be considered in a general program of early diet and minimum meddling. If the patient is given no water, his lung, skin and urine losses will produce dehydration; therefore, the intravenous administration of water (with glucose to render it isotonic to red cells) should be provided if low fluid intake by mouth must persist 24 hours or more. The antidiuretic tendency helps to reduce the amount of water that need be given. It is unnecessary to give more than 1,000 to 1,500 cc. intravenously per day to an individual unless there is hyperpnea, fever or extrarenal losses, all of which greatly increase the water requirement.

Some surgeons feel that sodium chloride should not be given at all during this period; others, that a small amount should be. The onset of sodium conservation after surgery is variable, and there is no great choice between the two alternatives. All are agreed that the intravenous or the oral administration of large amounts of sodium (75-250 mEq.) in the early postoperative days will result in excessive sodium accumulation in the body with a tendency to hypoproteinemia and edema. Of course, pathologic renal or extrarenal losses increase the need for sodium.

The use of potassium is unnecessary unless the outlook is for a prolonged absence of oral intake. If such persists over 3 days, the use of intravenous potassium as the chloride (40 mEq. per day) is advisable until feeding starts.

Oral diet should be advanced as peristalsis and the passage of feces or flatus permit. When a gastrointestinal anastomosis has been done, it is our general aim to have the patient at the level of 500 calories and 5 Gm. of protein (oral) by the 5th day. When there is no anastomosis and insignificant peritoneal reaction, advancement may of course be more rapid. And, when there is any delay, distention, tenderness or fever, the diet should be held up until clinical signs of digestive function are propitious. Lack of diet at this stage will not interfere with wound healing or recovery; distention may be the forerunner of wound dehiscence or pulmonary complications. The nutritional objective at this stage of surgical convalescence is a scaphoid abdomen.

PROLONGED INTRAVENOUS FEEDING

When dietary advancement cannot occur and prolonged intravenous feeding is necessary, certain general rules are helpful. These are:

1. Frequent check of the patient's weight is vital.

2. Weight gain means water accumulation, and is undesirable.

3. Sudden weight loss of more than 500 Gm. means dehydration, and is undesirable. The only exception is when high fever is present and catabolic weight loss is greatly accelerated.

4. A weight loss of 150 to 250 Gm. per day should be expected, as evidence of the fat oxidation inevitable until anabolism is established.

5. Total water intake should equal losses by all routes, allowing for renal output of 1,000 cc.

6. Total salt intake (Na, Cl, K) should balance all losses accurately, allowing for daily urine excretion of 40 mEq. of each ion. Do not try to replace daily urine losses of Na and Cl quantitatively!

7. Maximum carbohydrate intake is desirable to lessen nitrogen losses in the chronic situation, so long as the carbohydrate is utilized and intense glycosuria is avoided. From 50 to 150 Gm. of glucose is easily given (200-600 calories). By caval catheter much larger amounts may be used.

8. Intravenous amino acids are useful in the chronic situation so long as the calorie: nitrogen ratios in the 200 range are obtainable. It is much easier to give nitrogen than the calories adequate to support protein synthesis from that nitrogen.

9. Intravenous fat and alcohol can be used to provide additional calories.

10. At least one whole blood transfusion should be given each week to provide whole protein and red cells.

11. Need for additional blood, plasma or albumin is determined by blood volume and serum-protein concentration.

Most of the above maxims are self-evident. The reason for avoiding quantitative replacement of urine Na and Cl losses lies in the normal renal regulation of the extracellular phase. As a patient with large intestinal sodium losses gradually returns to "zero balance," his renal excretion of sodium gradually increases as his need for sodium decreases; then, as the intensity of sodium therapy diminishes during recovery as a bowel tone increases with resorption of luminal fluid, there may even be a brisk diuresis of sodium. Clearly, it would be a mistake to persist in replacing all this renal loss. Therefore, the rule is to replace extrarenal losses quantitatively, allowing a "modicum" (40 mEq. of each ion) for renal coverage. In an elderly patient or one with edema, even this "modicum" should be omitted.

POTASSIUM LOSS AND ALKALOSIS

The loss of potassium which follows surgery is ordinarily well tolerated, if not unduly prolonged: the serum potassium remains normal or becomes slightly elevated, despite the loss of potassium from the body. This is not the case if the patient is losing gastrointestinal secretion and is developing a metabolic alkalosis. Such an example is commonly to be found in pyloric obstruction. In this circumstance the potassium concentration may drop precipitously after surgery and the patient develops "hypokaliemic alkalosis." The effects of operation have produced retention of sodium (with an acid urine) and loss of potassium with a resultant severe exacerbation in alkalosis and a lowering of the serum potassium due both to the alkalosis and to the increased rate of potassium excretion.

This clinical and chemical syndrome is characterized by fever, lethargy, distention, absent peristalsis and a high CO_2, low potassium, normal sodium and a low chloride in the plasma. Electrocardiographic changes are marked and constitute a valuable warning sign and therapeutic guide, even though they are not a direct index of the serum-potassium concentration.

If the patient is alkalotic prior to surgery, the most important step with reference to hypokaliemic alkalosis is prevention of the syndrome by correction of the alkalosis prior to surgery. The administration of a 1 per cent ammonium chloride solution in the amount of 500 to 1,000 ml. suffices to lower the CO_2 combining power approximately 4 to 8 mM./L. in a normal-sized adult. Such therapy (plus KCl) should be continued until normal acid-base balance is restored, preferably before surgery. Then, when surgery is carried out, potassium-chloride therapy should be resumed and carried out with vigor until acid-base balance, dietary intake and serum potassium are shown to be maintained and normal.

Should the patient be operated upon when alkalotic, or should a metabolic alkalosis due to chloride loss ensue after surgery, then the situation of postoperative hypokaliemic alkalosis is almost inevitable unless treatment is well calculated and active. This treatment should consist in the intravenous administration of both potassium chloride and ammonium chloride. Frequent electrocardiograms are of great assistance in therapy. The electrocardiographic changes of hypokaliemia (low T-wave, appearance of a U-wave, depressed S-T segment) are not determined solely by the serum-potassium concentration, yet they provide a good danger signal and are more easily performed than serum-potassium determinations. When a patient is in critical condition because of hypokaliemia, it is good practice to study the serum-potassium concentration daily and to take more frequent electrocardiograms to assure one's self that the cardiac toxicity of hypokaliemia is not becoming more pronounced.

Hypokaliemic alkalosis most commonly occurs in patients with large extrarenal losses; the management should include the general procedures mentioned on page 274 (intravenous maintenance) and on page 278 (extrarenal salt losses).

HYPERKALIEMIA AND ACIDOSIS IN RENAL INSUFFICIENCY

The normal postoperative endocrinology and metabolism result in the release of potassium (100-300 mEq. in the 1st week) from the body's muscle mass. As mentioned above, this usually produces an increased renal excretion of the ion.

When renal function is impaired, as in post-traumatic renal insufficiency, lower nephron nephrosis, chronic renal disease or obstructive uropathy, a metabolic acidosis results, and the excess potassium released from the muscle mass by the trauma accumulates in the extracellular phase, producing hyperkaliemia.

The rise in serum potassium which occurs after injury when renal insufficiency is present may be quite rapid and will, in general, be much more rapid than the rising potassium seen in chronic renal failure without antecedent trauma. Acidosis accentuates the rise just as alkalosis accentuates a fall. After massive wounds with renal failure, the rise in serum potassium will occur at a rate of between 0.5 and 1.0 mEq./day. Within 3 days the serum potassium may be as high as 8 mEq./L. Ventricular fibrillation and sudden death may occur as a result.

It is beyond the scope of this chapter to discuss in detail the treatment of renal insufficiency and its attendant hyperkaliemia. Potassium intake should be avoided, and frequent electrocardiograms again provide a sensitive index of the degree of cardiac toxicity which is the dangerous feature of the situation. Potassium may be removed from the body by gastrointestinal suction, the use of resins, peritoneal lavage and the use of some sort of external dialysis such as the artificial kidney. The important point here is that the endocrine change which follows surgery greatly accelerates the release of potassium from cells, so that, when kidney function is inadequate, serum potassium rises much more rapidly than it would be in the nontraumatized state.

WATER METABOLISM

The fact that the postoperative patient does not excrete water normally means that he should not be given more water than he can lose. If he does not go to surgery in a dehydrated state, his water administration in the first few days should correspond to a summation of his losses by lung and skin, plus his expected urinary excretion. In the normal afebrile adult male, insensible loss (lungs and skin) is about 750 ml. per day; the urinary loss the first day is about 500 ml., and the second day about 750 ml. For this reason, amounts of electrolyte-free water totaling between 1,000 and 1,500 ml. on the 1st day are quite adequate. If there is some electrolyte loss through the gastrointestinal tract, the addition of a moderate amount of salt to this water (for example, 75 mEq. of sodium and a like amount of chloride) is well tolerated by the patient, and a transient positive sodium balance will not harm him.

The female tends to have lesser rates of lung and skin loss, and in the adult female these may not total much more than 500 ml. per day if afebrile.

The factors which most rapidly increase the loss of water by lungs and skin are fever and rapid respirations. A patient with a fever of 103° who is breathing rapidly with his mouth open may lose as much as 2,000 ml. of water a day through his lungs and skin. Clearly, an educated guess as to his losses must be made, and, if the situation is critical, daily weights should be taken.

The most accurate check of water metabolism in the postoperative patient is provided by his daily weight fluctuation. Because of the loss of nitrogen and the oxidation of fat, we expect the postoperative patient to lose from 150 to 350 Gm. a day for the first few days until anabolism becomes established again. If he does not lose weight or if he gains, or if he loses weight much more rapidly than this, we can assume on the one hand that he is being given too much water, or on the other that he is becoming dehydrated.

The administration of too much electrolyte-free water produces plasma hypotonicity recognized by low sodium, low chloride, low serum protein and a washed-out appearance of the patient. The administration of inadequate water in a patient with high insensible losses or large extrarenal losses from the gastrointestinal tract produces appearances which are familiar to all as extracellular dehydration, consisting of apathy, lethargy, thirst, a dry, coated tongue, loss of skin turgor and a glassy expression.

The adjustment of water therapy to requirements is best carried out by accurate measurements of water losses, an educated guess as to insensible loss and, in severe instances, the use of frequent measurement of body weight. When extrarenal loss or prolonged starvation is a part of the picture, loss analyses are essential.

PLASMA HYPOTONICITY, THE LOW SODIUM SYNDROMES

As already mentioned, one of the expected sequelae of a surgical operation is a slight fall in the serum sodium concentration. As recovery progresses, the sodium concentration returns to normal with little need for therapy. The cause of this normal hyponatremia is not fully understood. It is not wholly accounted for by the accumulation of water on the basis of fat oxidation and antidiuresis, although such a mechanism is of major importance.

In a wide variety of circumstances, this normal slight hyponatremia (sodium falling to 130-135 mEq./L.) is replaced by a profound hyponatremia with the sodium falling as low as 120 or even lower, and of long duration. The hyponatremia may be slow to occur, coming on a week or two after surgery if complications are severe. In certain instances, particularly heart disease, kidney disease and liver disease, the low sodium may be present prior to surgery, in which case operation will accentuate the defect. Since the osmolarity of the serum is largely determined by the serum sodium concentration in those instances in which there is not an excessively high blood sugar or blood urea, the presence of a low serum sodium is accompanied by marked plasma hypotonicity and, presumably, dilution of cellular constituents.

A low serum sodium concentration denotes a sick patient: if preoperative, it carries a bad prognosis for the outcome of surgery; if postoperative, it suggests that convalescence is far from complete. This suggestion is usually quite obvious from the presence of other defects, the most common of which are continued open wounds, continued infection and lack of caloric intake.

There are usually multiple causations in the production of a very low serum sodium, but in any given instance one mechanism may predominate. The accumulation of water, accentuated by antidiuretic mechanisms, is often of importance. Also important are lack of adequate caloric intake, loss of sodium from the body through either renal or extrarenal losses and, in some instances, disease of liver and kidney, as well as heart and adrenals. By an orderly process, the surgeon should seek out the predominant cause of the low serum sodium concentration, since certain causes are remediable, and, when remedied, convalescence is accelerated.

The possibility that the patient has been given *too much water* may be checked by history, by his weight and by the presence of edema. Current water intake should be markedly restricted, and, when water has been overadministered and serum sodium is low, minimal water administration for a day or two, permitting the patient to blow off water by lungs and lose it by kidney, is a reasonable procedure. Characteristically, edematous states are accompanied by a low serum sodium.

Excessive *urinary* loss should be sought out. The urine should be analyzed for its sodium content very early in the course. If, in the presence of a low serum sodium concentration, the urine sodium concentration is higher than 30 mEq./L., one may be confident that either renal or adrenal disease exists.* In such a case, the patient's care must be based on unregulated renal salt loss. This requires daily urine sodium analyses and, unlike the urine from a normal kidney, accurate salt replacement, and hormone therapy if adrenal function is found to be low.

If it is discovered that the patient's urine sodium concentration is extremely low, and if no edema is present, so that renal mechanisms as well as the excessive accumulation of water are ruled out, one is left with plasma hypotonicity as a complication either of *visceral disease* or *caloric starvation*. The presence of heart failure, liver diseases, unhealed wounds and starvation tends to produce plasma hypotonicity. The administration of moderate amounts of hypertonic saline (300 ml. of 3% sodium chloride) may be carried out cautiously for a few days, the infusion being given every other day, to study the response. In occasional instances, the sodium concentration will start upward with a good water diuresis and gradual mending of the plasma hypotonicity. However, if such does not occur, it is dangerous to continue hypertonic saline administration, since further edema production will be the result.

If the patient is taking a very low caloric intake but his surgical convalescence other-

---

* This test should be based on an overnight collection, taken when no sodium is being given intravenously.

wise is progressing satisfactorily, it is safe to give one or two infusions of hypertonic saline and then concentrate on caloric intake, confident that as caloric intake increases serum sodium concentration will return to normal. We have seen instances in which the administration of adequate calories alone has produced a restoration of the serum sodium concentration. An explanation of this is lacking, but, as a working hypothesis, one may assume that it requires energy at the cell surface to exclude sodium from the cell and that in the face of starvation, sodium tends to leak into the cellular mass.

EXTRARENAL SALT LOSS

Finally, there are those hypotonic syndromes associated with extrarenal salt loss such as vomiting, diarrhea, intestinal or pancreatic fistulas. If the loss is very high in sodium concentration (pancreatic juice sometimes runs as high as 185 mEq./L.), it is not remarkable that loss of only a liter or two produces drastic reduction in the serum sodium concentration with lowering of the extracellular volume and, in some cases, a shocklike state, with hemoconcentration. When the sodium concentration of the lost fluid is lower, as, for instance, in gastric or duodenal contents, other events must take place for this loss to lower the serum sodium concentration. As mentioned in the preceding section, the three most common complications are (1) the administration of excessive amounts of electrolyte-free water through error, (2) the accumulation of sodium-free water by the lysis of cell material and the release of cellular water and (3) caloric starvation with the accumulation of the water of oxidation of fat.* Therefore, the treatment of extrarenal losses of salt must take into consideration all these factors, as well as replacement of external loss and the regulation of acid-base balance.

In discussing plasma hypotonicity, the center of attention is on the sodium ion. Of course, chloride is important, and its differential loss or accumulation produces metabolic alkalosis or fixed acid acidosis, respectively. But under conditions of external loss and serum dilution, the chloride changes tend to

* It is not generally realized that the oxidation of a kilogram of fat releases more than a liter of water.

parallel sodium, and it is the sodium ion which is dominant in determining the serum osmolarity, because small differential losses or retentions of chloride are compensated for osmotically by respiratory mechanisms. When sodium is lost from the system, nothing else can accumulate in the cation column; when chloride is lost, bicarbonate accumulates through respiratory adjustments. Alkalosis, rather than hypotonicity, is the result. The lungs and the kidney conserve acid-base balance at the expense of tonicity in almost all instances seen in surgery.

The detailed management of the patient with large gastrointestinal losses of sodium, chloride, potassium and other electrolytes through vomiting, fistula, diarrhea, etc., is beyond the scope of this chapter. The management of sodium, chloride and potassium loss has already been mentioned. The general principle may be summarized by stating that the patient should be carried "in balance." One of the remarkable things about the biochemical and metabolic management of sick surgical patients is that such good results may be attained by the use of fairly simple salt mixtures, including sodium, chloride, potassium and water. This is especially true in dealing with extrarenal loss.

The use of hypertonic salt solution (300 ml. of 3% sodium chloride, for example) is extremely useful in the repair of salt deficit accompanied by low serum concentration, and due to extrarenal loss. The effectiveness of 1 per cent ammonium chloride in treating extrarenal chloride loss with alkalosis should be re-emphasized.

HYPOPROTEINEMIA

The commonest cause of hypoproteinemia in surgical patients is the overadministration of salt and water. The postoperative tendency to retain salt and water, if not properly evaluated by the surgeon, may result in the overadministration of these substances and the production of hypoproteinemia.

Clearly, the best step is prevention. If overadministration has occurred and hypoproteinemia results, the steps to take must be balanced carefully between avoidance for a few days of much fluid therapy, the use of diuretic agents or the use of concentrated albumin. A nice choice between these depends upon the cardiac reserve, ventilatory capacity and renal function of the patient.

Starvation alone, without water-and-salt loading, is remarkable for the preservation of normal serum protein and oncotic pressure, even though body protein is markedly depleted. Chronic and acute parenchymatous liver disease are important causes of hypoalbuminemia. If surgery has to be done, concentrated albumin is of use in temporary passive support of the albumin concentration.

Eosinophil Changes and Endocrine Failure

The occurrence of outright adrenal failure after surgery with the persistence of a high eosinophil count is a rare cause of shock and hypotension in surgery. Much commoner causes should be sought with care, not only because they are commoner but also because they are frequent causes of death. Examples are inadequate blood replacement, massive infection, pulmonary, embolus, coronary occlusion, unsuspected pneumothorax, hemopericardium and mediastinal emphysema. These are the commonest causes of so-called "irreversible shock" in man; yet, despite its rarity, adrenal failure should be considered in the differential diagnosis of postoperative hypotension because therapy is specific and effective. As part of this diagnosis a high eosinophil count may be observed.* But before passing on to a discussion of adrenal failure it is appropriate to review some of the other abnormalities of the eosinophil count.

By far the commonest abnormality of the eosinophil count in surgical patients is the maintained low count late after surgery, when recovery is expected. An example might be found in a patient having a combined abdominoperineal resection in whom oral intake has not been resumed at quite the speed one might hope, some distention has persisted and some fever has continued. By the 5th to the 7th day the eosinophil count should be high and rising. If it is still found low or at zero, it is highly suggestive that a pathologic process

ess is present, and it should be sought out and corrected. An example in such a case would be partial intestinal obstruction, undrained sepsis in the posterior wound or phlebothrombosis. As a general rule, a low eosinophil count 4 days or more after surgery, when the wound is closed, suggests the presence of a continuing surgical complication, which should be sought out and corrected. On the contrary, in the patient whose recovery seems slow but the eosinophil count is normal, complications are absent and the prognosis is good.

The time at which a rising count should be expected depends upon the nature of the surgery. In ordinary soft tissue surgery or elective skeletal surgery involving a primarily sutured wound, the eosinophil count should be on its upward course between the 4th and the 7th days. A continued low count after this time means trouble.

In the instance of fractures or burns, the eosinophil count remains low for a longer time. The maintenance of a low eosinophil count more than 3 weeks after an extensive body burn suggests that some pathologic process is present which is uncorrected, and this continued low count holds a very ominous prognosis. In the case of burns the commonest example would be infection or renal failure.

When patients have been ill for prolonged periods of time, their eosinophil counts may be rather high (500-2,000 per cu. mm.) and may then rise paradoxically with trauma. A common example is to be found in a patient with a burn whose count has risen normally at the 2nd week but who still has some wound to be closed as late as the 6th or the 8th week. In such circumstances the eosinophil count may be found to be between 600 and 800 per cu. mm., and it may rise well over 2,000 with surgery. In our experience, this paradoxical eosinophilia of chronic disease has not been associated with any other evidence of adrenal failure, and it should not be regarded as such.

Finally, resting abnormalities of the eosinophil count may be mentioned briefly. A resting high count over 1,000 per cu. mm. suggests the presence either of allergy or of borderline adrenal insufficiency. The differential diagnosis should not be difficult, the standard tests being employed for both conditions. A resting low count under 50 per cu. mm. suggests that the patient is under some psychological stress,

---

* Even in the presence of a low eosinophil count, one may encounter individuals with unregulated urinary salt loss. In occasional instances this is due apparently to borderline hypoadrenalism, since the renal tubule will respond to DOCA or other salt-retaining hormones.

that he is harboring unsuspected disease or that he has hyperadrenocorticism.

Surgery or acute infection in Addison's disease has been known for years to result in a shocklike state and a fatal outcome in most instances. The recognition of the need of the postoperative patient for steroid hormones in adequate quantity makes it possible to carry addisonian patients successfully through surgical experiences, and has given rise to a whole new era of surgery in which the adrenal glands themselves are removed for the treatment of hyperadrenocorticism, carcinoma or, in rare instances, of other diseases such as hypertension.

The spontaneous occurrence of postsurgical hypoadrenalism, or what might better be called post-traumatic endocrine failure, is very rare. It has been observed in patients with disease around the pituitary gland, in the thyroid or in the adrenals.

Patients with an inadequate endocrine response often do very poorly after surgery. The clinical picture will consist of some or all of the following:

1. Failure to maintain blood pressure and the appearance of clinical shock

2. Failure to maintain urine output

3. A high sodium concentration in what urine is formed

4. A tendency to fall in the serum sodium concentration

5. A tendency to rise in the serum potassium concentration

6. A maintained normal or high eosinophil count in the early post-traumatic phase

7. Lack of elevation of blood or urine steroids

The commonest causes of adrenal failure are adrenal tuberculosis and acute adrenal hemorrhage, often associated with the use of anticoagulants. The recognition of this rare syndrome is important, because a very ominous clinical situation may readily be restored to normal convalescence by the administration of adrenal hormones. In an acute situation of this type, the administration of compound F intravenously, in doses of 75 to 150 mg., followed in a day or two by the administration of compound E or F by mouth in the dosage of 50 to 100 mg., suffices. There are only a few situations in surgery in which short periods of cortisone therapy are harmful. For this reason,

"blind therapy" occasionally is needed, though never excusable if precise diagnostic methods can be undertaken.

In no circumstances should massive cortisone therapy be continued for more than 5 days in such a situation. It should be tapered off and replaced with ACTH, which in turn should be tapered off and stopped within a few days. If the patient does not do well on cessation of therapy, and blood and urine steroid levels establish that adrenal function has been completely lost or abolished (as by adrenal hemorrhage or previously undiagnosed Addison's disease), then continued cortisone replacement therapy at a low dosage, between 25 and 50 mg. per day, may be continued.

Hemorrhage from the gastro-intestinal tract is the most dangerous complication of cortisone or ACTH therapy in surgical patients, and it should be guarded against by using such therapy only for short periods and by covering the patient with ordinary antacid therapeutics during the period of therapy.

CALORIE AND NITROGEN FACTORS IN THE DIET

The administration of an adequate diet as soon as feasible after surgery is a first rule of surgical care. Its most common abuse arises from the unjustified assumption that the administration of caloric intake immediately after surgical operation will somehow alter or reverse the metabolic processes which follow surgery, and that such reversal is desirable. The premature administration of calories by mouth or by tube to a patient whose gastro-intestinal tract is not yet functioning produces gastric distention and vomiting. The results of these complications are decreased diaphragmatic excursion, discomfort, distention and, at the worst, aspiration pneumonia. For this reason, a realistic appraisal of the need and the acceptance of the patient for diet after surgery is of front-rank importance. It is in this sphere that an understanding of the dynamic aspects of surgical convalescence is of such importance. A patient who in the first 3 days after surgery needs or requires very little in the way of caloric or nitrogen intake, by a week or two after surgery literally craves intake, and an intake of calories and nitrogen in a well-balanced oral diet is an indispensable aid to recovery. No general rules may be made. Hunger, the presence of audible peristalsis and the anal expulsion of swallowed air are the most important signals for dietary advancement in the care of the surgical patient. Patients who are in the late postoperative period but are in coma may have to be fed by tube, and, if this is done carefully, it may produce recovery. In other instances, when diet cannot be taken because of gastrointestinal disease, one must weigh carefully the possible usefulness of gastrostomy, jejunostomy or high caloric intravenous feedings with glucose, alcohol or fat. When tube feedings are used, adequate water intake must be provided. In all circumsances, an adequate supply of vitamins must be provided.

The administration of glucose intravenously kills hunger; in a patient in whom the transfer to oral intake is a matter of concern, it is of critical importance to omit the "morning intravenous" and give warm, appetizing tasty fluids and soft solids.

The ratio of calories to nitrogen in the intake is of importance because of the fact that protein synthesis will not occur in the absence of adequate caloric intake. The calorie:nitrogen ratio is defined as the ratio of nonprotein calories to protein nitrogen in the diet. A normal resting individual consumes a calorie:nitrogen ratio of about 200 (2,400 calories and 12 Gm. nitrogen per day). As large workloads are imposed, this calorie:nitrogen ratio rises. Early caloric supplementation in the diet must be viewed with reservation because of the limitations on gastrointestinal function already mentioned. As convalescence progresses, the calorie:nitrogen ratio required for anabolism decreases progressively until at about the 7th day after operation such as cholecystectomy, prostatectomy, gastrectomy, pneumonectomy, a calorie:nitrogen ratio of about 150 will suffice for beginning anabolism. An example would be found in a caloric intake of 1,200 per day with 8 Gm. of nitrogen. As oral intake increases the calorie:nitrogen ratio will naturally increase to about 200, where anabolism is most satisfactory. The problem of calorie:nitrogen ratios arises particularly in intravenous feedings. Prolonged caloric lack produces bodily depletion and cachexia, a special endocrine and metabolic picture.

THE SYNDROME OF DEPLETION

A complete account of the body compositional changes of depletion is beyond the scope of this chapter. However, since depletion produces an accumulation of water and salt by endocrine mechanisms, it is appropriate to mention it briefly.

As used here, the word *depletion* denotes cachexia due to starvation of a variety of causations, the most common causes in surgery being gastrointestinal carcinoma, intestinal obstruction of other sources, chronic sepsis, ulcerative colitis, regional enteritis, long-standing obstructing duodenal ulcer.

Common to all these conditions is loss of tissue, loss of energy and loss of social effectiveness. There is a loss of muscle mass and of fat which is quite obvious to the onlooker, and it is noticeable to the patient, not only when looking in the mirror but when trying to carry out his work. Much thinking on this subject has been devoted to the selection of *"deficits"* which the patient has. It is also important to emphasize that the syndrome of depletion includes several very important *"excesses."*

In the *deficit* column should be included fat and muscle mass. This lack of muscle mass means that the total body protein, as well as the total body potassium, magnesium, sulfate and other intracellular ions, is low. But the most important deficit might be defined as a "chronic energy deficit." This is traceable to lack of caloric intake which has produced gradual combustion of body tissue.

The most important relative *"excesses"* are those of water and extracellular salt, of which sodium has been studied most extensively. These patients have too much water in their body, both in relative and in absolute terms. As fat disappears, the relative proportion of the body which is water of course rises because of their inverse relationship to each other. In addition, patients with chronic depletion show a marked antidiuretic tendency, and they will retain much of the water that they are able to drink. Since they frequently are unable to take solid foods but still have access to liquids, the accumulation of water is very marked. The renal tendency to retain sodium appears to be steroidal (aldosterone) in character. Therefore, the body compositional defect is summarized as being to little fat and too little muscle, with too much water, too much of which is extracellular water, and too much sodium.

In congestive heart failure (as in mitral stenosis), this defect is especially pronounced as regards excessive accumulation of water and salt. Decreased caloric intake, so characteristic of the later phases of the disease, and poor tissue oxygenation associated with low cardiac output both contribute to the defect.

The serum concentrations of sodium and potassium show an interesting inverse relationship to the body content. The serum potassium tends to be high (4.5-5.5 mEq./L.) despite the obvious depletion of body cellular mass and, therefore, potassium. The serum-sodium concentration tends to be low (125-135 mEq./L.) despite the measurable excess of body sodium. An understanding of the metabolic and endocrine defect in the depletion syndrome is basic to good surgical management.

Surgery in this depleted condition can be carried out successfully, and wound healing often is remarkably good. However, it is important in managing such patients to avoid infusions of further salt or water. The patient should come to surgery (1) dry, (2) with normal osmotic and oncotic pressure, (3) in normal acid-base balance and (4) with a store of liver glycogen. He cannot be "rebuilt" before surgery, but these objectives can be attained, along with a liberal supply of water-soluble vitamins.

Blood-volume changes in late depletion have been the source of much misunderstanding: the concept has become current that such patients always have low volumes because of their low hematocrits. In our experience such has not been the case unless hemorrhage has been a significant feature of the disease process. In the absence of significant blood loss (carcinoma of the esophagus, the stomach, the left colon), the typical picture is a low red cell mass and a high plasma volume, the latter especially marked if edema is present. The hazards of indiscriminate overuse of preoperative transfusion are obvious.

On the credit side of the ledger is the fact that these depleted patients rebuild their body stores with great readiness if they are given food and are able to absorb it. The depleted patient's tissues are "thirsty" for nitrogen. All workers who have studied such patients have noted the very low calorie:nitrogen ratios required for positive nitrogen balance in these patients. If they are operated upon with gentleness and care, with vitamins provided and infection avoided, the postoperative course may be most gratifying. But they are "sensitive and brittle," and their immediate preoperative and postoperative management must be condtioned by the facts that they have very little fat to burn for oxidative energy after surgery, that they already have too much water in their bodies and are extremely vulnerable to further water infusions, and that they have too much salt and are on the verge of generalized and pulmonary edema at the time of surgery. If tissues are handled gently and edema is avoided, wound healing will be solid.

SUMMARY

This chapter has covered a wide variety of factors important in the care of surgical patients. No extensive summary is possible.

An understanding of normal surgical endocrinology and metabolism is the first requirement in good surgical care.

BIBLIOGRAPHY

Albright, F.: Cushing's syndrome: its pathological physiology, its relationship to the adreno-genital syndrome, and its connection with the problem of the reaction of the body to injurious agents ("alarm reaction" of Selye), Harvey Lect. 38:123, 1942-1943.

Ariel, L. M., and Kremen, A. J.: Compartmental distribution of sodium chloride in surgical patients pre- and postoperatively, Ann. Surg. 132:1009, 1950.

Bland, J. H.: The Clinical Use of Fluid and Electrolyte, Philadelphia, Saunders, 1952.

Cannon, W. B.: Bodily Changes in Pain, Hunger, Fear and Rage, New York, Appleton, 1915.

Coller, F. A., Campbell, K. N., Vaughan, H. H., Iob, L. V., and Moyer, C. A.: Postoperative salt intolerance, Ann. Surg. 119:533, 1944.

Cope, O., Nardi, G. L., Quijano, M., Rovit, R. L., Stanbury, J. B., and Wight, A.: Metabolic rate and thyroid function following acute thermal trauma in man, Ann. Surg. 137:165, 1953.

Cuthbertson, D. P.: Observations on the disturbance of metabolism produced by injury to the limbs, Quart. J. Med. N.S. 1:233, 1932.

————: Post-shock metabolic response, Lancet *1*:433, 1942.

Dudley, H. A., Boling, E. A., LeQuesne, L. P., and Moore, F. D.: Studies on antidiuresis in surgery: effects of anesthesia, surgery and posterior pituitary antidiuretic hormone on water metabolism in man, Ann. Surg. *140*:354, 1954.

Elman, R.: Minimum postoperative maintenance requirements for parenteral water sodium, potassium, chloride and glucose, Ann. Surg. *130*: 703, 1949.

Forbes, A. P., Donaldson, E. C., Reifenstein, E. C., Jr., and Albright, F.: The effect of trauma and disease on the urinary 17-ketosteroid excretion in man, J. Clin. Endocrinol. *7*:264, 1947.

Franksson, C., Gemzell, C. A., and Euler, von, U. S.: Cortical and medullary adrenal activity in surgical and allied conditions, J. Clin. Endocrinol. *14*:608, 1954.

Gamble, J. L.: Chemical Anatomy, Physiology and Pathology of Extracellular Fluid, Cambridge, Mass., Harvard, 1952.

Goldenberg, I. S., Lutwak, L., Rosenbaum, T. J., and Hayes, M. A.: Thyroid-adrenocortical interrelations following operation, Surg., Gynec. & Obst. *98*:513, 1954.

Hardy, J. D.: Surgery and the Endocrine System, Philadelphia, Saunders, 1952.

Howard, J. E.: Protein metabolism during convalescence after trauma. Recent studies. Arch. Surg. *50*:106, 1945.

Hume, D. M.: The neuro-endocrine response to injury: present status of the problem, Ann. Surg. *138*:548, 1953.

————: The role of the hypothalamus in the pituitary adrenal cortical response to stress, J. Clin. Invest. *28*:790, 1949.

Hume, D. M., and Nelson, D. H.: Corticoid output in adrenal venous blood of the intact dog, Fed. Proc. *13*:73, 1954.

Ingle, D. J.: Permissive action of hormones, J. Clin. Endocrinol. *14*:1272, 1954.

Ingle, D. J., Ward, E. O., and Kuizenga, M. H.: The relationship of the adrenal glands to changes in urinary non-protein nitrogen following multiple fractures in the force-fed rat, Am. J. Physiol. *149*:510, 1947.

Krieger, H., Abbott, W. E., Levey, S., Babb, L. I., and Holden, W. D.: Metabolic alterations in surgical patients: III. The influence of peritonitis on nitrogen, carbohydrate, electrolyte and water balance, Surgery *36*:580, 1954.

LeQuesne, L. P., and Lewis, A. A. G.: Postoperative water and salt retention, Lancet *1*:153, 1953.

Lockwood, J. S., and Randall, H. T.: The place of electrolyte studies in surgical patients, Bull. New York Acad. Med. *25*:228, 1949.

Merrill, J. P., Levine, H. D., Somerville, W., and Smith, S., III: Clinical recognition and treatment of acute potassium intoxication, Ann. Int. Med. *33*:797, 1950.

Moore, F. D.: Bodily changes in surgical convalescence. I. The normal sequence—observations and interpretations. Ann. Surg. *137*:289, 1953.

————: Bodily changes in surgical convalescence, a 1954 revision, p. 172, *in* Selye, H., and Heuser, G., eds.: Fourth Annual Report on Stress, Montreal, Acta Inc., 1954.

————: Isotope dilution. A theory, a method, a pathway to new horizons. Tr. & Stud. Coll. Physicians, Philadelphia *21*:106, 1954.

————: Metabolic Care of the Surgical Patient, Philadelphia, Saunders, 1959.

Moore, F. D., and Ball, M. R.: The Metabolic Response to Surgery, Springfield, Thomas, 1952.

Moore, F. D., Haley, H. B., Bering, E. A., Jr., Brooks, L., and Edelman, I. S.: Further observations on total body water. II. Changes of body composition in disease. Surg., Gynec. & Obst. *95*:155, 1952.

Moore, F. D., McMurrey, J. D., Parker, H. V., and Magnus, I. C.: Body composition: total body water and electrolytes; intravascular and extravascular phase volumes, Metabolism *5*: 447, 1956.

Moore, F. D., Steenburg, R. W., Ball, M. R., Wilson, G. M., and Myrden, J. A.: Studies in surgical endocrinology. I. The urinary excretion of 17-hydroxycorticoids, and associated metabolic changes, in cases of soft tissue trauma of varying severity and in bone trauma. Ann. Surg. *141*:145, 1955.

Moyer, C. A.: Acute temporary changes in renal function associated with major surgical procedures, Surgery *27*:198, 1950.

————: Fluid Balance: A Clinical Manual, Chicago, Year Book Pub., 1952.

Reddy, W. J., Jenkins, D., and Thorn, G. W.: Estimation of 17-hydroxycorticoids in urine, Metabolism *1*:511, 1952.

Reifenstein, E. C., Jr.: The metabolism of convalescence, p. 374, *in* Gordon, E. S., ed.: Symposium on Steroid Hormones, Madison, Wis., Univ. Wisconsin Press, 1950.

Rhoads, J. E.: Protein nutrition in surgical patients; collective review, Internat. Abstr. Surg. *94*:417, 1952.

Roberts, K. E., Poppell, J. W., and Randall, H. T.: Relation between renal oxygen consumption, carbon dioxide production and hydrogen ion secretion. Abstract submitted to American Physiological Society, 1956.

Roberts, K. E., Randall, H. T., Sanders, H. L.,

and Hood, M.: Effects of potassium on renal tubular reabsorption of bicarbonate, J. Clin. Invest. *34*:666, 1955.

Selye, H.: "Conditioning" various "permissive" actions of hormones, J. Clin. Endocrinol. *14*: 122, 1954.

————: The general adaptation syndrome and the diseases of adaptation, J. Clin. Endocrinol. *6*:117, 1946.

Steenburg, R. W., Lennihan, R., and Moore, F. D.: Studies in surgical endocrinology. II. The free blood 17-hydroxycorticoids in surgical patients; their relation to urine steroids, metabolism and convalescence. Ann. Surg. *143*:180, 1956.

Thorn, G. W., Jenkins, D., and Laidlaw, J. C.: The adrenal response to stress in man, p. 171, *in* Pincus, G., ed.: Recent Progress in Hormone Research, Proc. Laurenian Hormone Conf., vol. 8, New York, Acad. Press, 1953.

Tyler, F. H., Schmidt, C. D., Eik Nes, K., Brown H., and Samuels, L. T.: The role of the liver and the adrenal in producing elevated plasma 17-hydroxycorticosteroid levels in surgery, J. Clin. Invest. *33*:1507, 1954.

Wangensteen, O. H., and Zimmerman, B.: Observations on water intoxication in surgical patients, Surgery *31*:654, 1952.

Wilson, G. M., Edelman, I. S., Brooks, L., Myrden, J. A., Harken, D. E., and Moore, F. D.: Metabolic changes associated with mitral valvuloplasty, Circulation *9*:199, 1954.

Burns

Classification
Historical Considerations
Therapeutic Principles

CLASSIFICATION

Before the discovery of the principles of cutaneous grafting the care of those injured by heat devolved largely upon doctors of physic, the equivalent of the internist of today, and during the latter part of the 19th century the more especially upon the dermatologist. The discoveries that led to the inception of reconstructive surgery were the primary forces finally effecting the entry of the surgeon as the therapist of thermal and radiational injury.

Burns were once classified into 7 categories or degrees. Today some still employ a 4-degree classification, but lately a simpler one is being adopted. The 4-degree classification is as follows:

1st degree—erythema
2nd degree—death of epidermis while viable epidermal appendages remain within the dermis
3rd degree—death of the epidermis and all of its appendages in the dermis
4th degree—carbonification of the part.

The classification more recently advanced by surgeons is:

Partial-thickness cutaneous injury
Full-thickness cutaneous injury

Figure 64 shows the older and the newer classifications diagrammatically.

Often one is unable to determine for days whether a burn or a scald is a partial-thickness or a full-thickness cutaneous injury. It has been said that blistering denotes partial thickness; in truth, it is a good sign of partial-thickness injury should the person have been scalded, but it is often misleading should the injury have been caused by more than a momentary contact with hot metal, glowing coals, or flaming clothing. Under the latter circumstances the epidermal temperatures tend to rise above 100° C., and steam blisters may form while at the same time the dermis and all the epidermal appendages are killed. In other words, blistering may occur with a full-thickness injury. However, blistering after contact with hot water usually signifies that those parts of the hair follicles and the sweat glands lying below the superficial dermal capillaries are viable, and from them the epithelium will regenerate: a partial-thickness injury. The formation of blisters within or about a thermal cutaneous injury 12 or more hours after the exposure to heat is a sign of an infection within the dermis. Such belatedly formed blisters almost invariably contain large numbers of cocci, either staphylococci or streptococci, or both.

The retention of tactile and superficial pain sensibility (pin prick) and capillary pressure blanching in an area of burn are indicative of a partial-thickness injury. The combination of loss of tactile and pain sense to pin prick, the absence of pressure-blanching, the loss of cutaneous pliability, and visibility of small veins through the burned skin are indicative of a very deep partial or full-thickness burn or scald. However, a burn having all of the characteristics of a partial-thickness one when first seen may turn out subsequently to involve the whole thickness of the epidermis and its appendages. At times infection and other factors operating after the heat load has been dissipated evidently convert a partial-thickness into a full-thickness injury. What these factors are must await meticulous chemical studies of thermally injured skin of man.

In a few words, the depth of a burn or a scald cannot be estimated accurately for days

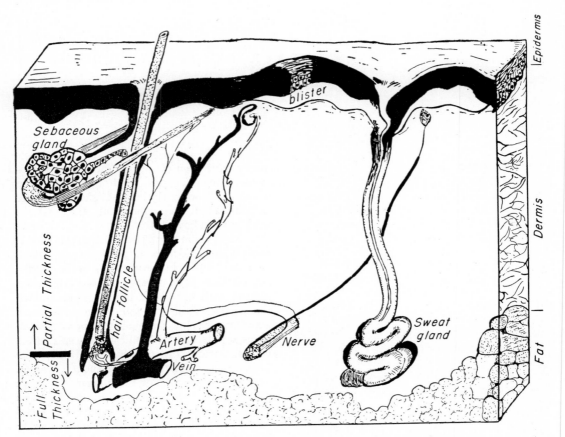

Fig. 16-1. The area of the skin is about 0.25 square meters at birth, and from 1.5 to 1.9 in adults. A standard formula for the calculation of surface area in man is as follows: surface area in square centimeters $= $ kilo-weight$^{0.425}$ $\times$ centimeter height$^{0.725}$ $\times$ 71.84.

The skin is primarily divisible into: (1) a superficial cellular ectodermal derivative, the epidermis and its appendages (sweat glands, hair follicles and sebaceous glands) and (2) a mesodermal derivative, the dermis. These two layers are underlaid by a layer of adipose tissue of variable thickness. The skin's thickness (epidermis and dermis) varies from 0.5 mm. over the eyelids and the ears to 3 to 6 mm. on the soles and the palms. The entire organ, exclusive of the fat layer, constitutes from 14 to 17 per cent of a lean adult's weight. In other words, it is one of the largest organs of the body. The thickness of the epidermis, exclusive of that on the palms and the soles, which is very thick (0.5 to 0.8 mm.), varies between 60 and 120 microns (0.06 to 0.12 mm.). A remarkably tough organ for all its thinness!

The dermis is from 5 to 10 times the thickness of the epidermis!

The epidermis contains no lymphatic or blood capillaries or nerve endings. These structures are contained especially within the superficial part of the dermis, and about the hair papillae, sweat glands, sebaceous glands and arrectores pilorum muscles. The capillaries are relatively few in the skin, numbering only 16 to 65 per square millimeter, while in skeletal muscle they number from 1,000 to 2,000. However, the skin contains numerous arteriolar venous shunts that constitute special structures, the cutaneous neuromyo-arterial glomera, that are important in regulating the radiational heat transfer from the body. When fully open, they are capable of shunting one fifth to one sixth of the resting cardiac output from the arterial to the venous system without passage of the blood through capillaries.

The structures affected in the old classification of burns are as follows:

First degree: (erythema) minor reversible damage to the epidermis with dilatation of the superficial dermal capillaries. (*Continued on facing page*)

after the injury; and the estimation of the depth of the burn soon after its sufferance often can be no more than an intelligent guess. If, with the passage of 2 to 4 weeks of time, a burn heals without grafting it was a partial-thickness injury. If the injured skin, the eschar, separates or is separable from the living tissue below the dermis, exposing fat, muscle, or bone, the injury was a full-thickness one.

The amount of heat needed to cause a full-thickness injury to the skin of man is remarkably small. Water at 85° C. will kill the whole skin in 10 seconds.[14, 22] The chemical changes within the cells of the skin accompanying heating just capable of killing it are unknown.[2, 30] Skin killed by heat takes up the dyes employed by histologists and pathologists in a fairly normal fashion for a day or two, and then the nucleoli, the chromatin granules and the nuclei disintegrate. However, the activity of a number of the enzymes involved in the Krebs cycle, namely, succinic dehydrogenase and fumarase decreases markedly in thermally injured skin very soon after the burn and long before any microscopic cellular changes have taken place.[5] The taking of multiple minute biopsies from burned skin and staining sections of them with tetrazolium dyes gives promise of permitting an earlier objective differentiation between partial and full-thickness burns than is now possible.

The formulation of therapeutic technics directed toward the reversal of heat injury to cells must await the time when the chemical changes associated with the heating of skin are known specifically and in detail. Until that day arrives, the primary objective of the treatment of the wound itself is—*above all, do no harm*. This adage has not always been followed in the recent past. Although the intellectual attitudes of Aristotle and Galen presumably have been our guides for centuries, they have been peculiarly ineffectual determinants of the therapy of burns and scalds. Sophisticated witchcraft better characterizes many of the past practices used in the treatment of the wound than does scientific objectivity. Often there has been practically no subjection of impressions regarding the supposed efficacy of a particular medicament or physical act to controlled experiment, though the steps requisite to the conduct of controlled experiment have been known for more than 2 centuries.

HISTORICAL CONSIDERATIONS

A historical outline* of the therapeutic practices directed toward the treatment of the burn wound during the 19th and the 20th centuries shows how far past therapeutic practices have strayed from the primary aim of *do no harm*.

The treatment of the thermal wound underwent a remarkable change about 1868. Listerism (antisepsis) then seized the minds of physicians. Consequently, one may divide the treatment of burns into two periods—one before Listerism and the other after.

The prevention of putrefaction was attempted before bacteria were discovered to be its cause. A mixture of mercuric chloride and lime water (aqua phagoedenical) was placed on burns in 1835, and even earlier silver nitrate was recommended. The idea of coagulating the wound arose, and the application of escharotics (silver nitrate) was begun about 1831. Tannic acid in water was employed for the same purpose in 1858, and turpentine in 1866.

The use of a pliable film as a dressing to

* Constructed from bibliographical references on burns and scalds in the Am. J. Med. Sc., Lancet, J.A.M.A., and Arch. f. Dermat. u. Syph. (Vols. 1 to current).

FIG. 16-1 (*Continued*)

Second degree: epidermal necrosis; variable dermal necrosis, but leaving viable deep parts of the epidermal appendages (hair follicles and sweat glands).

Third degree: complete epidermal and dermal necrosis (no viable epidermal appendages left).

The new classification lumps the older first and second orders into "partial thickness" and changes the term third degree to "full thickness."

The main structural components of the skin, excepting the lymphatics, are shown in this semischematic scale figure. The divisional level between partial and full-thickness injuries is shown in the left lower corner.

exclude the "harmful" air was adopted fairly widely on the Continent about 1830 when compound tincture of benzoin was used. In 1858 a mixture of castor oil and collodion was praised, the more especially because the film produced was transparent—*voilà* the modern Aeroplast.

The idea that the burn wound serves as a source of toxins gave rise to the wet dressing. A solution containing sodium and calcium chlorides was recommended by Lisfranc (1835); and Carron oil (a saturated solution of calcium hydroxide in linseed oil) gained so much favor after 1850 that it is used even today.

The bath was begun in 1845, using cold water to draw out the "caloric."* Oils and waxes have been placed on burns at least since Roman times—olive oil, the oil of flax (linseed oil), lard, tallow and beeswax are still used.

The idea that wounds healed the better if the raw area was fed by applying foodstuffs to it led to the application of flour in 1829 because of its high content of "animal gluten," and molasses (treacle) in 1847.

The dry cotton wool dressing was introduced into England from the United States, presumably via Charleston, S. C., between 1827 and 1831. Fine linen (gossamer) had long been placed upon the burns of the well-to-do. Syme[27] extolled the virtues of dry cotton wool in 1833, especially when applied "with a firm degree of pressure"—the pressure dressing.

The exposure of the wound long had been practiced on the Continent but had lost favor during the early 1800's. During the antiseptic, or post-Lister period, no new ideas regarding the care of the wound were introduced, but the emphasis changed. The dry cotton wool pressure dressing employed widely in England, Germany and France between 1830 and 1867 was superseded by a cotton dressing steeped in medicaments poisonous to bacteria and man alike. Physicians caring for burned individuals seemingly became bacteria-slayers and pus-eradicators who considered little that they might also eradicate the man as well as the bacteria.

Phenol first came into favor in 1867, a 14

* Caloric—the old term for heat that was supposed to stay in the burned area until withdrawn.

per cent solution in olive oil. This concentration of phenol kills unburned skin: what did it do to partial-thickness burns? Though the local and the general toxic propensities of phenol were soon recognized, a phenol-containing dressing was highly recommended at late as 1946.

The virtues of a saturated solution of boracic acid were extolled (1876) because it was cheap. It is still poured on dressings, even though it has been known to have poisoned man; toxicologically, bacteria seemingly tolerate it better than human beings.

Iodoform, soon recognized as a readily absorbable local and systemic poison, came along in 1887 and it is still to be found on the dressing carts of hospitals.

Picric acid, a more lethal agent, was dumped and sprayed upon burns after 1901. Recently, I had the opportunity of seeing an instance of acute picric acid poisoning attributable to the application of butesin picrate to a partial-thickness burn of the chest of a young man during December of 1953. The dressing had been applied by a recent graduate of a medical school.

The sulfonamides superseded picric and boracic acids as locally applied bacteria-killers in 1938, and the biologic antibiotics such as penicillin have won out over the sulfonamides since 1943.

The impervious dressing idea was extended after 1867; a combination of varnish, linseed oil, lead protoxide (litharge) and salicylic acid was compounded in 1881. It excluded air, kept the wound greased, killed organisms, and the salicylic acid separated the living tissue from the dead (chemical débridement. Gutta percha was praised in 1887. During World War I the English and the French almost came to blows over the priority rights to a paraffin dressing.

During the impetus of atomic fear Aeroplast has been born, although Edenbuizen's[6] experiments performed during the 1860's showed clearly that mammals cannot be covered over more than 30 per cent of the body's surface with materials impervious to fluid, such a gum arabic or linseed oil, without endangering life. In spite of this, the search still goes on for an easily applied spray-on dressing material. Should one be discovered that is not toxic and has the physical properties of epidermis, permitting the normal radiation of heat and the staying of the passage of water and salts as normal epidermis does, a significant contribution to the treatment of burns will be made. The likelihood of doing this, before much more is known about the skin, is rather remote. To our knowledge such a product is not available yet.

After 1925 the escharotics were raised from the dead. Tannic acid was reintroduced in 1925 when the modern medical tongue extolled it most fluently and persuasively. Somewhat belatedly (1942) it was found to possess few of the virtues claimed for it. In reality it is deadly: it is capable of converting a partial- to a full-thickness injury, it produces an impervious eschar that encloses infection, and it poisons the liver. During the late 1930's it was combined with silver nitrate, an agent long known to be inimical to healing of a wound.

The effects of therapeutic fadism upon the mortality attending thermal injury is shown in part in the plot of the burn mortality rates between 1833 and 1933 in the Glasgow Royal Infirmary (Fig. 16-2). The mortality rate between 1898 and 1910 was 3 times what it had been between 1853 and 1868.

THERAPEUTIC PRINCIPLES

Obviously, the therapeutic principles applicable to the thermal wound are:

1. Place nothing upon the wound having local or general toxic properties.

2. Provide for the free egress of pus if it forms.

3. Exclude the injured part from the bacteria carried by fomites, air, dressers and attendants.

4. Immobilize the injured part.

These aims can well be accomplished by the adoption of either one of two methods, or a combination of the two: exposure to air, or the application of an occlusive dressing.

In order that the occlusive dressing fulfill these aims it needs be made of a nontoxic material: vegetable fiber is suitable—cotton or linen; the innermost layer should be pervious to water. A thick coating of grease or wax tends to hold in pus and thereby may serve as the outer wall of an abscess.

The following reasons are advanced for greasing the inner layer of gauze: it stops pain the faster, it keeps the dressing from sticking. However, the severe phase of pain attending the contraction of a partial-thickness scald upon the arm of man has a duration independent of the type of dressing applied to it, and in my experience the lightly greased dressing sticks to the burned area when the dressings are first removed as firmly as the dry dressing does. A heavily greased gauze does not stick to the wound but macerates the skin, and should a pyogenic infection occur beneath it the greased gauze becomes an integral part of the wall of an abscess. A sticky dressing is preferable to an abscess.

The exclusion of the wound from airborne and spittle-borne bacteria can be effected with

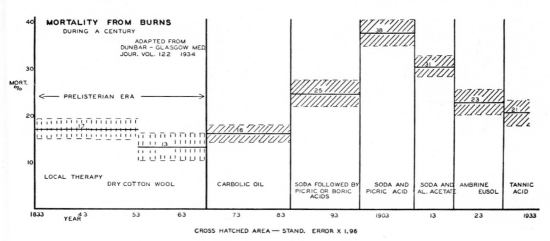

FIG. 16-2. Mortality from burns during a century.

the cotton or linen dressing by making it thick—this also serves to immobilize the part.

The massive occlusive cotton dressing, made of cotton wool or washed, sterile, mechanic's waste, has a few inherent dangers:

1. It reduces the rate of heat loss by convection and radiation and during warm or hot weather it may well endanger life by virtue of the burned individual's incapacity to lose his body heat fast enough. Heat exhaustion and heat stroke may be the consequences of the massive dressing during hot weather.

2. When applied to 3 or 4 extremities simultaneously, it effectively immobilizes the whole body, thereby increasing the chance for pressure necrosis, hypostatic pneumonia and the aspiration of vomitus.

3. Compressional atelectasis and pulmonary congestion may be caused by a tightly applied occlusive dressing covering the whole abdomen. Even anuria and hypotension may be induced by tight torsal occlusive dressings.

The reduction of fluid loss into the burned part has been advanced by some as the primary purpose of the pressure dressing. Controlled experiments show that the pressure dressing reduces the loss of fluid into an extremity little if at all when applied later than 30 minutes after the injury. Of course, it can hardly effect a reduction of transudation when applied at any time over a burn of the chest or abdomen—the abdominal viscera and chest are too yielding. A cheap, satisfactory elastic bandage can be made readily by cutting orthopedic stockinette cylinders spirally.

The dressing of a burned hand should separate the fingers and maintain the thumb, the fingers and the carpus in the handle-grasp position.

Recently, exposure of a burn or a scald to air has been revived. Exposure is especially applicable to burns of the face, a single surface of the torso and to the extremities *excepting the hands*. The maintenance of the burned hand in a fully functional handle-grasp position requires splinting—the occlusive bandage performs this function.

The care of a dangerously infected burn or scald is still a perplexing problem. Burned people still die of infections arising within the area of injury in spite of the use of antibiotics and special efforts to maintain asepsis. However, with burns covering less than 20 per cent of the body, infection of the burn wound now rarely causes death. Before the antibiotics and the sulfonamides were discovered, streptococcic wound infections known as burn erysipelas, caused an appreciable number of deaths among persons having small as well as large burns. Today, burn erysipelas is effectively prevented by giving penicillin, 50,000 to 300,000 units, 3 or 4 times daily. However, with burns covering more than 25 per cent of the body, infection is one, if not the most important, of major causes of death. Pathogenic strains of micrococci, especially *Staphylococcus aureus*, *Pseudomonadaceae*, *Enterobacteriaceae*, (*Escericheae* and *Proteae*) *Parvobacteriaceae* (Bacteriodes) and *Lactobacteriaceae* (*Streptococcus faecalis*) and *Streptococcus hemolyticus* (alpha viridans and beta pyogenes) are the predominant invaders of burn wounds. Excepting for the hemolytic streptococci, no satisfactory prolonged control of these organisms can be attained with antibiotics when they infect burn-wounds. The specific reasons for this are not apparent; the development of resistant strains of organisms while antibiotics are being given is one of the important factors; yet many others are likely to play parts such as the peculiarities of the tissue response to bacteria in a burned person, one of which is responsible for the actual growth of separate colonies of bacteria in the living tissue beneath burned skin with no cellular responses about the bacterial colonies.

Human gamma globulin fairly effectively controls infections with pyocaneous in burned laboratory animals,[17] though its effectiveness in human beings has not been completely established yet. Some measure of control of the growth of many organisms can be effected by coverage repeatedly, if necessary, of the open burn wound with living homografts taken from fresh cadavers. Within an hour after covering even bacteria-laden, pale, bleeding, edematous granulation tissue with living cutaneous homografts, the wound often becomes almost free of bacteria. The biologic mechanisms concerned in this are not known. To date no effective method has been devised for treating the massively infected, large, wet eschars of large full-thickness burns. We have attempted their excision with the immediate onlay of homografts while the patient was being given very large quantities of a broad-spectrum antibiotic and penicillin intravenously, but the sepsis continued and all 3 of the persons so treated died.

When this chapter was first written, the specific recommendation was made that from 200,000 to 1,200,000 units of penicillin be given daily for at least 5 days after the burn. Some persons believe that such specific recommendation cannot be made now because of the growing body of evidence that the "prophylactic administration of antibiotics" is without general merit and that what it does is to ensure that the bacterial flora of the burn wound is free of hemolytic streptococci but covered with penicillin-resistant strains of other organism most notably the staphylococci. The above statements are almost certainly true for the topically applied antibiotics, but it is questionable whether one may similarly indict the giving of penicillins, especially the newer forms, to a burned person for at least a few days after a burn. We believe that penicillin should be given parenterally for at least 5 days after a burn because it prevents invasive lethal streptococcic infections. After an invasive streptococcal infection develops in a burn wound the antibiotics are peculiarly ineffective at times. Of course, the antibiotics must be used for an actual infection in a burn wound; and insofar as it is possible to do, the antibiotics used should be those to which the bacteria are known to be sensitive (see Chap. 4, "Surgical Infections"). In brief, isolation of the individual from foreign strains of micro-organisms by the practice of aseptic technic, though especially difficult to attain with burns, is still the only known way of reducing the number of invasive infections in burn wounds, except the infections caused by the hemolytic streptococci; and penicillin prevents them.

Tetanus is still a threat with every burn. Give a booster dose of toxoid to those known to have been actively immunized and tetanus antitoxin (2,500 to 10,000 units) to those who are not. The amount of antitoxin given is determined by the size of the burn and the environment of the injury. A person who rolls or lies upon earth during or after a burn is given the larger dose. This upper limit of dosage is a larger amount of tetanus antitoxin than is recommended for the prevention of tetanus in a person not actively immunized excepting after multiple penetrating or massive injuries. A large burn that has had contact with earth or earth-soiled clothing is a massive injury as far as the danger of tetanus is concerned.

The signs of the birth of serious sepsis within a thermal wound are: an inordinately painful wound later than 24 hours after the accident, wetting through of the occlusive dressing, blistering of the burned skin adjacent to the wound, lymphangitis, painful lymphadenitis, and the general signs of sepsis. With and after the separation of the eschar the lack of visible evidence of a rim of epithelization about the edges of the wound, bleeding, and the formation of "pyogenic" crusts (crusts with pus beneath them) are the main local signs of a biologically significant infection. Pink, nonedematous granulation tissue with a rim of newly grown epithelium about it signifies an "uninfected" wound even though pathogenic bacteria may be found upon it.

Cleansing, free drainage, and inhibition of bacterial growth without interfering with reparative processes are the principles of treating infected burns. Cleansing and effecting free drainige are accomplished most safely with the repeated application and removal of thick compresses wet with saline solution. The cloth must be exposed to the air to permit evaporation at the external surface of the wet dressing. This moves bacteria from the wound surface into the dressing by capillary action. The covering of a wet dressing with an impervious cloth or plastic merely makes a fine incubator for organisms. The dressings are changed every 2 or 3 hours. The changing of an exposed wet dressing effects a continuous gentle scrub of the wound.

Parenterally administered bacterially appropriate antibiotics serve to effect inhibition of bacterial growth. The relative merits of antibiotics locally applied are yet unknown, although they have not effected miracles.

For a number of years "débridement" of the wound was practiced before the primary dressing was applied. Really, débridement in its true sense was rarely, if ever, practiced in that the excision of all dead tissue was not effected. The manner of performing a so-called "burn-débridement" amounted to medical mayhem in many instances; the injured individual, often while suffering from peripheral circulatory failure, was subjected to a general anesthetic. All blisters, whether broken or whole, dirty or clean, were cut off, and the whole surface of the injured area was *scrubbed* with a brush and a soft soap, and then washed with ether and saline.

We might look at this practice through the eyes of a physiologist, a bacteriologist and of a surgeon. The injured man was subjected to a powerful toxicologic agent, a general anesthetic, making him a weaker biologic object in every sense than he was before being subjected to it. The cutting away of the blisters exposed the denuded dermis and subjected it to desiccation, mechanical injury and the direct implantation of organisms. Undisturbed burn blisters go through a coagulative phase as a fibrin coagulum forms in them (24th to 48th hour); a desiccational or shriveling phase (48th to 120th hour); and a desquamative phase (120th to 240th hour). The color of the uninfected blisters changes from clear pink to yellow to gray to brown. Upon desquamating, a completely regrown, smooth soft epithelium becomes exposed. Controlled experiments performed recently by Gimbel[13] on human volunteers have demonstrated that the healing of a partial thickness burn takes place rapidly and uniformly when unbroken blisters are left intact.

The preparation of the wound for a dressing or exposure requires only the careful cutting off of clothing, the washing of dirty areas with saline-soaked pledgets of cotton, and the removal of grossly torn separated epidermis (burn blisters). All this can be accomplished without general anesthesia if care is exercised and morphine or demerol is given intravenously in dosage one third to one half that given subcutaneously in 5 to 10 ml. of saline when the procedure is begun. The entire procedure must be conducted under the identical conditions requisite to the performance of any operation, in an operating room with aseptic technic. The application of organic solvents, detergents, and antiseptics can only add to the injury—they are all protein denaturants.

The immediate excision of full-thickness injuries has been practiced sporadically for more than 50 years. Weidenfeld[32] began it in Vienna as a means of preventing "toxemia." It is performed readily without deep general anesthesia at any time up to the 5th day. The mode of its application in his words is:

With a thin transplantation knife (Thiersch knife) the eschar is cut away from the underlying tissue. One cuts so deeply that the underlying tissue bleeds, for only by this sign is one able to judge when sound tissue is reached. One needs recognize that the thickness of the eschar varies in an irregular manner and cut accordingly. . . . The undertaking of this procedure causes the patient only slight pain by virtue of the fact that the eschar is anesthetic and the subcutaneous tissues are scarcely sensible. Bleeding, however, is remarkable and one must conduct the process with foresight so that the patient is not inordinately weakened thereby.[32]

During World War II the procedure was reborn but has been practically abandoned again except for localized deep electrical burns (see Chap. 45). However, someday it may serve a useful function, especially in the treatment of small obviously deep burns; many surgical procedures have had to suffer a number of deaths and resurrections before finding acceptance.

The early treatment of the thermal wound may be summarized as:

1. Cleansing only the visibly dirty areas with saline under aseptic precautions.

2. The application of a dressing having a fine meshed dry cotton, linen or rayon gauze as a base *or* the exposure of the wound to air in as aseptic an environment as possible.

3. Meticulous attention to signs of local infection.

The human being burned or scalded to the extent of more than 70 per cent of the body's surfaces is in mortal danger of dying regardless of the manner with which the wound is dressed. 50 years ago a burn covering 40 per cent of the body was with few exceptions fatal within 5 days. Today, one so burned has 6 chances in 10 of recovering from his injury. Most of this therapeutic advance is attributable to the discovery of the physiologic deformations that follow the injury and the methods of grafting skin successfully.

The notation of the similarity of appearance and mode of death of victims of cholera and fire by Buhl (1855)[3] lead to the occasional administration of a solution of sodium chloride to burned individuals after 1850. The efficacy of a saline solution in reversing much of the illness attending cholera had been discovered by Latta[18] in 1831. Later, Tappeiner[28] found the blood of men dead of burns to have a much smaller proportion of water than normal blood. After experimenting with burned rabbits he surmised the water of the blood to have entered the burned tissue because the latter became edematous. It was he who first suggested that the transfusion of serum be employed in the treatment of the systemic illness attending burns and scalds.

Soon thereafter Lesser[19] found the mass of flowing red cells reducible by burning—the mass of red cells recoverable from animals by perfusion of the circulatory system was remarkably reduced after a large burn. Upon discovering that oligocythemia attended thermal injury he suggested that the transfusion of whole blood be entertained as a therapeutic measure.

In brief, most of the basic discoveries ultimately leading to the present treatment of burn shock had been made before 1880.

The general acute physiologic disturbances attending a thermal injury are at least 6 in number: hydrational, circulatory, hematologic, metabolic, endocrine and immunologic.

HYDRATIONAL DISTURBANCES

The hydrational disturbances associated with burns may be classified as early and late primary and secondary changes. Of the early primary disturbances the movement of extracellular fluid into the injured tissues and blisters is very important. This movement of interstitial fluid into the damaged tissues and blisters reduces the interstitial fluid mass in the uninjured tissues and blood. The fluid in the injured area has a lower content of protein than plasma but a higher content than nonvisceral lymph. It can be looked upon as a thin plasma.

The loss into the injured parts of fluid from the uninjured parts through blistering, edematous swelling and weeping proceeds with great rapidity and can well be life-endangering within an hour after an extensive partial-thickness burn or scald.[24]

The *intracellular fluid mass* of the uninjured tissues *does not move* across the cell membrane into the interstitial space to "buffer" the reduced volume of interstitial

fluid. This was observed by Tappeiner[28] during the late 1870's after an analysis of the water content of the plasma and the red cells of men following fatal burns. He found the content of water in plasma to be remarkably reduced (one fifth to one third) while at the same time the content of water in red cells was normal. These observations led him to write, "Why do the still water-rich cells not give up water to the water-poor serum?" Subsequent observations of Painter[15] show that intracellular fluid does not move out of body cells when extracellular fluid is lost into injured parts. In other words, the fluid-rich cells do not give up fluid to the impoverished extracellular compartment of the injured animal. Consequently, one must provide extraneous extracellular fluid for the seriously burned because there is no immediately available source of it within the body. In a physiologic sense a burn is somewhat like cholera: the normal parts of the body have lost extracellular fluid into and through the lumen of the gut with cholera and into and through the injured tissue with thermal injury.

Hyperkaliemia often occurs with severe burns within an hour or two after the injury.

The hyperkalemia is attributable to the egress of potassium from the injured cells (skin and red cells) and oliguria. At times the potassium concentration reaches "toxic" levels,[26] and hyperkalemia has been implicated as a possible cause of burn death since 1902.[31] Definite evidence is lacking regarding its actual contribution to the death of burned human beings, though it undoubtedly is a factor in death of burned rodents. However, the avoidance of potassium should be practiced during the acute phase of illness, the first 48 hours; fruit juices and meat broths should not be given.

Later and especially during the phase of the open wound hypokalemia may occur. This appears to be related to the rapid loss of potassium through exudation.

The early secondary hydrational disturbances are hypo-osmolality and acidosis. Both of these are often iatrogenic. The administration of more than 2 or 3 liters of water orally or 5 per cent glucose in water intravenously during the first 20 hours after a burn is attended by the retention of much of this water in the body and the dilution of all the body's solutes. The rapid reduction of the sodium concentration from normal to 120 to 125 mEq. per liter may precipitate the convulsive phase of water intoxication and anuria.

Early postburn acidosis is usually a chloride or dilutional acidosis. It arises whenever large quantities of noncolloid- or colloid-containing saline solutions made only of chlorides of Na or mixtures of chlorides of Na, K, Ca and Mg are given to a severely sodium-depleted organism before renal function is established. Briefly, this chloride acidosis arises because the concentration of bicarbonate buffer in the blood and extracellular fluid is reduced by the body's retention of the solution containing only chloride anions (see Chap. 5, "Fluid and Electrolytes").

Postburn dilutional or chloride acidosis does not occur when sodium bicarbonate containing Ringer's or sodium lactate containing Ringer's (Hartmann's) solutions are given because they sustain the oliguric burned body's base bicarbonate concentration; the bicarbonate-containing solution doing it directly and the lactate-containing one doing it indirectly by virtue of the catabolic degradation of the lactate anion.

Another secondary hydrational disturbance of burns is hypernatremia. It is especially prone to attend the daily forced feeding of burned children with large quantities (180 to 300 Gm.) of protein.[7] Serum sodium concentrations higher than 170 mEq./L. body temperatures over 39° C., and disorientation and coma have been observed to follow the forced feeding of high protein diets to burned human beings.

METABOLIC DISTURBANCES

The changes in metabolism that attend thermal injuries of mammals are an initial hypometabolism and a subsequent hypermetabolism. Both of these alterations are the greater the larger the injury. The hypometabolic period lasts for only 24 to 48 hours. Then it is followed by the period of hypermetabolism that lasts until the wounds are healed (see Fig. 16-3). With full-thickness burns, the hypermetabolism increases abruptly when the eschar is removed and an open wound is produced. The mechanisms concerned with the initial hypometabolic period have not

been fully elucidated. Extracellular fluid volume deficit amounting to 20 per cent of the normal original volume produced by depleting a normal human being of interstitial fluid by duodenal drainage is attended by a reduction of that individual's resting oxygen consumption amounting to 20 to 35 per cent. During the time that the metabolism is decreasing, the attendant oligemia is within the range of that which when produced by blood-letting is attended by no gross physiologic changes other than orthostatic hypotension. However, with burns the oligemia itself could also well contribute to the hypometabolism. The relationship between simple hemorrhagic oligemia and hypometabolism has long been known. The hypermetabolism that supersedes the initial period of hypometabolism is in large part, barring a serious infection, related to the increased rate of loss of water vapor through or upon the burned skin and later through the open wound. The most superficial layers of normal epidermis, and most importantly the stratum lucidum, has the remarkable property of staying the movement of water vapor through the skin. Although the water vapor pressure is high in a mammal (40 to 44 mm. of mercury per square cm.), normal epidermis permits only the passage of from 200 to 400 ml. of water as water vapor through the nonsweating skin of an adult daily. Caldwell has demonstrated that the hypermetabolism of the burned rat is practically entirely related to the increased heat loss secondary to the increased rate of movement of water vapor through the eschar as well as the open wound (see Fig. 16-3). Every gram of water lost from the body as water vapor represents the loss of a little more than one half of a kilocalorie of heat. The daily caloric expenditure by a severely burned man may reach 5,000 to 7,000 kilocalories daily. Caldwell and others have recently demonstrated that the maintenance of the air over only the burn wound at a temperature 2° to 6° C. higher than the temperature of the surface of the wound, or the coverage of the wound with a dressing impervious to water vapor, or the immersion of the body in warm Locke's solution, remarkably reduces the postburn hypermetabolism. Neither the hypometabolic nor the hypermetabolic postburn periods are thyroidal dependent.

They are not modified by thyropraevia when the burned animals' ambient temperatures are kept between 24° and 30° C.[4]

CIRCULATORY DISTURBANCES

The circulatory changes attending thermal injuries are local and general. Within the

thermally injured though still living tissues, red blood cells pack the widely dilated capillaries, and they flow only intermittently and slowly. This type of blood flow in capillaries is called stasic flow. The arterioles in the viable zone of injury are widely dilated and do not react to neural or hormonal stimuli

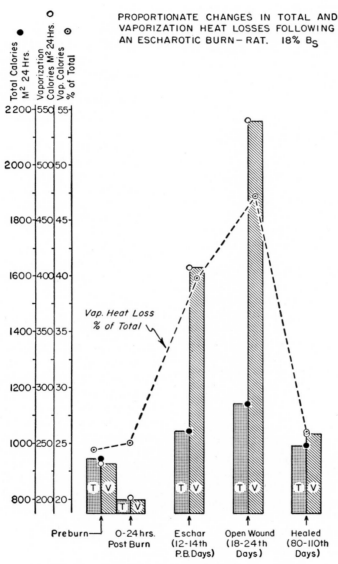

FIG. 16-3. T—total metabolism (O_2 consumption) V—vaporizational heat loss. The scales for the total and vaporizational heat loss are so constructed that 100 Calories of total metabolism is equivalent to 25 Calories of heat of vaporization because in the normal rat vaporizational heat loss is about 25 per cent of the total.

until the wounds are healed.[23] Within the lethally injured tissues blood flow stops, the capillaries being more or less destroyed, and thrombi fill the veins and the arteries.

The circulatory abnormalities in the unburned tissues may be classified as primary and secondary. The primary alterations are evidently at least in part cardiac in origin. With large thermal injuries in dogs cardiac output declines more than can be accounted for on the bases of oligemia and venous pressures (cardiac inflow). In such animals the cardiac output increases upon giving digitalis.[12] The secondary effects, such as diminished volume flow of blood, soft pulse, etc., are related to oligemia (see Chap. 7, "Shock"), and possibly to other factors such as the cellular metabolic effects of sodium depletion and burn auto-antigens or toxins.

HEMATOLOGIC DISTURBANCES

The hemic abnormalities associated with burns are (1) an immediate hemolysis, (2) a delayed hemolysis, (3) a faster than normal coagulation of the blood, (4) leukocytosis and (5) anemia.

Hemolysis occurs rapidly during the sufferance of the burn due to the direct action of heat on the blood in the capillaries beneath the burned surface and slowly for a week thereafter. The magnitude of the immediate hemolysis is directly proportional to the area of injury and its depth: as much as 6 Gm. of free hemoglobin per 100 ml. of plasma has been found in venous blood within 5 minutes after the immersion of two thirds of an anesthetized animal in water of 80° C. for 3 minutes. Hemolysis of the blood in burned men was first found by Lichtheim.[20] The delayed hemolysis seemingly affects red cells partially injured but not completely hemolyzed by heat during the sufferance of injury. There is some indication now that the delayed hemolysis and burn anemia may be related partially to sensitization.[10]

The origins of the anemia that almost universally follows large burns are not really known. It is not measurably controlled by giving iron and vitamin B_{12}. Until the mechanisms producing it are known all that can be done to control it is to treat it by the transfusion of packed red cells or whole blood.

ENDOCRINE DISTURBANCES

The endocrinal disturbances known to accompany burns are few in number. There is evidence of adrenocortical hyperfunction for a few days after a burn: the eosinophile numbers decrease precipitously and may almost reach zero. For 4 to 7 days the urinary secretion of 17-ketosteroids is supernormal or high normal, and then they decrease, becoming low normal; the urinary secretion of cortin increases and remains high for weeks.

There is no evidence that thyroid function is significantly altered by burns.

IMMUNOLOGIC DISTURBANCES

Burn toxins are thought to play a part in the production of burn sickness. Ever since the last quarter of the 19th century, a part of burn illness has been ascribed to the absorption of toxic substances from the thermally injured tissues. Until recently these substances were not characterizable. Within the past decade N. A. Fedorof and his associate in the U.S.S.R.[10] have found 2 toxic components in the burned skin of animals. One is thermolabile and thrombinlike and does not pass through a small-pored Zeitz filter. This quickly produces illness when injected into normal animals. The other passes through Zeitz filters and produces illness in normal animals from 3 to 8 days after it is injected into them. Fedorof[11] has also demonstrated a nonspecies specific antigenicity of the serum and the blood, and saline extracts of skin of burned animals. In the Soviet Union these discoveries have led to the treatment of burned persons with serum obtained from human beings who have recovered from burns ("reconvalescent" sera) and the sera of animals immunized to human burn antigens. Fedorof claims that giving 10 to 15 ml. of reconvalescent serum per kilo of body weight intravenously between the 3rd and the 20th days after the burn improves renal function, decreases pulse and respiratory rates, decreases the fever, decreases the oligemia and the rate of development of postburn anemia, reduces the leukocyte count, and in burned dogs reduces the total quantity of organic acids in the blood and the lability of the serum proteins. Plasma, serum and blood taken from human beings who have recovered from burns have been given to very sick burned persons by Rosenthal.[25] He claimed that their illnesses were ameliorated. However, the utility of convalescent or heterologus burn-immune sera in the treatment of burned human beings is still so poorly defined that at the time of revision of this chapter no definite recommendations can be made regarding their uses now. Nonetheless the demonstration of the autoantigenicity of thermally injured skin by Fedorof opens a new way to the investigation of burn toxins.

Burn Shock

It is now rather generally agreed that extracellular fluid volume depletion in the unburned tissues and in the blood by virtue of the movement of portions of their extracellular fluid into the edema and blister fluids of the burned parts is the major factor in the genesis of burn shock. This makes the shock attending burns differ somewhat from that attendant upon hemorrhage. With hemorrhagic shock the reduction in the volume of the blood, the oligemia per se, is a most important factor. With burn shock, in addition to the oligemia attendant upon the reduction of the mass of circulating red blood cells and the intravascular extracellular fluid (plasma) volume, the extravascular extracellular fluid volume of the unburned tissues is also reduced; this adds a cellular metabolic factor to the shock. Sodium depletion of vascularly isolated tissues reduces their oxygen consumptions; slight diaphoretic sodium depletion of normal human beings insufficient to produce any great impairment of the person's circulation or work capacity lowers their oxygen consumptions, sodium depletion of rats and man (see Fig. 16-4) of degree insufficient to lower their blood pressures reduces their metabolisms by as much as 25 per

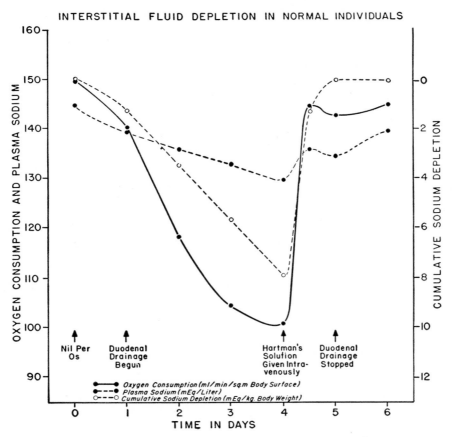

Fig. 16-4. Influence of sodium depletion with osmolal dilution upon the oxygen consumptions of normal men.

cent and the more especially when sodium depletion is attended by osmolal dilution which is often the situation with burns. In addition, sodium depletion is attended by a rise in the respiratory quotient from .72-.74 to .78-.82. This means that protein, and possibly carbohydrate (glycogen), constitute a greater part of the source of energy during fasting and sodium depletion than they do during fasting and sodium sufficiency. Sodium depletion also affects renal function peculiarly. In a normal man the depletion of about 20 per cent of the body's sodium during 4 days is associated with a 40 to 50 per cent decline in the glomerular filtration rate even when renal blood flow remains normal.

In other words, with burn shock in which sodium depletion of the unburned parts of the body plays a role, a number of peculiarities that distinguish it from hemorrhagic oligemic shock are to be expected. Furthermore, the direction of treatment only toward the restitution of the plasma and blood red cell volumes with colloid containing solutions or blood disregards the physiologic importance of extravascular sodium depletion.

Buffered Saline Solutions in Treatment of Burn Shock. During the past decade well-controlled investigations upon burned anesthetized animals[24] and accidentally burned human beings[21, 33] have demonstrated the effectiveness of buffered saline solutions in the treatment of burn shock. As stated previously, the giving of colloid-containing solutions alone or in combination with the buffered saline solutions has not effected demonstrable improvement in the effectiveness of treatment of burn shock over that attainable with the buffered saline solutions alone; *excepting in cases of badly burned children in which there has been a delay of 4 to 6 hours in treatment of shock*. In such cases of belatedly treated children the giving of a colloid-containing solution such as plasma or serum, in addition to the buffered saline solution, significantly increased the victims' chances of survival over that of similarly burned and belatedly treated children given buffered saline solution only.[21]

Should shock be mild or impending, the buffered saline solution (90 to 120mEq./Na/L.) may be given as a drink; 4 to 5 Gm. of table salt and 1½ Gm. of baking soda ($NaHCO_3$)

or sodium citrate dissolved in a quart or a liter of iced water is well taken and is effective in preventing the subsequent appearance of shock, water intoxication and acidosis, provided that it is retained by the patient.

In cases of profound burn shock, nausea and vomiting follow the drinking of anything; evidently, the stomach does not function properly. Consequently, in cases such as these, *no attempt at oral ministration of saline should be made;* instead, the buffered saline solution *must be given intravenously* until the shock has been largely overcome; then the oral solution may be used. Hartmann's solution (lactated Ringer's solution) is superior to any other saline solution for the intravenous treatment of profound burn shock, especially in children, because chloride acidosis does not attend its giving, while it almost always does the administration of 0.9 per cent NaCl or unmodified Ringer's solution.

The giving of the salt solution should be stopped as soon as the burned person begins to eat, a normal flow of urine is established, and the shock period (24 to 36 hours) is passed. Rarely, the wounds continue to weep large quantities of fluid for longer than 24 to 36 hours; in such cases some saline solution should be given orally in addition to food and water until the rapid transudation stops.

Vasoconstrictors and Hydrocortisone in Treatment of Burn Shock. The vasoconstrictors such as ephedrine and norepinephrine have no known place in the treatment of burn shock. On the contrary, hydrocortisone is occasionally very important. The adrenal cortical hormones play an important role in the treatment of shock in persons burned while taking corticoids, burned while chronically addicted to alcohol,* or suffering from thyrotoxicosis or subclinical adrenocortical insufficiency. A burned person in shock who does not respond well to saline and plasma therapy, especially if alcoholic or taking adrenal cortical hormones, should be given 100 to 150 mgm. of hydrocortisone intravenously after

---

* "Chronic alcoholics" behave after trauma as if they suffered from adrenal insufficiency; the concentrations of corticoids in their blood increase very little or not at all after an injury or an operation that, when experienced by normal persons, is followed by an increase in concentration of these substances in the blood of 2 to 5 fold their pre-injury levels.

having taken blood and urine samples for the ascertainment of the concentration of blood and urinary corticoids, and eosinophile numbers. A few such doses of corticoids do not constitute any known physiologic hazard to a badly burned person whose adrenals are sufficient, but not giving them to a burned person with insufficient adrenals is catastrophic.

COLLOIDS IN TREATMENT OF BURN SHOCK

Before 1940, the treatment of burn shock consisted of the administration of 0.9 per cent sodium chloride intravenously in relatively small quantities of 1.5 to 3 liters per 24 hours and the transfusion of whole blood in amounts rarely larger than 500 ml. With the development of blood-banks during the early 1940's, large quantities of plasma became available. Because it had been realized that fairly large quantities of plasma proteins were lost in burn blisters and into edematous burned tissues, large quantities of plasma were soon being given to very badly burned persons. With the giving of these large amounts of plasma, as much as 50 ml. per kilo of body weight, the mortality from burn shock dropped significantly (see Table 1). However, the functional significances of the colloids—serum albumin and serum globin and the carbohydrate polymer dextran—in the treatment of burn shock are still not clear. In untreated mortally scalded anesthetized animals the plasma protein concentration often rises significantly (1 to 2 Gm. %) before the animal dies. However, in similarly injured animals treated with sodium bicarbonate or sodium lactate buffered sodium chloride or Ringer's solutions (150 mEq./Na/L.) the serum protein concentration usually declines from 1 to 3 Gm. per cent. The addition of species specific serum in quantities sufficient to maintain the serum proteins of animals treated with the saline solutions did not measurably improve their biologic response to the injury; they died as soon as those treated with the buffered saline solutions alone. However, these experiments may have been too extreme to test the efficacy of colloid in the treatment of burn shock. Earlier, Rosenthal and associates[24] had found that colloid-containing solutions were no more effective in treating burn shock in mice than were the same solutions without colloid in them.

The effects of raising the plasma colloid concentration in sodium-depleted animals are peculiar: all of 40 rats died when acutely depleted of 20 to 24 per cent of their original extracellular fluid while their plasma colloid concentrations were being raised 2 to 4 Gm. per cent with human albumin or acacia; while none of 60 rats died after being depleted of 22 to 26 per cent of their extracellular fluid when no colloid was given to them. Increasing the concentration of albumin in blood changes its characteristics of flow in glass capillaries. The addition of from 1 to 3 Gm. per cent of human albumin to human blood completely changes the relationship of the flowing hematocrit to the static hematocrit in tubes smaller than 200 μ. With normal concentrations of albumin in blood the flowing hematocrit is always lower than the static hematocrit in tubes smaller than 200 μ, but with 1 to 3 added grams of albumin or acacia, the flowing hematocrit becomes higher than the static, and when it does the rate of flow of the blood driven by a constant pressure through the tube declines precipitously. The lower the static hematocrit of the blood, the smaller is the amount of added albumin needed to reverse the relationship of the flowing to the static hematocrit. In other words, the addition of albumin to blood (raising the cencentration of albumin) disrupts laminar flow in small tubes and greatly increases the resistance to flow through them. Whether this takes place in the small blood vessels of living mammals is not yet known, but the intense congestion of the lungs, the livers and the spleens, the enormously dilated hearts, the inordinately high hematocrits for the degrees of ECF volume depletion, and the bloody pleural effusions of rats dying with sodium deficiency and supernormal concentrations of albumin or acacia in their bloods, suggest that this phenomenon may take place in small blood vessels as well as in glass tubes.

Recently, various dextrans when given intravenously in small and large but not in intermediate amounts, have been found to produce massive edema and erythema of paws, snout, ears, genitalia and feet of unanesthetized rats. Antihistamines have no effect on the phenomenon.[16]

In brief, we do not as yet know enough about the physiologic and physical functions of the serum proteins or of the dextrans to use them intelligently in the treatment of burn shock *excepting in the treatment of belatedly treated, badly burned children for whom the addition of serum and plasma to the saline therapy is known to improve the chances of recovery from shock.*

BLOOD TRANSFUSION IN THE TREATMENT OF BURN SHOCK

For a time we believed that the hemolytic destruction of red blood cells and the entrapment of blood in the capillaries of thermally injured tissues played a definite role in genesis of burn shock. This belief was engendered by the discovery that transfusion of both a buffered saline solution and whole blood was the only way that anesthetized dogs, scalded by 30-seconds immersion of the hind legs and the torso up to their scapulae into water at 80° C., could be saved from dying of shock. Actually, the reduction of the circulating red cell mass may amount to one third of the original red cell mass within 1 day after a fire burn of one half of the body's surface.[8] However, Wilson[33] has collected data that indicates that the transfusion of blood is not requisite for the successful treatment of burn shock in man, provided that sodium chloride-sodium bicarbonate or lactate solutions and water are given by appropriate routes and in sufficient quantities. However, the transfusion of whole blood or washed red blood cells is important in treating the severely burned person whenever the postburn anemia appears. Postburn anemia becomes manifest with large deep scalds and burns between the 2nd and the 4th days after the injury. The transfusion of red blood cells then in sufficient quantities to maintain a normal hemoglobin, red count, or hematocrit prevents postburn anemia, keeps tachycardia at a minimum and prevents inordinate weakness.

A number of formulas have been used during the past 20 years as guides for the fluid therapy of burns. The one still extant is the Evans' formula: to wit, the fluids needed during the first 24 hours after a burn are: 1 ml. of plasma, plasma substitute or whole blood and 1 ml. of 0.9 per cent NaCl per kilo for each 1 per cent of body burned, and in addition enough 5 per cent dextrose in water to balance the insensible and urinary losses of water.

One-half of the estimated fluid is to be given during the first 8 hours, and one quarter of it during each of the 2 succeeding 8-hour periods.

This formula, like all the others that preceded it, is now relatively useless. Since it was first propounded almost 20 years ago it has been learned that the need for colloid-containing solutions such as blood, plasma, or plasma substitutes in treating burn shock is much smaller than Evans believed it to be. In addition, slightly hypotonic glucose containing buffered salines are now known to be physiologically superior to 0.9 per cent NaCl for the treatment of burn shock. Furthermore, when these slightly hypotonic buffered salines are used there is no need for the 5 per cent glucose in water.

In addition, it has been learned that burns covering less than 20 per cent of the body infrequently produce shock except among infants and very old people. Consequently, if fluid therapy is based on the Evans' formula it will usually lead to indiscriminate overtreatment of persons whose burns cover less than 20 per cent of the body. This means that if the Evans' formula is used indiscriminately, about 80 per cent of the burns treated in hospitals in the United States could be overtreated, because 70 per cent of all the burned persons treated in American hospitals have injuries covering 5 to 20 per cent of the body surface. Actually, considering only burns that are judged to be truly serious, namely, those covering 15 to 100 per cent of the body, only 55 per cent of them require more than a liter or two of orally taken buffered saline for supportive fluid therapy, because about 45 per cent of such serious burns cover only 15 to 24 per cent of the body, and shock has never been a major threat to life with burns of this size (see Table 1).

Another criticism of the formula is that it may lead to insufficient saline therapy of very large partial-thickness injuries. Large partial-thickness injuries involving the head, the neck, or the genitalia and the perineum swell very rapidly and greatly and may be attended, especially in children, with losses of extracellular fluid that are far larger than the saline replacement recommended in the Evans formula.

The amounts of interstitial fluid, plasma and analgesics needed to treat burn shock must be gauged by the individual's physiologic response to the physician's ministration. Formulary regulation of the therapy of burn shock is a manifestation of biologic naïveté. *Variance,* not constancy, is characteristic of the reactions of a population parameter to a change in environment. A burn of 30 per cent of the body's surface will be unattended by shock in a few individuals, moderate shock in many, and severe peripheral circulatory failure in some. To give all the same treatment would result in overtreatment of some, adequate therapy of some, and insufficient ministration to others.

Gauging therapy entirely on the basis of the rate of flow of urine disregards the variability of response of the kidneys of traumatized individuals to the administration of fluids. Rarely, some hurt men may excrete as much as 20 ml. of urine per hour while suffering from shock; while others will excrete very little, though they have not shock and are almost drowned with fluid. When nature has cast a man, she throws that mold away.

To regulate treatment solely upon the basis of the hematocrit is also unintelligent. Red blood cells are lost from the blood as the interstitial fluid (plasma) is; a rising hematocrit only signifies that the rate of reduction of the circulating plasma mass is more rapid than the rate of decrease of the red cell mass is. The employment of the hematocrit as the sole therapeutic gauge tends to lead to undertreatment, especially in the severely burned.

The repetitive examination of all vital signs while the person is being treated is the only means of regulating therapy to the needs of the individual. The signs of greatest value to the assessment of the therapy of a burned person are: the rate and the character of the pulse, the physical attitude assumed, the sensibility to the injury, hiccoughing and vomiting, the rate of flow of urine, the frequency of drinking, the rate and the character of breathing, the blood pressure and the mental reaction and attitudes. To illustrate:

Case a boy of 8 burned over one **half** of his body by having his clothing catch on fire

FIRST EXAMINATION—1 hour after injury
Pulse—76 and full
Attitude—quiet and apprehensive, says he has little pain
Orientation—normal

Respiration—30 per minute, of normal depth
Blood pressure—142/70
Urine—catheterized specimen, red, albumin ++
Vomiting—none
Hiccoughing—none
Thirsty and drinking often

SECOND EXAMINATION—2 hours after injury
Pulse—100, bounding
Attitude—threshing about and crying
Orientation—lost
Respiration—16 and deep
Blood pressure—112/40
Urine flow in 1 hour, 2 ml. of red albumin containing urine
Vomiting—once, blood-tinged fluid
Drinking—none
The supportive therapy has been inadequate. The rate with which the lactated Ringer's (Hartmann's) solution being given needs to be increased.

THIRD EXAMINATION—2 hours and 45 minutes after the injury
Pulse—120, bounding
Attitude—quiet
Orientation—partial return
Respiration—25 and less deep
Blood pressure—90/50
Urine flow—15 ml. in 45 minutes, less red, albumin ++
Vomiting—none
Drinking—asks for water
The treatment has changed things for the better, although the pulse rate has quickened, and the blood pressure has fallen. The rate of the infusions is maintained.

FOURTH EXAMINATION—4 hours after injury
Pulse—120, full
Attitude—fidgety and complains of smarting pain
Orientation—normal
Respiration—30
Blood pressure—110/80
Urine flow—30 ml. in 1 hour and 15 minutes, albumin +
Vomiting—none
Drinking—buffered saline solution frequently
The individual is now safely alive for the time being and the infusions are slowed.
2 HOURS LATER—all signs unchanged, rate of infusion maintained
2 HOURS LATER—breathing has speeded, and a few rales are heard—the rate of infusion is to be reduced or stopped and only the buffered saline solution is given to him orally.

Although the hematocrit used alone is an inadequate base for the regulation of therapy, it is of great value in adjusting the rate of administration of the lactated Ringer's solution with or without plasma. A rising hematocrit during the course of treatment denotes the need for increasing the rate of injecting the saline solution or the plasma.

Obstruction of the upper airway, by pharyngeal and laryngeal edema, and pulmonary edema are particularly dangerous complications of burns. Life-endangering pharyngeal and laryngeal edema are especially prone to occur soon after deep burns of the face and the neck. Should tracheostomy not be performed in such cases, pulmonary edema will soon kill the patient; partial obstruction of the trachea or the larynx, whatever its cause, is a sure way to pulmonary edema. Consequently, tracheostomy should be performed *for deep burns about the neck and the face* before signs of pulmonary edema appear. In fact, it can be said that tracheostomy is a very important early step in the treatment of deep burns of the head and the neck.

Pulmonary injury followed by pulmonary edema is a rather frequent complication of burns suffered within buildings or other confined spaces. The hot air or flames themselves do not injure the lung, because the water vapor generated in the upper air passages so cools the hot air that by the time it reaches the upper trachea it is no longer hot enough to injure tissue. Tracheobronchial and pulmonary injury associated with burns is caused by the inhalation of the many noxious gases associated with combustion of various building materials, furnishings and contents. Among these gases are nitric oxide and sulfur dioxide. Tracheostomy is also indicated for this chemical tracheobronchitis. The tracheostomy reduces the dead air space, lowers the respiratory resistance offered by the inflamed airway above the tracheotomy and permits the direct clearing of the trachea and the bronchi of the secretions coming from the distal bronchial tree that at times are so copious as literally to drown the patient unless direct suction aspiration of the trachea can be done through a tracheostomy.

Should the burned individual survive the period of burn shock with its associated dangers of attendant and subsequent renal insufficiency, and occasional acute myocardial failure, his illness becomes marked by manifold nutritional problems, infection and psychic disturbances.

For a few years overt emphasis was placed upon fighting the negative nitrogen balance by pouring progressively larger masses of protein into the organism through tubes placed in the stomach. As much as 300 Gm. of protein per diem has been recommended.[29] However, it was soon learned that a forced high protein diet led to trouble; a peculiar illness having many of the characteristics of diabetes was produced occasionally, and an illness characterized by progressive fever, hypernatremia, disorientation, and elevated concentrations of amino acid and nonprotein nitrogen attended the forced feeding of suspensions of partially digested or native proteins.[7]

Obviously, the care of a burned person constitutes one of the most difficult and complex duties that a surgeon can undertake. The problems he may face are many more than those sketchily considered here.

Delirium tremens and the illnesses caused by the withdrawal of morphine, heroin or barbiturates are often met because the drug and alcoholic addict is especially prone to suffer severe burns from bed fires. Acidosis is prone to occur in the severely burned child. Hypocalcemia occasionally bedevils the course of the burned person from the 2nd to the 4th weeks after injury.

Cardiac failure, myocardial infarction, pulmonary infarction, acute gastro-intestinal hemorrhage, the perforation of acute peptic ulcers (Curling's ulcer), venous thrombosis, gas gangrene, tetanus, encrustative pyoderma, surgical erysipelas, sensitivity reactions, especially to the antibiotics, abortion and infectious hepatitis will be encountered among burned and scalded people. In brief, the surgeon who undertakes the care of a burned man truly needs to be a physician in the broadest sense.

Little need be said about the treatment of the more frequent nonbacterial complications of burns. Vomiting needs to be treated with gastric intubation, because when it occurs soon after the burning, it is so often a sign of acute gastric dilatation. Water intoxication attending burns is easily treated: withhold water for the nonconvulsive form if the sodium mass within the uninjured tissue is normal, and give the appropriate hypertonic salt solutions

TABLE 1

% Body Surface	Expected Mortality		
	None 1902	Plasma 1946-50	Buffered Saline 1950-54
12-24	7.4	7.3	3
25-34	11.5	13	5.5
35-44	72.0	44	24
45-54	90	69	44
55-64	94	87	68
65-74	100	96	86
75-84	100	100	92
85-94	100	100	99
95-100	100	100	100

TABLE 2

Area Injured % Body Surface	Mortality %	
	Ages 2-60	Ages 61-85
5	0	5
10	0	10
15	1	54
20	2	92
30	10	98
40	30	99
50	54	100
60	78	100
70	93	100
80	99	100
90	100	100
100	100	100

intravenously for water intoxication with convulsions or whenever signs of sodium deficit exist (see Chap. 5, "Fluid and Electrolytes").

The prevention of starvation is a very pressing problem with severe burns. The daily caloric expenditure may be as high as 5,000 to 7,000 Calories. Unless tube feeding of high caloric liquid is used, such caloric demands cannot be met, largely because a sick, burned person will refuse to eat enough of any acceptable foods. Because a large part of the hypermetabolism associated with burns is related to the acceleration of water-vaporizational heat loss through the eschar or open wound, means may be developed to reduce the caloric needs of the burned person so as to do away with much of the nutritional problem. The means of doing this have not been sufficiently well developed to date to permit their description yet.

Inasmuch as the assessment of one's accomplishments is a most important part in the being of a surgeon, the inclusion in a surgical text of a basis for the assessment of one's treatment of burned and scalded individuals is deemed proper. The comparison of one's results with those of others without regard for the character or the size of the injuries or the ages of those treated is worthless. The relationship between the size of the injury and the mortality rate of burns and scalds in 1902 and 1950 is shown in Table 1. A cursory study of the table shows that there has been definite improvement in the effectiveness of burn therapy from a mortality standpoint during the last 50 years. However, the mortality rate attending injuries covering 5 to 20 per cent and 75 to 100 per cent of the

body's surface during 1902 and 1950 are essentially alike—the former being good in both instances, the latter poor in both instances. However, remarkable advance has been made in the treatment of burns and scalds covering 20 to 75 per cent of the body's surface.

Surgeons who deal largely with burned children have experienced lower mortality rates than others caring mainly for adults of all ages. As a consequence thereof they who deal with burned children have unjustifiably used their better gross mortality statistics as arguments for the superiority of therapeutic quirks. The remarkably deleterious effect of aging upon an individual's capacity to recover from a thermal hurt is readily seen in Table 2. The mortalities associated with burns and scalds of various sizes in persons of different ages is practically identical in England and the United States. Tables 1 and 2 are based on the Weidenfeld and Zumbusch*[32] statistics, and a burn population of 382 seriously burned individuals who were treated in the United States in the manner described in this chapter between 1946 and 1954.

In order quickly to assess one's capacity to treat burns all one needs do is derive the sum of the expected mortalities with the use of Table 2 and compare it with the actual number of deaths in the series. Treated a certain way, the expected chance of death from a burn or a scald for an individual depends upon his age and the size of his injury.

The estimation of the area covered by a thermal injury is readily accomplished with

* Statistics taken from Table 1, pp. 79-85 (patients not treated with infusions or baths) and Table V, p. 163. Arch. Dermat. u. Syph., Vol. 76, 1905.

TABLE 3. VIERORDT TABLE (1893)[30]

AREA	% OF BODY SURFACE
Head	5
Neck	2
Upper arm	5
Forearm	3
Hand	2
Thigh (with buttock)	14
Leg	6
Foot	3
Trunk	28

AGE	TOTAL SURFACE AREA (SQUARE METERS)	SURFACE AREA (SQUARE CM.) PER KG. OF BODY WEIGHT
1 day	0.2599	812
6 months	0.4381	626
1 year	0.5181	575
2 years	0.6028	533
4 years	0.7020	495
7 years	0.8552	450
10 years	1.0092	412
12 years	1.1505	386
14 years	1.3676	354
25 years	1.8936	301

fair accuracy with the aid of the Vierordt table (Table 3) derived from the data of Meeh and Funke or by simply applying the "rule of nines": head and neck 9%, each arm 9%, anterior trunk $2 \times 9 = 18\%$, posterior trunk $2 \times 9 = 18\%$, each lower extremity $2 \times 9 = 18\%$.

The Vierordt table (Table 3) is of special interest in view of the dependence of mortality upon the size of the burn. A burn of both legs and thighs is as large (40%) as one covering the entire trunk, head, neck, and one upper arm. A burn of the entire head, neck, upper extremities and entire chest (½ of trunk) involves only 40 per cent of the body's surface, while one spread over the abdomen to the belt line (⅓ of trunk) and the entire lower extremities excepting the feet covers 50 per cent. The relationship of surface area to body mass varies much with age. Consequently, the calculation of surface area from weight must take the patient's age in consideration (Table 4).

The Berkow method of estimating the surface area contributed by different parts of the body is similar to Vierordt's excepting that Berkow's estimate of the area of the trunk is larger than the actual measurements of Meeh and Funke indicate that it should be.

The treatment of thermal injury is a major health problem in the United States today. Roughly 6,000 hospital beds are occupied the year around by the burned and the scalded. Many more people die of thermal injuries than die of poliomyelitis and as many are hurt and crippled. Someday the existence of our nation may depend upon the capacity of the American physician to treat burns. Burns are a greater danger to modern armies and populations than are wounds from missiles.

Among 250,000 residents of Dresden no survivor has ever been found to tell of one night's incendiary bombing of that city. What will new atomic bombs do? Burns accounted for about one third of the deaths in Hiroshima.

The reconstructive surgery related to burns is discussed in Chapter 45.

REFERENCES

1. Bekkum, van, D. W., and Peters, R. A.: Change in enzymatic process in burns, Quart. J. Exper. Physiol. 36:127-137, 1951.
2. Beloff, A., and Peters, R. A.: Influence of moderate temperature burns upon proteinase of skin, J. Physiol. 103:461-476, 1945.
3. Buhl: Mittheilungen aus der Pfeufer'schen Klinik: Epidemische Cholera. Ztschr. Rationelle Med. (Henle and Pfeufer) 6:1-105, 1855.
4. Caldwell, F. T., Jr., Osterholm, J. L., Sower, N. D., and Moyer, C. A: Metabolic response to thermal trauma of normal and thyroprivic rats at three environmental temperatures, Ann. Surg. 150:976-988, 1959.
5. Cruickshank, C. N. D., and Hershey, F. B.: The effect of heat on the metabolism of guinea pig's ear skin, Ann. Surg. 151:419-430, 1960.
6. Edenbuizen, M.: Beitrage zur Physiologie der Haut, Ztschr. Rationelle Med. (Henle and Pfeufer) 17:35, 1863.
7. Engel, F. L., and Jaeger, C.: Dehydration with hypernatremia, hyperchloremia and azotemia complicating nasogastric tube feeding, Am. J. Med. 17:196-204, 1954.
8. Evans, E. I., and Bigger, I. A.: The rationale of whole blood therapy in severe burns, Ann. Surg. 122:693-705, 1945.
9. Evans, E. I., and Butterfield, W. J. H.:

Stress response in severely burned; interim report, Ann. Surg. *134*:588-613, 1951.

10. Fedorov, N. A., and Skurovich, S. V.: Experimental investigations on the immunotherapy of burn illness, Surgery (U.S.S.R.), no. 9, pp. 48-54, 1955. (In Russian)

11. Fedorov, N. A., Skurovich, S. V., Freeman, V. T., and Muzichenko, A P.: Experimental investigations on the burn autoantigen. Pathological Physiology and Experimental Therapy, Surgery (U.S.S.R.), no. 6, pp. 53-58, 1959. (In Russian)

12. Fozzard, H. A.: Myocardial injury in burn shock. Submitted for publication to Annals of Surgery.

13. Gimbel, N. S.: A study of epithelization of experimental burn blisters *in* Proc. First International Congress on Research in Burns, Washington, D. C., 1960. To be published.

14. Henriques, F. C.: Studies of thermal injury, Arch. Path. *43*:489-502, 1947.

15. Holmes, J. H., and Painter, E. E.: Role of extracellular fluid in traumatic shock in dogs, Am. J. Physiol. *148*:201, 1947.

16. Kato, L., and Gozsy, B.: Kinetics of edema formation in rats as influenced by critical doses of dextran, Am. J. Physiol. *199*:657-660, 1960.

17. Kefalides, N. F., Arana, J. A., Bazan, A., and Stastny, P.: Clinical evaluation of antibiotics and gamma globulin in septicemias following burns *in* Proc. First International Congress on Research in Burns, Washington, D. C., 1960. To be published.

18. Latta, Thomas: Documents communicated by the Central Board of Health, London, relative to the treatment of cholera by the copious injection of aqueous and saline fluids into the veins, Lancet *2*:274, 1831-32.

19. Lesser, von, L.: Ueber Todesursachen bei Verbrennungen, Virchows Arch. path. Anat. *79*:248-310, 1880.

20. Lichtheim: Ueber Periodische Hämoglobinurie, Samml. Klin. Vorträge *134*:1147-1168, 1878.

21. Markley, K., *et al.*: Clinical evaluation of saline solution therapy in burn shock, J.A.M.A. *161*:1465-1473, 1956.

22. Moritz, A. R., Henriques, F. C., Jr., Dutra, F. R., and Weisiger, J. R.: Studies of thermal injury, Arch. Path. *43*:466-488, 1947.

23. Ricker, G., and Regendanz, P.: Virchows Arch. path. Anat. *231*:1, 1921.

24. Rosenthal, S. M.: Experimental chemotherapy of burns and shock, U. S. Pub. Health Rep. *58*:513-522, 1943.

25. Rosenthal, S. R., Hartney, J. B., and Spurrier, W. A.: The "toxin-antitoxin" phenomenon in burns and injury, J.A.MA. *174*:957-965, 1960.

26. Rosenthal, S. M., and Tabor, H.: Electrolyte changes and chemotherapy in experimental burn and traumatic shock and hemorrhage, Arch. Surg. *51*:244-252, 1945.

27. Syme, James: Principles of Surgery, ed. 3, London, Baillière, Tindall & Cox, 1842.

28. Tappeiner, von, H.: Ueber Veränderungen des Blutes und der Muskeln Nach Ausgedehnten Hautverbrennungen, Centralbl. med. Wissenschaften *31*:385, 1881.

29. Taylor, F. H. L., Levenson, S. M., Davidson, C. S., Browder, N. C., and Lund, C. C.: Problems of protein nutrition in burned patients, Ann. Surg. *118*:215-224, 1943.

30. Vierordt, H.: Anatomische, Physiologische, und Physikalische Daten und Tabellen, ed. 3, p. 52, Jena, Fischer, 1906.

31. Weidenfeld, St.: Ueber den Verbrennungstod, Arch. Dermat. u. Syph. *61*:322, 1902.

32. Weidenfeld, St., and Zumbusch, L. V.: Weitere Beitrage zur Pathologie und Therapie Schwerer Verbrennungen, Arch. Dermat. u. Syph. *76*:163-184, 1905.

33. Wilson, B., and Stirman, J. A.: Initial treatment of burns, J.A.M.A. *173*:509-516, 1960.

CHAPTER 17

Radiation Injury from Local or Total Body Exposure

Certain Considerations in Radiation Exposure
Radiation Injury: Local or Total Body
Management of Wounds Contaminated with Radioactive Isotopes
Protection of Personnel in Radiology

CERTAIN CONSIDERATIONS IN RADIATION EXPOSURE

Many of the physical properties of ionizing radiation are discussed in Chapter 9, "The Principles of Isotope Technics in Surgery." In the case of radiation injury, particularly from total body exposure, it is important to delineate clearly the type of ionizing rays to which the individual has been exposed. Such factors as energy equivalents, penetration, duration of exposure and tissue sensitivity are among the essential considerations in estimating biologic effects. These qualities in turn depend upon the nature of radiations emitted and the source or sources involved. In the usual types of therapeutic radiation, the following particles may be emitted:[10]

Alpha Particles. These are nonpenetrating rays bearing a positive charge. They are stopped by the thickness of a single sheet of paper, and travel in air a distance of 2.7 cm. to 8.6 cm., depending upon their energy. Alpha particles are identified with the helium nucleus and eventually they annex 2 orbital electrons to become ordinary helium atoms. Because of their inability to penetrate tissue, they are essentially harmless.

Beta particles are actually electron particles of small mass and carry a negative charge. They are ejected from their parent atoms at much higher speeds than alpha particles, some with velocities approximating that of light.

Most of them do not penetrate 2 mm. thickness of brass or 1 mm. thickness of lead. In body tissue, they penetrate only thin layers of tissue and are therapeutically of value only when they can be employed under circumstances where this characteristic can be of advantage. The best example is I^{131}, wherein its diffuse concentration in the active thyroid allows ablation of the gland if desired, without harm to surrounding tissue. The measurement of beta emitters within the body is made possible with the Geiger counter because of the small amount of gamma radiation also emitted. Gamma radiation can be counted externally over deep-lying tissue containing largely beta particles; few or none of the beta particles may reach the surface. The decay rates of beta and gamma particles for a given isotope sustain their initial ratios; hence, the external measurement of gamma radiation reflects the local intensity of remaining beta radiation, thereby enabling calculations as to the residual concentrations of beta radiation at any one time.

Gamma rays travel with the speed of light, are electromagnetic and are not charged. They are capable of penetrating several centimeters of metal. Because gamma rays usually have a shorter wave length than x-rays, their penetrating power is generally greater. X-rays are also electromagnetic, uncharged and are considered identical with gamma radiation of other sources.

Natural radioactivity occurs for all elements with atomic weights above 209 or whose atomic numbers are greater than 83. Artificial radioactivity has been achieved for all elements in the periodic table. The characteristics of artificial radioactivity vary tremendously with the element involved. Half-lives range in time from miliseconds to millions of years. A radioactive element in the course of disintegration looses by expulsion a nuclear particle from its agitated unstable nucleus. This allows the residual components to settle down as a stable atom of another element. The decrease or decay in radioactivity for a given quantity of another element is gradual, but for the particular atom, the loss of the nuclear particle is instantaneous.

A number of units for biologic measurement of radiation have been devised to determine radiation exposure in biologic tissues. Each is defined for specific circumstances, and these are not subject for discussion here. The biologic response to a standard amount of radiation is remarkably constant for members of a given species, including man, although the interspecies tolerances vary greatly.

Technical developments in physics and radiology have been enormous during the past 15 years. X-ray machines currently employed in treatment include the 10-kv. machine used by the dermatologist, the 80- and the 250-kv. machine employed by the radiologist for therapy. Two-million volt x-ray generators are currently in use in many hospitals, and linear accelerators generating 6 million volts of x-rays are employed by some. Betatrons of various designs for x-ray and electron generation range upward from 30 million volts. More recently the proton beam of the cyclotron has been under test in the treatment of malignant disease after boron is introduced into the tissue to be treated. The proton beam produces neutrons from the localized interstitial boron, and these in turn radiate the area concerned.

Because the needs of the patient vary widely according to the sensitivity and location of the tumor under treatment, the radiotherapist must adjust the energies of his x-rays and electrons accordingly. This problem is complex and for the most part is regulated by variations in voltage aided by a variety of filters interposed between the energy source and the patient.

The limiting factor in portal radiation therapy is primarily the tolerance of adjacent normal tissues and secondarily the systemic response of the patient to his treatment. The patient's local and systemic response determine the amount of allowable radiation exposure. The third and equally important consideration is the radiosensitivity of the tumor or tissue in question. Some tumors are very sensitive, but all ranges of sensitivity and resistance are encountered. Some are extremely sensitive and respond well for a while, only to become increasingly resistant in time. Moreover, the magnitude of the dose of radiation that can be administered with the 2nd, the 3rd or the 4th course of therapy without engendering harm is reduced sharply. Thus, a tumor which cannot be totally ablated by the first course of treatment is not likely to be curable later on by radiation therapy. The malignant lesions responding to the highest percentage rates of cure are those of the skin and the cervix. They are often curable by the first series of exposures given under appropriate conditions. Basal and early squamous cell carcinomas generally are most amenable to this form of therapy, especially if less than 2 cm. in diameter. The malignant melanoma of the skin, on the other hand, is highly resistant to any form of radiation therapy. A sound understanding as to why some tumors are radiosensitive and others are resistant could prove to be of incalculable value to all types of treatment for malignant disease— not to radiation therapy alone.

CELLULAR DAMAGE FROM RADIATION

By no means is it possible at this time to define accurately or completely the effects of ionizing radiation upon the living cell. On the other hand, this is a subject of much study for many years, and its ultimate solution is basic to improvement in radiotherapy and to the prevention and the treatment of radiation injury in general.

Cellular changes or their death are functions of many variables, particularly dosage, time of exposure (single or multiple exposures) and the relationship of mitotic division to the time or the occasion at which the cell is radiated.

Dosage to tissue or to an organ is not uniformly distributed among cells, nor is the intensity of exposure constant for all cells within the same field. For example, if the concentration of the sulfur or calcium ion within one cell is elevated from that of another, the dosage in the former cell or tissue is significantly over that of the latter, even though the intensity of the energy output of the extracorporeal source of radiation is the same. For this reason the tissue immediately adjacent to bone is said to receive an exposure 60 per cent greater than the dose received by cells at distances of 1 mm. or more away from bone with 200-kv. x-ray.[25] These differences tend to be canceled out when one considers larger quantities of exposed tissue, i.e., a gram or more. Cellular dosage and damage then becomes a statistical concept wherein the total exposure of the individual cell is lost in the "crowd."

Most radiobiologists believe at present that certain acute chemical changes occur within the radiated cell but that these changes are essentially limited to the immediate electronic path of the electron entering or transversing the cell. This concept is not unlike the demonstrated or measured ionizing effects of particle radiation measured by the Wilson cloud chamber technic on photographic plates.

The chemical changes induced along the course or track of the bombarding electron in protoplasm are not well understood. Within the past decade, most studies have centered about the possibilities that the initial or primary effect was one of ionization of intracellular or "protoplasmic" water, and that the resultant products are at least as devastating as any direct physical effect which may also occur. Although it is probable that the amount of chemical toxins produced by ionized water along the immediate path of the electron particle is very great, this pathway is submicroscopic. Thus any of the chemical disturbances in a cell cerated by one electron traversing it are likely to be diluted rapidly in terms of the total intracellular protoplasm present. Many believe that any such toxins which might be present are of little consequence to the life of the cell unless countered by an increase in the total electron bombardment.

The biologic effects upon the cell are considered to be principally 2 in kind. One is the influence of the particle or ray upon the state of chromosomal activity or cellular division. The more active cellular division is, the greater the retarding influence of radiation upon its reproduction. The greatest retardation to cellular division is obtained when radiation is delivered just prior to its division. It is this effect which the radiotherapist desires to exploit in the treatment of malignant disease. The second effect is more specific and is the induction of chromosomal rearrangement with the result that mutant strains occur as demonstrated by the classic researches of Mueller.

An example of the first of the effects alluded to in the previous paragraph is the following. Griem and Stein (1960) found that L-triiodothyronine can be used both experimentally and clinically to produce a qualitative change in the radiosensitivity of certain selected tissues. This observation brings up the possibility of administering such drugs to increase temporarily the growth rate of tissue cells to render them more sensitive to irradiation.

Of course, the cellular changes induced by ionization do undergo substantial repair. It has been demonstrated[11] at slow rates of radiation that cellular repair may be able to keep pace reasonably well with the damages inflicted, at least for a while. At similar exposures, rapidly given, repair may not remain current with damage, and death occurs.

There are also quantitative differences to be considered in cellular damage which relate to the speed of the radiating particle. Fast-moving particles lose less energy than slow ones. The dose of radiation must be increased or decreased accordingly if one wishes to inflict comparable damage upon cells of similar structure.

The dosage may be altered in another manner. Lane, Mauderli and Gould (1960) tested the biologic effects of lead-grid focused telecobalt therapy with those of homogenous cobalt-60 irradiation. In white Swiss mice they found the latter to be 2.4 times as toxic, indicating a probable advantage of this type of grid irradiation.

It becomes quite apparent that the biologic response of the cell to ionization is a function of many variables; some of these are known and well established, others are not.

RADIATION INJURY

Reaction of the body to ionizing radiation depends upon the physical quality of the rays, the dosage administered, the extent of the body exposed, the systemic or general reaction encountered and the susceptibility of that portion irradiated. Because of the wide variety of exposure technics required in the treatment of human disease, the character of radiation injury assumes different patterns under different circumstances. The clinical syndromes produced by radiation conveniently fall into 2 classes: those associated with local or portal therapy and those which follow total body exposure to ionizing radiations.

Injury from Portal or Local Irradiations

Local radiation, applied externally, is capable of producing acute and/or latent injury and serious sequela, as well as systemic disturbances in the course of appropriate treatment. The systemic manifestations encountered in portal therapy differ from local reactions in regard to symptomatology, nature of the insult, its time of onset and host resistance.

Systemic Reactions (Radiation Sickness). Radiation sickness is the term generally applied to the syndrome of headache, anorexia, nausea, vomiting and diarrhea which occasionally develops in the course of portal therapy. If proper therapy is applied and administered over periods of time which are now well established by experience, these reactions are seldom of serious consequence. They are to be expected if sufficient carcinocidal radiation is to be administered to many patients. Radiation sickness of this type is a self-limiting disease. When the syndrome is full blown, its symptoms may necessitate permanent abandonment of the planned program of radiation therapy, or its interruption with a period of rest before resumption. In other patients, some modification of the therapeutic program may relieve the patient sufficiently to permit completion of treatment without interruption.

In general, 4 theories have been devised to account for radiation sickness: (1) the production of toxic products by the action of radiation on tissues; (2) toxic products arising from the breakdown of normal or tumor tissue in the course of radiation necrosis; (3) interference with ill-defined metabolic pathways with the potential that abnormal metabolites accumulate; and (4) emotional disturbances associated with the ritual of radiation therapy and the import of this form of treatment to the patient. Although many patients are benefited by reassurance, there remains sufficient indirect evidence in support of the toxic theories or disturbed metabolic pathways so that actual chemical or physical disturbances cannot be summarily dismissed

simply because they have not yet been demonstrated.

Because radiation sickness does present a troublesome problem in many patients, and its nature is not understood, many drugs have been tried blindly, seeking to minimize or abolish this complication. Good results have been claimed for the following drugs: epinephrine, Lobelin, corpus luteum, Nautixan, Cardiazol, morphine sulfate, calcium chloride, calcium lactate, sodium chloride, sodium bicarbonate, glucose, candy, cholesterol, histamine, Benadryl, phenobarbital-belladonna, amphetamine, pentobarbital, liver extract, thiamin chloride, nicotinic acid, ascorbic acid, inositol, riboflavin, choline chloride and the so-called tranquilizing drugs among others. Most writings in support of each of these agents claim that more than two thirds of the patients were improved after receiving the specific agent being reported. Even the most credulous soon come to entertain doubt that the results claimed can represent little more than cheerful and enthusiastic attitudes of the physician—possibly an improvement in his personal relationship with the patient more than an actual improvement in the patient's illness.

Local Reactions to Externally Administered Radiation. When radiation therapy is employed, it is inevitable that some degree of damage, however slight, will occur to the normal tissue exposed in the region under treatment. This is a fundamental fact to be considered in all forms of radiotherapy and, more than most other practical considerations, the threshold of damage of normal tissues or their tolerance to radiation is the central theme which determines the type of radiation therapy most appropriate and the quantity to be employed.

Radiotherapy is successful and the usual treatment of choice when the diseased tissue or organ is readily responsive to an exposure which provokes little damage or disorder in the surrounding normal tissue organs. If a substantial differential in radio-insensitivity between the tumor and the adjacent normal tissue included in the field of exposures does not exist, radiation is not the treatment of choice nor is it likely to serve a very useful purpose without inducing harm or at least carrying considerable risk. On the other hand, when the diseased tissue or the organ or the agent responsible for the pathology does respond to doses of radiation which are not harmful to normal adjacent structures, then radiotherapy is the treatment indicated, provided that a better form of treatment does not exist. Stated otherwise, it is the differential in the limits of tolerance of normal tissues for radiation compared with that of the diseased part which delineates those diseases amenable to radiotherapy from those which are not.

ACHIEVING EXTERNAL CARCINOCIDAL RADIATION WITHOUT SERIOUS LOCAL INJURY. The goal of radiation therapy is to deliver to the diseased part, often a malignancy, the largest possible percentage of the total radiation to which the normal tissues adjacent to the structures under treatment will tolerate very well. To this end, the radiotherapist strives to employ radiation of sufficient energy so that the skin and the underlying normal tissues receive the smallest possible percentage of radiation which does not also reach the depth of the diseased part under treatment. This may be accomplished by one or both of the following principles and technics:

External radiation may be directed to the deep-seated radiosensitive tumor from multiple portals, using the most energetic radiation suited for the particular circumstance. This practice assures penetration to the proper depth with as little extra and superficial exposure as is possible to any one adjacent area or portal of entry. The larger the percentage of ineffective penetration, the more heavily radiated will be the overlying normal structures and the smaller will be the dose delivered to the target depth. Thus in low-energy radiation, which means smaller percentages of depth penetration, the higher the exposure of superficial structures necessary to achieve a carcinocidal dose to the depths. To whatever extent the normal tissues are exposed above and beyond that of the deep-seated tumor, that is the extent to which any inherent differential in sensitivity between the tumor and the normal tissue is lost. Hence, with low-energy gamma or x-radiation, the effectiveness of radiotherapy is correspondingly diminished, and the likelihood of injury to superficial structures is correspondingly increased if an adequate depth dose is to be given.

How can a larger percentage of radiation therapy be delivered to a deep-seated tissue with the least injury to normal structures? Developmentally, the first principle to be employed was to increase the tumor dosage and to lessen skin or superficial damage by the practice of alternating the portals of external exposure. It is as though one were to move the external source along the rim of a wagon wheel with the beam of radiation always directed toward its hub—the site of the tumor. Thus, radiation to the peripherally located areas or normal tissue is correspondingly reduced; that of the axis or center is increased. Lead shielding of adjacent normal tissue by carefully placing such shields in different external locations each day of treatment so that a different external area or portal of entry is used to gain depth exposure has permitted much higher dosages to be delivered to the more centripetally located tumor site.

Continuous rotation or rotational therapy is carried out by some; this is an improvement upon the more laborious and less well-controlled technic of portal therapy. Rotational therapy is accomplished by rotating continuously the source of radiation 360° about the patient, placing the patient so that his tumor is located equidistant from the rotating source. In others the same is accomplished by rotating the patient continuously through a complete circle with the source remaining stationary. The results obtained by either rotational technic are similar. The chief factor in determining whether the source or the patient shall be rotated is whether the size of the source permits rotation.

A second and equally useful principle devised to increase the percentage of the total exposure to the tumor above that which is delivered to the skin and the superficial areas is accomplished by the use of more energetic radiation, often referred to as supervoltage radiation. Here again, two approaches are possible; they are generally employed in combination. First is the selection of the most energetic form of electromagnetic radiation practical to meet the patient's requirements. The second is the use of filtration. As most sources of such radiation emit a spectrum of wave lengths and energies, a portion of which has little or no penetrating power, these rays can be removed by the interposition of appropriate filters interposed between the external energy source and the surface of the patient. Filtration plays a more important role in low-energy radiation where the percentage of penetration is small. The alpha particles of radium are completely removed by the interposition of a thickness of a single sheet of paper. They present no problem for radium, as any container used effectively removes them. External beta rays are readily removed by the use of copper and/or aluminum filters; their elimination from the total dosage delivered to the skin is most important to the patient's safety. Although beta rays generally penetrate little more than the external or more superficial layers of the skin, the extent to which these rays do penetrate is just that much increase in skin exposure; hence, that much reduction in the quality of the more penetrating gamma or x-radiation that can be administered without harm to the interposed normal structures.

Even with ordinary x-rays, the skin may receive a considerably higher percentage of electromagnetic (gamma or x-ray) radiation than does the underlying tumor. More favorable relationships between the amount of radiation delivered to the tumor compared with that delivered to the skin has been obtained by increasing the energy or the penetrating powers of electromagnetic radiation. The greater their energy, the higher will be the proportion of the total dose reaching the skin, which will also reach the tumor depth. "Softer" gamma or x-radiation which are only capable of penetrating the skin and the superficial normal tissue and not the tumor are largely removed by filtration. There is a limit beyond which these practices cannot be extended, for there remains the principle that the quantity of radiation, light or heat diminishes at an exponential rate with the square of the distance from their sources.

Obviously, the problem of dosimetry, the technical know-how and the knowledge as to the sensitivity of the tissue under treatment, as well as that of the normal tissue also being exposed, are reasons enough to relegate or to confine the practice of radiation therapy to *those, and only those,* who are properly qualified in this field. Few forms of therapy carry greater potential risk of litigation and with a better chance for unfavorable judgment than radiation injury administered by those un-

skilled in its usage. Radiotherapy is no longer simply a matter of "button pushing," if indeed it ever was.

TISSUE INJURY FROM EXTERNAL RADIATION. Because normal tissue is damaged to varying degrees by radiotherapy, one must expect and accept within limits a certain amount of tissue injury if therapeutic or carcinocidal radiation is to be given. This damage the surgeon is likely to term "radiation injury"; the radiotherapist calls it "radiation reaction." This is a problem in semantics and is not unlike that presenting the patient and the surgeon discussing the risk entailed in the administration of an anesthetic agent and/or the performance of an operation. In either case, it is the duty of the physician to present to the patient or a responsible member of the family an accurate appraisal of the expected reaction as well as the risk involved prior to the institution of such forms of treatment. In most instances where gamma or x-radiation is to be used (properly employed), the damage to normal tissue is of little permanent or important consequence. In few patients, permanent damage to normal structures is the price known in advance, if treatment is to be successful, especially in malignant disease. Again, as in the planning of an operation, the risk entailed, the expected disability and its management must be weighed in terms of the result that one can reasonably expect. If these unpleasantries are anticipated, consultation with others experienced in the field is often useful to all concerned.

The following are some of the reactions and injuries to be expected from carcinocidal radiation, externally applied:

Skin reaction is a function of skin exposure and is not an indication of dose delivered to deep-seated tumors. On the other hand, cutaneous reaction should not pass unobserved, whether high- or low-energy radiation therapy is employed.

Erythema is the first reaction to appear with low-energy radiation. If sufficient gradients of radiation are administered to the skin, erythema progresses to desquamation, to superficial necrosis and to deep necrosis. Of the various qualities of radiation administered as a single dose, needed to produce the minimal erythema reaction, are the following approximate values as measured on the skin with back scatter:

Radium .... 1,000 r
250-kv. x-ray with 0.5 mm. copper
    filter .... 670 r
80-kv. x-ray (unfiltered) .... 360 r

As the intensity of external radiation is increased, the site at which the maximum dosage is delivered tends to move to deeper levels within the patient. This results from a phenomenon known as "forward scatter." For example, a 2-million volt x-ray source delivers the maximum dosage below the skin surface; it can produce destruction of the subcutaneous tissue and muscle with latent fibrosis without inducing any skin reaction. High-energy ray or particle radiation of this or greater magnitudes (supervoltage), delivered to the proximal surface of the arm, a theoretical example or model, may produce no demonstrable skin reaction at the portal of skin entry. Yet necrosis of muscle, subcutaneous tissue and skin at the portal of exit may occur due to the forward movement of the site of maximum dosage. Consequently, with the high-energy sources, the erythema reaction, so useful an indicator of dosimetry 10 years or more ago when only moderate radiation energies were possible, no longer serves as a valid indicator of exposure, especially when supervoltage radiotherapy is used.

Erythema, desquamation and superficial necrosis under proper radiation therapy are to be expected in many circumstances as part of the consequences of treatment. These will heal. Pigmentation usually occurs in carcinocidal dosages of these magnitudes and may or may not diminish or disappear over a matter of months.

Loss of skin appendages—hair and sweat glands particularly—is the rule in the skin at the sites employed for ordinary radiation administered in carcinocidal dosages. Telangiectasia also occurs occasionally which is a permanent cutaneous disorder in many patients given carcinocidal radiation. Occasionally it is unavoidable. If this is cosmetically a handicap, such skin often may be removed later and a graft applied.

None of these unpleasant results is a contraindication to carcinocidal radiation therapy provided that the dosage to be delivered is essential to the cure or the relief of a disease which is not otherwise amenable to less hazardous forms of treatment.

Skin necrosis and its latent complications at times represent evidence of unnecessary overexposure. In a few patients, however, the risk even of this complication is warranted, should the potential and ultimate achievement of tumor necrosis appear to be possible.

An example of unnecessary skin and subcutaneous fibrosis, musculature contractures and radiation-induced squamous cell carcinoma is illustrated in Figure 17-1. The hands and the feet of this 17-year-old girl, a concert pianist of promise, were treated for psoriasis by unmonitored x-radiation administered in a doctor's office by a technician without supervision. Repetition of treatment was carried out once a week over a 3½-year period. Dosimetry and other details have not been made available to the author. Ultimate amputation of both feet and amputation of portions of the hands and the fingers was necessary. No relief of the radiation contractures and fibrosis, involving the tendons and the joints, as well as the skin, was possible. Total disability of these structures persisted with moderate to severe degrees of flexion deformity and fixation resulting. The end result was a permanently and totally disabled patient at the age of 25, the mother of 4 children whose psoriasis continues as before. Already, 3 squamous cell carcinomas have been removed.

Wound healing is delayed when sufficient radiation has been administered. In acute but comparatively low doses (400 r or less) little change from the normal pattern of events is noted. More commonly encountered in surgical patients are the larger carcinocidal exposures. Under these circumstances, the healing process is impaired. Surgical incisions heal poorly if for no reason other than that the blood supply in radiated tissue is markedly impaired. It is likely that other disturbances also exist which interfere with healing.

Necrosis often follows incisions in the radiated skin and necessitates grafting or excision with closure by rotation or mobilization of flaps of full thickness nonradiated skin. So frequent is this a bad sequela of surgery performed in areas of heavily radiated skin that time and hospital costs are often saved the patient if the radiated area to be incised is also excised at the same time.

The crystalline lens and probably the cornea also are very sensitive to ionizing radiation.[11] If exposed to a few hundred roentgen units, the latent development of cataract is a good possibility. However, not all lens opacities so produced progress to permanent cataracts. Cataract formation has been observed among scientists exposed to external radiation acci-

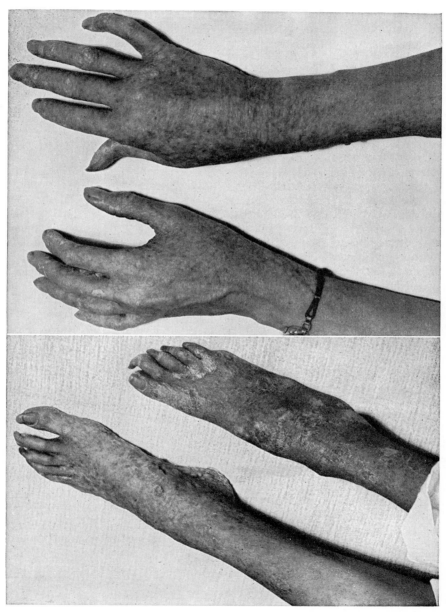

Fig. 17-1. Hands and feet 7 years after termination of an unknown amount of "soft" x-radiation in treatment of psoriasis. Fibrosis of skin and subcutaneous tissue with flexor deformities is evident. Note hyperkeratosis of skin which, along with avascularity, later necessitated amputation of both feet and some fingers. Multiple cutaneous carcinoma also developed.

dentally or incidentally. In the treatment of lesions about the face, particularly in the region of the orbit, every precaution should be taken to avoid injury to the eye. In malignant lesions, permanent damage to the eye may be unavoidable if radiotherapy offers potential benefit or cure and its usage is to be effective. This hazard should be explained to the patient and the immediate family before embarking upon treatment.

Necrosis of bone is a complication occasionally encountered from external radiation. This potential should be considered in planning the therapeutic dosage to be employed whenever intensive bone exposure is likely to occur. Fractures of the rib, the clavicle and the head of the humerus from aseptic necrosis have been observed in the course of therapy delivered in the postoperative treatment of carcinoma of the breast. In the growing child, the possibility of growth arrest of epiphyseal plates must be considered whenever more than 600 r are expected to be delivered to such areas. Aseptic necrosis of the head of the femur as well as the sacrum can occur among patients receiving radiotherapy for carcinoma of the uterus or the cervix, whether administered as radium therapy or x-radiation.

Radium- or x-ray-induced necrosis of the adjacent sigmoid colon or the bladder are other occasional complications of radiotherapy for pelvic cancer but these are avoidable in most patients when radiation is given properly.

Pneumonitis and occasionally *pulmonary fibrosis* are, respectively, relatively early and comparatively latent complications in some patients under external radiotherapy for carcinoma of the breast. Pneumonitis probably is observed more frequently than any radiation reactions other than those of the skin. Should intensive radiotherapy be necessary, pneumonitis of some degree may not be avoidable. Antibiotics are most useful in the prevention or the control of infection during its acute phases.

The avoidance or the treatment with benefit of minor degrees of pulmonary fibrosis after cortisone is claimed, but years of observation will be required to be certain. The development of other therapeutic methods to minimize radiation fibrosis of the lungs and other organs is under exploration.

MALIGNANCIES FROM RADIATION. Although radiation is second to surgical extirpation as the most effective form of therapy in the over-all cancer therapy program now available, improper exposure from ionizing radiation, on the other hand, is one of the most reliable means for the production of cancer, particularly skin cancer in man. As with all cancer, the nature of its pathogenesis is not understood; but of the fact that radiation can produce cancer there can be little doubt. Radiation-induced cancer is generally the result of excessive radiation therapy, but it is an occupational hazard as well.

Squamous carcinoma of the skin is already alluded to in the case report on page 312. Many physicians using the fluoroscope indiscriminately in the developmental early years of radiotherapy, prior to a knowledge of its hazard, eventually died of metastatic squamous carcinoma, particularly those arising from the skin of the hands. This complication was also observed fairly commonly among orthopedic surgeons employing fluoroscopic control without protection for the realignment of fractures.

Aside from cutaneous cancers among radiologists, there is radiation-induced *leukemia.* The incidence of leukemia among all physicians is said to be about twice that of the population at large. March[23] reports the incidence of leukemia to be 0.53 per cent among 26,788 physicians where the cause of death was known. Among the causes of death in 175 radiologists, the incidence of leukemia reached 4.57 per cent. This is an attack rate of about 10 times that of all physicians and approximately 20 times that of the population at large.

Recently, data have been presented which suggest that carcinoma in the *thyroid* in children and young adults may follow the radiation of the gland in infancy or early childhood. Duffy and Fitzgerald[7] reported in 1950 that, in 10 of 18 patients in the age group of 18 years or younger, radiation to the thymus had been administered some time between the 4th and the 16th months of life. Simpson, Hempelmann and Fuller[31] surveyed 1,400 of 1,722 children who had received x-ray therapy to the thymus between the years 1926 and 1951. The number of cases of thyroid cancer was markedly higher in the treated group than in either untreated siblings or the population at large.

Clark[5] uncovered a history of thymic radiation in 3 of 13 children under the age of 15 whom he observed for carcinoma of the thyroid. However, a careful check with parents and their physicians established that the remaining 10 had received radiation to the neck in the treatment of cervical adenitis, enlarged tonsils, adenoids, sinusitis, peribronchitis and pertussis. Thus, in all of his cases, radiation to the neck, including the thyroid area, was administered in infancy. The total roentgen dosage ranged from 210 to 725 r. Of the 13 patients, 12 were girls. The author has 3 cases.

Hempelmann's group compared the occurrence of all malignancies encountered in thymic radiation given to 1,400 children with the attack rates of that observed in 1,795 untreated siblings and in the general population of the same age distribution. Not only was the incidence of carcinoma of the thyroid increased, but so were some other types of malignancies, especially leukemia. The following data, taken from the Hempelmann report, would seem to introduce a serious note of caution regarding radiation in comparatively small doses administered to infants and children for benign disease.

TABLE 1. EXPECTED AND OBSERVED RATES
FOR MALIGNANT NEOPLASIA

TYPES OF CANCER	TREATED CHILDREN		UNTREATED CHILDREN	
	Ex-pected	Ob-served	Ex-pected	Ob-served
All cancers	2.6	17 (?19)	2.7	0
Leukemia	0.6	7 (?8)	0.6	0
Thyroid cancer	0.08	6	0.08	0

Osteogenic sarcoma, chondrosarcoma and *fibrosarcoma* have been reported by Hatcher,[13] Cahan et al.[4] and by others in association with externally administered roentgen administration. While these tumors are uncommon complications, their occurrence does argue against the use of radiation in the treatment of benign tumors which could be excised surgically without difficulty and with good results.

Reactions from Internally Administered Radiation. With the advent of isotope therapy in recent years, the potential hazard of over-exposure from internal radiation becomes a problem with which to reckon. In general, radioactive isotopes such as I^{131}, P^{32}, or Au^{198} have sufficiently short half-lives as to present little danger from chronic effects when properly used. They are capable, in excessive dosages, of producing acute radiation damage, especially those of aplasia of the marrow and even death. Excessive I^{131} can ablate thyroid function; in some patients this may be the desired result (see Chap. 26, "Thyroid Thymus and Parathyroids").

Chronic effects of isotope administration, which have long half-lives and are retained within the body, present other problems. Most prominent of these isotopes are the so-called "bone seekers." Within less than 2 decades of the discovery of radium, its soluble salts were administered parenterally or orally for numerous diseases. Salts of thorium X and radium were the small isotopes prescribed. Administration by inhalations of radon and thoron "gases" was also commonly practiced.

Unfortunately, because the early results for some of these diseases were interpreted as beneficial, such therapy was continued. It was only 10 to 20 years ago that toxic manifestations began to be apparent, particularly in patients receiving the bone-seeking salts of thorium, mesothorium and radium. To be included in this same group are the "dial painters" who touched the thorium X-containing paint brushes to their lips to draw out a fine brush point. The latent bone changes included necrosis, malignant disease and blood dyscrasias. These findings were first reported by Blum in 1924[2] and more extensively by Martland[26] and Hoffman.[16] By 1932, radium for internal administration was removed from the *New and Nonofficial Remedies* of the American Medical Association.[22]

Hatcher,[13] Hasterlik,[22] Marinelli[24] and others point out that hundreds and perhaps thousands of individuals in the United States were given radium or thorium salts orally or parenterally 20 or more years ago. They and others have examined many of these individuals and found them to be unaware that they carried radium or thorium deposits in their skeletal system. The hematologic findings also were neither striking nor diagnostic in most of these patients. 38 patients in Hasterlik's series[22] received radium salts therapeutically, and 6 had been employed as "radium" dial painters. Osseous lesions were readily demonstrated by roentgenograms in many. A general correlation existed between the amount of residual thorium and the frequency and the severity of osseous lesions observed. Bone sarcomas were observed in 6 patients in this series; all 6 probably received radiothorium and/or mesothorium; none was believed to have received radium alone.

Although the hazard from persistent radiation of bone-seeking radioactive isotopes is now well recognized and assiduously avoided in industry and medicine, the total problem or the ultimate end-result is not yet clear or evident. A similar potential and possibly uncontrollable hazard exists from the radioactive fall-out of strontium[90] in the event of atomic disasters and to a lesser extent from strontium[89] (see below) .

INJURY FROM TOTAL BODY RADIATION EXPOSURE

In the early dawn hours of July 16, 1945, on the Alamagordo range in the desert country of New Mexico, the first atomic bomb burst was witnessed some 7 miles away from ground "zero." This was to mark the hour, in fact, the milisecond of the beginning of a new era in human biology, if not also in history. Its arrival, for better or worse, is a matter to be settled by the course of human events—time alone will tell.

After the Hiroshima and Nagasaki bombings of August 6 and 9, and a few weeks later, there remained no doubt that for the duration of human existence, death from total body exposure to ionizing radiation would remain a threat.

The 16 years which have elapsed since then give every reason to believe that the radiation hazard from total body exposure is potentially greater than first expected, rather than less. Until the first thermonuclear explosion, March 1, 1954, at Bikini, hope remained among the less well-informed that the immediate blast effects and radiation exposure of the Alamagordo prototype would be largely limited to a radius of 10 miles or less. However, the thermonuclear detonation of 1954 clearly indicated to all that survival was more than a matter of local concern. This experience has disclosed a second and potentially more serious radi-

TABLE 2. CALCULATED EXPOSURE DATA OF RADIATION EXPOSURE 110 MILES AWAY FROM DETONATION OF THE THERMONUCLEAR EXPLOSION OF MARCH 1, 1954 (LAPP)

5 to 12 hours	1,000 r
12 to 24 hours	625 r additional
24 to 48 hours	545 r "
2 days to 1 week	815 r "
1 week to 1 month	720 r "
1 month to 1 year	840 r "
	4,545 r in the first year

ation hazard in that large numbers of the population hundreds of miles away could be exposed to lethal radiation, should they be victims of the "fall-out" or radioactive fission products from such a blast. The settling of radioactive dust upon the fisherman crew of the *Fortunate Dragon* 110 miles away from the 1954 Bikini explosion told its own story.

The fall-out phenomenon, while also occurring to some degree with the burst of the conventional atomic bomb, increases in "quantum" proportions when weapons of the thermonuclear variety are employed. In Table 2 are Lapp's[20] computations of the radioactive potential of the fall-out at 110 miles distance from the site of detonation in accordance with time. These are unofficial.

The geographic area in which fall-out radiation may have provided lethal exposure from a thermonuclear burst of the March 1, 1954, variety was largely elliptical in shape. Lapp computes it to have covered a ground surface ranging from 7,000 to 14,000 square miles. The "hottest" fall-out of the Bikini test he estimates as an "eternity dose of 15,000 r."

The location, the extent and the concentration of exposure from any one thermonuclear blast are functions of the size, the location of the burst (air, ground, etc.) and the nature of the explosion. Weather conditions, especially wind direction and rain, are also a variable to be computed for any one occasion. Lapp has enumerated the fall-out constituents of high-yield, long-lived fission products of uranium (Table 3).

These isotopes are chiefly beta emitters. In order to be of consequence to human biology other than as causing skin burns, they need to be ingested or inhaled in some quantity. Of these particular fission products, the bone-seekers Sr[89] and Sr[90] present the principal

TABLE 3

Strontium	Sr^{90}	28 year
Technetium	Tc^{99}	100,000 year
Ruthenium	Ru^{106}	1 year
Cesium	Cs^{137}	37 year
Cerium	Ce^{144}	0.8 year
Promethium	Pm^{147}	2.6 year

hazard because of their alleged high-fission yield, the character of their half-lives (both short and long) and their eventual biologic sequestration in bone with their immediate proximity to marrow. Strontium^{89} with a life of 26 days presents possibly a greater acute hazard than does Sr^{90}. "Gram for gram, Sr^{89} is 180 times more radioactive than its twin Sr^{90}." The chronic nature of the exposure from Sr^{90} suggests the potential hazard to be one which is similar to that of radium poisoning with the latent potential sarcomas of bone so produced.[13] Lapp quotes Libby that there will be about 2 to 3 Gm. of radiostrontium per square mile, or about 10 microcuries of Sr^{90} and 1.5 milicuries of Sr^{89} per square foot. How much of these materials may enter the body remains unknown.

Perhaps the other fall-out radioactive isotope of great potential threat is Iodine^{131}. With a half-life of 8.0 days, this isotope presents an acute problem in contrast with the chronic effects of Sr^{90}. Its tendency to localize within the thyroid under certain conditions is so well established that there can be little doubt as to the specific nature of its hazard. Much more information is needed before the I^{131} exposure risk can be assessed properly. Should the intensity of exposure from the fall-out of I^{131} assume proportions permitting radiation exposures equivalent to the thyroid of 200 to 800 r, is there the same thyroid carcinoma potential as Clark[5] and others have reported among children and young adults who have received x-radiation to the thyroid region in infancy?

The Civil Defense program may be made vastly more complicated and difficult if Lapp's calculations are correct. It is to be emphasized that his computations are derived from published but not necessarily official information. To the extent that his basic information may be correct or in error is the extent to which his conclusions may or may not be valid. Lapp's calculations may need to be revised—

downward and upward. It may well be that the era of shelter protection has come to an end as Lapp suggests.

The dreaded syndrome of total body radiation is like the sword of Damocles, poised and ready to strike at large segments of the world's population in event of atomic warfare.

Sublethal total body radiation or irradiation directed toward all of the bone marrow may be used intentionally in the following instance: patients requiring homografts (e.g., kidney) from a nonidentical twin donor may successfully accept such a graft if their immunity process is temporarily interrupted or diminished by such radiation. Such patients need all the diagnostic and therapeutic measures that must be used with accidental total body radiation.

Pathogenesis of Total Body Radiation Syndrome. Much more can be said of the pathogenesis of total body radiation injury than can be said of its treatment. The clinical picture of victims of an atomic explosion differs primarily from that induced by excessive isotope therapy in that the onset of symptoms in the latter case may not develop for weeks, as exposure from isotopic therapy is usually cumulative and not instantaneous. Also, in atomic disaster most of the surviving casualties suffer from thermal and flash burns, lacerations and fractures, as well as radiation. Otherwise, when the latent symptoms of radiation appear, they are similar in nature and largely reflect the physical character and quantity of the exposure encountered.

Nearly all of the observations on total body injury from ionizing radiation are based upon the reactions of different species of animals studied under controlled conditions. There is considerable variation from one species to another with regard to the magnitude of the lethal dose by single exposure, but the lethal exposure for members of any given species varies only to a slight extent.

The most complete clinical and pathologic report on radiation injury in man is that of Hempelmann, Lisco and Hoffman.[15]

In Table 4 are listed the LD 50 values established for some of the more common laboratory animals subjected to a single total body exposure. From what is known of the Japanese disaster and of the Los Alamos accident, the LD 50 single exposure to total body

TABLE 4. LD 50 TO 100 WITHIN 30
DAYS AFTER TOTAL BODY EXPOSURE
WITHOUT PROTECTION

Man	250 to 500 r (estimated)
Dog	200 to 350 r (established)
Rabbit	800 to 950 r "
Rat	500 to 800 r "
Mouse	600 to 750 r "

radiation for man is probably within the range of 250 to 350 r. Because the response of the dog to total body radiation is so similar to that observed for man, and the LD 50 values probably comparable, the presentation and the discussion that follow are derived primarily from observations and data obtained upon the dog.

One new method which may be applied to the prevention of infection in patients with partial bone marrow destruction from purposeful or accidental body radiation is the following. Levenson, Trexler, Malm, Horowitz and Moncrief (1960) have reported on the use of a disposable plastic isolator for operating in a sterile environment. Such an isolator is a modification of the germ-free chambers used in breeding germ-free animals. For use in the operating room, the patient is outside the isolator, which is sealed to the region of his internal wound. For use with irradiated patients, the entire patient could be kept in such an isolator during the period of his increased susceptibility. All air, water and food given to him would be entirely sterile, thus obviating *all* exogenous contamination.

Symptomatology. In case of a severe exposure from an atomic burst, nausea, vomiting and occasionally diarrhea may occur within minutes after exposure. These symptoms are transient, lasting usually less than 24 hours. This course of events generally does not occur, except in the near-lethal or lethal range of radiation exposure. However, the onset of early nausea and vomiting does not necessarily forecast a fatal outcome, although it is probably true that most of the fatally radiated will display some nausea and vomiting within the first few hours.

Between the 5th and the 20th days, anorexia, nausea, vomiting and diarrhea may develop again. This time there is adequate explanation, although that which is known may not represent the entire picture. Concomitant with

the onset of these complaints is the appearance of extensive desquamation and superficial ulceration of the gastrointestinal tract. Edema and petechial bleeding into these organs is also present in varying degrees and is associated with engorgement of the lymph nodes by blood as distinguished from hemorrhage. These blood-filled nodes appear to represent the filtration of the blood-filled lymphatic circulation. Interestingly, the spleen, with little or no lymphatic circulation, is atrophied and relatively free of blood and hemorrhage.

As the radiation syndrome progresses, weakness, anorexia and fever become prominent features. These are explained to some extent by malnutrition and infection. Weakness may continue for several months after fever and infection have disappeared. Characteristic of all serious total body exposures is pancytopenia (see p. 319).

Perhaps more important than total body radiation in the burst of the conventional atomic bomb are the complications that burns, lacerations and infections impose upon the radiated individual as well as the nonradiated. In a few instances, fatalities occurred in Japan from blast effects at distances in excess of 5 miles, whereas lethal radiation effects probably did not extend beyond 4,200 to 4,500 feet. These physical injuries are immediately evident, whereas the radiation effects may not be evident for 8 to 10 days. Consequently, any early surgical repair undertaken must take into account the possible ravages of total body irradiation that may make their appearance during the 2nd or the 3rd week. The over-all problem is not a simple one.

When the patient becomes ill from radiation, his tolerance to infection, physical exertion and other forms of stress is reduced sharply. Minor wounds and surgical procedures at the height of radiation effects assume major significance. This point is well illustrated in Figure 17-2, wherein a radiated dog, as late as 55 days after total body exposure, developed a fever of unknown origin. A sharp reduction in the formed elements of the blood occurred and was associated with anorexia, weight loss and listlessness. At the time of onset of fever, the animal was believed to have recovered. Following transfusion and antibiotic therapy, recovery was complete; 6 years later the animal remains alive and seemingly well. Similar observations frequently have been made by Evans,[3] wherein he noted that otherwise nonfatal injuries, administered to dogs given sublethal exposure of total body x-ray, had a cumulative effect with death occurring in more than 75 per cent of animals observed.

HEMORRHAGE is probably the most obvious disorder in the individual receiving total body radiation. Its time of onset and intensity vary in accordance with the severity of exposure as well as within members of the same species identically exposed. In man and in the dog, bleeding about the teeth and the mouth and from the gastro-intestinal tract are commonly observed after the 1st week when exposure has been within the near-lethal range. Petechial bleeding and ecchymoses are generously distributed over the body surface. Although the skin is the most common site of hemorrhage, evidence of bleeding may be found in any organ of the body. Hemorrhage into the lungs, the myocardium and the central nervous system frequently occur and occasionally is fatal in itself. Otherwise, the spectacular abnormal bleeding associated with total body radiation is more often a troublesome nursing problem than a fatal complication. If the individual survives, bleeding ceases spontaneously between the 3rd and the 4th weeks after exposure and before the peripheral platelet count is increased appreciably.

The pathogenesis of radiation hemorrhage is complex and poorly understood. The most consistent finding is thrombocytopenia which,

in the near-lethal range, develops without fail and is full-blown by the 8th to the 10th day. The platelet count remains near zero for 3 to 4 weeks; then it begins to recover slowly, reaching maximal values by the 6th to the 7th week (Figs. 17-2 and 17-3).

The clotting time is prolonged between the 7th and the 18th days (Fig. 17-4). To what extent the clotting abnormality is related to thrombocytopenia is not established. Certain features suggest these abnormalities to be unrelated, at least in part. For example, the clotting time may be increased before or after the onset of severe thrombocytopenia. Also, the clotting time always returns to normal or near-normal before recovery of platelet count can be detected. In the bloods of some animals a clotting inhibitor can be detected; the nature of this anticoagulant is unknown but probably is not heparin as commercially prepared. In some radiated animals, "heparin" or heparinoid substances can be detected and also in the course of blood transfusion where its occurrence may be the result of transfusion reactions.[1] In these animals, some improvements in the hemorrhagic tendency is brought about by the administration of protamine sulfate or toluidine blue. As yet, however, the most effective antihemorrhagic measure after radiation is the repeated transfusion of platelets. However, it is discouraging that the prevention of hemorrhage has no apparent beneficial effect upon mortality.[6]

Prothrombin and AG Globulin activities are not altered appreciably in total body radi-

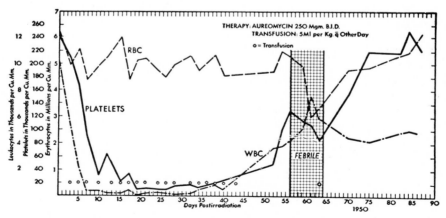

FIG. 17-2. Note unfavorable influence of infection and fever upon blood count as late as 2 months after heavy total body x-radiation exposure in dog.

ation, although the in-vitro conversion of pro-thrombin to thrombin is greatly impaired. This appears to be related to thrombocytopenia. To what extent the delay in prothrombin activation is responsible for the increased clotting time is not known.

The concentration of plasma fibrinogen is increased after irradiation. In the face of the systemic and local infections so frequently encountered in the irradiated subject, this is to be expected, but it is also said to occur in germ-free animals.

Vascular damage is suggested by petechial bleeding. However, this appears to be related primarily to the thrombocyte count and is largely prevented by platelet transfusions.[6] Transfused platelets with elevation of the platelet count do not abolish the increased clotting time.

Effective treatment of radiation hemorrhage is nonexistent at exposure levels approximately at the LD 100 range of untreated controls. Blood transfusions and the control of infection

have been suggested frequently as effective agents. An analysis of such reports discloses no important evidence to such contentions in severe radiation. There is ample proof that the liberal use of antibiotics has no beneficial effect upon the hemorrhagic tendency.[1] Also, the spectrum of clinical bleeding in species subject to this complication of radiation is not reduced in germ-free animals. These data lend generous testimony to the futility of these procedures as antihemorrhage measures. More alarming is the fact that when hemorrhage is largely prevented by the liberal transfusions of platelets, there is no reduction in either morbidity or mortality. It would seem then that there exist factors more significant than hemorrhage or infection as causes of death from total body radiation.

In exposure less than LD 100, antibiotics appear to be beneficial to some extent, but the extent of benefit is less than might be expected or hoped for.

INFECTION. An array of evidence exists to

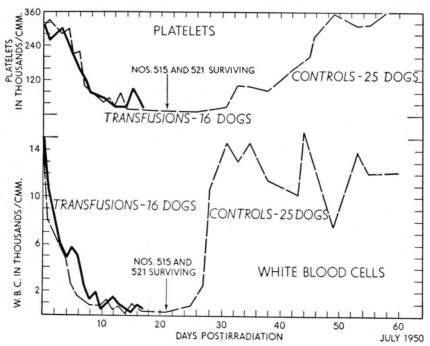

FIG. 17-3. Thrombocytopenia and leukopenia as they usually develop in range of an exposure of LD 50 or greater. Note that there is no numerical distinction between the degree of leukopenia and thrombopenia among those which die from those which survive.

demonstrate a reduced tolerance of the radiated individual to infection, but the control or the prevention of infection makes an unimpressive mark upon the mortality rate from radiation injury. Nevertheless, the control of infection is important to the welfare of the individual as well as to the community in the control and the prevention of epidemics following in the wake of disaster. Both hemorrhage and infection have been considered as serious factors in the mortality and the morbidity of radiation injury, but when both are eliminated, the individual's tolerance for total body radiation in the near-lethal range surprisingly is not increased materially. However, the great efforts which have been expended in these directions are probably more fruitful than is now apparent, for they have demonstrated that causes of death more subtle than either hemorrhage or infection undoubtedly exist and are yet to be identified.

Lethal or near-lethal total body exposures to ionizing radiation may reduce temporarily

the effectiveness of natural and acquired immune mechanism until the individual's defenses are seemingly too exhausted to cope with infection. These conditions impose a trying problem to the surgeon so far as any débridement and treatment of wounds and burns in the radiated individual are concerned, unless débridement can be performed early. If delayed a week or two, the patient becomes prey to both infection and bleeding. He is unable to eat or nourish himself, at least for 1 or 2 weeks. Thus, wounds that are of little consequence under ordinary conditions, assume serious proportions in the radiated subject after the 1st week.

When interpreting the harmful effects of ionizing radiation in terms of immunity, it must be remembered that the immunity of the host and the virulence of the invading organism are measured largely in terms of one another. In the case of radiation injury, infection is not due to any increase in the virulence of the organism but to the increased suscepti-

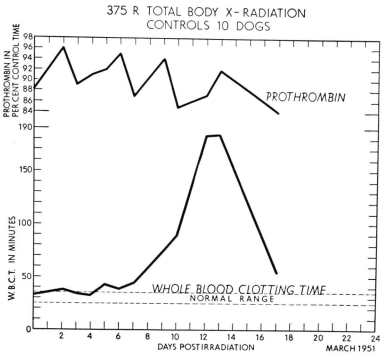

FIG. 17-4. Note abnormality of whole blood clotting time which can be detected by careful technic. Compare with Figure 17-3, and it will be noted that the clotting abnormality returns to normal before the platelet count begins to rise.

bility of the host to invasion and to his inability to isolate properly and destroy organisms once they enter the circulation. The ease with which bacteria may gain portals of entrance is not only the result of ulcerations, abrasions and burns immediately incident to an atomic explosion but also of the desquamation, the ulceration and/or the punctate hemorrhages so commonly noted in the gastrointestinal and the respiratory tracts in the late stages of intense radiation injury (1 to 4 weeks after exposure).

Similarly, once such organisms enter the blood stream, they are relatively unopposed by the natural factors of immunity. Leukocytes are nearly absent; those few remaining ones may be biologically inert. The antibody titer of the serum is reduced markedly.

Impairment of antibody production following total body radiation was observed by Hektoen as early as 1916.[14] Subsequent investigators have confirmed his observations repeatedly. Because of the variety of bacterial flora to which the individual is exposed, the passive transfer of antibodies for the present may be impractical in view of the comparatively rapid turnover of protein. There is no evidence that the daily administration of gamma globulin or plasma materially improves survival rate.

That total body radiation may act symbiotically with local radiation effects is supported by the following observation: Sikov and Lofstrom (1960) found that the amount of oncolysis produced by localized roentgen irradiation can be increased substantially by administering a small increment of total body irradiation. This increased oncolysis could be partially simulated by administering plasma from previously irradiated animals in conjunction with irradiation of the tumor. This was interpreted as indicating a possible substance in the plasma following total body irradiation which may be involved in the synergism.

It is to be expected that *antibiotic* therapy will be employed liberally in cases of total body radiation. Also, blood transfusion will be administered frequently to a few. There is at least no evidence that either is contraindicated.

PERIPHERAL BLOOD COUNT. Curiously, this does not reflect accurately the susceptibility of the individual to infection, nor does the leukocyte count determine which individual will survive. It is possible that there may exist certain qualitative differences in the remaining leukocytes of 2 individuals whose leukocyte counts are equally suppressed but from different quantities of radiation exposure. The leukocyte count in the near-lethal range is just as suppressed as when the exposure range has been lethal (Fig. 17-5). On the other hand, it must be admitted that an individual who maintains a near-normal leukocyte count almost surely will survive his exposure.

ANEMIA always develops in the total body-radiated individual who receives a near-lethal exposure, provided that he survives 10 to 15 days. Among the several factors contributing to anemia are: blood loss through hemorrhage, aplasia of the marrow, sequestration of blood by lymph nodes which filter the filled lymphatic circulation, and possibly hemolysis. Histologically, myelopoiesis is completely inactive by the end of the first week in near-lethal exposure. Evidence of regeneration does not reappear until the 3rd to the 4th week. Because the life of the circulating red cell is long (3 to 4 months), it is apparent that an accelerated rate of red cell destruction or anemia from blood loss or both must take place if one is to account for the rapid onset of anemia in the absence of blood loss. The red cell count also is the last of the circulating formed elements to return to normal concentration. It appears likely that the anemia of radiation has a dual pathogenesis and is biphasic in nature. The initial or early phase appears to be the result of blood loss and possibly hemolysis. The second phase is due to the lingering aplasia or hypoplasia which fails to correct the anemia of blood loss and destruction. There is also a failure to produce enough red cells at a rate sufficient to replace those lost through the normal course of metabolism; this appears to be an unimportant potential in the pathogenesis of this anemia, at least early anemia.

In spite of the extent of anemia, there is little evidence that its prevention or correction is of value unless severe *hypoxia* develops. Iron, B_{12} or liver extracts as therapeutic measures give no evidence of benefit in the refractory or aplastic phase. *Transfusion* accomplishes an increase in the rate or the extent of abnormal bleeding, if for no other reason that more blood is available to be disposed of by hemorrhage. There appears to be an increased rate of reactions to blood transfusion after total body radiation. In the dog, at least, their reactions cannot be predicted on the basis of matching. Immediately following transfusion, the blood in a small percentage of animals may become incoagulable.[6]

EXPERIMENTAL ATTEMPTS AT THERAPY. The observations and the experimental approach to the problem of prevention and treatment of total body radiation injury have been along 3 lines: (1) preconditioning prior to exposure, (2) shielding in part or *in toto* at the time of exposure, and (3) attempts at treatment administered after total body exposures.

POSTEXPOSURE TREATMENT is the evidence hoped for but to date the substance of which is not seen. While some degree of benefit has been derived from the use of transfusion combined with antibiotic therapy, any improvement obtained is sufficiently slight that it must be subjected to statistical analyses for appraisal of any benefit that may have occurred. Transfusions alone have given no evidence of any approved survival rate among dogs (Fig. 17-6). Negative results from this form of therapy tend to remove the premium that may be placed upon blood and its demands when it will be too scarce to treat but a small per-centage of the total injured in the event of atomic disaster. Even those who can be transfused have little or no assurance that its liberal use will be of value.

Transfusions of leukocytes have been employed and again with no evidence of definite improvement or response. One of the unusual features of an open and infected wound following an LD 50 or greater total body exposure is the absence of pus due to the severe leukopenia that develops. No leukocytes—no pus; thus one of the cardinal signs of local infection under ordinary conditions is missing.

The transfusion of platelet concentrates mentioned above will prevent much of the hemorrhage attendant to total body radiation, but disappointingly the control of hemorrhage bears little if any influence upon survival rates at LD 50 or greater ranges.

Many studies have been made as to the use of and the possible benefits to be derived from antibiotic therapy. It can be demonstrated that some benefit occurs from their usage when exposure dosages are less than an LD 50. Again, these changes are not sufficient to lend encouragement, but the results are very impressive. The studies of Miller have demonstrated that bacteremia may appear sporadically but that bacteremia is not necessarily an

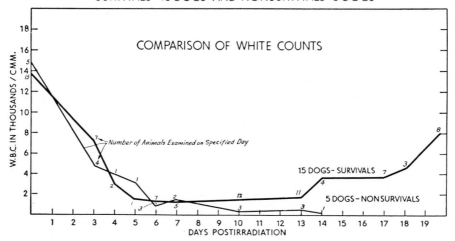

FIG. 17-5. Comparison of peripheral white cell counts in head-shielded animals, showing little difference in total residual counts among those which died from those which survived. The leukocyte response to single exposures of total body x-radiation offers no reliable clue as to prognosis.

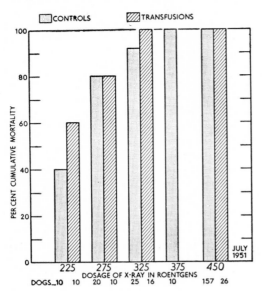

FOLLOWING SINGLE TOTAL BODY X-RADIATION – SURVIVALS 60 DAYS

FIG. 17-6. Data indicating the lack of any general or pronounced benefit over untransfused controls from blood transfusion, administered 3 times a week to dogs after total body exposures to x-radiation, ranging from 225 to 450 r.

indication of survival or of a fatal outcome. Further evidence along these lines is the observation that the LD 50 is not altered materially in species raised under "germ-free" conditions.

Thus the mechanism of death from total body exposure to ionizing radiation is unknown in most instances. Undoubtedly, both hemorrhage and infection may play a part, and at times may be the cause of death; but the prevention of either or both is not sufficient to alter statistically the spectrum of mortality among an exposed population.

PROTECTION AT THE TIME OF EXPOSURE— shielding of portions of the myelopoietic system has been demonstrated as an effective means of survival. Shouse, Warren and Whipple in 1931[29] reported that shielding as little as one vertebra in dogs materially altered survival rate.

The phenomenon of shielding has been studied extensively by Jacobson and collaborators[18] during the past decade. They have found that exteriorization of the spleen and its shielding doubled the tolerance for expo-

sure to ionizing radiation. Moreover, when shielding is carried out the usual delay in erythropoiesis is greatly shortened, and aplasia may not occur. Evidence of beginning marrow regeneration is detectable within a few days in contrast with several weeks required by the unshielded controls. Using homogenates of embryonic spleen injected intraperitoneally, Jacobson has been able to induce a similar beneficial reaction but only when the homogenates were administered within the first few hours following exposure. In this same connection it is of interest that the benefits continue if the animal whose spleen has been shielded during radiation is subjected to splenectomy only a few hours later. Herein lies a clue to the experimental approach to therapy, but as yet no one has been able to exploit the observation further. Nonetheless, the shielding experiments argue strongly in favor of shelter in the event of impending atomic disaster. The results to be expected from direct radiation should be commensurate with the excellence of the shelter available. However, the benefit of shelter protection may be lost should there prove to be a latent "fallout" of radioactivity (see p. 316).

PRECONDITIONING of animals prior to total body exposure has been studied extensively by many, particularly Patt.[27] On the theory that radiation is due to oxidation of water with resultant free radicals responsible for much of the injury, he has attempted to overcome this potential hazard by the administration of cysteine and similar compounds prior to exposure. This amino acid is a reducing agent by virtue of its sulfhydryl component. When cysteine was administered in advance of exposure, the tolerance of mice was increased from 550 to 1,000 r.

Anoxia or hypoxia also affords some degree of protection when employed just before radiation exposure. Hypoxia has been induced by direct oxygen deprivation as well as by the administration of compounds which compete more successfully for hemoglobin than does oxygen. Cyanide, para-aminopropriophenone and similar compounds have been tried with substantial benefit, but only when employed in advance of exposure.[32] In another interesting series of experiments, Patt employed refrigeration following exposure of frogs to lethal body radiation. As long as the frogs remained under refrigeration (often for months), they remained so far as could be determined in good health. However, once removed from the refrigerator and returned to normal temperatures, the syndrome of radiation injury appeared, and the animals died.

To date, the effects of total body radiation within the lethal range when experienced by the normal individual have proved to be irreversible. If full knowledge as to the reason for the protective action of pretreatment and/or shielding were at hand, possibly more promising leads than those in the past could be pursued with better results. Whereas preconditioning and/or shielding are important accomplishments, the fact remains that in the event of catastrophe, the therapy will be largely of the postradiation variety (Fig. 17-7).

MANAGEMENT OF WOUNDS CONTAMINATED WITH RADIOACTIVE ISOTOPES

Cuts, skin puncture wounds and abrasions are commonly encountered injuries among laboratory workers. These injuries may occur among those working with radioactive isotopes, whether in the laboratory or in industry, wherein the agent responsible for the break in the dermal layers is contaminated with one or more isotopes. The worker with an open wound incurred by other means may be exposed should he come into contact with a radioactive isotope at a time when the wound is capable of absorption of isotopes and the infliction of local and/or systemic radiation injury. Contamination in event of atomic warfare with the tens or hundreds of thousands of casualties whose wounds become contaminated presents a problem in civil defense. How serious is unknown.

These wounds deserve special attention which in principle may take one or more of several courses: local débridement or excision, prompt irrigation with agents which will bind a soluble isotope and hold it in the local area until it can be removed. Or it may be desirable to solubilize an insoluble isotope so that it may be removed more easily by careful irriga-

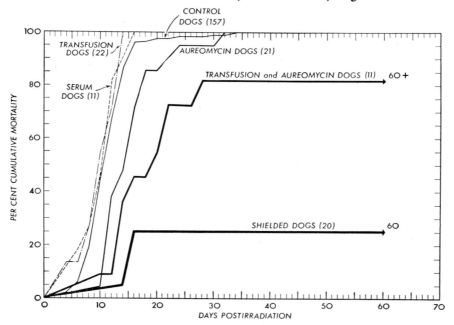

FIG. 17-7. Cumulative mortality curves of dogs subjected to various types of postradiation treatment. Included for comparison are the data obtained from head-shielding. The 450 r x-ray exposure is about 100 r above the LD 100 for this laboratory.

tion. Once the isotope has entered the body it may be desirable to accelerate its rate of excretion, if possible.

The choice of treatment most useful to the patient depends upon the character of the isotope(s) involved, the extent of contamination and the relative importance of the injury to any permanent functional or cosmetic defect that might be necessary should surgical excision of one type or another be required.

LOCAL SURGICAL TREATMENT

While the scrubbing of a wound will remove most bacteria, it does not follow that simple mechanical cleansing will necessarily remove radioisotopes, even from the unabraded surface.[8] Certain special precautions are necessary. Shaving of hair from the skin should be delayed until after "decontamination" has been accomplished satisfactorily, lest uncontaminated abrasions or cuts become contaminated from surrounding skin, and to that extent compound the seriousness of the problem already presented.

Arterial tourniquet may be applied promptly should the wound be on an extremity and the isotope be a soluble one. This procedure is not without the usual hazards of any tourniquet (necrosis or nerve injury) and is to be employed only when all precautions against the dangers of prolonged applications of tourniquets are borne fully in mind. Tourniquet should be used only when appropriate decontamination can be accomplished within less than an hour after its application.

Washing or irrigation should be more extensive than in the usual case of the ordinary wound. One of the detergents (sodium alkyl sulfonate, for example) is more useful than soap, as some detergents are more effective than soap in the formation of insoluble salts with many isotopes.

Nonsoluble isotopes contaminating the skin and the wound may not be absorbed for a matter of hours or days. When contamination is from an isotope of low solubility, a tourniquet is applied upon arrival at the doctor's office, and irrigations with a 1 per cent solution of sodium citrate is begun. Citrate is used as the irrigating fluid as a number of the heavy metals, including uranium, form soluble salts with citrate and hence may be washed away harmlessly. Many of these same metals

also form soluble chelates with edathamil (ethylenediaminetetra-acetate) which is an alternate irrigating solution that may be used (see below). Citrate is the less hazardous of the two, and more likely to be available.

In a few instances, cautery of an inconspicuous small area of skin or tissue may be employed with the aim of coagulating the blood and the lymph flow in the area, preventing or delaying absorption until the area can be excised; 8 normal concentrated hydrochloric acid or 14 normal nitric acid are suitable for this purpose, if the injured area is suitable for such treatment. Although both of these acids are available in most laboratories, it is the physician—not the scientist—who should decide as to the appropriateness of their use, and only the physician should employ them.

Then the usual surgical débridement is undertaken. The tissue removed is to be saved for monitoring and analyzing for its isotope content. Débridement may entail sacrifice of adjacent normal tissue if this is an important consideration to the potential of latent effects of residual isotope. This obviously is of greater concern in young patients than in the elderly and is also modified by the half-life of the isotope concerned and whether it probably will be retained in the body, e.g., radium and thorium.

GENERAL TREATMENT CONSIDERATIONS

Consultation with a competent health-physicist, acquainted with biology if not medicine *per se*, is imperative in any event. If the isotope is one likely to be absorbed, the patient should be admitted to a hospital equipped for metabolic studies and isotope measurements in tissue, blood, urine and feces.

Perhaps the most useful agent to bind certain of the heavy metal radioactive isotopes is intravenously administered edathamil calcium-disodium. This fairly nontoxic compound forms soluble chelates with yttrium, lauthanum, iron, cobalt, zinc, cadmium, lead, nickel, copper, plutonium and thorium.[9] These chelates are excreted unchanged in the urine; hence, the earlier this calcium-and-sodium-containing edathamil can be administered, the greater its benefits may be. The tetrasodium salt of edathamil should not be used as it may bind calcium and induce tetany.

Tritium may enter the body as HTO. Tritium quickly exchanges with the hydrogen of body water and thus enters to total water pool. Its elimination within less than 3 days can be accomplished by appropriate methods of diuresis[28]; otherwise it would remain for about 10 days. Similar exchanges of radio-sodium and potassium may be accelerated if required.[28]

PROTECTION OF PERSONNEL IN RADIOLOGY

Because of the potential hazards to personnel engaged in the practice of radiotherapy as well as diagnostic radiology, certain minimum standards are essential. Many useful suggestions have been published by the International Commission on X-Ray and Radium Protection.[17] In the United States, the National Bureau of Standards *Handbook 41 (X-Ray Protection)* and its *Handbook 23 (Radium Protection)* have been carefully compiled and should be consulted for details.

The outstanding feature of radiation injury to patients or personnel is its large percentage of instances wherein evidence of serious damages does not appear until many years have elapsed after the initial exposure. This applies to gamma and x-radiation as well as to poisoning from the internal ingestion of radium and other of the "bone seeker" radioactive isotopes. To the uninitiated, many of the regulations for protection set forth by those who have studied the subject may seem to be unnecessary.

The total exposure for any one week, whether acquired in a matter of minutes or uniformly distributed over the entire work week, carries essentially the same hazard for personnel in radiology. The International X-Ray and Radium Protection Commission originally adopted the permissible figure of 0.1 r per day exposure. In circumstances wherein the entire body is exposed to gamma or x-radiation, the maximum weekly permissible dose is 0.3 r per week as measured in air. More elaborate details are specified for other types of radiation and different qualities of radiation.[17] In exposure of the hands and the arms to gamma, x- or beta rays, the maximum permissible is slightly higher per week, 1.5 r or its energy equivalent. Among surgeons and internists, it is the orthopedic surgeon and

the fluoroscopist who are most likely to receive repeated exposures to radiation and encounter its injuries. They must adopt such precautions as necessary to maintain their own personal safety. However, the same precautions do not usually apply to patients undergoing radiation therapy or diagnostic x-ray procedures. Patients are exposed intentionally to dosimetries carefully calculated and prescribed under the immediate supervision of a competent radiologist.

Only the well-trained radiologist, functioning together with a health-physicist, can provide the greatest safety to the patient as well as to the personnel employed in radiology or allied fields.

REFERENCES

1 Allen, J. G., Basinger, C. E., Landy, J. J., Sanderson, M. H., and Enerson, D. E.: Blood transfusion in irradiation hemorrhage, Science *115*:523, 1952.

2. Blum, T.: Osteomyelitis of mandible and maxilla, J. Am. Dent. A. *11*:802, 1924.

3. Brooks, J. W., Evans, E. I., Ham, W. T., and Reid, J. D.: The influence of external body radiation on mortality from burns, Ann. Surg. *136*:533, 1952.

4. Cahan, W. G., Higinbotham, N. L., Stewart, F. W., and Coley, B. L.: Sarcoma arising in irradiated bone, Cancer *1*:3, 1948.

5. Clark, D. E.: Association of irradiation with cancer of the thyroid in children and adolescents, J.A.M.A. *159*:1007, 1955.

6. Cronkite, E. P., and Brecher, G.: Tr. Fifth Conf. on Blood Clotting and Allied Problems, pp. 171-212, New York, Macy, 1952; Allen, J. G.: *ibid.*, pp. 213-246.

7. Duffy, B. J., Jr., and Fitzgerald, P. J.: Thyroid cancer in childhood and adolescence: report on 28 cases, Cancer *3*:1018, 1950.

8. Finkel, A. J., and Hathaway, E. A.: Medical care of wounds contaminated with radioactive materials, J.A.M.A. *161*:121, 1956.

9. Foreman, H., Fuqua, P. A., and Norwood, W. D.: Experimental administration of ethylenediamine-tetraacetic acid in plutonium poisoning, A.M.A. Arch. Indust. Hyg. *10*: 226-231, 1954.

9a. Foreman, H.: Chelating agents, Indust. Med. *24*:287-292, 1955.

10. Glasser, O., Quinby, E. H., Taylor, L. S., and Weatherwax, J. L.: Physical Foundations of Radiology, ed. 2, New York, Hoeber, 1952.

11. Gray, L. H.: Biophysical basis: physical basis of the action of radiation on living materials *in* Carling, E. R., Windeyer, B. W., and Smithers, D. W.: Practice in Radiotherapy, London, Butterworth, 1955.

12. Griem, M. L., and Stein, J. A.: The effect of L-triiodothyronine on radiation sensitivity, Am. J. Roentgenol. *84*:695, 1960.

13. Hatcher, C. H.: Development of sarcoma in bone subjected to roentgen or radium irradiation, J. Bone & Joint Surg. *27*:179, 1945.

14. Hektoen, L.: Further studies on the effects of roentgen rays on antibody production, J. Infect. Dis. *22*:28, 1918.

15. Hempelmann, L. H., Lisco, H., and Hoffman, J. G.: The acute radiation syndrome: a study of 9 cases and a review of the problem, Ann. Int. Med. *36*:282, 1952.

16. Hoffman, F. L.: Radium (mesothorium) necrosis, J.A.M.A. *85*:961, 1925.

17. International Commission on X-Ray and Radium Protection: Recommendations of the Internat. Comm. on Radiological Protection and the Internat. Comm. on Radiological Units (Handbook 47), Washington, D. C., National Bureau of Standards, 1950.

18. Jacobson, L. O., Simmons, E. L., Marks, E. K., and Gaston, E. O.: Further studies on recovery from irradiation, J. Lab. & Clin. Med. *37*:683, 1951.

19. Lane, J. W., Mauderli, W., and Gould, D. M.: Biologic effect of grid cobalt-60 radiation, Am. J. Roentgenol. *84*:681, 1960.

20. Lapp, R. E.: Radioactive fall-out III, Bull. Atomic Scientist *11*:206, 1955.

21. Levenson, S. M., Trexler, P. C., Malm, O. J., Horowitz, R. E., and Moncrief, W. H., Jr.: A disposable plastic isolator for operating in a sterile environment, S. Forum *11*:306, 1960.

22. Looney, W. B., Hasterlik, R. J., Brues, A. M., and Skirmont, E.: A clinical investigation of the chronic effects of radium salts administered therapeutically (1915-1931), Am. J. Roentgenol. *73*:1006, 1955.

23. March, H. C.: Leukemia among radiologists, Radiology *43*:275, 1944.

24. Marinelli, L. D., Miller, C. E., Gustafson, P. F., and Rowland, R. E.: Quantitative determination of gamma-ray emitting elements in living persons, Am. J. Roentgenol. *73*:661, 1955.

25. Martin, H. E., Quinby, E. H., and Pack, G. T.: Calculations of tissue dosage in radiation therapy, Am. J. Roentgenol. *25*:490, 1931.

26. Martland, H. S., and Humphries, R. E.: Osteogenic sarcoma in dial painters using luminous paint, Arch. Path. *7*:406, 1929.

27. Patt, H. M., Tyree, E. B., Straube, R. L., and Smith, D. E.: Cysteine protection against x-irradiation, Science *110*:213, 1949.

28. Pinson, E. A.: Water exchanges and barriers as studied by the use of hydrogen isotopes, Physiol. Rev. *32*:123-134, 1952.

28a. Pinson, E. A., and Anderson, E. C.: **The Absorption, Distribution and Excretion of Tritium in Men and Animals,** Washington, D. C., U. S. Atomic Energy Commission, Doc. AECU-937, 1950.

29. Shouse, S. S., Warren, S. L., and Whipple, G. H.: Aplasia of marrow and fatal intoxication produced by roentgen radiation of all bones, J. Exper. Med. *53*:421, 1931.

30. Sikov, M. R., and Lofstrom, J. E.: Contribution of plasma constituents produced following whole body irradiation on the efficacy of local radiation therapy, Am. J. Roentgenol. *84*:705, 1960.

31. Simpson, C. L., Hempelmann, L. H., and Fuller, L. M.: Neoplasia in children treated with x-rays in infancy for thymic enlargement, Radiology *64*:840, 1955.

32. Storer, J. B., and Coon, J. M.: The Protective Effect of Para-Aminopropiophenone Against Lethal Doses of X-irradiation, TID-365, Univ. Chicago Toxicity Lab. Quart. Progress Rep. No. 5 on Radiology, pp. 16-19, 1950.

OSCAR P. HAMPTON, JR., M.D., AND WILLIAM T. FITTS, JR., M.D.

--- CHAPTER 18 ---

Fractures and Dislocations: General Considerations

FRACTURE MAXIMS

1. The saving of life comes first: treat impending asphyxia, hemorrhage, shock and other life-endangering conditions before treating a fracture.

2. Examine the injured part for signs of vascular and nerve injuries before searching for a fracture.

3. To minimize soft tissue damage and to avoid converting a closed to an open fracture, "splint 'em where they lie."

4. Obtain roentgenograms in at least 2 planes and examine them yourself.

5. Open fractures are contaminated wounds. Minimize the risk of infection by adequate débridement, open drainage or closure of the wound as indicated, and immobilization.

6. One measures the end-result of treatment of a fracture by the function of the part.

7. The chief aim in the treatment of fractures of the upper extremity is to ensure the proper functioning of the hand. Shortening and some malalignment are often acceptable.

8. The chief aim in the treatment of fractures of the lower extremity is to ensure painless, stable weight-bearing. Malalignment must be prevented, and full length is desirable.

9. Fractures involving joints require a perfect ("cabinet-maker's") reduction to minimize future arthritis.

10. To immobilize a fracture, both the joint above and below it usually must be immobilized.

11. Immediately activate all joints that are not immobilized for treatment of the fracture.

12. Throughout the treatment of a fracture, focus attention on the patient as a whole as well as on the injured part.

DEFINITIONS

A fracture is a break in the continuity of a bone. If it involves the entire cross section of the bone, it is a complete fracture; if it involves only a portion of the cross section, it is an incomplete fracture. Every fracture, therefore, is either complete or incomplete.

A closed* fracture is one which does not communicate with the outside air; an open* fracture is one which does communicate through a break in the skin or the mucous membrane and the underlying soft tissues— that is, through a wound. Therefore, every fracture is either closed or open.

Transverse, oblique and spiral are terms used to describe the direction of the line of fracture in relation to the long axis of the broken bone (Fig. 18-1).

* The terms *simple* and *compound* have been used to describe *closed* and *open* fractures until recent years.

329

A comminuted fracture has 2 or more communicating lines of fracture which divide the bone into more than 2 fragments.

Double fracture is present when the bone is broken at 2 levels without communicating lines of fracture.

An impacted fracture is present when one fragment is driven firmly into the other.

A greenstick fracture is a form of incomplete fracture, commonly seen in the forearm of children, in which one side of the cortex breaks and the other bends as a branch of a green tree bends.

A sprain or avulsion fracture is one in which a small piece of cortex is pulled away at the attachment of a ligament.

A depressed fracture, seen frequently in fractures of the skull and the facial bones, is one in which the fragments are in-driven.

A pathologic fracture occurs through an area of diseased bone, usually as a result of minimal trauma.

March (or fatigue) fracture results presumably from lack of normal muscle protection. It occurs in soldiers who have participated in long marches, especially when the troops are poorly conditioned. The second and the third metatarsal bones are the most common sites of march fractures.

An epiphyseal separation is a displacement of an epiphysis and signifies an injury through the epiphyseal line.

Dislocation signifies that a bone is "out of joint," that is, no longer in normal contact with the bone with which it articulates. Subluxation or partial dislocation is used to denote partial contact.

Nonunion of a fracture signifies that the

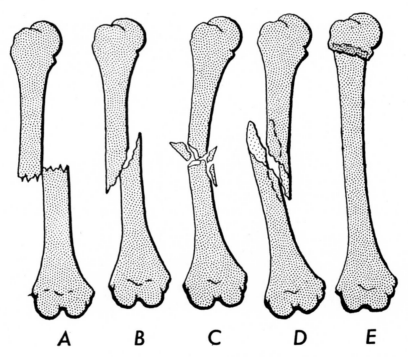

Fig. 18-1. Types of fracture, right humerus in the anteroposterior projection. (A) Transverse fracture of midshaft with medial displacement of the distal fragment. (The fragments are in poor apposition but good alignment.) (B) Oblique fracture with overriding. (The fragments are in partial apposition but good alignment). (C) Comminuted fracture with lateral angulation (apposition is not unsatisfactory). (D) Spiral fracture with lateral angulation (both apposition and alignment are poor). (E) Impacted fracture of the neck in good apposition and alignment.

process of healing has come to an end without union of the fragments.

Delayed union signifies that a specific fracture has not united in the time considered average for this fracture. The average time for healing of a fracture depends on many variables, and delayed union must never be considered non-union until the healing process has ceased without bony bridging.

Malunion signifies that the fracture has united with deformity sufficiently to cause impairment of function or a significant cosmetic defect.

Location. In locating a fracture in the shaft of long bones, it is usually described as being in the proximal, the middle or the lower third, or at the junction of 2 of these divisions.

A fracture of one of the bony prominences of the ends of long bones is described as a fracture of that prominence by name; for example, a fracture of the olecranon, a fracture of the medial malleolus, or a fracture of the lateral condyle of the tibia.

Apposition and Alignment. In describing the positions of the fragments, the terms apposition and alignment are used (Fig. 18-1). Fragments are in apposition when their ends are in contact. They are in alignment when their long axes parellel each other. Fragments may be in perfect apposition but angulated and therefore in bad alignment. They may be out of apposition and overriding but in good alignment if there is no angulation. In describing angulation, the direction of the point made by the fragments is given; for example, when fragments of the tibia and the fibula are angulated outward as in "bowlegs," they are in lateral angulation. The angulation of fragments may be lateral, medial, anterior or posterior. The position of the distal fragment in relation to the proximal is always described. For example, in a displaced fracture of the femoral shaft, a radiologist might report: "There is a transverse fracture of the shaft of the femur at the junction of the middle and the lower thirds with posterior and medial displacement and 3 cm. overriding of the distal fragment."

HEALING OF FRACTURES

The healing of fractures is primarily a local phenomenon. Adequate apposition of raw bone surfaces, adequate immobilization and a good blood supply to the fragments of bone are the most important prerequisites for the healing process. Local circulatory impairment, inadequate apposition of fragments, inadequate immobilization of fragments, interposition of material between the bone ends, extensive tissue necrosis, and infection have been shown to have a profoundly adverse effect on the healing effort. The most common sites of delayed union and nonunion—the neck of the femur, the lower shaft of the tibia and the carpal scaphoid—all have a precarious blood supply.

On the other hand, vitamin deficiencies, hypoproteinemia, osseous disease, debility and even a restricted calcium intake rarely cause an alteration in the sequence of healing of fractures, although senility and starvation may somewhat retard the rate of union. There really are no systemic causes of nonunion.

In general the healing of a wound of bone, a fracture, follows the same principles as the healing of wounds of other tissues. When a bone is broken, blood from ruptured medulary, periosteal and adjacent soft tissue blood vessels extravasates and forms a hematoma centered about the fracture site. With the ingrowth of capillaries and by the action of fibroblasts, the hematoma becomes organized into granulation tissue. This process is really the first stage of healing of a wound of any tissue.

In a wound of tissues other than bone (or cartilage) the fibroblastic action in the granulation tissue would continue to form mature fibrous scar. However, in a fracture, either because of the presence of bone ends in the granulation tissue or the specific action of osteoblasts upon it, the healing processes vary so that callus and eventually bone are formed to unite the fracture. Fibrous condensation of the granulation tissue takes place and then, apparently by metaplasia, areas of fibrocartilage and hyaline cartilage form in the young fibrous tissue. This seals the fragment ends together.

As the organization of the callus proceeds, the first new bone formation is seen subperiosteally at some distance from the fracture. The new bone spicules are bordered by large osteoblasts, presumably derived from the inner layer of the periosteum. This new bone forms a collar around each of the fractured segments and develops toward the fracture gap. At the same time, endosteal bone formation develops from the cells bordering the inner cortices and forms an inner core of new bone partly filling the medullary cavity and growing toward the fracture. The central area of cartilage tissue is replaced by bone as the advancing front of new bone reaches it. This latter process is similar to the endochondral ossification seen in normal growth.

The enveloping periosteal callus is usually more abundant in displaced fractures, where it acts as a scaffolding, uniting the separated fragments. The original callus is formed of rough, heavy-fibered, immature bone which is gradually replaced by more mature compact bone as the bulbous callus recedes and the new cortex and marrow cavity are formed. Fractures through bone which is primarily cancellous and flat, rather than cortical and tubular, usually show a more predominant endosteal phase with little subperiosteal new bone formation.

The exact process by which healing of a fracture is regulated is not known. Two theories have been widely discussed. These are the cellular theory (osteoblastic) and the humoral theory (physicochemical). The cellular theory holds that the osteoblast is a highly differentiated cell which has the specific function of forming bone either by actually secreting osseomucin and calcium or by secreting substances which precipitate bone-forming materials from the intercellular fluid. The humoral or physicochemical theory assigns the principal responsibility for the formation of bone to the tissue fluids and not to osteoblasts.

In the present state of knowledge these theories do not influence the treatment of a fracture. However, it is important to recognize the advantages of prompt, adequate and sustained reduction of the fracture so that healing processes may take place. The hematoma must become organized as the first step in the healing of a fracture. When a fracture is reduced within a few hours of injury before organization of the hematoma has begun, the healing process for the fracture has been given a good start. On the other hand, when reduction has been delayed, the manipulation of the fragment ends disrupts the healing process and in theory retards it. Certainly, repeated manipulations and inadequate immobilization of the fracture site may cause fresh bleeding, the formation of new granulation tissue and delayed healing. Healthy callus may never form, and the fracture may go to nonunion.

An optimum compression force across a fracture (contact-compression) appears to accelerate healing. Eggers, in experimental fractures of rats' skulls, noted an increased rate of healing when these fractures were subjected to compression forces. Whether the increased rate of healing was due to a stimulation of osteogenesis by the compression forces or was merely the result of close contact and rigid immobilization is not established. Friedenberg and French, in experiments on dogs, showed that excessive compression of fragment ends produced necrosis but that the optimum pressure for fracture healing is probably higher than that provided by the tone of muscles surrounding the fragments.

DIAGNOSIS OF A FRACTURE

The diagnosis of a fracture is made on symptoms furnished by the patient and on physical signs and x-ray examination. Usually, but not always, a history of injury is obtained.

SYMPTOMS

The characteristic symptoms of a fracture are (1) pain and (2) inability to use the part. Immediately following injury, a numb sensation may be present. After the initial numbness, pain becomes the outstanding symptom and continues with increasing severity until the fragments are immobilized. The patient usually is unable to use the part associated with most fractures. However, with impacted or incomplete fractures, function may be impaired only slightly or not at all.

SIGNS

The following signs indicate a fracture: (1) localized tenderness; (2) localized swelling; (3) visible or palpable deformity; (4) ecchymosis; (5) protective muscle spasm; (6) false motion; (7) crepitation (audible or palpable grating of bony fragments). Obviously, the most convincing signs are false motion and crepitation. They may be observed incidentally as the extremity is being examined, but testing for them is dangerous, as it may produce further tissue damage.

Every fracture is associated with some local soft tissue injury which may include injury to major blood vessels, peripheral nerves or tendons. These possible immediate complications (see p. 337) of a fracture demand a careful and complete examination of the entire part as an integral segment of the same examination to determine if a fracture is present.

As a routine in extremity injuries, the examiner must test for arterial pulsations distal to the injury (radial artery in the upper and the posterior tibial or dorsalis pedis artery in the lower extremity). Absence of the pulsation probably indicates interruption, partial or complete, of the arterial trunk of the extremity—a complication which takes precedence for treatment over the injury to the bone. Also as a routine, the examiner must test for the presence of nerve supply to the distal portion of the extremities. He must have the patient attempt to carry out movements of the fingers and the thumb or of the toes and test sensation of these parts. Loss of motor power in any muscle group or loss of sensation conforming to the known pattern of sensory nerve supply indicates injury to a major nerve trunk. Such a complication demands consideration as part of the entire injury and may modify the management of the fracture.

ROENTGEN EXAMINATION

The clinical diagnosis of a fracture always must be confirmed by adequate x-ray examinations. In possible fractures of the bones of the extremities and the spine, roentgenograms in both the anteroposterior and the lateral views should be made. Examination in 2 planes is essential, as a fracture may not be visualized in one view but may be obvious in the other (Fig. 18-2).

Roentgenograms of long bones always must include the joint above or below the injury and preferably the entire length of the bone in order that double fractures will not be overlooked.

However, routine roentgenograms in the 2 standard planes will not always visualize certain bone and joint injuries (Fig. 18-2). For example, a special oblique view is often re-

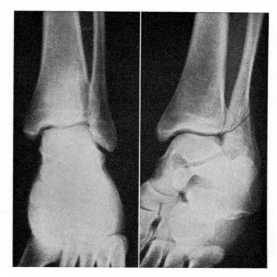

FIG. 18-2. Importance of special oblique roentgenograms in diagnosing injuries about the ankle. The standard anteroposterior view (*left*) and the standard lateral view disclosed no line of fracture. The oblique, or open mortise view (*right*) discloses an oblique fracture of the fibula.

quired to demonstrate a fracture of the carpal navicular. In injuries of the cervical spine, the classic anteroposterior and lateral views may show no evidence of bone or joint injury, whereas a lateral view with the head in flexion may demonstrate a subluxation of a cervical vertebra. A special axial view is often needed to demonstrate a fracture of the patella or a fracture of the os calcis. Frequently, x-ray examination of the contralateral uninjured side for comparison is exceedingly valuable in establishing the correct diagnosis, especially in fractures about the joints in children.

The physician who is to treat the fracture must know the views needed on x-ray examination to gain the maximum information about a fracture and he must examine the films himself to evaluate the problem before him. Good roentgenograms furnish information which is valuable in the selection of the method of management indicated for the fracture.

PRIORITY OF INJURY

Efforts to diagnose a fracture must not overshadow an accurate appraisal of the full effects of the injury on the patient and the injured part. These may be more important than the fracture itself. First attention always must be directed toward maintenance of an adequate airway and respiration, the control of hemorrhage and the treatment of shock, present or impending.

Consider a patient who has a cranial injury without signs and symptoms of increased intracranial pressure, a fracture of the mandible with some obstruction of the airway, an open sucking wound of the chest and an open fracture of the femur (Fig. 18-3). The patient has bled considerably and is in shock. Immediately an adequate airway is established, perhaps by an entotracheal tube, and the open thoracic wound is closed by an occlusive dressing. During these procedures

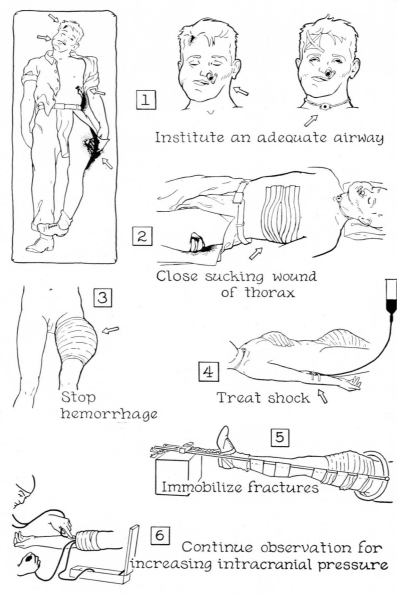

1 Institute an adequate airway

2 Close sucking wound of thorax

3 Stop hemorrhage

4 Treat shock

5 Immobilize fractures

6 Continue observation for increasing intracranial pressure

Fig. 18-3. Treatment of multiple injuries. Priority of injury. (See text.)

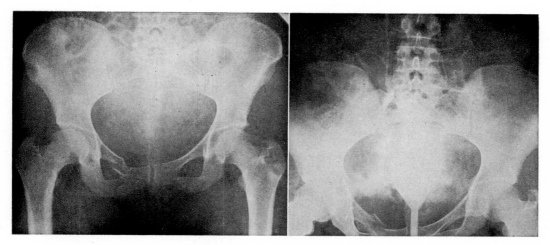

FIG. 18-4. Rupture of the bladder complicating a fracture of the pelvis with minimal displacement. (*Left*) Fractures of the pelvis with little or no displacement. (*Right*) Cystogram showing rupture of the bladder which is elevated, probably by hematoma formation.

whole blood transfusion has been started as therapy for shock. Without signs and symptoms of increasing intracranial pressure, the head injury needs only close observation for changing neurologic signs. The open fracture of the femur receives a sterile dressing to the wound and adequate emergency splinting which, incidentally, is further therapy for shock. Definitive therapy of the fracture of the femoral shaft must be postponed until the life-endangering injuries have been brought under control.

COMPLICATIONS OF FRACTURES

Complications of fractures may be divided conveniently into the immediate and the delayed. The immediate complications, such as hemorrhage and shock and intra-abdominal or intrathoracic injuries, may be life-endangering. The treatment of these complications takes precedence over treatment of the fracture.

IMMEDIATE COMPLICATIONS

Intra-abdominal. Fractures of the thoracic cage, the spine or the pelvis may be associated with intra-abdominal injuries. Blows to the upper abdomen which fracture the thoracic cage may rupture the spleen or the liver. Delayed splenic rupture always must be kept in mind by surgeons. Fractures of the

pelvis may be associated with injuries to the bladder, the urethra or the bowel (Fig. 18-4). Trauma to the pelvic region may cause only undisplaced fractures of the pelvis, yet a distended bladder may be ruptured. Bloody urine or the inability of the patient to void immediately alerts the examiner to the possibility of severe injury to the urinary tract. Every patient with a pelvic fracture who cannot immediately void clear urine must be catheterized at once. Severe crushing injuries to the left side of the trunk may cause the following triad of injuries—rupture of the spleen, the left kidney and the left diaphragm. Evidence of injury to any of these organs suggests injury to the others. All of these intra-abdominal complications of fractures are life-endangering and demand first consideration.

Intrathoracic. Hemothorax or pneumothorax may result from damage to the pleura and lung by the sharp ends of broken ribs or sternum (Fig. 18-5). Severe crushing injuries may fracture multiple ribs, creating a flail segment which causes paradoxical breathing. The "flail" area of the chest wall moves in on inspiration and out on expiration. Traumatic rupture of the major bronchi also occasionally attends crushing thoracic injuries. All of these complications are life-endangering and take priority for treatment.

Hemorrhage and Shock. Hypovolemic or

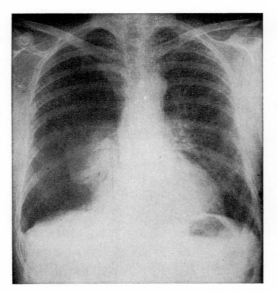

FIG. 18-5. Pneumothorax complicating fractures of the ribs. Anteroposterior roentgenograms of chest, showing complete collapse of the right lung with massive pneumothorax and slight shift of the mediastinum to the left with fractures of the ribs on the right. On admission to the hospital 16 hours before this roentgenogram was made, an admission roentgenogram showed the fractures of the ribs and only a very small pneumothorax. During the hours that followed, all of the clinical signs and symptoms of a tension pneumothorax developed. (Hampton, O. P., Jr.: Complications of common fractures *in* Hardy, J. D., and Artz, C.: Complications in Surgery, Philadelphia, Saunders)

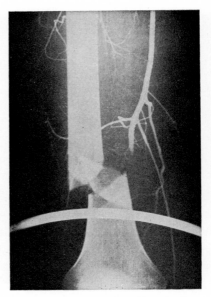

FIG. 18-6. Laceration of the femoral artery, complicating fracture of the shaft of the femur. An arteriogram demonstrates clearly the total interruption of the major arterial flow down the extremity at the level of the fracture of the femoral shaft. (Dr. James Stokes) (Hampton, O. P., Jr.: Complications of common fractures *in* Hardy, J. D., and Artz, C.: Complications in Surgery, Philadelphia, Saunders, 1960)

traumatic shock as a result of hemorrhage or hemorrhage plus loss of extracellular fluid into the traumatized soft tissues may accompany fractures of the extremities as well as those of the thorax, the pelvis and the spine. Loss of blood may stem from major vascular injury or merely from the broken bony fragments. It may be particularly severe in open fractures, but loss into the tissues in a closed fracture must not be underestimated. Fractures of the femoral shaft and the upper tibia are likely to result in considerable hemorrhage. The artery entering the tibia at the junction of the upper and the middle thirds is the largest nutrient artery in the body, and fractures at this level, particularly open frac-

tures, can lead to dangerous hemorrhage. Hemorrhage and shock are life-endangering and demand immediate therapy.

Injury to Major Arteries. Any of the major arteries of the extremities may be injured or occluded by a nearby fracture (Fig. 18-6). In some instances, collateral circulation will be adequate to maintain viability of the extremity. In others, the symptoms and signs of arterial insufficiency to the distal portion of the extremity will be present. Occasionally, fractures of the femur are associated with damage to the femoral vessels, especially those fractures in the supracondylar area in which popliteal vessels may be damaged by the sharp edge of the distal fragment which is pulled posteriorly by the gastrocnemius muscle.

If arterial insufficiency cannot be corrected

promptly by closed manipulation, which might free an artery merely occluded by the pressure of a fragment, continuity of the injured artery must be restored at once, if possible. The divided artery can rarely be repaired by end-to-end suture. A vascular graft is almost always necessary to repair arterial defects associated with fractures because of the extensive damage to the artery above and below the point of transection. End-to-end suture usually is attended by thrombosis if tension is used in bringing the ends together. In the extremities, venous autografts, arterial homografts and prostheses have been found to be satisfactory. When vascular repair is required, absolute fixation of the bone fragments must be effected with either an intramedullary nail or a plate and screws.

Injury to Major Nerve Trunks. Fractures of the bones of the extremities may have associated major peripheral nerve injuries. These are most likely to be present when a fracture occurs at a point where the nerve trunk is normally in close approximation to the bone. The most common nerve injuries as complications of fractures are (1) the radial nerve with fractures of the middle third of the humerus, (2) the peroneal nerve with fractures of the proximal portion of the fibula and (3) the ulnar nerve with fractures of the medial epicondyle of the humerus.

If the nerve has been merely contused, return of function may be rapid. On the other hand, if the nerve has been severed, end-to-end suture, either primarily or at a later operation, is indicated. Restoration of peripheral nerve function is often so important that it may be worth while to shorten the bone deliberately by excision of a portion of the fragments in order to get end-to-end approximation of the nerve.

A careful neurologic examination should be made in every injured extremity to determine if any evidence of nerve damage exists. The results of examination should be recorded before any effort at reduction of the fracture, either closed or open, so that it may be clear as to what part the original injury and what part the effort at reduction of the fracture played in damage to the nerve.

Injuries to the Spinal Cord. The seriousness of fractures of the spine is increased tremendously if the underlying spinal cord

receives even the most minimal damage. Fracture-dislocations of the cervical spine are particularly likely to cause damage to the cord. Transportation of patients with suspected injuries of the spine must be carried out in such a way as to avoid or prevent further damage (see "Emergency splinting," p. 341). Early reduction of fractures or dislocations of the spine may be of utmost importance in minimizing the permanent effects of damage to the cord.

Delayed Complications

Infection. Infection is not uncommon following open fractures and may follow open reduction of a closed fracture. All open fractures are contaminated and may become infected if the conditions are favorable. Such contributing factors are severe contamination, devitalized soft tissues, persisting exposure of bone, cartilage, tendon and fascia in the wound, retained foreign bodies, and poor reduction or immobilization of the fragments of bone. Clostridial myositis (gas gangrene), the most dreaded type of infection following open fractures, requires severely damaged and ischemic muscle for its development and often follows an open fracture complicated by an injury to a major artery. It is obvious, then, why thorough débridement is so important in preventing soft tissue and bone infection.

Nonunion and Delayed Union. The failure of a fracture to unite is due chiefly to local factors at the fracture site. Common sites of nonunion are the neck of the femur, the lower tibial shaft, the carpal scaphoid and the humeral shaft. These sites have in common a poor blood supply. Infection in the fracture site, interposition of soft tissues, inadequate immobilization and distraction (overpull) as part of treatment are common causes of delayed union and nonunion. Watson-Jones says, "There is only one cause of nonunion of fractures with continuous hematoma between the fragments—the cause of nonunion is inadequate immobilization."

The student must not think of a fracture in each location as having an exact time for healing, any prolongation of which means nonunion. The time required for a given fracture to heal with ideal treatment varies with many factors, known and unknown. Therefore, it is wrong to think that a fracture should be immobilized for a certain time and the immobilizing agent then removed, and, if union has not occurred during that time, that nonunion has resulted. While one may properly speak of "delayed union" if the time for union goes past a theoretical average for the site involved in a given patient, nonunion is a pathologic entity that may be recognized by gross and microscopic findings at the fracture site. These changes may be noted on roentgenograms by a rounding-off and sclerosis of the fragment ends (Fig. 18-7). Once nonunion has occurred, further immobilization is to no avail.

Loss of Motion of Joints. Probably the most frequent complication of fractures is some permanent restriction of motion in the joints adjacent to the fracture. Immobilization of joints necessary for the proper management of the fractures predisposes to this complication. The older the patient, the more likely that immobilization will result in some permanent restriction of motion. Loss of motion of joints may also result from injury to the soft tissues about them with resulting scar formation, from injury to adjacent muscles, which limits their subsequent function, or from injury to the articular cartilage of the joint itself with resulting traumatic arthritis. Loss of motion of joints must be minimized by as early mobilization of them as is compatible with good management of the fracture and by as much exercise of the adjacent musculature as is feasible during the period of immobilization.

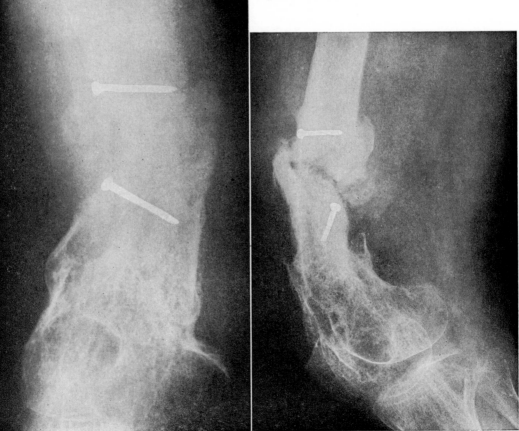

Fig. 18-7. Established nonunion of fracture of the lower femoral shaft. The anteroposterior roentgenogram (*left*) shows severe angulation, but the diagnosis of nonunion can be made only on the lateral view (*right*). When nonunion is suspected, multiple views are often necessary to make the diagnosis.

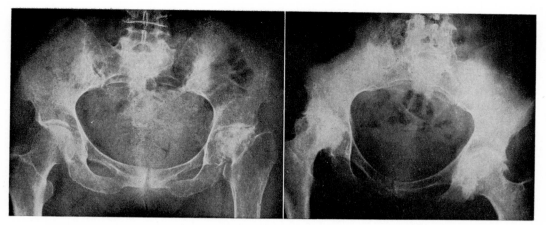

Fig. 18-8. (*Left*) Avascular necrosis of head of left femur, following fracture of the neck which united. (*Right*) Avascular necrosis of head of right femur, which developed several years after reduction of a posterior dislocation of the hip.

Causalgia. Fractures may be associated with causalgia (post-traumatic sympathetic dystrophy, Sudek's atrophy—see section on Causalgia). An injury to the major nerve trunks of the extremity usually has been associated with the fracture when causalgia develops. This condition is poorly understood. It must be treated by (1) the proper management of the fracture and (2) appropriate attack on the sympathetic nervous system.

Ossifying Hematoma. This is an ossification in the hematoma resulting from the fracture but occurring at a distance from the area of desired bone repair. Little is known concerning its cause and prevention. Some have postulated that the combination of hematoma and damaged muscle predisposes to its formation. Not infrequently it is seen complicating dislocations of the elbow associated with fractures of the head of the radius. It is especially serious when it occurs about the elbow because it usually restricts motion of the joint. In the forearm, it may cause a bony bridge between the radius and the ulna and prevent rotation.

Volkmann's Ischemic Contracture. This is a severe fibrosis with resulting contracture of muscles which have been rendered ischemic by obstruction of the arterial flow to the extremity. It most commonly involves the musculature of the forearm and the hand as a complication of fractures about the elbow in children (see p. 370). It may develop because of unrelieved swelling about the elbow,

impairing the arterial flow to the extremity as a direct result of the injury itself or because, in an effort to maintain reduction of the fragments, the elbow is immobilized in excessive flexion which causes occlusion of the arterial flow to the forearm and the hand. Volkmann's ischemic contracture is a complication that can be prevented by proper care. If allowed to develop, the results are disastrous.

Avascular Necrosis of Bone. Following injury, areas of bone may be isolated from their blood supply and die. This complication is called avascular or aseptic necrosis of bone in contrast with septic necrosis caused by infection. The process is recognized by a relative increase in density of the avascular area on x-ray examination. (Fig. 18-8). Avascular necrosis is observed most frequently in the femoral head following intracapsular fractures and dislocations of the hip, injuries which severely damage the already precarious blood supply of the head of the femur (Fig. 18-8). In some instances, the avascular necrosis may not appear for several years following injury. Avascular necrosis affecting the fragment deprived of its blood supply is often noted in fractures of the carpal navicular. It also may occur in the proximal fragment of a fractured talus. In general, this is an unpreventable complication.

Fat Embolism. Fat embolism following trauma is probably more common than is generally recognized. Free fat can be demonstrated in the urine of a high percentage of patients following injury. Fat embolism has been found most frequently after fractures but has also been noticed after soft tissue injuries. Considerable difference of opinion exists as to its clinical importance, and more study is needed to determine its role in the complications, chiefly pulmonary and cerebral, following fracture. Symptoms and signs suggestive of pneumonia or atelectasis may result from pulmonary fat embolism and changes suggestive of delirium tremens or cerebral trauma from cerebral fat embolism. At the present time no specific treatment is known for fat embolism. Vigorous supportive and symptomatic treatment should be carried out. Intravenous alcohol may be of value. Early tracheostomy to permit excellent toilet of the tracheo-bronchial tree may be livesaving.

Delayed and Late Nerve Paralysis. Whereas immediate nerve injury may be caused by a tearing of a nerve (e.g., radial nerve in fractures of the humerus) or pressure on a nerve (e.g., on the peroneal nerve in fractures of the fibular neck), nerve paralysis may occur many months or years after the fracture. An interesting but rare syndrome is late ulnar palsy caused by fractures of the lateral condyle of the humerus in childhood. Due to lateral epiphyseal damage, growth at the elbow is limited to the medial side, with the production of a relative medial protuberance and increased carrying angle. Years later (as many as 20 or more years), ulnar palsy may result from continued stretch and trauma of movement of the ulnar nerve over the relative protuberance of the medial condyle, even though the original injury was a fracture of the lateral condyle.

OBJECTIVES OF MANAGEMENT OF FRACTURES

The ideal to be achieved in the management of fractures may be expressed as a solidly united fracture in perfect alignment, the bone of full length and joints freely movable by strong musculature—all having been obtained in the shortest possible period of time. These objectives really mean the rehabilitation of the patient as quickly as possible with the patient as nearly whole as possible.

Unfortunately, in many fractures it is impossible to obtain a complete restoration of the part. For example, in some fractures, in order to obtain good contact of fragments so as to predispose to union, some shortening may have to be accepted. In others, particularly those about joints, the necessary immobilization to permit union of the fracture in good position may lead to some loss of motion in an adjacent joint. Necessary prolonged immobilization is likely to lead to some atrophy of the musculature of the part and it may be impossible for the patient to rebuild the muscle strength completely.

Moreover, the relative importance of each of the objectives outlined above varies with the location of the fracture. In the upper extremity, the most important objective in the management of a fracture is the maintenance or return of normal function of the hand. After the fracture has healed, stability of the fracture must be sufficient to permit the hand to function properly. While perfect alignment is desirable, union in slight angulation may be of no consequence. Certainly, the fracture may heal with some shortening without any real loss of function of the extremity.

In the lower extremity, on the other hand, stability without pain is the most important objective, but movable joints for locomotion and full length are highly desirable. In many fractures, however, mobility of the joints and full length must be sacrificed, at least partially, to ensure a solidly united fracture which will provide painless stability on weight-bearing.

The objectives in the management of fractures were well summarized by Darrach in his Presidential Address before the American Surgical Association in 1946. He listed these objectives as (1) reduction of secondary trauma to a minimum; (2) sufficient restoration of normal form to meet the requirements —this may be short of the ideal anatomic reduction; (3) immobilization of the bone fragments until healing has occurred—all joints should be mobilized immediately if their movement does not cause motion of the fragments; (4) restoration of function as early and as rapidly as possible and the atrophy of disuse minimized by the early institution of active motion; (5) sustaining of morale and physical and social rehabilitation.

The late Clay Ray Murray epitomized the principles of treatment of fractures in the following hypothesis:

The ideal way to treat a fracture would be to wish the fragments into place, hold them there by moral suasion and send the patient on about his business while the fracture healed. Comprehension of the implications of this hypothesis and adherence to its concept are mandatory to good fracture treatment regardless of the method used.

1. "To wish the fragments into place" means reduction without any additional tissue damage. It can't be done! Nevertheless, the best reduction is that most closely approximating this ideal, i.e., the earliest and gentlest reduction possible. For the same reason (prevention of secondary tissue damage) adequate first-aid care is essential to an optimum result.

2. To "hold them there by moral suasion" means maintenance of reduction without interfering with continued function of the associated structures. This is impossible! Nevertheless, the apparatus or method most closely approaching this ideal is best, i.e., that which provides adequate stabilization of the bone fragments coincident with minimum interference with local function throughout healing. A healed bone is of little use when the surrounding soft tissue has been ruined by overimmobilization or unnecessary disuse.

3. To "send the patient on about his business" means maintenance of all social, economic and other normal functions of the patient as a whole, throughout healing. This is rarely possible. However, the treatment method of choice is that which most closely approaches this ideal.

These principles cannot be taken as rules or blueprints for the treatment of fractures. Most fractures demand closed or open reduction and immobilization which must interfere with function, and for the surgeon to concentrate entirely on function in these would preclude reduction and immobilization. Other fractures require continued function of the part, even if this means accepting some bony deformity. As a rule, some compromise must be accepted. The best treatment for a fracture concentrates on the most important of the objectives at the expense of the least important.

EMERGENCY SPLINTING OF FRACTURES

Effective emergency splinting of fractures for transportation to and within a hospital is a highly significant procedure in the eventual rehabilitation of the patient. When emergency splinting is effective, the first objective outlined by Darrach—that is, the reduction of secondary trauma to a minimum—will have been achieved.

An injured part must be splinted when pain, loss of function, or deformity suggest a fracture. Efforts to elicit crepitus or false motion to prove a fracture are dangerous and contraindicated. The suspicion that a fracture is present is sufficient to justify emergency splinting for transportation of the patient to as hospital for adequate x-ray examination.

The objective of emergency splinting is, of course, not reduction of the fracture but the prevention of additional damage to soft parts by fragments of bone. When these fragments have been immobilized adequately, the other objectives in emergency splinting—namely, the relief of pain and the provision of comfortable and safe transportation—will have been achieved. When properly carried out, emergency splinting minimizes or prevents shock and is an important step in resuscitation of the injured.

Emergency splinting may be provided with standard or improvised splints. Standard splints, of course, are preferable but these are not always available. In such instances, various materials which are available may be employed to provide highly effective emergency splinting and achieve its objectives.

Effective emergency splinting may be provided as follows (Fig. 18-9).

Upper Extremity

Shoulder, Arm and Elbow

STANDARD. The extremity is placed in a sling, with the elbow usually at a right angle and is bound to the chest by means of a bandage or another sling. If an injured elbow has assumed a position of extension, no attempt is made to flex it to a right angle, but the extremity is bandaged to the body with the elbow in extension.

IMPROVISED. The individual's shirt tail may be turned up and pinned to the shirt so that it serves as a sling. The extremity may then be bound to the chest with any material that is at hand.

The full-ring hinged arm traction splint is mentioned only to condemn it. It has no

place in the emergency splinting of fractures of the upper extremity. This splint was given a trial during the early stages of World War II and was found to be totally unsuited for emergency splinting. It was promptly dis-

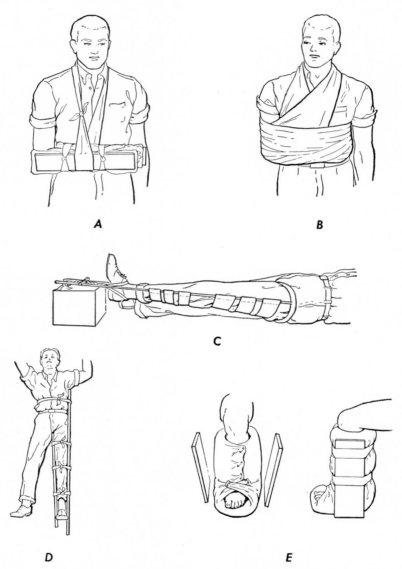

A   B

C

D   E

Fig. 18-9. Emergency splinting. (A) Coaptation splinting with boards for fracture of the forearm. (B) Sling and circular bandage about the thorax for fracture above the forearm. (C) Fixed traction in a Thomas splint for fracture of the femur. (D) Coaptation splinting with boards of fracture of the femur. Note that the lateral board extends to the axilla and is bound to the thorax. For fractures of the leg the lateral board need extend only to the hip. (E) Pillow and board splints for fractures about the ankle.

carded and is no longer standard equipment for emergency splinting on the battlefield.

Forearm, Wrist and Hand

STANDARD. The forearm and the hand are bandaged to a board or a metal splint placed on the palmar surface. The extremity is then placed in a sling with the elbow at a right angle.

IMPROVISED. As a rule the splinting will be improvised. An adequate substitute for a wood or metal splint is a magazine or even a heavy newspaper encircling the forearm and the hand and held in place with a bandage or adhesive tape. A sling is always indicated.

LOWER EXTREMITY

Standard. Traction splinting utilizing a Thomas or a hinged half-ring splint with traction being obtained by means of a hitch about the foot has been shown to be most effective for fractures of the femur. The slings on which the extremity rests may be towels, or bandages of any kind. The traction hitch is applied over the shoe if one is on the foot. Only moderate traction is desirable. The end of the splint always must be elevated sufficiently to lift the extremity so that it is entirely supported by the slings of the splint.

Improvised. The most common improvised splinting is obtained with board splints. For fractures of the lower two thirds of the leg and the ankle, the ideal improvised emergency splinting consists of 2 or 3 padded coaptation board splints which extend from the mid-thigh to below the foot. For injuries of the femur at any level, the knee and the upper third of the leg, the lateral board must extend to the axilla and must be bound securely to the walls of the abdomen and the chest. If the lateral board does not immobilize the hip joint, the splinting is entirely ineffective.

When board splints are applied to the lower extremity, padding must be arranged properly to protect the malleoli and the head of the fibula from painful pressure and, in the latter instance, to avoid pressure on the peroneal nerve which could cause peroneal nerve paralysis. For fractures of the bones of the leg a pillow bandaged securely about the leg, perhaps reinforced by boards extending to the mid-thigh, provides excellent emergency splinting. As a last resort when other materials are not available, the injured extremity should be tied to the uninjured counterpart.

SPINE

Cervical Spine. In suspected injuries of the cervical spine, the patient should be transported face up on a hard surface with sandbags or other heavy material placed on each side of the neck. Flexion and hyperextension of the neck must be avoided. If an appropriate neck brace is available, it should be applied.

Dorsal and Lumbar Spine. In suspected injuries of the dorsal and lumbar spine, the patient should be transported on a hard surface (a door removed from its hinges provides an excellent improvised stretcher) either face up with a small roll in the small of the back, or face downward. Flexion of the spine must be avoided. Particular care is necessary when lifting the patient on and off the support.

PELVIS

In suspected injuries of the pelvis, transportation should be provided on a hard surface with the patient on his back. Discomfort may be decreased if the thighs and the legs are tied together. If the thighs have assumed a flexed position and they cannot be extended easily, they should be kept in flexion. A record should be made as to whether or not the patient voids during transportation; if he does, it is important to note if the urine contains blood.

OPEN FRACTURES

An open wound should be covered promptly with a sterile dressing or the cleanest one available. If a fragment protrudes through the skin, it should be allowed to remain protruding and be covered with a sterile dressing.

In applying emergency traction splinting to the lower extremity, the amount of traction should be kept below a point which will cause the fragment to be pulled back into the wound. Information that the bone has protruded should accompany the patient in case traction inadvertently has been applied in an amount which will pull the exposed fragment within the wound.

Massive hemorrhage may take place through the open wound. Usually the bleeding can be controlled by a compression dressing, and a tourniquet is rarely if ever needed.

METHODS OF MANAGEMENT OF FRACTURES

There are 5 general methods of management of fractures (Fig. 18-10). Every means which is available for the treatment of any given fracture may be classified as one of these 5 methods. It must be clearly understood that management of the fracture includes not only the reduction of the fracture but also the maintenance of reduction, measures designed to obtain as much mobility of joints and strength of musculature as possible, and the rehabilitation of the patient as a whole.

The 5 general methods of management of fractures are:

1. Closed reduction (or maintenance of reduction if the position is satisfactory) and immobilization, usually with a plaster cast.

2. Continuous balanced traction, usually skeletal traction, less commonly skin traction.

3. Open reduction, usually with internal fixation.

4. External skeletal fixation.

5. No immobilization (perhaps a sling or a bandage).

CLOSED REDUCTION (OR MAINTENANCE OF REDUCTION IN FRACTURES IN SATISFACTORY POSITION) AND IMMOBILIZATION

In this method of management of fractures, the fragments, if displaced, are manipulated into satisfactory apposition and alignment and held in that position by some form of immobilization, usually a plaster cast. If the position of the fragments is already satisfactory, reduction is not required, and immobilization is all that is necessary. In accordance with a fundamental rule for the splinting of fractures, the joints above and below the fracture are immobilized.

Efforts at closed reduction usually should be instituted promptly after the diagnosis of a fracture is made. They are most effective while the hematoma about the fracture is still liquid and before the tissues have become inelastic and water-logged from swelling. This means that closed reduction will be easier if it is carried out within 3 or 4 hours after injury.

Reduction of a fracture is almost always accomplished under general, regional or local anesthesia. Only rarely can faulty position of fragments be corrected adequately without anesthesia.

The fundamental maneuvers of a manipulative reduction are strong manual traction on the portion of the extremity distal to the fracture with equally strong countertraction proximal to the fracture, combined with appropriate manipulation of the fragments. It is basic in closed reduction of fractures that the distal fragment be brought into approximation and alignment with the proximal fragment. When traction is slow and steady, only minimal direct manipulation of the distal fragment will be required as a rule; therefore, additional trauma to the soft tissues about the fracture will be minimal.

Closed reduction and immobilization is usually chosen when the contour of the fracture indicates that the reduction will be so stable that it will not be lost as long as good alignment is maintained by the immobilization. Under these circumstances this is a conservative method involving a minimum risk of complications. It is the most common method of management for fractures of the extremities. It is usually the method of choice for fractures about the wrist and the ankle in adults and for practically every fracture of the long bones in children, except those of the femoral shaft.

CONTINUOUS BALANCED TRACTION

By this method, continuous traction, usually over a period of weeks, is made on the portion of the extremity distal to the fracture against the countertraction furnished by the weight of the body. As a rule, the injured extremity is suspended in a splint; for example, a Thomas splint for fractures of the femur (Fig. 18-10).

The traction may be skin or skeletal. In skin traction, adhesive tape or moleskin is applied to the extremity, using a wooden block as a spreader just distal to the foot, as in Buck's traction. The theory of skin traction is that a weight pulling on the tape makes traction on the skin which in turn makes traction on the musculature and this in turn on the bone. In skeletal traction, rigid pins (Steinmann pins or Kirschner wires) are drilled through a bone distal to the fracture, and traction is applied to the pin or the wire. The pin or the wire may be inserted through the distal portion of the bone

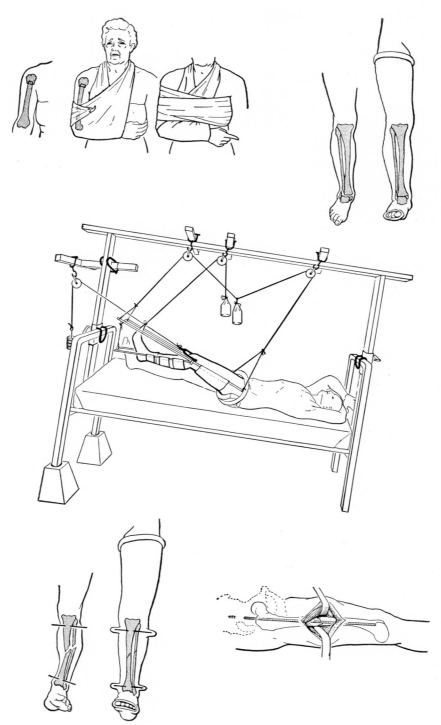

FIG. 18-10. Five methods of management of fractures. (*Top, left*) No immobilization. (*Top, right*) Closed reduction and immobilization with plaster cast. (*Center*) Continuous balanced skeletal traction. (*Bottom, left*) External skeletal fixation, Steinmann pins incorporated in a plaster cast. (*Bottom, right*) Open reduction and internal fixation with medullary nail.

which is fractured or inserted through one of the bones distal to the point below the fracture. For example, the pin or the wire may be inserted through the tibial tubercle for continuous skeletal traction for a fracture of the femur or through the os calcis for continuous skeletal traction for fractures of both bones of the leg. Obviously, skeletal traction is more effective than skin traction because it is traction applied directly to the bone. Moreover, the hazards of irritation and blistering beneath the tape and of slipping of the tape are obviated by the use of skeletal traction.

The rationale of balanced skeletal traction for the management of fractures is that the strong continuous traction applied in the long axis of the extremity will bring the distal fragment into apposition and alignment with the proximal fragment and therefore reduce the fracture. The strapping and molding effect of the musculature surrounding the fragments aids in the reduction. It may seem unnecessary to comment that the traction must be continuous, yet, in hospitals where this method is not used regularly, one is often distressed to find hospital personnel removing the traction weight when the bed is moved or the patient turned. Such a mistake may wreck the entire course of treatment.

Continuous traction is most likely to give adequate reduction of the fracture when it is instituted relatively soon after the injury. While traction need not necessarily be provided as early as closed reduction should be attempted, it must be instituted before the fragment ends have been fixed by early healing. The quicker traction is established, the more effective it will be. This means that it should be in effect within a few days after the injury.

Enough traction should be provided to obtain reduction and then to maintain it by avoiding the recurrence of overriding and angulation of fragments. With this amount of traction the normal muscle tone will maintain adequate contact-compression of the fragments. Overpull (or distraction) must be avoided as this predisposes to nonunion. The continuous traction method requires repeated roentgenograms to serve as indicators of the effectiveness of the method. Based on the findings on x-ray examination, repeated adjustments of the traction may be necessary.

Continuous balanced suspension skeletal traction was the method of management for the great majority of battle fractures of the femoral shaft during World War II. Until about 1950 this method was employed for the great majority of fractures of the femoral shaft in civilian injuries. Intramedullary nailing at operation, when applicable, is the preferred method of management for fractures of the femoral shaft in adults, but skeletal traction remains an excellent method for this severe skeletal injury.

Some form of continuous traction is frequently employed for fractures of the shaft of the humerus, comminuted fractures of both bones of the leg and in selected instances of fractures of the bones of the hand and the foot.

OPEN REDUCTION, USUALLY WITH INTERNAL FIXATION

In this method, the fracture site is exposed at operation, and under direct visualization the fragment ends are brought into approximation. Usually some form of metallic internal fixation (screws, plates, intramedullary nails, malleable stainless steel wire) is employed to maintain the reduction.

Open reduction, of course, affords the most exact reduction and offers many advantages. Perfect apposition and alignment and full length are usually obtained. The excellent reduction predisposes to rapid union. Internal fixation should prevent loss of reduction.

However, there are several objections to this method. In closed fractures it converts an uncontaminated fracture into an open fracture and thereby risks infection. The operation itself adds further damage to soft tissues and bone. Moreover, with some forms of internal fixation, as a rigid plate held by screws, the plate can serve to delay union of the fragments. Some absorption of fragment ends occurs in most fractures. If so, normal tone of the surrounding musculature cannot pull the fragment ends together, if they are strutted apart by a plate and screws. In an attempt to overcome this disadvantage of rigid plating of fractures and to effect continuous contact of the fragment ends, slotted bone plates have been developed to replace the rigid fixation. Although they appear to be advantageous, the relative effectiveness of slotted plates is yet to be proved.

In summary, open reduction and internal fixation of fractures is a calculated risk affording advantages and disadvantages. The method should be selected when the former outweigh the latter.

Open reduction is indicated primarily for many fractures—including separated fractures of the patella and the olecranon, fractures of the neck and the trochanteric region of the femur, displaced spiral fractures of the tibial shaft and, with the use of the intramedullary nail, for many fractures of the femoral shaft.

Stability of the fragments of bone sufficient to avoid the application of additional immobilization is not provided by internal fixation alone, with the exception of some intramedullary nailings of the femoral shaft. For practically every other form of internal fixation, a plaster cast for supplementary immobilization is required until union of the fracture has occurred. In certain fresh fractures notorious for their tendency toward nonunion, as an adjunct to the open reduction and internal fixation, autografts from the iliac crest may be added to speed union; e.g., in adults, fractures of the lower portion of the shaft of the tibia, fractures of shafts of both bones of the forearm.

External Skeletal Fixation

In this method, following closed or, at times, open reduction of the fragments, an effort is made to maintain reduction by means of strong metallic bars connected to rigid metal pins or half pins which are inserted through the skin and other soft parts into each fragment; hence, the name of the method external skeletal fixation. A plaster cast is not used as a rule. The Roger Anderson and Stader splints are examples of the apparatus employed.

This method is not recommended. It is mentioned for completeness and to warn against it. In the hands of most surgeons it has resulted in a too high incidence of malunion and nonunion, stiffness of adjacent joints and infection along the pin tracks.

A method of treatment which permits classification as external skeletal fixation is the use of one or two rigid pins inserted through both the proximal and the distal fragments and, following reduction, the incorporation of the pins in a full-length plaster cast. This method has been successful in certain fractures of the shafts of both bones of the legs. It has the distinct disadvantage of potentially "holding the fragments apart" as may occur with rigid plating as described above. In addition, ring sequestra may form about the transfixion pins. This has been attributed to excessive pressure by the pins on the bone from the various movements of the plaster cast that incorporates the pins and to devitalization resulting from heat generated at the time of introduction of the pins.

No Immobilization (Perhaps a Sling or a Bandage)

In the use of this method, chiefly applicable in impacted fractures, it is recognized that displacement will not occur with motion of the part. The position of the fragments is accepted, even though it may not be ideal. Immobilization is omitted in favor of early mobilization and this really is the keynote of the method. Actually, a sling or a bandage may be employed for a short period, but these do not produce real immobilization and merely provide some relief of pain during the first few days after injury.

This method should be employed in those fractures which do not require immobilization and in which early active exercise will lead to more functional restoration of the part in a shorter period of time than would immobilization. This technic is particularly indicated in impacted fractures of the neck of the humerus and in undisplaced fractures of the radial head. It is applicable in many chip fractures about the hand and the foot.

Selection of a Method

Each method of management offers advantages and disadvantages and these must be weighed carefully by the surgeon in selecting the method of management for any given fracture. The selection of a method to be instituted is based upon several factors. Of these, the contour of the fracture as revealed by the roentgenograms is probably the most important. Others are the age and the general condition of the patient, whether the fracture is open or closed, the presence of other significant injuries and, especially if open reduction is under consideration, the status of circulation to the soft parts, particularly the skin overlying the fracture, the equipment at hand and the experience and the ability of the surgeon.

In many fractures, one method will be employed, found to be ineffective and therefore another method must be selected. For example, Method I, closed reduction and immobilization, may be attempted for a fracture of both bones of the forearm. Postoperative roentgenograms may show a satisfactory reduction, but repeat roentgenograms a few days later may show that the fragments have slipped and are no longer in good position. Then Method III, open reduction, may be selected and the fragments stabilized in reduction by means of intramedullary fixation or slotted plates held by screws. Likewise, Method II, balanced skeletal traction, may fail to reduce a comminuted fracture of the femoral shaft adequately. Then open reduction may be employed, and the fragments fixed in good position by intramedullary nailing supplemented by other forms of internal fixation if indicated.

The student of fractures, as soon as he is confronted with any given fracture, is urged to consider these 5 methods of management and select the one which best fits the requirements. Many medical students despair of acquiring a thorough knowledge of fractures because of the multiplicity of gadgets and equipment seen in the fracture room and on the wards and the varying opinions expressed in the literature concerning the treatment of many fractures. This confusion arises from too great a concern for details of treatment and too little concern for the underlying principles of management. The details of treatment and the use of a profusion of splints and gadgets should not be the primary concern of the medical student. Rather, he should concentrate on the principles involved in the selection of 1 of the 5 methods of treatment for the particular fracture with which he finds himself concerned.

OPEN FRACTURES

An open wound communicating with the fracture site adds considerably to the seriousness of the injury and complicates management of the fracture for several reasons. The hematoma from the fracture site may be lost through the wound, and this loss may retard union of the fracture. Blood loss may cause shock and seriously delay management of the fracture. The damage to soft tissues is greater in open fractures, resulting in more scarring and limiting the eventual return of function. However, the principal hazards of open fractures are those of secondary infection and failure of healing of the wound.

Infection of the wound may result in several ways. There may be a true invasive infection by bacteria, primarily or secondarily implanted in the wound. Gas gangrene is an example of such an invasive infection. More often, however, infection of the wound results from the bacterial decomposition of devitalized soft tissue and blood clot with resulting suppuration. The suppurative process may lead to further destruction of soft tissue and bone which in turn leads to more suppuration. In other instances, a true infection is not present in the beginning, but the loss of soft tissue or a gaping open wound may leave bone, fascia or tendon exposed. The superficial cortex of bone, cartilage, fascia and tendon cannot survive if they remain exposed in a wound. They soon die and serve as the nidus for wound suppuration. The end result of an open wound in which these vulnerable tissues remain exposed is wound infection.

Regardless of how and why a suppurative process develops in an open wound of a fracture, it is a most serious complication. Union of the fracture is almost always delayed and may be prevented. Massive sequestration of bone may occur. Adjacent joints may become involved and be destroyed. The infection may become so extensive as to warrant amputation as a lifesaving measure. At best, there will be slow wound healing with excessive scar formation which probably will lead to a diminished functional restoration of the part.

The objectives of management of open fractures are rapid healing of the open wound without infection and healing of the fracture in good position. It readily follows that to achieve these objectives underlying factors leading to wound infection must be overcome. The depths and the recesses of the wound must be thoroughly cleaned of foreign material and debris during the so-called contaminated period before active infection can develop in the wound. Dead and devitalized tissue, including old blood clot, must be excised surgically before it decomposes and forms pus. Those tissues which will die if they remain exposed in a wound must be covered with soft parts at the proper time. Adequate drainage must be provided for residual dead space or, if indicated, to provide a means of egress for the possible septic decomposition of bits of devitalized tissue which could not be excised.

TREATMENT OF THE WOUND OF OPEN FRACTURES

First-aid treatment of an open fracture is, as mentioned above, merely the application of a sterile dressing and proper splinting. Cleansing the wound with so-called antiseptics is definitely contraindicated. Protruding fragments of bone should not be replaced in the wound but should be merely covered with a sterile dressing. It follows that in applying emergency traction splinting to an open fracture of an extremity with protruding fragments only minimal traction should be employed. Of course, immediate hospitalization is indicated. Antibiotics should be administered systemically as soon as possible.

Open fractures are true surgical emergencies. They deserve investigation, appraisal and treatment in a fully equipped operating room. However, before definitive surgery is begun, several things are necessary. First, any systemic effects of hemorrhage must be overcome by whole blood transfusions. Plasma or plasma expanders may be a temporary "stopgap" measure, but they cannot replace whole blood transfusions for the severely wounded. When the general condition of the patient warrants, roentgenograms should be made. The patient must be satisfactorily anesthetized, the part surgically cleaned and prepared and the wound thoroughly examined. An appraisal of the degree of contamination of the wound and the amount of damaged tissue probably remaining in it is the basis for determining the surgical procedure that is indicated (Fig. 18-11).

In order that all devitalized tissue may be removed, exposure of the depths of the wound must be ample. As a rule the wound must be extended. These extensions are made in the direction which will afford adequate access to the depths of the wound without injury to important structures such as nerve trunks. The extension must avoid unnecessary exposure of tissues likely to die when they remain uncovered and facilitate closure by suture. In the extremities, incisions usually are made parallel with the long axis of the limb.

In the technic of wound débridement, only the devitalized skin of wound margins should be excised. A long incision in the fascial layer gives free access to foreign bodies and devitalized muscle, the excision of which is a major objective of wound débridement. Healthy muscle is not discolored, bleeds freely and contracts when pinched; muscle which does not meet these requirements should be excised. Foreign bodies and dirt should be removed. Thorough irrigation of the wound with a saline solution will cleanse it of small, free particles. Bleeding vessels should be ligated. Small fragments of bone completely free of soft tissue attachment should be removed; bone which has some muscular attachment should be left in place, as it is usually viable.

Closure of the wound of an open fracture by suture at the proper time is highly desirable. However, the decision to suture the wound must be based on sound surgical judgment. Much has been said about the immediate closure of the wounds of open fractures so as to convert quickly each open fracture into a closed one. Of course, an immediate successful suture of the wound is most advantageous, but an unsuccessful suture of the wound because of abscess formation or necrosis of skin margins is worse than if the wound had been left open.

In civilian surgery suture of the wound is usually feasible, particularly if the time-lag after injury is not more than 4 to 6 hours, if the cleansing and the débridement of the wound have been thorough, and if closure appears to be surgically feasible without excessive tension. On the other hand, if the surgeon cannot be reasonably certain that he has rid the wound of the pabulum for sepsis, or if closure by suture would produce excessive tension likely to cause death of skin margins, then an open wound is preferable, despite its inherent hazards.

Closure of an open wound over a fracture

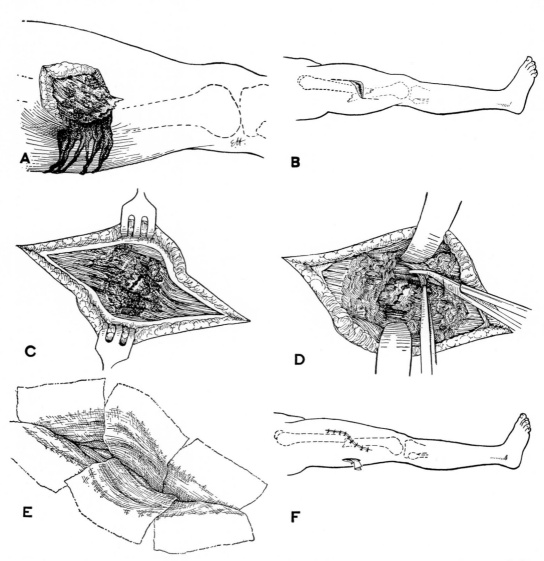

Fig. 18-11. Drawings of débridement of an open fracture. A. Open fracture of the shaft of the femur with the distal end of the proximal fragment protruding through the jagged open wound on the lateral surface of the thigh. B. The protruding bone and the exposed soft tissue are well cleaned, and any obvious tags of dead muscle are excised. Then the fragment is reduced into the depths of the wound. An important step in débridement is adequate enlargement of the wound by incision. A transverse or near-transverse wound should be enlarged by longitudinal extensions proximally and distally at opposite ends of the open wound as is illustrated by the dotted lines. Almost without exception an incision should not be made across the center of a wound so as to create a cruciate-type of wound. C. The fascia is split so as to facilitate exposure of the depths of the wound and excision of destroyed muscle tissue. D. Devitalized tags of muscle tissue are excised. Excision of muscle with scissors is highly acceptable technic, but only a knife should be used on the skin. E. Proper dressing of a wound which is to remain open with a fine mesh dry or petrolatum impregnated gauze. F. If primary suture of the wound is selected, dependent drainage for a few days through the posterolateral fascial plane as a safeguard against deep abscess formation. (Hampton, O. P., Jr.: Complications of common fractures *in* Hardy, J. D., and Artz, C.: Complications in Surgery, Philadelphia, Saunders, 1960)

versus the advantages of an open wound for drainage as a safeguard against deep infection (including anerobic infection) presents a problem which may severely tax the judgment of even the most experienced surgeon. If the decision is made to leave the wound open, delayed primary closure should be performed if surgically feasible between the fifth and the tenth days, provided that the wound is clinically clean. Delayed closure of clinically clean wounds is surgically sound, provided that dead space is obliterated or dependently drained and excessive tension is avoided.

Much has been written concerning the greater danger of infection in open fractures in which the wound is opened from "without-in" in comparison with those opened from "within-out." On a theoretical basis, the degree of contamination is always more in the former. Not only is foreign material more likely to be introduced into the wound but usually a greater degree of damage to the soft tissues occurs. It should be kept in mind, however, that considerable dirt and foreign material can be introduced into the wound of a fracture which is opened from within-out. For example, a child can fall on the outstretched hand so as to break both bones of the forearm in the middle third. A fragment of either the radius or the ulna may tear through soft tissues, usually on the palmar surface, and actually dig into the ground. As the child arises he may grab the injured forearm and cause the protruding fragment end to go back into the wound carrying with it considerable dirt. Such a case serves to illustrate the hazard of a false sense of security concerning contamination in fractures opened from within-out.

On the other hand, there will be many open fractures, usually opened from within-out but sometimes from without-in, in which the surgeon can be sure from the circumstances of the accident and the appearance of the wound and the clothing about the site of injury that no foreign material has been carried into the wound and that soft tissue damage is minimal. Under these circumstances, he may feel that the features discussed above which predispose to wound infection are not present and surgical investigation is not indicated. In such instances he may elect to irrigate the wound thoroughly with sterile 0.9

per cent saline solution, apply a sterile dressing, reduce the fracture by traction and manipulation and apply immobilization. While such practices cannot be condemned, it should be pointed out that they involve a real risk. In the majority of open fractures some cleansing and débridement of the depths of the wound will be definitely indicated.

Insofar as the fracture is concerned, the same methods of management are applicable in general to open as to closed fractures. In open fractures, however, the question of employing internal fixation at the time of wound excision often assumes paramount importance. As the wound is débrided, the fracture site may be exposed. If the contour of the fracture is such as to permit adequate stabilization by internal fixation, then the decision must be made as to whether or not that method will be employed. This, too, is a problem which requires expert judgment.

As a practical matter, when the time-lag after injury is not too prolonged, when the wound has been well débrided and when it can be closed by suture without excessive tension, there need be little hesitancy in applying internal fixation to the fracture through the open wound if the internal fixation is indicated otherwise. If, on the other hand, the factors predisposing to infection of the wound are present, internal fixation is probably too hazardous. In doubtful cases it is advisable to employ some method of management of the fracture other than internal fixation and to direct every effort toward obtaining early healing of the wound without infection. If, then, adequate reduction of the fracture has not been maintained, it will be possible to perform a delayed open reduction and internal fixation through a healed intact skin envelope with anticipation of success.

FRACTURES IN CHILDREN

Fractures in children are different. This often-repeated statement is true for several reasons. Incomplete fractures of the greenstick variety are common. Anatomically, the fracture line may cross an epiphyseal plate, or the injury may be a displacement of the epiphysis instead of a true fracture. Fractures in children unite rapidly; the younger the child, the more rapid the healing. For example, a complete fracture of the femoral shaft in a small infant may unite solidly within 10 days (Fig. 18-12).

Of greater significance are certain responses of growing bone which manifest themselves after a fracture during childhood has united. Even if malunion of the fracture has occurred, the normal contour of the bone is reconstituted by growth in accordance with Wolff's law which states that all changes in the function of a bone are attended by definite alterations in its internal structure. Bone will be laid down where it is needed to restore normal contour, and bone will be absorbed where it disturbs normal contour. This favorable response of growing bone to overcome what otherwise would be malunited fractures means, of course, that although precise reduction of a fracture in a child is desirable, it may not be necessary, and open operation to obtain perfect reduction is, for practical purposes, never justified (Fig. 18-13).

Another unique feature of some fractures in children is a tendency toward a subsequent increased rate of growth of the broken bone. Clinically and experimentally, it has been demonstrated that a fracture of the diaphysis in growing bone will stimulate activity of the epiphyses of that bone, and for a period of time there will be an increased rate of growth. This means, of course, that not only may fractures of the long bones in children be permitted to heal with slight overriding but that

such slight overriding is preferable. This is true because the increased rate of growth will enable the fractured bone to catch up in length with its counterpart in the other extremity, whereas if the reduction had been perfect, the increased rate of growth would produce excessive length of the bone which was fractured. However, rotational deformities are not so well corrected by growth processes and this should be taken into account in determining what is a satisfactory reduction of a fracture in a child.

In injuries of the extremities of children, it is often helpful to have roentgenograms of the normal extremity, especially in injuries near joints, because of the frequent difficulty in determining what is normal contour and degree of ossification of the epiphyses for the age of the injured child. Comparison of the roentgenograms of the injured and the uninjured sides may be quite valuable in establishing the presence and the extent of bony or epiphyseal injury.

The statement that open reduction of fractures in children is seldom justified deserves some modification. Open reduction is indicated in certain fractures in children especially in a group of fractures around the elbow. These include fractures of the medial or the lateral condyle of the humerus with rotation and significant displacement and fractures of the head and the neck of the radius with dis-

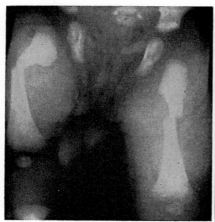 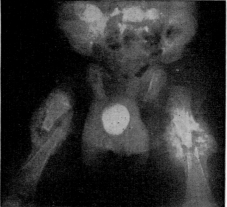

FIG. 18-12. Bilateral fractures of the femoral shafts from birth injury. (*Left*) Roentgenogram taken immediately after birth. (*Right*) Roentgenogram taken 10 days after injury, showing exuberant callus and satisfactory alignment. (From Dr. Robert Cram)

placement or severe angulation. Operative intervention is also indicated in irreducible epiphyseal separations such as those at the distal end of the femur and at the distal end of the tibia, although it should be pointed out that operative reduction is not necessary for those injuries when the displacement is minimal.

BIRTH FRACTURES

Fractures occurring at birth, usually from the trauma incident to a difficult delivery, are called birth fractures. These usually involve the clavicle, the humerus, or the femur. Those of the clavicle and the humerus require very little treatment. The extremity may be placed in a small sling, a small axillary pad placed between the arm and the chest and the extremity then bandaged to the chest snugly for a week or two. Fractures of the femoral shaft require more attention. They may heal with rotational deformity and 90° anterior angulation if untreated. They are best managed in overhead balanced skin traction (Bryant's traction, p. 412).

Multiple fractures may be seen at birth in osteogenesis imperfecta. Also, congenital pseudarthrosis of the tibia may be observed occasionally. The cause of this condition is not well understood; spontaneous union seldom occurs; and operative treatment at a later date is usually required.

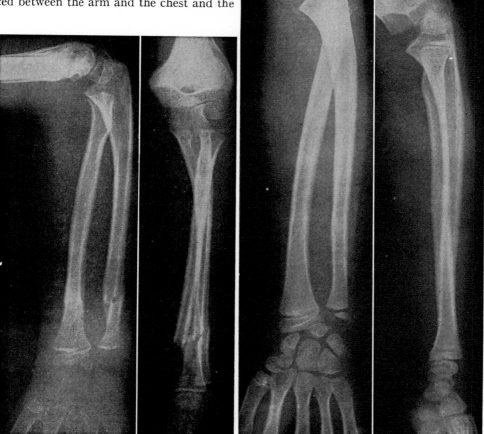

FIG. 18-13. (*Left*) Anteroposterior and lateral roentgenograms showing united fractures of both bones of the forearm in a 5-year-old child with fragments displaced and overriding. (*Right*) Anteroposterior and lateral roentgenograms 18 months later showing no residual evidence of the injury. (Case from Drs. Ward A. McClanahan and Charles K. Wier, Wichita, Kans.)

PATHOLOGIC FRACTURES

A pathologic fracture is one involving previously diseased bone and often occurs as a result of little or no trauma. Bone disease predisposing to fracture may be caused by nutritional or hormonal disturbances (hyperparathyroidism, senile osteoporosis) neoplasm, infection, or neurotrophic dystrophies. A fracture may be the earliest manifestation of generalized disease, and physicians treating fractures must be alert to the need for a complete history, physical examination and laboratory investigation. In general, pathologic fractures heal if the same principles of treatment are followed as with nonpathologic fractures.

Although cancer is widely considered as one of our most important medical problems, relatively little attention has been given to fractures caused by metastatic cancer. The incidence of cancer is increasing, and those interested in the surgery of trauma should anticipate treating an increasing number of fractures caused by cancer. Metastatic carcinoma of the breast accounts for the largest percentage of these pathologic fractures. The spine, the femur and the bones of the shoulder girdle are most frequently fractured. Metastases and therefore pathologic fractures distal to the knee and the elbow are uncommon. A hopeless "do-nothing" attitude is unjustified in fractures from metastatic cancer. Vigorous treatment of the fracture relieves pain, reduces hospitalization, simplifies nursing care and permits early ambulation. Open reduction and fixation with an intramedullary nail is often the treatment of choice, especially in fractures of the femoral shaft (Fig. 18-14).

PLASTER OF PARIS

Plaster of Paris* casts† or splints serve as the principal means of immobilization in the treatment of fractures and dislocations. As the student will learn with increasing experience, there is considerable art in the application of a good cast. It must fit snugly enough

---

* Plaster of Paris is anhydrous calcium sulfate.

† Plaster cast, strictly speaking, is incorrect terminology. Plaster encasement and a circular plaster splint are more nearly accurate terms. However, plaster cast, by prolonged and popular usage, has become part of our medical language and it is used throughout this discussion of fractures and dislocations.

---

to immobilize the part and yet not constrict circulation or cause localized pressure. It must be strong enough to avoid breaking, particularly across joints which are the vulnerable areas. Padding beneath the plaster must be smooth and evenly arranged. Point pressure on bony prominences must be avoided both during application of the cast by proper molding and while it is hardening by protection with soft pillows.

Plaster bandages for the application of plaster casts are made by impregnating the meshes of crinoline bandage with plaster of Paris. These bandages must be kept wrapped and not exposed to the air before they are put to use, as the plaster will take up moisture from the air with resulting impairment of its setting qualities.

Plaster casts (or splints) are either padded or nonpadded. A *padded* cast is applied over some material, usually sheet cotton, under which stockinette may or may not be used. The amount of padding varies. For snug-fitting casts, only 2 or 3 thicknesses of sheet cotton should be applied over the extremity. A heavily padded cast may have 6 or 8 thicknesses of sheet cotton; the heavier the padding, however, the less effective the immobilization provided by the cast. A lightly padded plaster cast is used most commonly in the management of fractures. A *nonpadded* or skin-tight cast is, strictly speaking, applied directly to the skin except perhaps for spot padding of bony prominences. Practically, a cast is considered as nonpadded when it is applied over stockinette but without sheet cotton, although bony prominences may be padded with a small portion of sheet cotton or felt.

Various names have been applied to plaster casts according to their location. A *forearm cast* extends from just below the elbow to, as a rule, the proximal transverse crease of the palm. A long *arm* cast extends from the lower level of the anterior axillary fold to the same level on the hand. The elbow is usually immobilized at a right angle. The degree of rotation of the forearm and the position of the wrist vary with the indications in each type.

A *boot cast* extends from just below the knee to the base of the toes. A long *leg cast* extends from the junction of the upper and the middle thirds of the thigh to the same

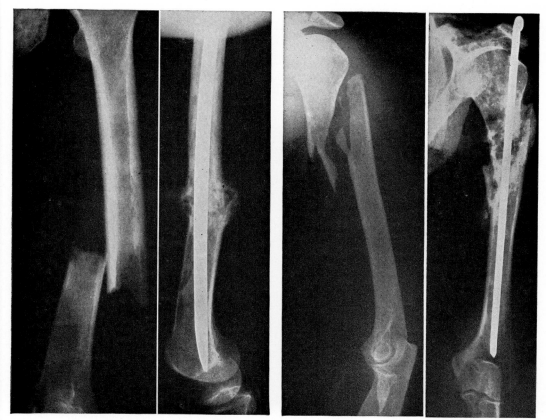

FIG. 18-14. Pathologic fractures of femur and humerus treated by intramedullary nailing. The patient had a radical mastectomy for cancer of the breast in 1949. In 1952 she fractured the left femur through an area of metastatic cancer. Fixation by an intramedullary nail allowed painless weight-bearing within 6 weeks. A year later she fractured the left humerus through another metastatic area. Fixation by an intramedullary nail relieved pain and allowed early motion. She remained comfortable until shortly before her death in 1954. (*Left*) Pathologic fracture of femoral shaft, anteroposterior view. Note metastases in pelvis. (*Center, left*) Four months after open reduction and fixation with an intramedullary nail, lateral view. Note callus and evidence of beginning bony union. (*Center, right*) Pathologic fracture of humeral shaft. (*Right*) Three months after open reduction and fixation with an intramedullary nail. Note evidence of union of the fracture despite multiple areas of metastasis in humerus.

level. Usually the foot is held at a right angle and in neutral version. In each type of leg cast, a plantar slab of plaster may be made to extend past the toes for their protection. This is at times advantageous and at other times disadvantageous. It protects the toes but prevents active plantar flexion of them.

A *spica cast* incorporates the trunk and an extremity. A *shoulder spica,* therefore, encloses the trunk and the upper extremity; a *hip spica,* the trunk and the lower extremity. A single hip spica covers only one leg; a double hip spica, both legs; and a one-and-one-half spica, one entire leg and only the thigh of the other.

A *body jacket* is a plaster cast applied to the trunk. All extremities remain free.

COMPLICATIONS OF PLASTER CASTS

These complications include constriction of circulation, pressure sores and pressure paralyses.

Constriction of Circulation. This may result because the cast was applied too tightly or because it becomes too tight as a result of swelling of the tissues beneath it, usually at the site of the injury. The tendency toward postoperative swelling may be minimized by elevation of the extremity and early active motion of the digits but, despite these precautions, excessive swelling may occur.

Constriction of circulation must not be allowed to persist. Following the application of every cast to an extremity, continuing observation of the color, temperature and sensation of the toes or the fingers and the patient's ability to move them is mandatory. Some swelling is permissible, but cyanosis and decreasing sensation, range of motion and temperature, together with increasing pain, demand that the cast be split or bivalved and then spread to some degree.

To *split* or *univalve* a cast, it is cut through over its entire length either along the front or the side. To *bivalve* a cast, it is split on each side over its full length into two halves. Whenever a cast is split or bivalved, the underlying sheet cotton should also be cut as it can shrink after being wet with blood and constrict the circulation. A split or bivalved cast must be spread sufficiently to relieve the constriction or circulation.

Pressure Sores (Decubitus Ulcers). These result from continuing pressure on bony prominences until necrosis of the soft tissue overlying them takes place. While special padding of bony prominences before the cast is applied is some protection, pressure sores may still occur. The most common sites are: in the lower extremity, the back of the heel, the malleoli, the dorsum of the foot, the head of the fibula and the anterior surface of the patella; in the upper extremity, the medial epicondyle of the humerus and the styloid of the ulna. With plaster body jackets or spica casts, the common sites of pressure sores are the sacrum, the anterosuperior iliac spines and the vertebral borders of the scapulae.

Pain at the location of a bony prominence is the warning symptom of an impending pressure sore. A patient with a fracture is entitled to some pain even after it has been immobilized in a plaster cast. However, when the patient complains of pain the surgeon and the nurse should make certain that the pain is at a site corresponding to the injury and not over a bony prominence. Too often, when a patient complains of pain, a p.r.n. medication is administered blindly without determining that the pain is at a location which justifies it. This error can easily be avoided by having the patient definitely locate the site of his pain.

Pain over a bony prominence may be relieved and the danger of a pressure sore eliminated by cutting the cast at this point in a crisscross fashion followed by slight elevation of each of the four flaps of plaster (Fig. 18-15). Definitely, this method of relieving the pressure is preferable to the removal of a circular window which allows the skin to bulge through the opening and risks further pressure along the circular margin. Pressure on a bony prominence may also be relieved by cutting the cast over it so as to form a tongue of plaster which is then elevated slightly away from the bony prominence. Pressure sores are preventable complications, as they may be avoided by proper investigation and relief of pressure before necrosis of the skin and other soft tissue occurs.

Pressure Paralyses. These result from prolonged pressure on a nerve trunk, usually at a point where the nerve is rather superficial and overlies bone. Nerve paralyses may occur with little or no evidence of pressure necrosis to the overlying skin.

Paralysis of the peroneal nerve where it encircles the neck of the fibula is the most common nerve palsy in the lower extremity as the result of pressure. The counterpart in the upper extremity is an ulnar paralysis as a result of pressure where the ulnar nerve enters the ulnar notch on the medial condyle of the humerus.

Paralyses from pressure beneath a cast can be avoided by proper padding of the bony prominences and by molding of the plaster while it is setting so as to avoid carefully any pressure which might cause this complication. After the cast has been applied, complaints of pain at a site where a nerve trunk is superficial, accompanied by paresthesias down the course of the nerve as, for example, pain at the head of the fibula and paresthesias down the course of the peroneal nerve, demand that the cast be cut immediately so as to relieve all pressure in this region. As a general rule, pressure paralyses clear up spontaneously, but recovery may be slow. Often the fracture under treatment is firmly united long before the complicating pressure paralysis has disappeared.

REHABILITATION

Rehabilitation of the injured patient with a fracture begins the moment he comes under treatment. Active motion of all joints that do not move the fragments of bone should be carried out frequently. Active contraction of muscle groups which normally move the immobilized joints—for example, the quadriceps group in the thigh—should be carried out many times daily. As soon as the fracture is healed enough so that immobilization is no longer necessary, the contiguous joints should be mobilized. The patient's nutrition and morale must be supported, and he should be encouraged to return to work as soon as this is feasible.

(For Bibliography, see pp. 451-452, at end of Chap. 21.)

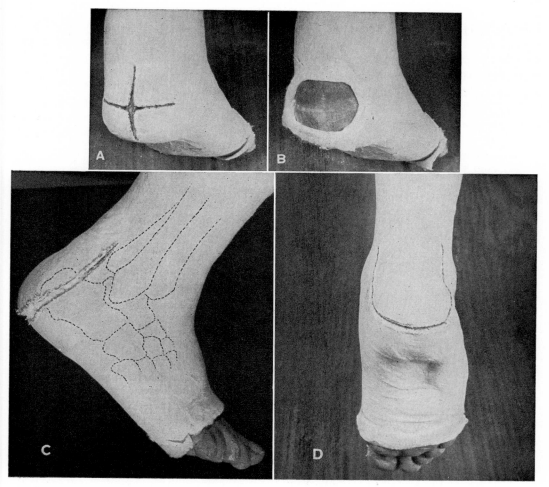

FIG. 18-15. Methods of cutting plaster casts so as to relieve excessive pressure on the prominence of the heel. A. The cruciate incision over the pressure area. Each quadrant of plaster should be elevated slightly so as to relieve the point pressure in the center. B. The circular window for relief of pressure. This is a somewhat undesirable method as it creates a circular rim against which the heel must rest so that other pressure points may develop. The bulging soft tissue may become edematous and increase the pressure on the circular rim. C. and D. The flap or tongue method for relief of pressure. The long tongue is merely sprung backward. (Hampton, O. P., Jr.: Complications of common fractures *in* Hardy, J. D., and Artz, C.: Complications in Surgery, Philadelphia, Saunders, 1960)

OSCAR P. HAMPTON, JR., M.D., AND WILLIAM T. FITTS, JR., M.D.

CHAPTER 19

Fractures and Dislocations
of the Upper Extremity

Fractures and Dislocations About the Shoulder

Fractures of the Shaft of the Humerus

Fractures and Dislocations About the Elbow

Fractures of the Shafts of the Radius and the Ulna

Fractures and Dislocations About the Wrist

As stated by Mason, "nature has developed in the hand a finely co-ordinated motor and sensory organ which has made possible our present civilization." Accordingly, the hand always must be considered carefully in the management of any fracture of the upper extremity. All therapy is designed to safeguard or restore its function even at the cost of some deformity at the site of the fracture. Full length and perfect alignment of the bones of the upper extremity are desirable, but they are not as essential in the upper as in the lower extremity. Mobility of the joints should be sufficient to permit the proper placement of the hand for its functions but only if this mobility can be obtained without impairment of the function of the hand.

FRACTURES AND DISLOCATIONS ABOUT THE SHOULDER

Skeletal injuries about the shoulder may be classified into (1) fractures of the clavicle, (2) fractures of the scapula, (3) fractures of the proximal end of the humerus, (4) dislocations of the shoulder and (5) acromioclavicular dislocations.

With each of these injuries, efforts must be made to avoid edema of the hand and to provide for active exercises of the fingers. As soon as practicable, pendulum exercises of the shoulder should be initiated in an effort to avoid or minimize restriction of motion in this joint (see Fig. 19-6D).

FRACTURES OF THE CLAVICLE

The clavicle serves as a strut for the shoulder and holds it upward, outward and backward from the thorax. It is frequently broken, especially in children. The injury usually occurs as a result of a fall on the shoulder or on the outstretched hand. The clavicle usually breaks in the middle third, probably because its two curves join at this point. In a complete fracture of the clavicle with overriding of the fragments, the outer fragment, along with the shoulder, falls downward, forward and inward (Fig. 19-1, *top*); the inner fragment is drawn upward by the sternocleidomastoid muscle. The diagnosis of a fracture of the clavicle is made by clinical examination and an anteroposterior roentgenogram. A lateral roentgenogram of the clavicle is impracticable.

Treatment. All methods of management of fractures of the clavicle aim at holding the shoulder upward, outward and backward until the fracture has united. Actually, there is no completely efficient and comfortable way to do this; accordingly, a multitude of methods have been devised. Practically all of them employ closed reduction and immobilization by external splinting (Method I). Open reduction and internal fixation is rarely indicated. A fracture of the clavicle is almost certain to heal solidly regardless of the position of the fragments. However, union usually occurs with some visible deformity which is accentuated by a visible and palpable mass of bony callus. In growing children, remodeling processes usually will eliminate the deformity and excess callus and restore normal size and contour of the bone within 6 months to a year.

Probably the simplest and certainly one of the most effective ways of obtaining adequate reduction and splinting of a fracture of the clavicle is with a figure-of-8 clavicular strap, such as those furnished by several splint manufacturers (Fig. 19-1, *bottom*). The clavicular strap is easily applied about the shoulders and may be tightened or loosened repeatedly as indicated. With an assistant holding the shoulders in the hyperextended position, the entire strapping may be removed for cleansing of the axilla as indicated and then be reapplied.

Alternative methods of splinting for fractures of the clavicle include a figure-of-8 plaster cast about the shoulders, a clavicular cross or T-splint and even a simple figure-of-8 roller bandage, all of which tend to hold the injured shoulder upward, backward and outward. Each may be used with good result. However, none has been found to be as simple and effective as the standard clavicular strap shown in Figure 19-1.

In children, greenstick fractures of the clavicle are common. No effort should be made to correct the deformity, which is usually one of upward (or superior) angulation. The fracture should be splinted as outlined above or with a sling and a Velpeau bandage and allowed to heal with angulation. The deformity will be corrected rapidly as growth proceeds.

Fractures of the clavicle must be splinted until union has occurred. The time for union varies with many factors, especially the youth of the patient. In children of 2 years, for example, the fragments may unite rapidly, in 2 weeks. In adults, it is advisable to maintain the strapping in place for 5 to 6 weeks.

Whatever the method of splinting selected for a fracture of the clavicle in adults, stiffness of the shoulder must be prevented by early active exercises. This is not a problem in children. In adults, unless exercise of the shoulder is adequate, a stiff shoulder may produce symptoms long after the clavicle has united.

FRACTURES OF THE SCAPULA

Fractures of the scapula are uncommon. At

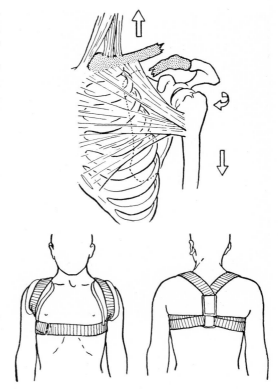

FIG. 19-1. Fracture of the clavicle. (*Top*) Anteroposterior view, showing typical displacement of midclavicle fracture. (*Bottom*) Method of immobilization with a clavicular strap.

times direct blows to the body of this bone produce comminuted fractures; blows to the point of the shoulder may result in fractures of the neck of the scapula. In fractures of the neck, the lateral fragment containing the glenoid is often driven medially and impacted firmly into the body.

Treatment. For fractures of the body, complicated treatment is not necessary. If the degree of pain requires some immobilization for its relief, the arm may be bound to the chest wall in a sling and a modified Velpeau bandage for a few days (Fig. 19-2). Then pendulum exercises should be started, followed shortly by active use of the extremity.

For the usual type of impacted fractures of the neck, the same regimen should be followed. Efforts to disimpact the fracture by lateral traction are not worth while. Excellent function of the shoulder may be obtained

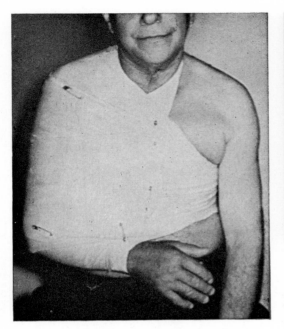

FIG. 19-2. Sling and swath bandage (modified Velpeau). A sling is first applied in the routine way. Then, 4-inch stockinet, 5 yards long, is split and rolled so as to provide an 8-inch bandage. This is used to bandage the extremity in the sling to the thorax. The stockinet is pinned to the sling at several points.

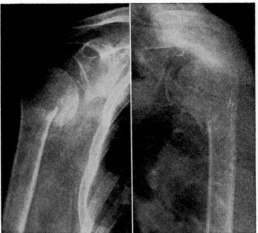

FIG. 19-3. Fracture of the neck of the humerus, adduction type. (*Left*) Anteroposterior view. (*Right*) Lateral view taken through the chest, the only method by which a satisfactory lateral view of proximal humerus may be obtained.

in these impacted fractures by minimal immobilization and early active exercise.

In those fractures of the neck of the scapula which are not impacted but are badly displaced, lateral skeletal traction using a wire in the olecranon may improve the position of the fragments. This method of therapy keeps the patient recumbent. The surgeon must be sure that the traction offers enough improvement in the position of the fragments to justify the immobilization of both patient and extremity. Too often traction has been employed in such instances without actual improvement in the position of the fragments.

FRACTURES OF THE PROXIMAL PORTION OF THE HUMERUS

Fractures of the proximal portion of the humerus occur usually as the result of an indirect force. They are produced most often by a fall on the outstretched hand or arm in such a way that the head of the humerus is jammed against the glenoid and the overhanging, protecting acromion. The arm may be forced into abduction until either a fracture of the neck of the humerus or a dislocation of the shoulder occurs. A fracture occurring as the arm moves away from the body tends to be an abduction type of fracture with medial angulation at the fracture site. On the other hand, if the breaking force is transmitted into the shoulder as the arm moves into an abducted position, an adduction type of fracture with lateral angulation results (Fig. 19-3). Both abduction and adduction type fractures may have minimal or severe comminution.

While fractures of the proximal portion and the humerus may occur at any age, they are found principally in the elderly. Fractures about the neck of the humerus are comparable in the upper extremity in frequency with fractures about the hip in the lower extremity in the latter decades of life. Injuries in this region in children are more likely to be epiphyseal separations; they are discussed elsewhere (p. 362).

Treatment. From the standpoint of treatment, these fractures fall into 2 large groups: (1) those not requiring reduction and (2) those requiring reduction. Fortunately, the majority of fractures of the upper end of the humerus do not require reduction, as they are impacted fractures of either the anatomic or the surgical neck. Almost without exception, the position of impaction should be accepted and no effort made to disengage and improve the position of the fragments. The functional end results are better and are obtained sooner by accepting the position of impaction, even though the alignment is poor, than by breaking up the impaction in an attempt to improve the position.

Impacted fractures of the proximal portion of the humerus are managed by Method 5— the no-immobilization method of management. In order to afford the patient some relief from discomfort during the first few days after injury, the arm may be supported in a sling supplemented by a modified Velpeau bandage (Fig. 19-2). Within a few days—at the most a week—the Velpeau bandage is removed, and soon after—never more than 10 to 12 days after injury—the sling is discarded. Pendulum exercises are initiated as soon as the patient will tolerate them, usually less than a week after injury.

With this method of management of impacted fractures of the proximal portion of the humerus, the patient is generally using the arm fairly freely within 2½ to 3 weeks after injury. However, the patient must make continuous efforts to increase the range of motion during the following weeks and months. Obviously, with severely comminuted fractures of the upper end of the humerus and particularly in the aged, some degree of limitation of motion of the glenohumeral joint is to be anticipated. However, limitation of function will be less with the no-immobilization method of management, which permits early passive and active motion, than it would be with a method of management which immobilizes the shoulder for several weeks.

Unimpacted fractures of the proximal portion of the humerus in satisfactory position require no reduction and are managed by a regimen similar to that of an impacted fracture. It is advisable to leave the sling and modified Velpeau bandage in place for some 10 to 12 days after injury, at which time there will be sufficient fixation of the fragments to permit the substitution of a sling and the initiation of active pendulum exercises. There-

after, management corresponds to that for impacted fractures.

Fractures of the proximal portion of the humerus which are not impacted and in which the fragments are displaced sufficiently to require reduction need a more complicated program. However, before embarking on such a program, the surgeon should be certain that the degree of displacement warrants efforts at improvement. Even though these fractures are near the shoulder joint, anatomic reduction of the fragments is not essential for the return of normal, or almost normal, function. An excellent end result can be obtained with what appears to be a poor apposition of the fragments. Further displacement of the fragments from the position into which they are driven at the time of the injury usually does not occur, because the musculotendinous cuff of the shoulder and the tendon of the long head of the biceps muscle serve to retain them in the same relative position.

In displaced fractures of the proximal portion of the humerus, the proximal fragment usually will be drawn into abduction and external rotation by the strong muscles attached to the greater tuberosity, and the distal fragment will be drawn medially by the pull of the pectoralis major. At times a fragment of greater tuberosity will be drawn high into the shoulder by the supraspinatus tendon. Manipulative efforts at reduction of this group of fractures must take into account the cause of these displacements.

In some of these fractures a stable reduction may be obtained by manual traction and closed manipulation (Method 1). Traction on the distal fragment is made with the arm in some abduction against countertraction furnished by the pull of an assistant on a folded sheet looped through the axilla. Traction applied to the region of the elbow makes traction on the long head of the biceps which tends to overcome the abduction and external rotation of the proximal fragment.

If sufficient traction is maintained, the proximal end of the distal fragment usually can be forced outward so as to bring it into apposition with the proximal fragment. If the reduction is stable, apposition of the fragments may be maintained by the sling and the stockinet Velpeau bandage described above. In such instances, about 3 weeks of immobilization is needed to permit sufficient healing of the fracture to maintain reduction. Then pendulum exercises are initiated, either with the extremity free or with the forearm supported by a sling.

In other displaced fractures some form of continuous traction (Method 2) will be necessary to maintain adequate apposition and alignment of the fragments. This need may be demonstrated immediately after efforts at a manipulative reduction. Following manipulation, a roentgenogram is made with the arm held at the side and the forearm fixed across the abdomen—the position in which a stable fracture would be immobilized. Another roentgenogram is made with the extremity in the same position but with manual traction being maintained at the region of the elbow. By comparison of the 2 roentgenograms it can be determined whether traction affords better apposition and alignment of the fragments.

When traction is necessary, usually it may be adequately obtained and maintained by the use of a properly applied hanging plaster cast. The details of the application of such a cast and the maintenance of traction while the patient is recumbent for a few days are presented under fractures of the humeral shaft (see p. 367). The hanging cast, to be effective, requires that the patient be ambulatory. Therefore, when it is used, the patient must be able to walk or sit reasonably erect in a straight chair without resting the elbow. The hanging cast is a traction method—a type of Method 2, Continuous Traction—and not Method 1, Closed Reduction and Immobilization. A "collar and cuff" sling arrangement is an alternative to the hanging cast. The weight of the elbow region provides the traction on the proximal humerus.

The mechanism by which traction may improve reduction of displaced fractures of the proximal portion of the humerus is afforded by the "guy rope" action of the tendon of the long head of the biceps as it passes through the bicipital groove on the proximal fragment and continues downward alongside the distal fragment (see Fig. 19-6 A).

Traction in a hanging cast or collar and cuff sling is continued until sufficient union has been obtained to eliminate all danger of redisplacement and malalignment. During this time it is possible to carry out some degree of pendulum exercises for the shoulder by having the patient lean forward and allow the arm to abduct and rotate. Later, after removal of the cast some 3 weeks after injury, pendulum exercises are carried out.

In selected instances of displaced fractures of the proximal portion of the humerus, in which continuous traction is necessary, such traction may be provided as skeletal traction by means of a Kirschner wire inserted through the olecranon, or as skin traction by means of adhesive tape. Continuous traction may be employed with the arm abducted 90° and resting on the bed and with the forearm suspended toward the ceiling, or with the arm abducted 90° and forward flexed 90° so that the traction is in the direction of the ceiling. In such instances, the forearm is supported by a sling attached to an overhead frame.

Operative reduction (Method 3) is rarely indicated in these injuries, particularly in the elderly age groups. It may be indicated for severely displaced fractures in the young. Open reduction for this injury is usually an extensive operation and should not be selected lightly.

Fractures of the Greater Tuberosity. These fractures are seldom displaced unless they complicate a dislocation of the shoulder. Undisplaced fractures of the greater tuberosity are managed as impacted fractures of the upper end of the humerus and accordingly require very little treatment. Fractures of the greater tuberosity complicating dislocations of the shoulder may be a difficult problem. They are discussed below under dislocations of the shoulder.

FRACTURE-EPIPHYSEAL SEPARATION OF THE PROXIMAL PORTION OF THE HUMERUS

Fracture-epiphyseal separations at this location usually occur in the second decade of life. Some have minimal displacement and require only immobilization with the arm at the side. In others, there is complete displacement with the shaft usually being drawn inward, upward and forward.

These injuries do not require an accurate reduction. Some angulation and displacement may be accepted with the anticipation of a good functional result and, unless the adolescent is too near maturity, correction of any deformity by growth processes. Efforts at closed reduction should not be too vigorous because of possible damage to the epiphyseal cartilage plate. If closed manipulation does not give a satisfactory reduction, open reduction is required.

DISLOCATIONS OF THE SHOULDER

Dislocation of the glenohumeral joint is the most frequent dislocation of a major joint and occurs as a result of forced abduction and external rotation of the arm until the head of the humerus is levered downward out of the glenoid cavity. After the humeral head has torn through the inferior portion of the capsule of the shoulder joint, it may come to rest anteriorly beneath the coracoid process (Fig. 19-4 A) (subcoracoid dislocation, the most frequent position), beneath the glenoid (subglenoid dislocation) or posteriorly behind the glenoid (posterior or subspinous dislocation). The last is rare and is frequently difficult to diagnose. Posterior dislocation of the

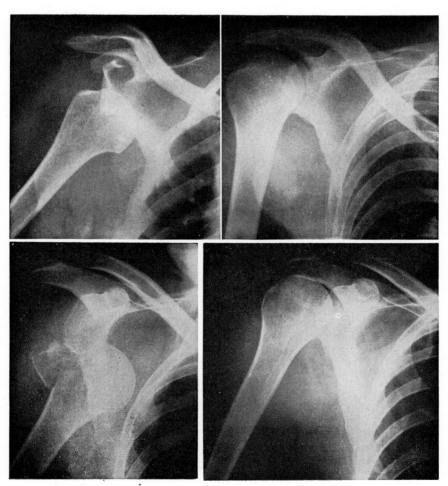

FIG. 19-4. Dislocation of the shoulder. (A, *top, left*) Roentgenogram of subcoracoid dislocation of the shoulder (the common type) without fracture of the tuberosity. (B, *top, right*) Roentgenogram after reduction. (C, *bottom, left*) Roentgenogram of fracture of the greater tuberosity associated with dislocation of the shoulder. (D, *bottom, right*) Postreduction roentgenogram, showing reduction of both fracture and dislocation.

shoulder should be suspected when routine roentgenograms are not diagnostic of a skeletal injury but pain and restriction of motion indicate a significant injury about the shoulder. In posterior dislocation, the tip of the coracoid process may be prominent. Stereoscopic roentgenograms in the anteroposterior view and conventional vertical views may confirm the diagnosis.

Following anterior dislocation of the humeral head, the arm ordinarily assumes a characteristic position which strongly suggests the diagnosis. The elbow is held forward and is abducted from the side. It cannot be approximated to the side. If the hand can touch the opposite shoulder with the elbow touching the side of the thorax, it may be assumed that an anterior dislocation of the shoulder is not present, unless there is an associated fracture of the humerus. With the humeral head dislocated, the normal contour of the shoulder is lost and is replaced by a shallow hollow. This causes the acromion to be unduly prominent.

While these signs often permit accurate clinical diagnosis, and while occasionally one may be justified in attempting manipulative reduction without roentgenologic confirmation, it is good policy always to obtain a prereduction roentgenogram. This not only confirms the diagnosis but also shows whether or not there is a complicating fracture of the greater tuberosity or other bony injury in this region. Occasionally, it will reveal the distressing complication of a fracture of the neck of the humerus combined with dislocation of the humeral head. This grave injury is discussed below.

Treatment. Manual reduction of the dislocation of the shoulder may be accomplished at times without anesthesia or under sedation provided by morphine. General anesthesia may be employed electively or after reasonable efforts at reduction without anesthesia have been ineffective, provided that conditions for anesthesia are favorable. The relaxation provided by anesthesia usually makes reduction of the dislocation easy and minimizes the hazard of the manipulations causing a fracture of the surgical neck of the humerus or further soft tissue damage.

TECHNIC OF REDUCTION. Dislocations of the shoulder may be reduced in several ways.

All methods attempt to return the head of the humerus to a point just inferior to the glenoid and by traction then to cause it to re-enter the joint through the rent in the capsule. Each method offers advantages and disadvantages.

In a great many instances reduction may be obtained without anesthesia (perhaps with an injection of morphine) by using the weight of the upper extremity to provide traction. The patient is placed face down with the injured extremity hanging over the side or the head of the table. A weight of 8 to 12 pounds suspended from the wrist provides traction. This position is comfortable to the patient. Since pain is relieved, spasm of the shoulder muscles subsides. After the extremity has dangled in this position for several minutes, reduction may occur either spontaneously or after the shoulder has been rotated gently a few degrees by the surgeon.

Traction without manipulation will reduce the majority of dislocated shoulders. The traction may be made at the wrist with the forearm extended or at the elbow with the forearm flexed. Countertraction is provided by pull on a folded sheet passed through the axilla and resting against the upper lateral chest wall. Traction is made first in the line of the position assumed by the humerus, i.e., slight abduction. While the traction is maintained the arm is brought into slight adduction. If reduction is not obtained immediately, the arm may be rotated inward and outward a few degrees while traction is maintained.

If straight traction does not result in reduction, Kocher maneuvers may be carried out. Fundamental maneuvers are traction on the flexed elbow in slight abduction, then external rotation, and then adduction of the arm followed by full internal rotation. During all the maneuvers, steady traction is maintained. Kocher maneuvers, while usually effective, are not without danger. They must be carried out without undue force lest the humerus be fractured through the surgical neck, an abominable complication.

An alternative traction method is known as the Hippocratic maneuver (heel-in-axilla method). In this method the shoeless heel of the surgeon is forced in the axilla, thereby providing countertraction while straight traction is made on the extremity at the wrist with the elbow extended. The pressure of the surgeons' heel against the humeral head is thought to be of some aid in forcing it back into the joint. The method is hazardous and is not recommended. It may injure the axillary vessels and nerves.

POSTREDUCTION MANAGEMENT. Authorities do not agree on postoperative management. Some consider immobilization of the arm and the shoulder of no value, while others insist on immobilization for 6 to 8 weeks. A middle-of-the-road course is 3 to 4 weeks of immobilization with the arm at the side, which may be provided by a sling and modified Velpeau bandage (Fig. 19-2). This is recommended for dislocations of the shoulder in individuals under 40 years of age, the age group in which recurrence of dislocation is the most common. For individuals over 40 years of age, a much shorter period of immobilization, 7 to 14 days, is recommended. Recurrent dislocation in the later decades of life is rare; therefore, all immobilization should be discontinued as soon as comfort of the patient permits, and active pendulum exercises should be initiated as a safeguard against stiffness of the shoulder.

Complications of Dislocations of the Shoulder. These include fractures of the greater tuberosity, fractures of the surgical neck with displacement, damage to the axillary nerve, damage to the axillary vessels and accompanying nerve trunks, and recurrent dislocation of the shoulder.

FRACTURES OF THE GREATER TUBEROSITY OF THE HUMERUS. This is not an infrequent complication of dislocations of the shoulder, as it occurs in about 20 per cent of cases. In the majority of instances when the glenohumeral dislocation is reduced, the greater tuberosity falls into good position (Fig. 19-4 C, D). In such instances treatment of the dislocation is sufficient treatment for the fracture also. Subsequent displacement of the greater tuberosity need not be feared because the fact that the fragment fell into reduction indicates that the musculotendinous cuff of the shoulder is intact.

In those instances in which the fragment of the greater tuberosity is not replaced when the dislocation of the shoulder is reduced, a more vigorous course of management is indicated. The fragment usually will remain displaced superiorly, and this position indicates that the musculotendinous cuff of the shoul-der has been torn. Unless the age and the condition of the patient contraindicate operation, open reduction (Method 3) is indicated. The fragment should be reduced accurately and fixed in position by suture or metallic internal fixation, and then torn musculotendinous fibers should be repaired. Postoperatively, the course of management is the same as for dislocation of the shoulder without fracture.

FRACTURE-DISLOCATION OF THE SHOULDER. A displaced fracture of the surgical neck with a dislocated humeral head is a highly complicated injury. Efforts at closed reduction are frequently unsuccessful but they may be made carefully. The method of attempted reduction employs traction and countertraction by assistants while the surgeon manipulates the humeral head with his fingers. If reduction can be effected, subsequent therapy follows that described for displaced fractures of the surgical neck. The fracture usually goes into reduction easily if the head can be reduced by closed manipulation.

In the majority of instances, open reduction of the humeral head will be necessary. Actually, the chance of a successful closed reduction is so poor that the effort should be made only after arrangements have been completed to proceed immediately with open reduction, if necessary, under the same anesthesia. Even at operation, reduction is often difficult.

INJURY TO BLOOD VESSELS AND NERVES. Damage to the axillary nerve by the humeral head as it leaves the shoulder joint is a not infrequent complication of dislocation, occurring in about 15 per cent of dislocations. It will manifest itself first by anesthesia in the sensory distribution of the axillary nerve. Later, when it is possible to test the power of the deltoid muscle it will be found that this muscle is paralyzed. Fortunately, the prognosis of this complication is usually good. The nerve is usually bruised but not torn, and spontaneous recovery takes place as a rule. Even if it does not, operative efforts to find and repair the nerve are not considered worth-while.

Occasionally there is evidence of trauma to the axillary vessels and the large nerve trunks. Usually these are merely bruised and not torn, and any motor or sensory deficit may be expected to disappear spontaneously.

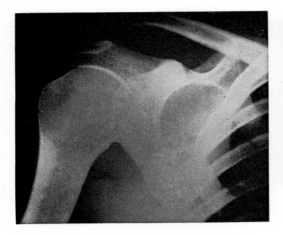

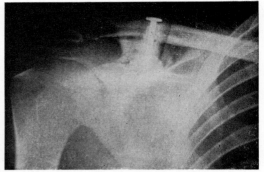

Fig. 19-5. (*Left*) Complete dislocation (or separation) of the acromioclavicular joint. (*Right*) Roentgenogram after operative reduction of a complete acromioclavicular separation. A lag screw passing through the clavicle and into the coracoid process stabilizes the reduction.

Arterial insufficiency persisting after adjustment of position is an indication for immediate operative exploration. If anesthesia or paresis has not disappeared within 4 months the problem is neurosurgical.

RECURRENT DISLOCATION OF THE SHOULDER. This distinct clinical entity is, of course, a delayed complication of acute dislocation of the shoulder. The diagnosis is made when the patient finds that he sustains repeated dislocations with minimal trauma which forces the arm into abduction and external rotation. There are several theories concerning the cause of recurrent dislocation. The most prominent, that of Bankhart, holds that the original injury to the labrium glenoidale and the joint capsule commits the patient to the syndrome of recurrent dislocation. He states that the labrium glenoidale and the capsule are so torn away from the anterior inferior rim of the glenoid that repair does not take place and, therefore, redislocation occurs easily. DePalma holds that the trauma to the muscular apparatus, particularly the rotator muscles about the shoulder, results in a loss of tonicity and efficiency which predisposes to recurrent dislocation. Regardless of the underlying cause, recurrent dislocation may be disabling. As pointed out previously, it is a frequent complication during the first 3 or 4 decades of life and uncommon during the later ones. When a fracture of the greater tuberosity complicates dislocation of the shoulder, recurrence of dislocation is most unlikely to occur. In other words, the presence of a fracture of the greater tuberosity is excellent evidence that the patient will not develop recurrent dislocation of the shoulder.

The treatment for recurrent dislocation of the shoulder is surgical. Several technics of repair are in general use. For a detailed description of them, the reader must consult more specialized texts.

ACROMIOCLAVICULAR DISLOCATION

Acromioclavicular dislocations or separations result from falls on the point of the shoulder. They may be either complete or incomplete. Complete lesions are described as complete dislocations or separations (Fig. 19-5, *left*). Incomplete lesions are called incomplete dislocations or subluxations.

The stability of the acromioclavicular joint depends upon the strong coracoclavicular and the acromioclavicular ligaments. In patients with complete dislocations, both of these are torn so that the outer end of the clavicle goes upward and backward. In incomplete dislocations or subluxations, the acromioclavicular ligaments are torn to some degree, but the coracoclavicular ligament is not torn, although it may undergo some stretching.

Treatment. Incomplete dislocations or subluxations require very little treatment. It is customary to attempt stabilization of the outer end of the clavicle with adhesive strapping over a felt pad applied just above the outer end of the bone and by a sling applied so as to lift the arm and the shoulder. Such measures are probably of little benefit, although they should be employed until pain about the injured joint has begun to subside. Prolonged immobilization is not necessary. The prognosis for an excellent functional result is good, although the outer end of the clavicle may remain somewhat loose and prominent in comparison with the opposite side. These lesions should be undertreated rather than overtreated.

Complete dislocations usually require operative management. Although many cumbersome pieces of apparatus and methods of immobilization have been described for nonoperative management of these injuries, none is highly effective, and all are uncomfortable. With open operation, chips of bone and cartilage can be removed from the joint, and tags of torn ligament released and sutured. Some method of internal fixation which stabilizes the reduction must be employed. With operative stabilization, minimal external immobilization, no more than a sling, is necessary, and relatively early pendulum exercises may be initiated. With early operative stabilization of complete dislocations of the acromioclavicular joint, the end result should be a normal or near normal shoulder.

In selected instances of old unreduced dislocations of the acromioclavicular joint, excision of the lateral portion of the clavicle may give a satisfactory final result.

FRACTURES OF THE SHAFT OF THE HUMERUS

The shaft of the humerus extends from a level a short distance above the insertion of the pectoralis major muscle distally to the supracondylar level. This portion of the humerus has a less abundant blood supply than the regions of the head and the neck and the condyles. A unique feature of the anatomy of the shaft of the humerus is the close proximity of the radial nerve as it partially encircles the humeral shaft in the musculospiral groove.

Fractures of the humeral shaft may be transverse, spiral, oblique, or comminuted, depending to some extent on the way the fracture is sustained. Obviously, these fractures may be caused in many ways, including a direct blow on the arm, excessive torsion of the arm, or undue leverage on the arm when the shoulder or the elbow is fixed.

Treatment. Despite the many ways by which these fractures may be caused, the several types which may be sustained, and the anatomic features tending to complicate management, the great majority respond highly satisfactorily to management in a hanging cast. This method, which at first glance appears to be an inadequate application of closed reduction and immobilization (Method 1), actually is a continuous traction method (Method 2) (Fig. 19-6). The hanging cast, applied with the elbow flexed to a right angle and extending from the level of the mid-humerus to or including part of the hand, furnishes continuous traction by its weight as it hangs. The continuous traction causes relaxation of the several muscle groups tending to displace the fragments and, with the muscles relaxed, it usually causes the fragments to drop into adequate apposition and good alignment. Obviously, the traction is really effective only when the patient is in the erect position. However, it is possible to provide some traction when the patient is recumbent as illustrated in Figure 19-7.

A satisfactory hanging cast usually may be applied without general anesthesia with the patient sitting on a stool or the edge of the table with the extremity held in the position in which it will hang later. The hanging position provides sufficient relief from pain. If general anesthesia is used, the cast should be applied with the arm as close as possible to the hanging position. The cast must not be so heavy that it will distract the fragments. A loop of plaster or wire at the wrist provides for a loop sling suspended around the neck, and another at the elbow provides for traction during periods of recumbency as mentioned above (Fig. 19-7).

During the first 2 or 3 weeks after application of the hanging cast, several check roentgenograms are made at intervals of 4 to 7 days to be certain that satisfactory reduction is being maintained. Anterior or posterior angulation at the fracture site is an indication to raise or lower, respectively, the wrist by changes in the length of the sling about the neck. Medial or lateral angulation can be corrected sometimes by moving the loop at the wrist inward or outward or by means of pads of sponge rubber or felt taped to the cast either on the inner side of the proximal end of the cast or at the inner side of the elbow as indicated. Sometimes to correct angulation of fractures at the junction of the middle and the lower thirds it is necessary to change the cast and either provide more pronation or more supination of the forearm and thereby to change the direction of muscle pull on the condyles. Occasionally, distraction of the fragments may necessitate substitution of a shoulder spica for the hanging cast.

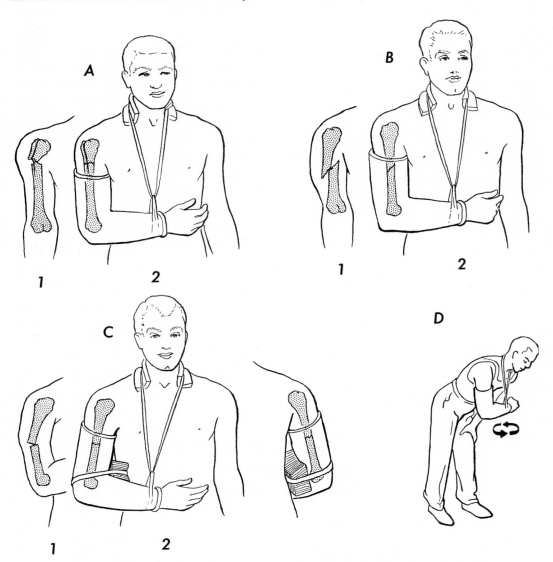

FIG. 19-6. Treatment of fractures of the shaft of the humerus with hanging cast. (A) Fracture of the proximal shaft: (1) abduction of proximal fragment and kinking of long head of biceps; (2) effect of application of hanging cast. (B, 1) Oblique fracture of midshaft with medial displacement and overriding; (B, 2) effect of hanging cast. (C, 1) Transverse fracture of humeral shaft with lateral angulation; (C, 2) after application of hanging cast with pad on medial side of elbow to correct angulation. (D) Circumduction exercises. (Note that the illustration shows the cast high on arm. It is not necessary and often inadvisable to bring the cast above the level of the fracture.)

As a rule, gentle swinging exercises of the shoulder should be instituted within a few days. If the patient leans well forward while the extremity remains suspended by the loop sling, the alignment of the fracture is not disturbed. The fact that these shoulder exercises can be carried out during the period of healing of the fracture is a distinct advantage of the hanging cast method, as other methods mentioned below which do not permit these exercises often are followed by considerable stiffness of the shoulder joint.

Other methods which may be considered for fractures of the humeral shaft include a shoulder spica cast, skeletal or skin traction with the arm abducted from the side and with the forearm suspended from above, and open reduction and internal fixation. About the only indication for a shoulder spica cast is, as mentioned above, when distraction of the fragments results from a hanging cast. Skeletal traction (preferable) or skin traction may be necessary when other injuries or diseases pre-

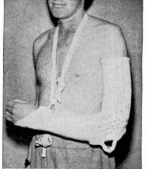

vent the patient's being out of bed. Open reduction with internal fixation occasionally is indicated when traction methods have not resulted in adequate reduction. This situation may develop when there is interposition of muscle between fragment ends or when the action of certain muscles causing displacement and deformity cannot be overcome. Signs and symptoms of a radial nerve paralysis may indicate early open reduction (see p. 411). Open operation and internal fixation with an intramedullary nail may be the treatment of choice for pathologic fractures of the humeral shaft. Pain is relieved, and x-ray therapy can easily be given to the lesion.

When the hanging cast is used, it is left in place until there is sufficient clinical and x-ray evidence of union to make traction by the weight of the cast no longer necessary. Then a cravat or collar-and-cuff sling may be substituted until union is solid. The usual period for healing of fractures of the humeral shaft varies from 6 to 12 or more weeks after injury. When skeletal or skin traction in recumbency is used, it is continued until other conditions permit the patient to be ambulatory, and then a hanging cast or collar and cuff sling is substituted. When internal fixation

Fig. 19-7. Hanging cast for fracture of the humerus. (*Top, left*) Patient ambulatory. (*Bottom*) Patient recumbent with traction maintained. (Hampton, O. P.: Wounds of the Extremities in Military Surgery, St. Louis, Mosby, p. 328)

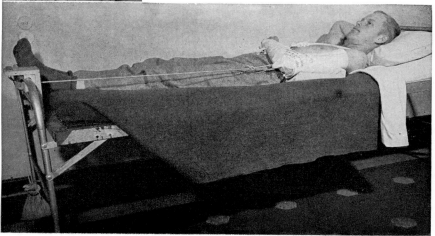

is employed, supporting external splinting in some form is usually necessary.

Nerve Injuries. The close proximity of the radial nerve as it winds about the shaft of the humerus in the musculospiral groove makes it particularly susceptible to injury when a fracture of the shaft of the humerus is sustained. In addition, the median and the ulnar nerves are not too far removed from the humeral shaft, and occasionally one of these is injured by a sharp fragment of bone. As in all extremity injuries, at the first examination the surgeon must determine by physical examination whether or not there is any deficit in the sensory and the motor functions of the major peripheral nerve trunks. This is easily done by having the patient carry out the various movements of the fingers and the thumb and also by testing for sensation on the hand. If there are signs of nerve paralysis when the patient is first seen, open reduction may be justified to appraise the extent of damage to the nerve and to make certain that it is free from impingement by the fragments, although the great majority will recover without operative intervention.

It also is important to retest the function of the major peripheral nerves, especially that of the radial nerve, throughout treatment of the fracture and especially after the extremity has been placed in a hanging cast or in traction. Signs indicating new nerve damage suggest the possibility of trauma to the nerve during manipulation of the fragments and may indicate early exploration by operation.

FRACTURES AND DISLOCATIONS ABOUT THE ELBOW

Fractures and dislocations about the elbow may be conveniently classified and discussed as (1) fractures of the lower end of the humerus in children, (2) fractures of the lower end of the humerus in adults, (3) fractures of the olecranon, (4) fractures of the head of the radius, (5) Monteggia or "parry" fractures, (6) dislocations of the elbow.

FRACTURES OF THE LOWER END OF THE HUMERUS IN CHILDREN

These common fractures of childhood may be classified as (1) supracondylar and trans-

condylar fractures, (2) fractures of the lateral condyle, (3) fractures of the medial condyle, (4) fractures of the medial epicondyle. Of these, the supracondylar and transcondylar fractures are by far the most common and comprise the typical elbow fractures in children.

Roentgenograms of the elbow of a child may be difficult to evaluate because of the many epiphyseal lines and ossifying epiphyses appearing successively as the age of the patient increases. The center of ossification for the capitellum, the first to appear, may be seen in roentgenograms at about 2 years of age. That of the medial epicondyle appears next, at about 5 years of age. The center for the trochlea become visible at about the 9th year, and that for the lateral epicondyle at the 12th year. These 4 centers fuse at about the age of 16 to form a single epiphysis which fuses to the shaft at about the age of 18. For the evaluation of roentgenograms of an injured elbow in a child, comparable views of the opposite uninjured elbow for comparison may be an invaluable aid to diagnosis.

One must remember that even though ossification of an epiphysis has not begun and it cannot be visualized on roentgenograms, the unossified cartilage can be injured and produce growth disturbances later. What appears to be only a small fragment on the roentgenogram may actually be several times larger because of the nonradiopaque cartilage which surrounds it.

Supracondylar and Transcondylar Fractures. These similar injuries vary only in the exact level of the fracture. The transcondylar level is slightly lower than the supracondylar. From the clinical standpoint, they are customarily considered together and called supracondylar fractures. They usually occur from a fall on the hand with the elbow extended.

Supracondylar fractures are true surgical emergencies. Swelling about the elbow begins promptly and progresses rapidly. Once considerable swelling has developed, manipulative reduction and maintenance of reduction become difficult and perhaps impossible. Massive swelling is likely to result in extensive bleb formation which will handicap proper therapy. Early reduction before excessive swelling has occurred is therefore essential, particularly if the fracture is to be managed by closed reduction and immobilization (Method 1).

As soon as the patient is seen and before any attempt at reduction of the fracture is made, the status of the radial pulse and the function of the major peripheral nerve trunks must be determined and recorded. These valuable prereduction observations must never be omitted.

TREATMENT. *Management by Closed Reduction and Immobilization (Method 1).*

Supracondylar fractures are preferably reduced by closed manipulation and held reduced in acute flexion (Jones position). Reduction is achieved as illustrated in Figure 19-8. The fundamental maneuvers are strong manual traction with the elbow in extension against equally strong countertraction applied to the arm by an assistant. Once the distal fragment has been unlocked and pulled distally by traction, lateral or posterior displacement, if present, is corrected by direct manual pressure. Then the elbow is flexed acutely. If the fragments have been reduced, acute flexion will maintain the reduction (Fig. 19-9).

Postreduction roentgenograms should be made before the elbow is immobilized. An important criterion of reduction is that in the lateral view the capitellum must extend well forward of the anterior margin of the humeral shaft. Another reduction must be attempted if the roentgenograms show faulty position of the fragments. Slight posterior displacement of the distal fragment may be accepted, but varus (inward) or valgus (outward) deformity resulting from lateral or medial angulation should be overcome if at all possible.

The degree of acute flexion which may be maintained safely is determined by the circulation of the hand. With a swollen elbow, flexion of the forearm may shut off the arterial flow and eliminate the radial pulse. The latter must be felt for at frequent, regular intervals. Only the degree of flexion of the forearm which permits a full radial pulse may be accepted. Moreover, the color of the hand must remain good as evidence that no obstruction of venous return exists. Such obstruction will lead to rapidly increasing swelling which eventually would obstruct the arterial blood flow. (See section on Volkmann's ischemic contracture below.)

The acutely flexed position of the elbow

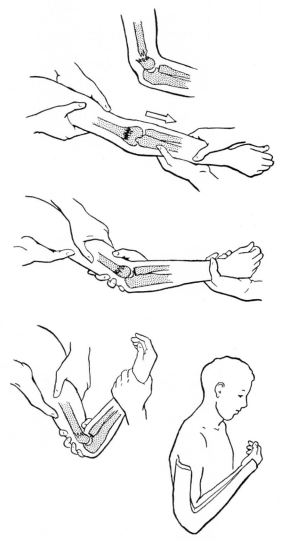

FIG. 19-8. Method of manipulative reduction of supracondylar fracture of the humerus. (See text.)

may be held in several ways. Circular adhesive (applied as several half circles) around the arm and the flexed forearm is highly effective. It is unyielding to later swelling, but if swelling becomes excessive, the degree of flexion can be diminished easily after cutting across the bands of adhesive. Then more adhesive can be applied easily in the new position without removing that which was applied originally. Instead of adhesive, a posterior molded plaster splint extending from the upper

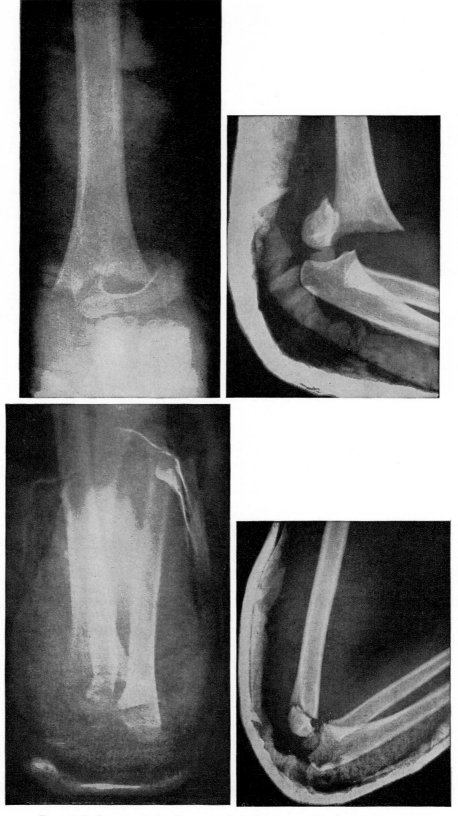

FIG. 19-9. Supracondylar fracture of the humerus. (*Top*) Anteroposterior and lateral roentgenograms before reduction. (*Bottom*) Postreduction views with elbow held in acute flexion by posterior plaster splint.

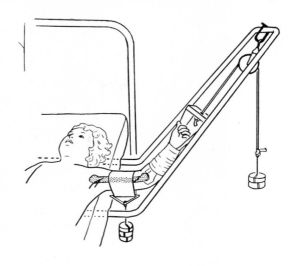

FIG. 19-10. Supracondylar fracture of the humerus. (*Top*) Dunlop's traction. The patient must lie near the edge of the mattress with the injured arm abducted so that it extends from the side of the bed. A loop about the arm which serves to make backward pressure on the proximal fragment may be easily constructed with a piece of felt threaded into stockinet. The skin traction on the forearm is applied in a direction which, with the aid of the weight attached to the loop over the arm, will maintain the elbow at about 135°. The amount of weight required to hold the arm down and to make sufficient traction on the forearm will vary from 2 to 4 pounds, depending upon the size of the patient. (*Bottom*) Skeletal traction with Kirschner wire through olecranon.

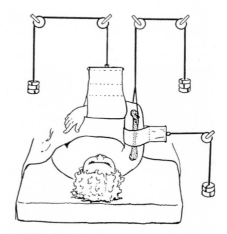

arm to the fingers may be used to hold the elbow in acute flexion. It is somewhat less effective than the adhesive strapping, as it may break and permit the elbow to extend enough to allow displacement of the fragments. However, it does have the advantage that with severe postreduction swelling, some extension of the elbow may be accomplished by slight adjustment of the plaster or may even occur spontaneously as the force of the swelling causes the plaster to give toward extension.

Careful postoperative observation of the circulation is mandatory. If it becomes at all impaired, flexion of the forearm must be decreased until a strong pulse at the wrist is palpable, even if reduction of the fracture is lost. If possible, the patient should be hospitalized for 2 or 3 days to gain the advantage of continuous and expert observation. Impaired circulation and its sequelae caused by the position of flexion are avoidable.

Volkmann's Ischemic Contracture (see p. 339). This dreaded complication of supracondylar fractures of the humerus in children results from impairment of the arterial flow to the forearm and the hand. The circulation may be obstructed as a result of hematoma and swelling from the injury itself or excessive flexion of the forearm on the arm. The possibility of Volkmann's contracture and the importance of maintaining adequate circulation to the forearm and the hand must be kept in mind at all times throughout treatment of these injuries.

Management in Balanced Traction (Method

2). Manipulative reduction and immobilization in acute flexion will not suffice for all supracondylar fractures of the humerus. Some of the patients with this injury will arrive with elbows already so severely swollen that flexion sufficient to maintain a satisfactory manipulative reduction will obliterate the radial pulse. In others, postreduction swelling will impair the circulation and require the release of acute flexion.

When, for any reason, a satisfactory reduction of the fracture cannot be maintained with the elbow in acute flexion, a traction method is indicated. Dunlop's traction is an excellent method for this injury (Fig. 19-11). It is a form of balanced suspension skin traction

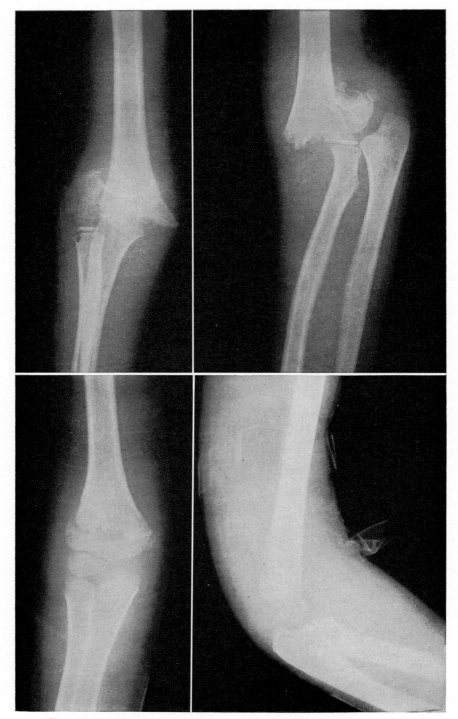

Fig. 19-11. Roentgenograms showing severely displaced supracondylar fracture of a child on admission and the position obtained promptly in Dunlop's traction. (*Top, left and right*) Anteroposterior and lateral views on admission to the hospital. (*Bottom, left and right*) Position obtained promptly and maintained until fragments united with no signs of embarrassment to the circulation of the extremity.

which usually gives adequate reduction of supracondylar fractures of the humerus even though the forearm is extended to an angle about 135°. In this position, circulation is almost never impeded.

The use of skeletal traction directed toward the ceiling with the patient recumbent, using a wire through the olecranon, is an alternative to Dunlop's traction (Fig. 19-11, *bottom*).

Dunlop's or skeletal traction is unlikely to provide as accurate a reduction of the fragments as is usually obtained with a manipulative reduction but, even so, an adequate reduction is usually obtained and maintained, and the hazard of ischemia is avoided. Swelling will usually subside within 1 to 2 weeks, and then the extremity may be immobilized in acute flexion as described above.

Supracondylar fractures of the humerus in children unite rapidly. While displacement of the fragments can recur during the first week, displacement thereafter is most unusual if ordinary precautions are taken. The length of time during which the position of acute flexion must be maintained varies with the age of the patient. In children below the age of 3, acute flexion may be discontinued after 10 to 12 days, and even in children up to the age of 14 the position of acute flexion may be discontinued after 3 weeks. After the retentive apparatus is removed and the position of acute flexion discontinued, it is usually advisable to place the arm in a sling with the elbow at 90° for an additional 7 to 10 days. During this time some active exercises should be carried out. Thereafter full active use of the extremity is allowed. The child should be encouraged to flex the elbow actively to the limit several times daily in order that the range of flexion may be maintained while the ability to extend is being regained.

The ability to extend the elbow completely may return slowly. However, the prognosis for complete or practically complete extension is good. Passive stretching is dangerous and is likely to do more harm than good. Even the carrying of weights to help force extension is inadvisable. Strenuous passive efforts may produce more injury about the joint and may retard or perhaps permanently prevent full extension. Increase in elbow motion may be slow, and the limits of motion which are to be gained may take as long as 2 years.

Fractures of the Lateral Condyle. In fractures of the lateral condyle in children the fragment includes the epiphysis of the capitellum. Any displacement distorts the articular surface of the humerus and, in accordance with the fracture maxim that fractures involving articular surfaces require exact repositioning, this injury requires the most precise reduction. Only in this way can one hope to prevent subsequent growth disturbances with the sequelae of limited elbow function and possible late ulnar nerve paralysis. The latter may occur as long as 20 to 30 years after the original injury from progressive increase in the carrying angle and resulting stretch on the nerve. The carrying angle, usually 10° to 15° of valgus, is formed by the arm and the forearm when the elbow is extended. The extensor muscles of the forearm attached to the lateral condyle tend to rotate the fragment to a variable extent. With full rotation the articular surface of the condyle may face the fracture surface of the humerus. The fragment must be returned to or near its normal position.

In undisplaced fractures of the lateral condyle, immobilization of the elbow in moderately acute flexion for 3 weeks will prevent displacement and is all that is necessary. Aspiration of the hematoma from the joint will minimize pain.

In displaced fractures closed reduction is difficult but is occasionally successful; therefore, an attempt is often worth while. The earlier the attempts at reduction the better the chance of success. The surgeon should flex the elbow slightly and then adduct the forearm forcibly to widen the lateral side of the joint. Direct pressure of the thumbs on the fragment is made in an attempt to rotate the fragment backward into place. Fluoroscopic visualization is advantageous. If a satisfactory position cannot be obtained by closed reduction, early open reduction with fixation by sutures or a pin is indicated. Failure to achieve accurate reduction by some method will lead to the complications listed above.

Fractures of the Medial Condyle. Fractures of the medial condyle in children are less common than those of the lateral condyle. The fragment includes the epiphyses for the trochlea and the medial epicondyle. Because the center of ossification for the epiphysis of the trochlea appears late, the size of the fragment is easily underestimated on the roentgeno-grams.

Management of this injury is comparable to that of fractures of the lateral condyle. For undisplaced fractures, immobilization in moderately acute flexion is sufficient. In displaced fractures, accurate replacement of the condylar fragment is necessary. If efforts at closed reduction are not successful, the fragments must be reduced by open operation and fixed with sutures or pins.

Fractures of the Medial Epicondyle. This injury of childhood and adolescence is really an epiphyseal separation rather than a true fracture. The common tendon of origin of the flexor muscles of the forearm arises in part from the medial epicondyle. When this epiphysis is avulsed, the entire tendon of origin may be torn also. When the tear is severe this muscle group tends to pull the medial epicondyle downward, at times into the joint cavity. This injury may occur at any time before the epiphysis for the medial epicondyle closes at about the age of 17 years. It is produced by a valgus strain at the elbow. It often complicates dislocation of the elbow. The ulnar nerve also may be damaged, particularly when the medial epicondyle is greatly displaced.

TREATMENT. With little or no displacement of the medial epicondyle, immobilization of the elbow in moderately acute flexion is sufficient. With considerable displacement as, for example, when the fragment is displaced into the joint, open operation must be performed and the fragment fixed with suture or pin. A guiding rule is that if the epiphysis is displaced less than a centimeter, only immobilization is necessary, but if the displacement exceeds a centimeter open operation is indicated. A careful repair of the torn tendon of origin is an important part of this operative procedure.

FRACTURES OF THE LOWER END OF THE HUMERUS IN ADULTS

For purposes of discussion, these injuries may be classified as fractures of the medial or lateral condyle, T-fractures of the distal humerus and fracture of the capitellum. Considerable comminution may accompany any of these types.

Undisplaced fractures in these groups require only immobilization in a plaster cast

extending from the upper arm to the proximal palmar crease of the hand with the elbow at a right angle and the forearm, as a rule, in mid-pronation. In displaced fractures of either the medial or the lateral condyle or T-fractures involving both condyles, precise reduction is necessary to restore the articular surface of the lower end of the humerus. In some instances, adequate reduction can be obtained by closed manipulation and maintained by plaster cast immobilization as in undisplaced fractures. In some T-fractures, traction provided by a Kirschner wire through the olecranon or by a hanging cast may suffice to give adequate reduction. In most displaced fractures involving the condyles, including the T-fractures, open reduction with internal fixation is necessary before adequate apposition and alignment of the fragments can be achieved and maintained (Fig. 19-12).

Capitellum. Fractures of the capitellum comprise a unique group peculiar to the elbow. They are usually vertical fractures separating the anterior projecting capitellum from the remainder of the condyle. They are produced by forces transmitted through a fall on the outstretched arm and hand and often are associated with fractures of the head of the radius. The fragment is usually displaced forward and upward anterior to the humerus.

If the fracture of the capitellum is not displaced, only immobilization in a plaster cast is necessary. Large displaced fragments must be replaced, if possible, by closed manipulation, using traction in complete extension combined with direct pressure of the thumbs on the fragment. If reduction cannot be maintained with the elbow in flexion, complete extension may maintain the reduction. The advantage of keeping this difficult fracture reduced by extension outweighs the risk of stiffness from immobilization in extension. If closed manipulation cannot effect reduction, open operation is indicated (Fig. 19-13). Large fragments should be replaced and fixed in position by a pin. Small fragments should be excised.

FRACTURES OF THE OLECRANON

The olecranon is usually broken by a direct fall on the elbow, although it is possible for the injury to result from a fall on the outstretched hand with the elbow slightly flexed,

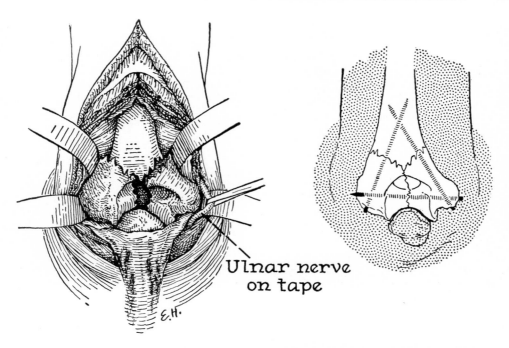

Ulnar nerve
on tape

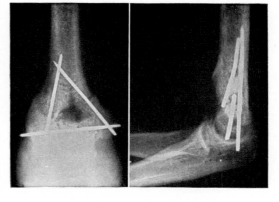

Fig. 19-12. Supracondylar T-fracture of the humerus in adults. (*Top, left*) Drawing to show displaced T-fracture of the lower end of the humerus and depicting the necessity for accurate reduction if the articular surface of the humerus is to be restored. (*Top, right*) Drawing showing internal fixation with multiple threaded pins. (*Bottom, left and right*) Anteroposterior and lateral roentgenograms showing "T" fracture of humeral condyles in an adult following open reduction and internal fixation with multiple threaded pins.

(*Top, left and right* from Hampton, O. P., Jr., and Fitts, W. T., Jr.: Open Reduction of Common Fractures, New York, Grune & Stratton)

which causes the tense triceps muscle to "snap" the olecranon over the articular surface of the humerus. Fractures of the olecranon are comparable with those of the patella in that each bone serves for the attachment of a powerful extensor muscle which also surrounds it. Just as the quadriceps muscle acts on the proximal fragment of the patella, so the powerful triceps muscle causes the proximal fragment of the olecranon to be drawn proximally.

Treatment. The objectives of management are to restore the extensor mechanism at the elbow and to maintain a normal range of motion of this joint. In undisplaced fractures of the olecranon, little active therapy is necessary. Since the fragments are not displaced, the tendinous expansion, including the fascial coverings of the olecranon, have not been torn, and subsequent displacement will not occur. The only treatment necessary is to apply a pressure dressing to the elbow and immobilize the arm in a sling with the elbow at 90° for 3 or 4 weeks (Method 5).

In separated fractures of the olecranon, the best treatment is open reduction and internal fixation by means of a large stainless steel lag type screw, intramedullary pin or loop of

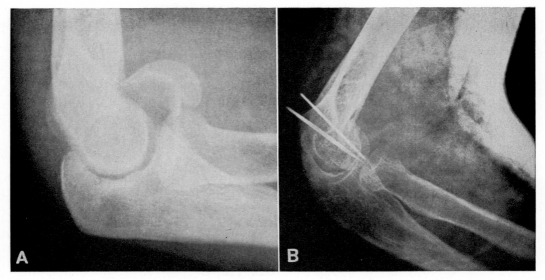

FIG. 19-13. Displaced fracture of the capitellum of the humerus. (*A, Left*) Lateral view, showing large fragment of the capitellum rotated and displaced proximally. (*B, Right*) Lateral view after open reduction and internal fixation with two unthreaded pins inserted from the posterior aspect of the lateral condyle. The pins were cut off just beneath the skin so that they could be removed easily under local anesthesia 4 weeks later.

strong malleable wire (Method 3) (Fig. 19-14). Some separated fractures of the olecranon may be reduced fairly well by closed manipulation and held in position with the elbow immobilized in extension (Method 1). However, this technic is unlikely to give a cabinetmaker's reduction of the articular surface, is likely to lead to considerable edema

of hand with some permanent restriction of motion of the fingers and may result in permanent loss of flexion of the elbow. For these reasons it is not recommended. Separated fractures of the olecranon are classical indications for the primary use of Method 3, the operative method of management. For severely comminuted fractures of the olecranon the frag-

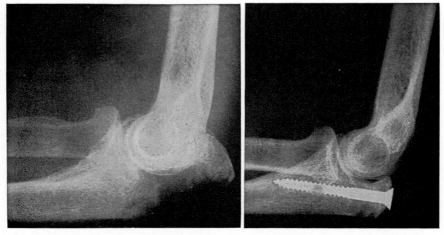

FIG. 19-14. Separated fracture of the olecranon. (*Left*) Roentgenogram taken before reduction. (*Right*) Three months after open reduction and fixation with a lag-type screw. Bony union is complete.

ments may be excised and the extension mechanism restored by suturing the triceps tendon to the periosteum and the fascia on the proximal part of the ulna.

FRACTURES OF THE HEAD AND THE NECK OF THE RADIUS

Fractures of the head and the neck of the radius usually are caused by a fall on the outstretched hand with the elbow in extension. The resulting force causes the radial head to be jammed against the articular surface of the capitellum. The injury causes limitation of motion of the elbow, pain in pronation and supination of the forearm and tenderness and swelling over the radial head. To determine the extent of damage, roentgenograms in several positions may be necessary, and even then the damage to the cartilage of the radial head and the capitellum is not demonstrated.

Apparently trivial fractures of the head and the neck of the radius can result in considerable disability. The head of the radius articulates both with the capitellum of the humerus (within the elbow joint) and with the proximal portion of the ulna at a groove along its radial surface. Malunion of fractures of the head of the radius or excess callus of fractures healed in good position can thus cause limitation of pronation and supination of the forearm as well as limitation of flexion and extension of the elbow. Fractures of the head of the radius, especially those associated with posterior dislocation of the elbow, may be complicated by ossifying hematoma.

Treatment. Fractures of the head and the neck of the radius either require practically no treatment, the "no immobilization" method (Method 5) or they require open operation (Method 3), depending upon the amount of displacement of the fragments. For fissure or crack fractures of the head and for impacted fractures of the neck with little or no displacement or angulation and for small marginal fractures of the lateral surface displaced away from the joint, the "no immobilization" method is indicated. A sling and sedation will also afford symptomatic relief. Aspiration of the hematoma from the joint decreases pain and allows better motion. Early active motion of the elbow and the forearm is encouraged and may be aided by hot wet compresses to the elbow.

For fractures of the head and the neck of the radius with displacement, open operation and excision of the radial head are required. Fractures requiring operation include comminuted fractures involving the articular surface of the head of the radius, marginal fractures of the head with displacement toward the elbow joint, large displaced fractures of the head including more than one third of the articular surface and fractures of the neck with significant angulation (Fig. 19-15). Operation and excision of the radial head should be performed as soon as is practicable, preferably within 1 or 2 days of injury. The entire radial head should be removed, and the neck made smooth. At operation, the injury usually is found to be more extensive than had been anticipated, and often there is evidence of injury to the articular surface of the capitellum. Following excision of the fragments, active motion of the elbow and the forearm is begun within a few days. In adults the disability following removal of the radial head is insignificant compared with the disability and the late complications attendant upon leaving it in place.

In children excision of the radial head following fracture is not indicated because severe growth disturbances would follow. For fractures or epiphyseal separations with severe displacement, open reduction is performed, the epiphysis being replaced and impacted if possible. No foreign material is used for fixation of the fragments unless the reduction is not stable.

MONTEGGIA FRACTURES

The term "Monteggia fracture" signifies a fracture of the ulna at about the junction of the proximal and the middle thirds with a dislocation of the head of the radius. The usual deformity is an angulation of the ulna toward the volar surface of the forearm with a forward dislocation of the head of the radius (Fig. 19-16, *Left*). However, a reverse Monteggia fracture can occur, with a dorsal angulation of the ulna and a posterior dislocation of the head of the radius. These injuries result from direct blows on the forearm, and as a consequence they are often open fractures. They are also known as "parry" fractures because the injury is often produced by attempts to parry blows with the forearm.

The dislocation of the head of the radius as an associated injury with a fracture of the shaft of the ulna has been overlooked frequently. This error has resulted because an obvious deformity of the ulna at the fracture site focused attention on this location, and roentgenograms did not include the elbow. It is technically easier, because of the way a patient with this injury holds his elbow and forearm, to make roentgenograms showing the bones of the forearm from just below the elbow down to and including the bones of the wrist. Such films show an angulated or overriding fracture of the ulna, but since they do not include the elbow joint, the dislocation of the head of the radius is not visualized. Such an error is disastrous.

The normal radius and ulna bear a constant relationship to each other at the elbow and at the wrist, and if either is intact and in position, it tends to prevent displacement of a fracture of the other. If one bone is broken so

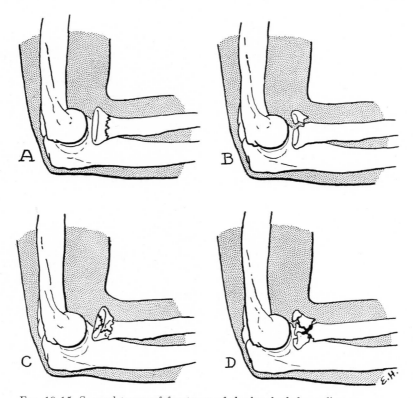

Fig. 19-15. Several types of fractures of the head of the radius.

(A) Undisplaced fracture which should be treated by early active motion of the elbow supplemented by aspiration of the joint.

(B)   A small displaced marginal fracture of less than one third of the articular surface for which early operation is indicated. Because this line of fracture is away from the radio-ulnar articulation, excision of merely the small fragment is acceptable.

(C) Comminuted radial head with minimal displacement. Regardless, excision of the radial head is indicated, as much more distortion of the articular surface of the radius is always found at operation than can be seen on the roentgenogram.

(D) Severely comminuted fracture with gross displacement of the fragments. Excision of all of the fragments (the entire radial head) is indicated.

(Hampton, O. P., Jr., and Fitts, W. T., Jr.: Open Reduction of Common Fractures, New York, Grune & Stratton)

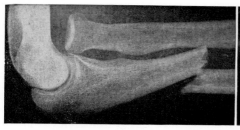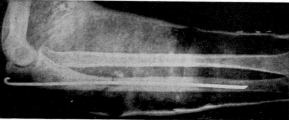

Fig. 19-16. Monteggia fracture. (*Left*) Lateral roentgenogram, showing anterior dislocation of head of radius and fracture of the shaft of the ulna at junction of proximal and middle thirds. (*Right*) Following open reduction of the ulna and fixation with an intramedullary nail. The dislocation of the radial head has been reduced.

that the fragments override or are angulated to any degree, there must be either a fracture or a dislocation of the other. If, therefore, the shaft of the ulna is fractured with overriding or angulation of the fragments so that there is in effect a shortening of the ulna, then either the radius is broken or dislocated at either its proximal or distal ends. Obviously, the radius would dislocate at the elbow because its attachments are weakest here. Conversely, if the radius is broken and is overriding or angulated, there must be a fracture of the ulna or a disturbance of its proximal or distal articulation. Obviously, this would be at the wrist joint because its attachments are weakest here. This guiding principle should serve as a warning to the surgeon when he sees a fracture of the shaft of the ulna which is angulated or overriding. He then may know that there is an associated fracture of the shaft of the radius or a dislocation of the radial head and he must make certain that x-ray films show the elbow joint. As a matter of fact, an excellent principle of radiologic technic is that when the shaft of a bone is broken, enough films should be made to visualize clearly the entire bone and its articulations proximally and distally.

Treatment. Occasionally a Monteggia fracture may be managed by closed reduction and application of a plaster cast (Method 1). In such instances the contour of the fracture in the ulna must be so near transverse that when the fragments are brought into apposition, the reduction will hold, and the full length and alignment of the ulna will be maintained. With such a fracture of the ulna properly reduced, it is then possible for the dislocation of the head of the radius to be replaced by manual pressure

over it. The extremity is then immobilized in a long arm cast with the elbow in at least 90° of flexion. Angulation of the ulna and redislocation of the radial head can take place in a cast. Therefore, serial roentgenograms at intervals of 5 or 6 days are necessary for a few weeks in order that such a situation may be detected promptly should it occur.

However, open reduction and internal fixation (Method 3) are indicated in most Monteggia fractures. With an intramedullary pin or a plate with screws, the ulna is stabilized in excellent apposition and alignment. This then usually permits closed reduction of the head of the radius (Fig. 19-16, *Right*). Subsequent immobilization of the extremity in a cast with the elbow at 90° will usually hold the reduction of the radius. If the radial head cannot be reduced adequately following stabilization of the ulna in reduction, the radial head must be reduced by open operation, and usually the torn orbicular ligament must be repaired.

DISLOCATION OF THE ELBOW

Dislocations of the elbow usually result from falls on the outstretched hand with the elbow in extension. The forearm is hyperextended until dislocation, usually backward, results. The injury occurs both in children and adults. In adults, associated fractures of the coronoid process of the ulna and of the head of the radius are often present.

Reduction is usually easy with traction on the extended forearm against countertraction by an assistant on the arm. If the dislocation has been medial or lateral, it usually is first manipulated into the posterior position, and then traction is made. When the coronoid process becomes disengaged from behind the lower end of the humerus, flexion of the forearm on the arm will reduce the dislocation.

After reduction of the dislocation the elbow is immobilized at 90° by a cast extending from the upper arm to the proximal palmar crease of the hand. The cast is removed after 10 to 14 days to permit some active motion of the elbow, but full extension is avoided for an additional 2 weeks by the use of a sling as a precaution against redislocation.

FRACTURES OF THE SHAFT OF THE BONES OF THE FOREARM

Fractures of the shaft of the bones of the forearm are common fractures in childhood and not uncommon in adults. Either the radius or the ulna alone or both bones may be broken at any level.

The forearm presents distinctive anatomic features. It is the only segment of the extremities where one bone rotates around the other (pronation and supination). For proper functioning of the forearm, the interosseus space between the radius and the ulna must be preserved, and the relative length of each bone must be maintained. The radius is the most important at the wrist, and the ulna at the elbow. Each bone of the forearm actually serves to splint the other.

The displacement of fragments following fracture of the shaft of one or both bones of the forearm is the result of the action of muscles which control pronation and supination, and the surgeon must know the anatomy and function of these muscles if he is to manage fractures of the forearm properly. They are the pronator teres, arising from the medial condyle of the humerus and inserting near the mid-point of the radius, the supinator arising from the shaft of the proximal ulna and passing posteriorly about the proximal radius to insert on its anterior surface, the pronator quadratus in the lower forearm passing transversely from the ulna to the radius, and the 2 muscles in the arm which act as supinators of the forearm, the biceps muscle inserting into the upper third of the radius, and the brachioradialis, sometimes called the supinator longus, arising from the external supracondyloid ridge of the humerus and inserting on the styloid process of the radius.

Relation of a fracture of the radius to the insertion of the pronator teres is highly significant in the deformity which results and the position in which the forearm must be immobilized to maintain reduction of the fracture. If the fracture of the radius is proximal to the insertion of the pronator teres, the supinating action of muscles described above is unopposed, and the proximal fragment of radius will be held in full supination, and the distal fragment will be held in pronation. To reduce and maintain reduction of such fractures, the forearm must be in full supination. In fractures of the radius below the insertion of the pronator teres, there is both pronator and supinator pull on the proximal fragment and, therefore, in theory at least, it will be held in mid-pronation. This means that such fractures are usually best reduced and immobilized with the forearm in mid-pronation.

FRACTURES OF THE SHAFTS OF THE BONES OF THE FOREARM IN CHILDREN

The majority of the fractures of the shaft of the bones of the forearm in children involve both the radius and the ulna. Fractures of the shaft of the radius alone are seen occasionally, but those of the ulna alone are rare and occur only as a result of a direct blow on the ulnar side of the forearm. Fractures of the forearm in children are usually greenstick of one or both bones (Fig. 19-17), although occasionally the fracture of one bone, usually the ulna, will be greenstick and that of the other complete with displacement and overriding. In rare instances the fractures of both bones are complete and overriding.

For practical purposes, all of these fractures in children are managed by closed reduction and immobilization (Method 1). Open reduction, the only reasonable alternative, is rarely, if ever, indicated (see Fig. 19-18).

In greenstick fractures, except for those with only minimal angulation, the surgeon should correct the deformity by a combination of traction and pressure against the point of angulation. While displacement of the fragments is to be avoided at all costs, there need be no hesitancy in completing the fracture (indicated by an audible and palpable snap) during the process of restoring alignment. When the fracture is completed and immobilized in good alignment there is no tendency toward recurrence of the deformity; whereas, when the fracture is not completed, angulation may recur in the cast as swelling subsides and the cast becomes loose. Following adequate reduction a long-arm plaster cast is applied from the upper arm to the proximal palmar crease of the hand with the elbow at a right angle and usually with the forearm in mid-pronation.

Anesthesia for children with greenstick fractures may be a problem. General anesthesia, while desirable from many standpoints, is hazardous unless the child's stomach is empty because of the danger of vomiting and aspiration with its dire consequences. If general anesthesia is used, it is best to wait for 8 or more hours after the last meal for the pa-

tient's stomach to empty. Actually, local anesthesia is not impracticable, and our recent experience indicates that it is applicable for the majority of these injuries. Of course, the child often resists and struggles, but, even so, adequate reduction of these fractures is often feasible without the hazards of general anesthesia.

When the fracture of one bone is greenstick and the other is complete and overriding, the problem of reduction is more difficult. For these general anesthesia may be necessary. The deformity of the greenstick fracture is first eliminated to restore full length of that bone and then, by a combination of traction against countertraction, leverage and direct pressure on the displaced fragments of

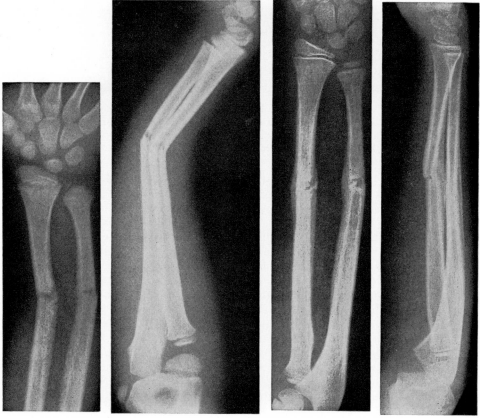

FIG. 19-17. Fractures of shafts of bones of forearm in a child. (Left) Roentgenogram of greenstick fractures of radius and ulna, anteroposterior view. (Center, left) Lateral view. (Center, right) Anteroposterior roentgenogram 1 month after closed reduction. (Right) Lateral roentgenogram 1 month after closed reduction. The slight anterior angulation of the radius is undergoing correction according to Wolff's Law.

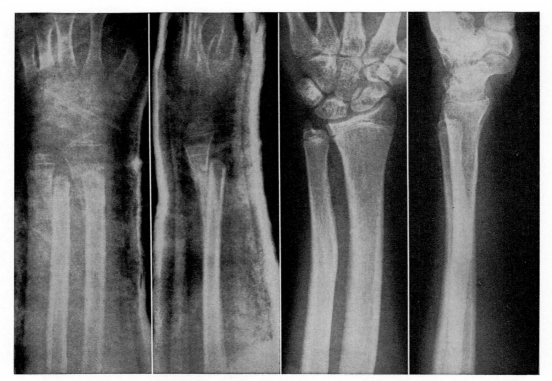

Fig. 19-18. (*Left*) Anteroposterior and lateral roentgenograms showing fractures of both bones of the forearm, uniting in poor position. (*Right*) Anteroposterior and lateral roentgenograms taken 4 years later. A perfect anatomic and functional result was obtained. (Drs. Ward A. McClanahan and Charles K. Wier, Wichita, Kansas)

the other bone, this bone usually can be brought into satisfactory apposition and alignment. Then a plaster cast as described above is applied.

In fractures in which both bones are displaced and overriding, reduction is still more difficult. Under anesthesia, by traction against countertraction, leverage and direct pressure, one bone is guided into reduction. Often the other will fall into reduction simultaneously but, if not, it then must be reduced by the same maneuvers. It is true that often the fracture first reduced will become displaced again while the other is being forced into position. This may be difficult to prevent, but cognizance of the level of the fracture in relation to the insertion of the pronator teres and the actions of other muscles will aid in reduction, because the manipulations can be made with the forearm held in the right degree of pronation and supination.

While perfect apposition and alignment of

the fractures of each bone are desirable, they are not absolutely necessary for a perfect functional result. At times it may be impossible to achieve complete apposition of the fragments of one bone or possibly of both bones. Even though malunion may follow, correction under Wolff's Law and a perfect end result may be anticipated (Fig. 19-18).

The board splint method of Key (Fig. 19-19) which is supplemented by a plaster cast may be highly advantageous in these injuries, not only in preserving the interosseous space but also in furnishing some degree of immobilization following the reduction during application of the plaster cast, thereby serving as a safeguard against redisplacement. The resulting cast appears bulky and cumbersome, but despite this, the board splint-plaster cast method of immobilization is worthwhile in managing these injuries, and it is particularly valuable to the surgeon who must work with relatively inexperienced assistance.

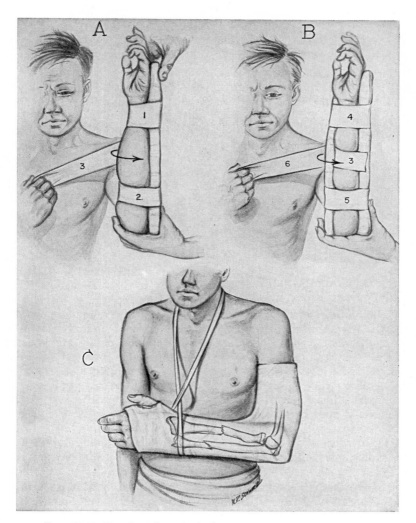

Fig. 19-19. Two-board method plus a plaster cast for fractures of the shaft of both bones of the forearm in children. With the forearm supported so that the fragments of each bone of the forearm are in good alignment, a long board slightly wider than the forearm itself is applied to the dorsal surface from the elbow to the metacarpophalangeal joints with 3 strips of adhesive tape. Then, a short board of the same width is applied to the volar surface from the elbow to the wrist with 3 additional strips of adhesive tape applied at the same point on the forearm as the first 3. Finally, a long arm plaster cast is applied from well above the elbow to the knuckles. The boards aid in maintaining good alignment of the fragments while the cast is being applied. The compression of the soft parts provided by the boards serves to compress soft parts between the bones and thereby help maintain the interosseous space. Because the boards are wider than the forearm itself and are applied individually, circulation is not embarrassed. The 2-board method may be a valuable aid in proper management of fractures of the shaft of both bones of the forearm in children.

Fractures of the bones of the forearm in children usually require from 4 to 8 weeks of immobilization in the long-arm plaster cast, depending somewhat, of course, on the age of the patient. The younger the patient the more rapid is the rate of union. If the fracture of either or both bones heals in any angulation, the plaster should remain in place until union is mature.

Refracture is especially common in fractures of the forearm in children, sometimes occurring years after the original injury, particularly if either bone shows any angulation. For this reason, the parents of the child should be urged to minimize the risk of additional trauma to the part as much as is reasonable.

Fractures of the Shaft of the Bones of the Forearm in Adults

Fracture of the Shaft of the Ulna Alone. This injury results from a direct blow on the forearm such as that described above in the production of the Monteggia or "parry" fracture. If the force is sufficient to angulate the fragments of the ulna significantly, the head of the radius must dislocate, producing a Monteggia fracture. It must be kept in mind, as outlined above, that with angulation or overriding of the fragments of the shaft of the ulna, the radius must either be broken or dislocated.

In fractures of the shaft of the ulna without fracture or dislocation of the radius, the fragments usually are not displaced, or if they are displaced, as a rule they are reduced easily by traction and manipulation. Following reduction the extremity is immobilized in a plaster cast extending from the upper arm to the proximal palmar crease of the hand with the elbow at 90° and the forearm in midpronation. Immobilization must be continued until the fracture has united, usually from 8 to 16 weeks, as fractures of the shaft of the ulna may unite slowly. Because of the relatively poor blood supply of the ulna, nonunion of these fractures is not rare.

Fractures of the Shaft of the Radius Alone. Fractures of the shaft of the radius without fractures of the ulna can occur at any level, but they are most common at the junction of the middle and the lower thirds. In fractures at this level, the pronator quadratus muscle in the lower third of the forearm usually pulls the distal fragment of the radius toward the ulna, a displacement which is difficult to overcome by closed reduction. Full radial length must be restored to prevent subluxation of the ulna at the wrist.

If the fracture is transverse, or near transverse, efforts at closed reduction are worthwhile. In some instances an excellent stable reduction will be achieved which can be maintained in a long-arm plaster cast. A plaster cast extending only to the elbow is *not* sufficient immobilization for this injury and must be condemned for any fracture proximal to the level of the Colles' fracture.

In many of these fractures at the junction of the middle and the lower thirds of the radius, the fracture line will be oblique so that a stable closed reduction cannot be achieved. Under these circumstances, open reduction and internal fixation of the fragments of the radius are indicated. Internal fixation may be obtained by an intramedullary pin or by a plate and screws. Because this fracture is an occasional site of nonunion, primary bone grafting supplementing internal fixation is likely to be advantageous.

Fractures of the Shaft of Both Bones. When both the radius and the ulna are broken in the adult, the fragments usually are displaced and overriding. Frequently, one or both fractures are comminuted. These fractures constitute a most difficult problem in management.

Efforts at closed reduction and immobilization may be successful in some instances. If the fractures are transverse so that when the fragments are brought into apposition and alignment the reduction will be stable, then efforts at closed reduction under general anesthesia are worthwhile and will be successful in some instances. Actually, the board splint method supplemented by the long-arm plaster cast described above, under fractures of the shaft of the bones of the forearm in children, may be highly advantageous in these fractures in adults.

However, in fractures of both bones of the forearm in adults, open reduction and internal fixation are often necessary. If there are no important contraindications, operative intervention is often selected primarily by surgeons experienced in fracture work. It affords ac-

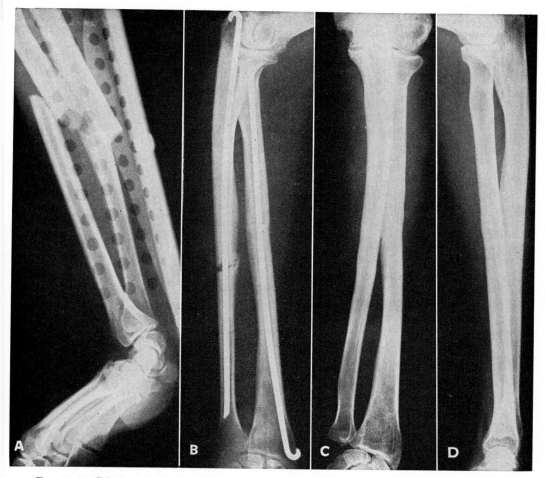

FIG. 19-20. Displaced fractures of the shafts of both bones of the forearm in adults managed by open reduction and internal fixation with intramedullary pins.

(A) Lateral roentgenogram, showing fracture of both bones of the forearm with displacement and overriding.

(B) Anteroposterior roentgenogram of bones of the forearm made immediately postoperative, showing excellent reduction of the fractures and stabilization with intramedullary Rush pins.

(C and D) Anteroposterior and lateral roentgenograms made after union of the fractures and removal of the intramedullary pins. Note that healing of the fractures has been obtained in perfect apposition and alignment.

(Hampton, O. P., Jr., and Fitts, W. T., Jr.: Open Reduction of Common Fractures, New York, Grune & Stratton)

curate reduction and permits stabilization of the fragments in reduction by means of intramedullary pins or plates and screws so that the position will not be lost later during the period of immobilization in a plaster cast (Fig. 19-20). It should be pointed out that nonunion of these fractures is not rare and, therefore, in an effort to prevent this complica-

tion by supplementary bone grafting at the time of the open reduction and internal fixation is a worthwhile procedure.

Fractures of the bones of the forearm in adults do not unite rapidly, and immobilization must be maintained until the fragments are united—at least 12 weeks and usually longer. It must not be discontinued until there is clinical stability and x-ray evidence of solid bony union of both fractures.

FRACTURES AND DISLOCATIONS ABOUT THE WRIST

Skeletal injuries about the wrist may be grouped for purposes of discussion as: (1) fractures of the distal end of the radius, (2) fractures of the carpus and (3) dislocations of the carpus.

FRACTURES OF THE LOWER END OF THE RADIUS

Fractures of the lower end of the radius are not only the most common fractures of the upper extremity but are also the most common fractures in the body in all age groups except small infants. Each is, to the laity, the typical "fracture of the arm" or "fracture of the wrist." These injuries may have an associated fracture of the styloid or at times of the distal end of the ulna. Even if bony injury of the ulna is not seen on a roentgenogram, the ulnar collateral ligament probably has been damaged. Management of the fracture of the radius suffices for any injury to the distal ulna.

Certain anatomic relationships of the distal ends of the bones of the forearm are important not only in determining the degree of distortion in each of these fractures but also in determining when a satisfactory reduction has been achieved. Normally, the tip of the styloid process of the radius extends distally about 1 cm. beyond the styloid of the ulna, and the distal articular surface of the radius is inclined toward the ulnar side of the hand at an angle of some 25° to 30°. These relationships, of course, are best observed in the anteroposterior roentgenogram of the wrist. The distal articular surface of the radius also inclines toward the palmar surface of the hand at an angle of some 10° to 15° as seen in the lateral roentgenogram. Unless the inclinations of the distal articular surface of the radius have been restored and full length of the radius has been regained, a fracture of the distal end of the radius has not been completely reduced (see Fig. 19-21).

Fractures of the lower end of the radius may be classified as hyperextension (Colles'), hyperflexion (reversed Colles' or Smith's), marginal (Barton's), and fracture-separation of the radial epiphysis.

Mechanism of Injury. Colles' fracture, Barton's fracture involving the posterior margin of the distal end of the radius, and fracture-separation of the distal radial epiphysis result from falls on the outstretched hand. Reversed Colles' (Smith's fracture) and Barton's fractures involving the anterior margin of the distal end of the radius result from a fall on the back of the hand forcing it into extreme flexion. In each of these fractures all degrees of displacement occur. In Colles' and reversed Colles' fractures, impaction of the distal into the proximal fragment may occur, or there may be severe comminution with lines of fracture entering the articular surface. In marginal fractures (Barton's fracture) displacement is usually not present or is minimal. Fortunately, in fracture-separation of the distal radial epiphysis in children, comminution does not occur.

Management. Closed reduction by manipulation is indicated in all except those that are undisplaced or only slightly displaced. As stated above, the objectives of reduction are the restoration of full radial length and the anatomic relationship of the distal articular surface of the radius. The fundamental maneuvers for closed reduction are strong traction against equally strong countertraction applied at the elbow with the forearm flexed, combined with manipulation of the distal fragment by pressure until it is brought into excellent apposition and alignment with the proximal fragment.

Anesthesia, either local or general, must almost always be employed. Efforts at closed reduction without anesthesia, particularly in adults, are likely to lead to the acceptance of inadequate reduction because of the painful resistance of the patient. Local anesthesia using about 15 ml. of 1 per cent procaine injected from the dorsum into the hematoma about the fracture of the radius is highly satisfactory in all fractures treated within a few hours after injury. A few milliliters of procaine injected about the distal end of the ulna makes the local anesthesia more effective. Local anesthesia is less likely to be effective in fractures 12 to 24 or more hours after injury because the blood about the fracture site will have clotted, and the procaine diffuses poorly. There is, of course, no objection to the use of general anesthesia if the patient has an empty stomach which minimizes the risk of aspiration of regurgitated gastric contents.

COLLES' (HYPEREXTENSION) FRACTURE. This, the most common fracture of the lower end of the radius, gains the name by which it is commonly known because it was first described in detail by Abraham Colles in 1814. It occurs principally in the middle and the latter decades of life.

In a typical Colles' fracture, all of the relationships of the distal articular surface are distorted (Fig. 19-22). The distal fragment is driven backward and into radial deviation so that the articular surface inclines dorsalward and radially. Radial shortening is present. The distal fragment may be impacted into the proximal fragment with crushing of cancellous bone and it may be severely comminuted. The characteristic displacements result in what is known as a silver-fork deformity because of the analogy of the hump

of the dorsum of the wrist to the hump of a silver dinner fork. The radial deviation of the distal fragment results in increased prominence of the distal end of the ulna.

Colles' fractures should be reduced as soon after injury as is surgically feasible. Closed reduction, as outlined above, is based upon a combination of traction and manipulation. In the usual closed reduction, the surgeon grasps the hand of the injured wrist in a handshake manner and applies traction while countertraction is provided by an assistant holding the lower arm just above the elbow with that joint flexed to about 90°. As the surgeon makes strong traction with one hand, he makes pressure against the dorsal surface of the distal fragment with the thumb of the other so as to force it into reduction. The hand is pulled in the direction of some palmar flexion and full ulnar deviation while the forearm is held in pronation. Reduction usually will have been obtained when the normal contour of the wrist has been restored and the tip

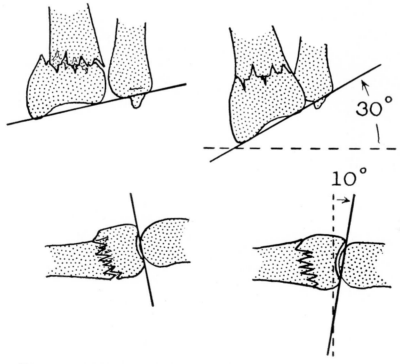

FIG. 19-21. Colles' fracture. (*Top*) Anteroposterior view: (*left*) showing typical displacement; (*right*) after reduction. (*Bottom*) Lateral view: (*left*) typical displacement; (*right*) after reduction.

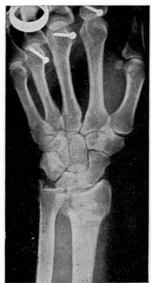

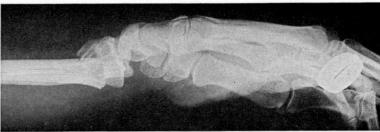

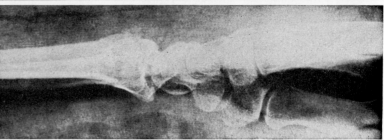

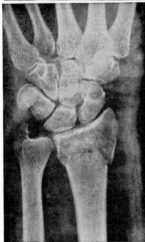

FIG. 19-22. Roentgenograms of Colles' fracture before and after reduction. Note normal inclination of articular surface of radius following reduction. (*Top*) Before reduction. (*Bottom*) After reduction.

fragment of the radius is molded into reduction.

Following reduction, the wrist is immobilized with the hand in moderate palmar flexion and full ulnar deviation and with the forearm in pronation by either a lightly padded plaster cast or anterior and posterior molded plaster splints. Full palmar flexion, the so-called Cotton-Loder position, is to be avoided. Any advantage to be gained in maintaining a better reduction of a difficult fracture is far overshadowed by the hazard of edema and stiffness of the fingers, which cannot be exercised in this position, and by permanent restriction of motion in the wrist. Either the cast or the splints extend distally only to the proximal transverse palmar crease in the palm and to just behind the metacarpal heads on the back of the hand so that full motion of the fingers is possible. Ordinarily, the plaster is extended proximally to just below the elbow, although in comminuted fractures there is some reason to extend the plaster to the upper arm with the elbow at 90° and the forearm in pronation. Of course, in undisplaced fractures, immobilization is provided with the hand in the neutral position of slight dorsal flexion and ulnar deviation.

of the styloid process of the radius extends distal to that of the ulna by about 1 cm.

The principles of traction and manipulation for closed reduction may be applied in another way. Traction may be applied to the hand in a strong steady fashion over a period of several minutes against equally strong countertraction. Strong pull on Chinese finger traps applied to the fingers is an acceptable way of obtaining traction in this method and makes application of plaster easier than when the hand is held by an assistant. After the fragments have become distracted as a result of traction the distal

Fig. 19-23. Lateral roentgenogram of reversed Colles' fracture (Smith's fracture).

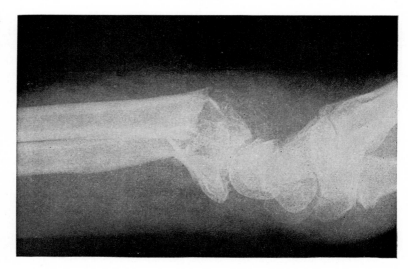

Check roentgenograms should be made as soon as the plaster has set (while the anesthesia is still effective) to make certain that adequate reduction has been achieved. If the reduction is not satisfactory, the plaster is removed immediately, and another closed reduction is attempted. While perfect reduction cannot always be obtained, certainly only the best possible reduction should be accepted. Reduction is measured by adequate apposition of the fragments, restoration of radial length and the proper palmar and ulnar inclination of the articular surface of the distal fragment.

The reduction achieved will not always be maintained even in a snug-fitting cast, especially if the distal fragment is badly comminuted. As swelling subsides, the immobilization is less effective, and some redisplacement of fragments may occur. Some telescoping of fragments often occurs, particularly in the aged. Therefore, it is advisable that check roentgenograms be made about the fifth postreduction day and, if all is well then, again about the tenth day. If some slipping of fragments has occurred, another reduction and cast may be indicated, depending upon whether the surgeon believes he can not only obtain but also maintain an improved position.

During postreduction management, objectives are to maintain a full range of motion of the fingers and the shoulder. Edema of the fingers must be minimized as much as possible. Measures to accomplish this include elevation of the hand almost constantly for a few days with strenuous exercises of the fingers. Throughout the period of immobilization, the patient must be encouraged to carry out a forceful full range of motion of the fingers. Similarly, the patient must repeatedly (every hour on the hour) put the shoulder through a full range of motion including full overhead reach and full internal and external rotation. Loss of motion in the shoulder joint following fractures of the distal end of the radius is a preventable complication; yet it occurs too often because these exercises of the shoulder have been poorly performed.

Immobilization of the wrist is maintained until union of the fracture has occurred. In adults, about 4 to 6 weeks of immobilization is required. A shorter period is necessary in children. In many patients, particularly in those in the latter decades of life, it is advisable to change casts at the end of 3 weeks in order to bring the hand out of palmar flexion into the neutral position or that of slight dorsal flexion. Obviously, no force should be used in obtaining this corrected position of the hand as displacement of the distal fragment might occur.

REVERSED COLLES' OR SMITH'S (HYPERFLEXION) FRACTURE (Fig. 19-23). In this fracture, much less common than the Colles', the distal radial fragment is displaced anteriorly, and the articular surface of the radius inclines forward excessively. Some degree of comminution is frequently present. The deformity is usually less pronounced than that of a Colles' fracture.

The principles of manipulative reduction are the same as with a Colles' fracture, except that the hand is brought into hyperextension, and the distal fragment is forced backward with the thumb. Immobilization is provided by a plaster cast or anterior and posterior molded plaster splints holding the hand in full supination and neutral or slight palmar flexion and ulnar deviation. Peculiarly, hyperextension of the hand after the reduction predisposes to volar redisplacement of the distal fragment. The postreduction management is comparable with that outlined for Colles' fractures.

BARTON'S (MARGINAL) FRACTURE. These fractures, which may involve either the anterior or the posterior margin of the distal end of the radius, usually include only a small portion of the articular surface. Displacement, if present at all, is always minimal. Because they involve the articular surface, reduction should be as accurate as possible. By direct pressure on the fragment under local anesthesia it usually can be forced into excellent position.

Immobilization should be provided for about 4 weeks by a plaster cast holding the hand in the neutral or slightly dorsal flexed position. Persistent exercise of the fingers and the shoulder throughout the period of postreduction management are as important as in the other fractures about the lower end of the radius.

FRACTURE-SEPARATION OF THE DISTAL RADIAL EPIPHYSIS. This injury, which occurs generally in children over 10 years of age, is quite comparable with the typical Colles' fracture in adult life. Separation usually occurs between the diaphysis and the epiphyseal cartilage plate so that following adequate reduction there is usually no disturbance of growth.

Reduction can almost always be obtained easily by the maneuvers outlined for Colles' fractures. It is preferable to employ a strong steady traction for several minutes so as to disengage the fragments completely. This permits the epiphysis to be molded into good reduction with a minimum of trauma. Although a perfect reduction is desirable, it is not absolutely necessary, as during subsequent growth slight malalignment will be corrected (Fig. 19-24).

Immobilization should be provided by a plaster cast holding the hand in slight palmar flexion and ulnar deviation for about 4 or 5 weeks. The end result in these injuries is usually excellent, provided that the epiphyseal cartilage plate was not damaged at the time of injury or during reduction.

FRACTURES OF THE CARPUS

The most important fracture of the carpal bones is a fracture of the navicular. Fractures involving the other carpal bones are usually mere chips or undisplaced cracks requiring at the most only a few weeks immobilization in a plaster cast with the wrist in the functional position of slight dorsal flexion. Fractures of the navicular, by far the most common fractures of the carpus, deserve special consideration.

Fractures of the Navicular. These injuries, like Colles' fractures, result from falls on the outstretched hand. They occur usually in young adult males whose strong musculature seems to prevent extreme dorsal flexion at the time of injury, thereby causing the navicular (carpal scaphoid) rather than the lower radius to receive the force of impact.

The navicular, the longest of the carpal bones and the only one not cuboidal in shape, has a precarious blood supply. The major blood supply comes from a small artery which usually enters the distal portion of the bone. When a fracture is sustained across the waist or the proximal pole of the navicular, the blood supply of the proximal fragment may be destroyed. The result may be avascular necrosis of that fragment.

The diagnosis of a fracture of the navicular is not always easy. Clinically, the patient complains of pain in the wrist, and slight swelling is present. Tenderness in the anatomic snuffbox is usually severe. With such a clinical picture, an oblique view of the wrist in addition to the routine anteroposterior and lateral views is indicated. Often a fracture of the navicular will be visualized in an oblique view when it has not been disclosed on the routine views (Fig. 19-25). Because of the ever-present possibility of an easily overlooked fracture of the navicular in every

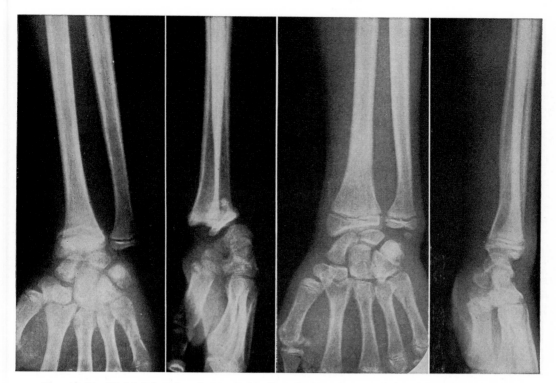

FIG. 19-24. (*Left*) Lateral and anteroposterior roentgenograms of unreduced united fracture, showing epiphyseal sepaartion with severe posterior displacement and anterior angulation. (*Right*) Lateral and anteroposterior roentgenograms taken 2½ years later. Complete correction by growth processes and perfect functional result. (Drs. Ward A. McClanahan and Charles K. Wier, Wichita, Kans.)

injured wrist, 3 views of the region are routine in many clinics.

A sprain of the wrist of significance is an exceedingly rare injury. Careful x-ray examination in 3 views usually will disclose either a fracture of the navicular or the distal end of the radius. Certainly, a sprain of the wrist which is not completely well in 10 days is likely to be a fracture of the navicular. In some instances, a fracture of the navicular may not be disclosed on x-ray films in all 3 views made soon after injury, and yet repeat films some 10 to 14 days later will show a fracture because the fracture line has become visible as a result of minimal absorption about it. There should be no hesitancy, therefore, in repeating x-ray films after 10 to 14 days if the patient's symptoms have not been completely relieved.

TREATMENT. As a rule, the fragments are in good position, and efforts at reduction are not necessary. If the fragments of a fracture of the navicular are displaced, an associated dislocation of another of the carpal bones is or has been present.

Fortunately the majority of fractures of the navicular will unite if they are immobilized adequately for a long enough period of time. Immobilization is obtained with a plaster cast which extends from just below the elbow to the proximal palmar crease of the palm and to the interphalangeal joint of the thumb with the hand in dorsal flexion and radial deviation. This position of the hand is important, as it tends to approximate the fragments more closely. Immobilization must be provided until the fracture has united as shown by repeat roentgenograms. At least 3 months of immobilization is to be expected, and at times from 6 to 9 months or even a year may elapse before the fragments have united. Watson-Jones has emphasized that all navicular frac-

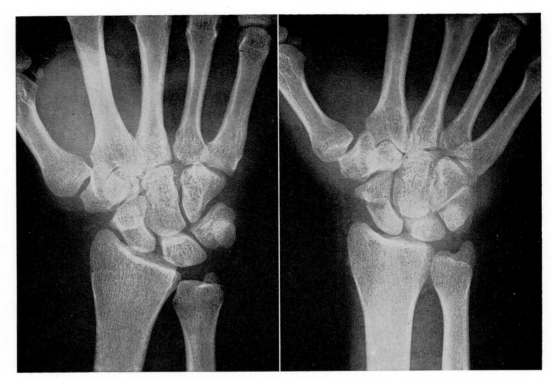

Fig. 19-25. Fracture of the carpal navicular. (*Left*) Roentgenogram in anteroposterior view. Fracture of the navicular is not prominent. (*Right*) Oblique view with hand in ulnar deviation plainly discloses fracture across the waist of navicular.

tures will unite if the immobilization is continuous and sufficiently prolonged. Failure of union is the result of delay in providing immobilization or its removal before union has occurred. As a rule the cast should be removed every 6 weeks, new roentgenograms made, and a new cast applied if it is indicated.

The outstanding complication of fractures of the navicular is avascular necrosis of one fragment, usually the proximal fragment (Fig. 19-26). In spite of this, union of the fracture can occur with prolonged immobilization, and the blood supply to the avascular fragment will be re-established so that a dead bone will be replaced by living bone by the process of creeping replacement. Immobilization should be continued until the revascularizing process is well established.

With nonunion of the carpal scaphoid, with or without avascular necrosis of the proximal fragment, traumatic arthritis of the wrist joint may develop. This may be an early or a late complication. Once traumatic arthritis has developed, operative fusion of the wrist joint in the position of function is likely to be necessary before the patient has a painless, stable wrist.

DISLOCATIONS OF THE CARPUS

Dislocations about the wrist include (1) dislocation of the lunate, (2) perilunar dislocation and (3) mid-carpal dislocation. A true dislocation of the wrist joint wherein all of the proximal carpal bones are dislocated out of articulation with the radius does not occur for practical purposes except as a complication of fractures of the distal radius.

All of these injuries result from forced hyperextension of the hand such as is sustained from a fall on the outstretched hand or when the hyperextended hand is jammed in attempting to protect oneself from impact against a fall. A miscalculated stiff arm in football could cause these injuries.

While clinically it can be determined from

examination that a significant injury has been received to the wrist, exact diagnosis is made by the findings on x-ray examination. The usual anteroposterior and lateral veiws may be sufficient, but in many instances oblique views will be helpful. Films of the normal uninjured wrist for comparison may be quite advantageous in establishing the exact diagnosis.

Dislocation of the Lunate. In this injury, as the hand is forced into hyperextension, the dorsal ligamentous attachments of the lunate are torn, and then the bone is rotated and extruded anteriorly to a point deep to the flexor tendons and the volar carpal ligament. Its only remaining ligamentous attachment is that to the anterior lip of the radius.

In the lateral roentgenogram (Fig. 19-27), the lunate no longer articulates with the radius and is displaced anteriorly. The capitate appears to be in articulation with the radius. In the anteroposterior view, the lunate appears

to be elongated and square or rectangular in comparison with its usual round appearance.

Closed reduction under general anesthesia should be attempted as soon as the diagnosis is made. While one assistant provides countertraction, another makes strong traction to open the space for the lunate and hyperextends the hand at the wrist. Pressure is made with the thumbs to replace the lunate, and then the hand is forced quickly into palmar flexion. When the lunate is reduced, the wrist assumes a more normal appearance and can be moved easily through practically a full range of motion. Reduction should be confirmed immediately by x-ray examination before application of the cast. Plaster immobilization with the hand in some palmar flexion is provided for about 3 weeks.

Efforts at closed reduction are not always successful even in fresh injuries. If not, either open reduction or excision of the lunate is indicated. Opinions vary as to the most de-

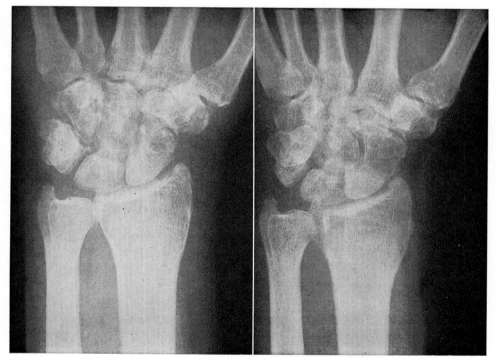

FIG. 19-26. Avascular necrosis of the proximal fragment of a fracture of the carpal navicular. Anteroposterior and oblique views of the wrist, showing a united fracture of the carpal navicular with avascular necrosis of the proximal fragment as indicated by the relative increase in density of this portion of the navicular bone in comparison with the distal fragment and other carpal bones.

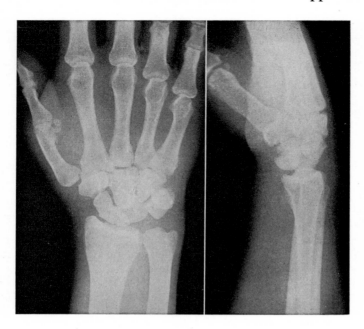

FIG. 19-27. Dislocation of carpal lunate. Anteroposterior and lateral roentgenograms, showing the carpal lunate displaced anteriorly. Note that the injury may be suspected in the anteroposterior view, and the diagnosis is confirmed in the lateral view.

sirable operative procedure. Following open reduction, there is a high incidence of avascular necrosis of the lunate, probably secondary to the further operative destruction of blood supply to the bone. On the other hand, with excision of the bone a weak wrist often follows and may require arthrodesis.

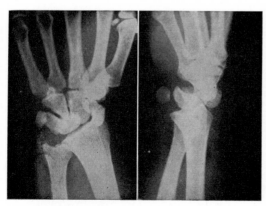

FIG. 19-28. Perilunar dislocation of the carpal bones. Anteroposterior and lateral roentgenograms, showing that the carpal lunate remains in normal articulation with the radius, but all of the other carpal bones have been displaced dorsalward. The proximal articular surface of the capitate now overrides the lunate rather than articulating with its distal surface.

Perilunar Dislocation. In this injury, instead of forward displacement of the lunate as the hand is hyperextended, it remains in normal relationship with the radius, and the remaining carpus with the hand are displaced backward. In some instances, the scaphoid is fractured. If so, the proximal fragment of the scaphoid usually remains behind in the joint with the lunate (Fig. 19-28).

Closed reduction under anesthesia is usually possible by strong traction and manipulation against countertraction. Immobilization by a plaster cast with the hand in slight palmar flexion is provided for 3 to 4 weeks, although, if the carpal scaphoid has been fractured, a much longer period of immobilization is indicated in the position previously described.

Perilunar dislocation at the wrist is a serious injury, and some permanent restriction of motion is to be anticipated.

Midcarpal Dislocation. In this injury, as the hand is hyperextended the distal row of carpal bones is dislocated dorsally on the proximal row. Frequently the correct diagnosis has been missed, presumably because the relationship of the carpus was not observed closely on the lateral view. This is a serious injury which can result in severe permanent limitation of function of the hand, particularly if it goes unreduced for any prolonged period of time.

Closed reduction under anesthesia is usually feasible, especially if it is attempted soon after injury. Reduction is maintained best by immobilization in a plaster cast with the hand in some palmar flexion for a period of 3 or 4 weeks. If efforts at closed reduction are unsuccessful, early open reduction is indicated.

Fractures and dislocations of the bones of the hand are discussed in Chapter 22, "Principles of Hand Surgery."

(For Bibliography, see pp. 451-452, at end of Chap. 21.)

OSCAR P. HAMPTON, JR., M.D., AND WILLIAM T. FITTS, JR., M.D.

CHAPTER 20

Fractures and Dislocations
of the Lower Extremity

The prime objective in treating fractures of the lower extremity is to obtain adequate bony union with full length and normal alignment and without rotational deformity. In addition, full restoration of muscle power and joint motion is highly desirable. In contrast with the upper extremity, stability, even at the expense of mobility, must be obtained in the lower extremity. Painless weight-bearing must be achieved if possible.

Edema is a troublesome accompaniment of almost all injuries of the lower extremities. Its prevention or reduction is often disregarded. In an injury of the lower extremity, elevation, or at least the avoidance of too much dependency, should be carried out from the beginning, provided that the arterial supply to the part is sufficient. Regular exercise of all joints which do not move the bone fragments, including even the small joints of the toes, helps to minimize edema. Following the removal of plaster casts, elastic bandages or elastic stockings should be worn to support the venous circulation. When the patient becomes ambulatory, intermittent elevation will minimize any tendency toward recurring edema.

FRACTURES AND DISLOCATIONS
ABOUT THE HIP

Skeletal injuries about the hip may be classified into (1) fractures of the hip (proximal portion of the femur); these are subdivided into fractures of the neck of the femur (intracapsular fractures), and fractures of the trochanteric region of the femur (intertrochanteric, peritrochanteric, subtrochanteric —all extracapsular fractures), (2) dislocations of the hip, and (3) fracture-dislocations of the hip.

FRACTURES OF THE HIP
(PROXIMAL PORTION OF THE FEMUR)

Fractures of the hip fall into two large divisions, depending on whether they involve (1) the intracapsular portion of the neck, or (2) the extracapsular trochanteric region of the femur (Table 1). Both groups have much in common. Both occur principally in the elderly. The mean age is in the 70's and almost a third occur in patients 80 or over. About 80 per cent occur in women. Factors which may make women more vulnerable are a natural tendency in the latter decades toward coxa vara deformity and osteoporosis, and a longer life expectancy than men. The hospital mortality rate is high for both types of fractures because of the age of these patients and because the fractures and their treatment demand sharp curtailment of activi-

TABLE 1. FRACTURES OF THE HIP

LOCATION	INTRACAPSULAR (NECK)	EXTRACAPSULAR (TROCHANTERIC)
Age	Usually 60 to 75 years	Usually 70 to 85 years
Operative treatment	Internal Fixation (Smith-Petersen nail or multiple pins) or Excision of head and insertion of hip endoprosthesis	Internal Fixation (Nail-plate with screws, such as Jewett, Mc-Laughlin, Neufeld, etc.)
Nonoperative treatment	Ineffective	Continuous traction effective but dangerous and inferior to operative treatment
Nonunion	Common	Very rare
Avascular necrosis of head	Common	Very rare
Mortality before weight-bearing is resumed	15 to 20%	30 to 35%
Expected period for union	4 to 12 months	3 to 4 months

ties in patients who tolerate inactivity poorly. However, these patients do not die from the direct effects of the fracture itself but from complications: such as, progression of cardio-vascular-renal disease, pneumonia and pulmonary embolism. It may seem paradoxical that the mortality in the group with trochanteric fractures is higher than in the group with intracapsular fractures, since fractures of the trochanteric region almost always heal and intracapsular fractures commonly result in nonunion. It is not the nonunion that causes the death of these patients but, as stated above, the complications chiefly related to senility. Trochanteric fractures have a higher mortality rate, probably because they occur, as a rule, in older patients. They also produce more trauma to soft tissues and blood loss than those of the neck of the femur.

Mechanism of Injury. Most fractures of the hip occur from a fall. As a rule the patient trips and falls onto the side of the hip. Not infrequently, however, a patient who sustains a fracture of the hip will have the sensation that the hip is broken by a misstep or stumble and that the fall is secondary to the fracture.

Diagnosis. Severe pain in the hip is the outstanding complaint. The patient is unable to arise. The injured lower extremity appears to be shortened and falls into external rotation. This position has been described as "helpless eversion."

The diagnosis always must be confirmed and the type of fracture identified by roentgenograms in two planes. A good lateral roentgenogram of the hip is difficult to make, but it is essential for accurate diagnosis and identification of a fracture of the proximal portion of the femur.

Treatment of Intracapsular Fractures of the Hip. For many years fractures of the neck of the femur as a group have been called the "unsolved fracture." This fracture is unsolved because it ends so often in nonunion or goes on to union only for the femoral head to reveal evidence of avascular necrosis many months or years after union has occurred. Furthermore, even under ideal conditions healing of the fracture takes so long. At one time, these fractures were treated by a "do-nothing" treatment; and, consequently, the great majority ended in nonunion. A great advance was made in 1897 when Royal Whitman advocated a careful manipulative reduction of the hip and immobilization in a plaster hip spica for 3 to 4 months. The next great advance came in 1931 with the introduction of internal fixation by the 3-flanged nail of Smith-Petersen after careful closed reduction and this remains the treatment of choice in most cases. In spite of these advances, the fracture frequently ends in nonunion (15 to 35% in reported series) and still must be considered as unsolved. In recent years, certain of these fractures, usually in the older age groups, have been treated by removal of the femoral head and replacement with a metal hip-joint prosthesis. This form of treatment represents a radical approach to the problem and needs further trial and observation before its permanent place in the treatment of fractures of the neck of the femur can be established.

The head and the neck of the femur have an extremely poor blood supply, and it is chiefly for this reason that nonunion is so common. The head and the neck receive blood from capsular arteries through periosteal and nutrient vessels and to a lesser extent from the small artery in the ligamentum teres. The capsular vessels may be torn by an intracapsular fracture. If so, the artery of the ligamentum teres alone is unlikely to provide a sufficient blood supply for the entire head. Following a fracture of the neck of the femur, aseptic necrosis probably will ensue unless some of the vessels of the capsule remain intact and patent.

Fractures of the neck of the femur may be impacted or unimpacted. The clinical findings and the method of treatment may vary accordingly.

Impacted Fractures of the Neck of the Femur. In some fractures of the femoral neck, the fragments become jammed or impacted together when the fracture is sustained. Under these circumstances, the patient has less pain and may arise from the fallen position and even walk unaided. The foot and the extremity do not fall into helpless eversion. The hip may be moved through a nearly normal range of motion in all directions, particularly if the fragments are firmly impacted. The degree and the position of impaction are determined by roentgenograms in 2 planes. Impacted fractures of the hip are subdivided into abduction or valgus impaction and adduction or varus impaction (Fig. 20-1).

In the abduction impacted fracture of the femoral neck, the fracture line tends to be horizontal, and the head assumes a slight upward or valgus position. In the lateral roentgenogram, the fragments usually are in excellent position. If the fragments are firmly impacted, the fracture is likely to go on to sound bony union with no treatment other than protection from weight-bearing by bed rest for a few weeks, followed by the use of a wheel chair or crutches for 3 months. Because an occasional fracture of this type changes position and becomes disimpacted, some authorities advise internal fixation as a safeguard against disimpaction. Certainly, if there is any doubt that the fracture is firmly impacted, internal fixation is indicated. Moreover, in those which appear to be firmly impacted, it is reasonable that internal fixation will permit the patient to be out of bed and

assume crutch walking in a shorter period of time without endangering the position of the fragments.

In the fracture impacted in adduction, the impaction is unlikely to persist. Disimpaction is the rule. These fractures should be managed as unimpacted fractures of the neck of the femur.

Unimpacted Fractures of the Neck of the Femur. The majority of fractures of the neck of the femur are not impacted and require painstaking, accurate reduction of the fragments under anesthesia with the patient, as a rule, on a fracture table. The reduction is followed by internal fixation with a Smith-Petersen three-flanged nail, a nail-plate combination or multiple pins (Method 3) (Fig. 20-2). Most surgeons prefer to perform this operation without exposing the fracture site, the so-called blind nailing. After closed reduction of the fracture confirmed by roentgenograms made in the operating room, the nail is inserted through a lateral incision below the greater trochanter, using additional roentgenograms to confirm the direction of the nail. Occasionally an accurate reduction of the fragments cannot be obtained by closed reduction. In these instances, an open reduction should be performed in order to ensure that the fragments are reduced adequately. Unless a good reduction is obtained, nonunion is to be anticipated even though the fragments are transfixed with a nail or pins.

Although patients with fractures of the neck of the femur are usually relatively poor risks, with prompt operation within 4 to 24 hours after admission, skillful anesthesia, adequate blood replacement and antibiotics, the immediate mortality rate should be low. Postoperatively, the patient may be turned from side to side and placed in a chair several times a day without endangering the fixation of the fragments. The majority of these patients do not have the strength in the arms to walk with crutches while avoiding weight-bearing. Weight-bearing should not be permitted until there is roentgenographic evidence of union of the fracture. This may require many months.

The operative method of treatment is by far the best for these fractures, not only because it gives the highest percentage of union, but also because it is the best form of treatment for the general condition of the patient.

If, for some reason the operative method is refused or cannot be carried out, the Whitman abduction cast method probably offers the best chances for union of the fracture. However, it does carry a high incidence of complications.

Because of the poor results often obtained with fractures of the neck of the femur (nonunion and avascular necrosis of the head) and the long period of time required to determine the end-result, some surgeons have aban-doned internal fixation of these fractures in patients over 70 or 75 years of age and when the line of fracture is subcapital. Instead of reducing and fixing the fracture by internal fixation, the head fragment is excised and replaced with an intramedullary type of metal hip joint prosthesis. Following insertion of a prosthesis for a fresh fracture of the neck of the femur, the postoperative management is essentially the same as if the fracture had

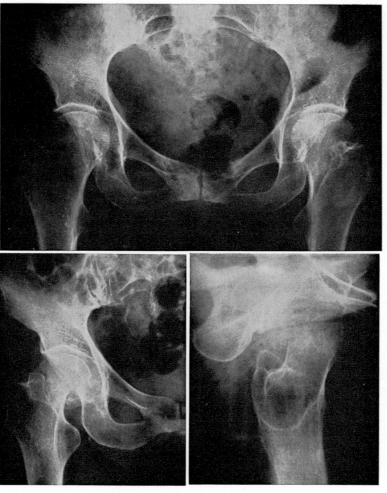

FIG. 20-1. Impacted fractures of the neck of the femur. (*Top*) Roentgenogram showing impaction of the neck of the right femur in abduction. Patient also had sustained an abduction-type impacted fracture of the neck of the left femur 2 years previously which healed with only protection from weight-bearing for 3 months. (*Bottom*) Anteroposterior and lateral roentgenograms of adduction-type impacted fracture of right femur. Since this impaction was unlikely to persist it was managed as an unimpacted fracture by reduction and internal fixation.

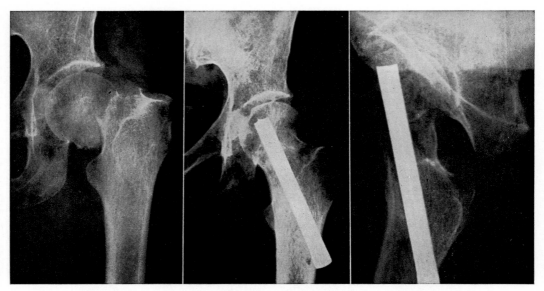

FIG. 20-2. Unimpacted fracture of the neck of the left femur. (*Left*) Roentgenogram before reduction and fixation with a Smith-Petersen 3-flanged nail. Anteroposterior view. (*Center and right*) After internal fixation. (*Center*) Anteroposterior view. (*Right*) Lateral view.

been reduced and fixed internally, except that weight-bearing may be permitted within a few days or at the most 2 weeks. This compromise treatment of fractures of the neck of the femur accepts a hip somewhat functionally inferior to one which would be obtained if the fracture united by bone but does offer a slightly inferior hip in a much shorter period of time. It should be anticipated that a cane will be used as an aid to walking and that the patient will experience mild discomfort in the hip, particularly during the first few steps after arising from the sitting position. The final place for this treatment of fractures of the neck of the femur has not as yet been determined, but results to date are most favorable. However, the fact that such a radical approach to the problem has been employed proves that the fracture remains unsolved.

Treatment of Trochanteric Fractures of the Femur. Fractures included in this group are those located between the neck of the femur and a level about 1 inch below the lesser trochanter. The fragments of a trochanteric fracture have an excellent blood supply and for this reason almost always unite if the patient survives and the fragments are held in a reasonably good reduction. The high mortality rate derives from the age of these

patients (70 to 85 years as a rule), their poor general condition, and the fact that these fractures, in contrast with those of the neck, result in considerable soft tissue trauma. Considerable blood is lost into the tissues with most trochanteric fractures (it has been estimated at about a liter), and much more blood is lost at operation than at operation on fractures of the neck of the femur.

Trochanteric fractures should be treated by the operative method utilizing a nail-plate type of internal fixation (Method 3) (Fig. 20-3). Union can be obtained with other methods, such as balanced suspension traction (Method 2), but the incidence of complications and the mortality rate are much higher with this method than with open reduction and internal fixation. A patient with this injury treated in traction must be kept constantly in bed on his back. This position predisposes to bed sores, thrombo-embolism, pneumonia, senile dementia, and residual loss of motion in the knee. The operative method permits the patient to be turned in bed frequently and to be out of bed in a chair promptly. The patient has less general discomfort and a much better mental attitude toward the restriction of activities imposed by convalescence. All of this tends to minimize complications. It should be

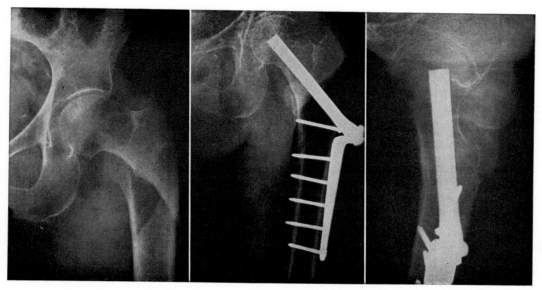

Fig. 20-3. Trochanteric fracture of the femur. Treatment by open reduction and internal fixation. The internal fixation must be of the blade (nail)-plate type, because a nail alone will not fix the fragments adequately. (*Left*) Roentgenogram before operation, anteroposterior view. (*Center*) Roentgenogram after operation and fixation with a Smith-Petersen nail attached to a McLaughlin plate, anteroposterior view. (*Right*) Lateral view.

pointed out that the fracture will unite without operative fixation, but that the operative method is indicated because it is the best for the patient. Weight-bearing must not be allowed until the fracture has united as shown by roentgenograms. Union is more rapid in trochanteric fractures than in fractures of the femoral neck and usually has occurred in 3 or 4 months.

DISLOCATIONS OF THE HIP

Traumatic dislocations of the hip may be classified as (1) posterior (iliac or sciatic notch) and (2) anterior (obturator or pubic), depending upon where the head leaves the acetabulum and comes to rest. Another form of dislocation, central dislocation of the femoral head through a fracture of the acetabulum, is really a fracture of the pelvis rather than a true dislocation and is discussed under fractures of the pelvis.

Posterior Dislocation of the Hip. Posterior dislocation of the hip occurs most frequently as the result of a strong force applied at the knee when the thigh is flexed and adducted, as when the knee strikes the dashboard after an automobile collision. Dislocation may

occur when a heavy weight drops on the low back of a stooping individual, as in a cave-in of dirt or the fall of a roof. A fracture of the posterior wall of the acetabulum frequently accompanies a posterior dislocation of the hip (Fig. 20-4).

DIAGNOSIS. The extremity immediately assumes the position of flexion, adduction and internal rotation at the hip and appears shorter than the opposite side. The position of flexion, adduction and internal rotation is the exact opposite of the position assumed by the extremity with a fracture of the neck of the femur. The position of the extremity and the type of trauma causing it practically establish the diagnosis but it must always be confirmed by an x-ray examination showing the pelvis and both hip joints.

In posterior dislocations, the sciatic nerve may be damaged by the head of the femur or a fragment of the acetabulum. Therefore, before attempts at reduction, a careful motor and sensory examination of the extremity should be made. Otherwise, if the symptoms and signs of damage to the sciatic nerve are found after reduction, it cannot be determined whether they are the result of the in-

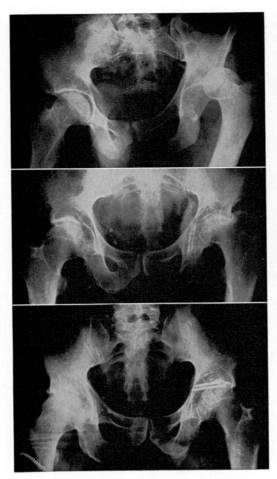

FIG. 20-4. Posterior dislocation of the hip. (*Top*) Roentgenogram of the left hip showing posterior dislocation *without* fracture of posterior wall of acetabulum. (*Center*) Roentgenogram of left hip showing fracture of posterior wall of acetabulum accompanying posterior dislocation of the hip. Note that the hip is displaced posteriorly but not so far superiorly as in *Top*. (*Bottom*) Roentgenogram following reduction of dislocation, and reduction and internal fixation of acetabular fragment.

jury or the trauma of reduction. Symptoms and signs of injury to the sciatic nerve found only after reduction indicate prompt surgical intervention.

TREATMENT. Reduction of a dislocation of the hip is a true surgical emergency. Prompt reduction is necessary not only to relieve pain but also to minimize the danger of avascular necrosis, the incidence of which is in direct ratio to the length of time that the femoral head remains dislocated.

Three standard methods exist for reducing a posterior dislocation of the hip. Each method probably offers certain advantages. Reduction at times is most difficult. In some instances one method will fail to give reduction but another will succeed. General or spinal anesthesia, sufficient to give real muscular relaxation, is essential. Ideally suited for the reduction is a one-sided spinal anesthesia with a small dose of the anesthetic agent.

1. Probably the most effective and safest method of reduction is strong traction in the axis of the femur with the hip flexed and slightly adducted, combined with gentle maneuvering of the thigh toward external rotation and mild abduction while an assistant provides countertraction by strong pressure against the pelvis. This, in effect, pulls the femoral head through the rent in the capsule in the reverse direction from that in which it left the joint. Reduction takes place with a satisfying snap or thump. For emphasis, it is repeated that traction is made with the hip flexed, not extended.

These maneuvers may be carried out with the patient on a pad on the floor. The surgeon stands over the patient as he reduces the dislocation. An alternative position is provided with the patient on an x-ray table and the surgeon in his stocking feet standing on the table. The latter position offers easy roentgenologic confirmation of the reduction.

2. The time-honored method of Bigelow may be used. In this method, the adducted thigh and leg are fully flexed and then, as traction is applied, the thigh is circumducted lateralward, then externally rotated and abducted. A disadvantage of this method is that excessive force can cause a fracture of the neck or the shaft of the femur. Moreover, a posterior dislocation may merely be converted into an anterior dislocation.

3. The Stimson method, used too seldom, is really a most atraumatic and effective method. The patient is anesthetized face down with the thighs flexed at the hip over the end of the table and with the legs supported in 90° of flexion at the knee. A heavy weight, up to 20 or 25 pounds, is applied to the affected leg just below the knee, thereby

making traction on the thigh. Traction is allowed to persist for several minutes until muscle spasm has been overcome, following which the operator merely rotates the extremity inward and outward. Reduction is sometimes obtained by this method after the two more popular methods described above have failed.

While reduction usually can be achieved with any of the methods just discussed, it is not always easy. Considerable force for traction is often necessary. In the rare instance when closed reduction is unsuccessful, open reduction must be used.

Postreduction Management of Posterior Dislocation of the Hip. Immobilization of the hip in plaster or prolonged traction on the extremity is not necessary. A few pounds of simple skin traction of the Buck's type may be provided for a few days to help overcome spasm of the muscles and thereby to contribute to the comfort of the patient. Redislocation is most unlikely to occur, but as a safeguard against it, the patient may be kept at bed rest without flexion of the thigh at the hip for a period of 3 to 4 weeks. The position of extension prevents pressure of the head of the femur against the rent in the capsule of the joint posteriorly.

Opinions vary as to when weight-bearing may be permitted following dislocation of the hip. One school of thought lays emphasis on the risk of avascular necrosis of the head of the femur and prefers as long as 6 months of crutch-walking without real weight-bearing in order that, if the early signs of this complication have developed, the patient may remain on crutches for a matter of several years anticipating creeping replacement of the dead femoral head. This concept seems to indicate that there will be full creeping replacement of the dead head and the subsequent return of function to the hip will be worth the prolonged period of time on crutches.

A second school recognizes that avascular necrosis of the head of the femur following dislocation may appear at any time after injury, even 4 or 5 years later. Since this is true, an arbitrary period of 6 months on crutches does not seem to be justified to this group. Weight-bearing and full function are permitted approximately 6 weeks after dislocation. This approach to the problem is by far the most practicable and is recommended.

Anterior Dislocation of the Hip. Anterior dislocation of the hip, which is rather rare, may occur when the thigh is forced into extreme abduction and external rotation. The head usually comes to rest in the obturator foramen. The extremity goes into abduction, external rotation and some flexion and appears to be longer than the uninjured limb. While the position of the extremity resembles that assumed when a fracture of the neck of the femur is present, it may be distinguished clinically from that injury because of the mild flexion and the increased rather than decreased length.

TREATMENT. Reduction usually may be achieved by traction in the axis which the femur has assumed, combined with internal rotation and adduction. The Bigelow method for anterior dislocations of the hip also may be used. This, of course, is somewhat the reverse of the maneuver for posterior dislocations of the hip. The thigh and the leg are flexed. Then, as traction is made, the extremity is circumducted toward adduction and brought into internal rotation and extension.

POSTREDUCTION MANAGEMENT. Only a few days of bed rest, avoidance of undue strain toward abduction, external rotation and hyperextension, and about 4 weeks on crutches are necessary. Avascular necrosis of the femoral head is unlikely to develop following anterior dislocation of the hip if reduction is performed within a few hours of injury.

Posterior Dislocation of the Hip with Fracture of the Acetabulum. A fracture of the posterior portion of the acetabulum frequently complicates a posterior dislocation of the hip, the femoral head driving a fragment or fragments ahead of it as it leaves the joint. This combination of injuries frequently results from automobile collisions as a knee of a front-seat occupant strikes the dashboard—hence, it is called the "dashboard dislocation." The fracture of the acetabulum can be diagnosed only by a roentgenogram.

TREATMENT. As the dislocation of the hip is reduced, the fragment or fragments of acetabulum usually fall into position. However, the important consideration in these injuries is the size of the fragments and the potential defect in the acetabular wall rather than whether or not the fragments go into good position with reduction of the hip. If the fragments are small, they may be ignored even if unreduced and the hip managed as a dislocation without fracture.

On the other hand, when the fragment or fragments are large, even though they are reduced, subsequent displacement and spontaneous redislocation of the hip can easily occur through the defect in the acetabular wall. Therefore, open reduction and internal fixation of large acetabular fragments are indicated to provide a stable posterior acetabulum (Fig. 20-4). Of course, operative reduction and fixation are necessary for unreduced large fragments.

After closed or open reduction of a dislocated hip with a fracture of the acetabulum, external immobilization is not necessary. Flexion of the thigh at the hip is avoided, as this would cause the femoral head to press against the weakened portion of the acetabulum. With the thigh in extension, normal muscle tone holds the femoral head against the intact superior portion of the acetabulum. All that is necessary, therefore, is to keep the patient at bed rest with the thighs in extension for a period of 4 to 6 weeks. So long as the injured hip remains in extension the patient may lie on either side, face down, or on his back.

Posterior Dislocation of the Hip with Chip Fracture of the Femoral Head. Occasionally, a piece of the head of the femur is sheared off as it leaves the acetabulum. This fragment may block reduction of the dislocation or it may fall into the acetabulum and prevent proper seating of the femoral head in the joint. If either situation cannot be overcome by manipulation, then excision of the fragment is necessary. On the other hand, if reduction of the dislocation is achieved without interference by the fragment, usually the latter may be ignored as it is unlikely to interfere with subsequent function of the hip. Early surgical excision is not indicated for 2 reasons: the operation itself may cause further damage to the arterial flow to the femoral head from capsular arteries and increase the chances of avascular necrosis. In addition, the operative trauma may predispose to myositis ossificans about the joint. In certain instances late operative removal of the fragment may be necessary.

FRACTURES OF THE SHAFT OF THE FEMUR

The shaft of the femur extends from a point about 1 inch below the lesser trochanter distally to the largely cancellous bone of the supracondylar area. The shaft of the femur is bowed slightly anteriorly and laterally. This lateral bowing is greater in females than in males. The shape of the femoral shaft is not cylindrical because of the ridge on the posterior surface, the linea aspera, which bifurcates in the distal third into two elevations which continue down to the condyles as epicondylar ridges.

In general the blood supply of the shaft of the femur is good, in contrast with the neck of the femur, and for that reason nonunion is relatively uncommon unless the fracture is not adequately reduced or immobilized or is held in distraction. Malunion is more frequent than nonunion. The most powerful muscles of the body attach to the femur and tend to cause angulation and overriding.

The femur is encircled by a tight muscular and fascial compartment. Collections of fluid inside this compartment are difficult to detect by physical examination. Consequently, a huge volume of blood or pus may go unrecognized. The large volume of blood usually lost from the circulation in closed fractures of the femoral shaft is contained within this tight fascial compartment.

Fractures in the proximal and the distal portions of the shaft show the greatest displacement and are the most difficult to reduce. In fractures in the proximal portion, the proximal fragment is usually flexed by the iliopsoas and abducted and externally rotated by the muscles attaching to the greater trochanter. In supracondylar fractures, the proximal end of the distal fragment is pulled posteriorly by the attachments of the gastrocnemii, causing posterior angulation. The sharp end of this fragment may occasionally injure the large nerves and blood vessels in the popliteal space. In fractures of the middle of the shaft, the strong adductor muscles tend to bow the fragments laterally.

IN ADULTS

Mechanism of Injury. Because considerable violence usually is required to break the shaft of the femur, extensive soft tissue damage, severe displacement of bone fragments and abundant blood loss usually accompany the injury. Such a fracture may result from a fall from a height or from direct violence, as in an automobile accident. Gunshot fractures of the femoral shaft are not uncomomn in warfare. In contrast with fractures of the neck and the trochanteric region of the femur, which occur principally in the aged, fractures of the shaft are seen more commonly in middle-aged and young adults and in children.

Diagnosis. Complete fractures of the femoral shaft are usually easy to diagnose because the powerful thigh muscles cause severe angulation and overriding, with an obvious deformity resulting. External rotation of the leg is usually present but not to the degree commonly seen when the hip is broken. Pain is usually severe. Traumatic shock may result from the severe soft tissue and bone damage with loss of blood and extracellular fluid into the tissues.

Clinical diagnosis must be confirmed by adequate roentgenograms (always after adequate splinting) so as to determine the exact location, type and contour of the fracture. The entire bone should be visualized so that double fractures will not go unrecognized.

Treatment. GENERAL. Treatment of fractures of the femoral shaft aims to prevent shortening, angulation and rotational deformity and to maintain apposition of the bone ends sufficient to effect union of bone. Exact anatomic apposition is not essential because satisfactory union usually will occur with only fair contact.

Restriction of knee motion is a common complication following fracture of the femoral shaft and may occur after any form of treatment. Every effort must be made to minimize loss of knee motion and atrophy of the quadriceps musculature, from the beginning of treatment. Quadriceps setting exercises must be started early, and active and passive knee exercises added when healing of the fracture permits. Foot and ankle exercises also should be started from the beginning of treatment.

EMERGENCY SPLINTING. Because of the large size of the femoral shaft and the huge muscular attachments, it is especially important to splint these fractures soon after injury, before the patient is transported, in order to prevent further tissue damage. Whereas a patient may "splint" a Colles' fracture by holding the injured hand and wrist with the other and thereby prevent further tissue damage while en route to the hospital even if

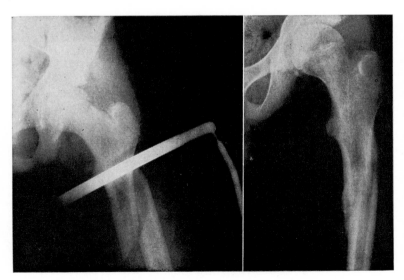

FIG. 20-5. (*Left*) Anteroposterior roentgenogram of fracture of femoral shaft in upper third soon after injury, and in an emergency splint. (*Right*) Anteroposterior roentgenogram after treatment in balanced suspension skeletal traction, showing good bony union. The position was equally good in the lateral view.

adequate splinting has not been provided, the patient with a femoral shaft fracture must have expert emergency splinting before and during transport. Such splinting may mean the difference between life and death, as was demonstrated by the British experience during World War I when splinting for transportation reduced the mortality by 25 per cent. A patient with a suspected fracture of the femoral shaft should be transported to the hospital with a Thomas or half-ring leg splint (Fig. 20-5, *left*), with traction on the foot or with good coaptation splinting with boards as described under the section on emergency splinting. In no injury is emergency splinting of more importance.

DEFINITIVE. Fractures of the shaft of the femur should be treated by one of the first three of the 5 methods of fracture treatment. The "do-nothing" method (Method 5) is never applicable. Although external skeletal fixation has been used by some surgeons, it has resulted in a high incidence of complications—nonunion, knee stiffness, infection along the pin tracts—and we do not recommend its use for fractures of the femoral shaft. The great majority are treated by Methods 2 and 3 (traction and operative fixation). Because of the powerful muscle pulls closed reduction and immobilization in plaster (Method 1) is rarely adequate, especially in comminuted, oblique, or spiral fractures. Dis-

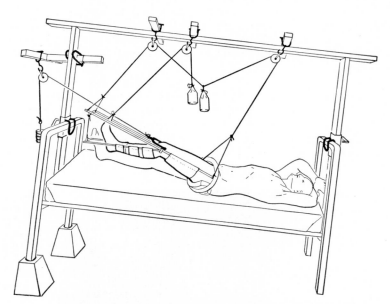

FIG. 20-6. Illustrating use of balanced skeletal traction for treatment of fracture of femoral shaft. The Pierson attachment is attached at the level of the upper border of the patella, with the knee in 170° to 175° extension. The angle of the attachment to the splint should conform to the normal valgus at the knee. The slings for the splint should not overlap, although they must be close to each other. They must support the thigh from the ring of the splint to just proximal to the posterior bulge of the femoral condyles. The slings for the Pierson attachment should support the leg from a point just distal to the posterior bulge of the tibial condyles to the tendo achillis. The foot is supported at 90° by suspension, using stockinet attached over the foot by tincture of benzoin. The ring is placed firmly against the ischial tuberosity. The suspension weights for the splint must not only support the entire splint and the Pierson attachment but also must aid in maintaining the ring against the tuberosity. Elevation of the foot of the bed to increase the countertraction of the weight of the body is essential.

placement and angulation tend to occur within the cast, even though a perfect reduction has been obtained, and the fracture is transverse.

Continuous Balanced Traction (Method 2). Before the introduction of intramedullary nailing for fractures of the femoral shaft, the most generally used method was continuous balanced traction (Method 2). Even now, balanced suspension skeletal traction by a Kirschner wire drilled through the upper tibia about an inch posterior to the tibial tubercle, or, in some instances, through the broad portion of the distal femur just proximal to the adductor tubercle, remains an excellent method of treating femoral shaft fractures. Skeletal traction is more efficient than skin traction: it allows better control of the fragments and is less apt to produce skin complications. Infection along the wire track is rare.

Figure 20-6 illustrates the use of balanced skeletal traction for treatment of a femoral shaft fracture. The Thomas leg splint with a Pierson attachment in balanced suspension from an overhead frame is the most generally employed method of balanced suspension skeletal traction. The splint must be long enough and wide enough for the extremity to rest comfortably in hammock slings.

A great danger in the use of continuous traction is overpull (distraction) of the fragments. Roentgenograms must be made frequently in the early stages of treatment to detect overpull and other deformities, and to allow the earliest possible reduction in the amount of traction and indicated adjustments of the traction apparatus. The distal fragment and accordingly the leg and the foot must be allowed to remain in sufficient external rotation to conform with the rotation of the proximal fragment.

In our experience, fractures of the upper half of the femoral shaft are treated best with the Kirschner wire through the distal femur although a wire through the proximal tibia may be satisfactory. An advantage in having the wire above the knee is that knee motion may be instituted earlier. In fractures of the upper third of the shaft, the proximal fragment usually is sharply flexed and abducted and externally rotated. In such instances traction must be made with the thigh flexed, abducted and externally rotated in such a manner as to bring the distal fragment into

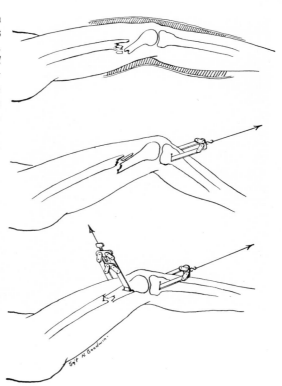

Fig 20-7. Diagrammatic representation of 2-wire skeletal traction for fracture of femur. (*Top*) Deformity on admission to hospital. (*Center*) Incomplete reduction in skeletal traction with wire in tibial tubercle. (*Bottom*) Adequate reduction when additional wire is inserted in lower femoral fragment and vertical left is secured. (Hampton, O. P., Jr.: Wounds of the Extremities in Military Surgery, St. Louis, Mosby, p. 273)

proper rotation and alignment with the proximal fragment.

Fractures of the lower half of the femoral shaft usually are controlled best with the Kirschner wire inserted through the proximal tibia posterior to the tubercle. It is difficult to control the short distal fragment if the wire is placed through the femur.

The posterior angulation of fractures of the distal end of the femoral shaft, caused by the pull of the gastrocnemii, is difficult to correct. One method is to insert two Kirschner wires: one at the level of the tibial tubercle for longitudinal traction and one just above the condyles for anterior or vertical traction to

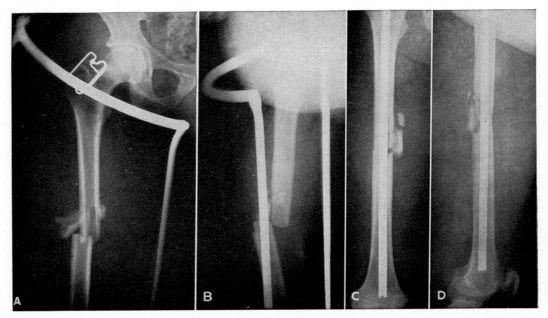

FIG. 20-8. Fracture of the shaft of the femur stabilized in reduction by an intramedullary nail.

(A and B) Anteroposterior and lateral views of a somewhat comminuted fracture of the shaft of the right femur in the upper portion of the middle third immobilized in a half-ring leg splint as emergency splinting.

(C and D) Anteroposterior and lateral views showing the fracture stabilized in excellent reduction with a cloverleaf (Küntscher) intramedullary nail. The fracture went on to solid union in excellent apposition and alignment.

(Hampton, O. P., Jr., and Fitts, W. T., Jr.: Open Reduction of Common Fractures, New York, Grune & Stratton)

correct the posterior angulation of the distal fragment (Fig. 20-7). Another method is the following: with the Kirschner wire at the level of the tibial tubercle and the hinge of the Pierson attachment at the level of the fracture site instead of at the knee, traction is made parallel with the leg which is kept horizontal with the floor. This is the only situation in which the line of traction is not made parallel with the shaft of the femur. If a satisfactory position cannot be accomplished by traction within 48 to 72 hours, then direct manipulation of the fragments in the traction apparatus should be done with the patient anesthetized.

Traction should be maintained until bony union has occurred, as shown by clinical and roentgenologic evidence. This may require from 3 to 5 months. Weight-bearing should not be allowed until union is solid. Patients with precarious union preferably should be kept in balanced suspension for an added length of time, during which active and passive knee exercises are instituted, or further immobilization may be provided by a plaster spica. Afterward in instances of precarious union, ischial bearing leg braces should be used until union is solid.

Open Reduction and Internal Fixation (Method 3). The other common method of treating fractures of the femoral shaft is open reduction and internal fixation. Until the introduction of intramedullary nailing for these fractures about 15 years ago, the operative method usually was reserved for those instances in which a satisfactory reduction could not be accomplished with balanced traction. The method of internal fixation then used was a metallic plate with screws (stainless steel or vitallium) which necessitated supplementary immobilization in a plaster hip spica. The incidence of nonunion was high

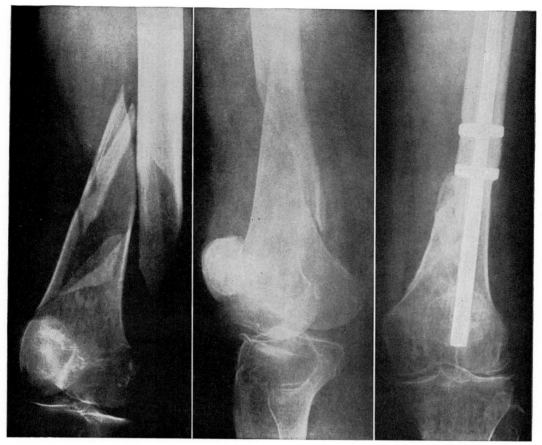

FIG. 20-9. Fracture of shaft of femur treated with Küntscher nail and supplementary Parham-Marten bands. (*Left and Center*) Anteroposterior and lateral roentgenograms before operation. (*Right*) Several months after operation, showing union progressing satisfactorily. The Parham-Marten bands were removed several months before the nail was removed.

when plates and screws were used and, even if the fracture united, the fact that plaster immobilization was necessary for several months must have contributed to knee stiffness and muscle atrophy. For these reasons internal fixation with plates and screws is not ideal, and intramedullary nailing has largely replaced it.

Fixation by intramedullary nailing is the preferable method for treatment of fractures of the femoral shaft if the contour of the fracture is such as to permit stabilization by the nail. It is especially applicable for transverse fractures of the middle three fifths of the femur (Fig. 20-8). In addition to an exceedingly high rate of union of the fracture, intramedullary nailing has the great advan-

tage of allowing early weight-bearing with better preservation of joint motion and less muscle atrophy. After a successful medullary nailing a patient with a femoral shaft fracture may be up on crutches with guarded weight-bearing within a few days and resume a sedentary occupation within a few weeks; whereas, if traction is used, he must spend from 3 to 6 months in bed. Intramedullary nailing in contrast with skeletal traction permits the patient to be transported about the hospital easily and therefore facilitates the care of other injuries.

Intramedullary nailing of femoral shaft fractures should almost always be done as an open operation. A single nail of adequate diameter is preferred. The Küntscher type of

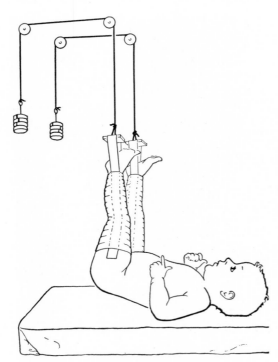

FIG. 20-10. Bryant's traction, a form of balanced suspension skin traction. Bryant's traction may cause ischemia of the feet and the legs (see text).

nail is strongly recommended. In certain comminuted or butterfly types of fracture, supplemental wire or screw fixation may be necessary to provide better stabilization of the fracture. (Fig. 20-9. See also Fig. 18-14).

The risk of the nailing operation is that an open operation on bone must be performed with all of its dangers and that technical difficulties may occur in the insertion of the nail. The nail may split, bend, or break. If driven too far distally, the knee joint may be injured. Fat embolism may occur, but serious effects from it are rare. The advantages of a good intramedullary nailing of the femur by far outweigh the disadvantages.

In open fractures of the femur the wounds preferably are débrided, perhaps closed, and allowed to heal while the extremity is held in balanced suspension skeletal traction. After sound wound-healing the advantages of intramedullary nailing may be obtained by operation. Occasionally, for good cause, the open fracture may be stabilized with an intramedul-

lary nail at the time of wound débridement, but this carries a definite risk of catastrophic sepsis.

In Children

Fractures of the femoral shaft in children always unite. In addition, children rapidly correct mild or even moderate degrees of angulation and shortening up to 1 inch. Accordingly, reduction does not have to be as precise as in adults.

Traditionally, these fractures in young children have been treated by Bryant's traction (Fig. 20-10), a form of skin traction. In Bryant's traction the thighs are flexed 90°, and enough traction is applied on both legs so that the buttocks are lifted just clear of the bed. Depending on the age of the baby, Bryant's traction is usually continued for 2 to 4 weeks, and then if necessary the extremity is immobilized in a plaster hip spica until union is solid—usually another 2 to 3 weeks. Studies by Nicholson showed that Bryant's traction is dangerous above the age of 2 years because this position is likely to cause ischemia of the legs. For children above the age of 2, traction should be skin (as a rule) or skeletal, with the thigh flexed to about 45° and with traction on only one leg.

Because children can easily correct some shortening and angulation, plaster immobilization can be used for many of these fractures as long as a reasonable position can be held. Restriction of joint motion and muscle atrophy, which usually follow such immobilization in the adult, are not problems in young children.

FRACTURES OF THE DISTAL END OF THE FEMUR

Supracondylar Fracture of the Femur

In almost all fractures of the lower end of the shaft and at the supracondylar level, the distal fragment is angulated posteriorly by the pull of the gastrocnemius, and shortening is usually severe. The sharp edge of the distal fragment as it is pulled posteriorly may injure the popliteal vessels and nerves.

Fractures of the distal femoral shaft and supracondylar fractures with severe posterior displacement may be difficult to reduce by closed methods. If reduction cannot be obtained by closed methods, satisfactory fixation may be effected at operation as described below under fractures of the condyles.

FRACTURES OF THE CONDYLES

In fractures of the femoral condyles, an anatomic reduction of the articular surfaces must be accomplished if traumatic arthritis is to be minimized. In most instances in which the fragments have been significantly displaced, open operation is necessary for proper reduction. Undisplaced fractures require only immobilization for 6 to 8 weeks.

"T" fractures of the femoral condyles are comminuted fractures in which a transverse fracture just above the condyles is continued into the articular surface by a longitudinal fracture between the condyles. The shaft of the femur is often wedged between the condyles. The preferred method of treatment is by open reduction and internal fixation (Method 3) (Fig. 20-11). The shaft is fixed to the condyles by a blade plate, after the condyles are fixed to each other by supplemental pins. In some instances 2 crossed intra-

medullary nails of the Rush type may be satisfactory.

Following internal fixation a plaster hip spica or at times a cylinder is applied until union is solid, usually 2 to 3 months after injury.

The next best treatment for these injuries is balanced suspension skeletal traction with a Kirschner wire inserted at the level of the tibial tubercle.

SEPARATION OF THE LOWER FEMORAL EPIPHYSIS

This is an injury of the second decade of life. In most instances, the displaced epiphysis lies medial and anterior to the shaft. Usually

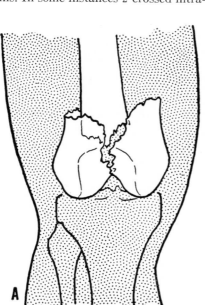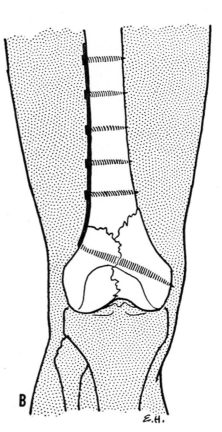

FIG. 20-11. Supracondylar T-fracture of the femur.

A. Drawing of fracture showing disruption of the articular surface and spreading and overriding of the condylar fragments.

B. Drawing showing excellent reduction of the fracture and stabilization with a blade plate and screws used for internal fixation.

(Hampton, O. P., Jr., and Fitts, W. T., Jr.: Open Reduction of Common Fractures, New York, Grune & Stratton)

reduction can be effected by closed reduction (Method 1), after which the extremity is immobilized in a single hip spica until union is solid, usually within 6 to 8 weeks. If a satisfactory reduction is not obtained by closed means, open reduction is carried out. Fortunately, open reduction is rarely necessary. It is best not to use internal fixation because thereby the epiphysis is further damaged and growth may be disturbed.

DISLOCATION OF THE KNEE

A true dislocation of the knee is a more serious injury by far than the injury which the layman calls a dislocation of the knee. The latter is one of the internal derangements of the knee, usually a torn semilunar cartilage. In a true dislocation of the knee the tibia is completely displaced so that it no longer articulates with the femur. This relatively rare injury is produced by direct violence to the proximal end of the tibia or distal end of the femur while the knee is extended or by forced hyperextension at the knee. For this dislocation to occur, both collateral and both cruciate ligaments must be torn. Probably momentary dislocation with spontaneous reduction occurs occasionally. In such instances, although a dislocation of the knee is not present when the patient is examined, there is marked instability in all directions.

Complications of a complete dislocation of the knee include damage to the popliteal artery and to a major peripheral nerve trunk posterior to the knee, usually the peroneal. The artery may be torn, or its flow of blood obstructed by pressure. This emphasizes the importance of a rapid appraisal of the circulatory status of the leg and the foot when the patient is first seen. Signs of vascular insufficiency demand immediate reduction of the dislocation which, at times, can be done without anesthesia. If after reduction of the dislocation the normal pulsations at the foot do not return, then surgical exploration of the popliteal fossa is indicated with appropriate arterial surgery being carried out, depending on the findings.

The peroneal nerve is much more likely to be injured in a dislocation of the knee than is the posterior tibial nerve. The ability to move the toes and the foot must be tested immediately. This prereduction observation may prove to be advantageous in evaluating the damage to the nerve trunk when a paralysis of the nerve supply to the foot is present after reduction of the dislocation. While the prognosis for eventual recovery is good, it is by no means certain. Even so, early exploration for repair of a damaged peripheral nerve trunk is not indicated.

TREATMENT

Closed reduction of a dislocation of the knee usually is obtained easily by traction and manipulation. Immobilization with the knee flexed 10° in a single hip spica for 4 weeks and then a snug long leg cast for 4 more weeks usually permits sufficient healing of the torn ligaments to give a stable knee and yet permit return of a good range of motion. A hip spica may not be necessary in thin individuals, as a long leg cast can be made to fit snugly; but in all others a hip spica during the first 4 weeks acts as a safeguard against abnormal mobility at the knee which can occur in a long leg cast.

In recent years the early operative repair of torn collateral ligaments has gained support, and operative repair of the torn structures following reduction of a dislocation of the leg at the knee has been advised by some authorities. While it is reasonable that a splendid end-result can be obtained faster by such an operative approach under the proper circumstances, many excellent knees have been obtained by closed reduction and immobilization for 2 to 3 months as described above.

INTERNAL DERANGEMENTS OF THE KNEE

The knee joint, a form of hinge-joint, depends on strong ligaments and the musculature of the thigh for its integrity and stability. The condyles of the femur and the tibia are held snugly in contact by these structures in all degrees of flexion and extension of the knee.

An internal derangement of the knee is a mechanical derangement of function of the joint caused by some lesion which eliminates the supporting strength of the major ligaments of the knee or mechanically prevents the constant snug contact and smooth gliding of the condyles of the tibia over those of the femur as the leg is flexed or extended. There are 4 principal internal derangements of the knee:

1. Tears of semilunar cartilages
2. Tears of collateral ligaments
3. Tears of cruciate ligaments
4. Loose osteocartilaginous bodies

All acute injuries of the knee without fracture are contusions, sprains (tears of the capsule of some degree, or possibly a tear or contusion of the infrapatellar fat pad) or true internal derangements. The surgeon must differentiate between these as well as is possible by means of the history of injury, the symptoms of the patients and the findings on physical examination. Unless the diagnosis of an internal derangement can be definitely established when the patient is first seen, the injury must be treated as a sprain by means of rest of the joint, compression dressings and possibly aspiration of the accumulated fluid. On the other hand, every acute injury of the knee must not be treated as a simple sprain, as many require specific treatment as outlined below in the discussion of the several internal derangements of the knee.

Tears of Semilunar Cartilages

Tears of the semilunar cartilages result from twisting injuries to the knee. Normally, the semilunar cartilages buffer any rotary grinding action of the condyles of the femur on the tibia. In some strains, however, one of the cartilages, usually the medial, becomes impinged between the condyles of the tibia and femur and is torn. The medial cartilage may be torn by an abduction-external rotation strain and the lateral cartilage by an adduction-internal rotation strain. The tear may take the form of a longitudinal split down the long axis of the cartilage (a bucket-handle tear) or a flap may be torn loose at any point along the inner margin. Occasionally, the lateral attachment of the cartilage is avulsed from the tibia. With each type, the torn portion of the cartilage may become caught between the condyles of the femur and the tibia to cause the symptoms of a mechanical derangement.

Diagnosis. In the classical case of a torn medial semilunar cartilage, the patient gives a history of a twisting injury and a painful snapping sensation on the inner side of the knee. Immediately the knee joint is locked* in slight flexion. This usually means a bucket-handle tear with the torn portion of the cartilage displaced into the intercondylar notch of the femur. Pain persists, and considerable effusion develops. Tenderness is fairly well localized over the medial joint line. Roentgenograms are negative, since the semilunar cartilages are not visualized by x-ray examination. This clinical syndrome establishes the diagnosis. However, it occurs in only a small percentage of patients with torn semilunar cartilages.

In the majority of instances, the diagnosis of a torn semilunar cartilage is made on the history of a twisting injury to the knee, perhaps with a snap and subsequent repeated episodes of painful, slipping, catching, near-locking sensations on the inner side of the joint. Tenderness over the cartilage is usually present, and a history of recurring effusions may be obtained. The history also is likely to reveal asymptomatic intervals between these episodes with recurrences brought on by additional twisting injuries of varying severity. Some atrophy of the quadriceps musculature may be discernible. Again x-ray examinations are negative. For diagnostic purposes, a history of repeated actual or impending mechanical derangements well localized to the inner side of the joint is more important than any other symptom or the findings on examination. In a few patients the diagnosis may be justified on only a history of twisting injury, persisting pain and tenderness on the inner side of the knee and a feeling of weakness in the joint, but the diagnosis is made on much sounder grounds if the symptoms of a true mechanical derangement such as locking are present.

The diagnosis of a torn lateral semilunar cartilage is made on comparable clinical symptoms and signs on the lateral side of the joint. This lesion is much less common than a tear of the medial cartilage.

Treatment. Once a semilunar cartilage is torn, it probably never heals. The cartilage has such poor blood supply that any healing efforts are usually ineffective. On the other

---

* In a locked knee, the leg cannot be extended completely because of a mechanical block. It can be flexed through a good range, although not necessarily a full range.

hand, if, instead of an actual tear of the cartilage, the coronary ligament, which attaches the cartilage to the tibia, is torn so that the entire cartilage is displaced, healing of the torn ligamentous attachment may occur readily if the cartilage is returned to its normal position and held there for a few weeks. With this exception, once a torn cartilage, always a torn cartilage.

Surgical excision of the torn cartilage, or, in selected instances, the torn portion of the cartilage, is the only definitive therapy once the diagnosis has been definitely established. However, surgery may be postponed until a time convenient to the patient, unless the knee remains locked.

Nonoperative treatment includes aspiration of the joint, compression bandages about the knee, the leg and the foot and protection from weight-bearing with crutches until most of the joint reaction has subsided. Actually, nonoperative therapy probably will be employed one or more times in those instances in which the joint is not locked, as the diagnosis cannot be established sufficiently to justify operation without a history of recurring episodes. Occasionally, in first episodes without true locking, a plaster cylinder may be used for 3 or 4 weeks. The rationale of the plaster cylinder in first episodes is based upon the possibility that the entire cartilage has been displaced and, if so, that healing of the coronary ligament as described above may permanently relieve the patient. With either operative or nonoperative treatment, strenuous quadriceps setting exercises throughout convalescence are highly important in rehabilitation of the patient.

Tears of Collateral Ligaments

Tears of the collateral ligaments result from the same type of abduction or adduction strains on the extended knee as those described as the mechanisms of injury for fractures of the tibial condyles (see p. 422). A tear of a a collateral ligament of the knee on one side and a fracture of the condyle of the tibia on the other side of the knee may result from the same trauma. Tears of the medial collateral ligament are far more common than those of the lateral collateral ligament.

Diagnosis. Tears of the collateral ligaments are acutely painful and are immediately disabling. In all but minor injuries, the patient cannot tolerate weight-bearing. Pain and tenderness are localized over the torn collateral ligament. Hemarthrosis develops rapidly. Within 12 to 24 hours, the skin overlying the torn ligament is likely to become discolored from subcutaneous hemorrhage seeping toward the surface.

The diagnosis is confirmed on physical examination. Normally, with the knee extended, abduction and adduction strains elicit little or no lateral movement. With a tear of a collateral ligament, this stabilizing function is impaired or lost so that the extended leg may be abducted (torn medial collateral) or adducted (torn lateral collateral) definitely more than the normal. This is the cardinal sign of a torn collateral ligament of the knee. The degree of abnormal mobility varies with the extent of tear of the ligament.

Treatment. Treatment varies with the extent of the tear which is determined principally by the amount of abnormal lateral mobility. The instability may be masked by the splinting effect of the spasm of the muscles of the thigh produced by the pain of examination as well as the injury itself. Therefore, examination under anesthesia, which relaxes the musculature, may be necessary to demonstrate the full extent of the ligamentous tear.

When the extended leg can be abnormally abducted (or adducted) only 10° to 15° or less, probably the injury is essentially a stretching tear rather than a true rupture of the ligament. Under these circumstances, immobilization in a plaster cylinder is indicated. In these cases the cast should be applied with the knee in 10° to 15° of flexion and with the precaution that the leg is held so as not to place any stretch on the torn ligament. The cast should remain in place for 4 to 6 weeks. During this time, in most instances weight-bearing should be avoided by the use of crutches. When the degree of tear is minimal and when the plaster cylinder remains snug and well fitting, weight-bearing without the use of crutches may be permitted.

When the degree of lateral instability on testing exceeds 15°, primary operative repair followed by 4 weeks of immobilization in a cast is usually the treatment of choice. This permits a thorough intra-articular inspection and, if the adjacent semilunar cartilage is torn, it can be removed. The accurate surgical repair of the torn collateral ligament predisposes to the optimal functional result for such a severe injury in the minimum period of time. If for any reason operative treatment is not selected, immobilization for 8 weeks should be provided in a plaster cylinder with the knee flexed 10° to 15°.

TEARS OF CRUCIATE LIGAMENTS

The cruciate ligaments are stretched or torn in injuries which cause excessive movement of the tibia on the femur in the anteroposterior direction. The anterior cruciate ligament, which becomes taut with the leg in extension and then limits hyperextension, is often torn in twisting-hyperextension injuries. This injury frequently occurs as a result of the extension of a force that ruptures the medial collateral ligament. The posterior cruciate ligament, which is taut in flexion and prevents backward displacement of the tibia on the femur, is often torn when the upper portion of the flexed tibia is thrown against a dashboard and as a result is driven backward on the femur.

Diagnosis. The diagnosis of a torn cruciate ligament is made on the basis of physical findings in a patient having all the symptoms of a severe sprain of the knee. Normally, when the knee is in about 90° of flexion, little or no passive movement of the proximal end of the tibia on the femur can be elicited in the anteroposterior direction. When the anterior cruciate ligament is torn, the proximal end of the tibia can be pulled forward excessively (the anterior drawer sign). In addition, excessive hyperextension of the leg may be found. With a torn posterior cruciate ligament, the proximal end of the tibia can be pushed backward on the femur excessively (the posterior drawer sign). Actually, with torn posterior cruciate ligaments, the proximal tibia may remain displaced backward, from which position it can be pulled forward to the normal position. When both cruciate ligaments are torn, the upper tibia can be pushed backward and pulled forward far in excess of the normal. Comparison with the range of passive movement in the anteroposterior direction of the opposite knee is always important in evaluating the findings in a suspected tear of a cruciate ligament. In the acute injury, these tests may be unsatisfactory because of pain; therefore, examination under anesthesia may be advisable.

Treatment. Whether a torn cruciate ligament ever heals spontaneously is subject to question. Many tears of this structure are stretching elongations so that after healing, the ligament remains lax. Complete tears seldom if ever heal so as to restore continuity without operative repair. When the anterior attachment of the anterior cruciate ligament has been avulsed from the anterior tibial spine, it can be held in place by a mattress suture of silk or wire passing through 2 drill holes in the upper tibia (see "Fractures of the Tibial Spine," p. 420). Such a repair is frequently a supplemental procedure to operative repair of a torn medial collateral ligament.

If the surgeon suspects a complete tear or an avulsion of a cruciate ligament in an acute knee injury, he is justified in examining the knee with the patient under anesthesia. If his diagnosis is confirmed, operative repair of the torn ligament is usually desirable. After repair the knee is immobilized in a plaster cylinder for about 4 weeks.

In an acute injury, without evidence of a tear sufficient to justify operation, therapy is the same as for a sprain of the knee. If the joint is distended, the fluid is aspirated. If a cruciate ligament has been damaged, the fluid usually contains a considerable amount of blood. A compression dressing is applied, and weight-bearing is restricted or avoided by the use of crutches. This regimen is usually followed until the reaction to injury about the joint has subsided. Occasionally, plaster cylinder immobilization for 4 to 6 weeks is justified. With anterior cruciate lesions, the cast should be applied with the knee in 15° to 20° of flexion. With posterior cruciate tears, the tibia should be held forward and in near complete extension during application of the cast. Strenuous quadriceps-setting exercises during convalescence are important in minimizing residual disability following all tears of the cruciate ligaments.

When a torn cruciate ligament is diagnosed as part of a chronic instability of the knee due to other than a most recent (up to 14 days) injury, about all that can be accomplished is strengthening of the quadriceps muscle by an intensive course of exercises. A strong quadriceps musculature compensates in a large measure for loss of the stabilizing effect of a cruciate ligament.

Loose Osteocartilaginous Bodies

The exact cause of these is not known. They are generally considered to be secondary to injuries which cause necrosis of a portion of articular cartilage and its subchondral bone. This piece of bone and cartilage is gradually separated from its bed until it falls free into the joint cavity. The most common site of origin of a loose body is the inner or anterolateral surface of the medial condyle of the femur. The condition leading to separation of such a body is called osteochondritis dissecans.

The symptoms of a loose body in the knee joint are some pain in the knee and recurring slipping, snapping, catching episodes, usually without true locking of the joint. The patient may experience frequent "giving-way" sensations. Recurring effusions are common. The patient actually may palpate a movable particle on either side or the front of the knee.

On examination the surgeon may feel the movable particle. There may be some atrophy of the quadriceps musculature. Otherwise, the physical findings are usually normal.

The diagnosis often is made (or confirmed, if a loose body has been palpable) by the x-ray examination which discloses the loose radiopaque particle varying in size from that of a pea to a large bean. It may lie in the intercondylar notch of the femur or in the knee joint bursa (quadriceps pouch). Occasionally, a loose body may be palpable and not show on x-ray examination. This indicates that the loose body is cartilaginous rather than osteocartilaginous.

Treatment. The indicated therapy is arthrotomy and removal of the loose body or bodies. If this is not done, nonoperative symptomatic therapy is the same as for a sprain of the knee.

FRACTURES OF THE PATELLA

The patella is a large sesamoid bone incorporated in the extensor mechanism of the thigh at the level of the knee. Practically full function of the extremity may be present with the patella removed, yet it does serve

several useful purposes. It protects the joint cavity and its contents from injury; it serves as a fulcrum for the extensor mechanism as the flexed leg is extended, thereby permitting better and smoother extensor action; and, cosmetically, it contributes to the contour of the knee.

Fractures of the patella are of real clinical significance only to the extent that the extensor mechanism is divided. An undisplaced or unseparated fracture of the patella on x-ray examination indicates that the surrounding tendon and the retinaculum patellae have not been interrupted. While these injuries are painful and cause some temporary loss of function, essentially the extensor mechanism remains intact, and the power of extension of the leg at the knee is not lost. On the other hand, displacement or separation of the fragments of a broken patella on x-ray examination demonstrates that the soft tissue structures about it have been severed to some extent. In these instances, the extensor mechanism has been interrupted and the power to extend the leg at the knee is lost.

Treatment

The objectives of management in fractures of the patella are: the restoration or maintenance of the extensor mechanism of the thigh; a smooth articular surface of the patella; strong musculature of the thigh, particularly the quadriceps muscle group; and maximum range of extension and flexion of the leg at the knee.

Without Separation of the Fragments

These fractures are accompanied by considerable hemarthrosis, for which aspiration followed by some form of compression dressing is desirable. Immobilization is not necessary if the patient will adequately protect the extremity against a sudden uncontrolled flexion of the leg at the knee which could tear the soft tissues about the patella, resulting in separation of the fragments. Usually, the use of crutches or perhaps only a cane will serve as an adequate safeguard against such a complication. Since early mobility of the knee joint is permitted, this application of the do-nothing method of management (Method 5) predisposes to the maximum return of motion in the knee and minimizes the duration of temporary disability.

When the patient cannot be trusted to protect the knee against additional injury or if he prefers to avoid the use of crutches, the undisplaced fracture of the patella may be protected by a plaster cylinder extending from the upper thigh to a short distance above the ankle with the knee extended to about 175°. The plaster cylinder should be applied over stockinet which is fastened to the skin by tincture of benzoin or some comparable preparation. With the distal end of the stockinet turned back and incorporated in the cast, the cast itself becomes fastened in place and does not tend to drift downward when the patient is ambulatory. With such a plaster cylinder in place, the patient may walk without the aid of crutches. From 4 to 6 weeks of such immobilization is sufficient.

WITH SEPARATION OF THE FRAGMENTS

These fractures present classical indications for primary open reduction (Method 3). Closed methods are inadequate. The operation is designed to repair the defect in the soft tissue portion of the extensor mechanism and in some instances (see below) accurately approximate the fragments of the patella.

Separated fractures of the patella may be classified as (1) fractures with two major fragments and practically no comminution, (2) one major fragment with comminution of the other—usually the distal fragment—and (3) comminuted fractures of the entire patella.

The operative technic varies in these 3 types of displaced fractures of the patella. In fractures with 2 major fragments, a circumferential loop of strong stainless steel wire properly woven in the tendinous tissue may be used to approximate the raw surfaces of bone accurately (Fig. 20-12). In fractures with comminution of the distal or proximal fragment, removal of the comminuted pieces is usually preferable, with approximation of the patella tendon to the raw distal surface of the proximal fragment or of the quadriceps tendon to the raw proximal surface of the remaining distal fragment by a loop of strong wire. In severely comminuted fractures of the entire patella, patellectomy is usually the procedure of choice.

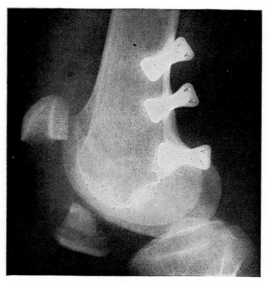

FIG. 20-12. Separated fracture of patella treated by reduction and fixation with a loop of stainless steel wire. (*Top*) Roentgenogram before reduction, lateral view. (*Bottom*) Roentgenograms after reduction, anteroposterior and lateral views. In this instance two additional fine-wire sutures were inserted through the anterior cortex of the patella to ensure perfect opposition of the fragments.

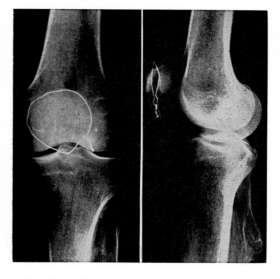

In all of these operative technics, the tears in the extensor mechanism—that is, the expansions of the quadriceps tendon and capsule —must be repaired accurately with interrupted nonabsorbable sutures. When a comminuted

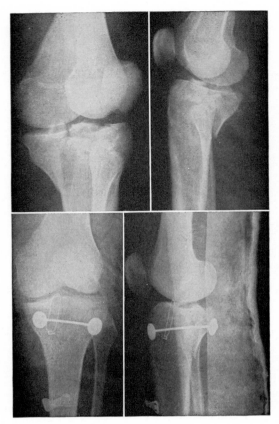

FIG. 20-13. Comminuted fracture of condyles of tibia, including fracture of tibial spine. (*Top*) Anteroposterior-oblique and lateral roentgenograms soon after injury. (*Bottom*) Anteroposterior and lateral roentgenograms after open reduction and internal fixation with tibial bolt. The elevated tibial spine was fixed in position with a loop of wire passed through drill holes.

fragment of the patella has been removed, often it will be advantageous to imbricate the torn tissues. An accurate repair of the torn tendon and capsule is an integral part of the operative treatment of fractures of the patella.

Postoperative immobilization may or may not be used. If the operative repair has been entirely satisfactory, immobilization is not really necessary, and after soft tissue healing early motion may be instituted. If there is some doubt about the operative repair, a plaster cylinder as described above may be employed for a few weeks.

FRACTURES OF THE PROXIMAL END OF THE TIBIA

Fractures of the proximal end of the tibia may be grouped as fractures of the (1) spine, (2) the lateral condyle, (3) the medial condyle and (4) both the medial and the lateral condyles. In each of these, one or more lines of fracture extend through articular cartilage and enter the knee joint. Objectives of management of each is to achieve as near perfect reduction as possible in order to restore accurately the contour of the articulating surface of the tibia and the stability of the joint.

The diagnosis of these fractures may be suspected by the symptoms and signs at the knee, but only by adequate x-ray studies can it be confirmed and the type of the fracture determined. At times, oblique views supplementing the routine anteroposterior and lateral views will be valuable.

SPINE

These are avulsion fractures, as the fragment of bones is pulled away by the anterior cruciate ligament to which it remains attached. They occur in adolescence as an isolated injury. In adults they may be the only significant injury at the knee or they may be part of a comminuted fracture involving one or both condyles of the tibia or complicate an essentially ligamentous internal derangement of the knee (usually a torn medial collateral ligament).

Treatment. When the fragment is not displaced or when a displaced fragment will drop into perfect position upon moderate extension of the knee, a long leg plaster cast is applied. The knee joint is aspirated if blood is present. As a rule, in displaced fractures open operation is indicated to fix the fragment in position. This may be accomplished by a mattress suture of catgut, silk or fine wire passing through 2 parallel drill holes beginning over the anterior medial surface of the tibia, emerging through the defect in the articular surface of the tibia and then passing through 2 comparable drill holes in the small bony fragment (Fig. 20-13). In this way, the loop of suture material becomes buried in the substance of the anterior cruciate ligament. Postoperatively, a long leg cast is applied with the knee extended to about 165°. The cast remains in place for 4 to 6 weeks.

LATERAL CONDYLE

These fractures may occur as a result of a force applied to an extended knee from the lateral side such as that provided by the bumper of a moving automobile (the common bumper fracture), or from above as might result in a fall from a height when the extremity is somewhat abducted at the hip. These mechanisms of injury force the leg into abduction at the knee. The lateral condyle of the femur and the tibia are suddenly compressed against each other. The same mechanisms of injury place a stretching force on the medial collateral ligament (see p. 416). A fracture of the lateral condyle of the tibia or the femur or a tear of the medial collateral ligament or some combination of these injuries may result. Also, the lateral semilunar cartilage may be torn by the same force when a fracture of the lateral condyle occurs, or the medial cartilage may be torn when a tear of the medial collateral ligament has resulted.

Fractures of the lateral condyle of the tibia may consist essentially of one large fragment or they may be severely comminuted. The fragments may remain in good position or be widely displaced. Several fragments, including portions of the articular cartilage, may be driven downward into the cancellous bone of the condyle.

Treatment. Considerable accumulation of blood in the joint is usually present. This is removed by aspiration of the joint before any form of immobilization is applied.

When the displacement is nil or minimal, a long leg plaster cast usually is provided for 5 or 6 weeks (Method 1). In some instances, when the fragments are so well impacted that further displacement will not occur, a cast may be omitted in favor of a compression dressing for 10 to 14 days. If so, active motion of the joint and quadriceps exercises are immediately instituted. Weight-bearing is avoided, but the patient can be up on crutches. This is an application of Method 5, No Immobilization.

When a large fragment of lateral condyle is displaced laterally or downward, it must be reduced accurately and held reduced until bony union has taken place. At times, reduc-

tion can be achieved by lateral compression, for which a carpenter's C-clamp is applicable. After accurate reduction is verified by immediate roentgenograms, a long leg plaster cast is applied. The cast should extend as far into the groin as possible.

However, open reduction of a displaced large condylar fragment is often preferable. The fragment can be reduced accurately under direct visualization and stabilized in excellent position by a bolt passing through it and the medial condyle. While the knee joint is open, any small chips of bone or cartilage and, if it is present, a torn lateral semilunar cartilage are removed. With the fragments firmly fixed in good position, plaster immobilization may be removed after only a few weeks or actually may be omitted altogether so that early active exercises are possible. Open reduction and internal fixation (Method 3) is likely to give the best result obtainable in this type of injury.

In comminuted fractures of the lateral condyle, several fragments are usually depressed downward and spread laterally. Therefore, the articular surface of the condyle is quite distorted. Adequate closed reduction cannot be obtained in most instances. Occasionally, side-to-side compression manually or with a carpenter's C-clamp will give a satisfactory reduction which may be held by a long leg plaster cast. Usually, however, particularly when several fragments including portions of the articular surface are depressed into the substance of the lateral condyle, open reduction is indicated. After the several fragments have been elevated and the articular surface of the condyle reconstituted as best possible, a defect remains in the condyle as a result of the compression of the cancellous bone. This is filled with bone chips removed from the adjacent tibia, the lateral condyle of the femur or the wing of the ilium so as to maintain the elevation of the articular fragments. Usually, supplementary internal fixation is advantageous. At best, a slightly irregular articular surface of the lateral condyle is likely to result. Postoperatively in comminuted fractures, from 6 to 8 weeks of immobilization in a long leg plaster cast is necessary.

In all fractures of the lateral condyle, whether they have been managed by closed reduction and immobilization (Method 1), by open reduction and internal fixation (Method 3), or by no immobilization (Method 5), prolonged protection from weight-bearing is necessary. While ambulation with crutches is permissible, weight-bearing must be avoided until there is solid bony union of the fragments. This usually requires from 3 to 6 months, depending upon the severity of the fracture. Too early weight-bearing while bony union is immature is likely to cause some depression of the lateral condyle with resulting knock-knee, instability and subsequent traumatic arthritis.

MEDIAL CONDYLE

These fractures may occur as a result of a force applied from the medial side to an extended knee, the opposite direction of the force which causes a fracture of the lateral condyle. A fall from a height is unlikely to produce a fracture of the medial condyle, as the extremity is seldom adducted at the hip at the time that the feet strike the ground; moreover, the slight normal valgus of the leg at the knee minimizes the chances of an impact causing a varus strain. The forces which tend to produce a fracture of the medial condyle of the tibia also may cause a tear of the lateral collateral ligament of the knee. Either or both of these may result.

Treatment. Treatment for fractures of the medial condyle of the tibia is entirely analogous to that of fractures of the lateral condyle (see p. 421). The same principles for obtaining reduction of the fracture, for providing immobilization when necessary, and mobilization and exercise as early as possible with prolonged protection from weight-bearing are applicable.

LATERAL AND MEDIAL CONDYLES (T-FRACTURES)

These fractures may occur as a result of a compression force which impacts the condyles of the tibia and the femur together while the knee is extended. They result from falls from a height or in vehicle accidents from the force of an uprising floor board which jams the condyles of an extended tibia against those of the femur. Each condyle may be essentially a large single fragment or both may be severely comminuted.

Treatment. Aspiration of blood from the knee joint is indicated. The choice of treatment for the fracture depends principally upon the degree of comminution of the fragments.

Occasionally, displacement of the fragments will be so minimal that reduction is not necessary. Mildly displaced fragments can be reduced in some instances by closed manipulation using manual traction applied at the ankle and side-to-side compression at the proximal end of the tibia. In either instance, immobilization is provided by a long leg cast. Much caution is required to make certain that the extremity is held so that neither a knock-knee nor a bowleg strain is made during application of the cast.

When the fragments are significantly displaced, open reduction or continuous traction is usually preferable. At times, a combination of these will give the best result.

When large condylar fragments are spread laterally and medially, they often can be approximated with a tibial bolt so as to restore the articular surface of the tibia (Fig. 20-13). The fixation of the condyles may provide sufficient stability at the fracture site to permit the use of a long leg plaster cast for immobilization. In other instances, continuous skeletal traction using a pin through the distal tibia will be necessary to avoid some telescoping of the shaft between the condyles and resulting shortening.

When the condylar fragments are severely comminuted and displaced, continuous skeletal traction is the preferable method of management. Traction must be maintained until sufficient healing has occurred so that the fragments will not telescope again. This usually requires from 6 to 8 weeks in traction. Then, further immobilization in a cast is usually necessary.

The period of immobilization in these fractures varies. It may be only a few weeks in impacted fractures. In severely comminuted fractures which are displaced, immobilization must be maintained for several months. When union has progressed to a point where redisplacement or angulation will not occur, removal of all immobilization is advisable in order to permit exercise of the knee. As with fractures of either the medial or the lateral condyle, however, weight-bearing must be avoided until bony union is solid and mature.

FRACTURES OF THE SHAFTS OF THE BONES OF THE LEG

Fractures of the shafts of the bones of the leg result both from direct trauma, such as the impact of an automobile bumper, and indirect trauma, such as the rotation or leverage strain incurred when an individual steps into a deep hole while running. One or both bones may be broken, and the fracture of either may be transverse, oblique, spiral, double or even triple, and minimally or severely comminuted. Because the tibia is entirely subcutaneous on its anterior and medial surfaces, open fractures of this bone are common.

Diagnosis of fractures of the shafts of the bones of the leg is usually established easily by the clinical symptoms and signs, especially when the tibia is broken. However, adequate roentgenograms are essential to determine the extent and the contour of the fractures so that the proper method of management can be selected.

A pitfall in diagnosis is the erroneous conclusion that only a fracture of the tibia is present when actually both bones are broken. This is important, not because the fragments of the fibula must be reduced, but because when the fibula is broken, its splinting effect on the tibia is lost, a factor which may be significant in the selection of the proper method of management for the tibia. Failure to recognize a fracture of the fibula is most likely to occur with a spiral or oblique fracture of the lower third of the tibia which on roentgenograms of the lower half of the leg is shown in fairly good position with minimal displacement and overriding. If a fracture of the fibula is not visualized, it may be wrongly concluded that the fibula is intact and that further displacement of the fracture of the tibia will not occur. Actually, the fibula may be broken in the unvisualized proximal third, a not uncommon location for such a fracture in association with spiral or oblique fractures of the tibia in the lower third. This combination of injuries is produced by a twisting trauma on the foot and the ankle. It is important that the entire shafts of both the tibia and the fibula be well visualized on roentgenograms before the diagnosis of a fracture of the tibia alone or even of the fibula alone is made (Fig. 20-14).

Fractures of the shafts of both bones of the

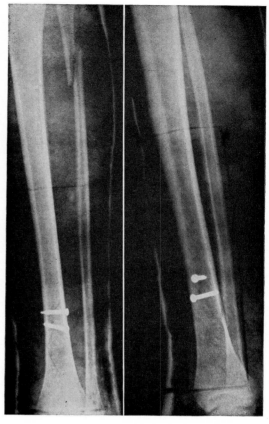

FIG. 20-14. Roentgenograms in 2 planes of spiral-oblique fracture of lower shaft of tibia with associated fracture of proximal fibula. Treatment by open reduction of fracture of tibia and internal fixation with 2 screws. Note the window in the cast made for dressing the wound and removal of the sutures. Replacement of the window minimizes localized edema. (*Left*) Anteroposterior view. (*Right*) Lateral view.

leg are problem fractures for several reasons. As stated above, many are open fractures so that the hazard of wound infection and prolonged drainage is introduced. Reduction is often not only difficult to obtain but even more difficult to maintain. Circulation to the soft tissues of the leg, particularly on the anteromedial surface in the lower third, is at times so precarious as to make operative intervention too risky. Nonunion of a fracture of the tibia occurs not infrequently, not only because of the reasons just enumerated but chiefly because this bone has meager muscle attach-

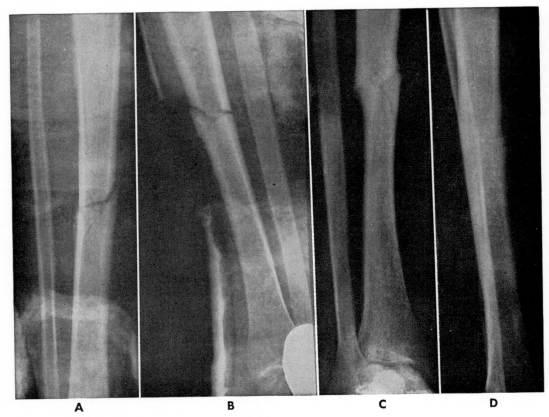

| A | B | C | D |

Fɪɢ. 20-15. Stable fracture of the tibial shaft. (A and B) Roentgenograms of stable near transverse fracture treated successfully by closed reduction and immobilization in a long leg plaster cast, utilizing the "3-way plaster" technic (see text). Anteroposterior and lateral roentgenograms taken at time of reduction. (C and D) Roentgenograms in 2 planes, showing united fracture.

ments and blood supply, especially in the lower half.

TREATMENT

Each of the first 4 methods of management —(1) closed reduction and immobilization, (2) balanced skeletal traction, (3) open reduction and (4) external skeletal fixation (usually by transfixion pins incorporated in plaster)—finds application for certain fractures of the shaft of the tibia. The fact that one of 4 different methods may be indicated is further evidence of the complexity of these injuries. Precise surgical judgment is often required for the selection of the best method of management.

The selection of the method of management is based upon several factors. Of these, the contour of the fracture as revealed by the roentgenograms is probably the most important. Others are the general condition and age of the patient, the quality of the circulation to the foot and the leg, the character of the skin overlying the fracture site, the presence of other injuries, the equipment at hand, and the experience and the ability of the surgeon.

Closed Reduction and Immobilization (Method 1). Closed reduction with immobilization in a long leg plaster cast is usually selected for fractures of the shaft of both bones of the leg when a stable reduction of the tibia may be achieved (or is already present in undisplaced fractures) (Fig. 20-15). A reduction is classified as stable when, because the contour of the fracture is transverse or so near transverse, displacement of the fragments is unlikely to recur so long as they are kept in good alignment. A stable reduction is not to be anticipated when the contour of the fracture is oblique, spiral or appreciably comminuted.

Reduction is achieved under general or spinal anesthesia by means of strong traction on the foot and the ankle against equally strong countertraction, usually applied at the knee, together with direct manipulation of the fragments at the fracture site bringing the distal fragment first into apposition and then into alignment with the proximal fragment. The stability of reduction is tested by gently compressing the distal fragment against the proximal fragment while good alignment is maintained. If the reduction is not sufficiently stable to withstand this compression force, it usually will not be maintained in a plaster cast.

When a satisfactory, stable reduction has been achieved (check roentgenograms at this stage are valuable) a lightly padded, long leg cast is applied. It extends from the upper thigh to the toes and holds the ankle at a right angle, the foot in neutral version, and the knee, as a rule, in 10° to 15° of flexion. The cast should be well molded, especially about the knee and the foot and the ankle.

The "three-way" plaster technic may facilitate the application of this method. By this technic one segment of plaster is applied from the groin to just above the fracture and another segment from the toes to just below the fracture. The fracture site itself is left uncovered. Then manipulation of the fracture is carried out using the 2 segments covered with plaster (Fig. 20-15). When reduction has been achieved the 2 segments are joined by applying plaster over the fracture site. The advantage of this method is that better control of the proximal and the distal fragments is effected, and one does not incur the risk of redisplacement while the cast is being applied about the knee and the ankle.

Closed reduction and immobilization in a plaster cast can be applied for a large percentage of the fractures of the shaft of both bones of the leg in adults and, for practical purposes, it is indicated for all of these fractures in growing children. It offers many advantages. It is a method with few pitfalls and complications. It entails no risk to life or limb. It makes the patient immediately ambulatory on crutches. It gives a very high percentage of good results, provided that the reduction is maintained in the plaster cast. However, if reduction is unstable, other methods must be used, even though they are more confining and may entail some risk. When an unstable rather than a stable reduction is to be anticipated from the contour of the fracture one of the other methods must be selected primarily unless there are complications. The choice between these will rest principally on the contour of the fracture, although the other factors mentioned above must also be evaluated carefully.

Continuous Traction (Method 2). This method may be selected for varying reasons. In comminuted fractures precluding a stable reduction by closed or open methods, traction will serve to maintain length and usually adequate apposition and alignment. In oblique or spiral fractures for which open operation might otherwise be preferable but which is contraindicated because of bad skin, the general condition of the patient, inadequate equipment or facilities, or inexperience on the part of the surgeon in the open treatment of fractures, continuous traction affords a highly acceptable method of management.

Skeletal traction using a Kirschner wire or a Steinmann pin through the lower tibia or the os calcis is far preferable to skin traction. The latter is, for practical purposes, ineffective for fractures of both bones of the leg.

Splinting for the skeletal traction may be provided in several ways. The extremity may be suspended in a Thomas splint with Pierson knee attachment or on a Böhler-Braun frame. More effective splinting, however, is provided by the use of skeletal traction combined with a plaster cast.

Skeletal traction in a cast is provided as follows: after insertion of wire or a pin and attachment of a traction bow, strong manual traction is applied, and the fragments are manipulated until good apposition and alignment are obtained. While the traction is maintained, a long leg padded plaster cast is applied. The padding is usually made rather heavy at the knee in order that the fixation there will not be absolute. The plaster incorporates the pin or wire and traction bow. The foot is immobilized at a right angle, and the

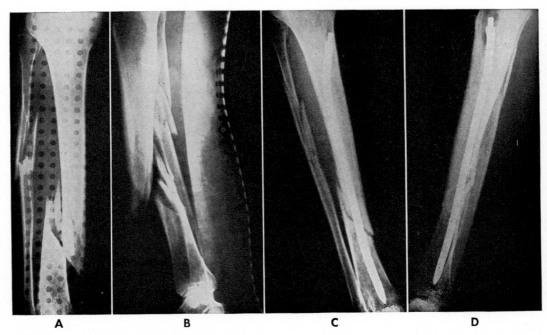

FIG. 20-16. Comminuted open fracture of both bones of leg in lower part of middle third. Treatment by débridement, internal fixation with a Lottes intramedullary nail and primary closure of the wound. (A and B) Roentgenograms in 2 planes with emergency splint in place. (C and D) Several months after operation, showing excellent apposition and alignment and early long union.

knee preferably in slight flexion. As the plaster is hardening, every effort is made to maintain perfect alignment of the fragments.

Postoperatively, the leg in the cast is placed on one or two pillows, and from 10 to 12 pounds of traction is provided. The patient may be turned to either side so long as the general direction of the traction remains the same. Traction is maintained until sufficient healing has occurred to maintain apposition and length. This usually requires from 5 to 6 weeks. Then, the wire or pin may be removed and perhaps a new cast applied for further immobilization. Throughout the period of traction, check roentgenograms in two views are made to ensure that the amount of traction is adequate but not excessive and that good alignment is being maintained.

Open Reduction and Internal Fixation (Method 3). This method may be selected for fractures having a contour permitting a stable internal fixation, provided that the equipment, the facilities and the experience of the surgeon are adequate. Oblique or spiral fractures of the tibia may be fixed with multiple screws (Fig. 20-14).

Intramedullary nailing of the tibia is being used increasingly for fractures of the shafts of both bones of the leg (Fig. 20-16). When the contour of the fracture will permit a reasonable stable fixation by an intramedullary nail, it is probably the best type of internal fixation. Fractures with enough comminution to prevent a stable closed reduction can often be stabilized adequately with this technic. Surgeons experienced in the use of intramedullary nails in the tibia can insert them "blindly" in closed fractures, that is, without an incision at the fracture site and thereby avoid any risk of wound complications at that level. Fractures with minimal comminution or with only a "butterfly"-shaped comminuted fragment also may be fixed with a plate, preferably slotted, held by screws (Fig. 20-17).

Supplemental immobilization in a plaster cast is essential following all forms of internal fixation, including intramedullary nailing. With the latter, earlier weight-bearing in a

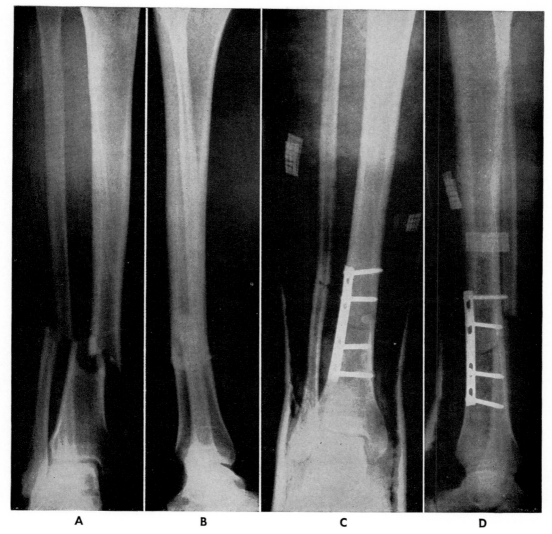

A   B   C   D

FIG. 20-17. Fractures of both bones of the leg in the distal third. Treatment by open reduction of the tibia and internal fixation with a slotted plate and screws. (A and B) Roentgenograms in 2 planes before operation. (C and D) After operation.

walking cast is feasible, and often this can be initiated a few weeks after operation.

External Skeletal Fixation (Method 4). This method has been used for unstable fractures of both bones of the leg. Its application with true external skeletal fixation apparatus (Roger Anderson or Stader apparatus are examples) is not a recommended procedure. Certainly, this method should be used only by surgeons with extensive experience with it.

An acceptable substitute is provided by a long leg plaster cast incorporating transfixion pins through the upper and the lower major fragments (Fig. 20-18). The pins are inserted, the fracture is held reduced, and the cast is applied. The pins are removed, and a new cast is substituted after enough healing of the fracture has occurred to prevent displacement and overriding of the fragments.

Period of Immobilization. The period of time required for solid healing of fractures of both bones of the leg will vary with the age of the patient, the contour and the location of the fracture of the tibia and the quality of the

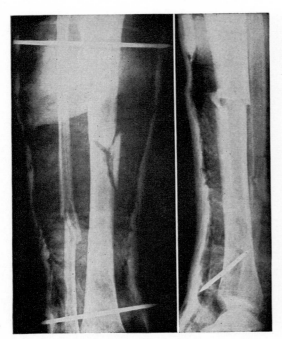

Fig. 20-18. Unstable fracture of both bones of the leg in the midshaft held in good reduction by a transfixion pin above and another below the fracture and incorporated in a long leg plaster cast. (*Left*) Anteroposterior and (*right*) lateral roentgenograms.

reduction and immobilization of the fragments. With all methods of management healing is slow and requires many months. While, in general, union is secured faster in closed than in open fractures and when apposition of the fragments is excellent and is maintained, even under these favorable circumstances, a long time may be required for solid union of the fracture of the tibia.

Older textbooks frequently have estimated the period of immobilization and for union of these fractures as from 8 to 12 weeks. This is entirely too short. The average period for adequate union is at least 4 or 5 months. Union does not take place in many for 8 or 10 months. Immobilization must be continued until the fracture of the tibia is solidly united, clinically and as shown on roentgenograms. The immobilization may be discontinued before union of the fracture is complete only in those fractures adequately stabilized by intra-

medullary nailing and, even with these, a walking plaster cast for several months is less hazardous than early removal of the immobilization.

FRACTURES OF THE SHAFT OF THE TIBIA WITH AN INTACT FIBULA

Fractures of the shaft of the tibia alone usually are not significantly displaced and require only immobilization in a long leg plaster cast (Method 1) with the knee in some 10° to 15° of flexion and the foot at 90° and in neutral version. The splinting effect of the intact fibula may effect a stable reduction of a fracture of the tibia with a contour which otherwise would indicate an unstable situation. Occasionally, however, significant displacement of a fracture of the tibia will occur even with an intact fibula. This often can be overcome and a stable reduction obtained by closed manipulation, following which the cast is applied. Infrequently, usually in spiral fractures in the lower third of the tibia, adequate apposition of the fragments cannot be maintained after closed reduction, so operative reduction and internal fixation (usually with 2 or more screws) are indicated. The perfect reduction obtained at operation avoids the slight shortening of the tibia which would result from overriding of the fragments. Such a shortening would cause permanent disturbance of the ankle joint relationship. Perfect reduction also shortens the healing time by providing excellent contact of the fragments. But even with internal fixation of the fracture, immobilization in a long leg plaster cast is essential.

The period of time required for solid healing of a fracture of the tibia alone, as with fractures of both bones of the leg, will vary with its contour and location and the age of the patient. In children, in whom fractures of the tibia alone are not uncommon, the period of immobilization should be from 3 to 4 weeks in very small children and from 6 to 8 weeks in young teen-agers. In adults a longer period of time is usually required. Certainly, from 8 to 10 weeks of immobilization is the minimum, from 12 to 14 the average, and from 16 to 18 not uncommon. The prognosis for union of a fracture of the tibia alone is excellent, but nonunion may occur, especially in

Fig. 20-19. Drawings to show bony and ligamentous support of the ankle mortise.

(A) The normal ankle, showing major ligamentous support of the ankle mortise.

(B) Bimalleolar fracture with lateral displacement of foot. The ligaments are intact.

(C) Fracture of the lateral malleolus and a disrupted deltoid ligament on the medial side of the ankle joint with lateral displacement of the foot. The injuries in (A) and (C) are quite comparable.

(D) Disruption of the deltoid ligament and the ligament supporting the inferior tibial-fibular synchondrosis with lateral displacement of the foot comparable in part to that in (C).

(Hampton, O. P., Jr., and Fitts, W. T., Jr.: Open Reduction of Common Fractures, New York, Grune & Stratton.)

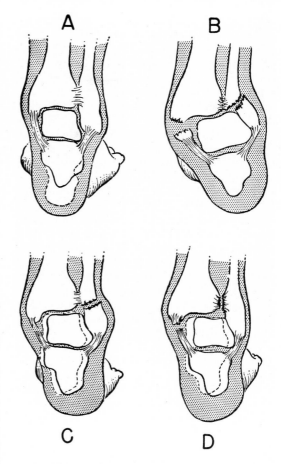

transverse fractures of the shaft of the tibia in the middle or lower thirds.

FRACTURES OF THE SHAFT OF THE FIBULA WITH AN INTACT TIBIA

Fractures of the shaft of the fibula are not important skeletal injuries. When this fracture accompanies a fracture of the shaft of the tibia, all efforts should be directed toward obtaining and maintaining adequate reduction of the latter, and the fracture of the fibula may be ignored. When the shaft of the fibula alone is broken, the intact tibia splints the fragments and they practically always remain in good position.

Fractures of the shaft of the fibula alone are usually immobilized in a plaster cast in order to minimize pain and maintain the foot in a good functioning position, although healing undoubtedly would occur without immobilization. A plaster cast applied for a fracture of the shaft of the fibula need not extend above the knee. The plaster need be kept on for only 3 to 4 weeks, although solid union of the fracture may not take place for 6 to 8 weeks.

FRACTURES AND DISLOCATIONS OF THE ANKLE

The ankle joint depends upon ligamentous as well as bony structures for its integrity. The ligaments supporting the inferior tibio-fibular synchondrosis contribute materially to the stability of the ankle by maintaining the ankle mortise, bony framework formed by the malleoli about the talus. The large deltoid ligament on the medial side of the joint and the calcaneofibular and the talofibular ligaments on the lateral side maintain the talus in the mortise and prevent abnormal lateral motion.

In evaluating and managing bony injuries about the ankle joint, it must be determined whether or not these ligaments have been torn (Fig. 20-19). A torn deltoid ligament, for example, is probably as significant as a fracture of the medial malleolus. Figure 20-19 B shows a bimalleolar fracture with lateral displacement of the malleolar fragments and the foot. Figure 20-19 C shows a fracture of the lateral malleolus only with the same displacement. For this to occur without fracture of the medial malleolus, the deltoid ligament must be torn. The injuries shown in Figures

20-19 B and 20-19 C then are entirely comparable insofar as the integrity of the ankle joint is concerned. Similarly, Figure 20-19 D shows a lateral dislocation of the foot without fracture. For this to occur, there must be disruption of both the deltoid ligament and the ligament supporting the inferior tibiofibular synchondrosis.

In addition to the malleoli and the strong ligaments of the ankle, the surgeon is concerned with the "posterior malleolus" of the tibia in injuries about the ankle. This posterolateral prominence of the tibia contains the posterior portion of the articular surface. It is frequently fractured and displaced away posteriorly or upward from the main body of the tibia. When a fracture of the posterior malleolus is the only injury about the ankle, it remains undisplaced. When it is associated with either a fracture of the medial or the lateral malleolus or of both, or a rupture of a major ligament, the foot and the posterior malleolus often are displaced posteriorly.

Fractures of the ankle result from strong abduction or adduction strains. They may be classified as those of (1) lateral malleolus, (2) medial malleolus or (3) posterior malleolus, and (4) bimalleolar (medial and lateral malleoli) or (5) trimalleolar fractures. As outlined above, any of these may be associated with dislocation. A trimalleolar fracture-dislocation of the ankle is not an uncommon injury.

TREATMENT

Treatment of fractures about the ankle varies with the degree of displacement of the malleolar fragments and the foot. The objectives of management of fractures about the ankle are: (1) to restore the talus to its proper place beneath the tibia; (2) to reduce accurately the fractures of all the malleoli; and (3) to maintain the reduction of the fractures and dislocation until all disrupted bony and ligamentous structures have healed. If any degree of dislocation of the talus or widening of the mortise is allowed to persist, instability, pain, early traumatic arthritis, and considerable disability are likely to follow.

FRACTURES OF THE ANKLE WITHOUT DISPLACEMENT

These fractures require only plaster cast immobilization (Method 1). Usually, the cast may extend only to just below the knee; but it should extend to the upper thigh if there is any question of subsequent displacement of the fragments in the cast, as in many trimalleolar and bimalleolar fractures. The ankle should be held at 90° and the foot in neutral version. Immobilization in plantar flexion and inversion is to be avoided, as this position predisposes to prolonged disability after the cast is removed. Usually, a walking type cast is advantageous.

Healing of a fracture of the lateral malleolus, even though it has not been displaced, is not rapid, and fracture lines may be visible on roentgenograms for several months. Usually, however, from 6 to 8 weeks of immobilization in a cast will permit sufficient union to make further immobilization unnecessary. A fracture of the medial malleolus unites more rapidly, and 4 weeks of immobilization is usually sufficient. The most rapid healing in fractures about the ankle occurs in those of the posterior malleolus. These fracture lines on roentgenograms have been observed to disappear in $2\frac{1}{2}$ to 3 weeks. Bimalleolar and trimalleolar fractures should be immobilized for 6 to 8 weeks.

FRACTURES OF THE ANKLE WITH DISPLACEMENT

These fractures require precise reduction. Usually closed reduction (Method 1) with immobilization in a plaster cast will suffice, but in many instances open reduction (Method 3) is necessary or advantageous.

Fractures of the Lateral Malleolus With Lateral Dislocation of the Foot (Fig. 20-20). Precise reduction of the dislocation and the fracture is essential. For this, general anesthesia or spinal anesthesia is necessary. The manipulative maneuvers are manual traction on the foot with pressure on the fragment toward its normal position. These should be carried out with the knee flexed from 45° to 90° to relax the gastrocnemius muscle. Flexion of the knee over the side or the end of the table will provide the necessary flexion.

This displacement cannot take place unless the deltoid ligament is torn. Some authorities strongly recommend operative repair of the torn deltoid ligament, which will ensure precise healing of that structure and is a safeguard against recurrence of the lateral dis-

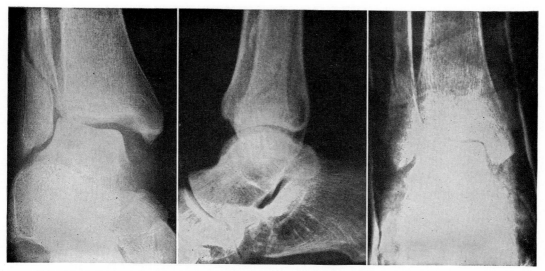

FIG. 20-20. Fracture of lateral malleolus with lateral dislocation of the foot. Treatment by closed reduction. (*Left and Center*) Anteroposterior and lateral roentgenograms before reduction. For this displacement to occur the deltoid ligament must have been ruptured. (*Right*) After closed reduction and immobilization in a plaster cast, anteroposterior view.

placement of the foot while in the cast. If precise reduction of the dislocation cannot be obtained by manipulation and maintained by a cast, it is likely that torn fibers of the deltoid ligament have become caught between the talus and the medial malleolus. Then operative intervention is mandatory. With removal of the intervening soft tissues, reduction of the dislocation is made easy, and if the deltoid ligament is repaired, dislocation will not recur.

In these injuries treated by closed reduction, the plaster cast should extend well above the knee so as to immobilize it and avoid rotation strains at the ankle. These might cause recurrence of the dislocation.

Fractures of the Medial Malleolus. WITH DISPLACEMENT OF THE MALLEOLUS BUT WITHOUT DISLOCATION OF THE ANKLE. The medial malleolus is frequently displaced distally. Usually, under anesthesia, an effort should be made to replace it by full dorsal flexion and perhaps slight inversion of the foot. If the raw edges can be well approximated, immobilization of the leg and the foot in a below-the-knee walking type plaster cast for 4 weeks will permit union of the fragment (Method 1).

In many instances, the raw surface of the medial malleolus cannot be approximated to that of the body of tibia because tags of the deltoid ligament have fallen into the fracture site. In such instances, operation is often indicated to permit removal of the ligament from between the fragments (Method 3). Operative fixation of the medial malleolus usually is obtained by means of a screw or a threaded pin. The internal fixation must be supported by a below-the-knee plaster of Paris cast for at least 4 weeks.

WITH DISPLACEMENT AND LATERAL DISLOCATION OF THE FOOT. As outlined above, this results from disruption of the inferior tibiofibular synchrondrosis. Under these circumstances, manipulative reduction may restore the fibula to its proper place and the medial malleolus into approximation with the tibia, but operative fixation of the malleolus is highly preferable (Method 3). With the malleolus fixed in accurate position, the fibula is pulled back against the tibia, and the ankle mortise is restored. The operative approach is on the medial side of the ankle in this injury, and operation on the outer side of the ankle usually is not necessary. On the other hand, screw fixation of the fibula to the tibia a short distance above the ankle is employed sometimes to aid in maintaining the mortise.

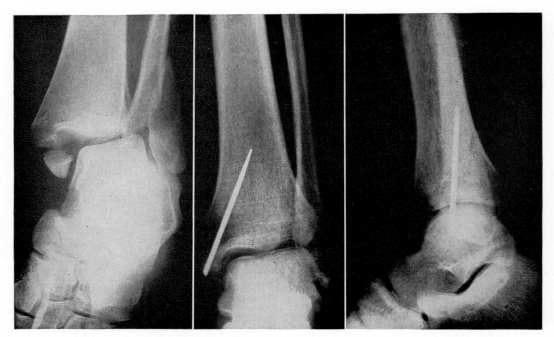

FIG. 20-21. Bimalleolar fracture of the ankle with lateral displacement of the foot, treated by open reduction and internal fixation of medial malleolus. (*Left*) Anteroposterior view before operation. (*Center and Right*) Roentgenograms in 2 planes showing position obtained at operation.

If a screw is used, it should be removed before full weight-bearing is allowed.

In this injury a long leg plaster cast for at least 3 weeks, followed by a below-the-knee plaster cast for an additional 3 to 5 weeks, is indicated. The use of a walking cast is hazardous, as the force of weight-bearing may tend to cause some spread of the mortise.

Bimalleolar Fracture-Dislocation. These injuries present a combination of the problems outlined above for displaced fractures of either malleolus. Usually closed manipulation will provide adequate reduction, which must be maintained in a long leg cast for at least 6 weeks. In many instances manipulation does not provide adequate reduction of the medial malleolus; then operative fixation of the medial malleolus is indicated (Fig. 20-21).

Trimalleolar Fracture-Dislocation of the Ankle. The addition of a fracture of the posterior malleolus to those of the medial and the lateral malleoli with dislocation of the foot creates a more complex problem. If the posterior malleolar fragment is of significant size, accurate reduction of this fragment must be maintained to provide for a smooth articular surface of the tibia (Fig. 20-22). In spite of a perfect closed reduction, displacement of the fragment and redislocation of the foot may occur in a cast.

Actually, the posterior malleolus may determine the preferable method of management. When it includes one third or more of the articular surface of the tibia, closed reduction usually will not be maintained in the cast; therefore, operative fixation of this fragment in reduction is indicated (Method 3). When the posterior malleolus includes less than one third of the articular surface of the tibia, reduction by manipulation may be attempted, and if precise replacement of the posterior malleolus is obtained, a long leg plaster of Paris cast may maintain the reduction (Fig. 20-23). Check roentgenograms every 4 or 5 days for 3 weeks are essential, since the posterior malleolus may become displaced again, thereby permitting redislocation of the foot. In such instances open reduction is then indicated (Fig. 20-24). If the posterior malleolus occupies only a small portion of the articular surface, perhaps 10 per cent, it requires no special attention. Even though reduction of this small fragment is not complete, there is likely to be little if any effect on future function of the ankle; therefore, operation for replacement of a fragment of this size is not justified.

FRACTURES OF THE BONES OF THE FOOT

Fractures of the bones of the foot may be grouped as fractures of (1) calcaneus, (2) talus, (3) midtarsals (navicular, cuboid and cuneiforms), (4) metatarsals and (5) phalanges of the toes.

FRACTURES OF THE CALCANEUS

These, as a group, are by far the most serious fractures of the bones of the foot. They are painful injuries. In all but minor fractures temporary disability is prolonged, and considerable permanent disability is to be anticipated in many instances. Disability often exceeds what would be expected from the findings on roentgenograms. Disability results from pain on weight-bearing, loss of inversion and eversion of the foot, and restriction of motion in the ankle joint. Fractures of the calcaneus are indeed serious injuries.

Mechanism of Injury. Fractures of the calcaneus result from falls onto the heels. In military experience, they are also commonly caused by explosion of land mines or the upsurge of the deck of a torpedoed ship. The same force which causes a fracture of the calcaneus is likely to cause a compression fracture of the spine. Therefore, fractures of the calcaneus routinely indicate a thorough clinical examination and, if at all suggested, roentgenograms of the back.

Fractures of the calcaneus are crush fractures. At impact, the calcaneus is crushed between the talus with the superimposed weight of the body on it and the object onto which the patient fell. Fracture lines may be created in many directions. Characteristic displacements are a downward crushing of the central portion of the calcaneus, including the posterior articular facet into the substance of the bone, lateral and medial spread of corti-

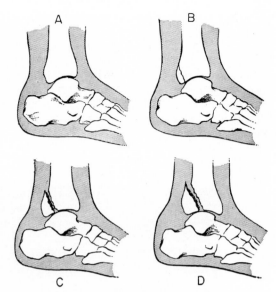

FIG. 20-22. Drawings of fractures of the posterior malleolus

(A) The uninjured ankle.

(B) The fragment of posterior malleolus makes up only about 10 per cent of the articular surface. Fragments of this size may be ignored even if they are not reduced.

(C) The fragment of posterior malleolus makes up about 25 per cent of the articular surface, and the foot is dislocated posteriorly. Fragments of this size must be reduced and held in perfect reduction. At times this can be achieved by closed reduction; however, many require open reduction and internal fixation.

(D) The fragment of posterior malleolus makes up about 35 per cent of the articular surface. Fragments of this size can seldom, if ever, be held in reduction by closed methods. Primary open reduction and internal fixation are preferable.

(Hampton, O. P., Jr., and Fitts, W. T., Jr.: Open Reduction of Common Fractures, New York, Grune & Stratton.)

cal fragments, and an upward displacement of a large posterior fragment to which the tendo achillis is attached. Böhler's angle (Fig. 20-25, *right*) is decreased and may even be reversed.

Diagnosis. Fractures of the calcaneus are characterized clinically by severe local swelling and ecchymosis. Swelling may be so severe as to cause massive bleb formation and even spotty necrosis of the skin overlying the bone.

Special roentgenograms are necessary to determine the type and the extent of the bony injury as well as to establish or confirm the diagnosis. In addition to a lateral view of the calcaneus, an anteroposterior view of this bone itself must be made as illustrated in Figure 20-25, *center* (axial view). At times, only this special view will demonstrate the fracture. It should be obtained routinely in all suspected fractures of the calcaneus.

Treatment. The principles of treatment of fractures of the calcaneus include: reduction of swelling prior to efforts at reduction of the fracture in most instances (fractures of the calcaneus are a definite exception to the rule of prompt reduction and immobilization); the best possible restoration of the contour of the bone, particularly of its articular surface and the tuber angle; immobilization of the foot and the ankle so long as immobilization is serving a useful purpose; mobilization of the foot and the ankle as soon as feasible in order

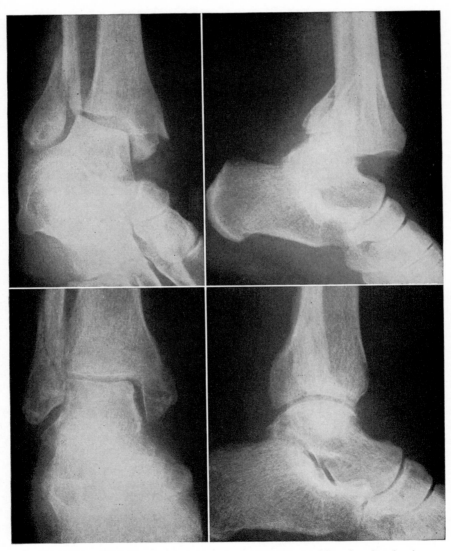

FIG. 20-23. Trimalleolar fracture of the ankle, treated by closed reduction and long leg plaster cast. (*Top*) Anteroposterior and lateral views before reduction. (*Bottom*) After partial healing of the fractures.

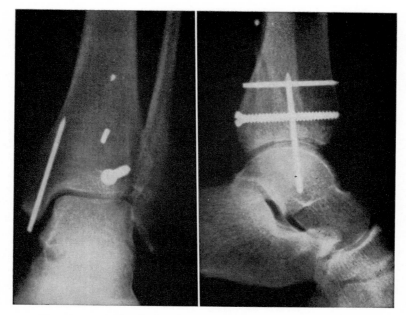

FIG. 20-24. Trimalleolar fracture-dislocation of the ankle after open reduction. Anteroposterior and lateral roentgenograms, showing that a fracture of the medial malleolus and a fracture of the posterior malleolus which contained about one third of the articular surface have been stabilized in excellent reduction so that the danger of redislocation has been eliminated. (Hampton, O. P., Jr., and Fitts, W. T., Jr.: Open Reduction of Common Fractures, New York, Grune & Stratton)

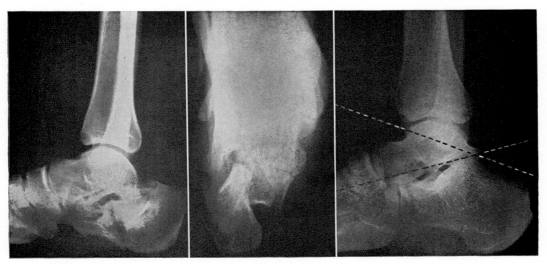

FIG. 20-25. Fracture of the os calcis. (*Left*) Lateral view, showing severe crush fracture with loss of Böhler's angle. (*Center*) Axial view. (*Right*) Normal foot with Böhler's angle demonstrated. This angle is that formed by two lines, one parallel with the superior surface of the tuberosity, and the other joining the anterior and the posterior articular facets. Normally, this angle is about 30°.

to minimize any permanent restriction of motion; freedom from weight-bearing until solid bony union has taken place; and prevention of edema as much as possible by elevation and, following removal of plaster, by adequate elastic support. These principles are applied by various means according to the type, the severity and the degree of displacement of the fracture.

Before reduction of the fracture is attempted or immobilization is applied, the severe swelling about the heel and the ankle should be allowed to subside so that the swollen and edematous soft tissues overlying the calcaneus will not be irreparably damaged during the reduction. When the patient is first seen, a large compression dressing is applied immediately to the foot and the ankle. Then the part is sharply elevated if the arterial circulation permits. Depending upon the severity of the fracture, from 5 to 10 days is usually required before swelling has decreased to a point where reduction should be undertaken. If it is attempted too soon, necrosis of the skin overlying the bone may be precipitated.

Fractures of the calcaneus may be grouped as (1) those requiring no reduction, (2) those which can be reduced reasonably well by closed methods, (3) those which will be benefited by open reduction and (4) those in which reduction is impossible.

Several steps are involved in the closed reduction of fractures of the calcaneus. When the fragments appear to be firmly impacted, this impaction must be broken up as a preliminary to reduction. This may be accomplished by strong manipulation of the heel with the hands or by forcibly striking each side of the padded heel with a large wooden or rubber mallet. Upward displacement of the posterior fragment must be overcome by downward traction on it. During this maneuver, the knee should be fully flexed to relax the calf muscles as much as possible. Traction on the heel may be made manually or on a Steinmann pin inserted through or just above the posterior fragment. After the posterior fragment has been pulled downward, traction is made in a posterior direction in an effort to restore the length of the bone. Downward and backward traction on the posterior fragment tends to restore the tuber angle toward normal. Medial and lateral bulging of comminuted fragments is overcome by side-to-side compression with the hands or preferably with a large C-clamp or a special calcaneus redressor made for this purpose. If a pin is used, it is removed after the fracture has been reduced.

Immobilization is provided with a padded plaster cast. In addition to sheet cotton, heavy felt pads are placed on each side of the calcaneus. As the plaster is setting, firm pressure is made with the heels of the hands over the felt pads. The persisting pressure by the cast serves to minimize exuberant callus beneath the malleoli. The ankle is immobilized in about 15° of plantar flexion and the foot in slight inversion, an exception to the rule of immobilizing ankles at 90° and feet in neutral version. In those instances where an upwardly displaced posterior fragment has been pulled downward, the cast must be extended to the mid-thigh with the knee immobilized in some 30° of flexion.

The duration of immobilization varies with the type of fracture, the degree of displacement and what has been achieved by efforts at reduction. In undisplaced fractures, 3 or 4 weeks of immobilization in a below-knee cast will suffice but, thereafter, all weight-bearing is avoided by the use of crutches until bony union is solid. Early removal of the cast permits active exercise of the foot and the ankle and tends to minimize the loss of motion in both the ankle joint and the subtalar joint. Actually, in certain impacted fractures immobilization serves no purpose and should be omitted in favor of early exercise.

When efforts at reduction have achieved little and the fragments remain unreduced, there is no reason to maintain immobilization for an extended period. It is better to remove the cast within a few weeks and initiate active exercises. In this way, permanent restriction of motion, especially in the ankle, will be minimized even though the fracture has not been reduced accurately.

Whenever the patient becomes ambulatory without a cast, elastic bandage support is provided from the base of the toes to just below the knee in an effort to minimize edema. Persisting edema itself tends to restrict motion of the foot and the ankle, and if edema can be prevented by the constant use of elastic support a better end-result will be obtained.

In those fractures consisting principally of a downward displacement of a fragment containing the posterior articular facet with impaction into the substance of the bone, efforts at closed reduction are usually not worthwhile. In these fractures, open reduction is often indicated. The fragment containing the articular surface is elevated into its normal position so as to restore the contour of the articular surface. A small block of bone from the ilium or the upper tibia is used to fill the defect and to maintain elevation of the fragment. In these instances plaster immobilization should be maintained for about 6 weeks.

In severely comminuted fractures in which it is certain that the contour of the bone, particularly the articular surface, cannot be restored by either closed or open methods, it is doubtful whether any effort to reduce them is worthwhile. It may be best to omit immobilization altogether and to start exercise immediately. In this group of cases, primary subtalar arthrodesis may give the best end-result. This operation is often indicated in late cases when persisting pain and disability warrant further effort at relief.

FRACTURES OF THE TALUS

These fractures result from injuries which produce excessive dorsiflexion of the foot. The fracture occurs across the neck of the talus when it is forced against the anterior rim of the lower end of the tibia.

Treatment. The fracture may remain undisplaced, but some upward displacement of the distal fragment is common. Accurate reduction is essential if a good result is to be obtained. Often closed reduction can be accomplished under anesthesia by strong plantar flexion of the foot. If, however, the fragments cannot be reduced accurately by closed methods, open reduction is indicated. When the fragments have been reduced accurately, a plaster cast is applied for 5 to 6 weeks. Thereafter, weight-bearing must be protected with crutches until union of the fracture is solid.

A displaced fracture of the neck of the talus may be complicated by a partial or complete dislocation of the body of the bone. Incomplete dislocations or subluxations may be overlooked unless the roentgenograms are studied

carefully. Closed manipulation for the fracture may effect reduction of the dislocated body but, if not, open reduction is necessary.

The outstanding complications of a fracture of the neck of the talus is avascular necrosis of the body of the bone (Fig. 20-26). The nutrient arteries for the talus enter through the distal portion of the bone. Therefore, in a fracture of the neck the major blood supply to the body has been destroyed. Avascular necrosis is unlikely to develop in undisplaced fractures but is a distinct possibility when the fracture has been displaced. Dislocations of the body, especially a complete or near complete dislocation in which ligamentous attachments to the bone are torn makes avascular necrosis a probability. When this complication ensues, prolonged protection from weight-bearing is necessary until new blood vessels grow into the body and the dead bone is replaced with living bone. This may require from 10 to 12 months or even more. Too early weight-bearing will cause the body of the talus to collapse, and then repair is impossible. Severe traumatic arthritis of the ankle will follow.

FRACTURES OF THE MIDTARSAL BONES (NAVICULAR, CUBOID AND CUNEIFORM)

These fractures are caused by side-to-side crush injuries or by a heavy weight falling on the foot. The skin and other soft tissues of the foot are often badly bruised or torn. After healing of these fractures, considerable disability often remains. This is caused by pain and soreness on twisting strains of the foot and the loss of motion in the midtarsal joints. Prolonged weight-bearing is usually painful.

Displacement of fragments may be corrected in some instances by manual manipulation. In others, open reduction and some form of internal fixation (Method 3) is advantageous. In still others, the midtarsal bones are so crushed that they can be molded only so as to restore the general contour of the foot.

Immobilization is provided by a plaster cast. This should be exceedingly well molded about the foot so as to conform to and support the arches. A walking heel may be added to facilitate ambulation. Weight-bearing in the cast during the period of healing tends to minimize demineralization and atrophy of the bones of the foot. Immobilization is discon-

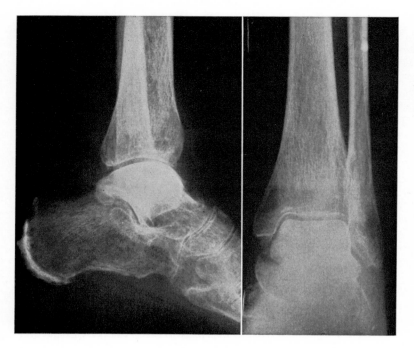

FIG. 20-26. Anteroposterior and lateral roentgenograms of the foot, showing avascular necrosis of the body of the talus, following a fracture through the neck, which had already united.

tinued after 4 to 8 weeks, depending upon the severity of the fracture or fractures.

FRACTURES OF THE METATARSALS

These may be considered as fractures of (1) the shafts or the necks of the metatarsals, (2) the base of the fifth metatarsal and (3) march fractures.

Fractures of the Shafts or the Necks of the Metatarsals. These result from compression injuries of the foot. The force may be front to back, side to side or top to bottom. The last includes a heavy object dropping on the foot. These injuries also result from falls onto the balls of the feet.

TREATMENT. Undisplaced fractures may be treated by merely a compression dressing and the use of crutches for 4 to 6 weeks. In many instances a walking cast will be preferable, as it will make the patient ambulatory without crutches and perhaps permit him to return to work. The cast should include a long plantar slab to protect the toes, as a subsequent blow on these might displace the metatarsal fracture. Occasionally the patient may be treated with a metatarsal pad taped to the sole of the foot, after which he is allowed to bear weight.

Fractures with significant displacement should be reduced. Precise reduction of frac-tures of the first and the fifth metatarsals is especially important so as to restore the weight-bearing heads of these bones to their normal position. Alignment of a fracture of each metatarsal must be restored so that after the fracture is united the head of the broken metatarsal will not project into the sole or the dorsum of the foot and result in painful callus formation.

In transverse or near transverse fractures, reduction can be achieved in many instances by closed manipulation. In oblique or comminuted fractures, continuous traction is often necessary to hold reduction (Method 2). Skeletal traction may be provided by a piece of small Kirschner wire through the tough tissue of the distal phalanx of the toe of the broken metatarsal. Traction is made on the wire by means of a rubber band connected to a loop of heavy wire incorporated in a cast. Skeletal traction may be applied to several toes simultaneously for fractures of several metatarsals. The traction must be maintained for about 4 weeks. In some fractures of metatarsals, open reduction and perhaps internal fixation with an intramedullary pin may be necessary to achieve adequate reduction (Method 3).

Fractures of the Base of the Fifth Metatarsal (Fig. 20-27). These relatively unimpor-

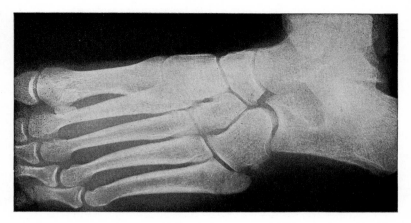

FIG. 20-27. Fracture of base of 5th metatarsal. This fracture should be treated by Method No. 5, no immobilization.

tant but common fractures usually result when the foot gives way into inversion as the patient is running or walking rapidly. As a rule they remain undisplaced, although occasionally the small proximal fragment is separated by the pull of the peroneus brevis muscle which attaches to the proximal end of the fifth metatarsal.

TREATMENT. Undisplaced fractures require little active treatment. Many may be treated by strapping with adhesive tape or by an elastic bandage, and immediate weight-bearing can be allowed. A few will require the use of crutches for 10 to 14 days because of pain. Rarely, a walking cast is justified. If there is any significant displacement of the proximal fragment, the cast should be used. The degree of displacement is seldom such as to predispose to nonunion, although the fracture line is often visible for many months.

March Fracture. A march or fatigue fracture results without any known trauma. It is usually seen in unconditioned military personnel who have been subjected to a long and fatiguing march and usually involves the second or the third metatarsal. Pain develops in the metatarsal region of the foot and persists. As a rule, the pain is relatively mild, and since there is no history of injury, x-ray films may not be made. If they are made, a faint line of fracture may be seen. Later, a palpable lump develops in the metatarsal region and this usually leads to roentgenographic examination. The findings on the roentgenogram are those of a healing fracture with some exuberant callus formation. It is important to recognize that a march fracture is present and not to consider the findings as indicative of a bone tumor.

A march fracture may be treated by immobilization in a walking cast for several weeks or, in many instances, by a metatarsal pad in the shoe or a metatarsal bar on the shoe, and restricted activity.

FRACTURES OF THE PHALANGES OF THE TOES

These result when some heavy object drops on the toes or when a toe is struck forcibly against an object. Fractures of the fifth toe occur frequently when a barefoot person catches it on a piece of furniture. Except for fractures of the great toe, fractures of the toes are not of great consequence.

Treatment. In undisplaced fractures, including those of the phalanges of the great toe, only protection from additional injury is necessary. Strapping of the injured toe to the adjacent toe or toes with small strips of adhesive tape affords some protection and tends to minimize discomfort. The use of a crutch or cane may make walking more comfortable for the first week or 10 days. With a metatarsal bar applied to the shoe, patients with these injuries often can resume activity long before the fracture is united.

In displaced fractures of the great toe, particularly in those of the proximal phalanx, reduction is necessary. At times this can be achieved by manipulation (Method 1). In some, continuous skeletal traction in a banjo cast, as described for fractures of the metatarsals, is advantageous (Method 2). Open reduction is seldom necessary. These fractures usually unite sufficiently in 3 or 4 weeks to permit the patient to resume weight-bearing without danger of displacement.

In displaced fractures of the small toes, efforts at reduction usually are not indicated. The bones are so small that even with perfect reduction redisplacement occurs easily. However, every effort should be made to restore good alignment, which usually can be maintained by strapping the broken toe to the toe or toes on each side of it.

DISLOCATIONS OF THE FOOT

Dislocations of the foot include (1) peritalar dislocation, (2) tarsometatarsal dislocation and (3) dislocation of the toes.

PERITALAR DISLOCATION

This corresponds to perilunar dislocation at the wrist. The talus remains seated in the ankle joint, but the remainder of the foot is dislocated medially. This means that the articulations between the talus and the calcaneus and between the talus and the navicular are disrupted. The injury may be closed or open.

Prompt reduction is indicated. General anesthesia is usually necessary. Traction and appropriate manipulation usually reduce the dislocation. A plaster cast should be applied to the foot and the leg, holding the ankle at 90° and the foot in neutral version for a period of about 4 weeks (Method 1). The prognosis is rather good for so severe an injury.

TARSOMETATARSAL DISLOCATION

In this injury, usually caused by some force which produces leverage at the mid-foot (as when the forefoot is caught and the body is forced medially or laterally), the metatarsals are torn loose from their articulations with the tarsus. Usually there are multiple chip fractures along these joints. This is a severe injury.

In many instances closed reduction may be successful by traction and manipulation. Then immobilization is provided by a plaster cast, including the leg and the foot (Method 1). When reduction cannot be obtained or maintained by closed methods, operative reduction and usually some form of internal fixation are necessary (Method 3).

DISLOCATION OF THE TOES

Dislocation of a toe without fracture is an unusual injury, but occasionally one of the toes, particularly the great one, is dislocated at the metatarsophalangeal joint. Reduction by traction and manipulation is usually easy and often may be done without anesthesia.

(For Bibliography, see pp. 451-452, at end of Chap. 21.)

Oscar P. Hampton, Jr., m.d., and William T. Fitts, jr., m.d.

CHAPTER 21

Fractures and Dislocations of the Spine, the Pelvis, the Sternum and the Ribs

Fractures and Dislocations of the Spine
Fractures of the Pelvis
Fractures of the Sternum
Fractures of the Ribs

FRACTURES AND DISLOCATIONS OF THE SPINE

Fractures and dislocations of the spine divide regionally for purposes of discussion into those of the (1) cervical spine, (2) dorsal and lumbar spine and (3) sacrococcygeal spine.

Injury to the Spinal Cord

The outstanding complication of fractures and dislocations of the spine is injury to the underlying spinal cord. For practical purposes, there must have been some dislocation of a vertebra for spinal cord injury to occur. Dislocations may show on roentgenograms, usually in association with a compression fracture of the body of a vertebra just below it, or it may have been reduced spontaneously so that only the compression fracture is visualized and the diagnosis of a dislocation made because of the cord injury. In fact, occasionally roentgenograms will show no fracture, and yet the patient will have a complete transverse lesion of the cord. It seems certain, in such instances, that there has been a temporary dislocation of a vertebra with crushing of the cord followed by spontaneous reduction.

Injury to the spinal cord may occur at any level between the first cervical and the second lumbar vertebrae, and below the level of the second lumbar vertebra the cauda equina may be damaged. Injury to the cord is most commonly found as a complication of injuries to the cervical and upper dorsal spine.

Injury to the spinal cord may produce either complete or incomplete loss of function of the nervous system below the level of the injury. In a complete lesion, motor power, sensation and bladder and rectal sphincter control are lost. In an incomplete lesion, varying degrees of these functions are retained. The seriousness of either a complete or an incomplete lesion of the cord demands an adequate neurologic examination as soon as the patient is seen with a suspected fracture of the spine in order that injury to the cord, if present, may be recognized promptly and every effort made to treat it properly. The ability to move the fingers and the toes fully, and the preservation of normal sensation and normal reflexes show that the function of the nervous system has not been impaired. Such an observation made early may be invaluable from a diagnostic standpoint should signs of injury to the cord develop.

Treatment. All that can be done for the neurologic lesion is to relieve pressure on the spinal cord. A Queckenstedt test may help to determine whether pressure is still present on the cord at the site of the injury. In many complete lesions, this test will show a patent spinal canal and absence of cord compression. Under such circumstances, considerable pressure on the cord must have been present at the time of injury and then spontaneously relieved. If the Queckenstedt is negative (patent spinal canal), surgical intervention is not indicated. On the other hand, with a positive Queckenstedt (a blocked spinal canal), either manipulation or open operation must be performed in an attempt to relieve pressure.

The operation of laminectomy may be employed. The cord is unroofed by removal of lamina to ensure that all pressure has been relieved. Occasionally, pressure on the cord may be relieved quickly by hyperextension of the spine. Relief of the pressure on the cord can be demonstrated by a repeat Queckenstedt test which would then be negative.

Because the cord has been so badly damaged the prognosis for recovery in complete lesions of the cord is usually poor even with laminectomy. This is particularly true in immediate complete lesions. The prognosis is better in complete lesions which come on several hours after injury and in all incomplete lesions. The management of paraplegia is discussed elsewhere.

FRACTURES AND DISLOCATIONS OF THE CERVICAL SPINE

Compression fractures and dislocations of the bodies of cervical vertebrae are flexion injuries. They usually result from a blow on the head, as from diving into shallow water, an automobile accident, or from a falling object. The extent of injury varies from a fracture of a small fragment of the anterior superior margin of a vertebra or a minimal forward subluxation of a vertebra to a severe compression fracture or a complete forward dislocation. The diagnosis and the extent of injury is determined by adequate roentgenograms.

Compression Fractures. TREATMENT. Minimal compression fractures require only the support of a brace or a Thomas collar for a period of 4 to 6 weeks. More severe compressions require reduction by hyperextension and immobilization usually for 8 to 12 weeks by a plaster cast incorporating the trunk and the head with the latter in hyperextension.

Reduction of a compression fracture may be obtained in several ways. The head may be allowed to lie unsupported in hyperextension over the edge of a table or a mattress. An excellent technic is that provided by 2 mattresses on the bed with the top mattress pulled toward the foot so that the patient's head may hyperextend over the top mattress. Halter traction on the hyperextended head for a few days is another method which may lead to reduction of the compression. A third method is hyperextension of the neck on a fracture

table. All modern fracture tables have arrangements for holding the head and the neck in hyperextension during application of a plaster cast to the head, the neck and the trunk. Hyperextension of the neck on a fracture table is the preferable method when the severity of the fracture warrants plaster immobilization because the other methods of reduction require that the patient be moved to such a table for application of the cast after the fracture has been reduced.

Dislocations of the cervical spine may be (1) incomplete, usually called subluxations, or (2) complete. In a subluxation, the inferior articular facets of a vertebra slide upward and forward on the facets of the vertebra below it, but not far enough for the sliding superior facets to become completely disengaged and to override those below. The body of the superior vertebra moves forward several millimeters on the one below it. In complete dislocations, the superior facets move upward and forward so that all contact with those below is lost and overriding occurs (Fig. 21-1). The body of the superior vertebra is displaced well forward on the one below and may override it. A complete dislocation of a cervical vertebra is often associated with a compression fracture of the vertebra below it. In these injuries, a complete transverse lesion of the spinal cord is common.

A subluxation of a cervical vertebra may be overlooked unless a special lateral view of the neck is made with the head flexed. The routine anteroposterior and lateral views are made with the head moderately extended with the patient sitting or recumbent. A subluxation of a cervical vertebra may have been reduced spontaneously so that with the routine positioning of the head and the neck, the films are negative. In such instances, the subluxation is most likely to recur with the head flexed to the limit of the patient's tolerance. Therefore, if the routine films are negative, it is necessary to obtain a lateral view with full flexion of the neck. In this way, subluxations which have been reduced spontaneously will not go undiagnosed, and proper therapy can be instituted.

TREATMENT. Dislocations of the cervical spine, complete or incomplete, require reduction and immobilization until the damaged capsular and ligamentous structures have

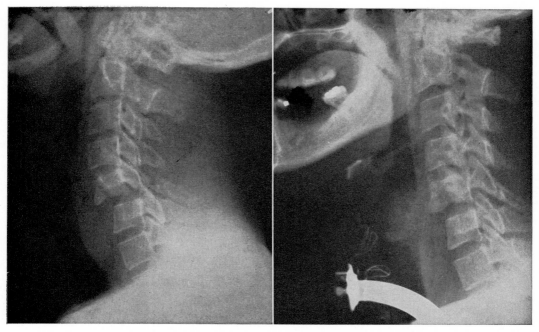

FIG. 21-1. Roentgenograms showing a fracture-dislocation of the cervical spine. (*Left*) Lateral roentgenogram showing a complete anterior dislocation of the 5th cervical vertebra with associated fracture of its body. (*Right*) Lateral roentgenogram showing the dislocation reduced by skeletal traction with Crutchfield tongs. Note the tracheostomy tube, which is often necessary to ensure an adequate airway and to permit aspiration of the tracheobronchial tree.

healed, so that dislocation will not recur. The basic measures by which reduction may be achieved are traction on the head and hyperextension of the neck. The way in which these measures are applied varies with the degree of dislocation.

In incomplete dislocations, the important maneuver is hyperextension of the head so that the facets and the body of the displaced vertebrae will go back into their normal position. Preliminary traction with a canvas head halter will aid in reduction and tend to relieve pain. Hyperextension may be obtained by any of the methods outlined above under Compression Fractures. If immobilization is to be by a plaster cast, obviously the preferable method of obtaining hyperextension is on a standard fracture table.

In complete dislocations, reduction is more of a problem. Traction is of equal and perhaps of greater importance. While head traction may be provided by a canvas head halter, skeletal traction with Crutchfield tongs or some modification of them is highly preferable. Traction at first is made with the head in slight flexion and continued until the facets are no longer overriding and locked. To effect this, as much as 25 to 30 pounds of skeletal traction may be necessary. When the facets are no longer locked, the head is gradually brought into hyperextension as the weights are reduced to about 8 to 10 pounds.

If displacement has been minimal, reduction may be maintained by a hyperextension neck brace which should be worn for 6 to 8 weeks. In more severe yet incomplete dislocations, reduction is preferably maintained by prolonged traction or by a plaster cast incorporating the trunk and the head and holding the head in hyperextension.

In complete dislocations of the cervical spine, the head must be immobilized in hyperextension for a full 3 months. Skeletal traction in some hyperextension may be maintained for a period of about 8 weeks, following which a hyperextension neck brace is worn for an additional 4 weeks. Usually, however, skeletal traction is maintained for only 1 to 3 weeks,

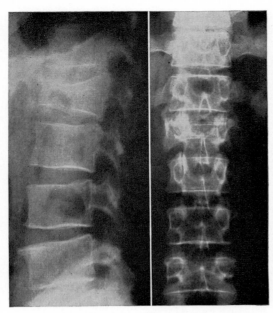

Fig. 21-2. Compression fracture of the lumbar spine. Lateral and anteroposterior views of a severe compression fracture of the 1st lumbar vertebra.

following which the trunk and the hyperextended head are immobilized in a plaster cast. Early operative fusion of the involved vertebrae after reduction is often indicated.

FRACTURES AND DISLOCATIONS OF THE DORSAL AND LUMBAR SPINE

Fractures of the dorsal and lumbar vertebrae may be considered as (1) fractures of the bodies, (2) fractures of transverse processes and (3) fractures of spinous processes. Lamina and articulating processes also may be broken. However, these are usually associated with severe compression fractures or dislocations of vertebrae and need not be considered as separate clinical entities.

Fractures of the Vertebral Bodies (Compression Fractures). Compression fractures of the dorsal and lumbar vertebral bodies are the typical fractures of the back and comprise some 60 per cent of the bony injuries to the spine. They are produced by hyperflexion or "jackknifing" of the spine as in falling from a height and landing on the feet (they often are associated with fractures of the os calcis), or on the buttocks. A compression fracture

may result when an automobile overturns, when an occupant is thrown out of the car following a collision, or when a heavy object falls on the shoulders of an erect or slightly stooped individual. In demineralized spines, as in postmenopausal osteoporosis, a compression fracture may occur merely from lifting strains or other minor trauma.

Compression fractures of bodies of vertebrae are often multiple. In such instances, 1 or at the most 2 vertebrae usually receive the most severe compression.

A compression fracture should be suspected when the patient complains of pain in the back associated with localized tenderness to deep pressure or fist percussion following any trauma which has caused sudden flexion of the back such as those described above. It is confirmed by adequate x-ray visualization in 2 views, the lateral view being the more important. Most compression fractures of the spine occur in the dorsolumbar region and therefore involve the 11th or the 12th dorsal or the 1st and the 2nd lumbar vertebrae (Fig. 21-2). By coincidence this is the region of the spine where x-ray visualization may be faulty unless the technic is precise.

Radiologic technic calls for a different exposure on different films for lateral views of the lumbar spine and the dorsal spine. An error in placement of a film may lead to failure to visualize either the 12th dorsal or 1st lumbar vertebra. The surgeon must be sure that the roentgenograms adequately visualize these vertebrae. Often a detailed view of this region is advisable.

Paralytic or adynamic ileus is usually a problem during the first few days after a compression fracture of the lower dorsal or lumbar spine. Hyperextension for reduction of the fracture, if it is to be used, should be postponed until the ileus has been controlled. It should be managed by the same measures as for adynamic ileus from any cause.

TREATMENT. For several decades, the accepted procedure in these injuries has been hyperextension of the spine in an effort to reduce the compression of the vertebral body or bodies, followed by application of a snug plaster jacket. Hyperextension has been obtained in several ways. With the patient placed on his back in an adjustable hospital bed so that his head is toward the foot of the bed, the knee rest is gradually elevated so as to provide a fulcrum at the level of the fracture and produce hyperextension of the spine. Watson-Jones introduced the method of placing the patient face down on 2 tables, one of them supporting the lower extremities and the other the head and the neck, so that the trunk dropped into hyperextension between them. Davis used a method which placed the patient face down on a table and then by means of a rope, tied about the ankles passing over an overhead pulley, raised the lower extremities so as to hyperextend the spine fully. All modern fracture tables have methods of hyperextending the spine to its limit of extension with the patient face down or face up.

All of these methods except hyperextension in bed permit application of a plaster jacket. The jacket should extend from the sternal notch to the pubic symphysis anteriorly and should make pressure at 3 points: the upper sternum, the pubic symphysis and the back at the level of the injury. In this way hyperextension of the spine is maintained. The best fitting and therefore the most effective plaster jackets are those applied with the patient in a face-up position. This permits the cast to be made snug-fitting at the 3 pressure points.

While hyperextension and plaster immobilization have not been employed in all compression fractures of the vertebrae by all surgeons, the method has gained wide application. In recent years, however, the method has been used less and less for several reasons. It has been recognized that as a spine is hyperextended most of the hyperextension has occurred at the lumbosacral joint, and maintenance of this position has predisposed to prolonged low back pain which often was much worse than any residual pain at the site of an unreduced fracture. In many instances prolonged immobilization has led to considerable permanent stiffness throughout the spine. The method is uncomfortable to the patient. Moreover, any improvement in the position of the fracture often has not been maintained in the cast when the patient became ambulatory. Particularly, it has been recognized that hyperextension is usually ineffective for compression fractures of the dorsal vertebrae above the level of the 9th dorsal vertebra. Certainly, it is reasonable to state that hyperextension and plaster immobilization (or

immobilization by new hyperextension braces to be described below) need be employed only in selected compression fractures of the lower dorsal and lumbar vertebrae. The following recommendations are made as guiding rules for the management of compression fractures of the dorsal and lumbar vertebrae.

MINIMAL COMPRESSION FRACTURES. These include compressions of about 10 to 15 per cent of the vertical height of the anterior portion of the body and also those chip fractures where the anterosuperior corner of a body is broken away. Effort at reduction of these fractures by hyperextension are seldom indicated regardless of the age of the patient. He should be kept at bed rest on a hard bed until acute reaction to the injury has subsided —that is, until the pain has decreased to the point where he wants to be out of bed. Usually from 2 to 3 weeks is required. If the compression fracture is in the lumbar region, he then is fitted with some kind of back support which may be a broad canvas back belt with strong stays or a full-length back brace. The former will suffice in many instances. The patient is made ambulatory with the support which may be removed when the patient is in bed.

If the fracture is higher than the 12th dorsal, a full length support (a brace or a full-length corset with shoulder straps and strong stays) becomes necessary if the region of the fracture is to be supported, but actually, for fractures above the 8th or the 9th dorsal, support often may be omitted if the patient is comfortable without it.

MODERATE COMPRESSION FRACTURES. These include compressions of from 10 or 15 per cent to about 35 per cent of the vertical height of the anterior portion of the body.

In individuals under 35 or 40 years of age, efforts at reduction by hyperextension followed by immobilization are often worthwhile if the fracture is in the last 3 dorsal vertebrae or the lumbar region. The immobilization may be provided in several ways.

As outlined above, the standard method of immobilization for several decades has been the 3-point pressure plaster jacket and this is still an acceptable way. However, there are several objections to it. Any reduction which was obtained by hyperextension may be lost in the cast as it loses its effectiveness in pro-

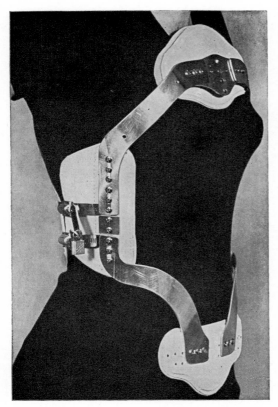

FIG. 21-3. Three-point pressure brace shown from in front (*top*) and behind (*bottom*). By tightening the set screws the pressure pad posteriorly is drawn tighter, and the sternal and the pubic pads are made to press more securely. The brace offers many advantages over a plaster jacket.

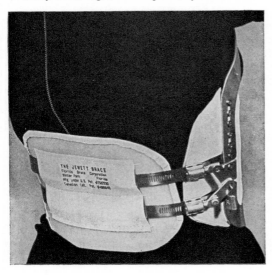

viding continuous 3-point pressure when it becomes loose as a result of atrophy of muscle and fat. This is unavoidable. The cast provides continuous immobilization of the spine, predisposing to stiffness. Plaster jacket immobilization is uncomfortable and becomes quite disagreeable to the patient as the cast becomes saturated with oil and perspiration from the skin.

The Jewett hyperextension brace (Fig. 21-3) (or an acceptable modification) is a distinct improvement over the plaster jacket. Continuous 3-point pressure can be provided. As atrophy of muscle and fat occurs, the brace is easily tightened to maintain effectiveness. After the first few weeks, the brace may be left off when the patient is in bed, thereby permitting some motion in the joints of the spine, especially in the lumbosacral region, which favors eventual recovery of motion in the back. This limited movement of the spine does not jeopardize the reduction of the compression fracture. A T-shirt under the brace may be changed every few days for cleanliness while the patient is recumbent.

In patients over 35 or 40 years of age, considerable judgment must be used in determining whether the end-result, as measured by a near pain-free useful back, will be obtained by hyperextension and prolonged immobilization or by minimal immobilization and early motion.

Certainly, in older individuals hyperextension which is maintained for any appreciable period of time predisposes to stiffness in the back which, in turn, predisposes to more pain. In this age group the best end-result is likely to be obtained by omitting efforts at reduction of the fracture and by providing just enough immobilization to minimize discomfort and yet permit enough movement in the back at frequent intervals to predispose to a maximum return of motion.

In moderate compression fractures above the level of the 9th dorsal vertebra, efforts at reduction by hyperextension are seldom worthwhile, regardless of the age group of the patient. After a period of bed rest, enough immobilization should be provided to minimize pain, but, as a rule, continuous or prolonged immobilization is not necessary.

SEVERE COMPRESSION FRACTURES. These include compressions of more than 35 per cent of the vertical height of the anterior portion of the body. This group, fortunately a small percentage of all compression fractures, is more likely than the less severe fractures to have associated damage to the spinal cord. Under such circumstances, of course, the fracture itself is of secondary importance, and specific measures to reduce it, as a rule, are indicated only when reduction of the fracture tends to eliminate compression of the spinal cord.

In severe compression fractures involving the last 3 dorsal or the lumbar vertebrae, reduction of the fracture by hyperextension by one of the methods outlined above is indicated except in the aged. Immobilization may be provided by any one of the methods discussed under moderate compression fractures. In individuals under 35 or 40 years of age, loss of reduction should be prevented as much as possible by maintaining 3-point pressure immobilization for at least 3 months and often longer, except where the patient is recumbent in bed. In individuals over 40 years of age, again, considerable judgment must be used in determining whether the advantage offered by prolonged immobilization in maintaining the best position of the fracture outweighs the disadvantages of immoblization in producing a stiff back. In this age group, regardless of the severity of the fracture, continuous immobilization and hyperextension by a plaster jacket for 3 months is hazardous. The Jewett hyperextension brace is preferable to the plaster jacket in this as in all age groups because it can be removed when the patient is recumbent in bed and therefore allows some motion in the spine without jeopardizing the reduction of the fracture.

Fractures of Transverse Processes. These injuries, for practical purposes, occur only in the lumbar region. They generally are avulsion fractures caused by a powerful contracture of the quadratus lumborum muscle which inserts into the 5 transverse processes as well as the 12th rib. The initiating factor in such injuries may be a fall from a height to the back or the side, a heavy blow from the side as when a man is struck by an automobile, or a crushing injury.

The diagnosis is made on the anteroposterior roentgenogram. The fracture may show as a mere crack, or the fragments may be widely separated. In the latter instances, fascia and muscles are torn, and a large hematoma develops. Considerable extracellular fluid may be lost into this severely traumatized area. A paralytic ileus may follow, as in compression fractures of the vertebral bodies.

TREATMENT. Fractures of transverse processes are treated symptomatically. Following a few days of bed rest on a hard bed, a broad canvas back belt with good stays is fitted to the patient. He may be ambulatory and allowed to resume some activity. For an undisplaced crack in one or two transverse processes, the belt may be needed for only a few weeks. Sometimes a simple adhesive strapping of the back for a week or two will suffice, without the belt. Activity is increased gradually, and practically no residual symptoms should remain after 2 months. When the fragments are widely displaced, however, signifying rather extensive soft tissue injury, the belt may be needed for 5 or 6 weeks. Some residual soreness is to be expected for several months and perhaps permanently as a result of scar formation in the traumatized area. Actually, nonunion of separated fractures of transverse processes is not unusual, but healing by scar reanchors the fragments.

Fractures of Spinous Processes. This relatively rare injury may result when a spinous process, made prominent and vulnerable when the spine is flexed, is struck "bulls-eye" by some falling object. It also may result in the low cervical or upper dorsal area by strong muscle contracture, as in laborers who are shoveling dirt. For this reason, the injury near the cervico-dorsal junction has been called "clay-shoveler's fracture."

Treatment is usually symptomatic. A Thomas collar for several weeks may benefit those in the lower cervical and upper dorsal area. A lumbosacral corset may help relieve pain for those in the lumbar region. Nonunion may occur. If so, and if pain persists, excision of the small fragment may relieve the symptoms.

FRACTURES OF THE SACROCOCCYGEAL SPINE

Fractures of the Sacrum. These injuries may occur following falls from a height in which the patient lands on the low back or as a result of severe direct blows, as when the patient is struck by an automobile. They

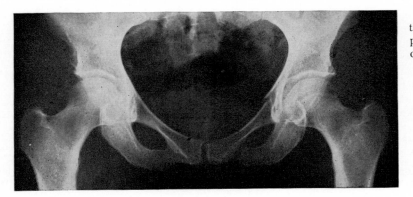

FIG. 21-4. Fracture of the pelvis. Fracture of superior and inferior rami of left pubis.

usually occur as linear fractures without displacement. Treatment is comparable with that for undisplaced fractures of the pelvis and usually consist of a few weeks of bed rest on a hard bed followed by the support of a good lumbosacral belt.

Fractures of the Coccyx. These result from falls into the sitting position. Usually there is a history that the region of the coccyx struck some protruding object, such as the edge of a step. Although the injury is not serious, it is painful.

If there is displacement of the distal portion of the coccyx, an effort should be made to achieve reduction by manipulation with one finger in the rectum, for which anesthesia is usually required.

Following reduction, or if the fracture is undisplaced, treatment consists of a rubber ring for sitting, the support of a girdle or a belt about the hips during ambulation, sitting in a tub of hot water several times daily and avoidance of reinjury. Pain on sitting is likely to continue for some time and may persist indefinitely. Under these circumstances, surgical excision of the coccyx may be indicated. At times, however, excision of the coccyx does not relieve the symptoms, particularly in neurotic and hypersensitive individuals. Therefore, the patient must be evaluated carefully before operation is advised.

FRACTURES OF THE PELVIS

Fractures of the pelvis are produced by direct violence, such as falls from a height, automobile accidents and crushing injuries of any kind. The fracture may involve one or both rami of the pubis (Fig. 21-4) or the ischium, or either wing of the ilium. Because of the framework of the pelvis, significant displacement of a fracture usually does not occur. However, with fractures involving both rami and the wing of the ilium on one side, upward and inward displacement of the outer fragment of that innominate bone may occur. With fractures through both rami on each side, as may occur in side-to-side crush injuries, the pelvis may collapse and the fragments override, or with such fractures following front-to-back crush injuries, separation of the fragments and spread of the pelvis may occur.

First consideration with fractures of the pelvis, particularly when the fragments are displaced, concerns not the fractures themselves but the contiguous soft tissues which may have been injured: the bladder, the intestine, or the iliac blood vessels. Unless the patient can void immediately, catheterization is indicated to determine whether or not the bladder has been damaged. This investigation is necessary even though the fragments are not displaced, because a full bladder may have been ruptured by the force of the impact. Absence of urine or the finding of bloody urine indicates injury to the bladder (see Chap. 48, Urology). Repeated examination of the abdomen is indicated to search for signs of injury to an intra-abdominal viscus. The absence of normal peripheral arterial pulsations in either lower extremity would indicate the probability of a torn iliac artery. The management of these life-endangering complications takes precedence over management of the fractures.

TREATMENT

Fractures of the pelvis with little or no displacement, which comprise the majority of these injuries, require nothing more than bed rest on a hard bed for a few weeks followed, perhaps, by the support of a canvas corset for a few weeks. With fractures of a single ramus or even 2 rami on the same side, the patient may easily become ambulatory on crutches in 2 to 3 weeks, but full weight-bearing should be postponed until about 6 weeks after injury. In undisplaced fractures involving rami on both sides, the period of bed rest should be prolonged to 4 to 5 weeks, and crutch-walking postponed until 7 or 8 weeks after injury. The prognosis in these undisplaced fractures of the pelvis is excellent for practically full function. Elderly individuals, in whom these periods of bed rest may be inadvisable, can be safely lifted into a chair after a few days.

In fractures through both rami and the wing of the ilium on the same side with upward and perhaps inward displacement of the lateral fragment of the innominate bone, strong traction, either skin or preferably skeletal, must be applied to the extremity early in the management of the fracture in an effort to pull the displaced fragment back into position. In some instances, efforts at reduction will be more successful if the patient is anesthetized for relaxation; while strong manual traction is being made on the involved extremity, a strong downward and rotary thrust is made manually against the upward displaced wing of the ilium. After reduction, traction must be maintained for several weeks (usually 5 or 6 weeks) to avoid recurrence of the upward displacement.

Those fractures with separation of the fragments and spreading of the lower pelvis require some compressing force. This is most easily accomplished by means of a pelvic sling which serves barely to lift the weight of the pelvis from the mattress and to supply a binding force which tends to mold the fragments back into place. Some caution is necessary to avoid converting a spreading type of fracture into a collapsing type as a result of excessive compression. Bilateral traction on the extremities may aid in obtaining reduction of the fragments and certainly, in the early

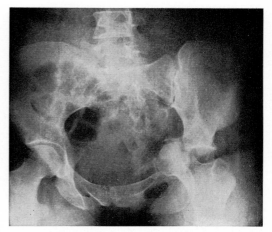

FIG. 21-5. Central dislocation of the hip.

stages, will contribute to the comfort of the patient.

In bilateral fractures of both rami with overriding and collapse of the pelvis, a pelvic sling is not indicated. Strong bilateral traction with the lower extremities in abduction may effect some improvement in the position of the fragments.

In all of these displaced fractures of the pelvis, the period of bed rest must be extended to 6 or 8 weeks, following which the support of a canvas corset should be provided for 1 to 3 months. Immobilization in a plaster cast is seldom worthwhile. When it is used, the cast must incorporate the trunk and one or both thighs.

FRACTURES ASSOCIATED WITH
DISLOCATION OF THE HIP

Fracture of Margin of Acetabulum. (This lesion is discussed on p. 405.)

Central Fracture-Dislocation of the Hip Joint (Fracture of the Floor of the Acetabulum). A blow in the line of the shaft of the femur, especially when the thigh is abducted, or a fall onto the greater trochanter may drive the head of the femur through the floor of the acetabulum and into the pelvis, pushing fragments of the acetabulum ahead of it (Fig. 21-5). The dislocated femoral head frequently can be reduced by skeletal traction. Often the acetabular fragments fall into good position but frequently they are not pulled back into place by traction so that the acetabulum remains distorted. Even so, open reduction of the acetabular floor is an extensive and dangerous procedure and should seldom be attempted in these circumstances, especially since a satisfactory functional result is often obtained even though the acetabular fragments are not reduced accurately. The explanation for this is probably that the weight-bearing part of the acetabulum is chiefly the superior undisplaced aspect rather than the central, displaced portion. If traumatic arthritis develops later, arthrodesis or arthroplasty may be performed.

FRACTURES OF THE STERNUM

Fractures of the sternum occur usually as the result of an automobile collision in which the driver is thrown forward so that his sternum strikes the steering wheel. Rarely, they occur in association with compression fractures of the dorsal spine following severe sudden jackknifing compression injuries, such as when a very heavy weight falls across the shoulders of a stooped individual.

The fragments, if displaced at all, may overlap slightly. The diagnosis is based upon pain, tenderness, discoloration and at times a palpable offset at the fracture site confirmed by visualization of the fracture on roentgenograms. The routine lateral view of the dorsal spine usually shows the sternum in the lateral projection.

TREATMENT

Efforts at reduction are seldom indicated as no impairment of function results even when the fragments unite in slight overriding. The patient is treated symptomatically, but the presence of a fracture of the sternum should serve as a warning for careful observation of the patient for signs and symptoms of intrathoracic injury. If reduction seems to be indicated, it may be attempted by strong hyperextension of the dorsal spine, or open operation may be employed.

FRACTURES OF THE RIBS

Fractures of the ribs result from direct trauma or compressions of the thoracic cage. The fractures cause pain, usually aggravated by respiration, localized tenderness, sometimes crepitus and perhaps subcutaneous emphysema. The diagnosis is confirmed by roentgenograms, but fractures of the ribs are at times difficult to demonstrate on roentgenograms, especially in the first 1 to 2 weeks after injury.

Although fractures of the ribs cause considerable pain, they are of little consequence in themselves. Even if untreated they will unite with no residual impairment of function. Their principal importance comes from the injury to the pleura and the lung and the impairment of pulmonary function which may accompany them. At the time of injury the pleura and the lung may be torn, resulting in pneumothorax or hemothorax or traumatic pneumonitis. These problems are discussed in Chapter 42, "Lung."

Even without damage to the underlying pleura and lung, fractures of the ribs may result in altered pulmonary function. The pain which they produce may decrease respiratory excursion and prevent coughing. Under these circumstances tracheobronchial secretions are not coughed up. As they collect in the tracheobronchial tree, aeration of the lung fields is minimized, and a predisposition to pneumonia and atelectasis is created. These considerations are exceedingly important in treating a patient with fractures of the ribs. An especially serious type of double fracture of several adjoining ribs results in a flail chest (see Chap. 42, "Lung").

TREATMENT

The pain of fractures of the ribs may be alleviated by adhesive strapping (adhesive straps should extend either about the entire chest or cover the involved side with extension onto the uninjured side; enough strips should be used to cover the chest wall from the level of the nipple downward to the belt line) or a wide elastic bandage applied around the lower thorax in circular fashion or a thoracic corset. A disadvantage of adhesive is that many patients are sensitive to it and develop painful blisters. While these time-honored methods may be employed for fractures of the ribs in selected instances, it should be kept in mind that each adds further restriction to the respiratory excursion and therefore may further impair the effectiveness of respiration, even though they do provide the patient with some relief of pain.

A more rational approach to the treatment

of fractures of the ribs is provided by posterior intercostal nerve block. Five cc. of 1 or 2 per cent procaine is injected in the region of the intercostal nerves on the inferior surfaces of each of the ribs involved (usually including 1 or 2 ribs above and below those obviously fractured) posterior to the fracture sites and usually at the posterior prominence of the rib some 2 inches from the mid-line of the spine. An adequate intercostal block relieves all pain of respiration, permits strong coughing to empty the tracheobronchial tree of its secretions and allows full inspiration so as to aerate the lung fields fully. Obviously, this procedure tends to restore the normal pulmonary function in contrast with strapping about the thoracic cage. It is surprising how often the patient remains pain-free long after the effects of the procaine have worn off. In many instances, however, the posterior intercostal nerve block should be repeated several times at intervals of 8 to 24 hours.

A combination of intercostal nerve block followed by strapping may be employed. The block serves to restore reasonably normal pulmonary function, leaving the tracheobronchial tree free of secretions and the lungs well aerated. Then, adhesive strapping will afford the patient some prolonged relief and any impairment of pulmonary function resulting from the compression will be minimal and probably insignificant.

The treatment of flail chest presents special problems and is discussed in Chapter 42, "Lung."

BIBLIOGRAPHY

Chapters 18-21

Bankart, A. S. B.: The pathology and treatment of recurrent dislocation of the shoulder joint, Brit. J. Surg. *26*:23, 1938.

Blount, W. P.: Fractures in Children, Baltimore, Williams & Wilkins, 1954.

Cave, E. F. (ed.): Fractures and Other Injuries, Chicago, Year Book Pub., 1958.

Committee on Trauma, American College of Surgeons: An Outline of the Treatment of Fractures, ed. 5, 1954.

Compere, E. L.: Banks, S. W., and Compere, C. L.: Pictorial Handbook of Fracture Treatment, ed. 3, Chicago, Year Book Pub., 1952.

Darrach, W.: Treatment of fractures, Ann. Surg. *124*:607-616, 1946.

DePalma, A. F.: Surgery of the Shoulder, Philadelphia, Lippincott, 1950.

Dunlop, J.: Transcondylar fractures of the humerus in childhood, J. Bone & Joint Surg. *21*:59, 1939.

Eggers, G. W. N.: The Internal Fixation of Fractures of the Shafts of Long Bones (Monographs on Surgery), Baltimore, Williams & Wilkins, 1952.

Essex-Lopresti, P.: Results of reduction in fractures of the calcaneum, J. Bone & Joint Surg. *33-B*:284, 1951.

Fitts, W. T., Jr.: Healing of fractures, S. Clin. North America *26*:1470, 1946.

Fitts, W. T., Jr., Roberts, B., Grippe, W. J., Muir, M. W., and Allam, M. W.: The treatment of fractures complicated by contiguous burns, Surg., Gynec. & Obst. *97*:551-564, 1953.

Fitts, W. T., Jr., Roberts, B., and Ravdin, I. S.: Fractures in metastatic carcinoma, Am. J. Surg. *85*:282, 1953.

Friedenberg, Z. B.: Recent advances in bone physiology, Internat. Abstr. Surg. *98*:313-320, 1954.

Friedenberg, Z. B., and French, G. O.: The effects of known compression forces on fracture healing, Surg., Gynec. & Obst. *94*:743, 1952.

Hampton, O. P., Jr.: Fundamentals of surgery in contaminated and infected wounds, J.A.M.A. *154*:1326-1328, 1954.

————: The prevention of gas gangrene and tetanus, Indust. Med. *23*:309, 1954.

————: Wounds of the Extremities in Military Surgery, St. Louis, Mosby, 1951.

Hampton, O. P., Jr., and Fitts, W. T., Jr.: Open Reduction of Common Fractures, New York, Grune and Stratton, 1959.

Hampton, O. P., Jr., and Holt, E. P., Jr.: The present status of intramedullary nailing of the tibia, Am. J. Surg. *93*:597, 1957.

Hanlon, C. R., and Estes, W. L., Jr.: Fractures in childhood, Am. J. Surg. *87*:312-323, 1954.

Key, J. A., and Conwell, H. E.: The Management of Fractures, Dislocations and Sprains, ed. 5, St. Louis, Mosby, 1951.

McLaughlin, H. L.: The Principles of Fracture Treatment, Committee on Trauma of the American College of Surgeons, 1954.

McLaughlin, H. L. (ed.): Trauma, Philadelphia, Saunders, 1959.

Magnuson, P. B., and Stack, J. K.: Fractures, ed. 5, Philadelphia, Lippincott, 1949.

Murray, C. R.: The timing of the fracture-healing process; its influence on the choice and application of treatment methods, J. Bone & Joint Surg. *23*:598, 1941.

Nicholson, J. T., and Heath, R. D.: Bryant's traction; a provocative cause of circulatory complications, J.A.M.A. *157*:415-418, 1955.

Palmer, I.: The mechanism and treatment of fractures of calcaneus; open reduction with the use of cancellous grafts, J. Bone & Joint Surg. *30-A*:2, 1948.

Rogers, W. A.: The treatment of fracture-dislocation of the cervical spine, J. Bone & Joint Surg. *24*:245, 1942.

Rush, L. V.: Atlas of Rush pin techniques, Mississippi Doctor (Book Section), March 1954.

Speed, J. S., and Knight, R. A.: Campbell's Operative Orthopaedics, ed. 3, St. Louis, Mosby, 1956.

Stewart, M. J., and Milford, L. W.: Fracture-dislocation of the hip. An end-result study, J. Bone & Joint Surg. *36-A*:315, 1959.

Watson-Jones, R.: Fractures and Joint Injuries, ed. 4, Baltimore, Williams & Wilkins, 1955.

LOUIS T. BYARS, M.D.

CHAPTER 22

Principles of Hand Surgery

A report of the National Safety Council indicates that injuries to the hand during 1951 constituted 25 per cent of all industrial accidents; 19 per cent of all compensation was paid for these injuries. This, considered with medical and hospital costs, totals an impressive figure but does not present the whole picture. The 1955 Compensation Laws of Illinois, for example, allow 70 weeks' compensation for the total loss of function of a thumb, 40 for the index finger, 35 for the middle finger, 25 for the ring finger, 20 for the little finger, or a total of 190 weeks for the loss of function of the hand. This compares with 140 weeks for the loss of vision of an eye, 155 weeks for loss of function of a foot, 150 weeks for the loss of both testicles. A week's compensation payment amounts to a minimum of $16.75, to a maximum of $40. The eventual cost to the patient and the taxpayer may be far in excess of the award set by law.

It should not be necessary to comment on the importance of the hand to the surgeon, who even owes the designation of his specialty to its significance (Greek, *cheiro*, meaning "hand"; French, *chirurgie*; English, surgery). Yet much of the disability from the trauma-tized hand results from failure to diagnose the extent of the injury and to treat it with the respect warranted.

EXAMINATION OF THE HAND

The hand, like a watch, is made up of small moving parts, working with little friction, confined to limited space and finely machined to small tolerances. It is contrived to permit perception undetected by the eye, manipulations of fine accuracy and the application of hundreds of pounds of force. Logically, the insignificant surface wound denotes possible disruption beneath. A few simple anatomic facts retained by the doctor undertaking the examination of the injured hand will enable him to recognize the less obvious but serious injury.

The examination should be systematic. Is the injury limited to the hand? Trauma between the spinal cord and the wrist may disrupt any of the 3 major nerves affecting the movement and the sensation of the hand.

IMPAIRMENT OF SENSATION

Laceration. HAND. If the hand is lacerated, test first for *sensory* impairment. In itself, anesthesia of the *palmar* surface of the fingers is a serious handicap. A numb finger is *useless*. A finger lacerated on the palmar surface may have *either or both sensory nerves severed*. These nerves are, one on either side, on the ventrolateral surface and pass under the points where the ventral flexion creases end. (Fig. 22-1.)

PALM. If the palm is lacerated, ascertain anesthesia distal to this point; *common digital* nerves may be severed, and several fingers rendered anesthetic. Unlike the anesthesia from finger lacerations, involvement here may presage *motor* nerve injury.

VOLAR WRIST. If the volar wrist is lacerated, the ulnar nerve may be severed, producing anesthesia of the ulnar third of the palm and of the little finger and adjacent one half of the ring finger. Although it is possible to have a partial injury of this nerve, in most instances there is associated serious motor loss.

The median nerve at the middle of the volar wrist provides sensation to the radial two thirds of the palm and to the thumb, the index, the middle and one half of the ring finger. Its severance produces a "dead" hand and serious motor loss.

IMPAIRMENT OF MOVEMENT

Having examined the hand for sensory nerve impairment, the next step is to test motor nerve function. This involves execution of hand and finger movements and is, therefore, a part of the examination for tendon injury. Since either nerve or tendon injury may result from a trauma and interfere with normal movement, the examiner must be aware of the effects of each and be able to differentiate between them. The diagnosis of a nerve or a tendon injury is often missed because the examiner asks the patients to move the hand and is satisfied with a few grossly executed, nonrevealing maneuvers.

Division of Long Flexor Tendons of Fingers. Long flexor tendons of the fingers originate from powerful forearm muscles and may be severed at any point.

THUMB. The thumb has a single long flexor. Test for its integrity by manually stabilizing the proximal phalanx and having the patient flex the distal phalanx in a normal manner.

REMAINING 4 DIGITS. The remaining 4 digits have 2 long flexor tendons each—the profundus and the more superficial sublimus. Both tendons are severed if the patient cannot flex the finger at the proximal interphalangeal joint; only the profundus has been cut if the finger can be flexed at the proximal interphalangeal joint but not at the distal joint. Severance of the profundus tendon leaves the distal phalanx subject to unopposed

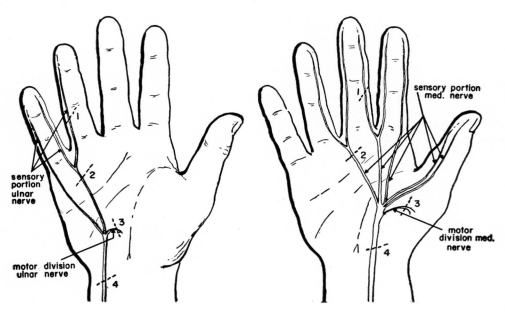

FIG. 22-1. (*Left*) Ulnar nerve supplies feeling to 1½ fingers on the palmar surface, but the small motor division innervates the major portion of the intrinsic muscles of the hand. (*Right*) The median nerve supplies sensation to 3½ fingers on the palmar surface. Its motor division innervates intrinsic muscles which bring the thumb to the front of the hand. Laceration 1 produces anesthesia of ½ finger on the volar surface; laceration 2, anesthesia of adjacent halves of 2 fingers; laceration 3, serious motor paralysis of intrinsic muscles; laceration 4, both sensory and motor sensory and motor paralysis.

extensor action so that, with use, this joint becomes less stable.

The finger movements just described may be absent consequent to nerve injuries in the arm but can result only from direct tendon severance if the laceration is in the volar wrist, the palm or the finger.

Muscle Group Paralysis. In addition to those muscles and tendons which originate in the forearm, there is an important array of muscles *intrinsic* to the hand. They bring about the countless maneuvers that allow the fingers to co-operate in opposition, grouping, rotation, combinations of flexion and extension and cupping of the hand. These muscles are so multiple that direct severance rarely results in gross disturbance of function; motor nerve section does so because it puts them out of action in groups.

Motor Ulnar Nerve. Paralysis of this nerve results from total or partial ulnar nerve division on the volar ulnar side of the wrist or from injury to the motor branch after separation into the sensory and motor components has occurred. Such an accident often follows a small stab wound over the hypothenar eminence. The ulnar nerve innervates the muscles of the *hypothenar* region, most of the *lumbricalis* and *interossei* muscles and the *adductor* muscle of the thumb. When seen early, the ulnar motor paralysis can be detected readily because the little finger lacks flexion at the proximal joint and side-to-side excursion, due to paralysis of the hypothenar muscle group. Paralysis of interossei and lumbricales muscles similarly affects action of the middle and the ring finger. The adductor of the thumb is flaccid, and the thumb cannot be "scraped" across the palm of the hand. When seen later, paralysis of these same muscles groups are detectable but, in addition, there is marked atrophy of the web muscles of the thumb, and the ulnar two thirds of the palm of the hand is shrunken. The hand is a "claw."

Severance of the Motor Median Nerve. This occurs from lacerations of the middle volar wrist or the base of the palm. The most crippling effect is on the muscles of the *thenar eminence*. The thumb cannot be swung forward in an arching manner in front of the palm to oppose the fingertips. When in doubt, compare the *quality* and the *range* of motion in the suspected part with that of the normal hand.

WOUNDS OF DORSUM OF HAND

The foregoing has dealt with the flexor mechanism and the muscles and the nerves contained within the palm of the hand and the wrist. The extensor mechanism of the fingers and the wrist is simpler of structure, weaker in power, easier to repair, and more apt to regain adequate function after repair. The nerve supply to the dorsum of the hand is sensory only. Nevertheless, anesthesia of the dorsum is annoying and subjects the patient to some danger from unconscious injury. These severed nerves regenerate readily if sutured. If the dorsum of the hand is lacerated, the involved digits must be examined for discrepancies in quality and range of motion, comparing with the uninjured member.

A forceful blow on the end of the finger, as from a baseball, often results in a rupture of the extension apparatus at the distal or middle joint with "dropped" or "baseball" finger.

PRINCIPLES OF SURGICAL PROCEDURE

Equipment. Operations upon the hand are seldom simple, and the "dressing room" operation is to be condemned. All facilities in the form of equipment and assistance must be readied. Preliminary treatment is limited to splinting and application of a sterile dressing.

Anesthesia. Operations other than minor surface procedures should be performed under general anesthesia or brachial block, thus permitting the painless use of a tourniquet. The extensive use of local infiltration within the hand is not satisfactory. Blocking the digital nerves at the base of the finger with procaine-adrenalin solution has resulted occasionally in gangrene and loss of the finger.

Tourniquet. All operations of any magnitude can be performed accurately only if the field is bloodless, and the use of a broad cuff type of tourniquet is essential. An exception is the situation where the blood supply to the member has been jeopardized through injury and the use of a tourniquet might further diminish the retarded flow.

Incisions. Most immediate tendon and nerve suturing will require that the skin laceration be enlarged by incisions placed to secure healing without the formation of hypertrophic, contracting scars. (Figs. 22-2 & 3.)

Skin Grafting. There is little excess skin on the hand, and even small surface defects should be covered with a skin graft rather than being permitted to heal secondarily with contracture.

Foreign Bodies. Foreign bodies within the hand are notoriously elusive, and every aid must be sought for their removal. Serious injury has often followed injudicious use of the fluoroscope.

Asepsis and atraumatic technic are mandatory. Scar from infection, tissue reaction or hematoma in the hand is the equivalent of rust in a fine watch; often it wrecks it forever.

Position of Function. The injured hand

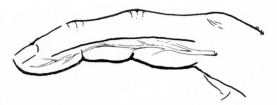

FIG. 22-3. Proper location of incision for approaching flexor tendons of finger or drainage of acute tenosynovitis. Mid-lateral incision such as this heals with minimal scarring. Small finger lacerations severing flexor tendons or nerves require further incision for exposure and repair. These lacerations should be extended as mid-lateral incisions.

must be placed in the position of function and this position maintained during healing (Fig. 22-4).

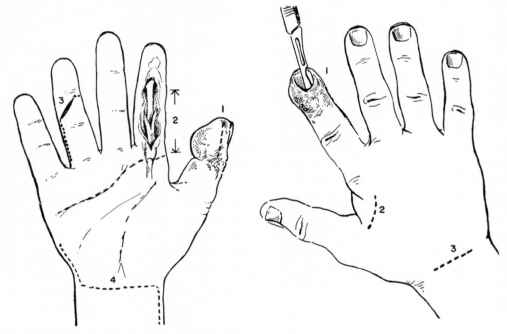

FIG. 22-2. (*Left*) (1) Incision for drainage of felon. Closed space of finger pad incised in front of bone of terminal phalanx. (2) "No man's land" from distal flexion crease of palm to mid-point of middle phalanx represents the area of the finger where repair of tendon injury is most likely to fail due to adherence within the tendon sheath. (3) Small lacerations which must be extended for repair of nerves or tendons should be enlarged as mid-lateral incisions and not across flexion lines for fear of subsequent contracture. (4) Incision for exposure of structures at wrist which tends to avoid secondary scar contracture. (*Right*) (1) Drainage of pus in "run around" by incision in nail sulcus. (2) Incision for drainage of thenar space. (3) Transverse incision for excision of ganglion leaves unnoticeable scar. Vertical incision causes prominent scar.

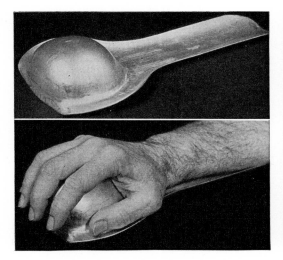

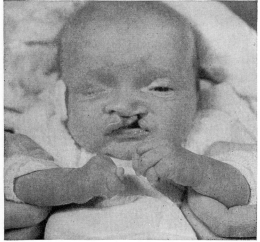

FIG. 22-4. (*Top*) Mason Universal Hand Splint. (*Bottom*) Position of function of the hand as maintained by the Mason Universal Hand Splint. This position of the hand must be continued during the healing period after operation or injury. This may be accomplished by the use of plaster of Paris, a bulky gauze dressing or by whatever means suits the need and the situation.

FIG. 22-5. Multiple congenital anomalies. Hand deformities are often hereditary. In this instance deformities seem to be hereditary but not of a specific nature. All digits of the right hand are fused. The left hand exhibits constriction bands and absent phalanges.

CONGENITAL MALFORMATIONS

BIZARRE AND VARIABLE

Congenital malformations of the hands are duplicated frequently to some degree in the feet of the individual. These are often hereditary—similar conditions cropping up in a family with greater or lesser regularity. They may also be an example of a familial tendency to nonspecific congenital deformity. As the hands are of complicated structure, the combinations of distortion may be many and bizarre—seemingly hopeless of classification. The hand itself may be basically normal but affected by malformation of proximal structures (Fig. 22-5).

As with all congenital malformations, the emotional impact on the parent creates the first problem, and an immediate answer as to the best time for correction is sought. It is well to remember that, when deformities are present from birth, the adaptability of the developing child is boundless and that dexterity is evolved to such a degree that even major distortions are overcome. As a consequence, improvement in appearance may be of most usefulness. Conditions hampering growth warrant early correction.

Each of the more complicated conditions is a problem requiring individual planning. Missing parts can rarely be added, but clefts may be deepened for grasping. Fused structures may be separated; often, crooked bones can be redirected by gentle, persistent splinting. Abnormal clefts may be made less deep, appearance being considered along with function.

In general, bone work, other than simple amputations, should be delayed until size of the structure permits accurate fixation after osteotomy or until interference with growth at the epiphysis is no longer a factor.

EXTRA DIGITS

If unrelated to the functioning hand, except by attachment, these may be removed at any time. When based on "Y"-shaped metacarpals or phalanges, an excision which protects other bones and joints can be done, a secondary contouring operation being planned at a later age when growth and function can be judged.

WEBBED FINGERS

Syndactylism may represent fusion of 2 or more fingers in an otherwise normal hand.

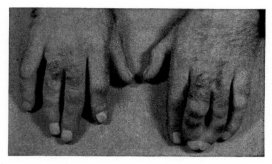

FIG. 22-6. Hands of an adult where webbing of the left hand is similar to that shown on the right hand in Figure 22-7. Marked distortion of the long finger because webbing was not released in childhood.

Correction always involves separation of the fingers and application of a free full-thickness skin graft, or a less desirable thick split graft, to the resulting raw surfaces. Any procedure other than grafting is likely to result in a distorting scar. If a long finger is attached tip to tip to a shorter finger, the separation should be accomplished under 2 years of age to prevent warping of the restrained long finger. Otherwise, the correction certainly should be completed well before school age. When more than 2 digits are involved, correction is planned in stages so that only one side of a finger is operated on at one time out of consideration for its blood supply (Figs. 22-6 & 7).

CIRCULAR CONSTRICTING CREASES

These annular grooves may adhere to skeletal structures and interfere with growth and function of an arm or a finger. They should be released, usually during the first year, by excising the crease from one half or less of the circumference of the part and suturing with the interdigitation of small local flaps to produce a "zigzag" scar with subcutaneous padding. The other half of the circumference is corrected after circulation has been established through the *repaired* segment (Fig. 22-5).

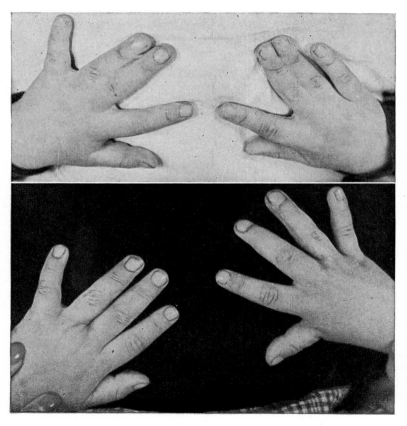

FIG. 22-7. (*Top*) Simplest type of syndactylism. Hand is normal except for fusion of 2 fingers, the long finger right hand being distorted since it is fused tip to tip with shorter finger. Early operation indicated. (*Bottom*) After separation of fingers with free full-thickness skin graft applied to raw surfaces.

A baby's hand is a small and flexible structure, subject to progressive distortion from scar tissue during its period of rapid growth. All open wounds resulting from surgery must be covered immediately with skin grafts to minimize this scar pull. Incisions must be planned so that the resulting scar does not cross flexion creases. Tight scars must be relaxed by skin grafts or by altering the direction of the scar.

INFECTION

Acute Pyogenic

The hands are vulnerable to injury, exposed to dirt, and prone to infection. Moreover, multiple fasciae and tendons, having poor resistance to infections, are superficial in position. The hand being made to withstand forceful usage is strengthened by the presence of many compartments, even within the subcutaneous tissue, and covered with tough skin matched only in the soles of the feet. These factors combine to prevent the outward spontaneous discharge of pus, and instead serve rather to confine it within the depths of the hand where untold destruction results if it is not liberated surgically.

Modern antibiotic drugs do not obviate surgical drainage of pus.

Paronychia results from the hangnail or from manicure trauma. It is an infection of the soft tissue adjacent to the nail, and when it encircles the nail has been termed a "run-around." The infection progresses to extend under the nail and thereby loosens it from its growth base. Incision in the sulcus adjacent to the nail or under the eponychium to liberate the pus and permit drainage is sufficient for the mild case. A vertical incision downward from one or both sides of the base of the nail with reflection of the eponychium may be required for the advanced case along with excision of any loosened segment of nail.

Chronic paronychia is often the result of the unremoved detached dead fingernail acting as a foreign body. If the infection persists after drainage and removal of the dead nail, cultures should be done for fungus.

Felon is an extremely painful, localized "closed space" infection trapped by the tough septa of the subcutaneous tissue of the pad of the tip of the finger. When neglected, it kills the bone of the terminal phalanx. A lateral incision the length of the fingernail but not encroaching on the tactile tip of the finger suffices for drainage if it passes just anterior to the bone to divide all septa. Advanced cases require incision on both sides (through and through) but only to be joined across the fingertip if there is extreme need, since a troublesome scar may result.

Collar-button abscess arises in the distal palm in the interspace between the fingers. Most of the swelling and pus is present on the volar side, but, because of the deep transverse fascia, there is also a narrow channel passing dorsalward to another pocket in the dorsal web. Adequate incision requires that both surfaces be opened, care being exercised to avoid the digital nerves when making the volar incision.

Palmar abscesses formerly often resulted in horribly prolonged and crippling illnesses with loss of hand function because the closed spaces containing the pus were not drained by the inadequate and inaccurately placed incisions then used. This tragic course usually is forestalled if the pus is drained adequately through anatomically correct incisions.

The closed spaces in the hand are *fascial compartments* and *tendon sheaths*. Infection may begin in either and spread to the other. When pus is present, it must be liberated early by diagnosing its position accurately and draining it through adequate incision, placed for proper access. The incision must be made in a bloodless field, and, since it is deep, care must be taken to avoid essential nerves and tendons.

Bunnell has pointed out that by careful observation and palpation of the swelling, hard edema, point tenderness and area of pain on movement, one can outline on the skin of the palm an ink drawing of the area of confined pus. The commonly described fascial spaces are the *mid-palmar,* the *thenar* and the *quadrilateral* space in the forearm. Since all of these are deep, the importance of careful dissection and a bloodless field during surgical drainage is obvious.

Tenosynovitis is a serious infection beginning in the flexor tendon sheath of a digit. If not relieved immediately, it extends further, necrosing tendons and breaking into the fascial spaces. The flexor sheaths of the index, the middle and the ring fingers usually terminate near the heads of their respective metacarpals. Those of the thumb and the little fingers extend into the forearm in the form of the radial and the ulnar bursae. The onset of this infection is rapid. Kanavel has outlined 4 diagnostic points: (1) the finger is held in slight flexion; (2) there is acute pain on extension; (3) uniform swelling of the volar surface of the finger is present; and (4) there is point tenderness along the course and the extent of the tendon sheath.

Treatment is immediate drainage through a mid-lateral incision the length of the proximal and the middle phalanges, the sheath being opened for this same distance, sparing the tendon sheath at the joint (retinaculum tendinum). The base of the sheath is opened in the palm by means of an incision paralleling a flexion crease (Fig. 22-3).

Antibiotics should follow surgery, but the operation is not delayed to see if antibiotics are effective.

Human Bites. The human bite (morsus humanus) presents a distinct problem because of the mixed and anaerobic bacteria inoculated into tendinous tissues of low blood supply through a bruising and ragged, penetrating wound. Usually it is sustained on the knuckles of a carelessly applied fist.

Treatment is early and thorough soap and water and saline cleansing with removal of devitalized tissues. Tendons are not repaired primarily. The wound is left open. The hand is dressed and splinted in the position it was in when the injury was received. This prevents the deeper parts of the injury from retreating under intact skin. Broad spectrum antibiotics are used (see Chap. 3, "Applied Surgical Bacteriology").

CHRONIC INFECTION

Tuberculosis of the skin of bone of the hand is the equivalent of a similar lesion elsewhere. However, this infection of the tendon sheaths may constitute a rather specific condition and often is not associated with generalized tuberculosis. It appears as a slowly progressing enlargement along the course of tendons. There is remarkably little pain and interference with function at first, and the casual examiner may confuse the early findings with a ganglion. Eventually, sinus forma-

tion, secondary infection and loss of function result.

Treatment is rest of the part and antibiotics. The progress of the tuberculous tenosynovitis may be stopped and the infection often cured. However, the treatment is always time-consuming. Radiation therapy was effective at times before antibiotics became available.

Surgery is effective only when complete excision of the infected tissue can be accomplished without ruining the hand. Partial excision or simple incision and drainage are ineffective.

Proliferative tenosynovitis of unknown etiology may be differentiated from tuberculous tenosynovitis only by microscopic examination in some cases. It is an extensive edematous thickening of the tendon sheath attended by few symptoms. It is amenable to excision. It may cause spontaneous rupture of a tendon. (Fig. 22-8.)

TRAUMA

LACERATIONS

Lacerations of the hand must be viewed with the suspicion that underlying nerve and tendon damage always exist (Fig. 22-1). (See p. 453, "Examination of the Hand.") Immediate treatment consists of the application of a sterile dressing and splinting. Then the best facilities are sought, and in an operating room the hand is cleansed without introducing further contamination into the wound. Finally, the wound is irrigated thoroughly, foreign material is removed, and devitalized tissue is excised.

In the absence of the full facilities of anesthesia and a fully equipped operating room and team, the skin is closed accurately, the hand dressed in the position of function, leaving the repair of deeper structures for a planned secondary operation later.

Immediate suture of all divided sensory and motor nerves and severed tendons is accomplished best if the patient can be operated upon with full facilities for anesthesia and the like within the proper time limit. This time limit has been set arbitrarily at 6 hours from the time of injury. If the injury were sustained under ideal conditions of cleanliness, this period might be extended. If the

FIG. 22-8. (*Left*) Soft semifluctuant tumor mass associated with spontaneous rupture of extensor pollicis longus tendon. Microscopic diagnosis was proliferative tenosynovitis. (*Right*) Extension terminal phalanx of thumb improved by tendon substitution, using extensor carpi radialis brevis tendon.

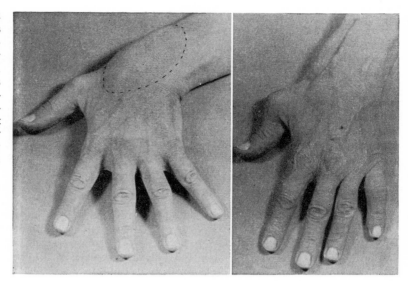

contamination were extreme, perhaps immediate deep repair is not warranted, or the safe time limit is shorter than otherwise.

Severed Sensory or Motor Nerves. Extend the wound if necessary by incisions which will not cause disability (Figs. 22-2 & 3). End-to-end approximation of nerve fibers is secured by joining the nerve sheath with stitches of finest arterial silk on atraumatic needles, taking care not to rotate either segment of the nerve. All such nerves should be repaired regardless of size.

Severed Tendons. IMMEDIATE REPAIR. Flexor tendons severed in the midpalm or the wrist regain good function when repaired carefully by direct suture, if healing is not retarded by hematoma or infection. Common digital nerves in the palm and median and ulnar nerves in the wrist are often cut at the same time and should be sutured. Both sublimus and profundus tendons may be repaired by direct suture in simple wounds. However, when the injury is extensive, it is better to join only the profundus tendons, trimming the ends of the sublimus away from the point of suture. An example of a wound where the nerves, the flexor pollicis longus and the profundus tendons only, should be sutured is the suicide attempt where all flexor structures are severed at the wrist.

Tendons severed between the distal flexion crease of the palm and the base of the middle phalanx of the finger must regain frictionless mobility through the tight channel formed by the sheath and the retaining bands which anchor the tendon in place in order to maintain function. The repair of such an injury is most complicated, and the prognosis is not consistently good. If the sublimus alone is cut at this point, it need not be repaired, because the remaining profundus action is more important and might be jeopardized by such an attempt. If both tendons are cut within this critical area of the finger, the retaining bands are severed laterally, the sublimus is detached at its insertion and removed from the finger. Only one tendon is repaired, namely, the profundus. In children of 5 years or under a meticulous end-to-end suture may be done. In others this repair is by means of a tendon graft. Both tendons are removed from the finger, the profundus is cut back to the palm well proximal to the point where the suture line would enter the retaining tunnel, and a single tendon is inserted as a free graft. This graft is joined proximally in the palm and distally to the terminal phalanx, avoiding a point of suture to freeze in the tight sheath. The removed sublimus tendon may serve as this graft if removed back to the wrist. However, a tendon graft must "take" the same as any other graft, and a structure of great bulk "takes" or assumes a blood supply less readily than one of lesser bulk. For this reason the smaller palmaris longus tendon is commonly used. As much of its paratenon as possible is transferred with it. The tendon graft may be sutured to the distal phalanx by drilling a hole in the bone and pulling the tendon into this with a wire suture. Proximally, the end of the profundus tendon is split and the smaller graft is inserted into this cleft. The point of suture is covered with lumbrical muscle.

The long flexor of the thumb may usually be repaired by direct suture, a graft being reserved for selected cases.

If the profundus tendon is severed distal to the bifurcation of the sublimus, it may be replaced immediately by a tendon graft, leaving the sublimus intact or, sometimes, if the division is quite distal, it may be sutured. If not repaired, the terminal phalanx not only loses the power of flexion but may go progressively into hyperextension. Fusion of this joint in slight flexion may be desirable at times. An alternate procedure is to use the distal stump of the profundus tendon as a checkrein to hold the terminal joint in a little flexion—the position of function.

DELAYED EARLY REPAIR. Immediate repair of flexor tendon lacerations permits surgery to be performed through normal structures free of inflammation, scar and edema, and before muscles shorten and tendon sheaths contract. However, in the absence of proper facilities and conditions, an attempt at primary repair may very well ruin all chances for subsequent salvage, and, under such circumstances, the skin should be sutured accurately under aseptic conditions, the finger splinted and the repair postponed. Occasionally, the tendon injury goes undiagnosed for a time. If there is prompt healing without infection, secondary repair may be done in 2 or 3 weeks, direct suture being done in appropriate cases; otherwise tendon grafts are used, and the result is not compromised unduly.

SECONDARY REPAIR. Extensive injury with many lacerations, crushing and perhaps the presence of fractures make primary repair impractical, and tendon replacement must be postponed until infection is absent, soft tissue replacement has been carried out if necessary, and scarring has softened. Such a finger must be evaluated carefully. An attempt at tendon repair is warranted only if the finger has promise of adequate sensation, is free from excess scar and edema, is not painful and has reasonable flexibility of the joints. No major

reconstructive procedure is of value when done on an apathetic patient—aggressive co-operation is essential, and youth is a great advantage. Physiotherapy may be more important prior to secondary repair than afterward. The skin must be put in good condition soon after injury by soap and water cleansing and removal of desquamating epithelium. The patient must be instructed in the use of warm soapsuds soaks, manipulation of the stiffened part many hours a day with the other hand and by overlapping the disabled finger with the tips of the 2 adjacent fingers so that the 3 fingers flex as a unit.

The principles of late flexor tendon repair are similar to those of earlier repair except that muscle shortening is always present, and direct repair is often impossible; most cases will require a tendon graft from midpalm to fingertip. Retaining bands and tendon sheaths will be contracted, and often new retaining bands will be required. Late repair necessitated by the severity of the original injury means a less hopeful outcome.

The common sources of tendons for grafting are the palmaris longus or the long extensors of the 2nd, the 3rd or the 4th toes. The sublimus is sometimes used. Paratenon should be included with the graft.

Extensor Tendons. These tendons are in every way more simple to repair than are the opposing flexors. The results from suturing are good.

Technic. Tendons should be sutured end-to-end, using the minimum of suture material in the form of fine silk or removable stainless steel wire. Catgut or excessive or heavy silk cause tissue reaction and proliferation with adhesion. Possibly the single most important point in the care of the hand is maintaining its position of function after injury, following surgery and during convalescence.

CHRONIC TRAUMA

This produces certain common tendon responses.

Trigger Finger or Thumb. This results from thickening of the retaining band at the base of the digit with a reduction of its lumen. A nodular thickening of the tendon forms. At first the nodule passes up and down with increasing difficulty, eventually becoming too large for the tunnel. The constriction is relieved by dividing the band on one or both sides to permit the tunnel to enlarge.

Stenosing tenosynovitis at the radiostyloid process is known as *de Quervain's disease.* This thickening of the sheath grips the extensor pollicis brevis and the abductor pollicis longus tendons, resulting in pain. It is treated by splitting the stenosed sheath.

Ruptured Tendons. LONG TENDONS, especially the extensors, may gradually wear thin and rupture in two with ordinary use. This is not to be confused with the rupture of tendons from severe trauma, such as being struck on the end of the finger by a baseball. The extensor tendon may be avulsed at its attachment to the distal phalanx, causing a dropped fingertip, or it may be torn over the middle joint. Immediate splinting in hyperextension may suffice to effect repair, inasmuch as this tendon does not retract from the point of severance. However, suturing may be required when splinting fails. Long tendons may be severed partially by laceration and pull apart later. Surgical repair is required.

PROLIFERATING TENOSYNOVITIS causes weakening of the tendon and eventually it may rupture. Repair by tendon transplant or substitution is necessary (Fig. 22-8).

TISSUE AVULSION

Replacement. As a part of the total injury, skin and subcutaneous tissue may be avulsed wholly or partially, and the question of whether or not replacement of this avulsed tissue as a graft should be done always arises. Avulsed tissue may be grafted successfully if the tissue and the wound fulfill the requirements for a free skin graft. The recipient area must have a minimum of infection and provide a blood supply to nourish the graft (open joints, bare bone and raw tendon do not provide such). The tissue to be grafted must be reasonably clean and free from contusion. It must be thin enough to be nourished for a time by diffusion of essential materials and to assume some blood supply within 48 hours. Its undersurface must be visibly free of fat. It is usually better to substitute a thick split-thickness or free full-thickness skin graft taken from an undamaged surface of the body. Partially avulsed tissue having no blood supply should be discarded and the wound

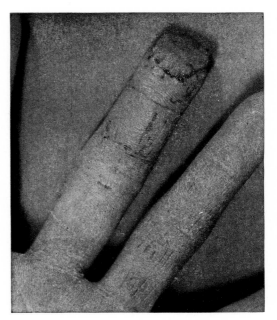

FIG. 22-9. Traumatic fingertip amputation repaired by immediate application of a small full-thickness skin graft. If available and suitable, the amount of finger severed at this accident usually can be restored successfully by suturing it back in place. To close the fingertip with conventional flaps would require further and wasteful amputation of the finger.

grafted. An exception to the above is the replacement of fingertips or the pads of fingers, a not uncommon childhood injury. If the raw surface from which this graft must receive nourishment is large in proportion to the bulk of the tissue, it may be replaced. Thus, if the excision is beveled, it is more favorable than if cut transversely. Completely free segments of finger, including one half the nail and a fragment of bone, have been restored permanently by suture replacement. If the effort to put back the cut-off part fails, a secondary repair can be done later. Further amputation of a finger to provide flaps for closure is wasteful. A repair of the defect by tissue transplantation preserves the maximum finger length (Fig. 22-9).

Even small areas of skin loss should be grafted. Denuded bone, compound fractures, open joints, bare tendons, or important nerves should be covered immediately with a pedicle

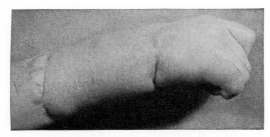

FIG. 22-10. Early result from the immediate application of an abdominal pedicle flap to denuded area of the hand and the wrist caused by the hands being trapped in the gears of a machine. No essential tendons or nerves were destroyed but were exposed and would have been lost if not covered immediately. The wrist joint was open in 3 places, which were covered with the flap. A free skin graft would not suffice here because bare tendon and open wrist joint would not provide proper bed for such a graft.

flap which carries its own blood supply. This flap may be of local tissue and its donor site covered with a free skin graft or it may be necessary to attach the hand to a skin flap from the chest, the abdomen, the clavicular region or the opposite upper arm (Fig. 22-10). In a few cases where the soft tissue of a thumb or finger has been avulsed, like the finger of a glove the denuded digit has been implanted to a subcutaneous pocket. In every such case, the digit survived probably because additional blood supply was introduced.

Specific Causes. CORNPICKER HAND INJURIES. These are among the most mutilating seen. The hand is horribly mangled, bones are fractured, tissues are avulsed, tendons are cut and torn, and nerves severed. Treatment consists of the painstaking cleansing, débridement and patient reassembling of viable portions of the hand. Partial amputation is frequently necessary because of loss of blood supply. The hand must be dressed and maintained at all times in the position of function.

MANGLE INJURIES FROM WRINGERS. These wounds usually present problems of skin avulsion and deep contusion. If the rollers are heated, the burn is deep in proportion to the pressure applied and the length of time the hand is trapped.

CONTUSIONS

Crushing injuries arising from the hand entering presses or pressure rollers are often complex. A simple example is the washing machine wringer injury. Often fractures are sustained, and the hand may have been burst like a crushed grape—the intrinsic muscles being spewed forth. Specific injuries are treated, and the hand is dressed and maintained in the position of function. Bulky dressings applied with springy compression limit edema. Permanent stiffening from fibrosis is likely to ensue after such injuries, especially in the older patient.

FOREIGN BODIES

Foreign bodies may be retained within the hand after an injury involving surface puncture or laceration. The seriousness of such retention varies according to their nature. Some, like the wadding in shotgun shells, predispose to gas gangrene or tetanus (see Chap. 4, "Surgical Infections"). Glass and many metallic particles cause little tissue reaction, but the presence of any foreign body should be diagnosed and it should be removed in most instances. All of the multiple particles from a shattered projectile cannot be removed. Foreign bodies, even those appearing to be superficial, as in the finger, may be most elusive. Every aid is sought in their removal. Careless use of the fluoroscope often has resulted in an acute radiation injury much worse than the foreign body.

BURNS

Thermal Burns. These injuries of the hand are treated locally by avoiding contamination, cleansing gently and excising thoroughly that tissue obviously dead, dressing the hand in the position of function and maintaining this position while splinting the hand with a voluminous springy pressure dressing to reduce edema.

The topical medicament must not injure crippled epithelial cells which otherwise would survive. No "fertilizer" has been discovered that will grow tissue. Mechanical injury is avoided by employing materials next to the wound which will not stick excessively and irritate further. One or two layers of "fine mesh," good quality bandage gauze, the interstices of which are just barely filled with petrolatum, is suitable. Coarse gauze inundated with grease does not qualify. Excess grease is harmful to healing.

SUPERFICIAL BURNS. These wounds heal within 10 to 14 days, if additional harm is not done in the treatment. Scarring does not result, because healing occurs from repair of existing skin. The second-degree burn may be converted readily into a third-degree loss by infection or harsh treatment or applications. The third-degree wound does not heal over with skin. The body cannot grow skin where it does not exist. It can only form scar epithelium of varying quality. This product does not possess skin appendages, is thinner than skin and less solidly attached to its base which is also scar. It is less elastic, less pliable, less strong than skin and always of less area than the original wound.

ACUTE BURNS. An acute burn causes edema in depth; a granulating wound is underlaid with a zone of inflammation. The finger joints are superficial and thus are readily involved in this inflammatory process, so that fixation must be feared. *The fibrosis of joints can be prevented only by covering granulating hand wounds with skin grafts at the earliest moment to gain a healed surface.* Obviously, these grafts must cover the wound totally if this is to be accomplished. Pinch or postage-stamp grafts eliminate part of the granulating wound but not all of it and, therefore, should not be used (Fig. 22-11).

After the first treatment every effort is directed toward early excision of dead tissue, prevention of infection by cleanliness, correct splinting and early grafting. The first dressing is changed in 2 to 5 days to eliminate purulent discharge and culture media. Subsequent dressings are delayed rarely more than 48 hours. Light anesthesia is often required. Grafting should be accomplished in from 10 to 21 days.

After healing, considerable time is required for the resolution of edema and inflammation and for skin grafts to become flexible. Subsequent to grafting, immaculate soap and water cleanliness is imperative. Early use of the hand to the point of tolerance is more desired than formal physiotherapy for a few moments several times weekly.

Secondary surgery may be required for re-

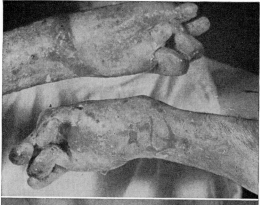

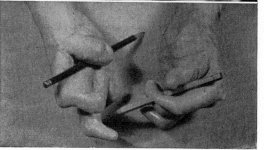

FIG. 22-11. (*Top*) Crumpled remnants of hands resulting from scar contracture, delayed graft, use of pinch grafts with slow healing and failure to preserve position of function. Hand still unhealed after 7 months. (*Bottom*) Final function less than could possibly have been given if hands had been grafted early with sheets of skin instead of pinches, and if position of function had been maintained.

sidual limitation of motion. When needed it should be delayed until movement is regained in reasonable amount and the tissues have softened.

Contractures are sometimes unavoidable. They are relieved by incision to relax tight areas followed by the insertion of additional skin. The occasional soft web of old flexible scar can be relaxed by shifting the position of existing tissue (Fig. 22-12).

Electrical injuries are localized and deep burns from intense heat generated at the point of contact. Pedicle flaps are more likely to be required for their coverage than they are for other burns. Occasionally, immediate débridement and application of such a pedicled flap may preserve important deep struc-

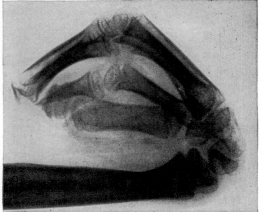

FIG. 22-12. (*Top*) Roentgenogram of deformity produced by a burn in infancy and worsened by being permitted to persist until 10 years of age. The fingers are flexed on the hand, the hand is flexed on the forearm, and the entire mass is enclosed in a single envelope of scar. (*Bottom, left and center*) After release of wrist contracture, lengthening of 11 flexor tendons and immediate application of pedicle flap. (*Bottom, right*) Separation of hand into 3 digits, with free skin graft.

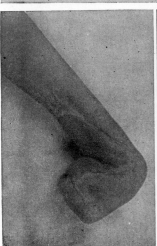
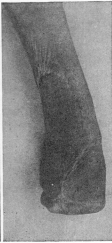
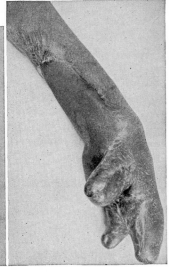

tures which otherwise would slough should the excision be delayed or the eschar be permitted to separate spontaneously.

Partial amputations of the hand are often required for electrical injuries because of the deep destruction that makes reconstruction impractical (Fig. 22-13).

Chemical burns differ from thermal injury only in the causative agent which may continue to act for an indefinite period. This must be removed by copious washing with water. If an antidote is used locally, it must not burn the area further, and immediate washing with water is mandatory while waiting for the more specific agent.

FROSTBITE

This is not unlike a burn in some respects. It results from cellular injury over a longer period of time, and there is likely to be a larger proportion of the tissue involved in marginal injury. The survival of this borderline tissue may hinge on blood vessel spasm and thrombosis. Prompt thawing without the application of heat above 40° C., procaine block of the appropriate sympathetic nerves and gentle wound cleansing and care are used. Such lesions infrequently require amputation, and the gangrene usually does not extend as far distally in the deeper tissues as it seem to on the surface, this being the opposite from arteriosclerotic gangrene.

IRRADIATION INJURIES

Permanent changes in the skin from exposure to radium, x-rays or other forms of irradiation are common and may be part of a calculated risk in the treatment of malignant tumors of the hand or due to accidental exposure or carelessness. They may be divided into the acute and the chronic forms. An acute inflammatory reaction accompanies the proper application of a total tumor dose of x-rays. This usually subsides rapidly after cessation of treatment, and hair growth usually is regained, and for a time nothing further may be noted other than dryness and inelasticity of the skin and a diminished amount of subcutaneous fat. However, the skin of certain individuals is more sensitive than that of others, or the exposure to x-rays may have been very heavy or protracted. In these, the acute reaction subsides, but the skin atrophy and inelasticity progresses, and an endarteritis of blood vessels in the treated skin develops, and telangiectases appear. These dilated, reddened, superficial vessels frequently thrombose with the subsequent appearance of keratoses and transient ulcerations. Such a condition is relentlessly progressive, and cancer of the skin almost invariably will develop in time. The patient is lulled into false security because of the slow development of this course. Malignancy may require from 5 to many more years to occur (Fig. 22-14).

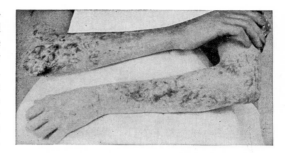

Fig. 22-14. Radiation effect on skin of hands and arms from attempted epilation by x-rays. Multiple areas of epidermoid malignancy present. Other areas may be expected to become malignant.

The acute injury may be very severe as a result of mechanical equipment failure or the prolonged use of a fluoroscope, such as may attend the search for an elusive foreign body in the hand. With acute radiation injuries blistering and indolent necrosis appear with a wide zone of marginal injury. The rate of healing is often so slow as to require excision and grafting before healing is gained. Such a heavy single exposure wound may heal with

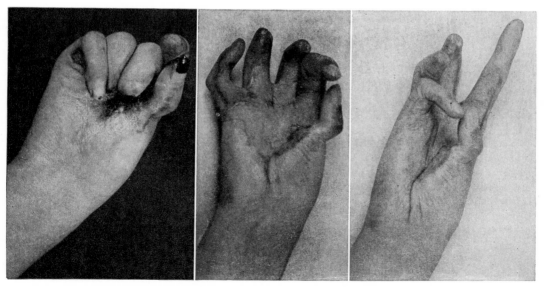

Fig. 22-13. (*Left*) Hand which was injured by an electrical burn and permitted to heal spontaneously. The destruction is localized but deep. The fingers are flexed tightly and bunched together, producing a functionless hand. Early grafting and preservation of position of function would have given a better result. (*Center and right*) Degree of function restored by excision of scar and replacement with skin grafts.

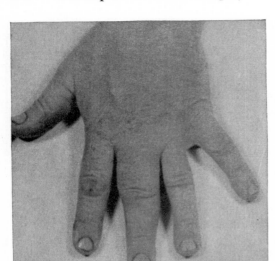

FIG. 22-15. Hand a few months after grease gun injury involving middle finger. Acute infection had followed the initial injury, and the finger is useless at this time. Grease has extended into the palm at the base of the finger. Eventual amputation of the finger was necessary.

chronic after-effects, necessitating later excision.

Typical chronic and progressive irradiation effect has most often involved the hands of radiologists and surgeons who use the fluoroscope frequently. The patient with a chronic dermatitis of the hands may be treated with x-rays by many different physicians over several years, the total dose eventually being very high before its cumulative effect is recognized.

Treatment. Medical treatment will suffice only for areas of chronic mild irradiation effect or as a temporary measure. Medical conservatism accomplishes nothing excepting jeopardy of the patients' life and must be abandoned in dealing with the well-developed radiation atrophy and keratoses unless the patient has a short life expectancy. Nonsurgical treatment consists of protecting the skin from sunlight with gloves and the use of bland, protective and ultraviolet-screening ointments.

Surgical excision of the acute ulcerative radiation injury which persists often necessitates the application of a pedicle flap carrying its own blood supply rather than free skin grafts because of fibrosis in the underlying tissues.

Chronic irradiation dermatitis of the hand should be excised and replaced with free split-thickness skin grafts before malignancy develops and before the entire part has become so avascular and avital as to develop progressive necrosis from superimposed trauma or infection.

GREASE GUN INJURIES

This trauma results when the lubrication nozzle used on automobile grease fittings comes in contact with the hand at the time of ejection. A tiny stream of oil propelled by air pressure is injected through a small perforation in the skin, sometimes filling a finger or the palm. There follows an immediate pressure ischemia and a chemical inflammation. Subsequently, infection occurs, and eventually a deep destructive ulotic granuloma arises of greater severity than the well-known paraffinoma because of the more liquid nature of the grease. The treatment is immediate wide incision, opening the tract of entry and the zone of extravasation, permitting evacuation of most of the foreign material, and relieving pressure and limiting further migration. Late removal is unsatisfactory, and partial amputation of the hand may be required (Fig. 22-15). *Air blast* may lacerate the soft tissues and fill the hand with air, resulting in pressure ischemia, inflammation and infection. Foreign bodies may be implanted. Cleansing and débridement, removal of foreign bodies and liberation of the gas under pressure by incision are indicated.

MOLTEN PLASTIC INJURIES

These injuries occur from accidental injection of the material during manufacturing processes. The heated liquid enters the hand, follows the path of least resistance and hardens as it cools. The injury is a severe internal burn.

MANUAL ATROPHY AND FIXATION

DISUSE FROM SPLINTING

The finger joints are susceptible to stiffening. The hand may become "frozen" (immobile), atrophic, or stiffened in some degree from any massive trauma, disuse, intrinsic or extrinsic nerve injury, arthritis or certain more or less specific conditions affecting circulation, nutrition and sensation. Disuse for a relatively short time may cause permanent fixation of the finger joints in the elderly patient or the individual having a propensity for periarthritic fixation. The simplest example is the stiffening of the uninjured fingers occurring following external fixation of a Colles' fracture. Any condition causing pain may produce disuse, and unfortunately many minor hand injuries have been followed by general stiffening because of improper splinting, neglect of soap and water soaks and care of the hand as a whole. Such neglect is often attributable to the failure to instruct the patient to use the hand after completion of treatment of the injury. The patient interprets the scruffiness and peeling of the skin and the presence of a newly healed scar as a warning not to use the hand. It is not unusual to see a healed hand which is filthy and covered with many accumulated strata of stale ointments. Soapsuds soaks and washing constitute the earliest stage of physiotherapy and never should be omitted.

SPECIFIC INJURIES TO TENDONS AND JOINTS

Specific injuries result in specific joints or tendons becoming frozen, and further surgery may be directed at the fault (Fig. 22-16).

Prevention of joint fixation consists of initially splinting and subsequently maintaining the hand at all times in the *position of function,* eliminating edema which begets fibrosis, continuing the movement of uninvolved structures and re-establishing total movement of the injured member at the earliest moment. The patient should perform everyday activities of increasing range. Washing dishes is one of the most valuable early forms of physiotherapy. Formal physiotherapy for a few moments several times weekly is wholly in-

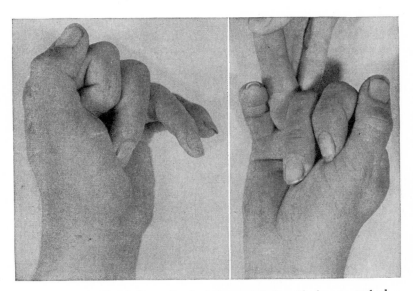

FIG. 22-16. (*Left*) Two distal phalanges of the 4th finger crushed, resulting in flexor tendons being anchored in position of extension. Although only 1 finger was injured there is also incomplete flexion of the 3rd and the 5th fingers because the tendons of these fingers cannot flex independently and are being checked by frozen tendons of the 4th finger. Amputation of useless distal and middle phalanges of the 4th finger, with retraction of flexor tendons into palm, restored flexion of the 3rd and the 5th fingers. (*Right*) Normal right hand of the same patient showing condition described at left of illustration reproduced by manually preventing flexion of the 4th finger. The effect of an adhered tendon in one finger handicapping function of a normal finger is often overlooked.

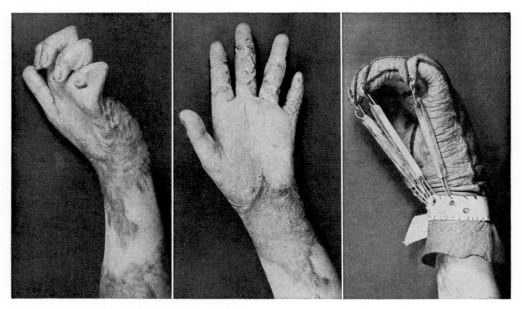

FIG. 22-17. (*Left*) Distorted hand with hypertrophic scar resulting from burns. This elevated scar is often incorrectly designated as a keloid. It is the result of irritation and infection associated with slow healing of a full-thickness loss of the skin. The scar contraction exerts tremendous force. Early complete grafting prevents this distortion and the inflammation attending an unhealed wound. (*Center*) Result soon after replacing hypertrophic contracting scar at the wrist with split-thickness skin graft and releasing the contraction of fingers by dissection of the scar and insertion of free full-thickness skin grafts. (*Right*) Residual stiffness in finger joints results from scar tissue immobilizing the joints in an abnormal position and inflammation which accompanies the unhealed wound and extends to the joint structures. A very simple dynamic splint is illustrated which is being used to restore flexion. Sometimes a dorsal splint is worn for a part of the day, alternated with a volar splint so that the fingers may be flexed and extended alternately.

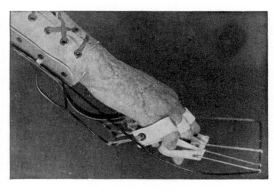

FIG. 22-18. Dynamic splint, the purpose of which is to gain extension of stiffened finger joints through gentle, continuous traction. This patient was given a simple description of what was needed and constructed his own splint. Most of such splints need not be elaborate or expensive.

adequate in itself; directing the patient in doing useful physiotherapy (or occupational therapy) 10 or 12 hours daily is effective.

Dynamic splinting means manufacturing and using a simple splint which employs constant gentle force. Such splints are made for the individual problem from sheet aluminum, felt, brads to attach the felt, web straps to buckle around the hand and arm and rubber bands or springs. Gentle constant traction tends to pull the part into position. A splint for flexion may be worn during the day and its opposite for extension during the night (Figs. 22-17 & 18).

MOTOR NERVE INJURIES

Operative mobilization of frozen tendons by surrounding the adherent part with fat or paratenon is effective. Surgery may place a joint in the position of function but is limited in its ability to restore motion to the ankylosed finger joint. Motor nerve injuries paralyzing forearm muscle result in characteristic deformities. Motor ulnar nerve palsy produces the characteristic "claw" hand.

SENSORY NERVE PARALYSIS

This condition produces anesthesia, painful paresthesias, disuse and trophic atrophy.

ARTHRITIS

Arthritis may be traumatic and even result from characteristic and repeated occupational movements. Tenosynovitis also occurs from this cause. Otherwise atrophic, hypertrophic or gouty arthritis is part of a general disease and is treated as such. Especially annoying or troublesome gouty deposits or enlargements may warrant surgical removal. A history of even mild arthritis symptoms should make the surgeon wary of complications following any injury or operation upon the hand or the arm.

An injury to the hand causes the patient to rest the entire extremity, and a "frozen" shoulder is prone to occur in such individuals.

CARPAL TUNNEL SYNDROME

Compression of the median nerve within its passageway beneath the volar carpal ligament is somewhat comparable with stenosing synovitis occurring elsewhere. The condition is most common in women. It is characterized by burning and tingling in the median nerve distribution. It is accentuated by flexing the wrist and may be elicited by tapping over the nerve at the wrist. The symptoms frequently come on at night, and the patient seeks relief by wringing the wrist or pulling on it. This condition appears to be rather common, and many patients with symptoms related to this compression have been regarded as having cervical spine disease or neuritis of some obscure nature. Tingling, burning and numbness are usual. Paralysis of the motor portion of the nerve is a late sign and results in atrophy of the thenar muscle group.

The treatment is surgical and consists of adequate decompression of the nerve by incision of the volar carpal ligaments under direct vision from the point of entry of the nerve into its tunnel to that of emergence in the hand.

POSTOPERATIVE OR POST-TRAUMATIC DYSTROPHIES

Injury to the hand or its vessels and nerves sometimes produces a degree of dysfunction the severity of which is out of proportion to the original injury. Edema, pain, atrophy, vasomotor and sudomotor abnormalities and joint fixation occur. The nature of this disturbance is not wholly understood. The patient may have reacted to the injury or the operation with an unusual degree of apprehension. Much has been written regarding its treatment. Blocking or cutting the sympathetic nerves produces vasodilatation and relieves blood vessel spasm. This is frequently helpful. The local injection of procaine hydrochloride to eliminate pain and spasm temporarily in the hope that this will permanently break some disadvantageous reflex is sometimes successful. Sudeck's atrophy is a far-advanced postoperative or post-traumatic dystrophy in which the atrophy of the bony structure of the hand or the foot is very marked and is seen readily by x-ray examination. Every dystrophy is an individual problem and must be treated on an individual basis. The surgeon must recognize the symptoms pointing to the onset of such a complication and institute active physiotherapeutic or other measures before joint fixation occurs. Stellate ganglion blocks with procaine may be of assistance.

DUPUYTREN'S CONTRACTURE

This is a progressive thickening and contracture of the palmar fascia. It is of unknown etiology and is often bilateral and familial. Men are affected more often than women. The fascia of the foot and the penis occasionally undergo similar contractures. The flexor tendons remain free and normal.

Pathogenesis. The onset is symptomless and often goes unnoticed by the patient. The first sign of the disease is a dimpling of the skin of the distal ulnar palm. After it begins its progress may be either rapid or very slow and is mainly a hypertrophy of the palmar fascia. Later contracture of the ring or the little finger appears as the palmar fascia contracts. Eventually, this may involve the middle

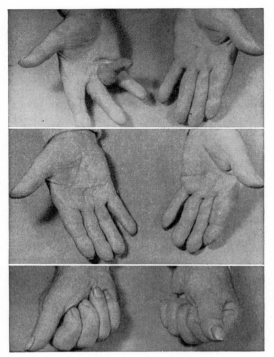

FIG. 22-19. (*Top*) Right hand shows typical Dupuytren's contracture of moderate severity in a 70-year-old man who works with his hands. The left hand is involved, but to much less degree. (*Center and bottom*) Result following extensive dissection and excision of the palmar fascia on the right and limited procedure on the left done at the same operation. The most common complication is the difficulty in obtaining a healed wound. A simple transverse incision near the distal flexion crease permits adequate exposure of the palmar fascia and ensures the best protection of the blood supply of the palmar skin. Often, additional finger incisions are required. Multiple incisions in the palm frequently jeopardize the blood supply to the thin skin overlying enlarged nodules of fascia.

and even the index fingers and the thumb web. Contracture of the proximal and middle joints draws the involved digits into the palm and interferes seriously with function of the hand (Fig. 22-19).

Treatment. The only effective form of treatment is the meticulous surgical excision of the palmar fascia and the extensions of this fascia into the 2 proximal phalanges of the involved fingers. This is immediately corrective and curative, although outlying nodules may form later and require other excisions when causing symptoms. The operation should be performed while the skin involvement is minimal. Waiting until the scar is very thick and the palmar skin very thin predisposes to the loss of the blood supply to the skin flap and the need for skin grafts. Because the advanced condition is always crippling, young or middle-aged people who develop it always should be advised to have the excision early. The active older person also should be so advised if the disease is progressing with sufficient rapidity so as to produce disability out of proportion to the patient's other infirmities. The early operation is simpler and attended by many fewer complications than is the attemped correction of the advanced contracture. In the opinion of the author, radiation therapy, cortisone, vitamin E and especially blind fascial transections are worthless therapeutic steps.

Operation. This is not to be undertaken lightly. The feared complication is the production of a stiff painful hand. This may come about through hematoma formation, loss of palmar skin because of avascularity, from excessive edema or prolonged immobilization following a too radical procedure.

The operative incision in the palm is planned to cope with the particular involvement present. No routine incision can be used. In general, a transverse incision near the distal flexion crease over the point of maximum skin involvement is safest. The skin flaps should be raised as thick as possible to expose the abnormal fascia. However, at certain points the skin may be very thin over this fascia and may be buttonholed in the course of the dissection. Midlateral incisions on the involved fingers will possibly be required, and, just proximal to the middle flexion crease, the skin must often be undercut, leaving it quite thin. This disposes to avascularity and skin loss with infection and delayed healing. The excision of the involved fascia is carried out to the point of relieving contracture and removing obviously thickened fibrous tissue. It is impossible to remove from the hand all fascia that could become involved in an advancing process, and an overaggressive approach is not justified.

Hemostasis must be complete. The operation is done with a tourniquet in place. After completion of the dissection the tourniquet is removed, and all bleeding is stopped by ligature with the finest of silk. Under no circumstances should the wound be closed and the dressing applied before the release of the tourniquet in the hope that a firm dressing will prevent a hematoma. Inspection of the wound after release of the tourniquet also permits evaluation of the blood supply of the flaps. It is better to trim away obviously non-viable skin and to apply an immediate skin graft than to permit necrosis and further inflammation.

In most cases it will be necessary to let the fingers and palm come into some flexion in order to suture the incision, because the fibrosis and the puckering have caused skin shortening. This will be overcome with use, and, if the progress of the finger contracture is stopped, it is not necessary for the fingers to have maximum extension.

Where the skin deficiency is severe, the palmar skin must be supplemented by grafts. The recipient area for these grafts is not the best. During the course of the fasciectomy all digital nerves have been dissected carefully, the strands of fascia attached to the metacarpals have been removed, and the bed to which the graft is applied is irregular and far from ideal. Full-thickness free grafts taken from the inguinal region or the upper inner arm where the skin is thin are cut carefully to pattern and fitted accurately into the defect. A grafted hand is likely to require a longer period of immobilization than is desirable. Extreme and long-standing flexion contractures of fingers, usually the fifth, are not released by fasciectomy, and straightening will require division of joint capsule. This is not rewarding, and often a partial amputation is better.

TUMORS OF THE HAND

There is no tumor, benign or malignant, which occurs only in the hand, although some are found here more frequently than elsewhere. The pathology of a specific tumor in the hand is the same as in other sites, and the principles of treatment are identical. The involved anatomy of the hand requires that surgery for tumors be done with the same meticulous care as other hand operations.

BENIGN

Benign lesions of frequent occurrence are:

Warts. These respond readily to simple treatment in children but may be resistant in adults, especially when about or under the nails.

Precancerous Lesions of the Skin. Degenerative changes occur most commonly on the areas of exposure of the skin of the face and the hands.

Implantation Cysts. Nodular, small cysts result from the subcutaneous implantation of a few epithelial cells as the result of a surface wound.

Ganglion. Degenerative connective tissue changes produce a cyst filled with clear mucoid material adjacent to joints. It is most common on the dorsum of the wrist and the flexor finger surface or the distal palm. A ganglion is important if painful. Treatment is excision utilizing a tourniquet to produce a bloodless field and through an incision so planned as to avoid contracture.

Xanthoma. This benign, painless, slow-growing tumor is one of the most common tumors of the fingers and the most frequent tumor of tendon sheath. Treatment is surgical excision.

Glomus Tumor. This is a very painful enlargement of normal terminal arteriovenous shunt apparatus. Small in size, red or purple in color, typically subungual in location, this characteristic tumor responds to complete surgical excision.

Enchrondoma is a cartilaginous tumor frequently found in the bones of the fingers.

MALIGNANT

Malignant tumors of frequent or characteristic occurrence are:

Epidermoid Carcinoma of the Skin. Occurring on the skin of the hand, it is in every way comparable with the same tumor of the skin of the face. It may be expected to develop in areas of irradiation dermatitis (Fig. 22-14).

Malignant Melanoma. This is a pigmented, radioresistant tumor of vicious potentiality; 13 per cent of them occur on an upper extremity. It may arise from a pre-existing mole, typically the junctional nevus. Frequently, it is subungual in position. Treatment is radical excision. Metastasis is by blood stream or lymphatics.

Sarcoma of all types may occur but is rare.

FRACTURES

Fractures of the metacarpals and the phalanges are common. Persistent displacement of the metacarpal fragments places the finger in an abnormal relationship, causes pressure prominences in the palm from irregularities and is likely to produce adherence of tendons at the point of fracture (Fig. 22-16). Stiffening of adjacent joints is also likely. Similar complications occur in the finger from fractures of the proximal and middle phalanges. Treatment is directed at normal realignment with minimal fixation of uninjured joints, thus avoiding the possibility of unnecessary stiffening.

Principles of treatment include diagnosis of displacement, reduction by pressure and traction and holding the reduction by splinting only the affected digits with the parts in midposition to relax muscle pull. Skin, finger pulp or skeletal traction is used to ensure against slipping when there is a tendency toward recurring displacement. Splinting the hand flat and straight with traction on the straight finger must be avoided. For metacarpal or proximal or middle phalanx fractures the position is much the same. The wrist is in slight extension and so held by a short forearm cast which stops at the distal flexion crease. The arch of the palm is maintained. The fractured finger or the finger attached to the fractured metacarpal rests on a padded wire extension incorporated within the cast; this extension is bent so as to flex the proximal phalanx 45° on the hand, the proximal interphalangeal joint 90° and the distal joint 45°. When one does this naturally with one's own hand the terminal phalanx comes comfortably into a position parallel with its metacarpal. Traction applied to the pad of the terminal phalanx pulls the finger around a curve holding good joint position and molding metacarpal and phalanges into anatomic form.

Direct wiring or transfixion of metacarpal fractures with Kirshner wires may be advisable when reduction cannot be retained by other means.

Mason's universal hand splint has many applications when recurrent displacement is not a problem.

Fractures of the distal phalanges usually result from crushing injury which produces painful tension of the sensitive pad and often subungual hemorrhage. Drilling the fingernail to evacuate blood gives merciful relief of pain. The fracture usually requires no treatment and is not amenable to much manipulation or splinting.

Bennett's fracture (fracture dislocation of the metacarpal of the thumb at its base) results from the metacarpal's being forced into flexion so that the anterior lip of the metacarpal is broken off. This lip forms a hook over the greater multangular carpal bone which gives stability to this joint. When the hook of bone is broken free, the metacarpal readily slides backward into dislocation, this movement being aided by the pull of the abductor pollicis longus. If the hook action is not re-established by reduction and fixation a very painful and troublesome situation results from loss of stability of the joint and later traumatic arthritis.

All authorities agree that this fracture may be reduced rather easily by manual traction on the thumb and forward pressure on the base of the metacarpal but that the reduction is very difficult to retain. Since it is oblique, splinting alone will not suffice. Bunnell recommends pin traction through the metacarpal head. A nonpadded cast including the forearm holds the wrist in radial flexion and supination to relax the abductor pull. The cast presses firmly forward against the back and the base of the metacarpal to prevent backward slipping. A rigid wire extension is incorporated for skeletal traction applied to the distal end of the metacarpal. Immobilization is required for 4 to 6 weeks. Criticisms of this method are: irritation and infection occur about the pin because of the web of the thumb; necrosis of the skin develops over the base of the metacarpal because of the pressure necessary to prevent backward dislocation; the traction requires frequent adjustment.

A more secure and less troublesome fixation recommended by Bunnell and by Wagner (Am. J. Surg. *80*:230-231) involves reduction and pinning of the small fragment to the metacarpal with removable Kirshner wires. The backward dislocation of the metacarpal

FIG. 22-20. (*Left*) Loss of a portion of the middle finger of a 5-year-old child from a lawnmower accident. (*Right*) Result 10 years after substituting a portion of the second toe.

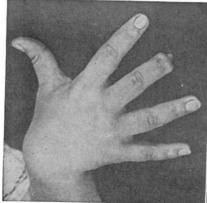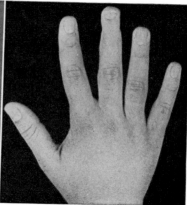

is prevented by the insertion of another wire obliquely through the metacarpal across the joint space and into the greater multangular carpal bone. This may be done blindly or by open operation.

Old fractures resulting in painful joints may require arthrodesis of the metacarpal joint.

AMPUTATIONS

Any amputation for a malignant tumor must have as its main objective the cure of the patient, and such amputations often cannot be done in a conservative fashion. Usually amputation is made necessary because of trauma, and conservatism is always the rule. Injuries to the dorsum of the hand and the wrist do not disrupt circulation, and essential sensation and some reconstructive procedure usually will suffice. Injuries to the volar surface are more serious, and it may appear that immediate amputation is the best solution but must never be done until the extent of the injury is evaluated carefully as to the possibility of salvage. Any surviving portion of a hand which is painless and has tactile sensation and some motion such as the palm on the wrist is superior to any prosthesis or will aid in the use of a prosthesis.

Loss of circulation is an indication for the removal of the affected part, but nerves and tendons may be repaired and skin replaced by immediate or delayed graft or pedicled flap. A structure can be removed later if necessary. It is a good rule in the hand not to excise viable tissue at the time of the injury.

Do not sacrifice additional tissue merely to provide a conventional flap for closure following amputation. Utilize that skin which is already present, supplemented by a graft or a flap. (See treatment of avulsion.) Do not sew finger tendons over the end of the amputated finger stump. Save the metacarpal head for stability. If the amputation is at the wrist, sew extensor and flexor tendons across the stump if necessary to ensure movement of the small remaining portion distal to the forearm. Secondary amputation for a given condition may be indicated in one individual but not in another who does different work or may be willing to undergo the long period of recovery necessary with certain correctable disabilities. The best that reconstruction can offer is useless in the face of apathy on the part of the patient.

RECONSTRUCTION FOLLOWING AMPUTATION

Hand prostheses are of 2 types. One is a lifelike prosthetic duplicate of the part over which a glove may be worn for good appearance. Little function is possible. The other is utilitarian and ranges from a post which may be strapped in place for existing fingers to work against or for a remaining thumb to pinch against, to a simple hook or a more complicated mechanical apparatus to which some motion for grasping can be imparted when the hand is totally absent. Prostheses cannot compete in usefulness with any fragment of a hand which is painless, movable and possessed of sensation.

Reconstruction of missing digits or a substitute is often feasible, but the finished product must be free from pain, not in the way and have tactile sensation to be of real value.

The thumb is the most useful digit and the one reconstructed most frequently. If the metacarpal remains, deepening the cleft between the first and the second metacarpals increases the usefulness of the hand. Building onto the end of the metacarpal by transplanting bone and skin provides a post but not sensation of a useful sort, and the structure is rigid.

Transposition of an adjacent digit to the thumb position provides a substitute which has some mobility and sensation with strength for grasping. The operation requires that the nerve, the tendon and the blood supply of the transplanted digit be left intact. When the fingers have been lost at the metacarpal phalangeal joints removal of appropriate metacarpals and the formation of a cleft between the remaining ones permits some grasping action.

Toes may be transplanted to the hand by attaching the hand to the foot for a suitable time—this can be accomplished only in children and contortionists. The procedure is of limited usefulness (Fig. 22-20).

JOHN M. HOWARD, M.D., AND I. S. RAVDIN, M.D.

—————————————— CHAPTER 23 ——————————————

Military Surgery

FUNCTION OF A COMBAT MEDICAL SERVICE

To understand military surgery one must appreciate the basic concept that the first principle of the military force is to win the battle. The functions of the medical services are secondary to this basic military principle.

The field medical service is designed with a twofold mission: (1) to help win the war; (2) to give the greatest support to the greatest number of casualties.

Obviously, the function of helping to win the war is important. Over the centuries, soldiers in the front line have developed great faith in the medical corpsmen and battalion aid surgeons, believing that in the event of their being wounded, medical assistance would reach them immediately, regardless of the danger to the medical personnel. By educating troops as to the value of the protective helmet or the armored vest, casualties can be prevented. Following thousands of cold injuries in North Korea, further casualties were prevented by the provision of better clothing

and the education of the troops as to their proper use. Sanitation and immunization are other examples of means of conserving troop strength. Finally, casualties with minimal injuries must be given appropriate treatment in the forward area and returned to combat duty.

The heritage of civilian medicine is that every conceivable support must be given the individual patient. This is based on the assumption that unlimited resources are available. Under combat conditions, this basic assumption may become untenable. Depending upon combat activities, the flow of casualties may vary from day to day between a dozen and a thousand. When the number of casualties imposes an overwhelming load on a medical unit, complete immediate care cannot be given each casualty. Under such conditions, the medical officers must decide who is to have immediate care and who can await delayed care. This function is designated "triage," the French word meaning "sorting; picking, choosing; selection, choice." Obviously, triage may necessitate compromises in the treatment of individual patients, but compromises that are designed to provide the greatest number of men with the best care.

ORGANIZATION OF A COMBAT MEDICAL SERVICE

Because of its nature as a supporting unit of a combat army, the medical service in a combat area must be organized so as to be mobile. The units in the front lines must be able to move under their own manpower at any time; a unit 10 miles behind the front lines must be able to move in a few hours; a unit 100 miles behind the lines must be able to move within approximately 24 hours. This prerequisite of mobility is basic in the

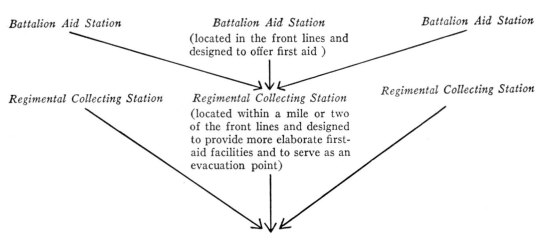

Battalion Aid Station

Battalion Aid Station
(located in the front lines and
designed to offer first aid)

Battalion Aid Station

Regimental Collecting Station

Regimental Collecting Station
(located within a mile or two
of the front lines and designed
to provide more elaborate first-
aid facilities and to serve as an
evacuation point)

Regimental Collecting Station

Divisional Clearing Station
(located within 5 to 10 miles
of the front lines and designed
primarily for triage. Casualties
with minimal injuries may be
held for short periods of time
and returned to duty. Those
more seriously injured may be
evacuated to evacuation hospitals in the rear. Those most
critically injured are sent to
adjacent mobile surgical hospitals for emergency surgical
care)

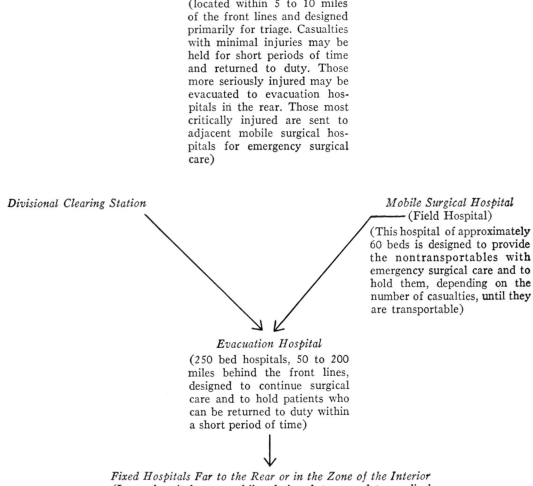

Divisional Clearing Station

Mobile Surgical Hospital
(Field Hospital)
(This hospital of approximately
60 beds is designed to provide
the nontransportables with
emergency surgical care and to
hold them, depending on the
number of casualties, until they
are transportable)

Evacuation Hospital
(250 bed hospitals, 50 to 200
miles behind the front lines,
designed to continue surgical
care and to hold patients who
can be returned to duty within
a short period of time)

Fixed Hospitals Far to the Rear or in the Zone of the Interior
(Large hospitals, nonmobile, designed to complete medical
care)

organization. Thus, a forward unit which must be capable of moving its personnel and equipment, without assistance and within an hour, cannot be elaborate nor can it contain at any time many critically ill, and thus immobilized, casualties. To a lessening extent, this characteristic pattern is true of medical facilities at increasing distances behind the front lines. Based on this need, the policy of evacuation was evolved. Since a forward unit cannot be large or elaborate, casualties must be evacuated toward the rear, being held at forward units only as their condition necessitates treatment or does not permit transportation.

The organization of a medical service in a combat theater varies, being adaptable to combat activity, but the diagram on page 478 is the basic pattern.

Such an organization necessitates that patients pass from one doctor to another without continuity of physician-patient relationship.

WOUNDING AGENTS

Military weapons are of 3 basic patterns:

1. **Small Arms.** Machine guns, submachine guns ("burp guns"), rifles and pistols. These weapons vary in range, velocity and rapidity of firing but fire a preformed missile which is not designed for fragmentation.

2. **Fragmentation Shells.** These larger missiles, consisting of mortar shells, artillery shells, conventional bombs, grenades and mines, are designed to explode into thousands of fragments.

Wounding Agent	World War II[3]	Korean Conflict[31]
Small arms	27%	23%
Fragmentation missiles	72%	76%

3. **Atomic and Thermonuclear Weapons.** These weapons are designed to produce blast, thermal and irradiation damage. In addition to the direct destructive effect of the blast, the target is fragmented, producing millions of secondary missiles.

The relative number of casualties produced by the first 2 types of weapons has been:

Burns accounted for approximately 1 per cent in each instance.

In World War II, approximately 23 per cent of men hit by small arms fire died, and approximately 18 per cent of men hit by fragmentation missiles died.[3] Thus, because of the

much higher incidence of injury, fragmentation missiles have been the chief cause of death.

WOUND BALLISTICS

Wound ballistics[34] is the science of the motions and the effects of projectiles, or other missiles, in the body upon and after impact.

Studies of wound ballistics have added materially to the knowledge of the nature of combat wounds. For the first time wounds can be described in terms of the amount of energy transmitted from the missile to the body rather than simply in terms of centimeters of tissue destroyed. By using bullets of known weight, investigators have measured the velocity of the missile as it struck the experimental animal and as it left the animal. Thus, the energy lost by the missile and transmitted to the animal could be calculated. These physical measurements of wounds permit description or classification on the basis of energy transmitted (Fig. 23-1). Thus, mechanical injuries can be compared quantitatively with each other, with electrical or irradiation injuries, or with the clinical course of the experimental subject.

As a high-velocity missile strikes the body, the resistance offered by the tissue results in

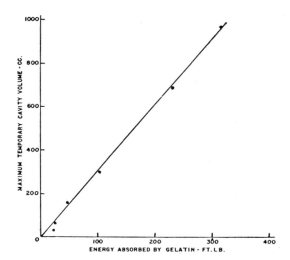

FIG. 23-1. Plot of energy absorbed in producing a "wound" in a gelatin body model (horizontal scale) versus maximum size of the temporary wound cavity (vertical scale). (Herget, C. M.: Wound ballistics *in* Bowers, W. F., Ed.: Surgery of Trauma, Philadelphia, Lippincott, 1953)

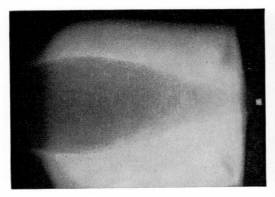

Fig. 23-2. Microsecond roentgenogram showing an early stage in the production of a temporary "wound" cavity in a gelatin body model by a 10-grain fragment which hit with a velocity of about 5,400 ft./sec. and is shown leaving the model. The maximal size of this "wound" cavity was much larger. (Herget, C. M.: Wound ballistics *in* Bowers, W. F., Ed.: Surgery of Trauma, Philadelphia, Lippincott, 1953)

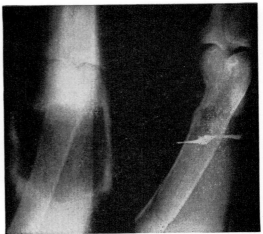

Fig. 23-3. On the left is a microsecond exposure roentgenogram showing the maximal size of a temporary wound cavity in an animal's limb. By comparison (*right*), a subsequent roentgenogram following the injection of a radiopaque fluid demonstrates the small size of the permanent wound tract. Note that the fracture is quite remote from the permanent wound tract. (Herget, C. M.: Wound ballistics *in* Bowers, W. F., Ed.: Surgery of Trauma, Philadelphia, Lippincott, 1953)

the transmission of energy to the tissues. Thus, every cell in the pathway of the bullet becomes a secondary missile traveling at right angles to the primary missile. As a result of these secondary missiles, the scope or size of the wound is increased greatly. Serial roentgenograms, taken with exposures of only a microsecond, demonstrate the transient development of a cavity that is far greater in size than that of the wounding agent (Fig. 23-2). The cavitation does not persist and would not be suspected by examination of the final gross anatomic defect (Fig. 23-3). During such studies, defects in large blood vessels, nerves, and even fractures, have been produced by the secondary force, even though the structures were not touched by the bullet. This concept of energy transmission as a measure of the magnitude of a wound can be correlated roughly with clinical experiences. A penetrating soft tissue wound is associated with a minimal absorption of kinetic energy. A bullet that encounters the resistance of bone and transmits enough energy to produce a compound fracture is a wound of greater magnitude. Finally, a traumatic amputation of an extremity, avulsing soft tissues and bone, requires a still greater force.

Wound	Number of Casualties	Mortality
Soft tissue penetration[32]	280	0
Compound fracture	82	1.2%
Traumatic amputation	32	9.7%

The correlation between this rough index of the magnitude of the wound and the resultant mortality in military surgery is not unexpected.

These basic studies of ballistics have confirmed and extended 2 well-recognized clinical observations: (1) that the wounds of entrance and exit do not depict the degree of damage to underlying structures; and (2) that the edges of the wound do not delineate the lateral extent of injury. This concept of lateral injury is the basis for the surgical principle of débridement.

THE BATTLE WOUND

The passage of a bullet through the body requires only a fraction of a second, and the combat soldier has sustained an injury. But lives, like wars, seldom are lost instantane-

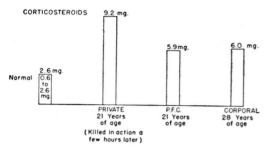

COMBAT STRESS
Urinary Excretion of Adrenal Steroids

Stress: On Front Line 40 days. Under heavy mortar
fire throughout this day of study.

FIG. 23-4. Demonstrating simultaneously the stress response of 3 soldiers who were sharing the same combat bunker.

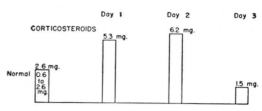

COMBAT STRESS
Urinary Excretion of Adrenal Steroids

Subject: Master Sergeant, 34 years of age
Stress: On Front Line 40 days. Under heavy artillery
fire during first day of the study

FIG. 23-5. Serial studies of individual soldiers revealed the continuation of the stress response throughout the 48-hour combat period.

ously. There is a struggle—an injury and a response—a continuing injury and a continuing response. Death may occur moments or weeks thereafter.

The missile has inflicted its damage, and then the wound itself exerts a deleterious effect on the body—as deleterious an effect, perhaps, as cancer. The injury is not a wound of the moment; it is a dynamic injury, progressive or regressive until death or healing results. Thus, it is a continuing injury, not just of the missile pathway, but of the entire body, which persists not for the moment but for days or weeks. Every system, every organ and, presumably, every cell in the body responds to this injury. Like the wound, this response continues for days or weeks. In general, it appears to be proportional to the magnitude of the injury.

Because of the stress of combat, the response in part may precede the physical

TABLE 1. COMBAT STRESS—ALL MEN ON FRONT LINE 40 DAYS. A STUDY OF 15 SOLDIERS

Day	Activity	AVERAGE CORTICOS-TEROID EXCRETION* (mg. per 24 hr.)
1st Day	Heavy artillery fire	6.3 mg.
2nd Day	Fewer incoming shells	3.7 mg.
3rd Day	Rain—quiet	—
4th Day	Quiet day	1.5 mg.

* Normal range 0.6 to 2.6 mg.

trauma. During 48 hours of an intensive artillery barrage by the enemy on the Eastern Korean Front in the spring of 1952, volunteers of an infantry division were studied by means of 24-hour urine collections and analyses of adrenal steroids. The first day the incoming artillery fire was intense. The second day the fire was less intensive but remained heavy; one of the subjects was killed, several others had their bunkers destroyed. The third day was quiet with rain so heavy that the collecting vessels for urine overflowed, and the specimens were lost. The fourth day was quiet.

The stress of such men is intense. Studies of the corticosteroid excretion of these men revealed a stress response comparable with that following major trauma.[19]

The first day every man demonstrated the stress response. The second day the stress response had subsided in some, not in others. The fourth day the stress response had subsided in every man (Table 1); Figs. 23-4, 23-5).

A wound is inflicted, and a compensatory response occurs. This response may be life-saving. The response is fully activated by the time the casualty undergoes operative treatment. Anesthesia blocks, in part, this response and, therefore, for the moment furthers the injury.

What is the nature of the injury of which a soldier may die?

TRANSMISSION OF ENERGY

The basic nature of the injury has been

described as the transfer of energy from the missile to the tissue. For the first time the magnitude of injury is being measured not in centimeters of tissue destroyed but in the amount of energy transmitted.

As described above, in clinical experience the magnitude of injury reflects the magnitude of injury from the physicist's measurements, especially when one limits the observations to nonvital structures, such as an extremity.

How does the passage of a missile exert its deleterious effect? Perhaps there is a transmission of energy to every cell of the body with a resulting deleterious effect, but at present at least the following 4 components of the battle injury are recognized. Any one of the components may predominate and result in a fatality, but the summation of injuries produces a distinct, continuing, deleterious effect.

1. Mechanical Defects

Defects such as an open chest, tracheal obstruction, cardiac tamponade, increased intracranial pressure or a perforated bowel carry an immediate threat to life that needs no elucidation here.

2. Destruction of Tissue

Destruction of tissue produces injury in 2 ways: (1) the acute injury—the loss of function of a vital organ; (2) the subacute injury—the production of necrotic tissue.

Only by seeing those killed in action can one appreciate the magnitude of a battle wound. A vital organ, such as the brain, can be destroyed, and death is inevitable. The destruction of such a vital organ is one of the two chief reasons why approximately 20 per cent of all men injured in battle die before reaching medical facilities. This figure has not been reduced appreciably during the 20th century. By contrast, the mortality rate of those casualties dying after reaching medical facilities has dropped steadily, reaching an all-time low of 2.4 per cent in Korea. These 2 categories are referred to in military statistics as "Killed in Action" and "Died of Wounds," respectively. Efforts to reduce the number of men killed in action have centered in the use of the protective helmet and the armored vest. Both have proved to be valuable in helping to offset the increasing de-

structiveness of modern weapons. Studies in Korea indicated that 68 per cent of missiles striking the vests were stopped. This does not imply that 68 per cent of casualties were prevented, since many casualties (and vests) were struck by multiple missiles. It does indicate, however, a degree of protection against fragmentation missiles. Most small arms missiles penetrated the armored vest.[15]

The second syndrome, centering in the subacute injury of necrotic tissue, is of historical importance in military surgery. One needs only to turn back to the medical history of the American Civil War[24] to appreciate the progress made in this field. The Surgeon General's report of the Civil War included 283 patients with wounds of the extremities who developed gangrene secondarily. The resultant mortality was 56 per cent.

The wound is dynamic. It is continuing to insult the body, and the body is continuing to respond. Dead tissue, contaminated with virulent bacteria, accentuates the injury, since this part of the wound is isolated from the blood stream. Serum collections and hematomas, like necrotic tissue, are isolated from the active circulation, and so behave like dead tissue in offering a springboard for infection. The fundamental principle of wound surgery is débridement—the removal of debris—so as to bring the defense mechanism, the blood supply, to the frontier of the continuing assault, the open wound.

If life is maintained, the dead tissue will be removed. Either the surgeon takes a few minutes to accomplish it with knife and scissors (débridement) or the body responds and takes 2 to 3 weeks to remove the dead tissue as a slough or metabolic débridement.

The shaggy, shredded tissue lining the missile pathway is identified easily as nonviable tissue, which must be removed. That immediately adjacent to the pathway may be obviously nonviable. But inevitably, as the surgeon débrides away from the pathway into the area of the indirect trauma, tissues become less obviously viable or nonviable.

The color of the muscle, the presence of bleeding on the cut surface, the contraction of the muscle bundles when pinched, may all suggest viability; yet often the surgeon simply cannot delineate, on the day of injury, the extent of devitalized tissue. It is for this paramount reason that the procedure of delayed closure of war wounds still is justified today. Thus, the basic principle of wound surgery is to excise the dead and foreign tissue and thus bring the blood supply to the wound frontier. Delayed closure is not a principle, only a means of ensuring the basic principle of débridement by providing drainage and the opportunity to reinspect the wound at a later time when any nonviable tissue has become obvious.

3. Blood Loss

Blood is lost, and thus the body's defense is injured seriously—its supply chain and communication system are disrupted. Death may result, as no part of the body is self-sufficient, each part being dependent upon the circulation for support. Thus, blood loss and systemic ischemia promote injury to the entire individual, so that the entire patient, not just the tissues of the open wound, is fighting for survival. Literally speaking, the wound then is the entire individual.

Three aspects of the problem are pertinent: control of bleeding; correction of blood-volume deficiency; and repair of damage from prolonged ischemia.

Control of bleeding is essential, and yet it constitutes one of the real challenges of surgery today. Usually, control of external bleeding is relatively simple, but control of intra-abdominal bleeding from major vessels or a large wound of the liver may prove to be difficult and sometimes impossible. When anesthesia is superimposed on deep or impending shock in an effort to control hemorrhage, death may result. This is the crucial problem today in the control of hemorrhage once the patient has reached the hospital.

The correction of blood-volume deficit in combat casualties in Korea reached a peak in efficiency. Never before in the history of military surgery was blood used so freely and so effectively. The concept of hopelessly severe injury did not exist except in an occasional patient with massive destruction of the brain. Instead, patients with massive traumatic amputations or massive intra-abdominal injuries were tackled with the concept of expectant salvage as blood was begun within seconds of arrival through 2 to 4 portals. Crossmatch was unnecessary, due to the universal donor

program of low titer Type O blood, and time and again patients received from 15 to 20 pints of blood without crossmatch and without transfusion reaction (Table 2). Transfusion was much more effective, of course, if hemorrhage could be controlled first. In lieu of whole blood or sterile plasma, plasma-volume expanders were introduced and used extensively in the front lines, for nature provides a relatively greater reserve in red cell mass than in blood volume.

The effects of prolonged ischemia, the third problem, are a matter of keeping the patient alive until he can repair the damage.

Postanesthetic, postoperative hypotension usually reflected a marked persistent blood-volume deficiency, although the body tolerates a deficiency of considerable magnitude at this time much better than it does immediately after injury.[30] Additional transfusion usually was the treatment of choice. Vasoconstrictors at this time were seldom of value; intravenous calcium gluconate occasionally produced a striking blood-pressure response. Irreversible cerebral damage in this age group, following shock without head injury, was not recognized.

Post-traumatic renal insufficiency carried a mortality of 80 to 90 per cent. Because of the gravity of the prognosis, a Renal Failure Center was established at an Evacuation Hospital in Korea to receive all casualties of the United Nations' troops in Korea with this complication. Slow, steady progress resulted in lowering the mortality to approximately 50 per cent.[37]

4. Bacterial Contamination

The open wound is a contaminated one. Studies by the Surgical Research Team in Korea re-emphasized several factors. The extremity wound, at the time of primary débridement, contains pathogenic aerobic and anaerobic organisms. In a study of 154 battle wounds,

TABLE 2. EXPERIENCES IN KOREA IN THE ADMINISTRATION OF TYPE O BLOOD, WITHOUT CROSSMATCH[17]

PINTS OF TYPE O BANKED BLOOD	HEMOLYTIC TRANSFUSION REACTIONS	INCIDENCE
10,000	3	0.03%

Policy:
High titer—Type O patients.
Low titer—All other patients.

a single bit of tissue from each wound revealed clostridia in 47 per cent, pathogenic clostridia in 27 per cent. In addition, 84 per cent of the cultures yielded aerobic organisms.[21] In a more detailed study of a smaller group of wounds, clostridia were found at the time of primary débridement in 82 per cent.[36] Blood cultures, taken from the most severely injured at the time of hospitalization, approximately 3.5 hours after injury, occasionally but infrequently revealed the presence of virulent organisms.[22] So, these wounds represent a break in the body's defense against bacteria and contain the virulent organisms necessary to produce life-endangering infections.

Because of the early débridement, the prevention of gangrenous tissue by the repair of severed arteries, and the consistent use of antibiotics, fatal infections almost disappeared from the Korean battlefield.

It is difficult to distinguish the effects of abdominal trauma per se from the effects of peritonitis. Abdominal trauma with peritonitis remains a major problem, although few patients died of abdominal wounds after the first 48 hours. Few in Korea died of peritonitis unaccompanied by severe hemorrhage.

In order to minimize the continuing nature of the injury, débridement is necessary. This can be performed only by blocking, in part, the lifesaving response as one introduces the fifth element of injury, anesthesia. The responses of the patient, particularly of the autonomic nervous system, are mobilized fully. Anesthesia depresses this response and so temporarily furthers the injury. This may be a critical moment, to be minimized only by correcting part of the injury, mechanical defects and *blood-volume deficiency* prior to

adding the anesthetic insult. To add anesthesia to the earlier insults prior to correcting the blood-volume deficit may be necessary sometimes, but it is comparable with shooting the bullet-ridden casualty one time more.

Finally, the day-of-combat injury is a day of continuing injury: combat stress, extremes of temperature, combat injury, painful litter rides, continued bleeding, repeated bacterial contamination, transfusion with cold blood, anesthesia, operation and fear of death. This is continuing trauma inflicted from without the wound. Korea saw this period of injury greatly shortened. The helicopter shortened the prehospitalization period in Korea to from 1.0 to 2.5 hours, the average time lag in the severely injured, combining helicopter and ambulance evacues, being 3.5 hours.

Because of continuing improvements in treatment, the mangling combat wound has continued its historic loss in its ability to kill and deform. Korea saw a new record in the low mortality rate of those wounded in action (2.4%, a drop of 4.5% in World War II). Wounds of certain anatomic areas showed marked decreases in mortality, especially those influenced by infection (Table 3).

RESUSCITATION AND EVACUATION

PRINCIPLES OF RESUSCITATION AND EVACUATION

Resuscitation includes emergency therapy designed to stop the injury and to correct its previous damage. The wound continues to exert its deleterious effect. The body continues to respond. Treatment also must be continuous. Within such a concept, it is diffi-

TABLE 3. COMPARATIVE STATISTICS FOR MORTALITY RATES WORLD WAR II*
(1942-45) AND KOREA† (1952-53)

	WORLD WAR II		KOREAN CONFLICT	
SITE OF INJURY	Number of Casualties	Mortality	Number of Casualties	Mortality
Abdomen	1,185	21%	402	12.6%
Colon	1,106	23%	140	9.3%
Jejunum and ileum	1,168	14%	134	3.0%
Stomach	416	29%	45	0 %
Liver	829	10%	102	9.0%
Spleen	341	12%	54	0 %

* Second Auxiliary Surgical Group.
† Surgical Research Team in Korea.

cult to define the point at which resuscitation ends. From the practical point of view, resuscitation includes first aid, correction of mechanical defects, control of hemorrhage, correction of blood-volume deficit, definitive surgery, including excision of the wound and continued supportive measures until the body, and especially the circulatory system, becomes stabilized. Most casualties who die are lost within the first 48 hours. It is during this period, and particularly during the first 24 hours, that resuscitation includes almost the total therapy.

Resuscitation is begun by the medical corpsmen or sometimes by a fellow combat soldier who first sees the casualty. The first responsibility is to stop the progression of the injury. In the front line, this consists of stopping hemorrhage by the application of a tourniquet if bleeding is profuse. The casualty either walks or is placed on a litter (Fig. 23-6) and carried the necessary distance, usually a

few hundred yards, to the battalion aid station (Fig. 23-7). Here, usually, he is seen first by a medical officer. The wounds are inspected, are covered with sterile dressings, and hemostasis is obtained by tourniquets, pressure dressings or, occasionally, by the clamping and the ligation of vessels. The most important responsibility of the battalion surgeon is to stop hemorrhage and correct any major blood-volume deficiency so as to make the soldier better able to withstand transportation to a forward hospital. The battalion aid stations often have to move and often are under artillery, mortar or small arms fire. As a result, they must be simple and improvised for protection. Only the most fundamental treatment can be carried out. Blood banks are impractical, due to the lack of electricity at this level. As a result, dried plasma, concentrated albumin and plasma volume expanders are maintained and used. Although these substances are not as beneficial as whole blood,

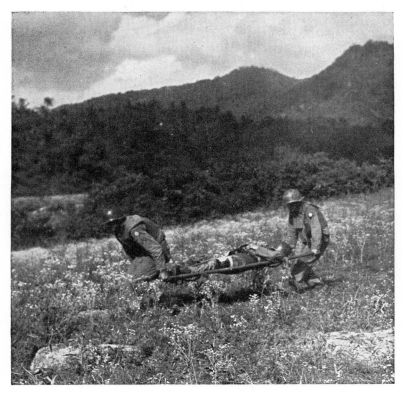

FIG. 23-6. Bringing a casualty off the front lines to the battalion aid station. The casualty will remain on the litter until he reaches the operating room at the forward surgical hospital.

they may be a life-saving compromise in the absence of blood. Coincident with the correction of blood-volume deficiency, mechanical defects are corrected. Sucking chest wounds are closed with occlusive dressings, and fractures are splinted. Occasionally, tracheotomy, thoracentesis or pericardiocentesis may be necessary. When the press of casualties permits, tetanus toxoid and antibiotics are administered at this time. When necessary, morphine is administered for the control of pain.

If the medical corpsman has not previously started the patient's record, it is begun at this level. The time of injury, the nature of the

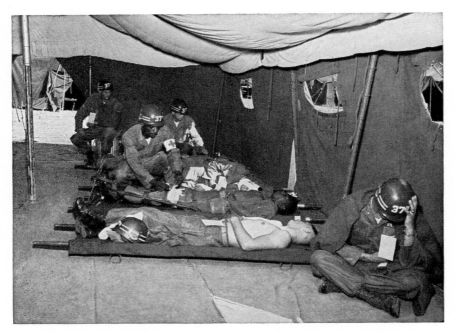

FIG. 23-7. Inside a battalion aid station. These simulated conditions lack the protective elements of sandbags and trenches. (Lt. Col. H. H. Ziperman, MC., U. S. A.)

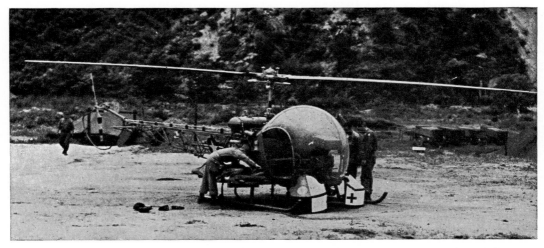

FIG. 23-8. Helicopters are invaluable in mountainous terrain in the rapid evacuation of the critically injured. This helicopter can carry 2 patients.

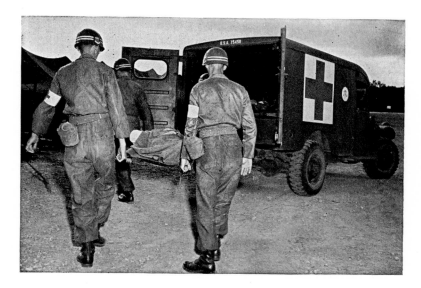

wounding agent, the description of the wound, vital signs and therapy are recorded.

When feasible, most casualties will be evacuated within 30 minutes. In Korea, the most critically injured were evacuated by helicopter (Fig. 23-8) directly to the forward hospital, but most casualties (and all casualties at night) are evacuated by ambulance (Fig. 23-9). From the battalion aid station, the casualty is carried approximately 1,000 yards to the company collecting station. The means of transportation is ambulance if roads permit; the other means are improvised as necessary.

At the collecting station, medical officers re-examine the patient and review and continue his record. If no additional first-aid treatment is necessary, the patient is evacuated farther to the rear. At the collecting station also, facilities are crude, and therapy is limited to correction of blood-volume deficiency and mechanical defects. By definition, the collecting station receives patients from several battalion aid stations. From this point they are evacuated by ambulance to the divisional clearing station several miles to the rear. The clearing station serves fundamentally as a triage or routing center, although resuscitation is continued when necessary. It derives its name from the organizational fact that a casualty who is evacuated to the rear of the clearing station leaves the control of the infantry division, the control passing to a higher headquarters. At the clearing station, a cas-

ualty may be examined and returned to duty (a function also served by the battalion aid station and the collecting station), may be held for observation, may be transported to an adjacent forward surgical hospital for emergency surgery (Fig. 23-10), or may be transferred to an evacuation hospital far to the rear for delayed care. These decisions depend not only on the casualty's condition but also on the combat activity and the number and the needs of the fellow casualties.

When the load of casualties exceeds the resources of the medical personnel, priorities for evacuation and definitive surgery must be established. These priorities represent a compromise based on the guiding principles of (1) promoting the greatest good of the greatest number and (2) the age-old surgical principle that life takes precedence over limb, function over anatomic deformity.

This function of triage, or sorting, of casualties requires mature surgical judgment, for occasionally many lives may depend upon proper immediate decisions as to the disposition of large numbers of casualties.

Priorities in the Surgical Management of Traumatic Casualties

Top Priority. Mechanical correction of defects that immediately endanger life:
    Control of external hemorrhage
    Relief of intracranial pressure

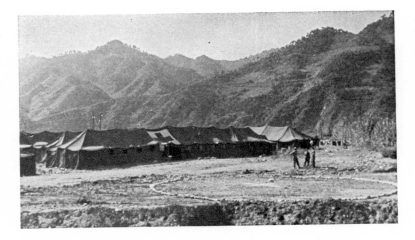

FIG. 23-10. A Mobile Army Surgical Hospital (Field Hospital) located within 10 miles of the front lines. This unit, containing 60 beds, consists of tents and sufficient equipment and personnel to perform definitive surgery. Helicopters land in the foreground; ambulances drive to the hospital entrance.

Closure of sucking chest wound or relief of tension pneumothorax

Control of internal hemorrhage

Relief of respiratory obstruction

Relief of cardiac tamponade

Shock, coma or evisceration, which places any casualty in this group as regards priority of medical attention

Second Priority. Correction of defect that ultimately endangers life:

Relief of progressive spinal cord pressure

Definitive repair of perforations of gastrointestinal tract or biliary-pancreatic tract

Débridement of cerebral wounds

Exploration of wounds of mediastinum

Surgical amputations following traumatic amputation (to control bleeding and prevent sepsis)

Third Priority. Correction of defect that immediately endangers limb or organ: Repair of major arterial wound

Fourth Priority. Correction of defect that ultimately endangers limb or organ:

Exploration of ocular injuries

Immobilization of compound fractures and reduction of dislocated joints

Fifth Priority:

Débridement of soft tissues

Realignment of fractures

Sixth Priority:

Closure of soft tissue wounds

Repair of peripheral nerves

CLINICAL EXPERIENCES IN RESUSCITATION

Military surgery has provided a few groups with the clinical opportunity of participating actively in the resuscitation of several thousand casualties. Valuable observations have resulted. The following discussion is based on such experiences in World War II and in the Korean War.

All major combat injuries are associated with significant losses of blood. To this loss the body responds by vasoconstriction and by increased cardiac activity. As the magnitude of blood loss increases, the clinical picture may change gradually as the body becomes unable to compensate for the loss. The basic concept is that all degrees of hemorrhage may be associated with these injuries. There is no magic point at which hypotension occurs or at which transfusion is required. "Shock" is not an end-point; instead, as the basic process of hemorrhage continues, vasoconstriction and increased cardiac activity cannot maintain a normal blood pressure. Hypotension results. A casualty may lose 1,000 ml. of blood and maintain a normal blood pressure. After he loses another 100 ml. he may be hypotensive and be described as "in shock." Actually, very little difference exists in his status in the 2 circumstances. With the loss of 1,000 ml. of blood he was in incipient shock. Hypotension might then follow evacuation, movement on a litter, change of position or the administration of morphine. Profound hypotension would follow the induction of anesthesia. It is absolutely essential to good surgery that this deficit be recognized, even though the blood pressure is normal. In the normotensive patient, the deficit can be estimated only by the other vital signs, the blood loss on the dressings and the magnitude of the wound. It is more difficult to estimate in the patient with intra-abdominal injuries. Because these patients are young and previously healthy, it is safer, when in doubt, to transfuse the compensated casualty with from 500 to 1,000 ml. of blood preoperatively.

The rapid loss of from 1,200 to 1,500 ml. (20 to 25% of the blood volume) is associated characteristically with a modest drop in systolic blood pressure from the normotensive level to a range of from 90 to 110.[4, 13] If the bleeding can be stopped, the patient's pressure responds immediately to transfusion.

Not infrequently, casualties arrive at a forward surgical hospital with a systolic blood pressure below 50 mm. Hg—even imperceptible. Such patients require immediate intensive transfusion. Transfusions must be started through 2, 3 or even 4 portals, large bore needles being used. Under careful supervision, air pressure is used to increase the rate of transfusion. Under the most careful supervision, a busy resuscitation team will inevitably encounter the grave therapeutic complication of air embolus unless a second bottle of blood or saline is used in continuity as an air trap. The inevitable occasional confusion of such a ward containing from 10 to 40 patients makes this precaution essential. Intravenous infusion appears to be as effective and as rapid as intraarterial infusion.

In the massively injured casualty, a therapeutic error encountered occasionally is to transfuse distally to a severed vein. Thus, if a laceration of the inferior vena cava is a possibility, the surgeon must not depend entirely upon transfusion portals in the lower extremities.

In Korea, where the evacuation time was short, the concept of hopelessly severe injury did not exist except in the presence of mangling injuries of the brain. Preoperative irreversible shock was not recognized, for, without exception, the blood pressure could be returned to normal in the preoperative period if bleeding could be controlled. Continued hypotension meant continued bleeding or inadequate transfusion.

Since the restoration of a normal blood pressure is a rough indication of the correction of the blood-volume deficit in the young subject, ideally this was a prerequisite to anesthesia and operation. So long as the pressure was rising toward normal, transfusion was continued, and anesthesia was postponed. The more difficult decisions arose when intra-abdominal bleeding continued during the period of transfusion. So long as the blood pressure continues to rise, vigorous transfusion should be continued and operation delayed. Should the bleeding be so profuse that the blood pressure fails to respond or stabilize at a subnormal level, operative control of the hemorrhage is the only recourse. The surgeon and the anesthetist must realize, however, that to block such a patient's compensatory mechanism with anesthesia carries the grave risk of immediate death. This problem of continued massive intra-abdominal hemorrhage has not been solved. Its solution probably will depend upon finding means of controlling hemorrhage without the use of general or spinal anesthesia. Hemostasis may be attained under local anesthesia when a single vessel has been injured, but it becomes more difficult when multiple missiles have produced many points of injury.

Operative correction of the wound, being necessary to stop the continuing injury, is a part of resuscitation. In itself, it is an added injury with added blood loss. Transfusion must be continued. In an analysis of a large military experience,[2] it was found that approximately 40 per cent of the blood was transfused preoperatively, 40 per cent during operation and 20 per cent during the first 24 hours after operation. Throughout this period, the seriously injured casualty was unstable and required active support—continuing resuscitation.

Patients with wounds of the central nervous system form a separate resuscitative group. These patients seldom lose large volumes of blood, yet they may be markedly hypotensive. Large transfusions are seldom useful, for the basic deficiency is not in the blood volume but apparently in the autonomic nervous system.

Experience has demonstrated several other points of clinical importance. The casualty seldom complains of severe pain. Unless severe pain exists, morphine often does more harm than good. Patients with intracranial injuries should not receive morphine, as the additional depression makes accurate evaluation difficult. The drug should be avoided also in patients with severe intrathoracic injuries, for the pharmacologic repression of respiration adds to the already embarrassed respiratory function. Finally, the drug should be administered with discretion in the presence of impending or incipient shock, as hypotension may result, presumably from the depression of the nervous system. As pointed out by Beecher, one of the rather frequent errors made formerly was the overdosage to patients in deep shock. In such patients, a single subcutaneous or intramuscular injection had little effect, as the circulation was so inadequate that the drug was not absorbed. When pain persisted, a second injection was given. Following transfusion and improvement in the peripheral circulation, increased absorption sometimes resulted in the signs of overdosage. When the drug is to be given to patients in shock, the intravenous route is preferable.

Unlike the civilian patient undergoing elective surgery, the battle casualty very often has a full stomach, with the inherent danger of vomiting and aspiration on the induction of anesthesia. In estimating this hazard, the critical period is not the duration between the last meal and operation but the time lapse between the last meal and injury, for gastric emptying is diminished greatly after injury. In fact, under the stress of active combat, gastric motility may be reduced greatly prior to injury. In such circumstances, food may be found occasionally in the stomach from 12 to 24 hours after eating. As a result of this stasis, the patient should be forced to vomit, or a gastric tube should be inserted and the stomach emptied prior to anesthesia when a full stomach is suspected.

The administration of antibiotics at the earliest feasible time was considered to be one feature of resuscitation in Korea. Studies of subsequent blood levels in the casualties and studies of the sensitivities of the bacterial flora of many wounds indicated that penicillin and Aureomycin or Terramycin probably were preferable to the penicillin-streptomycin regimen practiced during that conflict. Like morphine, the antibiotics are absorbed slowly while the patient is in shock.[31] In the face of peripheral vascular collapse, the intravenous route of administration probably is to be preferred.

As in all phases of surgery, the maintenance of good records is essential. This is emphasized here, for it is neglected frequently in the combat theater. The press of mass casualties occasionally makes the keeping of good records impossible. This compromise must not become standard practice or be acceptable when the flow of casualties is slow. Vital signs, therapy and response to therapy should be recorded in an orderly, continuous manner. Urinary output, measured on an hourly basis when feasible, is a vital sign of considerable importance in the critically injured man. It cannot be overemphasized that the compromises and the short cuts acceptable and advisable in the treatment of mass casualties must be recognized clearly as compromises, to be practiced when necessary but unacceptable when the casualty load is light. Combat medical records often reflect the need for this emphasis.

REGIONAL SURGERY: PRINCIPLES OF SURGERY

The distribution of total wounds over the body corresponds roughly with surface areas. The distribution of total wounds, however, is not representative of the problems in military surgery, for the professional requirements on the one hand and the resultant mortality on the other hand follow a far different distribution (Table 4).

The medical officer in the battalion aid station needs to be a surgeon with as broad a training in the field of trauma as is feasible, for he is without professional assistance. In the forward hospitals, slight specialization

TABLE 4. REGIONAL DISTRIBUTION OF WOUNDS[16]

LOCATION OF WOUNDS	"WOUNDED IN ACTION"*	"KILLED IN ACTION"†	"DIED OF WOUNDS"‡
Head	14%	42%	25.5%
Neck	3%	4%	3 %
Thorax	19%	36%	24 %
Abdomen	11%	9%	22 %
Upper extremities	25% }	6%	20.5%
Lower extremities	27% }		
Genitalia	1%	—	—
Buttocks	—	3%	5 %
Total	100%	100%	100 %
Multiple wounds	53%		

* Includes all fatal and nonfatal battle casualties.
† Battlefield deaths.
‡ Died after reaching medical units.

usually is possible if the flow of casualties is not overwhelming. Behind the forward hospital, specialization is rather complete, following in general the pattern of civilian surgery.

WOUNDS OF THE BRAIN

As shown in Table 4, approximately 14 per cent of all combat wounds occur in the head. Many of these involve the brain. Because of the resistance offered by the skull, most of the injuries are penetrating rather than perforating, the ratio being approximately 15:1.[16]

Many fatal wounds of the brain result from negligence in not wearing the protective steel helmet.

Most of the intracranial injuries are open injuries from penetrating missiles. These open wounds tend to decompress themselves, so that the rapid onset of increased intracranial pressure is unusual. As a result, operation may be less urgent than in many closed head injuries in which intracranial pressure may increase more rapidly. Because of the autodecompression, these patients tolerate transportation fairly well.

Blood loss from an intracranial wound is seldom of major proportion—a fact that adds to the relative stability and transportability of the preoperative patient.

At the battalion aid station, the primary concern centers in the problem of the care of the unconscious patient. First, attention should be directed toward maintaining an adequate airway, a tracheotomy often being required. Second, bleeding from scalp wounds or associated injuries should be controlled and relacement therapy instituted as needed. Then a neurologic examination should be *done* and *recorded*. A sterile dressing should be applied to minimize further contamination.

Transportation of the unconscious patient entails several real hazards. The most important is the mechanical obstruction of the airway by the tongue, by blood clots, by faulty positioning or by *vomiting* and *aspiration*. This hazard is minimized by performing tracheotomy prior to transportation when a reasonable doubt exists and by positioning the patient on his side with his head, shoulders and pelvis tilted ventrally. In such a position saliva, blood and vomitus may escape aspiration. Morphine and Demerol should be avoided, as pain seldom is a factor, and mental and respiratory depression is contraindicated. Helicopter transportation is highly desirable.

Because of the need for specialized care and because of the relative shortage of neurosurgeons, neurosurgical centers were established in the Combat Zone in World War II and were continued in Korea. Definitive surgery is performed at the neurosurgical center, usually within 6 to 12 hours of injury. Operation consists essentially of débridement. Bone fragments, devitalized brain tissue, foreign bodies and hematomas are removed meticulously by excision and irrigation. Hemostasis is obtained accurately, and the wound is closed primarily, because of the fear of secondary infection. Because of the rich blood supply in the scalp and the brain, secondary necrosis and residual infection are infrequent. Meticulous early surgery and consistent use of antibiotics made secondary abscesses rare and secondary meningitis almost unknown in the Korean Theater.

The deleterious effect of time lag before operation does not appear to be quite so pronounced in open wounds of the head as it does in wounds of other parts of the body, provided that the time lag does not exceed 24 hours. This factor should be considered in planning for mass casualties.

Matson,[23] summarizing the experience of World War II in the management of several thousand casualties with wounds of the brain, found an over-all mortality of 25 per cent among those reaching the hospital. Approximately 11 per cent were considered to be inoperable, due to the massive nature of the wound, or they died prior to operation; 14 per cent died postoperatively.

SPINAL CORD INJURIES

Therapy in these patients is designed (1) to minimize the effects of the local wound and (2)—often of more importance—to rehabilitate the paraplegic patient.

These patients have been handled in neurosurgical centers in the Combat Zone, as have the patients with wounds of the brain. Transportation to such centers is done best by helicopter, as was demonstrated in Korea. The patient may be placed in either a prone or a supine position for transportation, but every care must be taken not to increase the spinal cord injury by flexing or extending the vertebral column, thereby permitting bone fragments further to lacerate the cord.

Early laminectomy is indicated in almost every penetrating wound of the spinal canal and the spinal cord.[6] The aim of early intervention is to relieve pressure by bone fragments, hematoma or foreign bodies on the spinal cord, the cauda equina or the spinal nerve roots; to débride and close the wound primarily, and to determine the anatomic extent of injury. Laminectomy usually can be performed under local anesthesia. Only by direct visualization can anatomic transection be distinguished from physiologic transection.

The postoperative care of these patients determines the extent to which they can be rehabilitated. The surgeon who treats only an occasional paraplegic patient and adopts a fatalistic outlook may not realize the degree of success that has been developed in military centers in rehabilitating these men to useful creative positions.

There are several essential points in rehabilitation. At the very onset, and preferably beginning before operation, the neurologic defect, its possible or definite permanence, and the aims and the possibilities of rehabilitation should be discussed frankly with the patient, because his proper motivation is essential to recovery.

Transection of the spinal cord interrupts central control of the urinary bladder. A secondary center in the conus medullaris, governing the bladder through the sacral reflex arc, subsequently may assume control of bladder function. It is the aim of the surgeon to bring this secondary center into control and produce a reflex neurogenic bladder.[6] (See Chap. 48, Urology.)

To achieve this goal it is essential from the very first day to prevent overdistention of the bladder by the use of an indwelling catheter. Urinary tract infections also must be prevented. At a very early date, tidal drainage, as described by Munro,[25, 26] must be instituted. A successfully functioning bladder will result in most, but not all, patients.

Additional effort is necessary to prevent overdistention of the incontinent colon, decubitus ulcers and malnutrition. Physiotherapy should be instituted within the first week. Finally, leg braces, continued skilled assist-

ance and encouragement will result in subsequent ambulation of many of these patients.

WOUNDS OF THE FACE AND THE NECK

Treatment at the battalion aid station may determine whether these casualties live or die. With proper early care, almost all should survive.

These injuries are characterized by profuse hemorrhage and by a tendency to produce respiratory obstruction. Wounds of the scalp, the cheek, the tongue or the floor of the mouth may result in a surprising loss of blood, even though no single large vessel has been lacerated. Finally, the battalion surgeon may gain a false impression that a wound, such as the avulsion of the lower jaw, is of hopelessly severe magnitude. Final results justify no such fatalism.

The battalion surgeon first must ensure an adequate airway; next, control hemorrhage; and, finally, assess and record the neurologic status, since the incidence of associated injuries to the brain and the cervical spinal cord is high. In evaluating the factor of respiratory obstruction, the surgeon must consider the fact that the casualty is about to enter the chain of evacuation, during part of which time he will not be under direct medical observation. If he is in doubt as to the presence or the potential development of respiratory obstruction, tracheotomy should be done before the casualty leaves the battalion aid station. As a generalization it should be performed for wounds of the trachea and the pharynx and for large wounds of the floor of the mouth and the lower jaw. In addition, if the patient is unconscious, tracheotomy should be performed if the presence of intra-oral or pharyngeal bleeding predisposes to aspiration.

Because of the fear of respiratory complications, morphine should be avoided, thereby protecting the cough reflex and its resulting defense against aspiration of blood.

When endotracheal suction is required, it can be obtained by connecting a rubber catheter to a bulb syringe.

At the forward surgical hospital, the airway, hemostasis and neurologic status should be rechecked first. Any appreciable blood-volume deficiency should be corrected, and the stomach should be emptied by vomiting or by gastric tube prior to anesthesia. Loose teeth should be removed before or at the beginning of operation. Roentgenograms of the bones of the face and the skull should be obtained prior to operation.

Except in the patient with neurologic damage, primary repair should be attempted.

In the face and the neck, more than in any other part of the body, except perhaps the hand, loss of tissue or excessive scarring leads to serious functioning impairment as well as to disfigurement. The principles of treatment are the same as for wounds elsewhere. However, the rich vascular supply to the face and the neck limits the extent of lateral necrosis around a wound and minimizes infection. As a result of the excellent blood supply, it is possible to obtain good wound healing after minimal but meticulous débridement and primary closure. There are many exceptions when this is not possible, but the goal of therapy is to close the wound as soon as possible and thereby limit fibrosis and deformity. In general, every effort is made to conserve tissue, and, when feasible, primary closure offers the best cosmetic result.

When primary closure is not possible because of infection due to delay in reaching the hospital, secondary suture should be performed within the shortest feasible time. When primary suture is impractical because of the magnitude of the wound, the principle of early closure still holds, the wound being closed with a split thickness skin graft.

From the combat zone, these casualties are evacuated to the Zone of the Interior, where plastic centers, developed by the medical services, have contributed materially to the total knowledge of reparative surgery. The subsequent reconstructive surgery does not differ in principle from that of civilian practice. Obviously, the medical service has not discharged its full responsibility to such a combat casualty until the best possible functional and cosmetic result has been obtained.

Wounds of the Eye

Injuries of the eye constitute from 2 to 3 per cent of combat injuries. Tiny particles elsewhere in the body cause little difficulty, often hardly requiring medical attention, but, in the eye, penetration of a tiny particle may destroy the usefulness of the organ.

Superficial foreign bodies may be removed after the topical application of ½ per cent Pontocaine.

Major penetrating injuries of the eye should be treated by an ophthalmologist. In order to prevent movement of the injured eye with the possibility of secondary retinal detachment, both eyes should be bandaged. Antibiotic solutions should be applied topically, for blood-borne antibiotics penetrate the tissues of the eye poorly from the blood stream, and infection may mean the loss of vision. Mydriatics should not be used.

A principle of definitive surgery is to repair primarily any eye in which there has not been too great a loss of intra-ocular contents. Enucleation is not an emergency operation. One report from Korea indicated that 70 per cent of wounds of the eye were repaired.[10] Conservative management is especially important in bilateral injuries.

The general medical officer seldom is prepared to evaluate these injuries. Evacuation, if necessary, should be carried out to permit specialized attention.

Wounds of the Chest

Wounds of the chest constitute 19 per cent of all combat injuries. In 1 large series,[38] 70 per cent were penetrating in type, 28 per cent were perforating, and 2 per cent were due to crushing injuries.

Of all combat soldiers receiving wounds of the chest, many die from cardiac or major vascular injuries before reaching medical assistance. This constitutes 36 per cent of the total number "killed in action." Thereafter, only about 7 per cent of the group reaching the forward hospital are lost, but this constitutes a major problem, representing almost one fourth of the total hospital deaths. Body armor, as developed in Korea, covers the thorax as a vast and, by stopping many of the missiles, reduced the incidence of thoracic wounds after the vest was introduced.

The surgical management of most thoracic injuries differs from that of injuries to other parts of the body. The aims of management of intrathoracis injuries are (1) to correct the mechanical defects, (2) to replace the blood loss and (3) to prevent infection. These principles are not unlike those applied to other parts of the body, but the means of application differ.

The mechanical defects—pneumothorax, hemothorax, an open sucking thoracic wound, tension pneumothorax and hemopericardium—exert an immediate deleterious effect, and they should be corrected at the earliest possible time, often forward of the surgical hospital.

Operative control of hemorrhage seldom is necessary. Almost inevitably, bleeding from the pulmonary parenchyma will stop spontaneously. Usually, this tendency to self-limited bleeding is attributed to the low arterial pressure in the pulmonary system and its high thromboplastin titer. Only an occasional injury due to laceration of a large hilar vessel, an intercostal or internal mammary artery, or a subclavian vein or artery will continue to bleed and require operative hemostasis. Blood loss frequently is of major proportions, however, and vigorous transfusion may be necessary.

Efforts to prevent infection center in the prevention of atelectasis, the aspiration of blood and exudate from the pleural space, and the liberal use of antibiotics.

Débridement of the lung seldom is practiced. Occasionally, foreign bodies, such as bits of clothing or large metallic fragments, may have to be removed, but exploration rarely is advisable on the day of injury. Relatively few of these patients will ever require thoracotomy.

The practice of not débriding pulmonary wounds rests upon both a theoretic and a clinical basis. The elasticity of the lung permits the tissue to expand as the missile cavity forms, without secondary tearing. In contradistinction to hepatic wounds, stellate fractures of the parenchyma do not occur. Instead, the lung stretches with resultant minimal destruction of the parenchyma. Thereafter, the rich blood supply minimizes the extent of devitalization and infection and promotes healing. Clinical experience has demonstrated a lower mortality and a smoother clinical course since the more conservative management has been instituted (Table 5).

When the casualty with a penetrating thoracic wound first reaches the battalion aid station, the open wound in the chest wall should be closed. This can be achieved temporarily with several thicknesses of petrolatum gauze reinforced with a thick dressing and adhesive tape. Such a casualty retains a pneumothorax, but the sucking aspect of air moving in and out of the pleural space with each respiratory cycle is stopped. This has the advantage of overcoming the rhythmic shift of the mediastinum with each respiratory movement. After closing the wound in this way, the air and the blood in the pleural space can be aspirated, so that, temporarily at least, the positive (atmospheric) intrapleural pressure is relieved and the normal pressure relationships are restored. This not only permits re-expansion and function of the collapsed lung but restores the function of the thoracic pump mechanism in aiding the return of venous blood to the right side of the heart. Simultaneously, it may be necessary to begin transfusion of blood or of available blood substitutes. When respiratory obstruction is suspected, tracheotomy is mandatory.

Because the pneumothorax and intrapleural bleeding tend to recur, these casualties should

TABLE 5. WOUNDS OF THE CHEST

	WORLD WAR II		KOREAN CONFLICT	
WOUNDS	Number of Casualties	Mortality	Number of Casualties	Mortality
Thoracic wounds				
Immediate results				
Forward Surgical Hospital	2,000[11]	10%	33[32]	6%
Late results				
Army General Hospital	—	—	2,305	0.6%
Thoraco-abdominal wounds				
Immediate results				
Forward Surgical Hospital	903*	27%	29[19]	10%
Late results				
Army General Hospital	—	—	506[38]	0.8%

* Second Auxiliary Surgical Group.

not be delayed unduly in the evacuation chain. Experience in World War II suggested a significant increase in mortality as the time lag before definitive care increased.

At the forward surgical hospital, immediate reappraisal is necessary. As soon as the patient's condition warrants movement, roentgenograms of the chests should be made. These should be made with the patient sitting upright, both anteroposterior and lateral views being taken. The films demonstrate not only the degree of collapse of the lung and the degree of hemothorax and pneumothorax but also the nature and the location of retained missiles. The latter information may be of some assistance in estimating the pathway of the missile and possible damage to mediastinal or abdominal structures.

Repeated aspiration of the pleural space and continued transfusion often are necessary. It is essential that the expansion of the lung be maintained. If, after several thoracenteses, air and blood continue to collect, it is often advisable under local anesthesia to insert a fenestrated catheter into the pleural space and connect it to a bottle with an underwater seal. Respiratory movements then will expel the air and the fluid into the bottle. The catheter should not be inserted through the initial wound. The soft tissue wound of the chest wall should be débrided and closed primarily.

Occasionally, continued bleeding will require immediate thoracotomy. Such patients who bleed into shock in spite of transfusion, and repeatedly and rapidly refill their pleural space with blood, usually have a wound of a major systemic vessel (e.g., intercostal, internal mammary, subclavian artery or subclavian vein, or a large mediastinal vessel). Operative hemostasis may be lifesaving.

All patients with thoracic injuries should receive antibiotics parenterally in an effort to minimize pleural infection. Tracheal aspiration via the nasopharyngeal route is of assistance in preventing or overcoming atelectasis with its resultant parenchymal infection. Procaine block of intercostal nerves often is an adjunct to therapy in the relief of pain, especially when the injury includes rib fractures.

Preferably the patients should remain at the forward surgical hospital for several days to permit stabilization of their condition, as casualties with residual deficiency in pulmonary function do not tolerate well the high altitude of air evacuation.

Follow-up studies[38] of 1,395 casualties from Korea demonstrated that 80 per cent recovered completely after only thoracenteses, antibiotics and blood. Within a few weeks 68 per cent were returned to duty. The remainder were returned to the Zone of the Interior (U.S.A.) largely because of associated injuries to other parts of the body. Of the patients with residual hemothorax 2 weeks after injury, one fourth became infected and required surgical drainage or decortication.

Decortication was deemed to be necessary in approximately 10 per cent of the total group, and it was performed optimally within 3 to 5 weeks after injury. The operation was elected because of decreased pulmonary function or infection associated with large, clotted or organized, hemothoraces. Residual infection was the indication in three fourths of the patients.

Delayed thoracotomy was performed in 12 per cent of the casualties for removal of large foreign bodies, usually shell fragments. This indication has not been established clearly, but it rests on the belief that the incidence of infection and erosion of vessels is high when a large metallic foreign body remains.

Mediastinal Injuries

Five per cent or less of thoracic wounds will include mediastinal injuries. Injuries to the mediastinal trachea or bronchi may be suspected by the presence of mediastinal emphysema on the roentgenogram or occasionally by the presence of subcutaneous emphysema. Injuries to the esophagus can be suspected by the location and the pathway of the missile. An esophagogram, using Lipiodol, Diodrast or Urokon as a contrast medium, may demonstrate a perforation. In the absence of fluoroscopy, additional evidence of esophageal perforation may be obained by having the patient swallow a few cubic centimeters of dilute methylene blue prior to thoracentesis. The dye then may be demonstrated in the pleural fluid. Evidence of tracheal, bronchial or esophageal perforation in the mediastinum is an indication for immediate repair. These injuries are quite infrequent, but they must always be considered.

Cardiac Injuries

In contradistinction to civilian surgery, in which many cardiac wounds are due to stab injuries, most military casualties with cardiac injuries due to bullets or shell fragments die before reaching the hospital. Of those who reach the hospital alive, most will have small wounds with self-limiting hemorrhage. Immediate exploration and suture seldom are justified. This procedure should be reserved for the occasional patient with more massive hemorrhage. Most patients will have a small leak into the pericardial sac. If the pericardial laceration remains patent, the blood may pass into the pleural cavity, and the cardiac component of the injury may not be suspected. The more classic injury is that in which the pericardial wound closes or that in which the wound involves a part of the heart not covered by pleura. Blood then is retained in the pericardial sac. As the hemopericardium develops, the increasing pressure in the pericardial cavity results in cardiac tamponade. Pressure on the heart, especially the auricles, prevents adequate filling, the result being a decreased cardiac output. Clinically, the diagnosis can be made by the low systolic and pulse pressures, the faint heart sounds and the high venous pressure. Confirmatory evidence is obtained by the relatively slow pulse (in the absence of other injuries) and the reduction or the absence of pulsation of the heart shadow on fluoroscopy. Pericardiocentesis through the subxiphoid or the left 4th interspace route yields bloody fluid that does not clot because it has been defibrinated by cardiac motion.

Death usually is due to cardiac tamponade. Therefore, definitive therapy consists of blood transfusion and repeated pericardiocentesis as indicated by careful observation of the vital signs, venous pressure, arterial pressure and pulsation of the heart.

THORACO-ABDOMINAL INJURIES

Frequently, missiles penetrate the chest and reach the abdomen. These patients have thoracis wounds that usually are handled non-operatively and abdominal wounds that require laparotomy. The mortality of thoraco-abdominal wounds in World War II (Table 5) approximated that of abdominal wounds in contradistinction to that of thoracic wounds.

The thoracic component of the injury is treated as in other thoracic injuries. Care must be taken during anesthesia for laparotomy that the injured lung does not again undergo collapse and remain unrecognized. If catheter drainage of the pleural cavity is to be performed, sometimes it is well to insert the catheter at the beginning of operation or before laparotomy to assist in maintaining or restoring normal intrapleural pressures as the diaphragmatic wound is manipulated.

Unless thoracotomy is indicated for the specific wound of the chest, peritoneal exploration usually should be performed by the abdominal approach.

Most thoraco-abdominal injuries involve the liver. Less frequently, the spleen, the colon, the stomach and the kidney will be injured. Treatment includes closure of the diaphragm and proper management of the wounds of the abdominal viscera. Occasionally, exposure of small wounds of the diaphragm covered by the dome of the right lobe of the liver is so traumatic as hardly to justify the procedure.

In World War II, the mortality of thoraco-abdominal wounds of the left side of the body was greater than that of wounds of the right side. This presumably was due to the increased frequency of injuries to hollow viscera on the left side. Because of improvements in the treatment of infections, this difference apparently disappeared or was reversed in the Korean conflict.[5]

WOUNDS OF THE ABDOMEN

Physiologically, patients with abdominal injuries respond somewhat differently from those with wounds of the extremities. This appears to be due only in part to the increased prominence of the element of infection associated with intraperitoneal injuries. Patients with massive intraperitoneal injuries are not unlike the burned patient; they appear to lose plasma in large amounts into the peritoneal cavity. The hematrocit may remain stable or increase after injury and for a day or two after operation and transfusion. On the contrary, patients with massive wounds of the extremities tend to develop a falling hematocrit after injury, a trend that may persist in spite of massive transfusions. Casualties with moderate wounds of the extremities occasionally develop a hypertensive response, a finding seldom observed in patients with abdominal injuries (see Chap. 7, Shock). Patients with muscle destruction often excrete large amounts of creatine; presumably this is due to the destruction of muscle, since patients with abdominal injuries excrete much less. Paralytic ileus is much more marked in the presence of abdominal injuries. Furthermore, measurements of hepatic and renal function indicate greater impairment following abdominal injury. The incidence of demonstrable bacteremia appears to be about the same for the 2 groups. Finally, abdominal injuries result in a stormier clinical course and a higher mortality rate.

Although remarkable progress has been made in the treatment of abdominal injuries, these wounds remain one of the major problems in military surgery. In earlier wars penetrating wounds of the abdomen were treated nonoperatively. The surgeons of World War I began to wonder if laparotomy would not be a preferable form of treatment. During World War II, laparotomy was performed on all casualties with intra-abdominal injuries except the very occasional patient who was in so critical a condition that the surgeon felt that the additional operative trauma per se would be fatal. The mortality rate in World War II, as reported by the 2nd Auxiliary Surgical Group, was 23.5 per cent. The latter phases of the Korean conflict saw this mortality reduced by half, a morality of 12 per cent being reported by the Surgical Research Team in Korea during 1953.

Many abdominal injuries are of massive extent, involving multiple organs. The mortality rate is directly proportional to the number of organs injured, as indicated in Table 6.

A second factor that influences the mortality is the time lag before surgery. From the statistics of World War II, Beebe and DeBakey calculated an increase in mortality of approximately 0.5 per cent for every hour's delay before operation.

The reduction in mortality in Korea is attributable to the more liberal use of whole blood, the routine use of penicillin, the frequent use of wide spectrum antibiotics and the availability of helicopter evacuation for the more critically injured.

TABLE 6. COMPARISON OF MORTALITY RATES FOR ABDOMINAL WOUNDS BY NUMBER OF ORGANS INJURED*

NUMBER OF ORGANS INJURED	WORLD WAR II		KOREAN CONFLICT	
	Number of Casualties	Mortality Rate	Number of Casualties	Mortality Rate
0	98	5%	36	3%
1	496	10%	181	7%
3	132	42%	45	27%
5	13	92%	16	16%

* Casualties operated upon within approximately 7 hours after injury.

The goal in resuscitation and evacuation is to get the casualty into the operating room as soon as feasible.

Treatment forward of the surgical hospital is limited essentially to transfusion. The bleeding being intra-abdominal, hemostasis cannot be obtained at the battalion aid station; only supportive treatment is possible. No matter how vigorous the transfusion, the casualty with massive intra-abdominal hemorrhage will die unless evacuation is rapid. Helicopter evacuation truly was lifesaving for some of these patients.

Management at the Forward Surgical Hospital

Because hemorrhage is intra-abdominal and thus hidden, the inexperienced surgeon can be misled into underestimating the extent of blood loss in these patients. In such circumstances, anesthesia and laparotomy convert the patient from a state of impending shock to one of profound hypotension. As a result of this widespread experience, the maxim was developed of transfusing the patient with abdominal injuries "a pint or so more than he seems to need."

Preoperative evaluation and preparation include the insertion of an indwelling gastric tube and a urinary catheter, with attention to whether stomach or bladder contains blood. When injury to the rectum is suspected, the rectum should be checked for blood by digital and proctoscopic examination prior to operation.

Roentgenograms should be taken routinely. The demonstration of unexpected positions of missiles, multiple foreign bodies or vertebral fractures is occasionally of real assistance to the surgeon. Its aid in the evaluation of the individual patient cannot be predicted, but the experienced surgeon will utilize this adjunct to evaluation in most patients.

Principles of Abdominal Operations

Incisions. Almost always, vertical incisions are used for laparotomy in military surgery. Perhaps this is standardized unnecessarily, but the short time necessary to enter and close the abdomen, and the exposure offered to a wide area, have made the rectus splitting or the pararectus incision almost routine.

Because of the contamination of wounds of the abdominal wall, the incision is placed away from the wounds of entrance and exit. Like wounds of the thoracic wall, wounds of the abdominal wall should be excised and closed primarily. In extensive wounds, the skin and the subcutaneous tissues may be left open, but the peritoneum, fascia and, when feasible, muscle should be sutured.

Hepatic Wounds. These are among the most frequent and sometimes the most dangerous of intra-abdominal injuries. The surgical problem, primarily, is that of hemostasis and, secondarily, that of preventing bile peritonitis. In World War II and in Korea, the mortality remained from 9 to 10 per cent among patients whose only injury was of the liver.

The consistency of the liver is such that a high velocity missile produces extensive lateral damage resulting in stellate fractures that bleed profusely. Attempts to suture the wound sometimes increase bleeding, so that no single method of obtaining hemostasis is uniformly satisfactory. Hemostatic methods include ligature, suture, absorbable hemostatic agents, such as Gelfoam, and, when absolutely necessary, massive packs of nonabsorbable gauze. Because of inability to control bleeding, débridement at present is impractical. As a result, secondary necrosis and secondary hemorrhage occur occasionally. The latter also may follow the removal of large hemostatic packs.

Hepatic wounds must be drained, for, although the incidence is low, complications of bile leakage may occur. Drains permit the development of biliary fistulas; otherwise, bile peritonitis or subphrenic collections may prove to be fatal or near fatal. Almost invariably, such fistulas will close spontaneously.

Although complications of bile leakage are discussed most often, hemorrhage is the primary problem and the chief cause of death from hepatic injury.

Gallbladder. Almost always, injuries of the gallbladder are complicated by injury to the overlying liver. Cholecystectomy usually is followed by an uneventful course. Injuries to the extrahepatic bile ducts are seen infrequently, and usually they are associated with massive wounds and fatal hemorrhage because characteristically the wound traverses the hilum of the liver. Isolated injuries of the common duct should be repaired over a T-tube inserted through a separate opening in the duct.

Spleen. Injuries of the spleen are frequent and usually are accompanied by penetration of the adjacent abdominal organs and the overlying diaphragm and lung. Although splenectomy offers adequate therapy and few casualties of uncomplicated splenic trauma died in Korea, approximately 1 out of 6 casualties with splenic trauma died from associated injuries, accentuated doubtlessly by preoperative hemorrhage.

Stomach. Gastric injuries present few problems. Primary suture is followed by good wound healing due to the excellent blood supply of the stomach. Secondary leakage is almost unknown. The 29 per cent mortality in World War II for wounds that involved only the stomach was reduced to almost zero in Korea.[19]

Duodenum. Duodenal injuries are far more serious than gastric injuries. The retroperitoneal position of the duodenum is such that inevitably several other organs are injured. Bleeding often is profuse. Secondary necrosis of the suture line with the development of a duodenal fistula is not an uncommon complication. As a result, the mortality for all wounds involving the duodenum was over 50 per cent in World War II and approximately 40 per cent in Korea.

Jejunum and Ileum. Injury to the small bowel is the most frequent of abdominal injuries. Often the injuries are massive, involving from 10 to 20 perforations of the bowel and its mesentery. If multiple injuries are found closely approximated, localized resection with end-to-end anastomosis may be necessary. As a generalization, however, simple suture is adequate. The rich blood supply of the small bowel makes formal débridement of the wound edges unnecessary; healing usually is uncomplicated. When innumerable perforations are found, the experienced surgeon always counts his suture lines to be certain that an even number is found, for almost inevitably an odd count implies that a hidden point of entrance or exit has been overlooked. Injuries limited to the small bowel have a negligible mortality (Korea); yet wounds of the small bowel compounded by injury of other organs still resulted in the loss of 1 of every 8 casualties.

Colon. Injuries to the colon, approximately as frequent as those of the small bowel, have led to more numerous complications. The colon does not heal as well as does the small bowel. Secondary necrosis of a suture line leads to peritonitis, abscess or fistula. This presumably is due to a somewhat poorer blood supply, a greater distention from the accumulation of gas and feces, and a more virulent peritonitis resulting from the fecal spillage. Because of this complication, the wound usually is exteriorized as a colostomy. If the injuries are multiple, the distal wounds are closed, and the proximal wound is exteriorized, thus decompressing and defunctionalizing the distal bowel. Because of difficulty in exposing the rectum, a proximal sigmoid colostomy is performed, and from the perineum a presacral drain is inserted to the area of perforation.

The mortality from wounds limited to the colon fell from 23 per cent in World War II to 9 per cent in Korea. This mortality remains rather high, and colostomies require additional time and secondary operations during the period of convalescence. Re-evaluation of primary closure is being continued in civilian hospitals.

Pancreas. Like duodenal injuries, injuries to the pancreas usually include injuries to several other organs. Injuries to large or small pancreatic ducts are inevitable. Since the ducts cannot be repaired adequately, drainage is essential to prevent collections of pancreatic juice. Most pancreatic wounds drain for only a few days; it is rare that a persistent pancreatic fistula develops. Although most fistulas result from injuries to major ducts in the head of the pancreas, almost inevitably they will close spontaneously if given a prolonged period of time.

Urinary Tract. Approximately 3 out of 4 wounds of the kidney are associated with injuries to other organs; therefore, the management of renal injuries usually is carried out through the laparotomy wound used for the repair of the associated injuries.

The renal injury may be suspected by the presence of hematuria, which should be checked preoperatively, as occasionally the retroperitoneal position of the kidneys may obscure renal injuries.

Like the liver and the spleen, the kidney often fractures from the lateral force of a missile. Bleeding may be very profuse, and it is the chief cause of death.

Small penetrating wounds may simply be drained to prevent possible urinary extravasations and to demonstrate any secondary bleeding. Not infrequently, larger wounds require nephrectomy. The advisability of partial nephrectomy for injuries to one pole of the kidney is unsettled; many surgeons believe that the high incidence of late complications make such a conservative approach inadvisable, provided that the other kidney is present and uninjured. Small tears of the capsule or injuries to the renal pelvis may be repaired. In the future, it should prove to be feasible to repair injuries to the renal artery, but to date these injuries have required nephrectomy.

Injuries to the ureter are extremely rare. They should be treated by primary suture with drainage. (See Chap. 49, Urology.)

Wounds of the bladder are not rare; they occur most often when the bladder is distended with urine. Such wounds should be treated by primary repair and by decompression of the bladder by suprapubic cystostomy or by indwelling urethral catheter.

One of the more difficult injuries to treat is that of the posterior urethra. These injuries may be due to perforation by missiles or to the shearing force associated with pelvic fractures. Considerable progress has been made in the primary repair of these injuries, but it is probably too early to generalize as to the applicability of the procedure. The alternative is the insertion of an indwelling urethral catheter as a splint and the decompression of the bladder by the catheter or by a suprapubic cystostomy.

WOUNDS OF THE EXTREMITIES

In a study of the regional distribution of wounds among soldiers wounded in action in Korea, the Wound Ballistics Research unit found that over half of the wounds were of the extremities. Thus, although most men killed in action have injuries to the head or the trunk, most of the surgery done is for wounds of the extremities.

Soft Tissue Injuries

The principles of management of soft tissue wounds have been discussed under the heading, "The Battle Wound." These wounds are contaminated and may become infected if they are left untreated. Small wounds may require only incision, inspection as to the extent of damage, irrigation to remove loose debris and drainage by leaving the wound open. Larger wounds require extensive débridement (Fig. 23-11, A and B).

Almost all of these wounds are contaminated with virulent bacteria, many containing pathogenic clostridia. A group of battle casualties were studied by Strawitz and his associates in Korea by serial biopsies of the open wound over a period of the first week after injury.[36] At the end of débridement, culture of the remaining viable muscle revealed the presence of residual clostridia. Repeated biopsy cultures at 2-day intervals revealed the disappearance of the clostridia, provided the wound was free of necrotic tissue. If débridement had been inadequate, virulent clostridia remained in the wound. During the first 2 to 3 days after injury, histologic study (Vickery) of the open wound demonstrated an exudate and surface necrosis. About the 4th to the 6th day, granulation tissue and fibroblastic proliferation became evident, and the exudate and the necrosis diminished. This sequence of events is the basis for selecting the 4th to the 6th day as the time for secondary closure of the soft tissue wounds. The absence of residual necrotic tissue or spreading infection is evident then; healing has begun, and it will continue and be expedited by secondary closure.

Arterial Injuries

Few casualties with injuries to the aorta survive to reach medical assistance. An occasional patient with injuries of a large intra-abdominal artery, such as an iliac, reaches the forward surgical hospital alive, but he may die before or during operative hemostasis. The use of tourniquets and pressure dressings always has permitted most casualties with injuries of the extremities to reach the forward hospital. Until the Korean conflict, definitive treatment consisted of ligation of the severed artery. Under such a regimen, the area of the wound either had a collateral circulation sufficient to permit viability of the distal extremity or gangrene resulted.

The vascular pattern is similar in the upper and the lower extremities. A main arterial trunk gives off a deep branch to the arm and the thigh. The main artery divides at the knee or the elbow to form 2 smaller trunks. Thus, injury of the main trunk at the axilla or the groin, proximal to the origin of the deep branch, is associated with a poor collateral circulation and a graver risk of gangrene. Distal to the profunda branches, injury to brachial or femoral artery is associated with collateral circulation through the intact profunda. Distal to the elbow or the knee, ligation of 1 of the 2 arterial branches usually is not attended by gangrene. One of the most critical areas, however, is that of the popliteal artery. Here collateral circulation is poor, and, with the destruction of part of the collaterals by the wound and by the surgical incision, ligation is often disastrous.

In the American Civil War, 75 per cent of the casualties with injuries of the popliteal artery died because of the resulting gangrene, which probably had clostridial infection superimposed. In World War II, the incidence of gangrene and amputation following ligation of the popliteal artery was 73 per cent. In the Korean conflict, primary repair of the severed arteries was developed. As a result, the amputation rate following injury to the popliteal artery fell to 18 per cent. When feasible, the arterial wound was débrided and resutured directly. Such débridement should take cognizance of the fact that the damage on the inner walls of a large artery may extend from 2 to 3 mm. beyond the limits of that apparent on the outside. When the defect is too long to permit of primary suture, autogenous vein grafts (saphenous or cephalic veins) or stored homologous arterial grafts should be inserted. Neither sympathectomy nor anti-

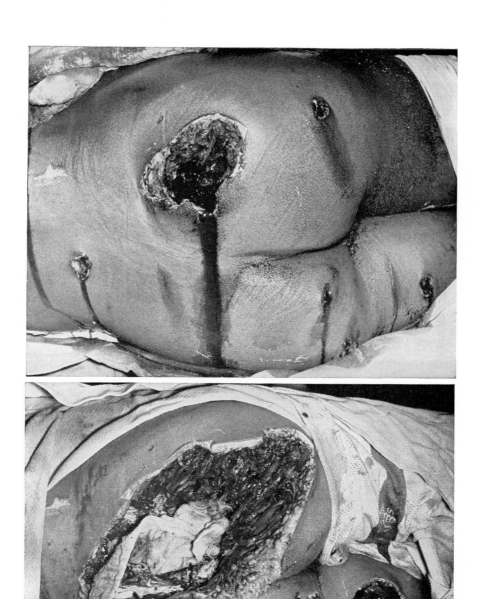

FIG. 23-11. (*Top*) Demonstrating the external appearance of penetrating shell fragment wounds of various sizes. (*Bottom*) Débridement includes adequate exposure and excision in order to prevent wound necrosis and infection. (Lt. Stephen Dittman, U. S. Army)

coagulants appear to be necessary. The overall results in Korea were excellent, as demonstrated in Table 7.

To date, wounds of the veins still are treated by ligation.

Peripheral Nerve Injuries

All patients with combat wounds of the extremities should be examined specifically prior to débridement for evidence of peripheral nerve injury. It is equally important that the findings be recorded, for the patient with peripheral nerve injuries has embarked on a prolonged course of evacuation, surgical treatment and rehabilitation by many surgeons, each of whom will find the record of inestimable value in determining treatment and prognosis. Management at the forward surgical hospital consists primarily of treatment of associated injuries, débridement, repair of arterial injuries and treatment of compound fractures. In addition, the record is of considerable assistance in the subsequent management of the patient if the extent of anatomic injury to the nerve can be ascertained; that is, whether the nerve is contused, severed or lacerated incompletely. In combat injuries caused by high velocity missiles, immediate peripheral nerve repair is contraindicated. This question was explored extensively in World War II; the casualties were followed for several years afterward, and no new evidence accrued to change this concept.[39]

Immediately following débridement, an active program of physiotherapy is begun. Unless necessitated by associated fractures, splinting is reserved for radial or sciatic nerve injuries. Such splints are not used continuously; they are removed intermittently to permit physiotherapy.

Definitive nerve suture is postponed for from 1 to 3 months, and the patients are transferred to specialty centers in the Zone of the Interior (U.S.A.). Within a month, the secondary degeneration of the nerve ends has occurred, allowing the extent of damage to be ascertained accurately. Meanwhile, the soft tissue wound has healed, and the danger of infection has lessened. If the wound has healed and if physiotherapy has protected joint motility, nerves known to have been divided should be repaired within 3 months after injury, and always within 6 months. These time limitations are based on the extensive follow-up studies from World War II.[39] Exploration appears to be advisable if, after 3 months, nerves injured in continuity or lacking a description of injury demonstrate no return of function. If tests of function reveal normally progressive regeneration, exploration should be postponed.

Regardless of the type of injury, the prognosis as to the extent of functional recovery must be guarded until progressive recovery is demonstrated.

Compound Fractures

The characteristics of compound fractures in combat surgery are their frequency, the massive destruction of bone and soft tissues that often is present (Fig. 23-12, A to D), the associated life-endangering injuries to other parts of the body and the repeated need for transportation of the casualty.

At the battalion aid station, a sterile dressing should be applied and immobilization begun. Various splints usually are available for the different parts of the body, but the battalion surgeon often finds himself forced to improvise to meet inevitable shortages of supplies or unpredicted combinations of injuries. His aim is to prevent further damage and to

TABLE 7. MANAGEMENT OF ACUTE ARTERIAL INJURIES. AMPUTATION RATE

ARTERY INJURED	LIGATION WORLD WAR II[8]		REPAIR KOREAN CONFLICT[20]	
	Number	% Amputated	Number	% Amputated
Axillary	74	43%	4	0%
Brachial	—	—	25	0%
Above profunda	97	56%	—	—
Below profunda	209	26%	—	—
Common femoral	106	81%	9	0%
Superficial femoral	177	55%	12	8%
Popliteal	502	73%	17	18%

minimize pain by immobilization. If splints are not available, the fractured leg may be bound to the uninjured leg. The fractured arm can be bound to the chest wall. Carbines or tent poles may become improvised splints.

At the forward surgical hospital, roentgenograms must be obtained prior to surgery, as the extent of bony injury from a high velocity missile cannot be predicted.

The aim of initial surgery is to prevent in-

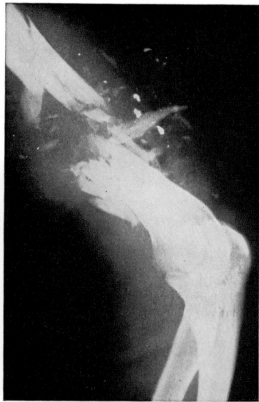

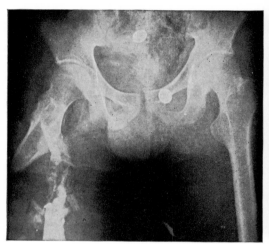

FIG. 23-12. Demonstrating the massive destruction of bone and soft tissues in compound fractures. (Lt. Stephen Dittman, U. S. Army)

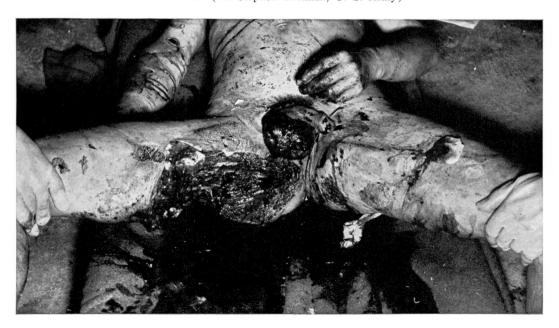

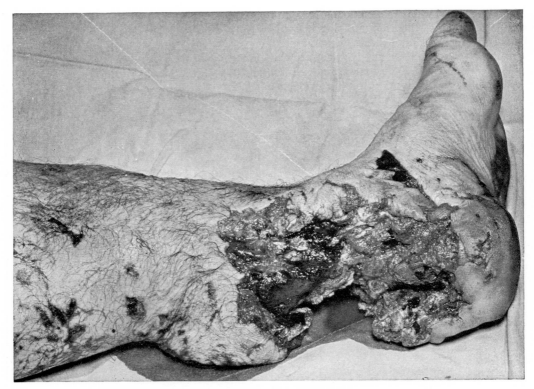

FIGURE 23-12 (*Continued*)

fection, for osteomyelitis results in a tremendous handicap to healing of a shattered bone. Débridement must be meticulous. Dead muscle and shredded fascia must be excised. Bone fragments attached to periosteum should be left in situ. Accessible shell fragments and all bits of clothing should be removed. Following hemostasis the wound should be irrigated copiously with sterile saline. Then the wound is left open.

A sterile dressing is applied, and the extremity is immobilized in a plaster cast. Immediately afterward, the cast and the underlying padding should be split longitudinally and spread to permit decompression. The injured extremity will swell, and, unless decompression is ensured, ischemia and gangrene may result. Experience has demonstrated the absolute need for this precaution in military surgery.

A line drawing of the site and the extent of the injury should be inscribed on the cast to assist personnel in the subsequent chain of evacuation.

The soft tissue wound is closed secondarily as soon as feasible after the first 4 to 5 days. Thereafter the needs of continued treatment are similar to those encountered in civilian practice.

Wounds of Joints

The objectives in treating wounds of joints are to prevent infection and to retain maximal function of the joint. These objectives can be obtained best by opening the wound and removing all foreign bodies, bone chips or devitalized cartilage. The joint cavity should be cleansed further by irrigation, after which the synovial membrane should be sutured primarily.[14] Then immobilization is maintained until the overlying tissues have been closed secondarily and have healed. At this point active movement of the joint is begun.

Wounds of the Hand

Wounds of the hand (Fig. 23-13) are handled as are other wounds of the extremities, except that débridement is very conservative. The wounds are left open, but secondary closure should be performed at the earliest possible time to prevent excessive fibrosis and damage to exposed joints and tendons. Reconstructive surgery, developed in specialty centers in the Zone of the Interior, has done much to rehabilitate these casualties.

Traumatic Amputations

Traumatic amputations may constitute the most massive injuries of the extremities ever seen by the surgeon. Such injuries result most frequently from the explosion of a land mine or the near-by explosion of an artillery shell (Fig. 23-14).

Casualties who have a hand blown off at the wrist or a foot at the ankle do not present difficult problems. Casualties with amputations more proximal than this are difficult to manage (Table 8). Tissue damage is extensive and may extend for proximal to the line

TABLE 8. TRAUMATIC AMPUTATION OF LOWER EXTREMITIES. MORTALITY—46TH SURGICAL HOSPITAL, KOREA (1952-53)

SITE OF TRAUMATIC AMPUTATION	NUMBER OF PATIENTS	MORTALITY
Below knee	64	5%
Above knee	16	19%

of amputation. A tourniquet must be applied immediately, because blood loss from the major vessels, as well as from the extensive muscular surface, may lead rapidly to exsanguination.

Reamputation through viable tissue is necessary in order to promote healing, obtain adequate hemostasis and prevent serious infections. The wound is left open and then closed from 4 to 7 days later.

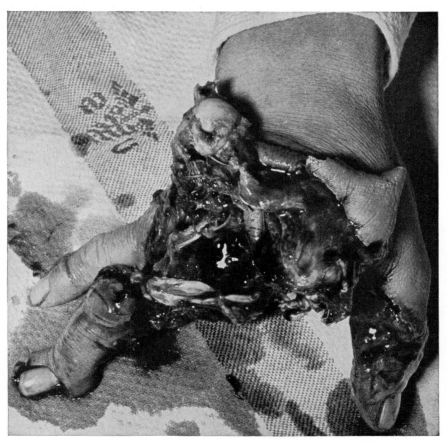

FIG. 23-13. A mangled wound of the hand. Initial conservation of tissue and subsequent reconstruction resulted in a useful hand.

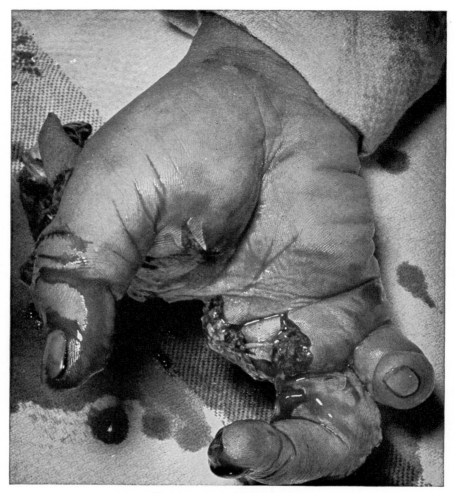

FIGURE 23-13 (*Continued*)

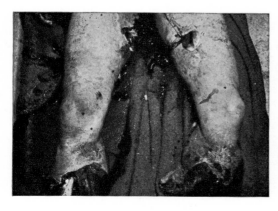

FIG. 23-14. Traumatic amputations. Both legs were blown off at the calf by an exploding land mine.

Skin traction should be applied after the first operation to prevent such extensive retraction of skin as will complicate secondary closure. In order to retain mobility of the patient for evacuation, yet permit continuous traction, traction is applied as shown in Figure 23-15.

Following secondary closure, these patients are returned to the Zone of the Interior for rehabilitation. The military prosthetic centers have devised many ingenious artificial limbs that can be effective in rehabilitating these casualties.

The cost of rehabilitation and the pension of a soldier with an amputation of a leg have been estimated by the Veterans Administration as $100,000.

TABLE 9. INCIDENCE OF TETANUS IN MILITARY CAMPAIGNS

WAR	YEARS	NUMBER OF CASUALTIES	INCIDENCE OF TETANUS (PER 1,000 CASUALTIES)
American Civil War	1861–65	246,172	2.07
Franco-German War	1870–71	—	8.0
World War I			
British troops			
Before antiserum	1914–15	—	8.0 ⎫
After antiserum	1915–18	—	1.0 ⎬ 1.47
World War I			
German troops	1914–18	4,000,000	3.8
World War II			
American troops	1941–45	2,500,000	0.006
World War II			
Manila civilians	1945	—	40.0*

* Estimated.

SPECIFIC COMPLICATIONS

TETANUS

Basic immunization, including a booster injection prior to entering the combat theater and followed by an emergency booster after injury, offers an effective prophylaxis against tetanus. The incubation period for tetanus is approximately 7 days; the antibody response to the booster requires only 4 to 5 days.

Edsall[9] collected only 15 cases of tetanus among the 2,500,000 wounded men in the U. S. Armed Forces during World War II. Only 6 had received the full scheduled immunization. All soldiers should be immunized and should receive a booster injection of the toxoid as soon as feasible after injury. Thus this complication of injury can be prevented.

In considering the possible mass casualties of atomic warfare, the problem must be reconsidered, for atomic casualties might include civilian (often nonimmunized) casualties. In World War I, the incidence of tetanus among the armies of the world varied from 2 to 8 per 1,000 wounded, falling to about 1 per 1,000 when wound surgery and tetanus antiserum became routine (Table 9). Deaths from tetanus among the German soldiers was estimated at 12,000. The problem of mass civilian casualties was described best by Glenn[12] in World War II. Among the untreated, malnourished civilian casualties of the siege of Manila (1945), the incidence of tetanus was about 40 per 1,000. Tetanus wards

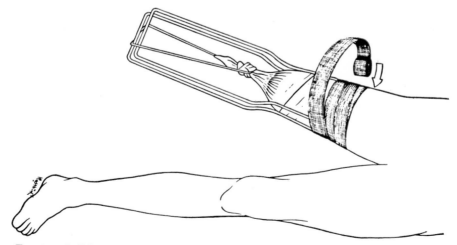

FIG. 23-15. Skin traction for amputees. The wire frame is incorporated in a plaster cast, thus permitting continuous skin traction during evacuation.

TABLE 10. GAS GANGRENE IN WORLD WAR I[1]

TYPE OF INJURY	NUMBER OF CASUALTIES	INCIDENCE OF GAS GANGRENE	MORTALITY
Soft tissue	128,265	1.1%	48.5%
Compound fractures	25,272	5.2%	44.6%

were established, and, of 473 patients treated, 82 per cent died.

GAS GANGRENE

Whereas tetanus can be prevented by prophylactic immunization, gas gangrene can be prevented by active surgical treatment. When the problem is applied to the situation of mass casualties, as from an atomic disaster, gas gangrene becomes a greater problem, for its prevention rests primarily on early adequate surgery.

As a generalizaion, almost all large battle wounds contain pathogenic clostridia that are capable of producing gas gangrene. However, gas gangrene develops only in necrotic tissue, and almost invariably it is preceded by proximal interruption of the main artery to the extremity. Altemeier described the average incubation period of gas gangrene (*Clostridium perfringens*) as 24 hours, and Trueta found in the Spanish Civil War that an untreated patient who survived 48 hours or longer without signs of anaerobic infection probably would escape gas gangrene. Once the infection has developed in experimental animals, penicillin prolongs life, but it does not affect the mortality if the wound is not treated.[1]

These facts explain the progress in military surgery in controlling gas gangrene, and they highlight the problem anew in terms of the management of possible atomic casualties.

In the latter half of the Korean conflict, gas gangrene almost disappeared. Among 4,900 consecutive casualties, 4 developed gas gangrene, and all 4 survived. This remarkable success was not due to lack of wound contamination; it was due to early consistent débridement, the repair of injured arteries and, perhaps, in part to the routine use of antibiotics. Antiserum was not used. In all 4 instances above, arterial injury had been followed by an unsuccessful surgical repair.

This represents quite a difference from the earlier experiences (Tables 10, 11) in World Wars I and II. Coupal[7] reported an incidence of gas gangrene of 1.1 per cent of soft tissue wounds and 5.2 per cent of compound fractures among American troops in World War I. Pettit[29] wrote of the more seriously injured of the Saint-Mihiel and Argonne-Meuse operations in World War I when a hospital received 4,377 casualties over a 2-month period, the time lag often being as long as 48 hours. These conditions as to time lag are pertinent to the problem of mass casualties. Pettit wrote that, of the 4,377 patients, 221, or 5 per cent, developed gas gangrene. This presumably represents approximately 10 per cent of the casualties with wounds of the extremities. The mortality of such infections was 27.6 per cent.

POST-TRAUMATIC RENAL INSUFFICIENCY

Among the massively injured casualties, post-traumatic renal insufficiency is a major

TABLE 11. CLOSTRIDIAL MYOSITIS (GAS GANGRENE)

	WORLD WAR I[29] Evacuation Hosp. No. 8 Sept. 10, 1918–Nov. 13, 1918	WORLD WAR II[27] Hospital, India	KOREAN CONFLICT[18] 46th Surgical Hosp. Jan., 1952–June, 1953
Number of casualties	4,377	4,600	4,900
Number developing clostridial myositis	221	32*	4
Percentage developing clostridial myositis	5.0%	0.7%	0.08%
Case fatality rate	27.6%	31.3%	0 %

* An additional 37 patients developed serious clostridial wound infections, making a total incidence of serious infection by *Clostridium perfringens* of 1.5%.

problem. Although its incidence approximated only 0.5 per cent among the surviving casualties in Korea,[37] the resultant mortality of the oliguric patient was between 80 and 90 per cent in World War II and in the earlier phases of the Korean conflict.

Studies by the Surgical Research Team in Korea demonstrated the gradation from the physiologic response of the kidney to trauma to the fatal syndrome of renal failure, in which the urinary output may be as little as 50 ml. per 24 hours. Renal failure is not an all-or-none phenomenon. There are innumerable stages, most of which are subclinical in extent.

The physiologic response to trauma, as represented by changes in renal function, includes the conservation of water and sodium, the increased excretion of potassium and nitrogen (urea) and albuminuria. Clearance studies by Ladd again indicated a marked reduction in renal blood flow and in the glomerular filtration rate. As the magnitude of injury increases, the metabolic response results in an increasing load of urea being presented to the kidney for excretion. The kidneys, with their blood flow reduced markedly, may not be able to excrete sufficient urea, even though the urinary volume remains in excess of 1,000 ml. per 24 hours. Azotemia without oliguria may result. Such patients may have a prolonged convalescence, but the mortality rate is not appreciable. A more striking degree of renal insufficiency is that characterized by azotemia and oliguria, the urinary output being from 200 to 500 ml. per 24 hours. These patients are quite ill, but after a few days of oliguria they develop a diuresis. A few such patients die, but usually it is of their original injury rather than of the renal complication.

Patients with the most severe degree of renal insufficiency excrete from 50 to 100 ml. of urine per day, the specific gravity being about 1.010. Azotemia, hyperkalemia and acidosis develop rapidly, and, given standard supportive care, almost inevitably the patient will die of cardiac failure about the 5th to the 8th day.

This complication cannot be predicted accurately when the casualty first is seen. As a generalization, he has suffered near-fatal injuries, is in profound shock and often responds rather slowly to the large transfusions that he requires. Hourly measurements of urinary volume may demonstrate a persistent "anuria" (2 to 3 ml. per hour) after his blood pressure has been returned to normal, or it may demonstrate a transient period of from 12 to 24 hours during which the urinary flow may remain almost normal.

The subsequent course of these patients is fulminating, having little counterpart in civilian practice. The blood nonprotein nitrogen rises about 50 mg. per cent per day. The plasma potassium rises steadily for several days, after which time it may rise precipitously to fatal levels. Hyperkalemia, accentuated by hyponatremia and hypocalcemia, produces a cardiotoxic effect that is demonstrated electrocardiographically by the peaking of the T-waves and the broadening of the QRS complex. Hypertension and anemia frequently develop in these patients, either or both developing within 2 to 4 days of injury.

Because of the extremely high mortality rate, a Renal Insufficiency Center was established at an evacuation hospital in Korea.[35] To this center, all patients of the United Nations' forces with post-traumatic renal insufficiency were taken by helicopter. Although critically injured, these patients could withstand helicopter evacuation within the first 72 hours. Thereafter, the effects of the renal failure increased the hazards of evacuation. Therapy consisted not only of fluid restriction and correction of the hyponatremia, hypocalcemia, acidosis and anemia but also hemodialysis by means of an artificial kidney. The results were encouraging, although not dramatic. The mortality gradually fell to 50 per cent, death resulting not from hyperkalemia but from complications of the original wound—infections, wound disruption or hemorrhage. Preliminary observations suggested that these complications resulted from compromises in initial surgery necessitated by the patient's critical status at that early time.

PERITONITIS

Death from abdominal injuries usually occurs within 48 hours after injury. The bacteriotoxic effect cannot be separated from the concurrent deleterious effects of blood loss and mechanical trauma. Hemoconcentration may be as marked as with severely burned patients.

At autopsy the peritoneal surfaces are

edematous and present a fibrinous exudate. An abdomen filled with pus, such as seen following a perforated appendix, seldom is encountered following trauma.

HEPATITIS

Because of the use in the forward areas of pooled plasma for resuscitation, homologous serum hepatitis was a frequent sequel. Sborov[33] reported an incidence of hepatitis (clinical and subclinical) as high as 22 per cent among the seriously injured who had received plasma. As a result of this high incidence and the resultant loss in life and hospital days, pooled plasma was withdrawn from the Korean Theater and replaced by concentrated human albumin and dextran.

COLD INJURIES

Because wars often are fought in cold climates, cold injuries have proved to be a serious, sometimes catastrophic, problem in military medicine. These injuries can be prevented under conditions of extreme cold if troops can be kept mobilized, can be provided with suitable clothing and can be taught how to wear their clothing properly. Enemy fire may immobilize large numbers of troops, or wounded men with inadequate circulation; they may be immobilized on the battlefield until aid can reach them. As a result, the American Army had over 55,000 cold injuries in World War II and over 7,000 in the Korean conflict—injuries resulting in 3 million hospital days.[28]

The fundamental injury, the loss of body heat resulting in a localized reduction in tissue temperature, does not appear to be unlike thermal burns, except that, after exposure to cold, injuries to the vascular and nervous tissue appear to be more prominent and more lasting.

Three syndromes have been described. All three have the same fundamenal injury—loss of heat with a resultant decrease in temperature which is most marked at the distal end of the extremities.

1. **Frostbite.** This, the most important injury, is described below. It results from exposures of relatively short duration (a few minutes to several hours) to temperatures of extreme cold ($+20°$ to $-80°$ F.). Exposure

to excessive moisture does not play as important a role as in the other 2 conditions.

2. **Trench Foot.** This injury results from longer exposures (several days or weeks) to milder temperatures (slightly above or below freezing) under conditions in which the feet remain on wet ground. It was a frequent injury of the trench warfare of World War I.

3. **Immersion Foot.** This injury, seen most frequently among naval personnel, results from prolonged immersion of the feet in cold water ($25°$ to $60°$ F.).

These syndromes are variations of the same injury and, like thermal burns, represent injury of varying degrees—superficial, dermal or deep (see section on Cold Injuries). Treatment is nonspecific. Unfortunately, the lesson that has had to be learned afresh in each war is that radical amputation is *unnecessary*. Conservative management offers the best results. The most difficult problem at present does not appear to be the treatment of the acute injury but rather the management of the sequelae, residual pain and sensitivity to cold.

The military problem with cold injuries is not primarily treatment; it is prevention. Prophylactic measures consist, in part, of ascertaining weather predictions and avoiding, when possible, undue exposure. When exposure is necessary, heat loss can be minimized by proper clothing, based on the principle of insulation by air spaces. Constricting clothes prevent air insulation, and moisture increases heat conduction. Because of the deleterious effect of moisture, many injuries have been prevented by the simple expedient of changing socks every day—something that under combat conditions can be achieved only by a continued educational program for the troops. Insulated rubber boots have been developed and have proved to be effective prophylactically, provided that the troops observe the above foot hygiene. No clothing can be completely effective in conserving heat if exposure and immobilization are prolonged unduly. Therefore, the prevention of cold injuries is as much the responsibility of commanding officers as it is of the medical officer. However, the medical officer must be responsible for teaching both command and troops the dangers and the preventive measures involved.

FAT EMBOLISM

The significance of fat embolism has not been established conclusively. Among the fatalities of the United Nations' troops in Korea, Scully often was able, at autopsy, to demonstrate fat emboli in the small pulmonary vessel. However, no clinical significance was evident except in the infrequent casualty in whom the emboli had passed through the pulmonary circulation to reach the brain or the kidney. Disturbances in sensorium and hematuria resulted.

Therapy is entirely nonspecific.

PRINCIPLES OF MANAGEMENT OF ATOMIC CASUALTIES

At Hiroshima and Nagasaki atomic casualties occurred in staggering numbers in a localized area in an exceedingly short period of time. Modern medicine seldom has faced such a catastrophe. Destruction of medical facilities and personnel, continuing fires, loss of electrical, water, transportation and communication facilities, panic and inadequate medical planning could nullify completely all that modern medicine has to offer at a time when it is needed most.

Few new problems were encountered at Hiroshima and Nagasaki; the problems were those of treating mechanical, thermal and irradiation injuries, all well known to medicine. However, the mass of casualties necessitate a new approach to the problems.

Although the hydrogen bombs have been described as being much more powerful, the smaller atomic bombs used in World War II offer the only base line in experience. The principles of care of mass casualties are apparently the same after the explosion of any weapon of this type.

A small atomic bomb similar to those exploded over Japan might be equivalent to 20,000 tons of TNT; therefore, the bomb might be called a "20 KT" or a "20 kiloton" bomb.

The detonation of an atomic bomb is followed immediately by a heat wave that lasts about a second. Initially, the heat produced has been estimated to be in the millions of degrees centigrade. In spite of this tremendous radiant energy, its destructive power is dissipated rapidly as the distance from the epi-

center (point on ground directly beneath the explosion) increases. Heat in excess of 8 calories per square inch will char clothing and skin; heat of 2 to 3 calories per square inch will produce first-degree burns. Ordinary clothing offers protection against the flash burn beyond a distance of from 3,500 to 4,500 feet; within this range, both clothing and skin are burned, so that unsheltered people would receive third-degree burns. Up to a range of 12,000 feet from the epicenter, unprotected people may receive first-degree and second-degree burns.

Other effects of the radiant energy include a temporary blindness, usually lasting a few minutes, due to staring at the fireball.

Whereas the initial flash will produce many primary burns, many other thermal injuries will result from secondary burns—burning clothing, houses, gas lines, overturned stoves, disruped electrical lines, etc.

The experience of Hiroshima and Nagasaki indicates that approximately 35 per cent of the casualties requiring medical care would suffer from uncomplicated thermal burns, and that an additional group would have thermal burns complicating mechanical injuries. This incidence of burns would have been lower in Japan had a warning period permitted the people to take cover.

Approximately 50 to 60 per cent of the casualties suffered from mechanical injuries secondary to the blast. Immediately after the explosion there is a tremendous surge of increased pressure. This blast wave is relatively sustained as it moves outward, carrying dirt, stones, tile, shingles—any and all articles, including millions of fragments of the shattered buildings. Following this primary pressure phase (blast), there is a secondary phase (suction) resulting from the return rush of air into the partial vacuum created by the explosion and by the loss of the rising hot air created by the fireball. This suction phase (2 to 3 minutes) exerts pressure on buildings from an opposite direction to the first pressure wave, thereby causing additional buildings to fall or disintegrate.

The blast per se produces few harmful effects upon the human body. Near by, it may be that eardrums will rupture, and some harm may accrue to the air-filled lungs and intestines, but the body withstands the pressure rather well. It is the secondary effects of the blast that are so devastating. A rock, a brick or a stick may be hurled with such force by the blast as to smash a man's skull. Window panes and roofs produce millions of "bullets." The devastating effect of this barrage of flying debris led to the descriptive expression that "the target becomes the missile."

It is probable that no casualties occur from the *direct* effect of the blast beyond a radius of 1,000 feet. Therefore, this effect is a minor factor in the total picture. From the epicenter to about 2,500 feet, most of the mechanical injuries from the *indirect* blast effect are fatal. From 2,500 to 7,000 feet, most of the injuries are serious; from 7,000 to 12,000 feet, minor injuries predominate. These distances apply only to the smaller bombs, but they offer a method of planning that can be adapted to larger weapons.

Radiation injuries, resulting chiefly from gamma radiation, constitute a moderate problem, although this factor is less important than the blast and the heat, particularly if the bomb bursts in the air, in contradistinction to bursting on the ground. In the latter type of explosion, millions of particles of dirt, contaminated with radioactive material, may be carried downwind to "fall out" over a radius of many miles. Nevertheless, irradiation illness is delayed; it is not crucial in the immediate management of the mass of casualties (see Chap. 17, "Radiation Injury").

The problem of atomic casualties cannot be appreciated unless one recalls that within a few seconds the small bombs over Hiroshima and Nagasaki produced the following casualties:

	Hiroshima	*Nagasaki*
Killed and Missing	70,000	36,000
Injured	70,000	40,000

Faced with responsibilities of such magnitude, the medical profession must plan, in generalities, its approach to therapy.

It is quite obvious that the hydrogen bomb has a much greater range of devastation. Perhaps very small atomic weapons may be utilized. In either instance, the principles remain unchanged.

On the basis of extensive military experiences and limited experience in civilian disasters, principles of management of mass cas-ualties can be outlined tentatively. These principles should include the following items, divided under several general headings:

GENERAL PRINCIPLE

1. The plan of treatment must be designed to accomplish the greatest good for the greatest number of people. The saving of a life takes precedence over the saving of a limb. However, it is conceivable that the return to military duty might, under conditions of total warfare, take precedence over either.

TRAUMA

2. Within the first 24 hours, most fatalities occurring after patients reach medical installations are due to hemorrhage, mechanical defects or thermal burns.

3. Traumatic wounds are contaminated wounds containing pathogenic aerobic and anaerobic organisms.

4. Primarily, the prevention of infection is dependent upon the adequacy of débridement. Antibiotics will not prevent infection in the presence of necrotic tissue. When débridement is not feasible because of the press of casualties, incision and drainage may be advantageous. Soft tissue wounds should not be closed under these conditions.

5. Gas gangrene develops primarily in patients with arterial injuries. It has an incubation period of from 24 to 48 hours. In the presence of gangrenous tissue, it cannot be prevented by antibiotics. Its prevention requires surgical removal of the mass of nonviable tissue.

6. Traumatic injuries are contaminated injuries, and in the presence of nonviable tissue they will become infected. In the absence of arterial injury, antibiotics probably will prevent early fatalities from these wounds. Under these conditions, infections will have to be treated rather than prevented.

SHOCK

7. Nature has supplied man with a relatively greater reserve in red cell mass than in plasma volume. A young man who loses rapidly 50 per cent of his whole blood is almost dead. The use of plasma or plasma volume expanders, while not restoring his red cell mass, restores his circulating volume and assists him materially to compensate for his

injury. Plasma or plasma volume expanders can be used as a compromise to replace blood loss in amounts of 1,000 to 2,000 cc. In greater amounts, units of whole blood and plasma substitutes may be administered alternately so as to extend the supply of blood.

8. When the supply of available blood is limited, it can be used most efficiently in patients in whom hemorrhage has been controlled. Therefore, a limited quantity of blood will save more patients with injuries of the extremities than with intra-abdominal hemorrhage.

BURNS

9. Burn wounds are contaminated, and, since immediate débridement is not feasible technically, immediate surgery has little to offer the patient with uncomplicated burns in mass casualty situations.

10. Since the burn wound is already contaminated, sterile dressings are not essential to the management of these patients.

11. The cause of early death in patients with thermal injuries is blood-volume deficiency. This deficiency is primarily in the plasma component. Whole blood is not absolutely essential in the immediate treatment of thermal injuries. Plasma or plasma volume expanders will suffice. Sodium chloride and sodium bicarbonate, given orally in isotonic solution, lowers substantially the mortality rate in the first 2 days.

12. Patients with burns of from 5 to 15 per cent of their body surface will survive if given oral fluids. Most patients with burns of from 60 to 100 per cent of their body surface will die in spite of intensive therapy. In the presence of mass casualties, first priority in the treatment of thermal injuries should be those casualties with burns of from 20 to 40 per cent.

HEAD WOUNDS

13. In the absence of increased intracranial pressure, patients with wounds of the brain tolerate transportation to fixed hospitals without greatly increasing the mortality.

THORACIC WOUNDS

14. Intrathoracic injuries, while seldom requiring formal thoracotomy, apparently result in a marked increase in mortality if treatment of the mechanical pulmonary defects and blood-volume deficiency is delayed. As a result, these injuries deserve a fairly high priority.

ABDOMINAL WOUNDS

15. Patients with perforating wounds of the bowel appear to deteriorate rather rapidly with the passage of time. They, too, deserve a fairly high priority.

SEDATION

16. Under conditions in which survival may depend upon one's ability to care for one's self, morphine or other sedatives may immobilize an individual to his ultimate detriment.

FLUID ADMINISTRATION

17. Limitations in personnel and supplies will make the routine use of intravenous fluids impractical. All patients should be given water or, better, a hypotonic saline solution orally, except those who are unconscious, in profound shock, have gastrointestinal perforations or are about to undergo anesthesia. Although the absorption of water is retarded after injury, thirst and fluid requirements often can be controlled by drinking.

EVACUATION

18. Evacuation of patients to hospitals in neighboring cities must be controlled in such a way that no single hospital is overcrowded while other hospitals are not utilized.

RADIATION INJURIES

19. Although experience is limited, radiation injuries appear to produce delayed manifestations and deserve little consideration during the immediate postdisaster period. Fatalities during the first few days result principally from thermal and mechanical injuries.

SUBMARINE MEDICINE

Until recent developments, the primary problem of submarine medical officers has been the control of carbon dioxide levels in the atmosphere of the submerged ship. This has now been controlled adequately, even under conditions of prolonged submersion (several months) in the atomic-powered submarines. Radiation hazards are minimal and are well controlled. The present problem is that of atmospheric toxins of a wide variety existing in the closed, limited environment for a long period: products of tobacco smoking, hydrocarbons from lighter fluids, solvents and polishes, decomposition products of lubricants, and even by-products of the processes used to "scrub" carbon dioxide and other contaminants from the atmosphere.

CHEMICAL WARFARE*

The medical problems of chemical warfare include the prevention of injury or the resuscitation after injury by several types of agents, which include the following.

LETHAL AGENTS

Anticholinesterases. Loosely referred to as "nerve gases," these chemicals block the action of acetylcholinesterase and therefore lead to muscarinic and nicotinic signs and symptoms. Treatment includes artificial respiration, the administration of atropine in large doses and the administration of one of several oximes.

Vesicants. Sulfur mustards, nitrogen mustards and certain arsenical compounds produce chemical burns of the skin and the eyes. Healing may be prolonged, but otherwise the surgical problem may be considered to be analogous to the treatment of thermal burns of comparable extent and severity.

Lung Irritants. The vesicants attack the respiratory tract when inhaled, producing severe tracheobronchitis and pneumonitis. Certain compounds, such as phosgene, have relatively little effect on the proximal tracheobronchial tree but produce pulmonary edema by damaging the alveolar membrane. Treatment is supportive (antibiotics, oxygen) and is disappointingly ineffective.

INCAPACITATING AGENTS

A wide variety of pharmacologic effects may be utilized to produce temporary, nonlethal impairment of purposeful activity. Such effects include paralysis, rigidity, tremors, convulsions, postural hypotension, physiologic blindness and other physical effects, or hallucinations, delusions, delirium, depersonalization and other psychological effects. Treatment will

* Lt. Col. Douglas Lindsey, M. C.

depend on careful diagnosis and the postulation of logical pharmacological counteraction.

ARCTIC MEDICINE†

Military commitments today include the deployment of troops to all climates. In arctic combat, man is the limiting factor; his success will depend upon his state of fitness, training, initiative and adaptability. A temperature of —30° F. is probably the lower limit for efficient, prolonged outdoor operations. At —40° F., even animal activity is markedly reduced. At —60° F., many kinds of outdoor activities become exceedingly difficult but by no means impossible.

The limitation of the soldier's ability to operate in a cold environment depends ultimately on his ability to maintain positive heat balance. This depends in turn on the severity of the environmental exposure, his heat production and his heat conservation, including insulation and clothing.

There are few, if any, specific evidences of general physiologic acclimatization in man. From a practical standpoint, such changes are in any case small compared with the importance of factors such as accustomization, experience, training and fitness. On the other hand, there may be some clear-cut evidence of local acclimatization to cold, such as the maintenance of high skin temperature and blood flow of the face and the hands during cold exposure in cold-acclimatized individuals.

The present military arctic uniform, providing somewhat less than 4 clo units, would offer adequate protection during moderate or light work at —40° F. when there is protection from the wind. During prolonged periods of exposure more severe than this, the soldier has to rely on physical exercise to augment heat production in order to maintain thermal balance. Therefore, a high level of physical fitness is essential in cold-weather operation, and simple, heated shelters should be provided whenever possible for troops who are resting. Casualties must be protected immediately.

The caloric requirements of troops in the Arctic are only slightly higher than those of soldiers stationed in temperate climates, the difference being due mainly to the hobbling

† Dr. Kaare Rodahl.

effect of the Arctic winter clothing and the greater energy expenditure required by movemen through snow, etc. The percentage of calories furnished by protein, fat and carbohydrate in the diet of American troops living in Alaska is not signicantly different from that reported for United States troops eating a garrison ration in temperate or tropical climates. There is no increased metabolism in the clothed man exposed to the Arctic environment under normal conditions of environmental protection. Nor is there any increase in thyroid activity under these conditions.

To a great extent, the success of the Arctic soldier will depend on his ability to adapt himself psychologically to the cold environment, to overcome his fear of the cold and to realize that snow is a very excellent protector against cold. Nevertheless, he must be aware of hazards such as hypothermia and frostbite. A severe degree of hypothermia may occur, especially in soldiers who are forced to remain inactive in extreme cold—for instance, while under fire in a foxhole. The recommended treatment is rapid rewarming. First-degree frostbite is a minor matter, commonly experienced by all who live or work in a cold environment. The treatment is simply to warm the frozen skin by applying heat.

MAN IN SPACE

Looking to the future, the military surgeon has a definite interest in the problems of space travel. Among the problems included are those of rapid acceleration and deceleration, low atmospheric pressure and the control of heat upon re-entry into the atmosphere. At this stage, the principles to be utilized remain incompletely developed.

REFERENCES

1. Altemeier, W. A., and Furste, W. L.: The problem of gas gangrene *in* Advances in Military Medicine, vol. 1, Boston, Little, 1948.
2. Artz, C. P., Howard, J. M., Sako, Y., Bronwell, A. W., and Prentice, T. C.: Clinical experiences in the early management of the most severely injured battle casualties, Ann. Surg. *141*:285-296, 1955.
3. Beebe, G. W., and DeBakey, M. E.: Battle Casualties, Springfield, Ill., Thomas, 1952.
4. Board for the Study of the Severely Wounded: The Physiological Effects of Wounds, Washington, D.C., U. S. Government Printing Office, 1952.
5. Bronwell, A. S., Artz, C. P., and Sako, Y.: Abdominal and thoraco-abdominal wounds *in* Recent Advances in Medicine and Surgery, Based on Professional Medical Experiences in Japan and Korea, 1950-1953, vol. 1, Medical Science Publication No. 4, Washington, D.C., Army Medical Service Graduate School, 1954.
6. Campbell, E., and Meirowsky, A.: Penetrating wounds of the spinal cord *in* Bowers, W. F. (ed.): Surgery of Trauma, Philadelphia, Lippincott, 1953.
7. Coupal, J. F.: Pathology of gas gangrene following war wounds *in* The Medical Department of the United States Army in the World War, vol. 12, section 2, U. S. Government Printing Office, 1929.
8. DeBakey, M. E., and Simeone, F. A.: Battle injuries of the arteries in World War II: an analysis of 2,471 cases, Ann. Surg. *123*:534-579, 1946.
9. Edsall, G.: Immunization of adults against diphtheria and tetanus, Am. J. Pub. Health *42*:393-400, 1952.
10. Edwards, J. E.: Practical considerations in the treatment of eye casualties *in* Recent Advances in Medicine and Surgery, Based on Professional Medical Experiences in Japan and Korea, 1950-1953, vol. 1, Medical Science Publication No. 4, Washington, D.C., Army Medical Service Graduate School, 1954.
11. Forsee, J. H.: Thoracic wounds *in* Bowers, W. F. (ed.): Surgery of Trauma, Philadelphia, Lippincott, 1953.
12. Glenn, F.: Tetanus—a preventable disease. Including an experience with civilian casualties in the battle for Manila (1945). Ann. Surg. *124*:1030-1040, 1946.
13. Grant, R. T., and Reeve, E. B.: Observations on the General Effects of Injury in Man. With Special Reference to Wound Shock. Medical Research Council Special Report No. 277, London, 1951.
14. Hampton, D.: Wounds of joints *in* Bowers, W. F. (ed.): Surgery of Trauma, Philadelphia, Lippincott, 1953.
15. Holmes, R. H.: Wound ballistics and body armor, J.A.M.A. *150*:73-78, 1952.
16. Holmes, R. H., Enos, W. F., Jr., and Beyer, J. C.: Medical aspects of body armor in Korea *in* Recent Advances in Medicine and Surgery, Based on Professional Medical Experiences in Japan and Korea, 1950-1953, vol. 1, Medical Science Publication No. 4,

Washington, D.C., Army Medical Service Graduate School, 1954.

17. Howard, J. M.: The battle wound, Mil. Med. *117*:247-256, 1955.

18. Howard, J. M., and Inui, F. K.: Clostridial myositis—gas gangrene. Observations of battle casualties in Korea. Surgery *36*:1115-1118, 1954.

19. Howard, J. M., Olney, J. M., Frawley, J. P., Peterson, R. E., Smith, L. H., Davis, J. H., Guerra, S., and Dibrell, W. H.: Studies of adrenal function in combat and wounded soldiers. A study in the Korean Theatre. Ann. Surg. *141*:314-320, 1955.

20. Inui, F. K., Shannon, J., and Howard, J. M.: Arterial injuries in the Korean War: experiences with 111 consecutive injuries, Surgery *37*:850-857, 1955.

21. Lindberg, R. B., Wetzler, T. F., Marshall, J. D., Newton, R., Strawitz, J. G., and Howard, J. M.: The bacterial flora of battle wounds at the time of primary débridement, Ann. Surg. *141*:369-374, 1955.

22. Lindberg, R. B., Wetzler, T. F., Newton, A., Howard, J. M., Davis, J. H., Strawitz, J. G., and Wynn, J. H.: The bacterial flora of the blood stream in the Korean battle casualty, Ann. Surg. *141*:366-368, 1955.

23. Matson, D. D.: The Treatment of Craniocerebral Injuries Due to Missiles, Springfield, Ill., Thomas, 1948.

24. Medical and Surgical History of the War of the Rebellion, Third Surgical Volume, Washington, D.C., Government Printing Office, 1883.

25. Munro, D.: The rehabilitation of patients totally paralyzed below the waist, with special reference to making them ambulatory and capable of earning their living. 3. Tidal drainage, cystometry and bladder training. New England J. Med. *236*:223-235, 1947.

26. Munro, D., and Hahn, J.: Tidal drainage of the urinary bladder: a preliminary report of this method of treatment as applied to "cord bladders" with a description of the apparatus, New England J. Med. *212*:229-239, 1935.

27. North, J. P.: Clostridial wound infections and gas gangrene, Surgery *21*:364-372, 1947.

28. Orr, K. D.: Developments in prevention and treatment of cold injury *in* Recent Advances in Medicine and Surgery, Based on Professional Medical Experiences in Japan and Korea, 1950-1953, vol. 2, Washington, D.C., Army Medical Service Graduate School, 1954.

29. Pettit, R. T.: Infections of wounds of war, J.A.M.A. *73*:494, 1919.

30. Prentice, T. C., Olney, J. M., Artz, C. P., and Howard, J. M.: Studies of blood volume and transfusion therapy in the Korean battle casualty, Surg., Gynec. & Obst. *99*:542-554, 1954.

31. Pulaski, E. J.: War wounds, New England J. Med. *249*:890-897 and 932-938, 1953.

32. Sako, Y., Artz, C. P., Howard, J. M., Bronwell, A. W., and Inui, F. K.: A study of evacuation, resuscitation and mortality in a forward surgical hospital, Surgery *37*:602-611, 1955.

33. Sborov, V. M., Giges, B., and Mann, J. D.: Incidence of hepatitis following use of pooled plasma. A follow-up study in 587 Korean casualties. A.M.A. Arch. Int. Med. *92*:678-683, 1953.

34. Silliphant, W. M.: Wound ballistics, Mil. Med. *117*:238-246, 1955.

35. Smith, L. H., Jr., *et al.*: Post-traumatic renal insufficiency in military casualties. II. Managament; use of an artificial kidney; prognosis. Am. J. Med. *18*:187-198, 1955.

36. Strawitz, J. G., Wetzler, T. F., Marshall, J. D., Lindberg, R. B., Howard, J. M., and Artz, C. P.: The bacterial flora of healing wounds, Surgery *37*:400-408, 1955.

37. Teschan, P. E., *et al.*: Post-traumatic renal insufficiency in military casualties. 1 and 2, Am. J. Med. *18*:172-198, 1955.

38. Valle, A. R.: An analysis of 2,811 chest casualties of the Korean conflict *in* Recent Advances in Medicine and Surgery, Based on Professional Medical Experiences in Japan and Korea, 1950-1953, vol. 1, Medical Science Publication No. 4, Washington, D.C., Army Medical Service Graduate School, 1954.

39. Woodhall, B., and Nulsen, F.: Peripheral nerve wounds *in* Bowers, W. F. (ed.): Surgery of Trauma, Philadelphia, Lippincott, 1953.

CARL A. MOYER, M.D., AND JONATHAN E. RHOADS, M.D.

CHAPTER 24

Skin and Subcutaneous Tissues

Introduction
Benign Tumors of the Skin
Malignant Tumors of the Skin

INTRODUCTION

The skin, as the dermatologists point out, is the largest organ of the body. It is a highly complex system of tissues capable of many and unexplained reactions. It is subject to immediate contact with the environment and hence to many types of trauma—mechanical, thermal, chemical or that due to ionizing radiation. It is a major defense against microorganisms but may become invaded by them. Likewise, it is a common site for tumors, both benign and malignant in type. Some of the skin elements extend into the subcutaneous tissue, and the subcutaneous fat and connective tissue layer is the site of an additional group of diseases, as well as being in a position to be involved early by many of the diseases of the skin.

It is not intended in this chapter to present a systematic review of the many conditions arising in the skin and the subcutaneous tissue because a majority of these are treated in other chapters. Cross references will be provided for a discussion of most of the injuries and infections of the skin, and brief statements of the more common tumors of the skin and their management will be presented:

Abrasions and lacerations (see Chaps. 2, 22, 23 and 45)

Avulsions of the skin (see Chaps. 22 and 23)

Burns of the skin, see Chaps. 16 (section on Chemical Injury) and 17 (including section on Ionizing Radiation)

The common infections of the skin and the subcutaneous tissues are discussed in Chapters 4 and 22.

Acne. Only a few afflictions of the sebaceous glands have surgical significance. *Acne conglobata* and *acne aggregata seu conglobata* are chronic inflammatory diseases of the sebaceous glands of males after puberty. They are characterized by scores of comedones, and their pitted scars spread over all of the body excepting the palms and the soles. Acne conglobata is separable from acne aggregata by virtue of the association of abscesses, cutaneocutaneous fistulas, and sinuses with the former. Acne conglobata is especially troublesome when located over the lower sacrum, the buttocks and the perineum. When it is widespread it produces chronic illness and septic wasting. The diagnosis is made by biopsy. Excision of the whole of the skin containing the abscesses, the fistulas and the sinuses and the immediate coverage of the denudation with split-thickness autografts is the only way known of ridding the person of acne conglobata.

Deep within the perineal segment of acne conglobata pictured in Figure 24-1, a squamous cell carcinoma was found. This case does not constitute evidence of a causal relationship between acne conglobata and cutaneous squamous carcinoma but it does tell us to suspect their co-existence and to look for cancers within the lesions of acne conglobata.

Acne rosacea ("brandy nose, drunkard's face") in its advanced form, rhinophyma, peculiarly affects the nose and the forehead, producing great facial disfigurement. The nose becomes bulbous and splayed, and all of its earlier contours are buried by nodules and ridges of hyperplastic epidermis containing acnelike pustules. A person having this disease may be the butt of malicious gossip, especially should he be a theologian, a doctor, or a lawyer. Its synonyms such as "brandy nose," "brandy face" and "rosy drop" are indicative of public misconceptions regarding the alco-

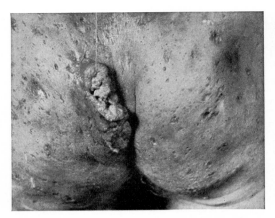

FIG. 24-1. Acne conglobata covering the sacral, the gluteal and the perianal regions of a man with a squamous carcinoma of the skin of the left buttock. All of the skin covering the buttocks and the perineum was excised with the carcinoma, and the cutaneous defect was covered immediately with split grafts that functioned successfully. (F.B., 52-5033)

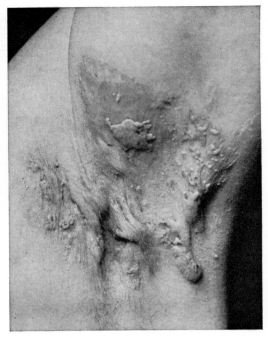

FIG. 24-2. Hidradenitis suppurativa of the right axilla. The skin of the entire axilla was excised and replaced immediately with split grafts. This cured the disease without cicatrix. (A.G., 52-4428)

holic origin of this disease. Actually, it afflicts both imbibers and abstainers just as the rain falls upon both the good and the evil. The diagnosis is made readily by inspection and biopsy. The treatment is simply shaving off the hyperplastic epidermis. One experienced with the procedure should do it because one must have sufficient experience so as to know when to stop shaving the skin from the bulbous member.

Diseases of the Sweat Glands. The diseases of the sweat glands with which the surgeon needs be concerned are hyperhidrosis, hidradenitis suppurativa, and tumors of the sweat glands. *Hyperhidrosis* is rarely a primary affliction but it is often associated with a number of diseases. The "dripping paw or hand" appears to be of congenital or familial origin. It often becomes intolerable to nonmanual workers and is a menace to mechanics and other manual laborers. Actually, it is a bar to some trades such as tool- and die-making, watch-making and repair and other skilled trades in which *dry hands* are required. Anxiety states and palmar hyperhidrosis are associated very frequently. Hyperhidrosis often is one of the symptoms of such ills as Sudeck's atrophy, Raynaud's phenomenon, chronic pernio, livedo reticularis, chronic

immersion foot or trench foot, and chronic dermatophytosis. A proper sympathectomy stops hyperhidrosis, whatever may be its cause.

Hidradenitis suppurativa (Fig. 24-2) is a chronic cicatrizing suppuration of apocrine sweat glands. Either staphylococci, streptococci, or both types of organisms are isolatable from the suppurating lesions. It tends to spread steadily, ultimately involving the whole of the region in which it began. The axilla, the pubic, the perianal and the mammary regions are the corporal areas affected by the disease. Rarely, large subcutaneous abscesses complicate it. No antibiotic cures or even controls the disease for any appreciable length of time. The excision of all of the skin containing the infected glands, followed by its replacement with split grafts, cures the disease.

The tumors of sweat glands are biologic oddities: mixed tumor of the skin is practically never malignant and is especially prone to occur on the face and the palms and the soles; the turban tumor is benign and often attains great surface extent, completely covering the scalp or large areas of the back or the arms; the syringomas are benign yellow, soft small nodules that appear in the skin of the eyelids, the thighs and the trunks of girls at puberty. The hidradenoma is benign and occurs most frequently in the skin of the labium majus and the perianal region. The sweat gland carcinoma is malignant. The vulva, the scrotum and the axilla are its principal loci. They are reddish-purple, smooth, polypoid tumefactions. The sweat gland carcinomas should be widely excised because they are prone to persistent and recurrent growth. The diagnosis of all sweat gland tumors requires biopsy.

Cutaneous blastomycosis is often mistaken for cutaneous cancer. It begins as a small papule, enlarges slowly, ulcerates and heals centrally as the papulopustular lesions spread circumferentially (Fig. 24-3). The diagnosis is best made from a biopsy. Treatment consists of surgical excision of the lesion if the area can be encompassed readily and if systemic blastomycosis does not exist. Stilbamidine and 2-Hydroxystilbamidine are very helpful. The prognosis is very good if the disease is localized.

Molluscum contagiosum is a viral disease of the pox group occurring mainly on the face, the arms and the genital regions.

It appears singly or in groups of small, discrete, firm, gray-white hemispherical nodules having umbilicated central areas. It is often mistaken for basal cell carcinoma.

The diagnosis is made by biopsy.

Surgical removal of the lesions is curative. Oxytetracycline has been reported to effect regression of the lesions.

BENIGN TUMORS OF THE SKIN

WARTS (VERRUCAE)

One of the commonest tumors of the skin is the ordinary wart (verruca vulgaris). It has been demonstrated that this lesion is due to a virus, and it is not uncommon to see groups of warts appear close together. They are especially common on the hands. Often they will persist for months or years and then may disappear inexplicably. Excision is sometimes followed by recurrence but may be successful in chronic lesions. Small doses of irradiation often lead to regression. Another

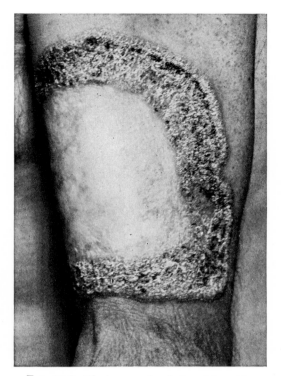

FIG. 24-3. Blastomycosis of the skin with central scarification.

method which has been successful at times is the injection of vaccinia virus beneath the lesion. This should not be done in a person who has not been vaccinated recently, lest a "take" occur in an unfavorable area.

Plantar warts often cause marked disability. Sometimes small doses of x-ray therapy have been helpful, but great care must be exercised in administering it. Large doses of vitamin A (50,000 units daily) for weeks or months have been regarded as helpful. The subverrucous injection of 1% procaine has also been followed by their disappearance in some instances. Surgical excision is sometimes necessary, but recurrence is not rare, and it should be remembered that plantar skin is specialized, and grafted skin tends to break down in this area under the stress of weight-bearing. Therefore, the amount of plantar skin which can be sacrificed with impunity is small. Furthermore, healing on the foot is slow, and use militates against primary healing so that a considerable period of rest (2 or more weeks) is often advisable if excision is carried out.

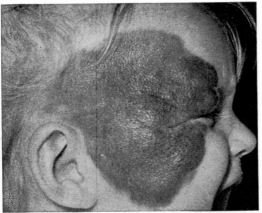

fied layer is very thin and that many of these lesions are rather vascular. In the past, many of these have been removed by electrocoagulation. This method is not advised because it affords no chance for histologic examination of the tissue, and there is always a real possibility that destruction of the lesion will be incomplete. These lesions are characterized by the presence of mole cells (see Fig. 24-5), and the color is determined by the amount of pigment or melanin which the particular lesion produces.

(For malignant melanomas see section on Malignant Tumors of the Skin.)

FIG. 24-4. (*Top*) Large hairy benign nevus in a child. This type of lesion is not prone to malignancy. (*Right*) Large blue benign nevus of the lower extremity. Note the intact covering epithelium. This type of nevus is **not** prone to malignancy.

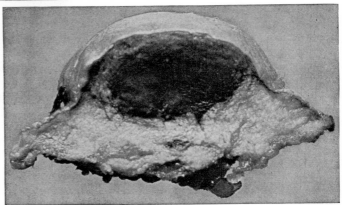

Venereal Warts (Condyloma Lata and Condyloma Acuminata) (see Chap. 38)

THE MOLE OR NEVUS

While the term "mole" is used rather indiscriminately for any elevated thickening of the skin, it usually refers to the nevus, which is a small tumor of the skin, ordinarily benign but capable of appearing in a malignant form, the melanoma. The nevus may occur in both a pigmented and nonpigmented form. It may present hair growth or absence of hair growth. The areas may be small and elevated or even pedunculated, or they may be flat. They may be as small as 1 or 2 mm. in diameter, or they may extend over an area of many centimeters (Fig. 24-4).

A typical one is about 1.5 cm. in diameter, somewhat raised from the surface of the surrounding skin, soft and pliable, brown to black in color, and subject to considerable bleeding on light trauma due to the fact that the corni-

VASCULAR TUMORS OR ANGIOMAS

These are sometimes hemangiomas and sometimes lymphangiomas, and sometimes are a mixture of the two. The "capillary" hemangiomas are red areas of the skin, with or without thickening, and these comprise the commonest form of birthmark. In the newborn these lesions sometimes show a tendency to decrease in size or to go away during the first year (Fig. 24-6). Many physicians prefer to wait 6 to 12 months before instituting definitive therapy unless the tumor is very large or becomes ulcerated and/or infected.

In infancy they are sometimes treated with x-rays in the hope of blanching them, but in view of the hazards of radiation in infancy which have been demonstrated in the cervical and the mediastinal areas (see Chap. 26), it is preferable to remove them surgically when they ulcerate or grow rapidly, or to neglect them if they are not seriously disfiguring. They have also been attacked by cryotherapy

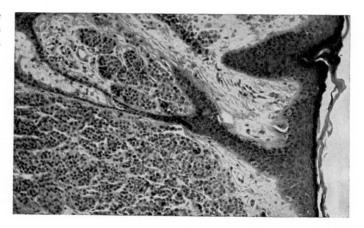

Fig. 24-5. Pigmented mole (compound type). Note "nevus cells" in dermis and at dermal epidermal junction.

(freezing), but it is doubful whether this form of destruction has material advantages over surgical methods. The risk of malignancy in these lesions is small, and a great many people carry them throughout their lives without difficulty. Small ones are very common and are present on close inspection of the body surface of a large percentage of individuals. The indications for removal are usually three: (1) cosmetic reasons; (2) confusion with moles in an area of the body which may be subject to irritation; and (3) suspicion of hemangioendothelioma which can occur in a malignant form.

Cavernous Hemangioma. Deeper angiomas containing large vascular lakes, are often called cavernous hemangiomas (Fig. 24-7). If they are large and extend deeply into muscles or between the structures of the hands and the feet, their removal may be a difficult or impossible task. Hemorrhage from them may be formidable.

A peculiar variant of the cavernous hemangioma is the diffuse dermal, subcutaneous, and intermuscular and intramuscular angioma attended by a remarkable overgrowth of the part of the body wherein it is located (Fig. 24-8). It most often involves the lower extremity, producing excessively rapid growth of the bones of the leg distal to the upper visible limits of the lesion. Extensive varicose veins and stasis ulceration appear very early. As time passes, grossly detectable arteriovenous communications with audible continuous bruits and systemic signs such as polycythemia and cardiac enlargement appear.

Treatment of the varicose veins is often attempted because they are so large. As a rule they cannot be eradicated completely by any suitable means.

The ligation of major arteries to the extremity effects only temporary benefit. Only

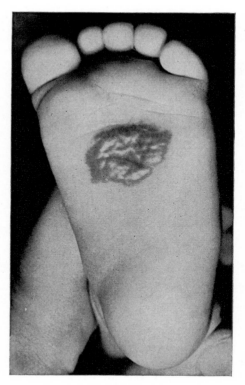

Fig. 24-6. Capillary hemangioma in an unusual location, on the plantar surface of the foot in a child.

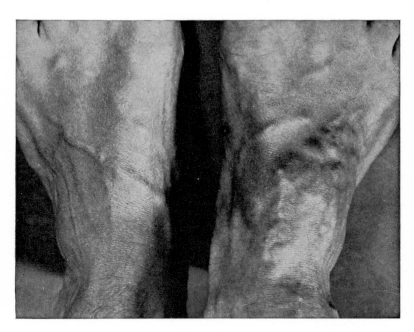

FIG. 24-7. Cavernous hemangioma of the dorsal surface of the ankle without overgrowth of the part.

excision of the lesion or amputation of the part will cure it. X-ray therapy is useless.

Lymphangiomas. There are 3 main varieties: lymphangioma simplex, lymphangioma cutis circumscriptum and lymphangioma cysticum. They are all benign tumors.

LYMPHANGIOMA SIMPLEX is a grayish pink, soft cutaneous nodule and often is associated with lymphangiectatic macroglossia. The tongue associated with lymphangioma simplex weeps lymph continuously from eroded dilated lymphatics that protrude above the mucosal surface and are covered by very thin epithelium. These lymphatic protrusions give the tongue, anterior to the circumvallate papillae, the appearance of being covered with hair.

Surgical excision of part of the tongue is requisite for the prevention of macrocheilia and chronic ulceration of the tongue.

Excision of the lymphangioma simplex is indicated solely for the improvement of appearance and effecting certainty of diagnosis.

LYMPHANGIOMA CUTIS CIRCUMSCRIPTA appear as soft warts. They may be removed for appearance's sake.

LYMPHANGIOMA CYSTICUM (Fig. 24-10) is a soft cystic tumor covered with normal skin

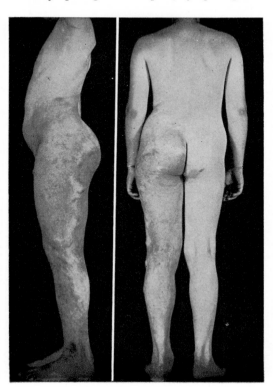

FIG. 24-8. Boy of 11 years with an extensive cutaneous hemangioma of the left leg, thigh and lower torso. He has extensive venous varicosities, overgrowth of the left femur, tibia, fibula, and bones of the foot, and an ulcer overlying the outer aspect of the left ankle.

FIG. 24-9. Superficial lymphangioma of the lower eyelid.

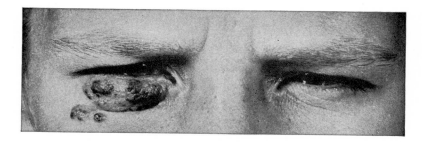

FIG. 24-10. Large complex cystic lymphangioma of the skin.

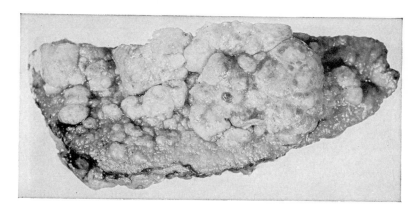

appearing predominantly in the neck, the mediastinum and the axilla. When limited to the neck it is called *hygroma colli*. Nine tenths of these tumors appear before the age of 2. Usually their growth period is limited, and they disappear from sight during late childhood. However, they may become infected and occasionally become so large as to interfere with deglutition and breathing. Drainage of infected tumors should be performed whenever a frank abscess occurs or antibiotics are ineffective.

Excision is indicated whenever they interfere with breathing or swallowing. Preparations for the transfusion of blood should be made before undertaking their extirpation. The operation is difficult, and blood loss is relatively large in many instances.

Juvenile nasopharyngeal angiofibroma (fibroid of adolescence) is a highly vascular nasopharyngeal lesion largely peculiar to adolescent boys. It is a smooth fibrous tumor which bleeds profusely when traumatized and at times may fill the nasal cavity (Fig. 24-11).

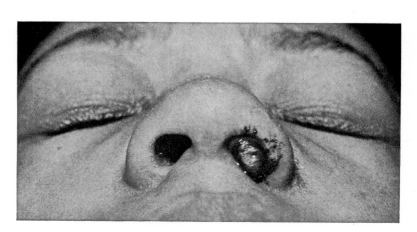

FIG. 24-11. Juvenile fibroma protruding from the nares.

When large they may erode contiguous bones and thereby be mistaken for sarcoma. However, with care patients can often live with these lesions for very long periods.

Biopsy is requisite for diagnosis. Because they have no malignant propensity and most of them regress spontaneously during the second decade of life, excision need not be performed unless recurrent exsanguinating epistaxis occurs or they are otherwise symptomatically very troublesome.

The excision of a juvenile nasopharyngeal angiofibroma is often a disquietingly, and at times, dangerously hemorrhagic affair. For this reason preparations for the transfusion of much blood should be made before the excision.

Glomus Tumor (see Chap. 22)

Lipomas

A very common subcutaneous tumor is the lipoma, which is sometimes difficult to distinguish from normal subcutaneous tissue. It is characterized by a thin, fibrous capsule and varying degrees of fibrous tissue, forming trabeculae which run through it. The trabeculae frequently extend somewhat beyond it, with the result that lateral displacement of the subcutaneous mass may produce a slightly dimpled or cobblestone appearance of the skin overlying the lesion.

By definition, a lipoma is a benign, fatty tumor, whereas the malignant forms are called liposarcomas. Fortunately, the benign variety greatly predominates, and liposarcomas, while not rare, are infrequent. Whether they represent malignant degeneration of a lipoma or a separate cell species from the beginning is uncertain.

The benign lipomas are especially frequent over the back and the shoulders and the interscapular area of the back. If a linear incision is made down to the fibrous capsule, many of them shell out quite easily. Others have firmer attachments to the surrounding tissues. Their removal often leaves a considerable dead space which may tend to collect serum, with the result that primary healing is not always obtained. Such tumors may range from a very small size to a very large size. Treatment consists of excision. Some physicians advise doing nothing when these lesions are asymptomatic and apparently not growing. However, they

may be confused with small sweat gland carcinomas, occasionally with sebaceous cysts, occasionally with neurilemmomas, granular cell myoblastomas and a few rare lesions such as malignant neurilemmomas, rhabdomyosarcomas, et cetera. For these reasons the authors are inclined to recommend their removal unless important contraindications are present.

Fat Necrosis. Localized traumatic fat necrosis is a benign lesion which is often grossly indistinguishable from an infiltrating neoplasm. Its sites of predilection are the breasts, the buttocks and areas subject to hypodermic injections. Characteristically, it appears some time after the injury or injection as a well-defined though indiscrete unencapsulated mass. It is often cystic. The skin overlying it is more or less fixed to it.

Excepting when located over points subject to pressure it is practically symptomless. By virtue of the impossibility of distinguishing fat necrosis within the breast from mammary cancer without a microscopic examination, its diagnosis should not be entertained excepting after biopsy.

Excision is curative.

Weber-Christian disease or idiopathic panniculitis is a peculiar lesion of fat involving the skin immediately over it. When located upon the legs, as it often is, usually it is mistaken initially for stasis dermatitis, acute thrombophlebitis, or cellulitis.

In the early phase, it is a painful, irregular, sharply circumscribed thick plaque covered by reddened, tender, slightly edematous, immobile skin. As the lesion resolves the involved subcutaneous panniculus practically disappears, leaving a crater lined by abnormally thin skin.

Biopsy is requisite for diagnosis. The removal of medications and salt containing iodine and the administration of cortisone usually effect a remarkably rapid resolution of the process. Should treatment with cortisone fail, excision of the involved skin and fat and the immediate coverage of the defect with a thick partial-thickness autograft of skin shortens the period of disability.

Xanthoma

A subcutaneous or intracutaneous deposit of a yellowish character not infrequently appears on the eyelid. These are called xantho-

FIG. 24-12. Classic example of a desmoid tumor of the abdominal wall. Note fibrous tissue replacement of muscle.

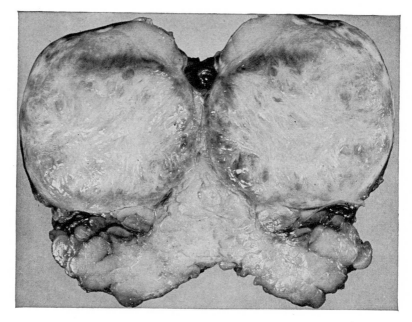

mata and are due to a deposit of cholesterol in the tissues. They sometimes, but not always, signify hypercholesterolemia and sometimes, but not always, indicate a tendency toward atherosclerosis. Occasionally, they will disappear in individuals who are successful in lowering their blood cholesterol concentrations by taking a very low fat diet. Usually, surgical treatment is not indicated.

MYXOMA

These tumors are of mesenchymal origin and are associated with a relatively large production of ground substance. They occur both in benign and malignant form and may arise in the subcutaneous tissues involving the skin or in the deeper tissues. Diagnosis is usually made microscopically subsequent to excision or biopsy. Treatment is excision where possible.

DESMOID TUMOR

The desmoid tumor is found in various areas such as the abdominal wall, usually in muscle. It consists of firm, fibrous tissue. Excision is apt to be carried out in order to establish the diagnosis, though it is not clear that the course might not be benign if it were not removed. However, occasionally the desmoid is locally invasive, and when located within the pelvis or about the hip or the axilla it may produce severe pain by virtue

of its growth into large nerves. When this is threatened, the tumor must be extirpated (Fig. 24-12).

NEURILEMMOMA

Neurilemmoma is a tumor arising from the sheath cells of Schwann and formerly was called a schwannoma. These tumors arise along nerve trunks but are not infrequent on the extremities, as well as within the interior of the body. Furthermore, they frequently arise from relatively small nerves. Characteristically, they do not produce much pain, so that the diagnosis should not be excluded because pain is lacking. Fig. 24-13.

Treatment is excision. A small proportion of these tumors show malignant changes. The author encountered one malignant neurilemmoma in the lower part of the back which recurred locally and metastasized to the lung on the opposite side of the body with a fatal issue, despite seemingly liberal resection of the original lesion and the surrounding tissue.

NEUROFIBROMA

These are subcutaneous masses of neurofibromatous tissue, usually multiple. They are soft and usually may be easily depressed into the subcutaneous tissue with a little pressure upon them. When pressed upon by a thin object such as a sharpened pencil, they deform

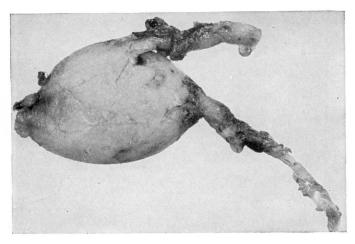

FIG. 24-13. A well-delimited neu-rilemmoma with nerve filaments expanding over its surface. This type of neurogenous tumor does not often become malignant.

only beneath the point of pressure, permitting the tip of the pencil to be depressed 5 to 10 mm. without deforming the contour of the mass. This has been termed pressure umbilication and differentiates cutaneous neurofibroma from fibroma, lipoma, and sebaceous cysts. In the multiple form, this condition is known as von Recklinghausen's disease. The masses sometimes cause protrusions of the skin which form hanging grapelike masses of tissue. These tend slowly to grow in the course of life and may become quite troublesome in the later years. These tumors are widely distributed within the body as well as in the skin. When located within osseously confined spaces they produce difficulty such as deafness and signs of cerebellopontine angle tumor when growing from the 7th or the 8th cranial nerves in the internal auditory canal and into the posterior fossa; they cause paralyses when growing from spinal nerve roots into the spinal canal and exophthalmos when arising from nerves within the orbit. Persons with neurofibromatosis are prone to develop certain other tumors, namely, meningioma; gliomas, including glioma of the optic nerve, especially in

FIG. 24-14. Neurofibromatosis (von Recklinghausen's disease) with multiple fibromata and café-au-lait spots. The tumors are soft.

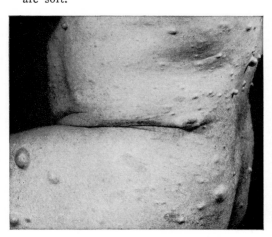

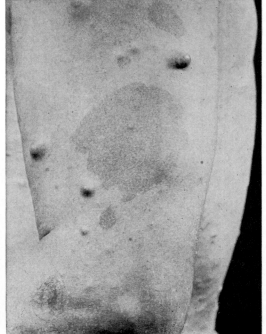

children; pheochromocytoma, (rarely) fibromas of colon (Chap. 37); and other diseases, such as localized gigantism, fibrous dysplasia, subperiosteal bone cysts, scoliosis and pseudoarthrosis. In addition, with von Recklinghausen's disease sarcomatous degeneration of one or more of the neurofibromas occurs in 5 to 10 per cent of cases. There is no effective treatment other than excision of particular tumors that are giving symptoms. (See Chap. 44, Carcinoma of Lung, page 1216.)

GRANULAR CELL MYOBLASTOMA

This tumor may present as a nodule under the skin or mucous membrane, particularly in the tongue. Histologically, it is composed of nests of large cells with small round nuclei and cytoplasm stippled with eosinophilic granules. The origin of these cells has not been definitely determined, although many sources have been suggested, such as striated muscle, nervous tissue, endothelial cells and fibroblasts. Most observers lean toward the former myogenic origin. A distinctive feature of this tumor is the characteristic pseudoepithelial hyperplasia overlying the lesion which may simulate squamous cell carcinoma. Many observers believe that this lesion represents the lowest grade of muscle tumors in which there may be a transition to the highly malignant rhabdomyosarcoma (Murphy, et al.*). Allen† feels that this transition cannot be substantiated and prefers to regard the tumor as a distinct and benign entity with its histogenesis still unsolved. Simple excision is the treatment.

Calcifying Epithelioma of Malherke. This peculiar tumor seemingly arises from skin appendage precursor cells. It is a benign tumor appearing most often on the face and the upper extremities and often occurs in children.

The lesion is a hard, rounded, well-demarcated nodule located in the deep dermis or the subcutaneous fat and frequently contains calcium, and rarely bone.

It is treated by excision.

Keratoacanthoma (Molluscum Sebaceum, Self-healing Epidermoid Carcinoma) (Fig.

* Murphy, G. H., Dockerty, M. B., and Broders, A. C.: Myoblastoma, Am. J. Path. 25:1157-1181, 1949.
† Allen, A. C.: The Skin: A Clinicopathological Treatise, St. Louis, Mosby, 1954.

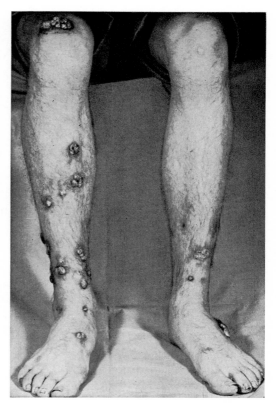

FIG. 24-15. Multiple keratoacanthoma of the skin. These lesions may be mistaken for epidermoid carcinoma, clinically and microscopically.

24-15). This is a benign, usually self-limited, cutaneous, tumorous affliction that is readily confused clinically and occasionally confused microscopically with epidermoid carcinoma.

The tumors tend to come and go singly or in crops over many years. Because a well-documented case of malignant transformation is lacking and the disease tends to be self-limited, excision of the lesions need not be practiced after the diagnosis is made.

Dermatofibrosarcoma Protuberans. This rare tumor arises within the connective tissue of the dermis (Fig. 24-16). It is a malignant tumor in that it is locally invasive, though it practically never metastasizes. It first appears as slowly growing, reddish, firm nodules which in time coalesce to form large multinodular masses that may ulcerate. It is curable by simple local excision without resection of contiguous lymphatic vessels or nodes. It may

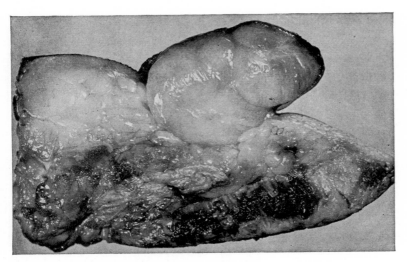

FIG. 24-16. Gross photograph of dermatofibrosarcoma protuberans with its typically multinodulated surface.

recur locally if excised inadequately. Distant metastases practically never occur.

Subepidermal Nodular Fibrosis (Sclerosing Hemangioma, Dermatofibroma Lenticulare, Histiocytoma). Subepidermal nodular fibrosis (Fig. 24-17) is a benign tumor of dermal origin occurring chiefly on the extremities and possibly incited by trauma. It usually appears as a small, nonpainful and nontender nodule or depressed area within the skin. The overlying epidermis is frequently pigmented. Often it is mistaken microscopically for fibrosarcoma or malignant melanoma.

Keloid (Fig. 24-18). When devoid of its cutaneous covering a keloid is practically indistinguishable cellularly from a desmoid. It is a fibrous tissue tumor that appears after traumatic or incisional disruption and healing of the skin. Attenuated epidermis practically devoid of lymphatics is closely attached to the tumor. Other than unsightliness and suscepti-

bility to injury, it has no clinical significance.

Subtotal excision with incision through the outermost limits of the tumor and meticulous suture of the skin to secure primary union usually will secure a significant reduction of the mass. Excision of the entire tumor with incision through the normal skin around the tumor is followed frequently by another keloid as large or larger than the first. The author's experience (C.A.M.) with subtotal excision and total excision leads him to prefer the subtotal.

SEBACEOUS CYSTS

These are retention cysts arising from the sebaceous glands about the hair follicles. They may grow to a surprisingly large size. The author has removed one from the posterior axillary fold which was approximately 6 inches in diameter. They are subject to infection and abscess formation. Malignant degeneration as

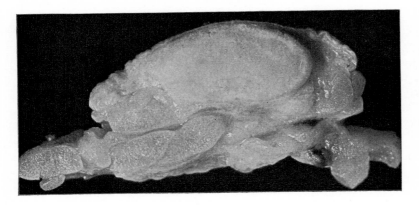

FIG. 24-17. Subepidermal nodular fibrosis (sclerosing hemangioma) of the dorsal surface of the leg in a young adult. This lesion was bright yellow in color on cross section.

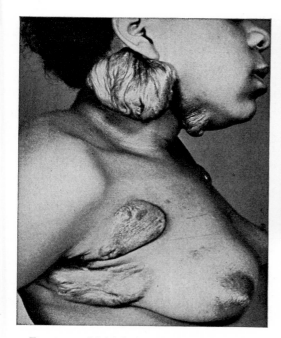

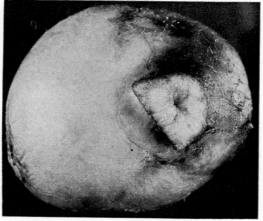

FIG. 24-19. Gross photograph of a slightly magnified epidermal inclusion cyst. Note the characteristic dimple in the piece of skin attached to the tumor.

FIG. 24-18. Multiple large deforming keloids in a Negress.

such occurs very rarely. Some of the instances of carcinoma supposedly arising with a sebaceous cyst represent cystic degenerations within squamous cell carcinoma; others, partially necrotic squamous cell carcinomas metastatic in superficial lymph nodes.

Treatment is excision, with care to remove the entire lining of the sac and the skin pore with which it is connected. On the scalp they are called wens and are frequently multiple. If they are infected, preliminary incision and drainage is often preferable, followed by excision a few weeks later after the acute inflammation has subsided.

INCLUSION CYSTS AND PILONIDAL CYSTS

While the commonest inclusion cyst of the body is the pilonidal cyst, thought by some authors to be due to the inclusion of epithelial remnants in the sacral region possibly early in fetal life, other inclusion cysts occur sometimes in the region of wounds due to small amounts of epithelium being carried into the depth of a wound or a needle tract; sometimes it appears in the webs between the fingers, where it apparently has been carried in through some previous injury, or occasion-

ally in other locations of the body (Fig. 24-19).

Treatment is excision, which in the case of the *pilonidal cyst* presents a rather special problem. These cysts always present at or very close to the mid-line between the buttocks. They are posterior to the rectum and seldom connect with it, though occasionally they may be confused with perirectal abscesses. Characteristically, close inspection reveals a pore with one or more hair shafts sticking out through it. These cysts, like sebaceous cysts, commonly become infected, and when acute inflammation supervenes it is best to open them with a mid-line incision which affords drainage and to defer any attempt to extirpate them until after the acute inflammation has subsided.

Three methods of treatment are then available. One is excision, leaving the wound open to heal by secondary intention. The other is excision with primary suture. By either method of treatment, completeness of excision is a prerequisite for success. If any of the epithelial elements are allowed to remain, recurrence is almost inevitable and frequently prompt. The first method (permitting healing by secondary intention) is more certain of success but usually requires 3 months or more for complete healing. The second method (primary suture) is generally employed. It requires technical competence and should not be attempted if the excision must be so wide

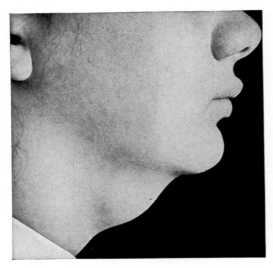

FIG. 24-20. A typically located thyroglossal duct cyst in a child.

that the resulting closure requires too much tension. Primary union may be obtained in upward of three quarters of the cases with a 10-to-14-day period of disability, followed by some protection of the area. If the wound does not heal primarily, the sutures may be removed and the wound opened widely which, in effect, constitutes the first method. The third method consists in excision of the cyst and suture of the skin edges down to the sacral fascia leaving a narrow strip (about 5 mm. wide) of the fascia exposed for a distance of 3 to 5 cm. This is more certain than the primary closure and takes a shorter time for healing than the first. Another method proposed is that of marsupialization in which the posterior wall of the cyst is left in place, and the skin edges are sutured to its edge. This seems less sound than the third method, and one of us has had 4 consecutive unsatisfactory results with it in chronically infected cases. Therefore, we do not recommend it in spite of the fact that there are some favorable reports in the literature.

Malignancy in pilonidal cysts is rare, but Weinstein, Roberts and Reynolds report a collected series of 11 cases (J.A.M.A. *170*: 1394-1395, 1959).

A thyroglossal duct cyst is considered to arise from an unobliterated part of the tract of descent of the thyroid anlage from the floor of the mouth into the neck. Characteristi- cally, it is located in the anterior mid-line of the neck inferior to the hyoid bone and is more or less attached to the pyramidal lobe of the thyroid inferiorly. Superiorly, it frequently passes into the base of the tongue as a narrow thin-walled tube piercing or notching the hyoid bone.

Patients having such a cyst often do not seek a physician's care until it becomes infected and painful or until it becomes obviously disfiguring (Fig. 24-20). Usually, no symptoms attend these cysts except when infected.

The treatment consists of the excision of the uninfected cyst and its superior tract through a transverse incision. A central segment of the hyoid bone may be removed with the duct in order to ensure its complete excision without fear of disturbing speech or swallowing. Therefore, removal of the central 6 to 10 mm. of the hyoid bone is a wise step unless the tract can be clearly demonstrated outside the bone and dissected from it completely. Infected cysts are simply drained, and the excision done after the wound has healed and all signs of infection have disappeared. Unless the superior tract is removed completely they are prone to recur. They have no neoplastic propensity.

Branchial cleft cysts (Fig. 24-21) presumably originate from unobliterated remnants of the fetal branchial clefts and the pharyngeal pouch. Like thyroglossal duct cysts they are rarely productive of symptoms unless infected. They appear as swellings mainly along the anterior border of the sternocleidomastoid muscle from the level of the mastoid process to the sternum, although they are usually located above the level of the thyroid cartilage. Cancer seldom arises from a branchial cleft cyst, but cystic swellings that contain cancer in areas often occupied by branchial cleft cysts are not uncommon and usually represent metastatic cancer within lymph nodes.

The treatment of branchial cleft cysts consists of drainage when they are infected and contain pus, and excision when uninfected.

HEMATOMA

A hematoma is a swelling produced by extravasation of blood. Such extravasations are apt to be associated with a considerable amount of ecchymosis within a few days following the injury, but subsequently a fibrous capsule may form around the main collection of blood, and this may persist for months or years unless it is evacuated. Such encapsulated hematomas in contact with bones of the head tend to erode the bone. Also, there is a tendency toward calcification in such lesions if they are permitted to endure for long periods.

In the abdominal wall, an occasional cause of hematoma is rupture of the *deep epigastric vessels*. In this case bleeding may be severe enough to result in shock. Also, it not infrequently produces sufficient irritation of the parietal peritoneum to give the symptoms of an acute abdominal catastrophe.

A rupture of the rectus abdominis muscle occasionally occurs as the result of severe coughing or straining. The torn end of the muscle contracts, producing a thickening that may present as a tumor. Other band-shaped muscles which are torn or severed may also form tumorlike masses where the unattached muscle contracts and thickens.

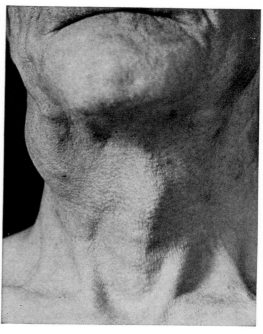

Fig. 24-21. A typically located branchial cleft cyst in an adult.

Tophi

These manifestations of gout consist in deposits of uric acid crystals. They are especially common about the ears and, while they constitute tumors, they are not to be thought of as neoplasms. Fig. 24-22.

Lymphoma

The *lymphomas* will sometimes affect the skin and the subcutaneous tissues by the invasion of these structures by collections of tumor cells. This is apt to be a late manifestation of lymphosarcoma or Hodgkin's disease.

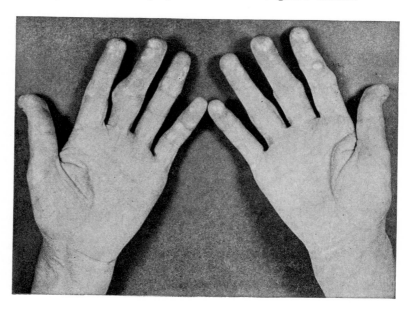

Fig. 24-22. Gout, involving the joints of both hands. Tophi.

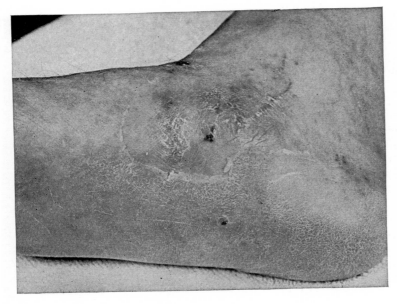

FIG. 24-23. Multiple black nodules of Kaposi's sarcoma involving the foot. Such lesions mimic melanocarcinoma.

FOREIGN BODIES

Occasionally, a subcutaneous tumor will prove to be the site of an old splinter or other foreign body. It should be remembered that common forms of glass are not very radiopaque, and one cannot be confident of detecting them by radiography, though examination is worth while and is sometimes positive. Wooden splinters are usually not radiopaque. The mass is formed not only by the foreign body itself but also by the surrounding inflammatory reaction or fibrosis.

MALIGNANT TUMORS OF THE SKIN

CARCINOMA OF THE SKIN

This lesion occurs in 2 forms: a *squamous cell carcinoma*, generally called an epithelioma, and a *basal cell carcinoma*. Both are slow to metastasize, the basal cell being somewhat less likely to metastasize than the squamous cell type. When metastasis occurs, it is apt to be to regional lymph nodes. The most frequent cutaneous sites of origin of epidermoid carcinoma are the ears, the temples, the dorsum of the hand and the mucous membrane of the lips, while the predominant sites of the basal cell carcinoma are the skin of the nose, the hair-bearing skin of the lips, the eyelids and the chin. All of these sites are on parts of the body directly exposed to air and sunlight. Epidermoid carcinoma is also the predominant cutaneous neoplasm arising in irradiated skin (x-rays, etc.) and old scars; basal cell carcinoma arises only rarely in these loci.

Epitheliomas of the skin and the mucous membranes frequently represent a malignant transition from various "precancerous lesions" such as kraurosis vulvae, xeroderma pigmentosum, senile keratosis, and keratoses caused by irradiation, arsenicals or exposure to tar.

Treatment is liberal excision, or deep x-ray therapy except for neoplasms arising in previously irradiated skin. Irradiation therapy is sometimes preferable in areas such as the eyelids, where the sacrifice of tissues is especially undesirable. Five-year cure rates as high as 95 per cent are claimed for skin carcinoma. However, if the lesions are not recognized early and dealt with accordingly, they can get beyond the range of curability and produce a high degree of destruction with great pain, sloughing, offensive odor, disability and slow death. Therefore, they always should be treated thoroughly and wholeheartedly at the outset.

Kaposi's disease or multiple idiopathic hemorrhagic sarcoma (Fig. 24-23) is possibly of reticuloendothelial origin. It occurs most frequently on the lower extremities. It is a slowly progressive malignant tumor. However, it may develop foci within viscera. It metastasizes late in its course to lymph nodes and distant organs and may be mistaken for malignant melanoma, especially when it appears on the lower extremities.

Multiple hemorrhagic sarcoma usually appears as discrete or grouped maculopapular to nodular, red-brown lesions of usually less than 1 cm. in diameter. It occurs predominantly in males and usually is associated with edema of the lower extremities.

Irradiational therapy is useful. Although the prognosis is poor insofar as control of the growth of the tumor is concerned, the afflicted person may live for many years by virtue of the tumor's slow natural growth.

MALIGNANT MELANOMA

The malignant melanoma (Fig. 24-24) is one of the most deadly of all tumors and is certainly the most deadly of the skin tumors. It metastasizes early, both through the lymphatics and often through the blood stream. Those arising within the upper part of the body, excepting those within the scalp, are more often curable than those arising in the lower extremity. The smaller the lesion is, when it is widely excised, the better the prognosis is. It used to be regarded as almost uniformly fatal. In recent years many 5-year survivals have been achieved through radical surgery and removal of regional lymph nodes and lymphatics. It is one of the few tumors that when widespread within the skin of an extremity, may often be temporarily controlled by the localized perfusion of the extremity with cancerocidal agents. The feeling that chronic irritation predisposes to malignant degeneration of a junctional nevus into a malignant melanoma is based on observations of various tumors in various parts of the body subject to irritation. Incomplete removal which may result from electrocoagulation is also thought of as a procedure which may increase the risk of malignant degeneration, although this has not been proved.

Diagnosis of this lesion requires a high index of suspicion. Juvenile moles (pre-puberty) are almost invariably benign. The junction mole as opposed to the intraepidermal or common mole is considered as premalignant. Suspicious signs include: a slate blue to black color (but it may be amelanotic), change in pigmentation, appearance after puberty, an increase in size, the presence of a pigmented ring around the primary lesion, and the location of lesions

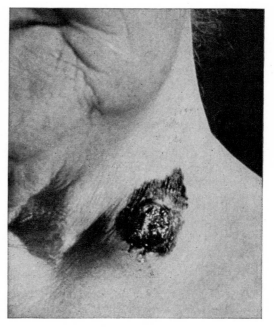

FIG. 24-24. Malignant melanoma.

on plantar or palmar surfaces where they are subject to excessive irritation. Preferred treatment is always excision biopsy rather than punch biopsy or electrodesiccation.

In excising moles, it should be remembered that the mole cells often extend to a considerable depth in the subcutaneous tissue, and that they not infrequently extend laterally, well beyond the visible confines of the lesion. In general, such lesions should be excised with a margin of skin equal to at least one half of the diameter of large lesions and equal to the diameter of small lesions of 1.0 cm. or less all around it, and excision should be carried down to the fascia over the muscle in most instances. Where such a procedure is likely to have especially unfortunate cosmetic or functional results, it is sometimes wise to remove the lesion with a narrowed margin for histologic study of the tissue. Then additional tissue is removed only if necessary. In removing these lesions, it is well to orient the specimen by inserting a black silk suture through one corner of the normal skin margin, so that if an extension of mole cells is demonstrated beyond the limits of the excision, the surgeon will know at what point to remove additional tissue.

Before undertaking a radical removal of lymphatics and other tissues for a malignant melanoma, one should exclude distant metastases insofar as possible by chest roentgenogram and thorough examination of the body surface. However, as long as there are no signs of distant metastases to parts of the body other than the skin, the excision of satellite lesions, appearing after the excision of the primary, should be performed even though it may require the denudation and the skin grafting of a large part of a leg, an arm, the neck or the thigh and the removal of appropriate deep lymph node chains and vessels such as the iliac and the deep cervical. This attitude is permissible because of the unpredictability of the growth characteristics of a particular melanoma.

LIPOSARCOMA

This is the fatty variety of malignant tumor arising from mesoderm. It has much the same potentialities as a fibrosarcoma and in many instances it does not metastasize until late. However, it is a very persistent tumor, and attempts at eradication frequently fail, so that local recurrence is not infrequent, even when the surgeon feels that a liberal excision has been done.

Both lipomas and liposarcomas often extend deeper than the subcutaneous tissues, sometimes lying between muscle bundles, and sometimes lying partly within the muscular tissue and partly in the subcutaneous area. They also occur within the body cavity and presumably may arise wherever fat is present. Very wide and deep excision is necessary to cure liposarcoma. Hemipelvectomy and scapulohumeral disarticulation are often necessary to cure such a tumor located in the upper thigh or the shoulder, respectively.

FIBROSARCOMA

These lesions may arise anywhere, and when they appear in the subcutaneous tissues or in the more superficial muscles, they are frequently slow-growing tumors capable of being eradicated by a wide resection. All too frequently, they recur. Whether this is due to failure to carry out a wide enough excision, to the secondary implants created at the time of operation, or to multicentric origin is not entirely clear. Ordinarily, amputation is not recommended for these tumors but it may have to be considered in some cases when an extremity is extensively involved and when there is no evidence on chest roentgenogram or physical examination of metastasis beyond the confines of the limb.

J. Garrott Allen, m.d.

Breast

The female breast is an organ subject to many disorders. Although the majority of these lesions are benign, the fact that cancer of the breast is one of the two most frequent primary sites of malignant disease in women underscores the importance of determining the nature of any breast lesion detected. Moreover, because of its physiologic change in menstruation, pregnancy, lactation and postmenopausal atrophy, the breast is subject to many alterations in gross and microscopic structure during these periods. These changes are to be distinguished from the disease encountered. The vestigial breast in the male is largely exempted from important pathologic disease, although not entirely.

The detection and the definition of breast lesions is not accomplished as readily as might be expected for an organ on the body's surface. In many instances, reliance upon biopsy procedures for final diagnosis is the only possible means for establishing an accurate diagnosis.

EMBRYOLOGY

The mammary gland is both ectodermal and mesodermal in origin. It is an analogue of the sweat gland and arises along the milk line or ridge which extends from the neck perpendicularly through the midclavicular line to the thigh, according to Gray. Generally, 7 papillae make their appearance embryologi-

cally along each line, but only one remains at birth. It is located in the 5th interspace and in the midclavicular line. Occasionally, one or more of these rudimentary structures persist as supernumerary nipples; they may secrete small quantities of milk during normal lactation. On occasion they have been the site of malignant disease.

ANATOMY

The anatomy of the breast is important to surgical pathology as it centers about the glandular and ductal structure. The ducts proceed in retrograde fashion from the nipple. As they radiate peripherally, they subdivide into primary, secondary and tertiary ducts, the last receiving the milk secretions during lactation.

The glandular tissue is firm in texture, convex anteriorly and concave posteriorly, thicker in the center than at the periphery. The superior part of each breast extends nearly to the axillary fold, deviating slightly laterally. This uppermost lateral part is known as the tail of Spence.

The gland is subdivided into lobes and these, in turn, into lobules enmeshed in areolar tissue interspersed with fat. Between the lobules course numerous fibrous strands known as Cooper's ligaments. These ligaments support the breast, running vertically from the deep fascia through the breast to the skin.

The epithelium of the mammary gland varies according to the physiologic state. Normally, in women, the alveoli are small and usually filled with masses of glandular cells. During pregnancy these cells undergo rapid multiplication. Near term, they undergo fatty degeneration and are excreted in the first milk as colostrum corpuscles. Fibrous tissue surrounds the entire breast and invests all structures of the gland.

The blood supply and the lymphatic supply are discussed under the section on radical mastectomy (p. 552).

The cutaneous nerve supply of the breast is segmental and arises from T-2 to T-6. The first interspace is usually supplied by the nerves to the subclavius. Two nerves are important to the radical mastectomy or other operations upon the anterolateral chest wall. The long thoracic nerve or the external respiratory nerve of Bell supplies serratus anterior muscles. It arises from the roots of the 5th, the 6th and the 7th cervical nerves to descend behind the brachial plexus and the axillary vessels to reach the serratus. It may be sacrificed if necessary but generally should be avoided in the course of operation. The other nerve is the thoracodorsal, arising from posterior cord of the brachial plexus after deriving its fibers also from the 5th, the 6th and the 7th cervical nerves. It passes behind the medial cord and the axillary vessels to touch lightly on the upper lateral chest wall before entering the anterior border of the latissimus dorsi. Its division or injury results in paralysis of a major portion of this muscle.

The nipple of the breast is perforated with a number of small ductal openings which drain various segments of the breast. Occasionally, these become important individually, as a bloody discharge may arise from a particular duct. The circular pigmented area surrounding the nipple is known as the areola, which contains from 12 to 15 elevations arranged in circular fashion. These mark the site of Montgomery's glands, which resemble sebaceous glands. During pregnancy these glands actively secrete sebum and at times become the site of low-grade and persistent infections.

INFLAMMATORY DISEASES

Chronic Cystic Mastitis (Schimmelbusch's Disease)

This is the most commonly encountered disease in the female breast. It is also known as Schimmelbusch's disease, cystic disease of the breast, fibrocystic disease, chronic interstitial mastitis and by other names, but is to be distinguished from chronic infections within the breast, such as suppurative mastitis.

Pathology. The histologic examination commonly discloses several variables including ductal hyperplasia or adenosis with the epithelium occasionally thrown into papillary folds. Ductal dilation from hypersecretion and occlusion occasionally gives rise to large cysts, very often to small ones. Periductal and interductal fibrosis are also commonly observed. In the active stages of the disease round-cell infiltration and evidence of old hemorrhage may be detected. Occasionally, cholesterol "slits" can be evident microscopically.

These changes may be noted in the late teens but are observed most commonly between 25 and 45 years of age. Generally, as the breast atrophies, the ductal hyperplasia abates to a large extent; so does the fibrous hyperplasia, too. But in some patients hyperplasia remains evident and active throughout life.

Etiology. The cause of chronic cystic disease of the breast is not known. It is believed by some to be associated with the estrogen cycle and to result from a failure of normal involution following menstruation or pregnancy, so that in time the hyperplastic phase predominates.

Symptoms. The symptoms are chiefly those of painful and tender lump or lumps in the breasts. Often the entire breast is painful. Pain is usually present intermittently, or at least not constantly of the same degree of intensity. It tends to be accentuated during menstruation. In others, pain is most prominent at the time of ovulation. Spontaneous nipple discharge occurs in at least 10 per cent of cases and is greenish yellow to brown in color but may be bloody. Pressure applied to the subareolar area and the nipple may elicit a slight secretion not otherwise known to the patient. When the discharge is bloody, usually it is associated with an intraductal papilloma and occasionally an intraductal carcinoma. Papanicolaou and others have examined these secretions for carcinomatous cells, making the diagnosis in 20 per cent of all cases by this technic.

The possibility that chronic cystic mastitis is a precursor to cancer has been the subject of much study, the results of which are discussed later (page 541).

Physical findings are those of a tender, firm, nodular breast, shotty to palpation. The edge of the breast tissue is often quite prominent when normally it is often difficult to make out. The greatest diagnostic problem these patients present is the differentiation of this disease from carcinoma. It is not sound teaching to imply that the finding of a cyst, whether of the blue dome variety or of the more commonly encountered greenish-yellow type, provides strong evidence against the diagnosis of carcinoma. It simply means that chronic cystic mastitis likely exists; the diagnosis of carcinoma or its exclusion must stand on its own merits—and it will come to light if overlooked —often too late.

Treatment. No very happy form of treatment exists. Mild sedatives and aspirin may give temporary relief. The use of estrogens is recommended by some, but the author has not found this form of therapy to be very useful. In most patients, operation is not likely to be indicated other than as biopsies dictate. In some, the pain experienced is disabling and may require partial or subtotal mastectomy, even bilateral. It is generally better to make a lateral incision at the periphery of the breast, removing as much tissue as necessary, than to perform a simple mastectomy, removing the nipple. These patients should be taught to practice breast examination by themselves and to report to a physician 2 to 4 times a year until after 50 years of age, as the incidence of carcinoma in this age group is considerably greater than in later life.

Mastodynia (painful breasts) usually is associated with chronic cystic disease of the breast. It may also occur without any demonstrable lesion and occasionally is associated with heavy and pendulous breasts. One or both breasts may be painful. In acute unilateral mastodynia, breast abscess or hemorrhage into a cyst should be considered; if present, it should be drained or excised. A solitary fibroadenoma is also occasionally found to account for unilateral mastodynia and should be removed; fibroadenomas occur largely in patients under 35 years of age.

Frequently, mild sedation, analgesics and reassurance are useful. If a mass is present, nothing is as reassuring to both patient and doctor as the exclusion of malignant disease with excision biopsy. Rarely, the surgeon may feel forced to perform a simple mastectomy to relieve the patient, but because emotional disorders often are associated with mastodynia and pain in the area may persist after operation he will do well to avoid mastectomy if possible.

ACUTE MASTITIS

This is an acute bacterial infection, usually resulting from the staphylococcus. Although it may occur in the adult female breast at any time, it is observed most frequently during lactation and in late pregnancy. It usually commences from abrasions about the nipple or the areolar tissue. By retrograde extension of a superficial infection along the ducts or the lymphatics it becomes deep-seated in breast tissue, forming an abscess. The local signs of heat, redness, tenderness and pain usually are associated with those of fever, malaise and occasionally a chill. Diagnosis can be difficult.

Its treatment should include the use of a suitable antibiotic, heat and analgesia until localization and suppuration warrant surgical drainage. Should the infection occur during lactation, breast feeding is discontinued immediately, and stilbestrol is given to induce involution and cessation of lactation. When symptoms persist several days without detectable localization, aspiration of suspicious deep areas of the breast may reveal the site of abscess which can then be incised and drained. Deep-lying abscesses often require counter-drainage if drainage is to be adequate. A persistent draining sinus may form in a few patients and require excision later.

TUBERCULOUS MASTITIS

This disease is rarely seen these days. It is usually of the bovine type. Occasionally, human tuberculous chondritis may spread to the breast with sinus formation, giving rise to tuberculous mastitis. Occasionally, it is associated with or arises from other nonpulmonary sites of bovine tuberculosis. Improved public health measures, especially pasteurization of milk, have effectively reduced the attack rate of tuberculous mastitis.

A tuberculous abscess usually opens spontaneously and drains chronically. Its treatment is the surgical excision of the sinus and the abscess wall, followed by primary closure. A course of PAS with isoniazid or streptomycin for a number of months is generally advisable, and the usual family and public health preventive measures should be observed.

FAT NECROSIS

Fat necrosis may occur from a blow to the breast, or from a breast abscess. It is an occasional sequela of a breast biopsy and is observed more frequently under these conditions in obese women. The necrotic area becomes soft and fluctuant; if aspirated, the fatty globules in the fluid resemble that in broth.

BENIGN TUMORS

FIBROADENOMA

Fibroadenoma is seen most frequently between the ages of 15 and 35, with a maximum incidence at approximately age 25. Only about 10 per cent of cases occur in the postmenopausal state. It is by far the most commonly encountered benign tumor in women under the age of 30 and almost the only tumor found under the age of 20. Usually the lesion is a solitary one, although several may exist independently within the same breast or in both breasts. The lesion generally ranges from 2 to 5 cm. in diameter, averaging closer to 2 than to 5. The lesion is generally mild to moderately painful but may be quite tender to the touch. It is firm, discrete and freely movable.

Pathologically, fibroadenomas may arise from the intraductal tissue (intracanicular fibroadenoma) or from that lying between the lobules (interductal fibroadenoma). They may undergo myxomatous degeneration and some are thought to be the source of origin for cystadenoma phyllodes (see p. 545). The treatment is their surgical excision.

INTRADUCTAL PAPILLOMA

This benign tumor of epithelial origin arises within the ducts, generally close to the nipple. There is no indication that it will become malignant; rather, most intraductal carcinomas are considered of that nature from the beginning. The significance and the treatment of lesions, benign or malignant, which give rise to bleeding from the nipple are discussed on page 546 and will not be elaborated upon here.

LIPOMA

Lipoma of the breast is encountered occasionally and is easily recognized by its soft rubbery consistency, its mobility and usual "cluster of grapes" contour when lying near the surface. Other benign tumors affecting the breast are those seen in the skin and the subcutaneous tissue elsewhere and need not come under discussion here (see Chap. 24, "Skin and Subcutaneous Tissue").

CANCER

Carcinoma of the breast is second in rank among all Caucasian women suffering from cancer. First is carcinoma of the uterus. In some reports,[31] carcinoma of the breast ranks first; such is the case in New York State.

Breast cancer is of special diagnostic significance because of the comparative ease with which the early diagnosis can be made by the physician alerted to its frequency. The goal is early diagnosis and early treatment. Self-examination of the breast at frequent intervals should enable earlier detection and treatment with resultant better survival statistics.

INCIDENCE

Statistics. A number of factors are known to affect the basic data gleaned from any particular series reporting the relative frequency of malignant disease. Some of these variables are common to all cancer; some are organ specific. Data relating to breast cancer must be scrutinized carefully lest the reported results be misinterpreted. Special considerations should be given to assessing the true frequency of the disease, its natural course and the influence of any and all forms of therapy upon its natural history when treated. The stage of the disease when first seen, the significance of its general histologic picture, the endocrine activity of the patient, the duration of history prior to treatment, the size of the tumor, the location in the breast, the site and the extent of nodal metastasis, the age of the patient when she contracts the disease, her normal life expectancy, geographic factors, the effect of infant mortality for the given country upon the over-all pattern or incidence for the area in question, local and geographic medical practices and available facilities, and the dominant socioeconomic status of the patients in the medical community from which data were collected, are among the more prominent factors to be considered.[9, 54] Some of these are organ specific data and relate to sexual maturity, pregnancy, lactation, premenopausal and postmenopausal states. Each may alter the end results in an otherwise fairly homogeneous population.[55]

Carcinoma of nearly all organs appears to be on the increase in the United States as well as in many other parts of the world. There are several facts to be considered before one can accept this conclusion as indicating an actual increase in frequency in contrast with an increase in the total number of cases being reported. First is life expectancy, which has nearly doubled in the past 100 years. The following data were assembled by the American Cancer Society.

Cancer is a disease encountered with increasing frequency with each decade in life. The lower the infant mortality rate the greater will be the percentage of those capable of reaching adult life. Lower infant mortality, coupled with an increasing life expectancy rate, increases the total number of a given population who live to enter the "cancer-age group." The number of the population under 15 years of age in 1900 in the United States was 26,145,000 compared with 13,480,000 who were 45 years or older. By 1950, 40,483,000 were under 15 years of age, and 42,907,000 were 45 years or older—a complete reversal of the age ratios in 50 years. We are well into the era of geriatrics!

Mortality from carcinoma of the breast in the United States today accounts for approximately 10 per cent of mortality from all cancer reported; the total mortality for all cancer in this country today exceeds 220,000; this is probably a conservative rather than excessive estimate. About 25,000 women die each year from breast cancer, or a crude mortality rate of 32.1 per 100,000 among the female population in Philadelphia and 24.6 per 100,000 for the United States at large.

The incidence rate per 100,000 women as opposed to the mortality rate is higher, as many breast cancers are "cured," allowing the patient to die of other disease. About 1,000 of every 100,000 females dying per year from any cause, die from cancer of the breast. About 500,000 new cases of cancer of all types are diagnosed each year in the United States; about 55,000 of these are cancer of the breast in the female. Cancer of the female breast occurs about 120 times for each cancer of the male breast.

About 70 per cent of all cancers in the female occur in the breast, the genital tract or the digestive tract. For every 100 females developing cancer, from 20 to 26 of these will be of the breast.

Data available[47] suggest that the incidence of carcinoma of the breast is lower among Japanese and Chinese women. Most series also show a higher frequency of breast cancer associated with a low birth rate, absence of marriage and nursing;[3, 8] these findings are interpreted by some as implicating breast cancer with possible endocrine disturbances. There also seems to be a reciprocal relationship between the incidence of breast and uterine cancer, whereas there is a negative correlation to cervical cancer. As there are no outstanding differences between the incidence of cancer of the breast and the mortality percentage from this disease for different age groups, the total number of patients for any age who develop breast cancer can be computed fairly well from the total number of those of the corresponding age who die from breast cancer. The reliability of such calculations then is largely a function of the accuracy in reporting causes of death. Approximately 40 per cent of patients *treated* for breast cancer will survive for 5 years with or without evidence of recurrence at the end of this time, whereas 18 per cent survive 5 years without treatment (p. 561 and Tables 12, 13 & 14).

Carcinoma of the breast does occur in children but it is almost unique among the age group under the age of 15. The author was able to find in the literature only 2 deaths reported in infants from 0 to 1 year of age and only 6 deaths from 5 to 14 years of age. Rhoads[43] informed the author of an unreported case, that of a 6-year-old male patient with carcinoma of the breast and pulmonary metastases. While carcinoma of most organs is rarely encountered in children, that of the breast is extremely so.

Organ-Specific Considerations. The frequency of carcinoma of the breast occurring during pregnancy and lactation may be slightly less than that of similar age groups. The reduction in frequency is real and not relative, for the percentage of women bearing children declines sharply after the age of 30. Steiner's series discloses that only 5 (1.6%) of the 315 cases of breast cancer he encoun-

TABLE 1. APPROXIMATE CUMULATIVE AGE DISTRIBUTION AS PERCENTAGES FOR CARCINOMA OF THE BREAST AT EACH 5 YEARS OF LIFE

AGE	PER CENT
Younger than 20 yrs.	0.09
" " 25 "	0.6
" " 30 "	2
" " 35 "	4
" " 40 "	9
" " 45 "	20
" " 50 "	32
" " 55 "	43
" " 60 "	55
" " 65 "	67
" " 70 "	78
" " 75 "	88
Over 75	12
	100

After the age of 30, however, the incidence of carcinoma of the breast in females steadily rises (Table 3).

tered occurred below the age of 30 and only 25 (8.0%) of the total were under 40 years of age. At the same time, the number of children born of women after the age of 30 begins to decline rapidly; after 40, pregnancy is encountered only occasionally, and very rarely occurs after 45. Hence on this basis alone, the incidence of carcinoma of the breast during lactation or pregnancy should be rarely encountered (Table 3), and its infrequent occurrence under these conditions in pregnancy and lactation is likely a function of biology rather than carcinogens. Finn[16] reported 46 cases of carcinoma of the breast among 62,561 pregnancies. Harrington[25] reported 92 patients among 4,638 patients with carcinoma of the breast who were either lactating or pregnant when their carcinoma was discovered. Mc-Whirter[35] encountered carcinoma in this group 26 times among his series of 1,882 patients.

In general, the prognosis is poor when the carcinoma is first detected in pregnancy or lactation. Several factors may contribute to this impression. First, the outlook for carcinoma of any type is generally less favorable in patients while they are pregnant. Second, breast engorgement tends to mask early detection of the tumor. The associated mammary hyperemia favors an early spread by the vascular route. Finally, is the unsettled effect of hormonal change with the pronounced elevation of estrogen levels encountered in pregnancy and lactation; most consider this hormonal effect to be adverse. Lest one consider surgery contraindicated in patients whose breast lesions are first detected during pregnancy or lactation, the reader's attention is directed to a 25 per cent 5-year survival at Memorial Hospital, New York,[1] and a 35 per cent 5-year survival reported by McWhirter.[35] The views of White[53] that coincident pregnancy and lactation should not serve as categorical reasons for inoperability of breast carcinoma seem to be sound.

Of 827 cases of cancer, the age distribution shown in Table 3 was encountered in Philadelphia.

Menopause may effect a slight change but if so, the magnitude of the increased incidence is not very persuasive.

Bilateral carcinoma of the breast is an infrequent occurrence among the female population. However, the chance that a patient with a carcinoma in one breast will develop one in the contralateral breast is in excess of 10 times

TABLE 2. INCIDENCE RATES PER 100,000 WHITE FEMALE POPULATION FOR CARCINOMA OF BREAST AND FOR LIVE BIRTHS ACCORDING TO AGE

Age	15–19	20–29	30–34	35–39	40–44	45–49	50–54	55–59	60–64	65–69	70–74
Carcinoma of Breast	0.7	11.6	28.9	59.1	97.9	139.1	163.1	182.0	225.0	242.7	266.4
Age	15–19	20–24	25–29	30–34	35–39	40–44	45–49				
Live Births*	7,640	21,890	18,180	11,120	5,560	1,470	100				

* Vital Statistics—Special Reports, Vol. 42, No. 13, Dec. 21, 1955, U. S. Dept. of Health, Education and Welfare.

TABLE 3. OCCURRENCE OF BREAST CARCINOMA ACCORDING TO AGE[13]

No. of cases	All ages	Under 15	15–24	25–34	Per cent 35–44	45–54	55–64	65–74	Over 75
827	100	0	0.6	4.2	14.6	23.0	24.1	20.9	12.6

that of the general population. From 1 to 9 per cent of patients develop carcinoma on the contralateral side. Bilateral cancer may be the result of cross metastases or from independent multicentric carcinoma. The relative frequency for each origin is not established, although in this author's experience, multicentric origin occurs more often. The decision as to metastatic versus multicentric disease is recognized fairly easily should both carcinomas be of the ductal variety; the independent origins in these are easily recognized but this is not easily established for other types. The breasts, as Dr. Eleanor Humphreys of the Department of Surgical Pathology at the University of Chicago Clinics points out, are in reality one organ split in two. Predisposing factors are likely to affect both rather than only one.

INCITING OR PREDISPOSING FACTORS IN CARCINOMA OF THE BREAST

Much is known about the pathogenesis of cancer, predisposing factors and treatment. However, all will agree that no assembled body of data exists today which allows an over-all understanding of its cause, its prevention or its cure by nonsurgical or nonradiation principles or technics.

Breast cancer has been one of the malignancies most extensively studied, both clinically and experimentally. The studies have provided a wealth of general knowledge, some of which has proved to be useful clinically and perhaps even more so to the experimentalist.

The clinical factors which seem to predispose to breast cancer are largely those of hormonal origin and those related to chronic cystic mastitis. In support of this contention is failure of these cancers to appear before the onset of sexual maturity, the increase in incidence among women who never have borne children or nursed them and the subsequent or simultaneous occurrence of independent cancer in the contralateral breast being greater than should be expected from chance alone. The possibly lowered incidence of carcinoma during pregnancy and lactation lends further indirect clinical evidence of a negative sort. In recent years, additional evidence of hormonal relationships have come from two other clinical sources: the palliative regression of mammary carcinoma following castration, adrenalectomy or hypophysectomy and the retarding influence upon its rate of growth in response to the administration of hormones, especially testosterone.

"Chronic mastitis," a noninfectious lesion, Warren[52] found to be a predisposing factor to breast cancer in that the incidence of carcinoma was 11.7 times the rate for the female population in the age group of 30 to 49 years of age in Massachusetts. It was 2.5 times greater in women over the age of 50. However, this is not considered sufficient reason to advise bilateral simple mastectomy as a precautionary measure in cases of cystic mastitis.

Aberrant or ectopic breast tissue is normally present in 1 to 5 per cent of the population.[13] The most frequent location is the upper, outer quadrant, although mammary ectopia occurs anywhere along the "milk line." Carcinoma arising in ectopic tissue near the upper, outer margin of the breast (the tail of Spence) is often considered as anomalous when in reality it arises within the breast. While many believe that carcinoma occurs with greater frequency in ectopic breast, there are insufficient data to prove this point at this time.

Experimentally induced mammary cancer in mice has been achieved by 3 general technics. As yet there is no evidence that any of these methods correlates well with the occurrence of the disease in man, unless it be in the hormonal relationships. By selective inbreeding and/or hybridization of certain strains of mice, a resultant high or low incidence of mammary cancer can be produced at will. While this type of controlled breeding study has provided a very useful experimental tool, there are no data in man to suggest conclusively that heredity plays more than a supporting role, if indeed it does even that.

That estrogens can produce mammary cancer in strains of mice which otherwise have a low incidence of spontaneously occurring tumors appears to be well established and documented by data from many laboratories. But again there is insufficient evidence to suggest that this exogenously administered hormone predisposes or induces mammary cancer in man.

Another interesting and important contribution to the experimental production of mammary cancer was the demonstration by the staff of the Roscoe B. Jackson Memorial

Laboratory[44] that a mammary tumor factor contributed by mothers of cancerous strains can be transmitted to offspring by nursing, by blood from an infected female fed tissue extracts and by coitus. The infective agent has many characteristics of a virus.[5] That virus disease plays a role in breast cancer in the human is unknown. Recent studies suggest that one of the causes of human carcinoma may be due to or related to certain virus agents.

PATHOLOGY

The students of breast cancer have gained little in their histologic classification based on the numbers of mitoses observed. However, the extent of anaplasia, the tendency to invade venules and lymphatics and the lack of fibrous tissue response or peripheral lymphocytic infiltration are important prognostic guides.

Classification of Malignant Tumors. In terms of a useful classification of malignant breast tumors, the author has found that employed by Stewart[48] to be very helpful. General histologic patterns are largely subordinated to the more meaningful prognostic dictates of the tumor behavior as disclosed by its localizing or infiltrating nature. If of the latter character, is the infiltration diffuse or local? What is the lymphoid response of the stroma? Does the tumor invade the microscopic lymphatic or venous channels? Are nodes involved? If so, what is their location in the axilla and what proportion of the total contain tumor? Is there an extension beyond the capsule? Thus histologic grading on the basis of scirrhous, adenomatous or medullary character of the tumor has proved to be of little value unless other factors are also reviewed. The important question to answer is: What is the tumor doing?

Predisposing lesions for carcinoma of the breast in the human female probably do exist but these are histologic conditions confined largely to the group wherein some doubt exists as to the exact nature of the lesion when biopsied. Stewart expresses the view that the change from a benign status to one of malignancy probably takes place before it is detectable under the microscope; he finds the term "premalignant" less and less appropriate as the years go by. Occasionally, it is applicable.

The question is "where or when." To this end, most will agree with the suggestions of Foote and Stewart that "the most frequent precancerous lesion of the breast is a cancer in the opposite breast," and that "the female breast is a precancerous organ." Cancer may and does occur in any postpubertal breast, whether "normal," the hyperplastic breast of pregnancy and lactation, the atrophic breast or in conjunction with chronic cystic mastitis. There are no barriers or inciting factors that breast cancer will respect.

Paget's Disease of the Nipple. This entity was described by Sir James Paget in 1874, only 2 years before his description of Paget's disease of the bone. It is characterized by an erythematous eruption of the nipple and/or the areolar tissue. A sensation of itching or burning about the nipple is often the first symptom.[43] It is to be distinguished only from bilateral eruptions about the nipple which generally connote some allergic or local irritant factor, although bilateral Paget's disease does occur. Paget's disease of the nipple is diagnostic of carcinoma within the breast. Generally, it is an intraductal carcinoma, although other types of carcinoma occasionally also produce the skin eruptions. The cutaneous eruption probably represents an extension of carcinoma cells into the skin from the underlying ducts, and most evidence is suggestive that the initial lesion aries within the ducts and often some distance from the nipple. The lesion is also to be distinguished from tuberculosis or syphilis, either of which may present at times gross appearances, which raise the question of Paget's disease but generally the differentiation is not a difficult one. There is no structural distinction relative to the changes in the ducts that would distinguish this clinical entity from that of ductal carcinoma unaccompanied by skin eruption. Often the nipple is enlarged, inflamed and granular in appearance, although late in the disease it may be destroyed.

The microscopic examination of the skin discloses the classic Paget cells which are large, round or "pavement stone" in appearance. Edema and some inflammatory response also may be noted. The Paget cells are present most abundantly in the malpighian layer of the skin but may extend to its surface.

In many instances, no tumor mass can be

felt in the breast, but should Paget cells be present in the skin, without exception the carcinoma exists within the breast. A radical mastectomy is indicated and without delay. At times axillary metastases are already evident in spite of the failure to feel the tumor. Careful sectioning of the breast will disclose the presence of a ductal carcinoma, often minute but infiltrative. Often extensive adenosis or intraductal epithelial proliferation, with piling up of cells, is noted. If there are any changes in the opposite breast, a biopsy generally is indicated, as ductal carcinomas account for most bilateral independent carcinomas of the breast, in the author's experience. The prognosis is generally good, provided that the physician recognizes the connotation of Paget's disease and does not wait for a palpable lump in the breast to appear.

Carcinoma of Mammary Ducts. Noninfiltrating ductal tumors or papillary carcinoma may display all gradients between benign and malignant disease. The features of adenosis and the piling-up of ductal epithelium usually are observed microscopically; the lumen of the duct is correspondingly reduced or obliterated. Usually, the cells are well differentiated, and mitotic figures are not abundantly noted. Carcinomas in this category may not extend beyond the basement layer. Indeed, the diagnosis of malignancy is often most difficult to make with certainty. On the other hand, if there is any one "benign" lesion likely to assume malignant characteristics at a later date, it is this one. Dr. Eleanor Humphreys has often advised breast amputation under these conditions, an opinion which the author in his earlier years of experience occasionally failed to heed. Without exception, subsequent malignancy developed, which indeed suggested that this lesion when first seen was cancerous and was not to be treated lightly. Intraductal hyperplasia, with the piling up of epithelium, is frequently found in the contralateral breast also. Should this be the case, a simple mastectomy should be performed on the opposite breast as soon as practical. In some instances, multiple foci of ductal carcinoma are found in the breast once the entire tissue becomes available for microscopic examination.

Intraductal carcinoma, if diagnosed early and treated by radical mastectomy, carries perhaps the best prognosis of any breast carcinoma. On the other hand, when operation is delayed until more positive evidence of carcinoma is available, prognosis is likely to be poor indeed.

Scirrhous carcinoma or carcinoma with fibrosis is among the more commonly encountered histologic variety. The term *scirrhous* is descriptive of its histologic pattern and has nothing to do with its site of origin within the breast. Grossly, these lesions usually are not well circumscribed and tend to radiate toward the periphery of the breast. They are unusually hard, and the cut surface discloses the striated appearance of tumor intermingled with fibrous tissue. It cuts with a hard and gritty feeling.

Microscopically, the pattern varies extensively between one of an orderly arrangement with the cells lying in columnar fashion between heavy strands of fibrous tissue and one of such extensive fibrous proliferation that the carcinoma cells are not always found readily.

Medullary Carcinoma with Lymphoid Infiltration (Circumscribed). In contrast with the fibrous qualities of scirrhous carcinoma, these are generally bulky tumors which cut with little resistance and tend to be circumscribed, although not encapsulated. The surface after cutting is pearly gray in color, often containing hemorrhagic and necrotic areas. Unlike scirrhous carcinoma which tends to be adherent to adjacent normal breast tissue, subcutaneous fat, skin or fascia, the medullary carcinoma is comparatively free from attachment and seems to metastasize later than the scirrhous tumors.

Medullary carcinoma generally is composed of large rounded cells with basophilic staining cytoplasma and large vesicular nuclei. The lymphocytic response at the periphery and indeed in some of the central areas of the tumor has been interpreted by some as a manifestation of "immune" response on the part of the host. This phenomenon often implies a better prognosis than is observed in the more infiltrative fibrous or scirrhous types of carcinomas.

Infiltrative lobular carcinomas are poorly demarcated grossly; they are tough and firm and frequently display the striations characteristic of scirrhous malignancies. From microscopic examination, it may not be readily evident that this form of infiltrating carcinoma is one arising within the lobules of the breast; nor is its infiltrating nature always apparent. Once infiltration has occurred, "threadlike strands of tumor" are fairly loosely dispersed throughout the adjacent fibrous tissue.

Intraductal infiltration carcinoma tends to metastasize early. Stewart points out that the metastases often may simulate lymphosarcoma. The author has had 2 personal cases wherein the final diagnosis from a biopsy of the axillary node in the absence of a palpable breast tumor could not be distinguished from a lymphosarcoma histologically until permanent sections were available.

Relatively Rare Carcinomas. Among these are the so-called "sweat gland" carcinomas, the intracystic carcinoma, the adenoid cystic carcinoma, the squamous cell carcinoma, the spindle cell carcinoma, and the carcinoma with osseous and cartilaginous metaplasia.

The *"sweat gland" carcinoma* involves the ducts with transitions ranging from typical apocrine epithelium to the hyperplasia of the intraductal carcinoma. It may or may not infiltrate as a cellular structure having the same cell type as apocrine epithelium. There is not sufficient evidence to justify the sweat gland as the site of origin for this tumor to the exclusion of the lobular epithelium as its origin. The fact that the breast is a sweat gland in embryonic origin has confused the picture of this tumor. In general, these cancers tend to grow slowly and to metastasize comparatively late.

The *intracystic carcinomas* are rare, possibly because the epithelium of most cysts is destroyed or lost as it enlarges. This tumor often arises within a residual portion of the epithelium in a fairly large cyst. Such cysts may be aspirated, obtaining as much as 30 to 50 ml. or more of the yellow cholesterol-bearing fluid occasionally tinged with blood. As the incidence of carcinoma in such cysts is probably less than 1 per cent, the practice of aspiration continues. In the occasional patient, however, a small carcinoma may be found within the wall of the cyst; if overlooked, it can metastasize with fatal consequence. Occasionally, the staining of the fluid aspirated by the Papanicolaou technic discloses suspicious cells, but more often these cells are either retained and destroyed or so

distorted as to defy diagnosis by this cytologic technic. (See abuses of aspiration, p. 549.)

The *adenocystic carcinomas* are extremely rare and probably need to be mentioned only because of their ability to metastasize in spite of their generally very slow-growing nature. Stewart states they are indistinguishable histologically from adenoid cystic carcinoma of the salivary glands as well as from those arising in the mucous glands of the tracheobronchus.

Squamous cell carcinoma connotes a tumor arising within the breast itself and not one from the overlying skin as the term might imply. In reality, it is an infiltrating ductal carcinoma with squamous metaplasia. However, its histologic structure is predominantly that of the squamous cell carcinoma with keratohyaline granules, intracellular bridges and epithelial pillars with transitional changes from ductal carcinoma also being detectable.

The *spindle cell carcinoma* is comprised microscopically of areas simulating sarcomatous tumors arising within the connective tissue. It may be difficult to distinguish from the malignant form of "cystosarcoma" phyllodes. Spindle cell carcinoma is rarely encountered. Stewart adroitly sums up the best methods for avoiding the controversy as to whether such tumors are carcinoma or sarcoma by acknowledging that "some doubt as to the ultimate accuracy of the diagnosis" may exist. However, these tumors metastasize to the regional lymph nodes unlike the usual expected behavior in sarcoma which, as a general rule, tends to metastasize via the blood stream. "As a general rule, applicable to neoplasms as a whole, it may be stated that it is much more common for an epithelial tumor to show pseudosarcomatous areas than for a connective tissue tumor to show pseudoepithelial areas" (Stewart).

Mammary carcinoma with osseous and cartilaginous metaplasia provides many unusual microscopic manifestations of metaplasia. Such aberrations may be limited to the tumor or arise in certain parts of the areas it infiltrates. In some parts osseous and cartilaginous tissue may predominate to the exclusion of most other histologic characteristics. The predominance of cartilage over osseous material or its reverse is an individual variant. It is most unlikely that these tumors represent either osteogenic or chondrosarcomas, but rather they are extreme examples of metaplasia occurring in epithelial tumors.

Cystosarcoma phyllodes generally attains enormous size and may actually burst. It usually behaves as a benign tumor, but occasionally a malignant variant is found. Its spectacular size and its infrequent occurrence undoubtedly is cause why this tumor is reported with the highest frequency of all rare tumors of the breast. It usually arises from a fibroadenoma of the intracanalicular type.

The malignant variant involves the connective tissue rather than the epithelium in most patients. Blood stream invasion, more characteristic of sarcoma than carcinoma, is the probable reason that when metastases occur from this tumor, generally they are discovered first in the lung or in some distant area instead of the regional lymphatics. More frequently than not, the tumor is benign. The choice of treatment is radical as opposed to simple mastectomy, as portions of the tumor may show malignant change not discernible from biopsy samplings.

Sarcomas arising from the fat, blood vessels, including the lymphatics, fibrosarcoma, leiomyosarcoma, osteogenic sarcoma are exceedingly rare. Carcinoma may also arise in the skin over the breast.

Metastatic Breast Cancer

Breast cancer may metastasize to any and all organs, and it may do so before the primary lesion is detected. Not infrequently a distant metastasis is the only presenting finding. As with any metastatic carcinoma, its microscopic structure may assume such unusual patterns of growth as to give no indication of its site of origin.

Occasionally, nodes are detected in the axilla or the supraclavicular region on the contralateral side when these same areas are apparently normal above the breast in which carcinoma is suspected. In some, perhaps the majority of cases, these are harbingers of bilateral carcinoma.

Metastases to bone is a prominent feature of advanced breast cancer. The lumbar vertebrae, the pelvis and the proximal femoral areas are the bones most commonly involved, but no bone is exempt. Occasionally, occult metastatic carcinoma is first detected upon the examination of a marrow smear, searching for the cause of an "unexplained" anemia.

The adrenal glands curiously are common organ sites of metastatic breast cancer, although metastasis to the lungs, brain and liver are encountered more frequently. Tumor extension to the parietal pleura from the chest wall is observed fairly regularly in advanced stages of breast malignancy. The lungs and the liver, when affected, generally receive tumor by lymphatic or hematogenous routes.

Direct spread of tumor through the intracutaneous lymphatics may occur over a fairly wide area of the chest wall (carcinoma *en cuirasse*). It is possible that skin metastases arrive at the distant areas by the same route. Metastatic carcinoma to the brain is frequently from the breast, but tumors of the thyroid and the lung are more likely to do so. The route and the nature of metastases for any particular breast cancer, and perhaps for all cancer are highly variable and factors influencing the route and extent are not understood.

Clinical Pattern of Carcinoma of the Breast

The course of untreated breast cancer invariably is fatal if intercurrent causes of death do not supervene the natural course of the disease. Death is rarely due to the localized lesion; almost always the fatality is from metastatic involvement of a vital organ(s) or from general debility too nonspecific to assign to any one organ alone.

History. There is no one factor or set of factors to be found in the past or family history which can be assigned an important role in the clinical history, except for a previously recognized carcinoma in the opposite breast. True, certain degrees of positive statistical correlation may exist, but none is specific or does more than to whet the intellectual appetite. Such minor abnormalities as menstrual or gynecologic disorders, celibacy, failure to nurse or to be able to nurse and familial background of cancer are of interest to note but cannot be taken as serious evidence contributing to carcinoma of the breast. However, these are somewhat useful and to be considered in a general way in patients whose complaint centers about gynecologic disorders, especially should an unexpected lump be discovered incidentally by the physician.

TRAUMA. An antecedent history of breast trauma is often spontaneously conjured up from the distant past by the patient seeking to explain why she should become victim of an established breast carcinoma. Moritz[36] attributes the patient's persistent attitude in desiring to involve trauma to claim value, especially that of compensation. The author of this chapter believes that this attitude of the patient persists from the fact that after trauma to the breast she may massage her breast and by this unintended "self-examination" find for the first time a breast mass. This she may choose to watch silently by herself. Often several months elapse before she seeks medical advice. Should a carcinoma be found at that time, she often assumes that the "bruise" has undergone spontaneous malignant transformation. It is important to disabuse patients of this concept, for they often waste the useful balance of residual life and expend much of their financial resources in the groundless litigation.

NIPPLE DISCHARGE, particularly a bloody discharge, alarms many patients. Its most likely cause is a benign intraductal papilloma. Occasionally an intraductal carcinoma causes a bloody discharge. Fitts and Horn[17] report nipple discharge to have been the only sign of an otherwise occult carcinoma.

Discharges that are yellow or dark green in color generally connote benign "cystic" disease of the breast. Study of this fluid may prove to be useful in the early diagnosis of cancer. Papanicolaou[38] examined the fluid obtained by gentle massage and has been able to detect carcinomatous cells. Of 560 patients entering the Strong Prevention Clinic for an asymptomatic check-up, he was able to express breast secretions in 19.3 per cent. By the use of an improved breast pump, secretions were obtained in 50 per cent of patients who had cancer of the breast.

BREAST PAIN as a dominant complaint usually arises from one of several causes, most of which are not malignant in nature. It is more important when unilateral. Bilateral breast pain (mastodynia) is observed fairly frequently prior to or during the early phases of menstruation and usually represents physiologic engorgement of the breast attending menstruation. It also occurs in pregnancy, particularly during the early part of the first trimester and in the last stages of the third trimester. Bilateral pain is often a severe complaint in women with heavy pendulous breasts; often pain of this origin radiates down the inner surfaces of the arms. Bilateral pain is also a frequent complaint of patients with chronic "cystic mastitis," but, as this disease may be more severe in one breast than the other, or limited to one breast, the complaint may refer to one side only. The duration of pain in this disease is often long and one of slowly growing worse until after the menopause. Complete remissions are not uncommon, but generally some recurrence at or just prior to menstruation is noted.

Pain of recent origin and localized to one breast is an important complaint. It is found in 15 to 25 per cent of patients with carcinoma with or without a lump or a mass in the breast noted by the patient. It is more suggestive of carcinoma in the postmenopausal period than in the premenopausal era. Reassurance of the patient as being free of cancer simply because her breast is painful is not warranted.

In patients under 30 years of age, a painful and tender discrete hard lump is most commonly a fibroadenoma. An acute or chronic abscess of the breast may simulate a fibroadenoma in some ways but generally can be excluded readily on other grounds. Occasionally, fibroangiomata, a breast scar, or fibrosis secondary to fat necrosis may also be painful.

The sudden onset of pain often indicates hemorrhage into a pre-existing cyst; a hemorrhagic cyst is rare but when present is strong supporting evidence that it may contain a carcinoma. Acute distention of a benign cyst from the rapid accumulation of fluid may suddenly become painful. Both of these lesions are generally very tender.

Thus pain is an important complaint and one to be evaluated and its cause diagnosed. Its presence does not exclude malignant disease.

LUMPS. The lump is the complaint most commonly heard. Generally, the patient has noted a mass or a lump in her breast while bathing, massaging after trauma or painful injury, or by the practice of frequent self-examination intended for this protection.

Lumps found in this manner are previously painless, although occasionally slight pain is the factor initiating self-examination. The physician is surprised by the frequency with which the patient may find very small masses in spite of obese breasts. It is equally surprising how large some masses may become without the patient's knowledge. Often, malignancies of the latter variety are discoid or flat, occurring in an obese female. Occasionally, however, they are rounded or oblong and actually affect the contour of the breast to a degree that seems impossible to escape the patient's attention. Perhaps, it really has not; fear of the truth can prove to be fatal.

Examination of the Breast. The normal texture of the breast varies considerably in accordance with the age of the patient, whether or not previous pregnancies have occurred, the strength of the suspensory (Cooper's) ligaments of the breast, atrophy or lobular separation which often give the impression of a granular or shotty nodularity. Previous disease such as chronic cystic mastitis, breast abscess or fat necrosis may distort the breast as well as the normal direction that the nipple should point. None of these variations is in itself necessarily significant but may create difficulties in detecting the presence of a lesion and in suspecting its nature. The obese or lactating breast is especially difficult to examine satisfactorily; fairly sizable lesions can escape attention although examined carefully and methodically.

Both breasts should be equal in size, the nipples pointing in isometric directions and protruding to a comparable extent. Any particular area more prominent than others should arouse suspicion. The nipples and the areolar tissue should be inspected closely for evidence of scaling, desquamation, retraction or asymmetric tilting. Skin retraction is searched for and usually is detected best with the patient in the normal sitting position, placing both outstretched arms above the head. Skin retraction implies skin invasion or involvement of Cooper's ligaments and more often than not tumor spread to the regional lymphatics as well (Fig. 25-1). Generally, this is a late manifestation of cancer. The same applies to the orange-peel or "pigskin" appearance of the skin, often referred to as *peau d'orange*. This appearance is created

by intracutaneous lymphostasis, causing intradermal pores to be widely separated. Often *peau d'orange* is associated with intracutaneous metastasic nodules locally or even at great distances from the primary site. Compared with the minor skin retraction, *peau d'orange* carries generally a much less favorable prognosis, although in neither instance is the prognosis good. Both are late signs.

Carcinoma *en cuirasse* is the classic example of widespread intracutaneous dissemination of cancer through its lymphatics with brawny induration being more prominent than *peau d'orange*. Often the entire breast, shoulder and upper abdomen may be involved. Discoid or rounded nodularity is present. When the skin is red and appears to be inflamed, the term "inflammatory carcinoma" is applied. The prognosis in such patients is especially poor or hopeless.

Upon palpation, generally one lump may prove to be more prominent than others if carcinoma is present. It is prominent because of one or more of the following features: it is generally firm to hard, often nontender and may be fixed to adjacent tissue. The lump may be adherent to the skin, producing dimpling or it may be adherent to the fatty tissue, or to the fascia and not affect the skin, depending upon the depth of its origin and whether it introduces traction of Cooper's ligaments. Advanced local carcinoma may be fixed to all four of the structures; an early cancer may be fixed to the skin should its site of origin be close to the dermal structures. Occasionally, the tumor is relatively soft and extends over a wide area and does not arouse much suspicion. Too much manipulation is to be avoided as this may disseminate tumor.

Examination of the axilla is carried out best with the forearm of the patient resting upon the examiner's arm or with one hand supporting the elbow of the patient. With his other hand, the axilla is examined gently, beginning at its base along the margin of the pectoralis major. The fingers are introduced gently into the truncated portion of the axilla, depressing the skin and the underlying subcutaneous tissue gently against the thoracic cage, trying to reach the apex. Any suspicious nodule encountered is rolled gently under the finger against the thoracic cage. Its size, consistency and freedom of mobility are noted.

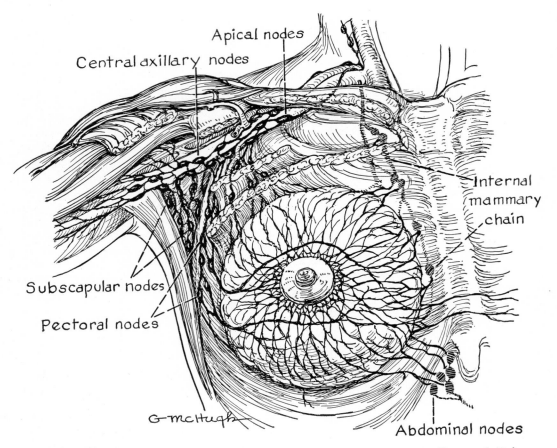

FIG. 25-1. Principal channels of the lymph drainage from the breast are illustrated. It is evident that carcinoma of the breast may spread in any direction, although metastases are more likely to follow the course of the dominant channels for the area of the breast in which the tumor arises. When nodes are involved, in about two thirds of the operable cases, the spread is to axillary lymph nodes; in the remaining third the internal mammary chain is involved. When axillary nodes are involved, the tendency to drain to substernal nodes may be increased.

Obviously, perfectly innocent lymph nodes are palpable in many patients; such nodes may be palpable to a similar degree in the contra-lateral axilla. Failure to detect nodes in the axilla is no assurance that nodal involvement does not exist, as only the larger and more laterally situated ones can be reached. Some lymph nodes may be replaced completely by carcinoma and remain fairly soft and freely movable. Others may be small, shotty and create little suspicion when extensively involved. Hence, in examination of the axilla, errors are fairly common, even among the most experienced clinicians.

The supraclavicular areas along the lower neck on both sides should be examined gently but firmly, searching especially for nodes lying just below the posterior margin of the mesial third of the clavicle and along the jugular vein and carotid artery.

Examination of the opposite breast will often reveal masses in patients with or without breast cancer. From 3 to 9 per cent of patients with carcinoma of one breast may be expected to have or to develop tumor in the opposite breast, simultaneously or within a year or two. Occasionally, carcinoma of the breast is multicentric in one breast so that more than one "dominant lump" may be found. When there are other signs raising suspicions as to the presence of a malignant lesion in one breast, the presence of a similar lesion perhaps without fixation should not delude the examiner into the belief that he is dealing with widespread benign disease, such as chronic cystic mastitis. Search is made for metastases in the abdomen, especially the liver. Roentgenograms of the chest and the pelvis may be helpful.

Breast Biopsy

Indications for Biopsy or for Repeated Observations. The examiner's findings are not always easily evaluated. He may experience even more difficulty in articulating the reasons for his recommended course of action, even to himself.

The consideration which most reliably favors a benign lesion is the patient's age. Breast cancer is seldom encountered under the age of 30 and it is all but unknown under the age of 20. If the physician is not completely satisfied that the lesion is benign, either it should be biopsied or the patient should be observed at frequent intervals. If the diagnosis of carcinoma of the breast is to be made early, the only attitude that the surgeon can assume is early biopsy of any lesion, even if it is only remotely suspicious. Unfortunately, this course of action will force him to perform biopsy on a considerably larger number of patients whose ultimate diagnosis proves to be benign compared with those who will prove to have malignant disease. However, he cannot afford a course of delayed action in suspected cases. Waiting for fixation, skin retraction or *peau d'orange* is to be avoided assiduously, as so often these are late manifestations of the disease.

Admittedly, the problem facing the family doctor is a different one. He may not encounter a carcinoma more than once in several years, as there are nearly 160,000 practicing physicians in the country and about 55,000 new cases of breast carcinoma annually encountered. The family physician often has the advantage of previous examinations he has performed for comparative purposes, as well as the opportunity afforded by an established rapport with the patient, which is so essential to a program of repeated examinations at frequent intervals. The surgeon, on the other hand, sees a different part of patient population. His patients often are those who are screened by referral from the family doctor. Understandably, the surgeon needs to recommend biopsy more frequently, as the preliminary screening by the referring doctor concentrates the population of positive or very questionable breast masses in the office of the surgeon.

If the surgeon is not entirely satisfied that the lesion under suspicion is benign, he has no recourse other than to advise *biopsy*. The sooner this is carried out, the better. Delay of one week is often necessary for the patient to arrange for the care of her family. Should the patient be refractory to the suggestion of biopsy and refuse consultation after careful explanation, additional reappointments should be made. For those patients whose lesions are not suspicious the following schedule is a reasonable one: 3 weeks, return again in 6 weeks, then 3 months and thereafter at 4-month intervals for at least 3 to 5 years. Additional safety is gained by instructing the patient thoroughly in self-examination to be carried out between her visits to the doctor's office.

Technics of Biopsy. Three types of procedures are practiced fairly commonly, but only one is recommended for most patients; that is excision biopsy. *Needle biopsy* should not be performed unless the tumor mass is fluctuant, transilluminates readily and the patient is under 35 years of age. Solid tumor should not be subjected to needle biopsy lest this manipulation disseminate tumor or transplant it along the track made by the needle.

Incision biopsy is to be avoided in most patients. Occasionally, this technic is necessary, especially if the tumor mass is so large that its removal amounts essentially to a simple mastectomy. Therefore, in large, soft tumors whose clinical nature is not decisive, incision biopsy may be advantageous. A small incision is made parallel with and equidistant from the elliptical incision planned if radical mastectomy should prove to be necessary. The wedge of tissue is removed, noting whether it grates when stroked with the scalpel blade. The incision should not extend to the pectoral fascia. Once the tissue is removed, its bed should be closed carefully and the skin reapproximated with closely placed stitches, sealing the skin from any possible seepage from beneath.

While closing the biopsy wound, the frozen section is performed. In more than 90 per cent of the cases, the diagnosis can be established accurately on the combined basis of gross appearance and frozen section microscopic examination. If the pathologist is unable to reach a definite decision by this technic, no further operation should be performed until the permanent sections can be reviewed a few days later; otherwise, the breast should be removed as soon as the frozen section information is decisively positive. In the interest of avoiding tumor implants, the biopsy instruments are discarded, the surgeon and his assistants don another pair of gloves, the wound is "re-prepped" and redraped before starting the radical mastectomy. The mastectomy incision should be wide of the biopsy wound not only at the surface but also in the depths of the wound and should never enter into the biopsy wound at any point—tumor asepsis.

Excision biopsy is the procedure of choice and most commonly performed. The tumor is removed, giving it a fairly wide berth, so that noncancerous breast tissue surrounds the excised tumor. This avoids tumor implantation. The wound is closed carefully, and if the biopsy is positive for carcinoma, then radical mastectomy is performed.

Two points of caution should be mentioned. Surgical biopsy should not be performed in the office or under local anesthesia. Breast biopsy is a procedure to be carried out under general anesthesia and with the patient's thorough understanding and permission that a radical mastectomy is a distinct possibility at that time, depending upon the biopsy findings.

TREATMENT OF OPERABLE CARCINOMA OF THE BREAST

The treatment of choice for operable carcinoma of the breast is radical mastectomy. Operability is a clinical term used to imply that cancer may either be curable or that its removable will be of definite palliative value. Curability, too, is a relative matter which implies to most surgeons that the patient will survive at least 5 years free of disease. A few patients may remain free of disease for 25 years only to develop actively growing metastasis at that late date; for at least a quarter of a century these patients have been cured in the practical sense.

We shall see a little later on that there is very good reason to perform radical mastectomy on nearly all patients whose disease clinically is limited to the breast or to the breast plus the axilla. For those with distant metastasis already established, simple mastectomy may be desirable if the local tumor is ulcerating or threatening to do so.

The Lymphatics of the Breast and Their Relation to Operation. There are few, if any, organs within the body where knowledge of the lymphatic circulation and its drainage is more important to the surgeon than that of the breast. In recent years, the excellent studies of the surgeon, Handley,[23] have greatly increased our information on this subject and that which follows is largely a summary of his writings.

There appears little reason to believe that the lymphatic vessels of the skin over the breast are different from those in the skin elsewhere. Normally, this skin is comprised of four lymphatic plexuses, the small lymph channels from the dermal papillae, the subpapillary intradermal plexus into which the lymph vessels from the dermal papillae drain, the intermediate plexus deep in the dermis and the deep plexus coursing over the surface of the deep fascia.

The breast lies between the deep dermal plexus and the deep fascial plexus. Communications between these two plexuses exist, permitting carcinoma to metastasize in either or both directions.

Handley believes that the subareolar plexus of Sappey is less important than was described previously and concludes that it drains away from the areolar tissue. Grant, Tabah and Adair[18] came to the opposite conclusion from their studies.

The lymphatic nodal system of the axilla is fed by numerous lymph channels arising about the neck, the arm and the pectoral girdle, in addition to those from the breast. The lateralmost nodes in the axilla drain primarily the arm and are not frequently involved in metastatic disease of the breast unless higher lymphatic channels to the axilla have been blocked. The subscapular nodes course along the anterior surface of the latissimus dorsi, the teres major and the subscapularis muscles in close proximity to the subscapular blood vessels. These should be identified and removed along with the corresponding blood vessels and fascia of these muscles, particularly for inferior-lying and lateral-lying breast lesions.

The pectoral nodes follow the course of the lateral thoracic blood vessels close to the margin of the pectoralis minor. They drain principally the upper and outer quadrants of the breast, terminating in the same central nodes of the axilla as do the subscapular channels. Between the pectoralis major and minor is a small group of nodes which ascend along the course of the acromiothoracic artery, draining both the inner and the outer upper quadrants of the breast to empty into the apical nodes of the axilla.

The central lymph nodes of the axilla are numerous. Fortunately, they are mostly situated below the axillary vein between the lateral thoracic and subscapular vessels. Often they are imbedded in axillary fat. These are the nodes usually detected clinically when enlarged. They receive lymph drainage from the pectoral, the subscapular and the lateral groups and in turn drain more centrally to the apical nodes.

The apical or subclavicular nodes lie between the lateral margin of the first rib and the mesial border of the pectoralis minor muscle. They tend to lie behind the axillary vein and the clavicle. These are probably the last nodal barriers of any significance, draining the pectoral girdle and the breast before the lymph enters the subclavian or internal jugular veins. These apical nodes are biopsied (also internal mammary chain) by Haagensen (1959)[20] as a preliminary step in determination of operability.

The internal mammary chain of lymph nodes, although recognized and described nearly 200 years ago, has received little attention surgically until recent times. Their efferent channels arise from the anterior pericardial nodal system, ascending in close proximity to the internal mammary artery and vein on the posterior surfaces of the upper 6 costal cartilages. They receive drainage from the adjacent chest wall, including the parietal pleura and the pectoral muscles. They may enter directly into one of the neighboring large veins be-

neath the clavicle or converge upon another lymphatic channel near the apex of the axilla. There is little evidence of cross communication with the contralateral internal mammary chain, which again is suggestive evidence that a carcinoma appearing in the contralateral side is more likely a primary tumor than a secondary one.

As these nodes receive much of the lymphatic drainage from the mesial aspect of the breast, lesions lying within this area tend to metastasize to this system. Such metastases in the patient have been overlooked. The reawakening of an interest in this drainage system is explained by the surgeon's efforts to improve his 5-year survival rates following radical mastectomy. However, because of difficulties encountered in resecting this channel, some surgeons prefer to biopsy the nodes in the second and the third interspaces adjacent to the internal mammary blood vessels and, finding the nodes positive in either of these areas, prefer less radical procedures. Others consider such findings a challenge for more radical surgery (Urban).[50] However, both the biopsy and the resections of the internal chain procedures are still in the experimental stage.

Handley has demonstrated the lymph drainage from the lower portion of the breast, particularly its mesial side, may enter the fascial lymphatics of the abdominal wall and from these to the liver via lymph channels of the round ligament. Fortunately, tumors in the lowest portion of the breast are comparatively rare, but when present one should consider removing the central portion of the anterior rectus sheath and the round ligament, in addition to the usual radical mastectomy procedure.

Although the lymphatic circulation as described above does segregate itself into groups draining more prominently one area of the breast, the skin or the fascia than another, nonetheless they intercommunicate fairly freely. In consequence, there is no one route that metastases may be expected to follow simply because the tumor lies predominantly in a particular region of the breast. However, a surgeon's approach to a radical mastectomy should be governed in part at least by the location of the tumor and its likely course of drainage, spending perhaps more time in certain areas than others. However, in all radical mastectomies, the central, the subscapular, the pectoral and the apical nodes of the axillary system should be removed *en bloc*.

The Radical Mastectomy Operation. As this operation is designed to remove the breast and the entire axillary contents *en bloc*, leaving no known tumor behind, the choice of the initial incision should be tailored to needs of the particular patient. Various types of incisions have been developed to serve these purposes (Fig. 25-2). For the most part, the surgeon generally employs only one as the incision of his preference. The author prefers the Deaver incision, a modification of the Meyer type. At times I employ a modification of the Stewart or the Orr incision, should the lesion lie on either the lateral or the mesial side of the central portion of the breast.

The tumor is ellipsed by the incision of choice, allowing at least 1½ to 2 inches of normal skin to be taken on all sides of the tumor. The subcutaneous tissue is undermined generously, leaving an estimated ¼ to ⅜ inch of subcutaneous tissue on the underside of the skin flap. The author prefers to leave this amount of subcutaneous fat in nontumor-bearing areas to avoid direct adherence of skin to the chest wall after the wound heals. This small amount of subcutaneous fat allows a small degree of gliding motion of the undermined skin edges which seems to be more comfortable to the patient later on. If the amount of skin ellipsed in the course of operation creates too large an area to be closed by approximating the undermined mesial and lateral flaps without undue tension, the remaining defect is closed with a split-thickness skin graft at the end of the operation, Fig. 25-3 B.

The superior aspect of the elevated skin flap is retracted to expose the tendinous attachment of the pectoralis major, which is then divided. One may leave the clavicular portion of the pectoralis major if the tumor does not lie in the upper quadrants of the breast. Generally, a little better exposure of the apical portion of the axilla is obtained by its removal. The pectoralis minor now comes into view, and its tendinous process is divided

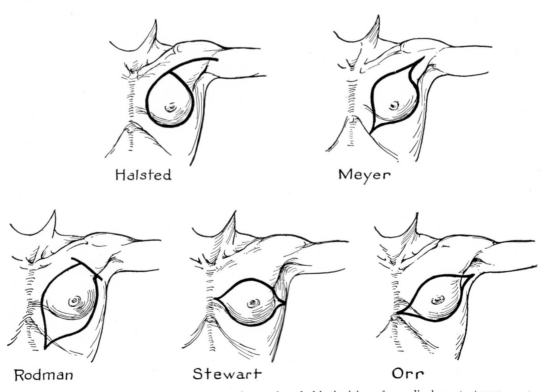

Halsted   Meyer

Rodman   Stewart   Orr

Fig. 25-2. Some of the more commonly employed skin incisions for radical mastectomy.

as it inserts into the coracoid process of the scapula. If the insertions of these two muscles are cut sufficiently close to the bone, little or no bleeding occurs from the residual ends. Together, these two muscles are retracted gently downward and mesially, exposing the

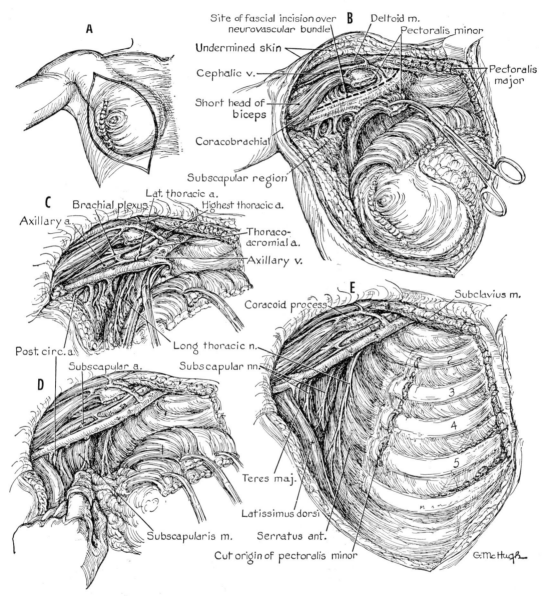

Fig. 25-3. Illustrations of operative principles in radical mastectomy (see text, p. 552). (A) Skin incision after excision biopsy. (B) Reflections of pectoralis major and minor after dividing at their respective insertions. Axillary contents are exposed. (C) Central and superior portions of axillary neurovascular bundle are cleaned of fat, fascia and lymph nodes. (D) Subscapular dissection of lymph nodes and fat. (E) Residual incision; note the perivascular fat and lymphatics along the long thoracic and thoracodorsal nerves have been resected. Resection of internal mammary lymph channels is not yet an established procedure and hence is not shown.

axillary fat, the brachial plexus, the axillary artery and vein, and the lymphatics of the area. Then the fascia enveloping the neuro-vascular bundle of the axilla is incised on its uppermost margin, and the incision is carried laterally from the apex to the base of the axilla. This permits dissection of the fascia and the overlying fatty tissue to be carried out from above downward over the entire anterior surface of the neurovascular bundle to its lowermost margin, at which point the subscapular artery and vein and the lateral thoracic vessels come into view (Fig. 25-3 B, C and D).

The axillary artery and veins, like the lymphatics, are of surgical importance and deserving of special attention in radical mastectomy. For convenience, the axillary artery and vein are arbitrarily considered in three portions (Fig. 25-3 C). The *mesial* portion is a direct continuation of the subclavian artery and runs from the outer margin of the first rib over its superior surface to the mesial border of the pectoralis minor. One small artery, the superior artery, is encountered in this segment as it passes to the second intercostal space. In this area also is the apical group of lymph nodes. This artery is divided and ligated. The second or *middle* portion of the axillary artery and vein lies behind the pectoralis minor. The thoraco-acromial and the lateral thoracic arteries and veins lie in this segment. The thoraco-acromial vessels constitute the axillary blood supply to the pectoralis major and to a lesser extent that of the minor. The lateral thoracic vessel descends perpendicularly for about 2 cm. along the long thoracic nerve of Bell and is one of the surgical landmarks of this nerve. This vessel supplies the anterior serratus, the intercostals and the mammary gland. Lymphatic channels ascending from the upper and more centrally located portions of the breast often are encountered in close proximity to these two vessels. They are carefully resected in mastectomy. The third or *lateral* portion of the axillary vessels emerges from behind the lateral margin of the pectoralis minor and extends laterally to the surgical neck of the humerus. Three arterial branches are derived from this portion of the axillary artery; the largest is the subscapular and then the anterior and posterior circumflex humeral ves-

sels which mark the distal end of the lateral segment of the axillary vessels. Paralleling these vessels are the ascending lymphatic circulation and nodes draining the corresponding areas. The circumflex vessels generally are the only ones of the 6 axillary vessels herein described which the author does not routinely divide and resect in the course of *en bloc* axillary dissection. The subscapular vessels along with the subscapular lymphatics and the underlying subscapular fascia are carefully resected in all cases.

The cephalic vein carries the venous return from most of the subcutaneous and cutaneous areas of the lateral portion of the arm. Entering the axilla, it lies in the deltopectoral groove passing along the upper margin of the pectoralis major in the axilla, serving as a surgical landmark to identify the cleavage plain between these muscles. Its mesial extremity pierces the costocoracoid membrane covering the subclavius muscle and then enters the first portion of the axillary vein just mesial to the pectoralis minor. This vein is generally preserved in mastectomy, for it may prove to be a useful channel for collateral venous return if tumor-bearing nodes are adherent to the second or the third portions of the axillary vein and necessitate its resection.

The 5 branches of the axillary vessels are clamped separately and ligated close to their parent vessels, thereby permitting the posterior aspect of the neurovascular bundle to be cleaned of its fascia and fatty contents (Fig. 25-3 E).

Once again the surgeon turns his attention to the area of the axilla, dissecting away the fascia of the anterior serratus muscle from the center laterally. Care is taken to avoid injury to the long thoracic nerve and the more laterally placed thoracodorsal nerve which respectively supply the anterior serratus and the latissimus dorsi muscles. Then the subscapular dissection, beginning with the division of the subscapular artery and vein from the axillary artery and vein, is carried out from above and downward by undermining the underlying fascia for a distance of at least 1 to $1\frac{1}{2}$ inches on either side of these vessels. The axillary vein should be spared, but if tumor is attached to it, a segment of this vein can be removed safely—with little increased danger of arm edema—so long as the cephalic vein is spared.

At this point, it is generally more convenient to clamp the sites of origin of the pectoralis major along its mesial border as it arises from the lateral half of the anterior portion of the sternum and the anterior surfaces of the first 7 or 8 costal cartilages. Its nerve supply, the lateral and the mesial thoracic nerves, are divided. The breast and the pectoralis major and minor are now elevated and rotated laterally until the origin of the pectoralis minor is encountered arising from the 2nd to the 5th ribs anteriorly. The few slips of muscle encountered beneath are clamped separately and ligated against the bared thoracic cage before being divided.

Finally, the inferior portion of the pectoralis major and its fascia (continuous with the rectus sheath below) are clamped and divided adjacent to the chest wall. All tissue lateral to the pectoralis major and extending to the anterolateral margin of the latissimus dorsalis is removed *en bloc,* avoiding, if possible, injury to the long thoracic and the thoracodorsal nerves.

This effects complete removal of the breast with the axillary and lateral contents attached intact. Then final inspection of the axilla follows to make certain that the dissection has been carried above and behind the neurovascular bundle of the axilla, that the retroclavicular area has been cleaned of its normal contents and the brachial plexus with the axillary artery and veins have been cleaned carefully of small bits of fat and adventitia which may contain nodes. A soft rubber drain of the Penrose type is introduced through a laterally placed stab wound in the axilla, carried posteriorly to the neurovascular bundle and allowed to lie in the denuded subscapular space. Suction may be attached later.

Next, the wound is closed, suturing the subcutaneous tissue to the chest wall whenever possible to obliterate dead space insofar as possible. If a skin graft is required to effect closure without tension, it is cut and applied at this time. The studies of Conway et al.[10] suggest that the routine grafting does not reduce the incidence of cutaneous metastasis appearing later as frequently as originally believed by Halsted.

The operative mortality should be no greater than that from the administration of anesthesia. Early morbidity may occur largely as the result of one of two problems. If the axillary dissection has been carried too far down into the arm, lymphedema may result because of interference with the return of its lymphatic supply which enters the lateral-most group of the axillary nodes. Only rarely does arm edema result from venous obstruction. The second complication, more easily avoidable, is skin necrosis; this complication is nearly always caused by attempting to close the skin under too much tension rather than to use a skin graft under these circumstances. Skin grafting to avoid tension is time and effort well spent. Making the skin flaps too thin is also a cause of postoperative necrosis. It is better to apply split-thickness grafts initially than to utilize skin flaps too thin.

Simple Mastectomy. A simple mastectomy is not an operation designed for the surgical cure of cancer of the breast. Its use should be limited to those patients requiring mastectomy for other reasons. It may be employed palliatively in the removal of an ulcerated carcinoma, when distant metastases are already recognized, simply to avoid stench. In some patients with intraductal adenosis where carcinoma has been found in the opposite breast, simple mastectomy of the uninvolved side employed *prophylactically* may avoid development of an independent carcinoma in the remaining breast. In a few patients with extensive abscesses of the breast, granulomatous disease of the breast, especially tuberculosis and certain of the mycotic infections, simple mastectomy may be the most effective form of therapy; in other words, it is used *curatively* for some benign lesions. The same holds true for the rarely encountered patient with crippling mastodynia, but only as a last resort.

Many surgeons performing a simple mastectomy do not appreciate the extent to which the superior and lateral portions of breast tissue may reach. Consequently, occasionally the tail of Spence (the upper outermost breast tissue) may be cut across and left behind. Stated otherwise, a *complete* simple mastectomy is difficult to perform and is seldom accomplished except by those keenly aware of these anatomic extensions of the breast tissue.

Postoperative Radiation. Many methods for the application of postoperative radiation have been used in the past, and a review of this material reveals discouraging results in many instances.[32] In general, however, the reports of poor response center about series of patients who received comparatively small doses of radiation therapy, 2,000 r or less tumor dose. When more intense radiation has been employed, tumor dosage of 5,500 to 6,000 r, more encouraging results have been obtained. The latter dosage ranges are more safely administered over a time interval of 8 to 12 weeks (McWhirter's report, see below). This somewhat longer time-spread generally avoids desquamation and the "wet epidermis," as well as other serious sequelae.

At the University of Chicago currently patients with breast carcinoma receive postoperative radiation of 5,500 to 6,000 r as estimated or measured in potentially tumor-bearing tissues.[32] Treatment is now given to 2 tangential breast portals, 2 opposing portals to the axilla and the supraclavicular areas. For breast lesions in the mesial half of the breast, a direct portal to internal mammary areas is also used. This author believes that it may be worthwhile to include the internal mammary chain in the majority if not all cases receiving x-ray. The tangential radiation to the chest wall largely spares the underlying lung. Postoperative radiation should begin as soon as the wound is healed.

Most surgeons employing postoperative radiation limit its use to those patients whose axillary nodes were shown to be positive for tumor metastasis. In the University of Chicago series, about half of those whose axillae were apparently free from metastatic disease also received this course of therapy. Concerning the latter group, the decision to radiate postoperatively has been based largely on the histologic nature of the tumor and its degree of invasiveness. In others this decision has represented personal choice on the part of the surgeon who recognizes that the failure to demonstrate tumor in the axilla does not necessarily imply that none was present or left behind.

X-ray therapy delivered to painful and localized metastases, particularly those in bone, may give a surprising amount of relief for a few months and in rare instances for even a few years. This should be considered as a palliative measure before attempting more radical forms of palliative treatment.[7]

Preoperative radiation has been advocated many times. Interest in this type of radiation ebbs and flows. For the most part, the dosage acceptable to the surgeon has been too slight to be considered beneficial. Larger dosages hamper subsequent surgical resection; therefore, this technic is not used extensively. Prevailing opinion is one of discouragement toward preoperative radiation; this is the dominant conclusion of most surgeons and radiotherapists at this time.

Lymphedema of the upper extremity is one of the unpleasant after-effects of radical mastectomy. It may result from resection of the axilla being carried too far laterally, from postoperative wound infection with obliteration of the lymphatic and/or vascular return, or from tumor invading the lateral lymph channels and nodes, from phlebitis or excision of too long a segment of the axillary vein. In some patients, careful dissection of the axilla and avoidance of wound infection eliminates or greatly reduces the extent of such swelling. The progressive increase of edema suggests local axillary recurrence occluding the residual lymph channels and/or the axillary vein. When edema is severe, the arm becomes less and less useful to the patient and may be so painful that narcotics are required or surgical transection of the posterior roots of the brachial plexus is needed. Neither of these forms of treatment is pleasant to contemplate. Infection, acute sunburn or trauma are to be avoided if possible as they may result in further edema.

Postoperative radiation may produce transient edema when it did not exist previously but does not constitute a contraindication to extensive radiation unless pronounced edema exists prior to treatment.

Sleeping with the arm elevated and carrying it in a sling during waking hours may afford some relief, but generally the amount of improvement is not an impressive one.

Postoperative limited exercises should be encouraged, beginning as early as the first postoperative day, to avoid restriction of motion of the arm and the shoulder on the affected side. At the beginning this may require considerable encouragement, especially among timid patients. It is therefore important that any pressure dressing applied at the conclusion of operation be placed about the shoulder girdle and the chest wall so as not to restrict early shoulder and arm motion.

A variety of exercises have been suggested, such as extending the arm above the head with the elbow flexed across the top of the head, touching the ear on the opposite side. Using the hand of the affected arm to comb the hair is another simple and early exercise to perform. Once the stitches are out and the wound healed, from 10 to 14 days after operation, the patient should be encouraged to abduct her arm and swing the arm in a circular fashion. With the arm abducted and the patient standing within reach of the wall, she should be encouraged to move her fingers stepwise up the wall as high as possible. If a certain amount of subcutaneous fat can be safely left under the skin flaps, motions of this kind are usually accomplished more easily.

Palliative Forms of Treatment for Metastatic Cancer. The procedures under discussion here relate primarily to hormonal control, including the administration of sex or corticoid hormones, oophorectomy, adrenalectomy and hypophysectomy. The effectiveness of these forms of therapy is based on the concept that many breast carcinomas are in part hormonal-dependent. Precise knowledge is lacking.

The extent of palliation accomplished varies considerably; in some the results are occasionally so striking as to permit a bedridden patient to return to work for several years entirely free of symptoms. Eventually, the disease always escapes hormonal control and the patient dies, usually very rapidly. Thus there is to be considered not only the possible duration of benefit from this form of therapy but, more important, the fact that frequently considerable or complete relief is obtained for months to several years. Fortunately, when benefit no longer is maintained, death usually follows rapidly—often within a few days or weeks, avoiding prolonged and painful final stages of the disease. The percentage of useful and happy life is increased considerably, albeit the increase of mean duration of survival, is not as long as desired.

OOPHORECTOMY. As early as 1896, Beatson[4] demonstrated the beneficial response from oophorectomy in a 33-year-old patient with recurrence of cancer in the surgical scar. She responded well, though temporarily, to oophorectomy. As this antedated the recognition of hormones, Beatson's report was subject to severe criticism, and the idea did not take hold. Nonetheless, periodically others tried the procedure and found benefit in about 20 per cent of patients with such metastases.

Ablation of ovarian function by x-radiation in patients with carcinoma of the breast was suggested by Courmelles in 1905[11] but was little pursued until 1930 and thereafter. The results of these experiences have been summarized recently by Huggins[27] in Table 4. Castration appears to be beneficial even when the urinary secretion of estrogen is low, although the best response seems to occur among premenopausal women and those with excessive estrogen excretion. Bony metastases respond better and more frequently than those in soft tissue.

ESTROGEN THERAPY. Although these substances are carcinogenic in certain species and strains, they are capable of inducing tumor regression in the human female with breast cancer and metastases. Haddow et al.[22] were the first to report beneficial results with this form of therapy. In some patients, the results have been striking for a while, generally doubling the mean survival time for similar cases receiving no estrogen. This effect is not limited to any particular product; a patient who fails to respond to one estrogenic substance is very unlikely to respond to another. In general, the results are better for the postmenopausal group than for those of younger age.

TESTOSTERONE THERAPY. Although several workers noted some degree of tumor regression as early as 1939 with the administration of testosterone, it was the report of Adair and Herrmann in 1946[2] which awakened a keen investigative and clinical interest in this subject. Methyltestosterone administered orally in large doses seems to be nearly as effective as intramuscular testosterone propionate, although long-acting depotestosterone affords more certainty of response. In this author's experience, this form of therapy has produced a higher percentage of good results, lasting generally longer than oophorectomy, x-ray castration or estrogen administration. One patient who developed pathologic fractures of several bones, including the hip, experienced complete remission the last $4\frac{1}{2}$ years without other forms of therapy. This is the exception and not the rule. Generally, improvement lasts only a few months. Peters,[41] in her experience, comes to the opposite conclusion, namely, that

TABLE 4. ENDOCRINE MODIFICATION IN ADVANCED MAMMARY CANCER:
PERCENTAGE OF IMPROVEMENT

AUTHORS	TOTAL CASES	OBJECTIVE IMPROVEMENT		REMARKS
		NUMBER	PER CENT	
Ovariectomy				
Thomson, 1902 (*3*)	80	18	22	16 Premenopausal and 2 postmenopausal
Lett, 1905 (*4*)	75	22	29	Premenopausal
	24	1	0	Postmenopausal
Adair *et al.,* 1945 (*5*)	31	4	12	Premenopausal
Sicard, 1947 (*6*)	5	5	0	Premenopausal
	1	1	0	Postmenopausal
Dargent, 1949 (*7*)	10	2	20	
Ovarian Irradiation				
Ahlbom, 1930 (*8*)	16	0	0	
Dresser, 1936 (*9*)	30	9	30	Premenopausal
Taylor, 1939 (*10*)	50	20	40	
Adair *et al.,* 1945 (*5*)	304	47	15	Premenopausal
Douglas, 1952 (*11*)	175	36	20	2 Postmenopausal improved
Testosterone				
Adair and Herrmann, 1946 (*12*)	11	4	36	Premenopausal
Cutler and Schlemenson, 1948 (*13*)	19	8	42	
Adair *et al.,* 1949 (*14*)	48	9	19	Bone metastasis
	54	8	15	Extraskeletal metastasis
A.M.A. Council on Pharmacy and Chemistry, 1949 (*15*)	82	15	18	Bone metastasis
	77	15	20	Extraskeletal metastasis
Segaloff, 1952 (*16*)	48	13	27	
Douglas, 1952 (*11*)	30	8	36	
Estrogen				
Haddow *et al.,* 1944 (*17*)	40	16	40	
Ellis *et al.,* 1944 (*18*)	100	14	14	Age less than 60 yrs.
	68	27	39	Age over 60 yrs.
Adair *et al.,* 1949 (*14*)	35	8	23	
A.M.A. Council on Pharmacy and Chemistry, 1949 (*15*)	144	36	25	Postmenopausal
Douglas, 1952 (*11*)	322	98	30	Majority postmenopausal

(From Dr. C. B. Huggins and the National Cancer Institute)

estrogens are more often effective than androgens. As the recent literature is replete with experiences favoring one or the other group of sex hormones, even among the same age group, one is left with the conclusion that both are helpful to many patients. If estrogens fail to give relief, try androgens and vice versa. There appears to be no rational basis other than clinical trial in the individual patient and possibly age as to which to employ.

The unpleasant side effects of testosterone are those of masculinization, salt retention, with edema, and an increased libido. This hormone increases the 17-ketosteroids in the urine and diminishes urinary gonadotropins.

The therapeutic dosages recommended for the various estrogenic and androgenic substances in the palliative treatment of metastatic carcinoma of the breast as listed in 1954 by the Council on Pharmacy and Chemistry of the American Medical Association* are as follows:

A. Estrogens
  1. Oral
     a. Ethynyl estradiol, 3 mg. daily
     b. Conjugated estrogenic substances, 30 mg. daily
     c. Dienestrol, 15 mg. daily
     d. Dimethyl ether of diethylstilbestrol, 30 mg. daily
  2. Parenteral (For the patient who cannot tol-

* J.A.M.A. *156*:1581, 1954.

erate oral medication, injectable estrogens may be substituted)
  a. Estradiol benzoate, 5 mg. 3 times a week
  b. Estradiol dipropionate, 5 mg. twice a week
B. Androgens
  1. Oral
     Methyltestosterone, 100 mg. daily, preferably 25 mg., 4 times a day
  2. Parenteral, short duration
     Stanolone,* 100 mg. 3 times a week
  3. Parenteral, long duration
     a. Testosterone cyclopentylpropionate, 200 mg. every 2 weeks
     b. Testosterone phenylacetate, 200 mg. every 2 weeks

The following dosage schedules for these two groups of hormones is employed at the University of Chicago:

INTRAMUSCULAR
A. Estrogen
   Estradiol benzoate, 5 mg. 3 times a week
B. Androgen
   Testosterone propionate (Depo preparation), 200 mg. every 2 weeks

ORAL
A. Estrogen
   Diethylstilbestrol, 10 to 15 mg. daily
B. Androgen
   Methyltestosterone, 100 mg. daily

BILATERAL ADRENALECTOMY was first accomplished successfully by Huggins and Scott[29] in 1945 as a means of palliative relief for advanced carcinoma of the prostate. These observers found the urinary excretion of 17-ketosteroids to be essentially abolished following the combination of orchiectomy and adrenalectomy (see Chap. 27, "The Physiologic Role of the Pituitary and the Adrenal Glands in Health and Disease," Part 2). Huggins[28] reported that adrenalectomy alone was beneficial in many patients with metastatic breast cancer when maintained on corticoids.

After bilateral adrenalectomy, the patient's general condition improves rapidly if she is to improve at all. She becomes animated, possibly from cortisone or possibly from relief of pain, her appetite improves, and she looks happily to the future. Osseous lesions heal,

* The Committee has had much experience with this level of dosage. There is some evidence to suggest that a lower dosage schedule may be effective; however, experience with such lower dosage is inadequate.

and so do some pathologic fractures. Fluid may disappear from the chest, the local tumor and even some of the cutaneous metastases may diminish or may disappear entirely. She literally may arise from her death bed, walk and resume a full and active normal life, sometimes for several months to several years.

Of course, adrenalectomy is no cure, but the excellence of palliation, if for only 6 months, seems to warrant the use of this procedure in many patients. In general, the subjective improvement tends to outstrip the objective changes; this is better, however, than the reverse. Profound improvement has persisted in 8 such patients for 2½ to 5 years at the University of Chicago; 3, still alive and well after 5 years, were in each instance bedridden at the time adrenalectomy was performed. It is regretted that more patients do not respond and that the mean palliative and survival time is not increased by years rather than months.

Methods for the selection of patients in whom there is a chance of improvement after

TABLE 5. CHANCES OF BENEFIT FROM ADRENALECTOMY

AGE OF PATIENT	FAIRLY GOOD 40 TO 65 YRS.	LIKELY TO BE POOR UNDER 40 AND OVER 65
Duration of breast carcinoma	3–5 yrs.	Less than 2 yrs. and longer than 6
Type of Carcinoma		
1. "Carcinoma en cuirasse"	+++	
2. "Adenocarcinoma"	++	
3. "Ductal carcinoma"	+	
4. Highly anaplastic	0	
Location of metastases		
1. Bone	+++	
2. Skin	++	
3. Lung	++	
4. Liver	0	
Increased estrogen excretion	++	
Calcium balance	Not yet sufficient data to evaluate	

Key: 0 Essentially no change
  + Slight chance for improvement
  ++ Moderate chance for improvement
  +++ Good chance for improvement

adrenalectomy have been studied seriously. Probably there is no absolute single criterion, but there are certain "straws in the wind" which are helpful.

Emerson and Jessiman[15] recently reported two tests which they believe to be of value in selecting patients for adrenalectomy. Sex hormones are administered, and if this results in an increased calcium excretion under metabolic conditions, a favorable response to adrenalectomy is predicted. The other is called the "cortisone-inhibition test"; should calcium excretion be diminished by cortisone therapy and the patient improve, adrenalectomy is advised. More data and experience are necessary to assess their results.

HYPOPHYSECTOMY was first performed by Perrault[40] for the treatment of metastatic breast cancer in 1951, and by Luft, Olivecrona and Sjögren (1952)[33] at about the same time. The reasoning behind this procedure was that the ablation of the pituitary removed the trophic hormones and hence theoretically could diminish more effectively hormonal activity and production in the target organs.

Rasmussen and Harper[42] have accomplished the same end by the implantation of yttrium[90] beads in the pituitary gland (Fig. 27-4). Illingworth and colleagues[30] implanted radon seeds into the pituitary for the same purpose. The early results of both groups appear to be encouraging.

Most impressive results from hypophysectomy have been reported by Pearson and Ray.[39] These authors reported on 109 patients with advanced carcinoma followed for at least 17 months. About 50 per cent of the patients obtained objective remissions, and 35 per cent had remissions of 6 months or longer. The average remission was over 15 months, and the average survival was over 21 months. The question still remains whether hypophysectomy is superior to adrenalectomy or combined adrenalectomy and oophorectomy. At the present time, hypophysectomy seems to be a worthwhile procedure in the palliative treatment of patients with metastatic breast cancer when adequate facilities are available to carry out this technic.

SUMMARY OF PALLIATIVE ENDOCRINE INTERFERENCE WITH ADVANCED BREAST CANCER. The benefits of the appropriate utilization of endocrine therapy in relieving the patient's symptoms are well stated in an editorial in the New England Journal of Medicine:[14] "The doctor who regards the complex endocrinology of carcinoma of the breast as 'just a confusing fog' had best do some reading and studying so that he can find a few landmarks in the fog." Perhaps this overstates the facts but not the principles.

The surgeon today has a much better chance than 5 years ago to relieve his patients with advanced carcinoma of the breast and to prolong their lives. Hormonal therapy, endocrine ablation and better technics of radiotherapy all are useful tools. The fullest possibility of each alone or in combination is not yet known, but surely substantial progress has been made.

Results of Treatment. Many scientific debates could be avoided were the opposing forces both in possession of all of the facts. Important differences in experimental plan and methodology may escape detection for many years, creating problems rather than solving them.

Seldom can clinical data be controlled as substantially as those in the laboratory. Upon many occasions, results attributed to a specific form of treatment have been proved to be inconsequential or due to the factors not yet considered. In many respects, this seems to characterize today's confused status regarding the end results of treatment for carcinoma of the breast.

IN UNTREATED CANCER. It is fundamental that the course of the untreated patient should be established before it can be assumed that any benefit has been derived from the treatment applied. Greenwood[19] collected data from several British hospitals relative to the eventual outcome of 651 patients who were known to have carcinoma of the breast which for one reason or another were untreated. This study covered the years 1882 to 1924. This was when life expectancy ranged from 44 years of age to 60, compared with today's 69 years. 50 per cent of Greenwood's patients were dead within 6 months after onset of symptoms. Another 25 per cent had died by the 46th month. The remaining 25 per cent died over the next 10-year period. The mean survival time was 38 months. Shimkin[45] arranged the mean survival time of Greenwood's patients according to the age of the patient when each

TABLE 6. SURVIVAL IN UNTREATED BREAST
CARCINOMA RELATIVE TO AGE

AGE RANGE	NO. OF PATIENTS	MEAN SURVIVAL TIME IN MONTHS
25–34	40	35
35–44	105	42
45–54	159	37
55–64	152	38
65–74	130	41
75 and older	37	36

developed carcinoma. These are tabulated in Table 6.

Daland[46] reported the mean survival time for 100 untreated patients with cancer of the breast, seen in 2 Boston Hospitals. The mean survival time for his group was also 38 months, with a similar spread in time of the percentage of patients surviving at many particular months. Later, Nathanson and Welch[37] reported almost identical data once again. Tabulated in Table 7 are the percentages of untreated patients surviving each year after the onset of symptoms.

The average percentage of patients surviving in each of the 3 groups of untreated patients is 19 per cent, being 18, 19 and 20 per cent in each instance and remarkably similar. Stated otherwise, 80 per cent of patients with untreated breast cancer will be dead in 5 years after apparent onset of the disease. With the natural course of the disease so well agreed upon, let us look at the results of treatment; remember one point: duration of survival is calculated from the time of apparent onset of disease until death.

RESULTS FROM RADICAL MASTECTOMY. There is perhaps no field in surgery today wherein the results from a particular operation are more difficult to assess than those reported for radical mastectomy in the treatment of cancer of the breast. Perhaps the outstanding variable is the character of the patient population that the particular institution serves. In general, indigent patients seek medical help late in the course of the disease, whereas private patients are more likely to seek help earlier. It is not practical to compare results from one institution with those of another unless it can be established that the patient populations are essentially identical.

If the student wishes to make a survey of results reported on carcinoma of the breast to date, he will be distressed to see the lack of uniformity in reporting. The data presented in Table 8 have been selected carefully from many reports, the basis of selection being determined by the presence of common data presented which would permit some degree of comparison. A number of reports wherein better results were claimed have been omitted as not suitably complete to be included in Tables 8 and 15.

It should be pointed out that, in computing survival time after treatment, one is using a different yardstick than that employed for the untreated series. In the latter, the duration of survival is measured from onset of the first symptoms; in the treatment series, survival time is computed from the time treatment was initiated (Tables 6, 7 and 15). To be correct, both should be computed from the date of apparent onset of the disease.

The points that stand out from the above table are very few. First, results are obviously better when no axillary nodal involvement is found. Second, the total 5-year survival is double that which follows no form of therapy. It is actually better than doubled for the duration of history ranged as averages from 7 to 12 months before treatment was begun. It is also apparent that the surgical results of today are better than those of Halsted, probably because of earlier operation. Many argue that the 20 per cent who survive for 5 years without any treatment are among the 40 to 50 per cent over-all postoperative 5-year survivals. They probably are. But it is clear that the high percentage of 5-year survivals among those without metastases should serve to en-

TABLE 7. PER CENT OF UNTREATED PATIENTS WITH CARCINOMA OF THE BREAST
ALIVE EACH YEAR AFTER ONSET OF SYMPTOMS

1 yr.	2 yrs.	3 yrs.	4 yrs.	5 yrs.	6 yrs.	7 yrs.	8 yrs.	10 yrs.	15 yrs.
75%	58%	40%	25%	18%	15%	10%	7%	4%	0%

(Nathanson and Welch, 1936[33])

TABLE 8. FIVE-YEAR SURVIVAL RESULTS FROM SELECTED HOSPITALS
(TREATED CARCINOMA OF THE BREAST)

	LOCALIZED TO BREAST		REGIONAL METASTASIS		DISTANT METASTASIS		OVER-ALL 5-YEAR SURVIVAL (Per Cent)
Untreated cases:							
1. Greenwood							
2. Forber } averages							19
3. Nathanson & Welch							
	Cases	% Survival	Cases	% Survival	Cases	% Survival	
Halsted, 1907	60	75%	160	18%	77	0%	26
Johns Hopkins Hospital, 1935–1940	78	64%	126	32%	?		41
University of Michigan	197	83%	217	41%	?		40
University of Chicago, 1946–1951	72	78%	91	45%	23	17%	54.3
Code Identified U. S. Hospitals, 1945–1951 (data averaged)	498	68%	521	30%	346	16%	41
McWhirter, 1942–1947	1,063	58%	546	30%	273	4%	42

courage every effort to effect an earlier diagnosis. It is also very apparent that the majority of patients are not seen or their disease recognized until metastasis has occurred.

Most radiologists and surgeons are disinclined to believe x-radiation as used in the past has materially affected the 5-year survival rate over that of radical mastectomy alone. Bryant, Lampe and Coller[6] concluded from their data that the routine use of x-ray therapy is not indicated when a complete radical mastectomy is performed. Unfortunately, the reports are too few to be certain of the role of radiation in breast cancer. Of those that are available, there is good evidence to believe that the dosage employed was ineffective and that considerably higher dosage rates could be given without harm under proper circumstances. Moreover, the conclusions of McWhirter[35] based on results from simple mastectomy plus x-radiation are striking but how much of that which he has accomplished is from radiation and how much if any is from the simple mastectomy remains to be established. By the time any sizable series of pa-

tients treated by x-radiaiton can be collected, improvements in the physics and the technics of radiotherapy have often been made. So, the problem continues to go unanswered. It would appear wiser to upgrade radiation therapy rather than to downgrade surgery (Table 16).

The comparison of radical mastectomy with and without postoperative radiation therapy results at the University of Chicago and the University of Michigan are presented in Table 9. The Chicago data show an arithmetical advantage to combined therapy, although the series is too small to weigh heavily in favor of radiation at the 5,500 to 6,000 r used.

Before departing from the subject of radical mastectomy and selected use of x-ray therapy, Harrington's series at the Mayo Clinic should be mentioned.[26] As there is little likelihood that their patient population experience corresponds with that of the institutions tabulated in Table 10, Harrington's data should be viewed separately. These data showing the increase in salvage rate with each 10 years until the current decade, are equaled by few reports.

TABLE 9. FIVE-YEAR SURVIVAL AFTER RADICAL MASTECTOMY WITH AND WITHOUT X-RAY THERAPY (DOSAGES 4,000 TO 6,000 R) REGIONAL METASTATIC GROUP ONLY

	MASTECTOMY ONLY		MASTECTOMY PLUS RADIATION	
	NO. TREATED	5-YR. SURVIVAL	NO. TREATED	5-YR. SURVIVAL
University of Chicago, 1946–1951	34	44%	42	62%
University of Michigan, 1954	54	39%	189	38%

TABLE 10. INCREASED PERCENTAGE OF 5-YEAR
SURVIVALS OVER 4 DECADES[24a]

	WITHOUT NODAL METASTASES (Per Cent)	WITH NODAL METASTASES (Per Cent)	TOTAL SURVIVING (Per Cent)
1910	62.7	23.4	39.7
1920	71.4	26.2	41.2
1930	77.2	32.5	47.9
1940	81.8	40.5	60.0

Other relationships are seen in Tables 11, 12, 13 and 14.

THE MALE BREAST

GYNECOMASTIA—"PHYSIOLOGIC" HYPERTROPHY

In the course of sexual maturity, enlargement of one or both breasts often occurs in the male, generally between the ages of 12 to 15 years. Enlargement is encountered so frequently that it might well be considered a variant lying within the normal range. These little subareolar buttons of tissue disappear before the age of 20, and their entire duration of existence is usually only a matter of a few months to a year or two.

The term gynecomastia generally has been applied to those patients in whom the breast enlargement at puberty does not subside. More often this type is unilateral and to be differentiated from fibroadenoma, lipoma and dermoid cysts.

Although the breast may be slightly painful

TABLE 12. DOMINANT COMPOSITION OF RACIAL AND ETHNIC GROUPS COMPRISING THE AUTOPSY POPULATION OF THE LOS ANGELES COUNTY HOSPITAL 1918-1947[42]

Caucasoids	26,515	75.1%
"Mexicans"	6,150	17.4%
Negroids	2,236	6.3%
Mongoloids	392	1.1%
Total	35,293	99.9%

As the total Mongoloid population is by comparison small, this group is not discussed further here.

and moderately tender, the two reasons for seeking medical advice are that the lesion creates embarrassment and that the parents of the boy are often concerned about the hypertrophied breast representing a malignancy or at least a premalignant lesion.

The etiology is related to the hormonal changes occurring with puberty. These are aptly described by some pediatricians as "the hormonal confusion of adolescence." In some

TABLE 13. RANK IN FREQUENCY OF OCCURRENCE OF CARCINOMA OF THE BREAST AMONG 6,072 PATIENTS AUTOPSIED AT LOS ANGELES COUNTY HOSPITAL, 1918-1947 INCLUSIVE[42]

DOMINANT RACE OR ETHNIC GROUPS	BOTH SEXES		FEMALES	
	Rank	Per Cent of All Tumors	Rank	Per Cent of All Tumors
Caucasoids	8th	5.4	2nd	13.8
"Mexicans"	9th	3.2	6th	6.6
Negroids	5th	6.5	2nd	12.1

TABLE 11. TABLE OF 5-YEAR CLINICAL CURE RATES IN CANCER OF THE FEMALE BREAST
ACCORDING TO SIZE OF THE PRIMARY TUMOR (PATHOLOGIST'S DIMENSIONS, MEMORIAL HOSPITAL)[1]

Based on 1,335 Primary Operable Cases Treated by Radical Mastectomy with
Determinate End Results (1935-42 Admissions)

LARGEST DIMENSION OF PRIMARY TUMOR	CASES AND PERCENTAGE	BREAST ONLY INVOLVED	BREAST AND AXILLA
Less than 2 cm. No. of cases	201	121	80
5-year clinical cure rate, per cent	74.1%	87.6%	53.8%
2.0 to 2.9 cm. No. of cases	396	185	211
5-year clinical cure rate, per cent	60.2%	74.6%	47.9%
3.0 to 3.9 cm. No. of cases	318	119	199
5-year clinical cure rate, per cent	47.8%	68.9%	35.2%
4.0 to 4.9 cm. No. of cases	183	65	118
5-year clinical cure rate, per cent	41.5%	60.0%	31.4%
5.0 cm. and over. No. of cases	257	57	200
5-year clinical cure rate, per cent	33.5%	75.4%*	21.5%

* "This figure may appear peculiar. It is somewhat elevated, because in the 5.0 cm. and over group there are included some of the bulky medullary carcinomas with lymphoid stroma which carry a better than average prognosis."

TABLE 14. DISTRIBUTION OF 315 CARCINOMAS OF THE MAMMARY GLAND BY RACE AND AGE (LOS ANGELES COUNTY HOSPITAL, 1918-1947)[42]

RACE	21-30	31-40	41-50	51-60	61-70	71-80	81-90	Totals	PER CENT OF ALL NECROPSIES IN FEMALES	PER CENT OF ALL TUMORS IN FEMALES
Caucasoids	3	17	59	67	69	47	13	275	2.9	13.8
"Mexicans"	2	2	5	5	3	2	0	19	0.7	6.5
Negroids	0	1	3	8	7	0	0	19	1.8	12.1
Japanese	0	0	0	2	0	0	0	2	3.3	20.0
Total	5	20	67	82	79	49	13	315	2.3	12.8

patients, especially with bilateral gynecomastia first appearing after ages 18 to 20, more important aberrations in endocrinology should be considered, particularly the estrogen-producing tumors. Of these, teratoma of the testis is perhaps the most commonly encountered; certain of the hormonally active adrenal tumors, benign or malignant, also should be considered. Enlargement of the male breast is also noted in many patients in the advanced stages of liver disease and is explained on the basis of impaired or faulty metabolism of the sex hormones due to the derangement of liver function. Testicular atrophy, from orchitis or trauma, may be followed by the appearance of bilateral hyperplasia of the breasts in the male. These days, bilateral hyperplasia is commonly seen in the adult male, as many men with carcinoma of the prostate are receiving stilbestrol as part of their treatment. Often the breast in this group of patients is painful and tender.

Treatment depends upon the cause of gynecomastia. In patients receiving stilbestrol for prostatic cancer, toleration of the associated gynecomastia is the lesser of the two evils. When due to an estrogen-producing tumor, breast enlargement subsides when the tumor is removed. In the adolescent, reassurance with observation is the only rational course in most instances. Occasionally, persistence of pubertal gynecomastia may require excision, largely because of the psychological and social

disturbances it may create. However, the surgical cosmetic result must be better than that created by gynecomastia and involves removal of the hypertrophied gland, but with preservation of the nipple. Finally, removal of the enlarged breast is essential should breast carcinoma be suspected (see below).

CARCINOMA OF THE MALE BREAST

Malignant disease of the male breast is rarely encountered. Most reported series disclose that cancer incidence of the female breast is at least 100 times greater than that of the male. The average age of males with this disease is slightly higher than that found for women.

The symptoms are variable; pain and tenderness and bloody discharge from the nipple are among the more common ones. Most frequently, the complaint is that of a painless lump. The occasional patient does not present himself until the skin over the lesion becomes ulcerated.

Examination of the breast will disclose the lump readily. It is much more commonly fixed to the nipple and the skin than is carcinoma of the female breast. Nipple retraction or distortion likewise is more frequently evident, as the amount of normal breast tissue is small and usually lies directly beneath the areolar tissue. Involvement of the axillary nodes in resected specimens occurs in a higher percentage of breast malignancies of the male,

TABLE 15. YEARLY PERCENTAGE SURVIVAL RATES OF UNTREATED BREAST CANCER*

				YEARS				
	Zero date	1	2	3	4	5	6	7
PERCENTAGE SURVIVING	100%	75%	58%	40%	28%	22%	17%	13%

* Composite data of Greenwood, Daland, Nathanson and Welch.

TABLE 16. COMPARISON OF THE UNIVERSITY OF EDINBURGH DATA WITH THAT AT THE UNIVERSITY OF CHICAGO AS TO 5-YEAR SURVIVAL RATE FOR CARCINOMA OF THE BREAST

STAGE OF DISEASE	Total	No. Alive	Per Cent Alive
A. Total operated (includes distant metastasis)			
1. Edinburgh* (1941–47)	1,882	786	42%
2. Chicago† (1946–51)	186	101	54%
B. Confined to breast			
1. Edinburgh	1,063	612	58%
2. Chicago	72	56	78%
C. Locally advanced with axillary metastases			
1. Edinburgh	546	162	30%
2. Chicago	91	41	45%
D. Distant metastases			
1. Edinburgh	273	12	4%
2. Chicago	23	4	17%

* Taken from McWhirter's Table V (Reference 35). All cases treated by simple mastectomy and x-ray therapy. No cases lost to follow-up.

† All cases treated by radical mastectomy, except for a few wherein simple mastectomy was performed to remove an ulcerated carcinoma. Both groups included together. Of the 179 patients treated between January, 1946, and December 31, 1950, 168 were followed (94%). The 13 not followed are tabulated as dead of their disease, although in 4 of these, no axillary nodes were found. All who died of intercurrent disease are also listed as having died of cancer.

but these nodes may go undetected on physical examination, particularly if the pectoralis musculature is well developed.

The pathologic findings encountered in malignant tumors of the male breast are similar to those of the female breast. The rare occurrence of this tumor prevents a reliable evaluation as to the frequency of the various types.

Treatment is radical mastectomy unless distant metastases already can be demonstrated. A skin graft is nearly always necessary to close the defect. In the event that distant metastases are established, simple mastectomy should be performed to avoid likely ulceration later on.

Hormonal therapy and adrenalectomy should be considered, but experience is too limited to evaluate either at present. In one patient, aged 73, osteolytic metastases became osteoclastic with relief of pain for 15 months under stilbestrol therapy. In another 34-year-old male at the University of Chicago Clinics, pulmonary and bony metastases receded surprisingly well for more than 24 months after bilateral orchiectomy was performed.

The prognosis in general is poor, being less favorable than for carcinoma of the female breast.

OPERABILITY AND CURABILITY FOR CARCINOMA OF THE BREAST

The term "operability" does not connote curability, but operability does imply more than a surgical exercise. (1) The operation must do no harm, *primum non nocere*. (2) The operation should provide a good chance that the patient will receive substantial palliative relief despite the recognized possibility that it may not prolong life. For example, the removal of an ulcerated carcinoma of the breast may abolish only the stench of necrotic tumor and its soiling of clothing; but the relief from these troubles will allow the patient to regain her social acceptability and lessens her burden to some extent. (3) Operability may accomplish an extension of her expected survival period, although any increase in survival time is of little merit unless it is accompanied by relief from or the avoidance of distressing symptoms.

Some of the criteria for operability are obvious and undebatable; hepatic metastases or spread of the tumor to the brain are not likely to respond to any form of therapy. Pulmonary and osseous metastases may respond very well for a while to one or more of the endocrine attacks upon the disease (see p. 558). Certain of the local findings often considered indicative of inoperability in the past may also need to be revised in view of the substantial relief afforded some patients by adrenalectomy and allied procedures. True, these patients may not survive a great deal longer, but if such ancillary procedures are effective, their residual life is a much happier one. Take the case of a young mother with carcinoma; an operative procedure may enable her to run her home effectively and to teach her children much longer without necessarily increasing her survival period. How can one evaluate these benefits if the only yardstick for measuring results is that of the "5-year" survival?

A number of years ago, Haagensen and Stout[21] set up certain criteria for operability of carcinoma of the breast, based upon the 5-year survival rates obtained from 1,040 patients operated upon at the Presbyterian Hospital in New York during the years 1915 and 1934. Their purpose in reviewing the experience at that hospital was to establish criteria wherein it could be concluded that patients with these findings could be classified as *categorically inoperable*. They believed that any one of the following criteria was cause to consider a patient with carcinoma as "categorically inoperable":

1. When the carcinoma is one which developed during pregnancy or lactation
2. When extensive edema of the skin over the breast is present
3. When satellite nodules are present in the skin over the breast
4. When intercostal or parasternal tumor nodules are present
5. When there is edema of the arm
6. When proved supraclavicular metastases are present
7. When the carcinoma is the inflammatory type
8. When distant metastases are demonstrated
9. When any two, or more, of the following signs of locally advanced carcinoma are present:
   a. Ulceration of the skin
   b. Edema of the skin of limited extent (less than one third of the skin over the breast involved)
   c. Fixation of the tumor to the chest wall
   d. Axillary lymph nodes measuring 2.5 cm. or more, in transverse diameter, and proved to contain metastases by biopsy
   e. Fixation of axillary lymph nodes to the skin or the deep structures of the axilla, and proved to contain metastases by biopsy

Unfortunately, these criteria make no distinction between operability and curability. These two terms may have entirely different meanings and in some patients operability may have little bearing upon curability; yet an operation may be very worthwhile from the patient's point of view. Certainly one could not assemble a group of criteria in which the 5-year survival could be lower. On the other hand, certain important exceptions exist and have been reported. Perhaps this classification should be modified to serve as a guide to operability rather than as a firm rule connoting "categorical inoperability."

Finally, Haagensen and Stout conclude from the study of their patients that the duration of the postoperative period among those listed in the category of inoperability was actually shortened because of the operative procedure performed. This conclusion may be an erroneous one, for it was based on the fact that their patients did not survive as long after treatment as those of Daland's untreated group.[12] In reality, the survival periods for both groups seems to be the same if the survival time is computed on the same basis, i.e., the date of apparent onset of disease which, for the era covered by their survey, was generally 10 to 12 months earlier than the time at which treatment was begun.[37]

A patient may be alive and well 3 years after operation; recurrences may manifest themselves at that time and the patient be dead 6 months thereafter. She was operable but not curable. On the other hand, the result of her operation may represent a better one than the patient who is considered categorically inoperable but survives 3½ years, with the last 3 of these years being spent in misery. Hence, in the field of carcinoma of the breast, the surgeon must evaluate each patient on an individual basis and plan his course of action accordingly. The results he obtains also must be individually evaluated, considering not only the duration of survival but also the degree of relief or lack of it that the patient may have experienced.

ATTEMPTS TO IMPROVE SURVIVAL RESULTS

Of all the known methods for increasing the survival and cure rates for carcinoma of the breast, those technics that assist in the establishment of early diagnosis are likely to be the most successful, provided that the establishment of the diagnosis is followed immediately by adequate treatment. The cooperative patient can be the greatest factor in assisting in the early diagnosis. She should be taught the art of periodic self-examination as well as the value of an examination by a competent physician at least once a year. Despite the use of both technics, some tumors will not be detected, and a few of those which are found early will be of such a nature that blood stream or lymphatic channel invasion will not enable a surgical "cure."

The so-called "super" radical operations in selected patients is currently under investigation. Many lesions situated in the mesial quadrants of the breast, particularly those in the upper mesial quadrant, tend to metastasize to the internal mammary chain. The extended radical operation has been largely concerned with the removal of this chain in addition to the axillary system. Three approaches to these parasternal nodes have been employed: splitting the sternum to expose the internal mammary chain, *en bloc* excision of the parasternal chest wall from the 2nd through the 5th ribs inclusive, followed by a grafting procedure, and the division of the costal cartilages of these same ribs to expose the chain. The last procedure carries the least risk insofar as increasing mortality and morbidity rates are concerned but in none are these prohibitive. To date, results obtained are insufficient to allow an adequate appraisal of the inclusion of this chain along with those of the axilla. Certainly more experience is required before such a radical procedure can be advised as routine for even selected series of patients. Its final evaluation must be made on the basis of comparing the end results with those of the standard radical procedure.

Some idea as to the location of the primary tumor site and the frequency of nodal metastases to various regions may be evident from the observations of Handley and Thackeray:[24]

Location of the Breast Lesion

	Inner Quadrants	Outer Quadrants
When all nodes were negative	16 cases	33 cases
When only the axillary nodes were positive	12 cases	40 cases
When only the internal mammary notes were positive	6 cases	2 cases
When both groups were positive	27 cases	14 cases

In Urban's series[51] of 300 cases in which surgical excision of the parasternal chest wall was carried out, the site of the primary tumor lay in the mesial quadrants 3 times more often

TABLE 17. NODE FINDINGS IN 300 CASES

	LATERAL PER CENT	MEDIAL PER CENT	TOTAL PER CENT
Number	61–20	239–80	300–100
All nodes clear	16–26	117–48	133–44.3
Internal mammary nodes +	2–3	21–9	23– 7.7
Axillary nodes +	21–34	40–17	61–20.3
Both int. mammary and axillary nodes +	22–36	61–26	83–27.7

If axillary nodes are positive, then internal mammary nodes are positive in:
    58% Over-all group
    61% Medial half
    51% Lateral half
If axillary nodes are negative, then internal mammary nodes are positive in:
    15% Over-all group
    15.2% Medial half
    11% Lateral half
(After Urban)

than in the outer quadrants among the 82 cases who proved to have positive nodal involvement along the internal mammary chain. In 100 cases of breast cancer in which there were metastatic internal mammary nodes, the most frequent involvement appeared in the 2nd interspace, and then in decreasing order, in the 3rd, the 1st, the 4th and the 5th interspaces. In Table 17 are the nodal findings reported for Urban's 300 cases.

The mortality for this series was less than 1 per cent. The 5-year survival of 100 patients with primary operable breast cancer treated by this method was 67 per cent, and the 5-year survival rate clinically free of disease was 61 per cent. These are excellent results, and continued evaluation of the technic is imperative.

REFERENCES

1. Adair, F. E.: Report of symposium at the sectional meeting of the American College of Surgeons, Feb. 11, 1952.
2. Adair, F. E., and Herrmann, J. B.: The use of testosterone propionate in the treatment of advanced carcinoma of the breast, Ann. Surg. *123*:1023, 1946.
3. Anderson, E., Reed, S. C., Juseby, R. A., and Oliver, C. P.: Possible relationships between menopause and age of onset of breast cancer, Cancer *3*:410, 1950.
4. Beatson, G. T.: On treatment of inoperable carcinoma of the mammae: suggestions for

a new method of treatment, with an illustrative case, Lancet *2*:104 and 162, 1896.

5. Bittner, John J.: Experimental aspects of mammary cancer in mice *in* Breast Cancer and Its Diagnosis and Treatment, Baltimore, Williams & Wilkins, 1955.

6. Bryant, M. F., Lampe, I., and Coller, F. A.: Cancer of the breast, Surgery *36*:863, 1954.

7. Cantril, S. T.: The care of the patient with advanced cancer of the breast, Radiology *66*:46, 1956.

8. Clemmesen, J.: On cancer incidence in Denmark and other countries, Acta Unio internat. contra cancrum *7*:24, 1951.

9. ———: Essentials of demographical studies in cancer, Brit. J. Cancer *4*:1, 1950.

10. Conway, H., and Neuman, C. G.: Evaluation of skin grafting in the technique of radical mastectomy in relation to local recurrence of carcinoma, Surg., Gynec. & Obst. *88*:45, 1949.

11. Courmelles, de F.: Quoted by Huggins.[25]

12. Daland, E. M.: Untreated cancer of the breast, Surg., Gynec. & Obst. *44*:264, 1927.

13. Deaver, J. B., and McFarland, J.: The Breast: Its Anomalies, Its Diseases and Their Treatment, New York, Blakiston Div. of McGraw-Hill, 1927.

14. Editorial: Carcinoma of the breast—endocrinology and statistics, New England J. Med. *254*:961, 1956.

15. Emerson, K., Jr., and Jessiman, A. G.: Hormonal influences on the growth and progression of cancer: tests for hormone dependency in mammary and prostatic cancer, New England J. Med. *254*:252, 1956.

16. Finn, W. F.: Pregnancy complicated by cancer, Bull. Margaret Hague Maternity Hosp. *5*:2, 1952.

17. Fitts, W. T., and Horn, R. C: Occult carcinoma of the breast, J.A.M.A. *147*:1429, 1951.

18. Grant, R. N., Tabah, E. J., and Adair, F. E.: The surgical significance of the subareolar lymph plexus in cancer of the breast, Surgery *33*:71, 1953.

19. Greenwood, M.: A report on the natural duration of cancer, Ministry of Health Reports on Public Health and Medical Subjects, No. 33, London, Her Majesty's Stat. Off., 1926.

20. Haagensen, C. D., and Obeid, S. J.: Biopsy of the apex of the axilla in carcinoma of the breast, Ann. Surg. *149*:149, 1959.

21. Haagensen, C. D., and Stout, A. P.: Carcinoma of the breast: II. Criteria of operability, Ann. Surg. *118*:859, 1943.

22. Haddow, A., Watkinson, J. M., and Paterson, E.: Influence of synthetic oestrogens upon advanced malignant disease, Brit. M.J. *2*:393, 1944.

23. Handley, R. S.: The anatomy of the breast *in* Breast Cancer and Its Diagnosis and Treatment, p. 8, Baltimore, Williams & Wilkins, 1955.

24. Handley, R. S., and Thackray, A. C.: Invasion of internal mammary lymph nodes in cancer of the breast, Brit. M.J. *1*:61-64, 1954.

25. Harrington, S. W.: Carcinoma of the breast—results of surgical treatment when cancer occurred in the course of pregnancy or lactation and when pregnancy occurred subsequent to operation (1910-33), Ann. Surg. *106*:690, 1937.

26. Harrington, S. W.: Results of surgical treatment of unilateral carcinoma of the breast in women, J.A.M.A. *148*:1007, 1952.

27. Huggins, C. B.: Endocrine methods of treatment of cancer of the breast, J. Nat. Cancer Inst. *15*:1, 1954.

28 Huggins, C., and Bergenstal, D. M.: Surgery of the adrenals, J.A.M.A. *147*:101, 1951.

29. Huggins, C., and Scott, W. W.: Bilateral adrenalectomy in prostatic cancer: clinical features and urinary excretion of 17-ketosteroids and estrogen, Ann. Surg. *122*:1031, 1945.

30. Illingworth, C. F. W., Forrest, A. P. M., and Brown, D. A. P.: A simple method of implanting radon seeds into the pituitary gland in treatment of advanced breast cancer, S. Forum *6*:406, 1956.

31. Lewison, E. F.: Breast Cancer and Its Diagnosis and Treatment, Baltimore, Williams & Wilkins, 1955.

32. Lochman, D. J.: Dosage in tangential radiation therapy of the postoperative breast portal, Am. J. Roentgenol. *73*:803, 1955.

33. Luft, R., Olivecrona, H., and Sjögren, B.: Hypofysektomi pa människa, Nord. med. *47*:351, 1952.

34. McGregor, J. K., and McGregor, D. D.: Paget's disease of the breast: twenty year survey of cases presenting at a large general hospital, Surgery *45*:562, 1959.

35. McWhirter, R.: Simple mastectomy and radiotherapy of breast cancer, Brit. J. Radiol., New Series *28*:128, 1955.

36. Moritz, A. R.: The Pathology of Trauma, ed. 2, Philadelphia, Lea & Febiger, 1954.

37. Nathanson, I. T., and Welch, C. E.: Life expectancy and incidence of malignant disease: I. Carcinoma of the breast, Am. J. Cancer *28*:40-53, 1936.

38. Papanicolaou, G. M.: The value of exfoliative cytology in the early diagnosis and con-

trol of neoplastic disease of the breast, CA (Bull. Cancer Progress) *4*:191, 1954.

39. Pearson, O. H., and Ray, B. S.: Results of hypophysectomy in treatment of metastatic mammary carcinoma, Cancer *12*:85, 1959.

40. Perrault, J.: Discussion, Bull. et mém. Soc. méd. hôp., Paris *68*:209, 1952.

41. Peters, M. V.: The influence of hormonal therapy on metastatic mammary cancer, Surg., Gynec. & Obst. *102*:545, 1956.

42. Rasmussen, R., Harper, P. V., and Kennedy, T.: The use of a beta ray point source for destruction of the hypophysis, S. Forum *4*:681, 1953.

43. Rhoads, Jonathan: Personal communication.

44. Roscoe B. Jackson Mem. Lab. Staff, Bar Harbor, Maine: Existence of nonchromosomal influence in the incidence of mammary tumors in mice, Science *78*:465, 1933.

45. Shimkin, M. B.: Duration of life in untreated cancer, Cancer *4*:1-8, 1951.

46. Simmons, C. C., Daland, E. M., and Wallace, R. H.: Delay in the treatment of cancer, New England J. Med. *208*:1097, 1933.

47. Steiner, P. E.: Cancer: Race and Geography, Baltimore, Williams & Wilkins, 1954.

48. Stewart, F. W.: Tumors of the Breast, Washington, D. C., Armed Forces Inst. Path., 1950.

49. Urban, J. A.: Extended radical mastectomy *in* Breast Cancer and Its Diagnosis and Treatment, p. 295, Baltimore, Williams & Wilkins, 1955.

50. ———: Radical mastectomy in continuity with en bloc resection of the internal mammary lymph-node chain: a new procedure for primary operable cancer of the breast, Cancer *5*:992-1008, 1952

51. ———: Clinical experience and results of excision of the internal mammary lymph node chain in primary operable breast cancer, Cancer *12*:14, 1959.

52. Warren, S.: The relation of chronic mastitis to carcinoma of the breast, Surg., Gynec. & Obst. *71*:257, 1940.

53. White, T. T., and White, W. C.: Breast cancer and pregnancy, Ann. Surg. *144*:384-393, 1956.

54. Willis, R. A.: Pathology of Tumours, ed. 2, St. Louis, Mosby, 1953.

55. Wynder, E. L., Bross, I. J., and Hirayama, T.: A study of the epidemiology of cancer of the breast, Cancer *13*:559, 1960.

CHAPTER 26

Thyroid, Thymus and Parathyroids

The Thyroid Gland

The surgery of goiter has been an integral part of the development of modern surgery. The peculiar anatomic and physiologic difficulties have stubbornly challenged the surgeon. Their conquest has contributed much to the technic of surgery, and the effect of the surgical removal much to the understanding of the physiology of the gland. A colorful phase of this surgical history is to be found in Halsted's *Story of Goiter*.[18]

In the latter part of the 19th century and the first portion of the 20th, surgery emerged as the only successful treatment of the various types of goiter. The middle third of the 20th century finds much of the therapy of goiter in transition from surgical to medical.

First, the establishment in 1917 that lack of iodine was the cause of endemic goiter provided an opportunity for preventive medicine.[22] The introduction of iodized salt has steadily reduced the incidence of endemic goiter throughout the world, and the need for operative care in this condition is vanishing.

Next, two effective medical therapies have appeared since 1941 for the control of hyperthyroidism. The earlier use of external irradiation and iodine had been only sporadically or incompletely effective. Radioactive iodine was the first adequate medical therapy. Its use started in 1941.[19] The second was the antithyroid drugs initiated by Astwood in 1943.[1] However, surgery is still advisable in younger patients and in those whose goiter is suspected of containing a tumor.

In sporadic nonhyperfunctioning goiter, surgery still holds sway. In spite of much new knowledge regarding the pathogenesis of such goiters and the occasional success of medical therapy, tumor is the problem, and surgery the treatment.

The study of the effects of the antithyroid drugs has occasioned new concepts of the pathogenesis of goiter. These concepts are described initially as an introduction to the subsequent sections on hyperthyroidism and nontoxic goiter.

The chapter includes short accounts of

thyroiditis and of attempts to alleviate heart disease by reduction of the activity of the normal gland. It is completed by remarks on the examination of patients with goiter, and pointers on surgical technic.

PATHOGENESIS OF GOITER

Hyperplasia was recognized as a part of both goiters and was considered by some to be the primary etiologic stimulus of tumor formation. Experiments with iodine by Marine in 1912 and its clinical introduction by Plummer in 1923 in the treatment of hyperthyroidism gave rise to the concept of iodine involution as a cause of tumors.[21, 28] Recent experiments using the blocking agents or antithyroid drugs have recapitulated the gamut of human goiters to a striking degree and have led to a possible consolidation of our ideas regarding the pathogenesis. The newer knowledge can be construed to reinforce the concept that hyperplasia is the basis of all goiter. If reasonable, the concept is to be used to guide the therapy of goiter. The following three processes are to be considered.*

HYPERPLASIA: THE PRIMARY PROCESS

Primary hyperplasia of the thyroid gland has been classically described both clinically and experimentally. There are 4 aspects recognizable by clinician, surgeon and pathologist.

1. The epithelial cells of the follicles are increased in number. The mitotic figures are visible on microscopic section, and there are papillary infoldings due to crowding of the cells. The process is diffuse throughout the gland, all areas taking part. Clinically, the thyroid gland increases in size.

2. The secretory activity is increased. Microscopically, this is seen as resorption of the colloid of the follicles. Clinically and experimentally, there is an increased turnover of radioactive iodine. The cells of the follicles change from cuboidal to columnar form, and there are large secretory droplets.

3. The blood flow through the gland is increased. The examiner recognizes this as a

* During the first half of this century, observation of the life history of endemic goiter and of the goiter associated with acute hyperthyroidism led to a number of theories regarding the pathogenesis of goiter.

bruit and sometimes a thrill in the gland. The surgeon sees it as enlarged, engorged major vessels and unusual prominence of the minor vessels.

4. Hyperplasia of the lymphoid follicles takes place both in the thyroid gland and in the lymph nodes surrounding the thyroid. This is still an incidental finding, the meaning of which is not clear.

These 4 changes appear to be due to an increased secretion of the thyrotropic hormone of the anterior pituitary. On clinical grounds this is believed to be true because sometimes the same findings are encountered in patients with acromegaly. The identical changes have been produced in several experimental animals and more recently in man by thyrotropic extracts of the anterior pituitary. An iodine-deficient diet is accompanied by the same changes. The thyroid-blocking agents or antithyroid drugs also produce them, but here a direct effect of the antithyroid drugs upon the thyroid gland cannot be excluded absolutely. The effect of iodine deficiency and of these drugs can be canceled by the simultaneous administration of desiccated thyroid or one of the synthetic thyroid hormones such as thyroxin or tri-iodothyronine.

IODINE INVOLUTION

The 4 manifestations of primary hyperplasia of thyroid gland can be reversed by iodine. This action of iodine has been termed "involution." Although it has been postulated that part of this involuting effect may be due to a direct inhibiting effect of the iodine upon the anterior pituitary gland, it is more probably due to a local effect on the thyroid itself. In patients with the spontaneous hyperplasia of acute hyperthyroidism, as a rule the involution does not return the gland to normal. In experimental animals the involuting effect varies with the dosage of the anterior pituitary extract. The involution is only moderate when the stimulus is intense.

Iodine has no visible effect upon the normal gland, either clinically or experimentally. Therefore, a demonstration of the involuting effect depends upon the existence of a pre-existing hyperplasia. The involution represents restraint rather than stimulation.

The involution may be accompanied by some disturbance in the architecture of the gland.[30] This disturbance has been mistaken for the beginning of early nodule formation. It is more likely, on the basis of recent evidence, that the storage of iodine within the follicles and the consequent expansion of the thyroid tissue, together with the loss of vascularity, may bring about an exaggeration of the normal lobulations of the thyroid, resulting in apparent nodule formation. Historically, iodine involution has provided the oldest explanation of nodule formation, and now it is probably of little importance. Nodules are more apt to be due to continued hyperplasia.

Continued Hyperplasia

The life history of endemic goiter first gave rise to the concept that continued hyperplasia was the reason for tumor formation. The initial process of formation of goiters in people living in an iodine-deficient area was hyperplasia. With continued iodine deficiency, a variety of nodules appeared, scattered here and there in the hyperplastic tissue. All sorts of tumors formed, including adenomas, cysts and, in later life, carcinomas.

Recently, the entire sequence of hyperplasia and a variety of tumors, including malignant ones, has been recapitulated in experimental animals given the antithyroid drugs.[5] [17, 24, 25, 27] Rats and mice have been fed thiouracil or other antithyroid drugs over a period of from many months to 2 years. The drug promptly initiates an intense hyperplasia. If the drug is continued, in 3 to 4 months tumors begin to appear. Their occurrence may be expedited by the simultaneous administration of a carcinogen.[6] Some adenomas are composed of embryoniclike cells, some of fetal cells, and others are typical papillary tumors. More differentiated follicular adenomas may occur with central necrosis and healing by fibrosis. In later months, cysts of inactive cuboidal epithelium appear immediately adjacent to the continued hyperplastic tissue. The apparent inactivity has given rise to the concept of cellular exhaustion.[24] Comparable cysts have been encountered in the pancreas of dogs and cats injected with large doses of a suitable anterior pituitary extract.[29] Eventually, after 18 months to 2 years of continued stimulation, malignant tumors appear. The simultaneous use of the carcinogens does not seem to make these appear any

earlier. The tumors metastasize and eventually grow to a size sufficient to kill the animal. They can be transplanted to other animals.[6]

In the pathogenesis of goiter, 3 other factors are to be considered: the endocrine phases of normal life, diet and the nervous system. Puberty and pregnancy are associated with an enlargement and increased activity of the thyroid gland. Diffuse goiter and thyroid nodules are apt to appear as abnormal accompaniments of both these phases of endocrine change. The menstrual cycle and the menopause may normally be associated with slight changes in thyroid stimulation and activity. Though the menstrual cycle has not been incriminated, at the time of the menopause a pre-existing goiter is commonly prone to renewed or intensified growth. These relationships to ovarian function are believed to be the reason why goiter is so much more frequent in woman than in man.

Certain foods contain thiocyanates and other goitrogenic substances.[2] Such foods have been suggested as possible causes of sporadic goiter, but beyond the occurrence of goiter in a number of monks of a monastery whose diet had been limited to cabbage for 2 or 3 years, such an origin has not been substantiated.

Because of the occurrence of the hyperplastic goiter of hyperthyroidism in patients subjected to undue emotional stress, the central nervous system has been suggested as the stimulator of the anterior pituitary's thyrotropic secretion, thus making it the primary cause of thyroid enlargement. Experimental proof of the pathways of such a stimulation has recently been offered by Harris.[18a]

HYPERTHYROIDISM

Hyperthyroidism occurs both as an acute disease and as a secondary complication of a pre-existing goiter. Acute hyperthyroidism is the most dramatic disease of the thyroid gland. It is generally known as exophthalmic goiter because of its frequent association with a characteristic form of exophthalmos. The disease was first recognized by Parry, a physician of Bath, England, in 1825.[26] Later it was described more fully by Graves of Ireland in 1835, and 5 years later by von Basedow of

Germany.[3, 16] In English-speaking countries it is commonly known as Graves's disease and on the continent of Europe as Basedow's disease.

Pathogenesis. Exophthalmic goiter is generally acute in onset because the enlargement of the thyroid, the initial symptoms from hypersecretion, and the appearance of the eye signs have a date of onset known by patient, family and friends. The disease is 4 times as common in women as in men, and it characteristically occurs during the phase of active ovarian life. It occasionally occurs in childhood before puberty, when the sex incidence is approximately equal. It also occurs, but less commonly, in both men and women after the age of 50. In the older group the exophthalmos is often absent.

Clinical evidence indicates that the acute form of hyperthyroidism is a psychosomatic disease.[20] The people from childhood to older age who succumb to this disease are emotionally anxious. Shortly before or at the time of onset of the hyperthyroidism a history of an additional emotional insult is almost always found. There is nothing specific known about the character or the type of emotional insult. The insults are the kind frequently encountered in other individuals who do not succumb to any psychosomatic disorder or may be afflicted by another type of organic disease. Therefore, it is probable that some predisposition exists. The disease has been encountered occasionally in several members of the same family, and it has been postulated, therefore, that there is a genetic factor.[8] At least the stimulus seems to fall upon fertile ground.*

An intact anterior pituitary gland and an excess of its thyrotropic hormone are prob-

---

* Objection has been raised to the psychosomatic concept of Graves's disease on the very ground that emotional conflicts are common and Graves's disease relatively rare. The occurrence of Graves's disease may be likened to that of lobar pneumonia. A large portion of our population in winter harbors the pneumococcus in the upper respiratory tract; only an occasional person develops lobar pneumonia, and only when the balance between virulence of the organism and immunity of the host provides the right conditions. Pneumococcus lobar pneumonia never occurs in the absence of the pneumococcus. Does acute hyperthyroidism ever afflict emotionally adjusted people living in a stable environment? The author has not seen such a case.

ably essential to the development of hyperthyroidism. Clinically, several arguments point to this. Sometimes exophthalmic goiter is encountered in patients in the initial phase of acromegaly. Reports of its occurrence in patients without intact pituitary tissue are open to question. Sometimes the disease can be arrested by x-ray irradiation of the anterior pituitary, much as Cushing's disease of the adrenal cortex is sometimes relieved by pituitary irradiation.[14, 33] The disease is prone to blossom in women at times when the anterior pituitary is undergoing abrupt changes in function; namely, during or at the termination of pregnancy and at the menopause. The cells of the anterior pituitary of patients dying with hyperthyroidism are consistent with increased anterior pituitary function.[31] Experimentally, the only known way of producing a comparable hyperplasia of the thyroid and increased activity of the thyroid gland is by an anterior pituitary extract or antithyroid drug. Hypophysectomy, or the administration of thyroid, prevents the effect of the antithyroid drug but not of the extract. Therefore, the full clinical concept of the genesis of acute hyperthyroidism is that emotional stress in a susceptible person stimulates the anterior pituitary to secrete an increased amount of thyrotropic hormone which in turn stimulates the thyroid to grow and oversecrete. The thyroid gland is the end organ of abnormal function, not the origin of the disease.

Signs and Symptoms. The prominent, characteristic eye signs of exophthalmic goiter have a dual origin. The exophthalmos is independent of the thyroid level and stems apparently from a pituitary secretion closely related to the thyrotropic hormone, while the stare and the lid lag depend upon the excess of thyroid.[15] Usually the eye signs develop coincidentally with the goiter and hyperthyroidism. Sometimes, however, the eye signs antedate by weeks or months the development of the goiter. Occasionally one eye may be involved first and the other eye only many months later or not at all. The eye signs may be absent even after prolonged enlargement and hypersecretion of the thyroid. Finally, the exophthalmos may become worse if treatment of the thyroid reduces the function to below the normal level.[23]

The eye signs usually come into abeyance

with therapy of the hyperthyroidism. The stare and the lid lag are the first to disappear. The recession of the eyeballs may be slow. Occasionally, the exophthalmos is increased after therapy, and the eyes may be endangered by the forward displacement of the eyeballs—so-called progressive exophthalmos. Hypothyroidism is to be avoided. Surgical decompression of the orbital cavities may be necessary to save the eyes.

Hyperthyroidism developing in a patient with a pre-existing goiter generally is termed "toxic nodular goiter." In contrast with exophthalmic goiter, it occurs principally in patients of the older age group, both sexes being involved, but with a continued preponderance in the female. It often develops insidiously and is characteristically slow in onset. The degree of hyperthyroidism usually is less severe. In those patients in whom the activity of the goiter has been studied and found to be normal prior to the development of hyperthyroidism, there usually has been a slow increase in size of the goiter coincident with the onset of hyperthyroidism.

The intimate pathology of the nodular goiter often fails to show any hyperplasia. Because of the increase in size prior to the recognition of the hyperthyroidism, it is felt that accretion in size gives rise to the hyperthyroidism rather than increase in activity of any part. In many women, the onset of renewed growth of the goiter and the development of the hyperthyroidism follow closely on the menopause, an argument that the anterior pituitary is an essential etiologic link in this type of goiter as well.

Differential Diagnosis. Much has been written differentiating the 2 types of hyperthyroidism, but basically the 2 are probably the same disease. The extremes are not alike, but there are transitional forms where one melts into the other. For example, long-standing acute hyperthyroidism without exophthalmos cannot be differentiated from toxic nodular goiter because nodules develop gradually in any hyperthyroidism of long standing. The intensity differs, and this may be related to the difference in age. The acute disease arises in flamboyant form; in the secondary nodular type the etiologic stimulus appears to be less virulent. In acute hyperthyroidism cardiac signs are less prominent because the patients are younger and more elastic; the nervousness and the irritability of the excessive thyroid hormone dominate the clinical picture. In the older age group, a modicum of hyperthyroidism quickly uses up the cardiac reserve, and signs of cardiac insufficiency are prominent. The absence of exophthalmos in the nodular type may well be due to loss of sensitivity of the orbital tissues with advancing age. The eye signs are absent in older people with no previous goiter and acute hyperthyroidism.

Treatment. SURGERY. Surgery was the first successful therapy of hyperthyroidism. In its initial years the therapy was faltering largely because of the vascularity of the gland and the precarious cardiac and physiologic status of the hyperthyroid patient. Therefore, external irradiation by x-rays was tried and was successful in about one third of the patients. In 1923 Plummer discovered that iodine, with its involution of the hyperplasia, induced a partial remission of the hyperthyroidism, thus opening the surgical era of therapy.[28] The iodine-induced remission made it possible for the operation to be carried out when the patient was less toxic, and the success of operation rose precipitously. From 1923 to 1941, refinements such as staged operations, attention to nutrition and the regaining of strength during remission under iodine brought mortality and complications to the level of other major surgical procedures.

The introduction of the thiouracil compounds by Astwood in 1943 enabled the surgeon to do even better.[1] The metabolic rate could now be brought to normal, the nutrition of the patient restored, and the operation carried out without urgency on an essentially normal person. Thus, it is now possible to operate under controlled conditions without fear of any mortality or complications such as hemorrhage, recurrent nerve palsy, or parathyroid insufficiency. Surgery, therefore, remains today as one of the 3 successful therapies of hyperthyroidism. Less often used in acute hyperthyroidism, it is still to be preferred in many patients with nodular goiters and secondary hyperthyroidism. The slightly higher frequency of a concomitant malignant lesion in such goiters and the size of the goiter itself with the complications of pressure make surgery preferable.

RADIOACTIVE IODINE was introduced by

Hertz in 1941 in the therapy of hyperthyroidism.[19] In principle, it is like surgery; instead of surgical extirpation of the larger part of the goiter, it eliminates the excess thyroid tissue by radiation necrosis. With experience, the right amount of radiation can be landed in the thyroid cells, and the desired necrosis accomplished.[9] Sometimes repeated doses are needed. It is as controlled a procedure as the surgical extirpation, but it takes more time to accomplish the desired result. Surgery brings an abrupt ending to the hyperthyroidism; radiation necrosis may take from 4 to 6 months or even longer, but it is equally sure, and it is far easier for the patient. Aside from the disadvantage of the length of time required to achieve the results, there is only one real disadvantage to this therapy—a theoretic one. Necrosing irradiation in other tissues has been followed after a latent period of many years by malignant degeneration of the tissue.[10] On the basis of experience with other tissues, the minimum latent period is 18 to 20 years, and the nature of this hazard cannot yet be appreciated. Therefore, in many clinics, an age limit has been placed upon the use of this therapy. Radioactive iodine has been given in therapeutic doses only to patients whose life expectancy is no greater than 25 years, or in whom a previous operation had failed to achieve the desired result or had been followed by a complication, such as parathyroid tetany or recurrent nerve palsy. If the bad dream of malignant degeneration can be dissipated, radioactive iodine probably will be the best of the therapies directed at the thyroid itself.

ANTITHYROID DRUGS. The second successful medical therapy is that of the antithyroid drugs, introduced by Astwood. These drugs eliminate hyperthyroidism by blocking chemically the elaboration of iodine into the thyroid hormone. There are 3 forms of drugs, each apparently acting at a different chemical phase—the thiocyanates, the thiouracils and perchlorate. Propylthiouracil, Tapazol and potassium perchlorate are the drugs now used most commonly. If a sufficient dosage of the drug is given, thyroid activity can be reduced to normal in all patients and can be so maintained with suitable adjustment of dosage. An excessive dose produces hypothyroidism.

The use of antithyroid drugs has been disappointing as definitive therapy for hyperthyroidism. If the metabolic rate is maintained at the normal level for only a few months and the drug then omitted, the hyperthyroidism returns in a large percentage of patients. If the drug is administered for a 2-year period, somewhat more than half of the patients have no recurrence. The disease process, being self-limited, apparently has run its course.* In those who do have a recrudescence of hyperthyroidism, a subsequent prolonged period of drug therapy may be followed by a permanent remission in another half. Such prolonged therapy means close care of the patient and is a nuisance to patient and physician; therefore, some of the clinics which at first advocated the use of the antithyroid drugs as the definitive therapy have abandoned it in favor of radioactive iodine.

PSYCHOSOMATIC CONSIDERATIONS. Evidence is accumulating that attention to the psychosomatic aspect of acute hyperthyroidism may lead to greater success with the prolonged drug therapy. If attention is paid to the emotional origin of the disease and irritating influences eliminated during the course of the drug therapy, it is more likely to be followed by a successful remission. Thus, the drug therapy has the additional advantage of calling to the physician's attention those very aspects of the patient's life which have been troublesome. Whether the emotional stress is etiologic or not becomes academic, for the combined use of drug and psychosomatic therapy brings to the patient relief that is more nearly complete. Such psychosomatic therapy also can be linked to the surgical and the radiation methods.

NODULAR GOITER

Nodular goiter includes a heterogeneous group of clinical entities, from small to large goiters, from single nodules to multiple, and from benign to malignant. The causes are obscure. Some case histories reveal only the rav-

* In 1926, Friedrich von Mueller, Professor of Medicine in Munich, advocated sending patients with exophthalmic goiter to the Tyrol Mountains for a minimum of 2 years. He stressed the need for a 2-year stay. The reason for the success of his therapy is now clear. The deficiency of iodine in these mountains deprived the thyroid gland of iodine as effectively as the use of the antithyroid drugs.

ages of just living, of bearing babies, or working hard and living long. Many people go to their graves not knowing that they had a lump in their thyroid. Since lumps are tumors, and tumors are still the concern of the surgeon, nodular goiters, with exceptions to be mentioned, are cared for largely by surgical methods.

Nodular goiter is a descriptive term. In some communities, "adenomatous goiter" is preferred. The use of "adenomatous" implies that the nodules in the goiter are adenomas, that is, benign neoplasms. Since there is often doubt regarding the true nature of the nodules, the use of the descriptive word is to be preferred. The term "adenoma" should be reserved for those nodules in which there is substantial evidence that the growth is both anatomically and physiologically independent of the remainder of the gland.

CLASSIFICATION

A number of classifications of nodular goiter have been proposed. The differences between the classifications depend upon differences of opinion regarding the nature of the origin and the character of the nodules. The following classification is in use in the Thyroid Clinic of the Massachusetts General Hospital. In relation to tumors it follows most closely that of Warren and Meissner.[34]

Diffuse nodular goiter means that the disease process involves to some extent the entire thyroid apparatus, that the entire thyroid is enlarged, and that at least one or more areas are nodular. Endemic goiter and sporadic goiter encountered in nonendemic, noniodine deficient areas are such goiters. The goiter of a patient with burned-out Graves's disease is also such a goiter. Secondary hyperthyroidism occurs in these goiters when growth is renewed, for example, after the menopause.

The nodules are of a variety of types, varying from exaggerated lobulations without clear-cut capsules through cysts to localized adenomas and occasionally carcinomas. They are comparable with the isolated tumors described below, and they are the variety of tumors mimicked in the experimental animals exposed to prolonged thiouracil therapy described above under Pathogenesis of Goiter.

A single goiter may have nodules of one or more types. Two or 3 types are common.

When several are present they have been called pudding-stone goiters. Approximately 4 per cent of such goiters coming to operation at the Mayo Clinic and at the Massachusetts General Hospital harbor a carcinoma as one of the nodules.[4, 13] The incidence of cancer in diffuse nodular goiter in the population at large must be considerably smaller.

Localized goiter is the term applied to those goiters in which the enlargement and the nodularity are limited to one area of the gland, the remainder of the gland being essentially normal. By definition, the nodules of these goiters are likely to be adenomatous, since they fulfill the definition of autonomous growth. It is not surprising, therefore, that such goiters have a higher incidence of definable neoplasms, including carcinomas, than the diffusely involved glands.[13]

The nodule of the diffuse or localized nodular goiter may be any one of the following varieties:

Exaggerated Lobulation. In the embryologic development of the normal thyroid, the lateral lobe is rarely fused into a smooth mass. The surface is frequently indented by 2, 3 or more sulci. A hyperplastic process increases the depth of such sulci, the adjacent tissue bulging out to form a rounded nodule. Separately encapsulated pieces of thyroid, which occur in at least 10 per cent of normal people, also enlarge under a stimulus and push forward, mimicking an adenoma. On cut section these exaggerated lobulations have no capsule separating them from the body of the lobe. Desiccated thyroid is effective therapy when the nodular goiter is limited to this lobular phase of development. The medication suppresses the anterior pituitary's thyrotropic action, and the goiter shrivels. Such therapy is not effective in eliminating true neoplasms described below, for they have developed an autonomy and an integrity independent of the thyrotropic stimulation.[12]

Cysts filled with colloid and lined by low cuboidal epithelium are not infrequent. The probability that such cysts represent exhaustion phenomena has been described already. They grow slowly and are to be differentiated from papillary cystadenomas.

Adenomas. PAPILLARY CYSTADENOMAS are uncommon. They usually have a thick, well-demarcated capsule. The cystic proportion of the tumor varies from largely cystic to essentially solid, in which case they may be called a papillary adenoma. There is no absolute line which can be drawn between papillary adenoma and papillary carcinoma described below. A locally benign-appearing papillary adenoma may have been accompanied by metastases to the regional lymph nodes.

EMBRYONAL ADENOMA denotes a localized, encapsulated tumor consisting of cords of cells similar to the cells of the thyroid in the embryonic stage of development. These are considered by some to be potentially malignant.

FETAL ADENOMA is a circumscribed, encapsulated tumor consisting of cells arranged in a rudimentary follicular configuration, with little or no colloid in the follicles. The cells resemble those of fetal thyroid, being somewhat more differentiated than the embryonal but less so than those of the follicular adenoma. The fetal adenoma is also considered by some as potentially malignant, though most surgical pathologists classify them as benign.

HÜRTHLE ADENOMA is a rare tumor with cells having a special staining reaction. The cells are arranged usually in the fetal or embryonic manner, the tumor probably being a variant of the relatively undifferentiated adenoma. Occasionally, it gives rise to distant metastases, particularly to bone, and therefore is potentially malignant. Probably less than 10 per cent of such adenomas are actually malignant.

FOLLICULAR ADENOMA is the most common of all adenomas and is a frequent lesion of the thyroid. Always encapsulated, it may grow to considerable size. When it reaches the size of a lemon, it usually is necrotic in the center with evidence of healing by fibrosis. Hemorrhage sometimes occurs into such adenomas. The cells form well-differentiated follicles with varying amounts of colloid secretion. Occasionally, such an adenoma gives rise to a blood-borne metastasis, usually to bone, even though the local lesion appears to be benign. Blood vessel invasion may be found if diligently searched for. Rarely do these adenomas spread their cells in the lymphatics. When a locally benign adenoma has given rise to a distant metastasis, perforce it must be called a carcinoma. The German pathologists have tried to combine both features by the awkward term of "benign metastasizing struma or adenoma." Since the follicular adenoma is a common tumor, and bone metastasis from such a tumor is rare, it is obvious that the vast majority of such adenomas are benign in keeping with their local appearance. The benign form are the tumors most commonly found incidentally in the thyroid at autopsy in the majority of people over 65 dying from any cause.[32]

All of these benign lumps are encountered more frequently in the female than in the male, and probably more often in women who have had one or more pregnancies. Their incidence increases with each decade in both sexes. Some are subject to physiologic influence. Their rate of growth may be slowed occasionally by thyroid medication, and frequently the rate is accelerated by pregnancy. Thyroid medication has not been proved to dissolve any of the adenomas.[12] Therefore, the only known effective therapy is surgery, and it is indicated if the diagnosis is in doubt or the growth is rapid.

Carcinoma. The carcinomas are of 3 general types: the papillary carcinomas, the adenocarcinomas and the undifferentiated. In contrast with the benign adenomas of the thyroid, which are common lesions in the population, the carcinomas are rare. Thus, they constitute a very small proportion of the nodules of the thyroid.

The carcinomas probably start *de novo*, as do the adenomas. The engrafting of a carcinoma on a part of a follicular or other benign adenoma has been described, but it is probably a rare occurrence. Only twice has the author encountered findings consistent with such a development. Mixed types of carcinomas are encountered not infrequently, the biologic behavior of the tumor following both types. It is believed that sometimes metastases deviate from the primary type.

PAPILLARY CARCINOMA is the most prevalent malignant lesion, representing approximately 60 per cent of the carcinomas. Biologically, no other tumor in the body is quite like these papillary lesions. They occur in all decades of life, as frequently in the later teens and twenties as in any other decade. They are no more malignant in the child or the adolescent than in any other age group. In other words, they do not follow the classic age distribution of malignancy. They have a sluggish growth, and this in spite of a wildly growing appearance of many on microscopic section. They are slow to invade surrounding tissues. If they have not invaded the cartilage of the larynx, for example, extirpation is easy and curative. They spread early through the lymphatics to the lymph nodes, and here the cells may stay for years without metastasizing through the blood stream. The cells grow luxuriantly in the lymph nodes so that the lymph node metastasis frequently outgrows the primary lesion. Only when the lymph node capsule is overdistended does the papillary growth spread into the neighboring tissue. The life span from initial lesion to lymph nodes to neighborhood spread may extend over several years.

A number of the papillary carcinomas have an occasional well-developed follicle containing colloid. Because of such follicles pathologists call them "papillary adenocarcinoma," a term describing their microscopic appearance rather than their biologic behavior. Studies with radioactive iodine reveal very low secretory activity, and in only an occasional metastasis has the activity been increased even a little by total thyroidectomy.

The papillary carcinoma is the type of malignancy encountered in an occasional patient with Graves's disease or nodular goiter of long standing. The clinical occurrence in Graves's disease indicates that long-continued hyperplasia is a dominant stimulus giving rise to the tumor. Usually the patients are above the age of 40 and have had long-standing Graves's disease. The youngest patient in the Massachusetts General Hospital series with hyperthyroidism, complicated with papillary carcinoma, was a girl of 15 who had had Graves's disease certainly since the age of 8 and probably since the age of 4.*

ADENOCARCINOMAS. The adenocarcinomas are more like carcinomas of other organs such as the stomach or the breast. They have the typical age distribution and, except for the well differentiated, are locally invasive. Lymph node metastases are less prominent than

---

* In a number of the patients in whom a papillary carcinoma has been found as the only lesion in the thyroid, there has been an antedating stress. This has been particularly true in the young males. It is hard to escape the conclusion that the trigger mechanism is hyperplasia following a stress.

blood-borne; bones and lungs are particularly fertile ground for seeding. If the cells of the metastasis are well differentiated to begin with or become biologically so by the total thyroidectomy, significant therapeutic restraint may be obtained with radioactive iodine. This form of radiation is most useful in the well-differentiated tumor described in the previous section under Follicular Adenoma. Their metastases may be held in abeyance for a number of years, although no radiation cure has been reported as yet. The metastases grow so slowly with or without radiation that if single and accessible, surgical excision should be considered as the most desirable therapy.

UNDIFFERENTIATED CARCINOMAS. These are a highly malignant group. Usually they are subclassified according to their cell type and include the small cell, the giant cell and the epidermoid. When first recognized, ordinarily they have spread beyond the limits of surgical extirpation; they have a bad prognosis. The cells are biologically undifferentiated and do not concentrate any radioactive iodine. Therefore, external irradiation is the sole therapy available beyond the effort at surgical extirpation. They follow the usual age distribution of malignancies.

Lymphoma has been reported arising in the lymph follicles of the thyroid. This tumor is difficult—sometimes impossible—to differentiate microscopically from the undifferentiated small cell carcinoma and from sarcoma of the thyroid. Malignant tumors of other organs metastasize occasionally to the thyroid, producing a goiter as the patient's first symptom and sign. Hypernephroma, myeloma and carcinomas of the gastro-intestinal tract are such tumors.

THYROIDITIS

Included under the term "thyroiditis" are a small group of poorly understood goiters. An occasional streptococcus abscess forms in the thyroid gland following an acute throat infection. In rare cases, a tuberculous abscess is encountered. The origin of these is clear enough. They are abscesses like those in any organ, the bacteria being blood-borne.

ACUTE THYROIDITIS

There is an acute inflammation which behaves like a virus infection, called acute thyroiditis. Sometimes the patients are encountered in waves, as if there were a mild epidemic. The thyroid becomes acutely tender and swollen in a few hours, to subside a week or 10 days later. Usually there is a moderate fever. The acute attack is characteristically recurrent once or twice after intervals of a month or two. Efforts to culture a virus have thus far failed. There is no residuum and no proven treatment, although many have been claimed. Often the inflammation is localized to one lobe of the gland; the alternate lobe may be affected in the subsequent attack.

CHRONIC THYROIDITIS

Three types of chronic goiter enlargement are included under chronic thyroiditis: non-specific lymphoid, Hashimoto's and Riedel's. Each has its characteristic cell picture. Hashimoto's thyroiditis is associated with destruction of the thyroid follicles. It is spongy and bulging and often grows over a period of many months, with increasing compression of the trachea and the esophagus. Its etiology is debatable. The only established therapy is surgical decompression if the size of the goiter warrants intervention. The isthmus and the anterior portion of the lateral lobes are removed, providing mobility for the remaining tissue. The process usually burns itself out and may leave the patient with an inadequate amount of secreting thyroid tissue and a consequent hypothyroidism. Thyroid therapy is indicated.

Riedel's struma is characteristically hard and has been termed *ligneous thyroiditis*. The gland is fibrosed, contracts and may constrict the trachea. Surgical decompression also may be indicated. Some think that this process is the end result of the Hashimoto type, but against this concept is the fact that Hashimoto's thyroiditis is common, and Riedel's struma is rare.

THE NORMAL GLAND

Surgical resection of the normal thyroid gland has been practiced in patients with decompensated heart disease. Benefit was only occasional—occurring in some of the patients with angina. Recently the same program has been advocated, using radioactive iodine to ablate the thyroid.[7] Limited use by cardiolo-

gists suggests a limited benefit. Success, presumably, depends on the wisdom used in selecting the patients. The failure of most hearts to improve under the diminished load of hypothyroidism may be due to the effect of the hypothyroidism on the action of the heart muscle.

SUGGESTIONS ABOUT THE INVESTIGATION OF THE PATIENT

Comprehensive investigation of the patient suspected of thyroid disease includes taking the history, and making the physical, the behavior and the laboratory examinations. The diagnosis usually can be established with surprising confidence by the history and a knowledgeable physical examination; the laboratory examination is needed only for confirmation. The behavior examination contributes, for the most part, to the therapy.

The principles of diagnosing hyperthyroidism are well established. The elevated metabolic rate of the tissues, even when only of

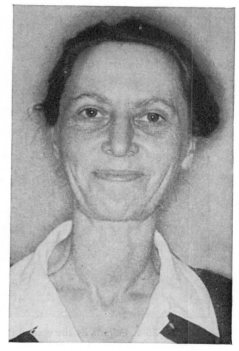

FIG. 26-1. Examination of the thyroid gland. Inspect as the first step. Watch as the patient swallows. Asymmetries and mediastinal extensions are readily picked up.

mild degree, increases the circulatory load and the irritability of the entire nervous system—peripheral, autonomic and central. In more extreme forms it undermines strength and disturbs organ function. In anyone with such symptoms or anyone with a goiter, hyperthyroidism is to be considered. Confirmation of the clinical impression is secured through determination of the basal metabolic rate, the radioactive iodine tracer and the protein-bound iodine of the blood serum.

A painstaking physical examination of the thyroid itself is most telling in relation to tumors. The basic principle of the examination is that a neoplasm is a localized disease and that a goiter, if it contains one, must give evidence of a localized change, one area out of line with the rest. Confusion between the diffuse process of hyperplasia and the localized neoplasia occurs when the original thyroid is unusually asymmetric or irregular. Such a gland enlarged by hyperplasia exhibits the asymmetry or the irregularity in exaggerated form. The right thyroid lobe is most often confusing in this regard. The normal right lobe averages 25 per cent heavier than the left. In a diffuse goiter the right lobe is expectedly larger than the left. The difference in size does not necessarily indicate a neoplasm in the right lobe. Corollary-wise a left lobe larger than the right should arouse suspicion of neoplasia in the left.

Refinements of the local examination include the mobility of a nodule within the thyroid substance, the smoothness of the capsule, tenderness and hardness. If a lump is stuck, rough, hard and not tender, it is suspicious of malignancy. Care must be taken not to render a lump tender by overpalpation.

Lymph nodes are to be sought. Normal

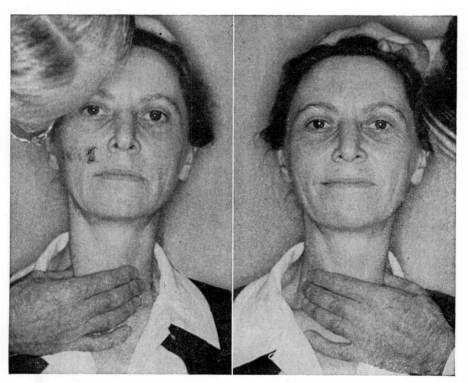

FIG. 26-2. Palpate as the second step, and always from in front of the patient. Examine one side at a time. Use the thumb to displace the goiter toward the examining fingers. Steady the patient's head with the nonexamining hand, relaxing the sternocleidomastoid muscle by slight rotation of the head. A small goiter may be felt by insinuating the fingers between the thyroid and the muscle; a large one must be felt through the muscle.

nodes are rarely large or firm enough to be felt. The easiest place to pick up initial enlargement is in the Delphian and the pretracheal groups.[11] The Delphian node lies in the mid-line just above the thyroid isthmus. It can be identified against the firm background of the cricoid cartilage. Always there is one node in this position and often two. The pretracheal nodes lie below the isthmus and can be felt against the trachea. Their position is not so constant and they are harder to find. Nodes of the jugular chains have to be palpated against the soft background of the jugular veins. They have to be larger to be felt. When the Delphian or the pretracheal nodes are palpable, then the thyroid disease is to be differentiated between thyroiditis and malignancy.

Many physicians examine the thyroid from behind the patient, using both hands. This approach has two disadvantages. First, the fingers are disadvantageously placed for palpation of the deeper parts of the gland. Only the anterior surface can be well felt. Stand to the side, slightly in front. Examine the right thyroid lobe with the left hand. The bulb of the fingers can feel the front and also slide around to the side and posteriorly. Place the right or nonexamining hand on the patient's head. Rotate the head slightly toward the examiner, thus relaxing the right sternocleidomastoid muscle. The fingers of the left hand can now be pushed in medial to the sternocleidomastoid to closer contact with the lateral and the posterior surfaces of the lobe. The thumb of the examining hand is placed against the left or contralateral lobe. Pressure pushes the right lobe out where it can be felt better. The left thyroid lobe is to be examined in comparable fashion by standing to the right side of the patient, using the right hand on the thyroid and the left hand on the patient's head.

The second reason that the position somewhat in front of the patient is to be preferred is that the patient's expression can be watched. Tenderness and the presence of anxiety are picked up readily. In examining from behind these two important points may be entirely overlooked. Besides, it is more comforting to the patient to be able to watch the physician's face. The hidden position behind does not consider the patient's concern. Too often physicians examining the thyroid from behind look off into the ceiling dreamily, inattentive of the patient, as if they were playing the piano.

Much of the emotional pattern can be learned by observing the patient during the taking of the history and the making of the physical examination. This is the behavior examination. During the talk the reaction of the patient rather than the specific answer to a question may be informative. The way the patient hesitates or talks voluntarily should be noted. The patient's attitude or reluctance during the physical examination may be revealing. These reactions should be looked for particularly at the first interview. Later, when the patient is accustomed to the physician, there is less to be noted.

What is observed of the patient's behavior is more than mental status, that final designation of the customary physical examination. It appraises his equanimity as well as his anxieties including his fear of the disease. It contains matters relating to the genesis, if the

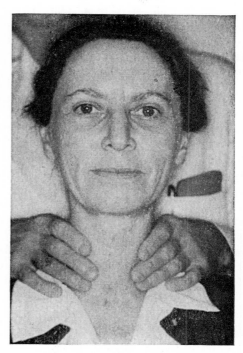

FIG. 26-3. The blind approach from behind, both hands at once. Only the front of the goiter is readily palpated from this position, and the patient's expression cannot be watched. Tenderness and anxiety are missed.

disease is considered to be psychosomatic. It also yields the clue to much of the management of the patient. It tells the sore points of the patient with hyperthyroidism that are to be rectified if possible during the course of the therapy of the thyroid. It tells the amount of anxiety about a possible cancer, which is to be taken into account in advising the removal of a tumor. Its thorough consideration and use will end in making the patient happier.

POINTERS ON SURGICAL TECHNIC

The technical approaches to thyroid operations may be classified as either dashing or deliberate. Which is chosen is a matter somewhat of training and somewhat of temperament of the surgeon. In the days before means were available to control the hyperthyroidism, the surgeon was forced to operate when the goiter was vascular, the nutrition poor, the anesthetic uncertain, and the procedure perilous. Time was precious, and the surgeon hurried, thinking that he would lose less blood. He contented himself with a subtotal resection, leaving a thick wad of gland to protect parathyroids and recurrent nerves. These were the horse-and-buggy days when the surgeon knew little of what he did.

The use of the antithyroid drugs and iodine in those patients with hyperthyroidism, attention to nutrition, and collaboration with a competent anesthesiologist provide all the time needed to carry out exactly the operation desired. Parathyroids can be identified and laid aside safely if they lie in the path of the dissection; so also with the recurrent nerves. Now, total excision of a lateral lobe can be accomplished with the same avoidance of complications or protection of the patient formerly sought by partial removal of the lobe. It is now possible to follow the precepts of Halsted, but it still takes curbing or self-

discipline on the part of the surgeon inclined to be vigorous.

Hemorrhage, a dreaded complication of thyroidectomy, can be eliminated by deliberate care. The vessels in the thyroid bed along the trachea, the esophagus and the larynx deserve the most attention. Tie every vessel, lay all knots down squarely. Do not cut the ends too short; otherwise the knots will untie when the larynx goes up and down with swallowing after operation.

Drains in a thyroid wound are a relic of the dashing days. If care is taken with the size of the bites and the hemostasis, there is no need to drain. Infection will not be introduced, and the scar will heal much better. If the bites behind the snaps are big, and oozing here and there is not controlled, do not try to get away without a drain.

Parathyroid tetany and laryngeal nerve palsy can be avoided by forethought, training and attention at operation. There are two ways of not falling down a mountain. One is never to go near a mountain, and the other is to walk carefully when climbing. The surgeons of a generation ago got around these complications by avoiding the areas where parathyroids and nerves lurk. Satisfactory surgery today demands that the surgeon approach these danger spots, but he must recognize them and deal with them. To do this he must prepare himself. Parathyroids are hard to identify. Dissections at the postmortem table provide excellent schooling. There also the surgeon can learn the vagaries of the inferior laryngeal nerves, including the nonrecurrent anomaly on the right side. He will also learn of the variations of the normal thyroid gland. It is gratifying to note how normal these tissues appear on fresh postmortem material. The effort will be well repaid in technical competence at the operating table.

The Thymus Gland

At the turn of the century the thymus gland was considered to be an organ important only to fetal development, becoming vestigial early in postuterine life. If it persisted in the child, it was a dangerous thing. Since 1901 when

Laquer and Weigert described a thymic tumor in a patient dying with myasthenia gravis, it has slowly become accepted that the gland survives with a function, is sometimes the seat of tumor and the instigator of mischief.[40]

Composed of epithelial and lymphoid cells, there is neither a comprehensive nor a detailed idea of its role or function.

SURGICAL ANATOMY

The thymus gland develops embryologically from the 3rd branchial clefts.[42] Each lateral component descends during fetal life behind the lateral lobe of the thyroid gland to rest in the anterior mediastinum. Each component usually leaves a thin tongue behind in the neck, stretching downward from the lower pole of the thyroid, broadening out as they pass the left innominate vein. The two components fuse in front of the ascending aorta, forming the body of the thymus. Sometimes driblets are left behind the thyroid lobe, well above the tongue of each component. The left tongue is normally a little longer, reaching higher in the neck. The left side of the body of the thymus is a little larger than the right. Sometimes the fusion in the midline is only partial, since there is a long or a complete cleft in the mid-line. Usually the thymus passes in front of the left innominate vein, sometimes behind, and occasionally it splits, with the vein running through the middle. In its final resting place each component lies against the pleura laterally, stretching down in front of the lung root and medially along the ascending aorta down over the upper pericardium. The gland receives its arterial supply locally. The larger part of venous return is directly to the left innominate vein.

The bulk of the thymus is composed of lymphoid follicles and fat. Here and there, scattered in the lymphoid tissue, are so-called Hassall's corpuscles, characteristic whorls, presumably of epidermoid origin.[42]

The lower pair of parathyroid glands also develop embryologically from the 3rd branchial clefts and descend along with the thymus in the neck to their usual position behind the lower pole of the thyroid lobes.[43] Not infrequently, during their descent they are carried down beyond the thyroid with the thymus. In 10 per cent of normal people one or more of this pair is contained within the thymic capsule, usually in the upper tongue In resecting the thymus or in looking for a parathyroid tumor, this frequent relationship is to be remembered.

PATHOLOGIC PHYSIOLOGY

No clear physiologic role as yet has been proved for the thymus gland. A specific substance with a curarelike action has been sought but not found. Because of the lymphoid tissue, it has been postulated that it is the site of immune body production. The one substantial fact that is known about the thymus is that it enlarges when lymphoid tissue generally is hyperplastic and shares in the atrophy when lymphoid tissue atrophies.[37] Thus, it is hyperplastic in patients with Graves's disease when lymphoid tissue generally is hyperplastic.* It waxes with the lymphoid hyperplasia of Addison's disease or experimental adrenal insufficiency and wanes with the lymphoid atrophy following cortisone or ACTH. It has not been proved how much of these changes are due to the adrenal hormone secreted in response to the anterior pituitary stimulation or how much directly to the anterior pituitary itself. The thymus atrophies following experimental hypophysectomy.

STATUS THYMICOLYMPHATICUS

Infants, children and adolescents dying suddenly in accidents or during operation sometimes were found at autopsy to have had a swollen thymus gland and generalized lymphadenopathy. So firmly was it believed that the sudden death was due to the thymic hypertrophy that as late as the middle 1920's many hospitals routinely x-rayed the chests of children below the age of 10 before undertaking an operation of any sort. If evidence of an enlarged thymus was found, it was treated with a small dose of x-rays before the operation. This dose of irradiation usually was followed by shriveling of the thymus. Although so-called status thymicolymphaticus never has been resolved to the satisfaction of everybody, it is no longer the practice to take chest roentgenograms and to carry out irradiation of the thymus. The sudden deaths are generally held to have been due to some cause other than the enlarged thymus.

---

* European clinicians speculated concerning the relation of the thymic hyperplasia in Basedow's disease to the myasthenia. As early as 1911 von Garré and Sauerbruch resected the thymus but without definitive relief of the myasthensia.[45]

AS A SEAT OF TUMOR

Thymus tissue is the not-infrequent source of benign and malignant tumors arising in the anterior mediastinum. Primary tumors include both lymphomas and epithelial neoplasms. Teratomas also are encountered. The tumors are often silent until they have reached considerable size, sometimes beyond surgical extirpation. The thymus is a rare site for a metastasis to settle from malignancy in another organ.

Although the early growth of malignant tumors of the thymus may be silent, when they have reached a relatively massive proportion, symptoms and signs of myasthenia gravis not infrequently appear as a harbinger of early death. External irradiation of high voltage may achieve considerable but temporary relief, including remission of the myasthenia gravis.

In general, whenever a tumor in the region of the thymus is diagnosed, immediate surgical exploration is indicated, since early eradication is considered at present to be the only possible chance for cure. Irradiation is palliative only.

AS AN INSTIGATOR OF MYASTHENIA GRAVIS

On the basis that thymic enlargement is the cause of myasthenia gravis, 3 different therapeutic approaches have been used attacking the thymus—x-ray irradiation, surgical extirpation and ACTH. Although hundreds of patients with myasthenia gravis have been treated by one or a combination of these methods, it must be admitted that success is sporadic and unpredictable, and that the relationship between the thymus and the myasthenia is poorly understood.

In 1921 Pierchalla reported that irradiation of the thymus improved patients with myasthenia gravis.[44] Two years later Mella recorded 2 patients similarly benefited.[41] The therapy attracted little attention and soon was abandoned. In 1936, Blalock excised a thymic tumor from a man with myasthenia gravis.[36] The patient improved, and the surgical era was initiated. In subsequent patients whose thymus was resected at the Johns Hopkins Hospital the good effect was obtained only

sometimes, and enthusiasm for this approach has waned.[35]

Thymectomy has been carried out in several centers; large groups of cases have become available for appraisal of the success of operation at the Mayo Clinic, Keynes of London, and the Masachusetts General Hospital.[38, 39, 46] At the Mayo Clinic enthusiasm for the operation has risen and fallen, alternately practiced and abandoned. Recently, there has been renewed interest. Sir Geoffrey Keynes is the most enthusiastic exponent of the therapy. He believes that success depends upon its early application. His results are criticized by those who have observed the life history of the disease in many patients without operation. Spontaneous remissions are common, and particularly in those patients in whom the disease has been of short duration. It is argued that many of his successful cases might have recovered without operation. The experience with Case 1 is a case in point.

Case 1. A married woman of 42, mother of 3, complaining of lower abdominal pain, was found to have a simple cyst of an ovary and erosion of the uterine cervix. An ovariectomy and hysterectomy were performed under ether anesthesia. Upon regaining consciousness the patient noted diplopia. This persisted, generalized weakness appeared, and 5 days after operation the diagnosis of myasthenia gravis was established with Prostigmine. In 1 month the disease had increased to moderate severity; the patient was incapacitated in spite of frequent Prostigmine tablets. Thymectomy was considered.

The patient had noticed occasional transient diplopia in the previous 5 years. The husband reported that the episodes were always at times when the patient was under stress. Recently she had been increasingly worried over the illness of the oldest daughter. It became obvious that much could be done to help the patient with her emotional problems. Therefore, thymectomy was delayed, and a series of interviews was undertaken by an interested physician.

By the 10th month after the pelvic operation, the patient had gained some understanding of her problems and a return of confidence in her doctors. Her daughter was also in better health. All signs of the myasthenia gravis disappeared. She has remained well for the ensuing year.

At the Massachusetts General Hospital 116 patients have undergone thymectomy for myasthenia gravis since 1939. Appraisal of the benefit of operation is difficult, since it involves the opinion of what would have happened if operation had not been performed. The author has the following general impression: $\frac{1}{3}$ of the patients were significantly improved; a few of them were completely relieved (Case 2 is an example); $\frac{1}{3}$ were somewhat improved; and in $\frac{1}{3}$ the severity of the disease was not influenced by thymectomy (Case 3 is an example of the last).

Case 2. The 25-year-old wife of a physician rapidly developed fulminating myasthenia gravis. She was almost totally dependent upon a respirator for 6 weeks, after which period slight improvement set in, enabling her to breathe unaided. The dosage of Prostigmine and atropine was maximal. Thymectomy was carried out; the thymus showed the lymphoid hyperplasia typical of myasthenia gravis. Following operation, improvement was rapid; within the first 2 weeks it was possible to halve the dosage of Prostigmine. By 4 months, from 2 to 4 15-mg. pills a day sufficed for reasonable activity. Within a year of operation Prostigmine was no longer needed. Five years after thymectomy she continued to be free of symptoms of myasthenia gravis.

She and her husband came from a country now behind the Iron Curtain. The myasthenia gravis developed at the time she first became shut off from her family. Now she and her husband have made a place for themselves in the United States. A much desired, successful pregnancy was started 2 years after thymectomy.

Case 3. At the age of 20, and 10 years before first being seen at the Massachusetts General Hospital, a woman became pregnant out of wedlock. When she first realized her predicament, she noticed transient difficulty in talking and swallowing and some generalized weakness. She was angry with the father of the child, refused marriage and moved from her home in a small town to a large city. Three months after the baby's birth she was prevailed upon by her family to return home, bringing the baby. She felt very awkward at home and 10 days after her return came down with full-blown myasthenia gravis which persisted unremittingly to the time of thymectomy 9 years later.

The surgical resection of a moderately hyperplastic thymus failed to improve her status during the first 12 months. She continued to live in the small town of her childhood where she was withdrawn, feeling that all eyes were cast upon her. As soon as she began to take a course in practical nursing with a view to moving away and building

a new life, she noticed an immediate, moderate improvement in the myasthenia gravis.

Keynes and Schwab agree that the most favorable group are the younger women with disease of short duration. The disease is less likely to be influenced favorably when in men, in older patients or when a thymoma is present. There are exceptions to each of these groups among the author's cases. For example, a 40-year-old man with a malignant thymoma and severe myasthenia was nearly completely relieved by resection of the thymoma. A year later with regrowth of the tumor from an implant the myasthenia rapidly recurred, and the patient died in crisis. The implant was found only at autopsy in the lower chest behind the heart.

What one advises about thymectomy in an individual patient depends upon one's concept of the disease. It is like an endocrine disease in that it is found most commonly in women and in the childbearing, active ovarian phase of life. Like acute hyperthyroidism and Cushing's disease, it appears to be a psychosomatic disease. Its onset is frequently coincidental with psychological trauma and emotional upset. It also bears a curious relationship to pregnancy and ovarian function. Pregnancy may induce a complete remission. The origin may be associated with resection of an ovary.

Thymectomy is indicated in any patient with myasthenia gravis with evidence of a tumor of the thymus. The tumor in itself demands the exploration. It is also to be carried out in any patient, man or woman, who is getting worse and in whom all other efforts fail. Adjustment to the problems of life are to be attended to in all patients.

ACTH is the newcomer to the field of therapy, having been tried first in 1948 by Soffer *et al.* and Torda and Wolff.[47, 48] There is still disagreement as to its efficacy and the advisability of its use. Certainly in some patients it induces a remission. For the first few days of injection the disease may be worsened, to be followed by remission. Its use is worth a try except in those patients with evidence of a thymic tumor in which the question of malignancy is unsettled.

In patients with a severe degree of myasthenia gravis, operation is hazardous. Everything that can be done to improve the myasthenia before undertaking the operation is wise. Roentgen-ray therapy to the thymus is such a measure. In the last 8 years it has been the author's rule to irradiate all patients, waiting at least 3 weeks before operating.

There has been good correlation between those improving with irradiation and those benefiting from thymectomy. Such irradiation emerges as a prognostic test of the benefit to be expected from thymectomy.

The Parathyroid Glands

INTRODUCTION

Disease of the parathyroid glands is a latecomer to the endocrine field. Not until 1925 was a primary disease established. For the 45 years from the time of their discovery until 1925, their sole interest for the surgeon was as danger spots, areas to be avoided when operating upon the thyroid gland. Since 1925, gradually it has dawned that disease of these glands is not uncommon, and their relation to the metabolism of calcium and phosphorus has made them a subject of wide interest to physiologist and biochemist, as well as clinician. In spite of the wide interest in these glands there is still little but speculation regarding the etiology of the disease, and nothing is known regarding the counterbalancing, reciprocating physiologic forces.

HISTORY

The parathyroid glands were discovered by the Swedish anatomist, Sandström, in 1880.[79] They were anatomic curiosities until Gley, the French physiologist, 11 years later proved that their removal led to tetany, disclosing the etiology of the tetany that sometimes followed thyroidectomy.[67] The relation of the calcium level of the blood to this tetany was demonstrated experimentally by MacCallum and Voegtlin in 1908.[73] These 3 discoveries established the effect of the removal of the normal glands.

Discovery of disease of the parathyroid glands came about more slowly. Overactivity of the glands was the first disease described. The story of how overfunction became recognized is important because it led at first to an overemphasis on the associated bone disease. Knowledge first came from the European pathologists. In 1891 von Recklinghausen described the generalized disease of bone which now bears his name.[76] Askanazy, in 1903, found a parathyroid tumor at autopsy in a patient who had died of this disease.[52] In the next few years other examples of this association were described. In the meantime, Erdheim in a clinical and experimental study showed that the parathyroid glands were slightly enlarged or hyperplastic in conditions such as rickets, osteomalacia and even pregnancy.[65, 66] These enlargements, he felt, represented a compensatory hyperplasia in response to the changes in the bones. Because of Erdheim's influence, it was assumed by most pathologists that the parathyroid tumors encountered clinically were secondary to the bone disease. Schlagenhaufer, another pathologist, suggested that the reverse might be true—that the parathyroid tumor might be the cause of the bone changes.[80] This was in 1915. Not until 10 years later did a surgeon, Mandl of Vienna, test this concept.[74] After failing to benefit a patient with von Recklinghausen's disease of bone by engrafting parathyroid tissue, he explored the patient's neck, removing a parathyroid tumor. The patient's bones improved, and the parathyroid enlargement as the cause of the bone changes was established. Hyperparathyroidism and von Recklinghausen's disease of bone were considered as synonymous.

On the west side of the Atlantic, knowledge of disease of the parathyroids grew from the physiologic rather than pathologic point of view. This difference had far-reaching consequences since it led eventually to a broader recognition of the disease. The first step was the successful extraction of the hormone from the parathyroid glands of animals. Hanson and Collip independently, in 1924, succeeded in obtaining a potent extract.[60, 69] Collip showed that when the extract was injected into dogs in sufficient quantity the serum calcium rose, even doubled in concentration with thickening of the blood and the death of the animal. The serum phosphorus level was reduced, and he observed calcium pouring out in the urine. The same effects on blood levels of calcium and phosphorus and of calcium excretion were found by Aub in patients with lead poisoning.[70] He employed Collip's extract to hasten the elimination of lead from the bone. Thus, the effect of an excess of parathyroid hormone upon calcium and phosphorus metabolism was established in the experimental animal and in man.

The next step came when DuBois found the same metabolic abnormalities in a patient with a widespread bone disease.[68] He postulated overactivity of the parathyroid glands as the cause and sent the patient to Aub for further study.[53] The changes in blood levels of calcium and phosphorus and the outpouring of both through the kidney were confirmed. In April, 1926, 8 months after Mandl's operation in Vienna, surgical exploration of the parathyroid glands was undertaken at the Massachusetts General Hospital. Unfortunately, the Americans were unaware of the discoveries of the German pathologists and of Mandl, and the surgeon had little idea of what he should look for. No abnormal parathyroid gland was found. It was not until 6 years later that the parathyroid tumor was found in this patient.[58]

Blocked at the beginning by lack of knowledge of pathology, the physiologic point of view has led eventually to a more comprehensive view of the nature of hyperparathyroidism. Albright, student of both Aub and Erdheim, first realized that the renal stones frequently found in patients with hyperparathyroidism were also a complication of the metabolic disorder. The excess of calcium in the urine, he reasoned, must lead to the precipitation of calcium and the production of stones. Calcium metabolism was investigated in patients entering the hospital with renal stones. Soon the diagnosis of hyperparathyroidism was made in such patients, and as more were encountered, evidence of bone disease was frequently absent.[50] It was realized for the first time that bone disease was not an essential part of hyperparathyroidism. Both the bone changes and the renal stones presumably were complications of the disordered metabolism, not primary effects.

The first patient with kidney stones and no bone disease was operated on in 1932, starting a new era of hyperparathyroidism. Albright's

disclosure led to the recognition of 2 clinical forms of hyperparathyroidism—von Recklinghausen's disease of bone, and renal stones. Of the 2, the classic bone disease has proved to be the less common; it is the severe and neglected form (Table 1). The patients usually have renal stones as well. In the more common form with the renal complication, the majority of the patients show no bony abnormality. The disease generally is milder in intensity, and an adequate dietary intake of calcium presumably protects the bones from being depleted. Since some of the patients with the classic bone disease have no renal stones and many of the patients with renal stones have no demonstrable bone disease, from the clinical point of view both the bony depletion and the renal stones must be complications of the parathyroid activity rather than primary sites of hormone action. It is also logical to deduce that there must be a form of the disease in which neither bone changes nor renal stones are present. The diagnosis of such a form has been made twice and will be described under Diagnosis (Case 107).

Two further complications of hyperparathyroidism have been recognized recently—peptic ulcer and pancreatitis.[63, 77] It is probable that peptic ulcer is a clinically significant form of hyperparathyroidism, although the incidence of the glandular dysfunction is not as yet established among patients with peptic ulceration. Surgical relief of the hormonal activity has already been demonstrated to be followed by prompt healing of the peptic ulcer.

HYPOPARATHYROIDISM

Hypoparathyroidism is of 2 types—the spontaneously occurring disease and that in-

TABLE 1. CLUES TO DIAGNOSIS OF HYPERPARATHYROIDISM IN 230 CASES AT MASSACHUSETTS GENERAL HOSPITAL

DISEASE MANIFESTATION	NO. OF CASES
Renal stones	130
Bone disease	63
Peptic ulcer	19
Pancreatitis	4
Fatigue	4
Hypertension	3
Mental disturbance	2
Central nervous system signs	3
No symptoms	2

duced by the surgeon. The spontaneous disease is extremely rare. The first case was diagnosed and studied by Aub and Bauer in 1927. Very few have been reported. The symptoms are those of chronic unremitting tetany of low calcium origin. Marble stones have been postulated as an accompaniment but this postulate is unproved. Cataract is common.

The disease is easily confused with pseudo-hypoparathyroidism, a bizarre condition with frequent convulsions and characteristic physical changes, including a moon face, stubby fingers and toes. This condition has been described by Albright who believed that it was due to immunity to the parathyroid hormone.[51] The parathyroid glands are normal grossly and microscopically. It is probably a genetic or microsomal disease.

Hypoparathyroidism complicating thyroidectomy is due either to damage to the parathyroid glands or to their resection. If the glands have merely been bruised by operative trauma, the function will return, and the tetany will be of short duration. If 3 glands have been removed and the 4th one remains *in situ* undamaged, the tetany will also be of short duration. Only if the remaining 4th has been damaged or its life endangered by interference with its blood supply will the tetany endure. If parathyroid tissue remains intact, the hypoparathyroidism will be reduced gradually as the remnant undergoes hyperplasia. If there was insufficient tissue for adequate regeneration, the hypoparathyroidism may be permanent.

The tetany of hypoparathyroidism should be treated by a high calcium and low phosphorus intake. In the severe acute phase the calcium is to be given intravenously in order to preclude laryngeal spasm. Calcium chloride, because it is highly ionized, is most promptly available for the relief of tetany; calcium gluconate, more slowly. Calcium gluconate may be given intramuscularly.

If the tetany is mild, oral intake will be adequate. The most readily available calcium salt by mouth is the gluconate. Calcium lactate is absorbed slowly. It is believed that the addition of vitamin D to the diet is useful to increase the absorption of calcium from the intestinal tract. AT 10* is a variant of high

* Dihydrotachysterol.

vitamin D therapy. Overdose of either vitamin D or AT 10 may result in hypercalcemia and loss of calcium in the urine, with renal calcification and damage.

HYPERPARATHYROIDISM

Hyperparathyroidism is proving to be a not uncommon disease. Although it exists as a disease without complications, nevertheless from a practical point of view, it is diagnosed only by one of its complications. The recognized complications, in order of their frequency, are calcification in the urinary tract, decalcification of the bones, peptic ulceration of the duodenum or the stomach, and pancreatitis. Almost never is the diagnosis made by the presence of a tumor in the neck; this is because the parathyroid glands are so small that tumors of them are not large enough to be recognized by patient or examiner. The diagnosis is made only by keeping hyperparathyroidism in mind when caring for patients with renal and bone disease, peptic ulceration and pancreatitis. Before describing each form of the disease fully, it is essential to understand the pathologic physiology.

PATHOLOGIC PHYSIOLOGY

The parathyroid glands dominate calcium metabolism and influence strongly aspects of phosphorus metabolism. There are differences of opinion about the intimate function of the glands. Some think there is evidence for 2 hormones; others, only 1. The best evidence indicates that the hormone (or hormones) affects the integrity of bone, the sensitivity of nerves and the excretory function of both kidney and large bowel. The following are generally accepted as actions:

The calcium level of blood plasma and extracellular fluid is regulated by the parathyroid hormone. A decreasing function lowers the calcium level, and an excessive function induces a rise. No other endocrine gland exerts a comparable effect.

The calcium in the plasma and the extracellular fluid can be isolated into 2 fractions— the protein-bound and the free or ionized. It is about equally divided in the plasma, but because of its low protein concentration, the spinal fluid normally contains about half as much as the plasma. The parathyroid hormone presumably influences the concentration of the ionized fraction only. In diseases such as myeloma associated with an elevated plasma protein, the calcium of the plasma is elevated. Conversely, the plasma concentration is low in patients with hypoproteinemia. In diagnosing hyperparathyroidism it is always wise to measure the serum protein concentration simultaneously with that of the calcium.

It is believed that it is the ionized fraction that affects the sensitivity of nerves and muscles. A low level is associated with hyperactivity or tetany, and a high level with a reduced sensitivity, producing fatigue and lassitude. The Q-T interval of the electrocardiogram is lengthened when the calcium is low and shortened when elevated.

The inorganic phosphate level of the blood plasma and the extracellular fluid is affected in a reverse direction to that of calcium. The level goes down with increasing function and rises with less than normal activity. If renal damage is present the level may be normal or elevated in the presence of continued parathyroid hyperfunction.

Calcium excretion is raised by hyperfunction of the parathyroids. In the absence of renal impairment the increased excretion is through the kidney. The elimination from the bowel may be slightly decreased compared with the expected normal. It is the increased excretion of calcium through the kidney that may lead to supersaturation of the urine and deposition of calcium somewhere in the urinary tract. The deposition may start in the renal tubule, the kidney pelvis, the ureter, the bladder or the prostate. If oxalates are present, the stones may be of calcium oxalate. Most commonly they are of calcium phosphate, since there is always an excess of phosphate in the urine.

If the pathologic calcification is extensive in the renal tubules, impairment of renal function ensues. The urine has a fixed, low specific gravity, and the excretion of calcium may be reduced to the normal level or even less than normal. In the face of continued hyperparathyroidism the bowel takes over the excessive excretion of calcium. Therefore, in a patient whose blood level of calcium indicates hyperparathyroidism but whose renal excretion is within normal limits, the fecal calcium should

be measured if the urine specific gravity is continuously low.

Phosphorus excretion is increased by hyperparathyroidism. Excretion is through the kidneys, except when damage has occurred; then phosphorus is retained. With such retention, the level of phosphorus rises to normal or even above normal.

The action of the parathyroid hormone on bone has long been a question and is still unsettled. The European pathologists felt that the primary action of the hormone was in decalcifying bone with a resulting rise in the blood level. The presence of patients with hyperparathyroidism without demonstrable bone disease suggested that the effect upon bone might be secondary, since the primary force is a disturbance of the fluid equilibrium of calcium and phosphorus. Most recent studies by Krane, using radioactive calcium, indicate a rapid turnover of calcium in bone in hyperparathyroidism.[72] A turnover more rapid than normal also occurs in hyperthyroidism so the exact specificity in relation to the parathyroid hormone still remains to be elucidated.

The excessive loss of calcium through the kidney or from the bowel if the kidney is damaged, probably is paid for either from the skeleton or from the food intake. If the amount of calcium in the food is adequate to meet the extra loss, the skeleton remains normally calcified. If the intake is less than the excretion, that is, if the balance is negative, the calcium comes from the bones, and the bones slowly become depleted.

The alkaline phosphatase activity of the blood serum is not directly affected by the parathyroid hormone. In patients with hyperparathyroidism and no bone disease, the activity is within normal limits. Only when there is bony depletion with active regeneration is the phosphatase elevated. The activity is proportionate to the osteogenesis and is a good indicator of the amount of calcium which the skeleton will absorb immediately following operation. Patients with a high activity (10 Bodansky units or more) are to be warned that after operation they will be prone to the tetany of the recalcification period. Such patients need large amounts of calcium postoperatively.

No physiologic reciprocating mechanism has

been established for the parathyroid glands comparable with that of the thyroid and the anterior pituitary, or the adrenal cortex and the anterior pituitary. There is suggestive evidence that the parathyroid glands respond with increased activity if the blood calcium level falls below normal, that the parathyroid balance is influenced by blood calcium level much as the islet cells of the pancreas are to changes in blood sugar level. There are also indications that at least a part of the parathyroid effect on both calcium and phosphorus levels is through control of renal function. However, there is no sound evidence that the kidney or any other organ secretes a counterbalancing hormone.

The absence of evidence of a reciprocating force leaves no clue regarding the etiology of hyperparathyroidism. A secondary form is known to be the sequel of chronic renal disease,[56] but a history of pre-existing renal disease is seldom disclosed in patients with hyperparathyroidism of the primary type.

ANATOMIC PATHOLOGY

Demonstrable anatomic changes of hyperparathyroidism are confined to the parathyroid glands, the bones, and certain tissues which become pathologically calcified.

THE PARATHYROIDS

Proof of the presence of hyperparathyroidism depends upon finding a clearly defined abnormality in one or more of the parathyroid glands. Hyperplasias involving all of the glands and neoplasias involving one or more have been found.[54, 57] Neoplasias are the more common (see Table 2).

Neoplasia. Hypersecreting neoplasms of the parathyroid glands are both benign and ma-

TABLE 2. PATHOLOGIC TYPES OF
HYPERFUNCTIONING TISSUE IN
HYPERPARATHYROIDISM
MASSACHUSETTS GENERAL HOSPITAL SERIES

ADENOMA (BENIGN NEOPLASIA)		193
1. Single Adenoma	183	
2. Double Adenoma	10	
CARCINOMA		9
HYPERPLASIA		28
1. Clear Cell	15	
2. Chief Cell	13	
TOTAL		230

lignant. The benign form, an adenoma, is found in nearly 90 per cent of patients with hyperparathyroidism. In approximately 90 per cent of the cases due to adenoma only one gland is affected. In the other 10 per cent, 2 adenomas have been found, 1 in each of 2 glands. Often there is considerable disparity in size between the 2 adenomas.

The cell type is variable, the chief cell being the commonest variety. Usually adenomas are of a single cell type. The clear cells have not constituted an entire adenoma, although they may appear here and there in either a chief cell or an oxyphil cell adenoma.

Carcinoma is an occasional form. It was encountered in 9 of 230 cases.[64, 78] Since 2 of these patients were referred after establishment of the diagnosis of carcinoma, it is probable that the incidence is not over 3 per cent. The growths are sluggish, the cells well differentiated. All of the primary tumors have been large. They have been locally invasive. They spread both by the lymphatics and the blood stream. After local eradication of the tumor, a metastasis may carry on hyperfunction. A single metastasis in the liver has been found in at least 2 patients at autopsy.[49, 64] If the capsule of the tumor is broken at the time of the initial resection, there is a high incidence of seeding throughout the wound. Local recurrence is stubborn.

In an occasional case the malignant process may be a degeneration of a benign adenoma. A carcinoma was found growing in one area of an adenoma, invading the adenoma. A benign adenoma was found subsequently in this same patient in a parathyroid gland of the opposite side of the neck.[64] It too was associated with hyperfunction.

Hyperplasia. The hyperplasias associated with hyperparathyroidism are both primary and secondary. Of the primary type, clear cell hyperplasia was recognized initially and was at first thought to be the more common.[57]

Clear cell hyperplasia of the parathyroid glands is the type of hyperplasia comparable with that of the thyroid in Graves's disease. In contrast with disease of the thyroid, it is found less often than the neoplastic form, constituting slightly less than 10 per cent of all the patients. The size and the configuration of the clear cells is so characteristic that generally these hyperplasias can be recognized on frozen section. The cells are huge compared with the chief cell of the normal gland or adenoma and for this reason Castleman adds the term hypertrophy to this type.[55] The cells are usually concentrically arranged with basally oriented nuclei. At first sight, the concentric grouping suggests follicles of thyroid without any colloid in the center. Also, the huge clear cells have been mistaken for those of renal cell carcinoma.

Clear cell hyperplasias are usually recognizable grossly. They are a darker chocolate brown than the adenoma; they have an irregular surface, frequently with pseudopod projections. The upper pair is nearly always larger than the lower.[55]

Chief cell hyperplasia, as a cause of primary hyperparathyroidism, is a newcomer to the field of parathyroid pathology. It was not encountered until the 142nd case at the Massachusetts General Hospital. Its exact nature remains to be established. Each of the enlargements resembles a benign adenoma. However, all of the glands are so characteristically involved in the process that it is difficult to assume that each constitutes a separate adenoma. In one of the 13 patients of this type there were 5 such enlargements, the 1st case with 5 enlarged parathyroids on record. In this case 4 were found at the first operation. Resection of 3 and $\frac{2}{3}$ of the 4th failed to relieve the hyperparathyroidism. Search of the mediastinum at a 2nd operation disclosed a 5th within the thymic capsule. It weighed 1.9 Gm., as much as the previous 4 together. Its resection was followed by a prompt drop of the calcium level to below normal with reversion of the calcium balance (Case 172).

The 13 patients with chief cell hyperplasia consist of 2 clinical groups. Ten were of the usual clinical types: 1 with osteoporosis and 9 with renal complications. However the parathyroid enlargements were much bigger than the relatively mild chief cell hyperplasia found secondary to renal disease or in vitamin D deficiency. The other 3 patients had associated endocrine abnormalities: an older man a pituitary enlargement; his daughter a pancreatic islet-cell adenoma; and the 3rd was a woman who bore her only child in the middle of a many-year period of amenorrhea.

Secondary chief cell hyperplasia is found in patients with long-standing chronic nephritis and in an occasional patient with rickets and osteomalacia.[56] The parathyroid enlargement is much less than in the previous group. The enlargements are bulbous and vascular and usually not more than 4 to 5 times the size of the normal gland.

THE BONES

The resorption of calcium from the bones under an excessive action of the parathyroid hormone results in 2 general types of anatomic change: simple decalcification and the classic disease of von Recklinghausen. In the first, the decalcification is diffuse, all bones sharing to some degree. It may be mild and presumably is present more often than is recognized because of the difficulty of diagnosis, so considerable is the variation in density of normal bones. Occasionally, the decalcification is sufficient to lead to pathologic fractures. The vertebral bodies of the thorax and the lumbar region not infrequently crumple, giving the fishbone type of vertebral body. At times, the bones of the feet also give way under the weight of the body.

The classic type of bone disease described by von Recklinghausen, *osteodystrophia fibrosa* or *osteitis fibrosa cystica generalisata*, is so characteristic that there is no mistaking it by roentgenogram or often by physical examination. In addition to a generalized demineralization, cysts and giant cell tumors are diffusely distributed throughout the skeleton. The cysts apparently start in the marrow and swell with cortical necrosis and pathologic fracture. The giant cell tumors probably start in the bone trabeculae. The microscopic picture of the trabeculae is diagnostic. In an orderly arrangement on one side there is active bone resorption with large numbers of osteoclasts, and here and there one finds osteoclastomata. On the opposite side there is active bone regeneration.

The giant cell tumors appear to be adenomas of the giant cell osteoplasts. There may be a hundred or more distributed throughout the skeleton. They often attain considerable size. In one patient, there were 2 the size of grapefruit, 1 on either side of the pelvis.

The tumors are distinguishable microscopically from the single giant cell tumors occasionally found in adolescence. Although the latter may be malignant, no case of malignancy developing in the giant cell tumors of hyperparathyroidism has been recorded. This is peculiar, because the cellular activity is often intense.

Following correction of the hyperparathyroidism, the giant cell tumors resolve quickly. First, they lose their vascularity with disappearance of the majority of the giant cells in a week. By 2 weeks, there are numerous islands of calcification. By 2 years, all evidence of the former tumor may have been eradicated by bone growth and re-formation of the normal bony contours. The vacuoles of the cysts, in contrast, do not recalcify, but the cortex surrounding the original cystic area is thickened.

The marrow is characteristically fibrosed. An anemia is usually present when the bone disease is advanced; it is believed to be due to the fibrous displacement of the cellular marrow. The anemia disappears spontaneously following correction of the glandular overactivity.

PATHOLOGIC CALCIFICATION

During the active phase of hyperparathyroidism, pathologic calcification occurs in a number of organs and tissues. The most common is the kidney. It is believed to be due to supersaturation of the urine with calcium, but the deposition of calcium occurs not only within the lumen of the tubule but also in the surrounding tubular cells. There are calcium-containing casts in the tubules. Stones are formed throughout the urinary tract.

Small, stonelike bodies form in the prostate, the pancreas and the salivary glands. Whether or not these are due to an increased concentration of calcium in the secretions of these glands has not been demonstrated.

Pathologic calcification also occurs in a number of other tissues, principally the gastric mucosa in the acid-secreting cells. There is deposition of calcium in the conjunctivae and the cornea of the eye.[59, 81] These deposits are in contrast with the cataracts which form in hypoparathyroidism. Thick calcification of the capsule of the parathyroid adenoma itself has been encountered in 2 instances.[58]

DIAGNOSIS

It is rarely possible to make a diagnosis of hyperparathyroidism before the onset of one of its complications. Although an excess of the hormone offsets the calcium equilibrium and affects the nervous system, the symptoms produced are so common or so easily mistaken for other conditions that the diagnosis has been made only twice on these alone. With the hormone overactivity and elevated calcium level, neuromuscular tension is decreased. Patients commonly feel fatigued. Their muscles and joints are relaxed. Their feet flop along, and they trip more easily. They are subject to backaches, presumably being unable to hold themselves erect. They may notice some mental perturbation, perhaps irritation, or failure to concentrate. In short, all these symptoms are so common among the population that they are quite uncharacteristic. Yet, the diagnosis has been made twice when these were the sole symptoms. The following case is illuminating.

Case 107. A man, aged 45, was seen first by Dr. Resnick of Stamford, Conn., in November, 1949. Dr. Resnick made a diagnosis of hyperparathyroidism in the following manner.

A resident of suburban New York, the patient had a desk job in the Navy in Washington, D. C. during World War II. He felt lackadaisical, without his usual energy. He ascribed this to the uprooting of his wartime job. With the cessation of hostilities, he returned to his old life. He continued to feel out of sorts and was checked over by his physician in New York. All tests were negative. A prominent right thyroid lobe was felt, and a right thyroidectomy was carried out in 1946. No nodule was found. The right lobe was larger than the left; therefore, part was resected. For 3 months following operation he felt better, then lapsed back into his previous state. He described his feelings as nothing in particular, simply no energy. Before World War II, when he returned home from work he repaired screen doors, did odd jobs about the house, and frequently played tennis. Now when he returned home all he wanted to do was sit and do nothing.

Discouraged, in 1949 he changed doctors. Dr. Resnick too found nothing on physical examination, but his laboratory routine included the Sulkowitch test for calcium content of the urine. The test was 3+, a definitely elevated concentration. Dr. Resnick asked the patient to return, and the check test was the same. He then obtained a fasting blood for calcium and phosphorus levels. The day following, in the late afternoon, the laboratory reported 12.0 mg. and 2.5 mg. per 100 cc., respectively. He intended to recall the patient for a check blood analysis.

That very night the patient was awakened by severe left flank colic and called Dr. Resnick who told the patient that he had a left ureteral calculus and to go directly to the hospital.

A stone passed spontaneously. The blood calcium and phosphorus levels were persistently altered. The patient was referred to the Massachusetts General Hospital for parathyroid exploration. On December 20, 1949, a single benign adenoma was excised. The patient's phosphorus and calcium metabolisms returned promptly to normal. In 3 months the patient had noticed a return of well-being and has remained well during the ensuing years.

Examination of the slides of the thyroid tissues resected in 1946 revealed normal thyroid gland. Presumably the usual preponderance of the right thyroid lobe, perhaps exaggerated in this patient, had been mistaken on physical examination and at operation as representing an abnormality.

Polydipsia and polyuria are occasionally present. In 4 of the Massachusetts General Hospital patients, a diagnosis of diabetes insipidus had been entertained. Apparently these symptoms are occasioned by the increased excretion of calcium and the need for water. They are more suggestive than those due to muscular relaxation.

For practical purposes, the presence of a complication is needed to call attention to the diagnosis. The deposition of calcium in the renal tract is the commonest source of symptoms. In all patients with renal stones, or calcification in the region of the kidneys and the prostate, hyperparathyroidism is to be considered. In the population served by the Massachusetts General Hospital, hyperparathyroidism constitutes approximately 5 to 8 per cent of all renal tract stones. Confirmation of the diagnosis depends upon careful chemical analysis and metabolic study. Many of the patients with renal stones have mild or borderline degrees of the disease. Therefore, the blood levels are borderline and need to be repeated at intervals, perhaps of weeks. It must be borne in mind that many endocrine diseases fluctuate in intensity with exacerbations and remissions. The number of cases that have been diagnosed at the Massachusetts General Hospital and more recently by Keating at the Mayo Clinic depend upon painstaking effort on the part of the internist

with repeated observation of the patients.[61, 71] In addition to the blood levels, the calcium excretion must be measured on a controlled diet. In view of the usual absence of bone disease, particularly in the mild cases, the phosphatase level of the blood is normal and is of no help diagnostically. Serum protein is always to be measured for correction of the calcium level if the protein concentration is low.

Chemical analysis of the stone is also helpful if a stone is available. Calcium phosphate is the commonest; calcium oxalate stones constitute approximately 10 per cent. The absence of calcium is against hyperparathyroidism.

The presence of decalcification is also helpful. Hyperthyroidism and Cushing's disease must be excluded, since they too decalcify the skeleton. Cushing's disease also causes renal stone. However, the thyroid and adrenal diseases do not disturb the blood levels of either calcium or phosphorus.

The classic form of bone disease can be diagnosed by roentgenogram alone. In the typical advanced case, chemical confirmation really is not needed. The bone disease is distributed throughout the skeleton and more or less evenly. Fibrous dysplasia of the bone, which in any one bone may give a picture mimicking exactly hyperparathyroidism, is distributed irregularly throughout the skeleton, following the distribution of peripheral nerves. Roentgenograms of sufficient areas of the skeleton must be taken in all patients to make sure that the disease is not a localized one. No other endocrine disease gives the picture of diffuse calcification with cysts and giant cell tumors.

Diffuse osteoporosis without cysts and giant cell tumors has a much wider differential diagnosis. It can be associated with hyperthyroidism, Cushing's disease and older patients, particularly women past the menopause. Hyperparathyroidism is the sole one of these endocrine conditions affecting the blood levels of calcium and phosphorus. Acromegaly affects the skeleton, producing some diffuse osteoporosis with a negative calcium balance. However, it does not simulate the classic bone disease of hyperparathyroidism. The overgrowth of the extremities of bones, and the widening of the jaw should not be mistaken for the resorption and the fracture

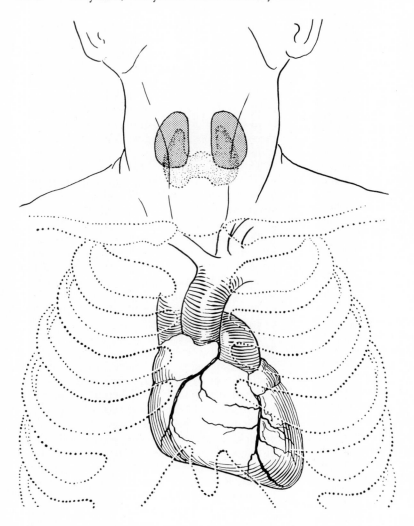

FIG. 26-4. Surgical anatomy. Lateral and anterior views of the upper parathyroid (IV) due to embryology. The shading shows the extent of possible positions of the normal upper parathyroids due to differences in development during fetal life. The limited area facilitates the surgical identification of these parathyroids. (Cope, O.: Ann. Surg. *114*:706)

of the terminal phalanges of the fingers and the loss of lamina dura and vacuolization of the jaws seen in hyperparathyroidism.

Patients with peptic ulcers of the duodenum and the stomach also should be screened for hyperparathyroidism;[77] likewise patients with acute pancreatitis.[63] The most difficult differential diagnosis lies in patients with peptic ulceration and renal calcification who have received a high calcium and alkali intake. The renal damage is much like that encountered with primary hyperparathyroidism and secondary renal damage with a normal or elevated phosphorus level of the blood. Differential diagnosis lies in evaluation of the calcium level of the blood and the fecal calcium excretion. In hyperparathyroidism both are elevated.

TREATMENT

Medical and irradiation therapies of hyperparathyroidism have not proved to be successful. A high calcium diet has spared the skeleton but has ruined the kidneys. No antiparathyroid drug has emerged, and the high incidence of neoplasia in parathyroid disease, in contrast with that of the thyroid, lessens the advisability of such a therapy, were it available.

Irradiation too has failed. The tumors perhaps are radioresistant, but also their variable position and number make it hard to focus sufficient irradiation upon the offending glands.

The treatment of hyperparathyroidism is still surgical.[62] It must be precise to meet the

FIGURE 26-4
(*Continued*)

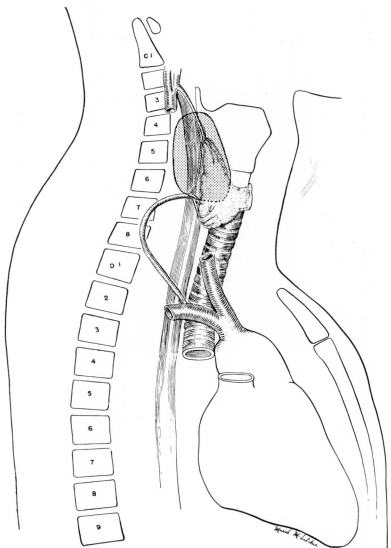

challenge of the diagnostician. The problems involve the nature, the number, the site and the size of the tumors.

It is essential to recognize the nature of the offending glands. The surgeon must keep in mind 7 types of glands. Prompt recognition of the pathologic type expedites the exploration and the judgment concerning resection.

First comes the normal gland; it must not be resected. It varies considerably in size and shape. The gland is soft and conforms to its surroundings. It is like a flat pancake when on the surface of the thyroid but, caught in a sulcus, it may be triangular or bulbous. It varies normally in color according to age. In children and older people it is browner because it contains less fat. With adolescence and early adult life, there is a larger proportion of fat to epithelial tissue, and the glands are yellower. Maximum fatty infiltration is found in people 30 to 35 years of age.

Second is the atrophic parathyroid. When the disease is of long standing and due to a single adenoma, the other 3 parathyroids, although not diseased, are not really normal. They are atrophic and therefore yellower than

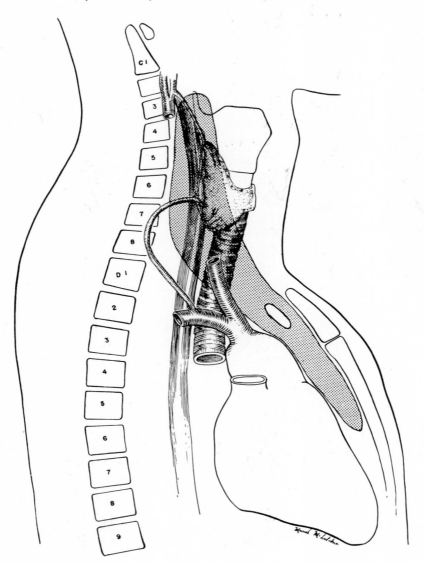

Fig. 26-5. Surgical anatomy. Lateral and anterior views of lower parathyroid (III) due to embryology. The shading shows the extent of possible positions of the normal lower parathyroids due to differences in development during fetal life. The extensive area accounts for the surgical difficulty frequently encountered in identifying these glands. The glands may lie anterior or posterior to the left innominate vein. (Cope, O.: Ann. Surg. 114:706)

the normal gland. They may be hard to see in the fatty tissue and recognizable only by their form and vascular pattern rather than by their color. They too are not to be damaged or resected. An atrophic parathyroid, when recognized as the first gland found, indicates that an adenoma must be present in 1 or 2 of the others.

Next are the pathologic glands. Their types have been described under Anatomic Pathology. Surgically, the following aspects are to be kept in mind. The adenoma is the commonest. Grossly, it is smooth, vascular, reddish brown and contains no fat. If the adenoma is only 1 or 2 mm. in diameter, there may be a rim of normal tissue surrounding it or a piece at one pole. Two adenomas are found in 10 per cent of the patients having the adenoma type. The importance of size will be described below.

The clear cell hypertrophy and hyperplasia is identified by its darker chocolate color and by the irregularity of its surface and pseudopod projection. It is essential in this pathologic type to identify all 4 glands. Generally, it is wise not to remove any one until all 4 have been found. Three of the enlargements should be resected, and a small piece of the 4th left

FIGURE 26-5
(*Continued*)

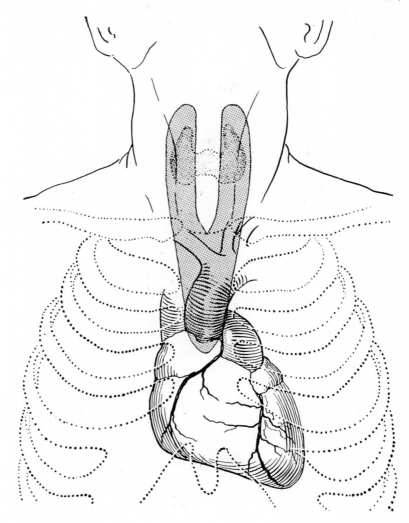

with its blood supply intact. A 40 to 100 mg. remnant has sufficed in 14 of the patients of the Massachusetts General Hospital series. It is sound practice to use the most accessible enlargement for the subtotal resection so that if too large a remnant is left and there is residual hyperparathyroidism, it can be uncovered readily at a secondary operation.

Realization that the hypertrophied upper gland usually is considerably larger than the lower should facilitate the search for a missing enlargement. If the upper has not been found in the usual position, it will have been displaced downward and posteriorly. If the lower is the missing gland, the neck having been searched, it will lie in the anterior mediastinum.

The chief cell hyperplasias resemble the adenomas. The clue that the patient has this type of the disease lies in finding 2 enlargements when the first 2 parathyroids have been identified. Then the search should be continued until an undiseased gland is found or until all 4 hyperplastic glands have been uncovered. The same principle as that used for the hypertrophied glands applies to the subtotal resection.

In order to establish the diagnosis of hyperparathyroidism, sometimes it is wise to explore the parathyroids in patients in whom the character of the disease is not clear. Trouble in differential diagnosis frequently lies between patients having minimal primary hyperparathyroidism with severe renal impair-

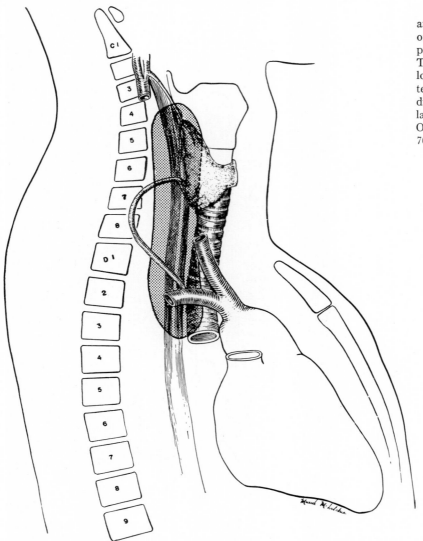

FIG. 26-6. Surgical anatomy. Lateral view of enlarged upper parathyroid (IV). The area of embryologic occurrence is extended by downward displacement of enlarged glands. (Cope, O.: Ann. Surg. *114*: 706)

ment and patients with primary nephritis with secondary hyperparathyroidism. In this latter condition, the parathyroid enlargements, the secondary chief cell hyperplasias, are only 4 to 5 times as large as the normal gland, much smaller than the primary chief cell hyperplasias. The importance of size is well illustrated.

The surgeon should be suspicious of carcinoma if a single tumor is unexpectedly large for the degree of the disease and also if it is stuck. All the carcinomas encountered at the Massachusetts General Hospital have been encased by a fibrous chronic inflammatory re-

action. This reaction has not been encountered surrounding a benign adenoma or hyperplasia and therefore is characteristic.

The normal parathyroid glands may be distributed over a wide area of the neck and the mediastinum, and when enlarged they may be shoved to a new position. The upper pair usually have the more confined distribution; therefore, they are the easier pair to isolate. Embryologically, the upper pair arise from the 4th branchial cleft along with the thyroid anlage.[75] They descend during embryonic life, together with the thyroid, to their final position in the neck. These upper glands are gen-

FIG. 26-7. Surgical anatomy. Lateral view of enlarged parathyroids (III) displaced from their original position in the neck. Glands having had embryologic position posterior to thyroid after enlargement may be displaced into the posterior mediastinum; those having had embryologic position caudal to thyroid in a more anterior plane may be displaced into the anterior superior mediastinum. (Cope, O.: Ann. Surg. *114*:706)

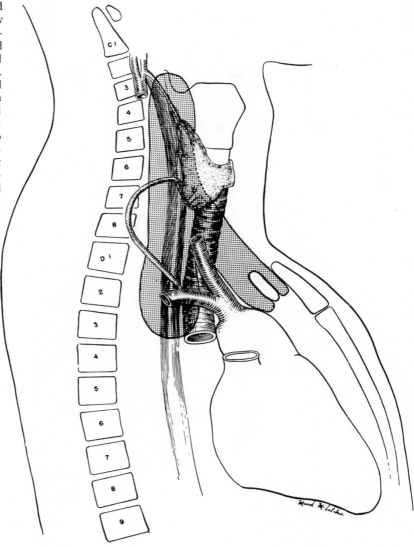

erally in close association with the lateral thyroid lobes.

When enlarged, the gland may be displaced from its final embryologic position. The parathyroid gland is attached solely by its vascular pedicle. It does not have a fibrous attachment to the trachea and the cricoid cartilage comparable with that by which the thyroid gland is held firmly in place. As it enlarges and bulges out, it is pushed by the motion of the thyroid on swallowing and also sucked down by negative intrathoracic pressure. It drags its vascular pedicle with it. Some-

times the upper gland is caught on the recurrent nerve or on a branch of the inferior thyroid artery. When it does move past the inferior thyroid artery, generally it is drawn posteriorly into the posterior superior mediastinum. The upper gland is to be found anywhere from above the upper pole of the thyroid, the length of the thyroid lobe, and down into the posterior superior mediastinum.

The lower pair of parathyroids normally have a wider distribution. They arise from the 3rd branchial cleft along with the thymus and descend with the thymus. Usually they

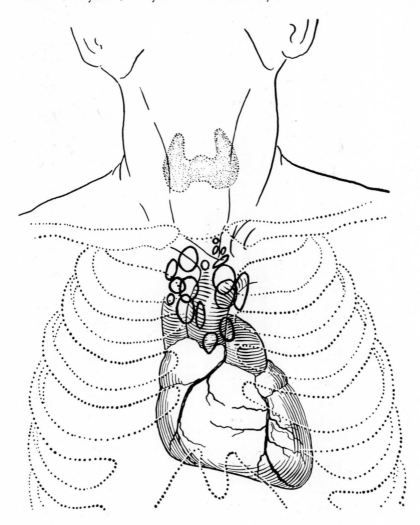

FIG. 26-8. Surgical anatomy. The position and the size of the parathyroid adenomata recovered from the anterior mediastinum in 17 patients.

stop off somewhere behind the thyroid gland or at the lower pole of the thyroid, the thymus continuing its descent. Sometimes they pass further down with the thymus into the anterior superior mediastinum. In 10 per cent of normal persons, one or more of the lower parathyroids is in the anterior mediastinum, and frequently one or more is within the thymic capsule, usually near the upper end of the tongue of thymus which stretches up from the body toward the neck.

The lower gland when enlarged also may be displaced by swallowing and suction into the chest. Because of its more anterior position at the level of the lower pole of the thyroid, it may be displaced into the anterior mediastinum. It lies usually in front of the

innominate vein, but like the thymus it also may lie posterior to the innominate vein. Because of their close association with the thymus, Norris has suggested that this pair should be called the *parathymus gland*. The lower pair of parathyroids has a considerably wider distribution and are found anywhere from the upper pole of the thyroid into the anterior mediastinum to a point as low as the pericardium.

The size of the tumor often directs surgical management. It has been referred to already in relation to carcinoma and secondary chief cell hyperplasia. It is perhaps most significant in relation to the adenoma type. Here, the size of the adenoma is roughly proportionate to the intensity of the disease. In the patients with the classic type of bone disease with a calcium level of 14 mg. or higher, and due to a single adenoma, the adenoma is recognized readily, since it will be at least 2 cm. in diameter and may be considerably larger. In the patients with mild disease, particularly those with the renal stones and no bone disease, the adenoma may be small, no larger than the normal gland itself. The volume of the hyperplasias also varies somewhat with the intensity of the disease, although the total volume of tissue in the primary hyperplasias is greater for the degree of the disease than those due to an adenoma. If a patient has a moderate or severe degree of the disease and the adenoma found is a small one, search should be continued until all 4 glands have been identified in order to exclude the presence of a second adenoma. Because of the large variation in size from case to case, if an adenoma has been found on the first side of the neck explored, generally it is wise to identify the other gland on that side before terminating the operation to make certain that it does not contain a second adenoma.

The number of parathyroids for practical surgical purposes is assumed to be 4. On embryologic grounds, Norris doubts that there can be more than 4 in over 2 to 3 per cent of normal people. In those reports claiming 6 and many more, the identification is questionable. In a careful series of dissections at the postmortem table, the author identified 5 glands in 2 of 30 cases. In only 2 patients has it been necessary to invoke the presence of a 5th gland to settle satisfactorily the hyperparathyroidism (see Case 172 under Anatomic Pathology). The surgeon never should be content that he has excluded disease if he has found only 3 normal-appearing glands.

The first exploration is the golden opportunity to identify parathyroid tissue. Scarring always makes re-exploration more difficult.

It is obvious that the surgeon must be tutored in what parathyroids look like before embarking on a parathyroid exploration. Many cases technically are easy, but a minority are difficult, and in a number of patients the surgeon has had to retreat and let somebody else try again. The postmortem room is a place in which the surgeon can tutor himself. The parathyroid glands of people recently dead are remarkably like the living, and their

lurking places become familiar to the surgeon who goes after them.

The tutored surgeon approaches the exploration with care and restraint. His hemostasis is painstaking, because only a little blood may so discolor the areolar and fatty tissues that he may overlook an undiseased gland or small tumor.

A swallow of barium sometimes reveals a nick on one side of the esophagus if a large enough mass is pressing against it. If no such evidence is available to indicate where an enlargement may be, where does the surgeon start? In the neck, obviously, but on which side? The number of tumors has been equal on the 2 sides in the Massachusetts General Hospital series and as many in the upper as in the lower gland. In choosing the side to start on, it has seemed wise to palpate the thyroid regions after the skin and the platysmal flaps have been elevated. Due allowance is to be made for the normally larger right thyroid lobes (see Case 107 under Diagnosis).

Sometimes the parathyroid exploration should be divided into 2 stages. This is the case if the search in the neck has been prolonged by scarring of a previous operation or if the offending gland is judged to be in the anterior mediastinum. It is not possible to see very far into the anterior mediastinum from a collar thyroid incision in the neck, and blind dissection is not likely to turn out the desired gland.

REFERENCES

THYROID

1. Astwood, E. B. Treatment of hyperthyroidism with thiourea and thiouracil, J.A.M.A. *122*:78, 1943.
2. Astwood, E. B., Greer, M. A., and Ettlinger, M. G.: The antithyroid factor of yellow turnip, Science *107*:631, 1949.
3. Basedow, von, C. A.: Exophthalmos durch Hypertrophie des Zellgewebes in der Augenhöhle, Wchnschr. ges. Heilk. *6*:197, 1840.
4. Beahrs, O. H., Pemberton, J. de J., and Black, B. M.: Nodular goiter and malignant lesions of thyroid gland, J. Clin. Endocrinol. *11*:1157, 1951.
5. Bielschowsky, F.: Experimental nodular goitre, Brit. J. Exper. Path. *26*:270, 1945.
6. Bielschowsky, F., Griesbach, W. E., Hall, W. H., Kennedy, T. H., and Purves, H. D.:

Studies on experimental goitre: transplantability of experimental thyroid tumours of rat, Brit. J. Cancer *3*:541, 1949.

7. Blumgart, H. L., Freedberg, A. S., and Kurland, G. S.: The treatment of incapacitated euthyroid cardiac patients by producing hypothyroidism with radioactive iodine, New England J. Med. *245*:83, 1951.

8. Boas, N. F., and Ober, W. B.: Hereditary exophthalmic goitre—report of 11 cases in one family, J. Clin. Endocrinol. *6*:575, 1946.

9. Chapman, E. M., and Maloof, F.: The use of radioactive iodine in the diagnosis and treatment of hyperthyroidism: 10 years' experience, Medicine *34*:261, 1955.

10. Cope, O.: Diseases of the thyroid gland, New England J. Med. *246*:368, 408, 451, 1952.

11. ———: The surgery of the thyroid *in* Means, J. H.: The Thyroid and Its Diseases, Ed. 2, pp. 507-509, Philadelphia, Lippincott, 1948.

12. Cope, O., and Barnes, B. A.: Nodular goiter: the 13 year experience in the treatment of 160 cases with desiccated thyroid. In press.

13. Cope, O., Dobyns, B. M., Hamlin, E., Jr., and Hopkirk, J.: What thyroid nodules are to be feared, J. Clin. Endocrinol. *9*:1012, 1949.

14. Cope, O., and Raker, J. W.: Cushing's disease: the surgical experience in the care of 46 cases, New England J. Med. *253*:119, 165, 1955.

15. Dobyns, B. M.: Present concepts of pathologic physiology of exophthalmos, J. Clin. Endocrinol. *10*:1202, 1950.

16. Graves, R. J.: Clinical lectures, London M. & S. J. (Part II) *7*:516, 1835.

17. Griesbach, W. E., Kennedy, T. H., and Purves, H. D.: Studies on experimental goitre: thyroid adenomata in rats on Brassica seed diet, Brit. J. Exper. Path. *26*:18, 1945.

18. Halsted, W. S.: Surgical Papers, The Operative Story of Goitre: The Author's Operation, vol. 2, p. 257, Baltimore, Johns Hopkins Press, 1924.

18a. Harris, G. W., and Woods, J. W.: The effect of electrical stimulation of the hypothalamus or pituitary gland on thyroid activity, J. Physiol. *143*:246, 1958.

19. Hertz, S., and Roberts, A.: Radioactive iodine in the study of thyroid physiology; VII. The use of radioactive iodine therapy in hyperthyroidism, J.A.M.A. *131*:81, 1946.

20. Lidz, T., and Whitehorn, J. C.: Psychiatric problems in thyroid clinic, J.A.M.A. *139*:698, 1949.

21. Marine, D.: The anatomic and physiologic effects of iodine on the thyroid gland of exophthalmic goiter, J.A.M.A. *59*:325, 1912.

22. Marine, D., and Kimball, O. P.: The prevention of simple goiter in man, J. Lab. & Clin. Med. *3*:40, 1917.

23. Means, J. H.: The Thyroid and Its Diseases, ed. 2, pp. 415-423, Philadelphia, Lippincott, 1948.

24. Money, W. L., and Rawson, R. W.: Experimental production of thyroid tumors in rat exposed to prolonged treatment with thiouracil, Cancer *3*:321, 1950.

25. Morris, H. P., Dalton, A. J., and Green, C. D.: Malignant thyroid tumors occurring in mouse after prolonged hormonal imbalance during ingestion of thiouracil, J. Clin. Endocrinol. *11*:1281, 1951.

26. Parry, C. H.: Collections from the Unpublished Papers of the Late Caleb Hilliel Parry, vol. 2, p. 111, London, 1825.

27. Paschkis, K. E., Cantarow, A., and Stasney, J.: Influence of thiouracil on carcinoma induced by 2-acetaminofluorene, Cancer Res. *8*:257, 1948.

28. Plummer, H. S.: Results of administering iodine to patients having exophthalmic goiter, J.A.M.A. *80*:1955, 1923.

29. Richardson, K. C., and Young, F. G.: Histology of diabetes induced in dogs by injection of anterior-pituitary extracts, Lancet *1*:1098, 1938.

30. Rienhoff, W. F., Jr.: Involutional or regressive changes in the thyroid gland in cases of exophthalmic goiter and their relation to the origin of the so-called adenomas, Arch. Surg. *13*:391, 1926.

31. Russfield, A. B.: Histology of the human hypophysis in thyroid disease—hypothyroidism, hyperthyroidism and cancer, J. Clin. Endocrinol. *15*:1393, 1955.

32. Schlesinger, M., Gargill, S. L., and Saxe, I. H.: Studies in nodular goiter; I. Incidence of thyroid nodules in routine necropsies in a non goitrous region, J.A.M.A. *110*:1638, 1938.

33. Thompson, W. O., and Thompson, P. K.: Treatment of toxic goiter by irradiation of pituitary, J. Clin. Invest. *23*:951, 1944.

34. Warren, S., and Meissner, W. A.: Tumors of the thyroid gland *in* Atlas of Tumor Pathology, Washington, D. C., Armed Forces Institute of Pathology, 1953.

THYMUS

35. Blalock, A.: Thymectomy in the treatment of myasthenia gravis; report of 20 cases, J. Thoracic Surg. *13*:316, 1944.

36. Blalock, A., Mason, M. F., Morgan, H. J.,

and Riven, S. S.: Myasthenia gravis and tumors of the thymic region, Ann. Surg. *110*:544, 1939.

37. Dougherty, T. F.: Effect of hormones on lymphatic tissue, Physiol. Rev. *32*:379, 1952.

38. Eaton, L. M., and Clagett, O. T.: Thymectomy in the treatment of myasthenia gravis; results in 72 cases compared with 142 control cases, J.A.M.A. *142*:963, 1950.

39. Keynes, G.: The results of thymectomy in myasthenia gravis, Brit. M.J. *2*:611, 1949.

40. Laquer, and Weigert: Beiträge zur Lehre von der Erb'schen Krankheit, Neurol. Centralbl. *20*:594, 1901.

41. Mella, H.: Irradiation of the thymus in myasthenia gravis, M. Clin. North America *7*:939, 1923.

42. Norris, E. H.: The morphogenesis and histogenesis of the thymus gland in man: in which the origin of the Hassall's corpuscles of the human thymus is discovered, Contrib. Embryol., no. 166, pp. 191-207, May 31, 1938.

43. ———: The parathyroid glands and the lateral thyroid in man: their morphogenesis, topographic anatomy and prenatal growth, Contrib. Embryol., no. 159, pp. 249-294, January 30, 1937.

44. Pierchalla, L.: Über die Röntgenbehandlung der hyperplastischen Thymus bei Myasthenia pseudoparalytica, Therap. Halbmonatsch. Heft *16*:504, 1921.

45. Sauerbruch, F.: Chirurgie der Brustorgane: Die Chirurgie des Thymus, vol. 2, pp. 512-514, Berlin, Springer, 1925.

46. Schwab, R. S., and Viets, H. R.: Thymectomy in myasthenia gravis (Scientific Exhibit), Interim Session of the A. M. A., Boston, Mass., Nov. 29—Dec. 2, 1955.

47. Soffer, I. J., Gabrilove, J. L., Laqueur, H. P., Volterra, M., Jacobs, M. D., and Sussman, M. L.: The effects of anterior pituitary adrenocorticotropic hormone (ACTH) in myasthenia gravis with tumor of the thymus, J. Mount Sinai Hosp. *15*:73, 1948.

48. Torda, C., and Wolff, H. G.: Effects of adrenocorticotrophic hormone on neuromuscular function in patients with myasthenia gravis, Proc. Soc. Exper. Biol. & Med. *71*:432, 1949.

PARATHYROID GLANDS

49. Albertini, von, A., Koller, F., and Gaiser, H.: Functioning parathyroid tumor with liver metastasis, Acta endocrinol. *12*:289, 1953.

50. Albright, F., Baird, P. C., Cope, O., and Bloomberg, E.: Studies on the physiology of the parathyroid glands; IV. Renal complica-

tions of hyperparathyroidism, Am. J. M. Sc. *187*:49, 1934.

51. Albright, F., Burnett, C. H., Smith, P. H., and Parson, W.: Pseudohypoparathyroidism —an example of Seabright's bantam syndrome, Endocrinology *30*:922, 1942.

52. Askanazy, M.: Über Ostitis Deformans ohne ostoides Gewebe, Arb. a. d. Geb. d. path. Anat. Inst. zu. Tübingen Leipzig *4*:398, 1903.

53. Bauer, W., Albright, F., and Aub, J. C.: A case of osteitis fibrosa cystica (osteomalacia?) with evidence of hyperactivity of the parathyroid bodies: metabolic study II, J. Clin. Invest. *8*:229, 1930.

54. Castleman, B.: Tumors of the parathyroid glands *in* Atlas of Tumor Pathology, p. 74, Washington, D. C., Armed Forces Inst. Path., 1952.

55. Castleman, B., and Cope, O.: Primary parathyroid hypertrophy and hyperplasia: a review of 11 cases at the Massachusetts General Hospital, Bull. Hosp. Joint Dis. *12*:368, 1951.

56. Castleman, B., and Mallory, T. B.: Parathyroid hyperplasia in chronic renal insufficiency, Am. J. Path. *13*:553, 1937.

57. ———: The pathology of the parathyroid gland in hyperparathyroidism: a study of 25 cases, Am. J. Path. *11*:1, 1935.

58. Churchill, E. D., and Cope, O.: Parathyroid tumors associated with hyperparathyroidism: 11 cases treated by operation, Surg., Gynec. & Obst. *58*:255, 1934.

59. Cogan, D. G., Albright, F., and Bartter, F. C.: Hypercalcemia and band keratopathy: report of 19 cases, Arch. Ophth. *40*:624, 1948.

60. Collip, J. B.: The extraction of a parathyroid hormone which will prevent or control parathyroid tetany and which regulates the level of blood calcium, J. Biol. Chem. *63*:395, 1925.

61. Cope, O.: Hyperparathyroidism: 67 cases in 10 years, J. Missouri M. A. *39*:273, 1942.

62. ———: Surgery of hyperparathyroidism: the occurrence of parathyroids in the anterior mediastinum and the division of the operation into 2 stages, Ann. Surg. *114*:706, 1941.

63. Cope, O., Culver, P. J., Mixter, C. J., Jr., and Nardi, G. L.: Pancreatitis, a diagnostic clue to hyperparathyroidism, Ann. Surg. *148*: 857, 1957.

64. Cope, O., Nardi, G. L., and Castleman, B.: Carcinoma of the parathyroid glands: 4 cases among 148 patients with hyperparathyroidism, Ann. Surg. *138*:661, 1953.

65. Erdheim, J.: Über Epithelkörperbefunde bei

Osteomalacie, Sitzungsb. d. k. Akad. d. Wissensch. Math. naturw. Cl. *116*:311, 1907.

66. ———: Rachitis und Epithelkörperchen, Aus der Kaiserlich-Königlichen Hof- und Staatsdruckerei, Vienna, 1914.

67. Gley, E.: Sur les fonctions du corps thyroïde, Compt. rend. Soc. biol. *43*:551, 567, 583, 841 and 843, 1891.

68. Hannon, R. R., Shorr, E., McClellan, W. S., and DuBois, E. F.: A case of osteitis fibrosa cystica (osteomalacia?) with evidence of hyperactivity of the parathyroid bodies: metabolic study I, J. Clin. Invest. *8*:215, 1930.

69. Hanson, A. M.: The hydrochloric x sicca: a parathyroid preparation for intramuscular injection, Mil. Surgeon *54*:218, 1924.

70. Hunter, D., and Aub, J. C.: Lead studies: XV. The effect of the parathyroid hormone on the excretion of lead and of calcium in patients suffering from lead poisoning, Quart. J. Med. *20*:123, 1927.

71. Keating, F. R., Jr., and Cook, E. N:. The recognition of primary hyperparathyroidism —an analysis of 24 cases, J.A.M.A. *129*:994, 1945.

72. Krane, S.: Unpublished data.

73. MacCallum, W. G., and Voegtlin, C.: On the relation of the parathyroid to calcium metabolism and the nature of tetany, Bull. Johns Hopkins Hosp. *19*:91, 1908.

74. Mandl, F.: Klinisches and Experimentelles zur Frage der lokalisierten und generalisierten Ostitis Fibrosa (unter besonderer Berücksichtigung der Therapy der letzteren), Arch. klin. Chir. *143*:245, 1926.

75. Norris, E. H.: The parathyroid glands and the lateral thyroid in man: their morphogenesis, topographic anatomy and prenatal growth, Contrib. Embryol., no. 159, pp. 249-294, January 30, 1937.

76. Recklinghausen, von, F. D.: Die Fibröse oder Deformirende Ostitis, die Osteomalacie und die Osteoplastische Carcinose in ihren gegenseitigen Beziehungen, Festschrift f. Rudolf Virchow, Berlin, 1891.

77. Rogers, H. M., and Keating, F. R., Jr.: Primary hypertrophy and hyperplasia of the parathyroid glands as a cause of hyperparathyroidism, Am. J. Med. *3*:384, 1947.

78. Sainton, P., and Millot, J. L.: Malignant degeneration of eosinophil adenoma of the parathyroids in the cause of von Recklinghausen's disease, Ann. anat. path. *10*:813, 1933.

79. Sandström, I.: On a new gland in man and several mammals (glandulae parathyreoideae), Upsala läkaref, förh. *15*:441, 1879-80.

80. Schlagenhaufer: Zwei Falle von Parathyreoideatumoren, Wien. klin. Wchnschr. *28*(2):1362, 1915.

81. Walsh, F. B., and Howard, J. E.: Conjunctival and corneal lesions in hypercalcemia, J. Clin. Endocrinol. *7*:655, 1947.

Dwight J. Ingle, ph.d.

—————————— CHAPTER 27, SECTION 1 ——————————

The Physiologic Role of the Pituitary and the Adrenal Glands in Health and Disease

Known Hormones of the Pituitary Gland (Hypophysis Cerebri)

Hormones of the Adrenal Glands

Role of the Anterior Pituitary-Adrenal Cortex Axis in the Response to Stress

Role of the Anterior Pituitary-Adrenal Cortex Axis in the Etiology of Disease

The purpose of the author is to summarize in this chapter some of the facts and the ideas which relate to the role of the anterior pituitary and the adrenal cortical hormones in maintaining homeostasis during health, stress and disease. To set this discussion in proper perspective the names and the functions of most of the known pituitary and adrenal hormones are reviewed briefly.

Hormones affect the rate of metabolic processes, but they are not known to create new processes. No metabolic process is known to be affected solely by any one hormone.

KNOWN HORMONES OF THE PITUITARY GLAND (HYPOPHYSIS CEREBRI)

Anterior Lobe (Pars Distalis or Pars Anterior)

The action of some anterior lobe hormones is to stimulate other endocrine organs. Some of the metabolic effects of growth hormone and lactogenic hormone are not mediated by other glands.

Growth hormone (somatotropin, somatotropic hormone or STH) is so called because its most dramatic overt effect is upon somatic growth. When the anterior lobe is destroyed in either laboratory animals or in man, skeletal growth is suppressed markedly but not com-

pletely. Other forms of growth can occur in the absence of growth hormone, such as tumor growth, wound healing, growth of hair and teeth, and regeneration of liver. Crude and highly purified preparations of growth hormone will stimulate skeletal growth in either normal or hypophysectomized laboratory animals but fail to stimulate growth in man unless the hormone has been extracted from the pituitary glands of primates (monkey or man). In addition to its dramatic effects upon protein anabolism in laboratory animals, the presently available preparations of growth hormone have marked effects upon the metabolism of water, electrolytes, carbohydrate and fat, the effects varying in different species and according to experimental conditions. The role of growth hormone in the adult is not known.

Thyrotropin is also called **thyrotropic hormone, thyroid-stimulating hormone or TSH.** Following removal or destruction of the anterior hypophysis, the thyroid undergoes atrophy and suppression of its secretory activity. These changes can be corrected by the administration of TSH. When an excess of thyroid hormone is administered to the laboratory animal or to man, the release of TSH by the anterior hypophysis probably is suppressed. A state of hyperthyroidism can be caused by the administration of an excess of exogenous TSH or by hypersecretion of TSH by the anterior hypophysis. The secretory activity of the thyroid does not fail completely in the absence of hypophyseal TSH; apparently the function of the thyroid can be modified to some extent by factors other than TSH.

Corticotropin is also called **adrenocorticotropic hormone or ACTH.** Following removal or destruction of the anterior hypophysis, the adrenal cortex undergoes extensive atrophy, but its secretory activity is not suppressed completely. The size and the secretory activity of the atrophic adrenal cortex can be restored to normal by treatment with ACTH, or a state of hypercorticalism can be induced by the prolonged administration of an excess of ACTH. When an excess of exogenous adrenal steroids is administered to laboratory animals or to man, there is compensatory atrophy of the adrenal cortices due to suppression of the release of ACTH by the anterior hypophysis. This can be prevented by the concomitant administration of exogenous ACTH. During any type of severe stress there is an increase in the secretion of ACTH, causing an increase in the size and the secretory activity of the adrenal cortex in order to meet the increased requirement of the body for adrenal cortical hormones. When the secretory response of the adrenal cortex is normal, a state of hypocorticalism probably is never caused by naturally occurring stress in either laboratory animals or in man.

The gonadotropic hormones are commonly called follicle-stimulating hormone (FSH) and luteinizing hormone (LH). These hormones act upon the gonads of the male and the female, influencing maturation of these organs in the young and morphology and function in adults. The gonads of either sex atrophy following removal of the anterior hypophysis. Replacement therapy with gonadotropic hormones of hypophyseal origin is effective in restoring size and secretory activity of the gonads of hypophysectomized animals, but these hormones have been little used in man because of the nonavailability of potent preparations. Administration of an excess of either estrogenic or androgenic steroids causes compensatory atrophy of the gonads in either sex by suppressing release of hypophyseal FSH.

Lactogenic hormone, or prolactin, is probably identical with luteotropin. This hormone participates in the initiation of lactation in mammals and promotes the secretion of progesterone by formed corpora lutea in the rat, but it has not been proved to have a luteotropic function in the human female. Prolactin elicits a variety of other metabolic and behavioral responses, depending upon the species and other conditions of study, thereby indicating that it may play a broader role in the economy of the body. Thus, the anterior hypophysis is an important regulator of thyroidal, adrenal cortical and gonadal functions, some of them homeostatic and others cyclic in nature. The mechanisms regulating the secretion and the release of hormones by the anterior hypophysis are not understood, but it seems probable that hypothalamic and perhaps other brain centers are involved which are sensitive to neural and humoral signals arising in the peripheral tissues.

POSTERIOR LOBE
(PARS NERVOSA OR PARS NEURALIS)

Two hormones have been isolated as pure polypeptides from posterior pituitary extracts, the structures of which were determined and confirmed by synthesis. Vasopressin, a powerful pressor principle, is identical with the antidiuretic hormone (ADH) of the posterior lobe. Oxytocin is a uterine-stimulating principle. Following removal of the posterior lobe, a severe diabetes insipidus ensues which tends to abate with time. It is probable that vasopressin and possibly oxytocin are secreted in cells of the hypothalamus, as well as in the posterior lobe, and that there is a compensatory increase in extrahypophyseal secretion of these hormones following removal of the posterior lobe. Section of the infundibular stalk or lesions in certain parts of the hypothalamus cause diabetes insipidus.

INTERMEDIATE LOBE (PARS INTERMEDIA)

A principle called intermedin, melanophore-stimulating hormone or MSH, has been isolated from the intermediate lobe. This hormone has a tropic influence upon the pigment cells of fishes, amphibians and reptiles and affects the extent of pigmentation in man. It is probable that the increase in pigmentation following destruction of the adrenal glands in man is caused by an increase in the secretion of intermedin.

HORMONES OF THE ADRENAL GLANDS

ADRENAL MEDULLA

Epinephrine, sometimes called Adrenalin or adrenin, has well-known cardiovascular effects and a number of more obscure but important effects upon metabolism. A second hormone from the adrenal medulla is called **norepinephrine or noradrenalin.** It differs from epinephrine in some of its pharmacologic properties. In most instances in which the 2 compounds have similar actions, norepinephrine is less potent than epinephrine. However, due to its vasoconstrictor action and property of supporting blood pressure, norepinephrine is a clinically important pharmacologic agent. Norepinephrine is secreted in postganglionic sympathetic fibers, as well as in the adrenal medulla. Adrenal demedullation does not seriously interfere with the economy of the body when the remainder of the sympathetic nervous system and the adrenal cortices remain intact. The only known disease of the adrenal medulla causing overproduction of its hormones is the tumor, pheochromocytoma.

Adrenal Cortex[5]

A large number of steroids have been isolated from extracts of adrenal glands and from adrenal vein blood. Only the few compounds which are important in the current practice of medicine and surgery will be considered. The formulas are shown in Figure 27-1.

Cortisone was once called 17-hydroxy-11-dehydrocorticosterone or **Compound E.** Apparently it is not a major secretory product of the adrenals of either laboratory animals or man, but it is a potent therapeutic agent.

Hydrocortisone, also called **Cortisol** and once called 17-hydroxycorticosterone or **Com-**

pound F, is a major secretory product of the adrenal glands of man and of at least some laboratory animals. Its biologic properties are essentially identical with those of cortisone, but it is somewhat more potent per unit weight.

Corticosterone, once called **Compound B,** is a minor secretory product of the adrenal cortex in man but apparently a major secretory product in certain laboratory animals. This steroid is of no practical clinical importance because its therapeutic value is less than that of other more readily available adrenal steroids.

Aldosterone (once called **electrocortin**) is a powerful sodium-retaining principle which apparently represents the active hormone present in the "amorphous fraction" of adrenal extracts of an earlier day. It is a natural secretory product of man and of laboratory animals. There is a degree of autonomy in the secretion of aldosterone. It continues to be secreted in significant amounts following hypophysectomy, and its rate of secretion is less responsive to ACTH than is the secretion of other steroids. It seems probable that the adrenal cortical secretion of aldosterone is responsive to changes in intake of electrolytes in the absence of the hypophysis.

The compound **11-desoxycorticosterone** is also called **DOC,** and its acetate is called **DCA.** It has not been found to be an important secretory product of the adrenal cortex,

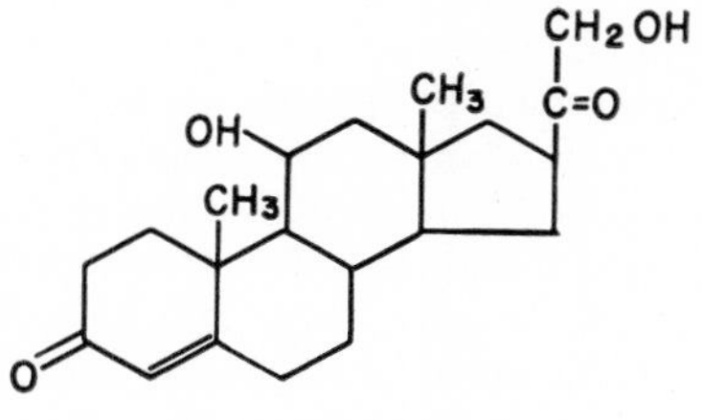

Corticosterone

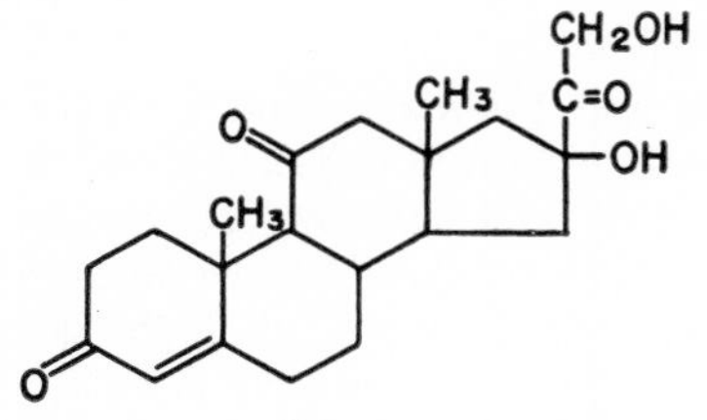

Cortisone

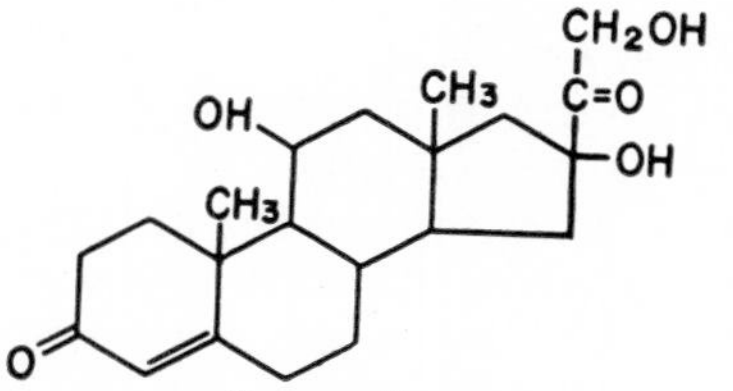

Hydrocortisone

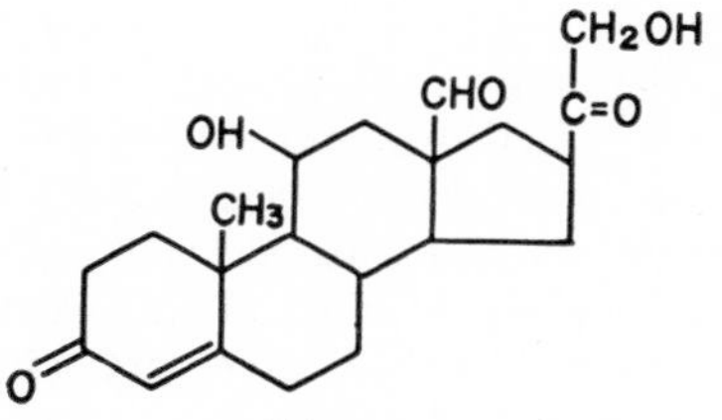

Aldosterone

Figure 27-1

but it is an important therapeutic agent due to its property of correcting the sodium and chloride loss of patients with adrenal cortical insufficiency.

A number of synthetic analogues of naturally occurring steroid hormones are of biologic and clinical importance, because of increased potency. Among them are 9-alpha-fluorohydrocortisone, 1-dehydrohydrocortisone, and 1-dehydro-9-alpha-fluorohydrocortisone.

The adrenal cortex also secretes biologically important amounts of androgenic and estrogenic steroids. Although the role of these adrenal steroids in normal body economy is not understood, there are signs of their action in certain syndromes of hypercorticalism, and there is evidence that these hormones can stimulate the growth of some tumors of the breast and of the prostate.

At a time when the supply of adrenal steroids was limited and few of their biologic effects were known, an oversimplified concept of their actions developed. According to this concept, those adrenal steroids bearing an oxygen at position 11 on the steroid nucleus, such as cortisone, hydrocortisone and corticosterone (Fig. 27-1), regulate the gluconeogenesis of carbohydrate from protein, and those steroids lacking an oxygen at position 11, such as 11-desoxycorticosterone, regulate the metabolism of electrolytes and water. It is now known that the cortical hormones can affect almost every tissue and function of the body. It has also become apparent that the mechanisms whereby these effects are produced are unknown.

Cortisone and hydrocortisone do have important effects upon the metabolism of carbohydrate, fat and protein, and they suppress the inflammatory response to several kinds of injury when administered in high dosage. Aldosterone (an 11-oxygenated steroid) and 11-desoxycorticosterone have powerful effects upon the excretion and the distribution of sodium, chloride, potassium and water. But there is overlapping in the biologic effects of these steroids. Cortisone and hydrocortisone can affect the metabolism of electrolytes and water; aldosterone and, to a lesser extent, 11-desoxycorticosterone affect organic metabolism. Corticosterone has moderate effects upon both organic and inorganic metabolism.

Patients with Addison's disease and most,

but not all, adrenalectomized animals waste sodium and chloride by excretion and retain abnormal amounts of potassium. There is a decrease in serum sodium, chloride and bicarbonate with a rise in serum potassium, and there is an accompanying loss of water so that hemoconcentration ensues. Some of the water lost from the blood is excreted, but there may also be a shift of water from the extracellular to the intracellular sites. Adrenally insufficient animals and patients fail to show a normal diuresis following the ingestion of water. Adrenal cortical insufficiency is characterized by hypotension and by an incapacity to make adequate circulatory adjustments in situations of stress. As adrenal cortical insufficiency progresses during nonstress conditions, an oligemia develops due to the excretion of water and internal fluid shifts. However, a mildly insufficient animal or patient may show sudden circulatory collapse during exposure to stress without oligemia.

In adrenal cortical insufficiency the carbohydrate content of the blood and the tissues is decreased below normal, especially during fasting. This is due in part to changes in food intake and absorption, but there is also a decrease in the amounts of carbohydrate formed from protein, and there are other changes in the utilization of carbohydrate. Not only are most forms of growth suppressed by adrenal cortical insufficiency, but also there is a decreased capacity to catabolize the tissue proteins when mobilization of the tissues is needed to meet energy requirements during fasting.

Adrenal cortical insufficiency cannot be fully corrected by any single steroid available to the physician at this time. Cortisone and hydrocortisone tend to normalize the defects in organic metabolism but do not fully correct electrolyte balance. This can be achieved by the additional administration of 11-desoxycorticosterone, a powerful sodium-retaining steroid, which by itself does not correct the defects in organic metabolism and does not fully support vigor.

All surgery is stressful and causes an increase in the secretion of steroids by the adrenal cortex to meet the increased need for these hormones. There are a number of clinical situations in which the surgeon needs to be familiar with the physiology of the adrenal cortex and with the biologic and therapeutic actions of its hormones. Patients having any degree of adrenal cortical insufficiency require careful preoperative and postoperative treatment with adrenal steroids, such as hydrocortisone. Adrenalectomy or subtotal adrenalectomy for any purpose requires postoperative therapy with adrenal steroids. Intravenous administration of hydrocortisone during surgery makes it possible to perform adrenalectomy in man without preoperative therapy with adrenal steroids. Large numbers of patients are now being treated with adrenal steroids in order to suppress the symptoms of rheumatoid arthritis or other inflammatory disease. If it is necessary to perform surgery upon a patient who is being treated with an adrenal steroid or has recently completed a prolonged course of therapy, the physician should assume that the adrenal cortices of the patient have undergone some degree of compensatory atrophy and may be incapable of a normal secretory response to the stress of surgery. It is probable that treatment with adrenal steroids will be required. The surgeon should be familiar with all of the clinical complications attributed to prolonged therapy with these steroids,[5] for some of them, such as peptic ulcers and fractures, may require surgical intervention. Intensive therapy with hydrocortisone and related steroids or with ACTH may decrease the resistance of the patient to infection and permit it to spread silently.

The author is not a physician. The details of therapy and the management of patients will not be discussed in this chapter.

ROLE OF THE ANTERIOR PITUITARY-ADRENAL CORTEX AXIS IN THE RESPONSE TO STRESS

CHANGES IN ANTERIOR PITUITARY FUNCTIONS DURING STRESS

During nonstressful conditions the anterior pituitary controls the cyclic activity of the gonads and possibly that of other target organs by changes in the amounts of tropic hormones released into the blood. During severe stress there is an increase in the secretion of ACTH and possibly of TSH, so that the adrenal cortex and sometimes the thyroid enlarge and secrete increased amounts of their hormones. There is a concomitant decrease in the secretion of hypophyseal gonadotropic

hormones, so that gonadal functions are decreased, and atrophy may occur. The effect of stress upon the secretion of growth hormone and lactogenic hormone is not established. Somatic growth is inhibited during severe stress, but this may be due to changes unrelated to the secretion of growth hormone.

This general pattern of pituitary response to severe stress was first emphasized and best elucidated by Selye. This is a part of his concept of the "alarm reaction."[6] The concept is of great importance in biology and medicine, for it means that demonstrable changes in the morphology and the secretory activity of the endocrine glands may not be the cause of a disease with which these changes are associated but rather may represent a normal response of the anterior pituitary-adrenal cortex axis to the stress of a disease arising from nonendocrine causes. The need for adrenal steroids is increased during any type of severe stress; an increased secretion of thyroid hormone may be needed during some types of stress, such as that induced by cold, and it is understandable that the functions of growth and reproduction should be suppressed as the organism struggles for survival. Thus, the changes in secretion of anterior pituitary hormones during stress is thought to support homeostasis.

ROLE OF THE ADRENAL CORTEX IN THE METABOLIC RESPONSE TO STRESS

The steroids of the adrenal cortex cause dramatic changes in metabolism when they are administered in excess. Cortisone and hydrocortisone are each capable of inhibiting growth and causing a negative nitrogen balance, stimulating gluconeogenesis, inhibiting some phases of carbohydrate utilization, etc. Aldosterone can cause the retention of sodium, chloride and water and the excretion of potassium to the extent of seriously disturbing the metabolism of electrolytes and water.

What are the metabolic consequences of the increased secretory activity of the adrenal cortices during severe stress? Some of the metabolic responses to injury (including surgery) resemble the metabolic responses to an excess of one or another of the adrenal steroids. Those responses which fail to occur in the adrenally insufficient animal or patient have been thought to be mediated by the change in secretory activity of the adrenal cortices. It is now known that the situation is more complex. In a number of instances it is possible to remove the adrenal cortices, substitute for them a steady maintenance intake of adrenal cortical hormones, and then elicit characteristic metabolic response to injury.[3] For example, the intact rat develops a negative nitrogen balance following multiple fractures of bone, but the response does not occur in the adrenally insufficient animal. However, when the adrenalectomized rat is maintained by adrenal cortical extract, the catabolic response to fractures is full blown. Similarly, the retention of sodium and chloride, which is a common response to injury, occurs following multiple fractures in adrenalectomized rats maintained by adrenal cortical extract. What is the relationship of the adrenal cortical hormones to the metabolic response to injury? For several of the responses studied 2 points are clear: (1) the response can occur in the absence of the adrenal glands; but (2) adrenal cortical hormones must be present in order to support normal responsiveness to the stress. The response is not likely to become overt in the absence of the cortical hormones. There are 3 hypotheses to explain the dependence of the metabolic response upon the presence of the cortical hormones: (1) in the presence of a fixed intake of cortical hormones, stress causes a decrease in their catabolism so that the titer in the body fluids increases and a state of hypercorticalism ensues. (2) In the presence of a fixed titer of cortical hormones in the body fluids, the stress sensitizes the tissues to give greater response to the hormones. (3) The cortical hormones play a permissive role in the metabolic response to injury. Herein it is supposed that the presence of the cortical hormones is necessary to normalize the responsiveness of cells to extra-adrenal stimuli. In support of the last concept, favored by the author,[2] are the facts that increased amounts of cortical hormones are required to maintain life during severe stress; in no case does exposure of an animal or a patient to stress produce a full-blown syndrome of hypercorticalism; and some feeble metabolic responses to stressors can be detected in the adrenally insufficient animal.

ROLE OF THE ANTERIOR PITUITARY-ADRENAL CORTEX AXIS IN THE ETIOLOGY OF DISEASE

PRIMARY DISEASES OF THE PITUITARY AND THE ADRENAL GLANDS

When the pituitary gland is removed or destroyed by disease, hypopituitarism (Simmonds' disease) develops. Growth, gonadal, thyroidal and adrenal cortical functions are decreased markedly. Various hypophyseal deficiencies may develop which represent hyposecretion of one or more of these hormones. Certain types of human dwarfism are assumed to be due to failure of growth hormone secretion. Hypogonadism, hypothyroidism and hypoadrenalism (Addison's disease) may be due to a decreased secretion of a tropic hormone or may be caused by destruction of the target organ itself. Overproduction of growth hormone is assumed to be the principal cause of gigantism or acromegaly. Hyperthyroidism can be caused by the hypersecretion of TSH. Some cases of Cushing's disease and virilism are assumed to involve the overproduction of ACTH, but proof is lacking. It is now believed that virilism can result from an enzymatic defect in the adrenal cortex so that there is increased secretion of androgenic steroids and decrease in the synthesis of hydrocortisone. Consequently, there is increased release of ACTH which stimulates the adrenal cortices to greater size and secretory activity without correcting the imbalance in secretory products. Such patients can be treated successfully with cortisone or hydrocortisone, which corrects the adrenal cortical insufficiency, inhibits release of ACTH and thereby suppresses the size of the adrenals and their secretion of virilizing steroids.[7]

Cushing's disease and virilism also can be caused by tumors of the adrenal glands which overproduce steroids, frequently in an abnormal pattern, without depending on ACTH. Indeed, these self-running tumors may secrete an excess of steroids which suppress the secretion of ACTH so that the normal contralateral gland undergoes compensatory atrophy. When the tumor is removed, it is necessary to treat the patient with steroids, such as hydrocortisone and DCA, to prevent adrenal cortical insufficiency. A syndrome of primary aldosteronism caused by tumors of the adrenal cortex has been described recently in man.[1]

Pathologic Changes Caused by an Excess of Adrenal Steroids or ACTH

It is easily possible to administer amounts of adrenal cortical steroids and synthetic derivatives of natural steroids which cause functional and morphologic abnormalities in laboratory animals and in man.[3] Similarly, it is easily possible to activate the adrenal cortices by exogenous corticotropin to secrete damaging amounts of hormones. Steroid diabetes can be induced in normal animals and in man, but it does not fully simulate diabetes mellitus. Overdosage with cortisone, hydrocortisone or ACTH can cause stomach ulcers in normal animals. Stomach ulcers also occur in the untreated adrenalectomized animal. Overdosage with 11-desoxycorticosterone can cause hypertension and cardiovascular damage in normal animals. This steroid is not known to be secreted in biologically important amounts. The more potent naturally occurring steroid, aldosterone, resembles 11-desoxycorticosterone in its actions upon electrolyte metabolism, but its overdosage effects are less than first anticipated.

Effects Upon Certain Diseases of Removing the Adrenal and the Pituitary Glands

Experimentally induced diabetes and hypertension are ameliorated by either adrenalectomy or hypophysectomy. In certain cases clinical diabetes and hypertension also can be ameliorated by removal of either the adrenals or the hypophysis. A significant number of patients having cancer of the breast develop a temporary remission following removal of either the adrenals or the pituitary gland.

Role of Adrenal Cortical Response to Stress in the Etiology of Disease

Selye is the principal protagonist of the hypothesis[6] that either an increase in the secretion of certain adrenal steroids or an imbalance in their secretion during stress can cause a variety of diseases which he has termed "adaptation diseases." There are signs

of alterations of adrenal and hypophyseal functions in many diseases, but, as noted above, these changes may be caused by the disease. Some patients with acromegaly or Cushing's disease, each rarely occurring, may have diabetes or hypertension or both.

Some experimentally induced and clinically occurring diseases are ameliorated by either adrenalectomy or hypophysectomy. Other diseases, such as arthritis, classified as diseases of the connective tissues, are suppressed by treatment with such steroids as hydrocortisone or by activation of the patient's own adrenal cortices by treatment with ACTH. The therapeutic effects of these hormones may be pharmacologic in nature. There is no convincing evidence that patients with arthritis or any other disease of connective tissues are adrenally insufficient or have stress-induced hormonal imbalances. However, the hypothesis that such is the case has some support and is worthy of further study.

Much of the evidence for a possible role of the adrenal cortical hormones in the etiology of disease is based upon the use of the rat which has been sensitized by the removal of one kidney and by the administration of an abnormally high intake of sodium chloride. In the sensitized rat the administration of 11-desoxycorticosterone causes a number of interesting cardiovascular and renal changes resembling diseases of man. Similar results can be obtained by overdosing sensitized rats with adrenal cortical extract,[4] indicating that some naturally occurring principle from the adrenal cortex will simulate the effect of 11-desoxycorticosterone when administered in excess to the sensitized rat. Suspensions of powdered anterior hypophysis cause cardiovascular and renal damage of this sort, but ACTH does not.

Overdosage with the hormones of other glands, especially those extracted from the anterior hypophysis, contributes to the development of cardiovascular and renal pathology in intact and in sensitized rats.

If Selye's hypothesis as to the etiology of the adaptation diseases is correct, it should be possible to cause these diseases experimentally by exposing normal animals to naturally occurring forms of stress. Evidence of this sort is lacking, although this phase of the problem has not been studied exhaustively. However, researchers at the Wistar Institute have reported that rats exposed to sound developed hypertension. If diseases could be caused by exposure to nonspecific stress, it would remain to be proved that the damage is mediated by the hormones of the adrenal cortex, and further proof would be required that this is the mechanism for the genesis of any of the diseases of man.

The author has suggested[3] that hormones of the adrenal cortex play a permissive or supporting role in the manifestation of clinical diabetes and hypertension, for it has been shown that these diseases can be induced in experimental animals without the mediation of the adrenal cortices.

The role of nonspecific stress and consequential hormonal imbalances in causing disease is not settled, but it is the hope of medical scientists that all such questions can be answered by the scientific method rather than by persuasion and debate.

REFERENCES

1. Conn, J. W.: Presidential address: Part 1—Painting background. Part 2—Primary aldosteronism, a new clinical syndrome. J. Lab. & Clin. Med. 45:3-17, 1955.
2. Ingle, D. J.: Permissibility of hormone action; a review, Acta endocrinol. 17:172-186, 1954.
3. ———: The relationship of the adrenal cortex to the manifestation of certain metabolic changes and to certain diseases, Am. Pract. & Digest Treat. 4:628-635, 1953.
4. Ingle, D. J., and Baker, B. L.: A consideration of experimentally produced and naturally occurring pathologic changes in the rat to the adaptation diseases in Recent Progress in Hormone Research, vol. 8, pp. 143-169, New York, Acad. Press. 1953.
5. ———: Physiological and Therapeutic Effects of Corticotropin (ACTH) and Cortisone, Springfield, Ill., Thomas, 1953.
6. Selye, H.: Stress, Montreal, Acta, Inc., 1950.
7. Wilkins, L.: The diagnosis of the adrenogenital syndrome and its treatment with cortisone, J. Pediat. 41:860-874, 1952.

J. Garrott Allen, m.d.

Pituitary and Adrenal Glands in Man

Their Interrelationships, Hyperplasia, Endocrine-producing Adenomas and Carcinomas

Pituitary Gland
  The Anterior Lobe
  Hypophysectomy, Its Complications and the "Posterior" Lobe Hormones
Adrenal Gland
  General Considerations
  Adrenal Cortex
  Adrenal Medulla

Pituitary function and its interrelationships with those of other endocrine organs and its broad influence upon many metabolic functions of the body place this organ in a category of unusual interest. In recent years, its interaction and interdependence upon adrenal cortical functions have caught the imaginations of many. The developments in the fields of pituitary-adrenal relationships have occurred so rapidly that it is still impossible to discuss the general subject with any degree of finality at this time. This point of view and caution are also emphasized by Ingle and by Moore in their respective writings in this textbook.

PITUITARY GLAND

The Anterior Lobe

The anterior lobe of the pituitary is known to produce at least 6 different hormones. With the exception of ACTH, TSH, and growth hormone, the rest have not been sufficiently purified to permit their repeated injection in man without risk of sensitization. Thus far, these hormones appear to be proteins or polypeptides. Therefore, antigenicity may be en-countered unless future developments in their purification eliminate this potential hazard. The question as to whether the corresponding hormones of the anterior pituitary derived from different species are chemically and biologically identical remains an unsettled one. The known pituitary hormones are:
  Growth or somatic hormone
  Adrenocorticotropic hormone (ACTH)
  Lactogenic hormone
  Follicle-stimulating hormone (FSH)
  Luteinizing hormone (LH) or Interstitial Cell-Stimulating hormone (ICSH)
  Thyrotropic hormone (TSH)
Those conditions resulting from excessive hormone production may call for surgical consideration directed toward partial or total hypophysectomy. Of particular concern at present are excesses in production of ACTH and the growth hormone. With the exception of growth hormone, the other 5 trophic hormones appear to direct their action toward specific organs. However, there is an increasing evidence that some systemic responses, as well as those of the "target" organs, may occur with some of the other hormones also.

Growth Hormone

This hormone probably is produced by the eosinophilic cells of the anterior pituitary, but other pituitary components also may take an active part in its elaboration, directly or indirectly. Growth or somatic hormone appears to regulate growth of the skin and of bone and cartilage. Visceral growth and to a lesser extent growth of the vascular system also are affected. Growth hormone has little effect upon growth of the brain.

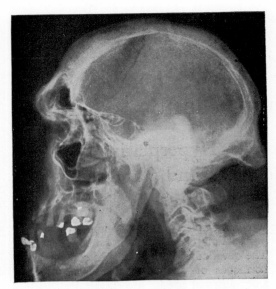

Fig. 27-2. Roentgenogram (14 × 17 in.) of skull in acromegaly. Note (1) enlarged sella, 32 × 25 mm.; (2) huge paranasal sinuses; (3) prognathism; (4) increased thickness but not increased density of tables of skull; (5) exostosis of occiput.

Growth hormone favors a positive nitrogen balance, characteristic of growth and other anabolic states. However, in order that a positive nitrogen balance may be obtained with growth hormone, insulin appears to be essential and may act in a cofactor role. Carbohydrate metabolism is also profoundly affected by growth hormone. In the absence of the hypophysis, extreme sensitivity to insulin develops, and the individual is unable to maintain his glycogen stores during the fasting state; he is unable to develop severe diabetes mellitus after pancreatectomy, as pointed out 25 years ago by Houssay.[21] Growth hormone appears to be synonymous with the diabetogenic hormone or to be closely allied with it; its influence upon carbohydrate metabolism appears to be independent of that governed by the adrenal cortex (see below).

Acromegaly and Gigantism. These syndromes are generally the result of an adenoma of the pituitary, usually of its eosinophilic tissue. In some patients, eosinophilic hyperplasia without adenoma may be responsible. In still others, more than one cell type and more than this hormone alone may be involved in the primary disease so that the clinical picture may become mixed and less well-defined.

Much of the information remaining in question would be clarified were there suitable methods for assay or analysis of growth hormone. Such technics would help especially in determining how often the disease totally destroys the pituitary and leaves the patient ultimately with moderate to severe hypopituitarism; whether in such patients there is cyclic function with periods of "rest"; or whether the disease continues to progress slowly with growth hormone continuing to be elaborated in excess of normal.

The enlarging pituitary eventually will exert its pressure upon the sella turcica. Several changes in this bony structure may then be demonstrated roentgenologically. By no means, however, is the absence of these findings to be considered as excluding pituitary disease when there are other sound grounds to suspect its presence. However, as the pituitary enlarges the sella generally does also. Usually its floor is depressed, and its cavity is ballooned out. Its dorsum may be displaced somewhat posteriorly and in time may be eroded and destroyed along with the clinoid processes. When this state of affairs obtains and is demonstrated roentgenographically, it is diagnostic of abnormal pituitary enlargement, regardless of cause. On the other hand, fairly wide ranges of variations in the size of the normal sella occur—8 to 12 mm. in depth and 9 to 16 mm. in length, respectively, are the usual extremes of normalcy as measured on the skull roentgenogram. Figure 27-2 is a roentgenogram of an acromegalic patient with a pituitary tumor in which the sella measures 32 mm. in length and 25 mm. in depth. This film also demonstrates the huge excavations of the paranasal sinuses, the increase in length and breadth of the mandible with blunting of its angle and thickening of the orbital ridge, so characteristic of acromegaly.

Among the somatic changes occurring in acromegaly and/or gigantism are the following:

Changes in bony structure which occur from growth hormone-producing tumors are modified considerably by the age of the patient at the time the onset of its excessive secretion begins. If the onset occurs prior to ossification of the epiphyseal plates of the long bones, the rate of growth is accelerated and the duration of growth prior to epiphyseal closures usually is prolonged by several years beyond that of the normal. Until epiphyseal ossification takes place, the excessive rates of growth are fairly uniform. Thereafter, growth continues in isolated skeletal areas, particularly, the mandible, the maxilla, the orbital ridges, the bones of the hands and the feet, with thickening of the long bones and of the vertebrae (Fig. 27-3). Later, the characteristics of acromegaly may be superimposed upon those of gigantism, should the patient with gigantism live long enough. When excessive elaboration of growth hormone does not occur until after full and normal growth has been attained with epiphyseal closures effected, only acromegaly occurs. More often the latter is observed; such patients often survive beyond 50 years of age.

With the continued growth of the mandible, prognathism becomes a prominent feature of acromegaly. The teeth protrude beyond the incisors of the maxilla, and the mandibular overgrowth causes a separation of its teeth. The bones of the hands and the feet are generally enlarged in pronounced acromegaly and are associated with tufting of the terminal phalanges. However, part of the enlargement or "spading" of the digits is due to thickening of the skin, subcutaneous and periarticular tissue.

Although the rate of osteogenesis is accelerated, so also is that of bony resorption. The end result is that the enlarged bones contain less calcium per gram of tissue rather than more.

The epiphyseal plates, if still active, continue to promote longitudinal growth. Ossification of cartilages is normally favored by sexual maturity because of the increased production of sex hormones and gonadal activity at this time. In excessive production of growth hormone, however, gonadal activity and the sex hormones are reduced; hence, the delayed ossification may be explained upon the hypogonadism, permitting further growth than might otherwise occur. Thus the skeletal growth of the pituitary giant is in part the result of diminished gonadal activity, but to a greater extent it is likely the response of excessive production of growth hormone.

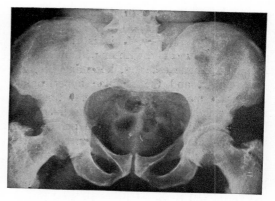

FIG. 27-3. This picture demonstrates the increased width of the bony pelvis, the 17-inch roentgenogram being scarcely large enough to contain both iliac wings. Note ossifications at sites of attachments of abductor muscle to greater trochanters, the increase in width of L-5, and the osteoarthritis of lower spine and hip sockets.

Enlargement or growth of the cartilaginous structures of the ears, the nose and the larynx add further to the grotesque features that these patients eventually display. Aside from disfiguring enlargement of the ears and the nose, caused by the cartilaginous overgrowth, the voice is deepened, often rasping in character, due to an overgrowth of the cartilaginous structures of the larynx. The growth of the costal cartilages is excessive, causing an abnormal enlargement of the bony thorax which, along with the usual dorsal kyphosis and elongated extremities, imparts the gorilla-like features that many of these patients display.

Skin Changes. Enlargement of the soft parts of hands, feet, face, nose and lips often is nearly as disfiguring as are the skeletal changes. The skin thickens, and hypertrichosis is commonly noted. The total mass of sweat glands is said to be increased. Connective tissue is excessive within the skin, as well as in the subcutaneous and submucosal areas. The brow and the face often take on the "bulldog" appearance. The fibrous proliferation about the joints contributes to the arthritic complaints that many of these patients express. The ligamentous attachments (Sharpey's fibers) likewise increase, favoring immobility; actually they may become encased or ossified at their sites of attachment to bone as the bones increase in diameter, particularly the spine (Fig. 27-3).

Organ Hypertrophy. This is the rule in advanced acromegaly, with or without gigantism. The tongue enlarges, becoming broader and thicker, and the papillae hypertrophy. The heart may exceed by several times its normal weight. The weight of the liver may be increased by more than 100 per cent of its normal limits. Similar increases are frequently noted in lungs, adrenals, pancreas, intestine, thymus and kidneys. However, the brain does not increase in weight, although the perineural tissue of the peripheral nerves often proliferate, contributing to the paresthesia and the numbness often encountered. Enlargement of the ganglia also usually occurs. It is suspected that some of the neurologic complaints are due to vascular insufficiency and tension upon the nerves in gigantism, caused by the stretch effect of unusual longitudinal growth. Personality changes may occur.

Physiologic disturbances created by the enlargement of organs are related primarily to the heart, the skeletal muscle and possibly to the unusual stretch of arteries and nerves when gigantism is present. Fragmentation of the individual muscle fibers of the heart and hypertension (probably not related) are fairly common findings. Diabetes mellitus is detectable in 15 to 20 per cent of patients, presumably from the demonstrated degeneration of islet cell tissue from the diabetogenic effect of growth hormone. It is insulin-resistant.

Many patients display an increase in basal metabolic rate; findings of plus 20 to 30 or more are not uncommon. Exophthalmos also may occur along with other features of hyperthyroidism, including tachycardia and goiter. These occur with sufficient frequency to present a confusing diagnostic picture at times. Presumably the thyroid changes result from coexisting excessive secretion of thyrotropic hormone (TSH).

In some patients with acromegaly, muscular strength even in fairly advanced stages of the disease may remain excellent for many years. For example, the roentgenographic illustrations of acromegaly in Figures 27-2 and 27-3 are those made of a professional wrestler who continued several engagements a week for many years after severe skeletal and cutaneous manifestations of his disease first appeared. He abandoned his wrestling career only 2 years prior to death at the age of 50. In others, however, muscular strength, while pronounced and perhaps greater than that of the normal in the early stages of the disease, is eventually superseded by weakness, the explanation of which is wanting.

CLINICAL FINDINGS AND DIAGNOSIS. If uncomplicated and other concurrent abnormalities such as hyperthyroidism or myxedema (latent) are not marked, skeletal and cutaneous changes together usually make the diagnosis of acromegaly obvious. Confirmation of this clinical picture by roentgenographic demonstration of erosion of the posterior sella, with ballooning of the sella and destruction of the clinoid processes, establish the diagnosis beyond question.

In patients in whom such changes are less severe or those who are seen early in the stages of their disease, the diagnosis may not be established so easily. Often the first complaints are those of paresthetic hypesthesia, pains about the joints associated with headaches, and impotence. These are the complaints so often associated with functional disorders or other ill-defined entities that acromegaly may not be considered. Moreover, the sella may appear perfectly normal in spite of the presence of an adenoma. In other patients with similarly mild complaints, the sella may be enlarged beyond average size but still remain within the normal range, causing one to suspect acromegaly, when in reality some other disorder may be at fault, especially hyperthyroidism or functional complaints.

Visual fields may be distorted in time if the tumor ruptures the diaphragm above the sella and exerts pressure upon the optic chiasm. Classically, loss of color vision precedes loss of the ability to recognize shape and form. Bitemporal hemianopsia, when present, is usually a latent development and eventually total blindness may occur in a few of these patients. Visual field disturbances are found in about 20 per cent of patients. Choking of the optic disks is seldom encountered, presumably because the tumor is slow-growing and is small by comparison with other intracranial tumors. The adenoma may become cystic.

Laboratory aids are not specific. Technics for the measurement of growth hormone are ill-defined and indirect. The increase in metabolic rate and the diabetic type of glucose tolerance curve, often with frank diabetes which is frequently insulin-resistant, are valuable diagnostic aids when in the presence of physical findings and x-ray observations compatible with acromegaly.

TREATMENT of acromegaly with or without gigantism centers about the ablation of pituitary function. This has been pursued historically along 3 lines: hypophysectomy, external x-radiation, and more recently local radiation.

Hypophysectomy as performed by Cushing was incomplete. This was necessary not only for technical reasons, but it now appears that total hypophysectomy in man creates an addisonian state requiring exogenous cortisone or ACTH to sustain life. As the clinical usefulness of these substances was not explored until a decade after Cushing's death, hypophysectomy probably was doomed to fail in his time, irrespective of the development status of surgical technic.

Recent experience with hypophysectomy suggests that once again its usage may be explored. However, most of the good results reported are in patients with normal glands in whom its removal is employed as a palliative measure in the management of breast carcinoma. Removal of pituitary tumors presents more difficulty and is not performed so readily.

X-radiation therapy to the pituitary has proved to be partially effective in the treatment of acromegaly and gigantism in many patients. Fortunately, brain tissue and the optic nerves are fairly resistant to radiation. Dosages of 3,000 r administered over a period of 3 to 4 weeks are generally employed.

Local Irradiation Implants. More recently, stereotaxic placement of yttrium[90] beads throughout the pituitary has been employed, especially by Evans[16] and Rasmussen,[27] with Harper (see Chap. 9, "The Principles of Isotope Technics in Surgery"). Radon seeds have been similarly employed by Illingworth and colleagues.[22] The dosages of such radiation are designed so as to ablate completely all pituitary tissue without damage to the neighboring hypothalamus and optic nerves. The ultimate place of this combined form of radiation and surgery remains to be determined (Fig. 27-4).

The urgency of diagnosis, particularly in

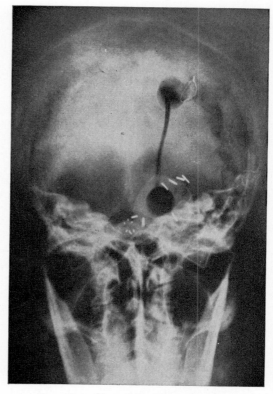

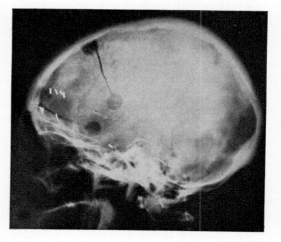

FIG. 27-4. Six yttrium[90] beads placed in the pituitary are shown in (*above*) the A-P and (*below*) the lateral roentgenograms of the skull. Large opacities are silver clips.

the presence of gigantism among the young, cannot be stressed too strongly. This disorder, even more than that of untreated acromegaly, is likely to lead to serious social maladjustment, with the creation of difficulty and intense psychological problems in the short-ened life span. Death usually occurs before the age of 30 in serious gigantism. These are a lonely lot of patients—almost outcasts. Therefore, the treatment to be undertaken should be effective and carried out as soon as the diagnosis can be made.

Pituitary Dwarfism. In the absence or severely diminished production of growth hor-mone, dwarfism results. As this is of no surgi-cal consequence, here it is referred to only briefly because it appears to be the counter-part of gigantism.

If the growth functions of the pituitary tissue are interfered with in infancy or child-hood, growth is retarded uniformly. The time of epiphyseal closure usually is delayed in dwarfism as well as in gigantism. Usually, but not always, other endocrine activities depend-ent upon the pituitary trophic hormones are also present.

Cushing's Syndrome (Pituitary Basophi-lism). The symptomatic and physiologic dis-turbances of this disease are mediated through the adrenal cortex. When the initial disturb-ance is from excessive ACTH production, hypersecretion of the adrenal corticoid hor-mones occurs. This syndrome was referred to earlier as basophilism, for it was presumed that ACTH arose from the basophilic cells of the pituitary. Until more is known of the exact origin of ACTH, perhaps it is better to con-tinue the designation of Cushing's syndrome.[10] Should the increase in corticoids be from an active adenoma or hyperplasia of the adrenal cortex, the same systemic changes occur as noted in Cushing's disease of pituitary origin. Therefore, it is useful to discuss these two entities together and more logically under the section on the Adrenal Cortex (see p. 621). In either case, the clinical end result is the same; only the cause of hypercorticism differs.

HYPOPHYSECTOMY, ITS COMPLICATIONS
AND THE "POSTERIOR" LOBE HORMONES

Surgery upon the hypophysis was first per-formed by von Eiselberg of Vienna in 1901.[17] This amounted to the drainage of a cyst of the pituitary and was not a hypophysectomy. The patient died. Cushing[12] first operated suc-cessfully upon the pituitary and developed the field. As mentioned above, the early ex-periences were frequently associated with injuries to the optic chiasm and to the neuro-hypophysis. The procedure soon was largely abandoned and was cause for the surgeon to compromise his operative attempts, settling for incomplete hypophysectomy with multiple operations if needed rather than the total removal of the gland.

Hemorrhage. The development of surgery of the pituitary is one of the many important contributions of Cushing and one that en-couraged him to develop other fields in neuro-surgery as well. Cushing soon found that the dangers of hypophysectomy were not limited to optic nerve trauma alone. Uncontrolled hemorrhage and diabetes insipidus were also serious problems and not infrequently fatal complications which beset him and continue to plague the neurosurgeon of today. The con-trol of hemorrhage in such deep wells as required in many neurosurgical operations caused Cushing early to focus his attention sharply upon the problems of neurosurgical hemostasis. He introduced the use of bits of muscle fragments obtained from the exposed temporalis muscle, recognizing its thrombo-plastic action; he may have been informed of this potential by the physiologist, William H. Howell, Professor of Physiology at Hopkins at the time Cushing began his experimental and clinical neurosurgery in that institution. At that time, Howell was studying problems in blood coagulation. Bone wax to plug the bleeding of cut bone edges was introduced by Victor Horsley but was used infrequently by Cushing. At Cushing's instigation, Ernest Grey[18] explored the use of fibrin clots placed at the bleeding site, but this technic proved to be of little value. The silver clip applied to bleeding points or to vessels before transec-tion was developed by Cushing in 1910 with his first report on its use being made in 1911.[11] (Note x-ray appearance in Fig. 27-4).

In 1926 Cushing explored the hemostatic effect of high-frequency current in cerebral surgery but not upon the hypophysis. This technic had been employed as early as 1911 in urologic surgery. Working with W. T. Bovie,[4] Cushing first employed electrocoagu-lation in neurosurgery on October 1, 1926. The patient suffered from a highly vascular "myeloma." Although nearly all methods cur-rently in use for the control of intracranial hemorrhage were either developed or first employed in this field by Cushing, many hemostatic problems remain to be solved. Uncontrolled hemorrhage continues to plague the neurosurgeon and especially in his operative attempts at removal of the hypophysis. Hypotensive anesthesia has been used in recent years and has proved to be helpful, but there is as yet no perfect answer.

Antidiuretic Hormone and Diabetes Insipidus. The second disquieting complication of hypophyseal surgery is the complication of diabetes insipidus, first described by Claude Bernard. Originally, this operative complication was attributed to injury to the posterior pituitary. Later it was realized that injury to the pituitary stalk, the hypothalamus or the supra-optic nuclei likewise could induce this disorder. With hypophysectomy being reintroduced in recent years, many of the earlier interpretations appear to need reconsideration. Re-examination of the newer evidence is necessary for it becomes increasingly evident that the original simple explanations of a few years ago do not satisfy all observations being encountered in patients today.

Many surgeons believe that total hypophysectomy performed by clipping the stalk as near the gland as possible is least likely to produce diabetes insipidus. However, no one procedure appears to avoid this complication completely, nor can any one procedure be relied upon to induce the disorder consistently. Fortunately, the magnitude of this complication often improves to some extent over that immediately observed after hypophysectomy.

The physiologic disorder believed to be responsible for diabetes insipidus is the interference with the production or release of an antidiuretic hormone (ADH) known also as *vasopressin*. This hormone appears to be under the nervous control of the posterior neurohypophysis. The identity of the chemical structure of the antidiuretic hormone is of added interest because it marks for the first time that a polypeptide hormone was identified chemically and synthesized. This feat was accomplished by du Vigneaud in 1953,[15] for which he became the Nobel laureate in 1955. Du Vigneaud also identified and synthesized a second hormonal polypeptide believed to be associated with the function of the posterior pituitary—*oxytocin*.

The physiologic action of the antidiuretic hormone (vasopressin or ADH) appears to be directed specifically toward resorption of water from the distal renal tubules. It promotes water absorption in some manner without much apparent influence upon electrolyte resorption. Thus it enables the body to conserve essentially osmotically free water. Should excess salt need to be disposed of in the urine, this may be accomplished without the serious losses of water which otherwise might occur were salt and water resorption not under separate means of control.

As the name "vasopressin" implies, the antidiuretic hormone also affects arteriolar tension as well as cardiac function. This action favors an increase in arterial blood pressure and diminishes renal blood flow.

In diabetes insipidus, ADH is of indispensable aid; it is administered best, at present, as a crude extract by nasal insufflation, 40 mg., several times daily. Pure ADH may be administered in oil, each dose generally lasting several days. Because of its current expense, this product is not yet widely used.

ADH increases intestinal tone and promotes peristalsis and may be of some therapeutic value in the treatment of adynamic ileus (see Chap. 36, "Anatomy, Physiology and Treatment of Intestinal Obstruction").

Oxytocin appears to be concerned primarily with uterine contraction in late pregnancy. The oxytocin content of the neurohypophysis is said to be diminished during lactation, when this hormone is believed to be elaborated to assist the periductal myoepithelium of the mammary ducts in expressing milk.[28] Oxytocin appears to depress vasomotor responses of the heart and the arteriolar vessels, lowering blood pressure. To this extent, its action seems to oppose mildly the vasopressor effects of ADH.

Again it seems essential to caution the student about the changing status and knowledge about the pituitary gland, and for that matter endocrines in general. Recent evidence tends to demonstrate that many of the views held earlier as fact may not be true. At least many of the well-accepted interpretations of a few years need to be re-examined, as a number of the pituitary functions now appear to be much too complex to support unitarian points of view.

ADRENAL GLAND

GENERAL CONSIDERATIONS

Anatomic and Surgical Considerations. The adrenal glands lie on the upper mesial aspect of the pole of each kidney which they cover as a cap. Normally, each gland weighs between 1 and 1.5 Gm.

Small accessory adrenal tissue occasionally is said to be found in the connective tissue adjacent to the adrenal itself; such an occurrence is rare in the writer's surgical experience.

The adrenal cortex is derived from celomic epithelium and hence is of mesodermal origin; the medulla is of ectodermal derivation, arising from the neural crests. Microscopic examination shows the cortex to consist of glandular epithelium enmeshed loosely in a fine stroma of connective tissue. The cortical architectural structure suggests 3 areas or zones stratified one upon another. The *zona glomerulosa* has its cells arranged in rounded clusters and is situated just beneath the thin external fibrous capsule. The cells are fairly large, polyhedral in shape and contain many granules. Just beneath the zona glomerulosa is the *zona fasciculata* with its cells arranged in columnar fashion, radiating toward the glomerulosa. Their cytoplasm also contains granular and much lipoid material. Most mesially situated is the *zona reticularis*. Its distal contact is with the fascicularis and mesially with the adrenal medulla. The cells of the reticularis often contain pigment granules in their cytoplasm which are not seen in those of the glomerulosa of the fasciculata.

The recent demonstration by Cooper and his associates that medullary tissues and, to some extent, the catechol amines themselves enhance the production of the steroids of the cortex supplies a logical explanation of the intimate anatomic relationship of the medulla and the cortex of the adrenal. These effects were demonstrated by incubating fresh tissue slices of human and of bovine adrenals.[7]

The adrenal arteries usually arise from the aorta, the inferior phrenics and/or the renal arteries. The lymphatic circulation terminates for the most part within the lumbar nodes.

The adrenal veins pass centripetally to form the left and the right adrenal veins, respectively. Generally, the vein from the left adrenal enters either the left renal or the vena cava; that on the right more frequently enters the vena cava directly. More than one vein leaving each gland is frequently found. Their walls are thin and easily torn; when this happens at operation, severe retrograde bleeding occurs from the vena cava and/or from the renal veins. Unless the surgical field is one of excellent exposure, control of this type of hemorrhage may be both difficult and dangerous, especially if one attempts blindly the placement of hemostats in the puddle of blood which continues to flood the field at a rate which is usually more rapid than can be cleared. The vena cava or renal veins also may be torn in attempting hemostasis, inviting not only more extensive hemorrhage but air embolism as well. Unless small sutures can be easily placed under direct vision, packing may be the safer hemostatic procedure to employ. The pack must not occlude the flow of blood in the vena cava, as this may create the acute vena cava syndrome with shock from the intravascular pooling of blood in the distal veins. Should shock appear an hour or so after packing, when there is insufficient evidence of continuing extensive blood loss, and be associated with distention of the veins of the legs as well as cyanosis of the distal extremities, the patient should be returned to the operating room, the wound reopened and the pack gently loosened until improvement in color of the distal extremities occurs. Transfusions under these conditions should be administered through the antecubital veins of the arms and not into the saphenous veins because of the diminished distal venous return. The acute vena cava syndrome, however, is a complication which generally can be easily avoided by careful dissection carried out under direct vision with good exposure.

In the performance of adrenalectomy, many surgeons prefer to apply silver clips (Cushing), cutting between the distal and the proximal clips. As these veins are small and not easily recognized as such, the author places 2 clips on any periadrenal thread of tissue which conceivably might be mistaken in identity as a nerve or a bit of fibrous tissue. As might be expected, many of the clips are placed upon the nerve plexus entering the adrenal as well as on the veins. These nerves are numerous and are derived principally from the celiac and the renal plexuses and probably also from the phrenic and the vagal nerves as well.

Adrenal Cortex

Physiologic and Pharmacologic Actions of Corticoid Hormones. The cortical hormones have in common with the sex hormones the steroid nucleus. About 30 such compounds have been isolated from cortical extracts, and of these about 7 are known to possess sufficient biologic activity to sustain life and good health after bilateral adrenalectomy as well as to treat successfully the patient with Addison's disease. Over a period of years, Kendall and associates and others have methodically isolated and identified the chemical composition of many of these compounds prior to much knowledge as to their biologic activity or therapeutic importance. A number of these compounds probably are parent substances from which the active hormones are biosynthesized. It is also possible that a few may have been created artificially in the course of chemical extraction procedures.

The gland seems to elaborate and to dispense these hormones so rapidly in meeting the body's normal needs that little storage is undertaken by the gland itself. Thus the adrenal cortex is a relatively poor commercial source of these compounds.

As Ingle points out, the original concepts as to the biologic functions of cortical hormones were oversimplified. It was early suggested that those hormones bearing oxygen at the 11 position of the steroid nucleus, such as cortisone, hydrocortisone and corticosterone, regulated gluconeogenesis of carbohydrate derived from proteins. Those lacking in oxygen at position 11 were believed to be concerned essentially with the metabolism of water and electrolytes. It is now known that the cortical hormones may affect nearly all of the body's tissues and functions, but until these mechanisms are better understood, it serves no useful purpose to classify them at this time. Some of the known metabolic functions that they influence will be discussed with the realization that these, too, are complex, incompletely understood, and that many may be either interdependent or interrelated.

Cortisone and hydrocortisone probably have the greatest influence of all natural cortical hormones upon metabolic functions under partial or complete adrenal control.

Protein Metabolism. The patient with Addison's disease or the animal subjected to adrenalectomy without replacement therapy encounters difficulty in mobilizing and metabolizing endogenous protein. As the normal human or mammal derives a certain amount of glucose from protein metabolism (gluconeogenesis), the addisonian patient and the adrenalectomized animal are prone to develop hypoglycemia. In the case of exogenous protein, as Ingle has pointed out, there is a much less demonstrable defect of metabolism. When the adrenal-insufficient patient or animal is fed protein and allowed a normal caloric intake, nitrogen is excreted in normal amounts, and the hypoglycemic tendency is reduced materially. However, the decreased potassium excretion in the addisonian is not affected unless cortical replacement is employed. The ease of fatigue upon exercise has been demonstrated most dramatically by Ingle in adrenalectomized rats without corticoid supportive therapy.

When excessive amounts of cortisone and/or hydrocortisone are present, whether from excessive cortical activity or administration, the nitrogen excretion is increased materially. This is a response about which much is known, but the information available is not sufficient to establish whether it results from an accelerated rate of catabolism or a diminished rate of anabolism or both.

Carbohydrate metabolism and its dependence upon cortical function in the adrenalectomized rat in the fasting state was first demonstrated by Cori and Cori in 1927.[9] They showed that neither the normal blood sugar nor the stores of liver glycogen could be maintained under these conditions. This phenomenon occurs in many species, including man. Diabetes mellitus may be ameliorated by adrenalectomy but may be produced by hypercorticism when diabetes did not previously exist.

Two factors appear to play a role in the diminished ability of the addisonian patient or the adrenalectomized animal to maintain the normal level of blood glucose. One is the retarded rate of gluconeogenesis from protein. The other is the apparent acceleration in the rate of glucose utilization after adrenalectomy in the fasting state. Presumably, the latter phenomenon is due to an antagonism between certain of the cortical hormones and insulin but further study is needed for elucidation.

In hypercorticism, the effect upon carbohydrate metabolism is reversed. Glycosuria, decreased glucose tolerance, frank diabetes and an increased insulin tolerance characteristically occur. Again, it should be remembered that in addition to an increased insulin tolerance[33] more carbohydrate is also made available from the accelerated rate of gluconeogenesis from protein when excesses of cortisone and hydrocortisone occur.

Fat metabolism is disturbed in that a diminished transport of fat to the liver as well as a reduction in the total lipid content in this organ occurs. Ketonuria and ketonemia are observed with less frequency and to a lesser extent than in the normal; this is not yet explained. In the addisonian, the respiratory quotient is reported to be increased, and to be diminished in hypercorticism. The cause of abnormal distribution of fat in the Cushing's state is unknown.

Water and electrolyte metabolism are among the more dramatic and acute disorders created by either the hypocortical or the hypercortical state. There are many internal factors and mechanisms which can alter water and electrolyte balance; those of hormonal origin are as important as any (see Chap. 5, "Fluid and Electrolytes"). Whereas the types of these disorders in the hypocortical and the hypercortical states are well known, the exact mechanisms by which they occur are not.

So far as the mineral electrolytes are concerned, sodium and potassium are among those subject to the most apparent and most important changes noted (see p. 628, Aldosteronism.) In hypocorticism, sodium excretion in the urine is increased; in hypercortical states, sodium tends to be retained. These changes are thought to reflect differences in tubular rates of absorption due to corticoid activity.

The first progress in the treatment of the addisonian patient resulted from the recognition that such patients required large quantities of salt.[20, 25] The synthetic desoxycorticosterone acetate (DOCA) was introduced as a therapeutic agent 20 years ago. Its administration favored sodium retention in the normal

patient as well as in the addisonian. The brilliant researches of Simpson and his discovery of the naturally occurring, potent, salt-retaining hormone, aldosterone, may lead to the explanation of many of the unknowns in mineral and water balance. Aldosterone, milligram per milligram, exerts more than 20 times the effect upon sodium retention exerted by DOCA.

It is probable that the excessive loss of sodium in the addisonian patient accounts for many of the well-established features of this disease: hypovolemia, reduction in extracellular water, the increase in hematocrit reading and in plasma protein concentration and blood viscosity, all of which render these patients very susceptible to the development of hypovolemic shock.

In hypercorticism, sodium is retained abnormally and along with this are the excesses in extracellular water with edema. Soon after the hypercortical state occurs, sodium equilibrium is established at a slightly higher level than normal, but in some it remains unchanged and at the normal level. The hyponatremia of the hypocortial state is usually much more alarming and serious than is the sodium retention in hypercortical activity. Certainly, the latter is not to be considered lightly, especially in the elderly patient or in those with pre-existing or concurrent cardiovascular, renal or hepatic disease.

The urinary excretion of potassium and its concentrations in the body fluids are also influenced considerably by the state of adrenal cortical function. In the addisonian or untreated adrenalectomized patient, potassium rentention is the rule. Many believed earlier that death in these patients was due primarily to potassium intoxication. Undoubtedly in some patients this was true, but as many other important and vital changes also occur in adrenal insufficiency, it is possible that these associated disorders each in themselves or in combination, can be lethal at times.

In hypocorticism, the potassium concentrations of serum, extracellular and intracellular water are increased. As the concentration of potassium in heart muscle increases, changes in the electrocardiogram occur which are believed to be characteristic of impending potassium intoxication. ECG tracings are often useful aids in the management of the hypocortical and the hypercortical states. However, these findings are not entirely reliable.

The mechanisms involved in the altered potassium metabolism from abnormalities in cortical activity are probably more intricate than those that affect sodium. Aside from considerations of disordered tubular absorption and internal fluid shifts are also the disturbances in protein metabolism. Normal concentrations of potassium are usually essential to normal protein metabolism; the reverse also is true and probably of equal importance. To what extent the abnormalities in protein metabolism are responsible for the altered potassium responses in adrenal cortical disorders is not established. Favoring the altered metabolism of protein is the reported observation that aldosterone, which has no known influence upon protein metabolism, appears to exert less influence upon potassium excretion than upon sodium retention.[26, 32]

The changes in water metabolism caused by some adrenal cortical hormones are in part due to the electrolyte shifts, especially sodium. In part they may also result from the ill-defined changes in tubular resorption assigned to the cortical hormones. In the addisonian patient there is a diminished diuretic response to water (Keppler water test). If large quantities of water are administered, water intoxication may occur. This abnormality appears to be more amenable to the administration of the 11, 17-oxysteroids than to the 11-desoxysteroids or to aldosterone. There is also considerable evidence to suggest that the antidiuretic hormone of the neurohypophysis and some of the adrenocortical steroids are antagonistic.

Surgical Diseases of the Adrenal Cortex. CUSHING'S DISEASE (HYPERCORTICISM). Harvey Cushing recorded in 1912 his first observations of the disease which now bears his name. This patient was a young woman who suffered from headache, pain in the back, obesity about the face, the neck and the trunk but not of the extremities, and from hirsutism and hypertension. The dorsal kyphosis and "buffalo hump" obesity that she displayed, with hirsutism, florid complexion, ease of bruising and purple striae of the lower trunk, along with diabetes mellitus, were to characterize this syndrome which he did not encounter again until 1932.[10] Cushing's first patient,

he believed, suffered from a pituitary disorder; his second patient, a male, received pituitary radiation and improved promptly.

Clinical Course and Diagnosis of Cushing's Syndrome. As others entered this field of study, additional clinical and metabolic disturbances were noted. The round "moon facies" was noted frequently. Weakness was commonly encountered. Hypertension was detected in about 75 per cent of cases. Osteoporosis was an important finding and to this was attributed the skeletal pain, the backache and the dorsal kyphosis often experienced by many of these patients. Negative calcium balance is the rule, and about 25 per cent develop renal stones, presumably due to the excessive quantities of calcium appearing in the urine.

Diabetes mellitus or a diminished glucose tolerance curve was encountered less commonly in Cushing's cases than the known physiology of hypercorticism might suggest. The syndrome occurs about 3 times more often in females than in males.

Perhaps the most characteristic and constant finding revealed by careful physical examination is the loss of muscular mass. This can be overlooked in the presence of the unusual obesity. It seems reasonable to explain the patient's muscular weakness on the basis of this finding alone, although other factors also may be involved.

The skin is thin, especially the corium, and sometimes is decribed as having a marble-like appearance. The wasting of fascial and fibrous connective tissue probably accounts for the striae of the skin so often noted over the areas of the abdomen where the skin may be stretched from obesity. These striae are usually "purple" in color and are attributed to the thinning of skin, allowing the color of blood contained in the underlying vessels to be transmitted more readily than in the striae of pregnancy or other types of obesity wherein the skin thickness is normal. Cope[8] states that these vessels are often enlarged, lacking in resiliency and strength; the latter may account for the ease of bruising often noted.

Associated with wasting of the skin, is wasting of most, if not all, organs, including occasionally also the brain.

The frequency of occurrence of the various complaints that Cope's patients present is tabulated in Table 1.

TABLE 1. COMPLAINTS OF THE 46 PATIENTS*

SYMPTOM	PRESENTING COMPLAINT No. of Cases	AS ADDITIONAL SYMPTOM No. of Cases	TOTAL OCCURRENCE No. of Cases
Fatigue and weakness	16	19	35
Weight gain and obesity	6	28	34
Changed appearance	2	31	33
Amenorrhea or irregularity	3	26	29
Bruising	. .	18	18
Nervousness, depression, irritability	4	11	15
Back pain and bone pain	5	9	14
Hirsutism	3	10	13
Headache	1	9	10
Ankle and hand edema	1	8	9
Libido (females); impotence (males)	. .	8	8
Paresthesias	1	3	4
Lower voice	. .	4	4
Blurred vision	1	2	3
Poor wound healing and leg ulcers	1	2	3
Cessation of growth	1	. .	1
Difficulty in walking	1	. .	1
General aching and malaise	1	. .	1

* Cope, Oliver, and Raker, J. W.: Cushing's disease, the surgical experience in the care of 46 cases, New England J. Med. *253*:119, 1955.

Prior to our understanding or interpretation of these findings, Albright and Bloomberg[3] attempted the use of testosterone as a means of re-establishing positive nitrogen balance with some reported success. The rationale of this approach was based upon the gonadal atrophy that these patients display and the demonstration by Kenyon in 1937[23] of the anabolic effect of testosterone with the increase in nitrogen balance when this hormone was given to the eunuchoid patient. In a few of Albright's cases, the negative calcium balance was restored to one of equilibrium or to a slightly positive balance; in only one was there suggestion that remission of the disease occurred.

The electrolyte disturbances tend to be those of a hypokalemic alkalosis with an elevated content of serum carbon dioxide. Lowered serum sodium is encountered infrequently. Despite the negative calcium balance and its increased rate of excretion, the values of serum calcium, phosphorus, phosphatase activities and chloride are usually found to be within normal range.

Specific laboratory diagnostic findings, including roentgenographic observations, exist but are not always present. Arterial hypertension is detectable only in approximately three fourths of these patients. Although its cause is not understood, it usually returns fairly promptly to normal after adrenalectomy.

Glycosuria and/or frank diabetes are by no means a constant finding. Blood sugar was normal more often than not in Cope's series.

The urinary 17-ketosteroid excretions are also variable. They are generally elevated in malignant cortical tumors but less constantly so in the benign ones. When the disease appears to be due to adrenal hyperplasia, the ketosteroids are usually increased in the urine. The studies which have been made to identify more specifically the chemical nature of the increased steroid excretion, those bearing the oxygen atom in the 11-position, appear to be increased more frequently than others.

Urinary ketosteroids as usually measured in urine represent the "total neutral" 17-ketosteroid. It may be useful to summarize the usual ranges under different conditions wherein no original adrenal pathology has existed. Slightly different values may be obtained by different methods of urine extraction. The following 24-hour values are usually obtained:

Young adult males .... 10 to 15 mg.
Aged adult males .... 3 to 8 mg.
Adult females .... 5 to 15 mg.
Children under 10 .... 0 to 1 mg.

Children 12 to 16	2 to	5 mg.
Late pregnancy	15 to	20 mg.
Castrated males	7 to	24 mg.
Castrated females	10 to	15 mg.
Postmenopausal females	10 to	15 mg.
Castration and adrenalectomy .	2 to	4 mg. on
		cortical extracts

Additional fractionation and separation into the ketonic and nonketonic fractions is possible; about 10 to 15 per cent or slightly more of the total is nonketonic normally. The larger ketonic fraction portion is comprised of alpha and beta fractions. The beta fraction comprises about 5 per cent normally but may be increased to 50 per cent or more in patients with adrenal cortical tumors with hypercortical secretory activity, in cortical hyperplasia and in patients with the adrenogenital syndrome (see p. 626). Abnormally low values are usually found in patients with hypopituitarism (Simmond's disease), hypophyseal infantilism, Addison's disease, myxedema and occasionally in anorexia nervosa.

The increased calcium and nitrogen excretions in Cushing's disease, with resultant negative balances they entail, have been alluded to above. Potassium excretion also is increased and probably relates to the general wasting of body protein; Albright reported its restoration to normal in some patients given testosterone as their only form of treatment. The fact that neither sodium balance nor the sodium "space" appears to be distinctly abnormal, in this disease generally, eliminates consideration of Addison's disease from the differential diagnosis. However, there are other clinical features that are more decisive in the elimination of Addison's disease than muscular weakness, for example—hypertension and obesity in the "Cushing" patient.

Thyroid function as revealed by the basal metabolic state is generally somewhat hypoactive; protein-bound iodine measurements are usually within normal range.

Origin of the Endocrine Disorder and the Pathology of Cushing's Disease. Cushing's original concept was that the primary pathology lay within the anterior lobe of the pituitary and was concerned chiefly with adenomatous formation of the basophilic cells. Soon the term "basophilism" was employed as descriptive of the presumed pathology for this syndrome; for it connoted the site which he

believed to harbor the primary disturbance as well as the cell type. His report in 1932[10] was so convincing that when others observed patients with the same phenomenon but with normal pituitary histology at autopsy, faith was shaken as to the validity of Cushing's concept and interpretations. Most patients failed to respond to pituitary radiation. As a number of these patients came to autopsy, a new phase of its historical development began to unravel. Many died of primary adrenocortical tumors, benign or malignant— more often the latter. In a smaller group, cortical hyperplasia, usually bilateral, was observed.

Final proof as to the nature of the hormonal disturbances did not come about until 1948 when ACTH and cortisone were first employed clinically. These agents, particularly ACTH, seemed to duplicate almost completely the Cushing picture. Although excessive and prolonged cortisone therapy produced many of these manifestations, acne, the moderate degree of virilism and the florid complexion were less striking and seemingly less frequently encountered than with ACTH administration. However, the question as to whether or not these are the only hormonal disturbances of the adrenal cortex in Cushing's disease remains an unsettled one. The demonstration of primary pituitary disorders in this disease is infrequent; in fact, the paucity of such pathologic material has been cause for some to conclude that the pituitary is seldom the site of the primary disturbance. With bilateral adrenalectomy or the removal of a unilateral tumor being so effective a form of treatment, these patients survive and return to normal life. Hence it may be many years before enough autopsy material is available from pituitary examinations to establish how often the origin of the disease lies within the pituitary. In most patients, the primary pathology appears to arise within the adrenal cortex.

Treatment. As the hypersecretory activity of cortical adenomas or tumors generally are not suppressed by the administration of cortisone or ACTH, complete unilateral adrenalectomy is performed with removal of the cortical adenoma or carcinoma if possible. Although multiple adenomas are found occasionally, they are usually located within the same gland; it is indeed rare that adenomas or tumors occur bilaterally.

When one adrenal is the cause of the Cushing syndrome, the activity of the contralateral one is always depressed; its cortex atrophies. Hence, unless such patients are maintained on cortisone after unilateral adrenalectomy, addisonian crisis is likely to develop postoperatively. In the postoperative period, ACTH therapy is administered to awaken cortical function in the remaining adrenal; cortisone therapy is reduced cautiously while ACTH is administered until finally both can be discontinued—generally within 8 to 10 days.

Subtotal adrenalectomy for bilateral adrenal hyperplasia would seem to be the ideal treatment of Cushing's syndrome of this origin. It is the treatment generally preferred and most commonly employed. It is not always possible to resect the proper amount of adrenal tissue to control completely the course of the disease. On the other hand, subtotal adrenalectomy is preferable to total removal of both glands despite the fact that replacement therapy in the bilaterally adrenalectomized patient poses a less serious problem than was anticipated earlier. Should more adrenal tissue need to be removed, this can be done at a later date.

Prognosis. Except for huge adrenal tumors and the technical difficulty that they may pose in removal, surgical mortality in adrenalectomy for this disease should be less than 5 per cent. Total cure is effected when the cortical tumor is benign or due to hyperplasia. Should cortical carcinoma be the cause, the prognosis is generally poor. These tumors tend to metastasize early, frequently to the liver, the lungs, the brain and bone. In this respect they appear to follow the similar metastatic pathways to the organs of predilection, which are also those characteristic for hypernephroma.

ADRENOGENITAL SYNDROME (ADRENAL VIRILISM). To appreciate the pathogenesis of the adrenogenital syndrome, it becomes necessary to describe the biologic effects of androgens insofar as currently established. In general, two types of reactions or clinical responses are observed from excessive androgen production or administration. The *precocious sexual development,* while striking, is nearly equaled by those characteristics associated with the *anabolic effects* of androgens. There is an increase in total muscle mass. The general appearance of these children is one of Herculean strength. The nitrogen balance is strongly positive. Bone growth is facilitated, in part from the anabolic effects of androgen. It is not yet established whether the normal production of growth hormone is altered or remains normal. The combination of sexual precocity and the increase in muscle mass in the child creates the appearance of a "little giant." The result is a freak, often serving as a source of torment by the child's playmates and of misunderstanding by his parents and the family associates.

Three pathologic states may account for the excessive androgenic activity: bilateral adrenal hyperplasia, androgen-producing adenomas, or carcinomas.

Although a number of androgenic steroids have been isolated by extraction procedures applied to urine, some may represent artifacts or chemical changes incident to extraction.[13] Of these, *androsterone* is generally the most abundant to be found and possesses potent biologic activity. When this substance is esterified with acetic acid, androstandiol is produced, having several times the activity of androsterone. The other natural androgen normally found in the urine is dehydro-iso-androsterone whose biologic activity is much less than androsterone.

Testosterone is the steroid of testicular origin. It is many times as potent as androsterone in promoting comb growth of the cock and seminal vesicular activation in the castrate rat. It is possible that much of the androsterone and dehydro-iso-androsterone in urine represent the end metabolites of testosterone. In the castrate human male or female, however, androsterone and dehydro-iso-androsterone continue to appear, but the quantity is less than normal. When adrenalectomy is added to castration, the 17-ketosteroids essentially disappear from the urine unless corticoids are administered. It was upon this observation that adrenalectomy in combination with orchiectomy was explored by Huggins in the palliative management of the partially dependent tumors of the breast or the prostate (see Chap. 26, "Breast").

There is a close quantitative correlation

between urinary androgens and the biologic activity that the patient displays clinically. Their excretion is diminished in castrates and is increased in hypercorticism, interstitial tumors of the testes or the ovary, n pregnancy and in acromegaly or gigantism of pituitary origin.

Androgens, in addition to effecting an increase in nitrogen balance, favor the retention of potassium and phosphorus. Although the metabolism of these two minerals is an intricate and complex one, their response in connection with androgen activity is believed to be related to or to be associated with the anabolic effects. Both of these minerals are associated with protein metabolism and indeed appear to be essential to the anabolic effect. In protein starvation, potassium and phosphorus are excreted in excess of normal; thus in addition to the negative nitrogen balance of protein depletion is also the occurrence of negative potassium and phosphorus balance. Estrogens do not appear to alter materially the excretion of either nitrogen or these two minerals.

Clinical Considerations of the Adrenogenital Syndrome. This is a masculinizing syndrome which occurs principally in females, and its clinical pattern is that due to the excessive production of androgens, especially androsterone. The cause of excessive androgen production is cortical hyperplasia or tumors. The latter may be benign or malignant and need not always arise from adrenal cortical tissue, as the testis and the ovary also produce androgens and in a small per cent of cases are the site of origin of androgen-producing tumors. There are on record about a dozen cases in which estrogen-producing adrenal tumors have created feminizing features in males—the counterpart of the masculinizing tumors in females.

The clinical picture of excessive production of androgens in the female is striking. Clinical studies of these patients have played an important role in the understanding of androgen activity and functions. The fact that the results of androsteronism have been those of "masculinizing" the female has caused these patients to be the subject of public curiosity and ridicule, especially in new surroundings. The syndrome may appear at any stage of life —infancy, childhood, or in adult life.

Most frequently, the disease begins in in-

fancy or childhood in the female. The types of disorders generally observed are those of precocious sexual development (usually heterosexual characteristics) and those which are related to the anabolic effects of androgenesis. When precocious sexual development in the preadolescent male occurs, the genitalia assume adult characteristics; in the female it is characterized by heterosexual development with beard, enlarged clitoris and deepening of the voice. Should the male patient suffer from an estrogen-producing tumor, the clinical picture is one of feminization, with the female distribution of fat, the development of breast tissue and diminution or loss of beard.

BILATERAL ADRENAL HYPERPLASIA AND THE ADRENOGENITAL SYNDROME IN INFANTS AND CHILDREN. Adrenal virilism at birth is due most often to adrenal hyperplasia. Whether the hyperplasia is from hyperpituitary (ACTH) activity or from idiopathic adrenal hyperplasia is not yet settled. The latter possibility seems to be a bit remote, as endocrine hyperplasias more often are the result of an overactive pituitary than self-induced. The adrenal hyperplasia is bilateral and often limited largely to the zona reticularis in this disease.

Often these patients respond to the administration of cortisone, presumably because of its depressing effect upon ACTH production. This fact also argues in favor of the primary disorder being one of pituitary origin. In some patients with bilateral hyperplasia, cortical exhaustion may occur, and an addisonianlike status may develop later on.

CORTICAL ADENOMAS AND CORTICAL CARCINOMA PRODUCING ADRENOGENITAL SYNDROME. These tumors usually arise in adult life. They produce the clinical picture of androgen excess which, of course, is more obvious in the female who tends to develop heterosexual characteristics. Virilism will occur in the male, but in adult life this change is less evident than in childhood. In either case, the 17-ketosteroid urinary excretion is increased; this laboratory finding coupled with roentgenographic evidence of a mass in or above the kidney strongly suggests the diagnosis of an adenoma or a carcinoma. These carcinomas are highly malignant, usually metastasizing to the lung and the liver in much the same manner and route as the hypernephroma and the cortical carcinoma of Cushing's disease. Adrenal hyperplasia is seldom responsible for the adrenogenital syndrome occurring in adult life.

Lesions in the pineal body, the hypothalamus, the interstitial cells of the testis or the ovary, the arrhenoblastoma, luteoma, or adrenal ectopic tissue may produce the same clinical picture, as each is capable of inducing androgen production. Those tumors which may lie within the abdomen are to be sought for at the time of laparotomy for exploration of the adrenals.

Treatment of virulizing tumors is surgical removal. As hypersecretion of one adrenal often suppresses the function of the other, the patient should be prepared for operation and managed in the early postoperative period in the same manner as is the Cushing's patient or the bilaterally adrenalectomized patient (see p. 629).

Aldosteronism. Aldosterone (electrocortin) is a corticoid with a potent influence upon sodium retention.[30] Its identification clarifies one of the important mysteries regarding adrenal function. Although desoxycorticosterone acetate (DOCA) has a moderate influence upon sodium retention and has been useful to a limited extent in the treatment of Addison's disease, DOCA is a synthetic compound which is probably not a hormone normally produced by the adrenal cortex. Thus, until the discovery of aldosterone as a normally produced hormone with at least one of its functions being directed toward sodium conservation, this function of the adrenal cortex had not been understood. Yet it has been clear that some factor[30] was needed to explain satisfactorily the incompleteness of corticoid replacement therapy after bilateral adrenalectomy, if salt and water were to be normal.

Excessive amounts of aldosterone have been reported in the urine in nephrotic edema, congestive failure, decompensated cirrhotics and in eclampsia.[26] Conn[6] believes that a metabolic event common to all of these conditions triggers the excessive production of aldosterone; the occurrence of edema and aldosteronism of these types he believes to be secondary to some more central disorder.

PRIMARY ALDOSTERONISM. Conn[6] infers this to be a disease entity due primarily to the excessive production of aldosterone. Cortical tumors are the principal causes. This syndrome also differs from that of secondary aldosteronism in that edema does not develop. The electrolyte disorder is comparable if not identical with that of the disease known as "potassium-losing nephritis."

To date, 13 cases have been recognized, 9 have been cured by removal of a cortical adenoma, 1 by bilateral adrenalectomy; 3 were classified as suffering from potassium-losing nephritis; a cortical adenoma was found in each at autopsy.[6] In the last 3, the diagnosis is *post hoc* reasoning. The most elaborately studied was Conn's patient, in whom this clinical entity was first recognized.

The clinical pattern of primary aldosteronism should be suspected in patients complaining of periodic muscular weakness, intermittent tetany, paresthesia, polyuria and polydipsia, and hypertension. There is no edema in contrast with those suffering from secondary aldosteronism; this difference is not understood.

Blood electrolytes reveal hypokalemia, hypernatremia and alkalosis. Serum calcium is reported as normal, as are the urinary 17-hydroxycorticoids and 17-ketosteroids. The hyposthenuria does not respond to pitressin (oxytocin). Serum potassium concentrations appear to be resistant to potassium administration.

There is no evidence at this time to relate or to deny pituitary control of aldosterone. However, this corticoid does not appear to be under the control of the usual pituitary hormones or at least in the usual sense.

Once the adenoma was removed in each of these 9 patients, the symptoms of primary aldosteronism disappeared, the normal electrolyte pattern returned, and after a few weeks the normal blood pressure was re-established.

Pathology is not well defined. In Conn's case, an adenoma of the right adrenal cortex 4 cm. in diameter was found, the left adrenal appearing grossly normal. On the basis of some degree of atrophy of the cells of the zona fasciculata of the left adrenal tissue, Conn suggests that these cells may be the source of aldosterone.

Treatment is limited to surgical exploration of both adrenals with removal of the adenoma. If no adenoma is found, adrenalectomy should be considered, provided that sound evidence of primary aldosteronism exists. If the adenoma can be found and removed, complete recovery appears to be likely.

Corticoid Therapy in Surgical Patients. As corticoid therapy is employed in a variety of medical disorders, in due course some of these patients may require operation, either for the disease under cortisone treatment (ulcerative colitis) or for independent disorders. In either case, certain adjustments in cortisone dosages appear to be necessary in the immediate preoperative and postoperative periods. A report from the Mayo Clinic in 1953[29] suggested that the causes of 3 deaths which occurred within a few hours after operation, were due to the failure to resume cortisone therapy or to increase the dosage during the time of operative "stress." As a result, they have recommended that any patient previously on cortisone therapy be given the drug again the day before operation, the operative day, and for 1 to 3 days thereafter, even when the patient's cortisone therapy had been discontinued many months previously. This same phenomenon was observed to occur in a similar manner when bilateral adrenalectomy was first performed, for originally cortisone therapy was not instituted until after the operation was completed.

Early studies implicated cortisone therapy as an agent disposed toward poor healing in surgical wounds. Certainly there are some patients whose wounds do not appear to heal well when they have received large doses of cortisone for weeks to months. In doses of 50 to 100 mg. of cortisone per day, however, there is little evidence of impaired wound healing when the total period of therapy is less than 2 weeks in duration.

The claim has been made by Grey et al.[19] that cortisone and/or ACTH therapy produce peptic ulcer. This view seems to be an unsettled one, as it appears from the studies of Dragstedt[14] that peptic activity and gastric secretion are not affected immediately by the administration of either ACTH or cortisone. Kirsner[24] reports only 1 perforating peptic ulcer among 224 patients under long-term corticoid therapy.

Because ACTH and cortisone increase the appetite for food, Cole,[5] as well as others, including the author, have administered cortisone for a few days to postoperative patients able to eat, in need of food but without appetite. Daily dosages beginning with 300 mg. of cortisone, tapered down each day, are generally used to this end, but for no longer than 5 to 6 days. Although the corticoids have a catabolic effect at these dosage levels, the benefit of the increased caloric intake appears to offset this disadvantage. Often the patient may consume in excess of 4,000 calories within a few days. After the drug has been discontinued, the patient usually continues to display an active interest in his diet and appears to recover more rapidly than otherwise. However, this is not a practice widely employed or one to be used indiscriminately.

Corticoid and Salt Management of the Adrenalectomized Patient. It is remarkable how easily the bilateral adrenalectomized patient can be managed; the problem appears to be more simple than that of many diabetics. Thus, the ability to maintain such patients in good health poses no contraindication to adrenalectomy, should the operation be necessary. Just as the diabetic must be advised about his insulin dosage, so must the adrenalectomized patient be instructed and advised about his corticoid and salt therapy and seen at regular intervals to guide his course.

The following schedule has been devised by Huggins and associates for corticoid hormonal therapy during the preoperative, the operative, the early postoperative and the subsequent maintenance periods.

A METHOD OF MANAGEMENT FOR PATIENTS
SUBJECTED TO ADRENALECTOMY

Preoperative 24 hours
Cortisone, 50 mg., IM each 6 hrs. until midnight (6 A.M., 12 N., 6 P.M., 12 M.)
DOCA, 5 mg., IM at 9 A.M.
NaCl, 4 Gm., at 6 P.M.
Day of operation
Cortisone, 150 mg., IM—given on call to O.R.
DOCA, 5 mg., IM given on call to O.R.
Immediately after operation
Cortisone, 50 mg., IM and then every 4 hrs.
Fluids: Slowly intravenous infusion of
     5% glucose in NS 1,000 cc.
     5% glucose in water 1,000 cc.
     Often it is desirable to give less saline than indicated above.
     Blood transfusions and plasma as needed
Blood pressure, pulse and respiration every 10 min. immediately after operation (the interval can be lengthened on judgment)
Temperature: every 2 hrs.

Measure hourly urinary output (by indwelling catheter) if catheter has been used.

First postoperative day

Cortisone, 50 mg., IM every 6 hrs.

DOCA, 5 mg., IM at 9 A.M. if blood pressure is low

Blood pressure, pulse and respiration every hr. or every 2 hrs., according to judgment

Temperature every 4 hrs.

Second postoperative day

Cortisone, 50 mg., IM t.i.d. (orally if not nauseated)

DOCA, 3 mg. IM (by judgment only)

Regular diet

Initiate NaCl, 1 Gm. t.i.d. or q.i.d. orally or by vein (NaCl is more important during hot weather)

Third postoperative day

Cortisone, 50 mg., IM, b.i.d. (orally, if not nauseated)

Blood pressure, pulse every 4 hrs.

(Blood pressure is taken in both the sitting and the lying positions—with a 5-min. interval—and recorded in graph form in chart.)

NaCl, 1 Gm., t.i.d.

Fourth postoperative day

Cortisone, 25 mg., b.i.d. (maintenance)

NaCl, 1 Gm., b.i.d. (maintenance)

DOCA is indicated in patients with significant orthostatic hypotension (more than 20 mm. Hg in systolic pressure). Implantation of DOCA pellets (225 mg. subcutaneously is advisable. OR: DOC-trimethylacetate (25 mg. IM) once every 4 weeks also is of benefit.

Adrenal Medulla

Chromaffin tissue, wherever found, is so named because it is stained yellow or brown with chromium salts. This tissue is associated with the ganglia of the sympathetic nervous system, of which the adrenal medulla embryologically is a part. The size of the autonomic system is proportionately much larger in fetal life than after birth, when it is reduced remarkably, except for a few areas. The remaining structures in adult life are the paraganglionic areas which connect with the principal sympathetic trunks, i.e., the celiac, renal, adrenal, aortic and hypogastric plexuses and the carotid body. The adrenal medulla is the largest single site of chromaffin tissues.

It is not surprising that factors which affect the autonomics may also affect the adrenal medulla and vice versa. The major hormone elaborated by the medulla is epinephrine, the first natural hormone to be isolated in crystal-line form. Its biologic activity was recognized by Abel in 1897.[1] Epinephrine and norepinephrine were synthesized by Stolz in 1904.[31] More than 45 years elapsed before norepinephrine was to be employed clinically. Both hormones are normally found in medullary tissue, epinephrine being predominant. In postganglionic nerves, norepinephrine is present in larger quantities than epinephrine and is usually present in larger quantities in pheochromocytoma (see p. 632). Both adrenergic hormones are stable in blood, although they are destroyed rapidly *in vivo*, probably by either conjugation or oxidation or both. Most, if not all, tissues appear to be capable of inactivating them.

It has long been known that the adrenal medulla is not essential for life. However, this is not justification to conclude that its 2 vasopressor hormones are unessential, for they are produced generously by other pheochromaffin tissues as well as by the adrenal medulla; therefore, removal of the adrenal medulla does not abolish all of their sources of production.

Pharmacologic Action of Epinephrine and Norepinephrine. The action of these hormones appears to be upon effector cells of specific organs and not to be mediated to any great extent through autonomic pathways. Many of the actions ascribed to epinephrine are also common to norepinephrine; but there are also major differences. These differences play an important role in the ultimate decision as to which is the most suitable preparation for use in the particular surgical patient. Among the important sites of actions of these agents are the heart, the arterioles and the kidney. A rise in pulse rate and an elevation of arterial blood pressure occur. Pulmonary circulation and bronchial musculature are also quite responsive. Gluconeogenesis may be sufficiently stimulated to overcome insulin shock and may produce frank diabetes in some patients with tumors producing these hormones over prolonged periods of time.

Cardiac response is one of an increase in rate and in stroke volume. The heart beat is more forceful and may be very distressing symptomatically to some patients during the systolic thrust. The minute volume output of the heart is greatly increased over that of normal. Ventricular irritability is exaggerated; extrasystoles and fibrillation may occur. The effect upon ventricular irritability is the chief reason why these agents should not be used in "cardiac arrest," hypoxia, hypothermia, in hyperthyroidism or in conjunction with cyclopropane anesthesia, all of which may also create an increased irritability of the ventricles. To superimpose the irritant properties of these drugs under conditions wherein an increase in ventricular irritability already exists may lead to fatal ventricular fibrillation.

Vascular effects are largely limited to the small arterial vessels, especially the arterioles. Vasoconstriction is the rule if one limits consideration to those of the skin and the splanchnic bed. However, vasodilation is the general response of the arteriolar vessels in the myocardium and the skeletal muscles.

Arterial blood pressure is elevated promptly. Within limits, this response is usually in proportion to the quantity of epinephrine or norepinephrine administered. Some state that the diastolic pressure is reduced in man, but this is not in accord with the observations of many, including the author. More often than not, the diastolic pressure is also elevated; so is the mean arterial pressure. When the vasopressor effect of epinephrine "wears off," transient hypotension may occur as a rebound phenomenon.

Renal blood flow is generally reduced by more than 50 per cent and is accompanied by an increase in peripheral arteriolar resistance. Glomerular filtration and tubular resorption are not consistently altered, although excretion of sodium and chloride is said to be decreased.

Pulmonary arterial pressure is elevated, but it is not certain that this effect is due to vasoconstriction alone. Bronchial musculature is relaxed by epinephrine; hence, the usefulness of this agent in the relief of bronchial spasm of asthma.

Intestinal tone is diminished, but the sphincters of the pylorus and the ileocecal areas contract. Gastric secretion is inhibited.

Contraction of the Spleen. In man the volume of blood contained in the spleen is small, but in the dog and the rabbit, when the spleen contracts, considerable quantities of blood are expressed into the circulation. In these species, the effect is that of an autologous transfusion; in man this seems to be of little consequence.

Gluconeogenesis promptly follows the administration of epinephrine. The glucose obtained is derived from glycogen stores, and for this reason the administration of epinephrine has been employed upon occasion in the treatment of hypoglycemia when exogenous sources of glucose were not available.

Blood and plasma volumes are unchanged.

The distinctions between epinephrine and norepinephrine are largely those related to specific functions of the cardiovascular response. These are summarized in Table 2.

Should norepinephrine be administered for many hours or for a day or two as a continuous intravenous drip, vasoconstriction along the venous subcutaneous channel of the extremity may be so intense as to cause cutaneous and fat necrosis on either side of the vessel

TABLE 2. COMPARISON OF THE EFFECTS OF INTRAVENOUS INFUSION OF EPINEPHRINE AND NOREPINEPHRINE IN MAN*

INDEX	EPINEPH-RINE	NOREPINEPH-RINE
Cardiac		
Heart rate	+	—**
Stroke volume	++	++
Cardiac output	+++	0, —
Arrhythmias	++++	++++
Coronary blood flow	++	+++
Blood Pressure		
Systolic arterial	+++	+++
Mean arterial	+	++
Diastolic arterial	+, 0, —	++
Mean pulmonary	++	++
Peripheral Circulation		
Total peripheral resistance	—	++
Cerebral blood flow	+	0, —
Muscle blood flow	++	0, —
Cutaneous blood flow	——	+, 0, —
Renal blood flow	—	—
Splanchnic blood flow	++	0, +
Metabolic Effects		
Oxygen consumption	++	0, +
Blood sugar	+++	0, +
Blood lactic acid	+++	0, +
Eosinopenic response	+	0
Central Nervous System		
Respiration	+	+
Subjective sensations	+	0, +

(After Goldenberg, Aranow, Smith, and Faber, Dec., 1950. A.M.A. Archives of Internal Medicine.)
* 0.1 to 0.4 microgram per kilogram per minute.
+ = Increase.
0 = No change.
— = Decrease.
** After atropine, +.

for a distance of several centimeters. From a practical point of view it is best that a transfusion of blood or plasma be administered into a vein of another extremity while norepinephrine is given *only* by a venous cannula, lest the rate of flow of the blood transfusion be sharply curtailed, or norepinephrine leak into the tissues.

LIMITATIONS AND CONTRAINDICATIONS OF EPINEPHRINE AND NOREPINEPHRINE IN HYPOVOLEMIC SHOCK. Epinephrine, its rebound hypotensive effect, its tendency to cause ventricular fibrillation and other side reactions virtually eliminate this drug from serious consideration in most cases of hemorrhagic, burn or traumatic shock. The author has not used this agent for the treatment of shock for many years.

Norepinephrine, while seemingly capable of "raising the dead" in some instances, should rarely be used in hypovolemic shock unless blood and/or plasma are immediately at hand and can be administered rapidly to expand blood volume. The peripheral collapse in hypovolemia results from the diminished circulating blood volume—not from lack of peripheral resistance. In reality, physiologic peripheral vasoconstriction is already almost maximal and no longer capable of sustaining the arterial pressure without blood replacement. Although admittedly exogenous, norepinephrine administered under these circumstances can induce the smaller arteries and arterioles, and possibly the veins also, to squeeze down a bit further in the agonal state; this is not a practice to follow. The agent that is needed in hemorrhagic shock is that which has been lost—blood—and very quickly!

On the other hand, occasionally after prolonged and complicated surgery or following extensive trauma, loss of peripheral tone does occur and norepinephrine may be indicated. Although almost always such patients require and may have received adequate blood replacement, further transfusion in volumes greater than needed can easily lead to cardiac failure and pulmonary edema, especially in patients with marginal cardiac reserve. These are the few patients in whom the use of an intravenous drip of norepinephrine is strongly indicated, and its administration may be lifesaving. To recognize when the continued use of blood or plasma may be harmful in shock and when the powerful vasoconstrictor, nor-

epinephrine, should be employed, may tax the judgment of the most experienced observer. Generally after a few hours (often less), norepinephrine administration may be slowed or discontinued. However, one should wait several hours longer before removing the cannula from the vein, in case norepinephrine therapy should need to be resumed.

Norepinephrine administration has proved to be more useful in the treatment of the normovolemic shock of toxemia—septic or chemical. Here the primary circulatory problem is usually one of loss of peripheral tone, although plasma loss may also occur. A vasoconstrictor as the definitive treatment in the hypovolemic shock of hemorrhage, burns or dehydration is contraindicated.

A specific effect of epinephrine and of norepinephrine is the stimulation of the thyroid to release protein-bound iodine, including triiodothyronine, into the blood stream. This was demonstrated in the dog by Ackerman and Arons.[2]

Pheochromocytoma (Adrenal Medullary Hyperfunction). This tumor produces another series of spectacular disorders in hormonal physiology. The symptoms and signs are those which result from the excessive epinephrine and norepinephrine that these tumors produce. The tumor is of pheochromoblastic tissue and most often located within the adrenal medulla; hence, the origin of its name. They may also arise occasionally from the chromaffin tissue of the paraganglia. They are comparatively rare.

CLINICAL PATTERN. In pheochromocytoma the course of the patient is that resulting from excessive production of epinephrine and norepinephrine, usually more norepinephrine than epinephrine. Both agents may be found in the urine. The patient may experience paroxysms or bursts of extreme hypertension, due to sudden releases into the circulation of large amounts of these powerful drugs. These attacks may last for minutes to several hours. Anxiety, throbbing headache, palpitation, blurring of vision, nausea and vomiting, perspiration, dilation of pupils, and prostration are among the patient's complaints. Hyperglycemia is often present, and hypercalcemia may occur in some. Generally, such bursts of adrenergic activity are associated with body motion, such as flexion or hyperextension of the spine, or from a tight belt or girdle which causes mild pressure on the adrenal area. The systolic pressure may exceed that which can be measured by the usual sphygmomanometer. Death from a cerebrovascular accident, cardiac arrest from ventricular fibrillation, or pulmonary edema may occur; occasionally, a shocklike state develops with high fever as the terminal pattern.

In about half of the patients encountered, however, a base line hypertension is present and is not readily distinguished from that of essential hypertension. Some clue is to be found in the elevated basal metabolic rate and the diabetic state which frequently are also present. It is thought that the patients in this group are those in whom hypersecretion of the longer-acting norepinephrine occurs rather than epinephrine.

DIAGNOSIS. In considering pheochromocytoma, one may try to produce an attack or paroxysm deliberately by palpating the adrenal areas or by asking the patient to perform such activities as he knows to precipitate an attack; however, this procedure is not without risk. Routine laboratory work is of little value other than in a negative way. An elevated basal metabolic rate is often found which is not usually accompanied by the expected avidity for thyroid uptake of iodine[131] or the usual expected altered relationships between the free and the bound serum iodine. Should the tumor be large, it may be detected by intravenous pyelography or the retroperitoneal insufflation of air.

Other lines of evidence for or against the diagnosis of pheochromocytoma may be uncovered through the application of certain pharmacologic tests. One may try to provoke a paroxysm by the administration of several types of drugs which incite the adrenergic hormones. Among them are histamine phosphate and methylcholine hydrochloride. Normally, these drugs produce slight hypotension and flushing. A rise in blood pressure, greater than that noted when the cold pressor test is applied, usually occurs in patients with pheochromocytoma. Neither test is free of the fairly frequent occurrence of false negative or false positive responses.

More useful diagnostically, as well as in the management of the paroxysms, are the so-called adrenergic "blocking agents." They should not be used excepting under resting conditions; preferably the patient should remain in bed for at least 24 hours to secure adequate blood pressure readings under basal conditions. Of these, benzodioxane and Regitine are the most helpful. The former is chemically related to epinephrine. While it retains certain of the pharmacologic actions of epinephrine, it also loses some. Instead of inducing hypertension, it produces hypotension in a remarkably high percentage of patients with pheochromocytoma. Benzodioxane, in dosages of 10 mg. per square meter of body surface, is administered intravenously over a period of about 2 minutes. At this rate and dosage, a fall in arterial pressure of to 50 mm. Hg or greater usually occurs when pheochromocytoma is present. False positive responses are rarely encountered. This same dosage similarly administered to the normal subject usually induces a slight rise in pressure.

Regitine (phentolamine) reacts similarly but with less side effects; 5 mg. of this compound given intravenously produces a lowering in blood pressure, should pheochromocytoma be present. At the University of Chicago, Regitine is preferred to benzodioxane, although both are occasionally used (Fig. 27-5).

PATHOLOGY. Although the incidence of pheochromocytoma is rare, in about 15 per cent of patients with this disease, multiple tumors are found. A like number is found to lie outside of the adrenal glands, as paragangliomas of the retroperitoneal or retropleural areas along the sympathetic chains, and at the periaortic plexes at its bifurcation and in the carotid body. The vast majority of these tumors are benign; only a few are malignant.

Usually these tumors are well encapsulated, highly vascular and relatively small. Hemorrhages and cystic degeneration are fairly common; the cut surface is usually brown in color.

SURGICAL TREATMENT. When the diagnosis seems to be reasonably well established or carries a sufficiently high index of suspicion, surgical exploration of the adrenal glands and the paraganglionic tissue is indicated. In fact, it is mandatory in most patients, as no other effective treatment exists.

From 1927, when C. H. Mayo removed successfully the first of these tumors, until the advent of the "blocking agents," surgical exploration was extremely hazardous. There was no means available to control the releases of epinephrine and/or norepinephrine induced by surgical manipulation of the adrenals essential to their surgical exploration and removal. Fatal cardiac arrest or cerebrovascular accidents from the hypertensive bursts were often caused by surgical exploration and proved to be discouraging to many surgeons. Still others attempted to ligate the adrenal veins and the usually numerous collaterals to and from the tumor, prior to palpating for the tumor. Often this could not be accomplished successfully and usually entailed prolonged anesthesia under the most unfavorable of circumstances.

With the introduction of the blocking agents, carefully and continuously administered and regulated according to need throughout the operation, the risk of operation is greatly reduced. Should the surgeon's manipulations cause a burst of epinephrine to enter the circulation, the elevation of arterial pressure is controlled promptly and readily. An example of this type of control of blood pressure change during the operative phase in a patient with pheochromocytoma during operation is demonstrated in Figure 27-6.

Opinions differ among surgeons as to the operative approach to be employed. Many prefer a transverse abdominal incision in order that both adrenals may be explored, as well as the paraganglionic area. Others prefer the extraperitoneal flank approach, each adrenal being explored separately. These tumors are seldom situated bilaterally; if multiple, they are usually within the same gland. When possible, ligation of their blood supply should be carried out before the tumor is removed.

A precipitous fall in blood pressure often occurs as soon as the tumor is removed. This response presumably is a rebound one and due to release of the arteriolar vasospasm formerly caused by the excess of adrenergic hormones. A solution of norepinephrine should be prepared in advance and the cannula for its administration already inserted into an appropriate extremity vein. Should the sudden onset of hypotension occur, control of rebound hypotension and the prevention of other untoward effects are easily accomplished. Usually after a few hours, the drip of norepinephrine can be slowed and discontinued when the patient's pressure and circulatory dynamics stabilize. In some, administration of norepinephrine may need to be continued for a day or two. The risk of a skin slough is real; Howard states

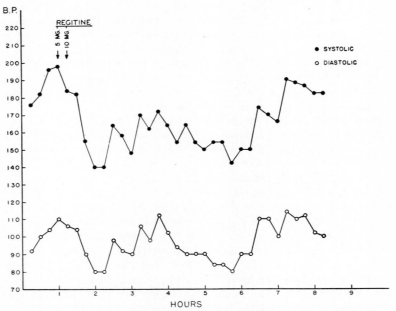

FIG. 27-5. A positive Regitine response in a patient in whom subsequently a pheochromocytoma was removed. (Chart from Dr. Dwight E. Clark)

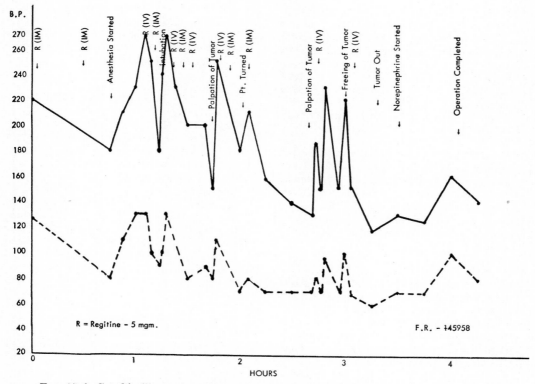

FIG. 27-6. Graphic illustration of the blood pressure increases in the course of operative manipulation of pheochromocytoma. Note response to Regitine and that after tumor was removed, norepinephrine was administered. (Chart from Dr. Dwight E. Clark)

that Regitine may be given subcutaneously in small amounts to avoid slough.

The surgical results, as well as the low mortality experience since the advent of the blocking agents and norepinephrine, have encouraged physicians to search more diligently for the presence of this syndrome among their patients with hypertension, especially those with hypermetabolism without hyperthyroidism.

Nonfunctioning Medullary Tumors of the Adrenals. The sympathogonioma, the ganglioneuroma and the neuroblastoma are nonhormonal tumors which may also arise from paraganglionic tissue, including the adrenal medulla. The first is rare and usually malignant, with early metastasis being the rule. The ganglioneuroma is essentially benign; it is well encapsulated and slow-growing, often producing few, if any, symptoms. The neuroblastoma, on the other hand, is highly malignant; it is a fairly commonly encountered tumor in the retroperitoneal area in children.

As none of the 3 is a hormone-producing tumor, their symptoms and detection depend upon pressure displacements and metastasis.

Treatment is surgical removal when possible, followed by intensive radiation therapy, although most are fairly radioresistant. Except for the ganglioneuroma, the prognosis is usually poor. (See Pediatric Surgery, Chapter 46.)

REFERENCES

1. Abel, J. J., and Crawford, A. C.: On the blood-pressure raising constituent of the suprarenal capsule, Bull. Johns Hopkins Hosp. *8*:151, 1897.
2. Ackerman, N. B., and Arons, W. L.: Effect of epinephrine and nor-epinephrine on the thyroidal release of thyroid hormones in dogs, J. Clin. Endocrinol. *16*:926, 1956.
3. Albright, F., Parson, W., and Bloomberg, E.: Cushing's syndrome interpreted as hyperadrenocorticism leading to hypergluconeogenesis: results of treatment with testosterone propionate, J. Clin. Endocrinol. *1*:375, 1941.

4. Bovie, W. T.: Electro-surgery as an aid to the removal of intracranial tumors; with a preliminary note on a new surgical-current generator, Surg., Gynec. & Obst. *47*:751, 1928.

5. Cole, W. H., Gross, W. J., and Montgomery, M. M.: The use of ACTH and cortisone in surgery, Ann. Surg. *137*:718, 1953.

6. Conn, J. W., and Louis, L. H.: Primary aldosteronism; a new clinical entity, Ann. Int. Med. *44*:1, 1956.

7. Cooper, D. Y., Rosenthal, O., Foroff, O., and Blakemore, W. S.: Action of noradrenalin and ascorbate on hydroxylation of progesterone by bovine adrenocortical homogenates, S. Forum *11*:127, 1960.

8. Cope, O., and Raker, J. W.: Cushing's disease: the surgical experience in the care of 46 cases, New England J. Med. *253*:119, 1955.

9. Cori, C. F., and Cori, G. T.: The fate of sugar in the animal body. VII. The carbohydrate metabolism of adrenalectomized rats and mice, J. Biol. Chem. *74*:473, 1927.

10. Cushing, H.: The basophil adenoma of the pituitary body and their clinical manifestations (pituitary basophilism), Bull. Johns Hopkins Hosp. *50*:137, 1932.

11. ———: The control of bleeding in operations for brain tumors, with the description of silver clips for the occlusion of vessels inaccessible to the ligature, Ann. Surg. *54*:1, 1911.

12. ———: Sexual infantilism with optic atrophy in cases of tumor affecting the hypophysis cerebri, J. Nerv. & Ment. Dis. *33*:704, 1906.

13. Dorfman, R. I.: The metabolism of androgens, Rec. Progress in Hormone Res. *2*:179, 1948.

14. Dragstedt, L. R., Ragins, H., Dragstedt, L. R., II, and Evans, S. O.: Stress and duodenal ulcer. Ann. Surg. *144*:450, 1956.

15. du Vigneaud, V., Lawler, H. C., and Popenoe, E. A.: Enzymatic cleavage of glycinamide from vasopressin and a proposed structure for this pressor-antidiuretic hormone of the posterior pituitary, J. Am. Chem. Soc. *75*:4880, 1953.

16. Evans, J.: Personal communication, 1956.

17. Frohlich, Alfred: Ein Fall von Tumor der Hypophysis cerebri ohne Akromegalie, Wien. klin. Rundschau *15*:889 and 906, 1901.

18. Grey, Ernest: Fibrin as a hemostatic agent in cerebral surgery, Surg., Gynec. & Obst. *21*:452, 1915.

19. Grey, S., Benson, J. A., Reifenstein, R. W., and Spiro, H. M.: Chronic stress and peptic ulcer: I. Effect of corticotropin (ACTH) and cortisone on gastric secretion, J.A.M.A. *147*:1489, 1951.

20. Harrop, G. A., Weinstein, A., Soffer, J. L., and Trescher, J. H.: Diagnosis and treatment of Addison's disease, J.A.M.A. *100*:1850, 1933.

21. Houssay, B. A., and Biasotti, A.: Hypophysis, carbohydrate metabolism and diabetes, Endocrinology *15*:511, 1931.

22. Illingworth, C. F. W., Forrest, A. P. M., and Brown, D. A. Peebles: A simple method of implanting radon seeds into the pituitary gland in treatment of advanced breast cancer, S. Forum *6*:406, 1956.

23. Kenyon, A. T., et al.: Urinary excretion of androgenic and estrogenic substances in certain endocrine states: studies in hypogonadism, gynecomastia and virilism, J. Clin. Invest. *16*:705-717, 1937.

24. Kirsner, J.: Personal communication, 1956.

25. Loeb, R. F.: Effect of sodium chloride in treatment of patient with Addison's disease, Proc. Soc. Exper. Biol. & Med. *30*:808, 1933.

26. Luetscher, J. A., Jr., and Johnson, B. B.: Observations on the sodium-retaining corticoid (aldosterone) in the urine of children and adults in relation to sodium balance and edema, J. Clin. Invest. *23*:1441, 1954.

27. Rasmussen, T., Harper, P. V., and Kennedy, T. The use of a beta ray point source for destruction of the hypophysis, S. Forum *4*:681, 1953.

28. Richardson, K. C.: Contractile tissue in the mammary gland, with special reference to the myoepithelium in the goat, Proc. Roy. Soc., London, ser.B. *136*:30, 1949.

29. Salassa, R. M., Bennett, W. A., Keating, F. R., Jr., and Sprague, R. G.: Postoperative adrenal cortical insufficiency, J.A.M.A. *152*:1509, 1953.

30. Simpson, S. A., Tait, J. F., Wettstein, A., Neher, R., von Euw, J., Schindler, O., and Reichstein, T.: Konstitution des Aldosterons, des neuen Mineralocorticoid, Experientia *10*:132, 1954.

31. Stolz, F.: Ueber Adrenalin und Alkylaminoacetobenzcatechin, Ber. Deutsch. chem. Ges. *37*:4149, 1904.

32. Swingle, W. W., Maxwell, R., Ben, M., Baker, C., LeBrie, S. J., and Eisler, M.: Effect of aldosterone and desoxycorticosterone on adrenalectomized dogs, Proc. Soc. Exper. Biol. & Med. *86*:147, 1954.

33. Thorn, G. W., Emerson, K., Jr., Koepf, G. F., Lewis, R. A., and Olsen, E. F.: Carbohydrate metabolism in Addison's disease, J. Clin. Invest. *19*:813, 1940.

K. ALVIN MERENDINO, M.D.

Esophagus

ANATOMY AND PHYSIOLOGY

The esophagus is a muscular tube approximately 25 cm. long, extending from the pharynx to the stomach. It begins in the neck at the inferior border of the cricoid cartilage at the level of the 6th cervical vertebra and descends in front of the vertebral column through the posterior mediastinum, passes through the diaphragm and upon entering the abdomen ends at the cardiac orifice of the stomach at the level of the 11th thoracic vertebra. It is narrowest at its beginning and a few centimeters proximal to the point where it passes through the diaphragm. In addition, while not narrowed, it may be compressed anteroposteriorly in two additional areas, viz., at the level of the aortic arch and the left main bronchus (Fig. 28-1).

The esophagus consists of 4 coats: an outer fibrous, a muscular, a submucous and an inner mucous coat. The muscular coat consists of 2 layers, an outer longitudinal and an inner layer which is in part circular, elliptical and spiral. The upper fourth of the esophagus is made up of striated or skeletal muscle, a continuation from the constrictor pharyngei, which in the second fourth is gradually supplanted by smooth muscle. The lower half of the esophagus possesses only smooth muscle with few exceptions; racemose glands of the mucous type are lodged in the submucous tis-

sue, and each opens upon the surface by an excretory duct. The inner layer consists of stratified squamous epithelium.[9]

The cervical esophagus receives its blood supply mainly from the inferior thyroid artery. Esophageal arteries may arise from the ascending pharyngeal and the common carotid arteries. In approximately 13 per cent of cases, the esophageal arteries to the cervical esophagus originate from sources other than the inferior thyroid artery. The blood supply to the thoracic portion of the esophagus is mainly from the thoracic aorta with the major supply being derived from the bronchial arteries; most frequently, there are 3 bronchial arteries: 2 on the left and 1 on the right. In addition, the thoracic portion of the esophagus receives blood supply from the right intercostals in 20 per cent of cases. Exceptional origins of esophageal arteries occur rarely from the internal mammary, the costocervical trunk and the subclavian artery. These vessels tend to course longitudinally and to anastomose with vessels which supply the abdominal portion of the esophagus coming up from below. The arterial supply to the abdominal portion of the esophagus is mainly from the left gastric and the left inferior phrenic arteries. These arteries extend upward through the esophageal hiatus of the diaphragm. In approximately 10 per cent of cases, esophageal arteries originate from an accessory left hepatic and splenic arteries and from the celiac axis.[27] The venous drainage tends to follow the arterial supply. Consequently, it is apparent that the thoracic esophagus between the jugular notch and the aortic arch is the most avascular segment. It is for this reason that if the esophagus must be transected in this area, thus depriving the organ of any arterial supply from the bronchial arteries, the anastomosis should be done at the apex of the chest. Thereby, the surgeon

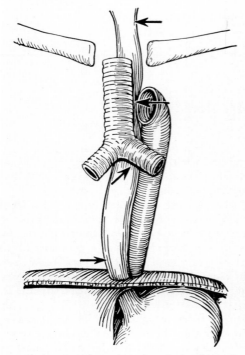

Fig. 28-1. The anatomic relationships of the intrathoracic esophagus indicating its relative inaccessibility and proximity to vital structures. Two normal sites of apparent narrowing of the esophagus exist at the beginning of the esophagus immediately below the cricopharyngei at the cricoid cartilage level and immediately above the diaphragm. This latter is variable from individual to individual and likewise variable in location. In addition, the esophagus is compressed by the aortic arch and also between the left main bronchus and the descending aorta.

can take advantage of the blood supply to the proximal segment from the inferior thyroid arteries.

The nerves are derived from the vagi and from the sympathetic trunks. These form a plexus in which are groups of ganglion cells: one between the 2 muscular layers, and a second in the submucous tissue.

The function of the esophagus is concerned with the conduction of food and liquid from the pharynx to the stomach during the third stage of deglutition. X-ray studies including cinefluorography have contributed greatly to our understanding of the actual behavior of the esophagus in man. The mechanism by which food reaches the stomach varies with the consistency of the food and the position of the patient. Three forms of esophageal contractions are noted: primary and secondary peristaltic waves and apparent purposeless tertiary contractions. The primary peristaltic wave is initiated by the act of swallowing and is largely responsible for the progression of the bolus along the esophagus. In the standing position the passage of the bolus is assisted by gravity. A liquid bolus drops quickly through a relaxed esophagus and collects above the contracted cardiac sphincter. Here it awaits the arrival of the primary peristaltic wave. With the approach of this wave the sphincter relaxes, and the contents are passed into the stomach. If the patient drinks rapidly, the entire length of the esophagus and the cardiac sphincter may remain relaxed, so that the fluid drops abruptly from the mouth into the stomach without interference. Apparently, the relaxation of the esophageal muscle is caused by waves of inhibition which precede the waves of contraction. The waves of contraction, which would be initiated by rapid swallows of liquid, find the esophagus in a phase of inhibition and, therefore, do not occur. If the bolus is firmer in consistency and dry, the wave of contraction is the primary factor in its transport. With the patient horizontal or in Trendelenburg's position, the force of gravity is eliminated, leaving the peristaltic waves as the sole propelling force. The wave initiated by the contraction of the pharyngeal muscles continues in an unbroken pattern down the esophagus. This is referred to as the primary perstaltic wave. The "law of the intestine," viz., contraction behind the bolus with relaxation ahead, applies here also. The speed of the wave of contraction is more rapid in the upper than in the lower portion of the esophagus. This difference is attributed to the nature of the muscular coat. Striated muscle is more rapidly contractile than is smooth muscle.

In some patients, particularly those having either a physiologic or an organic obstruction of the lower esophagus, another form of peristaltic wave is sometimes observed. This wave is termed the secondary peristaltic wave. It is thought by some to be set up by sensory stimulation of the walls. These waves are rarely seen during x-ray examination. When observed, they arise in the region of the aortic arch. Here a segment of the esophagus undergoes spontaneous contraction and forces barium toward the mouth and toward the stomach. The secondary wave, once initiated, progresses as does the primary wave described earlier. Barium that flows toward the mouth may enter the pharynx where its presence may cause the patient's swallow to initiate another primary wave. The inhibitory phase of the primary wave may overtake and inhibit the secondary before it reaches the diaphragm. Primary peristaltic waves sometimes cease at the level of the aortic arch, and secondary waves begin at this point, continuing down the esophagus. This may be due in part to the apparent break in peristalsis resulting from changes in the musculature at that level. Tertiary waves are minute indentations which are observed throughout the esophagus, particularly in its lower portion. These waves simulate the segmental contractions observed in the intestine. These contractions frequently are seen in patients with cardiospasm and, particularly, in older individuals without any diseases of the esophagus. Their true significance is unknown.[27]

The harmony of sequence as food passes from the pharynx along the upper esophagus depends upon an extrinsic nervous mechanism and not upon a simple conduction of contractions from one portion of the wall to the next. The exact innervation and nervous control of the act in man is not definitely known. From animal experimentation it is presumed that the motor impulses come through the vagi and that the sensory impulses pass over the 5th, the 9th and the 10th (vagus) cranial nerves. Clinical evidence for the dependence of peristalsis on extrinsic innervation can be observed in patients with large carcinomas of the esophagus. In these cases, when a primary wave progresses down to the tumor, it ceases but continues down the esophagus distal to the tumor an instant later. The coordinating mechanism lies in the medulla; apparently, the nucleus ambiguus supplies the striated, and the dorsal nucleus the unstriated muscle. In the lower portion of the esophagus, the wave apparently is independent of the extrinsic nerves. This difference is attributed to the presence of smooth muscle.

At the esophagogastric junction esophageal mucosa is immediately adjacent to gastric mucosa. Because of the sensitivity of esophageal mucosa to acid-peptic damage, considerable interest has been evidenced concerning the mechanism here which normally prevents the regurgitation of gastric juice into the lower esophagus. While there is some anatomic support that a sphincter is present, the muscular arrangement is unlike other areas of the enteric tract where true sphincters exist.[16] Some believe that a valvelike mechanism exists because of the oblique entrance of the esophagus with the stomach. This obliquity may be accentuated by the slinglike arrangement of the diaphragm and the oblique muscular fibers of the esophagus itself. Others stress the importance of a rosette of gastric mucosal folds which act as a valve mechanism. The exact nature of the protective mechanism is unclear. but few would deny its presence in function if not in actual substance.

FOREIGN BODIES

INCIDENCE

The incidence of esophageal foreign bodies is approximately equal in children and adults. Carelessness is responsible for the majority of instances in children. Most cases occur in unattended children who have easy access to pins, coins, buttons, etc. Under the age of 2, children instinctively put everything in their mouths; those between 2 and 5 years will do likewise unless under careful observation. In adults, foreign body ingestion is almost always accidental; however, some psychotic patients swallow objects intentionally. Artificial dentures are the underlying cause of many of these accidents in adults. The hard palate is rendered insensitive by the dental plate, and the swallowed object is under the reflex action of the constrictor muscles before it is detected. The presence of pathologic conditions of the esophagus (e.g., stricture) is sometimes responsible for the impaction of foreign bodies which ordinarily would create no difficulty.

The most common foreign bodies are fish, chicken and meat bones, metals, including safety pins, buttons, and a miscellaneous category which covers a remarkable variety of items. The commercial practice of chopping chicken rather than disjointing it, is another contributing factor. This custom, while time saving, creates many dangerous bone splinters which otherwise would not be present. The majority of bones will be impacted in the cervical esophagus. However, if this area is passed, they may be located anywhere in the esophagus and, particularly, at the sites of natural narrowing of the esophagus.

DIAGNOSIS

The history of a swallowed foreign body is easy to obtain from an adult but is often missed in children. If the initial symptoms of gagging, choking or coughing are not observed, a foreign body may not be suspected until obstructive symptoms, mediastinitis or an unexplained grave illness occurs.[3, 5] While vomiting is common, often dysphagia or the overflow of oral secretion into the trachea are the first symptoms noted. Children often hold their heads to one side and keep their necks stiffened.

Adults are usually immediately aware of the accident by the discomfort produced and often can locate the level at which the foreign body is lodged. Persistent pain and tenderness over the point of lodgment in the neck, the accumulation of saliva in the hypopharynx and evidence of oropharyngeal trauma may be the only important physical signs. A sticking sensation, particulary with fish bones, is not uncommon. On occasion, cervical crepitus may be present.

When the foreign body cannot be seen by examination of the hypopharynx, anteroposterior and lateral cervical x-ray studies are in order. The lateral view is the more important.[8] Opaque foreign bodies create no difficulty. The diagnosis can be made readily by x-rays in about 75 per cent of patients. While more difficult, with care and overexposure of film, certain types of fish bones may be seen. If complications are present, widening of the cervical area between vertebrae and esophagus, and/or air may be noted.

If after routine x-ray studies no final conclusion can be drawn, a swallow of opaque material should be given. Barium is best, unless perforation is suspected; then Lipiodol should be used. A filling defect or an obstruction to flow may be evident. The material may be divided into two streams and go around the obstruction. Radiotranslucency is the one

common quality of foreign bodies that go undetected for periods from weeks to years. The plastic materials are characteristically difficult in this regard.

X-ray studies always should precede esophagoscopy; however, on occasion endoscopy may be necessary as a diagnostic and therapeutic endeavor.

COMPLICATIONS

Foreign bodies may be complicated by periesophagitis, with or without abscess, mediastinitis or actual perforation. In long-standing cases, stricture and proximal diverticula may develop. The latter tend to recede in size after removal of the foreign body.

TREATMENT

Speedy removal of the foreign body is the best treatment. The operation should be done as an emergency when damaging objects are at fault. The procedure may be delayed a day or two with smooth objects, such as coins, when they are asymptomatic, as many of these pass safely out of the esophagus. If the foreign body is not arrested or impacted in the esophagus, or is accidentally pushed into the stomach at esophagoscopy, these objects, even open safety pins, frequently will pass through the intestinal tract without difficulty. Occasionally, external incision is necessary.

BENIGN STRICTURE

LOCALIZED

Benign strictures are relatively common. They may occur after gunshot wounds, lacerations of the throat or foreign-body ingestions. Strictures may follow operations for tracheoesophageal fistula, diverticulectomy and any operation in which an esophagogastrostomy has been performed (see reflux esophagitis).

The major symptom is dysphagia of varying degree. X-ray studies are important. Esophagoscopy and biopsy are essential for a histologic diagnosis.

Treatment ordinarily consists of simple periodic dilatation by bougies over a previously swallowed thread. However, in selected cases more extensive procedures are indicated. If localized, excision of the area with end-to-end esophageal anastomosis can be performed (Fig. 28-2). Unfortunately, recurrent stenosis may occur. Other measures consist of esophageal substitution for localized areas by means of a jejunal segment or a by-pass of the block by means of a jejunal segment en-Roux-Y as shown in Figure 28-6. Yudin's use of the jejunum as a bypass conduit deserves special mention.[32] Excision with esophagogastrotomy also has been utilized. Reflux esophagitis may follow this procedure.

EXTENSIVE

The largest group of benign strictures is comprised of patients who have swallowed strong alkalis, acids, or phenols, either accidentally or with suicidal intent. These lesions are apt to be extensive. In addition, there may be component areas of injury in the oropharynx and the stomach. The treatment is especially important.

Management of the Acute Burn. The history usually reveals the nature of the material that has been ingested. Weak antidotes, such as vinegar after alkalis, alumina gel or soda after acids, and milk or egg white after phenols, rather than strong agents are advised. Close observation for possible laryngeal edema is important in children. Occasionally, tracheotomy within the first 24 hours may be necessary. In adults the possibility of a chemical mediastinitis or perforation of the stomach due to the ingestion of a large amount of caustics must be considered. Fluids and nourishment must be administered intravenously if the patient is unable to swallow liquids. Gastrostomy should be considered early if there is a complete inability to swallow fluids or saliva. Formerly, the esophagus was placed at complete rest, and no further treatment was considered. During recent years, however, active treatment is advised within 24 hours after the caustic is ingested. This aggressive approach is considered as prophylactic treatment in the prevention of stricture formation.

Well-lubricated, mercury-filled bougies are

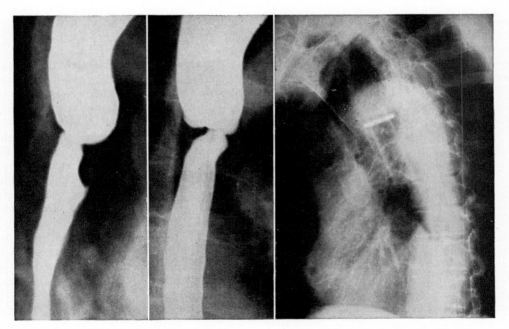

FIG. 28-2. This benign stricture (*left*) was treated unsatisfactorily by bougie dilatation. Local excision was carried out with an end-to-end esophageal anastomosis. An adequate full-sized lumen was obtained. A few weeks later restenosis occurred (*center*) which again could not be dilated adequately. The patient was an elderly severe arthritic and was considered a poor risk for any extensive surgical operation. Consequently, (*right*) a Teflon tube ¾ in. in diameter was inserted surgically through the stricture by an esophagotomy and held in position by a multiple-point fixation ring of stainless steel. This procedure is not advocated for benign lesions but was utilized for this unusual situation.

utilized. Bougies are allowed to pass through the esophagus into the stomach by their own weight. Generally, 3 bougies are passed each day, beginning with a No. 16 French and increasing the size as one determines what the lumen will accept. Usually, the 1st day No. 16 or 18 French bougies are passed. The size is increased gradually until No. 30 to No. 40 French mercury-filled bougies are accepted readily by the esophagus. The size depends upon the age of the patient. Usually, an infant 1 year of age can accept a No. 30 bougie fairly easily, while in adults the sizes are carried up to as high as No. 40 or No. 50 French. When the maximum size has been reached, treatment is reduced from daily dilatations to dilations every 3rd or 4th day. After the 1st month, bouginage is continued at intervals of 1 week, then once every 2 weeks, and finally once a month. In the absence of stricture formation, dilatations can be performed at greater intervals. Occasional dilations should be done during the remainder of the patient's life at intervals of 1 or 2 years to prevent the possibility of a tight stricture at a later date. A chronic stricture may develop weeks, months or even years after the initial burn. *It is extremely important to stress the fact that once the esophagus has been burned, stricture formation may develop at any time in the life of the patient. Under no circumstances should treatment be discontinued when normal deglutition returns.*[12]

Management of Chronic Strictures. Simple dilatations may be satisfactory for most chronic strictures. These dilatations are accomplished with olive-tipped bougies passed over a previously swallowed thread. In cases of multiple tight strictures, the patient should be treated by an early gastrostomy followed by retrograde or peroral dilatation. If a No. 6, 8, or 10 bougie can be advanced through the esophagus either from below or above, the bougie can be grasped at the opposite end, either in the stomach or in the mouth, and brought to the outside. Then a string is attached to it and drawn through the esophagus. Thus, with a string in the lumen, periodic dilations can be carried out rapidly over a relatively short period of time. When adequate stabilization in luminal size has been established, dilatations may be carried out in the usual peroral manner.

In certain cases, more extensive procedures may be in order. These operations are similar to those discussed under localized strictures and differ only in extent.

SPONTANEOUS RUPTURE OF THE ESOPHAGUS

INCIDENCE

The syndrome of spontaneous rupture of the esophagus presumably occurs unassociated with esophageal disease, foreign body, manipulation of the esophagus or any external force. However, many reported cases have shown evidence of pre-existing esophageal disease, viz., esophagitis. Usually such disease has been asymptomatic prior to perforation. Suffice it to say, spontaneous rupture can occur in the presence of a normal or an abnormal esophagus. This catastrophe is seen predominately in males in the ratio of 8:1, mainly between the age of 35 and 55 years. Although this condition has been recognized for over 200 years, successful treatment has occurred largely in the last few years.

ETIOLOGY

Esophageal rupture nearly always occurs in the terminal 3 or 4 inches of the esophagus. Experimentally, this area represents the weakest portion. In the human cadaver an average pressure of 7 lbs. per square inch is necessary to rupture the adult esophagus. Approximately 4 times as much pressure is required to rupture the esophagus of a child below 12 years of age. The rapidity of the rise in intraluminal pressure rather than the total pressure may be an important factor in perforation. Certain anatomic explanations have been made concerning the propensity of the lower esophageal wall to rupture. It has been stressed that the esophageal muscles at the lower end are tapered and extremely thin; these muscles are relatively weaker than the muscles of the stomach, and segmental defects are found occasionally in the circular muscle layer.

Whether the esophagus is normal or abnormal, the fact that rupture usually occurs in that portion of the esophagus, which experimentally and anatomically has proved to be the weakest, leads one to believe that internal force plays an important role as a causative factor. Because vomiting is observed frequently in spontaneous rupture, some believe that vomiting precipitates rupture by the sudden increase in intraluminal esophageal pressure. Consequently, the term postemetic rupture has been suggested.[24] However, vomiting is not always present until after rupture has occurred, suggesting in certain cases that the vomiting may be the result of rupture and not its cause. Actually, some patients never vomit.

PATHOLOGY

In 90 per cent of the patients with spontaneous rupture of the esophagus, the tear occurs on the posterolateral wall of the left side in the lowermost 8 cm. of the esophagus. It is usually vertical. When the stomach wall is involved also, severe bleeding may occur. However, perforation of the middle third of the esophagus and complete disruption of the lower esophagus have been described. These situations are unusually rare. In "true" spontaneous rupture no disease process, either gross or microscopic, is demonstrable at the site of tear. Esophagitis of varying degree has also been observed. It is difficult to be certain whether these changes are the result or the cause of the rupture.

DIAGNOSIS

The attack often is preceded by a large meal or an alcoholic bout. The acute onset is usually marked by a sudden severe pain. It may be preceded, followed, or unassociated with vomiting. The pain may be substernal, epigastric, or abdominal, and it is severe. The pain characteristically is unrelieved by ordinary doses of morphine. From minutes to hours, the epigastric or abdominal pain becomes substernal, occasionally radiating round into the back and between the scapula. Pleural pain may occur on either side.

The triad of rapid respiration, with or without cyanosis, abdominal rigidity and subcutaneous emphysema has been emphasized as being diagnostic.[2]

X-ray examination may reveal a hydrothorax and, occasionally, mediastinal air. Under fluoroscopic examination, a swallow of Lipiodol (not barium) often will delineate the perforation or reveal a para-esophageal pocket with a direct communication into the pleural cavity.

Thoracentesis may yield turbid or blood-stained fluid. It should be examined for food particles and hydrochloric acid, using Toepfer's solution as an indicator. Methylene blue may be given by mouth, and if immediately recovered in the chest aspirate, the presence of a fistulous communication is proved beyond doubt.

It is apparent that this clinical picture could be confused with many different disease entities, viz., ruptured peptic ulcer, acute pancreatitis, coronary thrombosis, dissecting aneurysm, pulmonary embolism and spontaneous pneumothorax. However, if the patient relates the usual history, exhibits the diagnostic triad and has fluid in the chest and lacks free air under the diaphragm, most of the other conditions can be ruled out quickly. Most diagnostic failures are due to the fact that the examiner is unaware of the symptoms of spontaneous esophageal rupture or simply fails to consider it a possibility.

TREATMENT

This condition is a surgical emergency. Treatment may be divided into conservative and radical management or, better, by surgical drainage of the pleural cavity versus thoracotomy with direct surgical repair of the site of rupture.

If the diagnosis is established, the patient should be operated upon as soon as possible.[13] Shock is almost always present and is attributable to fluid sequestration in the areas affected, which rapidly become very edematous, to blood loss, hypoxia, and pain (see Chap. 7, "Shock"). With proper attention to these factors, operation may be carried out. A left thoracotomy is performed, and the pleural cavity is cleansed. The opening in the mediastinal pleural is readily apparent. The pleura should be opened widely above this area in order to decompress the mediastinum into the pleural cavity. The esophageal rent is identified immediately, and the defect is closed in layers, with nonabsorbable sutures, utilizing finally the mediastinal pleura locally. A nasal tube is passed through this area beyond the perforation into the stomach. The chest always should be drained anteriorly and posteriorly in order to ensure proper drainage and complete pulmonary expansion. Ordinarily, the nasal tube is left in place for approxi-

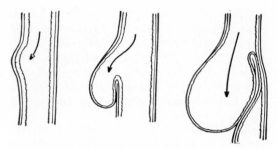

FIG. 28-3. Early, intermediate and late phases in the development of pharyngo-esophageal diverticulum. When fully developed, the diverticulum is in a completely dependent position, and its orifice appears on esophagoscopy to be the continuation of the esophagus. At the same time, compression of the esophagus by the sac containing food and fluid compromises the distal esophageal orifice. It can be understood that the blind passage of a nasal tube or esophagoscopy, unless expertly performed, may result in perforation of the diverticulum.

mately 1 week. Healing is sometimes retarded. Therefore, a prolonged period is required before peroral feeding is safe. Postoperative complications are empyema, mediastinitis and break-down of repair.

Conservative therapy may be reserved for those patients who have been seen 24 to 48 hours or longer after the onset of rupture. If the patient has survived this period, closed thoracotomy drainage may suffice, combined with nasogastric suction and prolonged parenteral feeding. Furthermore, exploration at this time may reveal edematous and friable tissue at the rupture site. Attempted closure at this stage may be harmful. If the patient survives with conservative management, residual fistulae and empyema usually require subsequent thoracotomy.

ESOPHAGEAL DIVERTICULA

Two varieties of diverticula occur in the esophagus: (1) pulsion and (2) traction types. These descriptive terms indicate the mechanism of formation. A pulsion diverticulum is thought to develop because of a force from within the esophagus pushing outward. Pulsion diverticula frequently develop in areas of muscular weakness existing naturally or ac-

quired. Consequently, they are mainly false diverticula in that the sac usually is made up of mucosa and submucosal elements and deficient in a complete muscular layer. On the other hand, traction diverticulum develops on the basis of a force pulling on the esophageal wall from without. Therefore, all layers of the esophagus are involved, and a true diverticulum occurs.

PULSION TYPES

Pulsion diverticula may occur anywhere in the esophagus. However, the most common site is at the pharyngo-esophageal junction; the second most common site is just above the diaphragm. These lesions are encountered in older patients for the most part.

Pharyngo-esophageal Diverticulum (Fig. 28-3). The propensity of diverticula to occur at the junction of the pharynx with the esophagus presumably is due to the relationship of the inferior constrictor muscle and the obliquely passing fibers of the cricopharyngei as they descend on the posterior wall of the esophagus to become longitudinal. Posteriorly at the junction of these muscular layers there is a relative weakness of the surrounding muscular coat of the digestive tube, probably more marked in some individuals than in others. The neuromuscular co-ordination, which brings about propulsion of food from the pharynx into the esophagus, acts normally when with contraction of the constrictors the cricopharyngei relax to permit the propelled food to pass into the esophagus. When there is in-co-ordination in this neuromuscular effort, the pressure from the constrictors above, combined with the obstruction below created by the unrelaxed cricopharyngei, may result in a posterior bulge, known as the pharyngeal dimple. Recurring pressure on this point eventually creates a sac.[11, 15]

DIAGNOSIS. Usually no symptoms are observed in the initial stages of pharyngo-esophageal diverticulum. In the intermediate stages there may be few if any symptoms. However, when symptoms are present, there may be minor difficulty in swallowing, although most complaints are referrable to a regurgitation of undigested food particles into the mouth with saliva when assuming the horizontal position, or with "gurgling" and unexpected belching. This latter symptom may be embarrassing to the patient; if severe, the patient frequently eats away from the company of other people. In the final stages of the development of a diverticulum, these symptoms become more marked, and dysphagia becomes prominent. In time the patient may be come severely malnourished.

On physical examination, the diagnosis occasionally can be made with the patient's mouth open and pressure exerted by the examining fingers at the base of the neck immediately above the clavicles. With backward pressure against the cervical muscles, gas and fluid may be compressed so that a belch can be heard very audibly, not only by the patient, but by any other individuals in the room.

The final diagnosis is made by x-ray studies following a barium swallow. On a straight anteroposterior view, an esophageal "web" in this area may give an x-ray picture similar to a diverticulum directed posteriorly. Therefore, to avoid this error, an oblique film should be taken which differentiates the two (Fig. 28-4).

Esophagoscopy is contraindicated in the ordinary case because of the danger of perforation of the diverticulum with mediastinitis. For the same reason, any attempt to pass blindly a nasal tube into the stomach should be avoided. In the presence of severe starvation, if a feeding vent is considered to be important, a nasal tube often may be guided into the stomach under direct vision by means of the esophagoscope.

TREATMENT. This disease is a progressive one. Surgery offers the only means of cure. However, surgical therapy is reserved for symptomatic patients. When symptoms are present, the diverticulum is at least in the intermediate stage. It appears best to advise surgery at this stage prior to the development of the final stages when surgical therapy is more difficult.

The surgical approach is dependent upon the side to which the diverticulum presents. In any event, the incision right or left is identical. Usually the operation is carried out by a vertical incision extending along the anterior border of the sternocleidomastoid muscle. A transverse cervical incision is preferred by some. The omohyoid muscle is severed, and the thyroid gland and the strap muscles are retracted medially and the sternocleidomastoid

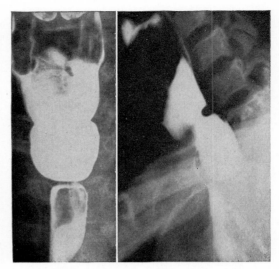

FIG. 28-4. (*Left*) Anteroposterior view of patient with a pharyngo-esophageal diverticulum. In this view this situation could be confused with a congenital esophageal web or the Plummer-Vinson syndrome. (*Right*) Lateral or oblique views are necessary for proper diagnosis. Here the diverticulum is clearly profiled with a spillover of barium into the distal esophagus.

laterally. It is necessary to retract laterally also the common carotid artery and the internal jugular vein. Care must be taken to avoid undue trauma to these vessels and inadvertent obstruction of the cerebral circulation. Usually, without great difficulty, the sac can be demonstrated protruding lateral to the esophagus and dissected free of its loose attachment. If any difficulty is encountered in identifying the sac, it may be packed with gauze through the mouth, transilluminated with an esophagoscope, or if local anesthesia is being used it can be distended by having the patient drink water. As the neck of the sack is approached, the wall of the diverticulum may be attached intimately to the esophagus proper. This part of the procedure is clean, unless there has been severe infection in the diverticulum or a previous rupture has occurred.

If a nasal tube is desired in the stomach for early postoperative decompression and, perhaps, later for feeding purposes, it should be passed at this stage. With the sac elevated and by direct palpation of the esophagus, the nasal tube is passed from above with ease.

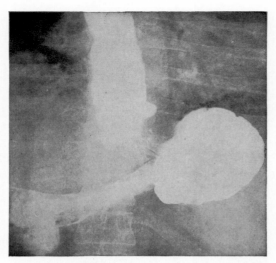

FIG. 28-5. Patient with free reflux of barium from the stomach up the esophagus during the Mueller maneuver (chalasia). A small epiphrenic diverticulum is demonstrated. While some have stressed that an obstructive mechanism usually exists distal to this type of diverticulum, its presence in this patient indicates that other mechanisms also are responsible for the development of epiphrenic diverticula.

The neck of the sac should be amputated flush with the esophageal wall. Care must be exercised to assure removal of all the sac and at the same time to avoid esophageal narrowing at this site. The presence of a nasal tube in the esophagus will help to avoid these dangers.

The neck of the sac may be closed by running or interrupted sutures of the mucosal and the submucosal layers with interrupted non-absorbable sutures in the muscular layer. Some have advocated transverse closure of the neck and longitudinal closure of the esophageal musculature. A sterile gauze pack may be placed in the defect created by the diverticulum if large and a portion removed daily until all has been removed by the fourth postoperative day. This irritation causes an obliterative reaction which tends to seal off the fascia planes of the neck which communicate with the mediastinum. A Penrose drain may be inserted down to the site of esophageal closure and be led out by a separate stab wound in the inferior portion of the neck.

Others advocate a 2-stage procedure. In the first stage, the diverticulum is elevated and sutured to the strap muscles of the thyroid so that the sac, rather than being dependent, drains by gravity into the esophagus. At a second stage, usually performed from 7 to 12 days later, the sac is amputated, and the repair is done in the usual manner. The 2-stage method was thought to protect the patient from a descending mediastinitis but has been used very little since antibiotics became available.

In a small number of cases, an esophago-cutaneous fistula will develop. However, these are treated by continued suction drainage and close spontaneously. In good hands, the operative mortality should be in the neighborhood of 1 to 2 per cent and the recurrence rate extremely small.

Epiphrenic or Supradiaphragmatic Diverticulum. Such diverticula are uncommon. In general, the symptoms, the x-ray findings, the stages of development and the indications for operation are similar in all respects to a pharyngo-esophageal diverticulum (Fig. 28-5). The major differences relate to the level of the lesion and the fact that some cases are associated with lower esophageal spasm or fibrosis immediately distal to the diverticulum. The mechanism of formation may be related to these obstructive factors and localized muscular weakness. In general, the same surgical principles apply to the treatment of these lesions as with the pharyngo-esophageal diverticulum. The procedure of choice is 1-stage transthoracic removal of the lesion. However, at the time of surgery one must be satisfied that no other obstruction mechanism exists below the diverticulum which might affect the result. If present, attention must be directed to this lesion as well.

TRACTION TYPES

Traction diverticula are likewise uncommon. They are seen characteristically about the tracheobronchial bifurcation. In contrast with the globular shape of the pulsion type, the traction diverticulum is cone-shaped. The apex of the cone usually is pointing directly to the inflammatory attachment of cicatrizing and healing bronchial lymph nodes. The esophageal opening is open-mouthed and dependent. Therefore, such diverticula empty readily, are usually small, and ordinarily produce no symptoms. They are frequently an incidental x-ray finding.

REFLUX ESOPHAGITIS (PEPTIC ESOPHAGITIS)

This clinical entity is characterized by the chemical irritation of the lower esophagus and is believed to be secondary to the regurgitation of acid-peptic gastric chyme. While an alkaline-tryptic esophagitis occasionally occurs following reconstructive surgery for total gastrectomy, the most common and troublesome type of reflux esophagitis is of acid-peptic origin.

ETIOLOGY

Considerable controversy exists concerning the exact mechanism at the junction of the esophagus and the cardia of the stomach which normally prevents the regurgitation of gastric chyme into the lower esophagus. Some believe that a sphincter is present in the area, others deny its presence and offer various explanations for the valvelike competence observed. However, it is generally agreed that some protective mechanism exists, otherwise peptic lesions of the esophagus probably would be more common than in the stomach and the duodenum.

When this mechanism is incompetent for any reason, reflux esophagitis develops. This entity has been observed in association with congenitally short esophagus, sliding esophageal hiatus hernia, repeated vomiting, prolonged use of indwelling nasogastric tubes, and following surgical procedures which destroy this mechanism either by incision or excision of this area with restoration of gastro-intestinal continuity by esophagogastrostomy. In addition, reflux esophagitis is observed in individuals with normal anatomic relationships in this region unassociated with any other apparent lesion.

PATHOLOGY

Peptic esophagitis usually is limited to the lower esophagus and, particularly, immediately above the cardiac orifice. The esophageal mucosa is the most sensitive of the entire gastrointestinal tract to acid-peptic digestion. The irritation produced by contact with acid-peptic juice results in varying degrees of injury.

In its early stages, a granular erythema with edema is manifest. As the disease progresses superficial ulcerations develop and may eventuate in large ulcers which penetrate with localized fixation or perforate into the mediastinum or the pleural cavity. With periodic irritation alternating with periods of healing, stricture may develop with or without the formation of proximal pulsion diverticula. On microscopic examination there may be epithelial necrosis and hyperplasia with marked polymorphonuclear infiltration and hypertrophy of the muscularis above the stricture. With advanced stages local fibrotic changes become prominent.

DIAGNOSIS

Lower substernal discomfort on swallowing, associated with heartburn, regurgitation and hemorrhage, may be presenting symptoms. Dysphagia may progress until liquid foods are substituted for solids. Physical signs are absent, although in later stages inanition may be manifest.

X-ray studies may be diagnostic. The findings will be dependent upon the stage of the disease. Early in the course of the disease there may be fine irregularity without clear delineation of the mucosal pattern. At times, spasm of the lower esophageal segment occurs also. In advanced cases, lower esophageal stenosis is prominent. The transition from the proximal esophagus which may be dilated to the strictured area usually is gradual and symmetrical. There may be esophageal ulcer or other associated pathology, e.g., short esophagus, hiatal hernia, etc. At times, reflux esophagitis in its final stages may be difficult to differentiate from cardiospasm and carcinoma.[31]

Esophagoscopy with biopsy is indicated in all cases in order to establish the correct histologic diagnosis.

TREATMENT

Medical treatment is similar in many respects to the treatment of the ordinary patient with peptic ulcer of the stomach or the duodenum. This consists of small frequent feedings of a bland, nonirritating diet, antacids at intervals of 1 or 2 hours during active phases and less frequently during quiescence. Some advise a conventional Sippy diet. Anticholi-

nergic drugs are of considerable help. In severely symptomatic cases, therapy must be
continued in modified form throughout the
night as well as during the daytime.

In addition, to minimize reflux, patients
should be advised to avoid intra-abdominal
pressure by garment compression, and to sleep
with the head and the chest elevated at least
8 inches, stooping by bending the knees and
the hips and not by spinal flexion.

Where symptoms of esophagitis are associated with a sliding hiatus hernia in an obese
individual, weight reduction is important.
With reduction in weight, the hernia sometimes reduces itself with amelioration of symptoms. However, if this combined with other
medical measures is of no avail, surgical repair
of the hernia is indicated. With the restoration of normal anatomic relationships, the
symptoms of esophagitis usually disappear.

When stricture formation is present, bouginage in the usual fashion over a swallowed
string may be necessary. Such dilatations must
be carried out at periodic intervals for the
remainder of the life of the patient. It should
be pointed out that dilatation of the stricture,
while allowing food to pass more readily into
the stomach, also may allow extension of the
lesions by permitting easier regurgitation of
gastric juice to more proximal levels. Consequently, bouginage is a complement to and
not a substitute for medical measures.

Major surgical procedures for esophagitis
and its complications without an associated
correctable lesion have left much to be desired. In order to be successful, such procedures must be directed not only to the relief
of obstruction but also to the reduction of
gastric secretion. Therefore, operations concerned with excision of the strictured area
with re-establishment of continuity by esophagogastrostomy are followed not infrequently
by recurrent esophagitis. If this procedure is
combined with vagotomy and a Finney pyloroplasty or gastrojejunostomy, the chances of
success may be improved. Experimentally, it
has been suggested that the reflux of gastric
contents following esophagogastrostomy may

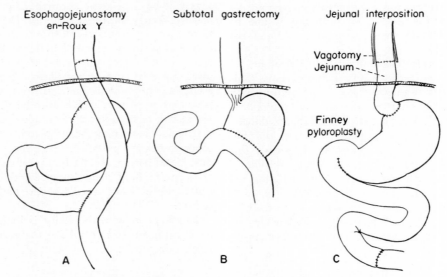

FIG. 28-6. These procedures may be considered acceptable surgical measures
in the therapy of reflux esophagitis. (A) An esophagojejunostomy en-Roux Y
with the stomach out of circuit has been done. Thus, there no longer exists the
possibility of contact of gastric chyme with the esophageal mucosa. (B) A subtotal gastrectomy has been performed in order to reduce acid-peptic secretion,
thereby protecting the esophagus. The stenotic segment is left in situ. (C) An
interposed jejunal segment which behaves as a substitute sphincteric mechanism
has been utilized. This is accompanied by a bilateral vagotomy and a pyloroplasty (see text).

be prevented by implanting the esophagus into a submuscular tunnel in the gastric wall.[22]

Another physiologic approach involves the use of the conventional subtotal gastric resection identical with that performed for peptic ulcer of the stomach or the duodenum.[30] The stricture is left in situ and treated by bouginage. In some patients, dilatations may be discontinued without recurrent stenosis (Fig. 28-6). In order to prevent the contact of gastric secretion with the sensitive esophageal mucosa, excision of the stricture with esophagojejunostomy en-Roux Y with the stomach out of circuit has been used successfully.[1] More recently, it has been proposed that the

surgical need is a new sphincter mechanism. A jejunal segment interposed between the esophagus and the stomach with excision of the stenosed area combined with vagotomy and a Finney-type pyloroplasty has been found to be satisfactory[17, 28] (Fig. 28-7).

CARDIOSPASM

Synonyms: Achalasia, mega-esophagus, phrenospasm, esophagospasm.

This disease is a concise clinical entity with definite but not completely understood anatomic abnormalities. It is characterized by spasm of the lower esophagus and the cardia,

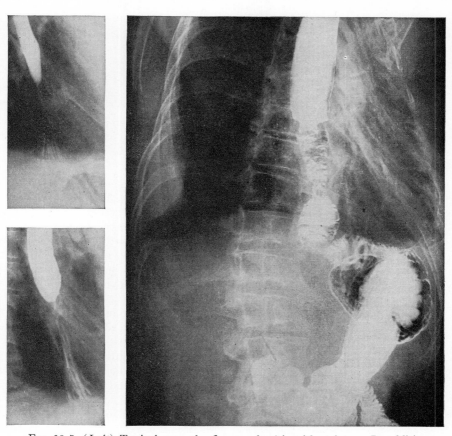

FIG. 28-7. (*Left*) Typical case of reflux esophagitis with stricture. In addition, a hiatus hernia is seen with gastric mucosal folds extending up to the stenotic area. Several years previously while this patient was hospitalized for pulmonary tuberculosis it was noted that he had a hiatus hernia. (*Right*) A jejunal segment has been interposed between the esophagus and the cardia of the stomach with vagotomy and pyloroplasty following resection of the stricture. An old left thoracoplasty can be noted as well as a healed empyema of the right pleural cavity. This patient is now asymptomatic.

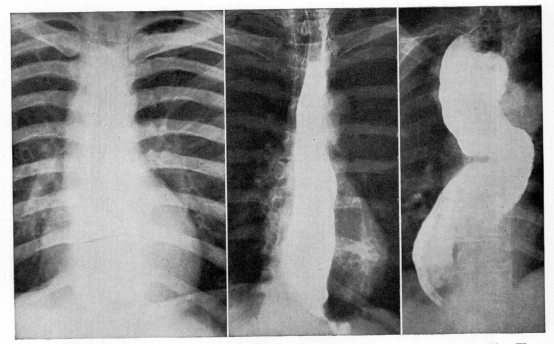

FIG. 28-8. (*Left*) The diagnosis of cardiospasm may be suggested on an ordinary chest film. The outline of the dilated esophagus can be seen behind the heart shadow. (*Center*) A relatively early case of cardiospasm. (*Right*) S or sigmoid contour of the esophagus typical of the late stages of this disease.

delayed passage and retention of food with dilatation of the proximal esophagus. The etiology is unknown. One theory suggesting autonomic imbalance seems to be the most acceptable. This imbalance may be due to degenerative changes either in the vagus or the sympathetic (Auerbach's plexus) nerves. Because no organic lesion can be found distal to the dilated esophagus, one must consider this disease to be due to a disordered neuromuscular mechanism. A strong psychosomatic overlay is noted in most patients.

DIAGNOSIS

Cases of cardiospasm divide themselves into 2 groups: (1) those starting early in life, in children even below the age of 5, and (2) those starting commonly after middle age. Males predominante in the ratio of 3:2. The characteristic symptoms are dysphagia, epigastric or substernal pain and regurgitation. This disease is the most frequent cause of dysphagia in the female and the second only to carcinoma as a cause in the male. The pain usually occurs immediately upon the ingestion and the swallowing of food and may be referred upward to the throat. The majority of patients are emotionally unstable and have many other unrelated complaints. Dysphagia and pain may occur long before the patient has difficulty with regurgitation. In the early stages of regurgitation it is prompt and partial and accompanied by a marked weight loss. As the tone of the esophagus decreases and esophageal dilatation ensues, regurgitation may be delayed for hours, and the emesis may contain material ingested many hours before.[10]

X-ray examination reveals the characteristic findings or spasm of the lower esophagus with dilatation above. The contour of the esophagus may be fusiform, flask-shaped or the S or "sigmoid" type, depending upon the stage of the disease (Fig. 28-8). Many cases are discovered accidentally during routine roentgenography with advanced changes in the esophagus while symptoms are slight, if present at all.

COMPLICATIONS

There exists no tendency toward natural cure, and, if neglected, the disease progresses steadily to a fatal termination over a prolonged period of time. The complications are concerned mainly with pulmonary difficulties and malnutrition. In the later stages of the disease a hugely distended esophagus may be present. Because of lower esophageal spasm, the esophagus fails to empty and consequently becomes a storage bin for food and saliva. At times, and particularly during sleep, overflow may occur into the posterior pharynx with tracheal aspiration. This results in recurring pneumonitis and lung abscess.

TREATMENT

There are neither drugs nor other medical means of ameliorating the patient's symptoms or the course of the disease.

Minor Surgical Procedures. BOUGINAGE is the most conservative method for the alleviation of the obstruction due to cardiospasm.[29] All dilatations should be carried out over a previously swallowed heavy silk thread. By the passage of a size No. 60 French bougie through the area of spasm, complete temporary relief of all symptoms occurs in approximately 10 per cent of patients. About half of these remain well for prolonged periods. When bougies are used, repeated periodic dilatations are necessary. However, bouginage may be dangerous, particularly in the large S-shaped esophagus, in spite of taking the precaution of attempting dilatation over a prepassed guide thread. Mercury-weighted dilators also have been used. In the late stages of the disease, the esophagus is frequently edematous and friable.

Hydrostatic Dilatation. Either as the primary therapy or if bouginage is unsuccessful, hydrostatic dilation of the lower esophagus and the cardia may be attempted. Such dilation should be done only after a No. 60 French bougie has been passed. Pressures of 20 to 30 ft. of water generally are held to be safe, although pressures of this magnitude in the cadaver may produce lower esophageal rupture. It is reported that 70 per cent of the patients treated in this fashion will be asymptomatic. Some patients will require subsequent treatment by the hydrostatic method. In ex-

perienced hands, hydrostatic dilatation appears to be dependent upon the uncontrolled rupture of the muscular coat in the area of cardiopasm. Among surgeons there is growing support for the management of cases refractory to or unsatisfactory for bouginage by direct surgical means, thereby avoiding hydrostatic methods.

Major Surgical Procedures. It is apparent that a group of patients remains in which the above-mentioned methods are unsuccessful. Currently, major surgical procedures are reserved mainly for this group. Most surgical procedures involve destruction of the cardiac sphincteric area by either incision or excision of this area or an attempt to bypass the area of narrowing.

While it is agreed that cardiospasm is unrelated to acid-peptic disease, the destruction of the cardiac sphincter allows gastric secretion to reflux into the lower esophagus. Because the esophageal mucosa is extremely sensitive to acid-peptic digestion, the patient frequently traded his original disease, viz., cardiospasm, for the more serious entity— reflux esophagitis. Consequently, certain procedures previously advocated for cardiospasm are performed less and less frequently. A list of these operations is included for historical purposes only.

Mikulicz (1904). Gastrostomy with retrograde manual or instrumental dilatation.

Wendel (1910). Longitudinal incision through all layers of the cardiospasm with cardoplasty by transverse closure.

Heyrovsky (1913). Side-to-side anastomosis of the distal portion of the dilated esophagus with the dome or fundus of the stomach.

Gröndahl (1916). Longitudinal incision through all layers of the lower esophagus and the upper stomach with reconstruction similar to a Finney-type pyloroplasty.

Other operations concerned with reconstruction of the esophageal hiatus and on the autonomic nervous system also have been attempted without success and have been abandoned.

Presently, the following operations are thought to possess some merit in the surgical treatment of cardiospasm recalcitrant to more conservative measures:

The Heller operation (1913) originally included longitudinal incision, both anteriorly and posteriorly, through the muscular layers of the area of cardiospasm, thus allowing the submucosa of the area to bulge outward. In current practice, only an anterior incision is utilized (Zaaiger-Heller). This operation is similar in concept to the *Fredet-Ramstedt operation* for congenital hypertrophic pyloric stenosis. *The Zaaiger-Heller operation* was discarded many years ago presumably because of unsatisfactory results. However, some proponents of this procedure have reported numerous successes. For this latter reason and the discouraging results with other operations, the Zaaiger-Heller operation has been revived. It is a simple procedure and probably should be attempted if conservative measures are unsuccessful (Fig. 28-9).

Merendino (1955)[17] suggested that the true surgical need in cardiospasm is a new sphincter. He has advocated excision of the area of spasm with restoration of gastrointestinal continuity by means of a segment of jejunum interposed between the proximal esophagus and the cardia of the stomach. This procedure is accompanied by a bilateral vagotomy and a Finney pyloroplasty. The clinical results to date in a few patients have been excellent.

TUMORS OF ESOPHAGUS

Tumors of the esophagus are primarily malignant. Carcinoma is the most important tumor of this organ.

CARCINOMA

The average age of the patient with carcinoma of the esophagus is 63 years. The majority of patients fall into the 5th and the 6th decades of life. The next important decade is the 7th, and a poor fourth is the 8th. Males predominate in the ratio of 10:1.

Pathology. Macroscopically, two varieties exist. The most common type produces stenosis (90%) and, eventually, occludes the esophageal lumen. Nonstenosing tumors (0 to 20%) do not occlude the lumen, even in the terminal stages of the illness. Typically, carci-

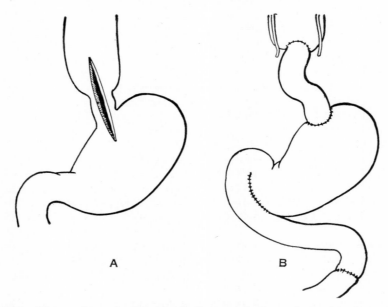

A   B

FIG. 28-9. These schematic drawings indicate procedures that might be considered acceptable in the therapy of surgical cardiospasm. (A) Zaaiger-Heller anterior cardiomyotomy is considered to be of value. Because the complications of the modified Heller operation when they occur are related to acid-peptic reflux c̄ esophagitis, some have suggested the addition of bilateral vagotomy and pyloroplasty in order to decrease gastric acidity and volume and to allow a larger gastric efferent outlet. (B) The interposition operation, utilizing a jejunal segment as a substitute sphincter with vagotomy and pyloroplasty (Merendino). This procedure has been carried out in a few patients with success; however, it is not recommended as the primary operation.

noma of the esophagus is of a squamous cell type. Primary adenocarcinoma of the esophagus accounts for less than 5 per cent of all cases. In the lower esophagus where an adenocarcinoma is contiguous with gastric mucosa, it is frequently impossible to determine whether such a tumor is primary in the esophagus or the stomach.

Carcinoma of the esophagus tends to spread locally by direct infiltration and widely by the lymphatics in the wall of the esophagus, as well as by metastasizing to regional nodes and distantly. Because of the intimate relationship of the esophagus to other important structures passing through the posterior mediastinum, direct extension of the tumor may result in the development of fistulae between the trachea, the bronchi, the pleura, or the aorta. Perforation locally may occur without the development of a fistula. The site of regional metastases will be dependent upon the location of the lesion. Carcinomas of the lower third of the esophagus tend to metastasize to the para-esophageal nodes at the diaphragmatic level, to the left gastric artery and the celiac axis. Lesions of the middle third tend to involve the para-esophageal nodes locally and the hilar lymph glands at the tracheal bifurcation and downward as well. Carcinomas of the upper third of the intrathoracic esophagus involve superior mediastinal and cervical nodes, tending to follow the venous drainage of this area.

Because of its potential surgical significance, considerable attenion has been directed to the incidence of localized esophageal carcinoma without nodal involvement at the time of autopsy. In large series of cases, the incidence of localized carcinoma without nodal involvement varies from 19 to 48 per cent. On the other hand, in one series of 50 cases, all had involvement, either regionally or distantly.

The anatomic location of the tumor conditions not only the probable site of regional metastases but also the magnitude of the operative procedures which might be necessary. When only squamous carcinoma of the esophagus is included for study, thereby excluding adenocarcinomas of questionable primary site, the mid-portion of the esophagus is the most frequent site for carcinoma of the esophagus. When one includes those adenocarcinomas thought to be primary in the esophagus, the lower esophagus becomes the most frequent area for carcinoma.

Diagnosis. Ordinarily, the history is invaluable in directing the attention of the physician to the esophagus. 90 per cent of the patients complain of dysphagia at the time of their initial visit. 63 per cent complain of pain, usually associated with swallowing, and 30 per cent complain of vomiting or regurgitation of food immediately ingested or of the regurgitation of salivary juice. Pain may be described as dull, burning, pressure, sharp, or anginal. It may be retrosternal, in the chest, the epigastrium, subcostal, in the back, or in the cervical area. Hematemesis rarely may be the presenting complaint. Rarely, aural pain aggravated by swallowing may be present. This symptom is ascribed to the reflex irritation of the tympanic branch of the 5th and the 9th cranial nerves or the auricular branch of the 10th.

A typical history usually reveals progressive dysphagia, together with voluntary restriction of solid foods to the point where only liquids are taken. Occasionally, early dysphagia is followed by a free interval, subsequent to which a recurrence of the difficulty makes its appearance. Consequently, transient dysphagia has the same implication as does permanent progressive dysphagia. With nonstenosing carcinomas, dysphagia may be absent, even at the time of death.

Many common digestive complaints have been said to represent early symptoms of esophageal carcinoma; none is specific. Although dysphagia is a relative late symptom, nonetheless, from the practical viewpoint it is the earliest symptom which directs attention to the esophagus. Dysphagia, whether transient or permanent, when combined with the rejection of solid food or a liquid diet, should suggest the diagnosis of carcinoma in the patient over 45 years. Obviously, other benign conditions can produce this symptom complex; nevertheless, carcinoma of the esophagus should be suspected, and every diagnostic measure explored until carcinoma is proved or excluded.

The correct diagnosis can be made by the roentgenologist in about 75 per cent of the patients. The roentgenograms should suggest the possibility of esophageal carcinoma in almost all cases. Esophagoscopy with biopsy is the final step in making the definitive histologic diagnosis.

Starvation and dehydration are extremely common in patients with carcinoma of the esophagus. These complications are related to dysphagia, which produces either a lack of desire or the inability to swallow. Many patients, with starvation only, die because they are thought to exhibit terminal stages of the disease with widespread metastases. In the absence of any evidence that distant metastases are in fact present, severe weight loss must not be construed as evidence of inoperability.

Prognosis. After the appearance of dysphagia, with few exceptions, untreated carcinoma of the esophagus appears to be a rapidly fatal disease. The patient with carcinoma of the esophagus has an average life expectancy varying from 7 to 12 months from the onset of symptomatology until death. These time relationships pertain to untreated patients or patients given palliative therapy only. Palliative procedures exert no significant prolongation of life, although their value in certain instances is unquestioned.

In the average patient the time of the onset of symptoms until the diagnosis is established varies between 4 to 6 months. Consequently, about half of the patient's survival time is dissipated in making the diagnosis. Unfortunately, undue delay is created by the physician as well as by the patient.[18]

Treatment. Intrathoracic carcinoma of the esophagus poses a serious problem for the surgeon and the elderly patient. Because of the age of the average patient with esophageal carcinoma and the presence of other stigmata associated with normal aging, one must make a meaningful evaluation of the patient's ability to tolerate the rigors of major surgery. The location of the lesion will dictate the magnitude of the operation necessary and should be an important consideration in the final decision. In view of the fact that the hope for cure is presently relatively small, one should not indiscriminately subject all patients to major surgery, even though there is no clinical evidence of tumor spread beyond the local lesion. Obviously, the general condition of the patient may contraindicate a direct surgical attack. For this group of patients and those with evidence of distant metastases, only palliative measures are available. In all other pa-

tients an exploratory thoracotomy is indicated.

For purposes of discussion, the treatment of carcinoma of the esophagus will be considered under the headings of palliative and curative methods.

PALLIATIVE METHODS
1. Bouginage
2. Intubation (metal or plastic)
3. Gastrostomy
4. Plastic prosthetic substitution with excision of the lesion
5. Bypass procedures using the jejunum or right colon
6. X-ray therapy

Periodic bouginage or dilatation is one of the better means of palliation. Most intubation tubes are of metals or plastics. They are usually funnel-shaped. The flange rests upon the proximal tumor mass with the stem extending through the lesion. This allows a passageway for the ingestion of food by mouth. Fixation of the tube is used by some. Gastrostomy establishes a feeding vent below the obstruction, thus bypassing the esophageal lesion. Gastrostomy in the starved individual is accompanied by some mortality, does not greatly prolong life and, in general, is unsatisfactory to the patient in that he is unable to eat by mouth. Recently, the use of a plastic prosthesis has been advocated with and without excision of the lesion.[4] The risk is great, and the value of this procedure is questionable.

The jejunum has been used to by-pass the obstruction. The esophagojejunostomy has been effected in the neck, and a jejunojejunostomy en-Roux Y has been performed in the abdomen with the stomach out of circuit. This intestinal segment may be placed subcutaneous or via the anterior mediastinum.[23] The surgeon then has the option at a second stage of attempting excision of the lesion if the situation looks favorable. For the most part, however, this has been used as a palliative method.

X-ray therapy as a means of treating carcinoma of the esophagus has been utilized for decades. Discarded in the past, it has been revived as a means of palliation. X-ray therapy is capable of sterilizing squamous cell carcinoma on the surface of the body. Unfortunately, the esophagus is disadvantageously placed in juxtaposition to other important structures. Consequently, to destroy the tumor one runs a simultaneous risk of destroying adjacent tissues, for x-rays are relatively unselective with regard to the tissues affected. The revival of this method of therapy is based upon the development of higher voltage machines and the concept of rotational therapy. By rotation of the patient a more nearly accurate and uniform dosage of x-ray with a higher cancerocidal potentiality may be delivered with less damage to the skin and other organs situated radially to this lesion. In addition, the renewed interest has come about because of the morbidity, the mortality and the small cure yield of radical surgery. While carcinomas of the cervical esophagus have been cured by x-ray therapy on rare occasions, this method must be considered mainly as palliative. It has been the experience that if the tumor has spread to regional nodes, a cure by means of x-ray therapy is impossible.

CURATIVE METHODS. Radical surgical procedures involve the wide excision en masse of the esophageal lesion, together with the nodal areas to which the lesion tends to spread.

Radical surgical excision with restoration of gastrointestinal continuity.

Esophagogastrectomy with esophagogastrostomy.[7, 25]

Carcinomas of the lower esophagus ordinarily are approached through the bed of the left 7th rib. Because of the propensity of esophageal lesions to spread in the submucosa, the esophagus should be transected just distal to the aortic arch (Fig. 28-10). Distally, the upper one third to one fourth of the stomach should be removed, including the left gastric artery at its origin from the celiac axis. Restoration of gastrointestinal continuity is made by esophagogastrostomy. Because the vagi must be sacrificed, a pyloroplasty should be performed also.

For lesions of the midthoracic esophagus, a 2-incision approach is gaining favor among

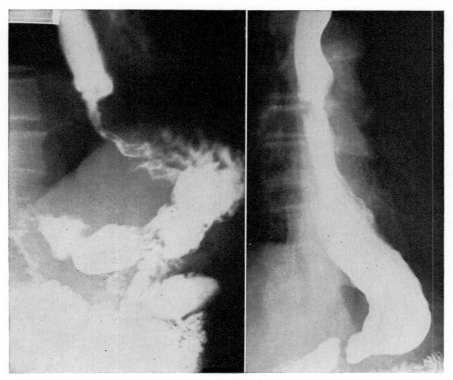

FIG. 28-10. (*Left*) Typical carcinoma of the lower third of the esophagus. (*Right*) Resection of almost the entire lower two-thirds of the esophagus, combined with an upper gastrectomy, has been carried out. Restoration of intestinal continuity has been effected by esophagogastrostomy immediately below the aortic arch. The indentation of the esophagus by the aorta is seen readily.

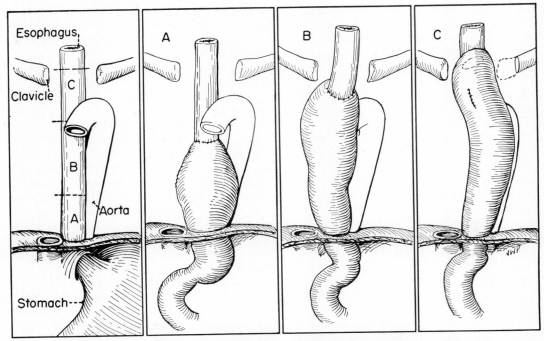

FIG. 28-11. The intrathoracic esophagus can be divided into approximately equal thirds. The location of the esophageal carcinoma conditions the surgical approach and the procedure to be done. (A) Lesions of the lower third may be approached by a left thoracotomy with a transdiaphragmatic component. In order to enhance the chances of cure, most of the lower two-thirds of the esophagus should be excised. This also is combined with upper gastrectomy. (B) Lesions of the middle third should be treated by separate abdominal and right thoracic incisions. The esophagogastric anastomosis is made at the apex of the thorax. (C) Few lesions in this area have been handled successfully. Separate abdominal, right thoracic and cervical incisions are necessary. Removal of the medial clavicular head aids in exposure.

If during surgery it becomes apparent that the operation is only palliative and/or the patient a poor risk, many surgeons presently prefer to terminate the operation. Rather than subject the patient to the high risk of a definitive resection, they depend upon lesser surgical procedures or x-ray therapy for palliation.

surgeons; one incision involves a mid-line supra-umbilical approach. This allows easy access for freeing the attachments of the stomach, leaving intact the right gastric and the right gastroepiploic arteries. By severance of the duodenal attachment to the posterior peritoneum, the duodenum and the pancreas may be mobilized sufficiently for deliverance of the stomach high in the chest. The second incision is a right-sided thoracic one. This incision may be made anteriorly through the 4th or the 5th intercostal space with severance of the costal cartilages or by a posterolateral thoracic incision with removal of the 4th or the 5th rib. With the anterior thoracic approach, the patient's position need not be changed; the posterolateral approach is more direct and gives wider exposure, but the patient's position must be changed. There are advantages and disadvantages inherent in either method. After excision of the primary lesion, the freed stomach is displaced into the chest, and the esophagogastrostomy is made at the apex of the chest.

For lesions above the aortic arch, one may combine the abdominal incision, a separate right thoracic incision, and a separate cervical incision for the deliverance of the stomach into the cervical area. This maneuver is facilitated by resection of the medial portions of the left clavicle and the left first rib (Fig. 28-11). Because of the high mortality rate with lesions in the upper third of the thoracic esophagus, most surgeons now feel that carcinomas in this location should not be resected and should be treated by x-ray therapy. Others feel that only carcinoma of the lower third of the esophagus is primarily a surgical disease, and that carcinoma of the esophagus at all other levels should be treated by x-ray therapy.[20]

For carcinoma of the cervical esophagus without evident lymph nodal involvement on examination or at the time of exploration, resection of the area with reconstruction by means of a full-thickness skin tube manufactured from cervical skin is considered as the procedure of choice. This operation must be staged. Recently, a split-thickness skin graft over a tantalum gauge splint has been used to bridge the gap.[6] In the absence of nodal cervical metastases where direct extension to the larynx may be present, a laryngectomy with a distal tracheotomy may be necessary. While this appears to be the best operative approach for uncomplicated lesions of the cervical esophagus, such lesions are frequently complicated by early cervical metastases. In this situation, x-ray therapy offers the best means of palliation.

Results. While radical surgical measures have been termed curative, unfortunately, the results to date indicate that such measures are mainly palliative. In general, approximately 60 to 70 per cent of the cases seen by the surgeon are operable. This implies that some cases already have been screened prior to the request for surgical consultation. Of those explored, approximately 85 per cent of patients with lesions of the lower esophagus and 70 per cent with midesophageal lesions are resectable. The mortality for lower esophageal lesions is approximately 15 per cent, while the mortality with anastomoses above the aortic arch varies between 25 and 30 per cent. An inadequate number of cases involving the upper third of the thoracic esophagus in the superior mediastinal area have been treated surgically for the establishment of a definite mortality.

It is apparent, even at the time of intervention, that most operations for carcinoma of the esophagus are palliative. However, in situations where a cure was thought to be possible at the time of surgery, the results in terms of

5-year cures after resection and reconstruction are about 14 per cent for carcinomas of the midesophagus and 34 per cent for carcinomas of the lower esophagus and the cardia, whether the growth is epidermoid or adenocarcinoma.[25]

In summary, of 100 cases coming to a hospital many will evidence distant spread of tumor when first seen. With additional screening, others for medical reasons will be unsuitable candidates for major surgery. Of these considered operable some will be unresectable. Of those surviving resection, some will be cured. Only about 7 per cent of the total number of cases seen result in 5-year cures. While this is a discouraging picture, the curability of esophageal carcinoma closely parallels the curability of carcinoma of the stomach and carcinoma of the lung. However, in order to gain this yield the patient must be subjected to a higher morbidity and mortality than in the case of gastric and pulmonary lesions.

BENIGN TUMORS

Benign tumors of the esophagus are rare. In one autopsy series of approximately 7,500 consecutive cases only 44 benign tumors of the esophagus wer found.[19] None were symptomatic. Approximately 60 such tumors have been treated surgically. The lower third of the esophagus is the most common location for such lesions. Histologically, leiomyoma is the most frequent benign tumor found in the esophagus. In addition, other histologic types, such as myoma, fibromyoma, papilloma, neurofibroma, endothelioma, bronchogenic and esophageal cysts have been described. While a great variety have been reported on a histologic basis, macroscopically all fall under one of two main groups:[14]

Classification

MUCOSAL OR INTRALUMINAL. These tumors arise in the submucosa, grow into the lumen and stretch the esophageal mucosa before them as they grow, being at first sessile, later becoming pedunculated. They nearly always arise at the upper end of the esophagus. These tumors are commonly fibromyxomyomata or fibrolipomata. Some tumors have been described as cystic. It is probable that cystic changes are noted in tumors which have undergone extensive degeneration. They are of all sizes and, if large, become sausage-shaped, conforming to the contour of the esophageal lumen. They rarely become malignant, but may do so.

EXTRAMUCOSAL OR INTRAMURAL. This group is more common than the first. These tumors originate from the smooth muscle, the connective tissue, the nerve sheath elements and the cysts developing from bronchial or esophageal cell rests. Unlike the intraluminal group, they are usually sessile but rarely may become pedunculated. Occasionally, leiomyomata will become malignant, or they may have been malignant from the beginning. Second to leiomyomata, cysts of esophageal and bronchial origin are the second most common benign esophageal tumors. Embryologically, esophageal and bronchial cysts have a gross relationship and histologically the lining mucosa shares common characteristics which makes differentiation difficult. Since the embryologic esophagus has ciliated epithelium, cysts of either origin may have a respiratory-like mucosal lining. The single distinguishing characteristic microscopically is that whereas bronchogenic cysts may contain cartilage, true esophageal cysts do not.

Diagnosis. Usually, benign esophageal tumors are asymptomatic. If there is some obstruction, dysphagia may be present. One should consider the diagnosis of a benign lesion, if dysphagia has been present for several years. Dysphagia may be intermittent and slowly progressive. Some patients may complain of substernal distress, tightness or fullness, or pain in the chest. In addition, with intraluminal types regurgitation of the tumor sometimes occurs after violent expulsion efforts, such as vomiting or coughing. If the neoplasm is regurgitated into the larynx, choking and coughing may ensue. Death due to suffocation has been reported.

Significant physical findings are usually absent. The diagnosis rests on fluoroscopic and contrast roentgenographic examination of the esophagus. The demonstration of a smooth, dome-shaped cap of barium adjacent to a rounded protrusion into the lumen of the esophagus suggests a benign intramural tumor. Esophagoscopy should be done and serves chiefly as a means of evaluating the esophageal mucosa overlying the tumor. Biopsy is usually of no value since, with the exception of tumors located near the cardia which may

ulcerate, the overlying mucosa is intact. Biopsy through the intact mucosa is dangerous and may jeopardize easy enucleation by introducing infection into the tumor bed.

Treatment. For pedunculated intraluminal tumors, particularly of the upper esophagus, removal may be accomplished by means of a long snare, with or without diathermy. Should the pedunculated tumor be very large, an external incision may be necessary.

With the exception of the relatively uncommon intramural lesion of the cervical esophagus, the transpleural approach to these tumors is preferred. In most instances, the simple enucleation is uniformly successful in true cysts. Less frequently, the tumor may be firmly attached to the mucous membrane. In such situations, the tumor-bearing mucosa should be excised with closure of the defect.[21] More extensive lesions may require resection of the esophagus and reconstruction. Once the diagnosis of tumor is established, a definite histologic diagnosis seems to be imperative in view of the danger of possible malignancy.

REFERENCES

1. Allison, P. R.: Peptic ulcer of the esophagus, J. Thoracic Surg. *15*:308-317, 1946.
2. Anderson, R. L.: Rupture of the esophagus, J. Thoracic Surg. *24*:369-383, 1952.
3. Barrett, J. H.: Foreign bodies in the air and food passages; observations in 108 private patients, A.M.A. Arch. Otolaryng. *54*:651-665, 1951.
4. Berman, E. F.: Carcinoma of the esophagus: a new concept in therapy, Surgery *35*:822-835, 1954.
5. Boyd, G.: Oesophageal foreign bodies, Canad. M.A.J. *64*:102-107, 1951.
6. Edgerton, M. T.: One-stage reconstruction of cervical esophagus or trachea, Surgery *31*:239-250, 1952.
7. Garlock, J. H.: Surgical treatment of carcinoma of the esophagus, Arch. Surg. *41*:1184-1214, 1940.
8. Goldman, J. L.: Fish bones in the esophagus, Ann. Otol. Rhin. & Laryng. *60*:957-973, 1951.
9. Goss, C. M.: Gray's Anatomy, ed. 26, Philadelphia, Lea & Febiger, 1954.
10. Gray, H. K., and Sharpe, W. S.: Benign lesions at the lower end of the esophagus, Am. J. Surg. *54*:252-261, 1941.
11. Harrington, S. W.: The surgical treatment

of pulsion diverticula of the thoracic esophagus, Ann. Surg. *129*:606-618, 1949.

12. Holinger, P. H., and Johnson, K. C.: Benign strictures of the esophagus, S. Clin. North America *31*:135-152, 1951.

13. Kinsella, T. J., Morse, R. W., and Hertzog, A. J.: Spontaneous rupture of the esophagus, J. Thoracic Surg. *17*:613-631, 1948.

14. Korkis, F. B.: Benign tumours of the oesophagus, J. Laryng. & Otol. *65*:638-645, 1951.

15. Lahey, F. H.: Esophageal diverticula, Arch. Surg. *41*:1118-1140, 1940.

16. Lerche, W.: The Esophagus and Pharynx in Action, Springfield, Ill., Thomas, 1950.

17. Merendino, K. A., and Dillard, D. H.: The concept of sphincter substitution by an interposed jejunal segment for anatomic and physiological abnormalities at the esophagogastric junction; with special reference to reflux esophagitis, cardiospasm, and esophageal varices, Ann. Surg. *142*:486-506, 1955.

18. Merendino, K. A., and Mark, V. H.: An analysis of 100 cases of squamous-cell carcinoma of the esophagus: Part I. With special reference to the delay periods and delay factors in diagnosis and therapy, contrasting state and city and county institutions, Cancer *5*:52-61, 1952; Part II. With special reference to its theoretical curability, Surg., Gynec. & Obst. *94*:110-114, 1952.

19. Moersch, H. J., and Harrington, S. W.: Benign tumors of the esophagus, Ann. Otol. Rhin. & Laryng. *53*:800-817, 1954.

20. Morrison, D. R.: The treatment of carcinoma of the esophagus, Surgery *46*:516-520, 1959.

21. Myers, R. T., and Bradshaw, H. H.: Benign intramural tumors and cysts of the esophagus, J. Thoracic Surg. *21*:470-482, 1951.

22. Redo, S. F., Barnes, W. A., and Oritz della Sierra, A.: Esophagogastrostomy without reflux utilizing a submuscular tunnel in the stomach, Ann. Surg. *151*:37-46, 1960.

23. Robertson, R., and Sarjeant, T. R.: Reconstruction of the esophagus, J. Thoracic Surg. *20*:689-701, 1950.

24. Samson, P. C.: Postemetic rupture of the esophagus, Surg., Gynec. & Obst. *93*:221-229, 1948.

25. Sweet, R. H.: Carcinoma of the midthoracic esophagus: its treatment by radical resection and high intrathoracic esophagogastric anastomosis, Ann. Surg. *124*:653-666, 1946.

26. Swigart, L. L., Siekert, R. G., Hambley, W. C., and Anson, B. J.: The esophageal arteries: an anatomic study of 150 specimens, Surg., Gynec. & Obst. *90*:234-243, 1950.

27. Templeton, F. E.: X-ray Examination of the Stomach, Chicago, Univ. Chicago Press, 1944.

28. Thomas, G. I., and Merendino, K. A.: Jejunal interposition operation—analysis of thirty-three clinical cases, J.A.M.A. *168*:1759-1766, 1958.

29. Vinson, P. P.: Diagnosis and treatment of cardiospasm, Postgrad. Med. *3*:13-18, 1948.

30. Wangensteen, O. H., and Leven, N. L.: Gastric resection for esophagitis and stricture of acid-peptic origin, Surg., Gynec. & Obst. *88*:560-570, 1949.

31. Winkelstein, A., Wolf, B. S., Som, M. L., and Marshak, L. H.: Peptic esophagitis with duodenal or gastric ulcer, J.A.M.A. *154*:885-889, 1954.

32. Yudin, S. S.: The surgical construction of eighty cases of artificial esophagus, Surg., Gynec. & Obst. *78*:561, 1944.

CHAPTER 29

Stomach and Duodenum

Some physiologists will have it that the stomach is a mill; others
that it is a fermenting vat; others again, that it is a stew pan, but
in my view of the matter, it is neither a mill, a fermenting vat, nor
a stew pan—but a stomach, gentlemen, a stomach.—John Hunter

INTRODUCTION

The stomach and the duodenum have important functions and at the same time are
the frequent site of serious diseases. In few
organs that are diseased so frequently can the
majority of affections be attributed to only
3 pathologic conditions. These 3 are peptic
ulcer, gastric carcinoma and hypertrophic
pyloric stenosis—an inflammatory, a neoplastic and a congenital condition, respectively.
Together these 3 conditions are a major cause
of morbidity (about 10,000,000 persons in the
United States alone are affected during their
lifetime) and of mortality (34,000 deaths per
year or 2,400,000 of those persons now alive
in the United States alone). All other affections of the stomach and the duodenum, while
important, are so dwarfed in relative significance by the 3 major conditions cited above
that they are listed separately at the end of
this chapter so as not to interfere with the
main discussion. Before proceeding with the
description of the individual diseases of the
stomach and the duodenum, a brief basic
background description will be given.

EMBRYOLOGY

The stomach appears as a spindle-shaped
dilatation of the foregut during the 4th week
of embryonic life. There are at this stage both
dorsal and ventral mesenteries, the latter extending only as far as the umbilicus. A rotation occurs because the dorsal and the cardiac
portions of the stomach grow more rapidly
than the ventral and the pyloric portions. The
result of this uneven growth is that the dorsal-
cardiac portions turn to the left and the
ventral-pyloric portions to the right. The
dorsal portion thus becomes the greater curvature with the dorsal mesentery forming part
of the lesser sac and the greater omentum.
The ventral portion becomes the lesser curvature with the ventral mesentery forming the
lesser omentum and the falciform ligament.
The vagus nerves go along with the rotation
of the stomach, the left becoming anterior
and the right posterior (rule to remember:
"LARP").

ANATOMY

The stomach lies between the cardiac and
the pyloric sphincters and includes the fundus,
the corpus and the antrum (see Fig. 29-1).
The lower part of the antrum is loosely termed
the "pyloric" or "prepyloric" region. The lesser
and the greater curvatures are of some surgical significance, the former being the site of
most benign gastric ulcers, while most ulcers
on the latter are malignant. The lesser curvature is also referred to as the *Magenstrasse*
or gastric pathway; it is the shortest route
through the stomach, being the course traveled
by ingested liquids. The term *Magenstrasse*

was introduced by Waldeyer (1908) and popularized by Bauer (1923).

The arteries to the stomach are plentiful. This excellent blood supply has the advantage that healing is prompt after operation (cf. esophagus and colon, which are the opposite in this respect), but, at the same time, the disadvantage that bleeding is difficult to control. Bentley and Barlow (1952) demonstrated that while in the rest of the stomach the mucosal arteries come from a rich submucosal plexus, along the lesser curvature they arise directly from long slender branches of the right and the left gastric arteries which pierce the muscularis directly. This apparently more precarious arrangement of the vascular supply may explain the predisposition of the *Magenstrasse* to develop gastric ulcer. The presence of arteriovenous anastomoses in the stomach was demonstrated by Barlow, Bentley and Walder (1951) and was confirmed by Sherman and Newman (1954). Glass spheres of maximum diameters of 100 to 180 μ were passed through the gastric circulation of living dogs by the latter authors.

The veins and the lymphatics tend to follow the arteries (Fig. 29-2).

The nerves include the vagi, a left anterior and a right posterior (which stimulate gastric secretion) and sympathetic fibers which probably inhibit gastric secretion.

HISTOLOGY

The most important cells in the stomach are the parietal (oxyntic) cells which are

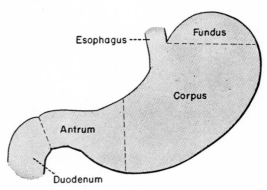

FIG. 29-1. The anatomic divisions of the stomach.

especially plentiful in the corpus. There are essentially *no* parietal cells in the antrum. The parietal cells secrete HCl; the chief cells secrete pepsin. Recent studies have shown that there is a relationship between the size of the parietal cell mass and acid output (Bruce, Card, Marks and Sircus, 1959; Card and Marks, 1960). In the proximal duodenum there is a special layer of cells, the so-called Brunner's glands, which secrete mucin that may protect the duodenum against peptic digestion. It is of interest that Moffat and Anderson (1955) reported an adenoma of a Brunner's gland. Such tumors are said to comprise 10 per cent of benign duodenal tumors.

PHYSIOLOGY

The physiology of the stomach and the duodenum is of great importance in studying

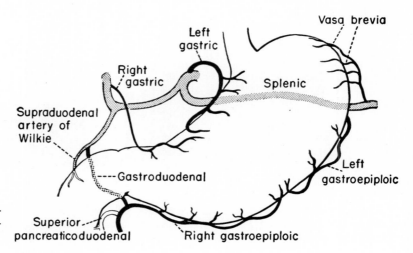

FIG. 29-2. The arterial blood vessel supply to the stomach.

and understanding the different affections of this region, not only peptic ulcer but the others as well. The following factors will be considered separately: (1) gastric acid secretion, (2) neutralization, (3) gastric pepsin and mucin secretion, (4) altered resistance of gastric and duodenal mucosa, (5) variations in mucosal resistance at different levels in the intestinal tract, and (6) gastric motility.

Gastric Acid Secretion. The secretion of hydrochloric acid is of especial importance clinically. The rule may be given: *No acid, no ulcer.* Acid activates the enzyme pepsin which works best at a pH below 4.0.

Acid secretion may be expressed in clinical units (numbers of cc. $^{N}/10$ NaOH to neutralize 100 ml. gastric juice using Töpfer's reagent as indicator) or in volume of secretion in liters. We prefer to express it as the product of these 2 factors, or the number of clinical units of free hydrochloric acid $\times$ the volume of secretion in liters = mEq. of free hydrochloric acid, usually using an overnight (12 hours) specimen.

Acid secretion is *stimulated* by the following factors:

CEPHALIC (NERVOUS OR PSYCHIC) PHASE by action of the vagi. This usually acts early in the course of a meal, occurring even at the sight or the smell of food. Hypoglycemia sufficient either to reduce the blood sugar level to below 50 mg. per cent or to produce definite symptoms of hypoglycemia acts upon the vagal centers, producing an increased secretion of gastric acid. This action is the basis of the so-called insulin or Hollander test for vagal function. If the test shows no increase in free hydrochloric acid secretion after administration of sufficient insulin to fulfill the requirements listed above, vagotomy has been complete. Because of the importance of the vagal factor in gastric secretion, representative experimental studies upon which our modern concept are based will be listed below:

1. Vagotomy eliminates the secretory response of the stomach to sham feeding (Pavlov, 1910).

QUANTITATIVE EFFECT OF VAGOTOMY ON GASTRIC SECRETION IN TOTAL POUCH DOG

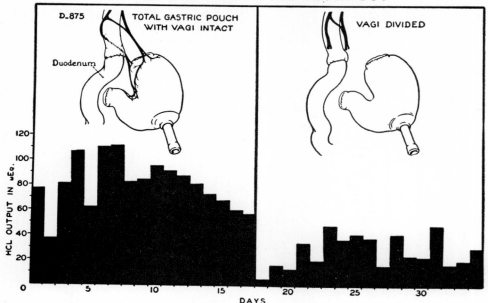

FIG. 29-3. The effect of vagotomy on gastric secretion in the total pouch dog. At the left the control 24-hour secretion of free HCl in mEq from the total gastric pouch is shown over a 17-day period. At the right the same is shown after vagotomy, demonstrating the marked decrease (Dragstedt, L., *et al.*: Ann. Surg. *140*:397).

2. Sectioning of the vagi to an isolated total stomach pouch or to a Pavlov pouch* causes a marked reduction in acid secretion from that pouch (Dragstedt, Woodward, Storer, Oberhelman, and Smith, 1950) (Fig. 29-3).

3. Sectioning of the vagus nerves to the stomach in the Shay rat preparation (if the pylorus is ligated in the fasting rat, an average of 22 gastric ulcers per rat develop within 24 hours) prevents the formation of gastric ulcers (Harkins, 1947).

4. Sectioning of the vagus nerves to the stomach in the Mann-Williamson preparation (see below) markedly lowers the incidence of marginal ulcer formation (Harkins and Hooker, 1947) (Fig. 29-4).

5. Sectioning of the vagus nerves to the stomach pouch in the Sauvage pouch preparation (Fig. 29-5) decreases the incidence of

stomal peptic ulceration in the connecting jejunal loop (Sauvage, Schmitz, Storer, Kanar, Smith, and Harkins, 1953).

6. To show that the action of the vagi is not a simple one, it was demonstrated that cutting the vagi to the *main stomach* causes an *increase* in the acid output of a Heidenhain pouch,† possibly because of secondary stimulation of the hormonal phase (Storer, Schmitz, Sauvage, Kanar, Diessner, and Harkins, 1952).

7. Stimulation of the anterior hypothalamus (Porter, Movius, and French, 1953) produces a prompt rise in the acid secretion of the stomach of monkeys. This response is believed to travel over the vagi, is blocked by vagotomy, but not by adrenalectomy, and is related to the acute stress ulcer of the Cushing's type (see p. 674 and Fig. 29-6).

*Pavlov pouch = a partial stomach pouch with the nervous connections still intact.

† Heidenhain pouch = a partial stomach pouch with no vagal fibers leading to it.

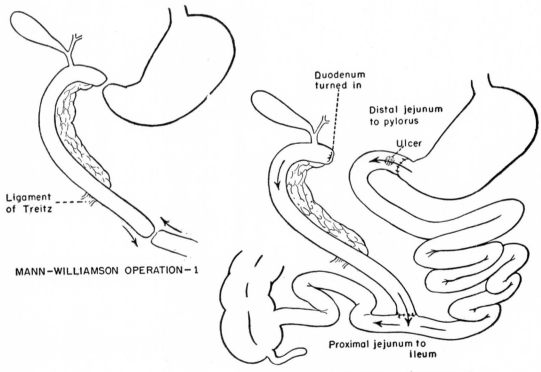

Duodenum
turned in

Distal jejunum
to pylorus

Ulcer

Ligament
of Treitz

MANN–WILLIAMSON OPERATION–1

Proximal jejunum to
ileum

MANN–WILLIAMSON OPERATION – 2

FIG. 29-4. The Mann-Williamson preparation for the production of experimental ulcer. On the left the lines of division of the bowel are shown. On the right, the reconstituted intestinal tract is demonstrated. The diversion of the neutralizing biliary and pancreatic juices away from the gastrojejunal anastomosis leads to ulceration at the point shown.

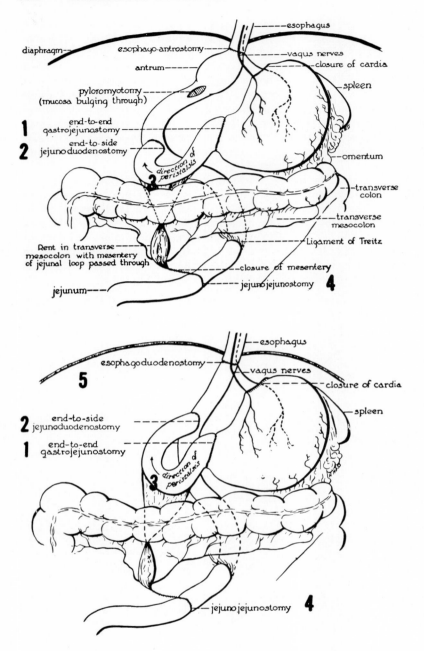

FIG. 29-5. The Sauvage pouch preparation for the production of experimental peptic ulcer. (*A, Top*) The 3-phase total parietal cell pouch with antrum and vagi intact and with the pouch connected to the duodenum for internal drainage by a jejunal loop. (*B, Bottom*) The 2-phase cephalic pouch: vagi intact but antrum excised.

ANTRAL (GASTRIC OR HORMONAL) PHASE by stimulation of the antrum to produce gastrin which travels by the blood stream acting as a hormone to stimulate the parietal cells of the corpus and the fundus to secrete, in turn, more gastric acid. There is some evidence that the cephalic phase exerts its full effect in the presence of an intact antrum and vice versa, indicating some interdependence of the two stimulating mechanisms. The hormone gastrin is an internal secretion of the antral mucous membrane, which contains no parietal cells, and acts on the rest of the stomach which secretes no gastrin.

Representative points demonstrating the importance of the antrum are as follows:

Fig. 29-5. (*Cont.*) (*C, Top*) The 2-phase hormonal pouch: antrum intact but vagi cut. (*D, Bottom*) Intestinal phase pouch: both antrum excised and vagi cut, only the intestinal phase of the 3-food-stimulated phases still being present.

In this procedure there are 4 anastomoses, denoted by the numerals in the figures: the first two, (1) end-to-end gastrojejunostomy and (2) end-to-side jejunoduodenostomy, are connected by (3) the jejunal loop. The other two are (4) jejunojejunostomy and (5) either an esophagoantrostomy or an esophagoduodenostomy, depending on the preparation.

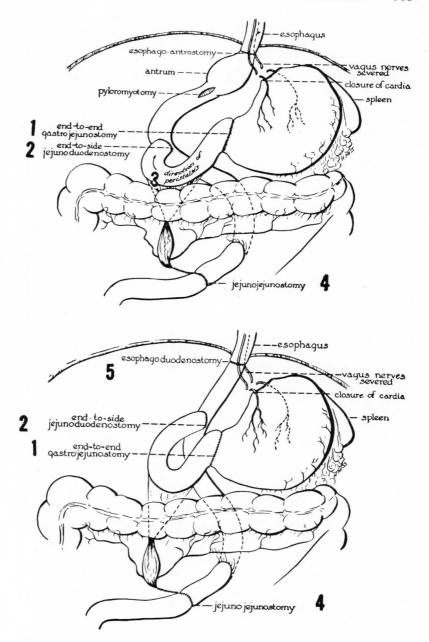

1. Antral extract injected intravenously causes increase in acid secretion (Edkins, of England, 1906).

2. The hard-learned clinical fact that if the excluded antrum is left in place after a partial gastric resection, marginal ulcer is more apt to occur (see below).

3. The fundamental observations of Dragstedt, Woodward, Storer, Oberhelman and Smith (1950) relative to transplantation or removal of the antrum. As shown in Figures 29-7 and 29-8, when the antrum is in contact with intestinal contents, it stimulates the secretion of hydrochloric acid from Pavlov or total stomach pouches in dogs. When it is isolated, excised, or transplanted subcutane-

SCHEMA FOR THE ACTION OF STRESS ON GASTRIC SECRETION

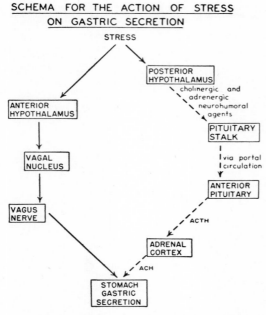

FIG. 29-6. A diagrammatic representation of two types of hypothalamic stress stimulation of gastric secretion (Cushing's type on the reader's left and Curling's type to the right). (Shay, Harry: Gastroenterology *26*:318)

ously, it does not act in this stimulatory manner.

4. Foods and other chemicals placed in the isolated antrum of dogs stimulate acid production of Heidenhain pouches (Oberhelman, Woodward, Zubiran, and Dragstedt, 1952).

5. Physical stimuli, including distention, to the antrum attached to the colon of dogs, causes an increase in Heidenhain pouch acid secretion (Dragstedt, Oberhelman, Evans and Rigler, 1954).

6. Antrumectomy in the Sauvage pouch preparation is a more potent factor than vagotomy in reducing the incidence of marginal ulcer in the connecting jejunal loop (Sauvage, Schmitz, Storer, Kanar, Smith, and Harkins, 1953).

7. *Effect of portosystemic shunting on gastric secretion:* That gastrin or other acid-stimulating substances which reach the parietal cells via the blood stream may normally be partly destroyed or inactivated while passing through the liver was postulated by Clarke, Ozeran, Hart, Cruze and Crevling (1958). Experiments indicated that portacaval shunts caused an increase in Heidenhain pouch production. Recent reports on this subject are those of Irvine, Duthie and Waton (1959) and Irvine, Duthie, Ritche and Waton (1959).

INTESTINAL PHASE. A hormone similar to but less powerful than gastrin may be secreted by the intestinal mucous membrane when in contact with food. This hormone is not believed to be enterogastrone, an inhibitory hormone.

PITUITARY-ADRENAL PHASE. Stimulation of the posterior hypothalamus may act on the stomach by way of the adrenal cortex as an intermediary. This type of hypersecretion is related to acute ulcers of the Curling's type (see p. 674). Porter, Movius and French (1953) demonstrated that in monkeys such

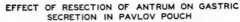
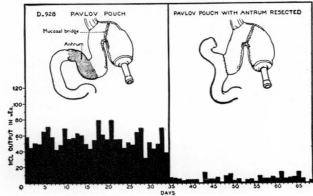

EFFECT OF RESECTION OF ANTRUM ON GASTRIC SECRETION IN PAVLOV POUCH

FIG. 29-7. The effect of antral resection on Pavlov pouch secretion of free HCl in the dog. (Dragstedt, L., *et al.:* Ann. Surg. *132*:629)

COMPARATIVE EFFECT OF ANTRUM TRANSPLANTATION INTO COLON AND DUODENUM

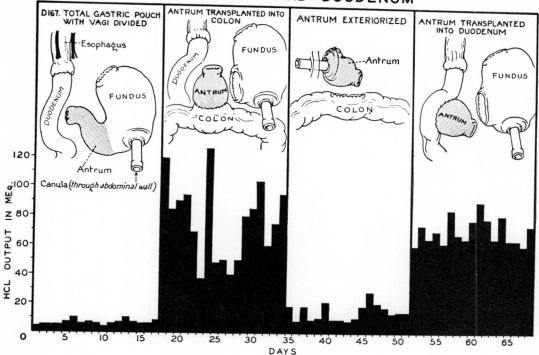

FIG. 29-8. The effects of the antrum in different situations on gastric pouch secretion in the dog. *Phase 1:* Antrum in contact with acid but not with intestinal contents-very low secretory rate. *Phase 2:* Antrum in contact with intestinal contents but not with acid-very high secretory rate. *Phase 3:* Antrum in contact with neither acid nor intestinal contents-quite low secretory rate. *Phase 4:* As Phase 2, except antrum is attached to duodenum instead of to colon. (Dragstedt, L., *et al.*: Ann Surg. *134*:333)

responses are blocked by adrenalectomy but not by vagotomy, and the response is slightly more delayed than that to anterior hypothalamic stimulation acting by way of the vagi (Fig. 29-9). Villarreal, Ganong, and Gray (1955) similarly found that in the dog ACTH stimulates gastric acid secretion after a latent period of 3 to 4 hours and despite antrumectomy or vagotomy, but that its action is blocked by bilateral adrenalectomy.

PANCREATIC PHASE. The pancreas plays a double role in the etiology of peptic ulcer. The first depends upon the fact that exclusion of the external secretion of the organ increases the tendency to ulceration of the duodenum. This observation is the main basis of the Mann-Williamson preparation to produce experimental ulcer.

Elman and Hartmann (1931) found that complete diversion of the pancreatic secretion away from the duodenum resulted in duodenal ulcer in all of the 6 dogs they studied. Dragstedt (1942) reported that external drainage of the pancreatic secretions produced peptic ulcer in 100 per cent of dogs, but that in 300 pancreatectomies the incidence of ulcer was only 1.3 per cent, indicating a curious difference. Poth, Mankoff, and De Loach (1948) further helped to establish the role of the pancreas in the production of peptic ulcer. Dogs with either pancreatectomy or pancreatic duct ligation developed numerous duodenal ulcers when given doses of histamine-in-beeswax which would give control dogs only occasional ulcers. It was concluded that the presence of alkaline pancreatic juice in the

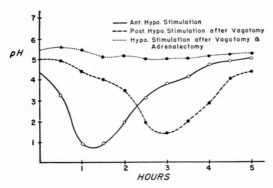

FIG. 29-9. Gastric HCl secretion induced by hypothalamic stimulation in the monkey. (Porter, R., Movius, H., and French, J.: Surgery *33*:876)

duodenum is of great importance in the prevention of ulcers.

The importance of the internal secretions of the pancreas in gastric secretion is more complex. The administration of insulin is the basis of the well-known Hollander test for completeness of vagotomy. Poth, Fromm, De Young, and Aldridge (1950) found that dogs given commercial insulin in an attempt to maintain the blood sugar level below 50 mg. per cent developed peptic ulcer in 50 per cent of the control animals and in the same percentage of animals that were also pancreatectomized. These authors postulated that such results might be explained on the basis that the H-G (hyperglycemic-glycogenolytic) factor (glucagon) of the pancreas, secreted by the alpha cells of the islets, which supposedly exists as an impurity in commercial insulin, is the cause of the ulcer formation rather than the insulin itself. This might also explain why in their individual dogs there was essentially no relationship between the development of ulcer and the degree of hypoglycemia maintained. This theory did not entirely stand the test of experiment, since Poth and Fromm (1950) found that the over-all incidence of peptic ulcer in pancreatectomized dogs receiving sufficient insulin to reduce the blood sugar level below 50 mg. per cent was the same whether or not that insulin contained the H-G factor.

Another important observation is that patients with hyperfunctioning islet cell tumors seldom develop peptic ulcer. The report of

Janowitz (1951) represents one of the few in the literature of coexistent peptic ulcer and hyperfunctioning islet cell tumor. Furthermore, in their case, removal of the islet cell tumor, while restoring the blood sugar values to normal, did not affect the clinical course of the ulcer.

Porter, Movius, and French (1953) reported that in monkeys the administration of insulin leads to an increased gastric acid secretion beginning within ½ hour and reaching a peak within 1½ hours, but not returning to normal for 4 to 5 hours. They concluded that this curve exhibits features of the responses to both anterior and posterior hypothalamic stimulation (Fig. 29-10). After vagotomy, however, the gastric acid response to insulin administration was delayed and followed a curve similar to that seen with posterior hypothalamic excitation; contrariwise, after adrenalectomy, the gastric response to insulin was limited to the curve seen with anterior hypothalamic stimulation.

These basic studies on the role of the pancreas indicate that its external secretion may prevent marginal ulcers, and its internal secretions may be a factor in (1) stress ulcers of both the Curling and the Cushing types, and (2) intractable ulcer (q.v.).

Acid secretion is *inhibited* by the following factors:

1. *Nervous Factor.* The action of the sympathetic fibers may either affect the stomach directly, or hold the vagal stimuli in check (Cushing, 1932, and Gregory and Tracy, 1960).

2. *"Antral Acid-Inhibition."* It is believed that when excess acid strikes the antrum, this acts as a signal to the parietal cells to slow down in the production of acid. It is of interest that one organ, the antrum, can be active in both stimulating and inhibiting the production of acid.

A. Oberhelman, Woodward, Zubiran and Dragstedt (1952) demonstrated that in the dog the flow of acid gastric juice through an antral pouch attached to the colon markedly diminishes the secretory stimulating effect of the antral pouch.

B. State, Katz, Kaplan, Herman, Morgenstern, and Knight (1955) demonstrated that after wedge resection the incidence of histamine-induced ulcers in dogs is significantly less when the antrum is preserved and anastomosed to the residual gastric pouch than when it is excised and continuity restored by Billroth I or II anastomosis.

C. Brackney, Campbell, and Wangensteen (1954) performed a modification of the Sauvage pouch experiment, except that in one variant the antrum was in contact with the acid secretions of the stomach. In such an instance the incidence of ulcer was much less than when the antrum was not bathed by acid.

D. Shapira, Morgenstern and State (1960) studied antral inhibition with twin antrum pouches.

3. *"Antral Inhibitory Hormone."* The presence of an antral inhibitory hormone, produced by the antrum was postulated by Harrison, Lakey and Hyde (1956). More recent studies of Jordan and Sand (1957); Woodward, Trumbull, Schapiro and Towne (1958) and of Dragstedt, Kohatzu, Gwaltney, Nagano and Greenlee (1959) tend to cast doubt on this hypothesis. However, the extraction of an inhibitor substance from human gastric juice has been reported by Smith, DuVal, Joel and Wolf (1959) and Smith, DuVal, Joel, Hanska and Wolf (1960).

4. *"Duodenal Acid-Inhibition."* This is a postulated mechanism similar to antral inhibition except that the excess acid acts upon the duodenum rather than on the antrum to cause a supposed hormonal warning which passes to the stomach which, in turn, cuts

down on the production of acid. Enterogastrone, a possible inhibitory hormone produced by the duodenum, may be the factor in duodenal inhibition. Evidence for duodenal inhibition is as follows:

A. Sokolov (1904) reported that the instillation of 0.5 per cent HCl into the duodenum inhibits gastric secretion.

B. Day and Webster (1935) and Griffiths (1936) confirmed this observation. Pincus, Thomas and Rehfuss (1942) reported that acid inhibition resulted only if the pH in the duodenum was 2.5 or lower. The extent of inhibition was dependent upon the level of pH produced.

C. Dragstedt, Oberhelman, and Smith (1951) and later Harkins, Schmitz, Nyhus, Kanar, Zech, and Griffith (1954) performed subtotal gastric resections in dogs after attaching the antrum to the colon. In half the animals (Fig. 29-11) the continuity was restored by gastroduodenal and in half by gastrojejunal anastomosis. In the former, 22 per cent of the dogs developed stomal ulcer (as shown in Table 1) while in the latter, 82 per cent developed ulcer. In other, and almost similar experiments, Harkins, *et al.*, used histamine-in-beeswax as the stimulus to excess gastric secretion. With this preparation, 25 per cent of the animals developed ulcer after gastroduodenal anastomosis and 100 per cent after gastrojejunal anastomosis. These experiments can be used to argue either for a greater

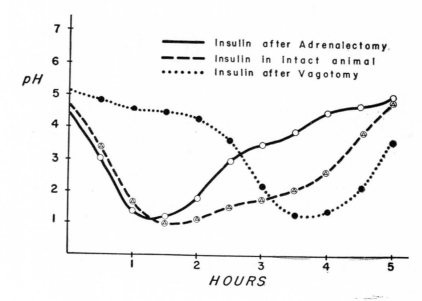

Fig. 29-10. Gastric HCl secretion induced by insulin in the monkey. (Porter, R., Movius H., and French, J.: Surgery *33*:877)

TABLE 1. EFFECT OF TYPE OF ANASTOMOSIS ON INCIDENCE OF EXPERIMENTAL ULCER PRODUCED BY ANTRAL TRANSPLANT TO COLON (COMBINED RESULTS OF DRAGSTEDT, ET AL., 1951, AND HARKINS, ET AL., 1954)

TYPE OF ANASTOMOSIS	NO. OF DOGS	NO. WITH ULCER	% WITH ULCER
Billroth I	18	4	22
Billroth II	17	14	82

resistance of the duodenum, as compared with the jejunum, for duodenal acid-inhibition, or for both.

D. The experiments of Brackney, Thal, and Wangensteen (1955), Sircus (1958), and Jones and Harkins (1959) are more clear cut in indicating the presence of duodenal acid-inhibition. Resection of the duodenum and transplantation of the bile and pancreatic ducts into the jejunum, or transplantation of the duodenum lower into the intestinal tract—both resulted in a definite increase in Heidenhain pouch secretion in dogs.

5. *Enterogastrone*. This chalone is prepared from the first 6 to 8 feet of fresh hog intestine. The colorless product is easily soluble in water, and 25 mg. will suppress histamine-induced gastric secretion in the total pouch dog. Greengard, Atkinson, Grossman and Ivy (1946) reported that only 25 per cent of 8 Mann-Williamson dogs injected with purified enterogastrone daily for 1 year developed ulcer, whereas 100 per cent of 10 such dogs given hog muscle extract injections as controls developed ulcer. Preliminary clinical trial by these authors is suggestive of benefit, but the drug is not commonly accepted as being of clinical benefit at present.

Interrelations Between the Phases of Gastric Secretion. Recent studies (Oberhelman, Rigler and Dragstedt, 1957; Woodward, Robertson, Fried and Shapiro, 1957; Thein and Schofield, 1959; Chapman, Nyhus and Harkins, 1960; and Nyhus, Chapman, DeVito and Harkins, 1960) indicate that vagal action probably releases gastrin. These interrelationships may explain the confusing reports concerning antral inhibition and antral inhibitory hormones. Since recent studies (Gillespie *et al.*, 1960) indicate that gastrin, besides its acid-stimulatory property, is able to influence the "reactivity" of the parietal cells to other

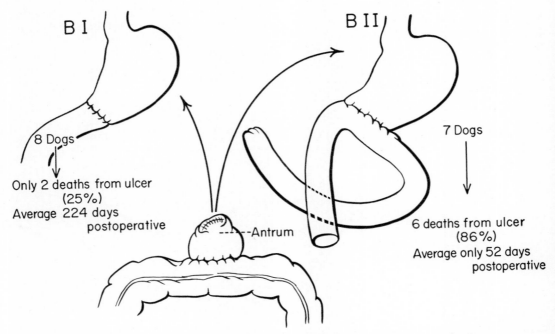

FIG. 29-11. The relative mortality from stomal ulceration following gastroduodenostomy and gastrojejunostomy in dogs with gastric hypersecretion on the basis of antrum transplant to the colon. (Author's animals only; Table 1 includes also those of Dragstedt, *et al.*)

stimuli, including vagal action. Apparent acid inhibition may be nothing other than removal of this facilitatory influence. Also, Gillespie (1959) showed that acidification of the antrum is capable of reducing the response of the parietal cells to histamine. A study on the final common pathway of gastric secretion is that of Peters and Womack (1958).

Neutralization. Since acid causes peptic ulcer, attempts at treatment within the stomach, both medical (Sippy powders) and surgical (gastrojejunostomy) have been partly based on an attempt to neutralize the acid. Both attempts have resulted in partial failure. Alkaline powders are followed by a "rebound phenomenon" and gastrojejunostomy has been followed by a high incidence (34%, Lewisohn, 1925) of marginal ulceration. In the duodenum, however, the normal alkaline bile and pancreatic juice plays an important neutralizing role. (See pp. 663 and 672 relative to [1] the Mann-Williamson preparation which is based upon deflecting these secretions away from the pylorus and [2] studies on the decrease in acid-buffering capacity of the intestine proportionate to the distance from the ampulla of Vater.)

Gastric Pepsin and Mucin Secretion. Although these two substances have different purposes, the one to act as the enzyme of protein digestion in the stomach, the other to lubricate the organ and to protect its wall from the digestive action of the more active constituents of the gastric juice, the two will be considered together here.

PEPSIN is believed to come from the body chief cells of the gastric glands. Unlike hydrochloric acid, its secretion is believed to be essentially continuous, although, of course, it cannot act in the absence of acid. Alterations in pepsin production after different surgical operations have been studied by Farmer, Burke and Smithwick (1954). Book, Chinn and Beams (1952) reported that in patients with duodenal ulcer there is no reduction in the secretion of pepsin per unit of volume of secretion following vagotomy, unlike the finding for free hydrochloric acid which is reduced following vagotomy. However, since vagotomy reduces the total volume of secretion, the total amount of pepsin secreted in 12 hours is reduced.

MUCIN. The surface epithelial cells, the

neck chief cells of the glands of the corpus, and the cardiac and the pyloric glands all secrete mucus. Mersheimer, Glass, Speer, Winfield and Boyd (1952) reported that in patients, mucin secretion, similar to hydrochloric acid, no longer responds to insulin hypoglycemia after vagotomy. Following partial gastric resection, on the other hand, the acid response to insulin was largely lost, while the mucous response was maintained at its preoperative level.

Altered Resistance of Gastric and Duodenal Mucosa. This factor has been brought forward repeatedly as an explanation for certain types of peptic ulcer. Overaction of the sympathetic fibers may not only decrease acid secretion but also by producing local ischemia may produce a lowered resistance to peptic digestion. A decrease in the mucin secretion of the gastric mucosa may cause a comparable decrease in its resistance. Friesen (1950) reported that hemoconcentration, with "its resultant mucosal congestion," is a factor in the causation of gastroduodenal ulceration following burns. Lillehei, Roth, and Wangensteen (1952) extended this hypothesis to demonstrate "that a number of stress-provoking agencies in experimental animals fail to influence gastric secretion or even depress gastric acidity; but nevertheless, they exert a powerful ulcer abetting effect by reducing the resistance of the gastroduodenal mucosa to autodigestion." (See also section on "Acute Ulcer," p. 674.)

Variations in Mucosal Resistance at Different Levels in the Intestinal Tract. In the duodenum of man, Brunner's glands extend as a dense sheet immediately below the muscularis mucosae from the pylorus to or beyond the ampulla of Vater (Fig. 29-12), but never beyond the ligament of Treitz. These cells are capable of secreting an abundant alkaline mucus which may be a leading factor in the protection of the normal duodenum, as shown by Griffith and Harkins (1956). It is of interest that the distribution of Brunner's glands in man and the pig are almost identical, whereas these glands are almost absent in the dog, upon which animal so much experimental work relating to ulcer has been done.

In the dog, below the level of the upper duodenum where the only Brunner's glands are present, Kiriluk and Merendino (1954)

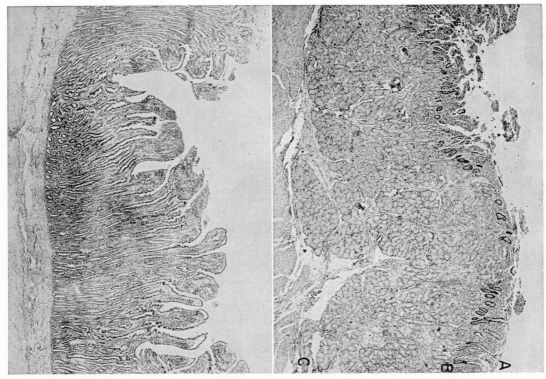

Fig. 29-12. (*Left*) Normal jejunum of man (8 cm. distal to ligament of Treitz) without Brunner's glands. (*Right*) Normal duodenum of man (3 cm. distal to pylorus) with solid mass of these glands (layer BC) lying below the muscularis mucosae. (Griffith, C., and Harkins, H.: Ann Surg. *143*:161)

have shown that there is little variation in inherent sensitivity between the lower duodenum, the jejunum and the ileum. In unpublished experiments, Merendino demonstrated that the colon might be added to this list. Two factors are involved in these studies: one is the inherent resistance of the part being tested, and the other is the buffering capacity of the corresponding lumenal contents which depends on the distance from the ampulla of Vater. Merendino and his associates controlled the distance factor—which had not been done by previous investigators—and found that the inherent resistance from lower duodenum to colon did not vary.

At the same time, the esophagus, which is lined with squamous epithelium, is *much* less resistant than any portion of the intestinal tract from cardia to pectinate line.

Gastric Motility. Alterations in gastric motility are known to be a factor in hunger and also may be responsible for some of the pain of peptic ulcer. Section of the vagi decreases gastric motility—does not decrease tone as is popularly believed—as well as gastric secretion. Rowe, Grimson, and Flowe (1953) devised a gastrometric balloon test for the completeness of vagal section which they stated is more reliable than the insulin test of Hollander.

PHARMACOLOGY

The possible compound effect of neutralizing drugs has been cited above. The important role of the antisecretory drugs (atropine, banthine, etc.) will not be elaborated upon here. Other drugs are also useful, and the pharmacologic aspects of gastric secretion are important. The introduction of histamine-in-beeswax as a method of experimental study of peptic ulcer by Code and Varco (1940) has been of great importance.

BACTERIOLOGY

In the presence of normal acidity the stomach is the least contaminated portion of the main intestinal tract. When acid is reduced after operation, or in many patients with carcinoma of the stomach, bacterial contamination increases. After vagotomy, not only the lowered acidity but also the decreased motility with resultant stasis tends to increase bacterial contamination of the stomach.

PATHOLOGY

The typical chronic peptic ulcer is surrounded by thickened, scarred gastric or duodenal wall. Acute ulcers are punched out, and there is little fibrous tissue between them and the surrounding intestinal wall. Two rules are of some practical significance: (1) Gastric ulcers are quite apt to be malignant; duodenal ulcers almost never so. (2) Perforated duodenal ulcers are *usually* anterior and do not bleed; bleeding duodenal ulcers are *usually* posterior and do not perforate (they penetrate into the pancreas and erode the gastroduodenal artery).

PEPTIC ULCER

Peptic ulcer is a medical and surgical problem of great significance accompanied by a considerable morbidity and, because of its complications, is a major cause of death. By definition, peptic ulceration involves the autopeptic digestion of the patient's own tissues. This is rendered possible by either an excess acidity—which enables the pepsin secreted by the chief cells to act at its optimum pH—or by the reduced resistance of the tissues in question.

Peptic ulcer occurs in a number of special types according to etiology and location. Each of these headings with its various subheadings will be considered, after which a separate account of duodenal ulcer, the most common and most important of all the peptic ulcers will follow.

SPECIAL TYPES OF PEPTIC ULCER ACCORDING TO ETIOLOGY

In this section, 5 special types of peptic ulcer will be considered, each with a special etiology according to present concepts. These include: (1) gastric ulcer, (2) duodenal ulcer,

(3) Cushing's acute ulcer, (4) Curling's acute ulcer and (5) intractable ulcer.

Gastric Ulcer. Such ulcers are undoubtedly peptic but have several differentiating features from duodenal ulcers. They tend to occur in older individuals. They may be associated with chronic atrophic gastritis, whereas there is no such atrophic gastritis in cases of duodenal ulcer. There is a different geographic distribution, gastric ulcer being more common on the continent of Europe and duodenal ulcer being more common in Great Britain and America, especially in the latter. Persons who eat rough foods are probably more susceptible to gastric ulcer, whereas persons living under conditions of emotional tension may be more liable to develop duodenal ulcers. The 12-hour night secretion of free hydrochloric acid is normal (average 18.6 mEq.) or on the average less (12 mEq.), as opposed to the elevated value in duodenal ulcer patients (average 63 mEq.) (Dragstedt, Oberhelman, Evans and Rigler, 1954). These authors and Dragstedt (1954) attributed gastric ulcers to an overproduction of gastrin by the antrum, possibly due to stasis.

Another factor pertaining to the etiology of gastric ulcer relates to why the majority of such ulcers occur along the lesser curvature, the *Magenstrasse*. Dragstedt (1955) pointed out that the lesser curvature is relatively fixed, and the mucous membrane is relatively smooth and has less rugae than the remainder of the corpus. Other factors to consider are the different anatomic arrangement of the end-arteries and the drinking of liquids which may wash the mucus off the lesser curvature, since they pass directly along it.

Additional differences are based on responses to treatment. After a minimal gastric resection, e.g., 40 to 50 per cent, including the entire antrum, however, for gastric ulcer, stomal ulcer seldom develops. Duodenal ulcer, on the other hand, responds well to vagotomy plus a drainage procedure and frequently (about 12% or more) is followed by a stomal ulcer when a 40 to 50 per cent gastrectomy is performed.

Duodenal Ulcer. Such an ulcer seems to be due to an increased cephalic phase of gastric secretion, possibly due to the tensions and strain of modern life. It responds well to either vagotomy-drainage procedure or to subtotal gastrectomy.

Acute Ulcer (Curling's Ulcer, Stress Ulcer, Posterior Hypothalamus-Stimulated Ulcer). In 1842, Curling described acute ulcers of the stomach or the duodenum following burns. More recently such ulcers have been noted following various types of trauma. Fletcher and Harkins (1954) reported 42 such cases at the King County Hospital, Seattle, during the 7-year period 1946-1953. The 42 cases occurred in 4,102 autopsies, an incidence of almost exactly 1 per cent. Of the ulcers 20 were gastric, 14 duodenal, 6 both gastric and duodenal, 1 gastrojejunal and 1 esophageal. The ulcer was not the cause of death in all of these cases, but in at least 15 cases there was perforation, massive hemorrhage, or both. Only 1 of the 42 cases occurred following a burn. These authors concluded: "The nature of the primary conditions usually includes an element of stress, so that a possible mechanism of production of the ulcers involves, as a final pathway, the action of an adrenal cortical hormone on the stomach, increasing gastric secretion." Bogardus and Gustafson (1956) reported a somewhat similar series wherein 28 cases (4.9%) of 566 consecutive autopsies revealed a coincident duodenal ulcer. Not all of these ulcers were acute, but a number of them were.

Other workers have approached this problem from the aspect of mechanism. Gray, Benson, Reifenstein, and Spiro (1951) postulated that in stress the cells of the anterior hypothalamus secrete a humoral substance which stimulates the pituitary gland to release corticotropin which in turn acts on the adrenals to liberate cortisone. A somewhat similar mechanism is described by Porter, Movius, and French (1953). Zubiran, Kark, Montalbetti, Morel and Dragstedt (1952) showed that cortisone stimulation of gastric secretion occurs even when both the antrum is removed and the vagi are sectioned, thus indicating a direct action on the parietal cells. Dragstedt (1953) utilized this evidence along with the recognized relief of duodenal ulcer by vagotomy to indicate that chronic duodenal ulcer, unlike the stress or acute ulcer under consideration here, cannot be due to this mechanism. Risholm (1956) postulated that

"acute portal hypertension" may be a factor in these acute stress ulcers.

Acute Ulcer (Cushing's Ulcer, Anterior Hypothalamus-Stimulated Ulcer). Such ulcers may be due to acute or chronic involvement of the central nervous system, especially the anterior hypothalamus, and were first described by Rokitansky in 1846 and by Cushing in 1932. Such ulcers also may be related to gastromalacia (see p. 706). They are especially apt to occur in acute bulbar poliomyelitis; Schaberg, Hildes and Alcock (1954) reported that in 480 cases of acute bulbar poliomyelitis, there were 34 instances (7%) of upper gastro-intestinal tract hemorrhage, of which 23 cases (5%) resulted in death. In addition, 2 patients died of perforation of the duodenum. Cabieses and Lecca (1955) reported 10 cases of acute gastro-intestinal hemorrhage following neurosurgical operations. Rupture of the esophagus was observed in 19 of 1,590 autopsies during a 4-year period by Maciver, Smith, Tomlinson and Whitby (1956). Seventeen of the 19 (89%) were associated with lesions of the central nervous system. While these authors favored a mechanical tear as the most common explanation, erosion could not always be ruled out.

As discussed previously in the section on gastric physiology, Porter, Movius and French (1953) reported experiments on monkeys demonstrating that injuries or stimulation to the anterior hypothalamus act upon the stomach by way of the vagus nerves, their effects are blocked by vagotomy, and the peak of response is prompt. In the 5 cases of such ulcers reported by King and Reganis (1953) the onset was also prompt.

The relationship between these 2 types of acute ulcer is portrayed graphically by Shay (1954) according to his concept as shown in Figure 29-6.

Intractable Ulcer (Ulcer Diathesis, Strøm-Zollinger-Ellison Ulcer). For a long time it has been observed by those doing a considerable amount of gastric surgery that an occasional patient—possibly 1 in 100 or 200—will have repeated recurrences despite supposedly adequate medical and surgical therapy. A typical history might run as follows: perforated duodenal ulcer, simple closure; intractable duodenal ulcer, gastrojejunostomy; marginal ulcer, subtotal gastrectomy; second marginal ulcer, vagotomy plus reresection; third marginal ulcer, thoracic revagotomy; finally total gastrectomy. These cases, although rare, present a serious situation.

In 1952, Strøm reported a case of peptic ulcer with "insuloma." In his patient no preoperative studies were made before the removal of the 8-Gm. tumor. Before the removal of the tumor the 32-year-old male patient had presented the following history: onset of ulcer symptoms in 1947, gastric resection for duodenal ulcer in 1948, recurrence of pain in February, 1950, with roentgen evidence of stomal ulceration, transthoracic vagotomy in July, 1950, recurrence of pain in 1950, reexploration on April 6, 1951, with finding of nonhealing of the stomal ulcer and of the tumor on the tail of the pancreas. A reresection and tumor removal were performed with complete relief of symptoms. The tumor contained "atypical beta-cells." Strøm made a thorough review of the literature and postu-

lated the possible relationship of the tumor to a possible increase in gastric secretion.

Recent observations of Zollinger and Ellison (1955), Ellison (1955), Ellison (1956), and Oberhelman, Nelsen, Johnson and Dragstedt (1961), reporting their own cases and collecting other cases and suggestive reports from the literature, may have furnished the solution to this problem. In their first paper these authors reported 2 personal cases plus 7 collected cases and in the second and third papers increased these figures to 7 and 24, respectively, in which islet cell tumors were related to peptic ulcer, especially the intractable type. Because of the nonspecific nature of these tumors, they believed that in these cases the hyperglycemic-glycogenolytic factors of the pancreas (glucagon) may have been the factor stimulating the gastric secretion to abnormal levels (Fig. 29-13). In a personal communication, Ellison (1956) stated that he now has collected 43 cases of this syndrome.

Zollinger and Ellison concluded: "A clinical entity consisting of hypersecretion,

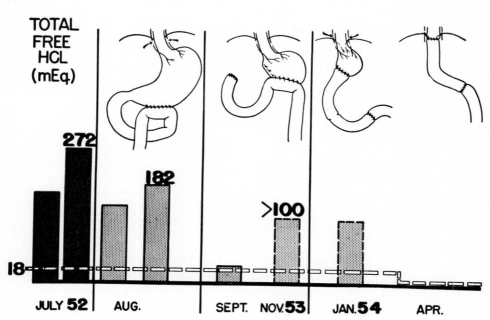

Fig. 29-13. Total mEq. of free HCl found in repeated 12-hour nocturnal gastric aspirations of patients with intractable ulcer (36-year-old married white female), showing the effects of a succession of operative procedures utilized to reduce the hyperacidity. The normal value is indicated by the broken horizontal line. (Zollinger, R., and Ellison, E.: Ann. Surg. *142*:712)

hyperacidity, and atypical peptic ulceration associated with non-insulin-producing islet cell tumors of the pancreas is suggested." The therapeutic implications are twofold and clear: (1) examine the pancreas more often in cases of peptic ulcer; and (2) in cases of intractable ulcer or ulcer in atypical locations (e.g., third portion of duodenum or jejunum) make a meticulous search of the pancreas. Some of the basic studies upon which these observations are based are discussed in the section on gastric physiology (see p. 667, Pancreatic Phase of Gastric Secretion).

It is of interest in this connection that 4 cases of ulcer, 2 coincident with parathyroid tumor and 2 with hyperplasia, have been reported (Rogers, Keating, Morlock and Barker, 1947; Robinson, Black, Sprague and Tillisch, 1951; Albright and Kerr, 1952). Since Ellison (1955) reported that some of the cases with islet cell tumor he studied also had "nodules in the parathyroids and hypophysis, it is possible that the parathyroid nodules reported by Rogers, *et al.*, Robinson, *et al.*, and by Albright and Kerr were only incidental. None of these reports mentioned exploring the pancreas.

SPECIAL TYPES OF PEPTIC ULCER
ACCORDING TO LOCATION

No matter where it occurs, peptic ulcer is due to the acid-peptic autodigestion of the lining of some portion of the alimentary tract. There are 7 special types of peptic ulcer according to the various locations in the alimentary tract in which they may occur, as follows:

1. **Ulcer from Ectopic Islands of Gastric Mucosa in the Upper Esophagus.** This type of ulcer is essentially theoretical and, to the author's knowledge, has not been reported in the literature. However, it is mentioned for completeness and to emphasize the contrast with Type 2, discussed below.

In the esophagus ectopic gastric mucosa occurs most frequently in the postcricoid region of the upper esophagus. Islands of such mucosa range in size from microscopic dimensions to 1 or 2 cm. in diameter were found in 70 per cent of autopsied cases (Schridde, 1904). These islands probably do not cause ulcer for the following reasons: (1) they are small; (2) in reports with a

histologic notation, they have been recorded as not containing oxyntic cells; and (3) they are located so close to the mouth that the saliva continually washes their secretion away. Barrett summarized this by stating: "I cannot believe that the tiny volume of acid, diluted by pints of salvia, would be likely to harm the lower reaches of the gullet."

2. **Ulcer From Heterotopic Sheets of Gastric Mucosa in the Lower Esophagus (Peptic Ulcer of Gastric Mucosa-Lined Esophagus, Barrett's Ulcer).** Unlike the theoretically possible, but never yet described, ulcers postulated in the first type, these ulcers, while rare, represent a distinct and important entity, especially in older people. They occur in heterotopic gastric mucosa in the lower esophagus which is continuous with the gastric mucosa of the stomach. Jackson (1929) reported gastric mucosa in 7 of his 21 personal cases of peptic ulcer of the lower esophagus. Such mucosa is smoother, has fewer rugal folds and, unlike the stomach proper, has no parietal cells. The gastric mucous membrane in the esophagus may have islands of esophageal mucosa in it and its upper border, or junction with the squamous mucosa-lined esophagus above, is irregular rather than a straight line.

Barrett (1950, 1954) believed that such a portion of the esophagus is part of the stomach, while Allison and Johnstone (1953) preferred to call this condition "esophagus lined with gastric mucous membrane" because the outer walls are typical of the esophagus. Whether the presence of the gastric mucosal sheet is always congenital and a part of the syndrome of congenitally short esophagus (see Chap. 28, "Esophagus") or whether it may result from an eccentric healing of a marginal squamous membrane ulcer (the gastric side healing more readily so that the gastric mucous membrane gradually "climbs" into the esophagus) is not yet settled. Also, it is not settled whether the Barrett's ulcers within this gastric mucosa-lined segment or possible peptic esophagitis in the squamous mucous membrane above it, if present, are caused by secretion of acid from the segment in question or due to reflux from the stomach proper below. The absence of oxyntic cells in the gastric mucosa-lined segment would tend toward the latter view, as would also the fact that most of the patients with gastric mucosa-lined esophagus do not get into trouble until later life, when a sliding hiatal hernia and consequent reflux occur. In all of Allison and Johnstone's cases of Barrett's ulcer a sliding hernia was present. Thus we have a paradox wherein a condition which presumably is congenital affects patients almost entirely in later life.

Barrett's ulcer behaves like an ulcer of the abdominal stomach. It may bleed profusely, it may perforate, and it usually does not cause stenosis, and then only if it is circumferential. If it is localized to one segment of the circumference, it may heal on medical treatment unlike peptic esophagitis (see below) which seldom regresses once a rigid tube is present. Perforation of Barrett's ulcers may occur into the mediastinum or the pleural cavity. When stenosis is present with Barrett's ulcer, it is usually a marginal stenosis in the squamous mucous membrane-lined esophagus immediately above.

Treatment of Barrett's ulcer is complicated and includes that of the almost always associated sliding hiatal hernia below, and of the squamous mucous membrane-lined esophagus above. The most radical treatments include: (1) complete excision of the affected segments with jejunal interposition between normal esophagus above and stomach below (see Chap. 28, "Esophagus") and (2) complete excision with esophagojejunal anastomosis by-passing the stomach. Less radical procedures include: (3) complete excision with esophagogastric anastomosis (this may lead to secondary marginal reflux esophagitis) and (4) local excision of a strictured or ulcerated segment, preserving the cardia and anastomosing the normal squamous mucous membrane-lined esophagus above to the stump of gastric mucous membrane-lined esophagus below. Morris (1955) performed this last procedure in 2 cases with success. It should be accompanied by repair of the hiatal hernia if possible to prevent recurrence. The success of this operation may depend on the possibly greater resistance of the gastric mucosa-lined esophageal segment than of the squamous mucosa-lined esophagus to peptic digestion (see p. 671, immunity of different segments of the gastrointestinal tract).

All of these procedures should be coupled with a drainage procedure to the stomach, preferably of the Finney pyloroplasty type. Treatment of patients with perforation or massive hemorrhage is urgent and in some instances of the former may involve drainage of the mediastinum or the pleura only as a temporary procedure pending more definitive treatment when the patient is in better condition.

3. **Reflux (Peptic) Esophagitis (Esophagitis and Peptic Ulceration of Squamous Mucous-Membrane-Lined Esophagus).** This condition was first described by Winkelstein (1935) and frequently has been elaborated upon since (see Chap. 28, "Esophagus"). It is the most common nonspecific inflammatory condition of the esophagus. There are several varieties (see below) of the condition, but they have certain features in common. This condition is secondary to regurgitation of gastric contents, and competence of the cardia is lost. Ulcerations are not as characteristic of the syndrome as is the esophagitis. Ulcerations tend to be superficial and serpiginous (Jones, 1955). There is a nonpenetrating ulceration with thin yellow surface slough, slow blood loss from the surface, and progressive fibrosis and stenosis. The submucous fibrosis which is present leads to stenosis and stricture formation which is much more severe than with Barrett's ulcer. Perforation, on the other hand, almost never occurs, and bleeding, while frequent, is usually not massive. However, De Vito, Listerud, Nyhus, Merendino, and Harkins (1959) have reported 3 cases with massive hemorrhage. The response to medical treatment is poor, but bouginage is useful so long as the main cause of obstruction is spasm and a rigid tube does not exist. In the latter instance, surgical treatment is required.

Esophagitis occurs in three quarters of the cases of sliding hiatal hernia but may exist in the absence of such hernias. Reflux is usually present but is not always demonstrable. The small superficial ulcerations which may be present are seldom seen on roentgen examination.

Carver and Sealy (1954) pointed out that in their series of 130 cases of peptic esophagitis, the following 3 factors were causative: (1) hiatus hernia, 76 per cent; (2) surgical excision or destruction of the cardiac sphincter, 13 per cent; and (3) persistent vomiting,

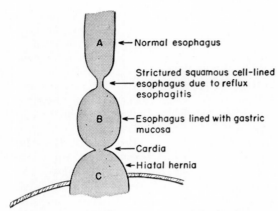

FIG. 29-14. Diagram of triple barium shadow above diaphragm indicative of heterotopic sheet of gastric mucosa at lower end of esophagus. (A) Normal esophagus. (B) Gastric-mucosa-lined esophagus. (C) Hiatal hernia.

11 per cent. The important symptoms in descending order of frequency included dysphagia, substernal pain, regurgitation, weakness and anemia, and hemorrhage and hematemesis. Related to these factors in causation, reflux esophagitis may be divided into the following 4 types:

TYPE 1. Cases which follow intubation or persistent vomiting or are associated with duodenal ulcer. Such cases are apt to be severe and acute. Hiatal hernia is often absent.

TYPE 2. The usual milder variety associated with sliding hiatal hernia. In such instances, at least in the early stages, roentgen signs of esophagitis are lacking. When stenosis does occur it is present immediately above the cardia.

TYPE 3. Marginal ulceration occurring in the squamous mucous-membrane-lined esophagus immediately above a segment lined with gastric mucosa. Bosher and Taylor (1951) reported such a case (without a hiatal hernia), but Allison and Johnstone (1953) and Morris (1955) have elaborated their reports into an elucidation of a definite and interesting syndrome in which the reflux esophagitis and associated stenosis, unlike that in Type 2, are usually high in the chest and are associated with hiatal hernia. Wolf, Marshak, Som and Winkelstein (1955) discussed a special type of this syndrome in which the segment of gastric mucosa-lined esophagus is short, discrete ulceration is more apt to occur in the area of esophagitis above it (possibly because it is nearer the source of reflux), the associated hiatal hernia is more triangular in shape than usual, the condition may occur in childhood, and the prognosis is especially poor.

Allison and Johnstone (1953) collected all the cases of esophageal stenosis seen in their clinic and found that 115 patients had stenosis from squamous ulcer of the esophagus and 10 from gastric (Barrett's) ulcer of the esophagus. Of the 115 patients with squamous ulcer and stenosis there was definite evidence in 11 of a segment of esophagus lined with gastric mucosa between the stenosis and the hernia. Thus, in these 125 cases, 21 had gastric mucosa in the esophagus, 10 had Barrett's ulcer of that mucosa (roughly half), and the relative chances of a peptic stenosis being squamous or gastric were about 10 to 1.

When the combined condition of esophagus lined with gastric mucosa and (squamous) peptic esophagitis at its upper end exists, a very interesting picture is present (Fig. 29-14). The stricture marks the lower limit of squamous epithelium. The esophagus below this, lined by gastric mucosa is normal or a little dilated. The position of the cardia can be identified as the place where the lumen widens out again to form the sac of the herniated stomach. As Allison and Johnstone pointed out, this gives a triple segmentation of barium in the chest, from above downward: (1) normal esophagus, (2) esophagus lined by gastric mucosa and (3) sliding hiatal hernia. The first is separated from the second by the stricture, and the second from the third by the cardia. As these authors stated, "When this picture occurs it can be concluded that the intermediate tubular stricture is esophagus lined by gastric mucous membrane." To complicate the situation further, sometimes typical Barrett ulcers are present in this intermediate tubular stricture below.

TYPE 4. Marginal ulceration following operations in which the cardiac sphincter has been sacrificed. This is a common clinical occurrence and has been studied experimentally by Hoag, Kiriluk and Merendino (1954). Esophagogastrectomy, in dogs, with or without vagotomy, led to a high percentage of fatal esophageal ulceration, as did the Grön-dahl esophagocardioplasty and the long Heller extramucous esophagocardiomyotomy procedures.

Treatment of reflux esophagitis varies according to the type and the stage of the disease but involves bouginage and/or repair of the associated hiatal hernia when the main obstruction is spastic, and surgical excision when it is present because of a rigid tubelike obstruction. Surgical repair, as discussed previously under the consideration of Barrett's ulcer, should include that of an associated hiatal hernia in some cases and, since in cases with resection preservation of the cardiac sphincter usually is not possible, esophago-gastrostomy with jejunal interposition is the ideal procedure in advanced cases.*

4. **Gastric Ulcer.** As stated previously, gastric ulcer may be of different origin than duodenal ulcer. The acute gastric ulcer or erosion may heal on medical management, but the typical chronic gastric ulcer is very apt to recur. Wangensteen (1953) reported that 11 of 12 gastric ulcers thought to have healed on roentgen examination were found to be still present at subsequent operation. Swynnerton and Tanner (1953) concluded that the healing of gastric ulcer by medical treatment was followed by recurrence in 75 per cent of the patients, while in the surgically treated patients, 80 per cent had very successful results, 10 per cent satisfactory results, and only 10 per cent poor results. Tanner (1951), in discussing the special indications of gastric resection for gastric ulcer, stated: "Gastric ulcer is a disease of wear and tear and will not be cured medically until wrinkles will be." The repeated and chronic healing of a chronic gastric ulcer can cause considerable shortening of the lesser curvature (Tanner, 1951). Dolphin, Smith and Waugh (1953)

* The student may wonder why so much space is given to the elucidation of this complicated subject of peptic ulcer of the esophagus and reflux esophagitis which may involve such major surgical procedures. This is done for the following reasons: (1) These conditions are far more common than is generally realized. (2) Their recognition by medical men, as well as by surgeons, is important. (3) Prompt simple treatment may eliminate the necessity for more radical therapy later. (4) This subject has advanced so rapidly within the past 5 years, in large part because of contributions of Allison, Barrett, etc., that no up-to-date textbook account has been available.

reported that multiple ulcers are present in 21.9 per cent of stomachs removed with benign gastric ulcer and in only 5.6 per cent of the specimens removed with malignant gastric ulcer, a ratio of 4:1.

The symptoms of gastric ulcer are quite similar to those of duodenal ulcer. There is a little less tendency to periodicity, the pain is sometimes a little more on the left side, and the patients are usually about 8 years older at the time of onset. Sometimes an older patient with gastric ulcer will present a history of a duodenal ulcer in his youth, now healed. This substitution of one ulcer for another is based on the lowered acidity yet increased susceptibility of the gastric mucous membrane due to a degenerative gastritis (Tanner, 1951). Johnson (1956) observed coincident gastric and duodenal ulcer in 10 per cent of his patients with peptic ulcer. In 130 cases of combined ulcer, the following facts were observed: (1) in 93 per cent the duodenal ulcer appeared first, and (2) in 64 per cent there was associated pyloric stenosis and retention, possibly indicating an antral hyperstimulation as postulated by Dragstedt (1954).

Other differences are that gastric ulcer seldom leads to stomal ulcer following gastric resection (not once in 700 gastric resections for gastric ulcer—Tanner, 1952), and that the differentiation between gastric ulcer and gastric carcinoma is difficult. This last point deserves special emphasis on two scores.

The question as to whether gastric ulcer becomes carcinomatous, or gastric carcinomas ulcerate is still not settled. Notkin (1955) reported 2 resected cases in which the pathologic findings strongly suggested the possibility of subsequent malignant degeneration in a previously benign ulcer. However, the author ascribes to the views of Palmer (1950) and others who stated that for all practical purposes gastric ulcers do not turn into carcinoma, but that carcinomas regularly ulcerate.

The differentiation between gastric ulcer and gastric carcinoma brings in an application of Hippocrates' dictum, because, in such instances, truly "experience is fallacious and judgment difficult." In general, about 10 per cent or more of gastric lesions thought to be ulcer turn out to have carcinoma at operation (Table 2).

TABLE 2. PER CENT OF PREOPERATIVELY DIAGNOSED GASTRIC ULCERS WHICH TURN OUT TO BE MALIGNANT AT OPERATION

AUTHOR	TOTAL CASES	PER CENT MALIGNANT
Allen and Welch (1941)	277	14.0
Allen and Welch (1953)	295	10.8
Walters (1942)	. . .	10.0
Ransom (1947)	246	10.1
Marshall (1953)	411	15.8

Jones and Doll (1953) reported that 11 per cent of their patients with simple closure of a perforated gastric ulcer were dead of carcinoma of the stomach after an average follow-up period of 6.3 years.

Differentiation on the basis of roentgen examination, gastroscopy and determination of acidity are all helpful but seldom definitive in borderline cases. Cytologic studies are promising and are useful when performed by one experienced in this technic.

Cytologic studies of the stomach involve specimens that are obtained by mechanical means (brush technic, etc.) or by aspiration after the instillation of mucolytic agents. This latter technic is less traumatic, and good results have been reported by Traut, Rosenthal, Harrison, Farber and Grimes (1953) and Rubin and Benditt (1955). These latter authors found that papain lavage is simple and rapid but does not regularly yield well-preserved cells. Chymotrypsin (a freshly prepared solution of 7 μg. of crystallized d-chymotrypsin in 500 ml. of 0.1 M acetate buffer) is instilled into the stomach with a Levin tube and removed in 10 minutes. The stained sediment shows well-preserved cells, and the test was positive in 19 of 20 patients who proved to have cancer.

While the decision is difficult as to whether or not a gastric ulcer is malignant, the results of surgical treatment in such cases are encouraging. Both Ransom (1947) and Lampert, Waugh and Dockerty (1950) reported that resection in such instances resulted in a 41 per cent 5-year survival rate which is almost twice that of preoperatively diagnosed carcinoma of the stomach. Olsson and Endresen (1956) also compared the results in a series of 25 "ulcer cancers," i.e., those thought to be ulcer before pathologic examination with 176 ordinary gastric cancers, both series including only cases with no metastases. The 3-year survival figures were 64 per cent and 42 per cent, respectively.

Amberg and Rigler (1956) approached this subject in a different way by comparing a series of 39 cases of gastric cancer, selected because the roentgen diagnosis was made after an earlier negative one, thus indicating relatively early or small lesions, with a control group of 866 cases. In the special series the incidence of cases without positive nodes was 46 per cent as compared with the 15 per cent in the control group.

The decision as to whether to operate for gastric ulcer is based on the known high recurrence rate after medical therapy and the danger of unrecognized carcinoma. Some advise gastric resection for all gastric ulcers. As will be shown below, this has some logical basis. In the large clinics, from 37 to 95 per cent of gastric ulcers are treated by resection. The present author believes the higher figure is more nearly correct but that under certain circumstances routine resection is not advisable. Acute ulcers, if *prompt* improvement, occurs within 3 weeks, corroborated by roentgen studies may be followed medically. The aid of a competent internist and an expert cytologist is also of help. (See section on "Carcinoma of the Stomach," p. 687.)

An analysis of the problem of whether or not to do routine gastric resection for gastric ulcer is taken from Moore and Harkins (1954) and is as follows:

If we consider 2 hypothetical series, each composed of 100 clinically benign gastric ulcers, and if we treat 1 series using subtotal gastric resection and the other using only medical measures, the outcome can be predicted with reasonable assurance based on available statistics. In each series it will be assumed that 10 patients will have carcinomatous ulcers. Other assumptions will be considered when the outcome of each separate series is discussed.

In the surgical series, all of the 100 patients will be benefited except the following; 6 of the 10 patients with carcinoma will die despite operation, 2 of the total series will be expected to die from operation, and 9 patients will develop disabling postgastrectomy symptoms. (Whereas some other patients will develop nondisabling postgastrectomy symptoms, we are assuming that these will be balanced out by the group of 6 carcinomatous ulcer patients which, even though counted as mortalities, will receive definite palliation.) Thus, a total of 17 of the 100 patients treated surgically will not be benefited (including 8 deaths) and 83 will be.

In the medical series, all of the 10 carcinoma patients will die; 20 of the remainder will have difficulty with medical management in the form of intractability, hemorrhage, perforation, or obstruction, and approximately 2 of these 20 will die of such complications. Thus, a total of 30 of the 100 patients treated medically will not be benefited (including 12 deaths), and 70 will be. Such is the case for subtotal resection for gastric ulcer.

This type of reasoning (see page 183) would tend to support the use of routine gastric resection for gastric ulcer; however, individualization of each patient has certain advantages which cannot be denied.

The technical aspects of the surgical treatment of gastric ulcer involve the following: (1) Resection should include the ulcer but need not be more radical than is necessary for this technical requirement. However, it should always include the antrum. (2) Because of the normal duodenal stump, after resection gastroduodenal anastomosis is preferable. (3) In cases where carcinoma is suspected, gastrotomy and observation and biopsy of the ulcer from within the stomach may be of help in deciding on the extent of resection. Care must be taken not to scatter the cells from the biopsy wound. (4) In similar cases, the omentum should be removed with the stomach, and an attempt to include the lymph-node-bearing mesentery should be made.

Gastric ulcer high on the lesser curvature ("juxta-esophageal gastric ulcer") presents 2 special problems. (1) There is the relatively high chance of malignancy in such ulcers. Figure 29-15 shows data from Plenk and Lin (1954) which indicate that a preponderance of such ulcers, including those in the fundus, is malignant. Marshall (1953) also reported that in his series of 411 gastric ulcers, despite the fact that only 15.8 per cent were malignant, this was *one* part of the stomach where the malignant tumors outnumbered the benign 6:4. Since these figures include the fundus, they may not apply strictly to the high lesser curvature, but the danger of malignant lesions in this region is to be borne in mind. The

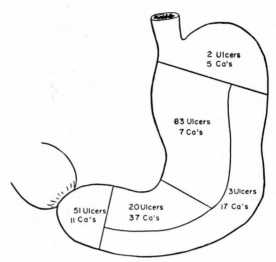

FIG. 29-15. Distribution of benign and malignant gastric lesions in Utah series. (Plenk, H., and Lin, R.: Am. Surgeon 20:351)

second point concerning these ulcers is that they are technically difficult to remove. For this reason some (Editorial, J.A.M.A., 1954) advise a longer than usual trial with medical management. However, before such a policy is adopted, the other factor, namely, the increased hazard of malignancy, must also be considered.

Treatment of gastric ulcer high on the lesser curvature involves the following: Subtotal distal gastric resection, including the ulcer, should be the intended procedure. If certain technical steps listed below are utilized, this can be attained more often. Total gastrectomy is not desirable, while the Kelling-Madlener operation (distal resection leaving the ulcer in place) is a compromise. The left gastric artery should be doubly ligated and divided as well as the associated vagus nerve (the latter for purposes of mobilization, not to affect the cephalic phase). If at any time during the operation it becomes obvious that a high-lying ulcer is malignant, a carcinoma-type of operation is done which is usually a proximal subtotal resection—seldom a total— and involves removal of the lower end of the esophagus above and a pyloromyotomy below.

Since most high gastric ulcers are slightly on the posterior surface, Tanner (1952) advised rotation of the stomach in such cases, bringing the lesser curvature forward and to the left so that the ulcer is now where the lesser curvature was. After resection, the closure of the lesser curve and the anastomosis are made in this rotated position. In removing a high gastric ulcer it is also best to do the operation by the open method without clamps, cutting the stomach above the ulcer with scissors. During closure of the lesser curve after resection, the surgeon should check the cardia frequently from within to be sure that it is not impinged upon too much.

Other points of importance in the treatment of gastric ulcer are as follows: (1) Massive hemorrhage from gastric ulcer is more dangerous than from duodenal ulcer. Therefore, if the diagnosis is known, an earlier operation is indicated in such instances. (2) Perforation of a gastric ulcer is more dangerous than of a duodenal ulcer. Also, the danger of carcinoma makes a definitive resection operation more strongly indicated. (3) Vagotomy has not been found suitable for the treatment of gastric ulcer. On theoretical grounds, if one accepts the theory that antrum hyperfunction is the cause of gastric ulcer, one would not expect vagotomy to be the treatment of choice.

5. **Duodenal Ulcer.** Since duodenal ulcer, the most common and most important of all peptic ulcers, will receive further elucidation in an entirely separate section below, only a few points of its relationship to the other types of peptic ulcer will be listed here. Duodenal ulcer is believed to be caused by an exaggerated cephalic phase of gastric secretion. Therefore, it can be approached both from the standpoint of eliminating this phase (vagotomy) or of cutting down on the source of acid from the parietal cells (gastric resection). Duodenal ulcer has a very high incidence of recurrence, and operations for duodenal ulcer are the main cause of stomal ulcer. Thus, from this standpoint, any surgical treatment to be successful must be thorough and radical. At the same time the danger of unrecognized malignancy is almost nil in duodenal ulcer, so that from this standpoint surgical therapy need not remove the omentum or lymph-gland-bearing mesentery.

6. **Stomal Ulcer (Marginal Ulcer).** Stomal ulceration is the most serious late complication of gastric surgery. Its one favorable feature is that with an additional major operative procedure it can be remedied, whereas some less severe complications tend more to persist despite therapy. The usual stomal ulcer is in the jejunum following a gastrojejunostomy (incidence 34%, Lewisohn, 1925) or a Billroth II gastric resection (incidence 2 to 6% or more). The ulcer may be at the actual stoma (stomal or gastrojejunal ulcer) or on the adjacent or opposite wall of the jejunum, in which case it is termed a jejunal ulcer. If it has broken into the adjacent colon, the more serious gastrojejunal-colic fistula results.

Whenever a surgeon performs a gastrojejunostomy he identifies the upper jejunum to be used for the anastomosis by its proximity to the ligament of Treitz. He always fears that he will mistake the ileocolic fold for the ligament of Treitz and perform an inadvertent gastro-ileostomy. This serious surgical error is evidenced by loss of weight, passage of recently eaten material in the stools, and general cachexia. Treatment is always surgical and involves takedown of the gastro-ileostomy with performance of a gastrojejunostomy in the proper place, or if the stomach has not been resected, an ulcer is present, and the patient is in reasonably good condition, performance of a gastric resection with correct anastomosis. The far rarer inadvertent gastro-colostomy is an unforgivable technical error and is never performed by a trained surgeon (Landry, 1951).

Stomal or marginal ulceration also occurs in the duodenum, or more often at the stoma itself, following the Billroth I type of gastric resection. The incidence of such ulceration, for the same extent of resection, is probably at least as low as for the Billroth II resection. Ulceration on the gastric side of the anastomosis was found to be much more common after Billroth I than Billroth II resections by Ordahl, Ross and Baker (1955) and by Goligher, Moir and Wrigley (1956). Other observers have not found these ulcers on the gastric side of the anastomosis except in rare instances. The results in our own patients have been summarized by Kanar *et al.* (1956).

Marginal ulcerations following esophagogastrostomy have been considered already. Stomal ulceration is more liable to occur under the following circumstances:

1. Original operation for duodenal rather than for gastric ulcer.

2. Original operation for perforated ulcer.

3. Inadequate resection (less than 70%, or less than 45% if done with vagotomy).

4. Incomplete vagotomy if the intended original procedure was a hemigastrectomy plus vagotomy.

5. Excluded remnant of antrum (for the acid-potentiating capacities of such a stump, originally advocated by Devine, 1925, 1928, see Kelly, Cross and Wangensteen, 1954, Nyhus, 1960, Thompson and Peskin, 1961.

6. Too long (> 15 cm.) jejunal loop.

One interesting point is that it takes a stomal ulcer much longer to show up after gastro-jejunostomy than after gastric resection. Walters, Chance and Berkson (1955) reported the mean interval in 186 cases of the former until subsequent surgical repair was 11.2 years, while in 115 cases of the latter it was 3.7 years. (These intervals were 8.0 and 3.9 years, respectively, Edwards, Herrington, Cate and Lipscomb, 1956.) Thompson (1956) reported that 75 per cent of marginal ulcers following gastrectomy occurred within 5 years as opposed to only 20 per cent of those following gastroenterostomy. Similarly, only 7 per cent of those following gastrectomy occurred after 10 years as opposed to 66 per cent following gastroenterostomy. In Walters, *et al.,* series 91 per cent of patients were men. Gastrojejunocolic fistula was present in 20 of their 301 cases (6.5%) and 16 of these (80%) followed an original gastrojejunostomy.

Complications of stomal ulcer include intractable pain, obstruction, hemorrhage and perforation, as with the original ulcer. However, the treatment is surgical in a much higher percentage of cases than with primary duodenal ulcer. In fact, operative management should be used unless there are definite reasons to the contrary in any case of stomal ulcer which has been diagnosed positively and persists after a few weeks of medical treatment.

If the original operation was a gastrojejunostomy, the preferred surgical treatment is an adequate gastric resection after takedown of the anastomosis. If the original operation was a gastric resection of known adequacy, transthoracic vagotomy, or abdominal vagotomy with reresection should be tried. As shown in Table 3, the results are much poorer if vagotomy is not used in such cases. On the other hand, the data of Walters, Chance and Berkson (1955) also demonstrate that the use of gastric resection or reresection reduces the chance of subsequent hemorrhage after operation for stomal ulcer as opposed to procedures in which vagotomy alone is used, the percentages being 3.4 as contrasted with 10.4 per cent.

If the stomal ulcer follows a previous gastrojejunostomy plus vagotomy, an insulin test to determine the completeness of the vagotomy is indicated. In all of 13 such cases, Everson and Allen found the test to indicate incomplete vagotomy. In such instances, another attempt at vagotomy, or a vagotomy plus resection should be utilized.

Schirmer and Bowers (1955) give an excellent review of secondary surgical indications for stomal ulcer following inadequate surgery. In all cases in which the original resection was of unknown adequacy, abdominal exploration should be made with a check as to length of loop, possible presence of an excluded antral stump, and adequacy of the extent of resection. Depending on the find-

TABLE 3. RESULT IN 301 CASES OF GASTROJEJUNAL ULCER TREATED SURGICALLY*

SECONDARY OPERATION	GASTROJEJUNOSTOMY			GASTRIC RESECTION		
	Total Cases (186)	% Mortality	% Good Results	Total Cases (115)	% Mortality	% Good Results
Vagotomy alone	29	0	77.8	88	1.1	70.5
Vagotomy with resection (or reresection)	3	0		14	14.3	100.0
Vagotomy with other operations	9	0		..	..	..
Resection (or reresection)	145	0.7	86.5	13	15.3	57.1

* From Walters, Chance and Berkson: Surg., Gynec. & Obst. *100*:1-10, 1955.

ings, a decision as to election of abdominal vagotomy, reresection, adjustment of the loop length (preferably less than 4 in. from the ligament of Treitz), or removal of an antral stump should be made. In all such cases the pancreas should be examined for the possible presence of tumor.

7. **Peptic Ulcer of Meckel's Diverticulum.** Heterotopic gastric mucosa occurs in 54 per cent of Meckel's diverticula (Gross, 1953). This congenital anomaly, in turn, is present in 1.4 per cent of autopsies (Harkins, 1933). The gastric mucosa may involve part or the entire diverticulum and may be grossly similar to that in the stomach with rugae. The usual ulcer develops in the diverticular or jejunal epithelium adjacent to the gastric mucosa, and hence is similar to a marginal ulcer. Most cases of peptic ulcer occur before the 6th year, involving boys 3:1. Pain and dyspepsia do not occur, but hemorrhage does occur frequently, and perforation rarely.

In 149 Meckel's diverticula which Gross removed, 50 (33%) were the site of ulcer and hemorrhage. This latter figure did not include 18 other cases with inflammation with or without perforation, in some of which the diverticulum contained gastric mucosa. In a series of 25 consecutive cases of symptom-producing Meckel's diverticulum, Berman, Schneider and Potts (1954) found 14 with bleeding, 2 with perforation, and 2 with both bleeding and perforation. Of the 4 other cases in which satisfactory sections were made, gastric mucosa was present in 2. The hemorrhage may be severe and recurrent. It is followed by melena, but we have never seen hematemesis. While this gastric mucosa is probably not under vagal control, it undoubtedly responds to gastrin, and the secretion is especially dangerous because the acid-buffering capacity of the ileal contents is much less than that of the upper jejunum or duodenum. Diagnosis usually is made only by exploration. Removal of the Meckel's diverticulum whenever found on laparotomy is advised, both therapeutically and prophylactically.

DUODENAL ULCER; INDICATIONS FOR OPERATION

Duodenal ulcer is not only an important factor in morbidity, but also in mortality.

According to the most recent published Vital Statistics of the United States for 1953 (Dunn, 1955), there were 4,511 deaths from ulcer of the duodenum. In the records of 2,837 of these, there was no mention of perforation while in 1,674 there was a mention of perforation. In 1,036 additional deaths, gastro-jejunal ulcer, duodenitis, etc., were cited which might have been related to ulcer of the duodenum.

Duodenal ulcer is the most common form of peptic ulcer. It affects particularly males between the ages of 20 and 50, but individuals of both sexes and all ages are susceptible. Persons with blood-group O are more prone to duodenal ulcer (Aird, Bentall, Mehigan and Roberts, 1954; Wright, Grant and Jennings, 1955).* The symptoms include postprandial pain, usually coming on more than an hour after meals and often temporarily relieved by food, milk, or alkali, and with a definite periodicity and remissions and recurrences. Physical signs are usually absent in uncomplicated cases, but often the patient will point to the epigastrium with one finger to indicate the location of pain. Roentgen examination of the upper gastro-intestinal tract is very important in the diagnosis. Gastroscopic studies may show mild hyperplastic gastritis. Gastric analysis usually reveals an elevated level of free hydrochloric acid. The more nearly accurate 12-hour night secretion study indicates both an elevated acidity and volume of juice, so that the mEq. of free hydrochloric acid excreted in 12 hours (clinical units $\times$ volume in liters = mEq.) is usually higher than the average normal value of 18, being in the range of 60 on the average. Most duodenal ulcers are in the first portion of the duodenum, but postbulbar ulcers are more common than is generally recognized (Clark, 1956).

Uropepsin, or the inactive proenzyme pepsinogen, is normally found in human urine. In a study of 72 patients with a history of definite duodenal ulcer, Nyhus (1957) found a definite tendency to increased excretion of uropepsin in the urine.

Most (about 75% or more) of duodenal ulcer patients should be treated medically.

* Group O is also more common in their siblings without ulcer—Clarke, Brit. M. J. 2:725, 1956.

During the first attack without complications, medical management almost always should be given a trial. Patients who do not respond to medical management or develop complications should be treated surgically. There are thus 4 indications for the surgical management of duodenal ulcer which will be considered separately below:

Obstruction. True organic obstruction at the pylorus or below it is rare, but a combination of stenosis due to scar with edema is common. If the history is of short duration, medical management almost always should be tried. On the other hand if the obstruction is of long standing, operation is indicated. The surgeon has a choice of operations in the following order of preference: (1) hemigastrectomy plus vagotomy with gastroduodenal (or gastrojejunal) anastomosis; (2) vagotomy plus drainage procedure; (3) subtotal (75%) gastrectomy with gastroduodenal (or gastrojejunal) anastomosis; (4) gastrojejunostomy, in aged or seriously ill patients, and (5) some of the newer experimental operations, such as the wedge or longitudinal tubular resections. (See section on Operative Procedures on the Stomach.)

Perforation. The perforation of a peptic ulcer is a surgical emergency. The standard treatment is simple suture closure of the perforation, covered by an attached omental tag to act as a plug. Including this method, there are 3 methods of treatment, each with special indications: (1) simple suture closure of the perforation (Byrd and Carlson, 1956), (2) primary subtotal gastric resection (Moore, Harkins and Merendino, 1954 and Jordan and DeBakey, 1961) and (3) conservative or medical treatment by suction (Seely and Campbell, 1956). In the United States, in 1953, there were 3,440 deaths from perforated peptic ulcer, 1,766 from perforated duodenal ulcer and 1,674, or almost as many, from the much rarer, but more dangerous perforated gastric ulcer.

A study of our own material at the King County Hospital, Seattle, and that of the Central Middlesex Hospital, London, leads us to the following conclusions and method of managing these cases based on these conclusions:

Certain patients will be too sick for operation, either because of associated disease or advanced peritonitis and shock. In these instances, we use the third method mentioned above, paying especial attention to seeing that the gastric suction tube is working at all times. Supportive treatment, including blood transfusions, is also given.

It appears that patients with perforated peptic ulcer requiring surgical intervention can be divided into 3 roughly equal groups on the basis of future possible difficulties, history of their disease, and the pathologic findings at operation:

GROUP 1. Patients who will have no further difficulty with ulcer symptoms following simple closure of a peptic perforation.

GROUP 2. Patients who satisfy the criteria for primary gastric resection. These criteria will be given later. Simple closure in these patients is followed by recurrent symptoms requiring further surgery.

GROUP 3. Patients who may have mild or moderate recurrent ulcer symptoms following simple closure of a perforation but do not satisfy the criteria for resectability at the time of exploration.

It is evident that two thirds of the patients with peptic ulcer perforations should be treated by simple closure of the perforation even though some of the patients in Group 3 may require subsequent surgical treatment. The patients falling into Group 2 should be treated by subtotal gastrectomy, provided that these factors of safety are observed: (1) satisfactory general condition of the patient; (2) adequate operating facilities are available; (3) the operation is performed by a competent surgeon experienced in gastric surgery; (4) proper facilities for satisfactory postoperative care are present; (5) consideration of the patient's physiologic rather than chronologic age; (6) sex of the patient. Female patients should have more of the preceding factors in their favor than males.

The criteria for placing the patients in Group 2 are as follows:

1. History of ulcer symptoms for over 1 year

2. Presence of a previously diagnosed peptic ulceration

3. Failure of adequate medical treatment or unreliability of patient's co-operation in following such treatment (alcoholics)

4. History of a previous perforation

5. Perforation of a large calloused peptic ulcer

6. Presence of multiple peptic ulcers

7. Perforation with concomitant or previous hemorrhage

8. Perforation which is less than 12 hours in duration

9. Perforated gastric ulcer—fear of later gastric carcinoma

10. Perforated gastric carcinoma with ulceration

11. Perforation of an ulcer associated with a fixed pyloric obstruction

Primary partial gastric resection for peptic perforation is technically easier to perform than an elective procedure for a chronic penetrating type of ulceration because the perforation is usually anterior. The morbidity and the mortality for primary subtotal gastrectomy are comparable with the morbidity and the mortality of simple surgical closure of a peptic perforation. In addition, one third of the patients with perforation will be saved the morbidity and the mortality of additional operative procedures if the criteria of selectivity for primary subtotal gastrectomy are observed.

We favor the use of the Billroth I type of resection for 3 reasons: (1) The operation is technically easier to perform; (2) the gastroduodenal anastomosis is more nearly correct physiologically, and (3) the patients have more satisfactory results with the Billroth I type of operation.

Massive Hemorrhage. Massive hemorrhage is defined as hemorrhage with a resultant hematocrit of 25 or less and usually with fainting or shock. It is of interest that the onset of bleeding often impels the patient to go to the bathroom, and often he faints there. Massive hemorrhage is the most frequent cause of death from peptic ulcer, causing 46 per cent of ulcer deaths (Wangensteen, 1954). The patient with massive hemorrhage should be seen by the surgeon from the beginning of the attack.

Bleeding duodenal ulcers, unlike perforated ulcers, are usually posterior, have penetrated into the pancreas and often erode the gastroduodenal artery. The duodenum and the stomach become filled with clots, and the jejunum and remainder of the intestine below have a bluish appearance at operation due to the contained blood.

Two important questions must be answered: (1) Is the bleeding from an ulcer? (2) Is it continuing? With regard to the first question, it is indeed fortunate when a patient enters the hospital during his bleeding attack with a well-verified history backed by roentgen diagnosis of old duodenal ulcer. Not all cases present this advantage. Carcinoma of the stomach, bleeding from esophageal varices, and other causes of upper gastro-intestinal hemorrhage should be ruled out. Bleeding gastric ulcers and esophageal varices tend to have more hematemesis than melena; bleeding duodenal ulcer is the opposite. Palpation of an enlarged spleen may indicate varices, but most cases of varices do not have a palpable spleen. A barium swallow is in order to arrive at a diagnosis, although it is usually not advisable to wash out clots in the stomach. On the basis of probability, upper gastrointestinal hemorrhage is due to duodenal ulcer (80% of all cases).

With regard to the other question, a useful positive sign is continued hematemesis after admission to the hospital. Blood volume studies, if available, should be utilized and are far more helpful than blood counts alone, or pulse and blood pressure changes alone (Stewart, Sanderson and Wiles, 1952). A positive head-up "tilt test" may be of value (Wechsler, Roth and Bockus, 1956). A falling blood volume despite adequate blood replacement indicates continued hemorrhage. Gastroscopic examination just before operation may be helpful (Tanner, 1951).

Additional factors which *tend* to influence the decision in favor of operation include the following: generalized arteriosclerosis, age over 50 years or especially over 60 years, history of previous massive hemorrhage, history of long-standing ulcer or many previous mild hemorrhages, and a history of previous perforation. If the bleeding is from a gastric ulcer or from a "stress" ulcer, it is less apt to stop without operation.

Medical management should be tried in almost all cases of bleeding peptic ulcer. The essential feature of medical management is also the best preoperative preparation, namely, adequate blood replacement. If bleeding continues, operation should be performed *before* the patient's condition deteriorates further.

Allen and Oberhelman (1955) have classified surgical intervention into 4 categories:

GROUP 1. INTERVAL SURGERY carried out after the patient has fully recovered from his hemorrhagic episode.

GROUP 2. EMERGENCY SURGERY when blood transfusion fails to keep up with blood loss and shock is neither circumvented nor corrected.

GROUP 3. URGENT SURGERY where shock is corrected but bleeding slowly continues. These patients cannot be weaned from their bottle of blood.

GROUP 4. ELECTIVE INTERVENTION because of the likelihood of a recurrent bout of bleeding during the same episode.

Surgical therapy requires that the patient come to the operating room in as good condition as possible, particularly so far as blood replenishment is concerned. As Allen and Oberhelman (1955) emphasized, the error in these cases is almost always in giving too little blood. Because of the clots in the stomach, gastric suction may be deficient, and if general anesthesia is used a cuff around the tracheal catheter is advisable to prevent aspiration of gastric contents.

The operation of choice is subtotal gastrectomy. The duodenum should be divided below the ulcer if possible, and if an artery is seen with pulsatile bleeding in the ulcer bed in the head of the pancreas, it should be oversown. Palliative operations, such as gastrojejunostomy, ligation of the major arteries supplying the stomach, or even subtotal gastrectomy leaving the ulcer in place and without suturing the bleeding point, are not advised.

The stomach stump should be anastomosed by the open method so that all clots can be removed and a careful search made for additional ulcers.

If no ulcer is found, and if the portal vein pressure is normal, and if the bleeding is obviously from the upper gastrointestinal tract, and if a thorough abdominal exploration has been done, a so-called "blind" gastric resection is indicated.

Intractability Despite or Incompatibility With Medical Treatment. Either of these situations is an indication for operative treatment. Incompatibility with medical treatment involves those patients whose lack of intelligence, lack of stick-to-itiveness, alcoholism,

or job requirements make adequate medical therapy impossible. After a thorough trial, sometimes including psychiatric assistance, the operations of choice are the same as those listed above under "Obstruction."

The mortality of operations for duodenal ulcer varies with the indications, being higher with massive hemorrhage or with perforation treated after 8 hours. Generally speaking, it is 1 to 3 per cent for gastric resection and 0.5 per cent for vagotomy plus drainage procedure. Acute complications are those of the operation in question and include blowout of the duodenal stump (in resection with gastrojejunostomy), wound infection, pneumonia, etc. Chronic complications are listed in the previous section. About 65 per cent have an excellent result, 27 per cent a satisfactory result (mild dumping but no pain, etc.), and 8 per cent have a poor result (operative mortality, stomal ulcer, severe dumping, etc.).

CARCINOMA OF THE STOMACH

Carcinoma of the stomach is a leading cause of death in this country today. The death rate from this cause will tend to increase as the average age of the population is elevated, unless either new methods of treatment are found or those currently known are given a wider application. Approximately 24,000 patients die of cancer of the stomach in the United States each year; in other words, of those persons now alive in this country, 1,700,000 will die from this disease.

ETIOLOGY

The cause of cancer of the stomach is essentially unknown. Recent studies indicate that the idea of Konjetzny (1913) that chronic gastritis is a precursor of cancer (which idea was discredited by Guiss and Stewart, 1943) may be important. Morson (1955) studied the occurrence, distribution and relation of "intestinal metaplasia" of gastric mucosa, a form of chronic atrophic gastritis, to gastric carcinoma. Intestinal metaplasia is a condition in which the stomach glands take on the appearance of colonic glands with goblet cells (which stain red with mucicarmine), and Paneth cells (which are low columnar cells with basal nuclei and cytoplasm packed with coarse granules that stain brightly with eosin).

TABLE 4. INCIDENCE OF INTESTINAL METAPLASIA
IN DIFFERENT SITES IN THE STOMACH
IN SURGICAL SPECIMENS*

SITE	D.U.(%)	G.U.(%)	CARCINOMA (%)
Antrum	59.6	71.4	87.1
Lesser curve	15.4	57.1	79.5
Greater curve	9.6	39.3	66.7

* From Morson, B. C.: Brit. J. Cancer *11*:369, September, 1955.

Such intestinalization was present in at least a portion of the stomach in patients operated upon for duodenal or gastric ulcer or carcinoma in 78.2 per cent of stomachs. Its presence was most common in carcinoma, least common in duodenal ulcer, while gastric ulcer took an intermediate position. In all cases it was most common near the pylorus (antrum), but in gastric ulcer and carcinoma this preponderance of location was not so marked (Table 4).

Morson also related the "signet ring" cells in colloid carcinomas to the goblet cells seen in intestinal metaplasia. He also pointed out that most gastric carcinomas originate in areas where intestinal metaplasia also is most common. In pernicious anemia, on the other hand, as shown by Schell, Dockerty and Comfort (1954), carcinoma is especially apt to occur in the cardiac and fundic portions of the stomach, and in pernicious anemia this is the site of predilection for intestinalization of the mucosa. Morson concluded his discussion by showing examples of gastric carcinoma which appeared to arise from epithelium of the intestinal type and by stating, "Evidence has been considered which suggests that about 30 per cent of gastric carcinomas arise from areas of intestinal metaplasia in the gastric mucosa."

PATHOLOGY

The pathology of carcinoma of the stomach includes a variety of primary tumor forms which can be divided roughly, in ascending order of malignancy, into polypoid, ulcerating and infiltrating varieties, of about equal frequency. Microscopically, they can be divided, also in ascending order of malignancy, into adenocarcinoma, colloid carcinoma, carcinoma simplex and undifferentiated carcinoma.

Local Spread and Invasion of Contiguous Organs. Such spread is apt to be far more extensive than can be detected with the naked eye or the palpating finger at the operating table. In the stomach wall it is most extensive and at the same time least conspicuous in the submucosal and subserosal layers, but it also occurs in the intramuscular layer. As shown by Zinninger (1954), spread into the duodenum is chiefly by the muscular and subserosal layers, while spread to the esophagus is chiefly by the submucosal route. In 101 cases, spread to the duodenum occurred in 43 per cent (Coller, Kay and McIntyre, 1941, reported a figure of 26.4% for duodenal spread). In only 3 of 43 cases (7%) was such spread for more than 3 cm. In 9 of the 101 cases (9%) there was extension to the esophagus; in only 1 case was the spread for more than 3 cm. In no instance did a carcinoma of the cardia extend into the duodenum or a carcinoma of the prepyloric or the antral regions extend into the esophagus. Fundic lesions, however, spread both to the duodenum (28%) and to the esophagus (8%). Therefore, the rule of removing at least 3 cm. of duodenum in low-lying carcinomas and 3 cm. of esophagus in high-lying carcinomas would seem to be in order.

In many instances not sufficient stomach is removed. Berne and Freedman (1951) reported an incidence of "recurrence" in the gastric stump in 78.6 per cent and in 10.7 per cent in the duodenal stump in autopsies. Coller, Kay and McIntyre (1941) reported that in 24.5 per cent of operative specimens the carcinoma had extended to the upper limit of the resection. McNeer, Sunderland, McInnes, VandenBerg and Lawrence (1951) reported recurrence in the gastric remnant in 50 per cent of 92 patients. Helsingen and Hillestad (1956) reported the interesting finding of development of carcinoma in the gastric stump after 11 of 229 gastrectomies for histologically verified peptic ulcer (4.8%). A breakdown of this incidence indicated 10.5 per cent in the 95 gastric ulcer cases and only 0.8 per cent in the 125 duodenal ulcer cases. (In the 9 cases with combined gastric and duodenal ulcer there was no development of carcinoma.)

Even when total gastrectomy is performed, there is a tendency to leave carcinoma behind at the ends of the resection. Ransom (1956) reported that in 38 histologically studied total gastrectomy specimens, the operations being all performed for carcinoma, there was cancerous involvement of one or both ends of the specimen in 26 (68%). Since in 19 of the cases the proximal end was involved, this would argue for resecting the lower esophagus more often in such cases.

Spread by way of the blood stream to lungs, brain, etc., does occur but is rare. Spread by way of the peritoneal cavity also occurs (the involvement of the greater omentum, of the bottom of the pelvis—"Blumer's shelf"—and the Krukenberg tumor of the ovary from colloid carcinoma of the stomach are examples).

Lymphatic Spread. This is extremely common. In the classical study of Coller, Kay and McIntyre (1941), evidence of metastases was present microscopically in 75.5 per cent of cases (plus 12.5% additional in which only a palliative operation was done, total 88%). The 4 zones of lymph node involvement are shown in Figure 29-16. The most commonly involved are Zones I and III. Of the sessile neoplasms, 95.4 per cent had metastasized in comparison with only 60 per cent of the polypoid carcinomas. The authors concluded: "Whether palpable lymph nodes are present or not, the 4 zones of lymphatic metastases

TABLE 5. INCIDENCE OF METASTASES TO THE HILUM OF THE SPLEEN IN 46 CASES OF GASTRIC RESECTION FOR CARCINOMA*

GROSS TYPE OF TUMOR	METASTASES TO HILUM OF SPLEEN	
	Number	Per Cent
Polypoid (21 cases)	1	4.8
Ulcerating (6 cases)	0	0.0
Infiltrating (19 cases)	9	47.4
Total (46 cases)	10	21.7

* From Eker, R.: Acta chir. scandinav. *101*:123, March 22, 1951.

should be included within the resection to increase the likelihood of cure."

Metastases to the hilum of the spleen are frequent. Eker's series (1951) contained 46 stomachs with the attached spleen. The high over-all (21.7%) incidence of metastases is shown in Table 5. It is true that these cases were selected, since in only those cases in which it was thought necessary was the spleen removed. However, 16 of the 46 carcinomas were in the lower part of the stomach, including 8 on the lesser curve. Fly, Dockerty and Waugh (1956) found the splenic hilar nodes involved in 36.3 per cent of 102 resected stomach specimens. Furthermore, in the

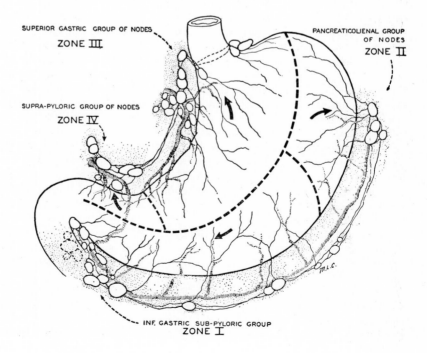

FIG. 29-16. Diagrammatic representation of zonal lymphatic metastases of carcinoma of the stomach. (Coller, F., Kay, E., and McIntyre, R.: Arch. Surg. *43*:751)

group of 20 carcinomas involving the distal half of the stomach, the percentage of splenic hilar involvement was almost as great, namely 30 per cent. Because the spleen is an "expendable" organ and also easily removed, it should be included en bloc with the stomach in resections for carcinoma.

Eker also reported that the frequency of histologically verified metastases in all locations was 70 per cent in his 100 subtotal resections and 82.9 in his 70 total resection specimens. Incomplete removal of nodes in Zone III seemed to be apparent in the subtotal resections as compared with the total resections.

Arhelger, Lober and Wangensteen (1955), during "second look" operations for gastric cancer, obtained positive findings in 11 of 26 patients in the hepatic pedicle and retropancreaticoduodenal areas (Zones IV and I, respectively). On the basis of these observations, a more nearly complete dissection of these areas was done in 24 patients. In 11 of these latter patients positive nodes were found in Zone IV and in 4 patients in Zone I. These authors concluded, "It is apparent that the lymph node dissection in present-day operations for cancer of the stomach is incomplete. An extension of the operation to include dissection of the hepatic pedicle and retropancreaticoduodenal area is recommended."

Classification. The importance of classification of carcinoma of the stomach is of especial significance from the standpoint of prognosis. Most classifications consider only the local lesion, while that of Hoerr (1954) takes into account both the element of metastases and of invasion, as follows:

Metastases. The extent of metastases is estimated preoperatively (as for example for osseous or pulmonary metastases) and at the time of operation. Capital letters (A, B and C) are used to denote 3 stages in descending order of favorableness.

Stage A. No metastases.

Stage B. Regional metastases to lymph nodes that usually are resectable.

Stage C. Distant metastases, connoting incurability.

Invasion. Invasion and local extension are determined at the time of laparotomy and are classified according to the degree to which the primary growth has penetrated the walls of the stomach. Three stages of invasion are recognized by Roman numerals (I, II and III), once more in descending order of favorableness.

Stage I. The growth is superficial and is confined to mucosa and muscularis.

Stage II. All gastric layers are involved, including the serosa, but there is no extragastric extension.

Stage III. The tumor has extended in continuity to neighboring structures, such as mesocolon, colon, liver, or pancreas.

In Stages I and II the primary lesion is resectable, but in Stage III only if the involved neighboring structures also are resectable.

Hoerr summarized the application of this classification by pointing out that at the time of operation the situation may be expressed by a combination of the two symbols: *metastases* represented by a letter A, B, or C, and *invasion* by a numeral I, II, or III. For example, superficial cancer with no clinical or pathologic evidence of metastases would be grouped as A-I, the most favorable type. On the other hand, the most serious would be C-III, with metastases to the liver and invasion of neighboring structures. (Hopeless carcinoma, e.g., with proved supraclavicular lymph node metastases and a gastric filling defect, but *no* laparotomy would be designated as Stage C-NX.) A pictorial representation of the six individual stages is shown in Figures 29-17 and 29-18.

In a series of 100 patients with 1- to 4-year followup in 100 per cent of the cases, Hoerr summarized the mortality. He found a progressive and marked decrease in the percentage of patients still alive as they were listed according to the different stages from A to C and from I to III.

DIAGNOSIS

The very important subject of the differential diagnosis between gastric ulcer and carcinoma has been covered in the section on ulcer. In summary, and extending the criteria of McGlone and Robertson (1953), malignancy is suggested by any of the following:

1. Roentgen evidence of malignancy, as determined by competent roentgenologic investigation

2. Gastroscopic evidence of malignancy

3. Cytologic evidence of malignant cells in the gastric aspirate

4. The presence of histamine-proved achlorhydria

5. Location of lesion

A. Greater curvature

B. Prepyloric portion of lesser curvature

C. Fundus

6. Failure of a lesion in any part of the stomach to heal within 3 weeks. (Not all agree even to giving medical treatment a trial, Edwards, 1950, stating, "Such a therapeutic test should be completely eliminated from practice.")

There are no typical symptoms of gastric cancer. Epigastric pain, loss of weight, ano-

rexia, tiredness, or even a protracted siege of "flu" (Wangensteen, 1951) may herald the onset of this most serious of all cancers. The physical examination is of limited value, because once a mass is palpable, cure is extremely unlikely. Among the simple laboratory tests, the determination of achlorhydria in the gastric contents, of normochromic or hypochromic anemia, and of occult blood in the stools are all helpful.

Males are affected about 3 times as often as females, and the average age of the patients is about 63 years, but neither of these two is of help in the diagnosis in an individual patient.

Boyce (1953) decried the fact that a com-

Fig. 29-17. Three stages of carcinoma of the stomach according to extent of metastasis. A fourth stage, C-NX, is listed as a variant of stage C. (Hoerr, S.: Surg., Gynec. & Obst. *99*:282)

Stage A. No metastases, grossly or microscopically.

Stage B. Regional metastases, usually resectable. Must be verified histologically since involved nodes may appear normal grossly, and enlarged nodes may represent only chronic inflammation. These metastases will be resectable unless fixed to aorta or in gastrohepatic ligament.

→

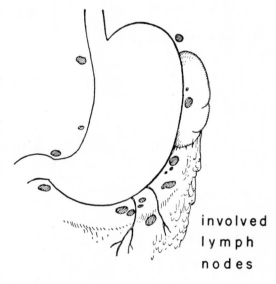

involved
lymph
nodes

→

Stage C. Distant metastases. Included are metastases to supraclavicular nodes, peritoneum, liver, lung, or bone. Usually will be verified histologically. At the present time they mean incurability.

Stage C-NX. Distant metastases. No operation. Distant metastases without surgical exploration of the stomach. A special case of stage C, such as might occur in a patient who has cancer in a biopsied supraclavicular lymph node, x-ray evidence of a gastric neoplasm, but no abdominal operation. "NX" is "no exploration" for grouping of invasion.

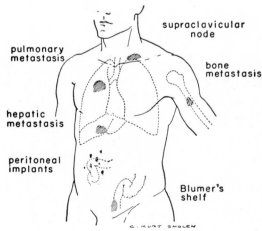

pulmonary
metastasis

supraclavicular
node

bone
metastasis

hepatic
metastasis

peritoneal
implants

Blumer's
shelf

parison of a recent series of cases of carcinoma of the stomach with other series he reported in 1933 and 1941 indicated that while the surgeon was doing his share of improvement by greatly lowering the operative mortality, the patients were still seeking treatment late. He advised more vigor in the prosecution of the diagnostic routine and a prompter and far more general resort to exploratory laparotomy in doubtful cases. He also stated: "An alarming tendency was noted in this most recent analysis, i.e., the invocation of psychosomatic medicine to explain symptoms and signs caused by gastric cancer."

TREATMENT

The only curative treatment of cancer of the stomach known at present is complete surgical excision of the tumor and its metastases. Roentgen therapy is of no curative value and of little, if any, palliative benefit. There is a

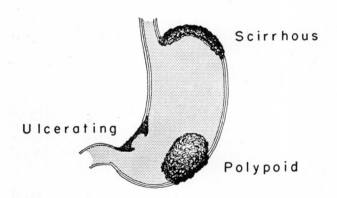

In polyp

Ulcerating

Superficial spreading

Polypoid

FIG. 29-18. Three stages of carcinoma of the stomach according to extent of invasion. (Hoerr, S.: Surg., Gynec. & Obst. *99*:283)

Stage I. Superficial cancer. Growth confined to mucosa and muscularis, irrespective of extent within the stomach. All are resectable.

Scirrhous

Ulcerating

Polypoid

Stage II. All gastric layers. Penetration to serosa but not involving extrinsic structures. Growths may extend into duodenum or esophagus if there is no external invasion. All are resectable.

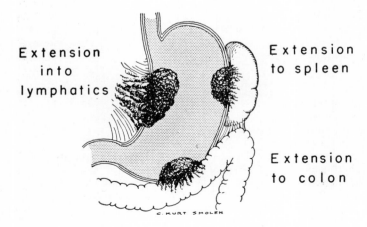

Extension into lymphatics

Extension to spleen

Extension to colon

Stage III. Extragastric invasion. Direct invasion of neighboring structures. These structures may be omentum, mesocolon, colon, pancreas, liver, spleen, diaphragm, aorta, adjacent lymphatics, or lymph nodes, or any combination of these. Resectability depends upon the structures that are invaded.

general trend toward more radical operation, going in two different but parallel directions. The first is the trend toward more frequent total gastrectomy (Lahey, 1950; Lahey and Marshall, 1950; McNeer, Sunderland, McInnes, VandenBerg and Lawrence, 1951). The second is toward a more radical subtotal gastrectomy, avoiding total gastrectomy in most pyloric or antral lesions, but including a more radical removal of lymph-node-bearing areas or portions of contiguous organs, especially the spleen, which are involved (Boyden, 1953; Fretheim, 1955; Arhelger, Lober and Wangensteen, 1955, and Hoerr, 1961).

The operations for gastric cancer can be listed as follows:

1. Radical subtotal distal gastrectomy for lesions of the distal stomach).

2. Radical subtotal proximal gastrectomy (for lesions of the upper stomach). The lower portion of the esophagus also is removed along with the spleen. A combined thoraco-abdominal incision is used.

3. Total gastrectomy (for lesions of the body, or extensive lesions of the lower or upper stomach). An abdominal apprcach is possible, but a thoraco-abdominal one is preferable.

A. With esophagojejunostomy by anastomosis to a jejunal loop coupled with enteroenterostomy

B. With esophagojejunostomy Roux-en-Y

C. With esophagoduodenostomy:
    a. Direct anastomosis
    b. With ileocolic segment as pouch (Hunnicut, 1951)
    c. Jejunal segment as pouch (Hunt, 1955)

4. Palliative operations: gastrojejunostomy, gastrostomy, etc. (of little or no value).

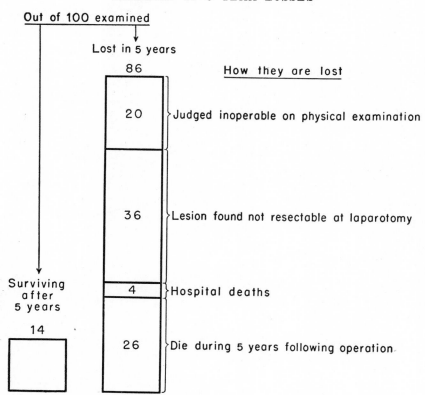

FIG. 29-19. Analysis of 5-year losses from cancer of the stomach. (Berkson, J., Walters, W., Gray, H., and Priestley, J.: Proc. Staff. Meet., Mayo Clin. 27:150)

PROGNOSIS

While the prognosis of carcinoma of the stomach could be improved markedly, the outlook is far from hopeless. It is true, as Berkson, Walters, Gray, and Priestley (1952) reported, of 100 patients examined with carcinoma of the stomach, that only 14 will be alive at the end of 5 years (Fig. 29-19). However, if one takes 100 patients who survive gastric resection for carcinoma of the stomach and in whom no metastases are found, 48.5 will be alive in 5 years. The differences in survival between resection, palliative operation and exploration only are shown in Figure 29-20, and the effect of metastases in Figure 29-21. In these charts the entire survival curve is included for as long a period as the follow-up of a sufficient number of

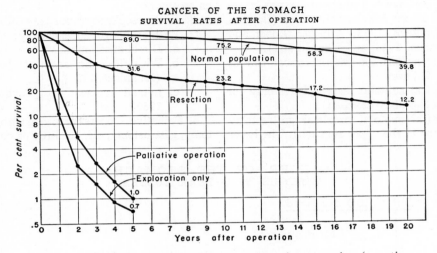

FIG. 29-20. Survival rates in successive years after operation (resection, palliative operation, or exploration only) for cancer of the stomach. (Berkson, J., Walter, W., Gray, H., and Priestley, J.: Proc. Staff Meet., Mayo Clin. 27:143)

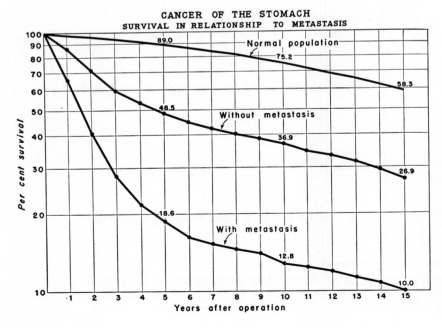

FIG. 29-21. Survival rates in successive years after gastric resection for cancer of the stomach, according to absence (middle line) or presence (lower line) of metastases. (Berkson, J., Walters, W., Gray, H., and Priestley, J.: Proc. Staff. Meet., Mayo Clin. 27:144)

patients allowed. The actuarial method of calculation of the curves was used.

Other authors have reported somewhat similar figures. Landelius (1948) found 31 per cent of 62 resected patients who survived operation were still alive in 5 years. In 343 resections for cure with survival after operation, Ransom (1953) found 28 per cent still alive at the end of 5 years. (26 per cent if the 31 palliative resections are included.) In 91 with negative nodes there were 49.5 per cent still alive at the end of 5 years and in 184 with positive nodes, only 15.8 per cent (nodes not recorded in 68). Shahon, Horowitz and Kelly (1956) presented more recent figures, namely, 57.1 per cent 5-year survivals in cases without nodes and 14.5 per cent in those with nodes. Beal and Hill (1956), after 133 definitive subtotal resections, reported similar figures of 48.6 and 15.9 per cent (33.1% in the entire group). The figures of Brown, Cain and Dockerty (1961) indicate an even more hopeful outlook.

HYPERTROPHIC PYLORIC STENOSIS

This condition, while one of the 3 most important lesions of the stomach and the duodenum will not be discussed here (see Chap. 46 where the story of hypertrophic pyloric stenosis and its treatment by the very effective Fredet-Rammstedt operation will be given in detail).

OPERATIVE PROCEDURES ON THE STOMACH

In the following compilation, only those surgical procedures which are currently in use

PYLOROPLASTIES

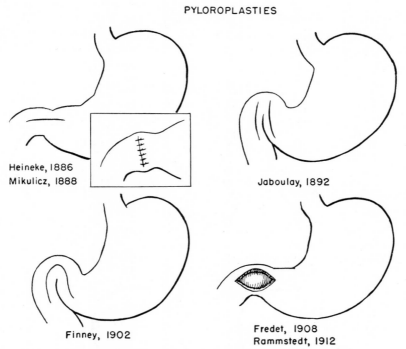

Heineke, 1886
Mikulicz, 1888

Jaboulay, 1892

Finney, 1902

Fredet, 1908
Rammstedt, 1912

FIG. 29-22. Different types of pyloroplasty procedures. The Heineke-Mikulicz involves the principle of longitudinal incision with transverse closure to enlarge the lumen. The Jaboulay involves an anastomosis of 2 longitudinal incisions. The Finney involves a closure of an inverted U-incision. Finally, the Rammstedt involves a longitudinal incision of muscularis down to but not through the mucosa; after separation of the muscle layer the mucosa should pouch out to a level even with the adjoining serosa. (Redrawn from Waugh, J., and Hood, R.: Quart. Rev. Surg. 10:205)

today will be discussed. Such operations as gastropexy and wedge resection of the stomach for *gastric* ulcer are not listed because it is believed that these procedures are obsolete. Some other rare or optional operations also are not listed.

When any operation is performed on the stomach or the duodenum, a careful preoperative and postoperative regimen must be followed as described in Chapter 5. Special attention must be directed toward getting the stomach as empty as possible before operation. Aspiration and irrigation with the large tube may be necessary in cases of pyloric obstruction. In most cases the patient comes to the operating room with a Levin tube in the stomach. Such a tube is left in the stomach a varying period after operation, usually less than 5 days, and the present tendency is to use the tube for a shorter period postoperatively than formerly, except after vagotomy.

DRAINAGE PROCEDURES

These are utilized either alone or with vagotomy to drain the stomach.

Pyloromyotomy (Fredet-Rammstedt). This operation is used not only in cases of hypertrophic pyloric stenosis for which it is almost specific but also in conjunction with certain upper and wedge gastric resections (see Chap. 46, "Pediatric Surgery").

Heineke-Mikulicz. This is used as a drainage procedure in conjunction with vagotomy or wedge resection. It involves a longitudinal incision through the pylorus which is then closed transversely, usually with one layer of interrupted sutures. Its plastic principle gives added diameter to the lumen (Fig. 29-22).

Finney Pyloroplasty. This involves a more extensive longitudinal incision than with the Heineke-Mikulicz. Then this is closed separately for the lower and the upper leaves of the incision in an inverted-U fashion. It has the same uses as the Heineke-Mikulicz but is used when one desires a bigger opening.

Gastrojejunostomy. This procedure anastomoses the jejunum, preferably within 4 inches of the ligament of Treitz, to the stomach. The loop of jejunum can be brought up either anteriorly or posteriorly with relation

BILLROTH I GASTRIC RESECTION

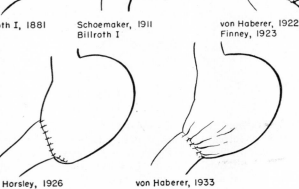

Billroth I, 1881   Schoemaker, 1911   von Haberer, 1922
                    Billroth I   Finney, 1923

Horsley, 1926   von Haberer, 1933

FIG. 29-23. Different types of gastroduodenostomy following subtotal gastric resection (Billroth I).

to the colon. Some surgeons do not realize that an anterior anastomosis can be performed with a loop shorter than 4 inches, but if the transverse colon is pulled to the right and the loop brought up toward the left side, this can be done easily in most cases.

GASTRIC RESECTIONS

Billroth I (Gastroduodenostomy Anastomosis After the Resection). This operation has the advantage of restoring normal continuity. It is especially applicable to the treatment of gastric ulcers or perforated duodenal ulcers (which are usually anterior). With adequate mobilization of the duodenum and preparation of the duodenal stump surgeons with experience in doing this operation can perform it in almost all instances where subtotal resection is indicated and without sacrificing the extent of resection. Harkins and Nyhus (1956).

1. The Finney-von Haberer variety of this operation anastomoses the end of the cut stomach to the side rather than to the end of the duodenum.

2. Another variant is "gastrectomy with replacement" (Henley, 1952) in which a jejunal loop connects the end of the stomach to the end of the duodenum, obviating tension on the anastomosis.

(*Application:* Gastric or duodenal ulcer or carcinoma of the lower stomach. See Fig. 29-23.)

Billroth II (Gastrojejunostomy Anastomosis After the Resection). There are several varieties of this operation, depending upon whether the jejunal loop is brought up anterior or posterior to the colon, and whether the entire stomach opening is anastomosed to the jejunum (Polya) or only its lower half (Hofmeister or Schoemaker), after closure of the duodenal stump (Fig. 29-24) in either instance.

(*Application:* Duodenal, or gastric ulcer, or

DUODENAL STUMP CLOSURE

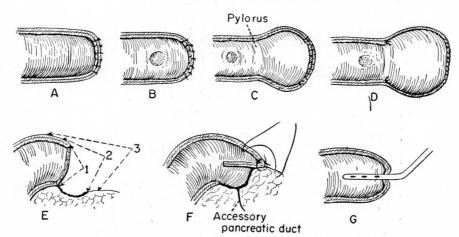

FIG. 29-24. Different methods of duodenal stump closure. (A) Routine closure distal to the removed ulcer. (B) A similar closure proximal to the ulcer which is left in situ. (C) The Devine exclusion of the distal stomach with the antral mucosa in place. (D) The Bancroft-Plenk exclusion with the antral mucosa excised. (E) The Nissen-I with the anterior duodenal flap sutured as follows: (1) Inner layer to distal edge of ulcer in situ in the bed of the pancreas. (2) The inner serosal sutures to the proximal edge of the ulcer bed. (3) The outer serosal sutures to the capsule of the pancreas. (F) The Nissen-II for ulcers which not only are left in situ but also may contain the opening of the duct of Santorini. The anterior edge of the duodenal stump is sutured in 2 layers to the proximal edge of the ulcer. (G) Closure over a tube which is brought out through a stab wound in the abdominal wall. (Modified from Dr. John A. Duncan)

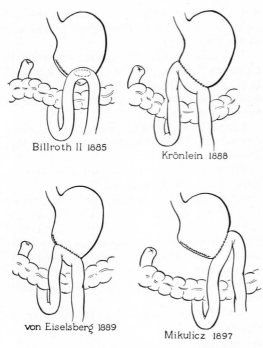

FIG. 29-25. Different types of gastrojejunostomy following subtotal gastric resection (Billroth II). (Waugh, J., and Hood, R.: Quart. Rev. Surg. *10*:212)

carcinoma of the lower stomach. See Figs. 29-25 and 29-26.)

Segmental Resection. This procedure has the advantage that it leaves the antrum in place and removes more parietal cells, at the same time leaving a larger stomach. It has been popularized by Wangensteen (1952) and reported on by MacLean, Hamilton and Murphy (1953). Because of the vagal interruption to the distal segment, a Heineke-Mikulicz pyloroplasty is necessary for drainage.

(*Application:* Duodenal ulcer in which instance it is a sound procedure and also a safe one since the duodenum is not touched.)

Longitudinal Tubular Resection With Transverse Gastroplasty. This operation, introduced by Wangensteen (1953), involves the longitudinal removal of the greater curvature portion of the stomach, followed by transverse closure of the defect. Since the vagal supply to the pyloric region is not interfered with, no pyloroplasty is necessary. A more recent evaluation of the procedure is that of MacLean and Lillehei (1954). The operation

has now been abandoned by its proponents. (*Application:* Duodenal ulcer.)

Proximal (Upper) Gastrectomy. This operation, a type of esophagogastrectomy, involves an end-to-end anastomosis between the lower esophagus and the remaining lower stomach. Usually it must be supplemented by a pyloroplasty (Tanner, 1954, 1955).

(*Application:* Tumor of the upper stomach. Not suitable for high-lying ulcer because of the danger of peptic esophagitis.)

Total Gastrectomy. A thoraco-abdominal approach is advised (Tanner, 1951).

(*Application:* Carcinoma of body or fundus of stomach.)

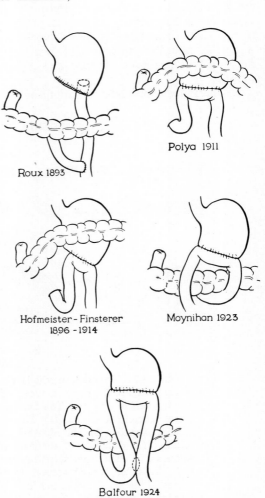

FIG. 29-26. Billroth II gastrectomies (*Cont.*) (Waugh, J., and Hood, R.: Quart. Rev. Surg. *10*:213)

Vagotomy

Vagotomy, introduced by Dragstedt and Owens (1943), is used for duodenal ulcer, not for gastric ulcer. It also requires a drainage procedure or a coincident resection.

1. *With drainage procedure* (gastrojejunostomy), Dragstedt, 1945; Holt and Robinson, 1955; Hoerr, 1955; Heineke-Mikulicz pyloroplasty, Weinberg, 1953

2. *With hemigastrectomy* (45 to 50 per cent, removing all of the antrum)

A. Billroth II anastomosis (Farmer, Howe, Porell and Smithwick, 1951; Stock, Hui and Tinckler, 1956, and others)

B. Billroth I anastomosis (Harkins, Schmitz, Harper, Sauvage, Moore, Storer and Kanar, 1953; Zollinger and Williams, 1956; Harkins, Jesseph, Stevenson and Nyhus, 1960; Herrington, Classen and Edwards, 1961, and Harkins and Nyhus, 1961)

3. *Selective gastric vagotomy.* With either drainage procedure or hemigastrectomy (Griffith and Harkins, 1957; Griffith, 1960). This technic spares the celiac and the hepatic branches of the vagi, sectioning only those to the stomach, and purportedly eliminates diarrhea and other complications that sometimes follow total abdominal vagotomy.

Miscellaneous Operations

Gastrostomy. These are more applicable for feeding below an obstruction in an attempt to maintain or get the patient in better shape than they are for palliation of a malignant process (Connar and Sealy, 1956).

Tube (Temporary) Gastrostomy (Stamm). Such a gastrostomy of the Stamm type involves introduction of a catheter into a hole in the stomach around which the wall is closed with 3 overlapping purse-string sutures. The catheter is brought out through the omentum and then through a stab wound in the abdominal wall (Farris and Smith, 1956). Use such a catheter as a temporary measure in place of nasogastric suction after many major operations.

Gastric Wall-Lined (Permanent) Gastrostomy (Spivack). While there are several varieties of permanent gastrostomy, the author prefers the Spivack variety which has a mucous membrane-lined valve to prevent leakage. Another type of gastric mucous membrane-lined gastrostomy is that of Glassman (1939) as modified by Gibbon, Nealon and Greco (1956). For a permanent type of gastrostomy, an interposed jejunal loop (Nyhus, Stevenson, Jones, DeVito and Harkins, 1958) is useful.

Simple Closure of a Perforated Peptic Ulcer. About 3 sutures are placed across the defect, without inversion and then are tied loosely over the tip of an attached omental tag.

LATE COMPLICATIONS OF GASTRIC SURGERY: THE POSTGASTRECTOMY SYNDROME

Mortality is the most serious complication of all surgery. Fortunately, for most of the common gastric operations it is relatively low (gastrojejunostomy, 0.5%; subtotal gastric resection for ulcer, 1 to 3%; subtotal gastric resection for carcinoma, 3 to 7%; total gastrectomy, 5 to 12%, and vagotomy with gastrojejunostomy, 0.5%).

In those patients who recover from a technically correct gastric operation, a number of late effects are observed in a varying proportion of patients. Sometimes these are lumped together as the "postgastrectomy syndrome"; sometimes this term is used to include only "dumping," and sometimes it is used to include all but recurrence. In the following discussion, the 5 main late complications of gastric surgery will be considered.

Stomal Ulcer

Such a complication is often called a recurrence. This involves a matter of definition since a stomal ulcer after a Billroth II gastric resection for duodenal ulcer is situated many inches away from the original ulcer and, from this standpoint, is hardly a recurrence. This type of complication has been considered previously under special types of ulcer according to location and will not be discussed further here.

"Dumping Syndrome"

Dumping may be defined as the occurrence of sweating, unpleasant warmth, subjective flushing, nausea, palpitation, or explosive diarrhea, with onset during or within 15 minutes after eating and lasting up to 45 minutes and partially or completely relieved by lying down. Parenthetically, it may be observed now, in connection with the discussion which will follow, that most if not all of these symptoms are similar to those of mild hypovolemic shock. These symptoms are more common following gastric resection, particularly when the resection has been radical in extent, but they occur following any gastric procedure. Since most of the symptoms are subjective, the incidence of dumping has been reported variously as ranging from 0 to 100 per cent following the same procedure, partly depending on the thoroughness of the follow-up studies. After gastric resection, 4 per cent severe or moderate dumping and an additional 15 per cent slight dumping is a reasonable average incidence.

Many theories have been postulated to explain the dumping syndrome. Among these are the following:

Theory 1. Secondary hypoglycemia following initial hyperglycemia due to rapid passage of food into, and absorption by the jejunum (Gilbert and Dunlop, 1947)

Theory 2. Nervous reflex from rapid overdistention of the jejunum (Hertz, 1913)

Theory 3. Loss of supporting structures holding the gastric remnant in place (Butler and Capper, 1951)

Theory 4. Alimentary hyperglycemic shock (Glaessner, 1940)

Theory 5. Reflex pooling of blood in the splanchnic vascular bed due to rapid entrance of food into the intestine, with secondary decrease in cerebral blood flow (Hoffmann, 1939)

Theory 6. Hypopotassemia (Smith, 1951; Kleiman and Grant, 1954)

Theory 7. Allergy to partially digested food (Zeldis and Klinger, 1951)

Theory 8. Hypovolemic shock due to osmotic inflow into the jejunum of plasma constituents (Roberts, Randall and Farr, 1954)

Theory 1 represents a satisfactory explanation of the late hypoglycemic dumping syndrome (see below) but does not explain the early dumping syndrome now under discussion and in which the symptoms may be at their maximum in the presence of hyperglycemia. Several of the theories agree in postulating that the rapid entrance of food into the jejunum is the initiating factor. Until recently Theory 2, the mechanical distention theory, was the most popular. At present, Theory 8, the shock theory (Fig. 29-27), seems to be most logical. As seen in Figure 29-28, there is a marked drop in plasma volume coincident with the administration of hypertonic solution sufficient to produce symptoms of dumping. Also, as seen in Figure 29-29, the electrocardiographic alterations, blood volume changes and symptoms occurred concurrently. On the other hand, the changes

PHYSIOLOGY OF THE DUMPING SYNDROME

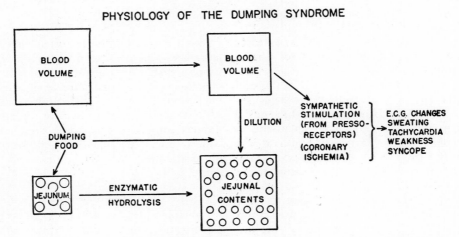

Fig. 29-27. The postprandial-hypovolemia concept of the dumping syndrome. (Walker, J. M., Roberts, K. E., Medwid, A., and Randall, H. T.: Arch. Surg. *71*:546)

FIG. 29-28. Changes in plasma concentration of the dye (upper half) and in plasma volume (lower half) following the administration of hypertonic solutions to a gastrectomized patient. (Roberts, K., Randall, H., and Farr, H.: S. Forum 4:302)

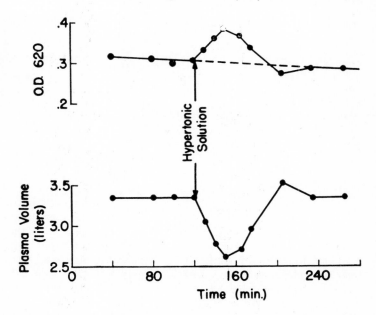

in potassium (see Theory 6, above) and phosphate levels occurred later.

Fisher, Taylor and Cannon (1955), advocates of Theory 2, devised a test for dumping involving the onset of symptoms after drinking of 150 cc. of 50 per cent glucose in water, while seated. In 53 postoperative patients, the incidence of clinical dumping was 36 per cent, and the incidence of test dumping 34 per cent. After either vagotomy and pyloroplasty or the Billroth I resection, the incidence of test

dumping was 29 per cent, and after the Billroth II it was 48 per cent.

The treatment of the dumping syndrome is largely medical. Many patients lose their symptoms after several months. Others learn to eat less at one time. In severe cases a "conversion operation" (Billroth II to Billroth I) can be tried, or an attempt can be made to narrow the anastomotic stoma (Woodward, Desser and Gasster, 1955; Zollinger and Williams, 1956).

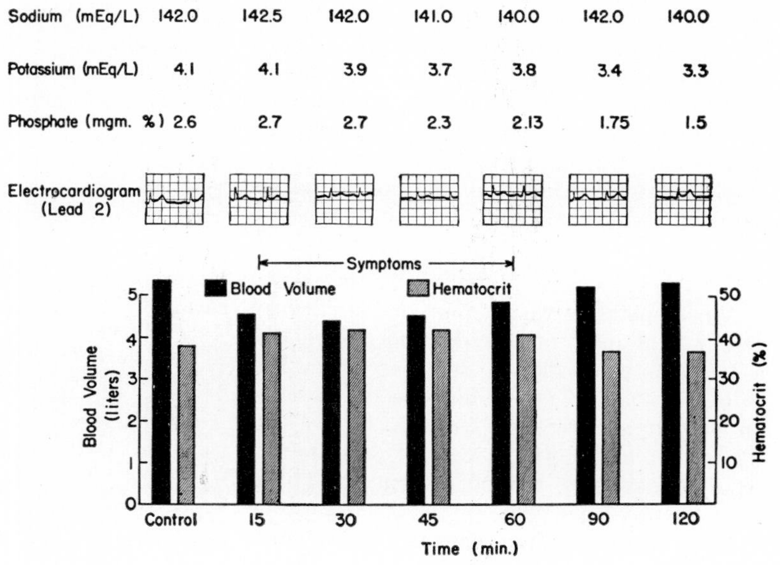

Sodium (mEq/L)	142.0	142.5	142.0	141.0	140.0	142.0	140.0
Potassium (mEq/L)	4.1	4.1	3.9	3.7	3.8	3.4	3.3
Phosphate (mgm. %)	2.6	2.7	2.7	2.3	2.13	1.75	1.5

FIG. 29-29. The relationship between changes in blood volume, electrocardiogram, plasma electrolytes and symptoms in a gastrectomized patient at 15, 30, 45, 60, 90, and 120 minutes following the oral ingestion of 200 ml. of 50 per cent glucose. (Roberts, K., Randall, H., and Farr, H.: S. Forum 4:305)

Late Hypoglycemic Dumping Syndrome

This syndrome is believed to be due to a secondary hypoglycemic phase occurring 2 to 3 hours after the initial hyperglycemic phase. The treatment involves the use of proteins, avoidance of carbohydrates, and the use of other measures to prevent the initial hyperglycemia. In such patients the syndrome involves an abnormal glucose tolerance curve, but in cases with recurrent ulcer as well, the pancreas should be examined for the presence of islet cell tumors.

Postgastrectomy Anemia

Owren (1952) emphasized that poor absorption of iron following subtotal gastrectomy is related to the rapid emptying of the gastric remnant. Postgastrectomy anemia has been reported in from 0 to 39 per cent of men and from 17 to 82 per cent of women. The fact that menstruating women normally lose comparatively more iron from the body stores than other individuals explains why they comprise such a large proportion of postgastrectomy anemias. Fortunately, this anemia is usually amenable to oral or intravenous iron therapy and causes very little disability to the patient. Because sufficient intrinsic antianemic factor is produced in the residual stomach pouch following subtotal gastrectomy, it is rare to observe a macrocytic anemia in such cases.

The interrelationship between the various types of postgastrectomy syndrome was shown by Wallensten (1955). He found a definite correlation between postcibal symptoms, including dumping, and the existence of anemia and especially of sideropenia. Furthermore, intravenous iron therapy relieved the postcibal symptoms in many of the postoperative patients with sideropenia.

Weight Loss

A postoperative weight loss, or inability to gain weight in those already underweight, is a frequent complication. In this respect the Billroth I type of anastomosis seems to have an advantage over the Billroth II. In the former, from 8 to 42 per cent of patients are reported as losing weight, and in the latter from 16 to 75 per cent.

Experimental studies indicate that almost

TABLE 6. Fecal Fat and Nitrogen Losses in Dogs Following Various Types of Gastrectomy*

	LOSS IN FECES, PER CENT	
OPERATION	Fat	Nitrogen
Billroth II	27.7	24.4
Billroth I	10.6	19.3
Segmental	6.4	12.6
Control	4.9	14.9

* Everson, T. C.: Surgery 36:525-535, 1954.

any kind of gastric operation decreases fat and protein absorption, but that, in general, this impairment is less with the Billroth I than with the Billroth II. Everson (1954) compared these two procedures along with segmental gastrectomy as shown in Table 6. It is seen that the Billroth I was distinctly superior to the II regarding both fat and nitrogen loss but was inferior to the segmental resection. The work of MacLean, Perry, Kelly, Mosser, Mannick and Wangensteen (1954) who performed metabolic studies on patients after various types of gastric resections was referred to in the section on Operative Procedures on the Stomach (see p. 698).

Javid (1955) also performed metabolic studies on 5 series of dogs as shown in Table 7.

The treatment of excessive weight loss following gastric operations is partly prophylactic, as shown by Zollinger and Ellison (1954) who advised avoiding extensive resections in patients who have had difficulty in maintaining weight before operation. From the therapeutic standpoint the treatment is largely medical but includes surgical measures to over-

TABLE 7. Fecal Fat and Nitrogen Losses in Dogs Following Various Gastric Operations*

	LOSS IN FECES, PER CENT	
OPERATION	Fat	Nitrogen
1. ⅔ Polya gastrectomy	17.1	26.2
2. Vagotomy, transthoracic	5.0	21.7
3. Vagotomy plus gastro-enterostomy	16.2	13.8
4. Gastroenterostomy	5.6	8.4
5. ⅔ Polya gastrectomy + vagotomy	32.1	31.5
Control	5.0	13.6

* From Javid, H.: Surgery 38:641-651, 1955.

come underlying stomal ulcer, etc. If weight loss persists, a conversion, without additional resection, from a Billroth II to a Billroth I may be tried.

The increased tendency to tuberculosis following gastrectomy may well be a secondary phenomenon due to the malnutrition which frequently occurs following gastrectomy (Waugh, 1956). Stammers (1955) and Boman (1956) pointed out the importance of this complication.

MISCELLANEOUS SURGICAL DISEASES OF THE STOMACH AND THE DUODENUM

A number of miscellaneous affections of the stomach and duodenum, including benign tumors and malignant tumors of the stomach other than carcinoma, are listed below alphabetically with brief discussions.

STOMACH

Benign Tumors of the Stomach. The comprehensive review by Palmer (1951) on this subject is outstanding. The relative incidence of reported cases of such tumors collected from the literature is shown in Table 8.

This table does not represent the true incidence, if the smallest tumors are to be considered but does signify the relative incidence of those intramural tumors large enough to be reported. Certain tumors such as neuromas, leiomyomas, fibromas, "gastritis cystica," etc., may be very frequent and are often multiple. One statement to emphasize the frequency of

TABLE 8. RELATIVE INCIDENCE OF BENIGN INTRAMURAL TUMORS OF THE STOMACH AS COLLECTED FROM THE WORLD LITERATURE*

TYPE OF BENIGN INTRAMURAL TUMOR OF THE STOMACH		NO. OF REPORTED CASES	PER CENT
1. Aberrant pancreatic tumors		215	13
2. Vascular tumors		93	6
A. Gastric angioma	59		
B. Gastric endothelioma	34		
3. Fatty tumors (lipoma, 95)		103	6
4. Neurogenic tumors		263	16
5. Leiomyomas		610	37
6. Fibromas		289	17
7. Cystic tumors		87	5
Total		1660	100

* Palmer, 1951.

benign tumors can be made, namely, that if all sizes of tumor are included, the leiomyoma probably is the most frequent intramural or nonepithelial tumor of the stomach (q.v.). If both epithelial and nonepithelial tumors of the stomach are considered, the polypoid adenoma is probably the most common benign gastric tumor (Woodruff, 1961).

Bezoars and Concretions. Such foreign bodies are similar to the hair balls occurring in long-haired domestic animals. In human beings, certain types of foreign bodies are more common in children or in the mentally deranged, while others occur more generally. A brief classification is as follows:

1. INDIVIDUAL OBJECTS (single or multiple): coins, bobby pins, etc. Most of these will pass into the jejunum if given sufficient time.

2. BEZOARS: Concretions resulting from the repeated ingestion of swallowed material which is unable to pass the pylorus:

A. *Trichobezoars:* hair balls (more common in female children)

B. *Phytobezoars:* vegetable fibers (persimmons—"diospyrobezoars," dried apricots, (etc.). (More common in male adults)

The diagnosis is based chiefly on the history and roentgen confirmation. Symptoms ranging from poor appetite to those of complications such as obstruction, hemorrhage, or perforation may be present. In the 14 cases of diospyrobezoar reported by O'Leary (1953), most were associated with gastric ulcer, 5 with bleeding, 4 with penetration, and 1 with perforation. In some instances, however, no symptoms may be present, even though the foreign body be large enough to indicate potential danger. Morey, Means and Horsley (1955) reported a diospyrobezoar removed 8 years after a subtotal gastrectomy.

Treatment of patients with single objects in the stomach includes: close observation with immediate operation for complications, bulky diet, mineral oil, and removal by gastrotomy if the object does not pass within 96 hours (a longer trial may be given if the object has no sharp edges or points). Multiple foreign bodies and bezoars almost always require laparotomy, gastrotomy and removal. If marked chronic ulceration is present, gastric resection occasionally may be necessary. The results of nonoperative treatment of bezoars results in a mortality of about 60 per cent (DeBakey and Ochsner, 1938-39) as opposed to 6 per cent in the operative cases.

Dreiling and Marshak (1956) recently pointed out that while ingestion of indigestible foreign bodies is always to be avoided, it is particularly hazardous in patients that already have duodenal obstruction from peptic ulcer. These authors reported 2 cases with chronic duodenal obstruction resulting from the impaction of ingested fruit pits in an area of duodenal stenosis resulting from chronic peptic ulcer.

Congenital Malformations. Unless the relatively common congenital hypertrophic pyloric stenosis is included, it can be said that congenital malformations of the stomach occur less frequently than in any other part of the intestinal tract. This is of interest in view of the fact that the stomach stands high in the list of organs with acquired abnormalities. Another condition that should not be included with the stomach is congenital diaphragmatic hernia containing the organ. Rare abnormalities include atresia at the cardia or the pylorus, congenital hourglass stomach, and aberrant pancreatic tissue near the pylorus.

Acute Dilatation of the Stomach. This condition usually occurs as a postoperative or post-traumatic complication, especially after abdominal operations and when peritonitis is present. It may be present even though the patient vomits frequently (generally in small amounts) and in such instances is similar to the urinary bladder retention present despite repeated small urinations. The upper abdomen is tympanitic and distended. Careful observation as to which part of the abdomen is distended is important, as some cases have been treated with a rectal tube or with enemas. The dangers of acute dilatation are: (1) aspiration of vomitus into the lungs, (2) disruption of operative suture lines and (3) occasionally rupture of the stomach. Continuous or repeated aspirations of the stomach, maintenance of fluid balance, and prevention of aspiration pneumonia by avoidance of narcosis are important in the treatment. In one postoperative patient following partial gastric resection for carcinoma of the stomach, the author saw a measured 5,200 ml. (approximately half air and half liquid) aspirated from the stomach during a 1 hour period 5 days after operation.

Diverticulum of the Stomach. In a series of 1,750 gastroscopic examinations, Tanner (1952) found 5 gastric diverticula, 4 being in the upper stomach. Treatment is medical unless the diverticulum is very large, retains barium more than 24 to 48 hours, or causes symptoms. Inversion is a satisfactory treatment unless the diverticulum is near the cardiac orifice, in which instance it may produce obstruction if inverted. In these cases, as well as in some others, it should be excised. Hillemand, Patel and Lataste (1955) have written a good recent review of this subject.

Eosinophilic Granuloma of the Stomach. This condition, described by Booher and Grant (1951), includes a granulomatous infiltration of the wall of the stomach and occasionally of the jejunum and the ileum. The patient may have an eosinophilia suggesting an allergic basis, possibly with sensitivity to certain foods. An eosinophilia was present in 2 of the more extensive cases collected by Booher and Grant and in 1 of the 2 reported by McCune, Gusack and Newman (1955), being 34 per cent in the latter. Also the condition may be due either to the traumatic introduction of food particles into the gastric wall or to the necrotizing effect upon the patient's own gastric wall tissues of gastric juice which has extravasated. At present this is not a surgical condition.

Booher and Grant pointed out that the most common manifestation of the disease, on the basis of the 10 cases they collected, is the formation of a poorly circumscribed submucosal nodule which tends to become pedunculated and polypoid and occurs most frequently in the pyloric antrum. In their own case such a tumor intermittently prolapsed through the pylorus.

McCune, Gusack and Newman also reported a case of generalized eosinophilic gastroduodenitis with an eosinophile percentage of 59 per cent.

Acute Gastritis. Behrend, Katz and Robertson (1954) divided acute gastritis into 5 types: (1) simple (due to alcohol, irritating foods, drugs, or allergens), (2) corrosive (due to strong caustics, acids, or other chemicals), (3) infectious (associated with influenza, pneumonia, scarlet fever, etc.), (4) phlegmonous (due to suppurative infection by streptococci or the colon bacillus), and (5) necrotizing (due to infection by necrotizing bacteria, such as fusiform bacilli and spirochetes, but without occlusion of the major arterial supply to the stomach). Treatment of the simple variety involves avoidance of the causative agent, antacids, bland diet and parasympatholytic drugs. Treatment of the infectious variety includes that of the causative disease, and antacids, diet and drugs as in the simple type. Corrosive, phlegmonous and necrotizing gastritis will be considered separately.

Atrophic Gastritis. Atrophic gastritis occurs in older people and represents a lessened capacity to secrete acid. Young individuals with high gastric acids and duodenal ulcer, on reaching an older age, may have less acid and develop a gastric ulcer. The relationship between chronic atrophic gastritis and carcinoma of the stomach was studied by Konjetzny (1934, 1938), who believed that the relationship is a close one and that the gastritis is a precancerous lesion with 85 per cent of gastric carcinomas developing on the basis of pre-existing "gastritis hyperplastica atrophicans." Guiss and Stewart (1943) opposed this theory, but more recent studies have revived it (see p. 687).

Chronic Gastritis. A chronic condition possibly representing acute hypertrophic gastritis in a late stage. Postoperative gastritis is a variety of chronic gastritis and follows most stomach operations. Chronic gastritis is said to occur in 6 per cent of the general population.

Corrosive Gastritis. In some instances ingested caustic agents may produce a sufficiently localized lesion that recovery occurs, yet scarring with atrophy and achlorhydria results. If pyloric obstruction is present, gastrojejunostomy or partial gastric resection may be advisable.

Hypertrophic Gastritis. This condition is said to occur in 2 to 17 per cent of gastroscopic examinations and to comprise 18 to 57 per cent of cases of chronic gastritis. It does not occur in children and in adolescents, the majority of the cases being in the 4th to the 6th decades. The cause of the condition is not known. According to Fieber (1955), the cardinal symptoms are pain (74%), weight loss (60%), vomiting (42%), and hemorrhage

(20%). The average duration of these symptoms is 2 years. The use of the term "hypertrophic gastritis," as used by Fieber, in reality combines the 2 types of Menétrièr, *polyadenomes polypeux,* a hyperplastic variety, and *polyadenomes en nappe,* a hypertrophic variety. The classification of the hypertrophic gastritides and polyps is still uncertain.

Necrotizing Gastritis. This lesion is one of the 5 types of acute gastritis and usually is due to infection with fusiform bacilli and spirochetes from severe mouth infections. The necrosis results from the infection, despite the fact that the major arterial vessels to the stomach are not occluded. In the case reported by Behrend, Katz and Robertson (1954) death resulted despite antibiotic therapy and drainage of the peritoneal cavity.

Phlegmonous Gastritis (Gastric Phlegmon). This rare lesion may be diffuse or localized. It includes a suppurative involvement, usually by streptococci, of the submucosa with the occasional occurrence of fibrin and pus on the outside of the stomach. Males are afflicted 3 times as often as females, and over 80 per cent of patients are between 30 and 60 years of age. Most patients are seen on charity wards, and many are excessive users of alcohol. The condition is somewhat related to acute necrotizing gastritis but does not involve the mucosa. Sachs and Angrist (1945) compared phlegmonous gastritis with phlegmonous cholecystitis. Three of their 4 cases had no break in the mucosa of the stomach in the form of an ulcer, a neoplasm or an operative wound. They concluded that phlegmonous gastritis is a "manifestation of sepsis with localization in the stomach wall rather than a lesion following local invasion from the lumen." Complications include localized and subdiaphragmatic abscess and the results of general pyemia. Treatment involves drainage of secondary abscesses, maintenance of nutrition by jejunostomy feedings and adequate vitamin C intake (Cutler and Harrison, 1940), and antibiotics.

Postoperative Gastritis. Palmer (1953) reported that many instances of postoperative gastritis represent a continuation of a preoperative process; however, 22 of 45 postoperative patients, all with normal preoperative gastric mucosa, showed postoperative gastritis. Such gastritis, once it had developed, tended to remain static. It occurred following subtotal gastrectomy, simple gastro-jejunostomy, and gastrojejunostomy with vagotomy.

Gastromalacia. This condition has been defined as an acute, erosive phenomenon, manifested by a gelatinous softening of a poorly defined area of stomach wall, with little or no inflammatory response (King and Reganis, 1953). There may be multiple small mucosal ulcerations, or large areas of dissolution of the entire stomach wall. The condition is related to Cushing's ulcer and may be due to an interference with the central autonomic control mechanism (see section on Cushing's ulcer). Bell, Thomas and Skillicorn (1956) reported the first instance of recovery after repair of a 5-inch-long gastric perforation in a case of gastromalacia. The association with poliomyelitis in this patient is of interest, and these authors pointed out that in their hospital in 1953 there were 8 bulbospinal deaths from poliomyelitis. Five of these 8 had antemortem perforations of the upper gastro-intestinal tract (1 esophagus, 3 stomach, and 1 of the duodenum). Treatment will succeed only if applied promptly because of the large size of the perforations and large amount of leakage into the peritoneal cavity within a short time. If the perforation is low in the stomach, gastric resection may be done, but in Bell, Thomas, and Skillicorn's case, the necrotic area on the anterior wall was débrided longitudinally and closed longitudinally.

Glomus Tumor of the Stomach. These tumors, related to the hemangiopericytomas, are rare benign tumors similar to glomus tumors found elsewhere. Allen and Dahlin (1954) reported 2 such tumors.

Leiomyoma of the Stomach. This tumor probably is not only the most common benign tumor but also the most common tumor of the stomach. Meissner (1944) found an incidence of 46 per cent in 50 necropsies. Many of these tumors are small, and they rarely grow to a size that proves to be of clinical significance. As pointed out by Appleby (1950), those large enough to produce symptoms usually produce ulceration and hemorrhage, the latter sometimes sudden and severe. Many are discovered inadvertently on roentgen examination. Treatment includes removal, even when symptoms are absent, because the exact na-

ture of the tumor is uncertain until examined microscopically. If frozen sections reveal benign tissue, localized removal is permissible; if not, the treatment is as for leiomyosarcoma.

Leiomyoma of the duodenum is much rarer, but Campbell and Young (1954) collected 30 cases, including 2 of their own.

Lymphoid Tumors of the Stomach. Such tumors comprise about two thirds of all sarcomas of the stomach (q.v.) and are next to carcinoma, the most common gastric malignancy. In turn, about half the lymphoid tumors are true lymphosarcomas, the remainder being Hodgkin's disease, reticulum cell sarcoma and malignant lymphoma. In the present discussion, the lymphoid tumors are grouped together under the general term of lymphosarcoma. Approximately 2 per cent of malignant tumors of the stomach are in the group of lymphosarcomas. The average age is about the same as for carcinoma, and there is a preponderance of males of from 2:1 to 6:1. Since these tumors do not involve the gastric mucosa as much as does carcinoma, hemorrhage and secondary anemia are less common.

The life expectancy of patients with lymphosarcoma of the stomach is appreciably greater than for those with carcinoma. Surgical excision involving either subtotal or total gastrectomy, possibly combined with roentgen therapy, offers the best chance for prolonged survival. Snoddy (1952) recommended that roentgen therapy be used only when lymph nodes are involved and only postoperatively. He re-emphasized 2 important points: "Certainly some cases of lymphosarcoma of the stomach represent a solitary lesion which can be cured if adequately removed. Lymph node involvement reduces the chances of cure, but does not preclude the possibility of a 5-year survival."

Traumatic Perforation of the Stomach. Such perforation of the stomach, in the absence of other severe injury, is relatively rare. It can occur from overdistention (beer drinkers), accidental perforation from a gastroscope, and from stab and gunshot wounds. Perforation of the stomach should be considered not only in cases of upper abdominal but also in instances of lower thoracic trauma. The symptoms and signs include those of perforation of peptic ulcer, plus those of associated hemorrhage and other injury. Treatment by simple suture is usually adequate, although partial resection may be necessary.

Rupture of the stomach in the newborn infant is a special condition which, while rare, deserves more attention so that prompter treatment may be instituted. Vargas, Levin and Santulli (1955) collected 55 cases and added 11 of their own. In 30 cases in the over-all series, surgical repair had been attempted with 11 survivals (37%). No patients survived without operation. Gastric ulcer, muscle defects, sepsis and trauma were factors in the etiology. Prompt surgical repair offers the only hope for survival.

Polyadenoma en Nappe (*Polyadenomes en Nappe* of Menétrièr, 1888, giant hypertrophic gastritis, localized hypertrophic gastritis). This condition, first described by Menétrièr (1888) and recently clarified by Berne and Gibson (1949), is a rare but interesting condition. It is most likely a form of diffuse gastric neoplasm which may be an indication for subtotal or even total gastrectomy.

Polyps of the Stomach (*Polyadenomes Polypeux* of Menétrièr, 1888; gastric polyps). Polyps may be associated with similar lesions elsewhere in the intestinal tract or even in the urinary bladder. They are usually single but may be multiple and may undergo malignant change. Unlike polyps of the colon, there does not seem to be a hereditary factor, although they may be congenital or inflammatory. The incidence varies from 0.3 to 0.8 per cent in autopsy examinations and 1.6 per cent in gastroscopic examinations (Yarnis, Marshak and Friedman, 1952). Bleeding is a significant symptom. Achlorhydria and atrophic gastritis are quite common. Coincident hypertrophic gastritis is seldom present.

Treatment should include resection of the polyps with the underlying wall, at least down to the muscle, if the polyps are not too numerous. In localized cases of diffuse polyposis subtotal gastrectomy should be performed. Instances of diffuse polyposis which involve the entire stomach present a serious problem. There are no current conclusive data, such as there are for multiple polyposis of the colon, to help the surgeon reach the important decision as to whether or not he should do a total gastrectomy. Consequently, this serious decision must be reached separately in each individual case. If polyps are left behind, careful postoperative observations, including gastroscopy at frequent intervals, are mandatory.

Prolapse of Gastric Mucosa Through the Pylorus. Such prolapse was first described by Schmieden (1911). While it is agreed that severe degrees of prolapse will produce symptoms, there is some argument as to whether minor degrees of prolapse are of clinical significance. Peptic ulcer, polyps, and malignant change in polypoid gastric mucosa must be differentiated. Feldman, Morrison and Myers (1952) in a thorough review of the subject reported that the incidence of the condition is 1.8 per cent of patients subjected to upper gastro-intestinal roentgen studies. However, they concluded that "prolapse of the gastric mucosa is ordinarily a medical problem and in only the severe intractable cases and those with complications is surgery indicated." Medical treatment includes bland diet and particularly antispasmodics. If obstruction, hematemesis, severe pain or other complications exist, operation is indicated and includes gastrotomy, followed by removal of the prolapsed mucosa, or gastrojejunostomy, or often preferably gastric resection.

Sarcoidosis. Gastric sarcoidosis is rare. In most of the reported cases this condition is a part of the generalized disease. Pearce and Ehrlich (1955) pointed out that the gastric lesions of sarcoidosis may ulcerate secondarily (as in carcinoma), necessitating gastric resection for the complication of the ulcer.

Sarcoma of the Stomach. Such tumors, while rare, are more common than is generally realized. There are 2 chief classes of sarcoma: the leiomyosarcomas (possibly related to the benign leiomyomas) comprising about 1 per cent of all gastric malignancies, and the lymphomas (mainly lymphoid tumors including lymphosarcoma [q.v.], but also including some cases of Hodgkin's disease, comprising about 2 per cent of gastric malignancies. Eker and Efskind (1956) reported 21 personal cases of another rare malignant gastric tumor, namely, hemangio-endothelioma (1.2% of their resected malignant tumors). Thus, the total incidence of the sarcomas is about 3 per cent (Marshall, 1955). Usually, the diagnosis is not made before operation.

Treatment includes gastric resection. Postoperative roentgen treatment is not advised for leiomyosarcoma but is to be considered for lymphoma (q.v.). Marshall and Meissner (1950) reported that the over-all 5-year arrest rate in 41 cases of sarcoma of the stomach was 44 per cent as opposed to 27 per cent for carcinoma of the stomach. In the leiomyosarcoma group alone, the 5-year arrest rate is even better, 67 per cent.

Syphilis of the Stomach. This tertiary lesion, while never common, is becoming rarer. Males are affected about twice as frequently as females. Patients with gastric syphilis are apt to be 20 to 40 years of age. The onset of symptoms occurs on an average of 10 years after the primary lesion. The symptoms include epigastric pain, fullness and heaviness. The pain resembles that of peptic ulcer except that it lacks the periodicity and the relief by food of the latter. Pyloric obstruction, vomiting and emaciation may be present. The most common pathologic lesion is a broad, plaque-like, spongy thickening of the gastric wall, sometimes with superficial ulceration of the mucosa. The *sine qua non* of gastric syphilis is the importance of differentiating it from gastric cancer *before* definitive operation. The occurrence in a young age group, a positive serology, and the atypical nature of the lesion with the patient's emaciation being out of proportion to the anemia, and the size of the lesion to the general condition of the patient, all tend to indicate the presence of syphilis. A therapeutic test of antisyphilitic therapy may be helpful in those cases in which obstruction is not present.

Treatment includes a trial at medical therapy and the treatment of obstruction. Since syphilitic proliferative lesions tend to heal by cicatrization, gastroenterostomy is often necessary. Occasionally, gastric resection is required.

Tuberculosis of the Stomach. This rare condition usually is associated with advanced generalized tuberculosis of the intestinal tract in the presence of open pulmonary tuberculosis. Ulceration, usually on the posterior wall of the stomach near the pylorus, occasionally may reveal visible tubercles. Ulcers of the duodenum may lead to stenosis. Achlorhydria, palpable tumor and gastrointestinal hemorrhage are common. Differential diagnosis, particularly on the basis of the roentgenographic studies, should rule out ulcer or carcinoma.

Treatment includes a high protein diet, P.A.S., streptomycin, isoniazid and occasionally, if obstruction exists or the differentiation from carcinoma cannot be made, gastrojejunostomy or partial gastrectomy.

Volvulus of the Stomach. This condition, first described by Berti in 1866, probably is more frequent than is generally recognized. In all cases of upper abdominal symptoms, particularly when acute, and when a definite diagnosis cannot be made, volvulus should be considered, especially if the Borchardt-Lenormont triad of symptoms is present. This triad includes: (1) strong efforts to vomit without result, circumscribed epigastric pain, and impossibility of passing a stomach tube. Because of the excellent blood supply of the stomach, rotation up to 180° usually is tolerated without strangulation, often for prolonged periods of time, but more severe cases require urgent surgical reduction. The von Haberer (1912) classification of gastric volvulus is as follows:

TYPE A. MESENTERO-AXIAL. Rotation of the stomach from right to left or left to right about the long axis of the gastrohepatic omentum. In the series of Gottlieb and associates, all 3 cases of this type were idiopathic and also infracolic.

TYPE B. ORGANO-AXIAL. Rotation of the stomach upward around the long axis of the stomach, i.e., around the coronal plane. This is usually supracolic but rarely may be infracolic. In the series of 20 cases, reported by Gottlieb, Lefferts and Beranbaum (1954), 17 were of this type; and of these, 16 were supracolic. The organo-axial can be further divided into idiopathic and secondary, there being 6 and 11 cases, respectively, in the series cited. Among the causative factors in secondary organo-axial volvulus were eventration of the diaphragm (3), parahiatal hernia (3), ulcer or adhesions (3), diverticulitis coli (1), and carcinoma of the pancreas (1). (See Fig. 29-30.)

Because of the relationship of the colon, roentgen studies should include examination of this organ. Differentiation from "cascade stomach," a spastic deformity, is based on the following points: (1) one fluid level in cascade stomach, 2 in volvulus; (2) the greater curvature is uppermost only in volvulus; (3) only in volvulus does the greater curvature form a convex curve continuous with the duodenum;

and (4) in volvulus the cardia is apt to have a low position due to the rotation, whereas in cascade stomach it is in its normal position.

In general, the more common organo-axial type of volvulus of the stomach is seen in connection with parahiatal diaphragmatic hernia (see Chap. 40, Hernia), the so-called "upside-down stomach" being popularly associated with such a hernia. Treatment of chronic volvulus with symptoms includes removal of the causative factor and reposition of the stomach. If symptoms are not present, the decision will rest upon the size and the type of volvulus present. If acute symptoms are present, immediate operation is mandatory as advocated by Sawyer, Hammer and Fenton (1956).

Wounds of the Stomach. (See perforation, traumatic.)

Duodenum

Carcinoma of the Duodenum. Primary carcinoma of this organ is rare (about 0.04% of all autopsies). The condition was first described by Hamburger (1746). In 1932, Mateer and Hartman correlated the clinical and pathologic findings. The distribution of duodenal carcinoma is as follows: suprapapillary, 23 per cent; peripapillary, 59 per cent, and infrapapillary, 18 per cent. Brenner and Brown (1955) pointed out that while the older literature included ampullary carcinoma with duodenal carcinoma, they believe that the two are separate entities as regards mucosal origin (biliary versus duodenal) and clinical picture. Symptoms of duodenal carcinoma are those of high intestinal obstruction, hemorrhage, biliary obstruction and peptic ulcer-type symptoms. Roentgen examination reveals deformity or obstruction, but usually it is only at operation that the final diagnosis can be made. Metastases are frequent, and the results of operation are poor, resulting in only about 5 per cent 5-year arrests in those cases treated by resection. Burgerman, Baggenstoss and Cain (1956) recently reported 31 cases of primary malignant neoplasms of the duodenum, excluding those of the papilla of Vater. Barclay and Kent (1956) reported 8 similar cases. Sarcoma of the duodenum, while rare, is almost as frequent as carcinoma. Benign tumors of the duodenum are also rare

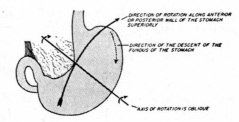

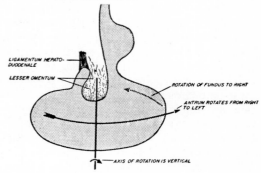

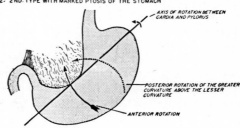

Fig. 29-30. Different types of volvulus of the stomach according to von Haberer classification. (A-1) Mesentero-axial volvulus with stomach in usual position. (A-2) Mesentero-axial volvulus with marked ptosis of the stomach. (B) Organo-axial volvulus with either anterior or posterior rotation of the greater curvature above the lesser curvature. (Gottlieb, C., Lefferts, D., and Beranbaum, S.: Am. J. Roentgenol. 72:611)

and include polyps, lipomas and heterotopic pancreas.

Cyst (Enterogenous) of the Duodenum. Enterogenous cysts of the duodenum are rare, 22 cases having been collected from the literature by Polson and Isaac (1953). Most of these cysts are believed to arise from a diverticulum with a constricted opening or from congenital abnormalities. Obstruction of the duodenum is a common symptom and requires excision.

Diverticula of the Duodenum. Two important points of discussion exist concerning such diverticula, namely, as to their true incidence and as to the proportion of them that should be treated surgically. Ackermann (1943) stated that the true incidence is far higher than the reported one, and that roentgenographic studies reveal only a small proportion of such abnormalities. Now it is recognized that primary duodenal diverticula of the pulsion type, as distinguished from diverticula secondary to traction of scarring, are found in 1 to 2 per cent of roentgenographic surveys and in 10 to 14 per cent of careful duodenal dissections. The true diverticula must be differentiated from the false or traction or scar diverticula of the upper duodenum, which most often evidence themselves by the clover-leaf deformity associated with duodenal ulcer.

True diverticula usually occur in the second portion of the duodenum, often are in the posterior wall in close association with the pancreas and the ampulla of Vater, and may produce diverticulitis. Blegen, Swanberg and Cox (1952) reported a case in which the common duct emptied into the diverticulum, which also was associated with a peptic ulcer, necessitating partial gastric resection with removal of the first and the second portions of the duodenum and reimplantation of the common duct.

If a diverticulum is asymptomatic, usually it should be left alone, although the rule of Zinninger (1953) may be applicable. This author stated that in addition to the rare cases of duodenal diverticula which cause symptoms, "in those instances in which the diverticulum is large and retains barium for 24 hours or longer and in which no other cause for the patient's symptoms can be demonstrated, operation for removal of the diverticulum is indicated." Invagination of the diverticulum into the duodenal lumen as advocated by Ferguson and Cameron (1947) may be advisable in some cases. If resection is elected, extreme care must be taken not to injure the closely associated biliary and pancreatic ducts and the duodenal blood supply.

In a series of 525 patients with a clinical diagnosis of duodenal diverticulum, 30 underwent surgical exploration of the upper abdomen as reported by Waugh and Johnston (1955). In only 8 of the explorations was the presence of the diverticula the basic reason for operation. Diverticulectomy was performed in 17 of these patients, and inversion of the diverticula in 2. Fewer than half of the surgically treated patients with adequate follow-up data were found to have relief of their symptoms. These authors concluded that, "Operative intervention is indicated in less than 1 to 2 per cent of the cases of duodenal diverticula noted on roentgenograms."

Duodenitis. Judd (1921) pointed out that in some patients thought to have a duodenal ulcer there is only a congestion and stippling of the serosal surface, a narrowing of the duodenum without scarring, or minute erosions of the mucosa or any of these 3 signs in combination. Such cases are thought to be chronic duodenitis, but an acute variety also has been described. The author does not dispute the existence of acute or chronic duodenitis but does believe that the majority actually represent various stages of the healing of a duodenal ulcer. In the past, most gastric resections have been performed by closing the duodenum over a clamp so that many surgeons do not see into the duodenum during this operation. When the open method of duodenal closure, or anastomosis, is used direct vision demonstrates small ulcer scars that otherwise might be missed.

Internal Duodenal Fistula. Such a fistula most commonly results from ulceration of a single large gallstone from the gallbladder into the duodenum. Cowley and Harkins (1943) reported that only 3 (12%) of the 25 cases of perforation of the gallbladder seen at the Henry Ford Hospital involved formation of a fistula into the bowel and, in turn, only 1 of these was into the duodenum. Such a fistula into the bowel is termed Class I perforation of the gallbladder according to the classification of Niemeier (1934). In such instances, of course, if the gallstone has not already passed the rectum, it may herald its presence by being impacted at the ileocecal valve with production of the classical syndrome of gallstone ileus (see Chap. 30, "Biliary Tract").

Duodenal ulcer occasionally may ulcerate into the biliary tract—usually the gallbladder —or into the colon, producing an internal fistula.

Treatment includes cholecystectomy, if this

organ is involved, with closure of the fistula and removal of the gallstone if still present.

External Duodenal Fistula. External duodenal fistulas are of two types: (1) the end type, in which there is leakage of duodenal contents from the duodenal stump following the different varieties of Billroth II gastric resections, and (2) the lateral type, in which there is no interruption of continuity of the duodenum, occurring usually after duodenotomy for exposure of the ampulla of Vater or other similar operations. Craighead and St. Raymond (1954) reported a 66 per cent mortality in the end type and only 40 per cent in the lateral type. Other authors have reported that the end type is less dangerous, probably because the peristalsis goes the other way in most of them. The average onset of the 2 types in Craighead and St. Raymond's series was 8 and 5 days respectively, after operation.

The end type of fistula should be treated prophylactically by utilizing a proper closure of the duodenal stump (see Fig. 29-24). As soon as a "blowout" is suspected, if an external fistula is not already present, the abdomen should be opened to permit reclosure of the stump, or secondary catheter drainage of the duodenum, or drainage of the perforation site. The first of these 3 measures is not often feasible; hence, one of the latter 2 usually must be adopted. In all cases of external duodenal fistula, whether end or lateral, the following measures should be adopted to keep the patient in as good general condition as possible. These measures include: (1) adequate fluids, electrolytes (including potassium), blood, protein and vitamins, (2) sump drainage and (3) jejunostomy feedings through a tube inserted either orally or abdominally. The fistula usually closes spontaneously in 3 weeks if the patient survives the 1st week and if there is no obstruction distal to the perforation.

Duodenal Ileus (Acute Arteriomesenteric Ileus). This syndrome usually is considered due to obstruction of the third portion of the duodenum where it passes around the superior mesenteric vessels. Because of the large volume of secretion of gastric juice, bile and pancreatic juice, vomiting is profuse and, unlike cases of pyloric obstruction, always contains bile. The head-down prone position may give relief, but if vomiting persists, a short-circuiting duodenojejunostomy should be performed as advised by Jones, Carter, Smith and Joergenson (1960).

Traumatic Perforation of the Duodenum. A special type of perforation, and the most common perforation of the duodenum, is that of the *retroperitoneal duodenum*. Such a perforation usually is the result of closed trauma—although it can result from penetrating wounds—and occurs at any point which is well fixed; i.e., the retroperitoneal duodenum, the jejunum where it crosses the spinal column just distal to the ligament of Treitz, and the lower ileum where it crosses the spine near its fixation to the cecum. Such fixed regions of the bowel are especially susceptible to transection or perforation because the organ cannot move in relation to the pressure exerted by the traumatic force. Such force may result from a steering wheel of an automobile. Diagnosis may be difficult because: (1) intestinal perforation may not have been considered in the list of possibilities; and (2) certain regions especially prone to perforate (retroperitoneal portion of the duodenum, Cottrell, 1954, and proximal jejunum) are in "blind" areas not readily visualized on exploration. (See also: Fistula, duodenal.) The diagnostic importance of retroperitoneal gas bubbles in the roentgenograms was emphasized by Rothchild and Hinshaw (1956). Treatment is surgical and is urgent.

Regional Enteritis Involving the Duodenum. The rare cephalad involvement of the small intestine by this disease has recently been emphasized. Segal and Serbin (1956) reported a case of their own and referred to 18 additional cases in the literature. Berk (1956) reported 3 cases. Treatment is more difficult than lower down in the small intestine because of the difficulties involved in either sidetracking or resection.

Duodenal Stasis (Chronic Duodenal Ileus). This condition may or may not be on an organic basis. In the latter instance therapy is usually unsatisfactory. The organic cases may be on the same basis as acute duodenal ileus. After thorough trial on medical management, treatment includes lysis of adhesions if present. Among the more definitive procedures, duodenojejunostomy is preferable to gastrojejunostomy.

BIBLIOGRAPHY

Ackermann, W.: Diverticula and variations of the duodenum, Ann. Surg. *117*:403-413, 1943.

Aird, I., Bentall, H. H., Mehigan, J. A., and Roberts, J. A. F.: The blood groups in relation to peptic ulceration and carcinoma of colon, rectum, breast, and bronchus: an association between the ABO groups and peptic ulceration, Brit. M.J. *2*:315-321, 1954.

Albright, H. L., and Kerr, R. C.: Primary hyperplasia of parathyroid glands: report of a case with coincident duodenal ulcer, J.A.M.A. *148*: 1218-1221, 1952.

Allen, J. G., and Oberhelman, H. A.: The problem of the bleeding peptic ulcer, Surgery *37*: 1019-1028, 1955.

Allen, R. A., and Dahlin, D. C.: Glomus tumor of the stomach, Proc. Staff Meet. Mayo Clin. *29*: 429-436, 1954.

Allison, P. R.: Reflux esophagitis, sliding hiatal hernia, and the anatomy of repair, Surg., Gynec. & Obst. *92*:419-431, 1951.

Allison, P. R., and Johnstone, A. S.: The oesophagus lined with gastric mucous membrane, Thorax *8*:87-101, 1953.

Amberg, J. R., and Rigler, L. G.: Results of surgery in carcinoma of the stomach discovered by periodic roentgen examination, Surgery *39*:760-775, 1956.

Appleby, L. H.: The outlook for patients with leiomyomas of the stomach, J. Internat. Coll. Surgeons *14*:512-516, 1950.

Arhelger, S. W., Lober, P. H., and Wangensteen, O. H.: Dissection of the hepatic pedicle and retropancreaticoduodenal areas for cancer of stomach, Surgery *38*:675-678, 1955.

Barclay, T. H. C., and Kent, H. P.: Primary carcinoma of the duodenum, Gastroenterology *30*: 432-446, 1956.

Barlow, T. E., Bentley, F. H., and Walder, D. N.: Arteries, veins, and arteriovenous anastomoses in the human stomach, Surg., Gynec. & Obst. *93*:657-671, 1951.

Barrett, N. R.: Chronic peptic ulcer of the oesophagus and "oesophagitis," Brit. J. Surg. *38*:175-182, 1950.

————: Hiatus hernia: a review of some controversial points, Brit. J. Surg. *42*:231-244, 1954.

Bauer, K. H.: Über das Wesen der Magenstrasse, Arch. klin. Chir. *124*:565-629, 1923.

Beal, J. M., and Hill, M. R., Jr.: An evaluation of the surgical treatment of carcinoma of the stomach, Surg., Gynec. & Obst. *102*:271-278, 1956.

Behrend, A., Katz, A. B., and Robertson, J. W.: Acute necrotizing gastritis, A.M.A. Arch. Surg. *69*:18-24, 1954.

Bell, L. G., Thomas, E. E., Jr., and Skillicorn, S. A.: Gastromalacia: a review and report of one case with recovery, Ann. Surg. *143*:106-111, 1956.

Bentley, F. H., and Barlow, T. E.: Stomach: vascular supply of in relation to gastric ulcer *in* Surgical Progress, 1952, London, Butterworth, 1953.

Beranbaum, S. L., Gottlieb, C., and Lefferts, D.: Gastric volvulus. III. secondary gastric volvulus, Am. J. Roentgenol. *72*:625-638, 1954.

Berk, M.: Regional enteritis involving the duodenum, Gastroenterology *30*:508-516, 1956.

Berkson, J., Walters, W., Gray, H. K., and Priestley, J. T.: Mortality and survival in cancer of the stomach: a statistical summary of the experience of the Mayo Clinic, Proc. Staff Meet. Mayo Clin. *27*:137-151, 1952.

Berman, E. J., Schneider, A., and Potts, W. J.: Importance of gastric mucosa in Meckel's diverticulum, J.A.M.A. *156*:6-7, 1954.

Berne, C. J., and Freedman, M. A.: Local recurrence following subtotal gastrectomy for carcinoma, Am. J. Surg. *82*:5-7, 1951.

Berne, C. J., and Gibson, W. R.: Giant hypertrophic gastritis, West. J. Surg. *57*:388-391, 1949.

Berti (1866): Cited by Gottlieb, Lefferts, and Berenbaum (see reference below), 1954.

Blegen, H. M., Swanberg, A. V., and Cox, W. B.: Entrance of common bile duct into duodenal diverticulum: report of a case corrected by surgery, J.A.M.A. *148*:195-197, 1952.

Bogardus, G. M., and Gustafson, I. J.: Gastroduodenal ulceration complicating other diseases, Surgery *39*:222-229, 1956.

Boman, K.: Tuberculosis occurring after gastrectomy, Acta chir. scandinav. *110*:451-457, 1956.

Booher, R. J., and Grant, R. N.: Eosinophilic granuloma of the stomach and small intestine, Surgery *30*:388-397, 1951.

Book, D. T., Chinn, A. B., and Beams, A. J.: Studies on pepsin secretion. II. Effect of vagal resection for duodenal ulcer, Gastroenterology *20*:458-463, 1952.

Bosher, L. H., Jr., and Taylor, F. H.: Heterotopic gastric mucosa in the esophagus with ulcer and stricture formation, J. Thoracic Surg. *21*:306-312, 1951.

Boyce, F. F.: Carcinoma of stomach; comparison of 3 series of surgical cases in large general hospital, J.A.M.A. *151*:15-20, 1953.

Boyden, A. M.: Radical gastrectomy for benign gastric ulcer, Surg., Gynec. & Obst. *97*:1-8, 1953.

Brackney, E. L., Campbell, G. S., and Wangensteen, O. H.: Role of antral exclusion in development of peptic stomal ulcer, Proc. Soc. Exper. Biol. & Med. *86*:273-277, 1954.

Brackney, E. L., Thal, A. P., and Wangensteen, O. H.: Role of duodenum in the control of gastric secretion, Proc. Soc. Exper. Biol. & Med. *88*:302-306, 1955.

Brenner, R. L., and Brown, C. H.: Primary carcinoma of the duodenum, Gastroenterology *29*: 189-198, 1955.

Brown, P. M., Cain, J. C., and Dockerty, M. B.: Clinically "benign" gastric ulcerations found to be malignant at operation, Surg., Gynec. & Obst. *112*:82-88, 1961.

Bruce, J., Card, W. I., Marks, I. N., and Sircus, W.: The rationale of selective surgery in the treatment of duodenal ulcer, J. Roy. Coll. Surgeons Edinburgh *4*:85-104, 1959.

Burgerman, A., Baggenstoss, A. H., and Cain, J. C.: Primary malignant neoplasms of the duodenum, excluding the papilla of Vater, Gastroenterology *30*:421-431, 1956.

Butler, T. J., and Capper, W. M.: Experimental study of 79 cases showing early post-gastrectomy syndrome, Brit. M.J. *1*:1177-1181, 1951.

Byrd, B. F., and Carlson, R. I.: Simple closure of peptic ulcer: a review of end results, Ann. Surg. *143*:708-713, 1956.

Cabieses, F., and Lecca, G. G.: Acute gastrointestinal hemorrhage in neurosurgical patients, Gastroenterology *29*:300-307, 1955.

Campbell, R. E., and Young, J. M.: Leiomyoma of the duodenum, Am. J. Surg. *88*:618-622, 1954.

Card, W. I., and Marks, I. N.: The relationship between the acid output of the stomach following "maximal" histamine stimulation and the parietal cell mass, Clin. Sci. *19*:147-163, 1960.

Carver, G. M., Jr., and Sealy, W. C.: Peptic esophagitis, A.M.A. Arch. Surg. *68*:286-295, 1954.

Chapman, N. D., Nyhus, L. M., and Harkins, H. N.: The mechanism of vagus influence on the hormonal phase of gastric acid secretion, Surgery *47*:722-724, 1960.

Clark, C. W.: Peptic ulcer of the second part of the duodenum, Ann. Surg. *143*:276-279, 1956.

Clarke, J. S., Ozeran, R. S., Hart, J. C., Cruze, K., and Crevling, V.: Peptic ulcer following portacaval shunt, Ann. Surg. *148*:551-566, 1958.

Code, C. F., and Varco, R. L.: Chronic histamine action, Proc. Soc. Exper. Biol. & Med. *44*:475-477, 1940.

Coller, F. A., Kay, E. B., and McIntyre, R. S.: Regional lymphatic metastases of carcinoma of the stomach, Arch. Surg. *43*:748-761, 1941.

Connar, R. C., and Sealy, W. C.: Gastrostomy and its complications, Ann. Surg. *143*:245-250, 1956.

Cottrell, J. C.: Nonperforative trauma to abdomen, A.M.A. Arch. Surg. *68*:241-251, 1954.

Cowley, L. L., and Harkins, H. N.: Perforation of the gallbladder: a study of 25 consecutive cases, Surg., Gynec. & Obst. *77*:661-668, 1943.

Craighead, C. C., and St. Raymond, A. H.: Duodenal fistula: with special reference to choledochoduodenal fistula complicating duodenal ulcer, Am. J. Surg. *87*:523-533, 1954.

Cushing, H.: Peptic ulcers and the interbrain, Surg., Gynec. & Obst. *45*:1-34, 1932.

Cutler, E. C., and Harrison, J. H.: Phlegmonous gastritis, Surg., Gynec. & Obst. *70*:234-240, 1940.

Day, J. J., and Webster, D. R.: The autoregulation of the gastric secretion, Am. J. Digest. Dis. *2*:527-531, 1935.

DeBakey, M., and Ochsner, A.: Bezoars and concretions, Surgery *4*:934-963, 1938; *5*:132-160, 1939.

Devine, H. B.: Basic principles and supreme difficulties in gastric surgery, Surg., Gynec. & Obst. *40*:1-16, 1925.

———: Gastric exclusion, Surg., Gynec. & Obst. *47*:239-243, 1928.

DeVito, R. V., Listerud, M. B., Nyhus, L. M., Merendino, K. A., and Harkins, H. N.: Hemorrhage as a complication of reflux esophagitis, Am. J. Surg. *98*:657-663, 1959.

Dolphin, J. A., Smith, L. A., and Waugh, J. M.: Multiple gastric ulcers: their occurrence in benign and malignant lesions, Gastroenterology *25*:202-205, 1953.

Dragstedt, L. R.: The etiology of gastric and duodenal ulcers, Postgrad. Med. *15*:99-103, 1954.

———: Gastric vagotomy in the treatment of peptic ulcer, Postgrad. Med. *10*:482-490, 1951.

———: Pathogenesis of gastroduodenal ulcer, Arch. Surg. *44*:438-451, 1942.

———: The role of the nervous system in the pathogenesis of duodenal ulcer, Surgery *34*: 902-903, 1953.

———: Sites of peptic ulceration, A.M.A. Arch. Surg. *70*:326-327, 1955.

———: Vagotomy for gastroduodenal ulcer, Ann. Surg. *122*:973-989, 1945.

Dragstedt, L. R., Kohatsu, S., Gwaltney, J., Nagano, K., and Greenlee, H.: Further studies on the question of an inhibitory hormone from the gastric antrum, A.M.A. Arch. Surg. *79*:10-21, 1959.

Dragstedt, L. R., Oberhelman, H. A., Jr., Evans, S. O., and Rigler, S. P.: Antrum hyperfunction and gastric ulcer, Ann. Surg. *140*:396-404, 1954.

Dragstedt, L. R., Oberhelman, H. A., Jr., and Smith, C. A.: Experimental hyperfunction of the gastric antrum with ulcer formation, Ann. Surg. *134*:332-341, 1951.

Dragstedt, L. R., and Owens, F. M., Jr.: Supradiaphragmatic section of vagus nerves in treatment of duodenal ulcer, Proc. Soc. Exper. Biol. & Med. *53*:152-154, 1943.

Dragstedt, L. R., Woodward, E. R., Storer, E. H., Oberhelman, H. A., Jr., and Smith, C. A.: Quantitative studies on the mechanism of gastric secretion in health and disease, Ann. Surg. *132*:626-640, 1950.

Dreiling, D. A., and Marshak, R. H.: Chronic duodenal obstruction from ingested fruit pits in patients with duodenal ulcer: report of 2 cases, A.M.A. Arch. Surg. *72*:411-414, 1956.

Dunn, H. L.: Vital statistics of the United States, 1953, vol. 2, Washington, U.S. Government Printing Office, 1955.

Editorial: The treatment of gastric ulcer, J.A.M.A. *154*:766-767, 1954.

Edkins, J. S.: The chemical mechanism of gastric secretion, J. Physiol. *34*:133-144, 1906.

Edwards, H. C.: Carcinoma of the stomach, Brit. M.J. *1*:973-990, 1950.

Eker, R.: Carcinomas of the stomach: investigation of the lymphatic spread from gastric carcinomas after total and partial gastrectomy, Acta chir. scandinav. *101*:112-126, 1951.

Eker, R., and Efskind, J.: Rare types of malignant gastric tumors. I. Hemangioendotheliomas, Acta path. et microbiol. scandinav. *38*:14-26, 1956.

Ellison, E. H.: Personal communication, October 30, 1955.

————: Personal communication, June 15, 1956.

————: Ulcerogenic tumor of the pancreas, Surgery *40*:147-170, 1956.

Elman, R., and Hartmann, A. F.: Spontaneous peptic ulcers of duodenum after continued loss of total pancreatic juice, Arch. Surg. *23*:1030-1040, 1931.

Everson, T. C.: Experimental comparison of protein and fat assimilation after Billroth II, Billroth I, and segmental types of subtotal gastrectomy, Surgery *36*:525-537, 1954.

Everson, T. C., and Allen, M. J.: Gastrojejunal ulceration, A.M.A. Arch. Surg. *69*:140, 1954.

Farmer, D. A., Burke, P. M., and Smithwick, R. H.: Observations upon peptic activity of the gastric contents in normal individuals and in patients with peptic ulceration, S. Forum *4*:316-325, 1954.

Farmer, D. A., Howe, C. W., Porell, W. J., and Smithwick, R. H.: The effect of various surgical procedures upon the acidity of the gastric contents of ulcer patients, Ann. Surg. *134*:319-331, 1951.

Farris, J. M., and Smith, G. K.: An evaluation of

temporary gastrostomy as a substitute for nasogastric suction, Ann. Surg. *144*:475-486, 1956.

Feldman, M., Morrison, S., and Myers, P.: The clinical evaluation of prolapse of the gastric mucosa into the duodenum, Gastroenterology *22*:80-102, 1952.

Ferguson, L. K., and Cameron, C. S., Jr.: Diverticula of the stomach and duodenum: treatment by invagination and suture, Surg., Gynec. & Obst. *84*:292-300, 1947.

Fieber, S. S.: Hypertrophic gastritis: report of 2 cases and analysis of 50 pathologically verified cases from the literature, Gastroenterology *28*:39-60, 1955.

Fisher, J. A., Taylor, W., and Cannon, J. A.: The dumping syndrome: correlations between its experimental production and clinical incidence, Surg., Gynec. & Obst. *100*:559-565, 1955.

Fletcher, D. G., and Harkins, H. N.: Acute peptic ulcer as a complication of major surgery, stress or trauma, Surgery *36*:212-226, 1954.

Fly, O. A., Jr., Dockerty, M. B., and Waugh, J. M.: Metastasis to the regional nodes of the splenic hilus from carcinoma of the stomach, Surg., Gynec. & Obst. *102*:279-286, 1956.

Fretheim, B.: Gastric carcinoma treated with abdominothoracic total gastrectomy, A.M.A. Arch. Surg. *71*:24-32, 1955.

Friesen, S. R.: The genesis of gastroduodenal ulcer following burns; an experimental study, Surgery *28*:123-158, 1950.

Gibbon, J. H., Jr., Nealon, T. F., and Greco, V. F.: A modification of Glassman's gastrostomy with results in 18 patients, Ann. Surg. *143*:838-844, 1956.

Gilbert, J. A. L., and Dunlop, D. M.: Hypoglycemia following partial gastrectomy, Brit. M.J. *2*:330-332, 1947.

Gillespie, I. E.: Influence of antral pH on gastric acid secretion in man, Gastroenterology *37*:164-168, 1959.

Gillespie, I. E., Clark, D. H., Kay, A. W., and Tankel, H. I.: Effect of antrectomy, vagotomy with gastrojejunostomy and antrectomy with vagotomy on the spontaneous and maximal gastric acid output in man, Gastroenterology *38*:361-367, 1960.

Glaessner, C. L.: Hyperglycemic shock, Rev. Gastroenterol. *7*:528-533, 1940.

Glassman, J. A.: A new aseptic double-valved tubogastrostomy, Surg., Gynec. & Obst. *68*:789-791, 1939.

Goligher, J. C., Moir, P. J., and Wrigley, J. H.: The Billroth-I and Polya operations for duodenal ulcer: a comparison, Lancet *1*:220-222, 1956.

Gottlieb, C., Lefferts, D., and Beranbaum, S. L.:

Gastric volvulus: Part I, Am. J. Roentgenol. *72*:609-615, 1954.

Gray, S. J., Benson, J. A., Jr., Reifenstein, R. W., and Spiro, H. M.: Chronic stress and peptic ulcer. I. Effect of corticotropin (ACTH) and cortisone on gastric secretion, J.A.M.A. *147*: 1529-1538, 1951.

Greengard, H., Atkinson, A. J., Grossman, M. I., and Ivy, A. C.: The effectiveness of parenterally administered "enterogastrone" in the prophylaxis of recurrences of experimental and clinical peptic ulcer: with a summary of 58 cases, Gastroenterology *7*:625-649, 1946.

Gregory, R. A., and Tracy, H. J.: Secretory responses of denervated gastric pouches, Am. J. Digest. Dis. *5*:308-323, 1960.

Griffith, C. A.: Gastric vagotomy vs. total vagotomy, A.M.A. Arch. Surg. *81*:781-788, 1960.

Griffith, C. A., and Harkins, H. N.: The role of Brunner's glands in the intrinsic resistance of the duodenum to acid-peptic digestion, Ann. Surg. *143*:160-172, 1956.

————: Partial gastric vagotomy: an experimental study, Gastroenterology *32*:96-102, 1957.

Griffiths, W. J.: The duodenum and the automatic control of gastric acidity, J. Physiol. *87*:34-40, 1936.

Gross, R. E.: The Surgery of Infancy and Childhood: Its Principles and Techniques, Philadelphia, Saunders, 1953.

Guiss, L. W., and Stewart, F. W.: Chronic atrophic gastritis and cancer of the stomach, Arch. Surg. *46*:823-843, 1943.

Haberer, von, H.: Volvulus des Magens bei Carcinoma, Deutsche Ztschr. Chir. *115*:497-532, 1912.

Hamburger, G. E. (1746): Cited by Brenner and Brown (see reference above), (1955).

Harkins, H. N.: Intussusception due to invaginated Meckel's diverticulum: report of 2 cases with a study of 160 cases collected from the literature, Ann. Surg. *98*:1070-1095, 1933.

————: The prevention of pyloric ligation-induced ulcers of the gastric lumen of rats by trans-abdominal vagotomy: a preliminary report, Bull. Johns Hopkins Hosp. *80*:174-176, 1947.

Harkins, H. N., and Hooker, D. H.: Vagotomy for peptic ulcer, Surgery *22*:239-245, 1947.

Harkins, H. N., and Nyhus, L. M.: A comparison of the Billroth I and Billroth II procedures: clinical and experimental studies, Bull. Soc. Internat. chir. *15*:111-118, 1956.

————: Surgery of the Stomach and Duodenum, Little, Brown, Boston, 1961.

Harkins, H. N., Jesseph, J. E., Stevenson, J. K., and Nyhus, L. M.: The "combined" operation for peptic ulcer, A.M.A. Arch. Surg. *80*:743-752, 1960.

Harkins, H. N., Schmitz, E. J., Harper, H. P., Sauvage, L. R., Moore, H. G., Jr., Storer, E. H., and Kanar, E. A.: A combined physiologic operation for peptic ulcer: (partial distal gastrectomy, vagotomy and gastroduodenostomy); a preliminary report, West. J. Surg. *61*:316-319, 1953.

Harkins, H. N., Schmitz, E. J., Nyhus, L. M., Kanar, E. A., Zech, R. K., and Griffith, C. A.: The Billroth I gastric resection: experimental studies and clinical observations on 291 cases, Ann. Surg. *140*:405-427, 1954.

Harrison, R. C., Lakey, W. H., and Hyde, H. A.: The production of an acid inhibitor by the gastric antrum, Ann. Surg. *144*:441-449, 1956.

Helsingen, N., and Hillestad, L.: Cancer development in the gastric stump after partial gastrectomy for ulcer, Ann. Surg. *143*:173-179, 1956.

Henley, F. A.: Gastrectomy with replacement—a preliminary communication; with an introduction by Rupert Vaughan Hudson, Brit. J. Surg. *40*:118-128, 1952.

Herrington, J. L., Jr., Classen, K. L., and Edwards, L. W.: Experiences with a Billroth I reconstruction following vagotomy and antrectomy for duodenal ulcer, Ann. Surg. *153*: 575-580, 1961.

Hertz, A. F.: The cause and treatment of certain unfavorable after-effects of gastro-enterostomy, Ann. Surg. *58*:466-472, 1913.

Hillemand, P., Patel, J., and Lataste, J.: A propos des diverticules gastriques, Presse méd. *63*: 1808-1810, 1955.

Hoag, E. W., Kiriluk, L. B., and Merendino, K. A.: Experiences with upper gastrectomy, its relationship to esophagitis with special reference to the esophagogastric junction and diaphragm, Am. J. Surg. *88*:44-45, 1954.

Hoerr, S. O.: Evaluation of vagotomy with gastroenterostomy performed for chronic duodenal ulcer, Surgery *38*:149-157, 1955.

————: A surgeon's classification of carcinoma of the stomach; preliminary report, Surg., Gynec. & Obst. *99*:281-286, 1954.

————: Carcinoma of the stomach, Am. J. Surg. *101*: 284-291, 1961.

Hoffman, V.: Klinische Krankheitsbilder nach Magenoperationen. I. Die nicht regulierte Sturzentleerung; II. Die nutritive Gastrojejunitis, München. med. Wchnschr. *86*:332-335, 1939.

Hollander, F.: The insulin test for the presence of intact nerve fibers after vagal operations for peptic ulcer, Gastroenterology *7*:607-614, 1946.

Holt, R. L., and Robinson, A. F.: The treatment

of duodenal ulcer by vagotomy and gastro-jejunostomy, Brit. J. Surg. *42*:494-502, 1955.

Hunnicut, A. J.: Replacing stomach after total gastrectomy with right ileocolon, A.M.A. Arch. Surg. *65*:1-11, 1952.

Hunt, C. J.: Subtotal versus total gastrectomy for gastric malignancy: with a discussion of the various technics advocated in the operation of total gastrectomy, West. J. Surg. *63*: 337-343, 1955.

Irvine, W. T., Duthie, H. L., Ritche, H. D., and Waton, N. G.: The liver's role in histamine absorption from the alimentary tract, Lancet *1*:1064-1068, 1959.

Irvine, W. T., Duthie, H. L.: and Waton, N. G.: Urinary output of free histamine after a meat meal, Lancet *1*:1061-1063, 1959.

Jackson, C.: Peptic ulcer of the esophagus, J.A.M.A. *92*:369-372, 1929.

Janowitz, H. D., and Crohn, B. B.: Hyperinsulinism and duodenal ulcer: a rare combination, Gastroenterology *17*:578-580, 1951.

Javid, H.: Nutrition in gastric surgery with particular reference to nitrogen and fat assimilation, Surgery *38*:641-651, 1955.

Johnson, H. D.: Associated gastric and duodenal ulcers, Surg., Gynec. & Obst. *102*:287-292, 1956.

Jones, F. A. (1955): Discussion of paper by Wolf, Marshak, Som and Winkelstein (see reference below), 1955.

————: Hematemesis and melena: with special reference to causation and to the factors influencing the mortality from bleeding peptic ulcers, Gastroenterology *30*:166-190, 1956.

Jones, F. A., and Doll, R.: Treatment and prognosis of acute perforated peptic ulcer, Brit. M.J. *1*:122-127, 1953.

Jones, S. A., Carter, R., Smith, L. L., and Joergenson, E. J.: Arteriomesenteric duodenal compression, Am. J. Surg. *100*:262-277, 1960.

Jones, T. W., and Harkins, H. N.: The mechanism of inhibition of gastric acid secretion by the duodenum, Gastroenterology *37*:81-86, 1959.

Jordan, G. L., Jr., and DeBakey, M. E.: The current management of acute gastroduodenal perforation: an analysis of 400 surgically treated cases, including 277 treated by immediate subtotal gastrectomy, Am. J. Surg. *101*:317-324, 1961.

Jordan, P. H., Jr., and Sand, B. F.: A study of the gastric antrum as an inhibitor of gastric juice production, Surgery *42*:40-49, 1957.

Judd, E. S.: Pathologic conditions of the duodenum, Lancet *41*:215-220, 1921.

Kanar, E. A., Nyhus, L. M., Olson, H. H., Schmitz, E. J., Scott, O. B., Stevenson, J. K., Jesseph, J. E., Sauvage, L. R., Finley, J. W., and Harkins, H. N.: The Billroth I subtotal

gastric resection: a follow-up report on 493 cases, A.M.A. Arch. Surg. *72*:991-1002, 1956.

Kelly, W. D., Cross, F. S., and Wangensteen, O. H.: The importance of the spatial relationship of the gastric antrum in the development of gastrojejunal ulcer in the dog, S. Forum *4*:339-345, 1954.

King, A. B., and Reganis, J. C.: Neurogenic erosions of the stomach and esophagus, Ann. Surg. *137*:236-244, 1953.

Kiriluk, L. B., and Merendino, K. A.: The comparative sensitivity of the mucosa of the various segments of the alimentary tract in the dog to acid-peptic action, Surgery *35*:547-566, 1954.

————: An experimental study of the buffering capacity of the contents of the upper small bowel, Surgery *35*:532-537, 1954. .

Kleiman, A., and Grant, A. R.: The role of K + in the pathogenesis and treatment of the postgastrectomy dumping syndrome, S. Forum *4*: 296-301, 1954.

Konjetzny, G. E.: Chronische Gastritis und Magenkrebs, Monatsschr. Krebsbekämpfung, pp. 65-78, 1934.

————: Eine besondere Form der chronischen hypertrophischen Gastritis unter dem klinischen und röntgenologischen Bilde des Carcinoms, Chirurg. *10*:260-268, 1938.

————: Ueber die Beziehungen der chronischen Gastritis mit ihren Folgeerscheinungen und des chronischen Magenulcus zur Entwicklung des Magenkrebses, Beitr. klin. Chir. *85*:455-519, 1913.

Lahey, F. H.: Total gastrectomy for all patients with operable cancer of the stomach, Surg., Gynec. & Obst. *90*:246-248, 1950.

Lahey, F. H., and Marshall, S. F.: Should total gastrectomy be employed in early carcinoma of the stomach?, Ann. Surg. *132*:540-565, 1950.

Lampert, E. G., Waugh, J. M., and Dockerty, M. B.: The incidence of malignancy in gastric ulcers believed preoperatively to be benign, Surg., Gynec. & Obst. *91*:673-679, 1950.

Landelius, E.: Results of partial and total gastrectomy in cancer of the stomach, Acta chir. scandinav. *96*:441-460, 1948.

Landry, R. M.: Gastroileostomy and gastrocolostomy, Surgery *30*:528-533, 1951.

Lefferts, D., Beranbaum, S. L., and Gottlieb, C.: Gastric volvulus. Part II. Idiopathic gastric volvulus, Am. J. Roentgenol. *72*:616-626, 1954.

Lewisohn, R.: The frequency of gastrojejunal ulcers, Surg., Gynec. & Obst. *40*:70-76, 1925.

Lillehei, C. W., Roth, F. E., and Wangensteen, O. H.: The role of stress in the etiology of peptic ulcer: experimental and clinical observations, S. Forum *2*:43-48, 1952.

McCune, W. S., Gusack, M., and Newman, W.: Eosinophilic gastroduodenitis with pyloric obstruction, Ann. Surg. *142*:510-518, 1955.

McGlone, F. B., and Robertson, D. W.: Diagnostic accuracy in gastric ulcer, Gastroenterology *25*:603-613, 1953.

Maciver, I. N., Smith, B. J., Tomlinson, B. E., and Whitby, J. D.: Rupture of the oesophagus associated with lesions of the central nervous system, Brit. J. Surg. *43*:505-512, 1956.

MacLean, L. D., Hamilton, W., and Murphy, T. O.: An evaluation of segmental gastric resection for the treatment of peptic ulcer, Surgery *34*:227-237, 1953.

MacLean, L. D., and Lillehei, R. C.: A comparative evaluation of tubular gastric resection, S. Forum *4*:285-291, 1954.

MacLean, L. D., Perry, J. F., Kelly, W. D., Mosser, D. G., Mannick, A., and Wangensteen, O. H.: Nutrition following subtotal gastrectomy of 4 types (Billroth I and II, segmental and tubular resections), Surgery *35*:705-718, 1954.

McNeer, G., Sunderland, D. A., McInnes, G., VandenBerg, H. J., and Lawrence, W.: A more thorough operation for gastric cancer, Cancer *4*:957-967, 1951.

Marshall, S. F.: Gastric tumors other than carcinoma, S. Clin. North America *35*:693-702, 1955.

————: The relation of gastric ulcer to carcinoma of the stomach, Ann. Surg. *137*:891-903, 1953.

Marshall, S. F., and Meissner, W. A.: Sarcoma of the stomach, Ann. Surg. *131*:824-837, 1950.

Mateer, J. G., and Hartman, F. W.: Primary carcinoma of the duodenum: clinical and pathologic aspects, with differential diagnosis, J.A.M.A. *99*:1853-1859, 1932.

Meissner, W. A.: Leiomyoma of the stomach, Arch. Path. *38*:207-209, 1944.

Menétrier, P.: Des polyadénomes gastriques et de leurs rapports avec le cancer de l'estomac, Arch. Physiol. Norm. et Path. *1*:32, 236, 1888. Cited by Yarnis, Marshak, and Friedman (see reference below), 1952.

Mersheimer, W. L., Glass, G. B. J., Speer, F. D., Winfield, J. M., and Boyd, L. J.: Gastric mucin—a chemical and histologic study following bilateral vagectomy, gastric resection and the combined procedure, Tr. Am. S. A. *70*:331-342, 1952.

Meyer, K. A., and Steigman, F.: The surgical treatment of corrosive gastritis, Surg., Gynec. & Obst. *79*:306-310, 1944.

Moffat, F., and Anderson, W.: Adenoma of Brunner's gland, Brit. J. Surg. *43*:106-107, 1955.

Moore, H. G., Jr., and Harkins, H. N.: The Billroth I Gastric Resection: With Particular Reference to the Surgery of Peptic Ulcer, Boston, Little, Brown & Co., 1954.

Moore, H. G., Jr., Harkins, H. N., and Merendino, K. A.: The treatment of perforated peptic ulcer by primary gastric resection, Surg., Gynec. & Obst. (Internat. Abstr. Surg.) *98*:105-123, 1954.

Morey, D. A. J., Means, R. L., and Hirsley, E. L.: Diospyrobezoar in the postgastrectomy stomach, A.M.A. Arch. Surg. *71*:946-948, 1955.

Morris, K. N.: Gastric mucosa within the oesophagus, Australian & New Zealand J. Surg. *25*:24-30, 1955.

Morson, B. C.: Carcinoma arising from areas of intestinal metaplasia in the gastric mucosa, Brit. J. Cancer *9*:377-385, 1955.

————: Intestinal metaplasia of the gastric mucosa, Brit. J. Cancer *9*:365-376, 1955.

Niemeier, O. W.: Acute free perforation of the gallbladder, Ann. Surg. *99*:922-924, 1934.

Notkin, L. J.: Carcinoma occurring on the basis of pre-existing gastric ulcer, Canad. M.A.J. *72*:288-296, 1955.

Nyhus, L. M.: Uropepsin excretion: its relation to duodenal ulcer disease in diagnosis and therapy, Surgery *41*:406-415, 1957.

————: The role of the antrum in the surgical treatment of peptic ulcer, Gastroenterology *38*:21-25, 1960.

Nyhus, L. M., Chapman, N. D., DeVito, R. V., and Harkins, H. N.: The control of gastrin release: an experimental study illustrating a new concept, Gastroenterology *39*:582-589, 1960.

Nyhus, L. M., Stevenson, J. K., Jones, T. W., DeVito, R. V., and Harkins, H. N.: Jejunal gastrostomy, Bull. Soc. Internat. de Chir. *17*:254-259, 1958.

Oberhelman, H. A., Jr., Nelsen, T. S., Johnson, A. N., Jr., and Dragstedt, L. R., II.: Ulcerogenic tumors of the duodenum, Ann. Surg. *153*:214-227, 1961.

Oberhelman, H. A., Jr., Rigler, S. P., and Dragstedt, L. R.: Significance of innervation in the function of the gastric antrum, Am. J. Physiol. *190*:391-395, 1957.

Oberhelman, H. A., Jr., Woodward, E. R., Zubiran, J. M., and Dragstedt, L. R.: Physiology of the gastric antrum, Am. J. Physiol. *169*:738-748, 1952.

O'Leary, C. M.: Diospyrobezoar: a review of 14 cases with an analysis of 46 collected cases from the literature, A.M.A. Arch. Surg. *66*:857-868, 1953.

Olsson, O., and Endresen, R.: Ulcer cancer of the stomach, Act. chir. scandinav. *111*:16-21, 1956.

Ordahl, N. B., Ross, F. P., and Baker, D. V., Jr.: The failure of partial gastrectomy with gastroduodenostomy in the treatment of duodenal ulcer, Surgery 38:158-168, 1955.

Owren, P. A.: The pathogenesis and treatment of iron deficiency anemia after partial gastrectomy, Acta chir. scandinav. 104:206-214, 1952.

Palmer, E. D.: Benign intramural tumors of the stomach: a review with special reference to gross pathology, Medicine 30:81-181, 1951.

————: Further observations on postoperative gastritis: histopathologic aspects with a note on jejunitis, Gastroenterology 25:405-415, 1953.

Palmer, W. L.: Certain aspects of benign and malignant gastric ulcer, Bull. New York Acad. Med. 26:527-537, 1950.

Pavlov, I. P.: The Work of the Digestive Glands, p. 54, London, Griffin, 1910.

Pearce, J., and Ehrlich, A.: Gastric sarcoidosis, Ann. Surg. 141:115-119, 1955.

Peters, R. M., and Womack, N. A.: Hemodynamics of gastric secretion, Ann. Surg. 148:537-550, 1958.

Pincus, I. J., Thomas, J. E., and Rehfuss, M. E.: A study of gastric secretion as influenced by changes in duodenal acidity, Proc. Soc. Exper. Biol. & Med. 51:367-368, 1942.

Plenk, H. P., and Lin, R. K.: Gastric ulcer and gastric carcinoma: a correlative study, Am. Surgeon 20:348-354, 1954.

Polson, R. A., and Isaac, J. E.: Enterogenous cyst of the duodenum, Gastroenterology 25:431-434, 1953.

Porter, R. W., Movius, H. J., and French, J. D.: Hypothalamic influences on hydrochloric acid secretion of the stomach, Surgery, 33:875-880, 1953.

Poth, E. J., Manhoff, L. J., and deLoach, A. W.: The relation of pancreatic secretion to peptic ulcer formation: effect of pancreatectomy, ligation of pancreatic ducts, and diabetes on the production of histamine-induced ulcers in dogs, Surgery 24:62-69, 1948.

Poth, E. J., Fromm, S. M., De Young, R., and Aldridge, M.: The relation of pancreatic secretion to peptic ulcer: II. effect of hypoglycemia with and without pancreatectomy, Proc. Soc. Exper. Biol. & Med. 74:514-518, 1950.

Poth, E. J., and Fromm, S. M.: The relation of pancreatic secretion to peptic ulcer formation: III. the influence of the hyperglycemic-glycogenolytic factor, Gastroenterology 16:490-494, 1950.

Ransom, H. K.: Cancer of the stomach, Surg., Gynec. & Obst. 96:275-287, 1953.

————: Cancer of the stomach: a report on cases treated by total gastrectomy, Gastroenterology 30:191-207, 1956.

————: Subtotal gastrectomy for gastric ulcer:

a study of end results, Ann. Surg. 126:633-652, 1947.

Risholm, L.: Acute upper alimentary tract ulceration and haemorrhage following surgery or traumatic lesions, Acta chir. scandinav. 110:275-283, 1956.

Roberts, K. E., Randall, H. T., and Farr, H. W.: Acute alterations in blood volume, plasma electrolytes, and electrocardiagram produced by oral administration of hypertonic solutions to gastrectomized patients, S. Forum 4:301-306, 1954.

Robinson, A. W., Black, B. M., Sprague, R. G., and Tillisch, J. H.: Hyperparathyroidism due to diffuse primary hyperplasia and hypertrophy of the parathyroid glands: report of a case, Proc. Staff Meet. Mayo Clin. 26:441-446, 1951.

Rogers, H. M., Keating, F. R., Morlock, C. G., and Barker, N. W.: Primary hypertrophy and hyperplasia of the parathyroid glands associated with duodenal ulcer, Arch. Int. Med. 79:307-321, 1947.

Rokitansky, C. (1846): Cited by Cushing (see reference above), 1932.

Rothchild, T. P. E., and Hinshaw, A. H.: Retroperitoneal rupture of the duodenum caused by blunt trauma; with a case report, Ann. Surg. 143:269-275, 1956.

Rowe, C. R., Jr., Grimson, K. S., and Flowe, B. H.: Comparison of insulin and gastrometric tests for completeness of vagotomy, S. Forum 3:1-5, 1953.

Rubin, C. E., and Benditt, E. P.: A simplified technique using chymotrypsin lavage for the cytological diagnosis of gastric cancer, Cancer 8:1137-1141, 1955.

Sachs, L. J., and Angrist, A.: Phlegmonous gastritis as a manifestation of sepsis, Ann. Int. Med. 22:563-584, 1945.

Sauvage, L. R., Schmitz, E. J., Storer, E. H., Kanar, E. A., Smith, F. R., and Harkins, H. N.: The relation between the physiologic stimulatory mechanisms of gastric secretion and the incidence of peptic ulceration: an experimental study employing a new preparation, Surg., Gynec. & Obst. 96:127-142, 1953.

Sawyer, K. C., Hammer, R. W., and Fenton, W. C.: Gastric volvulus as a cause of obstruction, A.M.A. Arch Surg. 72:764-772, 1956.

Schaberg, A., Hildes, J. A., and Alcock, A. J. W.: Upper gastrointestinal lesions in acute bulbar poliomyelitis, Gastroenterology 27:838-848, 1954.

Schell, R. F., Dockerty, M. B., and Comfort, M. W.: Carcinoma of the stomach associated with pernicious anemia: a clinical and pathologic study, Surg., Gynec. & Obst. 98:710-720, 1954.

Schirmer, J. F., and Bowers, W. F.: Operation for duodenal ulcer after inadequate surgery, A.M.A. Arch. Surg. 71:80-90, 1955.

Schmieden, V.: Die Differentialdiagnose zwischen Magengeschwür und Magenkrebs; die pathologische Anatomie dieser Erkrankungen in Beziehung zu ihrer Darstellung im Röntgenbilde, Arch. klin. Chir. 96:253-344, 1911.

Schridde, H.: Über Magenschleimhaut-Inseln vom Bau der Cardialdrüsenzone und Fundusdrüsenregion und den unteren, oesophagealen Cardialdrüsen gleichende Drüsen im obersten Oesophagusabschnitt, Virchows Arch. path. Anat. 175:1-16, 1904.

Seeley, S. F., and Campbell, D.: Nonoperative treatment of perforated peptic ulcer: a further report, Surg. Gynec. & Obst. (Internat. Abstr. Surg.) 102:435-446, 1956.

Segal, G., and Serbin, R.: Regional enteritis involving the duodenum, Gastroenterology 30:503-507, 1956.

Shahon, D. B., Horowitz, S., and Kelly, W. D.: Cancer of the stomach: an analysis of 1152 cases, Surgery 39:204-221, 1956.

Shapira, D., Morgenstern, L., and State, D.: Critical examination of the "acid-inhibition" phenomenon in dogs with twin antrum pouches, S. Forum 10:143, 1960.

Shay, H.: Stress and gastric secretion, Gastroenterology 26:316-319, 1954.

Sherman, J. L., and Newman, S.: Functioning arteriovenous anastomoses in the stomach and duodenum, Am. J. Physiol. 179:279-281, 1954.

Sircus, W.: Studies on the mechanisms in the duodenum inhibiting gastric secretion, Quart. J. Exper. Physiol. 43:114-133, 1958.

Smith, W. H.: Potassium lack in the postgastrectomy dumping syndrome, Lancet 2:745-749, 1951.

Smith, W. O., DuVal, M. K., Joel, W., and Wolf, S.: The experimental production of atrophic gastritis using a preparation of human gastric juice, Surgery 46:76-82, 1959.

Smith, W. O., DuVal, M. K., Joel, W., Hanska, W. L., and Wolf, S.: Gastric atrophy in dogs induced by administration of normal human gastric juice, Gastroenterology 39:55-61, 1960.

Snoddy, W. T.: Primary lymphosarcoma of the stomach, Gastroenterology 20:537-553, 1952.

Sokolov, A. P. (1904): Cited by Brackney, Thal, and Wangensteen (see reference above), 1955.

Stammers, F. A. R.: The complications of partial gastrectomy, Ann. Roy. Coll. Surgeons England 17:373-385, 1955.

State, D., Katz, A., Kaplan, R. S., Herman, B., Morgenstern, L., and Knight, I. A.: The role of the pyloric antrum in experimentally induced peptic ulceration in dogs, Surgery 38:143-148, 1955.

Stewart, J. D., Sanderson, G. M., and Wiles, C. E., Jr., Blood replacement and gastric resection for massively bleeding peptic ulcer, Ann. Surg. 136:742-748, 1952.

Stock, F. E., Hui, K. K. L., and Tinckler, L. F.: Vagotomy and pylorectomy in the treatment of duodenal ulceration, Surg., Gynec. & Obst. 102:358-368, 1956.

Storer, E. H., Schmitz, E. J., Sauvage, L. R., Kanar, E. A., Diessner, C. H., and Harkins, H. N.: Gastric secretion in Heidenhain pouches following section of vagus nerves to main stomach, Proc. Soc. Exper. Biol. & Med. 80:325-327, 1952.

Strøm, R.: A case of peptic ulcer and insuloma, Acta chir. scandinav. 104:252-260, 1952.

Swynnerton, B. F., and Tanner, N. C.: Chronic gastric ulcer: a comparison between a gastroscopically controlled series treated medically and a series treated by surgery, Brit. M.J. 2:841-847, 1953.

Tanner, N. C.: Cited by Allen and Oberhelman (see reference above), 1955.

————: The indications for surgery in peptic ulcer, Edinburgh M.J. 58:261-278, 1951.

————: Non-malignant affections of the upper stomach, Ann. Roy. Coll. Surgeons England 10:45-60, 1952.

————: Surgery of peptic ulceration and its complications, Postgrad. M.J. 30:448-465, 523-531, 577-592, 1954.

————: The treatment of carcinoma of the stomach, Ann. Roy. Coll. Surgeons England 17:102-113, 1955.

Thein, M. P., and Schofield, B.: Release of gastrin from the pyloric antrum following vagal stimulation by sham feeding in dogs, J. Physiol. 148:291-305, 1959.

Thompson, J. C., and Peskin, G. W.: The gastric antrum in the operative treatment of duodenal ulcer, Surg., Gynec. & Obst. (Intern. Abst. Surg.) 112:205-227, 1961.

Thompson, J. E.: Stomal ulceration after gastric surgery, Ann. Surg. 143:697-707, 1956.

Traut, H. F., Rosenthal, M., Harrison, J. T., Farber, S. M., and Grimes, O. F.: Evaluation of mucolytic agents in gastric cytologic studies, S. Forum 3:28-33, 1953.

Vargas, L. L., Levin, S. M., and Santulli, T. V.: Rupture of the stomach in the newborn infant, Surg., Gynec. & Obst. 101:417-424, 1955.

Villarreal, R., Ganong, W. F., and Gray, S. J.: Effect of adrenocorticotrophic hormone upon the gastric secretion of hydrochloric acid, pepsin and electrolytes in the dog. Am. J. Physiol. 183:485-492, 1955.

Waldeyer, W. (1908): Cited by Bauer (see reference above), 1923.

Walker, J. M., Roberts, K. E., Medwid, A., and Randall, H. T.: The significance of the dumping syndrome, A.M.A. Arch. Surg. *71*:543-550, 1955.

Wallensten, S.: The relation between sideropenia and anemia and the occurrence of postcibal symptoms following partial gastrectomy for peptic ulcer, Surgery *38*:289-297, 1955.

Walters, W., Chance, D. P., and Berkson, J.: The surgical treatment of gastrojejunal ulceration, A.M.A. Arch. Surg. *70*:826-832, 1955.

Wangensteen, O. H.: Cancer of the Esophagus and the Stomach, New York, Am. Cancer Soc., 1951.

————: Evolution and evaluation of an acceptable operation for peptic ulcer, Rev. Gastroenterol. *20*:611-626, 1953.

————: Segmental gastric resection for peptic ulcer, J.A.M.A. *149*:18-23, 1952.

————: The surgical treatment of peptic ulcer, J. Iowa M. Soc. *44*:356-373, 1954.

Waugh, J. M.: Quart. Rev. Surg. *13*:18, 1956.

Waugh, J. M., and Hood, R. T., Jr.: Gastric operations: an historic review, Quart. Rev. Surg. *10*:201-214, 1953; *11*:1-18, 1954.

Waugh, J. M., and Johnston, E. V.: Primary diverticula of the duodenum, Ann. Surg. *141*:193-200, 1955.

Wechsler, R. L., Roth, J. L. A., and Bockus, H. L.: The use of serial blood volumes and head-up tilts as important indicators of therapy in patients with bleeding from the gastrointestinal tract, Gastroenterology *30*:221-231, 1956.

Weinberg, J.: Personal communication, April 4, 1953.

Welch, C. E., and Allen, A. W.: Gastric ulcer: a study of the Massachusetts General Hospital cases during the ten-year period, 1938-1947, New England J. Med. *240*:276-283, 1949.

Winkelstein, A.: Peptic esophagitis: a new clinical entity, J.A.M.A. *104*:906-909, 1935.

Wolf, B. S., Marshak, R. H., Som, M. L., and Winkelstein, A.: Peptic esophagitis, peptic ulcer of the esophagus and marginal esophagogastric ulceration, Gastroenterology *29*:744-766, 1955.

Woodruff, J. F.: Personal communication, March 29, 1961.

Woodward, E. R., Desser, P. L., and Gasster, M.: Surgical treatment of the postgastrectomy dumping syndrome, West. J. Surg. *63*:567-573, 1955.

Woodward, E. R., Robertson, C., Fried, W., and Schapiro, H.: Further studies on the isolated gastric antrum, Gastroenterology *32*:868-877, 1957.

Woodward, E. R., Trumbull, W. E., Schapiro, H., and Towne, L.: Does the gastric antrum elaborate on antisecretory hormone, Am. J. Digest. Dis. *3*:204-213, 1958.

Wright, J. T., Grant, A., and Jennings, D.: A duodenal-ulcer family, Lancet *2*:1314-1318, 1955.

Yarnis, H., Marshak, R. H., and Friedman, A. I.: Gastric polyps, J.A.M.A. *148*:1088-1094, 1952.

Zeldis, A. M., and Klinger, J. R.: Sindrome postgastrectomia, Rev. méd. Valparaiso *4*:311, 1951 *in* Surg., Gynec. & Obst. (Internat. Abstr. Surg.) *94*:546, 1952.

Zinninger, M. M.: Diverticula of the duodenum: indications for and technique of surgical treatment, A.M.A. Arch. Surg. *66*:846-856, 1953.

————: Extension of gastric cancer in the intramural lymphatics and its relation to gastrectomy, Am. Surgeon *20*:920-927, 1954.

Zollinger, R. M., and Ellison, E. H.: Nutrition after gastric operations, J.A.M.A. *154*:811-814, 1954.

————: Primary peptic ulcerations of the jejunum associated with islet cell tumors of the pancreas, Ann. Surg. *142*:709-728, 1955.

Zollinger, R. M., and Williams, R. D.: Considerations in surgical treatment for duodenal ulcer, J.A.M.A. *160*:367-373, 1956.

Zubiran, J. M., Kark, A. E., Montalbetti, A. J., Morel, C. J. L., and Dragstedt, L. R.: Peptic ulcer and the adrenal stress syndrome, A.M.A. Arch. Surg. *65*:809-815, 1952.

JONATHAN E. RHOADS

CHAPTER 30

Liver, Gallbladder and Bile Passages

Surgery of the biliary tract includes the problems of the gallbladder and the extra-hepatic biliary ducts, and these will be considered first in this chapter. The surgeon should know the anatomic relationships between the gallbladder, the cystic duct, the common hepatic duct, the common bile duct, the portal vein, the hepatic artery and its branches, including the cystic artery, as they normally occur. He will require also an appreciation of the variability of these structures and their interrelationships and should bear in mind at least the more dangerous of the common anomalies which are illustrated in Figure 30-1. Many of the surgical catastrophies which have occurred during endeavors to benefit the patient with biliary tract symptoms have resulted from ignorance of or failure to recognize such anomalies.

He will also need to know the signs and symptoms of acute cholecystitis, the indications for immediate and delayed operation, and the basis on which a decision is made as to whether to do a cholecystectomy or merely to drain the gallbladder (cholecystostomy).

In the nonacute cases, he must learn the even more difficult problem of assessing the various signs and symptoms of cholelithiasis with chronic cholecystitis. Here, he needs to gain a practical knowledge of the uses of cholecystography and biliary drainage and of other laboratory aids in diagnosis. It is also of major importance for him to understand the accepted indications for opening and exploring the common bile duct (choledochostomy).

The jaundiced patient presents a complex problem in diagnosis which often calls for elaborate clinical and laboratory study and also requires as much knowledge as is available of liver physiology in order to assess the risks of operation and to prepare the patient as thoroughly as possible in order to diminish these risks. Biliary tract patients and especially those with common duct obstruction may be subject to certain special complications more or less peculiar to this field, such as the hemorrhagic tendency of obstructive jaundice (hypoprothrombinemia), liver shock, "pancreatic asthenia" and the hepatorenal syndrome.

The portion of this chapter devoted to the pathologic processes of the gallbladder and the extrahepatic bile ducts will be focused on these particular subjects. The surgery of the liver itself will be considered briefly, utilizing the material on liver physiology referred to in connection with obstructive jaundice.

It should be noted that there are two spe-

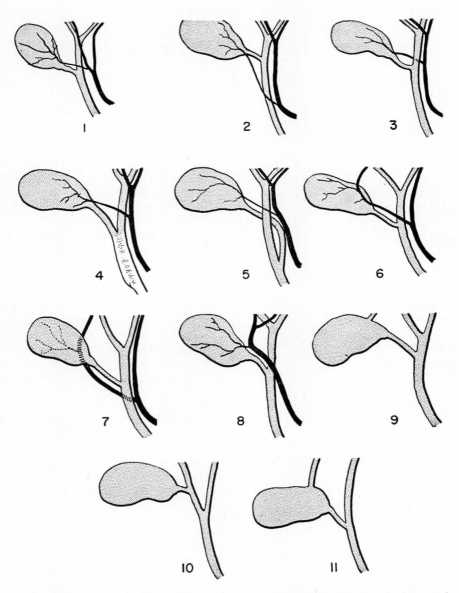

FIG. 30-1. Normal and anomalous arrangements of the extrahepatic bile ducts and their adjoining arteries.

1. Normal arrangement.

2. Caudad origin of cystic artery (frequent variation).

3. Placement of the cystic artery posterior to the common hepatic duct.

4. Long cystic duct attached to the common hepatic duct for some distance prior to the confluence to form the common bile duct.

5. Long cystic duct passing behind the common hepatic duct and joining it medially at a lower level.

6. Normal ductal system with anomalous right hepatic artery reaching the gall-bladder wall where it gives off the cystic artery and then turns into the liver. In this anomaly which is not rare, the right hepatic artery is often ligated either with the cystic duct or as a separate structure erroneously identified as the cystic artery.

7. Anomalous right hepatic artery in a posterior position presenting the same dangers as in No. 6.

(*Continued on facing page*)

cific hazards to the surgeon and members of his team who handle diseased gallbladders on the one hand and jaundiced patients on the other. The first is that of contracting typhoid fever, especially from adults who were alive before the decline in the incidence of this disease which occurred about 1910. The second is the danger of serum hepatitis in patients with jaundice. This disease may be contracted through any break in the skin.

The surgery of portal cirrhosis is considered in Chapter 33.

ANATOMIC CONSIDERATIONS

The common hepatic duct is formed by the union of the ducts draining the right and the left lobes of the liver. It runs from the transverse fissure of the liver inferiorly and posteriorly, lying in the right border of the lesser omentum. Here, it follows a course to the right of and anterior to the portal vein and also to the right of the hepatic artery. The duct is approximately 4 cm. long and is joined by the cystic duct to form the common bile duct.

The cystic duct runs a course of approximately 3.5 cm. from the neck of the gallbladder inferiorly, to the left, and posteriorly to enter the lesser omentum between the portal vein and the hepatic artery and finally to join the hepatic duct at an acute angle.

The common bile duct passes downward in the right border of the lesser omentum with the same relationships as the common hepatic duct. From here it passes behind the superior portion of the duodenum, entering the duodenum obliquely in its descending portion, and in over 50 per cent joining the pancreatic duct to form a terminal portion, the ampulla of Vater. The entrance from the ampulla to the duodenum is surrounded by a portion of the sphincter of Oddi which also surrounds the terminal pancreatic and the common bile ducts. Frequently, the common bile duct and the duct of Wirsung join to form a common channel for a significant distance before emptying into the duodenum. According to Howard and Jones (1947)[25], this amounted to 0.5 cm. or more in 17 per cent of cadavers, but they demonstrated reflux into the pancreatic duct of fluid injected into the common duct in 54 per cent of 150 cadavers.

The gallbladder is a pear-shaped sac, about 10 cm. in length, nestled against the inferior portion of the liver between the right and the quadrate lobes and covered with a layer of peritoneum which is reflected from Glisson's capsule. The gallbladder may be divided into 3 parts: the fundus, or superficial portion; the body; and the neck, or infundibulum, which joins the cystic duct. If the infundibulum has an abnormal sacculation, often it is referred to as Hartmann's pouch. Such a pouch may be adherent to surrounding structures, seriously obscuring important anatomic relationships at the time of dissection. The main arterial supply of the infundibulum is the cystic artery, which arises from the hepatic artery or the right branch of the hepatic artery. This may cross in front of, behind, or at some distance from the common duct to join the cystic duct and thus supply the gallbladder. (See Chap. 31, "Pancreas.")

Embryologically, the liver, the bile ducts and the gallbladder arise as a diverticulum from that portion of the gut which later becomes the second part of the duodenum. This diverticulum is lined by entoderm and grows upward and forward into a mesodermal mass called the *septum transversum*. Two solid

---

Fig. 30-1 (*Continued*)

8. A very dangerous anomaly of the entire hepatic artery which follows the cystic duct to the gallbladder before turning into the liver. Accidental ligation of the entire hepatic artery was almost always fatal before the development of penicillin and chlortetracycline and is still hazardous.

9. Anomalous bile duct entering gallbladder through its bed in the liver. Cholecystectomy in such instances is usually followed by profuse drainage of bile and is likely to result in fatal peritonitis unless external drainage is afforded.

10. Anomalous insertion of cystic duct into right hepatic duct. The section of the right hepatic duct caudad to its junction with the cystic duct can easily be mistaken for the cystic duct and ligated, thus shutting off the drainage of the right lobe of the liver into the intestine.

11. Anomalous arrangement of the right hepatic duct in which it enters the gallbladder so that all of the bile from the right lobe of the liver must drain through the cystic duct.

buds of cells then arise from it to form the right and the left lobes of the liver by growing into columns and cylinders called *hepatic cylinders*. They branch into a very fine network which invades the vitelline and the umbilical veins to form a series of tiny vessels called *sinusoids*. These capillarylike vessels ramify throughout the cellular network and finally develop into the venous capillaries of the liver. This growth and ramification continues until ultimately the mass of the liver is formed.

As this occurs, it gradually divides the ventral mesogastrium into 2 parts: the falciform and the coronary ligaments developing from the anterior part, and the lesser omentum from the posterior. By the 3rd month of embryonic life, the liver having differentiated from the septum transversum has grown downward and almost filled the abdominal cavity. The left lobe later degenerates somewhat and maintains a smaller size than the right lobe. Thereafter, the relative development of the liver is slower, but it maintains a relatively larger size during later fetal life and infancy than it does in the adult. At times, all or part of the extrahepatic biliary system fails to develop, which usually results in biliary atresia or agenesis. (See Chap. 46, "Pediatric Surgery," for this and other congenital anomalies of infants.)

PHYSIOLOGIC CONSIDERATIONS

The physiology of the liver parenchyma is so complex that a description of what is known about it could very readily fill several volumes. The liver has certain excretory functions. Beyond this, it is the central organ of intermediary metabolism. Despite its complex function, its cellular composition seems to be remarkably simple. In addition to its supporting stroma, capsule and 3 sets of blood vessels (portal vein, hepatic artery and hepatic vein systems), it has its excretory ductal system surrounded in the bile canaliculi only by the parenchymal liver cells which are the principal functional unit of the liver. The other cells of note are the reticuloendothelial cells situated in the vascular channels. These are not peculiar to the liver, but the liver is the site of the largest aggregation of them.

The liver also possesses an extensive and important lymphatic system. Among the substances which the liver excretes are the following: water, sodium, chloride, bicarbonate, calcium, bile pigments (bilirubin; biliverdin), bile salts (sodium taurocholate; sodium glycocholate), cholesterol, certain dyes (e.g., bromsulphalein, when this is injected into the circulation; tetraiodophenolphthalein, whether injected or absorbed from the gastrointestinal tract); and alkaline phosphatase of intestinal origin.

When injured, the liver's excretion of bile salts declines first—probably because of interference with their formation. When excretion is impaired by obstruction of the ductal system; bilirubin and alkaline phosphatase levels both mount in the blood. The itching which is so characteristic of obstructive jaundice has been attributed to the retention of bile salts. The disappearance of bromsulphalein from the blood stream is retarded when this drug is given in test doses.

The liver is largely responsible for the reduction of amino acids to urea and glucose. It is an important site of the conversion of glucose to glycogen, the storage of glycogen, and of the conversion of glycogen to glucose. It is one of the sites in which fat is converted to fatty acids and glycerol, and vice versa. It is a site of formation of uric acid. It is the principal site of formation of albumen.

It is vital for at least two major components of the coagulation mechanism, as it is the principal site of formation of fibrinogen and of prothrombin. It is the site of conjugation of benzoic acid with glycine, which is the basis for the hippuric acid conjugation test of liver function. It is the site of hydrolysis of certain sugars, and this is the basis of the galactose tolerance test of liver function.

It is the organ that removes certain steroids from the blood, preventing an excess. Thus, when the liver is damaged by cirrhosis, estrogens accumulate in the blood of male subjects to a degree which often causes mammary hypertrophy. Hydrocortisone is continuously metabolized in the normal liver with reduction to biologically inactive compounds and conjugation with glucuronic acid. The effective half life of this compound is of the order of 80 minutes. In the presence of liver damage the rate of inactivation is retarded with the result that administration of hydrocortisone may produce symptoms suggestive of Cushing's disease in such patients.

It is an important site of destruction of various drugs—notably morphine and several barbituric acid derivatives, so that serial doses of these agents in usual amounts may result in an accumulation to toxic levels in subjects with damaged livers.

As physiologic investigation continues more and more activities have been found to be attributable to the liver. The foregoing is by no means a complete list of known actions of hepatic cells, and there is a strong probability that additional hepatic activity will be revealed in the future.

The reticuloendothelial cells are important in removing particulate matter, such as carbon particles (as when India ink is injected intravenously experimentally), bacteria, et cetera, from the blood stream. Thus, they have an important function in resistance to infection. They are specifically involved with the conversion of hemoglobin derived from old erythrocytes to bilirubin which is carried in the plasma conjugated with albumen to the hepatic parenchymal cells, where it is separated from albumen and excreted in the bile conjugated with glucuronides. They are the site of accumulation of heparin which may be released by peptone shock. It was formerly thought that this occurred following exposure of the whole body to ionizing radiation and accounted for some of the hemorrhagic tendency found in radiation victims. It is now believed that this is not a major factor in this clinical picture (Hewitt, 1953;[24] DiLuzio, 1957[15]).

This brief list is sufficient to show that an individual whose liver has been severely damaged by acute poisoning, such as chloroform, by acute infection, such as hepatitis, or by chronic damage as in various types of cirrhosis, is liable to many physiologic derangements. Especially important among these are hypoalbuminemia, hypoprothrombinemia, intermittent hypoglycemia—which at times has been falsely attributed to hyperinsulinism, and failure to detoxify drugs at the expected rate with consequent overdosage. It is clear that the liver is an essential organ and cannot be sacrificed.

At the same time it must be borne in mind constantly that the liver has a large margin of reserve function, so that in the experimental animal four fifths of it can be sacrificed with survival. Hepatic lymph is peculiar; it contains almost as high a concentration of serum albumen as does plasma.

Bile in a quantity of 350 to 1,000 ml. per day is secreted by the liver. With the sphincter of Oddi closed, pressure relationships exist whereby most of this bile flows to the gallbladder. As has been stated, hepatic bile consists mainly of water, cholesterol, bile pigments, inorganic salts and salts of bile acids. In the gallbladder, water with chlorides and bicarbonates is absorbed, increasing the relative concentration of bile pigments and bile salts. The concentrate is stored in the gallbladder until it is expelled.

When gastric chyme comes into contact with the duodenal mucosa, a hormone, *cholecystokinin*, is released which causes the gallbladder to contract and the sphincter of Oddi to relax, thus making bile available for digestion.

In pathologic states, such as cholecystitis, the gallbladder very often loses progressively its capacity to concentrate bile salts and bile pigment. Figure 30-2, taken from the paper of Riegel, Ravdin, Johnston, and Morrison (1936)[47], demonstrates this graphically.

In the presence of jaundice or of liver damage without jaundice, the composition of hepatic bile will be altered also (compare section on The Jaundiced Patient).

TUMORS OF THE GALLBLADDER AND THE EXTRAHEPATIC BILE DUCTS

Benign papillomas occasionally occur in the gallbladder. At times the roentgenologist can suggest the diagnosis on the basis of fixation of an isolated shadow seen on a cholecystogram. The malignant potential of such lesions is not accurately known. Their removal by cholecystectomy is recommended because of the possibility of malignant degeneration, the possibility that they may cause symptoms—perhaps by acting like a ball valve, and the considerable doubt that surrounds their diagnosis by roentgenography. A shadow suggestive of such a papilloma may turn out to be due to stone or, conceivably, to carcinoma.

Carcinoma is the only primary malignant tumor occurring in the gallbladder with any frequency. It occurred in 1.41 per cent of a series of 3,842 gallbladders removed at the Hospital of the University of Pennsylvania. The survival rate of patients who develop carcinoma of the gallbladder is pitifully low—under 5 per cent in most series. Those few who do survive are apt to be cases in which the malignancy was an unexpected pathologic finding.

Since 73 per cent of gallbladder carcinomas are associated with stones, it has been suggested that all gallbladders containing stones should be removed for cancer prophylaxis. Certain authors have reported a 5 per cent incidence of carcinoma of the gallbladder among stone-bearing gallbladders. We do not believe that such a figure is representative but would analyze the problem as follows:

1. The incidence of gallstones increases in autopsy material each decade.

2. The average age of death from gallbladder carcinoma is between 50 and 60 years.

3. The incidence of gallstones in this decade (50 to 60) is 21 per cent.

4. Autopsy studies reveal that the incidence of gallstones in the presence of gall-bladder carcinoma is 73 per cent, and the over-all in- cidence of gallbladder carcinoma in long series of autopsies is only 0.39 per cent.

Therefore, if 73 per cent of the carcinomas occur in the 21 per cent of patients who have stones, the incidence of gallbladder carcinoma among stone-bearers in their fifties is 1.42 per cent—not far different from the figure of 1.41 per cent actually found in our clinic at operation. Thus, it appears that the incidence of carcinoma is about as high among the asymptomatic stone-bearers as among those who come to operation.

The average expectation that a person aged 59 will live 5 years is 89 per cent (Life Insurance Fact Book, 1959)[32]. Those who have gallbladder carcinoma can expect to live 5 years in only about 3 per cent of instances. Therefore, the salvage from gallbladder carcinoma death would be the incidence, $1.42\% \times (89\% - 3\%) = 1.22\%$ per 100 stone-bearers cholecystectomized. If the operative mortality can be held down to 0.5 per cent, one can theoretically justify removing the gallbladders of all stone-bearers at about age 50. However, the margin is rather narrow and, if due to mischance the mortality should rise to 1.5 per cent, one would lose more patients that he saved by such a policy. (Campbell, 1941[10];

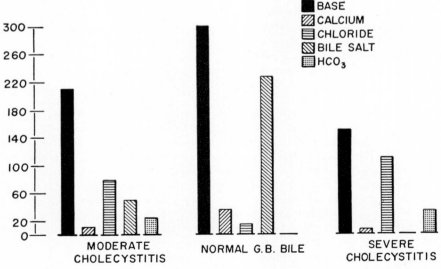

FIG. 30-2. Chemical differences in gallbladder bile from patients with moderate cholecystitis, patients with normal gallbladders, and patients with severe cholecystitis. Note particularly the profound diminution in bile salt concentration in the bile from diseased gallbladders. (Riegel, C., Ravdin, I., Johnston, C., and Morrison, P.: Surg., Gynec. & Obst. 62:933, 1936)

Cooper, 1937[13]; Illingworth, 1935[26]; Jankelson, 1937[27]; Kirshbaum, 1941[29]; Roberts, 1957[48]; Robertson, 1944[49]; Sainburg, 1948[50]; Sawyer, 1956[51]; and Swinton, 1948[52]).

The tumors of the common hepatic and common bile ducts are similar to those of the gallbladder. Benign papillomas occur but are rare. Carcinomas may produce early jaundice leading to operation and diagnosis. Those arising in the intrapancreatic portion of the common duct and the papilla of Vater may sometimes be saved and are discussed with the pancreatoduodenal carcinomas in Chapter 31. Those arising above the level of the duodenum have been uniformly fatal in the author's experience. Palliative relief of jaundice can sometimes be achieved by shunts of one type or another.

In a few instances, carcinoma of the gallbladder discovered at operation has been treated by right hepatic lobectomy as well as cholecystectomy and removal of lymph nodes about the common bile duct. This high risk procedure is not yet sufficiently well evolved to permit a recommendation but, at present, it seems doubtful if it will help to solve the problem of gallbladder carcinoma.

ACUTE CHOLECYSTITIS

Acute cholecystitis is a condition characterized by hyperemia, edema and polymorphonuclear cell infiltration and, in many instances, patchy or extensive necrosis of the mucosa of the gallbladder. Although the gallbladder is essentially a diverticulum of the main bile duct, an inflammatory process may not affect the other ducts in ways that are apparent. On the other hand, there is evidence in many cases that the inflammatory process does affect the biliary tract more widely. This is manifested by mild rises in serum bilirubin, typically 1.0 to 2.0 mg. per 100 ml. While stones usually are found in patients with acute cholecystitis, this is not always the case. Berk (1940,[7] 1946[6]) found calculi obstructing the neck of the gallbladder in 92 per cent of such cases. Acute cholecystitis can be produced experimentally in the goat by ligating the common channel formed by the common bile duct and the pancreatic duct, thus causing a retrograde flow of pancreatic juice into the gallbladder and stasis of bile (Bisgard, 1940[8]). Thus, it is postulated

that pancreatic ferments may contribute to an occasional case of acute cholecystitis in human patients.

Experimentally, Gatch (1946)[22] produced acute cholecystitis by injecting bile salts into the portal veins of dogs, increasing the concentration in the bile. The experimental production of cholecystitis seemingly has little relation to the clinical condition. Though infection often plays an important role in acute cholecystitis, this appears to be secondary to other factors such as stones. In addition to *Eberthella typhosa*, which characteristically gains access to the gallbladder and may persist there for many years, common bacteria found in this organ include *Escherichia coli*, other organisms of the coliform group, common pyogens, such as the streptococcus and the staphylococcus, and various representatives of the clostridium group.

SIGNS AND SYMPTOMS

The signs and symptoms of acute cholecystitis are usually rapid rather than sudden in onset. Fever and leukocytosis are well marked. Vomiting may be serious, leading to dehydration. Slight hyperbilirubinemia may be present. Local symptoms are striking; usually there is persistent pain in the right upper quadrant or the epigastrium. If the pain radiates to the back, in the region of the angle of the scapula or in the interscapular area, the diagnosis is strengthened. The pain is associated with tenderness commonly maximal just below the right costal margin. Rebound tenderness is often demonstrable and may be referred to the gallbladder area. Moderate to marked muscle spasm, generally more or less localized to the right upper quadrant, is the rule. Peristalsis diminishes somewhat; however, the sounds seldom cease for more than a minute or 2 unless the gallbladder ruptures. The gallbladder may be palpated in a third or more of the cases. Muscle spasm often prevents palpation; therefore, the gallbladder may become palpable for the first time after the attack has begun to subside or after anesthesia is induced.

While gallbladder pain is typically lateralized to the right, it may be bilateral or occasionally predominantly on the left side. The mechanism of this is not clear, but it is a fact to be reckoned with in diagnosis, as left-sided reference does not rule out the presence of an acute cholecystitis.

DIAGNOSIS

The diagnosis may be easy but at times can be confused with ruptured ulcer or necrotizing pancreatitis, which is often more severe, or with edematous pancreatitis, which frequently may coexist with cholecystitis.

Other conditions that may give rise to similar symptoms are acute appendicitis, coronary insufficiency with angina pectoris or coronary thrombosis, chronic passive congestion affecting the liver, pneumonia, pleurisy, renal colic, intestinal obstruction, tabetic crisis, lead colic, herpes zoster, phlegmonous gastritis, and gonococcal peritonitis with adhesions forming between the diaphragm and the liver (Curtis—Fitz–Hugh Syndrome). The diagnosis usually is confirmed at the operation if the symptoms do not improve fairly promptly, and by roentgenogram if improvement supervenes. Before operation an electrocardiogram and x-ray examination of the chest and the abdomen are frequently indicated.

After making the diagnosis, the decisions (1) when to operate and (2) whether to do a cholecystostomy (drainage of the gallbladder) or a cholecystectomy (removal of the gallbladder) have to be reached. If symptoms do not abate, complications may ensue, such as gangrene and perforation leading to internal biliary fistulas connecting with bowel or the common duct, pericholecystic abscess, or even spreading peritonitis, pylephlebitis (inflammation of the portal vein), cholangitis, pancreatitis, hepatitis or septicemia. In the acute case, edema and hyperemia are often so severe as to interfere seriously with safe dissection and exposure of the common duct and the cystic ducts. To insist on carrying out cholecystectomy under these circumstances is to risk injury to the main ductal system or the hepatic artery. Therefore, the safe surgeon sometimes will perform only a cholecystostomy when operating during the acute phase. A majority of these patients will require a second operation later for removal of the gallbladder. Donald and Fitts' follow-up study (1949)[16] indicates that it is wise to recommend elective cholecystectomy within several months in almost all patients having cholecystostomy. In general, three months is a suitable interval between a cholecystostomy and the subsequent cholecystectomy. Rarely, another acute attack will supervene within this period, but early reoperation is usually handicapped by the postoperative reaction to the first procedure.

PERFORATION OF THE GALLBLADDER WITH ABSCESS, PERITONITIS, OR BILIARY FISTULA

Rupture of the gallbladder is less frequent than rupture of the appendix. Nevertheless, it constitutes a grave hazard in acute cholecystitis, especially in elderly patients, and it is this danger that forces operation in a considerable number of poor-risk patients at times when they are acutely ill.

Rupture of the gallbladder is of 3 types: (1) it may rupture slowly into a previously prepared abscessed pocket—rupture with localized abscess; (2) it may rupture suddenly into the general peritoneal cavity—rupture into free peritoneal cavity; or (3) it may rupture slowly into an adjoining viscus attached by adhesions, especially the duodenum, the stomach or the colon—rupture with biliary fistula.

After rupture into the free peritoneal cavity, bile leakage through the cystic duct into the open gallbladder may lead to bile peritonitis. This is the only one of the 3 types of rupture of the gallbladder which causes bile peritonitis which, if untreated by early drainage, is apt to result in a fatal issue. Bile peritonitis is harmful not only because of infection but also because of the irritant action of the bile. This irritant action leads to shock due to plasma leakage from the peritoneal surfaces (see Chap. 7, "Shock") and also to fat necrosis due either to damage to the pancreas or to reflux of pancreatic enzymes (see Chap. 31, "Pancreas").

The third type of rupture of the gallbladder (rupture with biliary fistula) may lead to the interesting syndrome of gallstone ileus (see Chap. 36, "Intestinal Obstruction") if a large gallbladder stone passes through the fistula into the upper intestinal tract and then becomes impacted in the narrow lower ileum.

In modern hospital practice 2 per cent of the patients operated upon for disease of the biliary tract have rupture of the gallbladder, while the incidence rises to 10 per cent in cases of acute cholecystitis. The mortality rate among the patients with all types of gallbladder perforation averages about 20 per cent. The mortality for the type of perforation with localized abscess is usually less than this over-all figure. On the other hand, perforation with biliary fistula has a relatively low immediate mortality, but when the mortality of operations for cure of the fistula is included, the total mortality for cases with biliary fistula rises toward that for free perforation. References on incidence and mortality of gallbladder rupture which have been added to the bibliography are: (Stevenson, 1957[53]; Fletcher, 1951[19]; Pines, 1954[43]; Cowley, 1943[14]; Massie, 1957[37]; McCubbrey, 1960[33]; Becker, 1957[4]; and Morse, 1957[38]).

DIAGNOSIS

Typically, the attack of free perforation is similar to other attacks of acute gallbladder disease, but instead of subsiding, the acute symptoms spread—usually after 24 hours—and the local and systemic signs of peritonitis supervene. Unfortunately, the complication is prone to occur in elderly and debilitated persons and often is not attended by the amount of fever and/or leukocytosis which would be expected in a typical case of peritonitis. For this reason, persons over the age of 65 or persons who are weak and debilitated at any age should, in general, be operated on for an acute gallbladder attack if it persists over 24 hours without clear evidence that it is subsiding.

Unfortunately, not all cases of gallbladder perforation are preceded by sufficiently characteristic symptoms to lead to the diagnosis. In fact, some patients who develop fistulae into the intestine may seek medical advice only after the stone has passed down the intestine and caused an obstruction.

The diagnosis of biliary fistula can often be made preoperatively by a combination of the patient's history and the finding of air or barium in the biliary tract on x-ray examination.

PATHOLOGY

The gallbladder may have only a single point of necrosis, which gives way or becomes gangrenous with escape of bacteria through it, or the entire organ may rarely become gangrenous as though its blood supply had become compromised by distention or by thrombosis. As is usual when stones are present, bacteria usually are also, so that one is dealing with a bacterial as well as with a chemical peritonitis when the gallbladder ruptures.

TREATMENT

The objectives of the immediate treatment of free perforation are removal of necrotic material and stones and adequate drainage to the outside of the body. Thus, a cholecystostomy plus the placing of drains in the subhepatic space, and if the peritonitis is extensive, in the subdiaphragmatic space and the pelvis is usual. If the gallbladder wall is gangrenous, the gangrenous part should be removed even if this requires a cholecystectomy. However, one need not to be concerned with completing the cholecystectomy to within 5.0 mm. of the common duct but can stop it as soon as viable tissue is reached and drain the cystic duct or the infundibulum, as the case may be. These patients are actually or potentially very ill, and the procedure should be aimed solely at saving life with virtually no concern about the question of whether or not a subsequent operation may be required.

The treatment of perforation with localized abscess is little different from that of acute cholecystitis in a seriously ill patient except that an additional drain to the site of the abscess is generally required.

The treatment of perforation with biliary fistula is usually an elective procedure and, unless there is accompanying gallstone ileus, the patients are not acutely ill, although they may be seriously debilitated. However, the technical aspects of dealing not only with the diseased gallbladder but also with closure of the fistula into the intestine—all in scar tissue —make this a formidable operation. Furthermore, the fistula may be kept open by obstruction at the ampulla of Vater by a common duct stone—the bile draining through the fistula into the intestinal tract, so that the patient is not jaundiced. In such cases, when the fistula is closed, the common duct should be carefully palpated for the presence of stones and, if stones are present, they should be removed. It is essential to establish the patency of the common duct either by actual exploration or by operative cholangiography or both, when closing a fistula between the biliary tract and the intestinal tract.

Postoperative treatment is of great importance in the free perforation, as in any case of peritonitis, and consists in a regimen which includes gastrointestinal rest produced by nasogastric suction—nothing by mouth; support of blood volume—transfusions of blood and/or room temperature stored plasma; antibiotics— at first selected by guess and then chosen on the basis of bacterial sensitivity studies; and nutritional support by parenteral routes—to include water, sodium, potassium, chloride, glucose and, if the course is long, other nutritive substances. With timely intervention and vigorous but judicious support, a great majority of such patients can be saved.

CHRONIC CALCULOUS CHOLECYSTITIS AND CHRONIC NONCALCULOUS CHOLECYSTITIS

As in the case of acute cholecystitis, chronic cholecystitis can occur without stones. Unfortunately, surgical experience in treating noncalculous chronic cholecystitis has been exceedingly unsatisfactory. According to most authors, the majority of such patients have residual postoperative digestive complaints, frequently of greater magnitude than those for which the operation was carried out. From the surgical standpoint, therefore, the objective in studying patients suspected of having chronic cholecystitis is to establish the presence or the absence of cholelithiasis with reasonable certainty. The association of cholelithiasis with symptoms of discomfort after eating generally are considered as an indication for operation unless outweighed by contraindications, such as severe renal disease, etc.

There are 3 principal avenues through which a diagnosis of cholelithiasis is approached. First, there is the history and the physical examination. Most typically, the patient is a woman in middle life and inclined toward obesity who has intermittent attacks of severe pain in the right upper quadrant of the abdomen or the epigastrium, most often coming on in the evening or at night following a heavy meal. Often it is associated with radiation of the pain to the back in the region of the angle of the right scapula or the angles of

both scapulae, at about the level of the 8th dorsal segment and with nausea and vomiting. Often the patients have such severe pains that they call their physicians during attacks and are given morphine or other narcotics hypodermically. Many of them have been pregnant, and frequently the initial symptoms start during or immediately after a pregnancy. In addition to the severe attacks, such individuals often have postprandial fullness and distress in the epigastrium, accentuated by fatty foods and sometimes by cabbage or other closely related vegetables. Belching and sour eructations are common. Always it is important to inquire for a history of jaundice or of the appearance of especially dark urine, or of light-gray or putty-colored stools. Such symptoms, especially if they are of brief duration and intermittent, are highly suggestive of common duct obstruction due to stones. If the bouts of jaundice are ushered in by a fever and a chill, one has the classical picture of common duct obstruction due to stones described by Charcot (Charcot's intermittent hepatic fever).

Even without symptoms of common duct obstruction, if the patient has severe acute bouts of epigastric or right upper quadrant pain radiating to the right scapula with upper quadrant tenderness and a palpable mass, one can feel relatively certain that the patient has cholelithiasis. In fact, the existence of the above triad—typical pain, tenderness and mass —is indicative of the presence of gallstones 9 times out of 10. Babcock (1937) has stated that 94 per cent of patients with the typical clinical history have gallstones.

In the great majority of instances, however, the history is far less typical. It may consist only of some postprandial distress and upper abdominal discomfort. Under such circumstances, it is necessary to rely heavily on laboratory methods in order to reach a definitive diagnosis of cholelithiasis. Roentgenographic technics undoubtedly constitute the most valuable of these methods. A simple scout film of the abdomen will reveal gallstones in only about 10 to 15 per cent of patients having them. The amount of calcium necessary for a stone to show varies markedly with the distribution of the calcium in the stone. If it is evenly diffused through the substance of the stone, it may take much more

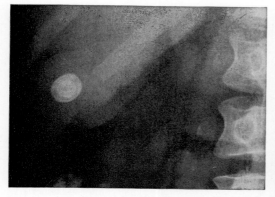

FIG. 30-3. Laminated gallstone.

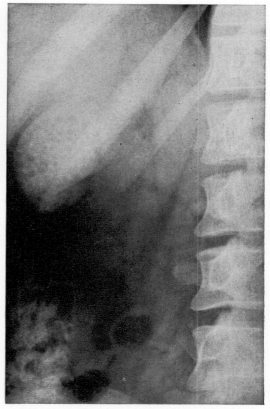

FIG. 30-4. Typical cholecystogram, showing
71 stones (nonopaque).

calcium to render the stone sufficiently opaque to be demonstrable on an x-ray film than if the calcium is deposited in a particular layer or lamina of the stone so that it forms ring-shaped shadows (Fig. 30-3).

Because such a small percentage of gall-stones are radiopaque, as contrasted with the urinary tract, where upward of 90 per cent may be demonstrated on a scout film, Graham, Cole, and Copher (1925)[23] successfully devised a method of demonstrating many of the non-opaque stones by the oral or intravenous administration of tetraiodophenolphthalein. This dye, absorbed into the blood stream, is excreted by the liver and is concentrated in the gallbladder. Thus, the functional gallbladder may be visualized roentgenographically, usually about 12 to 18 hours after ingestion of the dye. Nonopaque stones then stand out as negative shadows. The use of this dye intravenously was abandoned in many clinics because of occasional severe reactions, sometimes leading to death.

Other preparations, such as Priodax (beta-(4-hydroxy-3, 5-diiodophenyl)-alpha-phenyl-propionic acid), Telepaque (3-(3-amino-2, 4, 6-triiodophenyl)-2-ethyl propionic acid) and Biligrafin (di-sodium salt of N, N-adipyl-bis-(3-amino-2, 4, 6-triiodobenzoic acid) (Frommhold, 1953[21]) have been introduced and appear to have some advantages over the original material, although they are effective for the same reasons. Biligrafin is the first material to be excreted in sufficient concentration in hepatic bile to make possible more or less routine films of the common bile duct. This is obviously a real advance, although it is to be hoped that still further gain may be possible in this field. It is of considerable importance that a flat film be done as a routine before the dye appears, as a stone of density equal to that of the dye may blend in with the dye if only a cholecystogram is done.

Practical points to remember in connection with cholecystograms are: (1) that films should be taken in various degrees of obliquity in order to throw the shadow of the gallbladder away from the colon which, when containing pockets of gas, may suggest a gallstone if superimposed on the gallbladder shadow; (2) that some of the dyes induce vomiting or diarrhea. Therefore, if the gallbladder fails to visualize, it is important to inquire whether the patient did vomit or whether he had diarrhea after taking the tablets. It is important, of course, to be sure that the patient did take the tablets, and finally it is often best to give the patient

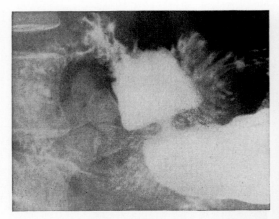

FIG. 30-5. Oblique film, showing radiopaque gallstones in gallbladder projected
over duodenal loop. Duodenum is opacified
with barium.

additional tablets and to make a second attempt at demonstrating the gallbladder if the
first attempt fails to do so. Tincture of paregoric in adult doses of 4 to 8 cc. may be
very helpful in preventing or diminishing the
diarrhea.

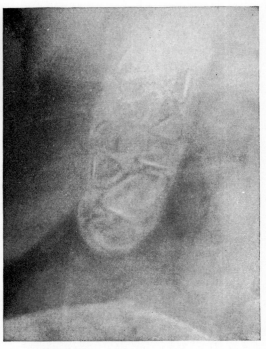

FIG. 30-7. Multifaceted stones in the gallbladder, showing peripheral calcification.

The results of such tests may clearly demonstrate gallstones (Fig. 30-4) or they may
show that the gallbladder does not visualize,
or that it visualizes very weakly. A well-
visualized gallbladder that shows no stones,
taken in conjunction with a flat film which
showed no opaque stones, is fairly strong evidence against cholelithiasis in the gallbladder.
Rarely, a stone may be small enough to be
overlooked on the cholecystogram and yet
large enough to block the cystic duct. If the
gallbladder is not visualized in either of 2
cholecystograms for which an appropriate dye
was given in recommended doses and retained
within the gastrointestinal tract satisfactorily, it is reasonable to suppose that cholelithiasis and gallbladder disease exist. This may be
in the form of an actual cystic duct obstruction, or it may be due to loss of the chemical
functions of the gallbladder (see section on
Physiology).

In many instances, the decision to operate
rests on failure to visualize the gallbladder in
the cholecystogram plus a suggestive but not
classical history of gallbladder symptoms.

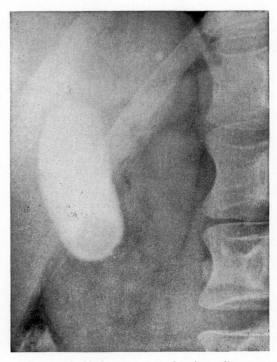

FIG. 30-6. Cholecystogram, showing solitary
large stone in fundus of the gallbladder.

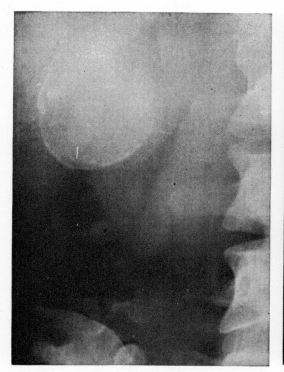

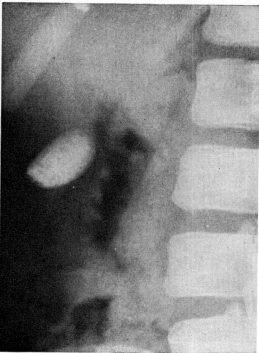

Fig. 30-8. Calcification in the wall of the gallbladder. A marble-sized stone was impacted in the cystic duct at the time of operation.

Fig. 30-9. Milk calcium bile and stones in 8-year-old patient with congenital hemolytic anemia. (Stones palpated during splenectomy.)

The direct demonstration of stones in patients with cholelithiasis is raised to the range of 55 or 60 per cent by means of the cholecystogram. In most of the remaining individuals who harbor stones, the gallbladder will fail repeatedly to concentrate the dye sufficiently for visualization. In other words, repeated failure of the gallbladder to visualize is good evidence that it contains stones (present in more than 85%).

It is important in assessing gallbladder function to recognize that severely impaired liver function may be a cause of the failure of the gallbladder to visualize. Thus, in patients with jaundice, no weight can be given to failure of the gallbladder to visualize, and usually the decision for or against operation is arrived at best without recourse to a cholecystogram. Additional examples of roentgenologic studies of the biliary tract are shown in Figures 30-5 to 30-20.

The 3rd method of diagnosis is biliary drainage. For this purpose, a rubber tube 3 or 4 ft. long and about 16 mm. in circumference is passed through the patient's nose, pharynx and esophagus into the stomach and from there is advanced so that the tip lies beyond the pylorus. Suitable tubes for this purpose have all of their openings close to the distal end of the tube, so that once this has passed the pylorus, aspiration will not withdraw material from the stomach simultaneously with that from the duodenum. In order to get the tube past the pylorus, the patient is placed on his right side, and sometimes a metal weight is used on the end of the tube. The position of the end of the tube must be checked, either by fluoroscopy or by aspiration of the tube and testing the samples aspirated with litmus paper—an alkaline reaction indicating that the tube has passed beyond the stomach. With the tube in this position, duodenal contents are aspirated, and this is designated as "A-bile." Then the gallbladder is stimulated to

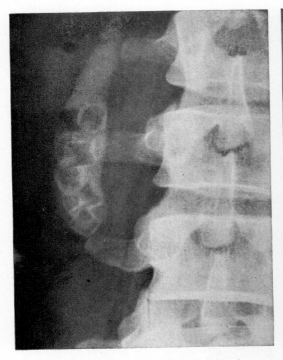

FIG. 30-10. Cholecystogram, showing faceted stones in a gallbladder that shows some function.

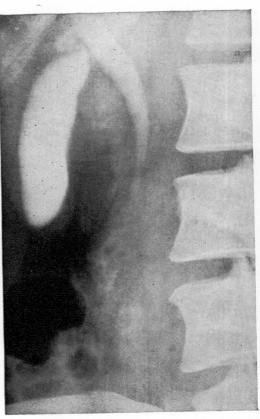

FIG. 30-11. Demonstration of the common bile duct and the cystic duct during a routine cholecystogram.

contract by the administration of either olive oil or concentrated magnesium sulfate. Most workers feel that the oil is unsatisfactory because it interferes with the microscopic examination of subsequent samples. In normal individuals, stimulation of the gallbladder is followed by the recovery of dark black-brown concentrated bile. This is the sample (B-bile) most likely to give evidences of cholelithiasis. The presence of amorphous aggregates of calcium bilirubinate and of the flat platelike crystals of cholesterol are indicative of cholelithiasis. These are illustrated in Figure 30-21. If both are present in fresh biliary drainage samples, the incidence of cholelithiasis, according to Bockus, Shay, Willard, and Pessel (1931)[9], is 90 per cent. Such findings, taken in conjunction with symptoms suggestive of biliary tract disease, are commonly used as an indication for operation when the roentgenogram is doubtful or difficult to interpret. Frequently, a 3rd sample of bile is collected following stimulation of the gallbladder and aspiration of the B-bile; this is spoken of as

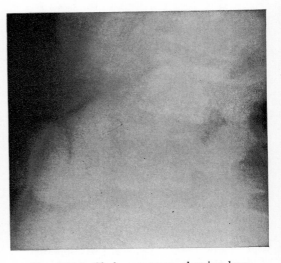

FIG. 30-12. Cholecystogram, showing long S-shaped gallbladder, a normal variant.

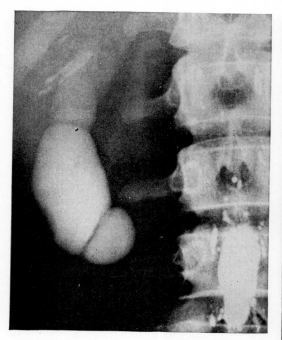

FIG. 30-13. Cholecystogram, showing functioning gallbladder with phrygian cap. (Note also contrast material in spinal canal introduced previously for myelography.)

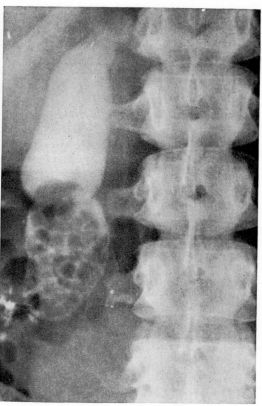

FIG. 30-14. Cholecystogram, showing a gallbladder with an hourglass constriction and stones appearing in the distal half only.

C-bile and is thought to represent hepatic bile as it comes from the liver. The results of biliary drainage studies have been strikingly related to the experience and the interest of the individual making the examination. Under most circumstances, negative findings should not be given much weight.

Therefore, it is readily seen that diagnosis of patients with chronic calculous cholecystitis may be difficult and that the diagnostic criteria on which we rely are not completely accurate. If an operation is undertaken on these criteria and the gallbladder appears entirely normal at operation, it is difficult for the surgeon to know what to do, or for the medical consultant to advise him. It has been the author's experience that if the gallbladder shows evidence of fibrosis, adhesions or thickening of the wall, generally it is best to remove it, for in most such instances small granular stones have been found in the region of the cystic duct. However, if the gallbladder really appears normal in every respect, at times he has preferred to do an exploratory cholecystostomy, and if no stones can be recovered by stone forceps and

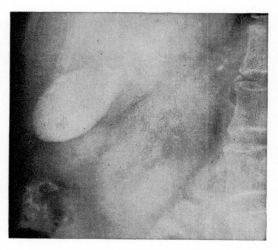

FIG. 30-15. Cholecystogram, showing stellate area of radiolucency due to a gas pocket within a stone.

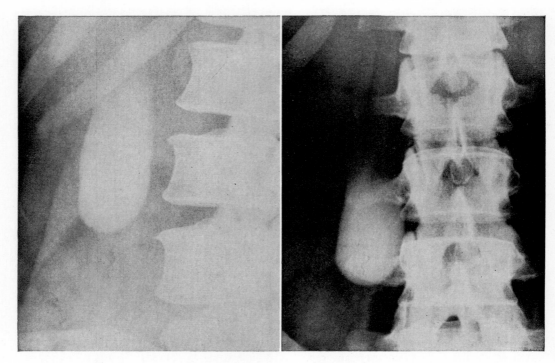

FIG. 30-16. Cholecystogram, of S. R. (*Left*) Film made with patient lying down. Functioning gallbladder. No stone shadow seen. (*Right*) Film made with patient erect. Note line of stones which have formed a radiolucent layer at the junction of the distal and the middle thirds of the gallbladder.

scoop and if no cholesterosis is present, the gallbladder has not been removed but has been drained to the outside with a catheter or a plain rubber tube for 1 to 2 weeks.

Cholesterosis, the deposit of cholesterol in the gallbladder wall, may be visible only from the mucosal side when it appears as a network of fine straw-colored lines. If the mucosa is hyperemic, the appearance is reminiscent of the surface of a strawberry (strawberry gall-

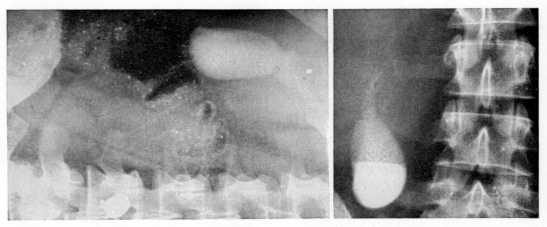

FIG. 30-17. Multiple stones wth layering of the contrast medium. (*Left*) Horizontal position. (*Right*) Erect position. Direction of x-rays was horizontal in both films.

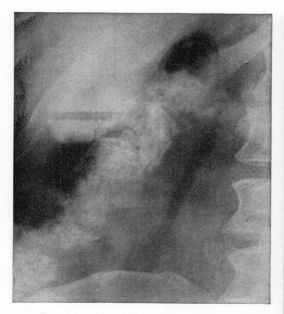

FIG. 30-18. Layering of nonopaque gallstones as seen on a cholecystogram. Film made with patient erect.

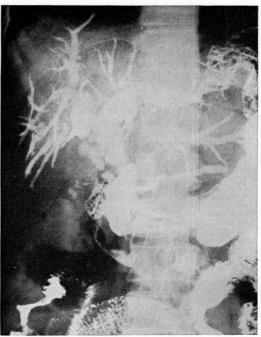

FIG. 30-20. The biliary tree filled with barium sulphate in a patient with a duodenobiliary fistula after administration of a water barium meal.

bladder). Such gallbladders should be removed when encountered at operation, even though no stone is found in the lumen. Whenever the gallbladder is opened and not removed, it should be drained.

Despite the many impressive series of cholecystectomies that have been done without drainage, the editors feel strongly that whenever the biliary tract is entered, drains should

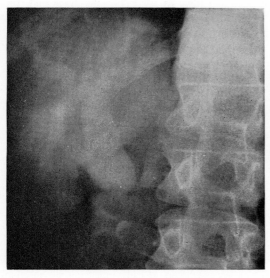

FIG. 30-19. Cholegrafin study, showing dilated common duct with stones (confirmed at operation).

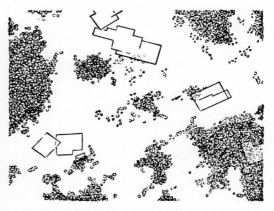

FIG. 30-21. Showing platelike crystals of cholesterol and masses of calcium bilirubinate sediment as they characteristically appear in specimens obtained by biliary drainage from patients with cholelithiasis.

be employed. (See section on Biliary Tract Operations.)

DIAGNOSIS OF COMMON DUCT STONE AND OTHER INDICATIONS FOR CHOLEDOCHOSTOMY

In a patient with cholelithiasis, jaundice is prima facie evidence of a stone in the common duct and, if there are indications for any elective biliary tract operation in such a case, choledochostomy is almost always indicated. The history of previous jaundice in a patient presenting other indications for operation on the biliary tract is accepted by most surgeons as an indication for choledochostomy. Palpation of a stone in the common duct at the time of operation is likewise an indication, and palpation should be carried out not only at the beginning of the procedure but also after the common duct is mobilized as fully as the surgeon feels is justified. The existence of a dilated common duct is generally accepted as an indication to explore it and to carry out a choledochostomy. Some allowance should be made for the physiologic dilatation that occurs if a cholecystectomy has been done some months previously. The existence of small stones in the gallbladder with a cystic duct which appears large enough to transmit them is accepted by many surgeons as an indication for exploration of the common duct.

A conservative policy, and one which is followed in the great majority of clinics, is always to drain the common bile duct with a T-tube if it is opened. In clinics in which operative cholangiography is carried out, a defect in the cholangiogram may well prove to be the indication for opening the duct. Great care should be taken in carrying out such cholangiograms to avoid the introduction of air bubbles which may cast a shadow similar to that produced by a calculus on the x-ray film. Injection through the cystic duct may be helpful (Fig. 30-29).

The proper role of operative cholangiography is by no means agreed upon. The author makes wide use of this technic, usually injecting the dye through the cystic duct. He uses the findings when positive as additional indications for opening the common duct. He does not use a negative operative cholangiogram as a basis for omitting choledochostomy and common duct exploration when other clear indications are present.

He also uses cholangiography performed through a T-tube in the common duct at times to check the completeness of the common duct evacuation, particularly when multiple stones were present. Proceeding in this way, it is only infrequently that common duct stones are found which would otherwise have been missed. However, this additional precaution adds only about 10 minutes to the operative procedure, so that there is little reason to withhold it in the average biliary tract case. He has not seen acute pancreatitis as a sequela, although this has been reported by Zeck (1949)[59] and others, and recently discussed by Bergkvist (1957-58)[5]. The injection of Diodrast should be made gently and not in a way that is likely to build up excessive pressure in the ductal system.

Other indications for exploring the common duct may be found in the existence of anomalies, the existence of strictures not tight enough to produce jaundice, etc. (See also section on The Jaundiced Patient and section on Biliary Tract Operations.)

THE JAUNDICED PATIENT

Jaundice is the yellow color of skin, sclerae and mucous membranes due to an increase in bilirubin in the plasma. This increase may be due to obstruction of the ducts which carry the bile from the liver to the duodenum (obstructive jaundice), to disease of the cells which excrete bilirubin (hepatocellular jaundice) or to an overproduction of bilirubin due to increased breakdown of erythrocytes (hemolytic jaundice).

Jaundice is to be differentiated from other yellow colorations of the skin. The most important of these are the lemon-yellow color of individuals with profound anemia in whom the color of the fat shows through the skin more than usual and carotenemia due to ingestion of excessive amounts of carotene, either as carrots or as vitamin A precursor in drug form. The gray color of argyria sometimes has given rise to confusion, especially with long-standing or declining icterus.

Frequently, obstructive jaundice is relieved by operation, whereas hepatocellular jaundice is apt to be made worse by anesthesia and operation. Thus, the differentiation between the two is often crucial to the survival of the patient. Hemolytic jaundice does not usually call for operation but may do so if the increased production and excretion of bile has led to the formation of gallstones, or if the hemolysis is largely occurring in the spleen when splenectomy may be helpful (see Chap. 32).

OBSTRUCTIVE JAUNDICE

The most common cause of obstructive jaundice during adult life is a stone in the common duct. A second common cause is carcinoma of the head of the pancreas (see Chap. 31). Metastatic carcinoma involving the liver is a third and fairly frequent cause, though usually it is one of the terminal events in malignant disease.

Other neoplasms which may cause obstructive jaundice are primary carcinoma of the liver, carcinoma of the gallbladder, carcinoma of the bile duct and carcinoma of the papilla of Vater. Rarely, jaundice may be caused by a benign polyp in the bile duct.

The author has seen obstructive jaundice resulting from abscesses pressing against the duct from the right side, from chronic pancreatitis, from penetrating ulcer of the duodenum, from primary carcinoma of the duodenum, from enlarged lymph nodes pressing against the duct, from congenital (or spontaneous) stricture of the common duct in a man of 18, from so-called chronic hypertrophic biliary cirrhosis and iatrogenic jaundice from various injuries to the duct—transection, excision of part of the wall, occlusion with sutures during cholecystectomy, occlusion during gastrectomy and after accidental clamping of the duct. Parasites, such as *Ascaris lumbricoides* or *Schistosoma japonicum*, have caused common duct obstruction. While this occurs very rarely in the United States, common duct obstruction due to parasites is by no means uncommon in certain geographic areas in which infestation with the parasites is more frequent. During the neonatal period the common causes of obstructive jaundice are atresia, agenesis and choledochal cysts.

Principal interest in the differential diagnosis is focused on cholelithiasis versus carcinoma of the head of the pancreas. The French surgeon, Courvoisier,* enunciated the law that bears his name: "When the common bile duct is obstructed by a stone, dilatation is rare; when the duct is obstructed in some other way, dilatation is common." A palpably distended gallbladder indicates carcinoma of the head of the pancreas, whereas in cholelithiasis the gallbladder is usually too shrunken and fibrotic to become palpably distended. Unfortunately, the exceptions to the law are so common as to permit only the most modest emphasis of it.

Jaundice is likely to be accompanied by pain when due to stone, and that accompanying carcinoma of the head of the pancreas is apt to be relatively painless at the time of onset ("silent jaundice"). Unfortunately, there are exceptions in both directions. However, painless jaundice is not very frequent with stones but does occur. On the other hand, pain is by no means rare in carcinoma of the head of the pancreas, even by the time the jaundice is noted (see Chapter 31).

Laboratory aids in differentiating between the 3 basic types of jaundice are summarized in Table 1.

Most important in the differentiation of hemolytic jaundice is the dark color of the stools. In severe anemia (< 6 Gm./100 ml.) patients with hemolytic jaundice may not

* While Courvoisier is identified with French surgery, he was born in Basel and for a period was Professor of Surgery at the University of Basel (Nissen, 1959)[39].

TABLE 1. CHARACTERISTIC FINDINGS IN LIVER FUNCTION IN THREE TYPES OF JAUNDICE

	OBSTRUCTIVE	HEPATO-CELLULAR	HEMOLYTIC
Bilirubin—total	+	+	+
1-minute reading	+	±	±
Cephalin cholesterol flocculation	±	+	±
Thymol flocculation	±	+	±
BSP retention	+	+	N
Alkaline phosphatase	+	N	N
Urine urobilinogen	0, if complete	±	+
Prothrombin response to vitamin K*#	>75% of N	<75% of N	

N = Normal   + = Increased   ± = Sometimes Increased   0 = None.

* = Response within 24 hours to 20 mg. of Synkayvite in afebrile patients whose initial prothrombin levels are below 75% of normal.

= Allen, J. G. (1940, 1943).

show these findings. Of outstanding value in differentiating obstruction from hepatocellular jaundice has been the alkaline phosphatase level in the serum. However, none of the tests has been infallible, and the experiments of Mann (1926)[35] indicate that large fractions of the liver can be resected without significant reductions in various of the function tests.

Differential diagnosis is, of course, most important when it involves the decision to operate. Thus, the diagnosis of hepatitis versus obstruction is tremendously important. However, if hepatitis can be excluded and the jaundice is clearly obstructive, it is often not essential to know whether stone or carcinoma is the cause, as both cases usually need to be explored surgically if only to relieve the jaundice.

If no satisfactory differentiation is reached by laboratory methods and the patient does not improve on supportive therapy within a reasonable time (usually about 3 weeks), laparotomy should be done. Some clinicians resort to needle biopsy of the liver, provided that the prothrombin concentration is above 75 per cent of normal. Occasional serious hemorrhages have occurred, either into the peritoneal cavity or into the bile ducts producing hemobilia. However, the principal objection to the procedure is the likelihood of missing significant areas by blind sampling and the difficulties encountered by the pathologist in interpreting the scanty material obtained.

Patients with hemolytic jaundice have a high incidence of gallstones, typically of the pure bilirubin type (jackstones).

THE PROGNOSTIC SIGNIFICANCE OF OBSTRUCTIVE JAUNDICE

Obstructive jaundice is a serious symptom. Cholelithiasis associated with jaundice is accompanied by a higher mortality than cholelithiasis alone. If it is due to carcinoma, the ultimate outlook is probably more than 99 per cent unfavorable. In the author's experience, all of the metastatic cases have gone on to die; all of the primary carcinomas of the liver have gone on to die; all of the primary carcinomas of the gallbladder have gone on to die within 5 years except 1, and all of the carcinomas of the bile ducts have gone on to die, except for a rare few involving the papilla of

Vater or the adjacent area of the duct who have survived several years and may possibly turn out in the final analysis to be cured. In a recent compilation from the literature, there were over 100 instances in which Whipple resections of the duodenum and the head of the pancreas for malignant disease have survived for 5 years or more. (See Chap. 31.)

As mentioned above, cholelithiasis with jaundice is accompanied by a much higher mortality than is cholelithiasis confined to the gallbladder. One can point to various series of cholecystectomies in which the operative mortality (death in the hospital within 30 days) was less than 1 per cent for cholecystectomy. Yet, the same clinics commonly report a mortality rate of 4 to 8 per cent for individuals with obstructive jaundice. This mortality represents a decided improvement from that of a few decades ago when it frequently ranged around 15 per cent higher.

The cause of the higher death rate is explained partly by certain special complications to which the jaundiced patient is subject. These are: the hemorrhagic tendency in obstructive jaundice, "pancreatic asthenia," "liver shock" and "hepatorenal syndrome." In the past the most important of these has been the hemorrhagic tendency. About 20 per cent of patients undergoing major operations for relief of jaundice used to have hemorrhagic episodes in the postoperative period as reported by Ravdin et al. (1939)[45] and Ulin (1943)[55].

This problem was solved by 2 discoveries: (1) the discovery of vitamin K, the coagulation vitamin, by Dam in 1935; (2) the discovery by A. J. Quick that prothrombin deficiency is the basic coagulation defect in obstructive jaundice. It was not until 1938, however, that E. D. Warner and his associates[56] demonstrated that hypoprothrombinemia in patients actually could be relieved in many instances by the oral administration of vitamin K with bile salts, to facilitate its absorption. In order to avoid this complication, it is customary to give vitamin K_1 or one of the synthetic preparations with similar action, such as menadione, preoperatively until the prothrombin level has returned to normal or has been brought up as well as possible (see Chap. 6). It is important to continue therapy into the postoperative period until the wound is healed.

Late hemorrhagic episodes have been reported 3 or 4 weeks after operation when vitamin K is stopped before wound healing has occurred. Experience rapidly showed that about 18 per cent of patients with obstructive jaundice and hypoprothrombinemia failed to respond to vitamin K therapy, and an additional 12 per cent or so responded only partially. Failure of the prothrombin level to respond adequately to vitamin K is seen more frequently in patients with jaundice due to malignancy or in people with very long-standing liver damage or infectious hepatitis than in other jaundiced patients.

Many bits of evidence combined to demonstrate that vitamin K is effective only in the presence of a functioning liver. Impairment of function can be produced by chloroform, or the liver can be removed surgically in animals after which the prothrombin falls progressively and at a much more rapid rate than fibrinogen, the level of which in the blood is also dependent on the liver (Warren and Rhoads, 1939)[57].

Further study of the coagulation mechanism indicates that the prothrombin, as measured by the Quick test, is not a single factor but is composed of at least 2 factors—one of which diminishes on storage of blood in a blood bank (accelerator globulin), whereas another is diminished by Dicoumarol (pure prothrombin). Both are diminished by chloroform anesthesia. When the prothrombin level does not respond to vitamin K, it is possible to give the patient some prothrombin through transfusion of fresh blood. Frequently, stored blood also can have a beneficial effect, if the deficiency as determined by the 1-stage method of Quick happens to be in the component which is not much affected by storage (prothrombin).

Vitamin K_1 prepared as an emulsion for intravenous use and given intravenously in doses of 50 to 100 mg. or more will often produce a brief rise not obtained by ordinary doses. This is specifically indicated in Dicoumarol poisoning or in patients under the influence of Dicoumarol who must have emergency operations. It can be tried in other situations.

The second of these complications, pancreatic asthenia (a term introduced by Whipple, 1923[58]), is now believed to result from prolonged bile drainage. The symptoms are anorexia and progressive weakness. A sodium and chloride deficiency may be part of the picture, but simple replacement of sodium and chlorides has failed practically always to bring about marked improvement. Refeeding of bile, however, in amounts of 150 ml. a day or up, usually will restore appetite and improve the patient greatly within 2 or 3 days. Because of the bitter taste, usually it is necessary to refeed the bile through a nasogastric tube introduced into the stomach. Sometimes hardy patients can drink it mixed with pineapple juice or some other flavoring.

Liver shock is a picture that can be reproduced experimentally in the dog by ligation of the hepatic artery close to the hilum of the liver. It has been seen occasionally in patients who had injury or thrombosis of the hepatic artery. Such injuries can occur easily during cholecystectomy in those instances in which the hepatic artery runs up along the cystic duct, giving off the cystic artery opposite the infundibulum of the gallbladder and then turning back into the liver. Here the main hepatic artery or the right hepatic may be ligated instead of the cystic artery.

Markowitz (1949)[36] showed that dogs receiving penicillin frequently do not develop liver shock after ligation of the hepatic artery. Fitts and his associates (1950)[18] confirmed this observation and found also that chlortetracycline would protect similarly; however, streptomycin did not.

The present concept is that death results from an overgrowth of anaerobes which are resident in the liver. Appropriate antibiotics may suppress the growth of these organisms until such time as the liver has established an adequate collateral arterial circulation.

As a result of the improvements that have occurred in the understanding of the pathology of jaundice, it is now possible to operate on simple cases of jaundice produced by common duct stones with a large probability of success.

The fourth of the complications listed, hepatorenal syndrome, is described sometimes as including a chronic phase. The acute phase is, in effect, liver shock. The chronic phase corresponds to liver failure with cholemia, frequently with evidence of renal irritation, so-called bile nephrosis and with coma. Recent studies by McDermott, et al. (1954)[34] indicate that hepatic coma is associated sometimes with a rise in the blood ammonia level. This change is observed routinely in Eck-fistula dogs fed on a meat diet. In the normal animal, ammonia concentrations in the portal vein are considerably higher than in the systemic circulation, and the ammonia is removed by the normal liver as the blood flows through it. In the experimental animal, a critical level is often reached at which the rise in blood ammonia is accompanied by coma (so-called meat intoxication). The level varies for different individuals but, according to McDermott, is fairly constant for any one animal. Therefore, it appears unwise to feed much protein to a jaundiced patient if coma is impending. McDermott and his associates have advised that, in patients with advanced cirrhosis of the liver, blood escaping from esophageal varices be aspirated from the stomach to reduce ammonia formation in the intestine. That the intestine is the actual site of the formation of free ammonia was reported by Folin in 1912[20]. Apparently, it is due to the activity of micro-organisms, and patients in hepatic coma have at times been brought out of coma by the administration of broad-spectrum antibiotics into the gastrointestinal tract (Stormont, 1958)[54].

PREPARATION OF THE JAUNDICED PATIENT FOR OPERATION

After the appropriate diagnostic studies are completed or where possible while they are being carried out, certain steps should be taken to be sure that the patient with jaundice is in as good condition as possible for operation. Menadione (vitamin K) should be given in doses of 5.0 mg. 2 to 4 times a day. In the event that this does not bring the prothrombin back to normal, vitamin K_1 emulsion may be given intravenously. Most surgeons prefer to give vitamin K to all patients with jaundice who are to undergo operation, even though the prothrombin happens not to be particularly depressed in advance of operation.

It also appears advisable to place the patient on a diet containing as close to 3,000 calories per day as he can be persuaded to take, and to supply about 70 per cent of these calories as carbohydrate, not less than 20 per cent as protein, and a relatively small portion as fat. There is some evidence that it may be suitable to go as high as 20 per cent of the calories from fat which, in general, permits a more palatable diet. When it is necessary to sacrifice one objective for another in planning the diet, the total caloric intake is probably the most important, and the relatively high protein intake next most important.

The studies of Ravdin et al. (1943)[46] suggest that when such a diet is actually ingested by patients for 5 to 7 days before operation, it is rare that one finds the high fat content of liver biopsy specimens which are encountered frequently in patients not prepared in this manner. It is believed that patients are better risks for anesthesia and operation as the result of such dietary preparation. Occasionally, the progression of symptoms, particularly of pain and tenderness in the upper abdomen, make it inadvisable to take the time required for such careful dietary preparation. Under these circumstances it is usually advisable to carry out the minimum procedure which will relieve the patient of his acute symptomatology.

Other aspects of the preoperative preparation of a patient with biliary tract disease are similar to the steps used in preparing other patients for major abdominal operations and are set forth in Chapter 14.

STANDARD OPERATIVE PROCEDURES ON THE GALLBLADDER AND THE EXTRAHEPATIC BILIARY PASSAGES

In the following paragraphs certain operations performed on the biliary tract for indications already discussed are described briefly. These include cholecystostomy, cholecystectomy, choledochostomy, duodenotomy with transduodenal exploration of the common duct, sphincterotomy, cholecystojejunostomy, choledochojejunostomy and choledochoduodenostomy and, finally, pancreaticoduodenectomy. The surgeon who opens the peritoneal cavity to perform biliary tract surgery should be capable of doing any combination of these procedures when indicated and therefore should have all of them available in his armamentarium. It is sometimes difficult, if not

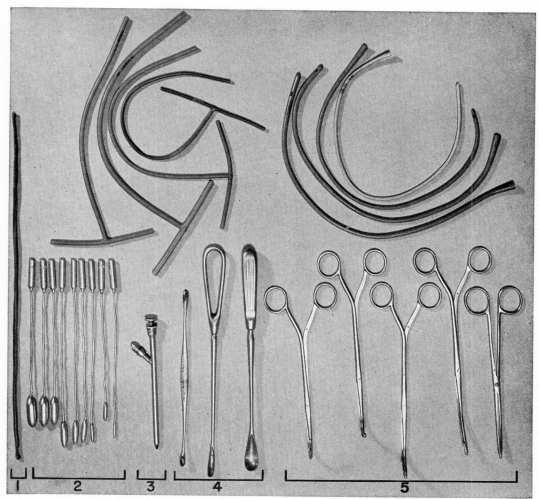

FIG. 30-22. Instruments commonly used in biliary tract surgery. (*Top, left*) Rubber T-tubes of various sizes. (*Top, right*) Straight rubber catheters of various sizes. (*Bottom, left to right*) (1) Malleable common duct probe. (2) Graduated common duct dilators (Bakes). (3) Trochar aspirator point for entering the distended gallbladder. Suction tubing fits on side arm and sharp point is withdrawn by drawing back plunger after the trochar has entered the gallbladder. (4) Three types of stone scoops. (5) Five stone forceps of varying degrees of curvature.

impossible, to differentiate before operation exactly which patients will need which of these procedures (see Fig. 30-22 which shows instruments commonly used in biliary tract surgery).

CHOLECYSTOSTOMY

The gallbladder is opened, usually through its fundus (see Figs. 30-23 and 24); an effort is made to remove all stones. Then a rubber tube, fenestrated near the end, is introduced into its lumen, and the gallbladder is closed tightly around it with purse-string and accessory sutures of catgut. The end of the tube leads outside the body wall where it is connected to a drainage bottle. The subhepatic space usually is drained to the outside with a "cigarette" or other soft drain.

The procedure can be done with local infiltration anesthesia, using 0.5 to 1.0 per cent

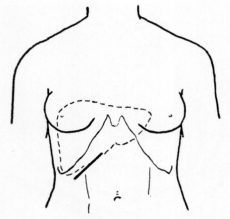

FIG. 30-23. Short subcostal incision suitable for cholecystostomy. Local, regional, or general anesthesia may be used.

procaine hydrochloride solution and is admirably adapted as a minimal procedure to prevent rupture of the gallbladder in very elderly or debilitated persons.

CHOLECYSTECTOMY

It is believed that the first cholecystectomy was performed by Langenbuch and reported in 1882[31]. The first such operation to be reported in the United States is believed to be that performed by Ohage (1886[41]; 1887[42]).

The gallbladder is removed, beginning either at the fundus or at the infundibulum (see Figs. 30-25 and 26). The great dangers are injury to the main bile ducts, injury to the hepatic artery or the right hepatic artery, and postoperative hemorrhage. Anatomic variations in the arrangements of the various structures account for a considerable proportion of the accidents which occur. While the possibilities of injury are as many as the anatomic variations which have been described (see Fig. 30-1), the main dangers are:

1. Clamping of the bile duct in a blind effort to control hemorrhage from the cystic artery or some other vessel at the hilum of the liver. Even though the clamp is removed, there is reason to believe that stricture may form in the crushed area. This is avoided best if, at the outset of dissection, the foramen of Winslow is identified, so that unexpected hemorrhage can be controlled by placing a finger through the foramen behind the hepatic

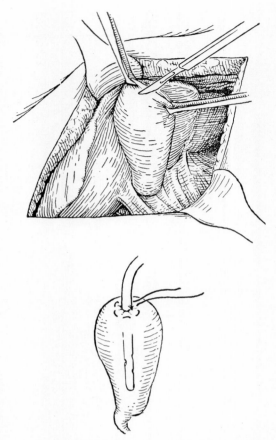

FIG. 30-24. Surgical exposure of the gallbladder for cholecystostomy, showing insertion of tube after evacuation of the organ by suction, stone forceps and scoops. The trochar aspirator tip shown in Figure 30-22 (3) is often used when the gallbladder is tense to diminish leakage of bile. Then the opening is enlarged as necessary with the scalpel.

artery and the portal vein, and then compressing these vessels digitally.

2. Tenting of the common duct upward by traction on the cystic duct with application of the cystic duct clamp across all or a part of the main bile duct (see Fig. 30-27).

3. Laceration or actual division of the common duct or of the right hepatic duct which may join the cystic duct or even the gallbladder before uniting with the left hepatic duct. The complications (2 and 3) are preventable by complete identification of the cystic duct, the common duct and the com-

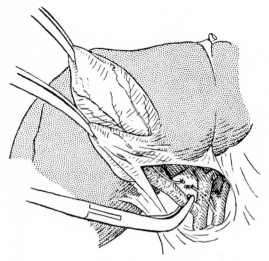

Fig. 30-25. Retrograde cholecystectomy, showing the application of a Shallcross clamp to the cystic duct after division and double ligation of the cystic artery.

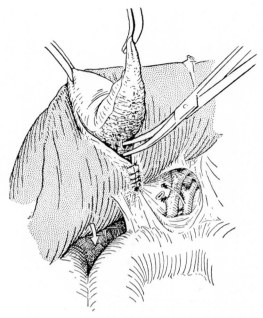

Fig. 30-26. A later stage in the retrograde removal of the gallbladder, showing the 2 ligatures on the stump of the cystic duct placed close to but not quite flush with the wall of the common duct. Note the interrupted sutures used in closing the liver bed. Arrow points to Morison's pouch. After removal of the gallbladder has been completed, the author employs a rubber tube drain in Morison's pouch and a Penrose drain which overlies the site from which the gallbladder has been removed. These drains may be exteriorized through the lateral end of the incision when the subcostal approach is used, or a separate stab wound may be made to accommodate them. Subsequently, they are removed in stages, usually in 3 to 7 days.

mon hepatic duct before ligation and division of the cystic duct.

4. Injury and subsequent ligation of the common hepatic artery or the right hepatic artery. First, one should identify the course of the hepatic artery by palpation. At operation, whenever that which appears to be the cystic artery looks unusually large, it is wise to dissect it up on to the gallbladder and make sure that it does not turn back into the liver before ligating or clamping or dividing it. These two steps help to avoid liver shock. The reliability of antibiotics in protecting against liver shock after these injuries is uncertain but, when injury occurs or is suspected, they certainly should be used in large doses (300,000 units of penicillin every 3 hours, and 250 mg. of chlortetracycline every 12 hours, by vein or 1 Gm. twice daily by mouth). If the structures at the infundibulum and the common duct region cannot be exposed easily, it is safer to begin the dissection at the fundus, gradually separating the gallbladder from the liver. This requires more time for hemostasis because the cystic artery is not secured until near the end of the dissection. The gallbladder bed is drained with a soft drain, and the kidney fossa (Morison's pouch) is drained in a similar manner.

CHOLEDOCHOSTOMY

Choledochostomy is employed not only to remove stones from the common duct but also to explore the common duct for possible stricture or tumor (see Fig. 30-28). After freeing the anterior surface of the common bile duct of fat for a short distance, it is finally identified by aspiration of bile through a fine 22-gauge needle. Then the duct is held forward by 2 guide sutures placed in its anterior surface for the purpose. It is opened longitudinally between the sutures for a distance of

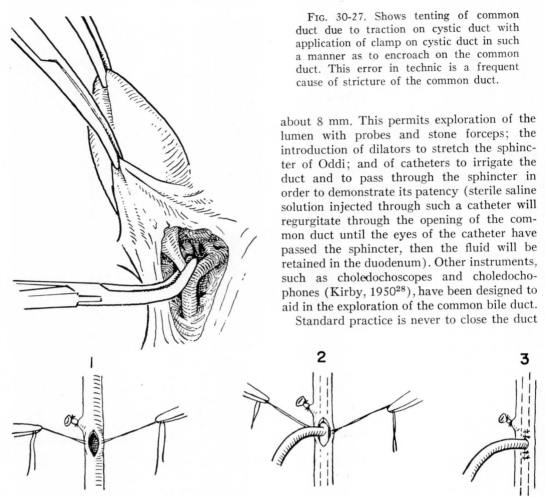

FIG. 30-27. Shows tenting of common duct due to traction on cystic duct with application of clamp on cystic duct in such a manner as to encroach on the common duct. This error in technic is a frequent cause of stricture of the common duct.

about 8 mm. This permits exploration of the lumen with probes and stone forceps; the introduction of dilators to stretch the sphincter of Oddi; and of catheters to irrigate the duct and to pass through the sphincter in order to demonstrate its patency (sterile saline solution injected through such a catheter will regurgitate through the opening of the common duct until the eyes of the catheter have passed the sphincter, then the fluid will be retained in the duodenum). Other instruments, such as choledochoscopes and choledochophones (Kirby, 1950[28]), have been designed to aid in the exploration of the common bile duct.

Standard practice is never to close the duct

FIG. 30-28. Shows an opening in the anterior wall of the common duct slightly caudad to the cystic duct. The opening is made in the long axis of the common bile duct between 2 sutures which are used to support the anterior wall of the duct, thus preventing the likelihood of injury to the posterior wall. Through this opening, the duct is explored with appropriate probes, scoops and stone forceps. Frequently, it is irrigated with a straight rubber catheter. The sphincter of Oddi in the lower end of the duct usually grips the Bakes dilators, so that the operator can tell when the duodenum is entered. By passing dilators of successively larger sizes, the sphincter may be gently dilated sufficiently to accommodate a small rubber catheter. Irrigation of this catheter determines quite accurately when the sphincter has been passed in doubtful cases. If the openings in the side of the catheter remain in the common duct, the irrigating fluid regurgitates; whereas if these openings have passed the sphincter into the duodenum, the fluid does not regurgitate.

When the operator is satisfied that the common duct is empty and communicates freely with the duodenum below and the hepatic duct above, a rubber T-tube is introduced. This provides drainage to the outside for bile which otherwise might leak into the peritoneal cavity. It also forms a splint which is helpful in preventing narrowing of the common bile duct by the absorbable sutures used to close the choledochotomy. After 12 days or longer, the stem of the tube is enclosed in a fibrous tract, and the T-tube can be removed by simple traction from the outside with the expectation that the common duct will seal off spontaneously and that bile will not drain into the general peritoneal cavity.

without a drain tube. The almost universally accepted type of drain is the T-tube, the cross bar of the T lying in the common duct and the stem extending out to the exterior of the body. The opening in the duct is closed with 2 or 3 fine sutures of swaged catgut about the stem of the tube. Care should be taken to take small bites so that the duct is not narrowed appreciably as the result of the suture. Such a tube is useful both at the operating table and subsequently, to introduce radiopaque material into the common duct and to obtain cholangiograms (Fig. 30-30). This should be done at the time of operation if the requisite x-ray equipment is available in the operating room and always should be done before removal of the T-tube. After about 12 days, the tube may be removed by simple traction, provided that the sutures have absorbed sufficiently. The wound in the duct then heals by itself, and there is little, if any, tendency toward stricture formation.

Although some have advocated complete closure of the duct after choledochostomy, this procedure should not be employed except by a few individuals who are studying the subject by special technics.

DUODENOTOMY WITH TRANSDUODENAL EXPLORATION OF THE COMMON DUCT

Mobilization of the duodenum by cutting the avascular peritoneal attachments to the right (Kocher, 1903[30]) not only renders duodenotomy more feasible but also permits palpation of the ampullary region to be carried out more definitively (see Fig. 30-31). Duodenotomy (see Chap. 32) is performed best by a short longitudinal or diagonal incision in the duodenum at a level determined by the location of the tip of a common duct probe inserted from above. After exposing the ampulla, a probe can be inserted from below. With the combined action of the 2 probes plus palpation, stones may be recovered which were not found with the use of probes from above alone. The duodenotomy incision should be closed transversely according to the Heineke-Mikulicz principle to avoid narrowing of the duodenal lumen.

SPHINCTEROTOMY

In certain very rare instances, an impacted

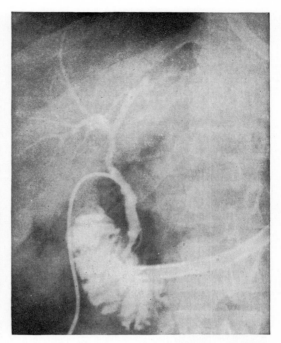

FIG. 30-29. Normal cholangiogram made at operation by use of a catheter introduced through the cystic duct. The large tube entering the duodenum from the left is a gastric suction tube introduced through the nasopharynx, which has slipped through the pylorus.

stone can be dislodged only after sphincterotomy. Other indications for this procedure are discussed in Chapter 32, "Pancreas."

CHOLECYSTOJEJUNOSTOMY

This procedure is used to sidetrack the common duct when the latter is obstructed and direct removal of the obstruction seems to be unwise for one reason or another. A 2-layer anastomosis is done between the inferior surface of the fundus of the gallbladder, and a loop of jejunum which is drawn up anteriorly in front of the transverse colon. The anastomosis should be placed as high as possible in the small bowel but not so high as to result in any tension. As demonstrated by Fitts (1948)[18] and others, the sphincter of Oddi mechanism is very important in preventing retrograde cholangitis from the bowel. None of the anastomoses of the extrahepatic biliary system to the intestinal tract have been entirely free of this complication.

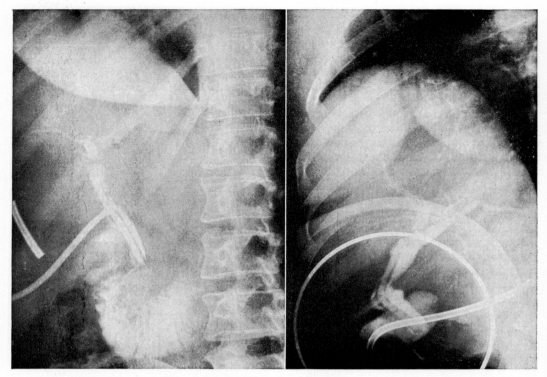

FIG. 30-30. The use of an inflated balloon in the duodenum to fill the hepatic radicals during a postoperative cholangiogram. (*Left*) Attempt without the balloon. (*Right*) Attempt with the balloon.

Allen (1945)[1] and Cole (1951)[12] independently have recommended defunctionalizing the loop of jejunum which is to be used for the anastomosis (see Chap. 32). This is done by means of the Roux-Y principle and probably is helpful to some extent in reducing the incidence of cholangitis. There is experimental evidence to show that the defunctionalized loop should be at least 30 inches long. The idea of taking tucks in one side or the other of the bowel to produce so-called valves has been advanced, but it is doubtful if it confers much advantage.

Now it is generally accepted that cholecystogastrostomy is a less satisfactory procedure, and this is seldom practiced.

CHOLEDOCHODUODENOSTOMY

This procedure was used formerly more than at present. Its decreased use is due to ascending infection and a tendency toward stricture of the anastomosis. However, experience with it has varied, and some surgeons have obtained encouraging results.

CHOLEDOCHOJEJUNOSTOMY

A defunctionalized loop of jejunum may be brought up and anastomosed either to the side of the common duct or the common duct may be transected and anastomosed end-to-end or end-to-side to a jejunal loop. This is a necessary part of a local resection for removal of the distal end of the common duct, the head of the pancreas, and the duodenum. The length of the loop should be not less than 30 inches.

PANCREATICODUODENECTOMY

In a small number of patients, usually those with surgical jaundice due to carcinoma of the region of the head of the pancreas or the ampulla of Vater, radical resection by the method of Whipple must be resorted to (see Chap. 31).

GENERAL PRINCIPLES FOR SECONDARY OPERATIONS ON THE BILIARY TRACT

Secondary operations are not infrequent in biliary tract surgery. These extend in magnitude and difficulty from cholecystectomy following cholecystostomy to very difficult procedures for recurrent stricture of the common duct. Adhesions form with great regularity in the region of the gallbladder and the subhepatic space as the result of previous operation and/or inflammation. The safe exposure of the parts of the biliary tract without injury to them or to other organs can be a very perplexing problem—especially to the novice.

There is one rule which has been of inestimable help to many surgeons: Find the anterior caudad edge of the liver and then keep the plane of dissection directly against Glisson's capsule as you separate the adherent organs from the undersurface of the liver. This plan is supplemented by periodic palpation for the hepatic artery, remembering that it is often not palpable if the blood pressure is as low as 80 mm. of mercury. Once the hepatic artery is located, it may be useful to locate the common duct by aspiration through a fine (22-24 gauge) needle, remembering that if complete obstruction of the common duct is present, only "white" bile looking like water or lymph may be found.

PATHOLOGIC CONDITIONS OF THE LIVER PARENCHYMA WITH NOTES REGARDING SURGICAL THERAPY

The problems of portal hypertension are discussed in Chapter 33 in connection with shunt operations. Portal hypertension may result from either intrahepatic obstruction to the portal flow or extrahepatic obstruction. Whereas the common cause of the latter is thrombosis, the common cause of the intrahepatic obstruction is cirrhosis.

Cirrhosis may be described as a progressive involvement of the liver with fibrous tissue, presumably resulting from progressive and repeated liver damage with replacement with scar tissue. The histologic picture is frequently one of both fibrosis and regeneration. In the Laennec's form, the fibrosis results in diffuse scarring with the lobulations of medium size. As judged by the irregularities in the surface of the liver, the trabeculae become

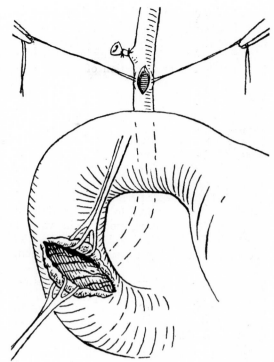

FIG. 30-31. Shows transduodenal exploration of the papilla of Vater. The author prefers a diagonal incision in the anterolateral wall of the duodenum which may be closed from side to side without danger of constricting the duodenum. Choledochotomy always is made in the supraduodenal position. The lateral attachments of the duodenum are also incised so that the duodenum may be mobilized and delivered into the wound. This also permits the operator's fingers to palpate posteriorly over the pancreas traversed by the common duct. Closure of the duodenal wound must be thorough. The author uses an inverting Connell suture of catgut as the first layer, followed by two layers of interrupted nonabsorbable sutures. In addition, a tag of omentum is held in place by other interrupted sutures so as to cover the suture line in the duodenum. A T-tube is placed in the choledochotomy. A sump drain is often used in Morison's pouch.

prominent at distances of the order of perhaps ¼ inch apart. In Hanot's cirrhosis, the trabeculation is finer, whereas in biliary cirrhosis the trabeculation is coarser. The latter form of the disease is apt to follow chronic or recurrent obstruction of the bile ducts and is more frequently associated with jaundice in its earlier stages than the other forms.

Whereas obstruction resulting in hematemesis from rupture or ulceration of dilated esophageal veins usually is treated by vascular shunts or direct attack on the affected portion of the esophagus, cirrhosis resulting in ascites primarily is less susceptible to surgical treatment. Many procedures have been recommended to increase anastomoses between the portal circulation and the systemic circulation. One of these is the Talma-Morison procedure in which the parietal peritoneum is scarified and the omentum sutured to it. The variations of this include forming pockets in various layers of the abdominal wall into which the omentum or other organs, such as the spleen, is fitted.

Another group of procedures involves removal of segments of the peritoneum or making apertures to allow the ascitic fluid to penetrate the peritoneum into other layers of the abdominal wall, especially the subcutaneous layer in the hope that it will be absorbed there. In still other procedures efforts have been made to anastomose the stump of the saphenous vein to the abdominal cavity in the hope that fluid actually will be pumped back into the vascular system. Another method is to anastomose the pelvis of one kidney to the abdominal cavity so that the fluid may make an exit via the urinary tract.

None of these procedures can be recommended with much enthusiasm. If any is to be undertaken, perhaps the removal of large segments of parietal peritoneum offers the most to recommend it. Such ascites usually represent a fairly advanced form of cirrhosis, and the average life expectancy is not long, although individuals sometimes exceed the average by a number of years. Treatment of this condition should be primarily medical along the lines of that recommended in the section on the preparation of the jaundiced patient but continued for many months. Such dietotherapy may be quite helpful.

A number of other processes involve the liver, such as actinomycosis, tuberculosis and syphilis. All of these conditions are now rare, and the reader is referred to special articles such as that by Ravdin (1941)[44].

Cysts of the Liver

With respect to cysts of the liver, there are 2 principal types: congenital cysts which may contain either bile or mucus, and hydatid cysts due to echinococcus disease. Both are rare in this country. The echinococcus cysts should be removed intact if possible. In the event of rupture, there is danger of an allergic reaction to the antigen in the cysts, and there is also great likelihood that daughter cysts will become engrafted in other viscera and grow, producing a series of secondary symptoms. The congenital cysts may require no treatment or, if they become infected, may require drainage as in the case of a liver abscess. Where feasible, excision is perhaps the best treatment for those that become symptomatic, but this is not always possible.

Echinococcus Cysts

Echinococcus cysts are still common among pastoral peoples who live with their dogs. The *Taenia echinococcus* or dog tapeworm uses the intestinal tract of the dog as a primary breeding ground and then may be ingested by man, penetrate the wall of his alimentary canal and lodge in various organs, of which the most common are the lung and the liver. Here the cysts are characterized by large fibrous envelopes (the false cyst) containing a soft lining or membrane (the true cyst). The latter contains fluid in which may float the scolices, which are the organs by which the future tapeworm will attach himself to the alimentary tract of a future canine host. Many of these will be embedded in or at least attached to the true cyst wall. In addition, the true cyst will often contain daughter cysts or smaller compartments made up of the same kind of walls as the true cysts.

Current practice in Iran, where echinococcus disease is frequent, is to aspirate the cyst through a hollow needle and then carefully to open the false cyst and dissect out the collapsed true cyst. The object is to remove the true cyst wall intact. After this is completed, the false cyst wall may be excised; or, if this is not feasible, it may be closed about drains.

Wounds of the Liver

Wounds of the liver are important because this is the most frequently injured of the solid viscera within the abdomen. Hemorrhage is apt to be profuse and not infrequently is attended by a slow pulse until late in the development of shock. Suture should be undertaken promptly, using a large blunt needle and coarse suture material tied over omentum or some absorbable hemostatic agent, such as gelatin foam. The abdomen always should be drained as the wounds frequently leak bile and not infrequently give rise to subhepatic or subphrenic abscesses. Often large amounts of blood must be transfused to save the lives of patients with large liver wounds, as these commonly bleed very rapidly.

With penetrating injuries, the vessels to the liver also may be injured, and here the chance of saving the patient's life is slight unless the patient is seen early, and intervention is prompt. The vascular channels should be restored by suture. Should it be necessary to tie off the hepatic artery or a major branch of the hepatic artery, penicillin or chlortetracycline are recommended to reduce the chances of liver shock.

The earlier literature contains much about ptosis of the liver and corset liver, but neither of these conditions requires treatment frequently enough to justify emphasis in a book of this length. The reader is referred to Ravdin (1941)[44].

HEPATIC BIOPSY

A biopsy of 0.5 or 1.0 Gm. of liver can be taken conveniently from the anterior edge of the liver, preferably remote from the gallbladder. Hemostasis can be obtained by swaged catgut sutures if they are tied judiciously and not so tight as to cut through the liver tissue. It is believed that this is a safer procedure than the use of needle biopsy. A needle biopsy is ordinarily done: (1) without visualization of the point at which the needle enters the liver; (2) without visualization of any organs or tissues which may be present between the skin and the liver at the site selected; and (3) without visualization of the amount of bleeding which follows the puncture.

PARTIAL HEPATECTOMY

Relatively large segments of the liver have been removed in man. Many times, most of the left lobe has been sacrificed, and various substantial proportions of the right lobe. At times, the entire right lobe has been sacrificed with survival. The indications for these procedures are not encountered very frequently because most of the malignancies of the liver are either metastatic from another site or are multicentric or diffuse in their growth. Therefore, it is seldom that a case presents in which there seems to be a worthwhile chance of eradicating a tumor by a partial hepatectomy. Multiple abscesses in a given localized part of the liver, echinococcus cysts and so forth occasionally may provide a sufficient indication for a partial hepatectomy.

Technically, the problem is mainly one of hemostasis. Clamping of the blood supply of the liver at its hilum is interdicted because this results in a pooling of blood in the portal bed which may be fatal. It also interrupts the blood supply to the liver for a period which is undesirable. The use of the electric knife and the electric cautery, the use of coarse catgut swaged on larger curved needles and absorbable sponge such as foam gelatin are valuable technical aids. Sutures must be placed deep and tied loosely. If they are tied over Gelfoam or omentum, they cut the tissue less.

If the dissection is begun at the hilum, the divisions of the hepatic artery and the portal vein going to the various parts of the liver may be identified. It is then best to ligate those branches going to the portion to be excised, e.g., the right lobe. With this done, blunt dissection through the liver with the handle of a scalpel will expose the larger communicating vessels in time to doubly clamp, divide and ligate them. The most hazardous part of the procedure is apt to be that which concerns the hepatic veins. These should be identified before they are entered. Vascular sutures may be required to close the junctions of these veins with the inferior vena cava.

DRAINAGE OF HEPATIC ABSCESSES

Liver abscesses may be drained transperitoneally through an incision below the costal margin. They may be drained transpleurally, but if this is to be done it is wise to utilize a 2-stage procedure which permits a 5-day period for the pleura to seal off in the costophrenic angle before one traverses the pleural cavity. Usually a resection of the 9th and the 10th ribs is carried out at the posterior axillary line. Packing is introduced against the pleura; and after 5 days, if the pleural surfaces appear to be glued together, an incision is made through the parietal pleura and then through the parietal pleura on the diaphragm, and thence through the diaphragm into the subdiaphragmatic space and on into the liver as necessary. To avoid possible air embolism, it is well to have the patient in a slight head-up position when the liver is transected.

Ordinarily, an aspirating needle of large gauge is utilized to locate the abscess, and frequently a cautery is used to form a larger tract along the needle into the abscess cavity. Then such a tract can accommodate rubber drain tubes. Care must be taken with this plan not to go too close to major vessels, such as the inferior vena cava or the main hepatic veins.

The lung itself does not present a problem with this approach, as it lies higher at rest, and the packing and the splinting of the diaphragm prevent its downward excursion after the first stage.

Another route by which abscesses of the liver can be drained is the so-called extraperitoneal route proposed by Ochsner (1938).[40] The 12th rib is resected, its bed is incised, care being taken not to enter the pleura above. One then dissects bluntly under the diaphragm, more or less at the top of the perirenal fat. This permits a plane to be developed between the reflected peritoneal surface and the muscle fibers of the diaphragm. This allows one to expose from the outside a clear area near the dome of the liver where there is no peritoneal covering. Sometimes, the abscess will present there. In other instances, it may be necessary to explore for it with an aspirating needle. This method has found considerable application where amebic abscesses are frequent. Greater experience with chemotherapy of amebic abscesses has reduced the frequency with which this operation must be done. However, it is still necessary occasionally for amebic abscesses which become secondarily infected and it may be useful in the approach to subdiaphragmatic collections of infected material occurring after operations of various kinds in the abdomen.

Where there are multiple small abscesses in the liver, effective surgical drainage seldom can be accomplished, and in general one must pin his hopes on chemotherapy which will sometimes effect recovery.

BIBLIOGRAPHY

1. Allen, A. W.: A method of re-establishing continuity between the bile ducts and the gastrointestinal tract, Ann. Surg. *121*:412, 1945.
2. Allen, J. G.: The diagnostic value of prothrombin response to vitamin K therapy as a means of differentiating between intrahepatic and obstructive jaundice; collective review, Internat. Abstr. Surg. *76*:401, 1943.
3. Allen, J. G., and Julian, O. C.: Response of plasma prothrombin to vitamin K substitute therapy in cases of hepatic disease, Arch. Surg. *41*:1363, 1940.
4. Becker, W. F.: Perforation of the gallbladder, Surg., Gynec. & Obst. *105*:636, 1957.
5. Bergkvist, A., and Seldinger, S. I.: Pancreatic reflux in operative cholangiography in relation to pre- and postoperative pancreatic affection, Acta chir. scandinav. *114*:191, 1957-1958.
6. Berk, J. E.: Chapter C *in* Bockus: Gastroenterology, vol. 3, Philadelphia, Saunders, 1946.
7. ———: Management of acute cholecystitis, Am. J. Digest. Dis. *7*:325, 1940.
8. Bisgard, J. D., and Baker, C. P.: Studies relating to the pathogenesis of cholecystitis, cholelithiasis and acute pancreatitis, Ann. Surg. *112*:1006, 1940.
9. Bockus, H. L., Shay, H., Willard, J. H., and Pessel, J. F.: Comparison of biliary drainage and cholecystography in gallstone diagnosis, J.A.M.A. *96*:311, 1931.
10. Campbell, D. A.: A clinical study of carcinoma of the gallbladder, Ann. Surg. *113*:1068, 1941.
11. Cole, W. H., Reynolds, J. T., and Ireneus, C., Jr.: Strictures of the common duct, Ann. Surg. *128*:332, 1948.
12. ———: Strictures of the common duct, Ann. Surg. *133*:684, 1951.
13. Cooper, W. A.: Carcinoma of the gallbladder, Arch. Surg. *35*:431, 1937.
14. Cowley, L. L., and Harkins, H. N.: Perforation of the gallbladder; a study of twenty-five consecutive cases, Surg., Gynec. & Obst. *77*:661, 1943.
15. DiLuzio, N. R., Simon, K. A., and Upton, A. C.: Effects of x-rays and trypan blue on reticuloendothelial cells, A.M.A. Arch. Path. *64*:649, 1957.
16. Donald, J. D., and Fitts, W. T., Jr.: Cholecystostomy: a study of patients 10 to 16 years later, Am. J. Surg. *78*:596, 1949.

17. Fitts, W. T., Jr.: Personal communication, 1948.
18. Fitts, W. T., Jr., Scott, R., and Mackie, J. A.: Antibiotics in the prevention of death following ligation of the hepatic artery in dogs, Surgery *128*:458, 1950.
19. Fletcher, A. G., Jr., and Ravdin, I. S.: Perforation of the gallbladder, Am. J. Surg. *81*:178, 1951.
20. Folin, O., and Denis, W.: The origin and significance of the ammonia in the portal blood, J. Biol. Chem. *11*:161, 1912.
21. Frommhold, W.: Ein neuartiges Kontrastmittel für die intravenöse Cholezystographie, Fortschr. Geb. Röntgenstrahlen *79*:283, 1953.
22. Gatch, W. D., Battersby, J. S., and Wakim, K. G.: The nature and treatment of cholecystitis, J.A.M.A. *132*:119, 1946.
23. Graham, E. A., Cole, W. H., and Copher, G. H.: Cholecystography: The use of sodium tetraiodophenolphthalein, J.A.M.A. *84*:1175, 1925.
24. Hewitt, J. E., Hayes, T. L., Gofman, J. W., Jones, H. B., and Pierce, F. T.: Effects of total body irradiation upon lipoprotein metabolism, Am. J. Physiol. *172*:579, 1953.
25. Howard, J. M., and Jones, R.: The anatomy of the pancreatic duct, Am. J. M. Sc. *214*:617, 1947.
26. Illingworth, C. F. W.: Carcinoma of the gallbladder, Brit. J. Surg. *23*:4, 1935.
27. Jankelson, I. R.: Clinical aspects of primary carcinoma of the gallbladder, New England J. Med. *217*:85, 1937.
28. Kirby, C. K.: Instrument for detection of stones in the bile ducts, Am. J. Surg. *80*:133, 1950.
29. Kirshbaum, J. D., and Kozoll, D. D.: Carcinoma of the gallbladder and extrahepatic bile ducts, Surg., Gynec. & Obst. *73*:740, 1941.
30. Kocher, T.: Textbook of Operative Surgery, London, Black, 1903.
31. Langenbuch, C.: Ein Fall von Exstirpation der Gallenblase wegen chronischer Cholelithiasis; Heilung, Berlin klin. Wchnschr. *19*:725, 1882.
    A case of extirpation of the gallbladder for cholelithiasis *by* C. Langenbuch (Trans. by S. Brandeis), Louisville M. News *15*:161, 1883.
32. Life Insurance Fact Book 1959, New York, Institute of Life Insurance, pp. 126.
33. McCubbrey, D., and Thieme, E. T.: Perforation of the gallbladder, Arch. Surg. *80*:204, 1960.
34. McDermott, W. V., Jr., Adams, R. D., and Ridell, A. G.: Ammonia metabolism in man, Ann. Surg. *140*:539, 1954.
35. Mann, F. C., and Bollman, J. L.: Liver function tests, Arch. Path. *1*:681, 1926.
36. Markowitz, J., Rappaport, A., and Scott, A. C.: Prevention of liver necrosis following ligation of the hepatic artery, Proc. Soc. Exper. Biol. & Med. *70*:305, 1949.
37. Massie, J. R., Coxe, J. W., III, Parker, C., and Dietrick, R.: Gallbladder perforations in acute cholecystitis, Ann. Surg. *145*:825, 1957.
38. Morse, L., Krynski, B., and Wright, A. R.: Acute perforation of the gallbladder, Am. J. Surg. *94*:772, 1957.
39. Nissen, R.: Personal communication, May 14, 1959.
40. Ochsner, A., DeBakey, M., and Murray, S.: Pyogenic abscess of liver: II. An analysis of 47 cases with a review of the literature, Am. J. Surg. *40*:292, 1938.
41. Ohage, J.: Report of case at meeting of County Medical Society, Sept. 27, 1886, Northwestern Lancet *6*:55, 1886.
42. ———: The surgical treatment of diseases of the gallbladder, Med. News Phila. *50*:202, 233, 1887.
43. Pines, B., and Rabinovitch, J.: Perforation of the gallbladder and acute cholecystitis, Ann. Surg. *140*:170, 1954.
44. Ravdin, I. S.: Surgery of diseases of the liver *in* Bancroft, F. W., ed.: Operative Surgery, New York, Appleton, 1941.
45. Ravdin, I. S., Rhoads, J. E., Frazier, W., and Ulin, A. W.: The effect of recent advances in biliary physiology on the mortality following operations for common duct obstructions. Surgery *3*:804, 1939.
46. Ravdin, I. S., Thorogood, E., Riegel, C., Peters, C., and Rhoads, J. E.: The prevention of liver damage, J.A.M.A. *121*:322, 1943.
47. Riegel, C. R., Ravdin, I. S., Johnston, C. G., and Morrison, P. J.: Studies of gallbladder function: XIII. The composition of the gallbladder bile and calculi in gallbladder disease, Surg., Gynec. & Obst. *62*:933, 1936.
48. Roberts, B., and Dex, W. J.: Primary carcinoma of the gallbladder *in* Proceedings of the Third National Cancer Conference, p. 802, Philadelphia, Lippincott, 1957.
49. Robertson, H. E., and Dochat, G. R.: Pregnancy and gallstones; collective review, Internat. Abstr. Surg. *78*:193, 1944.
50. Sainburg, F. P., and Garlock, G. H.: Carcinoma of the gallbladder; report of seventy-five cases, Surgery *23*:201, 1948.
51. Sawyer, C. D., and Minnis, J. F., Jr.: Primary carcinoma of the gallbladder, Am. J. Surg. *91*:99, 1956.

52. Swinton, N. W., and Becker, W. F.: Tumors of the gallbladder, S. Clin. North America 28:669, 1948.

53. Stevenson, J. K., and Harkins, H. N.: Acute perforations of the gastrointestinal tract, West. J. Surg. 65(5):286, 1957.

54. Stormont, J. M., Mackie, J. E., and Davidson, C. S.: Observations on antibiotics in the treatment of hepatic coma and on factors contributing to prognosis, New England J. Med. 259:1145, 1958.

55. Ulin, A. W.: Therapeutic trends and operative mortality in cases of obstructive jaundice, Arch. Surg. 46:504, 1943.

56. Warner, E. D., Brinkhous, K. M., and Smith, H. P.: Bleeding tendency of obstructive jaundice: prothrombin deficiency and dietary factors, Proc. Soc. Exper. Biol. & Med. 37:628, 1938.

57. Warren, R., and Rhoads, J. E.: Hepatic origin of the plasma-prothrombin observations after total hepatectomy in the dog, Am. J. M. Sc. 198:193, 1939.

58. Whipple, A. O.: Pancreatic asthenia as a postoperative complication in patients with lesions of the pancreas, Ann. Surg. 78:176, 1923.

59. Zech, R. L.: Acute pancreatitis following cholangiography, West. J. Surg. 57:295, 1949.

JONATHAN E. RHOADS

CHAPTER 31

Pancreas

ANATOMY

The pancreas, variously called by such eponyms as the "hermit organ" and the "abdominal salivary gland," is a yellowish, elongated, retroperitoneal gland situated at about the level of the 2nd lumbar vertebra on the posterior wall of the upper abdomen (Fig. 31-1). It is a transverse L-shaped organ about 15 cm. long, 2 to 3 cm. thick and approximately 65 to 125 Gm. in weight, consisting of a head, a neck, a body and a tail. The head nestles in the concavity of the duodenum with which it is intimately associated. The neck overlies the superior mesenteric vessels and the origin of the portal vein. The body and the tail extend upward and laterally to reach the hilum of the spleen. The uncinate process, an inferior extension of the head, is in apposition with the third portion of the duodenum and lies posterior to the mesenteric vessels. Thus, the pancreas is wrapped around the superior mesenteric artery and vein on 3 sides: anteriorly, to the right and posteriorly.

The arterial supply is derived from 3 princi-pal sources. The *superior pancreaticoduodenal* artery arises from the hepatic artery via the gastroduodenal artery and supplies the duodenum and the pancreas in part. It anastomoses with the *inferior pancreaticoduodenal,* which usually arises from the superior mesenteric, and the two vessels form an arcade between the duodenum and the pancreas and supply principally the duodenum and the head and the neck of the pancreas. The splenic artery, a branch of the celiac axis, courses along the posterosuperior border of the pancreas en route to the spleen. It is the principal source of supply to the body and the tail of the gland.

Numerous variations of the vascular supply may occur to plague the surgeon. Ligation of certain anomalous vessels may result in such catastrophies as necrosis of the liver or the transverse colon. The principal veins correspond to the arteries except that the superior pancreatoduodenal vein often empties into the terminal portion of the splenic vein.

There are 3 principal groups of lymph nodes closely associated with the pancreas.

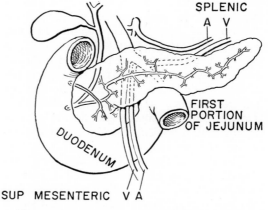

FIG. 31-1. Anatomy of the pancreas and its relation to surrounding structures.

These comprise the subpyloric group, the pancreaticolienal nodes and the group in proximity to the uncinate process and the superior mesenteric vessels at that level. Lymphatics accompany the major vessels and may terminate in the pancreatic nodes; they anastomose freely with lymphatics which terminate in the nodes about the stomach and the aorta. Branches of the sympathetic and the parasympathetic nerves accompany the vessels, terminating as fine filaments about the acini.

Duct System

The duct of Wirsung, coursing throughout the length of the pancreas, is the main pancreatic duct. In the head of the pancreas it becomes closely associated with the terminal portion of the common bile duct and, in the majority of cases, the 2 ducts terminate jointly at the papilla of Vater on the concave side of the second part of the duodenum (about 7 cm. from the pylorus). The ampulla of Vater is a channel lined by epithelium and formed by the confluence of the common bile duct and the main pancreatic duct. The sphincter of Oddi encompasses the ducts at their terminus on the papilla.

Since 1901 when Opie[58] first presented his common channel theory of the etiology of acute pancreatitis interest has centered in the termination patterns of the 2 ducts. In 29 per cent of cases (Rienhoff and Pickrell 1945[71]) the 2 ducts enter the duodenum through separate openings on a common papilla. However, in the majority of cases the 2 ducts communicate to form a single short channel before entering the duodenum. Various classifications have been employed using as a criterion the depth of the ampulla. In from 54 per cent (Howard and Jones 1947[39]) to 66 per cent (Cameron and Noble 1924[13]) of cadavers it was found that a stone impacted distally could divert the flow of bile into the pancreatic duct or vice versa. Millbourn (1949),[49] using cholangiographic technics in postmortem specimens, found a common channel in 91.5 per cent.

The duct of Santorini, the accessory pancreatic duct, is present in the majority of glands and drains a portion of the head of the pancreas. It opens separately, without a sphincter, into the duodenum proximal to the papilla of Vater. The 2 pancreatic ducts were found to communicate in 36 per cent (Howard and Jones[39]) and in 89 per cent (Rienhoff and Pickrell[71]) of cases.

Histology

The pancreas has no true capsule but is enveloped by loose connective tissue from which septa extend to divide the gland into lobules. It is covered on the anterior surface by the posterior parietal peritoneum. Both the exocrine and the endocrine secretory cells are derived from the finer ductules, although the latter lose their connection with the duct system. The exocrine gland cells form the main mass of the organ and form acini whose component secreting cells are characterized by basal nuclei and zymogen granules. Spheroidal aggregations of light-staining cells, the islets of Langerhans, are found scattered throughout the gland but are more numerous in the tail. The islets number from 200,000 to 2,000,000.

Annular Pancreas

Pancreatic tissue surrounding the second portion of the duodenum is termed annular pancreas. It represents a developmental defect and is occasionally symptomatic, causing the picture of high intestinal obstruction, especially in children, due to the formation of a constriction. It is usually best treated by anastomosis of the jejunum to the duodenum, proximal to the point of narrowing. (See Chap. 46, "Pediatric Surgery.")

Pancreatic Heterotopia

Another developmental abnormality is the occurrence of pancreatic tissue along various parts of the alimentary tract not connected with the main organ. These too are occasionally symptomatic.

PHYSIOLOGY

The pancreas is a dual gland, having both an exocrine and an endocrine function.

The Pancreas as an Exocrine Gland

Pancreatic juice, the daily production of which is about 1,500 to 2,000 milliliters, is a clear, limpid fluid with an alkaline pH. It contains trypsinogen, chymotrypsinogen, amylase, pancreatic lipase (steapsin) and maltase.

Pancreatic juice also contains a carboxypolypeptidase capable of digesting certain peptides.

Trypsinogen is activated (converted to trypsin) by the action of enterokinase, an enzyme found in the succus entericus and also by the action of trypsin itself. *Activated trypsin* splits proteoses, peptones and polypeptides to simple peptides in an alkaline medium. It is more potent than pepsin. *Chymotrypsinogen* is activated by trypsin and has a similar action but is a weaker proteolytic agent. *Amylase* converts long-chain carbohydrates such as starch and glycogen to dextrins and sugars. *Pancreatic lipase* splits fats into glycerin and fatty acids. *Bile salts* increase the efficiency of this process by helping to emulsify the fats. All these enzymes are apparently secreted by the acinar cells.

The rate of secretion and the composition of pancreatic juice is influenced by humoral and nervous mechanisms. It is not secreted at a uniform rate. When acid chyme comes into contact with the mucosa of the small bowel, a hormone, *secretin*, is released into the blood stream which stimulates the secretion of the acinar cells directly to secrete a watery pancreatic juice relatively high in bicarbonate content and volume and relatively poor in enzymes. Secretin also stimulates the flow of bile and the production of succus entericus. Vagus stimulation causes the secretion of a more viscous juice rich in enzymes. It can be inhibited by large doses of atropine or by vagotomy. There is some evidence that sulfa drugs and some of the antibiotics are excreted in pancreatic juice.

Pure pancreatic juice does not digest living tissue such as skin. Excoriation of the skin about abdominal fistulas implies that the pancreatic juice has become activated. Recently, aluminum paste and building cement powder (bentonite) have found favor in minimizing the skin excoriation. However, constant wound suction still remains the single most effective method of reducing skin damage from pancreatic enzymes.

THE PANCREAS AS AN ENDOCRINE GLAND

Insulin, a product of the beta cells of the islets of Langerhans, is the hormone which plays a vital role in carbohydrate, fat and protein metabolism. Without it men soon die.

Its exact mechanism of action has not yet been completely elucidated.

Recently, cells of the islets of Langerhans have been shown to produce a blood-sugar-raising principle (glucagon). Because it was found that completely depancreatized dogs, maintained on insulin, still died in a few months and at postmortem demonstrated fatty infiltration of the liver, it was postulated that the pancreas elaborated yet another hormone. Dragstedt[27] prepared an extract of the pancreas, which he called "lipocaic," that prevented fatty infiltration and permitted prolonged survival of depancreatized dogs maintained with insulin. The dose was about 1 Gm. daily. Lecithin, choline and methionine also have been found to possess similar properties.

Rhoads, *et al.,*[66] studied the effect of a lipotropic extract, produced by the method of Bosshardt, Ciereszko and Barnes,[8] on depancreatized dogs. They found that it was effective in preventing fatty infiltration of the liver, and the observations suggested that the material acted as an enzyme, since it was less effective in dogs that ate poorly (insufficient methionine?).

Haanes and Gyorgy[34] found that Bosshardt's extract contained a powerful proteolytic enzyme (probably trypsin), the action of which was masked by an excess of an inhibitor. Duodenal juice (from a depancreatized dog) destroyed the effect of this inhibitor, leaving the proteolytic enzyme free to liberate methionine from casein.

In certain depancreatized patients Nardi [56, 57] and his collaborators have found that no replacement therapy except insulin has been necessary. Marked differences apparently occur between species and probably between individuals so that replacement therapy is provided after total pancreatectomy until detailed studies show that digestion is reasonably complete without it.

ACUTE PANCREATITIS

Acute pancreatitis is an inflammation of the pancreas affecting all or, more rarely, a part of the gland. It may be evidenced only by edema and leukocytic infiltration, or by these signs and evidence of necrosis in the gland and necrosis of fat in the vicinity of the pancreas or even at a distance in the peritoneal cavity due to the escape of enzymes. In severe cases fat necrosis also has been observed in the thoracic cavity. Severe pancreatitis may be associated with hemorrhage into the gland or even hemorrhage from the gland into the peritoneal cavity (hemorrhagic pancreatitis) or by actual necrosis of macroscopic portions of the gland with sloughing (necrotizing pancreatitis). In the past, a considerable effort has been made to distinguish edematous pancreatitis from hemorrhagic and necrotizing pancreatitis. The mortality of those cases showing only edema is slight, whereas the mortality in the hemorrhagic and necrotizing forms has exceeded 50 per cent in some series. However, available evidence suggests that these are 2 stages of the same disease rather than separate entities. Some patients who have been operated on and the edematous stage found have recovered from that attack only to experience subsequent development of the hemorrhagic necrotizing form from which they died. Certainly the attempt to differentiate the two at the time of a hospital admission is uncertain unless operation or autopsy is performed. Men are afflicted by the severe forms of the disease more frequently than women.

In a series of cases reported from the Hospital of the University of Pennsylvania, the preoperative range and average for temperature, pulse rate, respirations and leukocyte count were almost identical for those cases in which edematous pancreatitis was found at laparotomy and for those cases in which necrotizing pancreatitis was found at laparotomy. Probably it is possible to pick out as hemorrhagic or necrotizing a few of the very severe cases on the clinical picture, but for the large majority differentiation can be made only on the basis of the course of the disease and the pathologic findings at operation or at autopsy.

The development of practical methods for the determination of the serum amylase and lipase have revolutionized the diagnosis of pancreatitis within certain limitations to be discussed below. However, it is not claimed that the studies of these enzymes at the time of admission to a hospital will effectively distinguish the edematous form of the disease from the hemorrhagic or necrotizing forms, as very high values frequently occur in edematous pancreatitis as well as with the more severe types of the disease.

CLINICAL PICTURE

The milder forms of pancreatitis are associated with pain in the epigastrium, frequently radiating to the back near the angles of the scapulae; this radiation may be to the left side of the back, to the right side of the back or to both sides. Vomiting may or may not occur. The chief differential problems in diagnosis at this stage are acute cholecystitis, peptic ulcer with a slow leak or a leak that is sealed off, or a penetrating ulcer that has given rise to inflammation without frank perforation. From this picture one sees various degrees of severity up to and including the patient who has had a rapid onset of severe abdominal pain, with prostration, marked tachycardia, high fever and a gray, shocklike appearance. Such patients often become distended early from adynamic ileus and not infrequently vomit profusely. The vomitus is sometimes fecal in character. Associated with these symptoms will usually be found very marked abdominal tenderness, rebound tenderness, diminution or absence of peristaltic sounds on ausculation of the abdomen, and marked muscle spasm and rigidity. Here the differential diagnosis includes ruptured peptic ulcer, renal colic, acute phlegmonous gastritis and possibly perforation of the gallbladder, mesenteric occlusion, volvulus, dissecting aneurysm of the abdominal aorta or myocardial infarction.

The most useful confirmatory studies from the laboratory are the serum amylase and the serum lipase. The amylase is of greater value in the first 48 hours of the disease, whereas the lipase remains elevated for a longer period, usually 5 to 7 days. Unfortunately, the elevation of the serum amylase is not absolutely pathognomonic for primary pancreatitis. Elevations occur frequently in patients in whom an ulcer penetrates against the pancreas, setting up a local inflammatory process. Elevations have also been noted in a miscellaneous group of patients undergoing operation and especially in patients with acute cholecystitis. The editors of this volume have seen marked elevations of amylase in high intestinal obstruction, volvulus of the small intestine, mesenteric vascular occlusion, trauma to upper lumbar and lower thoracic space (laminectomy), and acute renal insufficiency. The significance of this is that when one wishes to treat pancreatitis without operation, one would like to have a test which would remain unaffected by other diseases entering into the differential diagnosis which do require operation. Hence, in the present state of our knowledge, it is still frequently necessary to operate on patients suspected of having an acute pancreatitis because the picture is sufficiently compatible with that of a perforated peptic ulcer, a very acute cholecystitis with rupture, or mesenteric occlusion.

Determination of serum amylase by the method of Somogyi[74] requires approximately 1½ hours, whereas determination of lipase by most of the standard methods requires from 4 to 24 hours. Therefore, for emergency use the amylase test has been of greater value. The normal level runs up to about 200 Somogyi units; in the presence of acute pancreatitis, this value usually is exceeded by more than 100 units and not infrequently mounts as high as 1,000 units or more. Institutions caring for patients with acute abdominal disease should provide for the performance of this test on emergency admissions on a 24-hour-a-day, 7-day-a-week basis.

The concentration of serum calcium often falls from 36 to 48 hours after the beginning of an attack of severe pancreatitis. Levels as low as 7 mg./100 ml. have been seen. This is not known to occur in any other acute abdominal condition except occasionally in a leaking duodenal stump, a perforated peptic ulcer, or ulcerative colitis with ileostomy. The fall in serum calcium is commonly attributed to the binding of calcium with fatty acids to form insoluble calcium soaps in areas of fat necrosis.

Etiology

Acute pancreatitis can be reproduced experimentally in the dog by injecting bile into the main pancreatic duct under pressure. Opie[59] originally postulated that some instances of the disease in man might be due to the entrance of bile into the pancreatic duct as the result of a stone lodged in the papilla of Vater. This presupposes a common channel of sufficient length to permit the bile to move into the pancreatic duct behind the stone.

According to the studies of Jones and Howard,[39] there was a common channel of at least 0.5 cm. in 54 per cent in a series of 100 individuals examined at necropsy whom they had opportunity to study. It also presupposes a higher pressure in the biliary tract than in the pancreatic ductal system. However, experimental evidence does not support this presupposition with uniformity.

Also, it has been suggested that pancreatitis arises by virtue of bacterial infection coursing toward the pancreas from the gallbladder and the hilum of the liver through the lymphatics. Others have postulated that the infection is an ascending one through the ductal system into the pancreas from the duodenum. There are authenticated cases in which an acute pancreatitis has followed trauma. While this may be penetrating in type, it also has followed blunt trauma to the abdomen without a break in the skin. Another small group of cases has occurred after operation, particularly operations on the biliary tract or the stomach where, of course, there may be some disturbance or even trauma to the pancreas. A further occasional cause of pancreatitis is apparently the mumps virus, which attacks primarily the salivary glands but may attack the gonads and the pancreas also.

The frequency with which severe acute necrotizing and hemorrhagic pancreatitis occurs among alcoholics is so much higher relative to its frequency among the nondrinkers that alcoholic debauchery may be considered as a predisposing factor.

Mallet-Guy[48] and others of the French workers have produced pancreatitis in the experimental animal by electrical stimulation of autonomic nerves leading to the pancreas.

Treatment

The treatment of acute pancreatitis has gone through cycles, between operative and nonoperative treatment. In the severe forms of the disease attempts at drainage of the pancreas have been attended by mortality rates as high as 70 per cent (Babcock[2]). The present consensus is that wherever the diagnosis can be established safely, operation should not be done during the acute stage, though if the process goes on to the formation of abscesses or collections of necrotic material in the pancreas, usually these will require free drainage, perhaps, in the 2nd or the 3rd or subsequent weeks after the onset of the attack.

If early operation is done, as is not infrequently necessary in order to exclude the possibility of other serious intra-abdominal conditions, and if at the time of operation acute pancreatitis is found it is our practice to do a simple cholecystostomy in order to permit an easy route for bile to escape in the event that the common channel is occluded at its termination either by stone or spasm, and to lay drains down to the pancreas without injuring its substance in any way. Then the wound is closed, all unnecessary surgical manipulation being scrupulously avoided.

Nonoperative treatment includes antibiotics, which have had a profound effect on the course of acute pancreatitis. Penicillin is administered in divided doses totaling 1,000,000 units a day; one of the polyvalent antibiotics parenterally and possibly chlortetracycline by mouth or through a stomach tube may be given. According to the experiments of Fine[61] and his collaborators on the dog, chlortetracycline by mouth was especially beneficial in the reduction of the mortality rate in experimental pancreatitis. It also depends on the application of standard methods of treating peritonitis, hypotension and hypovolemia, including suction drainage of the stomach, water and electrolytes in sufficient amounts to maintain the internal environment of the body normal with respect to sodium, potassium, chloride and pH, and transfusions of blood or plasma sufficient to maintain blood volume, and hemoglobin and protein concentrations near the normal range. If the serum calcium is reduced, calcium gluconate should be given intravenously in doses up to 1 Gm. every 2 to 4 hours.

The role of paravertebral injections of local anesthetic agents deserves especial mention. This method of treatment in pancreatitis was advocated vigorously by Mims Gage[31] in New Orleans. From 10 to 20 cc. of 1 per cent procaine is introduced on each side of the body just below the level of the 12th rib along the anterolateral surface of the vertebral body. Often the procedure is followed by a striking relief of pain, even in patients whose pain has not been relieved by 15 to 30 mg. of morphine sulfate. Gage[31] believed that the procaine relieves vascular spasm and exerts a therapeutic as well as a symptomatic effect. The method was very widely practiced, although perhaps more on an empiric basis than anything else. It is now used chiefly for relief of pain. In our own clinic, it is customary to give 1 or 2 procaine injections on each side during the first 24 hours and to repeat them once a day for 2 or 3 days if pain persists.

The combined use of gastroduodenal suction and atropine constitutes a very important part of the treatment of acute pancreatitis by virtue of the fact that atropine prevents vagal stimulation of the pancreas, and the gastroduodenal suction removes the stimulus for the elaboration of secretin, the principal humoral stimulant.

PROGNOSIS

If one takes all patients diagnosed as having acute pancreatitis with the support of an elevated serum amylase, mortality is relatively low; Howard[65] reported 3 per cent. On the other hand, if one restricts the series to those cases known to have hemorrhagic or necrotizing pancreatitis on the basis of laparotomy, mortality rates are much higher, usually 20 per cent and up. A recent review of the statistics from the Hospital of the University of Pennsylvania by Kirby and Senior has yielded the following data (Table 1). Severe acute pancreatitis remains a serious disease despite all forms of present-day therapy, including antibiotics. Mortality rates are likely to reflect more the zealousness of an institution in establishing the diagnosis in a large number of mild or borderline cases than any other one factor. It should be remembered that be-

TABLE 1. ACTIVE PANCREATITIS*

Hospital of the University of Pennsylvania
Mortality Before and After 1946 (Per Cent)

	EDEMATOUS	NECROTIZING	TOTAL	POST-OPERATIVE
1922–46	11.9	76.2	28.8	...
1946–53	4.6	33.3	13.8	57.1

* Rhoads, J. E., Senior, J. R., Kirby, C. K., and Rhoads, D. V. Surgery of the Pancreas. Presented at the 66th annual meeting of the Mid-South Postgraduate Medical Assembly, Memphis, Tenn., Feb. 8–11, 1955.

fore the development of the amylase test, only the severe forms were recognized.

Early deaths from pancreatitis indeed appear to be much rarer than was the case before the advent of the antibiotics and other concomitant advances. In those days it was common for pancreatitis to be fatal in the first few days—sometimes in the first 24 hours. With the exception of a single case in our recent experience, all of the patients have lived for over a week, and most of the fatal cases have survived from 2 to 6 weeks. In these individuals a suppurative autolyzing process is set up in the pancreas, which it seems impossible to control by drainage or even by the removal of some of the necrotic tissue after an appropriate interval of some weeks. Activated pancreatic ferments apparently continue to be released, and the terminal event is frequently hemorrhage from a large artery, the wall of which is digested away. This may be the hepatic artery or some other major branch of the celiac axis or the superior mesenteric artery. Necrosis involves not only the pancreas but seems to extend some distance into the retroperitoneal fat. It is difficult to define what the factors of resistance may be to this process, but some individuals clearly have greater powers of localizing the process than do others.

Recent experience with acute pancreatitis in Moscow was reported by Bystrov (1959)[12] in a series of 810 cases. Of these, 60 patients or 7.4 per cent of the series were classified as having hemorrhagic necrosis of the pancreas. Twenty-three patients, including all of the 8 not operated upon, died, so that the per cent of mortality was 38.

It is evident that recovery from one attack of pancreatitis does not guarantee that the individual will not suffer a subsequent attack. In a series of 47 cases of acute pancreatitis followed by Howard,[41] 5 were found to have had subsequent attacks of pancreatitis, 2 of them fatal. Cholelithiasis is present in about 75 per cent of the patients in most series of cases of acute pancreatitis. In many clinics it is customary to investigate the gallbladder by cholecystography after the acute attack has passed and to remove those in which there is evidence of cholelithiasis. We believe this to be good practice, although we know of no body of statistics which would demonstrate conclusively whether or not this per se would reduce the chances of recurrent attacks of pancreatitis.

The use of dyes for visualizing the gallbladder after pancreatitis raises certain questions. When the original dye advocated by Graham and Cole,[32] tetraiodophenolphthalein, was employed in the presence of jaundice, several instances of acute pancreatitis were reported. Dick and Wallace[24] found that if the dye were given to an animal and the contents of the gallbladder aspirated at a time when the dye was concentrated there, this material seemed to be especially toxic when injected into the pancreatic duct. However, Howard[38] was unable to confirm this finding, with Priodax (iodoalphionic acid). So far biligrafin has not been incriminated but we have not studied it from this standpoint experimentally. A case of acute pancreatitis occurring immediately following an operative cholangiogram occurred in 1954 and was reported by Hershey and Hillman.[36]

Acute pancreatitis, apparently due to parasitic infestation, has been reported from Hanoi by Tong That Tung and his associates (1960).[76] Among 103 patients, there was one in whom the parasite was actually found in the pancreatic duct. In 19 patients ascarides were found in the bile duct without stones; in 17 patients ascarides and stones were found; and in the remaining patients (67) only "ascaridic" stones were found containing eggs of Ascaris, pieces of dead worms, or both.

These cases require operation, and the authors report that acute, severe "ascaridic cholecystic-pancreatitis" treated expectantly is accompanied by a mortality rate approaching 100 per cent. Operation usually included clearing the common bile duct, except in the sickest patients in whom cholecystostomy was used as a first stage.

The editors know of no matching experience in the United States with which to compare this unusual report.

TRAUMA

Injuries to the pancreas result, most commonly, from operations upon the pancreas or structures in close proximity to it, such as the biliary tract, the duodenum, the stomach and

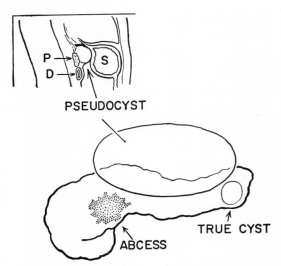

PSEUDOCYST

TRUE CYST

ABCESS

Fig. 31-2. Diagrammatic representation showing difference between true cysts, pseudocysts and abscess of the pancreas. P-pancreas; D-duodenum; S-stomach.

the spleen. In operations in this area, pancreatic parenchyma, ducts or vessels may be injured with resultant hemorrhage, escape of pancreatic ferments and necrosis. Obviously, prevention is the most important part of treatment.

Penetrating (gunshot and stab wounds), nonpenetrating (automobile accidents, falls and contact sports), abdominal and, less commonly, flank trauma may cause pancreatic injury. Penetrating pancreatic trauma usually is associated with damage to contiguous structures and nearly always requires exploratory laparotomy. If the gland is found to be injured, silk sutures are employed to stop hemorrhage but accurate suture of lacerated parenchyma is rarely feasible. Adequate drainage with sump or Penrose drains is mandatory. Continuous suction is instituted to prevent wound digestion from the pancreatic juice, in case it is activated.

Nonpenetrating abdominal or flank trauma need not necessarily be so severe as to cause extensive pancreatic injury. Injury of the smaller pancreatic ducts with escape of pancreatic juice may result in extensive pancreatic necrosis and severe hemorrhage from autodigestion of contused parenchyma. The most common clinical picture is that of pancreatitis which may be associated with surgical shock

by virtue of blood loss or with adynamic ileus as a result of widespread peritoneal irritation.

Treatment is similar to that of acute pancreatitis. Laparotomy will almost always be necessary to evaluate the extent of the damage and to establish the diagnosis.

The principal sequelae of pancreatic trauma are pancreatic abscess, pancreatic fistulas and the formation of pseudocysts (Fig. 31-2). The first two are treated with antibiotics and surgical drainage followed usually by continuous aspiration of the drainage tract; treatment of the last is discussed in the section on pancreatic cysts.

External pancreatic fistulas should be treated conservatively, with continuous suction, in the hope that the fistula will close. If the amount of drainage has not decreased significantly in several weeks, further treatment is indicated. The treatment of choice is excision of the tract down to and including the segment of the pancreas from which it arises plus excision of all pancreatic tissue distal to this point. If this is impossible, implantation of the tract into the gastrointestinal tract, preferably jejunum, may be performed.

As long as fluid balance can be maintained it is best to be quite patient as many of these fistulas will close spontaneously even after several months. Roentgen therapy (600 to 1,200 r) has been observed to reduce the trypsin content, although not the volume. This has led to early closure of such fistulas in a number of instances.[53]

ISLET CELL TUMORS

Tumors of the islet cells of the pancreas were first described by Nichols, a pathologist, in 1902. However, it was not until 1927, after the discovery of insulin by Banting and Best[3] and the elaboration of the concept of hyperinsulinism by Harris,[35] that Wilder, et al.,[83] first established the unquestioned correlation between clinical hyperinsulinism and a malignant islet cell tumor which they found at operation. Roscoe Graham[33] recorded the first surgical cure of organic hyperinsulinism in 1929 with the excision of an islet cell adenoma. The tumors may be benign or malignant, functional or nonfunctional. The majority of these circumscribed, vascular, reddish-gray tumors are about 1 to 2 cm. in diameter, although they have been described up to 15 cm. They occur in the head, the body and the tail of the pancreas with a somewhat higher incidence in the tail. Microscopically, the tumor cells closely resemble normal islet cells. It has been suggested that functioning tumors are composed of beta cells, while the nonfunctioning tumors are composed of alpha cells. This has not been established.

Howard, Moss and Rhoads[40] collected 388 cases and added 10 from the Hospital of the University of Pennsylvania. They found that 78.6 per cent were benign adenomas, 12.1 per cent were microscopically malignant but clinically benign, that is, there was no evidence of recurrence or metastasis, although histologically these tumors demonstrated anaplasia, blood vessel invasion or lack of well-defined encapsulation; and 9.3 per cent (37 cases) were carcinomas of which 22 were hyperfunctioning tumors. Of the 361 localized tumors, 200 were operated upon for hyperinsulinism, and 161 were found at autopsy. The incidence of multiple tumors was 12.6 per cent. Ectopic pancreatic tissue was found to be the site of islet cell tumors in 9 patients, 8 of whom presented clinical evidence of hyperinsulinism. This collected series has been extended recently to 1959 (Moss and Rhoads, 1960).[52]

SYMPTOMS

Nonfunctioning islet cell tumors are rarely diagnosed during life unless quite large or malignant. Functioning tumors manifest themselves by the symptoms of hyperinsulinism. These patients have periodic attacks of hypoglycemia which may present as weakness, anxiety, "nervousness," sweating, palpitation and syncope, convulsions and coma. Often they are admitted to the neurologic or neurosurgical service of a hospital. Misdiagnoses as functional hypoglycemia, epilepsy, encephalitis, psychoneuroses and brain tumor are not uncommon.

During an attack, the blood sugar frequently drops to 30 mg. per cent or lower, causing increased nervous excitability of central nervous system origin which in its severe form is manifested by epileptiform convulsions, followed by depression of the central nervous system which may be severe enough to cause coma. Prolonged episodes of hypo-

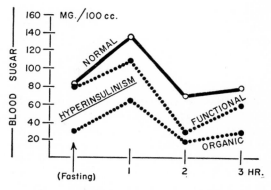

FIG. 31-3. Glucose tolerance curves differentiating functional from organic hyperinsulinism.

glycemia or repeated attacks may cause irreversible nerve cell damage leading to mental deterioration and death.

DIAGNOSIS

The criteria for diagnosis of a functioning islet cell tumor are as follows:

1. Signs and symptoms of insulin shock, frequently induced by the fasting state or during exercise

2. Repeated fasting blood sugar concentrations below 50 mg. per cent

3. Relief of symptoms by glucose administration

4. Lack of relief by low-carbohydrate, high-protein diet to exclude functional hypoglycemia as far as possible

The first 3 of the above criteria constitute Whipple's triad.

The principal differential diagnostic problem is functional hypoglycemia which is largely ruled out by the above criteria. Conn[20] believes that the latter is responsible for 70 per cent of cases with hypoglycemic manifestations. It is due to an exaggerated insulin response to an elevation of the blood sugar such as occurs with meals, especially carbohydrate foods, and excitement (adrenalin response) (Fig. 31-3). Tests based on the effect of insulin on blood sugar levels and the effect of epinephrine on blood sugar levels are no longer widely used in the diagnosis of organic hyperinsulinism.

Rare causes of hypoglycemia are due to the following: (1) biliary cirrhosis of the liver with decreased storage of glycogen, (2) Von Gierke's disease and (3) functional hypoglycemia after gastric operations.

TREATMENT

Carefully planned laparotomy with simple enucleation of the adenoma if found is the treatment of choice. Excision of surrounding normal pancreatic tissue is unnecessary, as there is no evidence that the adenoma is a premalignant lesion. A very careful examination of the entire pancreas must be carried out, even though one or more adenomas are easily found because multiple tumors occur in about 12 per cent of these patients.

If no localized adenoma is found in an individual having all the criteria requisite to a diagnosis of organic hyperinsulinism, a resection of all but a small section of the head of the pancreas is advocated by many surgeons. Occasionally, small adenomas are thus removed blindly (see below). The operative mortality should be below 5 per cent in experienced hands. Alloxan has been demonstrated to be ineffective and dangerous in the treatment of these tumors (Brunschwig and Allen[11]).

RESULTS

The results of surgical therapy have been remarkably good. In the 398 cases collected by Howard, Moss and Rhoads,[40] operative removal consisted of exploration and enucleation in 153 patients, and exploration and partial resection in 48 patients. The mortality was about 9 per cent, and end results were reported as good in 87.3 per cent of the survivors.

In 118 patients no tumor could be located at the time of exploration. Of these, 37 eventually were found to have an islet cell tumor, 12 having the adenoma removed at a subsequent operation, and 12 having it resected blindly during subtotal pancreatectomy. Adenomas were found in 13 cases at autopsy. In 81 patients the tumor never was found. Of these, 56 had a partial pancreatectomy with an operative mortality of 7.1 per cent and a satisfactory therapeutic result was obtained in 46.4 per cent. Only 1 of the 37 patients with carcinoma was alive when last reported.

PANCREATICODUODENAL CANCERS

Cancers of the lower end of the common duct, the papilla of Vater, the pancreas and the duodenum were termed pancreaticoduodenal cancers by Child.[17] Whipple emphasized that patients with these tumors have much in common in the insidious onset of symptoms and in their common confusion with digestive and biliary disturbances. Consequently, they frequently receive nonoperative symptomatic therapy for prolonged periods of time.

TABLE 2. TYPES OF PANCREATICODUODENAL CANCER

(1931–1950 Massachusetts General Hospital)
McDermott and Bartlett[46]

CANCER	NO. OF CASES 1931–1940	NO. OF CASES 1941–1950
Head of pancreas	112	136
Ampulla of Vater	9	24
Common bile duct	10	17
Duodenum	1	6
Totals	132	183

The Lahey Clinic group found 40 ampullary carcinomas and 105 carcinomas of the head of the pancreas in a series of 168 cases. The remaining 23 had carcinoma of the body of the pancreas.

CARCINOMA OF THE AMPULLA OF VATER

There are 2 principal types of ampullary carcinoma, the papillary and the ulcerating carcinomas. Microscopically, both are adenocarcinomas. The former arises from the ampulla itself and by its growth, edema and invasion tends to cause early obstruction of the terminal common bile duct and in some instances also of the pancreatic duct. The ulcerating variety arises from the epithelium of the papilla and invades the ampulla and the ducts secondarily. Cattell and Warren[15] stated that the gallbladder is distended in 90 per cent of these cases.

Spread of ampullary carcinoma occurs by direct extension and by lymphatic and vascular dissemination. The liver is the most common site of visceral metastasis. Carcinoma of the ampulla of Vater offers the best prognosis with radical surgery, perhaps because it tends to cause biliary tract obstruction early in the course of the disease and because the more common type, the papillary variety, tends to remain localized for a longer period than most other tumors in this area. The tumor tends to bleed and slough and thus may mimic the intermittent jaundice caused by a common duct stone. Whereas all types of pancreaticoduodenal carcinomas may give rise to occult blood in the stool, this symptom in a patient with jaundice should direct attention particularly to the possibility of ampullary carcinoma.

Carcinoma of the Duodenum

This rare adenocarcinoma is difficult to diagnose in an operable state unless it occurs near or in contact with the papilla of Vater, in which case the signs and symptoms resemble those of ampullary carcinoma.

TABLE 3. INCIDENCE OF CARCINOMA OF DUODENUM

Review of World Literature
Deaver and Ravdin[22]

1. Carcinomas of duodenum—0.033% of hospital autopsies
2. Inch for inch the duodenum is much more liable to undergo carcinomatous change than the jejunum or ileum
3. Relative frequency at various sites of duodenal carcinoma

1st portion	22.15%
2nd portion	65.82%
3rd portion	12.02%

Carcinoma of the Common Duct

This infiltrating, stenosing type of carcinoma has less tendency to bleed and slough than has the tumor of the papilla of Vater. Such tumors produce symptoms usually indistinguishable from those of carcinoma of the head of the pancreas, unless the duct is affected above the junction of the cystic duct when the gallbladder usually would not be dilated. The prognosis in these tumors has been very poor, especially if they occur above the level of the duodenum.

Carcinoma of the Pancreas

This tumor presents itself as a hard, irregular mass in the pancreas. In over two thirds of the cases it is located in the head of the

gland. Differential diagnosis with chronic inflammation is often difficult, as is the determination of the extent of the tumor, because of associated inflammation and fibrosis sometimes secondary to ductal obstruction.

Miller, Baggenstoss and Comfort[50] reported that 81.6 per cent of their series of carcinoma of the pancreas arose from ductal epithelium. A smaller number arise from acinar epithelium. The vast majority are adenocarcinomas; a few are squamous cell carcinomas. Pancreatic carcinoma also may arise from the islet tissue (see above).

The spread of these tumors occurs by direct invasion of the contiguous structures and by metastasis via the abundant lymphatic and vascular systems. Cattell and Warren[15] refer to 77 of 108 cases of carcinoma of the pancreas found to be inoperable because of metastasis or invasion of major vessels. Peripheral venous thrombosis not uncommonly accompanies carcinoma of the pancreas, especially of the body. Therefore, a search for signs of a neoplasm of the pancreas always should be made in persons with peripheral venous thromboses.

Pancreaticoduodenal cancer is found most frequently after age 55. Men are affected twice as often as women. The duration of symptoms before medical consultation is most commonly from 3 to 5 months. Only about 25 to 30 per cent are resectable by the time the patient is hospitalized. The disease runs a rapid course.

Symptoms and Signs of Pancreaticoduodenal Cancers

While the earliest symptoms are local pain, anorexia and weight loss, jaundice has attracted the most attention. Jaundice frequently may be the first sign, especially in ampullary or common duct cancers. Contrary to earlier opinion, painless jaundice is not a regular finding in pancreatic carcinoma, nor is a palpable gallbladder with intense jaundice found in most patients with operable cancer.

When the common bile duct is obstructed by a stone, dilatation of the gallbladder is rare (Courvoisier's Law). When the duct is obstructed in some other way, dilatation is frequent. This is valid in the majority of cases of carcinoma of pancreaticoduodenal origin, although its converse that a nonpalpable gallbladder with jaundice signifies choledocholithiasis is by no means always correct, as the gallbladder is not felt in some of the cases of carcinoma. The law is based on the finding that stones in the common duct generally are preceded by inflammation in the gallbladder with resultant fibrosis and shrinkage of the organ and its inability to dilate when the pressure in the biliary tract rises due to blockage.

Pain is one of the most common symptoms and is more frequent as the presenting complaint than is jaundice. The reverse is true for ampullary carcinoma where jaundice often without pain is the cardinal complaint. The pain may be paroxysmal or steady and deep in the epigastrium. Very frequently it radiates through to the back. On occasion it radiates to the right or even to the left upper quadrants or may be girdling in character. Biliary tract or peptic ulcer pain may be mimicked. Da Costa[21] noted relief of the pain by leaning forward. It may be aggravated by the dorsal recumbent position. As the disease progresses the pain may become excruciating.

Therefore serious consideration should be given to cordotomy if pain, anorexia and weight loss persist and cannot be relieved satisfactorily by careful study and treatment. Only about 75 per cent of the patients are icteric. Painless jaundice was present in 25 per cent of the Lahey Clinic series. If unrelieved, the biliary obstruction may cause intractable pruritus and will result in severe hepatic damage. In spite of the fact that jaundice is often not an early symptom, Cliffton[19] noted that in 75 patients it was the only symptom or sign actually bringing them for definitive treatment in an operable state.

Weight loss is probably the most common serious symptom and occurs early. It averages about 20 pounds by the time the patient is hospitalized.

Anorexia and weakness, nearly always present, are early symptoms, though nonspecific.

Constipation is frequent, although not helpful in diagnosis. Diarrhea is less common and tends to occur when the pancreatic duct is obstructed. However, typical foul, bulky stools are quite uncommon, and at times patients may have complete duct obstruction without any obvious changes in the stools. Nausea and vomiting are frequent. Occasionally, chills and fever may occur with neoplastic biliary obstruction and associated cholangitis, but more often they are associated with stones. Ascites and unexplained migratory phlebitis, particularly of the lower extremities, may occur. The appearance of mild diabetes has been noted occasionally.

PHYSICAL FINDINGS

There may be no physical findings, especially in the early operable cases (Table 4).

Jaundice is common, as noted above. Its absence does not rule out early carcinoma of the head and, of course, is not to be expected early in carcinoma of the body and the tail of the pancreas.

An enlarged palpable liver is fairly common, appearing in 75 per cent of the cases according to Berk.[7]

Palpable gallbladder with jaundice is frequently but not uniformly present. However, at operation the biliary tract and/or the pancreatic ducts are dilated in the majority of cases. As emphasized by Cattell and Warren,[15] resection is not carried out unless such dilatation can be demonstrated, since, in many cases, it is necessary to proceed without a histologic diagnosis because of the unreliability of biopsy of this area.

A palpable epigastric tumor is rare and must be regarded as of poor prognosis.

PANCREATIC BIOPSY

Frequently at operation an area of pancreas is found which is either thicker or firmer than one expects. A histologic diagnosis would be helpful. However, there are two cogent reasons for not undertaking pancreatic biopsies lightly. The first is that many of the lesions are in the head of the gland and one does not know where the common bile duct or the pancreatic ducts lie precisely. The result is that the biopsy obtained must be limited and therefore inconclusive if negative. The second danger is that sometimes incision into the pancreas is followed by acute pancreatitis or a pancreatic fistula. Therefore, pancreatic biopsies are to be avoided and should be undertaken only for well-considered reasons. In pancreaticoduodenal carcinomas sometimes a satisfactory biopsy may be obtained from inside the duodenum after duodenotomy.

TABLE 4. DIFFERENTIAL DIAGNOSIS OF COMMON DUCT OBSTRUCTION

	OBSTRUCTION DUE TO STONE	OBSTRUCTION DUE TO CARCINOMA OF HEAD OF PANCREAS
Symptoms		± early
Pain	+++ Colicky	+++ Aching later
Jaundice	++++ Often intermittent. Rapid onset	++++ Insidious onset. Persistent and progressive
Weight loss	++	++++
Fatigue	++	++++
Anorexia	+++	+++
Nausea, vomiting	++++	++
Chills, fever	+++	±
Physical Findings		
Jaundice	++++	++++
Hepatomegaly	++	+++
Palpable gallbladder	Rare	+++
Migratory phlebitis	Rare	Occasional
Laboratory Findings		
Bile pigment in stools	Usually present intermittently	Usually absent constantly
Occult blood in stools	0	±
Excess fat and undigested meat fibers in stool	0	+++
Hyperbilirubinemia	++++	++++
Serum alkaline phosphatase and cholesterol	Elevated	Elevated
Liver function tests indicate the presence of obstructive jaundice (usually) in both		
Pancreatic enzymes in duodenal contents	Normal	Often decreased
Anemia	±	+
Hyperglycemia and glycosuria	0	±
Glucose tolerance test (oral)	Normal	±
Plasma anti-thrombin titer	0	Occasionally elevated

Ackerman and his associates (1959)[1] have achieved considerable success in the diagnosis of specimens by frozen section of material obtained at laparotomy. At times, they have used needle biopsies.

LABORATORY DATA

A mild to moderate anemia is usually present. Elevated levels of serum bilirubin, alkaline phosphatase and cholesterol are present in pancreaticoduodenal carcinomas as they are in most instances of biliary tract obstruction. Liver function tests will indicate the presence of obstructive rather than hepatocellular jaundice in the earlier cases. However, in prolonged obstruction varying degrees of parenchymal damage may coexist. The prothrombin determination and its response to parenteral vitamin K is a valuable test.[63]

Serum amylase and lipase may be elevated, but usually the values are not significant. Stool examination for neutral fats and undigested meat fibers may show excessive amounts of both.

Aspiration of the duodenal contents with a double lumen tube as emphasized by Bauman[6] and stressed by Whipple[82] may be a valuable test for diagnosis and for differential diagnosis between choledocholithiasis and various types of pancreaticoduodenal tumors obstructing the pancreatic ducts near the duodenum (Fig. 31-4). Tumors of the body of the pancreas do not result, as a rule, in low enzyme levels in material aspirated from the duodenum.

The value of these studies depends on the expertness and the thoroughness with which they are carried out.

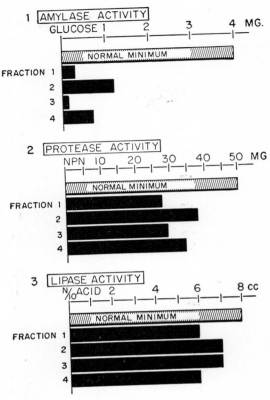

FIG. 31-4. Pancreatic function tests (from Bauman). Pancreatic enzyme determinations in a case of carcinoma of the head of the pancreas as compared with the normal minimums when no pancreatic disease is present.

ROENTGENOGRAPHIC FINDINGS

An upper gastrointestinal series may show, at times, enlargement of the duodenal loop or displacement, distortion or actual invasion of contiguous organs (Figs. 31-5 and 31-6). The inverted-3 sign of Frostberg[30] is suggestive but rare. The films are most often negative; in fact, Cattell and Warren[15] state that: "We have come to regard negative studies as one of the important indications of the presence of pancreatic disease in those patients who have dyspepsia, fatigue and progressive weight loss."

SUMMARY

The diagnosis of pancreaticoduodenal cancer is made most often if the possibility is kept in mind. A middle-aged patient who presents himself with persistent abdominal pain, anorexia and unexplained weight loss and in whom physical examination and an upper gastrointestinal series are negative should suggest immediately the possibility of carcinoma of the pancreas, even in the absence of jaundice. However, jaundice remains the symptom which most often leads to the diagnosis.

TREATMENT

The treatment of pancreaticoduodenal cancers by resection has been and remains relatively unsatisfactory. Prior to 1935, curative procedures had been given up. Then, Dr. Allen O. Whipple (1935)[80] reported a radical resection in 2 stages. He and other surgeons soon modified this to a 1-stage procedure (Trimble, 1941).[77] Only about 25 per cent of the lesions are resectable, and for the majority of individuals, the procedure has turned out to be palliative. Preoperative preparation includes parenteral vitamin K therapy to restore the prothrombin activity, a high protein, high carbohydrate diet and blood transfusions. A glucose tolerance test should be performed preoperatively since diabetes mellitus is present in 10 per cent of cases.

Essentially 2 general types of operations are available:

1. Strictly palliative procedures for inoperable carcinoma (Cattell and Warren)[15]

A. Cholecystojejunostomy with enteroenterostomy (Fig. 31-8, *Right*)

B. Pancreatojejunostomy

C. Ligation of the gastroduodenal and inferior pancreaticoduodenal arteries

D. Gastrojejunostomy

The majority of such patients are dead within 12 months after palliative operations.

2. Possibly curative procedures

A. Pancreaticoduodenal resection is the procedure most commonly employed. Essentially, this consists of the block resection of the head of the pancreas, the duodenum, the pylorus, the distal stomach, and the lower end of the common duct. Then the remainder of the stomach is anastomosed to the jejunum. The common duct and the pancreatic duct also are anastomosed to the jejunum proximal to the gastrojejunostomy. Failure to place the gastric anastomosis distally has led to fatal peptic ulceration of the jejunum. Some surgeons do not anastomose the pancreatic ducts but simply ligate them. The absence of the external secretion can be compensated by the oral administration of animal pancreatic enzymes when necessary; indeed, some patients without external secretion have apparently normal stools and regain their weight without such therapy. However, anastomosis is generally considered desirable because it is thought to reduce the incidence of fistulas and to preserve a part of the exocrine function of the gland (see Fig. 31-9).

Though the mortality of pancreaticoduodenectomy has been reported in the literature as about 30 per cent, now it is approaching 10 per cent or less in several of the leading surgical clinics.

B. Total pancreatectomy is similar to the

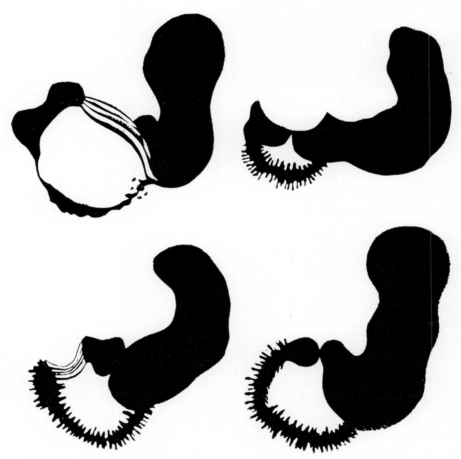

FIG. 31-5. Various x-ray changes sometimes produced by pancreaticoduodenal carcinoma. (*Top, left*) Diagrammatic representation of gastrointestinal series, showing widening of duodenal loop due to pancreaticoduodenal carcinoma. (*Top, right*) Diagrammatic representation of gastrointestinal series showing compression by dilated gallbladder on upper border of duodenum and pyloric antrum due to a pancreaticoduodenal carcinoma. (*Bottom, left*) Diagrammatic representation of gastrointestinal series, showing postbulbar impression due to pressure of the obstructed biliary tract due to pancreaticoduodenal carcinoma. (*Bottom, right*) Diagrammatic representation of gastrointestinal series showing distortion of mucosal folds on medial side of second portion of duodenum due to pancreaticoduodenal carcinoma. (From Dr. Philip J. Hodes)

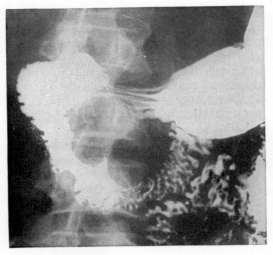

FIG. 31-6. The inverted 3-sign of Frostberg which is indicative (though not pathognomonic) of carcinoma of the pancreas when it occurs.

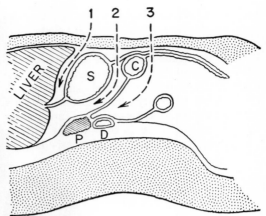

FIG. 31-7. Approaches to the pancreas: (1) Through the gastrohepatic omentum. (2) Through the gastrocolic omentum. (3) From below through the transverse mesocolon.

preceding operation except that all pancreatic tissue and the spleen are removed—the spleen because of the arrangement of the blood supply. The splenic vein and artery course within or immediately contiguous to the pancreas.

The author feels that for the present at least these two operations should be reserved for patients without evidence of distant metastasis or involvement of the major vessels. Brunschwig[10] recently reported 2 five-year survivals in patients who had lymph node involvement at the time of pancreaticoduodenal resection. Furthermore, Child[18] and others are investigating resection of the portal vein and have reported success in experimental animals and in a limited number of patients.

POSTOPERATIVE COMPLICATIONS

Pancreatic fistula is the most common complication; others are hemorrhage, biliary fistula, peritonitis, diabetes mellitus, and obstruction of the gastrojejunostomy.

(See also section on Metabolic Effects of Total Pancreatectomy.)

RESULTS OF TREATMENT OF PANCREATICODUODENAL CANCER

The reported results of radical pancreatic surgery were very poor at the time of the first edition of this text. There has been some improvement reported since. McDermott and Bartlett[46] have compared all cases treated at the Massachusetts General Hospital in the

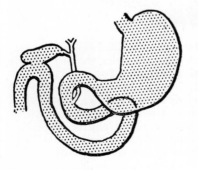

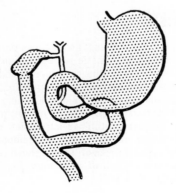

FIG. 31-8. Two palliative procedures for inoperable carcinoma of the pancreas: (Left) Loop cholecystojejunostomy. (Right) Cholecystojejunostomy en Y.

Fig. 31-9. Restoration of pancreatic, biliary and gastrointestinal continuity after radical pancreaticoduodenal resection. (*Left*) Poor method. (*Center*) Fair method. (*Right*) Satisfactory method.

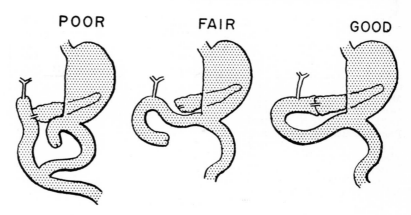

POOR   FAIR   GOOD

decade 1931 to 1940 (132 cases), when only palliative procedures were done, with all cases in the decade 1941 to 1950 (183 cases), when 35 per cent of the tumors were resected by pancreaticoduodenectomy with a 34 per cent mortality. The average duration of life after pancreaticoduodenectomy was 11 months. The average survival of resected and palliative cases between 1941 and 1950 was 6.2 months for carcinoma of the pancreas compared with 7.7 months in the preceding decade when only palliative procedures were done.

For carcinoma of the ampulla the survivals were 21 months in the first decade and only 18.5 months in the second decade. Of the 183 cases, there were only 2 five-year survivals among the 65 per cent resected. None of the cases with carcinoma of the pancreas survived 5 years.

Logan and Kleinsasser[43] have reviewed the literature and collected 123 cases of pancreaticoduodenal cancer for which pancreaticoduodectomy was performed from 1942 to 1949. Of the resections, 35 were for ampullary carcinoma. The operative mortality was 23 per cent, the average survival was 23 months, and 8 of 28 patients were alive at the end of 5 years. 62 of the resections were for carcinoma of the pancreas with a mortality of 31 per cent —an average survival of 13 months and only 1 patient of 30 was alive after 5 years. 23 of the resections were for all other cancers requiring pancreaticoduodenectomy, with a mortality of only 4.5 per cent, an average survival of 20 months, and 1 of 15 patients alive in 5 years.

Orr (1952)[60] was able to collect from the literature 17 patients who lived for 5 or more years after pancreaticoduodenectomy for cancer. Only 3 of these patients had carcinoma of the pancreas. Most of the remaining had ampullary carcinoma.

Cattell and Warren[15] reported 5 of 32 pattients (16%) living after 5 years.

Dennis and Varco (1956)[23] reported 13 5-year survivors of radical pancreaticoduodenal resection. Eight of these patients had primary lesions in the head of the pancreas.

Kaufman and Wilson (1955)[42] reviewed the American literature and reported 36 5-year survivors following pancreaticoduodenectomy, 8 of them having had carcinoma of the head of the pancreas and 21 ampullary carcinoma.

Muir (1955)[55] made inquiries in Great Britain and found 4 unpublished cases which had survived 5 years after pancreaticoduodenectomy. He also reported 2 5-year survivors who had carcinoma of the head of the pancreas.

A further series of radical operations for pancreaticoduodenal carcinoma was reported by Rhoads, Zintel and Helwig (1957;[67] 1960)[68] and several more recent reports have appeared, including one from the Lahey Clinic in two parts (Cattell, Warren, and Au, 1959;[16] Warren and Cattell, 1959),[78] reporting 41 5-year survivors (Table 5).

There have now been reported more than 100 5-year survivors of carcinoma in the pancreaticoduodenal region. Practically all of these invade pancreatic tissue to some extent. Those deemed to be primary in the head of the pancreas are decidedly less favorable than those arising at the papilla of Vater.

In conclusion, it now appears that if the pancreaticoduodenal carcinomas are consid-

TABLE 5. REPORTED 5-YEAR SURVIVALS OF CARCINOMA OF THE PANCREATICODUODENAL REGION AFTER OPERATIONS OF THE WHIPPLE TYPE

AUTHOR	YEAR	HEAD OF PANCREAS	BILE DUCT	DUODENUM	PAPILLA OF VATER	NOT STATED	TOTAL
Orr[60]	1952	3			11	2	16
Muir[55]	1955	1			1		2
Dennis & Varco[23]	1956	8		1	3	1	13
Smith[73]	1956	1		2	3		6
Rhoads, Zintel & Helwig[67]	1957		3	1	2		6
Ross[72]	1957	1					1
Waugh & Giberson[79]	1957	3		2	5		10
Porter[62]	1958			1	3		4
Warren & Cattell[78]	1959	7	3	7	24		41
Rhoads, Zintel & Helwig[68]	1960				1		1
Total		24	6	14	53	3	100

ered collectively, about 25 per cent of the cases are resectable, and about 25 per cent of those resected survive 5 years or longer. In the series from the Hospital of the University of Pennsylvania, the average survival was 30.5 months for the resected cases, 11 months for those undergoing palliative shunts, and 2.5 months for those who were merely explored. This, of course, reflects the fact that the most favorable cases were apt to be chosen for resection. Nevertheless, resection would seem to offer some hope of cure for the more favorable cases.

If a shunt for bile is decided upon, experience dictates that a gastroenterostomy be constructed also, as duodenal obstruction frequently follows bile duct obstruction by a short interval.

CYSTS

Cysts of the pancreas are uncommon but not rare. There are many etiologic varieties. Of the many classifications that have been proposed, a modification of that of Mahorner and Mattson (1931)[47] appears to be most useful.

1. Cysts resulting from defective development
   A. Fibrocystic disease
   B. Cysts associated with polycystic disease of other viscera
   C. Simple cysts
   D. Dermoid cysts
2. Cysts resulting from disruption of pancreatic tissue, either traumatic or inflammatory
   A. Pseudocysts
   B. Hemorrhagic cysts
3. Retention cysts
4. Neoplastic cysts
   A. Cystadenoma
   B. Cystadenocarcinoma
   C. Teratoma
5. Cysts resulting from parasites: echinococcus cysts

Two main types of non-neoplastic cysts are encountered—the true cysts which have an epithelial lining, and the false or pseudocysts which do not. Of the neoplastic cysts, the cystadenoma is the most common, although only 53 of these have been reported in the literature. Of a total of 46 pancreatic cysts of all types treated at the Lahey Clinic, 30 were pseudocysts.

PSEUDOCYSTS

Pseudocysts of the pancreas are the result of fluid accumulations about the pancreas which apparently do not undergo resorption. The exact mechanism of formation is not known; presumably, disruption of pancreatic tissue with hemorrhage and escape of pancreatic juice in addition to local exudation accounts for the accumulation of fluid. A proliferation of connective tissue forms a fibrous wall which may include parts of the pancreas or neighboring organs and tissues. Either trauma to the pancreas or acute and chronic pancreatitis may be the cause of disruption of the parenchymal tissue. The trauma is usually a severe blow to the epigastrium or the midabdomen, and the latent period before the cyst becomes evident may vary from a few days to a few years but usually it is a few months. Fallis and Plain[29] believe that pesudocysts occur as a sequel of acute pancreatitis in about 10 per cent of cases. The author's experience would not place the figure nearly so high.

The pseudocyst has no epithelial lining and usually has only a single cavity. The contained fluid is usually cloudy, and pancreatic enzyme activity may be demonstrable. It, as do most pancreatic cysts, presents most commonly in the lesser peritoneal cavity, displacing the stomach forward and up and the transverse mesocolon downward. Anteriorly, it is covered by the gastrocolic omentum.

CYSTADENOMAS

Cystadenomas are rare (Figs. 31-10 and 31-11). Generally, they are considered to be true neoplasms arising from the parenchymal cells. These coarsely lobulated, multicystic tumor masses are found most commonly in the tail of the pancreas. They usually vary in size from 2 to 8 cm. and though larger tumors have been reported, they are generally smaller than non-neoplastic cysts. The tumors have a definite semitranslucent capsule, and Brunschwig has likened them to a cluster of grapes. They feel cystic and when sectioned appear spongelike or honeycombed. The fluid contained in them is clear, yellow or brown and varies in viscosity. Microscopically, the cystic spaces are lined with cuboidal or flattened epithelium, and there may be papillary projections of epithelium into the spaces. Though these tumors are usually well encapsulated and grow by expansion, infiltration of surrounding tissue also may occur.

Mozan (1951)[54] collected 49 histologically verified cystadenomas from the literature. The ratio of females to males was 7 to 1. He found that a palpable tumor mass in the epigastrium was usually the first recognizable sign of the lesion. Zintel, Enterline and Rhoads (1954)[84] reported 4 cases of cystadenoma of which 3 were papillary. All patients had long survivals without metastases, and the authors reiterate that malignancy should not be diagnosed on the basis of papillary projection alone. However, though malignant degeneration is rare, these tumors should be considered as potentially precancerous and hence should be excised completely.

SIGNS AND SYMPTOMS OF PANCREATIC CYSTS

Though the symptoms and signs of pancreatic cysts are dependent somewhat upon etiology, size, location and duration, they are quite similar and are usually insidious unless associated with trauma or inflammation (pancreatitis).

Epigastric pain, which may radiate to the back or flanks, occasionally associated with sharp, darting pains in the abdomen, is the

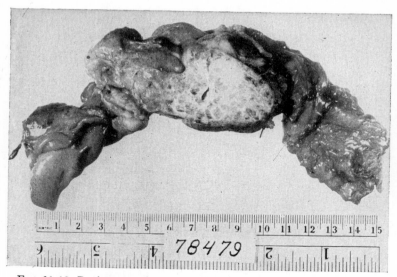

Fig. 31-10. Benign cystadenoma. Gross appearance of a sectioned lesion in relation to the duodenum.

most prominent symptom. It is usually dull and intermittent but may be severe.

Dyspepsia and anorexia are common, and icterus rare. When jaundice exists it may be due to pressure upon the common duct or to concomitant biliary tract disease.

Weight loss and fatigue are common symptoms. Constipation and a sense of fullness in the abdomen may be present. Chills and fever and glycosuria are uncommon. Steatorrhea is rare.

A palpable abdominal mass, usually epigastric, is present in 90 per cent of cases, according to Cattell and Warren. Often the mass is not tender to moderate pressure and may be mobile.

Laboratory findings are seldom very helpful in diagnosis.

ROENTGENOGRAPHIC EXAMINATION

A gastrointestinal series is usually negative but may reveal displacement and compression of contiguous organs if the cyst is large. In rare instances, calcification in the cyst wall may be visible.

DIFFERENTIAL DIAGNOSIS

Pancreatic cysts are to be differentiated from other pancreatic tumors and from tumors, cysts or enlargements of surrounding organs. These include retroperitoneal tumors and lymph node enlargement, splenomegaly, renal and hepatic masses, hydrops of the gallbladder, cysts of the omentum and the mesentery, tumors of the stomach and aneurysms.

TREATMENT

The treatment of choice of pancreatic cysts is complete excision if compatible with the extent and the size of the cyst and the condition of the patient. This may necessitate amputation of a portion of the tail and the body of the pancreas. Even pancreaticoduodenectomy has been done when the lesion involves the head of the pancreas or if differentiation from carcinoma is uncertain (see discussion of pancreatic biopsy above). It is doubtful, however, if pancreaticoduodenectomy is justified in the absence of malignancy. Ordinarily such cysts can be excised. Some

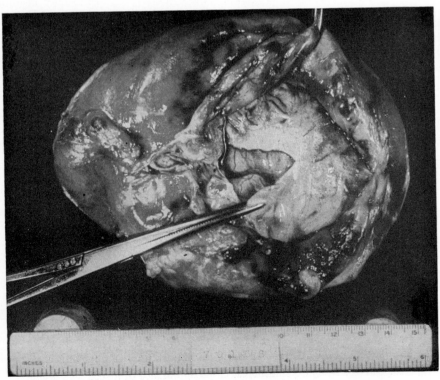

FIG. 31-11. Gross appearance of a large cystadenoma of the pancreas.

cysts, especially pseudocysts, may involve surrounding organs or tissues so extensively that excision is impossible. In that event, marsupialization has been advised. This consists of suturing the wall of the cyst to the abdominal wound with subsequent drainage. However, marsupialization is followed by a fair number of recurrent cysts and persisting fistulas, especially if the cyst is multilocular or contains a lining of epithelial cells. In the latter event, sometimes destructive chemicals are painted on the walls of the cyst to destroy secretory cells, but this is seldom entirely successful.

Other methods which have been employed are simple drainage, which is rarely indicated, and internal drainage by anastomosis of the cyst or persistent sinus tract to the gastrointestinal tract. The latter procedure should not be the initial treatment if excision is possible, because stenosis of the anastomosis is relatively common. Hemorrhage and perforation also may occur.

The operative mortality is relatively low, and the prognosis for life is good, although persistent pancreatic fistula and recurrent cysts may plague patient and surgeon for prolonged periods.

BENIGN SOLID TUMORS

Excluding islet cell tumors, solid benign tumors of the pancreas are very rare. In addition to solid adenomas, which may represent an early stage in the development of cystadenomas, lipomas, fibromas, myxomas and chondromas may occur in the pancreas. Hemangiomas of the pancreas also have been reported.

Signs and symptoms, when present, namely, dyspepsia and epigastric distress or pain, resemble those of cysts of the pancreas. The tumors may reach sufficient size to become palpable. Small benign tumors are asymptomatic unless compression of the ductal system occurs.

Treatment is surgical excision. The prognosis is good provided that the benign nature of the lesion is recognized before the surgeon subjects the patient to a high-risk procedure under the impression that the lesion is malignant.

PANCREATIC HETEROTOPIA

Aberrant or ectopic pancreatic tissue, subject to all the pathologic changes of the pancreas itself, has become of increasing clinical significance. Barbosa, Dockerty and Waugh,[4] of the Mayo Clinic, reported 41 histologically proved surgical cases, of which 61 per cent were of clinical significance. Such ectopic tissue was found about once in every 500 upper abdominal operations, the highest percentage of the total (70%) being in the duodenum, the stomach and the jejunum. However, its occurrence in the biliary tract, ileum, diverticuli of the small bowel including Meckel's diverticulum, spleen, liver, omentum, mesentery and mediastinum (teratoma) have been reported.

Symptoms produced resemble those of peptic ulcer, duodenal obstruction, biliary tract disease, intussusception, or indefinite gastrointestinal complaints. Pathologically, edema, ulceration, hemorrhage, fat necrosis and inflammation may be observed. It is believed that malignant change is more likely to occur than in normal pancreas. Since most of these lesions are not recognized preoperatively and the findings may be misinterpreted at operation, frozen section examination is very helpful.

The treatment of choice is local excision whether the lesions are symptomatic or are found incidentally at laparotomy.

Howard, et al.,[40] summarized 9 cases of ectopic islet cell tumors, 8 of which produced hypoglycemia. Autopsy incidence of pancreatic heterotopia in the literature as collected by Barbosa[4] ranged from 0.6 per cent to 5.6 per cent.

POSTOPERATIVE PANCREATITIS

Acute postoperative pancreatitis has been reported not only after surgical procedures in close proximity to the pancreas such as gastric resection, biliary tract surgery and splenectomy, but has also occurred following cholangiography, transurethral resection, thyroidectomy, appendectomy, cesarean section, dorsolumbar laminectomy and colon resection. Hotchkiss et al.[37] recently reviewed the literature of postoperative pancreatitis and studied the effects of intra-abdominal and extra-abdominal operations on the serum lipase and amylase. The following possible etiologic factors concerned in the mechanism of postoperative pancreatitis may be listed:

1. Mechanical injury to the parenchyma of the pancreas

2. Injury to pancreatic vessels

3. Injuries to the pancreatic ducts, especially the duct of Santorini

4. Obstruction of the pancreatic ducts associated with an actively secreting gland

5. Spasm of the muscles about the ampulla producing a common channel permitting a reflux of bile into the pancreatic ducts

6. An increase in the viscosity of pancreatic secretion induced by dehydration, atropine and ether during operation and by pancreatic manipulation (Dunphy, Brooks and Achroyd[28])

7. Postoperative infection in the region of the pancreas

8. Overzealous palpation of the pancreas at operation

Hotchkiss found that there is a moderate depression of serum amylase and a moderate and consistent depression of serum lipase in most postoperative patients. Elevations of serum amylase without significant elevations in serum lipase were found in some cases after both the intra-abdominal operations and extra-abdominal operations, especially after operations upon or near the pancreas. None of the patients he studied had clinical signs of pancreatitis, and the author concluded that such a diagnosis is hazardous on the basis of elevated serum amylase alone.

The author has seen several cases of postoperative pancreatitis of a severe degree (with hemorrhage and massive necrosis)—one following a common duct exploration which seemed to be uneventful at the time of operation.

METABOLIC EFFECTS OF TOTAL PANCREATECTOMY

At least 33 total pancreatectomies have been reported in the literature (Cattell and Warren[15]). These were performed for carcinoma, sarcoma, chronic pancreatitis, and for hyperinsulinism where no adenoma was found. The mortality was 36.4 per cent. A number of metabolic studies have been reported, a careful one being that of Nardi.[57]

INSULIN

The insulin requirement is relatively low, usually 40 units daily or less. The patient with pre-existing diabetes may have his insulin requirement slightly increased, unaltered or decreased following pancreatectomy. Thorogood and Zimmerman[75] found that pancreatectomy reduced the insulin requirements of alloxan-diabetic animals and postulated the presence of a diabetogenic factor in the pancreas. However, Mirsky, et al.,[51] have shown that fasting depancreatized dogs, previously rendered alloxan-diabetic, have an aggravation of the diabetic state.

The apparent mildness of diabetes following pancreatectomy is explained by Mirsky, et al., by the absence of external secretion, since these authors found that pancreatectomy produces a decrease in absorption of proteins and carbohydrates from the gastrointestinal tract.

Lukens[45] also believed that pancreatectomy produces the severest form of diabetes. However, Nardi's patient required only 10 units each of protamine zinc and crystalline insulin for adequate control of the diabetes. The usual experience has placed the requirement in the range of 30 to 40 units per day.

FATTY LIVERS

In contradistinction to dogs, fatty infiltration of the liver seldom has been reported in man. Brunschwig[69] reported one instance in a patient with diabetes prior to surgery. However, most patients have been protected by choline, methionine, or pancreatic extracts.

PHOSPHOLIPID METABOLISM

Barker, et al.,[5] working with pancreatectomized dogs, found a reduced ability of the animals to incorporated radioactive phosphorus into phospholipid and postulated that the post-pancreatectomy fatty livers may be related to this. However, Nardi repeated the experiment in his patient and found no such abnormality.

STOOLS

Whipple[81] reported 2 patients who showed no fecal disturbances after total pancreatico-duodenectomy. Nevertheless, some patients have bulky, soft, diarrheic stools. The nutritional status of Nardi's patient was better without pancreatin than with it. Thus, it appears that such supplements are not always necessary.

SERUM ENZYMES

Normal or low normal levels of serum amylase and lipase have been found in nearly all reported cases.

Despite the interesting studies reported, the author is impressed with the moderate and relatively constant insulin requirement of depancreatized patients, including one who survived 9 years and gained weight and remained active to the age of 71.

In the present state of knowledge a methionine supplement of 5 to 6 Gm. per day is recommended.

CHRONIC PANCREATITIS AND CHRONIC RELAPSING PANCREATITIS

CHRONIC PANCREATITIS

This term is reserved largely for fibrosis in the pancreas without acute symptoms, whereas chronic relapsing pancreatitis is marked by remittent symptoms with significant pain.

These two conditions are almost certainly different forms of the same process. Chronic pancreatitis may be relatively "silent" with vague digestive disturbances. Occasionally, it causes sufficient constriction of the lower end of the common bile duct to produce jaundice. It then is almost indistinguishable from carcinoma of the head of the pancreas. Biopsy of the head of the pancreas is difficult, uncertain and sometimes followed by severe reactions. Because it and the frozen section examination are unreliable, sometimes these patients are subjected to pancreatoduodenectomy. This is an unnecessarily extensive procedure, because these patients usually do very well with a simple sidetracking procedure such as a cholecystojejunostomy. Therefore, the more radical procedure should not be done unless it is believed that malignancy is present and resectable.

The decision to resect is a difficult one. There must be a tumor in the pancreas so situated as to explain the symptoms. Involvement of the entire gland is suggestive of chronic pancreatitis rather than malignancy. If there are enlarged lymph nodes adjacent to the pancreas, often one can be removed for frozen section. The finding of malignant cells would militate against resection. Age and debility may be deciding factors against resection. The existence of fat necrosis suggests inflammation but does not absolutely rule out neoplasm.

The experience cited by Rhoads, Zintel and Helwig (1960)[68] suggests that 7 per cent of hard, pancreatic swellings accompanied by jaundice probably were due to chronic inflammation rather than carcinoma.

CHRONIC RELAPSING PANCREATITIS

Whereas the diagnosis of chronic pancreatitis must most often be made at operation, that of chronic relapsing pancreatitis can be made preoperatively with a fair degree of accuracy.

A typical case is the following. A middle-aged man, a regular consumer of alcohol, began having epigastric pain of a dull aching character extending through to the back at about the 8th dorsal segment but not sharply localized. It tended to be accentuated by eating, and he noted anorexia but no vomiting. He lost 15 pounds in weight over a period of 6 months. The pain would flare up acutely for 1 to 3 days at a time. At such a period he would run a low-grade temperature, 99 to 101° F. He usually had mild tenderness in the epigastrium, and during exacerbations this became more marked but was not associated with much muscle spasm or rebound tenderness. Gradually, he had come to use codeine with increasing frequency.

Roentgenograms of the abdomen were first interpreted as showing only calcified mesenteric lymph nodes. Then the patient was referred to a psychiatrist with the impression that the symptoms might be psychosomatic.

Later x-ray studies showed calcification in the region of the pancreas (Fig. 31-12). A sugar tolerance curve was diabetic in type, and postprandial blood sugars were high. Finally, a tube was passed into the duodenum, and specimens were collected before and after stimulation of the pancreas by secretin. The specimens were analyzed for enzyme concentration, and marked reductions were found in fat, starch and protein-splitting activity. A diagnosis of chronic relapsing pancreatitis was made and confirmed at operation.

Some patients develop marked diffuse cal-

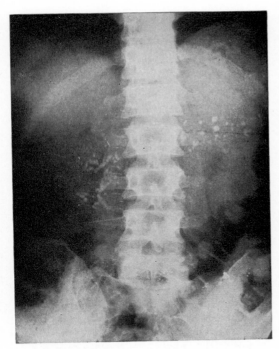

Fig. 31-12. Roentgenogram showing calcification in pancreas in chronic relapsing pancreatitis.

cification which delineates the whole gland. In others this may not be found. Some patients develop discrete calculi in the pancreatic ducts. Formerly, attempts were made to remove such stones, but at present the balance of evidence seems to be that they are usually a part of the picture of chronic relapsing pancreatitis and should be treated as such. Simple removal of the calculi rarely afforded lasting relief. Large solitary calculi constitute most of the exceptions.

Likewise, diabetes is not necessarily present, but as the disease progresses the sugar tolerance curve may go up, and eventually frank diabetes may appear.

The enzyme studies (lipase, amylase, trypsin) are at times very helpful but are very time-consuming. In addition to time required in obtaining specimens, nearly 2 days of the time of a trained chemical technician is demanded for a single study.

Another finding which may be helpful is a rise in blood amylase and/or lipase early in the exacerbations. Late in the course of the disease, however, the pancreas may act as

though it were "burned out," so that the absence of such rises does not exclude the diagnosis. In fact, low amylase values may be suggestive of chronic pancreatitis.

Except in very fully developed cases, the diagnosis requires confirmation at laparotomy. Grossly, the pancreas feels firm to hard and usually a bit enlarged. The surrounding tissues are edematous, fibrotic or rubbery, as the case may be, and generally show evidence of inflammation in adjacent tissues. If biopsy is done, it shows increased fibrosis and round cell infiltration. There may or may not be dilatation of the ducts, calcification, or polymorphonuclear cell infiltration. Occasionally, a cystlike area will mark the site of a subsiding abscess or focus of necrosis. Both the acinar cells and the islet cells are replaced to varying degrees by fibrous tissue.

While the chronic relapsing pancreatitis is not frequent, its chronicity makes it a pressing problem whenever it is encountered. One of the difficult features of this disease is the frequency with which patients seeking relief from its symptoms become addicted to narcotics.

Therapy is still at the stage where the number of the methods of treatment advocated indicates that none are ideal. The following are among those reported:

1. **Total Pancreatectomy.** This eradicates the disease process but leaves the patient diabetic and handicaps his digestion. Operative mortality has been high. Unexpected coma following the ingestion of alcohol has resulted in the death of a number of those individuals who have survived the operation.

2. **Sphincterotomy** (Doubilet and Mulholland[25, 26]). Good results have been claimed following division of the sphincter of Oddi, but it is not clear that the process is due to obstruction at the sphincter. Most follow-up reports have been short. Relief from symptoms has not been uniform by any means.

3. **Ligation of the Ducts** (Rienhoff). The objective here is to complete the process of fibrosis as observed in the dogs used by Banting and Best in the discovery of insulin. Little experience has been reported with this method as yet.

4. A. **Anastomosis** of the duct of Wirsung to the jejunum (Cattell[14]).

B. **Amputation** of the tail of the pancreas and anastomosis of the duct to a de-functionalized loop of jejunum.

These again are procedures to improve drainage of the ductal system.

5. **Vagotomy, Sympathectomy, Splanch-nicectomy** (Rienhoff and Baker[70]). The objective here is to relieve symptoms by interruption of the sensory nerve fibers. It appears that vagotomy is not necessary for this.

6. **Lumbodorsal Sympathectomy and Splanchnicectomy.** The studies of Ray[64] indicate that the afferent nerve impulses from the pancreas travel over the sympathetic system. They can be interrupted by bilateral removal of the sympathetic chain from D11 - L2 inclusive and resection of the greater, the lesser and the least splanchnic nerves bilaterally.

Next to vagotomy, this procedure is probably the one most often employed and gives good relief of symptoms in about 50 per cent of instances. It has certain disadvantages. It leaves the pancreas in situ, and there was evidence in some of Ray's cases that flare-ups of the inflammatory process continue. It also interrupts the sensory pathways from the gallbladder, the duodenum and part of the stomach so that intercurrent disease in these organs may develop quite far without the usual warning symptoms. Eventually, however, inflammation arising from any of these sources will reach areas such as the parietal peritoneum where sensory innervation is intact and symptoms will supervene. Finally, the procedure is apt to require 3 operations: (1) laparotomy to establish the diagnosis and to exclude other pathologic changes; (2) a right lumbodorsal sympathectomy; (3) a left lumbodorsal sympathectomy. Some cases have been relieved after the second step, but usually only temporarily.

At present exploration to confirm the diagnosis and transduodenal sphincterotomy probably are most popular as a first step. Unless symptoms are relieved, this step is followed by the sympathectomies.

Some surgeons have attacked the splanchnic nerves and the celiac ganglia at the time of laparotomy. The exposure is somewhat difficult, and the results thus far are hard to evaluate because of the paucity of reported cases and the brevity of the follow-up periods.

Longmire and his associates (1956)[44] have found it necessary to resect most of the pancreas in these cases, leaving a short segment of the tail to preserve some islet cell function. The widespread use of this logical approach to the problem would seem to depend on future mortality experience in the hands of various surgeons.

Recently, Ralph Bowers[9] has reported good results in 16 of a series of 17 patients with chronic relapsing pancreatitis by anastomosis of a defunctionalized loop of jejunum to the common bile duct.

FIBROCYSTIC DEGENERATION OF THE PANCREAS

This congenital malformation is discussed in Chapter 46, under "Meconium Ileus."

REFERENCES

1. Ackerman, L. V., and Ramirez, G. A.: The indications for and limitations of frozen section diagnosis; A review of 1269 consecutive frozen section diagnoses, Brit. J. Surg. *46*: 336, 1959.
2. Babcock, W. W.: Principles and Practice of Surgery, p. 1331, Philadelphia, Lea & Febiger, 1930.
3. Banting, F. G., and Best, C. H.: Internal secretion of pancreas, J. Lab. & Clin. Med. *7*:251-266, 1922.
4. Barbosa, J. J. DeC., Dockerty, M. B., and Waugh, J. M.: Pancreatic heterotopia, Surg., Gynec. & Obst. *82*:527-542, 1946.
5. Barker, W. F., Rogers, K. E., and Moore, F. D.: Effect of pancreatectomy on phospholipid synthesis in dogs, Arch. Surg. *61*:1151-1162, 1950.
6. Bauman, L.: The Diagnosis of Pancreatic Disease, Philadelphia, Lippincott, 1949.
7. Berk, J. E.: Diagnosis of carcinoma of pancreas, Arch. Int. Med. *68*:525-559, 1941.
8. Bosshardt, D. K., Ciereszko, L. S., and Barnes, R. H.: Preparation of a pancreas derivative having lipotropic activity, Am. J. Physiol. *166*:433-435, 1951.
9. Bowers, R. F.: Discussion of a paper by Longmire, W. P., Jr., Jordan, P. H., Jr., and Briggs, J. D.: Experience with pancreatic resection for chronic relapsing pancreatitis, Tr. Am. S. A., vol. LXXIV, 1956.
10. Brunschwig, A.: Pancreatoduodenectomy: "curative" operation for malignant neoplasms in pancreatoduodenal region; report of three over-five-year survivors, Ann. Surg. *136*:610-624, 1952.

11. Brunschwig, A., and Allen, J. G.: Specific injurious action of alloxan upon pancreatic islet cells and convoluted tubules of kidney: comparative study in rabbit, dog, and man; attempted chemotherapy of insulin-producing islet cell carcinoma in man, Cancer Res. 4:45-54, 1944.

12. Bystrov, N. V.: Clinical forms of acute pancreatitis, their diagnosis and treatment, Khirurgiia 35:7, 1959.

13. Cameron, A. L., and Noble, H. F.: Reflux of bile up the duct of Wirsung caused by an impacted biliary calculus, J.A.M.A. 82:1410-1414, 1924.

14. Cattell, R. B.: Anastomosis of duct of Wirsung; its use in palliative operations for cancer of head of pancreas, S. Clin. North America 27:636-643, 1947.

15. Cattell, R. B., and Warren, K. W.: Surgery of the Pancreas, p. 374, Philadelphia, Saunders, 1953.

16. Cattell, R. B., Warren, K. W., and Au, F. T. C.: Periampullary carcinomas, diagnosis and surgical treatment, S. Clin. North America 39:781, 1959.

17. Child, C. G., III: Advances in management of pancreaticoduodenal cancer *in* Andrus, W. D., ed.: Advances in Surgery, vol. 2, pp. 495-561, New York, Interscience, 1949.

18. Child, C. G., Holswade, G. R., McClure, R. D., Jr., Gore, A. L., and O'Neill, E. A.: Pancreatoduodenectomy with resection of the portal vein in the Macaca mulatta monkey and man, Surg., Gynec. & Obst. 94:31-45, 1952.

19. Cliffton, E. E.: Carcinoma of pancreas: symptoms, signs, and results of treatment in 122 cases, A.M.A. Arch. Surg. 65:290-306, 1952.

20. Conn, J. W., and Seltzer, H. S.: Spontaneous hypoglycemia, Am. J. Med. 19:460-478, 1955.

21. DaCosta, J. M.: Cancer of the pancreas, North American Med-chir. Rev. 2:883-909, 1858.

22. Deaver, J. B., and Ravdin, I. S.: Carcinoma of the duodenum, Am. J. M. Sc. 159:469-477, 1920.

23. Dennis, C., and Varco, R. L.: Survival for more than five years after pancreatoduodenectomy for cancers of the ampulla and pancreatic head, Surgery 39:92, 1956.

24. Dick, B. M., and Wallace, V. G. H.: Cholecystography: toxic effects of the dyes, Brit. J. Surg. 15:360-369, 1928.

25. Doubilet, H., and Mulholland, J. H.: Results of sphincterotomy in pancreatitis, J. Mt. Sinai Hosp. 17:458, 1951.

26. ———: The surgical treatment of pancreatitis, S. Clin. North America 29:339-359, 1949.

27. Dragstedt, L. R., Van Prohaska, J., and Harms, H. P.: Observations on a substance in pancreas which permits survival and prevents liver damage in depancreatized dogs, Am. J. Physiol. 117:175-181, 1936.

28. Dunphy, J. E., Brooks, J. R., and Achroyd, F.: Acute postoperative pancreatitis, New England J. Med. 248:445-451, 1953.

29. Fallis, L. S., and Plain, G.: Acute pancreatitis; report of 26 cases, Surgery 15:358-373, 1939.

30. Frostberg, N.: Characteristic duodenal deformity in cases of different kinds of perivaterial enlargement of the pancreas, Acta radiol. 19:164-173, 1938.

31. Gage, M.: Treatment of acute pancreatitis with report of cases, Surgery 23:723-724, 1948.

32. Graham, E. A., and Cole, W. H.: Roentgenologic examination of gallbladder, J.A.M.A. 82:613-614, 1924.

33. Graham, R.: Quoted by Howland, G., Campbell, W. R., Maltby, E. J., and Robinson, W. L.: Dysinsulinism: convulsions and coma due to islet cell tumor of the pancreas, with operation and cure, J.A.M.A. 93:674-679, 1929.

34. Haanes, M. L., and Gyorgy, P.: In vitro action of a new lipotropic fraction in the pancreas, Am. J. Physiol. 166:441-450, 1951.

35. Harris, S.: Hyperinsulinism and dysinsulinism, J.A.M.A. 83:729-733, 1924.

36. Hershey, J. E., and Hillman, F. J.: Fatal pancreatic necrosis following choledochotomy and cholaniography, A.M.A. Arch. Surg. 71:885-889, 1955.

37. Hotchkiss, D., Jr., Fitts, W. T., Jr., and Rosenthal, O.: The effect of abdominal operations upon the serum amylase and serum lipase, S. Forum, 1954. V, 490-495.

38. Howard, J. M.: Experimental studies on the toxicity of beta-(4-hydroxy-3,5-diiodophenyl)-alpha-phenyl-propionic acid (Priodax), Am. J. Roentgenol. 59:408-415, 1948.

39. Howard, J. M., and Jones, R., Jr.: Anatomy of pancreatic ducts; etiology of acute pancreatitis, Am. J. M. Sc. 214:617-622, 1947.

40. Howard, J. M., Moss, N. H., and Rhoads, J. E.: Hyperinsulinism and islet cell tumors of the pancreas, Internat. Abstr. Surg. (Surg., Gynec. & Obst.) 90:417-455, 1950.

41. Howard, J. M., and Ravdin, I. S.: Acute pancreatitis: a study of 80 patients, Am. Pract. 2:385-395, 1948.

42. Kaufman, L. W., and Wilson, G. S.: Carci-

noma of the head of the pancreas and periampullary region, Am. J. M. Sc. *230*:200-212, 1955.

43. Logan, P. B., and Kleinsasser, L. J.: Surgery of the pancreas: results of pancreaticoduodenal resections reported in the literature. Internat. Abstr. Surg. (Surg., Gynec. & Obst.) *93*:521-543, 1951.

44. Longmire, W. P., Jr., Jordan, P. H., Jr., and Briggs, J. D.: Experience with resection of the pancreas in the treatment of chronic relapsing pancreatitis, Ann. Surg. *144*:681, 1956.

45. Lukens, F. D. W.: Experimental diabetes and its relation to diabetes mellitus, Am. J. Med. *19*:790-797, 1955.

46. McDermott, W. V., Jr., and Bartlett, M. K.: Pancreaticoduodenal cancer, New England J. Med. *248*:927-931, 1953.

47. Mahorner, H. R., and Mattson, H.: The etiology and pathology of cysts of the pancreas, Arch. Surg. *22*:1018-1033, 1931.

48. Mallet-Guy, P., Jeanjean, R., and Feroldi, J.: Provocation expérimentale de pancréatites aiguës par excitation électrique du splanchnique gauche, Lyon chir. *39*:437-447, 1944.

49. Millbourn, E.: Excretory ducts of pancreas in man, with special reference to their relations to each other, to common bile duct and to duodenum, Acta anat. *9*:1-34, 1950.

50. Miller, J. R., Baggenstoss, A. H., and Comfort, M. W.: Carcinoma of the pancreas: effect of histologic type and grade of malignancy on its behavior, Cancer *4*:233-241, 1951.

51. Mirsky, I. A., Futterman, P., Wachman, J., and Perisutti, G.: The influence of pancreatectomy on the metabolic state of alloxan-diabetic dog, Endocrinology *49*:73-81, 1951.

52. Moss, N. H., and Rhoads, J. E.: Hyperinsulinism and islet cell tumors of the pancreas *in* Surgical diseases of the pancreas by Howard, J. M., and Jordan, G. L., Philadelphia, Lippincott, 1960.

53. Moyer, C. A.: Personal communication.

54. Mozan, A. A.: Cystadenoma of the pancreas, Am. J. Surg. *81*:204-214, 1951.

55. Muir, E. G.: Resection for carcinoma of the head of the pancreas; two five-year survivals, Brit. J. Surg. *42*:489-490, 1954-55.

56. Nardi, G. L.: Metabolic studies following total pancreatectomy for retroperitoneal leiomyosarcoma, New England J. Med. *247*:548-550, 1952.

57. ————: Phospholipid synthesis in patients with pancreatic disease, A.M.A. Arch. Surg. *69*:726-731, 1954.

58. Opie, E. L.: The anatomy of the pancreas, Bull. Johns Hopkins Hosp. *14*:229-232, 1903.

59. ————: Diseases of the Pancreas, ed. 2, p. 291, Philadelphia, Lippincott, 1910.

60. Orr, T. G.: Some observations on the treatment of carcinoma of the pancreas, Surgery *32*:933-947, 1952.

61. Persky, L., Schweinburg, F. B., Jacob, S., and Fine, J.: Aureomycin in experimental acute pancreatitis of dogs, Surgery *30*:652, 1951.

62. Porter, M. R.: Carcinoma of the pancreaticoduodenal area, operability and choice of procedure, Ann. Surg. *148*:711, 1958.

63. Ravdin, I. S.: Some recent advances in surgical therapeusis, Ann. Surg. *109*:321-333, 1939.

64. Ray, B. S., and Console, A. D.: Relief of pain in chronic (calcareous) pancreatitis by sympathectomy, Surg., Gynec. & Obst. *89*:1-8, 1949.

65. Rhoads, J. E., Howard, J. M., and Moss, N. H.: Clinical experiences with surgical lesions of the pancreas, S. Clin. North America *29*:1801-1816, 1949.

66. Rhoads, J. E., Liboro, C., Fox, S., Gyorgy, P., and Machella, T. E.: In vivo action of a new lipotropic fraction of the pancreas, Am. J. Physiol. *166*:436-440, 1951.

67. Rhoads, J. E., Zintel, H. A., and Helwig, J., Jr.: Results of operations of the Whipple type in pancreaticoduodenal carcinoma, Ann. Surg. *146*:661, 1957.

68. Rhoads, J. E., Zintel, H. A., and Helwig, J., Jr.: An evaluation of palliative and curative operations in the treatment of pancreatoduodenal carcinomas, Acta Un. Int. Cancr. *16*:1397, 1960.

69. Ricketts, H. T., Brunschwig, A., and Knowlton, K.: Effects of total pancreatectomy in a patient with diabetes, Am. J. Med. *1*:229-245, 1946.

70. Rienhoff, W. F., Jr., and Baker, B. M.: Pancreatolithiasis and chronic pancreatitis; preliminary report of case of apparently successful treatment by transthoracic sympathectomy and vagotomy, J.A.M.A. *134*:20-21, 1947.

71. Rienhoff, W. F., Jr., and Pickrell, K. L.: Pancreatitis; anatomic study of pancreatic and extrahepatic biliary systems, Arch. Surg. *51*:205-219, 1945.

72. Ross, D. E.: Cancer of the pancreas with two case reports of five-year survivals, Am. J. Surg. *93*:990, 1957.

73. Smith, R.: Long-term survival after pancreatectomy for cancer, Brit. J. Surg. *44*:294, 1956.

74. Somogyi, M.: Micromethods for estimation of diastase, J. Biol. Chem. *125*:399-414, 1938.
75. Thorogood, E., and Zimmerman, B.: The effects of pancreatectomy on glycosuria and ketosis in dogs made diabetic by alloxan, Endocrinology *37*:191-200, 1945.
76. Tong That Tung, Nguyen Duong Quang, and Hoang Kim Tinh: The diagnosis and treatment of acute pancreatitis caused by parasites, Vestn. Khir. Grekov. *84*:3, 1960.
77. Trimble, I. R., Parsons, J. W., and Sherman, C. P.: A one stage operation for the cure of carcinoma of the ampulla of Vater and of the head of the pancreas, Surg., Gynec. & Obst. *73*:711, 1941.
78. Warren, K. W., and Cattell, R. B.: Pancreatic surgery (concluded), N. England J. Med. *261*:387, 1959.
79. Waugh, J. M., and Giberson, R. G.: Radical resection of the head of the pancreas and of the duodenum for malignant lesions, S. Clin. North America 965, August, 1957.
80. Whipple, A. O., Parsons, W. B., and Mullins, C. R.: Treatment of carcinoma of the ampulla of Vater, Ann. Surg. *102*:763, 1935.
81. Whipple, A. O.: Radical surgery for certain cases of pancreatic fibrosis associated with calcareous deposits, Ann. Surg. *124*:991-1008, 1946.
82. ———: The radical surgery of pancreaticoduodenal cancer *in* Carter, B. N.: Monographs on Surgery, pp. 1-19, Baltimore, Williams & Wilkins, 1952.
83. Wilder, R. M., Allan, F. N., Power, M. H., and Robertson, H. E.: Carcinoma of the islands of the pancreas; hyperinsulinism and hypoglycemia, J.A.M.A. *89*:348-355, 1927.
84. Zintel, H. A., Enterline, H. T., and Rhoads, J. E.: Benign cystadenoma of pancreas, Surgery *35*:612-620, 1954.

J. GARROTT ALLEN, M.D.

———————————— CHAPTER 32 ————————————

Spleen

The spleen is of surgical importance because the majority of its diseases, whether primary or secondary, respond to splenectomy. On the other hand, the role of most surgeons in performing splenectomy for its nontraumatic diseases has been a passive one more often than not. They often must rely upon the judgment of the hematologist or the pathologist for the intricacies of the detailed examination of the blood, the marrow and the splenic pulp essential to the diagnosis.

HISTORICAL NOTE

Although the spleen has often been referred to as an "organ of mystery," a review of some of the early writings on the subject discloses no unusual deficiency in knowledge or lack of thought on the part of physicians. Among the writings of the laity, however, the spleen has been assigned bizarre, apochryphal and imaginary functions. Perhaps this accounts for some of the luster in folklore and fiction surrounding functions of the spleen.

Aristotle[2] recognized the spleen as belonging to the hepatic and portal circulations, but he erroneously believed it to be the "second liver." Galen,[25] who added much sparkle to earlier medical history but little to medical knowledge, believed "yellow bile" to be disposed of by the liver and "black bile" to be attracted to the spleen. Aretaeus of Cappadosa[1] may have been influenced by Galen's writings. He, Aretaeus, thought that the spleen "strained black blood," believing the spleen to

be porous and recognized that it often was enlarged. It is interesting to speculate why he found that the spleen was "often enlarged" among the Greeks and the Romans of 2,000 years ago; to what extent did parasitic diseases and perhaps Mediterranean anemia contribute to his conclusion?

Marcello Malpighi[39] was the first to study the spleen by means of the microscope. In 1659, he described its capsule, the contractile nature of its trabeculae and its lymph follicles later to bear his name. He proved that the spleen is essentially an organ of the vascular system, especially of the splanchnic bed.

Florian Matthis is said[41] to have performed the first splenectomy in dogs in the late 16th century. This feat was repeated a few years later by Paul Barbette (1629-1699)[3] in dogs but was not achieved in man until 2 centuries later.

An interesting sidelight relating to the history of surgery of the spleen is that found in the condemnation of John Blundell (see Chap. 8, "Blood Transfusion"). He was a bold surgeon for his day, and his exploits in blood transfusion in 1818 were soon to be followed by his performing "radical" intra-abdominal operations which proved to be the source of severe criticism resulting in his disrepute. The *Lancet* expressed the fear in 1825 that his next activity might well be the surgical removal of the spleen. 32 years later (1857), Gustav Simon (1824-1876) did perform the first human splenectomy,[53] and later Spencer Wells[57] exploited the operation to advantage.

As the physiologic, pathologic and clinical consequences of splenic diseases developed, the developments assumed many aspects of interest and importance. Some of these will be mentioned briefly in the appropriate sections which follow.

ANATOMY

The spleen arises embryologically from the dorsal mesogastrium just above the tail of the pancreas. When fully developed, it lies in contact with the lateral and the posterior margins of the diaphragm to which its superior pole is suspended by the phrenicolienal ligament. All of its ligaments are in reality reflections of the posterior parietal peritoneum upon the splenic surface as visceral peritoneum. Its posterior border abuts the abdominal wall in the regions of the 11th rib, where it is held by a continuation of the phrenicolienal ligament which attaches along the posterior parietal peritoneal wall. This ligament departs from the abdominal wall, the tail of the pancreas, the splenic vessels, the splenic flexure of the colon at its superior-posterior margin, to encapsulate the spleen as visceral peritoneum. The inferior and posteriolateral portions of the spleen are covered with peritoneum derived from that over the area of the kidney, forming the lienorenal ligament.

Thus, except for the posterior line of parietal reflections of peritoneum over the spleen, more than 90 per cent of its surface faces into the peritoneal cavity and is covered with serosa. In some patients its ligamentous attachments are fairly long so that the spleen may be somewhat mobile and subject to torsion. In others these peritoneal reflections are short, holding the spleen firmly in place. Should the spleen enlarge, it must do so in the anterior direction. Its posterior ligamentous attachments are stretched, and it may acquire more mobility. This increase in mobility often facilitates splenectomy, and for this reason the enlarged spleen at times is more easily removed surgically than the one normal in size.

The spleen is also held by the gastrolienal ligament which is a reflection of anterior and posterior visceral peritoneum of the stomach as they come together along the lateral uppermost part of the greater curvature. This omental ligament attaches to the splenic hilum. Between its leaves run several short arteries and veins from the distal portion of the left gastroepiploic vessels which supply the gastric fundus. Thus on its mesial surface the spleen receives both parietal and visceral ligamentous attachments. The major splenic vessels enter via the posterior visceral peritoneal reflection; the short gastrics enter through its anteromesial gastric attachments.

The color of the normal spleen is dark purple. The normal weight of the spleen in the adult is from 200 to 225 Gm., and it cannot be felt. In infancy the normal spleen weighs more in proportion to body weight; its greater weight in infancy is attributed to its hematopoietic activity at that time, especially in the formation of lymphocytes—the dominant leukocytic cell in this age group. The organ is normally palpable in most infants under the age of 2 years. The amount of blood contained within the normal human spleen is not great. Motulsky *et al.* (1958) found the normal spleen to contain from 1 to 2 per cent of the total circulating red cell mass. In normal man there is neither splenic sequestration of red cells of any significance nor a noncirculating reserve of red cells (Ebert and Stead, 1941). These latter observations are in contrast with findings in the dog. Reeve and his associates (1953) indicated that in the dog up to one third of the red cell mass could be sequestered temporarily in the spleen during barbiturate narcosis. These observations emphasize the important species differences in the function of this organ.

The splenic artery is usually the first and largest branch of the celiac artery. It is remarkably tortuous, the most tortuous artery normally within the abdomen. As it departs from its source, it passes horizontally to the left just above the superior margin of the pancreas in the retroperitoneum of the lesser omental bursa. Along its lateral half, the artery generally parallels the course of the splenic vein, which lies slightly below and anterior to the artery. Within 1 to 3 cm. of the spleen, the artery divides into 2 or 3 major branches before entering the splenic hilum. Venous drainage leaves the spleen through several branches which quickly converge to form the splenic vein.

The lymphatic drainage of the spleen is certainly grossly inconspicuous. The lymph channels converge upon the hilum from within the spleen and then drain into the nodes in the region of the tail of the pancreas; the author seldom has encountered them.

Accessory spleens, ranging from a few hundred milligrams to several grams in weight, are found in about 12 to 15 per cent of patients at operation, whether or not splenic disease is present. Usually they lie near the hilum, in the adjacent omentum, or to the left side of the esophageal hiatus. They are important in certain of the hypersplenic diseases; in some patients with these disorders, failure to respond to splenectomy is attributed to accessory splenic tissue left behind (see below). Accessory spleens are often multiple, 2 to 10 or more.

The splenic capsule is comprised of serosa and a subserosal fibro-elastic coat. The serosa is its visceral peritoneum derived from the peritoneal reflections described above. The fibro-elastic coat is easily torn at operation. This coat surrounds the spleen and on its internal surfaces interlaces its way toward the center, forming the trabecular network that Malpighi described. This is the basic internal structural architecture of the spleen in which is enmeshed the splenic pulp and its internal vascular system. The trabecular network with its fibro-elastic tissue converges upon the major splenic vessels.

PHYSIOLOGY

Although the spleen is not essential to normal childhood development or to adult life, it does partake in certain functions shared also by the "reticuloendothelial system," and at times may share some of those of the marrow, especially in fetal life and early infancy. In certain diseases that encroach upon the marrow space in adults, the spleen as well as the liver may resume their embryonal functions of hematopoiesis; in fact, under these circumstances, they may be the major portion of the blood-forming tissue. Hence, splenectomy under these circumstances can prove to be disastrous.

When the normal spleen is removed from man for acute trauma or to facilitate another surgical procedure, transient thrombocytosis and leukocytosis lasting several weeks is the rule. Platelet and leukocyte counts several times normal may occur. Several report definite but less conspicuous increases of the circulating red cells also. These observations usually are interpreted as implicating the spleen as an organ involved in the normal destruction of the formed elements of blood.

Jacobson and co-workers (1951) showed that shielding the spleen during fatal doses of total body radiation protected the animal from the lethal effects of the irradiation. Cole *et al.* (1952) showed that intravenous infusions of spleen cell homogenates also conferred protection from lethal irradiation. For a time the protective effect of the administered spleen cells was thought to be due to a humoral factor. However, Barnes and Loutit (1956) showed that the protective effect of spleen cells could be achieved only with living cells and was not due to a humoral or chemical agent. Lorenz *et al.* (1951) showed that bone marrow infusions would also protect against irradiation injury. It appears that the benefit of shielding the spleen is a general phenomenon, since shielding other portions of the hematopoietic tissue from lethal doses of total body radiation will produce the same protective effect. The protective effect of shielding hematopoietic tissue is related to the fact that the shielded tissue will quickly recover its normal function. The protective effect of the injected spleen or marrow cells is related to the fact that the injected cells live and multiply within the recipient and assume the functions of the destroyed hematopoietic tissue.

The spleen is intimately related to the production of antibodies, but its presence is not essential to this end. Other organs are also involved. King and Shumacker (1952) found no significant relationship between splenectomy in infants and children to suggest an increased incidence or susceptibility toward infection, despite the fact that antibody production is impaired. However, important differences conceivably could exist and not necessarily be reflected short of a very large clinical study unless carried out over a period of many years. Harkins' (1956) experience leads him to the clinical conclusion that such patients are more susceptible to intercurrent infections. This author has observed no postoperative infections which could not be explained upon technical errors, but he is not willing to discount the possibility of abnormal susceptibility to infection.

When the spleen alone is exposed to x-rays, Hektoen, as observed in 1916, found that the capacity for the body to elaborate antibodies during the next few weeks is diminished. Friedell *et al.* (1947) observed an even

A. Normal Splenic Circulation

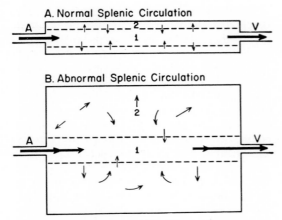

B. Abnormal Splenic Circulation

FIG. 32-1. Physiology of the normal (A) and the abnormal (B) splenic circulation. Normally, blood enters from the artery (A) and leaves through the vein (V) via channel 1: the rapid circulatory component. Some cells may enter compartment 2: the stasis compartment. Normally, compartment 2 is small and not significant physiologically.

In the abnormal circulation (B) formed blood elements may enter the enlarged stasis compartment (2). Delay in splenic transit results. Cells are subject to destructive influence in the stasis compartment. Splenomegaly per se is not necessarily associated with such a circulatory system. In many types of splenomegaly, the stasis compartment is not enlarged, as described in the text. (Motulsky, A. G., Casserd, F., Giblett, E. R., Broun, G. O., and Finch, C. A.: New England J. Med. *259*:1167)

greater depressed antibody production capacity after total body radiation in rabbits. The transient depression in antibody production following depressed antibody response of the spleen after splenic x-radiation in man has been used as a partial treatment in the past for various forms of hypersplenism in which the formation of auto-antibodies is believed to be their cause.

Rowley (1950) has studied antibody response in patients splenectomized for a variety of conditions, including trauma and surgical extirpation of normal spleens necessary to other surgery. His studies disclosed the same results regardless of whether splenectomy had been performed a few weeks to several years before. Compared with the capacity of his

normal human subjects to produce antibodies to a standard antigen, the ability of the splenectomized individual to produce antibodies was greatly diminished. Steiner (1956) has extended this type of study experimentally and demonstrated the enormous capacity of splenic tissue to form antibodies in tissue culture. Thus the relation of the spleen to antibody formation seems to be unquestioned, but the problem as to the susceptibility of infection in man is not.

The splenic pulp is comprised of reticular cells and splenocytes in which are enmeshed lymphocytes, granulocytes, erythrocytes and platelets. It is this structure that appears to be responsible for most of its physiologic functions. Lymphoid follicles (malpighian corpuscles) are numerous and located throughout the normal spleen. They are believed to be one of the sites of lymphocyte and monocyte production in adult life. In fetal life and early infancy, the spleen is also the site of normal hematopoiesis, an atavistic function observed in certain diseases, as mentioned above.

For centuries, the spleen has been considered as the "graveyard" for the formed elements of the blood. Observations suggest that splenic circulation differs from that of other vascular beds in its ability to trap and concentrate particulate matter. Circulatory delay appears to be a characteristic of the splenic circulation in many species. There is disagreement about the anatomic site of stasis. Adherents of the open circulation theory maintain that erythrocytes leave closed vascular channels and are delayed when traversing the open pulp. Those in favor of a closed circulation believe that stasis occurs within sinusoids (Björkman, 1947). Splenic blood flow, for purposes of clinical physiology, may be visualized as consisting of two components (Fig. 32-1). Flow from artery to veins may proceed rapidly as in most other tissues or may bypass the main stream of circulation and enter a more slowly flowing compartment. The stasis compartment is unimportant under normal conditions, and most blood flow occurs by direct channels. Under certain conditions associated with splenic enlargement, the stasis compartment enlarges, and this slow-circulating component assumes major clinical significance (Motulsky, *et al.*, 1958). Prolonged splenic mixing may be caused by either a greatly enlarged stasis compartment or certain types of abnormal blood elements such as hereditary spherocytes or antibody-coated red cells.

DISEASES OF THE SPLEEN
RUPTURE

Rupture of the spleen is a serious surgical emergency because of its attendant blood loss and hypovolemic shock. Trauma is the most common cause; rarely the spleen may enlarge rapidly in disease and rupture spontaneously, or it may do so because of torsion when its ligamentous attachments are long—the so-called "wandering spleen" (Davidson, 1948). In some patients with splenomegaly, the spleen may undergo torsion, or its weight may sheer it from its artery and/or vein with fatal hemorrhage if not recognized promptly and treated surgically. Splenosis may follow (p. 788).

Acute Traumatic Rupture from Nonpenetrating Injuries. Rupture of the spleen caused by nonpenetrating trauma generally tears its capsule or sheers the spleen from its vascular attachments. Knopp and Harkins (1954) and later Parsons and Thompson (1958) surveyed the literature and pointed out that the automobile was the most common etiologic agent. In Parsons and Thompson's series, 46 per cent of their cases resulted from vehicle accidents in which the victims were involved either as pedestrians or occupants of vehicles. In some instances, the trauma seemed to be surprisingly mild; generally, however, there is a history of a stout blow to the upper left abdomen.

The clinical pattern is fairly consistent. The symptom most frequently encountered is generalized abdominal pain. In about one third of cases, pain is limited or predominately located in the left upper quadrant. Pain radiating to the left shoulder (Kehr's sign) is present less often than might be expected (15% of cases).

Abdominal rigidity and hypovolemic shock are present in about 75 per cent of patients when first seen. Dullness to percussion in the flank and the "doughy abdomen" are usually observed if sought for. Nausea and vomiting are frequently noted. The association of other injuries is to be expected in many instances. These include head and chest injuries, especially fractures of the ribs of the lower left chest. Lacerations of the liver and the kidneys as alternate or co-existing diagnoses also must be considered and sought for at the time of exploration. Occasionally the gut may be torn.

Delayed Traumatic Rupture. Not all spleens rupture at the onset of injury. In some patients, the rupture may not occur until 48 hours or longer after injury. Baudet (1907) suggested that the term "delayed rupture" be applied as a means for emphasizing the latent possibilities of splenic rupture following injury. The incidence of traumatic rupture of the normal spleen in which the onset of symptoms is delayed ranges from 5 to 40 per cent of reported cases, averaging about 15 per cent. Although the onset of hemorrhage is delayed, possibly several days to a week, when it does occur the same serious set of consequences as those of acute rupture result.

Delay in rupture of the spleen after injury lies in the fact that there is no immediate complete tear in the capsule. Rather, there is an intracapsular or subcapsular tear into which blood continues to seep and dissect until the capsule is finally ruptured. At this point, blood flows freely into the abdomen. In others, a subcapsular tear or contusion of the pulp gives rise to a splenic hematoma which continues to distend the spleen until this is able to rupture the capsule. In some patients the capsular tear is slight and may be "self-sealing" in a short time only to reopen or to be torn further by the enlarging subcapsular hematoma. In a few the bleeding ceases, and the hematoma may form later a false cyst of the spleen and calcify or resorb. Such favorable responses are uncommon.

The syndrome of delayed splenic rupture is so hazardous because in the interval of time between trauma and the onset of rupture, the patient often is symptom-free. Many of these patients have been treated for their initial injuries and sent home before the first indication of splenic rupture is evident.

Treatment of rupture of the spleen is splenectomy as soon as the diagnosis is made and the patient can be prepared with blood transfusion. Often the rate of blood loss is faster than that which can be replaced; under these circumstances one is forced to operate, removing the spleen to secure hemostasis while continuing blood replacement. Once the spleen is out and hemostasis effected, blood transfusion should be continued until the patient is shock-free. Search for tears in the liver, the kidneys, the stomach, the bowel and the urinary bladder is mandatory. If these are found, they are repaired as indicated.

As the splenic bed in the traumatized patient may later be the site of abscess formation, the author prefers to employ routinely a broad-spectrum antibiotic. Because the tail of the pancreas also may be injured and its severed ducts secrete into the abdominal cavity, the author places a soft rubber drain in the region of the splenic fossa which is removed 3 or 4 days later; antibiotics are continued a day or two longer.

Needle biopsy of the spleen, a useful diagnostic procedure, occasionally has been followed by unrelenting bleeding from the site of needle puncture. In a few instances, the capsule has been torn also. Splenectomy occasionally has been necessary to control this complication. Spleen biopsy should not be undertaken lightly, but fear of this consequence is seldom warranted if the information expected is important and can be obtained in no other way. Needle biopsy of the spleen in the author's experience carries a greater risk of serious hemorrhage than does needle biopsy of the liver. Neither of these procedures should be undertaken when serious platelet or prothrombin deficiency is present.

Operative tears of the normal spleen occasionally occur incidental to other upper abdominal operations, particularly gastric resection, vagotomy, and surgery performed on the splenic flexure. Seldom are the major vessels torn. Usually unrealized tension upon the gastrolienal ligament in gastrectomy or vagotomy tears the capsule or, less frequently, the vasa brevia. The capsule of the lower pole may be torn in dissecting free the splenic flexure of the colon; again, this usually is encountered without realization.

Its treatment is splenectomy at the time, unless the tear is very minor and bleeding ceases promptly. Sutures seldom hold and usually tear the capsule further.

Splenosis is a clinical entity resulting from the autotransplantation of splenic tissue. It was first reported as related to rupture of the spleen by von Küttner in 1910, who regarded the implants as accessory spleens rather than implants (Küttner, 1954). 50 or more implants have been found in some of these patients in contrast with 1 to 10 accessory spleens (Buchbinder and Lipkoff, 1939; Cotlar and Cerise, 1959). Blood supply enters the capsule of such implants rather than through the hilum as in the normal or accessory spleens. Some report that splenosis does not follow the rupture of diseased spleen (Cotlar and Cerise). Experimenal implanation of splenic tissue is easily accomplished; even homologous splenic tissue will survive for a while (see Chap. 17, "Radiation Injury").

CYSTS

Cysts of the spleen are rare. They may be classified as true cysts, false cysts and those caused by parasites. True cysts are thought to represent an embryonal defect or rest. They are lined with flattened epithelium which may be cuboidal or squamous in nature. False cysts are thought to be the end result of intrasplenic hemorrhage. The wall consists of flattened epithelium and trabeculated or fibrous tissue. Occasionally, these cysts are multiple. Many true or false cysts give little or no distress and are found only at autopsy. Others become large and burdensome and occasionally are associated with signs of hypersplenism. In this latter circumstance, splenectomy is in order.

Echinococcus cysts may occur in the spleen, although they are found more often in the liver. The parasites may be alive; hence, splenic puncture and its tear at operation are to be avoided. The diagnosis may be suspected in patients with masses palpable in the splenic area, especially among those who have lived in areas where the disease is endemic. Eosinophilia of varying degree is generally found. Roentgenographic examination of the upper abdomen frequently discloses the rather large cyst whose wall is usually calcified. Intradermal injection of the echinococcal antigen usually gives a positive reaction.

Treatment is splenectomy when possible. Occasionally, the spleen is totally destroyed, and only the cyst remains. At times this can be excised without risk of spilling its contents into the abdominal cavity which may give rise to other cysts later on. Should splenectomy or excision of the cyst *in toto* be impossible, the wall of the cyst nearest the portion of the abdominal wall is marsupialized by suture. Then the cyst is punctured, and its contents are evacuated carefully. Its wall is sponged gently with formalin, and a gauze pack is placed in the cavity and is removed slowly over a few days. Usually it is necessary to reapply a clean pack, removing it, too, in piecemeal fashion over a period of several days. When the cavity is nearly collapsed, a cigarette drain is placed to its base and removed slowly while the entire cavity fills in from the bottom. This is the same form of treatment often employed in the drainage of echinococcus cysts of the liver.

INFECTIONS

Infections of the spleen are comparatively rare in the total consideration of its diseases. They may be bacterial, parasitic or viral in origin. The spleen may enlarge in the course of systemic infections without necessarily harboring the specific agent. The splenomegalic reaction must be distinguished from those in which the spleen is a host organ to infection.

Bacterial infections involving the spleen may give rise to abscess formation requiring splenectomy or drainage. Usually, splenic abscesses are secondary to pyemia with some other focus serving as the point of origin. In a few instances, splenic abscess may result from nearby bacterial infections in the upper abdomen of which the reports of perforated peptic ulcer are an example. Septic thrombi of arterial or venous origin may produce a splenic abscess. Splenic hematomas incurred in trauma may become infected at times and result in abscess formation. Among the organisms more commonly encountered as pathogens are the staphylococcus, the pneumococcus, *B typhosus* and the coliform group.

ABSCESS. The splenic abscesses induced by septic emboli or infarcts are largely confined within the spleen and may not be recognized readily. Should they not respond to antibiotic therapy or go unnoticed, the abscess cavity often continues to enlarge, and in time the capsule may be perforated with the formation of a subphrenic abscess, presenting its usual complications, including empyema of the left chest and bronchopleural fistula. Septic thrombi may form in the splenic vein as a result of splenic abscess. The clots may embolize via the portal vein to form intrahepatic

abscesses. In a few, rupture of the abscess occurs into the free peritoneal cavity, giving rise to peritonitis. Often the spleen is totally destroyed by the abscess, and its vessels are completely thrombosed. Once necrotic tissue develops, the abscess continues until drained. In about one third of cases, fragments of splenic tissue will be discharged through surgical wounds as "sequestra."

Clinical features of splenic abscess are as variable as is the nature of the antecedent history of infection responsible. Should a septic infarct be the origin and sufficient occlusion of the circulation occur to create perisplenitis, pain referred along the left phrenic nerve may be a complaint. In others, pain in the region of the spleen may be the only complaint and is perhaps the one most commonly encountered. A febrile course is the rule. The left diaphragm is generally elevated and is immobile as determined by respiratory excursions upon percussion or fluoroscopic examination. Its continuing presence unrecognized may lead to weight loss and the debility and the septic course common to any chronic but serious infection. Frequently, there is a palpable tender mass in the left hypochondrium; this may be spleen or the omentum.

Treatment depends upon the stage of abscess development at the time the diagnosis is first suspected. A heavy course of antibiotic therapy is indicated in any event, using a broad-spectrum agent such as a tetracycline. That many splenic abscesses subside without splenectomy or surgical drainage when antibiotics are used is an unsettled question. In the past, many continued to progress, and mortality was high. Splenectomy is still the treatment of choice in many patients, draining the splenic bed through a stab wound. The spleen may be so adherent to adjacent structures that the surgeon may be forced to drain the abscess through a lateral incision, leaving the spleen in place. In such cases the wall of the abscess should be sutured to the peritoneum at the point intended for drainage; in the case of abscesses of the upper pole, the left transpleural approach may be advisable. Drainage of the spleen involves the same principles as entailed in the surgical drainage of suprahepatic or intrahepatic abscesses (see Chap. 33, "Mesentery, Splanchnic Circulation, Portal Hypertension and Mesenteric Thrombosis"). Drainage is likely to persist for weeks to months, unless all sequestra of necrotic splenic pulp are expelled early. Once healed, delayed splenectomy is rarely indicated.

TUBERCULOSIS of the spleen occasionally requires splenectomy to correct the secondary manifestations of the hypersplenic states which may also develop. Otherwise, the patient should be treated for his systemic disease, realizing that the spleen, too, will heal in due course if medical therapy is successful. Calcifications form within the spleen, often giving the appearance of buckshot, each of the larger miliary tubercules becoming calcified. The same is the end result for histoplasmosis involving the spleen, which may be found roentgenographically. This fungus disease may also induce thrombocytopenic purpura when it involves the spleen, as may sarcoid. If healing occurs, miliary calcifications of the spleen are often observed on roentgenography of the upper left abdomen. The response of the thrombocytopenic purpura to splenectomy is excellent and may be lifesaving; the patient should not be deprived of the benefits afforded by splenectomy simply because of the systemic nature of tuberculosis, histoplasmosis or sarcoid (see p. 802).

Parasitic infections involving the spleen are comparatively rare in the northern half of the United States. Principally concerned are malaria, leishmaniasis (kala-azar) encountered overseas and echinococcal disease; the last is discussed under "Cysts of the Spleen."

MALARIA occasionally induces extreme enlargement of the spleen. When this occurs rapidly, the spleen may rupture spontaneously, requiring emergency splenectomy. If medical management of the acute phase is successful, the splenomegaly subsides, usually without further difficulty. When the disease has been chronic and untreated, the enlargement of the spleen also can be huge; its weight may be so great as to shear it from its ligamentous moorings, and in doing so tear the major splenic vessels at its hilum. Emergency extirpation of the spleen is necessary, with ligation of the severed vessels; such an event is likely to be fatal unless the accident occurs in the hospital and is recognized early. It is for this reason that elective splenectomy should be strongly considered when the spleen becomes huge, regardless of cause, unless life expect-

ancy is obviously very short. Three patients with chronic lymphoid leukemia and huge splenomegaly have experienced such an accident in the wards of the University of Chicago during the past 2 years. Prompt surgical intervention was successful in each instance; each patient survived comfortably for longer than a year after operation.

LEISHMANIA INFANTUM OR DONOVANI are parasitic diseases affecting the spleen, often causing huge splenomegaly similar to that seen in chronic malarial infections. Neither of these diseases is encountered frequently in this country. The diagnosis is made on biopsy tissue obtained by splenic puncture; portions of the biopsy material should be cultured. Antimony therapy or the more recently developed ethylstibamine (Neostibosan) are usually effective. But if the spleen remains very large, splenectomy may be necessary.

Among other rarely encountered parasitic infections which on occasion have been the origin of huge splenomegaly are *Toxoplasma pyrogenes* and *Cryptococcus farciminosus*. The spirochetal infections—syphilis, yaws and Weil's disease—generally respond to medical therapy; splenectomy is rarely required unless an associated uncontrolled hypersplenic disorder appears.

FELTY'S SYNDROME

This syndrome is characterized by splenomegaly, anemia, lymphadenopathy, osteoarthritis, cutaneous pigmentation and leukopenia of the neutropenic variety. It has been known by many names; among these are Chauffard-Still's disease and von Jackson's syndrome. Felty's report in 1924[23] was the first in the English language, and so in this country it bears his name, although Still's description antedates Felty's report by 28 years (1896). Felty's syndrome is a clinical rather than a pathologic entity.

The clinical pattern is one of chronic arthritis affecting few or many of the joints. Weakness and abdominal pain are frequent complaints. Brownish pigmentation of the skin may be noted, and lymphadenopathy is fairly general. Uusually, these nodes are not matted together, thus assisting in the distinction of Felty's syndrome from that of lymphoma or Hodgkin's disease. However, the nodes are generally fixed to the adjacent tissue and often tender to palpation. Gastric achlorhydria or diminished secretion is a common finding, but usually normal responses are elicited to Gastramine or histamine. Anemia is present, usually mild to moderate, and normochromic in character. The marrow is not usually abnormal to any particular degree, nor does it possess any distinct characteristics.

Some have reported the occasional finding of *Streptococcus viridans* on blood culture or cultures of biopsied nodes. Fever is generally present; more often it is low-grade than serious. The consensus today is that this disease is a form of rheumatoid arthritis.

Treatment is medical which, for the want of a better understanding as to its pathogenesis, is largely symptomatic. Corticoids and salicylates are commonly used.

Splenectomy has been performed in a number of these patients with reported improvement. Its rationale is that hypersplenic disorders may account for granulocytopenia and/or thrombocytopenia. The response to splenectomy is variable; an early good response often is not sustained. Operative results are often doubtful—more often disappointing.

SPLENIC TUMORS

Malignant tumors of the spleen unassociated with blood dyscrasia are extremely rare. A few patients suffering from primary sarcoma of the spleen have been reported. Fibroma, myoma, leiomyosarcoma and angiomatous tumors may occur. For the most part, however, any splenic enlargement is much more likely to be secondary to infection, cyst formation, lymphoma, Hodgkin's disease, portal hypertension, or chronic congestive failure than tumor. The positive diagnosis is made by needle biopsy or from the removed specimen.

Metastatic tumors to the spleen are also rare by comparison with metastases found in other organs. This may be due in part to the scanty lymphatic supply to the spleen. However, experimentally implanted tissues grow as well in the spleen as in other organs, implying that the infrequent occurrence of tumor metastasis is not likely due to any particular noxious influence that the spleen may have upon tumor cells. Apparently, the infrequency of metastasis to this organ is simply one of failure of significant quantities of tumor cells to arrive there.

HEMOLYTIC ANEMIAS AND THE SPLEEN

Interaction of Red Cells and Spleen. In certain diseases red cells are held for an appreciable period within the spleen, thus providing opportunity for cell destruction. This situation may be achieved by an abnormality either in the red cell or in the spleen.

Spleen-Susceptible Erythrocytes. The susceptibility of certain red cells to destruction by the normal spleen was first demonstrated by survival studies of hereditary spherocytes transfused to patients with and without spleens. Studies attempting to define types of damage leading to splenic destruction indicate a high degree of susceptibility of red cells coated with certain incomplete autoantibodies, cells coated with metallic cations, cells exposed to high temperatures, and the erythrocytes of patients with hereditary spherocytosis (Motulsky, *et al.*, 1958).

Plasma Iron Clearance in Plasma and Marrow and Its Significance in Splenic Disorders. Iron normally circulates within the plasma as a complex beta globulin. The total quantity of iron within the plasma normally is only about 0.1 per cent of the entire amount of the body; yet plasma iron is extremely important, for its represents the only means of transport of iron from one part of the body to another.

In recent years a number of investigators have employed radioiron (Fe^{59}) as a means of studying the turnover rates of iron in normal and pathologic hematopoietic states. Although there is evidence that the status of the iron stores within the body may influence to some extent the rate at which iron is incorporated into new hemoglobin, generally iron liberated by hemolysis is reutilized promptly in the formation of new hemoglobin (Figs. 32-5 and 6).

For the most part, those conditions that favor an increased rate of hematopoiesis disclose a high rate of plasma iron turnover. In those in which hematopoiesis is reduced in activity, the turnover rates of plasma iron are retarded correspondingly. Thus, there is a rapid clearance of radioiron from plasma in iron-deficiency anemias, hemolytic anemias and polycythemia vera, indicating true hyperplastic states of the marrow in these conditions. It should be pointed out, however, that many studies of iron metabolism are currently under way and that a thorough understanding of this mechanism is not yet at hand.

Congenital Hemolytic Anemia (Spherocytic Anemia or Familial Hemolytic Icterus). This is a hereditary disease whose basic disorder is attributed to the spherocytic shape of the patient's erythrocytes instead of their usual discoid character. The disease is inherited as a mendelian dominant characteristic and, as occurs under similar circumstances, does not imply that all progeny of a parent so afflicted will display this disorder. The abnormality is not sex-linked.

HISTORICAL CONSIDERATIONS. This disease was first described by Murchison in 1885; its familial nature was pointed out later by Minkowski (1886). Chauffard (1914) reported in 1907 the increased fragility of erythrocytes to trauma in this disease which he attributed to the spherocytoidal properties of the cells. Shortly thereafter osmotic fragility was reported and studied by several observers, especially Dawson (1931). However, it has been Haden's study in 1934 which serves as the basis for most of the present-day saline dilution tests employed. Splenectomy as its treatment was first employed by Spencer Wells (1818-1897) in 1887; the early results were not as good as those of today, probably because of inaccuracies in diagnosis.

CLINICAL PATTERN is one of mild icterus, with or without anemia, a slowly enlarging spleen, with the eventual formation of bilirubinate gallstones in many patients. Icterus may be present at birth or may not appear until later in life; pruritus and bradycardia do not occur. Generally, icterus is slight and often overlooked. There is a positive correlation between the degree of anemia, the serum level of bilirubin and the incidence of gallstones. The disease tends to be one of remission and exacerbation, although the sallow color of the skin tends to remain. Once severe anemia and intense icterus develop, there is little likelihood of spontaneous remission. Chronic leg ulcers are observed in this disease, as is true in a number of other chronic hemolytic states.

The most striking and unusual feature of this disease is the hemolytic crisis which may occur at any time in life. While these are characterized by severe abdominal pain, nausea and vomiting, fever, palpitation, dyspnea, and often the acute onset of profound anemia, serum bilirubin is not increased above its pre-existing levels; in fact, Owren (1948) reports a decline in serum bilirubin, urobilinuria and reticulocytosis, with the onset of acute aplasia of the marrow during crises. These findings led him to conclude that the cause of the crisis is one of acute suppression of erythropoiesis rather than that of a suddenly increased rate of red cell destruction. Leukopenia and thrombocytopenia also are usually present during these episodes.

Of interest is the observation reported by Marson *et al.* (1950) that crises may occur in several members of the family at the same time, suggesting a common trigger mechanism. Presumably such "epidemics" could result from the exposure to a common toxin or some other pathogen to which the family is exposed simultaneously. Owren's postulations as to the pathogenesis of these crises have subsequently proved to be true in some instances, although it seems that there are also occasions when a rapid increase in the rate of hemolysis may occur.

The presence of pigmented gallstones is reported in 40 to 70 per cent of cases. The range of such an incidence is undoubtedly influenced by the nature of medical practice, especially the frequency of or time lapse before splenectomy is performed. This varies from one community to another. After stones have formed, then these patients are subject to attacks of biliary colic to the same degree as patients with cholelithiasis from other causes. The formation of gallstones requires time: it is likely that the incidence of cholelithiasis will be higher among patients in communities where splenectomy is withheld until late in the course of the disease. Such stones in themselves are indications for operation in many patients.

Several infrequently encountered skeletal abnormalities have been described in association with the disease, including the "tower" skull, the one observed most commonly. Growth impairment and endocrine disorders occur in a few children if the disease is severe.

Roentgenographic changes of the skull and the long bones may disclose the striation changes of the former and evidence of increased marrow mass in the long bones. As these are the same findings of any severe anemia associated with hyperactive marrow activity, they are confirmatory and not diagnostic.

Iron metabolism has not been studied sufficiently well to permit firm conclusions as to the character of its disturbance in this disease. The current status of this metabolic problem is summarized by Bothwell *et al.* (1956).

All evidence suggests that greatly increased rates of red cell destruction and replacement occur in this disease. These augmented phenomena are always present, but the extent to which they are increased varies from patient to patient as well as from time to time in the same patient. The hyperplastic bone marrow and reticulocytosis are the cardinal findings of an increased rate of production of red cells. These observations, coupled with anemia, icterus, an elevation of serum bilirubin, urobilinuria, an increase in fecal urobilinogen and the formation of pigmented gallstones provide the classic pattern of an accelerated rate of red cell destruction. Spherocytosis, the increased red cell fragility and the familial history of the disease superimposed upon the above establish the cause of the hemolytic anemia as one of familial or spherocytic anemia. Whereas the usual life span of the circulating normal red cell is in the neighborhood of 3 to 4 months, studies employing tracer or other technics suggest that the life span of erythrocytes in familial hemolytic anemia is reduced markedly, often to a few days to a few weeks.

PATHOLOGY of familial hemolytic anemia is most interesting, although again neither its exact nature nor its entire mechanism is understood. The most logical and usual explanation of the augmented erythropoiesis is its stimulation by the increased rate of red cell destruction. Presumably the stimulus here is a nonspecific one and does not differ from the erythroid stimulation induced by blood loss from other causes, such as hemorrhage or hemolysis, except that in this disease its chronicity (years rather than days, weeks or months) may pose certain special problems in relation to hemosiderin deposits and the greater frequency of gallstone formation. Hemosiderosis is seen classically in the spleen, in or near its smaller blood vessels, occasionally forming deposits in the adventitia and the elastic coats of smaller arteries; sometimes the latter deposits are referred to as Gandy-Gamma nodules (Wells, 1931). Hemosiderin deposits are also found frequently in most other body tissues, particlarly in the Kupffer cells of the liver, the lymph nodes, the marrow and in the loops of Henle of the kidney. Fatty degeneration of the heart with brown atrophy is noted occasionally.

The marrow may be exceedingly hyperactive in severe cases. Cut sections of the vertebrae, the ribs and the long bones showing the beefy red character of marrow hyperplasia are strikingly impressive. Normoblasts are more numerous than megaloblasts, and mitotic figures are seen commonly. Leukopoiesis is less pronounced, but the number of mitoses may be increased in the myeloblastic elements, too. Extramedullary marrow activity may occur in severe cases, especially in infants and children.

For a time, hematopoiesis seems to be capable of matching the increased rate of red cell destruction, but as the disease progresses, marrow exhaustion may occur. Cellular hyperplasia becomes less and less efficient in erythrocytic replacement. The number of megaloblasts at this stage may exceed that of the dominant cell type, the erythroblast, found earlier in the disease.

As for the *circulating* blood, the most notable feature is microcytic anemia and the characteristic spherocyte. This abnormal shape of the circulating red cells is the primary disorder generally believed to account for the clinicopathologic aspects of the disease. To the increased fragility of spherocytic red cells after mechanical agitation has been attributed most if not all of the abnormalities associated with this disease. Although the fragility of these cells may be due in part to defects in stroma and possibly in the cellular membrane, most have entertained the possibility that the spheroidal shape itself posed certain mechanical problems in addition to the increased fragility. There has been no convincing evidence that there is a circulating antibody to account for hemolysis; this is of some assistance in the differential diagnosis of other hemolytic disorders associated with the splenomegaly.

Whipple *et al.* (1954) in a recent study presented observations which suggest that spherocytes may experience more difficulty traversing the splenic circulation than normal ones. Perfusing the normal spleens with mixtures of spherocytic and normal erythrocytes disclosed that a distinctly higher percentage of normal cells finally reached the venous side of its circulation. Microscopic sections of the spleen disclosed upon examination that the spherocytes were predominant among the cells retained. It is possible that the erythrocytic engorgement of the spleen in this disease is due in part to the impairment in cell transit across the splenic pulp. It is not known whether the capillaries of other organs pose similar problems; possibly they do. It would seem reasonable that cells that are more fragile than normal might well be broken up more rapidly, particularly if they encountered more trauma in passing through the capillary vessels. As pointed out in Chapter 8, "Blood Transfusion," the rate of destruction of red cells transfused to a normal recipient is increased exponentially in accordance with the age of the cells.

Testing for the increase in *red cell fragility* when exposed to diminishing concentrations of saline solution is not detected as easily as might be expected. Many suggest refrigeration storage of the blood sample overnight before testing for altered osmotic fragility.

DIAGNOSIS is usually fairly easy to establish, especially when hemolytic anemia, spherocytes and their increased osmotic fragility are demonstrated in multiple members of the same family who are mildly icteric and display splenomegaly. The accuracy of the diagnosis depends upon the certainty that spherocytosis and an increased osmotic fragility exist, plus the hyperplastic marrow. Measurements of fecal urobilinogen excretion or plasma iron "clearance" disclose an increase in both. These tests provide specific evidence of hemolysis, but they do not disclose its cause. Family history in the presence of the other classic findings establishes the diagnosis beyond much question. However, family history is not essential to the diagnosis nor is it always present, for occasionally the patient is the first member of his family to develop the mendelian mutant necessary for this disease. In this respect the situation is similar to the familial aspects of congenital hemophilia. The disease must start with some progenitor.

TREATMENT. Spencer Wells (1931) appears to have performed the first successful splenectomy for this disease in 1887 in a 27-year-old female with "bouts" of jaundice since the age of 9. The operation was performed 3 years before the disease was first described by Minkowski. The spleen weighed "11 lbs. 4 oz." Jaundice disappeared, and the patient survived at least 40 more years. Her only son developed jaundice, splenomegaly and gallstones at about the age of 14, was operated upon for obstructive jaundice as well as for his hemolytic spherocytic anemia; by this time the disease was known and the diagnosis clearly established in the boy.

Of all the nontraumatic indications for splenectomy, this is the one disease in which this operation has the most nearly perfect record in effecting a permanent cure. Conservative treatment is nonspecific and relies upon spontaneous remission. The few surgical failures reported are likely the result of diagnostic error.

Because of the prompt improvement after splenectomy, most hematologists believe that the operation may be carried out at the time of a crisis if required. In general, however, it is better to avoid crises, performing splenectomy prior to their onset if possible or during a quiescent interval. Blood transfusions during operation should be withheld until after the spleen's blood supply is ligated, as transfusion reactions are encountered more commonly in hemolytic anemias and are also more difficult to avoid.

The author prefers to perform splenectomy in most young people with icterus in whom the diagnosis is established. Should the disease not be detected or only give symptoms late in life, splenectomy is deferred unless crises or gallstones develop.

The finding of gallstones alone is usually an indication for cholecystectomy in most patients under the age of 60 in whom contraindications do not exist (see Chap. 30, "Biliary Tract"). Gallstones in the presence of familial hemolytic anemia greatly strengthen the operative indication for either disease. Most surgeons believe that cholecystectomy and splenectomy can and should be carried out through the same incision at the same time if the patient is in good condition.

PROGNOSIS is good provided that one can avoid the complications imposed by crises, cholelithiasis and endocrine disturbances. The author does not recommend splenectomy simply because the diagnosis of familial spherocytic anemia is made, nor does he condone expectant treatment when anemia, icterus and gallstones are present, unless strong contra-indications to any surgical procedure exist. In experienced hands, elective splenectomy carries the lowest mortality of all diseases for which the spleen is removed—generally less than 3 per cent. The operative mortality is much less than that of the untreated disease. Although icterus may be remitting in early life, over the years it tends to increase and to be associated with other complications.

The lessening of spherocytosis or its complete disappearance after splenectomy is reported occasionally. This has caused some to question the generally accepted concept that a primary constitutional defect is responsible for spherocytosis. Many also raise two unanswered questions about the primary nature of this disorder: does it lie within the spleen or is the spherocytosis dependent upon or mediated by some unknown activity of the spleen?

Sickle Cell Anemia. This interesting hereditary disease for which splenectomy occasionally is performed was first recognized by James B. Herrick (1910). It is predominantly a disease of Negroes and characterized by hemolytic anemia with the hyperplasia of the marrow of any hemolytic disease. The clinical pattern is that of chronic leg ulcers, attacks of acute abdominal pain, osteoarthritis, abnormal bleeding with remissions and exacerbations frequently encountered. The seriousness of the disease and its manifestations are variable. Should complaints appear in early childhood or early adult life, the eventual outlook is likely to be poor. Few in this group survive beyond the age of 30.

Among the causes of death are cardiac failure, often with cor pulmonale, thrombosis, hemorrhage, intercurrent infection, or shock in association with abdominal crises attributed to vascular stasis. The spleen is usually enlarged in children, but almost never palpable in adults, as it tends to fibrose and shrink below that of its normal size.

Sickle cell trait is to be distinguished from sickle cell anemia. The finding of the trait is seldom of consequence. The diagnosis of symptomatic sickle cell anemia is aided by the fact that studies indicate that the disease is limited to those in whom both parents bear the sickle trait. Most patients with the disease die within the first 2 decades of life.

The sickle shape is best demonstrated at 37° C. in an atmosphere devoid of oxygen, with the pH of the blood slightly reduced. A drop of blood mixed with a 2 per cent solution of sodium metabisulfite and examined 15 minutes after placing a cover slip over the slide usually shows that sickling is present.

The cause of sickle cell anemia is an abnormal hemoglobin (HbS) found in the red cells of patients with this disease (Pauling, et al., 1949). Hemoglobin S is less soluble than normal hemoglobin (HbA) and forms a gel more easily than other varieties of hemoglobin. When hemoglobin S is subjected to low oxygen tensions its solubility is reduced even more, and in such low oxygen tensions it assumes a sicklelike shape. These sickled cells are easily destroyed; they also increase the viscosity of the blood and somehow propagate the painful and destructive infarctions which are characteristic of the disease.

Sicklemia and the acute abdominal symptoms it may cause have occasionally led the physician erroneously to recommend abdominal exploration. This disease is among the differential diagnoses to be considered in patients with acute abdominal complaints, especially young Negroes. When acute abdominal pain with fever and leukocytosis occur, the diagnosis of a surgical condition within the abdomen is difficult if not impossible to exclude in some of these patients. However, the increased nucleated red cells, sicklemia and anemia are very helpful. Wilson (1950) tabulates the following "surgical features" of this disease:

1. Acute adbominal symptoms, more often simulating colic, intussusception or other forms of acute mechanical ileus

2. Jaundice

3. Bone and joint pains, occasionally simulating osteomyelitis, later showing evidence of aseptic necrosis of bone by roentgenography

4. Leg ulcers

5. Priapism

6. Hematuria may be associated with the clinical picture of renal colic

7. Cerebral accidents

Satisfactory treatment does not exist. Splenectomy has been performed without notable, if any, benefit. Any improvement is likely to be a misinterpreted spontaneous re-mission. Splenectomy, understandably, is not a cure. Splenectomy fails to correct the sickle shape, the abnormal protein moiety or the symptoms.

Many believe that the shape of the cells imposes difficulties upon its traversing the capillary bed throughout the body and not just that of the spleen. The tortuous vessels of the eye grounds leading to visual disturb-ances provide a direct opportunity to note this effect. It is also proposed that cardio-megaly with its cor pulmonale is another mani-festation of the same phenomenon of vascular stasis.

The surgeon needs to bear in mind that often the abdominal crises may simulate the picture of the acute abdomen except that peri-staltic activity usually persists. If he over-looks this disorder, he may perform a need-less abdominal exploration, particularly on the Negro patient.

Thalassemia (Cooley's Anemia). Cooley's anemia or thalassemia also has been reason for splenectomy in a few instances. Operation is performed primarily for relief of the dis-tress from splenomegaly; it has no apparent benefit upon the disease per se.

HYPERSPLENIC DISORDERS

The spleen, as part of the general reticu-loendothelial tissue is assumed to participate in the normal destruction of the formed ele-ments of the blood, but this function under ordinary circumstances is not measurable. However, there are certain conditions in which the enlarged spleen has the capacity to destroy increased numbers of the formed elements of the blood.

The theory or concept of hypersplenism was introduced by Eppinger in 1922 to describe the conditions resulting from an increase in the normal activities of the spleen: thrombo-cytopenia, neutropenia, anemia separately, to-gether, or in their various combinations. When all 3 elements are involved, the term panhyper-splenism is applied.

Splenic Thrombocytopenia. In general, two types are described; primary and sec-ondary thrombocytopenia. The term "sec-ondary" as employed here connotes the occurrence of thrombocytopenia secondary to some other abnormality within the spleen, usu-ally one or another of the splenomegalies, in-cluding that of portal hypertension.

PRIMARY IDIOPATHIC THROMBOCYTOPENIC PURPURA OR WERLHOF'S DISEASE (ALSO KNOWN AS ESSENTIAL THROMBOCYTOPENIA, PURPURA HEMORRHAGICA). This is a symp-tom complex characterized by petechial hem-orrhage, prolonged bleeding time, impaired clot retraction, normoplastic or hyperplastic marrow, all due primarily to thrombocyto-penia. This same clinical pattern is observed in patients with severe thrombocytopenia from aplasia of the marrow in the leukemoid dis-eases and in extensive replacement of marrow by tumor or obliteration in Albers-Schönberg disease. It is most important to distinguish these secondary states from Werlhof's disease in which the marrow is normal or hyperplastic and the thrombocytopenia results from an increased platelet destruction rather than a failure of their production.

Paul Gottlieb Werlhof (1699-1767) de-scribed in 1735 the disease that bears his name.

An adult girl, robust, without manifest cause, was attacked recently, towards the period of her menses, with sudden severe hemorrhage from the nose, with bright but foul blood escaping together with a blood vomiting of a very thick extremely black blood. Immediately there appeared about the neck and on the arms, spots partly black, partly violaceous or purple, such as are often seen in malignant smallpox. . . .

She recovered spontaneously.

As blood platelets were not recognized for another 100 years, the above case can only be presumed to have been one of thrombocyto-penia. Not until 1883 did Brohm describe the first case of purpura ascribed to a demon-strated thrombocytopenia.

Physiology of Platelets. The origin of platelets was clearly demonstrated by Wright in 1906 to be the megakaryocyte. The latter was first described by Howell in 1890 and shown by Wright to fragment. These particles enter the circulation as "platelets." Wright's observations were disputed by many, but no longer are they opposed.

Agglutination and disintegration of plate-lets occur rapidly where blood is shed, as first shown by Bizzozero in 1882. He believed them to be essential for coagulation and predicted that their absence might create a hemorrhagic state.

The ability of platelets to agglutinate and adhere to the site of an intravascular injury represents the earliest of the several complex hemostatic events occurring in mammals in response to vascular injury. Platelets rapidly collect about the point of trauma, piling up to form clumps intermingled with laminations of fibrin deposits.

Under some circumstances, circulating platelets are removed rapidly from the circulation when multiple sites of thrombi formation exist, with the result that severe thrombocytopenia develops. This phenomenon may occur in a variety of ways; one of the most commonly encountered is associated with numerous platelet deposits occasionally found along the surface of the aorta, extensively involved with atheromatous ulcerations or plaques. Similar minute and numerous platelet thrombi may occur from other coagulation disorders, such as those associated with the giving of a mismatched blood transfusion or from cobra venom. The pathologic state becomes a mixture of coagulation and abnormal bleeding known as *thrombotic thrombocytopenia*. It is unrelated to the activities of either the spleen or the marrow and caused by excessive platelet utilization.

More difficult to understand than the platelet's participation in coagulation is its normal role in the prevention of hemorrhage and in the maintenance of the normal hemostatic state, often referred to as the "integrity of the capillary walls." It seems to be fairly obvious that normal concentration of circulating platelets is essential to the prevention of petechial bleeding, as their absence or serious reduction in number nearly always results in purpura. Restoration of normal platelet concentration, whether by splenectomy or platelet transfusion, overcomes the bleeding tendency. The occasional exception noted is the symptomatic cure, either by spontaneous remission or following splenectomy wherein the platelet count remains at its previously low levels.

The platelets are likely very actively concerned with the normal maintenance of the capillary circulation as also seems likely for other clotting factors. It is only when their number is exhausted that their silent purposes and dynamic activities become evident with

the development of purpura. The same, of course, likely applied also to the other elements of coagulation, each performing an unknown function essential to life in the normal individual. Coagulation at the site of vascular trauma is interpreted fairly easily, although incompletely understood; that of spontaneously occurring abnormal bleeding is not. So far as can be established now, the abnormality in the thrombocytopenia appears to be largely one wherein diapedesis assumes hemorrhagic proportions.

Clinical pattern of the Werlhof syndrome is one of petechial hemorrhage, more numerously distributed over the more dependent portions of the body (Fig. 32-2). The increased venous pressure from gravity causes the number of petechial hemorrhagic points to increase. This phenomenon is simulated artificially by the so-called Rumpel-Leede or tourniquet test and in recent years has been demonstrated by the application of suction cups applied to the skin.

The petechial areas tend to become confluent, forming intracutaneous ecchoymotic areas. At autopsy, the organs of motion generally display more evidence of hemorrhage than those which are inactive. Ease of bruising is one of the prominent features noted (Fig. 32-2). Nonetheless, should the platelet count be seriously depressed, spontaneous extravasations can occur with fatal consequence in organs which display no motion and are not likely traumatized. The most common cause of death in these patients is spontaneously occurring intracranial hemorrhage; this complication may appear while the patient is lying in bed. Abnormal bleeding may be found in all organs and tissues in severe thrombocytopenia. The seriousness in symptoms varies generally in accordance with the degree of platelet depression. Massive gastro-intestinal hemorrhage, melena, hematuria, epistaxis and intracranial hemorrhage may occur together, or in various combinations. In mild cases, hematuria or a "skin rash" over the lower legs may be the patient's only complaint. Each of these symptoms upon occasion has been the first manifestation of hemorrhage to be encountered. Often the physician confronted with complaints of abnormal bleeding may center his attention so closely upon the organ source of bleeding that he overlooks the neces-

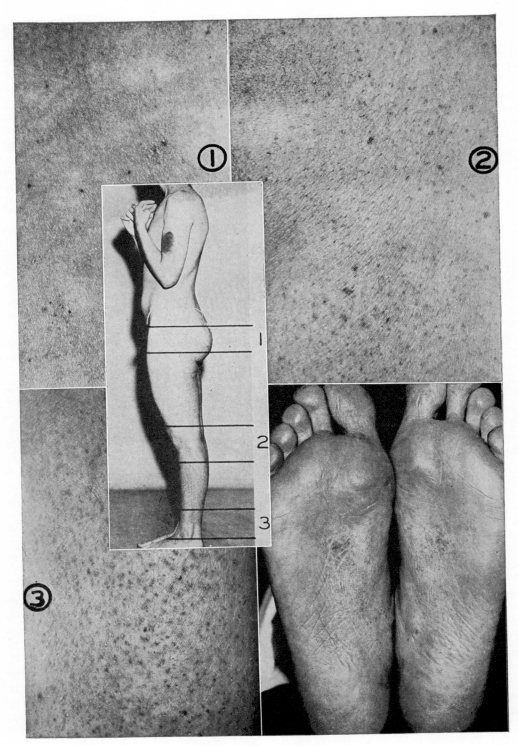

FIG. 32-2. Profile of ambulatory patient with idiopathic thrombocytopenic purpura. Note hematoma on arm which followed a hypodermic injection. Pictures 1, 2 and 3 are enlargements of correspondingly numbered skin segments and show an increase in numbers of petechiae in more dependent parts of the body. Note that petechiae on soles of feet are largely limited to nonweight portions of skin.

sity for a careful examination searching for the clotting abnormalities in general.

In many patients with Werlhof's disease, spontaneous remission occurs, especially in the group under 12 years of age. True Werlhof thrombocytopenia is seldom seen after the age of 30. It is encountered 4 to 5 times more commonly in females and is likely to have its onset at the time of menstruation. Curiously, in this connection, estrogen administration in the dog, followed about 10 days later by its sudden withdrawal, usually is followed promptly by thrombocytopenia and an abnormal bleeding state resembling that in man.

Diagnosis is not especially difficult in the hands of an experienced hematologist. Certain features are essential: (1) the demonstration of thrombocytopenia; (2) the demonstration of normal marrow aspirates which are much more meaningful and accurately interpreted if fixed and permanent sections are made, as described by Block (1947), than when examined by direct smear. The results following splenectomy for this disease at the University of Chicago have improved greatly during the past 8 years. During this time the section technic has been used in preference to that of the marrow smear. This author is inclined to attribute the improved end results to the better

histologic preparations for diagnostic studies and its influence upon case selection.

Classically, the marrow shows an abundance of megakaryocytes but few platelets. The erythroid elements are also normal or hyperplastic, seeming to be determined by the presence and the extent of hemorrhage. It is as important to establish that no other dysplasia of the marrow is going on; hypoplasia argues strongly against splenectomy.

The clotting time usually is described as being normal in this disease. From a practical point of view, this is true, as most who perform clotting times fail to obtain any increase. With the use of skilled technic, including the entrance into the vein with only one puncture, placing the blood gently in the series of glass test tubes which need not be lined by silicone or similar antiwetting agents, the clotting time is found almost always to be prolonged. It is not generally realized that all errors in measuring the clotting time of blood *in vitro* hasten coagulation. The values of 3 to 8 minutes, usually reported as normal, represent the summation effect of multiple errors, for a carefully performed clotting time of the Lee-White technic will yield normal values of 30 to 40 minutes in uncoated glassware. In Figure 32-3 are shown the differences in

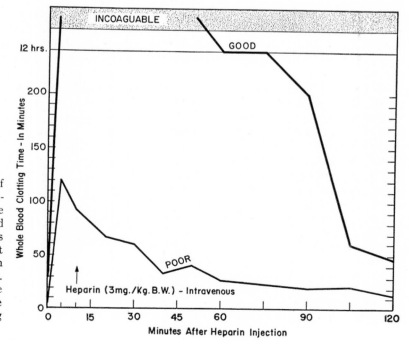

FIG. 32-3. Effect of good and poor venepuncture technics upon the Lee-White whole blood clotting time. Punctures for samples were made at the same time but from opposite extremity veins. Faulty venipunctures are prominent causes for the usually short clotting times reported.

whole blood clotting time after heparin when the only difference is one in excellence of venepuncture.

One other simple laboratory test also is positive; clot retraction (syneresis) is greatly impaired or lacking. Platelets appear to be essential to the occurrence of this phenomenon. To perform this test, 3 or 4 ml. of blood is added to a serology tube. After this blood has clotted, a small wooden applicator or glass rod is introduced at the edges to free the clot from the glass surface. Then the tube is placed in a refrigerator for a few hours and observed for evidence of clot retraction.

There are no findings upon physical examination which will disclose the nature of thrombocytopenic purpura except for the indirect supporting evidence of one negative finding. In the true Werlhof picture, the spleen classically is not enlarged and therefore not palpable. Should the spleen be palpable, the diagnosis is very frequently one of secondary hypersplenism which may also respond well to splenectomy, or it is one of a blood dyscrasia which is usually unresponsive to operation.

Two other major categories of diseases exist which can induce thrombocytopenia without splenomegalia and from which recovery is spontaneous if the patient survives. Splenectomy is not beneficial and often harmful in either instance and therefore to be avoided assiduously. These are the allergic purpuras usually seen in conjunction with infection or the administration of certain drugs, or following exposure to certain noxious agents, including ionizing radiation.

Pathogenesis. In January, 1949, work was presented from this laboratory by Bogardus, *et al.*, in which it was pointed out that a humoral factor probably existed in idiopathic thrombocytopenic purpura and that it was likely related to its pathogenesis. The basis of this contention was the observation that many newborn infants displayed a transient thrombocytopenia with purpura when their mothers suffered from the Werlhof syndrome. Within a matter of days to a few weeks after delivery the platelet count of the infant returns to normal, and its purpuric tendency disappears. We postulated a humoral factor to be present in the maternal blood and to be transmitted across the placental barrier to induce the disease in the infant while *in utero*. After

birth, the source of this factor being no longer available to the infant, its recovery was spontaneous. Later that year these observations were reported independently by Saltzman (1949).

In November of 1949, Evans pointed out that auto-antibodies to platelets could be demonstrated occasionally in patients suffering from idiopathic thrombocytopenic purpura. In his study he was unable to demonstrate the presence of auto-antibodies in many of his patients, a failure that he attributed to technical difficulties, plus the possibility that an excess of auto-antibody titer could be present and related to the cause of the disease but not necessarily be of sufficient titer to be demonstrable.

These observations were soon followed by that of Harrington *et al.* (1951) demonstrating that the infusion of 100 to 300 ml. of plasma obtained from patients with this disease induced significant thrombocytopenia in recipients. This effect lasted 4 to 6 days. In 1953, Harrington *et al.*[28] reported the same phenomenon previously described in the neonatal infant.

Stefanini (1952) reported upon attempts at typing platelets. Recently, Coombs *et al.* (1956) described a test for platelet antibodies which gave negative results in 34 patients studied. Occasionally, the Coombs' antiglobulin test (see Chap. 8, "Blood Transfusion") is positive in some of these patients, especially those who display a hemolytic component associated with thrombocytopenia. The Coombs' antiglobulin test is to be distinguished from his platelet test; they are entirely different (see Chap. 8).

In spite of the demonstration of auto-antibodies, their transmission across the placental barrier and the thrombocytopenic effect of transfused plasma obtained from such patients, the argument still persists as to whether the primary defect of the hypersplenic disorders—in this instance thrombocytopenia—is one of impaired maturation of the cellular components concerned or one of their increased rate of destruction. These two schools of thought have persisted for nearly 40 years without sign of resolution of the differences each maintains. Each still has proponents. To this author, the facts at hand seem to be compatible with either or both but favor destruction.

Two Forms of the Disease. Much has been written about the separation of idiopathic thrombocytopenic purpura into the acute and the chronic types. Persons who have the acute type are predominantly children. In them the onset of bleeding into the skin and from the mucous membrane is acute. In many instances a history of preceding infection can be obtained. The acute form of idiopathic thrombocytopenic purpura is very often a self-limited disease. For the chronic form of the disease splenectomy is the treatment most likely to succeed.

Treatment. Kaznelson (1916) of Prague persuaded Professor Schloffer to perform splenectomy on a 36-year-old female patient with thrombocytopenic purpura and splenomegaly in 1916. His suggestion was based on the possibility that the spleen was destroying platelets at an excessive rate. This concept he carried over from the established benefits of splenectomy in familial hemolytic anemia. An excellent result was obtained. That a medical student could persuade a professor of surgery to try something of this nature is remarkable in itself!

Three courses are open to the physician today in the management of Werlhof's disease. Should the disease be mild, watchful waiting with or without the administration of cortisone or ACTH is reasonable. These agents are employed because of their depressing effects upon antibody formation, in this instance the auto-antibody of Evans. Good results are often obtained in milder forms of the disease on this conservative therapy, especially in children. As the disease tends to diminish in recurrence rate after the age of 20, the remissions successfully induced in many young patients tend to be permanent as the child grows older.

In severe cases, serious consideration must be given to the possibility that a beneficial effect from cortisone or ACTH may not be obtained soon enough to avoid intracranial hemorrhage. Some deaths of this type have been reported under this form of therapy. Splenectomy should be strongly considered, as the beneficial response it induces is often almost immediate. Abnormal bleeding often ceases as soon as the splenic pedicle is ligated, although the rise in platelet count may be delayed several days to several weeks. Cortisone therapy as an adjunct to splenectomy should be considered and is a practice often employed today.

Platelet transfusions have been alluded to in Chapter 8, "Blood Transfusion." They can be exceedingly helpful, but, due to the enormous quantities of blood required, their usage often is delayed until the day of operation or employed only when the response to splenectomy is slow and bleeding continues. In the latter situation they tide the patient over until he makes a satisfactory response of his own.

Results of splenectomy for idiopathic thrombocytopenic purpura are contingent upon the accuracy of diagnosis, removal of accessory splenic tissue and possibly to some extent certain imponderable factors not yet described. Miller and Hagedorn (1951) reported 32 of 47 patients living and well after 5 years, although 4 had episodes of epistaxis and hematemesis too slight to cause the patient concern. These authors reported only 1 hospital death; 3 others died later. In one, the cause of death was Albers-Schönberg disease; in another the cause was chronic myeloid leukemia; and in the third, the cause of death was unknown. Thus in at least 2 of the 3 late deaths the initial diagnosis was incorrect, leaving 1 hospital death from hemorrhage in true Werlhof's disease failing to respond to splenectomy and 1 late death in whom the patient died 18 months after splenectomy of unknown cause.

Cole *et al.* (1949) reported no operative mortality among 26 patients with the Werlhof syndrome. Platelet response in 2 was slow at first but did return to normal later; 1 died of tuberculosis; 2 had good symptomatic relief but poor hematologic results.

Walter and Chaffin (1955) reported their experience with idiopathic thrombocytopenic purpura in infants and children conservatively managed for the most part. Of 41 patients in this age group, 31 responded to conservative management, and 5 died; 2 of these 5 deaths occurred on the day of admission; another died of pneumonia, nephritis and hemorrhage; 2 died of hemorrhage 1 and 2 months after coming under their care, and both of these deaths occurred prior to the cortisone–ACTH era. Splenectomy was performed in only 5, all of whom were cured; however, 2 of these continued with low platelet counts. The results of Walter and Chaffin from conservative treatment are similar to those of others and those at the University of Chicago.

ACCESSORY SPLEENS. Accessory spleens left behind are believed to be responsible for failure of improvement in many of these patients. To Curtis (1946) belongs the credit of alerting the surgeon to this possible hazard, although Morrison *et al.* called attention to this possibility in 1928. Curtis reported accessory spleens to be present in 56 of 176 patients subjected to splenectomy or an incidence of 31.8 per cent. Others report a somewhat lower incidence. The location of accessory spleens is usually in the following regions: the hilum, the pedicle, the omentum, the retroperitoneum, splenic ligaments (gastric and colic) and small bowel mesentery. The last 3 locations are rare sites of accessory spleens. A number of patients with recurrences of the disease after splenectomy are reported to be relieved completely by removal of accessory spleens found at re-exploration. Thus it is important to search for accessory spleens at the time of splenectomy.

SECONDARY THROMBOCYTOPENIC PURPURA WITH SPLENOMEGALIA. This term as referred to here is hemocytologically similar to those connoted as primary, except for the fact that the spleen per se is pathologic, often secondary to another disease. Platelet auto-antibodies in the plasma of some of these patients, too, have been identified (Harrington, *et al.,* 1953). The principal difference between primary and secondary thrombocytopenic purpura of the hypersplenic variety then is the enlarged spleen in the latter and that its enlargement results from a variety of causes. In many instances, the cause of the enlarged spleen is either its involvement in a more generalized disease or from any one of the various forms of portal hypertension. Among the diseases in which secondary hypersplenism has occurred are the following: cysts and tumors of the spleen, acquired hemolytic anemia, tuberculosis or histoplasmosis, leishmaniasis and ecchinococcal disease of the spleen, malaria and filariasis, the various leukemias and Hodgkin's disease, a number of the "storage" diseases of which Gaucher's disease is a common example, portal hypertension and chronic passive congestion, occasionally congenital hemolytic anemia, sickle cell anemia in early stages, Felty's syndrome, and, in fact, almost any disease at times should it affect the spleen.

Splenectomy is, of course, the treatment of choice if the purpuric manifestations are severe. At the same time, all workers in this field, including the author, recognize that many of these diseases that cannot be cured medically are in time fatal diseases. Therefore, splenectomy in this group is largely one of palliation, although in some instances curative. Hence, the palliation anticipated must be weighed against that of life expectancy should the problems of abnormal bleeding be relieved.

Of those causes of splenomegaly which more commonly and often provide a prolonged survival are Gaucher's disease, Banti's syndrome and acquired splenic anemia. Rarely in some of the cases of splenomegalies where the primary disease is often fatal, relief from the associated thromocytopenic purpuras may be required to permit survival. An occasional patient may survive indefinitely; therefore, withholding splenectomy should not be taken lightly or discouraged simply because of the poor prognosis that is implied by the primary diagnosis. Moreover, the diagnosis may be in error or at least carry less serious import than was believed at the time of hemorrhage. Death from hemorrhage may be more certain than is the course of the primary disease. A case in point is that which follows.

A 22-month-old male infant was admitted with the diagnosis of Letterer-Siwe disease (reticuloendotheliosis) involving the left scapula, the right ilium, the left femur and the skull. Radiophosphorus was administered, and local radiation was superimposed. The enlarged spleen was not altered. Petechial hemorrhages, present on admission, progressively worsened, and bleeding from the mouth and the alimentary tract appeared. ACTH and cortisone were to no avail. Pneumonia developed, and the child was placed in an oxygen tent. Anemia rapidly progressed in spite of transfusions. Severe neutropenia appeared, and the platelet count was less than 10,000 per cu. mm. Marrow studies revealed hyperplasia but with the characteristic "reticuloendothelial cells" also being present.

The infant was transported from his oxygen tent to the operating room where splenectomy was performed. The patient's general condition began

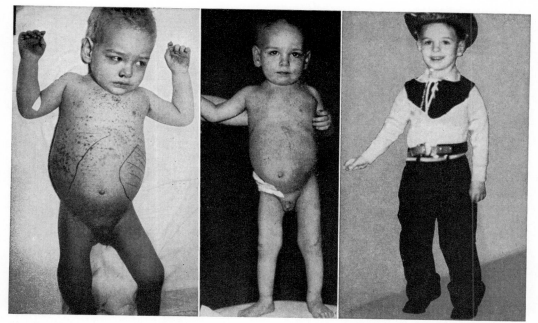

Fig. 32-4. Letterer-Siwe's disease and thrombocytopenic purpura. The photograph on left was taken 2 weeks prior to serious deterioration. The picture in center was on the 16th post-operative day. The photo on right was taken 4 years later when no evidence of disease remains. (53-78-00 U. of C.)

to improve at once; his fever promptly began to return toward normal. Bleeding ceased, and the platelet count 12 hours later was 31,000 and gradually reached 200,000 by the 6th day. He was discharged on the 43d postoperative day (Fig. 32-4).

Surprisingly, the bony lesion began to disappear, and 24 months later none remained. The child, now 7 years of age, appears to be well and free of disease. As Letterer-Siwe's disease is so frequently fatal, there is good reason to question the diagnosis which may have been eosinophilic granuloma.

In any case, however, to have concluded that the infant should have been spared splenectomy, in favor of the assumed fatal course that his diagnosis implied, almost certainly would have been in error. There are, of course, many clinical situations in which a less heroic course is indicated. In this child, such a course would have been a fatal mistake. The proper decision in many patients in such categories is not easily made upon a rational basis.

The Erythrocyte-Destroying Spleen. The term "splenic anemia" was introduced to describe cases of anemia attributed to splenomegaly. In the 90 years which have elapsed

since this term was first introduced, any anemia associated with splenomegaly from any cause has often been referred to as being of splenic origin. With the recognition of auto-antibodies and their probable relation to increased red cell destruction, the term "splenic anemia" today is usually restricted to patients with auto-antibodies and splenomegaly. In this group, the hemolytic process is curable by splenectomy. Unfortunately, knowledge is not advanced to the point wherein the presence of a hemolytic component can be expected simply because the spleen is enlarged in association with certain anemic states, although most cases of splenomegaly demonstrate a hemolytic component at one time or another.

The clinical picture is one of mild to moderate anemia, developing usually over a period of several years. Severe anemia is the exception but does occur. Icterus is seldom evident and when present is generally slight. These patients often live for many years with few or no symptoms related to the pathogenesis of the splenomegaly save for the distress of an enlarged or heavy spleen and anemia.

The anemia encountered is usually normo-

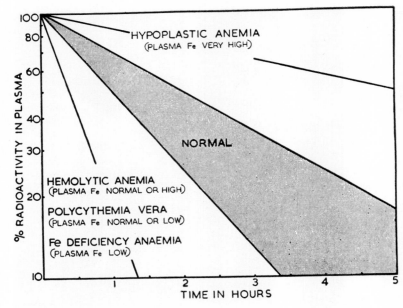

Fig. 32-5. The usual patterns of radioiron clearance from the plasma in normal subjects and in patients with various blood disorders. (Bothwell, T. H., Callender, S., Mallett, R., and Witts, L. J.: Brit. J. Haemat. 2:1)

cytic in type. If repeated bouts of blood loss are superimposed as in portal hypertension with bleeding varices, hypochromic anemia develops. It does not involve the marrow as in leukemia, the storage diseases, etc. Normoplastic and mildly or moderately hyperplastic marrow activity may be found. If hypoplastic, anemias of suppressed marrow activity should be searched for, and splenectomy is not indicated or may be contraindicated.

Once the marrow and peripheral blood studies have been concluded, splenic puncture should be considered in doubtful cases, lest the spleen prove to be an important source of extramedullary erythropoiesis. Should this be so, splenectomy is strongly contraindicated.

Plasma iron clearance rate may be an important diagnostic aid. The technics employed in such patients appear promising as an accessory means for establishing the diagnosis in this disease (Figs. 32-5 and 32-6; see also p. 791).

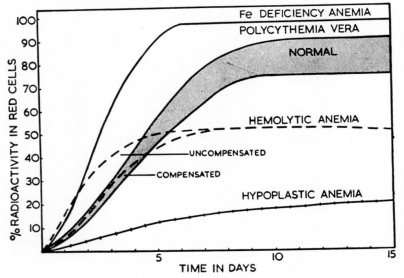

Fig. 32-6. The usual patterns of red-cell utilization in normal subjects and in patients with various blood disorders. (Bothwell, T. H., Callender, S., Mallett, B., and Witts, L. J.: Brit. J. Haemat. 2:1)

Auto-antibodies are demonstrated most reliably by the "diagnostic Coombs' test" (see Chap. 8, "Blood Transfusion"). Should this test be negative in the presence of splenomegaly and anemia, other causes of anemia should be considered more seriously. Whether the increased red-cell destruction is caused by a normally functioning but greatly enlarged spleen—that is, whether it is a quantitative rather than a qualitative abnormality—is not known.

Splenectomy is the treatment of choice and indeed of necessity when severe anemia of this origin is demonstrated. However, it should be restricted to those patients with normal or hyperplastic marrow activity and preferably also to those in whom a positive diagnostic Coombs' test can be demonstrated. As many of these patients survive for years or appear to live a normal life-span, splenectomy is not required unless anemia becomes profound. The following case illustrates the prolonged story and complications in a female patient observed for a number of years at the University of Chicago Clinics, beginning in February, 1940:

At that time she was treated for an unexplained anemia and nonthrombocytopenic purpura. Other than severe anemia ranging between 3 and 6 Gm. per cent of hemoglobin, no other blood or marrow abnormalities were noted. Her bleeding time, clotting time and prothrombin time were normal, although her Rumpel-Leed test was positive. Clot retraction was normal. She was 30 years of age when seen here in 1940.

Her history of abnormal bleeding dated back to the onset of menstruation and even in childhood as her parents forbade spanking because of her tendency to "bruise easily." Each menstrual flow had been excessive since adolescence, generally lasting for 1 to 2 weeks. In consequence, her severe anemia had been known and present for 15 years. An attempt to correct her hemoglobin concentration by repeated blood transfusion and iron therapy were met with little success. After transfusion of sufficient blood to elevate the hemoglobin concentration to 10 Gm. per cent, she complained of the symptoms of plethora and stated that she was more comfortable with her anemia, to which she had become accustomed. The platelet count remained normal during the periods of her observation in this hospital from 1940 until 1947, at which time mild thrombocytopenia developed, and for the first time the spleen became palpable that year. Over a 12-month

period the platelet count gradually fell to levels of 40,000 per cu. mm., and characteristic petechial hemorrhage appeared. On July 6, 1948, splenectomy was performed without incident. The platelet count promptly returned to normal, and for the first time her menstrual periods assumed a normal character. Her hemoglobin concentration slowly increased to its normal values at 15 to 16 Gm. per cent. Once this normal hemoglobin concentration was achieved, the patient again complained of the symptoms of plethora, and these complaints remained present and unpleasant for 18 months following splenectomy. Thereafter she began to feel better and for the last 6 years she has been well.

Comment: The nature of the initial purpura in this patient is not understood, nor is it known why the thrombocytopenic component should have finally appeared after more than 30 years of nonthrombocytopenic purpura. Perhaps she had two separate bleeding states, although after splenectomy no further bleeding has occurred in 8 years. Of special interest are the pronounced adjustments that she had made to her near-lifelong severe hypochromic anemia as well as the difficulties that she encountered once her anemia was corrected by the avoidance of further blood loss after splenectomy was performed.

Splenic Neutropenia and Panhypersplenism. Splenic neutropenia may also occur in conjunction with splenomegaly. It is much more frequently a part of thrombocytic or of hemolytic hypersplenism than an isolated form of hypersplenic disease. The more commonly encountered forms of neutropenia are those from drug reactions, especially the amidopyrine series, or from other hemocytologic toxins which also cause aplastic anemia. In others, neutropenia may be a manifestation of one of the malignant blood dyscrasias. In some individuals, moderate neutropenia (1,000 to 2,500 total leukocyte count per cu. mm. of blood) may exist without much difficulty being encountered other than the more frequent occurrence of upper respiratory infections. In time, some of the patients with splenic neutropenia may develop an aplastic anemia or a leukemia.

In profound neutropenia (250 to 800 leukocytes per cu. mm. of blood) from any cause (hypersplenism, leukemia or aplastic anemia) the clinical pattern is one of infection, cutaneous ulceration, poor wound healing and mucosal desquamation of the alimentary tract. These are the same symptoms frequently

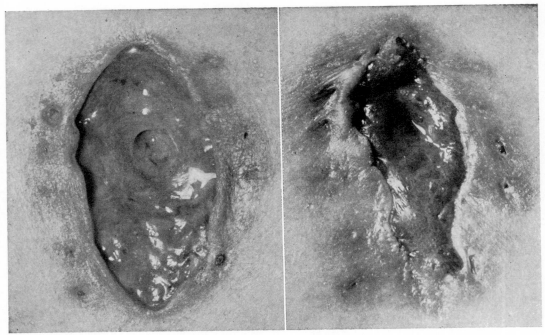

FIG. 32.7. Surgical biopsy of sternal marrow in patient with hypersplenism, predominantly of the neutropenic type. Picture on left shows grayish color of granulating wound after it separated. No pus is seen. Photo on right was taken 5 days after splenectomy and shows wound healthy and beginning to heal. Leukocyte response promptly followed operation.

noted in total body exposure to ionizing radiation in the near-lethal range. One is more impressed by the role of the leukocytes in the control or the prevention of infection when they are absent than by the usual and normal leukocytosis accompanying primary infections. Such was the case in the following patient who suffered from pancytopenia or panhypersplenism in whom the dominating picture was that resulting from her profound neutropenia.

The patient (40-65-32), a 50-year-old female, was admitted to the University of Chicago Clinics on April 20, 1947. Her chief complaints were weakness of 10 weeks' duration and daily fever ranging between 100° and 103° F. for the last 4 weeks. The remainder of her history was negative, and there was no history of exposure to drugs or known toxins. The lungs were clear, the heart and blood pressure normal, but the spleen was palpable, enlarged and firm. Laboratory findings revealed a hemoglobin concentration of 8 Gm. per cent, the leukocyte count was 1,050 with 7 per cent neutrophils, and the platelet count was 138,000. The urine was negative. A surgical biopsy of the sternal marrow was performed the day following admission. Although the incision was closed, it became infected, failed to heal, and broke down (Fig. 32-7). This open wound produced no detectable pus, presumably because there were so few neutrophils. During the first week of hospitalization, the patient's course was rapidly downhill. Her temperature increased from 102° to 105° F. Bronchial pneumonia developed, and the patient was placed in an oxygen tent. Her anemia and neutropenia became more pronounced. The diagnoses of primary splenic neutropenia and splenic anemia were made. Splenectomy was performed on the 9th day. Her improvement was remarkably rapid, and within 48 hours her fever disappeared, and the pneumonitis began to clear. The day of operation, her leukocyte count was 1,250; 18 hours after splenectomy the total white blood count was 10,000 with 44 per cent neutrophils. There was a sharp increase also in the lymphocytes as well. The surgical biopsy incision promptly changed its color from a grayish red to a bright red and was nearly healed by the 17th day, when the patient was discharged. When last seen 3 years later, she was in excellent health.

Comment: The patient's general condition was desperate by the time splenectomy was performed.

The operation was undertaken at this time only because a fatal outcome was expected unless splenectomy relieved rapidly the course she displayed.

Summary of Hypersplenic Disorders.
From the above discussions, it is evident that considerable overlap exists among these diseases. The one exception is primary idiopathic thrombocytopenic purpura of the Werlhof variety, which occurs principally between the 2nd and the 4th decades of life. This disease generally stands out as a single entity or at least the purpuric manifestations often become so serious that neutropenia and anemia are relatively unimportant should they coexist. Usually the spleen is not palpable.

Secondary thrombocytopenia may occur at any age and is commonly associated with mild to moderate leukopenia and anemia. The spleen is "always" enlarged and nearly always can be felt.

Marrow activity in all of the hypersplenic disorders is either normal or hyperplastic. A hypoplastic or aplastic marrow provides the most important evidence against the diagnosis of hypersplenism and is generally reason enough to abandon any consideration of splenectomy. One other important element of the marrow examination is that there be no abnormal or malignant cells of the hematopoietic series. The occasional patient with one of the chronic forms of leukemia may develop also signs of hypersplenism; the decision as to the value of splenectomy in the relief of his hypersplenism must be made on the best guess as to the probable life expectancy from his primary blood dyscrasia should his hypersplenic symptoms be deemed correctable by splenectomy.

Auto-antibodies, while likely present in most if not all forms of hypersplenism, are not easily demonstrated in many patients. The diagnostic Coombs' test, when positive and when Rh sensitization is not a presenting problem, provides supporting but not diagnostic evidence of hypersplenism.

Splenic puncture in the presence of splenomegaly may be indicated. It may provide evidence of other types of disease and serves to exclude secondary myeloid metaplasia wherein the spleen may be the dominant site of erythropoiesis. The risk is slight in view of its

diagnostic importance. However, there are no pathologic findings in the spleen that are diagnostic of the hypersplenic disorders.

With the above considerations in mind, splenectomy is the treatment of choice in severe Werlhof's disease, severe neutropenia of hypersplenic origin and in severe hypersplenic anemia. Cortisone and ACTH may be tried if the disease is not too serious, but their prolonged use in the face of advancing disease can lead to disaster, especially in severe thrombocytopenic purpura and profound splenic neutropenia. Often splenectomy is not considered until all methods of conservative therapy have failed and hope has been abandoned. Such delays seem to increase unnecessarily the risk of surgery entailed, but the surgeon must be willing to accept the patient. Brilliant results are the rule rather than the exception, provided that the diagnosis of hypersplenic disease is correct.

SUMMARY OF INDICATIONS AND CONTRAINDICATIONS FOR SPLENECTOMY

Indications. Splenectomy is the only effective treatment currently available in the following disorders:
1. Rupture or torsion of the spleen
2. Splenic abscess
3. "Wandering" spleen
4. Cysts and tumors of the spleen
5. Aneurysm of the splenic artery
6. Severe congenital hemolytic anemia
7. Severe forms of hypersplenism
  A. Primary or secondary thrombocytopenic purpura
  B. "Splenic" neutropenia
  C. "Splenic" anemia
  D. Panhypersplenism
8. In the performance of certain operations as a technical necessity
9. In Banti's syndrome (splenic vein block only), otherwise as a necessity in splenorenal shunts
10. In certain general diseased states when hypersplenic manifestations dominate the picture and threaten the life of the patient who otherwise might live in comfort many years with his disease. Gaucher's disease is an example (also see case example, p. 802).

Contraindications. The spleen should not be removed when it is an important organ of erythropoiesis as in secondary myeloid metaplasia, in hypoplastic and malignant disorders of the marrow, or in most infections amenable to medications.

1. Secondary myeloid metaplasia. Examples include

A. Sclerosing osteitis

B. Extensive marrow replacement by fibrous tissue or metastatic tumor

2. Aplastic or hypoplastic anemia

3. The "leukemoid" states, with few exceptions

4. In portal hypertension unless the surgeon is prepared to perform a splenorenal anastomosis or is satisfied that an anastomosis cannot be carried out satisfactorily by him or someone more experienced.

TECHNIC OF SPLENECTOMY

The experienced surgeon does not often find this to be a difficult operation, although numerous adhesions may be encountered, and extensive collateral veins may give rise to troublesome bleeding in some patients. Almost all technical difficulties can be attributed to one of two technical faults or both: inadequate surgical exposure and failure to secure adequate hemostasis. The best and surest means for securing hemostasis is the benefit afforded by sufficient exposure.

Two other points in technic contribute or are primarily responsible for the majority of the postoperative complications of splenectomy. One is surgical injury to the tail of the pancreas which often abuts or is included in the hilus of the spleen. The other is the inclusion in a hemostat or ligature of a small portion of the greater curvature of the stomach in the course of ligating the vasa brevia. As the greater curvature may have some temporary impairment of blood supply along its splenic margin after ligation of the gastro-epiploic and short gastric vessels (vasa brevia), gastric perforation with subphrenic abscess or peritonitis may occur. Both injury to the pancreas and the stomach are avoided best by gaining adequate surgical exposure before attempting splenectomy (Fig. 32-8).

A long left paramedian incision is made, beginning at the upper left portion of the xyphoid cartilage and extending below to at least half way between the umbilicus and the pubic symphysis, slanting to the left, and terminating over the midportion of the lower rectus muscle. The additional exposure provided by a "T" with the vertical arm to the left and extending horizontally for several inches is seldom necessary but nonetheless should be taken advantage of in difficult cases, especially when the spleen is huge. Some prefer the transthoracic approach as recommended by Stewart.

Once the abdominal exposure is obtained, the gastrocolic omentum is carefully dissected away from the anterior surface of the colon, beginning slightly to the right of the center of the transverse colon and proceeding gently to the left until the splenocolic ligament is divided and the entire left portion of the transverse colon is freed of its omental and splenic attachment.

At this point the following optional procedure may be carried out: The greater curvature of the stomach with its freed omentum is gently retracted upward and mesially, exposing the lesser peritoneal sac. This usually brings the tortuous splenic artery into view 5 to 10 cm. away from the splenic hilus as the artery courses above the pancreas in the retroperitoneum, from the celiac axis to the spleen. Generally a ligature can be easily slipped under the artery at this point and tied securely and cut after gaining access to it by incising a small area of its overlying peritoneum. However, the artery is not yet to be divided. Care is taken to avoid injury to the body of the pancreas and the splenic vein lying just below and often in direct contact with the artery. The ligature serves to reduce any loss of blood that may be entailed should the spleen be torn later in the course of its removal.

The next step is the cutting with scissors of the lateral peritoneal reflection along the posterior margin of the spleen. Gentle retraction is applied along the left costal margin and directed upward and laterally. This assists in securing the exposure necessary to extend the cut along the posterior peritoneum to the upper pole of the spleen and to its mesial aspect, thereby dividing the phrenicolienal ligament, which is the upper suspensory ligament of the spleen. Any adhesions between the lateral and/or the superior surfaces of the spleen and the diaphragm encountered in this maneuver are carefully clamped if necessary

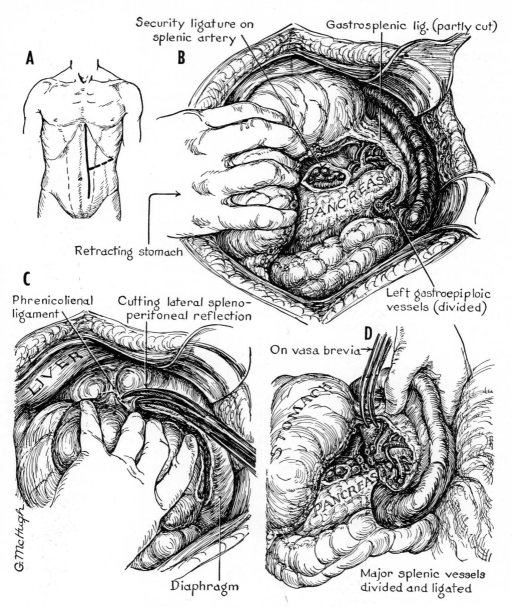

A

B
Security ligature on splenic artery

Gastrosplenic lig. (partly cut)

Retracting stomach

PANCREAS

Left gastroepiploic vessels (divided)

C
Phrenicolienal ligament

Cutting lateral spleno-peritoneal reflection

LIVER

Diaphragm

G. McHugh

D
On vasa brevia →

STOMACH

PANCREAS

Major splenic vessels divided and ligated

FIG. 32-8. Drawing A illustrates a long paramedian incision. The lateral extension of the incision is optional. (B) Security ligature placed about splenic artery after entering lesser peritoneal cavity. Lienocolic ligament has been divided to prevent tearing of splenic capsule. (C) Spleen is gently rotated mesially, exposing its retroperitoneal attachments; the lateral leaf is divided, extending upward to include the phrenicolienal ligament. Should the vasa brevia be readily accessible at this time, they, too, are clamped and ligated, being careful not to include any portion of adjacent wall of gastric fundus. (D) Cupped hand is introduced through the posterior lateral cut margin, and the fingers are advanced gently through the divided lateral margin into the retroperitoneum of the lesser peritoneal cavity, freeing the spleen with its pedicle and the distal third of the pancreas, permitting the spleen to be advanced safely to a forward position. With one hand supporting the mobilized spleen in its new position, the gastrolienal omentum is divided, exposing the splenic artery and vein at hilum. These vessels are divided and ligated separately. Finally, the vasa brevia are divided if not already cut.

and cut more closely to the diaphragm than the spleen.

Then the "cupped" hand is introduced through the incised lateral splenoperitoneal reflection, entering the retroperitoneum. The fingers gently dissect mesially beneath the spleen, the tail of the pancreas and the splenic vessels. This allows the spleen and its pedicle to be rotated forward and advanced to the anterior portion of the abdominal cavity. Several laparotomy pads are carefully placed in the splenic bed to support the spleen in its new forward position; this has the additional effect of hastening coagulation should there be a seepage of blood from the denuded retroperitoneum.

The pedicle is now easily exposed by the careful dissection of the retroperitoneum as it is reflected from the pedicle onto the mesial surface of the spleen covering anteriorly the splenic vessels. Then each branch of the splenic artery and vein are clamped separately, divided and ligated as encountered. With this accomplished (without injury to the tail of the pancreas), the surgeon rotates the upper pole forward a little more if need be, exposing the vasa brevia. The peritoneum along the anterior surface is cut *close* to the spleen. With these vessels thus exposed, each is clamped separately with small hemostats close to the spleen, divided and ligated under direct vision. Care is taken to avoid enclosure or encroachment upon the stomach at any point.

The spleen is now entirely free and is lifted from the abdomen. Then the greater curvature is inspected for hemorrhage, the packs are removed, and the denuded splenic bed is inspected for bleeding, as is the underside of the diaphragm. A final check is made for the presence of any accessory splenic tissue which may have been left behind. The distal portion of the lienalcolic ligament is sutured to a location similar to its original site, and the abdomen is closed without drainage unless the tail of the pancreas was injured or splenectomy was performed for an abscess.

Mortality for splenectomy is less than 3 per cent when the patients are presented to the surgeon before seriously ill or moribund. If not, mortality rates of 10 to 30 per cent may be expected; stated more accurately, 70 to 90 per cent of these moribund patients may be salvaged by splenectomy, especially those with splenic rupture or hypersplenism.

Anesthesia. The choice of the anesthetic agent and its method of administration deserve special consideration in patients with hypersplenic thrombocytopenic purpura. In some patients, liver or other systemic diseases pose special problems to be considered.

Intubation, spinal anesthesia or intercostal "blocks" are to be avoided lest the trauma entailed cause extensive local hemorrhage in the face of the generalized tendency toward abnormal bleeding. The use of cyclopropane is disapproved by many, as it is alleged to augment bleeding, a point not convincingly settled at this time. Third is the need for good relaxation which is essential to adequate exposure. Augmenting the general anesthetic agent with the very careful use of drugs with curarelike action is most helpful, but the anesthesiologist must bear in mind that in these patients intubation offers unusual risk; hence, the use of such agents is compromised if not contraindicated in the purpuric patient. Due consideration also must be given to the liver which is diseased in many, especially those with portal hypertension (see Chap. 33, section on "Portal Hypertension").

Blood transfusion in hypersplenism and congenital hemolytic anemia should be withheld if possible until the splenic artery has been ligated or, better, until the spleen has been removed. Blood should be "type-to-type" and Coombs' negative. Although these reactions are seldom serious if the patient is not critically ill, they may become so under these circumstances. If platelet transfusions are to be employed, they, too, should not be given until after the spleen is out; this author does not rely upon platelet transfusions but does not object to their usage, if available, especially should bleeding continue after splenectomy.

Complications after splenectomy are principally those of thrombosis and infection. Thrombosis of the splenic vein with extension into the portal vein was encountered more commonly in the days before splenorenal or portacaval shunting procedures. Two factors peculiar to splenectomy favor thrombosis. First is the thrombocytosis which often follows a few days after removal of the spleen. Platelet counts 3 to 5 times the normal value may occur. The second and likely the more important one is splenectomy performed for portal hypertension when the increased venous pressure is not relieved. This leads to venous stasis which always favors intravascular thrombosis. Thrombocytosis and stasis together provide such fertile soil for coagulation that it is amazing that this complication is not encountered more frequently. Pancreatitis also may occur and may contribute to splenic and portal vein thrombosis.

Subphrenic abscess may occur occasionally, and its prevention by drainage of the subphrenic space via a stab wound in the flank always should be considered before closing the abdomen. This possibility is obviously needed should splenectomy be performed for an abscess of the spleen. Drainage should be considered if the tail of the pancreas has been injured. If there remains some doubt, the author prefers to drain.

REFERENCES

1. Adams, F.: The Extant Works of Aretaeus the Cappadocian, London, 1856.
2. Aristotle: Quoted by Mettler, C. C.: History of Medicine, p. 358, New York, Blakiston Div. of McGraw-Hill, 1947.
3. Barbette: Cited by Mettler, C. C.: History of Medicine, p. 2, New York, Blakiston, 1947.
4. Barnes, D. W. H., and Loutit, J. F.: The immunological and histological responses following spleen treatment in irradiated mice. In: *Progress in Radiobiology,* Oliver and Boyd, London, 1956, p. 291.
5. Baudet, R.: Ruptures de la rate, Med. prat. *3*:565 and 581, 1907.
6. Bizzozero, J.: Ueber einen neuen Formbestandtheil des Blutes und die Rolle bei der Thrombose und der Blutgerinnung, Virchows Arch. path. Anat. *90*:261, 1882.
7. Björkman, S. F.: The splenic circulation, Acta med. scandinav., Supp. 191, 1947.
8. Block, M. H.: Personal communication, 1947.
9. Bogardus, G., Allen, J. G., Jacobson, L. O., and Spurr, C.L.: Role of splenectomy in thrombopenic purpura, Arch. Surg. *58*:16, 1949.
10. Bothwell, T. H., Callender, S., Mallett, B., and Witts, L. J.: The study of erythropoiesis using tracer quantities of radioactive iron, Brit. J. Haemat. *2*:1, 1956.
11. Brohm: Cited by Quick, A. J.: The Hemorrhagic Diseases and the Physiology of Hemostasis, p. 130, Springfield, Ill., Thomas, 1942.
12. Buchbinder, J. H., and Lipkoff, C. J.: Splenosis: multiple peritoneal splenic implants following abdominal injury, Surgery *6*:927, 1939.
13. Chauffard, A.: Pathogénie de l'ictere hémolytique congenital, Ann. méd. *1*:3, 1914.
14. Cole, L. J., Fisher, M. C., Ellis, M. E., and Bond, V. P.: Protection of mice against x-irradiation by spleen homogenates administered after exposure, Proc. Soc. Exper. Biol. & Med. *80*:112, 1952.
15. Cole, W. H., Walter, L., and Limarzi, L. R.: Indications and results of splenectomy, Ann. Surg. *129*:702, 1949.
16. Coombs, R. R. A., Marks, J., and Bedford, D.: Specific mixed agglutination: mixed erythrocyte-platelet anti-globulin reaction for the detection of platelet antibodies, Brit. J. Haemet. *2*:84, 1956.
17. Cotlar, A. M., and Cerise, E. J.: Splenosis: autotransplantation of splenic tissue following injury to spleen. Report of two cases and review of literature, Ann. Surg. *149*:402, 1959.
18. Curtis, G. M., and Movitz, D.: The significance of the accessory spleen, J. Lab. & Clin. Med. *31*:464, 1946.
19. Dawson (Lord of Penn): Hemolytic icterus (The Hume Lecture No. 1), Brit. M.J. *1*:921, 1931.
20. Dowidar, M. L.: Wandering spleen, Ann. Surg. *129*:408, 1948.
20a. Ebert, R. V., and Stead, E. A., Jr.: Demonstration that in normal man no reserves of blood are mobilized by exercise, epinephrine and hemorrhage, Am. J. M. Sc. *201*:655, 1941.
21. Eppinger, H.: Das retikulo endothelial system, Klin. Wchnschr. *35*:1078, 1922.
22. Evans, R. S., and Duane, R. T.: Acquired hemolytic anemia, Blood *4*:1196, 1949.
23. Felty, A. R.: Chronic arthritis in the adult is associated with splenomegaly and leukopenia; a report of 5 cases of an unusual clinical syndrome, Bull. Johns Hopkins Hosp. *35*:16, 1924.
24. Friedell, H., Sanderson, M., Kirschon, A., Milhan, M., and Allen, J. G.: A study of hemolysin titrations in sensitized irradiated rabbits *in* Quart. Rep. Biological & Medical Res. Div., No. 4078, pp. 78-93, Chicago, Argonne National Laboratory, 1947.
25. Galen: Cited by Walsh, J.: Galen's writings and influences inspiring them. III. Ann. M. Hist. n.s. *7*:428, 1935.
26. Haden, R. L.: The mechanism of the increased fragility of the erythrocytes in congenital hemolytic jaundice, Am. J. M. Sc. *188*:441, 1934.
27. Harkins, H. N.: Personal communication, 1956.
28. Harrington, W. J., Minnich, V., Hollingsworth, J. W., and Moore, C. V.: Demonstra-

tion of a thrombocytopenic factor in the purpura, J. Lab. & Clin. Med. *38*:1, 1951.

29. Harrington, W. J., Sprague, C. C., Minnich, V., Moore, C. V., Aulvin, R. C., and Dubach, R.: Immunologic mechanism in idiopathic and neonatal thrombocytopenic purpura, Ann. Int. Med. *38*:433, 1953.

30. Hektoen, L.: Further studies on the effects of roentgen rays on antibody production, J. Infect. Dis. *22*:28, 1918.

31. Herrick, J. B.: Peculiar elongated and sickle-shaped red corpuscles in a case of severe anemia, Arch. Int. Med. *6*:517, 1910.

32. Jacobson, L. O.: Evidence for humoral factors concerned in recovery from radiation injury: A review, Cancer Res. *12*:315, 1952.

33. Jacobson, L. O., Simmons, E. L., Marks, E. K., and Gaston, E. O.: Further studies on recovery from irradiation, J. Lab. & Clin. Med. *37*:683, 1951.

34. Kaznelson, P.: Verschwiden der hämorrhagischen Diathese bei einem Fälle von essentieller thrombopenie (Frank) nach Milzextirpation; splenogene thrombolytische Purpura, Wien. klin. Wchnschr. *29*:1451, 1454, 1916.

35. King, H., and Shumacker, H. B., Jr., Splenic studies: I. Susceptibility to infections after splenectomy in infants, Ann. Surg. *136*:239, 1952.

36. Knopp, L. M., and Harkins, H. N.: Traumatic rupture of the normal spleen, Surgery *35*:493, 1954.

37. Küttner: Discussion at Medical Section of the Silesian Society for Patriotic Culture in Breslau, Berlin klin. Wchnschr. *47*:1520, 1910.

38. Lorenz, E., Uphoff, D., Reid, T. R., and Shelton, E.: Modification of irradiation injury in mice and guinea pigs by bone marrow injection, J. Nat. Cancer Inst. *12*:197, 1951.

39. Malpighi, Marcello: De Pulmonibus Observations Anatomicae *in* a letter to Borelli, tr. by Foster, Lane Lectures on History of Physiology, London, Cambridge, 1901.

40. Marson, F. G., Meynell, M. J., and Tabbush, H.: Familial crisis in acholuric jaundice, Brit. M.J. *2*:760, 1950.

41. Matthis, Florian: Opera omnia medica et chirurgica, Leyden, 1672. Quoted by Mettler, C. C.: History of Medicine, p. 862, New York, Blakiston Div. of McGraw-Hill, 1947.

42. Miller, E. M., and Hagedorn, A. B.: Results of splenectomy: a follow-up of 140 consecutive cases, Ann. Surg. *134*:815, 1951.

43. Minkowski, O., and Naunyn, B.: Über den Icterus durch Polycholie und die Vorgänge in der Leber bei demselben, Arch, exper. Path. u. Pharmakol. *21*:1, 1886.

44. Morrison, W. Lederer, M., and Fradkin, W. Z.: Accessory spleens: their significance in essential thrombocytopenia purpura haemorrhagica, Am. J.M. Sc. *176*:672, 1928.

45. Motulsky, A. G., Casserd, F., Giblett, E. R., Brown, G. O. Jr., and Finch, C. A.: Anemia and the spleen, New England J. Med. *259*: 1164, 1958.

46. Murchison, C.: Clinical Lectures on Diseases of the Liver, Jaundice, etc., edited by Lander Brunton, London, 1885.

47. Owren, P. A.: Congenital hemolytic jaundice: The pathogenesis of the hemolytic crisis, Blood *3*:231, 1948.

48. Parsons, L., and Thompson, J. E.: Traumatic rupture of the spleen from nonpenetrating injuries, Ann. Surg. *147*:214-223, 1958.

49. Pauling, L., Itano, H. A., Singer, S. J., and Wells, I. C.: Sickle cell anemia, a molecular disease, Science *110*:543, 1949.

50. Reeve, E. B., Gregersen, M. I., Allen, T. H., and Sear, H.: Distribution of cells and plasma in normal and splenectomized dog and its influence on blood volume estimates with P^{32} and T-1824, Am. J. Physiol. *175*:195, 1953.

51. Rowley, D. A.: The formation of circulating antibodies in the splenectomized human being following intravenous infusion of heterologous erythrocytes, J. Immunol. *65*:515, 1950.

52. Saltzman, G. F.: Pregnancy in essential thrombocytopenia, Acta med. scandinav. *133*:221, 1949.

53. Simon, Gustav: Die Extirpation der Milz am Menschen, Giessen, 1857.

54. Stefanini, M., et al.: Studies in thrombocytopenic purpura, J. Clin. Invest. *31*:665, 1952.

55. Steiner, D. F.: The formation of antibodies *in vitro*. Recipient of Borden Student Award, University of Chicago School of Medicine, 1956.

56. Walter, L. E., and Chaffin, L.: Splenectomy in infants and children, Ann. Surg. *142*:798, 1955.

57. Wells, Spencer: (Quoted by Lord Dawson of Penn), Hemolytic icterus (The Hume Lecture No. 2), Brit. M.J. *1*:963, 1931.

58. Werlhof, Paul Gottlieb: Opera medica, p. 748, Paris, Wichmann, 1775.

59. Whipple, A. O., Parpart, A. K., and Chang, J. J.: A study of the circulation of the blood in the spleen of the living mouse, Ann. Surg. *140*:261, 1954.

60. Wilson, Harwell, Patterson, R. H., and Diggs, L. W.: Sickle cell anemia: a surgical problem, Ann. Surg. *131*:641, 1950.

61. Wright, J. H.: The origin and nature of blood plates, Boston M. & S.J. *154*:643, 1906.

CHAPTER 33

Mesentery, Splanchnic Circulation, Portal Hypertension and Mesenteric Thrombosis

Anatomic Considerations of the Mesentery and the Splanchnic Circulation
Portal Hypertension
Mesenteric Thrombosis

From the beginning of the modern era of intestinal surgery, surgeons have been acutely aware of the importance of relationships of the arterial and the venous blood supply to and from the small and the large bowel and of the considerable extent to which these relationships are determining factors in limiting any bowel resection undertaken. In recent years the venous drainage of the alimentary tract has received additional attention in connection with the surgical developments in the treat-

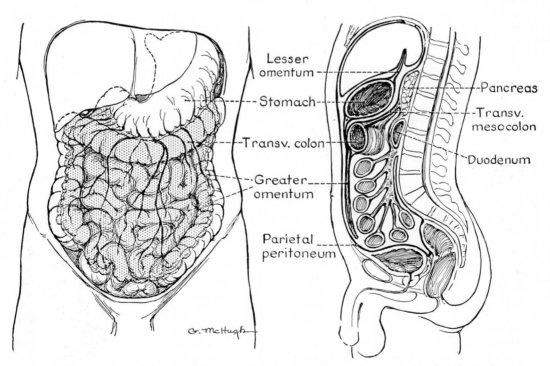

Fig. 33-1. Illustrates the effective manner by which the transverse mesocolon, in conjunction with the greater omentum, normally confines the small bowel to the midabdomen. See text on page 814.

ment of portal hypertension. In yet another direction, surgery of the alimentary tract has been extended in the treatment of malignant disease wherein the origin and the course of the lymphatic circulation also play an important role in the extent of bowel resection required. Finally, any discussion of the abdominal portion of the intestinal tract must consider the mesentery *in part* or *in toto,* not only because the blood and the lymphatic circulations to and from the bowel traverse the mesentery, but also because certain anomalies of the mesentery are responsible occasionally for acute surgical diseases. Hence, it is useful to consider the splanchnic circulation and the mesentery somewhat independent of the alimentary tract.

ANATOMIC CONSIDERATIONS OF THE MESENTERY AND THE SPLANCHNIC CIRCULATION

THE MESENTERY AND THE OMENTUM

The small bowel is attached to the anterior margin of its mesentery throughout its entire length and is confined principally within the midabdomen. Its restriction to this position of the peritoneal cavity is determined largely by length of the mesentery, its "encapsulation" by the omentum and the transverse mesocolon, and by the "picture frame" or peripheral position, of the abdominal colon within whose confines the small bowel tends to remain.

The superior boundary of the midabdomen is that of the undersurface of the transverse mesocolon. This mesocolon serves as a cupola and covers the small bowel superiorly. It continues anteriorly below the transverse colon, fusing with the greater omentum. These 2 structures essentially eliminate the possibility that the small bowel may wander into the upper abdomen; thus, there is little chance that the subcolic small bowel (not including the duodenum) will become adherent to stomach, duodenum, gallbladder, liver or spleen in acute inflammatory lesions affecting these organs (Fig. 33-1). Inflammation of the pancreas, which lies in the upper abdomen with its inferior margin located just above that of the superior leaf of the transverse mesocolon at its posterior attachment, is an occasional exception, in that inflammation of the pan-

creas may involve the small bowel secondarily. In acute pancreatitis, the adjacent mesocolon may become sufficiently inflamed to produce an inflammatory response in the loops of neighboring small bowel, causing them to become adherent to the underside of the mesocolon and perhaps to give rise to small bowel obstruction.

The mesentery of the small bowel is essentially a reflection of the parietal peritoneum from the posterior abdominal wall onto the mesenteric vessels and the surface of the gut. The parietal peritoneum becomes visceral peritoneum when it leaves the abdominal wall to encase the mesenteric vessels as they travel from the aorta to the intestinal tract. The free mesentery of the small bowel begins at the ligament of Treitz, located at the level of the body of the 3rd lumbar vertebra. From this ligament to the ileocecal valve the entire small bowel is suspended from its mesentery, which allows motion in any direction, bounded only by the limits of the mesenteric length. The root, or origin, of the small bowel mesentery at the posterior abdominal wall descends obliquely to the right, terminating in the iliac fossa near the right sacral joint. In doing so, it passes about 1.5 cm. to the right of the retroperitoneal course of the right ureter and the common iliac vessels on this side (Fig. 33-2).

The mesentery of the ascending and descending colon differs from that of the small bowel in that the lateral leaves of peritoneum adjacent to the ascending and the descending portions of the colon generally are short or functionally nonexistent. Usually the lateral portions of the posterior parietal peritoneum pass directly from the abdominal wall over the ascending and descending colon, respectively, in its course toward the mid-line and the root of the mesentery of the small bowel. When the parietal peritoneum reaches the centrally located mesenteric vessels, where it forms the peritoneum of the small bowel mesentery, it continues over the entire jejunoileum as visceral peritoneum. Occasionally, a freely moving mesentery is formed for the ascending and descending colon so that these structures may become as mobile as the small bowel. When this anomaly exists, these portions of the colon are subject to torsion and the resulting intestinal obstruction and ischemic necrosis if not promptly relieved.

The mesentery of the transverse colon is fully developed in contrast with those of the ascending and descending colon. This mesentery is known as the transverse mesocolon. The transverse colon is adherent anteriorly to the undersurface of the greater omentum, which suspends this part of the colon superiorly from the greater curvature of the stomach, in addition to its posterior suspension by the transverse mesocolon from the abdominal wall. Suspension of the transverse colon in 2 directions accounts for the rare occurrence of torsion of this part of the colon compared with that of its lateral portions, when unattached to the retroperitoneum; the sigmoidal colon is the most frequent site of torsion, especially when its mesentery is abnormally long.

The mesentery of the sigmoidal colon usually is well developed, and in this respect is like that of the small bowel, except for location. Normally, the sigmoidal mesentery begins at the end of the descending colon in the left iliac fossa, and from this point of origin its posterior margin runs diagonally upward and mesially along the left iliac vessels nearly to the bifurcation of the aorta, where it turns downward sharply into the sacral fossa and terminates in the pelvis, as the sigmoid-rectum leaves the peritoneal cavity to become the rectum (see Fig. 33-2).

The normal colon then is covered with visceral peritoneum, except for those portions lying in direct contact with the posterior abdominal wall, where no mesentery exists (see Fig. 33-2). Occasionally, the cecum also has little or no mesentery; its posterior portion

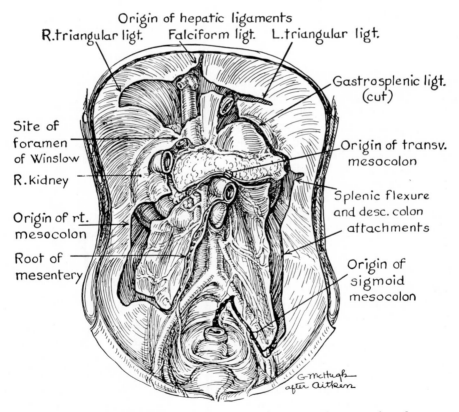

FIG. 33-2. The abdominal viscera and their mesenteric suspensions have been excised, including suspensory or triangular ligaments of the diaphragm and the posterior abdominal wall. Shown are the portions of the abdominal wall and the diaphragm not covered by parietal peritoneum as they are the sites of origin of the visceral peritoneum. (Drawn from Aitken)

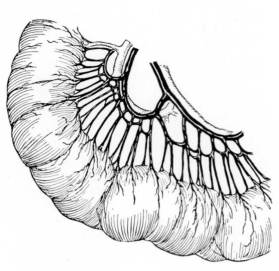

EARLY JEJUNUM

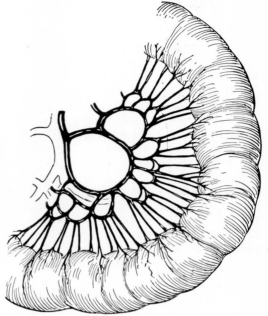

MIDILEUM

Fig. 33-3. Illustrations drawn from dissections of the arcades of the small bowel and its mesentery at different levels. The arcades increase in number from the upper jejunum to the terminal ileum, providing the lower ileum and its mesentery better collateral blood supply.

has a broad area of direct contact with the iliac fossa, and this area of the posterior cecum is free of peritoneum. On the other hand, the dependent cecum may have a fairly well-developed mesentery, causing it to be more mobile than usual; then it, too, becomes subject to torsion, although torsion of the cecum is encountered much less frequently than that of the sigmoid. In any case, torsion is not a frequent occurrence, even when such abnormalities of the mesentery of the various areas of the colon exist. (See Chap. 36.)

BLOOD SUPPLY OF SPLANCHNIC BED

The splanchnic vascular bed is the blood supply of the abdominal alimentary tract, the omentum and the spleen.

Arterial Supply

The small bowel from the ligament of Treitz to the ileocecal valve is supplied almost entirely by the 14 or 15 major branches of the superior mesenteric artery. A few inches of the 1st portion of the jejunum derives part of its arterial supply from the inferior pancreatoduodenal, which forms collaterals with the superior duodenal artery, hence the celiac, often enabling the proximal 6 to 12 cm. of

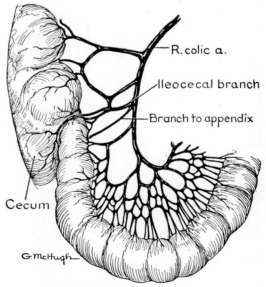

R. colic a.

Ileocecal branch

Branch to appendix

Cecum

G. McHugh

TERMINAL ILEUM

jejunum to survive when the superior mesenteric is occluded.

The superior mesenteric artery arises from the aorta about ½ in. below the origin of the celiac artery, opposite the level of the 2nd lumbar vertebra. It passes beneath the body of the pancreas, but anterior to its uncinate process. Then it crosses in front of the 3rd portion of the duodenum, which it may compress in some patients, causing symptoms of partial intestinal obstruction, a syndrome known as the "superior mesenteric artery syndrome."

The variant blood supply and collateral circulation between the branches of the superior mesenteric artery and the celiac axis is presented by Michels (1960). In careful dissection of 200 cadavers, he found that the vessels that supply blood to the upper abdominal organs conformed to the textbook description in only 55 per cent.

A more thorough knowledge of the most common variations is of utmost importance to the operating surgeon.

As each branch of the superior mesenteric artery courses through the mesentery to gain entrance to the bowel wall, it subdivides to form a series of 2 to 5 anastomotic arcades within the mesentery before their terminal branches reach their destination. These arcades provide alternate channels through which blood may reach the bowel wall should functional or permanent occlusions of minor or short arterial segments occur (Fig. 33-3).

At the point of arterial entrance into the bowel wall, the terminal portion of each artery ascends alternatingly on one side of the bowel wall and then the other (Fig. 33-4). Only occasionally does this terminal branch bifurcate and send a branch to both sides of the bowel. This arrangement largely prevents interference with blood flow in acute distention of the bowel or in the course of normal peristaltic activity. Each of these terminal arteries seldom supplies more than 1 or 2 cm. of the length of bowel wall; therefore, when any surgical anastomosis of the gut is performed, these small arteries must be preserved as near to the cut margins of the bowel as is compatible with the technical demands for obtaining an adequate suture line lest necrosis occur.

Within the intestinal wall, the smallest arterial branches and the arterioles are also

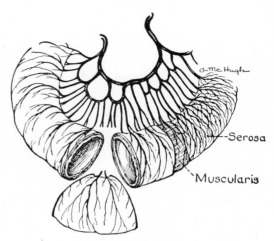

FIG. 33-4. Segment of small bowel depicting the tendency for the arteries to traverse the surface of the gut on either side, generally alternating from one to the other. Also indicated is the necessity of a wedge-shaped resection in preserving arterial blood supply to the antimesenteric border of the bowel. Note that the intramural distributions of the arterial and the venous plexuses follow a similar pattern.

of surgical consequence. Their competence must be considered in the preparation of the severed ends of the proximal and the distal segments for anastomosis of small and/or large bowel. The distribution of these vessels to and within a segment of small bowel is shown in Figure 33-4. The arteries pass from the mesentery into the wall of the bowel at a 90° angle to the direction of the lumen. The caliber of these small arteries diminishes as they cross the bowel wall to its antimesenteric border. Although they anastomose to some extent, the amount of blood available to the gut at its antimesenteric margin is considerably less than that at their points of entrance on the mesenteric side of the gut.[4]

In preparing the mesenteric edge of the severed bowel for anastomosis, it is usually necessary to trim back from the cut margin 1 to 1½ cm. of its mesenteric attachment. While this may reduce the blood supply at its mesenteric side, that of the antimesenteric portion is diminished to a hazardous proportion, as its blood supply often is impaired seriously. The neighboring, or adjacent, arteries remain but are unable to provide enough

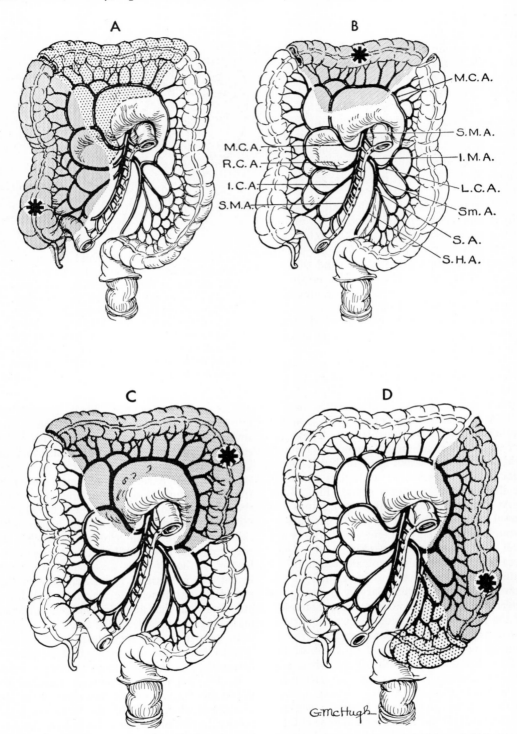

FIG. 33-5. Showing the extent of colon resection necessitated by the division of (A) the ileocolic artery, (B) the middle colic artery, (C) the middle colic and the left colic arteries and (D) the inferior mesenteric artery.

blood to the cut edges at the antimesenteric border other than to that portion which they normally serve. While these arteries are capable of developing a collateral supply of blood, generally this does not occur soon enough to prevent some degree of necrosis with possible perforation at the antimesenteric margin of a surgical anastomosis, should the bowel be divided at a 90° angle. To maintain and insure good blood supply at the antimesenteric margins of the divided proximal and distal ends of the bowel, the cut edges are trimmed back at a 60° to 70° angle rather than left at a 90° angle. This technic preserves the artery which normally supplies the cut edge of the antimesenteric border and eliminates its dependence upon collateral circulation from adjacent arteries (see Fig. 33-4).

The proximal colon from the appendix to the distal third of the transverse colon also is entirely dependent upon branches of the superior mesenteric artery. Save for the ileocolic and the sigmoidal mesenteries, which generally have secondary and even tertiary systems of arcades, the rest of the colon has only a primary system of vascular arcades in its mesentery (Fig. 33-5). *The ileocolic artery* is the most distal branch of the superior mesenteric artery and the only reliable source of arterial blood to the appendix, the cecum and the lower portion of the ascending colon. It anastomoses via arcades with the vessels of the more proximal ileum and, distally, with those of the right colic. *The right colic* artery passes just beneath the peritoneal surface and divides as it approaches the mid-portion of the ascending colon, sending anastomotic branches to the ileocolic and the middle colic arteries.

The distal portion of the hepatic flexure and the proximal two thirds of the transverse colon are supplied by the *middle colic* artery, which enters the transverse mesocolon just below the inferior margin of the body of the pancreas. This artery passes between the leaves of transverse mesocolon, dividing into a right and a left branch, whose primary arcades in turn anastomose with those of the right and the left colic arteries (see Fig. 33-5 A-D).

The distal colon, which includes the splenic flexure from its proximal side, the descending colon and the sigmoidal colon, and the upper rectum, receives its blood from the *inferior mesenteric* artery originating from the aorta opposite the 3rd lumbar vertebra. The principal branches of the inferior mesenteric artery are the *left colic* artery, which supplies the distal transverse colon, beginning near its splenic flexure, and most of the descending colon. The *sigmoidal* artery and its branches run obliquely to the sigmoidal colon in its mesentery; they anastomose with the primary arcades of the left colic artery above and the primary and the secondary arcades of the superior hemorrhoidal artery below. The *superior hemorrhoidal* artery is the terminal continuation of the inferior mesenteric and descends almost vertically in the sigmoidal mesentery to form usually 2 systems of arcades in its course before entering the wall of the lower sigmoid and the rectum. The superior hemorrhoidal artery also communicates with the *middle* and the *inferior hemorrhoidal* arteries, which are the near-terminal branches of the internal iliac artery, giving the rectum a dual source of arterial blood. However, the superior hemorrhoidal artery is the more important source of arterial blood to the rectum (Fig. 33-6).

Colon Resection and Arterial Supply

Knowledge of the arterial blood supply to the large bowel and the rectum is a *sine qua non* to the performance of safe operative procedures upon these structures. In resecting malignant lesions involving the cecum or the ascending colon, not only must the surgeon take into consideration the extent of the operation needed to remove potential sites of tumor spread within the mesentery and the segmental periaortic nodes, but also he must be certain that the remaining bowel has an uncompromised blood supply (see Figs. 33-4 and 5). It is for this reason that the extent of the bowel resection beyond the tumor site may sometimes be greater than that required to circumvent the tumor and its likely area of lymphatic spread.

Resection of the right colon necessitates the inclusion of about 6 in. of the terminal ileum, the appendix, the cecum, the ascending colon and the hepatic flexure to a point at which there can be no doubt that the remaining portion of the transverse colon can be well sustained by the blood flow of the middle colic artery. The extent of the resection is determined by position and adequacy of the blood flow from the middle colic artery. Resections of lesions involving the transverse colon require division of the middle colic artery at its point of origin from the superior mesenteric artery. Removal of the entire transverse colon is required in order that the remaining portions of the hepatic and the splenic flexures receive sufficient blood from the right and the left colic arteries, respectively (see Fig. 33-5 A-D).

Resection of the descending colon, the sigmoid and the rectum may be necessary should the removal of the inferior mesenteric artery and its mesenteric wedge be essential to elimination of probable sites of tumor spread.

Nonmalignant lesions, such as diverticulitis and polyps, may be removed by local bowel resection, only such segments being excised as required to eradicate the local area of bowel involved. In these diseases some conservation of colon may be possible, but generally the saving of a few inches of colon is an unimportant consideration, provided that previous bowel resection has not been performed and further resection at a later date does not seem to be a likely possibility. Excepting these circumstances, it may be easier to resect the bowel segment required after ligation of its arterial supply an inch or two from its point of origin from the superior or the inferior mesenteric artery than to attempt a less anatomic resection designed to conserve only small portions of colon (Fig. 33-7).

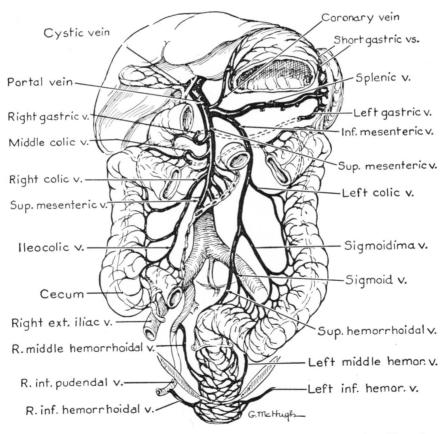

FIG. 33-6. Illustrates the major branches of the portal circulation. Note the portal communication with the systemic circulation at its superior end through the coronary vein and that of the terminal or inferior segment through the middle and the inferior hemorrhoidal veins.

The Small Vessel Circulation of the Mucosa and the Submucosa of the Intestinal Tract

One of the characteristics of many capillary circulations appears to be the coexistence of arteriolar venule anastomosis capable of shunting or bypassing a segment or a major portion of the capillary bed when the latter's function is not needed.[8] This intermittent shunting is to be suspected in most organs which have a phasic function and whose active phase depends in part upon blood flow. The alimentary tract is an example of such a system of organs whose principal functions are predominantly phasic in character.

The suggestion of arteriolar-venule shunts to bypass a capillary circulation is not new. In recent times renewed interest in this phenomenon can be credited to the studies of Spanner in 1931.[53] In a series of observations, Spanner demonstrated beyond reasonable doubt the existence of such shunts within the villi and the mucosa of the stomach and the bowel. Confirmation of Spanner's studies has been reported by Barlow,[3] Walder[57] and Grayson;[25] all studies to date, whether of anatomic, physiologic or pharmacologic nature, seem to come to the same conclusion, namely, that shunts exist within the villi and the

mucosa of the stomach and the intestine. They appear to shunt blood away from the villous mucosa during the fasting state, and are said to be under nervous rather than humoral control.

Evidence thus far demonstrates considerable lability of the intraluminal circulation of the alimentary tract, a lability comparable with that exhibited by the capillary bed of the skin. The control of the circulation of the gut and the skin is largely autonomic in nature; that of the striated muscle appears to be free of nervous control, responding chiefly to altered concentrations of serum metabolites, particularly those bearing upon CO_2 and pH values of the blood itself.

Venous Drainage, the Portal Circulation

The venous return from the splanchnic viscera recently has assumed a new role of surgical importance and of anatomic and physiologic consequence, due to the developments in the operative treatment of portal hypertension.

The venous drainage of the small bowel and the colon is through a confluence of veins that terminate ultimately in the portal vein, which drains into the liver. The portal tribu-

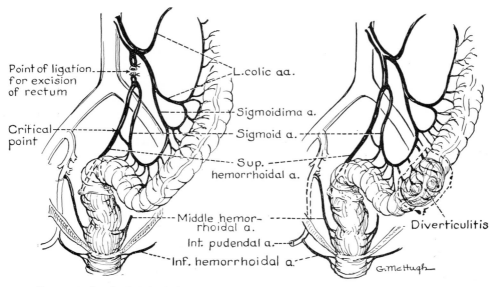

FIG. 33-7. On the left is designated the point of ligation of the superior hemorrhoidal artery for resection of the lower sigmoid for benign disease. Note that if the ligature were placed at the critical point shown, it would be necessary to resect not only the sigmoid but also the rectum as well.

taries correspond in nomenclature and location to those of the arterial supply of corresponding segments of the small bowel, the colon and the rectum. The primary arteries to the intra-abdominal alimentary organs, including the liver and the spleen, arise directly from the aorta as 3 separate vessels (celiac axis, superior mesenteric artery and inferior mesenteric artery) and at 3 distinct aortic levels. The venous return differs in that all of it culminates in the large solitary portal vein.

The portal circulation differs from that of the systemic venous circulation in at least 4 respects:

1. The normal venous pressure of the portal vein generally is 12 to 15 cm. of water compared with the normal pressure values of the inferior vena cava which fluctuate between a positive pressure of 1 to 3 cm. of water during the expiratory phase of respiration and a negative pressure of 1 to 3 cm. during inspiration.

2. When venous blood from the gastrointestinal tract finally is collected into the single common channel, it must circulate through the sinusoidal or capillary circulatory bed of the liver before reaching the inferior vena cava via the hepatic veins. In this respect, the venous return from the splanchnic bed resembles that of the arterial system between the right and the left sides of the heart, save for the fact that portal blood manages to pass through the liver by virtue of the much lower venous pressure at its point of exit through the hepatic veins compared with that of the portal vein.

3. The portal system, like the vena cava, has no valves, although valves are abundantly present in the veins of the extremities leading to the vena cava.

4. The venous drainage of the alimentary tract, along with that of the splanchnic lymphatic circulation return, is the only known source for the normal transport of ingested food products aside from the lacteals.

The portal circulation also receives venous return from the spleen. As the spleen has no known function related to alimentation, there is no very obvious physiologic explanation for its anatomic location within the splanchnic circulation (see Fig. 33-6).

The portal system begins with the capillary circulation within villus folds of the intestinal mucosa. After these coalesce to form the venules and the veins in the submucous layer, eventually they emerge alternatingly from the bowel wall about 1 cm. or so apart in a fashion corresponding to the small arteries entering the bowel. From here they pass directly into their respective mesenteric segments to converge upon a system of venous arcades corresponding in location and number to that of the mesenteric arteries. From these anastomotic arcades, blood enters the major branches of the superior or the inferior mesenteric vein and eventually into the portal vein. Usually the venous and the arterial channels in the corresponding areas of the gut and the mesentery run parallel and in close proximity.

The inferior mesenteric vein usually drains the distal portion of the transverse colon, its splenic flexure, the descending and sigmoidal colon, and the upper half of the rectum. The most distal portion of the inferior mesenteric vein is its superior hemorrhoidal branch, which begins at the superior margin of the venous plexus surrounding the mid-portion of the rectum. The lower portions of this plexus drain through the middle and the inferior hemorrhoidal veins into the "headwaters" of the internal iliacs, hence into the systemic rather than into the portal circulation (see Fig. 33-6).

The confluence of the superior hemorrhoidal, the sigmoidal and the left colic veins forms the inferior mesenteric vein, which then ascends along the psoas muscle beneath the parietal peritoneum, passing under the ligament of Treitz at its left margin to disappear beneath the body of the pancreas, where usually it joins the splenic vein as the latter passes in its mesial direction to unite with the larger superior mesenteric vein in the formation of the portal vein. From this junction the portal vein emerges and continues in an upward direction, leaning slightly to the right until it reaches its termination, the right and left branches at the porta hepatis, before entering the capillary and the sinusoidal network of the liver.

The superior mesenteric vein receives the venous return from the middle, the right and the ileocolic veins and drains the colon proximal to its splenic flexure. These veins are joined by 12 to 15 major tributaries from the small bowel; they account for all venous return of this portion of the colon and all of the small bowel short of a few centimeters distal to the ligament of Treitz. The superior mesenteric vein runs within the mesentery of the small bowel at the left of the superior mesenteric artery. As the two pass over the duodenum and the uncinate process of the pancreas, the artery is directed more posteriorly, allowing the vein to cross anterior to the artery. The vein deviates slightly to the right to ascend in the gastrohepatic ligament as the portal vein. Under the pancreas the superior mesenteric vein generally receives several pancreatic veins, some of which are major branches of the superior and the inferior pancreatoduodenal veins, and generally the gastroepiploic veins, which drain the greater omentum and the greater curvature of the stomach.

The coronary vein, which drains most of the blood from the lower esophagus, the fundus and the lesser curvature of the stomach, generally is of no unusual consequence in the course of surgical operations performed on patients without portal hypertension. However, should portal hypertension exist, it is largely the small branches of the coronary vein that become varicosities in the esophagus and the upper stomach, due to the increased portal pressure transmitted to them. To a lesser extent, the gastroepiploics and the short gastric veins also may contribute to esophageal and gastric varices (see Figs. 33-6 and 33-13).

The portal vein, from 6 to 9 cm. in length, passes in the posterior edge of the gastrohepatic omentum after emerging from behind the superior margin of the mesial portion of the head of the pancreas. Usually the common duct lies along the anterior right surface of the portal vein; to the posterior left of the vein is the hepatic artery. These relationships and positions are fairly constant, though not always so. Less constant anatomic relationships are found among some of the major tributaries to the portal vein, especially the gastroepiploics and the coronary veins, which may enter the portal vein directly or at the junction of the superior mesenteric with the splenic vein.

PORTAL HYPERTENSION

PATHOGENESIS, DIAGNOSIS AND TREATMENT

Portal hypertension is a clinicopathologic syndrome characterized by esophagogastric varices and splenomegaly, caused by the increase in portal pressure. Often it is accompanied by hepatomegaly and ascites. The varices may bleed with exsanguinary vigor, and frequently this is the first manifestation of the existence of portal hypertension. In some patients the splenomegaly may create serious problems in secondary hypersplenism (thrombocytopenia, leukopenia and anemia). Because there usually is serious impairment of liver function, hepatic coma and death may occur. The ascites, as well as the liver disease and the hemorrhaging varix, can contribute to severe nutritional and metabolic disorders, which are often lethal.

This syndrome of portal hypertension is associated most frequently with hepatic cirrhosis. As a clinical entity, portal hypertension is fairly easy to diagnose, although the primary nature of its pathology is not always clear or easily defined. Usually the diagnosis may be suspected, or it should be considered in any patient suffering from upper gastrointestinal hemorrhage; the history or the finding of liver disease should increase the index of suspicion that "silent" portal hypertension may exist in such patients, and that a bleeding varix is the source of blood loss. Bleeding varices account for the point of origin of acute upper gastrointestinal hemorrhage in approximately 15 per cent of all patients over the age of 30. This indicates the need for fairly elaborate diagnostic studies insofar as the patient's general condition and course permit, if the site of bleeding is to be established accurately and treated appropriately.

In children and young adults with massive gastrointestinal hemorrhage, the likelihood that the bleeding point is from a varix is much greater than in the older age group. One factor which seems to be responsible for this difference is that peptic ulcer accounts for about 80 per cent of all massive bleeding from the upper gastrointestinal tract in adults and that peptic ulcer is a comparatively rare disease among children and adults under 20 years of age. Another factor is that some of the causes of portal hypertension, hence the bleeding varix, either are congenital or are acquired in early life. Many of these young patients do not live to adult life or much beyond.

Pathogenesis

The vast majority of patients with portal hypertension have associated liver disease as its cause. However, in about 20 per cent of all cases, portal hypertension results from occlusion of the portal or the splenic vein before it enters the liver, and in an even smaller group portal flow is obstructed by certain diseases affecting the hepatic vein outflow above the liver.

The cause and the treatment of portal hypertension in any patient can be established most readily in the light of an accurate location of the point of obstruction of portal blood flow. The site of portal obstruction is the basis for the classification of portal hypertension to be followed here. The site of impaired venous return rarely is located above the liver (suprahepatic); most frequently it is within the liver (intrahepatic); and in children and young adults especially it may be obstructed below the liver (subhepatic). In most patients the cause of portal hypertension of intrahepatic obstruction is one of the various types of cirrhosis.

Suprahepatic portal hypertension may result from cardiac failure, pulmonary fibrosis and hepatic vein compression or occlusion. Impairment of blood flow between the right and the left heart chambers from any cause transmits the resulting increased venous pressure to the hepatic veins and the portal circulation, as well as increases the venous pressure within the systemic channels of venous return. Cardiopulmonary pathology of this variety creates generalized venous stasis, wherein cardiac cirrhosis and portal hypertension usually are relatively unimportant considerations in light of the seriousness of the primary disease. Should the primary pathology be amenable to medical therapy, cardiac cirrhosis and portal hypertension usually regress fairly quickly. Generally, this type of portal hypertension is recognized easily, as the venous pressure of the peripheral veins also is increased. Although esophagogastric varices may be demonstrated readily in some patients with cardiopulmonary disease, massive bleeding seldom occurs, for the disease either is amenable promptly to medical therapy, or, if not, death usually occurs before such varices present serious problems.

Obstruction of blood flow from the hepatic veins into the inferior vena cava is a most serious but rarely encountered cause of suprahepatic portal hypertension and bleeding varices. Obstruction to the outflow of hepatic veins may be complete, and its cause usually is hepatic vein thrombosis or their compression by tumor. This condition is known as the Budd-Chiari syndrome[10] and is characterized by the prompt appearance of extensive ascites and huge esophagogastric varices. The resulting increases in portal pressure are among the highest readings encountered in portal hypertension of any cause, in contrast with the relatively mild portal hypertension secondary to cardiopulmonary disease. The liver pathology in the Budd-Chiari syndrome generally is very similar to that of cardiac cirrhosis, for indeed the pressure influence upon the central veins of the liver lobules qualitatively is the same in both conditions. Systemic venous pressure measurements are elevated in cardiac cirrhosis but are normal in the Budd-Chiari picture, unless both conditions are present independently. The prognosis of patients with the Budd-Chiari type of obstruction is very poor. Moreover, in those patients whose hepatic vein obstruction is from thrombosis, the portal vein and many of its radicals often are similarly involved. Thus, there seldom is an opportunity to employ one of the portacaval anastomoses for the relief of this type of portal hypertension.

Intrahepatic portal hypertension is prevalent and accounts for approximately 80 per cent of all causes of portal hypertension requiring surgical treatment. As the portal blood flow through the liver in hepatic cirrhosis seldom is as completely occluded as in the Budd-Chiari type of hepatic vein obliteration, portal hypertension resulting from intrahepatic disease generally is not so high and usually ranges between 25 and 50 cm. of water. However, pressures within this range are sufficient to give rise to the development of varices in nearly all patients, and in due course many or most of the patients bleed seriously. Among the types of cirrhosis acquired in the adult which may give rise to portal hypertension are those of portal, periportal, pigment, posthepatic and biliary obstructive origin. In due course, ascites generally appears, but usually it is less rapid in development than that observed in portal hypertension of suprahepatic origin.

These same forms of cirrhosis also may exist in children, but certain additional types of liver disease not often seen in adult life also must be considered. Among these are hepatic agenesis or atrophy, including the so-called Cruveilhier-Baumgarten syndrome.[17] Hepatic atrophy in this syndrome is attributed to a congenital communication between the portal and the systemic circulations through the patent umbilical vein. The reduced flow of portal blood through the liver is believed to cause atrophy or agenesis of the liver. An explanation that is equally or more plausible to the author would seem to be the failure of the umbilical vein to undergo its usual postnatal fibrosis because of the existence of intrahepatic portal hypertension at the time of birth, presumably from hepatic agenesis or cirrhosis acquired *in utero.* Both of these conditions do occur and should favor the development of collateral venous circulation *in utero* at a time in life when the umbilical vein is still patent and in direct communication with the portal vein. Should agenesis or atrophy of the liver occur *in utero,* it may be anticipated that the channel most likely to shunt the portal circulation to the systemic circulation would be the umbilical vein, and in doing so it would form extensive communications with the systemic veins in the anterior abdominal wall. In a few adult patients with portal hypertension the recanalization of the umbilical vein and its ability to form collaterals with those of the abdominal wall also seem to occur.

The interesting and diagnostic clinical feature in this syndrome is the venous hum and thrill usually detectable in the veins of the abdominal wall near the umbilicus.

Subhepatic portal vein obstruction is encountered more commonly in children and young adults than in older patients. Generally it is referred to as Banti's syndrome. If portal vein occlusion alone is responsible for portal hypertension, the liver appears to be perfectly normal. In rare instances, only the splenic vein may be thrombosed, leaving the superior mesenteric and the portal veins intact and normally patent. It is in this small group of patients that splenectomy has proved to be curative at times.

The cause of portal vein occlusion in the young probably is inflammation, although no specific etiologic agent can be implicated. Much of the gross pathology observed at operation or autopsy suggests the basic disturbance to be one of a chronic phlebitis, with progressive obliteration of the major veins of the portal system. Cavernous segments of the portal vein or its major radicals are seen frequently. In many areas of the peripheral portal system, the veins appear to be relatively normal and uninvolved.

In most young patients with subhepatic portal hypertension, numerous enlarged and chronically inflamed lymph nodes are found along the course of the portal vein or adjacent to it, particularly in the upper abdomen at the junction of the superior mesenteric and the splenic veins, and in the retroperitoneum of this area. The peritoneum in these same regions usually is chronically inflamed.

Certainly, the causes of these inflammatory changes are not known; indeed, one cannot be certain that the phlebitis, the periphlebitis and the venous occlusion are the primary cause of this type of subhepatic portal hypertension or the sequelae of another. One may postulate a low-grade phlebitis arising shortly after birth from a postnatal omphalitis which extends from the umbilical vein into the portal as one possibility; another is that of a phlebitic process beginning in the portal system in childhood and secondary to some other intra-abdominal disease, such as mesenteric adenitis, regional enteritis or ulcerative colitis. At best these are highly speculative suggestions as to the otherwise unexplained origin of portal hypertension in early life.

Ascites, except for modest fluid accumulations found at operation, usually is not detectable by clinical examination in patients with subhepatic portal hypertension if the liver is otherwise normal and other causes do not exist. In adults, portal hypertension of the subhepatic variety also is seldom associated with ascites. Generally, subhepatic portal occlusion in middle or late life is from tumor invasion or its compression of the larger radicals of the portal system. Tumors of the kidney (the hypernephroma in particular), carcinoma of the stomach, the pancreas and the common bile duct, metastatic tumors, or tumors from the duodenum account for most of those producing portal obstruction. Abdominal lymphoma, especially Hodgkin's disease, accounts for obstruction in some patients. Tumor obstruction of the portal vein, even when complete, generally results in only mild increases in portal venous pressure and a moderate varix formation. Under these conditions the bleeding varix is seldom encountered, probably because death from the malignancy supervenes fairly soon. On the other hand, migratory phlebitis of the portal system may occur in the adult and end in as pronounced a portal hypertension as in children; in these instances, formation of esophagogastric varices is prominent and may bleed as seriously as in the child.

In any patient in whom the formation of ascitic fluid is rapid, or in any patient who has been subjected to repeated tappings, one must be on the lookout for the "low sodium syndrome" and other electrolyte disturbances.

Diagnosis

The diagnosis of portal hypertension always must include a search for liver disease and an evaluation of hepatic function, secondary hypersplenism, and a careful evaluation of renal function and of the patient's general health. As most effective operative procedures for the relief of portal hypertension are rather formidable in magnitude, all reasonable possibilities for evaluating the patient's general condition and hepatic function should be explored prior to the decision as to the treatment to be followed.

The onset of the clinical history in the patient with otherwise asymptomatic portal hypertension often has for its outstanding feature at least one massive bout of hematemesis. Patients who bleed from gastric or duodenal ulcer also may bleed massively (see Chap. 30, "Stomach and Duodenum"), but in the case of the bleeding duodenal ulcer the quantity of blood vomited is likely to be less than when bleeding is from either the esophageal varix or the gastric ulcer, even though the total quantity of blood lost is the same or greater. Generally this clinical pattern is explained on the basis that much or most of the blood lost from the bleeding duodenal ulcer tends to continue downward in the small bowel rather than to back up and enter the stomach. Blood from the hemorrhaging varix or a gastric ulceration tends to accumulate within the stomach and cause rapid distention and induce massive hematemesis.

The child with portal hypertension tends to develop a more efficient collateral circulation than the adult; for this reason, as well as because of his small size, the bleeding varix in the adult is more likely to be fatal for any given episode than in the child.

In other patients, especially those suffering from symptoms of heart or liver disease, diagnostic evidence of portal hypertension is obtained by searching for signs of portal hypertension in the course of the general work-up. Not infrequently patients with portal hypertension present themselves to the doctor because of unexplained weight gain in spite of a drawn facies or because of a recent increase in girth, obvious ascites or the recent detection of mild to moderate icterus. A few will have noted an enlarged liver and/or spleen, which may or may not cause distress, but such findings alarm the patient and prompt him to seek his physician's advice.

Preceding episodes of virus hepatitis, "toxic" hepatitis or cirrhosis can be elicited among a few patients with portal hypertension. Of some interest in this connection are the histories of 5 patients operated upon by the author for portal hypertension that developed several years after the onset of nonspecific ulcerative colitis. Four of these received multiple transfusions of blood in previous years; one did not. It is possible that the cirrhosis and portal hypertensive states in these patients represented latent manifestations of serum hepatitis, or that the virus of infectious hepatitis can and did enter the portal circulation more readily in ulcerative colitis than in the normal individual, or that the hepatitis and the cirrhosis were primarily a problem of malnutrition and possible an associated increased susceptibility to virus hepatitis.

The physical examination, when the portal hypertension is of the *suprahepatic* variety, almost always discloses 3 important corollaries. These are hepatomegaly, splenomegaly and massive ascites.

Ascites presents a special problem in diagnosis and treatment, as well as in establishing its etiology both clinically and experimentally. The association of ascites with suprahepatic portal hypertension is present so reliably that its absence, when other evidence of portal hypertension is present (hepatomegaly, splenomegaly and demonstrable esophageal varices), generally is sufficient evidence to question or to disqualify the Budd-Chiari syndrome from consideration. The prompt formation of experimental ascites in the dog can be accomplished only when the site of obstruction is one that constricts the hepatic vein outlet.[7] Complete occlusion of the portal vein in man or in dog below the liver usually does not induce ascites; it should be pointed out that acute subhepatic portal obstruction in either man or dog usually is incompatible with life. Other factors that may play some role in the formation of ascitic fluid is the increased serum concentration of the salt-retaining hormone aldosterone. The serum level of aldosterone in patients with heart and liver disease, glomerulonephritis and eclampsia is said to be increased.[10] Its actual role in the formation of ascitic fluid has not yet been established. The hypoproteinemia of liver disease is another etiologic or contributing factor in the formation of ascites, especially hypoalbuminemia.

Patients with portal hypertension of *intrahepatic* origin nearly always have splenomegaly, but they may or may not have ascites. Extensive ascites is a more common accompaniment of advanced portal cirrhosis in intrahepatic portal cirrhosis than when the liver disease is less severe. Admittedly, ascites may be encountered in all types and stages of liver disease. Extensive ascites is rare indeed in patients with subhepatic portal vein obstruction; the presence of moderate to large accumulations of ascitic fluid in patients with portal hypertension and without evidence of heart or renal disease, or of malnutrition, should direct attention first to the liver as its cause, second to the Budd-Chiari syndrome, and third, if at all, to the subhepatic as the causes of the portal hypertension.

The rapid formation of ascitic fluid may lead to dehydration and hypoproteinemia, for its sources of water, electrolytes and protein are chiefly tissues of the body. Hence, the loss of turgor of the skin, the drawn facies and the loss of muscle tone, prominent findings in many patients with advanced liver disease and extensive ascites, seem to be explainable.

Peripheral edema is not likely to be present in patients with a moderate degree of hepatic cirrhosis if they do not also have ascites or hypoproteinemia. In general, the cirrhosis is associated with sodium retention, hypoalbuminemia and possibly to some extent an increased intra-abdominal pressure from ascites. This combination can easily induce edema. Edema may involve the sacral area and that of the back, as well as the lower extremities, in patients who are bedridden.

Splenomegaly is present nearly always in portal hypertension, whether or not liver enlargement is present. However, before the enlarged spleen may be palpable, it usually must be enlarged from 2 to 3 times its normal size, except in infants. If it remains posterior as it enlarges, it may not be felt in spite of its increased size. In the abdomen distended with ascitic fluid, even very large spleens may not be palpable until the fluid is removed. Assessment of splenic size by percussion is subject to many errors and has little merit when evaluated in the face of operative or autopsy findings. Some have sought to determine the size of the liver or the spleen by the use of pneumoperitoneum, wherein air contrast about these organs outlines them upon roentgenographic films. Information provided by such ancillary procedures is seldom of great importance, either to the diagnosis or to the treatment to be followed.

Icterus may or may not be present in patients with long-standing portal hypertension from chronic liver disease. When present and of intrahepatic origin, it is a sign of need for caution. Generally, icterus infers the presence of an active or a subacute form of hepatitis or cholangitis; otherwise, it infers extensive replacement of liver cells by fibrous tissue. In either instance the patient's prognosis is likely to be poor unless obstructed by stones.

Cutaneous and subcutaneous venous collaterals may be evident in many patients with portal hypertension from any cause, especially in those who are thin and malnourished. As the circulating blood volume generally is reduced to 75 per cent or less its normal value during periods of active formation of ascitic fluid, the systemic veins, including the collaterals, may not seem to be as distended as they

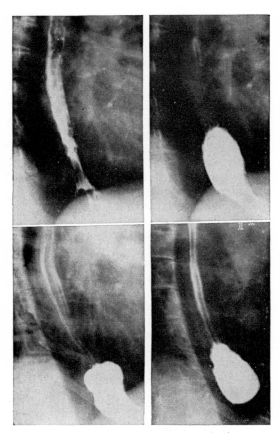

Fig. 33-8. Compares the preoperative demonstration of moderate esophageal varices with their total absence 4 years following splenorenal anastomosis for portal hypertension.

countered most commonly and giving rise to varices in these areas.

2. The cutaneous collaterals, which may develop in 1 of 2 areas, or both. More often they appear as varicosities along the hypogastric veins to the epigastrics and the internal mammary veins, and much less commonly they also may appear to arise largely from the umbilical area, as in Cruveilhier-Baumgarten syndrome, spreading out largely in radial directions toward the superior and the inferior epigastrics, a finding referred to as the caput medusae.

3. Finally, should intra-abdominal adhesions between the omentum or other organs be situated along the venous return of the portal circulation, collateral vascular channels may develop between these organs and the systemic veins of the abdominal wall via such adhesions (this is a spontaneous Talma-Morison omentopexy).

Roentgenologic Diagnostic Aids. The presence of portal hypertension is inferred diagnostically by the fluoroscopic demonstration of esophageal and/or gastric varices. During early phases of portal hypertension, esophageal varices may not be evident; thus a negative fluoroscopic result does not always exclude the possibility of portal hypertension. A series of films taken over a period of several months to a year or two often demonstrate clearly an increase in size and number of varices if the disease progresses and the patient is unrelieved of his portal hypertension. Varices disappear after successful shunting procedures. In reality, probably they remain but become inconspicuous once their intraluminal pressure is relieved (Fig. 33-8).

It is important to search for the presence of gastric varices at the time of fluoroscopy. Varices in this location can bleed as briskly as those in the esophagus. One of the reasons for failure of esophageal tamponade to control the bleeding of portal hypertension is the bleeding gastric varices beyond the reach of the balloon employed (see below). The oversewing of varices in the esophagus when hemorrhage continues from those of the stomach has accounted for some of the failures in this form of surgical treatment.

A second and more recent use of diagnostic roentgenography in patients with portal hypertension is the preoperative demonstration

did before ascites began to appear. The extent of collateral vein development can be demonstrated easily by means of infrared photography. The presence or the absence of internal hemorrhoids from the increased pressure transmitted to them through the superior hemorrhoidal vein seldom is cause for serious consideration of the existence of portal hypertension should other findings be absent. Patients with portal hypertension frequently also have hemorrhoids (see Fig. 33-5), but hemorrhoids are encountered so commonly that their presence without other evidence is no reason to suspect portal hypertension.

Collateral venous developments in portal hypertension are primarily along 3 channels:

1. The esophagogastric plexus, the site en-

FIG. 33-9. Demonstrates by splenoportography a communication between the portal vein and the vena cava. Note also that the portal vein appears partially obstructed at its point of entrance into the liver (Cruveilhier-Baumgarten syndrome).

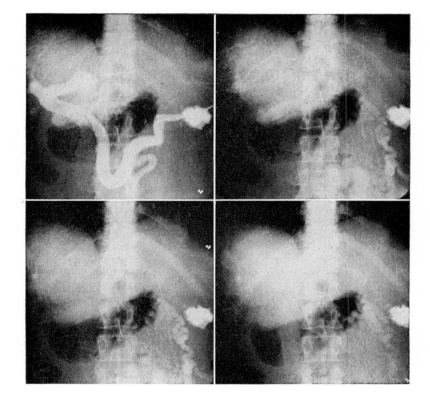

of the location of the venous obstruction in the portal system (Fig. 33-9). This procedure is known as splenoportography. It has proved to be a valuable diagnostic aid and of great practical help to the surgeon, as it may provide advance information as to the location of portal obstruction of the subhepatic type. This is a procedure that should be performed in the operating room just before surgical decompression of the portal system is to be carried out (Fig. 33-9). Prior to the splenoportogram, a splenic pulp pressure determination can be made which may confirm the clinical impression of portal hypertension. Rousselot (1960)[48] has utilized successfully splenic puncture for direct measurement of the portal pressure in patients with obscure hemorrhage from the upper gastro-intestinal tract.

Esophagoscopy may be used to detect the presence of esophageal varices and the bleeding site. While many favor and use this procedure, some are fearful that such an examination may induce bleeding should the varix be traumatized. In selected cases and in com-

petent hands, esophagoscopy is a procedure of diagnostic merit when other technics fail. Some have attempted to measure portal pressure by the insertion of a needle attached to a manometer, introduced through the esophagoscope into a varix. Such attempts to measure portal pressure are dangerous and also may yield variable results.

EVALUATION OF HEPATIC FUNCTION IN PATIENTS WITH PORTAL HYPERTENSION

Operations of any type performed upon patients with liver disease carry certain risks related to the extent of impairment of hepatic function. The complications arising from the operation and anesthesia employed are principally those of hepatic and renal failure (see below) and, less often, that of bile nephrosis known also as so-called hepatorenal syndrome.

Hepatic failure in patients with severe liver disease may be precipitated by an operation as minor as hemorrhoidectomy. This is an extreme example; generally in such patients more than three fourths of the hepatic parenchyma has been replaced by fibrous tissue, or an acute loss of function has occurred secondary to acute hepatitis, whether of bacterial, viral or chemical origin.

Recovery of hepatic function from acute hepatitis may be complete in many patients. In some, subacute hepatitis persists with exacerbations and remissions over periods of months to years, leading eventually to cirrhosis, ascites, hemorrhage, coma and death.

Recovery of hepatic structure from cirrhosis of any type, as determined by histologic study, seldom regresses unless its cause can be relieved early. Relief of chronic obstruction of the extrahepatic biliary tract at times will allow a remarkable degree of regression of biliary cirrhosis, provided that the latter is not of more than a few months' duration. Similarly, recovery from cardiac cirrhosis may be essentially complete if cardiac failure can be cured by either medical or surgical means. Although improvement in the histologic patterns of the liver is discernible in many patients whose biliary or cardiac cirrhosis is relieved, varying degrees of permanent fibrous change may remain. The extent and eventual consequence of the liver damage is often difficult to evaluate.

Recovery of hepatic function in patients with either hepatitis or cirrhosis over a period of weeks to months may be surprisingly good, but this recovery of function may not necessarily conform to or correlate closely with histologic recovery. If hepatic function continues to improve or returns to normal, the prognosis is usually good. Thus, in patients with hepatic disease, assessment of the liver's functional capacity often is as important to prognosis as the organic or the histologic findings obtained; both types of information are essential to the proper evaluation of surgical risk.

Evaluation of Hepatic Function

As the functions of the liver are numerous and diverse, no one test will disclose reliably the total functional capacity of this organ. Therefore, the best that can be hoped for at present is an estimation based upon data obtained from "tests" that attempt to appraise different types of hepatic function.

If a battery of tests are to be used, certain criteria should be considered in the selection of those that may be most practical. (1) They should be simple tests, performed easily and with reproducible accuracy in the average hospital laboratory. (2) The function each measures should be one performed only by the liver. (3) When an impairment in function is detected, it should have a high degree of correlation with the extent of organic hepatic disease present. Negative results from such tests need not exclude the presence of organic liver disease, but they should be of such nature as to indicate little chance of early hepatic failure. Thus, in selecting patients with liver disease for operation, the surgeon is searching for indications that suggest strongly the presence or the absence of seriously impaired hepatic function rather than for evidences of minor deviations from normal. For the most part the surgeon is already aware of some degree of hepatic dysfunction, but he needs additional information in order to appraise the ability of the liver and the patient to withstand the operation and the anesthesia that he plans.

A number of commonly used tests of hepatic function and the capacities that they appear to measure are listed in Table 1. Only a few of these are useful in solving the problems presented to the surgeon by patients with known liver disease. The author prefers the use of the serum bilirubin concentration and the bromsulphalein test as tests of the excretory function of the liver; the serum albumin and the prothrombin time as general indicators of the liver's ability to synthesize protein; and the free cholesterol and cholesterol ester ratio as a crude index of lipid metabolism within the liver. If all 3 of these functions appear to be good in patients with hepatic disease, the prognosis is likely to be favorable, and generally such patients withstand surgical operations well.

In the author's experience, the serum albumin level of these 3 groups of tests deserves more weight in assessing hepatic functional capacity than most other tests. On the other hand, in certain patients a positive bromsulphalein excretion test in the absence of icterus probably is the most important and reliable index of impaired hepatic function that we have, but in most patients a positive BSP test is not as reliable an indication of serious hepatic impairment as is the reduced serum

TABLE 1. TESTS OF HEPATIC FUNCTION USED COMMONLY IN PATIENTS WITH
LIVER DISEASE WITH SPECIAL ATTENTION TO SURGICAL PATIENTS

TEST	ORIGINATOR	VALUE TO SURGEON
Excretory Tests:		
Bromsulphalein	Rosenthal & White, 1924	Excellent in detection of liver disease in absence of icterus (moderate to severe liver disease)
Bilirubin excretion	von Bergman, 1927	Offers no advantages over BSP and is more difficult to perform
Detoxication Tests:		
Hippuric acid synthesis	Quick, 1932	Good but of limited value and too complex for simplicity. Positive in other diseases
Cholesterol and cholesterol ester ratio	Feigel, 1918	Excellent when positive but positive in diabetes and thyrotoxicosis also (advanced liver disease)
Galactose tolerance	Bauer, 1906	Excellent when positive (advanced liver disease)
"Flocculation" Tests:		
Takata-Ara	Takata-Ara, 1925	Of little value
Cephalin	Hanger, 1939	Of little value
Colloidal gold	Gray, 1940	Of little value
Thymol turbidity	Maclagan, 1944	Of little value
Prothrombin Assays and Response of vitamin K:	Bay: Allen & Julian, 1940	Good when observing course of hepatic disease. Excellent when positive as differential test of jaundice (obstructive versus nonobstructive)
Serum Protein Concentration:		
Albumin	Many observers	Excellent for advanced disease in absence of starvation or albuminuria
Globulin	Many observers	Excellent for advanced liver disease

albumin concentration with a reversal of the albumin and globulin ratio.

None of these tests can be relied upon entirely. As in most clinical situations, the information that they provide must be reviewed and interpreted in light of the data gleaned from the taking of a careful history, the physical examination, the routine blood and urine analysis, and other special tests.

The bromsulphalein test is performed by the intravenous injection of 5 mg. of this material per Kg. of body weight.[41] Normally, all of this dye will be excreted by the liver in bile within less than 45 minutes. The detection of its presence in excess of 10 per cent in the serum after 30 minutes indicates impaired hepatic excretion, as this is its major means of rapid escape. Usually the greater the percentage of dye retention, the more pronounced the disturbance in excretory hepatic function, and usually the more extensively diseased the liver if extrahepatic biliary obstruction is not present.

The BSP test serves no useful purpose if the serum bilirubin is elevated. Icterus is evidence enough that excretory function is impaired, provided that acute hemolysis has not occurred recently. Moreover, the elevated serum bilirubin level obscures the BSP color and invalidates the use of the latter.

The serum albumin level normally is about 4.5 Gm. per cent. A reduction in its concentration may come about from diseases other than of hepatic origin, but these are so conspicuous that they are not likely to be overlooked or to confuse the general picture; they are principally the various forms of starvation and the abnormal losses of albumin secondary to other diseases such as burns, cutaneous ulcers and the nephroses.

Some patients with ascites and liver disease may have a hypoalbuminemia only because of the loss of albumin in ascitic fluid, especially if they are tapped frequently; or they may be unable to synthesize albumin at a rate sufficient to sustain the normal serum concentration irrespective of ascites. When ascites is present, hypoalbuminemia is not so dependable an indication of the status of hepatic reserve, but it is reassuring indeed when the serum albumin level is normal in the presence of ascites.

Prothrombin activity may or may not be altered seriously in extensive liver disease.[1]

In general, the more depressed the prothrombin activity and its unresponsiveness to vitamin K administration, the more severe the liver damage. Exceptions, however, are encountered with sufficient frequency to disqualify the level of prothrombin activity as a good index of hepatic function. However, over a period of time a rise or a fall in prothrombin activity correlates fairly well with regression or advance of hepatic disease.[1]

The use of the prothrombin time as an index of hepatic function in patients with known liver disease is not to be confused with its employment to measure the response to vitamin K administration as a means of distinguishing between obstructive and intrahepatic jaundice.[1]

The prothrombin level has a 3rd connotation; it is a good indicator as to the likelihood of abnormal bleeding at the time of operation or needle biopsy of the liver from hypoprothrombinemia. Most observers agree that the prothrombin activity as measured by the Quick 1-stage technic should be in excess of 50 per cent of its normal value before operative procedures are undertaken.

Cholesterol ester formation appears to be a function performed only by the liver. Normally, from 25 to 40 per cent of the total serum cholesterol is so conjugated. Usually this function continues to be performed at a rate sufficient to maintain the normal ratio between free and esterified cholesterol; only in severe liver disease or hepatic failure does the percentage of esterified cholesterol begin to fall. It is a sound presumption that serious impairment of hepatic function may be present when less than 10 per cent of the total cholesterol is esterified, particularly if the total serum cholesterol level is not elevated materially.

As the drop in the percentage of cholesterol esters usually is a late occurrence in liver disease, normal values are not necessarily harbingers of good fortune.

Flocculation tests—the Takata-Ara, the cephalin flocculation, the colloidal gold and the thymol turbidity—are of some value in assessing surgical prognosis in patients with liver disease. They measure essentially an altered stability of serum protein solutions when mixed with these agents. The value of these tests is largely in the opposite direction of those mentioned above, in that the flocculation tests are designed to pick up comparatively minute disturbances in hepatic function, and for this reason they are of greater diagnostic consequence than of prognostic value. Since the chief concern of the surgeon is not so much whether or not liver disease is present but what it is likely to mean in terms of risk to the patient needing an operation, such tests are less important to the surgeon than those likely to be positive only in advanced liver disease.

Evaluation by Histologic Examination (Liver Biopsy)

The nature of the pathologic process responsible for the altered hepatic function can be established only by histologic examination of liver tissue. Until the development of the Silverman needle technic,[30] biopsy material could be made available only at the time of operation or autopsy. The needle-biopsy technic has largely overcome the need for surgical exploration as the means of establishing the diagnosis and the nature of liver disease. It is a procedure to be performed whenever the nature and the extent of liver disease are important in the choice of treatment. From the sample tissue obtained, it is usually possible to distinguish between intrahepatic and extrahepatic biliary obstruction to determine the presence and the nature of cirrhosis, the presence or the absence of hepatitis and, less frequently but occasionally, the detection of metastatic tumor within the liver. However, the biopsy material may not shed much information on the liver's functional capacity; hence the need to test liver function continues and is to be considered as an important separate series of studies to be carried out, even though the final diagnosis of hepatic disease is based on histologic evidence.

Bleeding from the needle site of liver puncture seldom is a serious problem, although undoubtedly some bleeding usually occurs in most instances. Most clinicians believe that the prothrombin time should be in excess of 50 per cent of normal if needle biopsy is to be performed. In the face of serious hypoprothrombinemia and/or thrombocytopenia, needle biopsy usually should be avoided; otherwise the author believes that the value of the information obtained from needle biopsy in selected patients outweighs the risk of bleeding, despite the fact that the bleeding encountered in a few patients may require surgical hemostasis.

Hepatic Coma

In a discussion of McDermott's paper[38] Eiseman points out rightly that a number of metabolic disorders in advanced liver disease can induce coma. Recently a series of studies culminated in a practical form of therapy for some patients when hepatic coma is due to an elevation of blood ammonia. This form of hepatic coma is characterized by lethargy, coma, convulsions and death.

As early as 1893 Hahn, Massen, Nenki and Pavlov[39] described a form of hepatic encephalopathy related to an increased intake of nitrogenous food in Eck-fistula dogs. Monguio and Kraus[39] detected elevated levels of blood ammonias in these circumstances and concluded that this type of encephalopathy was the result of ammonia intoxication. Several clinical studies 30 years ago related ammonia intoxication to hepatic coma in patients with cirrhosis of the liver. Bollman and Mann[38] demonstrated a rise in the concentration of ammonia in the peripheral blood after hepatectomy, again implicating the liver as the organ of ammonia detoxification.

Krebs[32] showed ammonia to be used in the synthesis of urea by the liver cells, and Foster et al.[23] demonstrated that ammonium nitrogen was converted rapidly to amide nitrogen, probably as the amide group of glutamine through an interaction of ammonia with glutamic acid. This reaction probably is the normal mechanism for preventing excessive accumulations of blood ammonia. These are the basic papers leading to our current understanding of ammonia intoxication and encephalopathy and their relationship to glutamic acid metabolism.

Based on Krebs'[32] observations that brain slices were able to synthesize glutamine from glutamic acid and ammonia at a fairly rapid rate in the presence of glucose, Sapirstein[39] demonstrated that convulsions in rabbits caused by the intravenous injection of ammonium chloride could be prevented if glutamic acid were given first. In 1952 Davidson et al.[39] and Stahl et al.[39] reported ammonia intoxication in patients with liver disease and

portacaval shunts. In 1954 McDermott and Adams[37] instituted a series of studies demonstrating a critical elevation of blood ammonia in the peripheral blood to be a constant finding in Eck-fistula animals with "meat intoxication." This Boston group[38, 39] and others claimed recently that the administration of L-glutamine acid (25 Gm. daily intravenously or orally) was an effective means of lowering the blood-ammonia concentration in patients with hepatic coma; apparently a number of their patients responded with the prompt disappearance of their neurologic symptoms. The glutamine formed from glutamic acid binds the circulating blood ammonia, and the end product, glutamine, appears to be excreted promptly in the urine.

This method of management of hepatic coma may be particularly useful when recovery depends primarily upon survival of ammonia encephalopathy. It does not appear to alter the course of liver disease. As other causes of coma exist in the terminal phase of hepatic disease, the relief of hepatic coma achieved by the administration of L-glutamic acid depends upon the importance of the etiologic role of ammonia intoxication in the production of the encephalopathy in the particular patient.

The normal peripheral blood-ammonia concentration is about 50 μg. per cent. Symptoms of intoxication begin to appear between levels of 150 and 250 μg. Most patients are comatose when the level exceeds 250 μg. per cent, and it may rise to 450 or 500 μg. before death, especially after hemorrhage into the alimentary tract.[39]

Indications for Operation

The 2 principal features of portal hypertension amenable to surgical therapy are the bleeding varix and the relief of portal hypertension itself. The major point of concern is the surgical decompression of the portal system: (1) When should it be performed? (2) And what does it offer in long-term gains to the patient? These questions beg 2 more: (1) What percentage of patients with esophagogastric varices will experience bleeding before death? (2) Is there any evidence that restoring the normal portal pressure reduces the extent of residual liver damage or retards

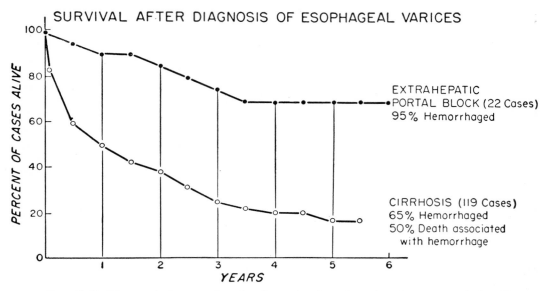

FIG. 33-10. The survival rates after the diagnosis of esophageal varices was made in 119 patients with an intrahepatic portal bed block and in 22 patients with an extrahepatic block seen at the Massachusetts General Hospital from 1934 to 1945 and treated by conservative measures without the benefit of shunt surgery. (Merendino & Volwiler: Northwest Med. 52:724)

or reverses its course? Neither can be answered with much assurance at this time.

Fate of Untreated Patients With Portal Hypertension. A number of reports are to be found from which it would appear that more than 50 per cent of patients with portal hypertension and varices die within a year or two, either from liver disease or hemorrhage, or both.[7, 34, 43, 52] Unfortunately, such reports may not be representative of a cross section of the patients at large who are suffering from portal hypertension. Those with subhepatic portal hypertension and no liver disease live longer; when death does occur in this group, usually it is from hemorrhage and its complications. The larger group of patients with portal hypertension are those of the intrahepatic variety. They die of liver disease as well as of hemorrhage and hepatic coma. Those with portal hypertension of the suprahepatic type may die of their primary disease, with liver failure and hemorrhage infrequently playing a major role in the death.

If one restricts his study to those patients with intrahepatic portal hypertension, death is said to occur in 50 to 80 per cent of cases within 1 to 2 years after the patient is first

seen; this does not answer well the basic question relative to duration of survival after the onset of liver disease or the first appearances of varices.

Mortality at the Massachusetts General Hospital between the years 1934 and 1945 inclusive[52] disclose that 54 per cent were dead within 1 year after the onset of hemorrhage; 65 per cent died in 2 years; and 77 per cent were dead after 4 years. Among those with subhepatic portal block and no liver disease, 5 per cent were dead in 1 year and 26 per cent died by the 4th year. In comparing mortality risk of repeated hemorrhage in patients with varices with and without cirrhosis, Merendino and Volwiler[43] found the mortality rate to be 5 times greater among those with cirrhosis; 17 per cent of their cases died after the 1st hemorrhage. Others report similarly discouraging results when portal hypertension is not relieved (Figs. 33-10 and 33-11).

The author agrees with Blakemore[7] that current data and experience warrant early shunting of the venous circulation to avoid the ravages of hemorrhage and its potential sequelae: aspiration pneumonia, ammonia intoxication and exsanguination. Whether or not

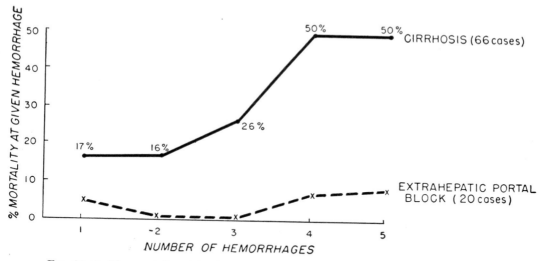

FIG. 33-11. The mortality risk of repeated hemorrhages from esophageal varices observed in 66 patients with an intrahepatic portal bed block and 20 patients with an extrahepatic block, taken from the records of the Massachusetts General Hospital from 1934 to 1945. (Merendino & Volwiler: Northwest Med. *52*:724)

regression in liver disease may occur in some patients after portal decompensation is not yet known. Thus, the presence of varices in portal hypertension is reason for a shunting procedure, provided that liver function is not disturbed seriously. Not all agree with this view.

SELECTION OF PATIENTS WITH PORTAL HYPERTENSION FOR SURGICAL TREATMENT

The same principles for evaluating surgical risk in patients with liver disease apply to patients requiring surgical decompression or hemostatic operations for intrahepatic or suprahepatic portal hypertension. Usually those with subhepatic portal hypertension are free of liver disease. However, tests of liver function, as well as needle biopsy of the liver, usually are as essential to the correct interpretation as to the pathogenesis and the general location of portal obstruction and the state of hepatic reserve. These studies are basic to case selection in the surgical treatment of portal hypertension.

Linton[34] has pointed out certain clinical features that he believes may play a role of equal or greater importance in case selection

than the laboratory tests of hepatic function. The clinical classification presented herein is modified from that employed by Linton. In each instance portal hypertension with demonstrated esophagogastric varices is presumed, with or without a previous episode of bleeding.

Excellent surgical risks are those patients with subhepatic portal hypertension and no evidence of cirrhosis or hepatitis. Varices with or without a previous history of bleeding are their only evidence of portal hypertension. Secondary hypersplenism may or may not be present. The one disappointing surgical feature in this group of patients that is of fairly common occurrence is splenic and/or portal vein thrombosis. These veins often are resolved in cavernous recanalization, leaving little or no opportunity for shunting the portal circulation. Operative mortality is minimal, and, so far as is known now, long-term survival is compatible with normal life expectancy if an adequate shunting procedure can be performed and maintained.

Good surgical risks are those patients with mild to moderate liver disease who are without jaundice, fever or ascites and in whom the serum albumin level is above 3.5 Gm. per cent. These are patients in whom cirrhosis is minimal to moderate and not complicated by hepatitis or cholangitis. A shunting procedure generally can be performed with less than 10 per cent mortality and with good reason to anticipate a 5-year or longer survival without difficulty.

Moderate surgical risks are those patients whose tests of hepatic function are not altered severely. The serum albumin remains above 3.0 Gm. per cent; these patients may have 15 to 25 per cent bromsulphalein retention but no icterus, or elevation of serum bilirubin or histologic evidence of active hepatitis. With these limitations the presence or the absence of ascites is not too important; in fact, the maintenance of the serum-albumin level above 3.0 Gm. per cent when ascites is present is good evidence that hepatic function is better than reflected by the serum-albumin level. Shunting procedures generally can be carried out in this group of patients with less than 15 per cent operative mortality and with an expectation that 4 out of 5 surviving will live a normal life for a number of years without ascites or hemorrhage.

Poor surgical risks are those patients with icterus, ascites and cirrhosis of long standing and increasing in severity, and in whom the serum albumin is less than 3.0 Gm. per cent with a reversal of the A/G ratio. An analysis of the course of such patients discloses that it is within this group that posthemorrhagic hepatic coma is most likely to develop, ascites is not relieved by shunting operations, and liver disease is most likely to progress with death from hepatic failure only months to a year or two away despite any form of treatment. A successful shunting operation may avoid subsequent hemorrhage, but generally it has little if any other influence upon the patient's course. Yet, within this group there are a few patients who may benefit from a shunting procedure with relief from ascites, avoidance of hemorrhage and survival for periods longer than 5 years. These are the patients whose general condition improves under conservative management over a period of time. Generally they are those whose hepatic function is impaired temporarily and disproportionately and whose liver disease is, by comparison, less severe than suggested by either clinical or other laboratory findings.

Some are patients with an exacerbation or superimposed bout of hepatitis. If operation can be delayed until the patient's general condition improves, then he may be operated upon as a moderate-risk patient and possibly with a good prognosis.

MANAGEMENT OF THE PATIENT WITH THE BLEEDING VARIX

Causes of Death in Patients with Bleeding Varices. There is little disagreement among surgeons that surgery should not be performed for the relief of portal hypertension when the patient is bleeding actively. This opinion has crystallized out of the bad experience of the past decade in surgical attempts at hemostasis or portal diversion carried out during active episodes of bleeding. In spite of the successful control of hemorrhage and hemorrhagic shock, 2 complications have not been avoided often or treated successfully in these circumstances. They are hepatic coma and aspiration pneumonitis.

Hepatic coma, already discussed, may arise from the digestion of blood remaining within the alimentary tract.

Aspiration bronchopneumonitis in the absence of hepatic failure is the major cause of death in patients with massive upper gastro-intestinal bleeding, short of exsanguination itself.[2] The bleeding varix or, for that matter, the bleeding gastric ulcer usually fills the stomach with blood fairly promptly, and about the time the stomach is distended sufficiently to induce vomiting the sensorium is dulled by the hypoxia of hypovolemic shock from blood loss. The patient feels faint and often becomes unconscious before he has a massive bout of hematemesis. Thus the stage is set for aspiration of some of the gastric contents into the tracheobronchial tree. The gastric aspirate is highly irritating and induces edema of the bronchial mucosa shortly after contact; generally this continues as a bronchopneumonia. The presence of blood in the gastric aspirate may neutralize partially the acidity of gastric juice, but this potential benefit is overcome by the numerous small clots of blood lodged in the periphery of the bronchial tree and the excellent culture media that they provide for prompt bacterial growth. Patients rarely recover from these misfortunes.

The patient with the bleeding varix preseiting himself for the first time is an unresolved risk in that his hepatic function cannot be assessed rapidly or accurately under such conditions. Conservative management with esophagogastric tamponade is strongly indicated. Later a shunting procedure may be indicated.

Esophagogastric Tamponade. Because of the high mortality rate in patients with cirrhosis and portal hypertension whose varix bleeds—75 per cent in the Sengstaken-Blakemore[50] series—nonoperative measures to control hemorrhage have been explored vigorously. To date the most successful is the employment of a balloon tamponade devised by these 2 investigators. This is a triple lumen tube: one arm of it serves to inflate a sausage-shaped balloon to compress against the esophageal wall; the 2nd arm leads to a globular-shaped balloon which, when inflated, remains in the stomach; the 3rd leads to the distal tip of the tube, serves to aspirate the stomach and enables the surgeon to wash it free of clots. To be effective in the arrest of hemorrhage, both balloons are inflated to a pressure of 25 to 30 mm. of mercury. When they are in proper position, as determined by fluoroscopic examination, traction is placed on the tube entering the patient's nasal passage or mouth. This in turn exerts its greatest point of pressure at the esophagogastric junction, occluding the veins in this area and often controlling bleeding. The tube leading into the stomach is irrigated at hourly intervals to be certain that bleeding does not recur. Within 48 to 96 hours the inflation pressures and traction are released. If further bleeding does not occur within 24 hours, the tube is removed. This is a very useful form of treatment, and it should be tried carefully in all cases of bleeding from the varices of portal hypertension. Bennett, *et al.*[5] in 1952 and Conn[13] in 1958 have clearly presented an intrinsic danger in the use of these tubes. Sudden rupture of one of the balloons while in position within the esophagus leads to a calamatous situation; the counterweight utilized for traction pulls the remaining intact balloon suddenly into the oropharynx with asphyxiation of the patient.

Injection of Varices with Sclerosing Solutions. Transesophageal injection of the esophageal varices with sclerosing solutions was introduced in 1930 by Crafoord and Frenckner.[15] The results were occasionally good, but usually only temporary, multiple repeated injection being required as a rule. This procedure still should be tried if bleeding is not controlled with tamponade and the patient's general condition does not permit of more elaborate surgery when seen.

Use of Drugs to Decrease Portal Hypertension. Intravenous pituitrin or pitressin have been demonstrated recently to be of value in the treatment of bleeding esophageal varices (Schwartz, *et al.*,[49] 1959). Twenty clinical units of either drug are diluted in 200 cc. of 5 per cent dextrose in distilled water and administered intravenously over a period of 20 to 30 minutes. This dose may be repeated in 4 hours if recurrent bleeding occurs. The authors suggest careful monitoring of the blood pressure during administration and also warn against use of this technic in patients with a past history of coronary thrombosis or angina pectoris. On the basis of their clinical observations, they recommend that this regimen be given an initial trial in control of bleeding from esophageal varices. Eiseman *et al.*[21] (1959) have presented experimental evidence that the decrease in portal pressure subsequent to use of surgical pituitrin or pitressin is due to closure of gastroenteric submucosal arteriovenous shunts.

OPERATIONS FOR THE RELIEF OF PORTAL HYPERTENSION AND THE THREAT OF BLEEDING

Direct Shunting of Portal Blood Around the Liver. This procedure was performed first by von Eck in 1877,[20] a side-to-side anastomosis being made between the portal vein and the vena cava. After the anastomosis was completed, the portal vein adjacent to the porta hepatis was ligated so that all portal blood circumvented the liver. Although this has been a useful physiologic preparation, the operation was used in patients only rarely prior to 1945 and then, with few exceptions, usually to anastomose smaller branches of the portal bed with the vena cava.

Whipple, Blakemore and Lord[62] attacked the problem of portal hypertension directly, beginning sixteen years ago. They anastomosed the splenic vein to the left renal vein. Within the following decade, various modifications of their procedure were introduced with the successful decompression of portal hypertension in suitable patients. Among the more prominent modifications are the end-to-side or the side-to-side portacaval anastomosis. The end-to-side anastomosis is the easiest to perform technically and is the least likely to thrombose; its disadvantage may be largely theoretical. It diverts all portal flow away from the liver, and in doing so may present a greater threat of ammonia intoxication. The lateral portacaval or the splenorenal anastomosis has in its favor the theoretical advantage that not all portal blood bypasses the liver. The author favors the latter 2 procedures and has experienced no serious difficulty or recurrence of bleeding in patients treated in this way. However, most surgeons prefer the end-to-side portacaval because of the ease with which it can be accomplished. When ascites is present, there is a marked difference of opinion as to the most efficacious method, i.e., end-to-end or side-to-side (Welch, et al.,[61] 1959; Madden,[40] 1959).

Shunting the superior or the inferior mesenteric veins may be all that can be accomplished in patients whose portal and/or splenic vein is thrombosed. These are less satisfactory procedures, as generally they do not divert sufficient blood to decompress the portal pressure

adequately. Merendino and Dillard[42] (1955) suggested the use of an interposed jejunal segment between the esophagus and the stomach to prevent regurgitation of acid onto the varix with subsequent erosion and hemorrhage in these unfortunate patients. Habif[26] (1959) has reported excellent results with this technic.

Portal pressure normally ranges between 10 and 15 cm. of water. Increases of the ranges of 25 to 65 cm. are generally found in portal hypertension. Most observers believe that portal pressure should be reduced below 20 cm. of water, preferably below 15, if recurrence of bleeding is to be avoided.

Omentopexy was introduced by Morison,[19] Talma[55] and others about 1900. It was their hope that suturing the omentum to the abdominal wall would promote vascular adhesions and thereby shunt some of the portal blood to the systemic circuit through such collaterals. Its failure is now understood in that the volume of blood such adhesions may carry is much too small to be effective in reducing portal hypertension.

Splenectomy crept into the treatment of portal hypertension originally because it afforded a means of relief of the discomfort produced by the enlarged spleen. Any benefits to portal hypertension soon were recognized as

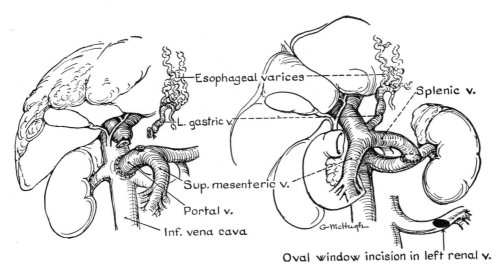

FIG. 33-12. (*Left*) Shows a portacaval end-to-side anastomosis wherein the coronary vein is divided and ligated in this particular instance in the treatment of portal hypertension. (*Right*) Illustrates the technics of end-to-side splenorenal anastomosis. Note the oval window made in the renal vein to ensure its continued patency.

being limited to patients without cirrhosis. It was not realized until recent years that the patients whose course splenectomy relieved were those few patients whose portal obstruction was limited primarily to the splenic vein. The concept of segmental portal occlusion was largely an outgrowth of the work of Whipple and Blakemore; this concept has done much to explain the heretofore random results obtained from splenectomy in portal hypertension.

The relief from the secondary hypersplenism that often accompanies enlargement of the spleen (see Chap. 32, "Spleen") is reason enough for removal of the spleen in portal hypertension. However, this procedure should not be carried out in this disease unless the surgeon is certain that he can perform either a splenorenal or a portacaval anastomosis at the same time. He may not do this later.

Surgical Hemostasis. Treatment of bleeding varices otherwise uncontrolled has been explored by many, and occasionally it is the only successful therapy that can be employed today. In general, it is not the primary surgical treatment of choice; nonetheless, in a few patients it may be the only treatment possible. In 1926, Flerow[22] attempted to devascularize in part the blood flow to and from the lower esophagus and the upper stomach by ligating the left gastric artery and vein, the short gastrics and the inferior mesenteric vein. These procedures have failed to prevent hemorrhage.

Esophagogastrectomy and Gastric Bisection. In 1945, Phemister and Humphreys[46] reported on esophagogastrectomy as a means of controlling bleeding varices. This procedure is reserved for patients whose portal and splenic veins are not suited for shunting operations. The results reported have been good. The development of collaterals later on with return of hemorrhage is anticipated but has been an infrequent event.

Tanner,[56] and later the author,[2] introduced gastric bisection, wherein the left gastric artery and vein are ligated and divided, splenectomy is performed, and the stomach sectioned completely at the level of its proximal fourth, and simply reanastomosed (Fig. 33-13). Occasionally, a sleeve of the distal segment of stomach is resected to avoid necrosis, in case the blood supply to this portion appears

to be impaired after bisection. This eliminates successfully all venous bridges between the major portal tributaries and the collaterals of the lower esophagus and the upper stomach. It has the advantage that it can be performed through an abdominal incision, if need be, without entering the chest. As neither this procedure nor the Phemister resection can be performed without a vagotomy, a gastroenterostomy should be carried out at the time of resection or bisection. The resulting hypoacidity should favor the healing of any peptic esophagitis,[58] and to date (6 years) experience with this procedure appears to warrant its use when shunting cannot be accomplished and hemorrhage otherwise is uncontrolled.

Suture of the bleeding varix by the transthoracic approach, exposing and opening the lower esophagus and the upper stomach, has been advocated by Blakemore,[50] Linton,[35, 36] Crile[16] and Cohn and Mathewson.[12] This procedure has given good temporary relief in bleeding patients whose hemorrhage is uncontrolled by tamponade. Its disadvantage is the transthoracic approach required. When performed during the active bleeding state, the patient's condition generally is poor, and already he may have developed aspiration or pneumonitis to compromise his air exchange, if the transthoracic approach is used. Linton's results are good.

Emergency Portacaval Shunting. There has been relatively little experience with this technic. Mikkelsen and Pattison[45] reported their experiences in 11 patients. They concluded that the operative mortality was little different from more temporizing procedures and that continued effective control of bleeding was more likely with portacaval shunt. Wantz and Payne[60] (1959) and Rousselot et al.[48] (1960) reported similar experiences.

Hepatic Artery Ligation. Ligation of the hepatic artery, wherein this vessel is ligated proximal to the gastroepiploic artery, thereby allowing some collateral arterial flow to enter the distal hepatic artery via the gastroduodenal artery, is a method devised in 1951 by Rienhoff[47] for the treatment of portal hypertension and bleeding varices. Its merits rest on the 1907 report of F. C. Herrick,[29] who believed that he demonstrated the development of abnormal arteriolar connections with the small portal radicals in cirrhosis; thus it

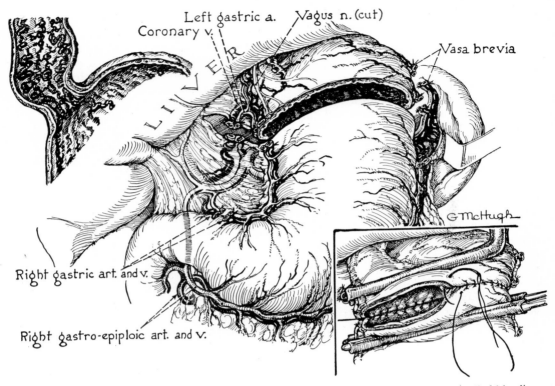

FIG. 33-13. Gastric bisection as employed by the author in the treatment of uncontrolled bleeding from esophageal gastric varices in the patient with portal hypertension. Note that the spleen is removed, the vagi are divided, as are the left gastric artery and the coronary vein, as well as the right gastric arteries and the vein to the lesser curvature of the stomach. The blood supply to the greater curvature is preserved. The stomach is re-anastomosed with 2 rows of continuous suture and a gastroenteroplasty or pyeloplasty is performed. Subsequently a portacaval anastomosis may be performed, if desired. Resection of 2 or 3 inches of upper end of distal segment of stomach should be considered if arterial blood supply to stomach seems to be in question. (Allen and Head: S. Clin. North America *36*:119)

is concluded that to reduce the arterial blood flow would lower portal pressure. The merits of both the concept and the therapeutic results claimed remain in controversy; some who have tried this operation report death from hepatic necrosis. The procedure is not advocated at this time.

MESENTERIC THROMBOSIS

Acute occlusion of the mesenteric vessels usually is thrombo-embolic in origin and may affect either the arterial or the venous side of the splanchnic circulation, or both. The superior mesenteric vessels or their major branches are involved more commonly than the inferior mesenterics; in either case this condition generally represents an acute surgical emergency. Its treatment is prompt resection of the segment of bowel involved.

ETIOLOGY

In acute mesenteric occlusion, thrombosis of the mesenteric arteries is rarely encountered; when thrombosis occurs, it is much more likely to be in the portal or its tributaries. On the other hand, embolism is the usual cause of acute occlusion of the mesenteric arteries but rarely the primary cause of acute mesenteric venous occlusion, though thrombotic extension distal to site of lodgment of the arterial embolus is a common occurrence. The factors favoring either arterial or venous thrombosis of the mesenteric vessels are similar to those also predisposing to thrombosis in vessels elsewhere.

Stasis in unrelieved portal hypertension is a common cause of portal thrombosis as exemplified by the occurrence of thrombosis of the splenic and the portal veins reported after splenectomy is performed for portal hypertension of any type. A patient with the Budd-Chiari type of portal hypertension, measuring 65 cm. of water, explored by the author and no possible site for a shunting procedure found, died on the 4th postoperative day of acute portal vein thrombosis. Presumably, the trauma of venous exposure plus portal stasis prepared the ground for the sequence of events that followed.

Phlebitis secondary to inflammatory diseases of the bowel, such as diverticulitis, appendicitis and secondarily infected carcinoma of the bowel, are the sources of septic mesenteric thrombophlebitis usually encountered. Such thrombi are extensive and may extend to involve the entire portal system; or they may fragment, giving rise to septic emboli that lodge within the liver, causing intrahepatic abscess formation. Dehydration with hemoconcentration or pronounced polycythemia with its elevated platelet levels is occasionally associated with either thrombosis or embolic disorders in the splanchnic vessels. The thrombotic tendency of Buerger's disease also affects the mesenteric vessels occasionally and can cause mesenteric thrombosis.

Arterial emboli to the mesenteric arteries arise from the usual sites of arterial emboli to other portions of the body. Vegetative endocarditis, mitral stenosis with auricular fibrillation, early postcoronary heart disease and the thrombi formed at the site of atheromatous plaques within the aorta or at sites of vascular aortic grafts interposed between the heart and the origin of the superior mesenteric artery are among the prominent causes of arterial emboli to the mesenteric vessels. Probably the reason that the inferior mesenteric artery seldom is the site of lodgment of an embolus is that only small emboli can enter this vessel, and when this occurs their lodgment is likely to be at the site of the division of the inferior mesenteric artery into the left colic, the sigmoidal or the superior hemorrhoidal vessels. The collateral flow of the arterial circulation from the middle colic and the middle hemorrhoidals, through the arcades of the inferior mesenteric arteries peripheral to the embolus, appears to be able to sustain the left colon in many instances (see Fig. 33-7). Emboli to the inferior mesenteric artery may occur with greater frequency than is believed, as many may produce few or no symptoms.

Occasionally, blunt trauma to the abdomen or a dissecting aneurysm of the aorta or the superior mesenteric artery may be the cause of mesenteric infarction.

PATHOLOGY OF INFARCTED BOWEL

Acute venous occlusion of the portal or the superior mesenteric vein is followed promptly by hyperemia, edema and subserosal petechial hemorrhages of the infarcted segment of bowel and its mesentery. In massive venous occlusion, death from hypovolemic shock occurs usually in less than 24 hours and is believed to be due to the continuing arterial blood flow into the splanchnic bed without adequate venous drainage or return. The bowel and the mesenteric surfaces are found "weeping" serosanguineous fluid, and the patient, aside from having abdominal pain, usually complains of bloody diarrhea, presumably due to venous engorgement of the intestinal mucosa. Should the patient survive long enough, thrombosis of the mesenteric artery is the likely sequela.

Acute occlusion of the mesenteric arteries produces bowel necrosis without the hypovolemic disturbances seen in extensive venous thrombosis. Bloody diarrhea is less commonly a complaint, although abdominal pain is generally present. Death from the gangrenous bowel and its peritonitis is the usual end-result if the bowel is not resected. Of these 2 types of vascular occlusion, arterial embolic occlusion is more likely to be amenable to successful surgical treatment than is venous thrombosis.

In some patients the clinical course of mesenteric thrombosis is comparatively mild, progressing for a week or 10 days before the patient is seen by his physician. If these cases could be diagnosed early, extensive bowel resection might be avoided in many instances.

DIAGNOSIS

Often the diagnosis is not made preoperatively unless the causes of arterial or venous mesenteric occlusion are evident. In major infarctions, the acute onset of severe abdominal or back pain, vomiting, bloody diarrhea, with progressive tenderness of the midabdomen, generally are observed. Bowel sounds are present, and during the early hours may be somewhat hyperactive. As ischemia progresses to necrosis, peristalsis becomes hypoactive and disappears if generalized peritonitis develops. Colicky pain is not observed unless, as happens occasionally, the proximal viable bowel intussuscepts with the distal infarcted segmen (Harkins, 1936; Hardy, 1960).

Gradual occlusion of the superior mesenteric artery may result in a syndrome characterized by intermittent abdominal pain, weight loss and intestinal malabsorption (Shaw and Maynard, 1958).

In venous occlusion a rise in pulse rate and a decline in blood pressure occur fairly early. Distention of the abdomen is not usually a prominent feature of either arterial or venous mesenteric occlusion.

TREATMENT

Early operative intervention with surgical excision of the nonviable segment of bowel involved is the only treatment that will prevent death. In those patients in whom occlusion is either incomplete or located in vascular segments which collateral circulation can sustain, resection is not necessary and perhaps contraindicated as the intact cyanotic bowel may recover. If such bowel is resected, the healing of the anastomosis may be impaired and leak a few days later. In cases of questionable viability, the bowel segment may be exteriorized and covered with a protective sterile dressing for a day or two to observe its course (Wangensteen, 1955). Black bowel does not always indicate dead bowel; the petechial subserosal hemorrhages of infarcted bowel may hemolyze, become confluent, and the hematin pigments turn black. In several patients in whom the infarcted bowel segment (generally the colon) was jet black but its peristaltic activity persisted, the author exteriorized the loops involved. A day or two later the color returned entirely to normal and the bowel was obviously viable. The loops were returned to the abdomen, and the patients recovered. With increasing awareness of the entity superior mesenteric artery occlusion, more cases can

be treated successfully by thrombectomy, endarterectomy and/or resection of the involved bowel (Glotzer and Shaw, 1959; Shaw and Maynard, 1958; Hardy, 1960; Stewart, Sweetman, Westphal and Wise, 1960).

Extent of bowel resection compatible with life varies considerably. Experience has shown that some patients with as much as three fourths of the small bowel resected survive to live a normal existence after a few months (Bierman, Ulevitch, Haft and Lemish, 1950). Generally such extensive resections are tolerated better by adults than by children. A number of successful resections of major portions of the small bowel, often with resection of the right colon, have been reported in recent years (Christensen, Musgrove and Wollaeger, 1950). Most of these patients suffer severe diarrhea for a few weeks but may appear to be able to compensate for bowel loss after a few months. Thereafter, they may have 1 to 3 liquid bowel movements a day and maintain or gain weight. On the other hand, some patients do not respond; diarrhea and malnutrition continue; and eventually after many months they die in spite of vigorous medical management.

Anticoagulant therapy may be of value in the management of acute arterial mesenteric occlusion, but it is not without greater hazard of hemorrhage than usual during the acute episode (Laufman, 1942; Wangensteen, 1955). Generally, anticoagulants should not be used in venous mesenteric occlusion unless the extent of the occlusion, edema of the bowel and hemorrhagic enteritis are minimal or absent. Subsequent to the patient's recovery from arterial embolic occlusion, the author prefers to maintain the patient on Dicumarol indefinitely if the potential sources of emboli from the heart or the aorta persist.

Aneurysms (mycotic or dissecting) may produce sufficient pain to encourage surgical exploration before bowel necrosis occurs. In some of these patients the aneurysm may have occluded the vessel slowly and, therefore, usually can be ligated or excised, as adequate collateral circulation will have been established. In others, the situation may be less favorable, and in a few patients rupture of the aorta or the superior mesenteric aneurysm results in death promptly from hemorrhage or from bowel necrosis caused by dissection of blood within the arterial wall, compressing the lumen of the mesenterics.

PROGNOSIS

Recovery of patients with acute mesenteric occlusion depends largely upon 3 conditions, singularly or collectively: (1) duration of time between onset of symptoms and surgical exploration; (2) the extent of bowel resection required; and (3) the seriousness of the predisposing factors responsible for mesenteric occlusion. These are largely clinical situations unlikely to be modified greatly within the near future. In 1955 Wangensteen[59] reported 100 per cent mortality among patients not resected and 33 per cent mortality when operated upon. Of 47 patients operated upon with this disease in 1904, only 4 survived (Jackson, Porter and Quinby, 1904). In 1935 Douglas[18] reported 4 survivals among 11 patients operated upon.

Most agree that early surgical therapy offers the patient his best chance of survival; the conservative forms of therapy, including the use of anticoagulants, should be considered only after the operation is performed.

REFERENCES

1. Allen, J. G.: The clinical value of the functional tests of the liver; a review with a special study of the plasma prothrombin, Gastroenterology 3:6, 1944.
2. Allen, J. G., and Head, L. R.: The diagnosis of portal hypertension with notes on treatment, S. Clin. North America 36:119-130, 1956.
3. Barlow, T. E.: Vascular patterns in the alimentary canal, in Visceral Circulation (Ciba Foundation Symposium), Boston, Little, Brown & Co., 1953.
4. Barlow, T. E.: Variations in the blood-supply of the upper jejunum, Brit. J. Surg. 43:473, 1956.
5. Bennett, H. D., Baker, L., and Baker, L. A.: Complications in use of esophageal compression balloons (Sengstaken tube), A.M.A. Arch. Int. Med. 90:196-200, 1952.
6. Bierman, L. G., Ulevitch, H., Haft, H. H., and Lemish, S.: Metabolic studies of an unusual case survival following resection of all but 18 inches of small bowel, Ann. Surg. 132:64, 1950.
7. Blakemore, A. H.: The portacaval shunt for portal hypertension with special reference to cirrhosis of the liver, Bull, New York Acad. Med. 27:477-494, 1951.
8. Boyd, J. D.: General survey of visceral vascular structures, in Visceral Circulation (Ciba Foundation Symposium), Boston, Little, Brown & Co., 1953.
9. Brandes, W. W.: The effect of mechanical constriction of the hepatic veins, Arch. Int. Med. 44:676-692, 1929. Quoted by Child, C. G.: The Hepatic Circulation and Portal Hypertension, p. 190, Philadelphia, Saunders, 1954.
10. Budd, G.: Diseases of the liver, Lancet 1: 654, 1850. Quoted by Child, C. G.: The Hepatic Circulation and Portal Hypertension, p. 120, Philadelphia, Saunders, 1954.
11. Christensen, N. A., Musgrove, J. E., and Wollaeger, E. E.: Extensive resection of bowel for occlusion of the superior mesenteric artery, Proc. Staff Meet. Mayo Clin. 25:449, 1950.
12. Cohn, R., and Mathewson, C., Jr.: Observations on patients during the surgical treatment of acute massive hemorrhage from esophageal varices secondary to cirrhosis of the liver, Surgery 41:94-99, 1957.
13. Conn, H. O.: Hazards attending the use of esophageal tamponade, New England J. Med. 259:701-707, 1958.
14. Conn, J. W.: Primary aldosteronism, J. Lab. & Clin. Med. 45:3, 1955.
15. Crafoord, C., and Frenckner, P.: New surgical treatment of varicose veins of the esophagus, Acta Oto-laryng. 27:422-429, 1939.
16. Crile, G., Jr.: Transesophageal ligation of bleeding esophageal varices, Arch. Surg. 61: 654-660, 1950.
17. Cruveilhier, J.: Traité d'anatomie descriptive, Paris, Bechet, 1834-6; ed. 2, Paris, Labe, 1843-5; ed. 4, Paris, Asselin, 1862-71.
18. Douglas, T.: Mesenteric vascular occlusion, Tr. Am. S. A. 53:155, 1935.
19. Drummond, D., and Morison, R.: A case of ascites due to cirrhosis of the liver, cured by operation, Brit. M.J. 2:728, 1896.
20. Eck, N. V. von: Ligature of portal vein, Voyemo-Med. J. 130:1, 1877.
21. Eiseman, B., Silen, W., Tyler, P., and Earley, T.: The portal hypotensive action of Pituitrin, S. Forum 10:286-291, 1959.
22. Flerow: Quoted by Child, C. G.: The Hepatic Circulation and Portal Hypertension, p. 225, Philadelphia, Saunders, 1954.
23. Foster, G. L., Schoenheimer, R., and Rittenberg, D.: Studies in protein metabolism. V. the utilization of ammonia for amino acid and creatine formation. J. Biol. Chem. 127: 319, 1939.

24. Glotzer, D. L., and Shaw, R. S.: Massive bowel infarction: an autopsy study assessing the potentialities of reconstructive vascular surgery, New England J. Med. *260*:162, 1959.

25. Grayson, J.: Observations on the blood flow in the human intestine, *in* Visceral Circulation (Ciba Foundation Symposium), Boston, Little, Brown & Co., 1953.

26. Habif, D. V.: Treatment of esophageal varices by partial esophagogastrectomy and interposed jejunal segment, Surgery *46*:212-237, 1959.

27. Hardy, J. D.: Surgery of the aorta and its branches, Am. Pract. & Digest Treat. *11*: 317, 1960.

28. Harkins, H. N.: Mesenteric vascular occlusion of arterial and venous origin, Arch. Path. *22*:637, 1936.

29. Herrick, F. C.: An experimental study into the cause of the increases of portal pressure in portal cirrhosis, J. Exper. Med. *9*:93-104, 1907.

30. Iverson, P., and Roholm, K.: On aspiration biopsy of the liver, with remarks on its diagnostic significance, Acta med. scandinav. *102*:1, 1939.

31. Jackson, J., Porter C., and Quinby, W.: Mesenteric embolism and thrombosis; a study of 214 cases, J.A.M.A. *42*:1469, 1904.

32. Krebs, H. A.: Metabolism of amino acids. IV. Synthesis of glutamine from glutamic acid and ammonia, and enzymic hydrolysis of glutamine in animal tissues, Biochem. J. 29:1951-69, 1935.

33. Laufman, H. F.: The effects of heparin on the behavior of infarction of the intestine, Surg., Gynec. & Obst. 74:479, 1942.

34. Linton, R. R.: Portacaval shunts in the treatment of portal hypertension, New England J. Med. *238*:723-727, 1948.

35. ———: Surgical treatment of bleeding esophageal varices by portal systemic venous shunt, Ann. Int. Med. *31*:794-804, 1949.

36. Linton, R. R., and Warren, R.: The emergency treatment of massive bleeding from esophageal varices by transesophageal suture of these vessels at the time of acute hemorrhage, Surgery *33*:243-255, 1953.

37. McDermott, W. V., Jr., and Adams, R. D.: Episodic stupor associated with Eck fistula in humans with particular reference to metabolism of ammonia, J. Clin. Invest. *33*:1, 1954.

38. McDermott, W. V., Jr., Adams, R. D., and Riddell, A. G.: Ammonia metabolism in man, Ann. Surg. *140*:539-556, 1954.

39. McDermott, W. V., Jr., Wareham, J., and

Riddell, A. G.: Treatment of hepatic coma with L-glutamic acid, New England J. Med. *253*:1093, 1955.

40. Madden, J. L.: Discussion, paper of Welch, C. S., Welch, H. F., and Carter, J. H.: The treatment of ascites by side to side portacaval shunt, Ann. Surg. *150*:442-444, 1959.

41. Mateer, J. G., Baltz, J. I., Marion, D. F., and MacMillan, J. M.: Liver function tests, J.A.M.A. *121*:723, 1943.

42. Merendino, K. A., and Dillard, D. H.: The concept of sphincter substitution by an interposed jejunal segment for anatomic and physiologic abnormalities at the esophagogastric junction: with special reference to reflux esophagitis, cardiospasm and esophageal varices, Ann. Surg. *142*:486-508, 1955.

43. Merendino, K. A., and Volwiler, W.: Medical and surgical aspects of portal hypertension, Northwest Med. *52*:724, 1953.

44. Michels, N. A.: Newer anatomy of liver-variant blood supply and collateral circulation, J.A.M.A. *172*:125, 1960.

45. Mikkelsen, W. P., and Pattison, A. C.: Emergency portacaval shunt, Am. J. Surg. *96*:183-190, 1958.

46. Phemister, D. B., and Humphreys, E. M.: Gastroesophageal resection and total gastrectomy in the treatment of bleeding varicose veins in Banti's syndrome, Ann. Surg. *126*:397-410, 1947.

47. Rienhoff, W. F., Jr.: Ligation of the hepatic and splenic arteries in the treatment of portal hypertension with a report of 6 cases: preliminary report, Bull. Johns Hopkins Hosp. *88*:365-375, 1951.

48. Rousselot, L. M., Gilbertson, F. E., and Panke, W. F.: Severe hemorrhage from esophagogastric varices—its emergency management with particular reference to portocaval anastomosis, New England J. Med. *262*:269-276, 1960.

49. Schwartz, S. I., Bales, H. W., Emerson, G. L., and Mahoney, E. B.: The use of intravenous pituitrin in treatment of bleeding esophageal varices, Surgery *45*:72-80, 1959.

50. Sengstaken, R. W., and Blakemore, A. H.: Balloon tamponage for the control of hemorrhage from esophageal varices, Ann. Surg. *131*:781-789, 1950.

51. Shaw, R. S., and Maynard, E. P.: Acute and chronic thrombosis of the mesenteric arteries associated with malabsorption: A report of two cases treated successfully by thromboendarterectomy, New England J. Med. *258*: 874, 1958.

52. Shull, H. J., Personal communication. Quoted

by Linton, R. R.: Portal hypertension, *in* Schiff, Leon: Diseases of the Liver, Philadelphia, Lippincott, 1956.

53. Spanner, R.: The arterio-venous anastomoses in the intestine, Anat. Anz., Supp., pp. 24-26, 1931.

54. Stewart, G. D., Sweetman, W. R., Westphal, K., and Wise, R. A.: Superior mesenteric artery embolectomy, Ann. Surg. *151*:274, 1960.

55. Talma, S.: Chirurgische Offnung neuer Seitenbahnen für das Blut der Vena Porta, Berlin klin. Wchnschr. *35*:833, 1898.

56. Tanner, N. C.: Hemorrhage as a surgical emergency, Proc. Roy. Soc. Med. *43*:147, 1950, and personal communication, 1954.

57. Walder, D.: Some observations on the blood flow of the human stomach, *in* Visceral Circulation (Ciba Foundation Symposium), Boston, Little, Brown & Co., 1953.

58. Wangensteen, O. H.: Discussion of Phemister and Humphreys.[46]

59. ———: Intestinal Obstructions, ed. 3, pp. 789, 790, Springfield, Ill., Thomas, 1955.

60. Wantz, G. E., and Payne, M. A.: The emergency portacaval shunt, Surg., Gynec. & Obst. *109*:549-554, 1959.

61. Welch, C. S., Welch, H. F., and Carter, J. H.: The treatment of ascites by side to side portacaval shunt, Ann. Surg. *150*:428-444, 1959.

62. Whipple, A. O.: The problem of portal hypertension in relation to hepatosplenopathies, Ann. Surg. *122*:449-475, 1945.

CHAPTER 34

Appendicitis and the Acute Abdomen

INTRODUCTION

At any age in life, the most common cause of acute inflammatory disease in the right lower quadrant of the abdomen in males, and probably in females, is acute appendicitis. This disease in the past has provoked more clinical studies and discussions centering about the differential diagnosis of acute inflammatory lesions of the abdomen and the management of their most serious complication—local or extensive peritonitis and abscess formation—than have been contributed by the writings on inflammation of all other abdominal organs combined.

In an extensive co-operative study involving a number of hospitals throughout the country, Castleton, Puestow and Sauer (1959) found that in these institutions whereas in 1941 appendectomy made up about 10 per cent of all surgical procedures, in 1956 this percentage had fallen to 2 per cent. The fall in the number of cases of *acute* appendicitis which were subjected to appendectomy was not quite so striking—the figures being 4 and 1.5 per cent,

respectively. Furthermore, during the 28-year period from 1911 to 1939, the death rate for appendicitis per 100,000 decreased only from 10.9 to 10.7, and in 1942 it had dropped to 5 and thereafter was progressively halved each year to 1956. The use of chemotherapeutic and antibiotic agents may explain part of this decrease in the treated cases and also may explain the actual decrease in incidence of the disease.

In some areas of the world, acute appendicitis is said to be unusual or rare; certain areas of Asia and Africa have been cited as examples. The explanation usually given is one pertaining to dietary habits of more primitive peoples. As a history of constipation is fairly frequent in patients with acute appendicitis in this country, the lack of it in countries whose inhabitants eat fruits and vegetables is believed to account for the reported differences in attack rates. However, all these reports do not take into account the high infant mortality rates or the poor quality of medical records in such areas. In consequence, these claims (low incidence of acute appendicitis and its explanation on dietary and bowel habits) cannot be accepted readily without greater assurance as to the validity of the original data.

Historical Note

Acute appendicitis probably is encountered with no less frequency than it was in 1759 when Mestivier[26] reported one of the first cases. This report is believed to be the first valid description of this disease, although Heister and Fernel may have been discussing appendicitis in their writings in 1581 and 1711 respectively. John Parkinson[29] in a case report published in 1812 is credited with the first description of a death from peritonitis following perforation of the appendix. Nearly

50 years earlier, de Lamotte[10] described autopsy findings wherein he attributed death to intestinal obstruction secondary to recurring attacks of appendicitis in which its lumen was occluded by "cherrylike" stones. Melier[25] in 1827 pointed out that perforating appendicitis was a frequent cause of peritonitis and death in the young adult, but the value of his observations and those of others were to be negated by the erroneous conclusions of the more influential Dupuytren who attributed the disease to the cecum rather than the appendix. Dupuytren persuaded Husson and Dance to accept his views, and they were expressing his views in their report of 1827.[17] Dupuytren[11] subsequently made known his own feelings in his lectures on clinical surgery in 1833.

It is not clear to this author that the indictment of Dupuytren in this connection should be as severe as generally quoted. True, Goldbeck[14] wrote his thesis at Heidelberg, expressing and adopting the French views in 1830; he coined the terms perityphlitis, attributing the disease to peri-inflammatory disease of the cecum (typhlon) in spite of the fact that his report contained also a recognized case of perforative appendicitis from fecal concretions and was associated with peritonitis. Burne[4] in 1837 recognized the fallacy of the French conclusions and made a strong appeal that their views be modified.

Boyce[3] credits Voltz in 1846 as reporting 38 cases of "intra-abdominal inflammation followed by perforation of the appendix as the result of fecal concretions." He is said to doubt that perforations of the appendix ever occurred in the absence of concretions except in tuberculosis and typhoid fever; he believed that perityphlitis is secondary to perforation of the cecum. Voltz distinguished between nonperforative and perforative appendicitis and subdivided the latter into those forming localized abscess and those which were not localized but progressed to generalized peritonitis. Boyce also states that Leudet concluded in 1859 that

Perforation of the ileocecal appendix is in itself more common than all other perforations of any part of the intestine whatever; it at least equals in frequency all perforations of the digestive tract taken collectively.

On the surface, these appear as convincing proof that acute appendicitis was generally recognized prior to 1886; but this was not true. This author examined several medical and surgical texts published between the years 1875 and 1885 and found no mention of appendicitis or that perityphlitis, typhlitis or paratyphlitis was considered as the result of appendicitis. As late as 1884, J. Graham Brown of Edinburgh, writing in *Birmingham's Medical Library,* discussed carefully the patient's attitude in acute peritonitis from "typhilitis," stating that "A patient with acute peritonitis lies with knees drawn up"; but nowhere is there reference in his writing to the fact that perforation of the inflamed appendix was a cause of this condition. That same year, 1884, Krönlein apparently first recognized a case of peritonitis as due to perforating appendicitis and performed the first planned appendectomy for this disease but the patient died.[18]

Hall of New York recorded in June of 1886 the first appendectomy performed in the United States. His preoperative diagnosis was in error, that of strangulated hernia. Thomas G. Morton of Philadelphia, according to Kelly and Hurdon,[18] appears to have performed the first successful appendectomy wherein the preoperative diagnosis was perforated appendicitis; the operation was performed for this disease; and the patient recovered. A concretion the size of a "cherry stone" was found near the appendix, both the concretion and the appendix lying in an abscessed cavity. Concretions, pins and other foreign bodies usually were reported to lie within the appendix or the abscess cavity in most of the early cases reported—from Mestivier's patient whose appendix contained a pin to that of Morton alluded to above.

The recognition of appendicitis as a clinical and pathologic entity, for which the surgical therapy was essential to recovery, was largely the result of the efforts of two men: Reginald Fitz, Professor of Pathologic Anatomy at Harvard, and Charles McBurney, a surgeon at St. Luke's Hospital in New York City. Fitz reported before the first meeting of the American Association of Physicians, held in Washington, D.C., on June 17, 1886, the general problem of perforated appendicitis and its sequelae—peritonitis and abscess formation.[12] He discarded the terms of typhlitis perityphlitis and paratyphlitis, calling attention "to the importance of the fact that in the vast majority of cases, the primary disease was an inflammation of the cecal appendix." He presented 257 cases of perforated appendicitis diagnosed anatomically and recognized that the one treatment which could be expected to give good results was an appendectomy performed early in the course of the disease. The Fitz report was convincing and was not allowed to lie dormant; he persisted in repeating his views and presented his data in an accurate and understandable manner. No one has succeeded in diminishing the importance of his contributions.

McBurney's contributions were those of formulating in an orderly and accurate arrangement the clinical features of early appendicitis, making possible the diagnosis prior to rupture.[23] He contributed to the operative considerations of appendectomy and insisted upon early appendectomy. The principles set forth by this surgeon continue as the basis for clinical and therapeutic practices of today.

ANATOMY OF THE APPENDIX

The vermiform appendix is the remnant of the apex of the cecum. The 3 longitudinal muscular bands (taenia coli) of the cecum arise at the base of the appendix and traverse the colon throughout its intra-abdominal length. Occasionally, the appendix is not easily located; if present it always will be found by following the taeniae downward to their point of origin at the apex of the cecum which conforms to the point of origin of the appendix. The appendix varies in length from 1 to 10 inches. It has its own mesentery, triangular in shape, in which course its blood and lymphatic vessels. The arterial blood supply is the appendicular artery, a branch of the terminal portion of the ileocolic artery.

The position of the appendix in relation to the caput of the cecum and the terminal ileum varies considerably. Some of these variations account for minor but important differences in the location of pain and tenderness which accompany an attack of appendicitis. The more commonly encountered positions of the course and the tip of the appendix in the abdomen are listed below in the order of the frequency generally found. These are also illustrated in Figure 34-1.

Positions in Which the Appendix Is More Commonly Found:

1. The right side of the false pelvis
2. The right iliac fossa beside the right iliac vessels
3. Mesially toward the sacral promontory
4. Posterior to the cecum, usually referred to as the retrocecal position
5. At the inferior angle of the ileocecal junction
6. Mesial or lateral to the cecum
7. Along the anterior surface of the cecum (infrequent)

The histology of the appendix is important to the cause of appendicitis in some patients, especially in the young (see below). The mucosa resembles that of the colon. In the submucosa are situated numerous lymph follicles which gradually atrophy with age. The muscular and serosal coats are also similar to those of the colon.

PATHOGENESIS OF ACUTE APPENDICITIS

The most frequent cause (about 90%) of acute appendicitis is occlusion of the lumen of the appendix. The usual cause is a fecal impaction or concretion and rarely a foreign body such as a seed. These concretions (fecaliths) may be solitary or multiple and may be located in the lumen at any point from appendiceal-cecal junction to its distal tip.

Locally, the concretion may produce ulceration of the mucosa with inflammatory response which, if allowed to continue, usually induces necrosis, gangrene and perforation. Occasionally, concretions are found in the appendix incidentally; thus, not all concretions produce appendicitis. Some of these may be calcified and identifiable by roentgenographic examination. At a later date, they may no longer be visible; presumably, in such cases, the fecalith has been expelled uneventfully into the cecum. Others may remain inactive indefinitely. Still others may lie dormant, sometimes for months to years, only to give rise to acute appendicitis at a later date. A case in point is that of a 62-year-old male who was on periodic medical management for the treatment of duodenal ulcer over a 20-year period. The roentgenogram in Figure 34-2 shows the presence of an appendiceal concre-

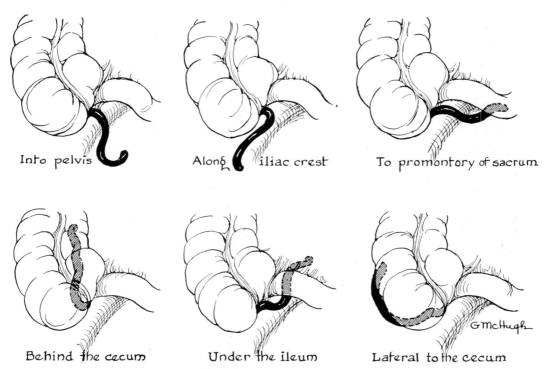

Into pelvis   Along iliac crest   To promontory of sacrum

Behind the cecum   Under the ileum   Lateral to the cecum

G McHugh

FIG. 34-1. The position of the appendix varies considerably; the more commonly encountered locations are illustrated. This factor of variation in its position can be important to the location of pain in general and of tenderness in particular.

tion present for at least 1 year prior to an attack of acute gangrenous appendicitis. Chemical analysis of the opaque concretion removed at appendectomy proved that it was largely barium sulfate. Presumably this resulted from one of the several barium meals administered in following the course of his duodenal ulcer. The last barium meal had been administered 12 months prior to the onset of acute appendicitis; the appendiceal concretion had been observed 18 months prior to that examination, or 30 months prior to his attack of appendicitis and appendectomy.

It is the author's impression as well as that of most writers, that constipation favors fecal impaction and therefore acute appendicitis. The occurrence of appendicitis in ulcer patients on calcium carbonate management in the author's experience seems to be encountered slightly more frequently than in the same age group at large. Constipation also is not a rare complication of pregnancy, at which time acute appendicitis also may be encountered.

Obstructive appendicitis may result from causes other than appendiceal concretions, fecaliths or foreign bodies. In children or young adults, the abundant lymphoid tissue in the submucosa of the appendix may undergo acute hyperplasia along with the lymphoid tissue elsewhere in response to systemic infections, especially those of the upper respiratory tract. The lymphoid hyperplasia may obstruct the appendiceal lumen temporarily, giving rise to appendicitis. In a large student population, the incidence of acute appendicitis increases at times of epidemics of respiratory diseases, possibly for this reason. In the older age patients, acute appendicitis may be a manifestation of carcinoma of the cecum obliterating or obstructing the appendiceal lumen. A carcinoma of the cecum should be searched for at the time of appendectomy if peritonitis is not present. A month or 6 weeks later the patient should be examined fluoroscopically and the stools examined at this time for the presence of occult blood.

As the individual ages, the appendix tends

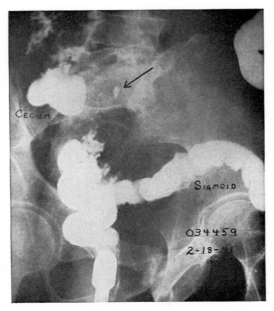

FIG. 34-2. Photograph of an opacity in the region of the appendix which had been interpreted as a probable appendiceal fecalith in a 62-year-old male. 30 months later appendectomy was performed for perforative appendicitis. The fecalith proved to be barium sulfate. The lumen was completely occluded by this barium concretion at the time of appendectomy, illustrating that some concretions within the appendix may remain dormant for long periods of time, but eventually some may produce trouble.

to atrophy; often this atrophy is not uniform, leaving certain areas in which the lumen is partially or totally obliterated and more distal ones in which the lumen remains. If the obliterated lumen involves only the proximal end of the appendix, the more distal portion remains patent and subject to subsequent infection. This is not an infrequently encountered setting responsible for acute appendicitis among older patients. Intestinal parasites, especially pinworms, may infest the appendiceal lumen, giving rise to acute appendicitis. Regional ileitis or ileo-ulcerative colitis at times also obstructs the proximal lumen and may cause appendicitis.

About 10 per cent of cases have no demonstrable or obvious cause to explain the attack. The author has seen one case in which a small

arterial embolus to the appendicular artery caused gangrenous appendicitis in a 69-year-old male. In this patient, the onset of pain began in the right lower quadrant; there was no epigastric distress.

The pathologic sequelae of acute appendicitis which occur within the first few days to few weeks after the attack are primarily those of peritonitis and abscess formation and septic thrombi of the portal tributaries which may in turn give rise to abscesses in the liver. Latent complications (months to years) are almost always those related to adhesions. The small bowel is either enmeshed in these adhesions from the beginning or a segment of bowel insinuates itself between adhesive bands, causing obstruction or volvulus. In either case, "closed loop" obstruction and ischemic necrosis of the bowel wall may occur.

NONPERFORATIVE ACUTE APPENDICITIS

There are several forms of appendicitis that should be distinguished. These include mild appendicitis, edematous and suppurative appendicitis, gangrenous appendicitis and perforative appendicitis.

CLINICAL ASPECTS OF ACUTE NONPERFORATIVE APPENDICITIS

Onset of Pain and Tenderness. The symptoms of nonperforative appendicitis were first described by Charles McBurney[23] of New York in 1889. He observed the early onset to be usually that of mild general abdominal pain beginning in the epigastrium; usually this is associated with acute loss of appetite and occasionally with nausea and vomiting. After a few hours, the pain localizes or "settles" in the right lower quadrant. Then the early and more generalized abdominal pain or distress may subside. A history of recent constipation is the rule, but the occasional patient may have experienced some diarrhea or no change in bowel habits.

Fever in nonperforative appendicitis, as McBurney pointed out, is slight, generally 99° to 100° F. The pulse rate is usually normal. The patient sometimes prefers to lie with flexion of the right thigh. Occasionally, reflex hyperesthesia is present along the cutaneous area supplied by the distribution of the right 10th, 11th and 12th intercostal nerves in the lower right side of the abdomen.

The point of greatest early *tenderness* usually is located in the region referred to as *McBurney's point*. This point he described as being "located exactly between an inch and a half and two inches from the anterior spinous process of the ilium on a straight line drawn from that process to the umbilicus." As subsequent experience accumulated, so exact a location is not always possible, nor is the point of maximum tenderness always so specific. This tenderness is a function of the position in which the appendix lies. In malrotation of the colon, the tenderness in acute appendicitis may not be in the right lower quadrant at all should the cecum lie elsewhere in the abdomen. If the inflamed tip of the appendix lies deeply in the pelvis, the point of greatest tenderness may be that elicited only high on the right side by rectal examination. Occasionally, the cecum is felt to be distended with gas.

The quality of the tenderness varies considerably. If the inflamed appendix lies anteriorly and in contact with the abdominal wall, tenderness is maximal. If the appendix is retrocecal, tenderness may be slight. If the tip lies deep in the pelvis, little or no tenderness may be elicited by abdominal examination. *The diagnosis may be missed unless rectal and pelvic examinations are made.*

Rebound tenderness, that is, pain referred to the region of the appendix when the examining hand releases its pressure suddenly from the abdomen, is commonly seen in appendicitis. In nonperforative appendicitis, the rebound tenderness is localized to the appendiceal area. Contralateral abdominal pressure with sudden release also may cause rebound pain in the right lower quadrant. This is highly suggestive of inflammatory disease confined to the region of the appendix but is noted less often than when the sudden release is from pressure applied directly over the cecum.

Muscle spasm of the right lower abdomen often is seen early. At first, this is a voluntary type of splinting which can be overcome by gentle pressure, particularly if the patient's attention is distracted. Muscle spasm tends to become involuntary as the disease progresses, especially if perforation occurs and peritonitis develops. However, as Cope[9] states, the appendix may be on the verge of perfora-

tion without the slightest evidence of rigidity being demonstrable. Thus, the absence of voluntary rigidity is not an all-important consideration.

The use of the stethoscope to determine whether or not bowel sounds are present is of the greatest importance in establishing the presence or the absence of generalized peritonitis. The stethoscope can be a very important instrument in the examination of the acute abdomen; in some instances, the information obtained may be decisive.

Laboratory Aids. An elevation of the leukocyte count is commonly found within a few hours after the onset of the first symptoms of appendicitis. As the disease progresses, the count continues to rise; minor changes may be due to error or to diurnal variation; and such changes do not constitute good reason either to wait or to intervene. Initially, a count of 10,000 to 12,000 per mm. of blood is found; at this level, the leukocyte count is not very helpful or necessarily reliable. When it reaches 14,000 or higher, it assumes a role of major diagnostic importance, especially when accompanied by other symptoms and signs suggestive of appendicitis. In debilitated or critically ill patients, as well as in the aged, the leukocyte count may not be elevated or is increased only slightly, even in acute perforative appendicitis. However, a blood smear in most instances shows an increase in the number of neutrophilic granulocytes even when the total leukocyte count is not elevated. Valuable as the leukocyte count has proved to be, failure to find an elevated white count in the face of other dominant clinical findings of appendicitis should not discourage or delay appendectomy. A blood smear should be done in connection with the diagnostic work-up for acute appendicitis for other reasons also. On occasion, it has been the first evidence for the presence of some blood dyscrasia or infectious disease. Such a finding indicates the need for further study but does not preclude the diagnosis of acute appendicitis or the need for appendectomy.

The sedimentation rate also may be elevated but is not diagnostic and is not usually employed by this author in most patients suspected of having appendicitis. A greatly accelerated sedimentation rate within a few hours after onset of symptoms should make one search for other causes or explanations, especially pelvic inflammatory disease.

Examination of the clean voided urine is essential. The finding of glycosuria, albumin, or casts suggests the presence of other important co-existent disease which may modify the program of fluid therapy and possibly the choice of anesthesia. Large quantities of red or white blood cells in the urine suggest that the symptoms attributed to acute appendicitis may be the result of urologic disease such as pyelitis, cystitis, renal tract tumor, renal calculi and renal tuberculosis. However, the presence of 10 to 30 erythrocytes per high-powered field in the uncentrifuged urine is an occasional finding in acute appendicitis should the inflamed appendix lie alongside the course of the ureter or be in contact with the urinary bladder. Bacilluria in fresh catheterized urine generally is not found in acute appendicitis; when present, it is cause to suspect renal tract infection as the basis of the patient's complaints.

A plane roentgenographic film of the abdomen occasionally may be desirable. The diagnosis of a radiopaque fecalith in the region of the appendix when other manifestations of appendicitis are present strongly supports the presumptive diagnosis of appendicitis. Also, a chest roentgenogram may be useful, as pain in the right lower abdomen may be referred along the 9th, 10th, 11th or 12th nerves irritated by pathology located in the lower right chest giving rise to pleurisy. The author does not employ either of these roentgen procedures routinely except for chest roentgenograms in young children but has utilized either or both roentgenographic procedures in puzzling cases, especially in the aged patient.

Diagnosis of Nonperforative Acute Appendicitis

The clinical features of early acute appendicitis are by no means as constant as may be implied above. Yet, in most cases, the diagnosis is made fairly easily. In the first place, the fact that acute appendicitis is the most commonly encountered inflammatory disease in the right lower abdomen of all age groups is reassuring. Acute pain and tenderness within this region always should alert the suspicion of the surgeon to the possibility of this diagnosis. Although there may be evidence to im-

plicate other sources for the origin of symptoms, such as a slow leak from a perforated duodenal ulcer, an inflamed gallbladder or pelvic inflammatory disease, often the possibility of acute appendicitis cannot be excluded readily.

When acute appendicitis is present, usually more than one complaint or finding is observed. Some of these findings are more important than others; given a patient whose history is of short duration with abdominal tenderness over the region of the appendix or rectal tenderness elicited on the right side by digital examination, this alone is sufficient evidence to make the diagnosis of appendicitis, barring indications of disease elsewhere. However, pain and/or tenderness may not always be pronounced or severe in acute appendicitis, especially should the appendix lie retrocecally or deep in the pelvis.

In the author's experience, the following are the findings most commonly observed in acute appendicitis; they are listed in the order of their importance to this diagnosis.

1. Point tenderness over the region of the appendix, whether from abdominal or rectal examination, in patients with a short history of epigastric or periumbilical distress and pain which localizes in the right lower abdomen a few hours later

2. The above findings with a slight fever (99° to 100.6° F.)

3. Co-existing moderate leukocytosis (12,000 to 18,000) or a pronounced increase in the percentage of neutrophiles in the blood smear should the total white count not be elevated

4. Normal urinary sediment

5. Absence of disease elsewhere

If any error is more common than others in making the diagnosis of acute nonperforative appendicitis, it is the tendency to be too precise as to the nature of the pathology present. It is more important to arrive at the conclusion that an acute surgical condition exists in the right lower abdomen and to explore promptly for its cause and surgical correction than to risk perforative appendicitis while waiting for better definition of symptoms. Some diagnostic errors cannot be avoided, but the percentage will not be high when the patient is examined thoughtfully and carefully. In doubtful cases, wherein the patient has little systemic or localized findings, repeated examinations by the same individual at intervals of 3 or 4 hours is a most useful practice, often saving the patient from needless operation on one hand and needless perforation on the other.

Certain alterations in pain and tenderness are thought to have special connotations; at times they may relate to the onset of gangrenous appendicitis, the occurrence of perforation of the appendix and to recovery from an attack.

The Significance of the Relief of Pain and Tenderness

Acute Gangrenous Appendicitis. In this type of appendicitis pain may abate temporarily and, in some cases, even disappear for a few hours. Tenderness, likewise, may be less pronounced. This may give the false impression that the pathologic process is improving. However, fever and leukocytosis are likely to persist or to increase during this same short period of time. The lessening of pain when the appendix becomes gangrenous generally is attributed to death of the intrinsic nerve plexus within the gangrenous appendix, and therefore the nerves no longer respond to the painful stimulus of stretch from the distention so often present in the whole nongangrenous appendix. As this temporary relief of pain is not a constant association with the onset of gangrene of the appendix, its occurrence in these patients has been interpreted (without much statistical evidence) as indicating death of the appendix prior to perforation. The onset of much inflammatory reaction of the parietal peritoneum could account for the cases in which pain does not disappear. Gangrenous appendices in which a brief respite of symptoms occur are likely to lie in the retrocecal or deep ileocecal areas or to be covered with omentum; thereby, to some extent, they are less likely to have ready access to the free peritoneal cavity.

Perforation of the Appendix. Should the distended and inflamed appendix undergo perforation, there may also be a sudden relief of pain for short periods of time, even though the remainder of the appendix is viable. In these cases, the relief of symptoms is attributed to the acute release of distention; perforation is thought to afford an avenue for the escape of the detritis responsible for the increased intraluminal pressure and hence the pain arising from the stretch reflex of the appendix. Tenderness also may abate temporarily in these patients, if the intraluminal discharge at the time of perforation is confined and does not have early access to the free peritoneal cavity. However, in gangrenous appendicitis, fever and leukocytosis are likely to increase after perforation, in spite of the apparent brief period of relief of symptomatic complaints. The relief of pain and tenderness following perforation or gangrene and so often alluded to in the surgical literature is not frequent in this author's experience; generally, pain becomes more pronounced—not less so.

Spontaneous Recovery from Acute Appendicitis. The relief of pain and tenderness is also associated with a recession of an attack of acute appendicitis. In such cases, fever and leukocytosis also diminish and may return to normal within a few days. Relief of symptomatic complaints in subsiding appendicitis is likely to be at a slower rate than when associated with the onset of gangrenous or perforative appendicitis.

Recovery from an attack of appendicitis in the author's opinion is more likely to occur when obstruction is incomplete and due to occlusion by liquid feces, or to obstruction from temporary lymphoid hyperplasia within the appendix associated with generalized or regional hyperplasia of lymphoid tissue.

Recovery can occur also when obstruction of the appendiceal lumen is from fecal concretions or other foreign bodies. Recovery in these cases may be only temporary. Should these concretions remain, *recurring appendicitis* is a good probability; recurring attacks may follow within a few weeks to several months, and for this reason the appendix should be removed electively within 6 to 8 weeks after the preceding attack if for any reason it has not been removed during the attack.

Treatment of Nonperforative Appendicitis

The treatment of acute appendicitis is appendectomy. This should be carried out as soon as the diagnosis is made, provided that any serous fluid or electrolyte imbalance is first corrected. When a short delay is necessary to meet these requirements, the author prefers to administer parenterally one of the broad-spectrum antibiotics or one of their combinations prior to operation, particularly if the leukocyte count and fever are sufficiently high as to suggest impending or actual perforation. If the patient has eaten within 8 hours, a stomach tube is passed, and the gastric contents are aspirated prior to the induction of anesthesia (see Chap. 13, "Operative Surgical Care").

Anesthesia. The choice of the anesthetic agent is conditioned by the age and the general state of the patient. In children or infants, an appropriate general anesthetic agent is employed, usually open-drop ether (see Chap. 12, "Anesthesia"). In the otherwise normal adult between the ages of 18 and 65 years, the author prefers a "single-shot" or continuous procaine spinal anesthesia. If the patient is elderly, debilitated or suffers from substantial cardiovascular disease, local infiltration with 1 per cent procaine along the lines of the incision may be used in the various layers of the abdominal wall, including the peritoneum. Regional blocks as the primary and only type of procaine infiltration have not often been successful in the author's experience. Before the incision is made, the surgeon should palpate the abdomen in the region of the appendix, as an occasional mass that otherwise would not be detectable may be felt when the patient is relaxed by anesthesia.

Incision. The muscle-splitting incision was designed originally for the purpose of performing an appendectomy and the lateral drainage of abscess so commonly present in latent cases. It remains to this day the incision of choice and is the one which all 4 editors of *Surgery: Principles and Practice* recommend for most patients.

The technic of this incision is as follows: The skin is incised parallel with its nerve supply. The author prefers to place the incision beginning just mesial to the anterior superior spine of the ilium. It is carried in a slightly curved line, crossing the lateral margin of the right rectus muscle for a distance of about ¾ in. The mesial end of the cut lies about ½ in. lower on the abdominal wall than does the lateral end. The entire length of the skin incision is 4 to 6 in.

The mid-portion of the edges of the skin with its subcutaneous fat is elevated above and below for a distance of about 2 in. in each direction. Retractors are placed at the centers of each skin flap, and the assistant pulls gently in both directions so as to expose the underlying tendinous portion of the external oblique.

Then these fibers are incised for a distance of 4 to 6 in. in the descending direction in which they run, passing about 1 in. mesial to the anterior superior spine.

The fascial incision should be placed so that one third of its length lies above a projected line from the anterior superior spine to the umbilicus and two thirds of its length lies below this imaginary line.

The internal oblique is now exposed and incised in the parallel horizontal direction at a level corresponding to that of the skin incision. At times it may be necessary to incise the fascia at the lateral margins of the rectus muscle to permit better mesial exposure. The transversalis fascia is similarly incised or separated with scissors.

The peritoneum is now incised obliquely but only for a short distance, beginning about 1 in. mesial to the anterior superior spine. The author prefers to stretch the incised peritoneum with the retractors rather than to incise the full length of the available area as this makes its upper and lower ends more easily seen when ready for closure after appendectomy. The end result of these 4 incisions is a "gridiron" effect, a term by which this incision occasionally is known.

Usually the appendix is located easily unless it is retrocecal or adherent to pelvic structures or the sacral promontory. The caput of the cecum is lifted gently out of the wound along with a short portion of the terminal ileum. If the tip of the appendix comes out easily, its arteries and veins are divided and ligated; the appendix then remains attached only to the cecum. Should the tip of the appendix be bound down too tightly to permit its gentle deliverance into the wound, or if it is too friable or necrotic to permit flexion without rupture, on such occasions the author has separated the base of the appendix from the cecum first. Then the clamped base of the appendix is lifted gently and separated from its mesentery, from its base to tip. Each vessel is individually ligated after being clamped adjacent to the appendix. In effect the appendix under these circumstances is removed in reverse fashion.

The management of the appendiceal stump is a point of considerable variance in practice. In general, there are 3 methods of closure that can be employed. Some prefer to crush momentarily the base of the appendix at its junction with the cecum and to ligate the short stump at this site and not to reinforce. Others prefer not to crush the base of the appendix; rather, they incise the appendix at its point of junction with the cecum. Then this opening is closed with interrupted fine catgut sutures. Still others prefer to ligate the base of the appendix and to bury the short ligated stump by means of a purse-string suture placed in the cecum. The author prefers the last technic, using No. 000 plain catgut to ligate the base of the appendix and No. 00 medium chromic catgut as the cecal purse-string suture. In theory, should an abscess form at the site of the buried appendix, it might rupture more easily into the cecum than into the peritoneal cavity as the plain catgut ligature should digest much more rapidly than the chromic purse-string ligature. Each of the proponents of these 3 methods sees more hazard in the 2 that he does not employ. The facts are that there is little reason to choose between them; all have produced consistently good results when properly used.

The question of the placement of a drain into the region of the amputated appendix to be led to the outside through a laterally placed stab wound has resolved itself largely as to whether or not there was rupture of the appendix or spillage of pus from an abscess which was encountered during appendectomy. In either of the latter instances, the author employs a small soft rubber drain of the Penrose type which is led to the outside through a laterally placed stab wound. Also, a small slip of a drain is placed in the subcutaneous tissue and emerges from the lower end of the skin incision. Clean cases are not drained.

Closure of the wound is then effected, gently approximating each layer separately. The one layer likely to be missed is that of the transversus muscle. This is found readily by turning back the edges of the internal oblique muscle. These two layers may be approximated as one.

Unless other factors contravene, ambulation is possible the day of operation. Oral feeding usually can begin the next day with liquid to soft to regular diet progressing over a period of 3 or 4 days. At this time the patient may be ready for discharge.

This "gridiron" incision has certain advantages: There is little blood loss. The nerves to the musculature of the abdominal wall are spared. It affords ready access for the drainage of an appendiceal abscess if this be present. Should adhesions form, they are likely to be lateral and of little consequence. Finally, the wound, because of its crosshatch nature, is stronger than any other type. Those objecting to its use do so on the basis that the exposure is limited in patients where pathology lies elsewhere, particularly in the left tube or ovary. Because the incision can be expanded or extended readily, this criticism seems to be unwarranted. Others believe it to be impracticable should the primary disease be that of a perforated gallbladder or duodenal ulcer. To this the author agrees, but such cases are rare and when they are encountered, it is simple to close this incision and to make another in a more appropriate area. The appendix is first removed, however.

Of historical interest is the question as to whom should go the credit for the introduction of the muscle-splitting incision for acute appendicitis. Undoubtedly, the first publication on this subject was that of McBurney, which appeared in the July issue of the *Annals of Surgery* in 1894.[24] He had employed this technic in 4 cases, the first being operated upon December 18, 1893. Also, in 1894, is the independent report of McArthur which appeared in the November issue of the *Chicago Medical Recorder* at which time he described the use of this incision in 59 cases.[21] From the published discussion it appears clear that McArthur had employed this incision for at least 18 months prior to its use by McBurney and certainly in many more cases. McArthur's report had been submitted to the secretary of the Chicago Medical Society in the Spring of 1894 but could not be read before that society until after the summer's vacation. While the students and the admirers of each of these men have debated the question as to whom priority should be given, it is to the credit of both of these great surgeons that this was never a point of concern to them.

MORTALITY IN NONPERFORATIVE ACUTE APPENDICITIS

Death from nonperforative acute appendicitis is nearly always from other causes: anesthesia, pulmonary embolism, cardiovascular accidents and bronchopneumonia. These are largely preventable deaths. Thus death from the operative procedure—appendectomy —is indeed rare, less than 0.3 per cent when the operation can be performed prior to perforation even when deaths from all other causes are included. The story is quite different for perforative appendicitis (see below).

PERFORATIVE ACUTE APPENDICITIS

Once perforation of acute appendicitis occurs, the essentially nonexistent operative mortality and morbidity of nonperforative appendicitis no longer obtains. Peritonitis and intra-abdominal abscesses are serious sequelae to be reckoned with; pulmonary embolism, pylephlebitis and miliary abscesses in the liver are another set of complications to be expected in some patients; bowel obstruction, fecal fistula and malnutrition are still other serious consequences which may appear. The folly of surgical delay or of the expectant management of acute appendicitis is so obvious as to point up sharply that any practice other than appendectomy prior to perforation has nothing to recommend and indeed much to be condemned.

CLINICAL ASPECTS AND COURSE

Prior to the time of perforation, the symptomatology from acute appendicitis which will rupture if left unattended cannot be distinguished from one which is removed prior to perforation. Hence, the history and the physical signs of perforative appendicitis are of 2 types: those which exist prior to perforation and those which come into the picture only after perforation has occurred. Only the latter course will be described here. The ruptured appendix is seldom if ever without some antecedent complaint in the conscious patient

or the child old enough to make known his distress.

Why does perforative appendicitis continue to occur? There can be only 2 possible explanations: either acute appendicitis is not recognized by the patient or his physician, or the patient is in a sufficiently isolated area that he cannot or does not seek medical counsel. It is better to educate the public and the medical profession alike. The dogma for practical purposes that all cases of acute appendicitis will perforate if not removed has much to recommend it, although there is the possibility that this disease may subside spontaneously. However, those that subside cannot be distinguished in advance from those that will perforate.

Much has been accomplished by public education; undoubtedly, it has brought many patients to the surgeon earlier than they might come otherwise. At the same time, there are certain patients who when seen by their physician exhibit minimal complaints in the face of advanced suppurative acute appendicitis; these are seen most often in the aged and in young children or infants.

For some reason appendicitis in the child is likely to progress more rapidly to the stage of perforation than is usually observed in adults. Perhaps the fairly frequent gastrointestinal upsets from dietary indiscretion or other causes lead parents to conclude that this is only another upset stomach or "belly-ache." While all agree that these may cause unnecessary delays in children, the fact remains that the time interval from onset of symptoms to perforation in the child is by comparison with the same course in adults, often relatively short. Moreover, peritonitis in children is believed to be tolerated less well than in adults. In part, this may be due to the fact that infection in the peritoneum of the child is not localized readily, possibly because his omentum is relatively scanty in size and structure. The child's systemic reaction also seems to be greater in response to deviations in electrolyte and water balance than when comparable changes occur in the adult; metabolic acidosis from any infection appears more likely to occur and seemingly with less provocation in the child than in the adult. All things considered, most surgeons prefer to operate for suspected appendicitis earlier in children when the complaints are suggestive of the diagnosis but perhaps not as fully confirmed as may be desired in adult patients.

The importance of perforation in acute appendicitis in children is attested to by Boles, Treton and Clatworthy (1959). These authors found that 30 per cent of the children in their series of 837 cases had perforation. Furthermore, in preschool children, this increased to 66 per cent. Also, the complication rate in the patients with perforation was 7 times that of those with simple acute appendicitis.

Acute appendicitis in the aged patient is also likely to have reached the stage of perforation prior to the physician's being aware that rupture may have taken place already. This situation may be attributed to several factors: the threshold to pain in the aged generally is increased, partly from tolerance by habit and partly from some loss of cerebral sensory interpretation. His febrile response develops more slowly, and his leukocyte count may rise surprisingly slowly, and in some there may be little or no rise. Atrophy of the abdominal musculature with advancing age and the accompanying loss of tone tends to obscure any muscle spasm that may be present. However, tenderness and a mass or abscess generally are detected more easily and reliably in the aged than in the young adult or child. Thus, the diagnosis of acute appendictis is not difficult to make, but the physician does not always remind himself that acute appendicitis is still the most common cause of acute right lower abdominal pain even in the aged. Many more causes for this symptom complex exist in the aged than in the young adult or the child; yet, for both age groups, acute appendicitis leads all the rest.

The clinical onset of perforation is said by many to be characterized by a lessening of complaints for a few hours after the appendix ruptures (see p. 853). This relief of pain is attributed to the sudden release of the increased intraluminal pressure that existed prior to perforation. However, in the author's experience, this diminished pain rarely has been observed; generally, pain is more severe and diffuse.

Although the debris and the feces contained within the lumen of the appendix at the time of perforation escape and cause local peritonitis, large quantities of feces are seldom found when the abdomen is opened. Occasionally, in removing a necrotic appendix adjacent to the cecum, the cecum is perforated, and the fecal flow which follows is interpreted as pre-existent. It is doubtful that a continuous flow of feces from the cecum occurs very often in spontaneous perforative appendicitis, as the site of perforation is generally distal to that of appendiceal obstruction. In this respect, the ruptured gallbladder, secondary to cystic duct obstruction, represents a similar mechanical problem in that when rupture occurs, cystic duct occlusion is seldom relieved; consequently, it is only the bile and the fluid contained in the gallbladder at the time of rupture that is released into the abdomen, and the continuous free flow of bile from the cystic duct is seen only occasionally.

Nonetheless, the discharge of pus and feces contained in the obstructed appendix at the time of perforation serves as an excellent source for a continuing and spreading infection—peritonitis. If this material is not localized promptly or if the appendix is not already involved in omentum or between loops of small bowel, generalized peritonitis is the likely eventuality and cause of death in untreated cases.

Tenderness in the abdomen immediately after perforation usually increases and continues at this intensity. If peritonitis spreads or becomes generalized, abdominal tenderness becomes more diffuse and generalized. If, on the other hand, perforation occurs into the omentum or between agglutinated loops of small bowel, it may remain restricted largely to the right lower abdomen. Thus, the fingerpoint tenderness of nonperforative appendicitis usually is no longer observed once perforation occurs. It is the diffuse character of the tenderness, even though it still may be limited to the right lower abdomen, that largely distinguishes clinically, spreading or general from local peritonitis, and all 3 from that of nonperforative appendicitis.

Rebound tenderness continues after perforation, but its localization is no longer as sharp as that of nonperforative appendicitis; rather, it is likely to conform to the extent of the area involved in peritonitis at the time that the examination is made, extending or receding in accordance with the progress or the recession of peritonitis.

The origin of pain and tenderness is possibly different in perforative appendicitis than in nonperforative appendicitis; in the latter, it is probably a reactive expression from irritation of the parietal and visceral peritoneal surfaces by infection. In nonperforative appendicitis, these symptoms are attributed largely to the compression by the examination of the tense and swollen appendix; adjacent peritonitis is thought to play a less important role. It should be pointed out quickly that these are theoretical conclusions which have a certain degree of logic in their support but little or no scientific proof. Moreover, it is the origin of pain and tenderness that may be different in perforative appendicitis from that of nonperforative acute appendicitis, not its character; there is no possible means known to this author by which reliable distinctions can be made clinically between the pain and the tenderness seen in the late stages of nonperforative appendicitis and that occurring in the early stages of perforative appendicitis. One can only suspect.

Palpation of the abdomen in perforative appendicitis generally reveals more intense and extensive spasm of the muscles of the abdominal wall, roughly corresponding to the area of the peritoneum involved in active inflammation. In the author's experience the "boardlike" rigidity, so often characterizing peritonitis of the perforated duodenal ulcer with its highly irritating contents, is not often observed early in peritonitis of bacterial origin, including that of perforative appendicitis. This, too, is not of strong differential diagnostic significance but rather is an observation which, with other considerations, may add or subtract a little from the over-all clinical picture in favor of one diagnosis over another (see Chap. 38 "Peritoneum and Peritonitis").

If peritonitis is spreading or generalized, the gentle palpation of the abdomen may reveal a certain degree of "doughiness" of the skin and the subcutaneous tissue. This sign is generally fairly distinct when present but requires some degree of skill and experience to detect its presence; it is nondiagnostic. The experience of most surgeons, including that of the author, is that the doughy abdomen is observed more commonly after intra-abdominal hemorrhage than in chemical or bacterial peritonitis.

The auscultatory findings of peritonitis are largely those of the adynamic ileus in that portion of the peritoneum involved. Bowel sounds are first hypoactive and, as the disease progresses, they may be entirely absent. Seldom, if ever, are bowel sounds hyperactive unless a portion of the bowel is uninflamed and proximal to this, mechanical obstruction exists. In most patients with less than a generalized peritonitis, all peristalsis ceases; this may be due in part to the reflex adynamic ileus, similar to that observed in the early postoperative stages following intra-abdominal operations and anesthesia; it is also from the local effects of peritonitis.

Laboratory Aids. Some of these are of considerable value in establishing the general condition of the patient with peritonitis but they are of little specific diagnostic consequence. The loss of plasmalike fluid into the peritoneal cavity and the subperitoneal spaces is likely to result in hemoconcentration relative to the preperitonitis values of the hemoglobin and the hematocrit reading; the degree of hemoconcentration is influenced also by the loss of fluids from gastric intubation, an essential part of the treatment of both adynamic and mechanical ileus (see Chap. 35, "Peritoneum and Peritonitis"). At the same time, early anemia from so extensive an infection may also occur; its cause is incompletely understood, but its presence tends to obscure to some extent the magnitude of hemoconcentration actually present. For further discussion of this subject, as well as the problems of mineral, water and plasma losses created by peritonitis, see Chap. 35, "Peritoneum and Peritonitis."

The leukocyte count generally rises fairly sharply in perforative appendicitis; it soars above that usually observed in the earlier preperforation stages of acute appendicitis. The infrequently encountered exceptions in the aged or debilitated patients should be mentioned once again. The sedimentation rate generally is increased considerably over that noted in nonperforative acute appendicitis, even when corrected for any pre-existing anemia and taking into account that the hemoconcentration of peritonitis is likely to yield normal or increased red cell volume also.

Roentgenographic examination of the abdomen in perforative peritonitis may disclose one of two features or both; neither is diagnostic. The first is the pattern suggestive of adynamic ileus, and the other is the disclosure of an intra-abdominal abscess. Save for the clinical history and physical findings upon which the diagnosis of perforative appendicitis depends, x-ray findings are largely confirmatory. In the author's opinion roentgenographic studies are of greater value in following the progress of the patient, particularly with reference to subsequent abscess formation in areas distal to the site of the appendix. Such examinations may be useful in connection with the initial diagnosis if certain other acute intra-abdominal conditions need to be evaluated and if possible to be excluded by this technic. This author never has seen a case of perforative acute appendicitis in which free intraperitoneal air has been demonstrated. Although this possibility does exist, the obstructive nature of perforative appendicitis seldom allows the free retrograde flow of feces or gas from the cecum.

Diagnosis of Perforative Appendicitis

The diagnosis of perforative appendicitis is largely one of the differential diagnosis of local, spreading or generalized peritonitis. Clinically, the events antecedent to perforation and peritonitis are most important to the conclusion of the origin of peritonitis.

The physical findings are largely those relating to peritonitis if the patient is seen for the first time after perforation has occurred. Two features of the examination may be useful to the diagnosis of perforative appendicitis: (1) the localization of the finding of peritonitis largely to the right lower abdomen; (2) the detection of a tender mass within the abdomen or the right pelvis, suggesting an abscess or agglutination of omentum or small bowel to the appendix. Finally, some consolation and possible confirmation is derived from the fact that appendicitis, more than any other inflammatory disorder, accounts for peritonitis limited to the right lower abdomen. Should peritonitis be full-blown and generalized when the patient is first seen, one may have only this statistical possibility in favor of acute appendicitis to aid in formulating his impression

of its origin. Should a mass be detectable in the right lower abdomen, the diagnosis of perforative appendicitis is nearly certain in younger people. The possibility of a perforating carcinoma of the cecum with abscess must be considered in older patients; the presence of occult blood in the stool favors the diagnosis of carcinoma. (See also regional enteritis and ulcerative colitis, Chap. 37).

Thus, 3 features favor the diagnosis of perforative appendicitis as the cause of peritonitis and form a reasonable basis for this presumptive diagnosis:

1. A history compatible with acute appendicitis prior to the onset of peritonitis

2. A mass palpable in the right lower abdomen or high on the right side of the pelvis as determined by rectal examination. This diagnosis is reinforced by the failure to find occult blood in the stool

3. The statistical probability of appendicitis in the absence of other disease, especially of peptic ulcer and diverticulitis.

Treatment of Perforative Appendicitis

Certain clinical facts should be made clear about abscess formation in acute perforative appendicitis as they bear upon the time at which appendectomy can be performed to the best advantage. One has been discussed already. By no means are all masses felt in the right lower quadrant in cases with appendicitis due to abscesses. Many of these are masses of omentum and/or small bowel agglutinated to an inflamed but not perforated appendix. Such masses often are misinterpreted as abscesses, and expectant treatment is pursued; the appendix may perforate, a fate which could have been avoided had appendectomy been carried out when the patient was first seen. Should the patient not be seen until the 4th to the 6th day and found to appear toxic with a fever of 103° to 105° F., such masses are very likely to be abscesses; this author believes these, too, should be operated upon at this time in many instances. Drainage through a laterally placed McBurney incision is the operation of choice and usually can be done with little risk. The appendix should be sought for and removed at this same time, provided that its identification does not mean that the surgeon must explore beyond the confines of the abscess cavity.

If no abscess has formed and if local or spreading peritonitis is found and the perforated appendix lies in the free peritoneal cavity, it must be found and removed. The earlier opening of the appendiceal abscesses with appendectomy under these circumstances is a more recent practice made possible primarily by the advent of chemotherapy and antibiosis.

In experienced hands, this change in attitude toward the treatment of appendiceal abscesses or spreading peritonitis has much to recommend it. In the past, some of these abscesses have ruptured into the peritoneal cavity. Others have dissected into the pelvic area or upward to the regions of the duodenum or have formed fistulae. Spreading peritonitis often has extended rather than receded on conservative management. The relief of fever and intoxication is in itself a desirable accomplishment if early drainage and/or appendectomy can be performed safely. Finally, it is possible but not proved that a reduction in incidence of intrahepatic abscess from migratory septic thrombi arising in the venous radicals of the appendiceal veins may result from draining the abscess with earlier surgical intervention. Pulmonary emboli, septic or sterile, arising from the iliac, the pelvic, or the more distal veins of the extremities, are also to be considered, as these account for a not inconsiderable number of deaths in perforative appendicitis and other inflammatory diseases arising within the lower abdomen.

Appendectomy for perforative appendicitis has been a subject of much discussion and of strong positions by surgeons since Day One June 17, 1886. Until the past 2 decades, the dominant school was that popularized by A. J. Ochsner:[27] namely, bed rest, opium "around the clock" and nothing by mouth. This was known as the "expectant treatment," awaiting a well-defined abscess to form and to drain it within 10 days of the initial onset of the attack. J. B. Murphy and others held the opposite view for most cases, referring despairingly to the Ochsner method as the "expectans mortans" regimen.

Those who advocated the expectant method were not without fairly sound grounds, at least for many patients seen in their time. They held that the silent abdomen was important to avoiding rupture of the abscess; to this

end they stopped feedings, the use of purgatives and enemas, and endorsed the use of opium to quiet bowel activity. They also maintained that time favored the development of an immune response, believing that in due course antibodies to the offending organisms would form. This latter view may be more substantial in theory than in fact, as its importance is not yet settled. To this end, Murphy maintained that the abscess wall and the immune response were very minor considerations compared with leaving the source of the infection within the abdomen, namely, the necrotic appendix.

Today the lines are drawn more in favor of early appendectomy for perforative appendicitis, as many of the older arguments favoring delay are not germane to current practice. The surgeon today has additional supportive measures not available in the days of Ochsner or of Murphy. These are, in the order of their development: intravenous fluid therapy, prompt intragastric intubation and the use of safe blood and plasma transfusion. Fowler's[13] positioning of the patient to favor the gravitational flow of pus into the pelvis still may be used, but it should be avoided in the presence of impending or actual shock. This author does not employ Fowler's position as frequently as before the days of antibiotic therapy as it favors stasis and embolism, theoretically at least.

Gradients of Conservative and Operative Intervention in Patients with Perforative Appendicitis First Seen After 48 Hours. It is better to decide for each patient the advantages and the disadvantages of operative management of perforative acute appendicitis, realizing that appendectomy must be performed in each case but that timing is the important consideration. This approach perhaps is the most useful and widely practiced method of treating cases of suspected perforative appendicitis at this time. It employs the sound principle of case selection, applying initially to each patient one treatment or the other or their combination once a careful clinical appraisal is made of his particular problem. Such an appraisal should include the possibility that the case is one in which nonperforative appendicitis exists surrounded by a mass of omentum or small bowel and that abscess formation or spreading peritonitis has not yet occurred. It also takes into account the possibility that the mass is really an abscess and that a spreading or full-blown generalized peritonitis is already present, and that these latter two complications do not necessarily imply that early drainage and appendectomy will be more harmful than beneficial in all instances. To individualize each case, considering each of these points separately at the time the patient is first seen is useful, but it must be recognized that an accurate clinical appraisal which will correlate with the actual state of the pathologic process at any one time is difficult. Yet this approach can be employed to good advantage, provided that thoughtful consideration is given to each patient. This may require several visits and examinations of some patients at hourly intervals before a basis for sound judgment can be reached to determine the early course of therapy best suited for these patients. For some patients the merits of the conservative approach over that of prompt appendectomy is quite as obvious as is the reverse, even when seen as late as a week after the onset of symptoms.

FAVORING PROMPT APPENDECTOMY in suspected perforative appendicitis soon after the patient is first seen, is the good general condition of the patient and the absence of serious complications. In the author's opinion the suspicion of an abscess and/or the presence of a local or spreading peritonitis are less important considerations, provided that the abscess and the appendix is to be approached from a laterally placed McBurney incision without entering the free peritoneal cavity. The purpose of appendectomy in these cases is the removal of this necrotic organ which, if left in place, continues as the active source for spreading infection. This more bold attitude assumes that appendectomy and lateral drainage will at least maintain the *status quo* and can be done without entering the free peritoneal cavity save in those cases in which no abscess has been formed. It is also predicated upon the vigorous use of appropriate antibiotic drugs, the willingness of the surgeon to use blood and plasma to combat shock, the use of gastric intubation and the near-constant vigilance on the part of the physician, resetting his therapeutic "compass" as the patient's course indicates.

Most surgeons adopted the plan of prompt appendectomy in perforative appendicitis in children many years ago, as they found that the expectant treatment did not allow, or seemed to favor, localization or abscess formation to the extent that it did in adults.

FAVORING DELAYED SURGERY in perforative appendicitis are 3 conditions. Foremost is the patient's clinical course prior to his being seen; if it is clear that this abscess or spreading peritonitis is receding, he should be managed conservatively. If there is evidence that more than one abscess has formed (subdiaphragmatic, intrahepatic, subhepatic or intermesenteric), primary concern generally centers about the drainage of these satellite abscesses after a vigorous use of antibiotic drugs having broad spectrum influence upon the usual organism found in perforative appendicitis (see Chap. 35, "Peritoneum and Peritonitis" and Chap. 4, "Surgical Infections"). Toxemia is in itself more often an indication for early appendectomy than a contraindication, unless the patient is moribund. The toxic patient should be transfused promptly with blood and plasma, and adequate fluids should be administered; also, he should be given massive doses of antibiotic drugs. The mineral and water balance should be assessed and corrected if deficiencies exist. After the few hours required for these procedures, the patient should be re-evaluated with respect to the continuation of conservative management or appendectomy, continuing all supportive measures in either case. Such judgments are not easy to make.

If the patient recovers from his attack of perforative appendicitis, how long should appendectomy be delayed? Barring the persistence of other sequela, his appendix should be removed within 2 months' time, as he is subject to recurring attacks, some of which may be more severe than the initial one. A case in point was a patient observed by Harkins[15] wherein the patient experienced 3 recurrent episodes of perforative appendicitis within less than 4 months before he would submit to an interval appendectomy. Interval appendectomy as soon as symptoms subsided was advocated by Fitz[12] in his original paper. A number of the fatalities that he reported in 1886 occurred from 2nd or 3rd attacks, some coming on within a matter of weeks after the initial one.

Thus, in perforative appendicitis, appendectomy is as important as in nonperforative appendicitis; the only difference is that in the latter there is no question but that immediate appendectomy is the only safe recourse open to the surgeon. The operation these days also should be performed promptly in many if not most cases of perforative appendicitis with certain of the above considerations weighing in favor of delay—but only temporary delay.

APPENDICITIS IN PREGNANCY

Acute appendicitis in pregnancy deserves special and separate consideration in that the diagnosis is often difficult because of the large uterus which usually displaces the cecum and the appendix upward and laterally, or the uterus may come to lie in front of the appendix, obscuring many of the signs normally found in appendicitis and thus presenting a confusing picture. In addition, a mild leukocytosis and an increased sedimentation rate are a normal occurrence in pregnancy; the surgeon must recognize these facts lest he place more diagnostic weight upon the finding of a mild leukocytosis than it deserves.

The pregnant woman with acute appendicitis carries a special hazard, pointed out first by McArthur[22] in 1895. Once an appendiceal abscess forms, it usually has for its mesial or posteromesial wall the adjacent enlarged uterus. If the inflammatory reaction of the untreated appendicitis continues, it may provoke uterine contractions and induce abortion or labor, following which shrinkage of the uterus often tears the mesial wall of an appendiceal abscess, allowing free flow of pus throughout the abdomen.

Conservative management of nonperforative appendicitis in pregnancy is likely to be more disastrous in pregnancy than in the population at large. The tendency of the patient to abort or miscarry is slight indeed when appendectomy is performed for acute appendicitis in pregnancy prior to perforation. There is no justification for delay. The removal of a normal appendix in a mistaken diagnosis under these circumstances cannot be condemned, because the risk of a nonoperative error when appendicitis exists is likely to be of much greater consequence.

Priddle and Hesseltine[30] reported a series of 51 cases of appendicitis subjected to appendectomy in Chicago Lying-In Hospital between 1930 and 1950 in which they found the diagnosis of acute appendicitis to be 0.07 per cent of all expectant mothers seen at that hospital during that 20-year period. The cases encountered were distributed essentially equally for each trimester. Five more occurred during early postpartum. All but 6 of the 51 patients were under 30 years of age. Only 2 of these patients underwent premature labor. Progesterone was used in none of the 51 patients.

One maternal death occurred—in 1931. This case is typical of many others reported for neglected appendicitis in pregnancy. The patient, a 32-year-old gravida VI, para V, was 5 months pregnant when seen for the first time. Her history was one of a 4-day history of nausea, vomiting, abdominal pain and tenderness. She was admitted promptly when first seen and, after rehydration, she was explored immediately for perforative appendicitis. An abscess was found behind the cecum; it contained about 60 ml. of pus arising from retrocecal perforative appendicitis. Drains were placed, and the appendix was removed. Hemolytic streptococci were cultured from this pus. Her recovery was slow, and she was discharged on the 25th day. Two days later she went into premature labor, delivering a 980-Gm. fetus which promptly died. On the 3rd postpartum day, a painful swelling appeared in the region of the previous drain site; this was reopened, and large quantities of pus escaped. Two weeks later a pelvic abscess was drained of 400 ml. of pus; this recurred and resulted in death from sepsis on the 41st postpartum day.

The practice regarding the treatment of suspected appendicitis at the Chicago Lying-In Hospital is appendectomy without delay and is that advocated by most obstetricians. The author has performed appendectomy in 2 patients in early normal labor in that hospital; in another patient whose symptoms did not occur until late in the second stage of labor, appendectomy was delayed 4 hours until after delivery was completed.

There is little fear of wound disruption should the patient go into labor soon after appendectomy. The McBurney incision always should be used, as this gives the strongest wound. The skin incision generally is placed higher and more lateral than usual, and that of the internal oblique may need to be longer than is generally applied to achieve adequate exposure.

RECURRENT APPENDICITIS

This type of appendicitis is another form of acute appendicitis and first was described by Fitz in 1886. A patient recovered from one attack is prone to recurring attacks. As mentioned above, it is for this reason that the appendix always should be removed within 2 months after perforation, should the judgment of the surgeon dictate delay or conservative treatment at the time of the initial attack of perforative appendicitis.

REMOVAL OF THE NORMAL APPENDIX IN THE COURSE OF OTHER INTRA-ABDOMINAL OPERATIONS

Opinion is not unanimous as to the wisdom of removing the normal appendix in the course of other intra-abdominal operations. This procedure is to be considered not only as an elective one but also as one which is prophylactic in nature. In favor of appendectomy under these conditions is the prevention of appendicitis at a later day; few surgeons can practice surgery for many years without encountering appendicitis among his own patients on whom he has operated previously for some other intra-abdominal conditions. It is probable that the older surgeons are more in favor of removal of the normal appendix, if it can be done without discernible increase in risk in the course of another procedure, than is the newcomer to the field. At times previous experience has been embarrassing in this regard. Those who have opposed this view do so on their considered grounds that any operative procedure in addition to the one currently at hand carries an unnecessary risk, however slight.

This author favors removal of the normal appendix in the course of another operation, provided that appendectomy can be performed through the incision already in use, especially if the patient's general health and operative condition are good, and if in the surgeon's judgment that appendectomy can be performed without threat, including wound soilage. It seems logical that appendectomy under these conditions is likely to carry less risk than that of a second anesthetic should a subsequent attack of acute appendicitis occur. This position seems to be reinforced at this writing as only 12 hours before writing this section the author removed a perforated appendix from a 30-year-old female upon whom he had performed a cholecystectomy for cholecystitis and cholelithiasis 6 years before. The studies of Boyce[3] at the New Orleans Charity Hospital showed the mortality rate for nonperforative acute appendicitis to be 10 times greater in patients over 40 years of age compared with similar cases operated upon in younger patients.

COMPLICATIONS OF ACUTE APPENDICITIS

The nature and the incidence of the common complications of acute appendicitis are largely conditioned by the character of an attack of appendicitis itself. Complications from appendectomy for *nonperforative* acute appendicitis are indeed rare; of those which have been encountered during the postoperative period, infection in the subcutaneous tissue or an abscess in the region where the appendix lay are the principal ones. Pylephlebitis with miliary abscess formation in the liver, pulmonary embolism and fecal fistula are seldom seen in simple appendicitis. Most complications from appendectomy for nonperforative appendicitis are from anesthesia, poor hemostasis, failure to observe the principles of aseptic surgical technic and sponges left inadvertently in the wound. Latent complications are largely limited to those of small bowel obstruction from adhesions; obstruction usually makes its first appearance years later but may occur at any time during the remainder of the patient's life.

The complications of *perforative* appendicitis, in comparison with those of the nonperforative form of the disease, are encountered much more frequently. Most of the complications of perforative appendicitis are inseparable and synonymous with those of bacterial peritonitis and/or of abscess formation. They also include adynamic ileus, hypovolemic shock and its fluid problems (see Chap. 35, "Peritoneum, Peritonitis and Intra-abdominal Abscesses"), intra-abdominal abscess formation at more distant sites, fecal fistulae, early and late mechanical obstruction, thrombophlebitic and embolic disease—sterile or septic, in both the portal and the systemic venous systems. Malnutrition, cutaneous ulceration or pressure necrosis (bed-sores) are also commonly encountered in obese and elderly patients.

PERITONITIS FROM PERFORATIVE APPENDICITIS

The onset of perforative appendicitis is generally also the onset of peritonitis. The extent to which peritonitis develops varies immensely; it may progress to involve the entire abdominal cavity or may be largely contained within the right lower quadrant, forming peri-appendiceal or residual abscesses and occasional cecal fistulae. The incidence and the extent of peritonitis from perforated appendicitis varies among hospitals. This is partly because of the type of patient encountered (charity or private) and in part from the lack of uniformity of well-defined or similar terminology when reporting this complication. As bacterial peritonitis may result from many intra-abdominal sites and causes, this subject and its sequelae are discussed more extensively under a separate heading (see below).

ABSCESS FORMATION FROM APPENDICITIS

Intra-abdominal abscesses from appendicitis are of 3 types: (1) those localized to the appendiceal area, (2) those situated more distally, as in the subphrenic spaces or pelvis, and (3) those located within other organs, especially the liver, and resulting from migratory pylephlebitis and embolism in the portal vein and from pyemia. In addition, subcutaneous or superficial abscesses may occur in the incision. None of these are peculiar to appendicitis, as they may come from any other cause of intra-abdominal infection. However, they are reported more frequently in acute perforative appendicitis, as this is the most commonly encountered cause of bacterial peritonitis.

The incidence of true abscess within the abdomen is difficult to assess, as many surgeons employ conservative management, and thereby distinctions between masses of omentum and a periappendiceal abscess are not known. Boyce[3] reports a mortality rate of 13.2 per cent from periappendiceal abscess at the Charity Hospital in New Orleans and believes that abscess formation is a fortunate outcome of perforative appendicitis only insofar as this is a lower mortality than that experienced with spreading peritonitis. Periappendiceal abscess is largely limited to the perforative form of appendicitis, but it may occur also in more instances from contamination during operation in patients with non-perforative appendicitis.

PYLEPHLEBITIS WITH PORTAL EMBOLISM IN APPENDICITIS

This is perhaps the most serious single complication of appendicitis, but its occurrence is comparatively rare, accounting for less than 8 per cent of fatal cases. In the portal system this is generally a septic thrombophlebitis with embolism into the venous channels from the appendix (generally perforative). These septic clots fragment and break away only to be trapped in the liver where they usually establish multiple intrahepatic abscesses; occasionally, solitary intrahepatic abscess is formed. The onset of chill and its recurrence, fever (usually fairly high and with multiple daily spikes), and a few days later mild icterus with tenderness over the liver lend strong evidence in favor of this diagnosis. Positive blood cultures may be obtained.

Treatment includes a therapeutic trail on massive doses of antibiotics as the first measure; should a positive blood culture be obtained; sensitivity studies may be run and a more appropriate antibiotic drug subsequently selected and given. If this proves to be inadequate and a mass can be felt in the liver, surgical exploration may be considered after several weeks. Two surgical possibilities exist: should the abscess be single or few in number, it (they) may be drained to good advantage. If the abscesses are limited to the left lobe, this lobe may be removed entirely. Two successful cases resulted from these surgical procedures in patients with liver abscesses from perforative appendicitis treated at the University of Chicago Clinics in 1955. Peripheral phlebitis and pulmonary embolism may be complications of peritonitis and abscess formation. The increased incidence of both in perforative appendicitis is considered by some to result largely from compression of the adjacent iliac vein, periphlebitis, shock, hypovolemia, malnutrition and infection in general; all are undoubtedly contributing factors.

ADYNAMIC ILEUS AND MECHANICAL OBSTRUCTION IN PERFORATIVE APPENDICITIS

Adynamic ileus often accompanies spreading or generalized peritonitis from any origin and may continue for a week or longer. As stated on p. 860, this may have protective value in assisting localization of peritonitis. The most effective treatment is gastric intubation with continuing suction until bowel tone returns and the patient expels flatus and has a bowel movement. Occasionally, suction through a long gastrointestinal tube is more advantageous. Recovery from adynamic ileus in children generally is more rapid than in adults. It is slowest to disappear in elderly or malnourished patients (see Chap. 35, "Peritoneum, Peritonitis and Intra-abdominal Abscesses").

Mechanical obstruction as a complication is observed much less frequently in the early weeks of recovery from perforative appendicitis and is usually a sequel of the increasing adhesions about an abscess or fecal fistula. If mechanical ileus occurs, it is more likely to do so several months or years later and is seen more often when right paramedian incisions have been used. Appendectomy for nonperforative appendicitis through the lateral McBurney's incision rarely produces adhesions of consequence due only to the operation.

WOUND INFECTION, FECAL FISTULA AND MALNUTRITION AFTER APPENDECTOMY

These comprise a complex series of events which may occur in perforative appendicitis with or without abscess formation. These also may be complicated by any other intraperitoneal infection. Abscess or fecal fistula may be the cause of the other, directly and reciprocally. Malnutrition may result from either or both as well as from other persisting serious complications of appendicitis. The fecal fistula is the least harmful of this group of complications and is more often the result of necrosis

of the adjacent cecal wall from periappendicitis or periappendiceal abscess than from blowout of the ligated or impacted appendiceal stump. Foreign bodies, especially sponges left at operation, should be searched for whenever bowel fistula persists.

MORTALITY FROM APPENDICITIS

INCIDENCE OF PERITONITIS FROM ALL CAUSES AND FROM APPENDICITIS IN PARTICULAR

The mortality in appendicitis is largely that of spreading or generalized peritonitis. The remarkable reduction in mortality from acute appendicitis is primarily a function of 2 factors: more and more patients being operated upon prior to perforation and (2) the improved therapeutic measures for the management of peritonitis. This author believes that earlier operation has done more to reduce mortality than have the advances made in the management of peritonitis; nonetheless, the improvement in the management of the latter is by no means inconspicuous or of little consequence.

Peritonitis from perforative appendicitis, although still a serious problem when present, carries a much lower morbidity and mortality rate than at the turn of the century (see below). Ochsner, Gage and Garside[28] reviewed this subject in 1930 and reported variations in the incidence of peritonitis to range from 7 to 78 per cent for perforative appendicitis. A decade later, the Commission on Acute Appendicitis Mortality in the State of Pennsylvania[1] reported 68 per cent of all cases of spreading peritonitis as due to perforative appendicitis. Five years later, 1945,[8] the incidence of peritonitis from all causes had fallen markedly; and only 9 per cent of the cases with perforative appendicitis developed spreading peritonitis. Similar reductions for this disease have been reported from the Cincinnati group at 5-year intervals for corresponding years.[31] The Charity Hospital of New Orleans, in a series of reports, also has indicated a decline in spreading peritonitis from perforative appendicitis,[3] and more recently Cannon[5] observed and reported the same phenomenon at the University of Chicago (Fig. 34-3).

DEATH FROM PERITONITIS

Cannon[5] has shown recently that death from peritonitis of any origin has been reduced. At the University of Chicago Clinics, the ratio fell from 32 cases of fatal peritonitis per 500 unselected autopsies in 1927 to 16 cases per 500 autopsies in 1951. This decline of 50 per cent in mortality rate has been steady and at no point has it shown a sharp drop. However, percentagewise, this improvement is of more consequence than may appear at first glance. The total amount of major surgery in this hospital has increased 400 per cent during the same period; and peritonitis arising from the surgical services has declined to a greater extent than those occurring on the medical services.

During the same 25-year period, improved fluid management, gastric intubation, increased use of blood and plasma and finally the sulfonamides and the antibiotics became realities and routine in therapy for peritonitis, not to mention the influence of public education during this same time. Each has played a contributing role in the improvement, but the mortality rate still remains high.

DEATH FROM APPENDICITIS

Death from appendicitis was frequent 45 years ago. This has rapidly changed until now it is very low among causes of death listed. At the University of Chicago Clinics, death occurred 17 times from peritonitis of appendicitis among 2,556 autopsies performed consecutively from 1927 to 1941, but only twice in 2,436 autopsies performed from 1941 to 1952. This is a reduction to one eighth that experienced during the first period (1927-1941).[5] This is a reduction 4 times as great as that occurring from bacterial peritonitis from any and all causes during the same period. These data are remarkably similar to those compiled by the Metropolitan Life Insurance Company wherein death from appendicitis in 1937 was 11.3 per 100,000 policyholders, and 1.3 in 1953. A still broader sampling discloses that there were 21,000 deaths from appendicitis in the United States in 1931; by 1946 this figure was 6,000, representing a saving of 15,000 lives per year. Extrapolating from these latter data, Harkins[16] points out that, if the 1931 mortality rate had continued for one complete genera-

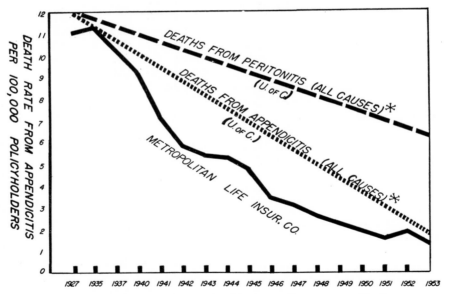

FIG. 34-3. Mortality trends in peritonitis from all causes, graphically compared with that of peritonitis from acute appendicitis. Decline in mortality rate for appendicitis percentages is about 4 times that of peritonitis from all causes over corresponding years. (Data compiled by Paul R. Cannon, University of Chicago, in 1955, and by the Metropolitan Life Insurance Company in 1953)

tion (65 years), 1,400,000 lives would have been lost from this disease. The 1946 figure, when similarly extrapolated and with the same assumptions made, would account for only 400,000 deaths from appendicitis over a 65-year period, a saving of 1,000,000 lives.

It is possible, in this author's opinion, to single out one factor in reducing the mortality rate from acute appendicitis over all others. While most credit antibiotics, blood plasma and better anesthesia and intravenous fluid therapy (and indeed they have done a great deal), the one which stands out as more important than the others is early operation. This was accomplished by education—education of both laity and the profession alike. A higher index of suspicion for this disease and a broad understanding of its consequences if untreated has led to earlier and earlier appendectomy, reducing the number of patients coming to operation after peritonitis has developed. It is likely to continue to play an important role in the future if further substantial reduction in mortality is to be achieved. Much credit should be accorded to such men as John B. Deaver (1855-1931) of Philadelphia, Mont Reid (1889-1943) of Cincinnati, and John Bower (1885-1960), formerly chairman of the Commission on Appendicitis of the Pennsylvania State Medical Association, for preaching early diagnosis and treatment in appendicitis.

MUCOCELE OF THE APPENDIX

This is a rare but interesting disorder of the appendix and is, in a sense, a form of sterile "appendicitis." It is essentially a hydropic enlargement of this organ which occurs when the proximal lumen of the appendix is occluded and the remaining lumen is bacteriologically sterile. An old abscess cavity may form part of the mucocele. The mucus secretions distal to the obstruction continue and result in its gradual distention which may exceed 2 in. in diameter and grow 6 to 10 in. in length. If unrecognized, it may rupture, seeding viable mucus-secreting cells throughout the peritoneal cavity. These cells become implants and reproduce themselves. The result is the accumulation of numerous tumors which actively secrete mucus into the free peritoneal cavity. These generally induce numerous adhesions throughout the abdomen. Intestinal obstruction and mucous ascites often develop. Because of the extensive and serious nature of these sequelae, this complication can be fatal. It is known as pseudomyxoma peritonei. Appendectomy should be performed, as this removes one source of cells.

Abdominal Pain and the Differential Diagnosis

CLINICAL CONSIDERATIONS

Acute appendicitis can be mimicked fairly successfully at times by certain other acute intra-abdominal diseases. Although there are many causes of pain and tenderness in the right lower quadrant of the abdomen with slight fever and moderate leukocytosis, acute appendicitis always should receive first consideration. Therefore, a working knowledge of the origin of abdominal pain is essential to the understanding of the nature of the patient's complaint.

Nature, Pathways and Clinical Interpretation of Peritoneal Pain

As abdominal pain is a subjective complaint and not readily analyzed objectively, any analysis of its nature, nervous pathways and interpretation is complicated by such vagaries as "threshold of complaint," the individual's capacity to make known the character of his pain, and the ability of the observer to record as well as reinterpret the patient's communications. Nonetheless, much is known about abdominal pain, the types of stimuli that provoke it, the difference between parietal and visceral peritoneal pain and the disorders most likely to produce many of the patient's complaints. Obviously, interpretation of abdominal pain is as much an art as a science and not easily acquired save by experience.

Capps initiated an important clinical study of parietal and visceral pain published nearly a quarter of a century ago.[6] His findings, along with the later ones of Lewis,[19] serve as the basis upon which most of our present-day knowledge is based. Capps's views as to the importance of abdominal pain are largely held today. He wrote: "Pain (peritoneal) is perhaps the most important evidence upon which we base our interpretation and diagnosis of abdominal disease."

Parietal Pain. The stimuli that provoke pain from the parietal peritoneum more nearly correspond to those causing pain when applied to the skin. They include contact with sharp or cutting instruments, pain of pressure, thermal pain, and pain from irritants, either chemical or bacterial in nature.

Visceral Pain. The only stimulus that appears to be capable of provoking pain from the visceral peritoneum of the alimentary tract is distention. Cutting, pinching, or cautery applied to this visceral peritoneum produce no pain.

The nature of the peripheral sensory nerve endings is not well known. However, it appears that these sensory origins are located in the peritoneum itself as well as in its ajacent subserosal tissue, particularly that of the parietal peritoneum. There is some reason to conclude that the sensory nerve terminals of the visceral peritoneum may arise largely from the subserosa and the muscularis of the alimentary tract rather than the visceral peritoneum itself.

Sensory Nerve Pathways. PARIETAL. These pathways of the parietal peritoneum are somatic in distribution. The peritoneum of the abdominal wall is supplied by sensory nerves which correspond to the overlying skin. Both enter the posterior roots of the thoracic sensory nerves from T-7 to T-12 inclusive. The diaphragm likewise is supplied by somatic nerves which enter principally C-4 and to some extent C-3 and C-5. Any appropriate painful stimulus to the parietal peritoneum is referred along to the corresponding cutaneous nerve(s); hence, diaphragmatic pain is characteristically refererd to the shoulder cap cutaneous distribution of C-3, C-4 and C-5. Pain from the abdominal peritoneum is referred to the corresponding cutaneous segment(s) of T-7 to T-12. In general, these cutaneous points of pain reference correspond fairly precisely to the site of parietal peritoneal irritation. Thus, pain from acute appendicitis generally is localized to the 10th or the 11th thoracic cutaneous nerve distribution on the right. Pain from the gallbladder usually is in the region of the 8th nerve distribution and follows its course to the back. The pain of acute salpingitis is generally bilateral and of 11th nerve distribution, and so on.

VISCERAL. Pain pathways from the visceral peritoneum of the alimentary tract are believed to be transmitted along somatic pathways, but in the course of reaching the dorsal root of the spinal nerves, they may find their way along the course of the autonomic nervous system. This intermingling of the afferent somatic sensory nerves and the efferent autonomic fibers usually is cited as the explanation for pain experienced when the central end of the divided splanchnic nerves are stimulated. Lewis[19] maintains that the painful response from stimulation of central end of the autonomic fibers is not reason for

regarding the pain nerves of the sympathetic system as distinct from those supplying the deeplying somatic structures . . . the fact that those (pain fibers) from the somatic structures at first use the channel of the spinal nerves and that those from the visceral structures at first use the channel of the autonomic system before entering the posterior roots is really immaterial.

This may be an oversimplification which will be elucidated later when more information becomes available. Lewis cites Barrington as observing that the pain of ureteral colic has the segmental distribution of somatic pain corresponding to the particular level at which the stone is lodged, provided that the stone remains above the bladder. In this author's experience, pain from the visceral peritoneum of the alimentary tract cannot be localized as precisely by the patient as the pain of parietal peritoneum irritation. For example, the pain (visceral) of distention in small intestinal obstruction usually is more diffuse, being localized to the anterior and the lateral portions of the abdomen of the patient. Similarly, distention of a colostomy by the finger causes the patient to experience cramplike pain of the abdomen which often is associated with pain in the back. However, this lack of preciseness is no reason to question the somatic origin of visceral pain; rather, it indicates certain possible differences in quality between parietal and visceral peritoneal pain.

Pain arising from stimulation of the parietal peritoneum often is associated with splinting of the overlying abdominal musculature. Should the stimulus and the pain be of mild intensity, guarding or muscle spasm is not great and generally can be overcome by gentle pressure of the examining hand; this is known as "voluntary muscle spasm." Should the painful stimulus be more intense, such as occurs when the highly irritating acid gastric juices escape into the peritoneal cavity from a perforation of a duodenal ulcer, muscle spasm is likely to be maximum, and the "boardlike" rigidity of the abdominal wall it produces is not overcome by the physician's examining hand and, for this reason, is commonly referred to as "involuntary muscle spasm." This difference between voluntary and involuntary splinting of the abdominal wall appears to be largely a quantitative one.

The skin surface location by the patient of his abdominal pain, when of visceral origin, is in general as follows: pain of gastric or duodenal origin is experienced above the region of the umbilicus. That of the small bowel and the appendix is often periumbilical; and that of the colon usually is localized below the umbilicus.

Certain experimental observations made by Lewis and Kellgren[20] are interpreted by these workers as indicating the somatic nature of visceral pain. They claim to have produced many types of pain by the injection of hypertonic saline into the regions of various interspinous ligaments. When injected into the proper interspinous ligament, they report that their subjects were unable to distinguish between the pain induced by saline and that experienced by the abdominal disorder producing the pain for which the patient was seen. For example, the injection into the first lumbar interspinous ligament caused pain resembling that of "renal colic." Injection of the saline solution into the 9th thoracic interspinous ligament caused pain in the back and over the distribution of the 9th intercostal nerve. An analysis of data from more patients similarly studied might be useful in providing more information as well as providing means for interpretation of the patient's localization of his pain.

The location of the patient's pain in general is of much greater practical value when it arises from the parietal peritoneum than from the visceral peritoneum. However, even for visceral pain, the physician may obtain information by a careful analysis of the patient's complaints, especially the location of his pain, which can play an important role in the differential diagnosis of the acute abdomen.

Operative Pain. Unless the patient is maintained in the 3rd plane of a general anesthesia or under a fairly high spinal anesthetic, the peritoneal stimuli attending the operation result in an involuntary spasm of the muscles of the abdominal walls and may interfere with both surgical exposure and surgical closure of the abdominal cavity. Two very useful additions in the technics and the principles of anesthesia have been devised to assist the surgeon when his procedure requires the maximum of muscular relaxation. The first is the transabdominal procaine block of the celiac ganglia which usually abolishes the transmission of stimuli induced by retraction or tugging upon the mesentery. It is often helpful to supplement this by infiltration of the parietal peritoneum about the wound edges. The second and more widely used technic is the temporary paralysis of somatic motor nerves at the myoneural junctions by the use of drugs having a curarelike action. These drugs are effective regardless of the persistence of perceptive painful stimuli and make possible a lighter plane of general anesthesia. As muscular relaxants they are useful indeed, but they also paralyze temporarily the action of all striated muscles, including those of respiration. Their use should be limited to experienced anesthesiologists and then only if the patient is properly intubated so that his respiration can be supported at all times if necessary.

DIFFERENTIAL DIAGNOSIS OF APPENDICITIS

Ruptured Graafian Follicle. This lesion may produce a picture like that of appendicitis. It is sudden in onset, usually producing mild abdominal distress localized to the lower abdomen and often to the right side. Acute loss of appetite, nausea and occasional vomiting may occur. Fingerpoint tenderness is absent or not well defined. If much blood escapes, the patient may experience phrenic pain referred to the shoulder with pain distribution over the 3rd, the 4th and the 5th cervical nerves when lying down, as blood may migrate to the under surfaces of the diaphragm. The most important diagnostic clue is to be found in the history; the sudden onset of pain occurring in the mid-term of the intermenstrual period. Hence, this syndrome is known as *mittelschmerz*. Anemia may be present, but leukocytosis and fever are mild or nonexistent in the first day or two.

Ectopic Pregnancy. Generally, this is associated with some irregularity of the recent menstrual cycle. This condition may produce pain simulating in part that of appendicitis. Maximum tenderness is lower than McBurney's point. A right tubo-ovarian mass may be felt on pelvic examination. If rupture has occurred, shoulder pain may be complained of, and shock may appear soon if operation is delayed. The abdominal wall develops the doughy consistency characteristic of intra-abdominal blood, and peristaltic activity may be reduced or absent. Fever, if present, is slight, although leukocytosis and anemia may be observed. Shock is often present.

Twisted Ovarian Cyst or Tumor. This lesion produces sudden and sharp lower abdominal pain and vomiting. In a few cases reference of pain may be to the medial aspect of the thigh. As with the ruptured ectopic pregnancy, the acuteness and the seriousness of the signs and symptoms make unnecessary a discussion of details, because soon the necessity for prompt exploration of the lower abdomen is obvious.

Acute Salpingitis. This condition is by no means always easily distinguishable from acute appendicitis. Pain is generally hypogastric in location. Tenderness is low and often bilateral. Motion of the cervix is usually very painful, and often bilateral tender pelvic masses can be felt. From the purulent discharge it may be possible to demonstrate the intracellular gonococcus by stained smear. Fever and leukocytosis are generally greater than for early appendicitis, and the sedimentation rate is substantially increased early over that seen in nonperforative appendicitis. Occasionally, appendectomy is necessarily resorted to simply because acute appendicitis cannot be excluded satisfactorily by any other means.

Mesenteric Adenitis. This occurs more commonly in children and young adults. This syndrome is characterized by generalized abdominal pain which may be more pronounced in the right lower quadrant. It usually accompanies or follows a respiratory infection and may or may not be associated with fever and leukocytosis. If this disease resembles too closely the symptoms of acute appendicitis, the diagnosis of the latter always should be made and appendectomy performed.

Regional Enteritis. This type of inflammation also may resemble appendicitis and indeed may give rise to the latter by obstructing its lumen. Its symptom complex in the acute and first attack so often resembles appendicitis that most patients whom the author has seen with regional enteritis have had appendectomy at the time of a previous attack of similar nature. In some patients the "sausage roll" swelling of the terminal ileum may be felt, but even though regional enteritis may be suspected, concurrent appendicitis is often difficult, if not impossible, to exclude.

Ureteral Stone. This condition occasionally simulates appendicitis, particularly if lodged in the right ureter and producing pain without colic. Reference of pain into the scrotum of the penis is often complained of. Hematuria, no fever and the absence of leukocytosis strongly suggest the presence of a ureteral stone. However, more often than not ureteral stone is associated with fever and leukocytosis. Cystoscopy and pyelograms usually produce the indisputable evidence necessary to eliminate the need for further concern about the appendix, barring the coexistence of both diseases.

Perforated Peptic Ulcer. Such an ulcer may simulate an attack of acute appendicitis, especially if the perforation is small and the leakage of gastroduodenal juices is at a slow rate. Pain in the epigastrium with nausea and occasional vomiting may mark its onset. As the fluid tends to flow down into the right iliac fossa, pain and tenderness in the right lower quadrant become prominent findings and may resemble acute appendicitis. Often the diagnosis is confused with perforative appendicitis, especially if rigidity of the abdominal wall is present and bowel sounds are absent. Leukocytosis and slight fever may be present early and tend to rise later on.

The differential points are chiefly the history of peptic ulcer. The fact that pain, tenderness and muscular rigidity are more pronounced than are seen in early appendicitis is helpful; the presence of air under the diaphragm on roentgenographic examination is usually diagnostic but it also may not be observed in small perforations (see Chap. 29, "Stomach and Duodenum").

On the other hand, a history of peptic ulcer, even of perforated ulcer, does not weigh too heavily against the diagnosis of acute appendicitis. It is the impression of this author that the incidence of the latter disease among ulcer patients on medical management is greater than that of similar age groups in the population at large. The author has seen one patient, in whom there was a history of 3 perforations of duodenal ulcer, who presented himself to the University of Chicago Clinics with a sudden attack of severe epigastric pain of 3-hours' duration and in whom the diagnosis of another perforation seemed to be much more likely than that of acute appendicitis. At operation, perforated appendicitis proved to be the correct diagnosis. The incidence of acute appendicitis and of duodenal ulcer is greater in men than in women. Fortunately, both conditions require early surgical exploration, at which time the correct diagnosis can be established.

Acute Cholecystitis. Occasionally, acute cholecystitis can and does simulate acute appendicitis in some patients. The pain onset is generally epigastric, which slowly localizes slightly to the right. Colic may or may not be present, and often the pain is referred to the right flank and/or the right subscapular area. Acute loss of appetite, nausea and vomiting are more prominent features than are generally seen in appendicitis, as is the associated fever and leukocytosis. If muscular rigidity is not pronounced, occasionally a dis-

tended gallbladder or a mass of surrounding omentum can be felt. However, in some cases the gallbladder lies lower than usual, and the distinction between acute cholecystitis and appendicitis is made more difficult. In doubtful cases early exploration is indicated.

Acute Pancreatitis. This is another condition to be considered, as it too may give rise to right lower abdominal pain in some patients (see Chap. 31, "Pancreas").

Pleuritis of the Right Lower Chest or of the Right Diaphragm. The pleuritis of the right lower chest or of the right diaphragm may be difficult to distinguish from appendicitis, especially in children. Loss of appetite, nausea and vomiting are infrequently present, although leukocytosis and fever are commonly present. Splinting of the abdominal muscles, hyperesthesia and voluntary rigidity are commonly present and to an extent greater than might be expected early in the course of appendicitis. Bowel sounds are nearly always present. A roentgenogram of the chest may or may not disclose evidence of pleuritis or pneumonitis. The most important single sign in the author's experience is that achieved by splinting of the lower chest by hand compression over the right lower chest cage and having the patient breathe deeply. This generally relieves his pain. If not, then the procedure is repeated, applying manual splinting to the abdomen below the thoracic cage. Thus thoracic motion is accentuated, and as a rule pleuritic pain is accentuated upon deep inspiration. (See also Chap. 35, "Peritoneum.")

Intussusception. (See Chap. 46, "Pediatric Surgery.")

Intestinal Obstruction. (See Chap. 36, "Intestinal Obstruction.")

In Table 1 are listed the sites of origins of

TABLE 1. PAIN IN ACUTE INTRA-ABDOMINAL EMERGENCIES

SITE OR ORIGIN OF PAIN	LOCALIZATION OR REFERENCE OF PAIN	CHARACTER OF PAIN
Subphrenic abscess, or irritation from blood, bile, or other irritating fluids in this area	Shoulder cap and at times also to the hypochondrium and the upper and the middle portions of the abdominal wall of the affected side	Made worse by deep inspiration and generally is diminished by splinting of the abdomen
Perisplenitis, abscess, infarct, or tear of spleen	Similar to that of left subphrenic abscess	Made worse by inspiration
Gallbladder disease: 1. Acute distention	Subscapular pain, 8th nerve	Fairly continuous unless distention is intermittent

TABLE 1. PAIN IN ACUTE INTRA-ABDOMINAL EMERGENCIES (*Cont.*)

SITE OR ORIGIN OF PAIN	LOCALIZATION OR REFERENCE OF PAIN	CHARACTER OF PAIN
2. Acute inflammation	Over the region of the gallbladder and generally along the course of T-8 sensory distribution	Continuous
3. Cystic or common duct stone	Right hypochondrium and right subscapular area. As gallbladder becomes inflamed, pain is also in the hypochondrium	Generally continuous, occasionally intermittent and often recurring
Penetrating duodenal ulcer	Anteriorly, over region of duodenum and generally to back in area of penetration	Continuous. Made worse by slight amount of hydrochloric acid, through Levin tube. Generally relieved by gastric drainage and milk or alkaline therapy
Appendicitis: 1. Early	Usually mild and in periumbilical or midepigastric area	Usually mild and ill-defined, tends to recede
2. Within a few hours	Right lower abdomen and generally conforming fairly well to location of appendix	Well localized and continuous. Mild to moderate in severity
3. With local or spreading peritonitis	More extensive and less sharply defined	Generally more severe and diffuse
Salpingitis or impending rupture of ectopic tubular pregnancy	Low in abdomen and lateralized to area involved	Dull to sharp and constant
Ruptured graafian follicle	Mild to moderate. Generally located to lower abdomen. If much blood escapes, subphrenic pain in recumbent position may be experienced. Onset sudden	Usually mild and somewhat ill-defined. Constant and may be of sudden onset, occurring in the midintermenstrual cycle
Ruptured ectopic pregnancy	First lateralized in lower abdomen, tends to become more diffuse and may give rise to subphrenic pain if in recumbent position	Sudden, moderate to severe, continuous. May be bilateral
Twisted ovarian cyst	Low in abdomen and may radiate also to upper mesial side of thigh	Sudden in onset and usually intense. Continuous
Sigmoidal diverticulitis	Generally left-sided or bilateral and located low in abdomen	Mild but progressing in intensity
Acute intestinal obstruction (mechanical ileus)	Pain at first may be diffuse and later tends to localize over region of obstruction	Early or sudden in onset. In the early stages is generally cramp-like, severe and intermittent; this remains, but as bowel becomes inflamed, a local persistence of pain appears in region on the inflamed bowel
Mesenteric thrombosis	Onset may be sudden; first is generalized and a little later may be associated with dull pain in upper lumbar area. As bowel becomes inflamed it may produce localization at site of necrotic bowel	Is mild to moderate. Is continuous and often ill-defined

pain, the location of reference of pain, and the character of pain frequently observed in many of these acute intra-abdominal emergencies.

Many other conditions must be considered which at times can resemble acute appendicitis. These are encountered less frequently and also confused less frequently with acute appendicitis. Among others are: spinal cord and vertebral diseases, tabes dorsalis, sickle cell anemia, porphyria (including lead poisoning), rheumatic fever, hepatic or subhepatic abscesses, herpes zoster, periarteritis nodosa with extraperitoneal hematoma, rupture of the abdominal musculature, intra-abdominal hernia, mesenteric thrombosis, torsion of the omentum or of an appendices epiploicae, coronary thrombosis, and last but not least is acute retention of urine in children.

If the diagnosis of appendicitis remains in doubt, take the appendix out.

REFERENCES

1. Boles, E. T., Treton, R. J., and Clatworthy, H. W., Jr.: Acute appendicitis in children, A.M.A. Arch. Surg. 79:447, 1959.
2. Bower, J. O.: Report on the second state-wide survey of acute appendicitis from state-wide hospital records of 1942, Pennsylvania M.J. 43:1145, 1940.
3. Boyce, F. F.: Acute Appendicitis and Its Complications, New York, Oxford, 1949.
4. Burne, J.: M. Chir. Tr. 20:219, 1837. Quoted by Fitz, 1886.[12]
5. Cannon, P. R.: The changing pathologic picture of infection since the introduction of chemotherapy and antibiotics, Bull. New York Acad. Med. 31:87, 1955.
6. Capps, J. A.: Pain in the pleura, Pericardium and Peritoneum, New York, Macmillan, 1932.
7. Castleton, K. B., Puestow, C. B., and Sauer, D.: Is appendicitis decreasing in frequency?, A.M.A. Arch. Surg. 78:794, 1959.
8. Commission on Acute Appendicitis Mortality: Report of the third state-wide survey of acute appendicitis mortality, Pennsylvania M.J. 55:449, 1952.
9. Cope, Z.: The Early Diagnosis of the Acute Abdomen, ed. 10, London, Oxford, 1951.
10. de Lamotte, J.: Observations made at the opening of a body of a person dead of tympanites, J. med., chir. et pharm. 22:65. Quoted by Major, R. H.: Classic Descriptions of Disease, p. 617, Springfield, Ill., Thomas, 1932.
11. Dupuytren, B. G.: Leçons orales, Clin. Chir. 3:330, 1833. Quoted by Fitz, 1886.[12]
12. Fitz, R. H.: Perforating inflammation of the vermiform appendix; with special reference to its early diagnosis and treatment, Tr. A. Am. Physicians 1:107, 1886.
13. Fowler, G. R.: Diffuse septic peritonitis, with special reference to a new method of treatment, namely, the elevated head and trunk posture, to facilitate drainage into the pelvis, with a report of 9 consecutively-treated cases of recovery, M. Rec. 57:617, 1900.
14. Goldbeck: Über eigenth. entz. Geschw, i.d. rechten Huftbeingegend, 1830. Quoted by Fitz, 1886.[12]
15. Harkins, H. N.: Personal communication, 1956.
16. ———: Unpublished data, 1956.
17. Husson, and Dance: Répertoire gen. d'anat., etc. 4:154, 1827. Quoted by Fitz, 1886.[12]
18. Kelly, H. A., and Hurdon, E.: The Vermiform Appendix and Its Diseases, Philadelphia, Saunders, 1905.
19. Lewis, T.: Pain, New York, Macmillan, 1942.
20. Lewis, T., and Kellgren, J. H.: Observation relating to referred pain, visceromotor reflexes and other related phenomenon, Clin. Sc. 4:47, 1939.
21. McArthur, L. L.: Choice of incisions of abdominal wall; especially for appendicitis, Chicago M. Rec. 7:289 and 330, 1894.
22. ———: Gestation complicated by appendiceal abscess, Am. J. Obst. 31:181 and 228, 1895.
23. McBurney, C.: Experience with early observative interference in cases of diseases of the vermiform appendix, New York M.J. 50:676, 1889.
24. ———: The incision made in the abdominal wall in cases of appendicitis, with a description of a new method of operating, Ann. Surg. 20:38, 1894.
25. Melier, F.: Mémoire et observation sur quelques maladies de l'appendice caecale, J. gen. med., chir. et pharm. 100:317, 1827.
26. Mestivier, M.: On a tumor situated near the umbilical region on the right side, produced by a large pin found in the vermiform appendix of the cecum, J. med., chir. et pharm. tom. 1:441, 1759. Quoted by Major, R. H.: Classic Descriptions of Disease, p. 617, Springfield, Ill., Thomas, 1932.
27. Ochsner, A. J.: The cause of diffuse perito-

nitis complicating appendicitis and its prevention, Chairman's Address, delivered before Section on Surgery and Anatomy, 55th
Annual Meeting, A.M.A., June 4-7, 1901.

28. Ochsner, Alton, Gage, M. I., and Garside, E.:
The intra-abdominal postoperative complications of appendicitis, Ann. Surg. *91*:544,
1930.

29. Parkinson, J.: Case of diseased appendix
vermiformis, Med. Chir. Tr. *3*:57, 1812.

30. Priddle, H. D., and Hesseltine, H. C.: Acute
appendicitis in the obstetric patient, Am. J.
Obst. & Gynec. *62*:150, 1951.

31. Reid, M. R.: The mortality of appendicitis—
a national disgrace, South. Surgeon *8*:404,
1938.

J. Garrott Allen, m.d.

CHAPTER 35

Peritonitis and Intra-abdominal Abscesses

Peritoneum
Acute Peritonitis
Intra-abdominal Abscesses

THE PERITONEUM

STRUCTURE AND SURFACE AREA

The peritoneum is a glistening, serous lining, enveloping all of the abdominal viscera and their mesenteries (the visceral peritoneum), as well as the peripheral confines of the abdominal cavity (the parietal peritoneum). The visceral peritoneum is attached loosely to its underlying structures by the subserosal areolar tissue, while the parietal peritoneum overlays the transversalis fascia and in places is rather firmly attached to it. The peritoneal surface consists of a single layer of flattened mesothelium moistened by a small quantity of serous fluid, which permits the viscera to glide about in the abdominal cavity.

The surface area of the peritoneum is approximately equal to that of the skin. Consequently, it is one of the largest absorptive, transudative and exudative surfaces of the body.

SUBDIVISIONS OF THE ABDOMINAL CAVITY

The anatomic subdivisions of the abdominal cavity are only 2: the greater and the lesser peritoneal sacs. They communicate through the foramen of Winslow, the epiploic foramen.

The Lesser Peritoneal Cavity or Omental Bursa. The boundaries of the lesser cavity are: anteriorly, the posterior wall of the stomach; inferiorly and left laterally, the superior surface of the transverse mesocolon; and posteriorly, the peritoneum over the pancreas and the diaphragmatic peritoneum above

the pancreas. Its right lateral limit is the mesial border of the gastrohepatic ligament which envelops the hepatic artery, the portal vein and the common duct. Because the gastrohepatic ligament is reflected onto the posterior surface of the stomach but not onto the posterior abdominal wall, a foramenal connection is left connecting the greater and the lesser peritoneal cavities. This opening between the greater and the lesser omental cavities is the foramen of Winslow.

The Greater Peritoneal Cavity. It contains most of the abdominal viscera. Each organ or vessel contained in or transversing this cavity is covered with peritoneum on its surface facing into the abdominal cavity. Where such organs as the liver, the kidney and pancreas lie against the abdominal musculature the visceral peritoneum of these organs passes onto the abdominal wall where it continues as the parietal peritoneum. Organs having portions of their surfaces not covered with peritoneum and other portions which are covered are said to be retroperitoneal.

That part of the greater peritoneal cavity which lies below the brim of the true pelvis is considered to be a somewhat separate division of the greater omental cavity because it contains most of the urogenital organs.

ACUTE PERITONITIS

Peritonitis is an inflammatory response of the peritoneum to bacterial, chemical, thermal, irradiation and physical injuries and to foreign bodies. The inflammatory response evoked is qualitatively similar to that induced by similar agents in other tissues. Because of the vast surface area of the peritoneum, generalized bacterial or chemical peritonitis is attended by the rapid movement of large quantities of extracellular fluid, plasma proteins and white blood cells into the peritoneal

875

cavity and into the soft areolar tissues beneath the visceral and parietal peritoneum. This intraperitoneal and subperitoneal sequestration of extracellular fluid is attended by a decrease in the plasma volume and consequently by an oligemia that contributes a great deal to the shock that at times soon kills. Related to the speed of absorption through its large surface area is the speed with which septic toxemia accompanies acute generalized peritonitis—a generalized peritonitis being somewhat analogous to a fulminant subcutaneous abscess underlying almost the entire skin.

Classification of Peritonitis

Although any classification of peritonitis is to some extent arbitrary, it can be effected on the bases of: temporal relationships, extent of the peritoneal surface involved, the nature and the sources of the pathogens responsible, and whether peritonitis is primary or secondary in origin.

The most frequent as well as the most dangerous form is that of *acute peritonitis*. This may cause death within a few hours or a day or two.

Acute peritonitis may be confined to a relatively small part of the abdominal cavity. This is *localized peritonitis*. At times it may spread quickly or gradually during a day or two and is then called *spreading peritonitis*. When the entire peritoneal cavity is involved it is called *generalized peritonitis*. Peritonitis may exist for a time as local peritonitis and then may spread and evolve in 12 to 48 hours through the spreading stage to a full-blown generalized peritonitis. These developments can transpire so rapidly that the local and intermediate stages are difficult or impossible, to identify.

Bacteria and Chemicals and Their Relationships. Both usually provoke extensive inflammation of the peritoneal cavity, cause extensive outpouring of fluid and generally incur an adynamic ileus. With perforation of a peptic ulcer into the peritoneal cavity large quantities of chemically irritating fluids pour into the peritoneal cavity within a matter of minutes. In such cases if the leak is not stopped, and if removal of the inflammatory chemicals is not effected, shock may ensue rapidly. Death from shock[1] may occur in such

cases before infection and septicemia assume serious or irreparable proportions. In many cases of secondary peritonitis, the inflammation is localized for a time; this is especially true with appendicitis, salpingitis and cholecystitis. The initial localized phase of peritonitis is associated with the inflammation of and about the sick organ; the peritonitis becomes a spreading one, often progressing to a generalized one, after the appendix or the gallbladder perforates or the tubal abscess ruptures. The time that elapses between the beginning of the localized peritonitis and the time it begins to spread is decidedly variable, being only a few hours in some cases of appendicitis, and weeks with tubal abscesses. In these cases, septicemia is more likely to cause death than is hypovolemia, although both are involved in any case.

The things that most often produce chemical peritonitis are gastric juice, bile, pancreatic juice and urine. With the exception of a sterile urine, all of these fluids very often, if not practically always, contain or become contaminated with intestinal bacteria; consequently, in practically all cases of chemical peritonitis, a bacterial peritonitis soon becomes imposed upon the chemical one unless the leak of the irritating chemicals is stopped very soon after it starts.

Primary and Secondary Peritonitis. Primary peritonitis, while rare, is most frequently due to pneumococci, hemolytic streptococci or gonococci and is often associated with recognizable infections due to these organisms elsewhere. Primary peritonitis is largely limited to children, young women and persons with ascites. The symptoms and signs are essentially identical with those of secondary acute bacterial or chemical peritonitis.

Primary acute chemical peritonitis occasionally occurs with certain systemic diseases, such as polyserositis and uremia.

Secondary bacterial peritonitis usually results from perforation of the alimentary tract, penetrating abdominal wounds, or from septic pelvic inflammatory disease. The distinction between primary and secondary bacterial peritonitis is often very difficult to make. Consequently, it is frequently impossible to avoid surgical exploration in some cases of primary bacterial peritonitis. Whenever the circum-

TABLE 1. BACTERIA COMMONLY ASSOCIATED WITH PERITONITIS

ORGANISMS	ANTIBIOTIC OF GREATEST EFFECTIVENESS*
*Escherichia coli**	Chloramphenicol†
Streptococci (Lancefield Group A)	Penicillin, erythromycin, tetracyclines
Pneumococci	Penicillin
Aerobacter aerogenes	Chloramphenicol,† tetracyclines
Staphylococcus aureus	Chloramphenicol, erythromycin, vancomycin, staphcillin (Dimethoxyphenyl penicillin)
Staphylococcus albus	Chloramphenicol, erythromycin
Streptococcus faecalis	Chloramphenicol, tetracycline, penicillin
Proteus vulgaris	Chloramphenicol† ⎫
P. mirabilis	Chloramphenicol† ⎬ tetracyclines
P. morgagni	Chloramphenicol† ⎪
P. rettgeri	Chloramphenicol† ⎭
Pseudomonas aeruginosa	Polymyxin B†
Paracolon bacilli	Chloramphenicol, gamma-globulin
Neisseria gonorrhoeae	Penicillin, tetracyclines
Anaerobic streptococci	Penicillin, erythromycin, chloramphenicol, tetracyclines
Actinomyces bovis	Penicillin, sulfonamides
Bacteroides	Tetracyclines†
Clostridia	Tetracyclines, penicillin, antitoxin
Tubercle bacilli	Streptomycin, isonicotinic acid hydrazide, para-aminosulfosalicylic acid
Alpha streptococci	Penicillin†

* Names in italics are generic terms.

† Usually the antibiotic of choice, but should be confirmed by sensitivity tests.

stances are such that one cannot make a distinction, the chance of overlooking an early case of secondary bacterial perforative peritonitis is too great, and the consequences of a mistake are too grave to warrant an expectant course hoping that the passage of time will permit a sure differentiation of whether the peritonitis is primary or not.

THE BACTERIOLOGY OF ACUTE PERITONITIS

A wide variety of organisms, many of which are not usually regarded as pathogenic, have been found within the peritoneal cavity in this disease. Table 1 summarizes the kinds of bacteria most often found in peritonitis. The author is indebted to Dr. Ross Benham, Director of Clinical Microbiology at the University of Chicago Clinics, for the compilation of, and permission to use, these data. Included in this table are the antibiotic agents in use against these bacteria. The organisms which have been found infrequently or rarely in peritonitis are listed in Table 2.

DIAGNOSIS OF PERITONITIS

The history, the physical examination of the chest and the abdomen, the differential white

TABLE 2. ORGANISMS INFREQUENTLY ISOLATED FROM CASES OF PERITONITIS

ORGANISM	ANTIBIOTIC OF CHOICE
Salmonella typhi	Chloramphenicol
Salmonella, other than typhi	Tetracyclines and chloramphenicol
Nonhemolytic streptococci ⎫	
Diphtheroids ⎬	Must be determined in each individual case
Rambacterium ramosus ⎭	
Lymphogranuloma venereum	Tetracyclines and chloramphenicol
Coccidioides immitis	Amphotericin-B
Treponema pallidum	Penicillin
Hemophilus influenzae	Streptomycin and sulfonamides
Pasteurella tularensis	Streptomycin
Brucella abortus	Tetracyclines
Monilia albicans	Mycostatin and amphotericin-B

blood count, the hematocrit, simple roentgeno-graphic examinations of the abdomen and aspiration of fluid from the peritoneal cavity are the bases for diagnosing the various forms of peritonitis.

Pain. The pain suffered with peritonitis is varied. With a chemical peritonitis secondary to rupture of an ulcer of the stomach or the duodenum; it usually comes suddenly without an antecedent illness; it is usually a severe burning and at times even an excruciating cutting agony; it spreads rapidly and within minutes or in an hour or two occupies the entire abdomen; it is aggravated by every sort of movement and immediately or very soon incapacitates the sufferer. The pain of peritonitis secondary to appendiceal or chole-cystic rupture usually follows preceding pains that were different in character from that of peritonitis. At times with appendicitis this first type or colicky pain suddenly decreases or even disappears, signaling rupture of the ap-pendix. Then the gradually increasing burn-ing ache of secondary bacterial peritonitis begins, first in the region of the site of the organ that perforates and from there may spread over the entire abdomen. The pain of secondary bacterial peritonitis is rarely ex-cruciating. The pain of acute primary peri-tonitis is preceded almost always by an acute febrile illness such as pneumonia, erysipelas, a streptococcal pharyngitis in children, or acute gonorrhea, a septic abortion or a puerperal sepsis in women. The pain is usually described by the ill person as a terrible soreness of the entire abdomen, though often excepting the epigastrium. Abdominal pain is usually almost lacking with chronic tuberculous peritonitis and the primary chemical peritonitis of uremia.

Tenderness. Abdominal tenderness tends to vary in severity with the pain. It is quick and severe with acute secondary chemical peritonitis, begins gradually and locally and spreads with acute secondary bacterial peri-tonitis, is diffuse from the beginning with pri-mary bacterial peritonitis, and practically lacking with chronic bacterial and uremic chemical (nonbacterial) peritonitis.

Muscle Spasm. Reflex spasm of the ab-dominal musculature is characteristic of all forms of acute peritonitis. With local peri-tonitis only the parts of the muscles supplied by the neural segments affected by the inflam-mation of the parietal peritoneum are spastic, but with a general peritonitis all of the ab-dominal musculature is affected. One must be able to distinguish reflex from "voluntary" muscle spasm. The latter is stimulated when-ever pressure is applied over any part of the abdomen overlying abscesses, closed loop intestinal obstructions, or acutely swollen lymph nodes and is not really a sign of peri-tonitis. In order to distinguish between volun-tary and reflex muscle spasm, the search for spasm is best made by placing one's fingers lightly upon the abdominal skin and shaking the fingers and the skin beneath them from side to side all the while the patient is breath-ing 3 or 4 times. If during the inspirations the sensation beneath one's fingers changes to or remains like that obtained by so shaking the skin of the cheek, the spasm is voluntary. If during the inspiration the sensation remains similar to that experienced by one's fingers when they deftly slide the skin overlying the malar imminence back and forth over the bone, the spasm is reflex.

Reflex muscle spasm comes immediately and is often so intense that the abdomen is rigid or "boardlike" with rupture of duodenal and gastric ulcers; it is there but less intense with acute bacterial peritonitis and is usually lacking with chronic tuberculosis and often so with uremic peritonitis.

Ileus. With all forms of acute generalized peritonitis, peristalsis soon becomes feeble and infrequent, and unless gastric intubation is done quickly, the intestine rapidly fills with gas and fluid. The ileus attending generalized peritonitis is in part reflex in origin because ileus does not attend a peritonitis induced in dogs by the intraperitoneal instillation of turpentine after the animal's splanchnic nerves are cut and its celiac ganglia are removed. However, bacterial toxemia also plays a role because adynamic ileus is prone to attend any sepsis, such as lobar pneumonia, or septicemia.

With localized and chronic peritonitis ileus may be lacking. In fact, with pelvic peri-tonitis there may be normal peristalsis or even hyperperistalsis with diarrhea.

Changes in Blood. Leukocytosis too is a variable accompaniment of peritonitis. An acute generalized massive peritonitis such as following rupture of the cecum is at times associated with a polymorphonuclear leukopenia—not leukocytosis; with tuberculous peritonitis the white blood cell count is often within normal range, and it may be almost anything with uremia. However, excepting tuberculous peritonitis and uremic peritonitis, a shift to the left of the neutrophils (shift to young forms) is characteristic of practically all cases of acute secondary, and primary bacterial, peritonitis.

A rising hematocrit regularly attends acute generalized chemical peritonitis. However, a falling rather than a rising hematocrit may go with severe acute bacterial peritonitis. In the case of a falling hematocrit the patient soon becomes jaundiced, presumably because hemolytic bacterial toxins absorbed from the peritoneal cavity lyse the red blood cells very rapidly. The falling hematocrit in such cases merely means that red blood cells were being destroyed more rapidly than the plasma volume decreased, even though the plasma volume itself may have dropped precipitously because of the escape of extracellular fluid into the inflamed abdominal tissues and into the peritoneal exudate.

Temperature. With all forms of bacterial peritonitis, even tuberculous, some fever is the rule. However, the body temperature is usually normal or subnormal during the first 3 to 6 hours after the perforation of gastric or duodenal ulcers. When hypothermia occurs with bacterial peritonitis, it is a sign of nearness to death; when it occurs during the first few hours of an acute chemical peritonitis, it is a sign of dehydrational (sodium deficit) shock.

Pulse and Respiration. Tachycardia accompanies all forms of peritonitis.

Tachypnea and restriction of abdominal respiratory movements are characteristic of all forms of acute chemical and bacterial generalized peritonitis.

Roentgenograms of the abdomen and the intestine are often very helpful in the differential diagnosis of peritonitis. Plain films of the abdomen taken after the patient has been sitting upright for 5 minutes often show an extragastric air-fluid level beneath the diaphragm whenever the peritonitis is secondary to the perforation of the intra-abdominal gastrointestinal tract. Because most of the very rapidly developing generalized secondary peritonitis arises from perforation of the stomach or the duodenum the oral giving of 50 to 100 ml. of a water-miscible iodinated radiopaque fluid such as Hypaque is a safe, quick and rather accurate way of roentgenographically ruling out rupture of gastric or duodenal ulcers as the cause of the generalized peritonitis, especially when there are indications that a primary bacterial rather than a secondary chemical peritonitis may exist. Barium should never be used for this purpose because, should it escape into the peritoneal cavity with gastrointestinal fluids, a disabling and life-endangering adhesive peritonitis will be produced.

Peritoneal Aspiration. For a number of years the aspiration of fluid from the peritoneal cavity has been sporadically practiced for the purpose of ascertaining the cause of an acute generalized peritonitis especially when there was doubt as to whether it was a primary or a secondary one, or an abortion or birth of a child had preceded the peritonitis by a few hours or days. It is a rather safe procedure when the aspiration is performed through a short-beveled, large-bored spinal-puncture needle and the needle is passed through the anterior abdominal wall away from fixed parts of intestine such as the cecum, the ascending and the descending colon. The fluid of peritonitis from rupture of a duodenal ulcer contains bile; that from an acute hemorrhagic necrotizing pancreatitis is serosanguineous and contains much amylase; that of a primary peritonitis contains only one type of bacteria such as a pneumococci, streptococci, or gonococci; that of acute secondary bacterial peritonitis from rupture of such organs as the appendix, the colon, or the ileum contains all sorts of bacteria and at times microscopical recognizable food debris. The tentative ascertainment of the type or types of bacteria in the fluid can be done quickly by centrifuging some of the fluid and staining the sediment with Gram's stain.

Actually, aspiration of the peritoneal cavity is a most important maneuver in a number of situations other than those alluded to above.

It is a most important step for ruling out peritonitis as a possible cause of any *prostrating acute illness of indeterminate nature with which there is abdominal distention and a silent abdomen that strikes: a severely burned person, one who is being given corticoids, has severe diabetic neuropathy, has a transverse myelitis anywhere above the mid-portion of the thoracic cord, is insane, is being given antibiotics, or is severely debilitated for any reason.* It is a most important diagnostic step in such cases because with these states the signs of peritonitis such as abdominal pain, tenderness and abdominal muscle spasm may be practically lacking, even though a fulminant generalized peritonitis exists. In the experience of one of the authors only once was peritonitis suspected in 5 cases of generalized peritonitis arising from perforations of duodenal or gastric ulcers in badly burned persons who were wrapped in occlusive dressings. All 5 died, and in 4 the peritonitis and duodenal or gastric perforation were uncovered only during the necropsy. None of these burned persons complained of abdominal pain, none had abdominal muscle spasm, but *all of them had meteorism, developed shock* long after the shock-stage of burns was passed, and *deteriorated very rapidly.* In none of these cases was an abdominal tap done! Somewhat similar experiences can be cited for all of the other conditions listed above.

Immediate Postoperative Peritonitis. Peritonitis that begins immediately or very soon after a celiotomy also often tends to be peculiarly lacking in muscle spasm, severe abdominal pain and tenderness. There is a rapidly progressing, febrile, shocking illness and often little else. In cases such as this a diagnostic abdominal tap is relatively useless in the author's experience, because fibrinous adherence forms very numerous and often isolated pockets of exudate that are readily missed by the needle. Whenever a prostrating shocking febrile illness immediately or quickly follows a laparotomy, and significant pulmonary consolidation indicative of a lobar pneumonia and E.C.G. changes of myocardial infarction are lacking, the abdominal wound should be opened in an operating room and should it be found normal, the abdominal cavity should be entered and exudate searched for. Postoperative staphylococci and chemical peritonitis from rupture of a closed duodenal stump after a gastric resection or leak of bile after operation on the biliary tract are especially prone to behave as described above.

A peritoneal aspiration that gets fluid is

often of great help; one that obtains none means nothing—peritonitis still may exist!

Differential Diagnosis. LOBAR PNEUMONIA. The differentiation of peritonitis from conditions which have a number of the same features that peritonitis has is usually rather easy, provided that the physician is astute. Lobar pneumonia in the lower lobes of the lungs is, during the acute pleuritic phase, often associated with continuous abdominal pain, *reflex spasm* of the abdominal musculature, abdominal tenderness, weak and infrequent peristalsis and even abdominal distention. However, the lower lobar pneumonic consolidation (x-ray and physical signs), the pleuritis, and the chill with which the illness began serves to differentiate a lobar pneumonia with abdominal signs from peritonitis.

SPIDER BITE. So too is the boardlike abdominal rigidity and severe abdominal pain caused by the bite of *Latrodectus mactans* (the black widow) easily distinguished from peritonitis. There is no fever or leukocytosis, and the muscles of the back, the legs and the neck are also spastic after the spider bite—but not with acute peritonitis.

ABDOMINAL CRISES. More difficult is the differentiation of the abdominal crises that occur with such things as sickle cell anemia, anaphylactoid purpura, spherocytic anemia, tertiary syphilis and Hodgkin's disease. However, with all of these crises the abdominal spasm, tenderness and pain wax and wane rather rapidly, shift from one place to the other and are not associated with the type of fever or the leukocytoses that peritonitis is. Nonetheless, the differentiation of these crises from peritonitis is too often so uncertain that celiotomy needs to be performed so as not to miss a spreading peritonitis.

From a practical point of view, the only differentiation between the various forms of peritonitis that is very important is that of the primary from the secondary. The former is now readily and effectively treated with appropriate antibiotics alone, while surgically stopping the enteric leak is often the most definitive step in the treatment of secondary peritonitis. The differentiation of primary from secondary peritonitis rests largely upon the history, the x-ray examination and peritoneal aspiration (see Symptoms and Signs section of this chapter).

At times one cannot surely differentiate primary from secondary without recourse to diagnostic celiotomy. When in doubt after exhausting diagnostic methods, it is better to commit a laparotomy error for primary peritonitis than to let a person die of secondary peritonitis without attempting to stop the leak.

TREATMENT OF PERITONITIS

The treatment of peritonitis may be divided into supportive and specific measures.

The supportive treatment consists of:

1. Preventing aspiration pneumonitis and meteorism, and relieving distention of the stomach and the intestines, when they exist, with proper intestinal intubation and drainage (see Chap. 36).

2. The alleviation of pain with the analgesics, morphine or Demerol.

3. Restitution of the extracellular fluid volume deficit produced by intra-abdominal exudation, the sequestration of edema fluid beneath the parietal peritoneum and in the intestinal wall, and the collection of fluid within the adynamic intestine. Because the body fluid aberrations with peritonitis are so similar to those of bad burns and intestinal obstruction, the principles of fluid therapy applicable to burns and intestinal obstruction are applicable to peritonitis (Chaps. 16 and 36).

4. In cases of peritonitis complicated by rapid hemolysis, septic shock, or anemia, the transfusion of blood is a very important supportive measure.

5. Feed the person parenterally something safe, such as glucose.

The specific therapeutic measures are: for *spreading or generalized secondary peritonitis —stop the leak, remove the exudate and the intra-abdominal debris* and *give antibiotics parenterally;* and for *primary peritonitis,* give the *appropriate antibiotics.* Stopping the leak that has produced the secondary peritonitis may consist of such things as appendectomy for appendiceal rupture, resection of ileum for Meckel's diverticular perforation, colostomy for perforation of the neoplastically obstructed colon, resection of the colon with perforated ulcerative colitis, choledochostomy or cholecystectomy for bile peritonitis, meticulously controlled continuous gastroduodenal drainage, omental or suture closure, or gastric resection for perforated duodenal and gastric ulcers, and

closure and external drainage for the rent bladder.

In all cases of spreading secondary peritonitis and of generalized peritonitis, the sooner the leak is assuredly stopped, the better is the person's chance of recovering (see Table 8, Chap. 11).

The principles of antibiotic therapy of established infections of Chapter 4 are immediately applicable to the use of antibiotics for peritonitis. Because of the heterogeneity of the bacteria associated with secondary peritonitis, large doses of penicillin (1,000,000 units every 4 hours) and 250 mgms. of chloromycetin should be used intravenously until the organisms in a particular case have been identified and their sensitivities to the various antibiotics ascertained. Then the principles of Chapter 4 can be readily followed.

The treatment of septic shock is partially discussed in Chapter 7. Buffered saline solutions, blood, large amounts of appropriate antibiotics and a judiciously used vasopressor agent such as norepinephrine constitute the basic materials for treating septic shock.[1]

Hypothermia, though sporadically used for the treatment of septic shock, has not been proved to be effective by itself. Until more is learned about its use for septic shock, reliance should be placed upon the factors listed above and, if hypothermia is used, saline solutions, blood, antibiotics and vasopressors must be used with it!

SOME SPECIAL FORMS OF PERITONITIS

Because of the peculiarities of peritonitis that are relatable somewhat to a particular etiology, some individual attention needs to be given them.

Bile peritonitis is a relatively rare cause of acute peritonitis. It is generally a chemical peritonitis, but infection will often supervene. Some of the chemical constituents of bile are very irritating and induce rapid exudation into the peritoneal cavity. Consequently, shock tends to occur soon and is more likely to be the cause of early death than infection.

Extensive bile peritonitis is seldom seen from perforation of the gallbladder. When this viscus ruptures, the cystic duct is usually obstructed by impacted gallstones. Thus, the spillage is limited in amount, unless the release of intracystic pressure attending rupture of the gallbladder dislodges the impacted stone.

Bile peritonitis is more commonly secondary to operation upon the biliary tract, and penetrating injuries or traumatic avulsions of the gallbladder than to perforation of the diseased gallbladder. Several types of surgical accidents account for most intraperitoneal extravasations of bile. During cholecystectomy an unrecognized small accessory hepatic or cystic duct may be cut and not ligated. Necrosis or "blowout" of the cystic duct stump or a dislodgment of its ligature may occur a few days after the operation, especially should the flow of bile into the duodenum be partially or totally obstructed by a stone lodged in the ampulla of Vater. Postoperative bile leakage may also occur from simple aspiration of the common ducts through a needle. When such a procedure is used for cholangiography, catheter drainage of the duct should be employed. Unrecognized operative injury to the common duct and spontaneous localized necrosis of this structure are additional causes of bile peritonitis.

Pancreatic peritonitis in its early stage is usually a sterile inflammatory process and is attributable to the effects of enzymatic activity and the cleavage products of pancreatic lipase and tryptase upon the peritoneal surfaces and the subserosal fat. (See Chap. 31, "Pancreas.")

Blood "Peritonitis." Blood in the peritoneum may produce a mild peritoneal inflammatory response which may not be detectable for a day or two. Common nontraumatic sources of intraperitoneal hemorrhage are ruptured graafian follicles or cysts and tubal pregnancies. Aside from the early appearance of mild distress in the lower abdomen in the former, the characteristic complaint is one of pain in one or both shoulder regions when lying down. The rate of blood loss in ruptured ectopic pregnancy may be rapid indeed. The blood loss may be fatal unless surgical intervention is prompt and blood replacement is adequate.

Urine peritonitis is generally at first a sterile one. Later, especially with rupture of the dome of the bladder, signs of peritonitis may be strangely lacking even though the bladder has been ruptured for 2 or 3 days and there are 6 or more liters of uriniferous ascites. In such cases, the urine is sterile, and presumably it is not so acid or hypertonic as to produce inflammation. After all, a sterile urine with a pH of about 7 and a specific gravity of 1.012 to 1.018 is a rather physiologic saline solution containing urea which is practically nonirritating to many tissues. Ruptures of the vesical urethra or the bladder are the usual frequent cause of urine peritonitis (see Chap. 48, "Urology").

CHRONIC PERITONITIS

Chronic bacterial peritonitis is exemplified almost exclusively by tuberculous peritonitis. This granulomatous disease generally involves the entire peritoneum (Fig. 35-1). When it complicates acute miliary tuberculosis the visceral and parietal peritoneal surfaces are often covered in their entirety by miliary tubercles and with fronds of fibrin. In these cases the peritoneal fluid is fibrinous and generally scanty.

When tuberculous peritonitis is associated with nonmiliary tuberculosis it assumes a somewhat different form. The peritoneal tubercles are larger and occasionally fibrotic; adhesions are numerous and occasionally cause intestinal obstruction. Fluid accumulations are large, low in protein content and contain little or no fibrin.

The prognosis of tuberculous peritonitis is good now since the advent of certain of the antitubercular drugs. The fibrotic form is often complicated by intestinal obstruction, and consequently, its ultimate outcome is seldom certain.

Chronic chemical peritonitis is perhaps best illustrated by the talc granulomata resulting from dusting of surgical gloves with this material. The disease smolders along for many years and may require many operations for release of intestinal adhesions causing obstruction. Barium sulfate perforating the bowel or entering the peritoneal cavity via an unsuspected perforation also causes a chronic inflammatory reaction similar to that produced by talc in the peritoneum. This can largely be avoided if the barium is removed promptly from the abdomen.

Meconium peritonitis occurs from the intra-abdominal perforation of the gut *in utero* or in the neonatal period. This is a sterile

Fig. 35-1. Photograph showing the adherence and the appearance of the omentum and the bowel in a 30-year-old man with tuberculous peritonitis.

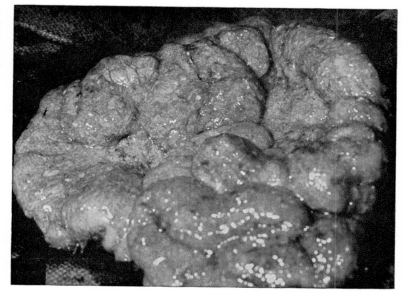

chemical peritonitis if it develops *in utero* (see Chap. 46, "Pediatric Surgery").

Idiopathic chronic peritonitis is observed occasionally in patients with long-standing ascites. It is not clear that the thickened serosa and its granular surface is the cause or the result of accumulations of ascitic fluid. This condition is observed more frequently in children or young adults in whom ascites and portal hypertension are the result of portal vein thrombosis than in adults with cirrhosis and ascites.

Chylous ascites and peritonitis are accompanied by a nonspecific inflammatory reaction to chylous lymph within the abdominal cavity. Most frequently, spontaneous chylous ascites is caused by the blockage of the flow of chyle in the region of the cisterna chyli by lymphomas and malignant tumors of the pancreas, the retroperitoneal connective tissue (sarcomas) and the kidney. However, chylous ascites may also be idiopathic and persist for many years with the patient otherwise remaining in good health, having only a swollen fluid-containing belly to plague him. Nitrogen mustard or radioactive colloidal gold have been used to treat chylous ascites with reported success.

COMPLICATIONS OF PERITONITIS

The most frequent complications or sequelae of peritonitis are intra-abdominal inflamma-

tory masses, abscesses, adhesions with mechanical intestinal obstruction, and enterocutaneous fistulas. Rarer sequelae are septicemia, septic thrombosis of pelvic and mesenteric veins, intrahepatic abscesses, empyema, and enterovaginal and enterovesical fistulas.

Inflammatory Masses. Intra-abdominal inflammatory masses must be distinguished from intra-abdominal abscesses because the former disappear without surgical intervention while the latter require drainage. Intra-abdominal inflammatory masses are made of fibrin-adherent edematous inflamed loops of intestine and parts of the omentum and do not contain pus. This inflammatory conglomeration of tissue is tender and readily felt through the abdominal wall or the rectum, depending upon its location. It is also attended by leukocytosis and some fever. The only way the inflammatory mass can be distinguished from an abscess without recourse to a diagnostic celiotomy is to repeatedly examine the mass and the patient, noting what is happening to the size of the mass and the overlying tenderness, and taking cognizance of the course of the illness. If within 24 to 48 hours the mass decreases in size, if the tenderness subsides, and if there is steady recovery from the general illness, the tender intra-abdominal tumor is an inflammatory mass, and nothing need be done about it. Should the lump increase in size, the tenderness not subside, and the patient remain septic, it is an abscess; drain it!

Adhesions and intestinal obstruction have been treated in Chapter 36. All that need be said here is: the long intestinal tube is a fairly effective way of treating adhesive mechanical intestinal obstruction should it occur within the first week or two after the peritonitis began. But celiotomy is usually the better treatment for adhesive mechanical intestinal obstruction that may occur later.

Pyelophlebitis is discussed in Chapter 34, and hepatic abscesses in Chapter 30.

INTRA-ABDOMINAL ABSCESSES

These are the most frequent complications of peritonitis. They are classified mainly on the basis of their anatomic locations: subphrenic, mid-abdominal and pelvic.

SUBPHRENIC ABSCESSES

The subphrenic space is that portion of the abdominal cavity bounded by the diaphragm above and the transverse colon and the mesocolon below. Barnard's (1908) description of the subphrenic spaces quoted for so many years is not anatomically correct. The subphrenic space is divided by the liver into the suprahepatic and the infrahepatic compartments. The falciform ligament further divides the space into the right and the left divisions. The triangular ligaments and the coronary ligament do not suspend the liver from its superior diaphragmatic surface but are actually dorsal mesenteries attaching the liver to the transversalis fascia overlying the base of the right crus and the posterior third of the right dome of the diaphragm. Consequently, on the right there is only one large space above the liver—the right suprahepatic space. The so-called posterior suprahepatic abscesses really occupy the posterolateral part of the suprahepatic space lying anterior and lateral to the coronary and the right triangular ligaments. Below the right lobe of the liver there is only one space, the right infrahepatic space; its most posterior recess is known as the pouch of Morison. On the left side of the abdomen the space above the left lobe of the liver is the left suprahepatic space. Because of the small size of the left lobe of the liver, this space freely communicates anteriorly and laterally with the space below the liver and

anterior and superior to the stomach and the spleen, and for this reason it is considered to be only a single space, the left anterior infrahepatic. The lesser peritoneal sac constitutes the left posterior infrahepatic space. Abscesses within these spaces rarely occupy more than a part of a particular space. Consequently, an abscess may be located either anteriorly or posteriorly, medially, centrally or laterally, in any of the spaces described above excepting the omental bursa; abscesses in it usually occupy it in entirety. Approximately two thirds of all the subphrenic abscesses are located on the right side, the suprahepatic spaces being occupied by them more frequently than the infrahepatic spaces. Approximately one sixth of the abscesses affect more than one of these spaces simultaneously, and about 6 per cent of them are so large as to be bilateral.

Diagnosis of Subphrenic Abscess. Subphrenic abscesses are often conspicuous by the lack of local signs of inflammation. After all, they are usually buried far away from the abdominal wall, the structures about them contain few somatic sensory nerves, and the ribs keep us from feeling them. Therefore, the old saying, "When there must be pus somewhere, but it is seemingly nowhere, there is pus under the diaphragm" is often remarkably appropriate. Pain and tenderness over the upper abdomen or the lower chest is most often inconspicuous; however, subphrenic or suprahepatic abscesses are frequently attended at one time or another by a pleuritic pain that may be referred to the shoulder. Widening and bulging of the intercostal spaces and edema of the skin are seen only rarely and then only late. Often about the only signs of a subphrenic abscess are: a septic temperature, an occasional chill (10 to 15%), tachycardia, anorexia, malaise, leukocytosis with a shift to the left, anemia and a pleural effusion. Most of these signs may be suppressed by antibiotics, and when they are, the subphrenic abscess may burst catastrophically into the free peritoneal or pleural cavities before the diagnosis is made.

RADIOLOGIC EXAMINATION is most important for the diagnosis and the localization of subphrenic abscesses. Demonstration of an air fluid level separable from the gastrointestinal tract is to be seen in approximately 25 per cent of the cases and is diagnostic. Elevation and loss of mobility of the affected diaphragm occur in approximately two thirds of the cases. A sterile pleural effusion on the affected side is present in 90 per cent. Occasionally, the stomach when distended with barium or carbonated beverage is found to be displaced, and with a barium enema the hepatic or the splenic flexures may be found out of place and distorted. Occasionally, a pneumoperitoneum (750 to 1,000 cc.) may be used to demonstrate obliteration of the normal spaces between the liver, the stomach or the spleen and the diaphragm. Diagnostic aspirations are somewhat hazardous because of the danger of contaminating the pleural space with them. In addition, they are unreliable because the abscess is readily missed by the needle. Once the presence and the localization of an abscess is established, it should be drained. The main consequences of an undrained subphrenic abscess, besides septicemia and death, is related to rupture of the abscess into the abdomen, producing a usually fatal generalized peritonitis, or into the thorax, followed by empyema, pyopneumothorax or bronchopleural fistula.

Treatment of Suprahepatic Abscesses. The approach used in the drainage of suprahepatic abscesses is important. Ever since the intro-

duction of the posterior extraperitoneal approach by Nather and Ochsner (1923), and the anterior extraperitoneal approach of Clairmont and Meyer (1926), the mortality from suprahepatic abscesses has been reduced to approximately half that associated with the previously used transperitoneal and transpleural routes. Suprahepatic abscesses may be drained under local or light general anesthesia.

Abscesses located posteriorly are generally drained by subperiosteal resection of the 12th rib on the affected side. Melinkoff found on cadavers that the pleura extended below the 12th rib in 62 per cent but never extended below the level of spinous process of the 1st lumbar vertebra. Therefore, after resection of the appropriate 12th rib, a transverse incision, *not one paralleling the bed of the rib,* is made at the level of the spinous process of L-1, thereby permitting assured entrance into the retroperitoneum below the diaphragm. With the index finger, the transversalis fascia is stripped from the diaphragm upward until the abscess is felt, perforated and drained.

For the drainage of abscesses located anteriorly, subcostal incisions located approximately 1 inch below the costal margin and extending from the middle of the rectus abdominus laterally and downward for 3 inches paralleling the costal margin are very satisfac-

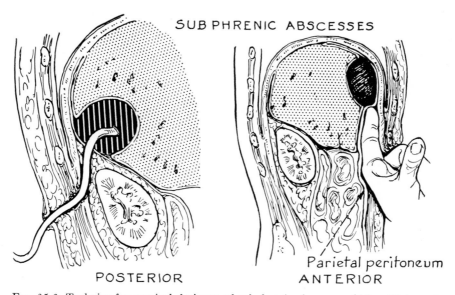

SUBPHRENIC ABSCESSES

POSTERIOR

Parietal peritoneum
ANTERIOR

FIG. 35-2. Technics for surgical drainage of subphrenic abscesses. (After Clairmont, Ochsner and DeBakey)

tory. The incision is carried down to *but not through* the transversalis fascia, and then with blunt dissection with a finger the transversalis fascia is separated from the diaphragm, taking care to keep out of the peritoneal cavity until the abscess cavity is located and drained. In a few instances when the location of the abscess is uncertain, particularly in subhepatic abscesses, it may be necessary to open the free abdominal cavity first in order to identify the limits of the abscess. Then this incision is closed, and another is made so as to drain the abscess without transversing the free peritoneal cavity. Recently, the transpleural approach has been resurrected for the drainage of posteriorly located suprahepatic abscesses. The 9th or 10th rib is resected in the posterior axillary line. The pleura is displaced superiorly when possible; when this is impossible, it is separated from the posterior chest wall, pushed against the diaphragm, and carefully sutured to the diaphragm all about the selected site for the diaphragmatic incision in order to seal off the pleural cavity before incising into the abscess. This is now a safer method than it used to be, presumably because of our having antibiotics.

Treatment of subhepatic abscess in a few instances may need to be located by exposing first the free peritoneal cavity away from the suspected site of the abscess. A counter incision is then made directly into the abscess without entering the peritoneal cavity, where the visceral and parietal surfaces adhere. Caution is necessary lest the exploratory intraperitoneal incision become contaminated; if possible, the skin area to be incised should be marked and the exploratory incision closed before attempting stab-wound drainage directly into the abscess cavity through the marked skin surface. More often, subhepatic abscesses can be entered directly from the overlying abdominal skin. Usually the site of location can be established by nonsurgical means and the drainage incision properly placed to ensure against transperitoneal drainage or contamination.

MID-ABDOMINAL ABSCESSES

Abscesses in the mid-abdomen may be located anywhere between the transverse mesocolon superiorly and the rim of the true pelvis inferiorly. The right colic gutter is the most

usual site, the left gutter the next, and between the folds of the small intestinal mesentery the rarest.

Abscesses in the mid-abdomen most often follow perforative appendicitis, diverticulitis and carcinoma of the colon, ulcerative colitis, traumatic perforations of large and small intestines, regional enteritis, and the leaving of sponges in the abdomen during laparotomy. Occasionally, perforations of the biliary tract or of a peptic ulcer are followed by a mid-abdominal abscess located in the region of the cecum. The diagnosis of abscesses lying in the gutters of the mid-abdomen is usually relatively easy. A septic fever and a tender growing mass in the abdomen that is easily felt, excepting in very obese persons, are the only signs requisite for diagnosis.

The diagnosis of intermesenteric abscesses lying between folds of the jejuno-ileal mesentery or below it (see Fig. 35-3) is much more difficult because abscesses thus located are usually small and multiple and do not come in contact with the anterior abdominal wall. Continued sepsis and partial mechanical obstruction of the small intestine are practically the only signs of intermesenteric abscesses unless they become so large as to be felt through the anterior abdominal wall.

Because of the paucity of signs that abscesses produce when located between folds of the mesentery, their existence must always be suspected when sepsis continues after the acute phase of peritonitis has passed and localizing signs of abscess cannot be found anywhere else. Especially in case of failure to find subphrenic abscess, when it is operatively searched for, should the mid-abdomen be explored for intermesenteric abscesses.

The treatment of mid-abdominal abscesses is drainage, using incisions that will permit a retroperitoneal or a direct approach into the abscess without transversing any open part of the peritoneal cavity. This is practically always possible with abscesses located in the colic gutters. It is impossible with abscesses located between folds of mesentery. The latter must be drained by the complete evacuation of their pus and the separation of the mesenteric folds one from the other.

At times the free peritoneal cavity must be opened first to delineate the boundaries of an abscess. When this is done this wound is closed, and then another is made to drain the pus from the abscess without permitting its entry into the peritoneal cavity.

All foreign bodies and dead organs such as the appendix or the gallbladder should be lifted out from the abscess should this be possible without breaking through the abscess wall or opening into the intestine that practically always makes up a part of the wall of the abscess.

PELVIC ABSCESSES

Pelvic abscesses most often follow pelvic inflammatory disease in women, perforative appendicitis and colonic diverticulitis. Pus draining into the pelvis from perforation of the upper or mid-abdomen may also lead to abscesses within the pelvis. It is said that should any patient with peritonitis be kept in Fowler's position (semisitting), the abscess that may form is more likely to do so in the pelvis making it easy to diagnose and drain. The symptoms of pelvic abscess include pain and tenderness in the lower abdomen and fever in women, and lower abdominal pain, frequency of urination, dysuria and fever in men.

Often the only symptom of a pelvic abscess in either sex is fever and a general feeling of being sick. The only way to keep from missing the "silent pelvic abscess" is to *perform a digital examination of the rectum every day after all appendectomies and during and after any acute peritonitis!*

Pelvic abscesses are tender masses that are readily palpated through the anterior rectal wall because they push this part of the rectum posteriorly and downward. The anterior rectal mucosa becomes thick and edematous, and the rectal sphincter becomes lax. One must be careful to distinguish between a pelvic inflammatory mass and a pelvic abscess. About two thirds of the tender pelvic masses felt through the rectum after peritonitis from perforation of a duodenal ulcer disappear spontaneously. Should an attempt be made to drain such a pelvic inflammatory mass through the rectum or the vagina all that may be accomplished is the creation of an enterorectal or enterovaginal fistula! In general, the inflammatory mass does not bulge into the rectum, while the abscess does; the inflammatory mass has indefinitely palpable limits, while the abscess is discrete and hemispherical; the inflammatory mass becomes smaller and less discrete over a day or two, while the abscess grows steadily larger; and the inflammatory mass is associated with an improving patient, while the abscess is associated with a continuing or worsening illness.

The treatment of a pelvic abscess is drainage into the rectum or the vagina (Fig. 35-4). Needle aspiration, once such an abscess is felt

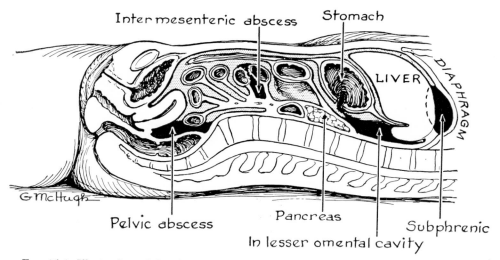

FIG. 35-3. Illustration of the dependent areas of the peritoneal cavity when the patient is in the supine position. These are the same areas in which intra-abdominal abscesses are encountered most frequently.

by rectal or pelvic examination, usually can be performed with reasonable safety. A 16-gauge, 4-inch needle is inserted through the posterior wall of the vaginal vault, or through the anterior wall of the rectum entering directly into the previously palpated abscess. Once pus is obtained, the site of needle puncture is enlarged by spreading with a hemostat or a pair of scissors inserted directed into the abscess cavity (Fig. 35-4). A soft but noncollapsible piece of rubber tubing is left in the abscess cavity and led to the outside. A piece of heavy silk is firmly secured to the tubing and appropriately attached to the adjacent external skin.

In all cases of spontaneous intra-abdominal abscess further studies should be made to determine its cause as soon as the patient's condition permits. Removal of the appendix should be carried out within 6 to 8 weeks after drainage of an appendiceal abscess. Carcinoma or other serious disorders which may require more surgery should be sought for and treated as required.

Occasionally, pelvic abscesses communicate with abscesses in the mid-abdomen; in these cases combined rectal or vaginal and abdominal drainage is often needed.

In all drainages of abdominal abscesses, wherever they may be, continuous drainage must be maintained until the cavity of the abscess has disappeared. The principles of drainage are discussed in Chapter 2 ("Wound Healing").

The persistence of an abdominal enterocutaneous fistula after the drainage of an intra-abdominal abscess complicating peritonitis is almost always relatable to one or more of six factors: (1) the persistence of an abscess between the abdominal wall and the intestine, (2) partial obstruction of the intestine distal to the fistula's enteral orifice, (3) a foreign body within the peritoneal cavity (usually a sponge), (4) a chronic granuloma within the intestine such as actinomycosis or tuberculosis, (5) a neoplasm of the bowel about the enteral orifice of the fistula, and (6) the juncture of skin with mucous membrane within the fistula. The injection of water-miscible radiopaque contrast media

FIG. 35-4. Drainage of pelvic abscess through the vagina or the rectum. (Kelly's Operative Gynecology, 1898)

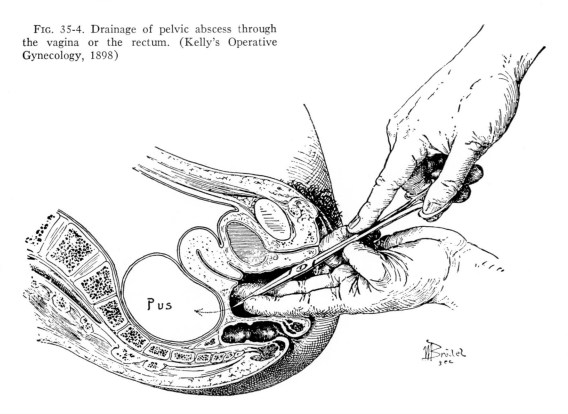

Pus

through a catheter into the fistula during fluoroscopy and subsequent filming of the region is the simplest and best means of ascertaining whether one or more of the first three causes are operative. Biopsy and proper culturing of scrapings from the depths of the fistula serve to examine whether causes 4 or 5 may exist, and close inspection of the fistula, which is usually very short, in cases of cutaneous mucosal juncture, serves to examine possibility 6. The treatment of chronic enterocutaneous fistulas rests upon removing the cause: e.g., wide direct drainage for residual abscesses, resections of the intestine and lysis of adhesions for distal obstruction, proper antibiotic therapy for actinomycosis and tuberculosis, resection for neoplasm, and separation of intestinal mucosa from the skin for cutaneous-mucosal juncture.

REFERENCES

1. Altemeier, W. A. and Cole, W. R.: Nature and treatment of septic shock. Arch. Surg. *77*: 498-507, 1958.
2. Clairmont, P., and Meyer, M.: Erfahrungen über die Behandlung der Appendicitis, Acta chir. scandinav. *60*:55, 1926.
3. Ochsner, Alton, and De Bakey, Michael: Amoebic hepatitis and hepatic abscess, Surgery *13*:635, 1943.

Other reading material on the subject of peritonitis is to be found in the bibliography of Chapter 34 on Appendicitis and the Acute Abdomen.

J. Garrott Allen, M.D.

CHAPTER 36

Intestinal Obstruction: Anatomy, Physiology and Treatment

GENERAL CONSIDERATIONS

It is estimated that approximately 8,000 deaths occur each year from intestinal obstruction. The mortality rates reported from a number of places vary from 5 to 20 per cent, which would imply that more than 160,000 cases of intestinal obstruction occur annually. An analysis of the fatal cases discloses that death is usually the result of the sequelae of intestinal obstruction, e.g., perforation, peritonitis, fluid and electrolyte loss, shock and aspiration pneumonitis. These are sequelae which for the most part are avoidable if treatment can be implemented early.

The mortality rate from acute intestinal obstruction over the past 50 years has diminished sharply due to earlier diagnosis, preoperative decompression as established by Wangensteen,[27] fluid and electrolyte replacement, blood and plasma administration, antibiotic therapy, earlier surgical intervention and improvements in operative technics. McKittrick and Sarris[14] demonstrated a decided reduction in mortality at the Massachusetts General Hospital when the patients were operated upon within 48 hours and nasogastric suction was employed concurrently.

Wangensteen's contributions to the reduction in mortality of intestinal obstruction are singularly outstanding. Prior to the use of nasogastric suction, the mortality rate for acute intestinal obstruction was approximately 45 per cent. Within the first decade that nasogastric suction of the Wangensteen type was widely employed, the mortality rates dropped from 45 per cent to about 18 per cent. In more recent years, mortality has been reduced further, now averaging about 10 per cent for the country at large which continues today. Most causes of death today are rightfully attributed to delay of the patient's seeking medical help, or to inadequate decompression and fluid replacement, old age and other infirmities.

ANATOMY

The jejuno-ileum or the "small bowel" extends from the ligament of Treitz to the ileocecal valve. It is about 20 feet in length. About 40 per cent of its proximal length is considered to be jejunum and the distal 60 per cent as ileum. It is all covered by serosa except on its mesenteric surface. There is no discernible gross anatomic feature which allows an accurate or exact separation of the jejunum from the ileum. The jejunum is generally of a little larger diameter, and its muscular coats are a little thicker than those of the ileum. The entire jejuno-ileum is attached to the anterior border of the mesentery in which courses its blood and lymph vessels. Situated about 3 to 4 feet from the ileocolic junction and on the antimesenteric border of the ileum, occasionally there is to be found a fingerlike projection, Meckel's diverticulum (see Chap. 46, "Pediatric Surgery").

Intra-abdominal Colon. The colon is about 5 feet in length and except during infancy is about twice the diameter of the small bowel. Its musculature differs from that of the small bowel in that the longitudinal muscle fibers are collected together in 3 bands, the *taeniae coli*. Each taenia is located equidistantly; one lies along the site of the embryologic attachment of the mesentery of the colon. The taeniae spread out over the colorectum and there disappear. The circular fibers of smooth muscle of the colon also are more or less collected together at intervals of 1 or 2 cm. apart and account for the haustra that give the colon its sacculated appearance.

The anatomy of the cecum and the appendix have been discussed in Chapter 34, page 848. The mesenteric relationships and the vasculature of the small and the large intestines have been presented in Chapter 33.

Lymph Drainage. The lymphatic circulation from the small bowel, the colon, the rectum and the anus must be known by the surgeon in planning operations upon malignant tumors arising from these organs. The lymphatic spread of tumors arising within these portions of the alimentary tract tends to be through the regional lymph channels and nodes draining the particular bowel segment involved. Consequently, the *en bloc* removal of the regional lymphatics and lymph nodes affords the patient his best chance for cure.

To a large extent, the lymph channels of the small bowel, the abdominal colon and the rectum correspond in location and distribution to those of the blood vessels of the same organs (see Figs. 33-5 and 33-6). However, when the lymphatics reach the root of the mesentery, this relationship no longer strictly obtains.

Lymphatics of the anus usually drain anteriorly, uniting with those from the scrotum or the labium majora and terminating in the superficial inguinal nodes.

Lymphatics of the anal canal drain the lower rectal mucosa and generally follow the course of the middle and the inferior hemorrhoidal blood vessels, to the hypogastric (internal iliac) nodes. These particular lymph channels are fairly diffuse and may course along the superior surface of the levator ani muscles, reaching the sacral nodes prior to entering the hypogastric lymph glands.

The lymphatics of the rectum and the colon are described in Chapter 37 (see Figs. 37-18 to 37-22).

Lymphatics of the jejunum and the ileum serve as conduits for chyle. These lymphatics pass through or around the preaortic nodes of the superior mesenteric region before entering the cisterna. The cisterna chyli is the central point of collection of all three preaortic nodal clusters (celiac, superior and inferior mesenteric). Thus it receives lymph from all of the intra-abdominal organs.

The cisterna chyli is an irregular, somewhat conical, saccular structure located on the anterior surface of the 2nd lumbar vertebra to the right side of and behind the aorta. From its cephalic end arises the *thoracic duct* which passes into the posterior mediastinum along the anterior surface of the thoracic vertebra between the right side of the aorta and the mesial side of the azygos vein. At the level of the 5th thoracic vertebra, the duct crosses to the left, where it continues its upward course, to empty into the left jugular or the subclavian veins or their point of juncture. Through this duct tumor cells from the alimentary tract may reach the systemic venous blood without passing through the liver. Virchow recognized that occasionally tumors (from the stomach especially) may reach lymph nodes in the left supraclavicular area via the thoracic duct route. Such nodes are often referred to as "Virchow's nodes."

Between the leaves of the mesentery of the small intestine and the intra-abdominal portions of the colon are large numbers of mesenteric lymph nodes. These are the nodes that are frequently the earliest sites for metastases from tumors of the bowel. The mesenteric nodes are frequently very prominent and enlarged in regional enteritis and ulcerative colitis.

PHYSIOLOGY

Intestinal Motility
(Including Peristalsis)

Four types of intestinal motion occur: peristalsis, segmental contractions, pendular movements and an undulating motion of the intestinal villi.

Peristaltic motions propel the bolus of food in the aboral direction; the segmenting and pendular contractions do not. Peristalsis is a contraction wave of the circular muscle that progressed in the aboral direction a few centimeters per second for distances of 5 to 30 cm. before stopping. Although the role of the long muscle coat in peristalsis is not known, some shrinkage in the length of the contracted segment of bowel appears to occur in man; this may represent the contraction of the longitudinal muscles. The distance traveled and the vigorousness of the peristaltic contraction are usually greatest in the upper jejunum. The contractions of the lower ileum are less vigorous.

The bolus of food is propelled forward and spread out by each peristaltic motion. It then remains stationary until another propelling wave of contraction comes along.

From time to time, a much more vigorous type of peristalsis occurs. These movements are known as *"peristaltic rushes"* and they swiftly sweep all that lies before them for distances of 20 to 50 cm. or further within a second or two before they die out.

Mechanical distention of the lumen appears to be the main stimulus to peristalsis. In the normal person, food is propelled most rapidly through the upper jejunum. Lower in the small bowel, peristaltic activity is less active, and the transit time is longer. The distance traveled by each peristaltic wave is less in the ileum than in the jejunum. Moreover, there is evidence that competitive antiperistaltic waves (damming back of intestinal contents) may occur normally in the lower ileum and oppose those traveling in the aboral direction. In the lower ileum the process of food transit becomes a "two steps forward—one step backward" sort of affair.

Segmental Contractions. These have no capacity to propel food. Cannon[3] described them as groups of simultaneous contractions, occurring at intervals, spaced fairly regularly throughout the small bowel. They occur more frequently than peristaltic waves, generally 6 to 15 a minute.

The segmenting movements appear to disseminate the bolus of food, in addition to turning the bolus over, thereby exposing fresh portions to the intestinal mucosa and facilitating absorption. These contractions also speed the flow of lymph through the lacteals. Some of these contractions may continue to occur in an adynamic ileus.

Pendular or oscillating motions are also annular contractions. They travel up and down a small segment of bowel for short distances. Because they may travel in both the oral and the aboral directions, their motion suggests the swinging of a pendulum, hence their name. They, too, knead and churn the food, spreading it forward and backward for short distances within the lumen of the small bowel.

Pendular motions are less obvious in man than peristaltic or segmenting contractions. Their function, when present, is very similar if not identical with those of the segmenting contractions.

The undulating motion of the intestinal villi may be most important in facilitating food absorption. Such motions constantly change the food environment at the absorptive surfaces, bringing into contact with each villus new fluid constituents. Each villus has its own capillary and lymph vessel and its own smooth muscle fibers. Contractions of the latter seem to account for the swaying or undulating motion of the villi.

Intestinal activity is under the influence of 2 sets of nerve plexuses; one is extrinsic and the other is intrinsic. At least pendular motion is capable of functioning independently of the functional integrity of either plexus; therefore, like the heart, it is myogenically activated. The student should consult standard anatomy texts for the details of the distributions of these nerve plexuses.

The motor functions of the extrinsic nerves are as follows: stimulation of the parasympathetics—the vagus nerves—increases the tonus and the motor activity of the bowel. Tonus is decreased and motility temporarily inhibited by stimulation of the sympathetics—the splanchnic nerves.

Experimentally, the stimulation of the sympathetics is believed to reduce intestinal tone and to stimulate contraction of sphincters; increase of parasympathetic activity is said to have the reverse effect. In man, vagotomy retards temporarily gastric motility but has little if any demonstrable influence upon intestinal activity. The removal of the coeliac ganglia, together with the cutting of the preganglionic fibers, is followed by an intractable diarrhea in the dog and in man.

The intrinsic nerves are comprised of Auerbach's and Meissner's plexuses—the myenteric plexuses. Auerbach's plexus lies between the longitudinal and the circular coats of the bowel. This plexus contains numerous ganglion cells whose absence is the primary defect in Hirschsprung's disease of the colon (see Chap. 46, "Pediatric Surgery"). The ganglia in Auerbach's plexus are believed to be the terminal connections of the vagus nerves and other parasympathetic nerves to the intestines.

Meissner's plexus lies in the submucosa and, compared with Auerbach's, contains relatively few ganglion cells. This plexus is said to be largely sympathetic in function; stimulation inhibits action of the smooth muscle.

Finally, it should be stated again that the churning and mixing motions (largely segmenting and pendular motions) of the intestine continue in the absence of either extrinsic or intrinsic nervous control and are not affected when strips of smooth muscle are suspended in solutions of cocaine or other ganglionic blocking agents. Therefore, this type of movement is considered to be myogenic in origin and to be independent of nervous control, though not necessarily unresponsive to nervous stimuli.

Defecation. As peristaltic activity gradually propels food through the small bowel and the colon, the feces distend the rectum. As the intraluminal pressure in the rectum rises to 40 to 50 mm. of mercury, the reflex of defecation is set in motion. This reflex is characterized by strong peristaltic contractions of all the smooth muscular coats of the descending and the sigmoid colons. Both longitudinal and circular contractions take place. Contraction of the longitudinal musculature (the taeniae coli) shortens the colon. These two contractions are associated with the simultaneous relaxation of the anal sphincters, and feces are expelled.

Additional forces are applied by certain of the striated muscles which seem to act automatically but are under voluntary control. The simultaneous contraction of the musculature of the abdominal wall exerts considerable increase in the intra-abdominal pressure when the diaphragm is held in the fixed position of deep inspiration.

Voluntary control of defecation is largely effected by relaxation of the musculature of the abdominal wall and the diaphragm, while maintaining the tonus of the external anal sphincter. The latter is supplied by the 4th sacral and the internal pudendal nerves. If these nerves are cut, voluntary sphincter control is lost.

INTESTINAL ABSORPTION

The absorptive surface of the small bowel in man is estimated to exceed 10 square meters or about 8 times the area of the skin of an average adult. The large surface of the bowel mucosa is made possible by its innumerable villus folds.

There is no disagreement as to the intestine's ability to absorb water, alcohol, glucose, amino acids and fat, but the mechanisms by which these various substances are absorbed are not well understood. Until such time that more precise information is available, perhaps it is best in a text such as this to state that foodstuffs are absorbed primarily in the small bowel and that the function of the colon is largely restricted to the absorption of water. The colon will also absorb certain aqueous solutions, such as isotonic or hypotonic solutions of glucose and saline; consequently, these substances may be administered by proctoclysis if administered slowly. Water absorption in the colon takes place mainly in the cecum and the right half of the colon. The descending colon, the sigmoid and the rectum are largely reservoirs for feces.

INTESTINAL SECRETIONS

Intestinal juice or succus entericus is comprised of water, electrolytes, glucose and urea essentially in isotonic concentrations.

In a normal man, enormous quantities of water pass into and out of the intestinal tract during 24 hours. Approximately 8,000 to 10,000 ml. enter the alimentary tract in the course of 24 hours, while normally less than 200 ml. of water is excreted in feces. In other words, more than 96 per cent is reabsorbed, a ratio of water salvage close to that of the normal kidney in its recovery of the glomerular filtrate.

Diarrhea and intestinal fistulae result in excessive losses of water and electrolytes from the alimentary tract and for this reason alone may be rapidly fatal unless water and salts are given rapidly and properly. The tragic but dramatic stories of John Snow and others about epidemics of cholera a century ago tell of progression of symptoms from onset to death in less than 24 hours. Snow recognized the lethal effect of uncontrollable purgation with its loss of water and salt and proposed their replacement as the most effective form of treatment.

Consider for a moment the result of losing most of the following intestinal secretions (see Table 1). It can be readily appreciated that the entire loss of any one of the secretory fluids which normally enters the alimentary tract could be rapidly fatal if uncorrected. Death was a common sequel to duodenal, pancreatic or biliary fistulae as recently as 20 years ago. Elucidation of the quantitative and qualitative aspects of water and mineral metabolism has enabled us to treat these abnormalities effectively (see Chap. 5, "Fluids and Electrolytes").

Mucus is an important constituent of intestinal secretions. It is a protein-polysaccharide complex whose function appears to be the maintenance of a "nonwettable" bowel surface, especially in the colon. Mucus is secreted in response to mechanical stimulation and does not appear to be under hormonal control.

The volume of intestinal juice is modified by a number of stimuli: mechanical, nervous, humoral, osmotic and chemical. Secretin increases its secretion, as does the intravenous injection of saline solutions and sympathetic denervation.

ORIGINS OF INTESTINAL GASES

The normal intestinal tract contains only small amounts of gas within the stomach and the colon. The small bowel of normal persons, excepting infants, is largely free of gas. Normally, about 300 to 500 ml. of flatus is expelled in the course of the day.

Much of the intestinal gas enters the gut through the esophagus during swallowing, deep breathing and coughing. However, some of it is formed in the intestine by chemical and bacterial action, namely, methane and carbon dioxide. Actually, about $7\frac{1}{2}$ liters of carbon dioxide is elaborated in 24 hours by the interaction of hydrochloric acid of gastric juice upon the bicarbonates of biliary and pancreatic secretions, but because CO_2 is absorbed readily, this gas is usually an unimportant cause of intestinal distention.

The enzymatic degradation of certain foods potentially may yield surprisingly large quantities of gas. Schwartz,[24] for example, calculated that 30 liters of carbon dioxide, methane and hydrogen could come from the digestion of 100 Gm. of cellulose. Since no mammalian enzymes can attack the cellobiose bond of cellulose and since bacterial hydrolysis of cellulose in man is not a prominent activity, this figure of Schwartz may be more theoretical than actual.

Portis[21] described the composition of intestinal gases with particular diets as follows:

TABLE 1. RATES OF TURNOVER OF WATER BY VARIOUS ORGANS IN A 70-KILO HUMAN INDIVIDUAL IN CUBIC CENTIMETERS PER 24 HOURS

ORGANS	MINIMUM	LIBERAL
Salivary glands	500	1,500
Stomach	1,000	2,400
Intestinal wall	700	3,000
Pancreas	700	1,000
Liver (bile)	100	400
Lymph	700	1,500
Total recovered by body	3,700	9,800

(Adolph after Wangensteen, O. H.: Intestinal Obstructions, ed. 3, Springfield, Ill., Thomas).

AVERAGE CONCENTRATION OF SODIUM, POTASSIUM AND CHLORIDE IN THE GASTROINTESTINAL TRACT SECRETIONS REMOVED BY INDWELLING TUBES, MILLIEQUIVALENTS PER LITER

	SODIUM	POTASSIUM	CHLORIDE
Through Gastric Tube			
Salivary ⎱ Gastric ⎰	59	9.3	89.0
Through Small Bowel Tube			
Bowel Wall ⎱ Bile ⎰ Pancreas	104.9	5.1	98.9
Through Miller-Abbott Suction			
Ileum	116.7	16.2	105.8
Through Ileostomy	129.5	20.6	109.7
Through Cecostomy	79.6		48.2

(Randall, H. T.: Surg. Clin. North Amer. 32:2, 457, 1952).

TABLE 2

	MILK DIET %	MEAT DIET %	LEGUMES %	NORMAL DIET %
CO_2	16.8	13.6	34.0	10.3
CH_4	0.9	37.4	44.6	0.7
H_2	43.9	3.0	2.3	29.6
N_2	38.4	46.0	19.1	59.4

Normally, gases are absorbed from the intestinal tract at rates that are directly proportional to their diffusibility, the latter property being related to the relationship of the partial pressures of the particular gas in the tissues and the intestine and in the plasma and in the air breathed. For example, under normal circumstances, the partial pressure of carbon dioxide is highest in tissues, intermediate in the plasma and very low in the air breathed. Consequently, there is a net diffusion of CO_2 from tissues to plasma to air. However, with nitrogen the partial pressures of this gas are the same in tissue, in plasma and in air; consequently, the net diffusion of nitrogen is zero as long as air is breathed.

Fine and collaborators[10] have employed this knowledge for treating patients with gaseous distention from intestinal obstruction. They recommend increasing the concentration of oxygen breathed by these patients. By so doing, the partial pressure of nitrogen in the air breathed is reduced, and some of the nitrogen of the plasma will move into the alveolar air

and be breathed out, lowering the partial pressure of nitrogen in the plasma below that in the tissues and the intestinal lumen; consequently, some of the nitrogen within the intestine will move into the plasma, thereby decreasing the intestinal distention. Obviously, if only 100 per cent oxygen is breathed for 3 hours, the partial pressure of nitrogen in the body and the lumen of the intestine will approach zero. This process is termed denitrogenation. This technic may be of practical value in the treatment of intestinal distention, particularly when it cannot be relieved by intubation.

DIAGNOSIS

Definitions. *Ileus* is a word derived from the Greek and literally means to twist. However, ileus is a synonym now for intestinal obstruction from any cause.

There are 2 rather distinct forms of ileus: the mechanical and the adynamic or paralytic. They may be functionally subclassified as they are in Table 3.

TABLE 3. INTESTINAL OBSTRUCTION (ILEUS)

TYPE	SUBTYPE		PREDOMINANT CAUSES
Mechanical Ileus	Without direct interference to intestinal flow of blood	(a) Intraluminal:	Bezoars, gallstones, foreign bodies, polyps, atresia, diaphragms
		(b) Mural:	Inflammatory, irradiational and neoplastic strictures, hemorrhage into wall of bowel (Dicumarol, hemophilia, crushing trauma)
		(c) Extraintestinal:	Annular pancreas, intra-abdominal congenital bands, perienterostomy strictures, incomplete dehiscence of laparotomies, nonstrangulating hernias, simple adhesional obstructions
	With direct interference to intestinal flow of blood	(a) Extraintestinal:	Strangulated hernias, intraperitoneal adhesions with closed loop obstructions
		(b) Mural:	Intussusception
Adynamic or Paralytic		(c) Mesenteric:	Volvulus
	Without direct interference to intestinal flow of blood	(a) Metabolic:	Potassium deficiency, severe sodium deficiency, diabetic ketosis
		(b) Reflex:	Handling of the intestine; injuries to the thoracic and the lumbar spine; obstructions of ureters, cystic duct, common duct or appendix; acute distention of the bladder; chemical and bacterial peritonitis
		(c) Septic:	Bacteremia, septicemia, lobar pneumonia, acute pyelitis, meningitis, bacterial peritonitis
	With direct interference to intestinal blood flow	(a) Mesenteric arterial occlusive:	Emboli, thrombi and ligatures
		(b) Venous occlusive:	Thrombi and ligatures

Mechanical intestinal obstruction is a structural occlusion of the intestine. There are 3 categories of obstructing mechanisms: (1) the closure of the intestinal lumen by occlusion from such things within it as polypoid tumors, congenital diaphragms, foreign bodies, gallstones, bezoars, or impacted feces; (2) the closure of the intestinal lumen by intramural abnormalities such as congenital atresia and duplications, intussusception, stenosing inflammations of the intestine (segmental enteritis, terminal ileitis), strictures from primary cancer or metastases to the intestinal serosa, and very rarely from intramural hemorrhage; and (3) the closure of the lumen by abnormalities outside of it and the intestinal wall by such things as hernial rings, adhesive bands and volvulus. Some of the mechanisms of mechanical intestinal obstruction are shown in Figures 36-2 to 36-5.

Nearly 80 per cent of all mechanical intestinal obstructions fall in the third causal category. Groin, umbilical, incisional and internal hernias alone account for about a third of all of them. The hernias and the adhesive bands collectively account for about 70 per cent of all mechanical intestinal obstructions (Table 4).

TABLE 4. CLASSIFICATION OF INTESTINAL OBSTRUCTION AND THE APPROXIMATE PERCENTAGES OF EACH TYPE USUALLY ENCOUNTERED AMONG ADULT PATIENTS IN A LARGE GENERAL HOSPITAL

	APPROXIMATE PERCENTAGE OF ALL CAUSES
Mechanical obstruction	
A. Simple obstruction	40 (of total)
a. Adhesive bands	25
b. Tumors and foreign bodies	15
B. Strangulated obstruction	45 (of total)
a. External strangulated hernia	30–25
b. Adhesive bands	20
C. Special types of strangulation obstruction	15 (of total)
a. Volvulus	7
b. Intussusception	5
c. Mesenteric thrombosis or embolism	3
	100

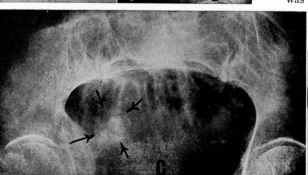

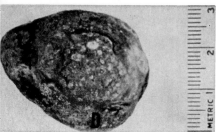

FIG. 36-1. Simple obturator obstruction caused by a gallstone in the ileum. Roentgenographic records depict the events in a 74-year-old woman with a large solitary gallstone which led to "gallstone ileus." (A) Shows the calcified gallstone in the gallbladder in May, 1946. (B) A roentgenogram 3 months later when she first experienced persistent right upper quadrant pain of 3-days' duration, associated with increasing upper abdominal tenderness, mounting fever and leukocytosis. Note that calcified gallstone is not seen on this film. (C) A roentgenogram of the lower abdomen taken 4 days after B showing small bowel distention and the calcified gallstone. This stone was removed from the terminal ileum. (D) Photograph of the calculus removed during operation.

Intraluminal Obstruction

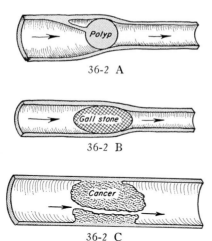

36-2 A

36-2 B

36-2 C

Mural Obstruction

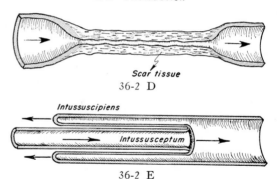

Scar tissue
36-2 D

36-2 E

FIG. 36-2. Varieties of mechanical intestinal obstruction. Intraluminal obstruction due to: (A) polyp; (B) gallstone; and (C) cancer. Mural obstruction due to (D) scar tissue, and (E) intussusception.

SYMPTOMS AND SIGNS OF INTESTINAL OBSTRUCTION

The symptoms and signs of intestinal obstruction are rather variable. Their variability depends a great deal upon the type of obstruction, its location within the intestine and when it occurs; for example: (1) cramping pains occur regularly with mechanical intestinal obstruction in which intestinal blood flow is not interfered with, while constant pain characterizes a strangulated obstruction; (2) abdominal distention is often great with simple mechanical obstruction and adynamic ileus and is small with closed loop obstructions, excepting sigmoid volvulus; (3) vomiting regularly and soon accompanies obstruction of the proximal jejunum and inconstantly and tardily attends mechanical obstruction of the sigmoid colon; and (4) simple mechanical obstruction of the small intestine during the first week after an abdominal operation is often relatively painless and crampless but is rarely so later. Obviously, the diagnosis of intestinal obstruction is often difficult.

The history is important. Questions relative to a previous condition in the past which could

FIG. 36-3. Volvulus with obstruction of small bowel due to a twist of a loop of small bowel about adhesions on its anti-mesenteric border. Note distended proximal loop and collapsed distal loop. Other mechanisms may produce volvulus.

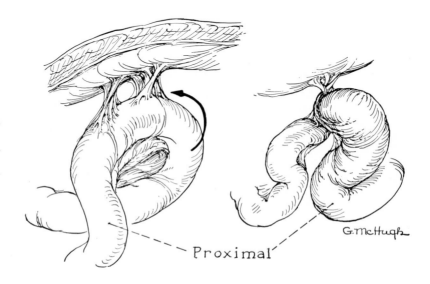

Proximal

Extra Intestinal Obstruction
Adhesive band — Closed loop

Hernial Obstruction

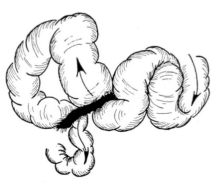

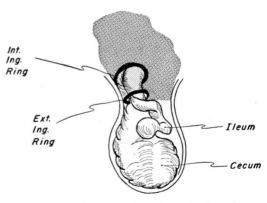

FIG. 36-4. Strangulated closed-loop obstruction with a loop of bowel under an adhesive band. As the loop of bowel that passed beneath the band distends, strangulation occurs.

FIG. 36-5. Strangulated mechanical intestinal obstruction of a sliding hernia of the cecum and terminal ileum.

produce intra-abdominal adhesions should be searched for in the history, and the answers should be evaluated critically. A history of an intra-abdominal operation or abscess, a bout of peritonitis or pelvic inflammatory disease, regional enteritis or diverticulitis can very readily provide the necessary intra-abdominal adhesions to account for acute mechanical obstruction.

Postoperative adhesions, especially following mid-abdominal or lower abdominal operations and pelvic peritonitis or inflammatory disease, are the most commonly encountered elements in the past history that give rise to adhesions causing acute mechanical obstruction. In the absence of an abdominal operative scar, external hernia, and with no history of nonoperative peritonitis or pelvic inflammatory disease, attention is directed toward tumor, volvulus, intussusception, fecal impaction, mesenteric thrombosis or embolism, or foreign body—the declining order of frequency in causes of intestinal obstruction in the adult.

Actually the problem of diagnosis may be approached best by discussing the variances of the symptoms and signs of ileus.

Pain With Intestinal Obstruction. Intestinal colic characterizes the pain of simple mechanical ileus (mechanical obstruction without inference with intestinal blood flow).

Intestinal colic is pain that comes and goes away coincident with the coming and the going away of intestinal peristalsis. The person having intestinal colic will often say that the pain comes while gurgling is heard and felt within the abdomen. Ascertainment of the coincidence of the pain with peristalsis is the only way of being certain that an abdominal pain that comes and goes is intestinal colic. *Ureteral colic comes and goes too, but the colics of ureteral obstructive pain are not associated with intestinal peristalsis but are disassociated with it.* At times the ascertainment of the coincidence of abdominal pain with intestinal peristalsis requires 15 or more minutes of continuous auscultation of the abdomen.

As the obstructed intestine becomes distended with fluid and gas, the colics and the peristalsis decrease in intensity and may even disappear. As this happens, a steady abdominal pain takes its place. This disappearance of peristalsis in intestines simply mechanically obstructed is ascribed to decompensation of the intestine. Presumably, the obstructed intestine becomes too distended to peristalt. The steady pain associated with decomposition of the intestine is rarely severe. Peculiarly, simple mechanical ileus occurring during the immediate postoperative period may *not* be accompanied by intestinal colic. *Severe steady or increasing abdominal pain that soon supersedes intestinal colic usually signifies that strangulation of the obstructed intestine has taken place.* With volvulus the pain may be so excruciating that the sick person may act maniacally and may even be wrongly judged to be insane.

During the height of paralytic or adynamic ileus, the abdominal pain is diffuse and steady and is rarely severe. However, during the recovery phase of adynamic ileus, typical intestinal colics occur—"gas pains" they are called. The steady pain that attends the adynamic ileus caused by occlusions of the mesenteric vessels by thrombi or emboli grows steadily worse until shock occurs, and then it abates. In fact, whenever shock complicates any type of intestinal obstruction, the pain partially or wholly subsides.

Meteorism. Some abdominal distention usually follows all types of intestinal obstruction. However, the amount of distention is highly variable. It is often very great with adynamic ileus, with simple mechanical obstructions of the ileum and the left colon, volvulus of the sigmoid colon and Hirschsprung's disease. It is often practically nonexistent with simple mechanical obstructions in the proximal jejunum, with closed loop obstructions of the small bowel and with mesenteric arterial obstructive ileus.

Nausea and vomiting usually attend most forms of intestinal obstruction sooner or later. When the obstruction is located within the proximal intestine, such as in the duodenum or the upper jejunum, nausea and vomiting occur almost immediately or soon after the intestine is obstructed; they tend to be oft repeated. In addition, the vomiting often *completely relieves the intestinal colic temporarily* when the obstruction is located in the proximal small intestine; just as it relieves the pain of pyloric obstruction. In general, the more distal in the intestine the obstruction is located, the longer time will be between the beginning of ileus and the inception of vomiting. Actually, a complete obstruction of the sigmoid colon may be unattended by vomiting for days and sometimes not at all.

CHARACTER OF VOMITUS. Before roentgenography was developed, the character of the vomitus was considered to be important diagnostically and prognostically. Today all that need be said about the significance of the character of vomitus with ileus is: feculent vomitus signifies that the bacteria normally largely restricted to the colon and the distal ileum are now growing freely throughout the small intestine. For this to take place the intestine usually needs to have been obstructed for days and widely distended with fluid and gas. Prognostically, it is still a dire omen.

Obstipation is a universal accompaniment of complete intestinal obstructions. To be sure, individuals may pass feces or gas either spontaneously or following an enema after the small intestine or the proximal colon has become completely obstructed, but this act only represents the passage of the gas and the excrement located distal to the obstruction. Consequently, the passage of feces or flatus after the intestinal colic has begun *does not mean that complete mechanical small intestinal obstruction does not exist.* The old test of the trial enema is worse than worthless; it is often misleading.

Diarrhea. Peculiarly, the frequent passage of liquid feces is often a sign of partial mechanical intestinal obstruction. Persistent diarrhea through ileostomies and colostomies is almost a certain sign of partial intestinal obstruction proximal to or at the site of the enteral stomata. Rectal fecal impactions are heralded by diarrhea. Partially obstructing neoplasms of the colon are often accompanied by alternate periods of alvine flux and obstipation.

Temperature With Intestinal Obstruction. Fever with mechanical intestinal obstruction is predominantly a sign that: (1) *the blood flow to the closed part of the intestine is obstructed and that part of the intestine is dead or dying (the obstruction is strangulated);* (2) *that the intestine is perforated;* or (3) that the obstruction is related to or associated with an infection within the intestinal wall and about it such as with diverticulus or deeply ulcerating neoplasms. Very rarely is fever with intestinal obstruction caused by hypernatremia and water deficit.

Hypothermia occasionally occurs with intestinal obstruction. When it does, it practically always means that the person has been severely depleted of sodium and is hyponatremic.

Concentration of Cellular Elements in the Blood. Just as fever is usually a sign of strangulation, so is leukocytosis. However, a slight degree of leukocytosis may be attributable to dehydration alone. However, dehydrational leukocytosis is not associated with increased numbers of immature forms of polymorphonuclear leukocytes. Consequently, a differential count of the leukocytes is very important with intestinal obstruction. This is especially true because a polymorphonuclear leukopenia will occasionally occur with such forms of intestinal obstruction as strangulating obstructions, volvulus and mesenteric vascular occlusions. When leukopenia occurs with such intestinal obstructions, practically all of the polymorphonuclear cells in the blood will be immature.

The hematocrit is often somewhat elevated in all forms of intestinal obstruction because of dehydration.* However, rapidly rising and very high hematocrits are practically certainly indicative of volvulus, mesenteric venous occlusion, or strangulation obstruction with peritonitis; all of these promote the rapid loss of plasma from the blood and thereby rapidly raise the concentration of red blood cells. This is one of the reasons why a person with intestinal obstruction and a very high or rapidly rising hematocrit is so often precariously ill and is so likely to die.

Localized Abdominal Tenderness. Tenderness that is restricted to a limited part of the abdomen of patients with mechanical ileus means strangulation of the mechanically obstructed intestine. Should this tenderness overlie a palpable mass, a strangulated, closed-loop intestinal obstruction almost certainly exists. Should the tenderness overlie a mass and the abdominal musculature over it is reflexly rigid, the obstructed intestine is most likely dead or perforated or both.

Serum Amylase and Serum Lactic Dehydrogenase. For reasons that are as yet poorly understood, the concentration of serum amylase rises very rapidly in some patients with only obstructed intestines and especially

* Dehydration refers to loss of water. It has been shown that one can add or remove water from blood and not change the hematocrit, based upon the fact that water is not only extracellular but intracellular. To change the hematocrit, a loss of colloid or saline is necessary. Water alone will equilibrate its increments or decrements between the intracellular and extracellular compartments proportionately, while colloid and saline remain for the most part extracellular and therefore affect the hematocrit. (H.N.H.)

so when the larger arteries and veins to a long piece of intestine are occluded. No evidence of pancreatitis can be found in such patients when operated upon or subjected to necropsy. Serum amylases higher than 3,600 Somogyi units have been found with small intestinal volvulus, strangulation of long segments of jejunum beneath adhesive bands and in internal hernias, and mesenteric arterial thromboembolic occlusions.

Lactic dehydrogenase, an enzyme contained in moderately large amounts within the normal intestine and its mucosa, recently has been found in amounts more than three times the normal in the sera of 8 of 11 human beings with *infarction of the intestine* (volvulus, strangulated closed-loops and mesenteric arterial and venous occlusions). The serum lactic dehydrogenase concentrations were normal in: 4 cases of peritonitis without intestinal infarcts, 2 infarcted herniated pieces of omentum, 18 cases of intestinal obstruction without death of intestine, and 5 cases of pancreatitis (serum amylases above 1,000 S. U. in 4 of them).[2]

DIFFERENTIAL DIAGNOSIS

The differential diagnosis of intestinal obstruction is 2-phased. One is concerned with the differentiation of intestinal obstruction from other conditions that mimic it, and the other pertains to the differentiation of the types of ileus one from the other.

The main conditions that mimic intestinal obstruction are: (1) acute bacterial and toxic enteritis; (2) the various abdominal visceral crises, such as tabetic intestinal and renal, the abdominal crises associated with porphyria and the hemolytic anemias and with Henoch's and the Schönlein-Henoch purpuras; (3) renal colic; (4) acute pancreatitis; (5) acute cholecystitis; (6) pseudocyesis and (7) the acute meteorisms that are suffered by persons having intractable asthma or disabling pulmonary emphysema or fibrosis. Clearly, the ascertainment of the existence of mechanical intestinal obstruction is often not easy, and the chance of making diagnostic errors is good unless the surgeon knows much about internal medicine.

Acute Bacterial Enteritis. The initial tormina (pains) of acute bacterial enteritis (such as dysentery and bacterial toxic) and toxic enteritis (such as lead and arsenic poisoning) are typical intestinal colics; the pains are synchronous with hyperperistalses. Initially, these tormina are accompanied by obstipation for variable lengths of time varying from a few minutes to hours. During the obstipational period of dysentery and toxic enteritis even the abdominal roentgenographic appearance may mimic mechanical obstruction of the small intestine. About the only thing which may serve to make one aware of the possibility of toxic enteritis during its obstipational period is the profundity of the general illness that develops so soon after the beginning of the colic. The student should consult appropriate texts of gastroenterology and toxicology to learn the rather peculiar gastroenterologic pictures of bacterial and toxic enteritis.

Abdominal Crises. The differential characteristics of the various abdominal crises are beyond the scope of this text. The diagnoses of renal colic, pancreatitis and cholecystitis are discussed in Chapters 48, 31 and 30, respectively. The differentiation of acute hemorrhagic pancreatitis from volvulus, large closed loop and mesenteric arterial occlusive intestinal obstruction is particularly difficult because adynamic ileus, fever, tachycardia, leukocytosis and shock attend both hemorrhagic pancreatitis and these forms of ileus *and so does hyperamylasemia.* Serum amylases higher than 3,600 Somogyi units have been observed in persons having only volvulus of the small intestine or mesenteric arterial vascular occlusion. In other words, a celiotomy may be the only way to differentiate with certainty acute hemorrhagic pancreatitis from volvulus, strangulating intestinal obstructions and mesenteric vascular occlusion.

Pseudocyesis or spurious pregnancy is an organic manifestation of hysteria that will often lead the unwary into performing laparotomies for what they take to be intestinal obstruction. The abdomen *appears to be distended, but true meteorism does not exist.* With pseudocyesis, breathing is fast, shallow and almost completely thoracic. The thoracic cage is chronically held in the inspiratory position even at the end of expiration. Fluoroscopically, the diaphragm is held in the inspiratory position, and it moves little with breathing. The lateral abdominal musculature is rigid, and the central part of the abdominal wall is pushed forward. With all this the sufferer complains of continuous or "crampy" pains in the abdomen, and of breathlessness. The abdominal walls of these patients are almost always "battle scarred," occasionally bearing as many as 10 to 15 scars of laparotomies. The diagnosis of pseudocyesis is easy: the ostensible abdominal distention disappears upon having the patient rebreathe into a tight-fitting quart-sized paper bag for 3 or 4 minutes, or having her breathe from a closed breathing system containing 5 per cent carbon dioxide in oxygen. True meteorism is unaffected by these maneuvers.

Meteorism. Acute periods of meteorism accompanied by intestinal colic occasionally bedevil the severely emphysematous and the so-called chronic pulmonary cripple. The differentiation of this meteorism from that of intestinal obstruction is usually easy. Obstipation does not accompany the abdominal distention and cramps. On the contrary, excessive amounts of flatus are passed; and the *entire intestine, including the colon and the rectum, contains gas.*

Types of Ileus. Concerning the differentiation of the types of ileus one from the other, the most important thing is the differentiation of ileus *without mechanical interference to the flow of blood to the obstructed intestine* from ileus *that is associated with mechanical interference to the flow of blood to the obstructed intestine.* This is very important because a delay of the operative correction of an ileus such as a volvulus, a strangulated obstruction, or that which accompanies mesenteric vascular occlusion leads very often to death of the obstructed intestine, and often to the death of the patient from overwhelming peritoneal sepsis and shock. For this reason, often one cannot safely await the analytical reports of the serum amylase or lactic dehydrogenase, the decision as to the state of blood flow to the obstructed intestine should and must be reached whenever possible upon the bases of other evidences that can be gathered more quickly. These have already been discussed or are listed in Table 5. In other words, ileus accompanied by occlusion of blood flow to the obstructed intestine is an immediate surgical emergency, and one cannot afford to delay making a decision for want of erudite chemical evidence. Frequent repeated examinations of the abdomen for localized tenderness, a mass, and changing character of peristalsis, the pulse, the temperature and the leukocytes constitute the main ways of determining whether or not an ileus has an intestinal vascular occlusive component. Often the signs of intestinal vascular occlusion will be few and meager during the initial hours of a strangulated ileus, although the blood vessels to the intestine are then already partially choked and may become completely occluded any moment. Consequently, one should *never* assume that an ileus which at first ostensibly has no evidences for vascular occlusion actually does not have or will not develop one. Therefore, a person with an ileus that lacks signs of intestinal vascular impairment must be examined at intervals not longer than 1 or 2 hours apart until the obstruction is removed.

Roentgenographic Examination. A relatively simple roentgenographic examination of the abdomen is very valuable for the differential diagnosis of ileus.

Stereoscopic filming of the abdomen with the patient in the *supine* position is the basis of all abdominal roentgenologic diagnosis. Examination should not be done with the patient prone because of the alteration of normal location of abdominal viscera due to external pressure against the abdominal wall in this position.

Prior to obtaining the supine abdominal film, it is important that no cleansing enema be administered. Not only may such an enema be painful and dangerous to the patient, but, in addition, it almost certainly will produce confusing collections of air and fluid on the abdominal x-ray examination.

Despite the popularity of the erect film of the abdomen, it seldom proves to be of significant diagnostic aid. Certainly gas-fluid levels within the bowel ("stepladder pattern") can be seen by this method, but no reliable information concerning location of or degree of intestinal distention can be obtained by this procedure. Such gas-fluid levels are not pathognomonic of mechanical ileus as is widely believed but may be seen also in cases of adynamic ileus, regional enteritis, ulcerative colitis, sprue or even in patients with normal abdomens following cleansing enemas. Nor does the finding of such a gas-fluid level insure that it is intraluminal in position; such

TABLE 5

		TYPE OF OBSTRUCTION CAUSE	CHARACTER OF PAIN	ABDOMINAL DISTENTION	PERISTALTIC SOUNDS
WITHOUT INTERFERENCE WITH INTESTINAL BLOOD FLOW	Mechanical	Bezoars, gallstones, foreign bodies	Severe sudden colics that often suddenly stop for days at a time	Variable	Hyperactive during pains
		Strictures inflammatory or neoplastic	Colics that are rarely severe and tend to increase over days or weeks	Usually great unless obstruction is high in gut	Variable if colic is severe, hyperperistalsis is great; if pain is weak, peristalsis is weak
		Hernias and adhesions	Severe colics that usually come suddenly	Variable	Hyperactive during colics
	Adynamic	K deficit, severe Na deficit, peritonitis, sepsis, handling of bowel	Diffuse soreness or discomfort	Usually great if ileus persists for more than a day	Few in number faint and tinkling
WITH INTERFERENCE WITH INTESTINAL BLOOD FLOW	Mechanical	Strangulation of hernias and intestine beneath adhesions	Continuous pain that is usually preceded or accompanied by colics	Variable	Few or absent usually
		Volvulus	Steady and severe until shock occurs, then it subsides		
	Adynamic	Mesenteric thrombotic or embolic occlusion		Usually small	

a finding is frequent, for instance, in subdiaphragmatic abscess in which the fluid is pus in the peritoneal cavity, and bacteriogenic gas caught under the diaphragm forms the level.

If the simple radiologic procedures outlined above indicate that there is a lesion of the colon, obstructive or otherwise, without evidence of perforations, then barium enema may be performed safely and is frequently diagnostic of not only the site but also the nature of the lesion. In cases of obstructive lesions of the colon, the oral administration of barium sulfate suspensions is contraindicated because of the tendency of this material to convert a partially obstructing lesion to a complete acute obstruction because of its tendency to become inspissated due to colonic water absorption. This leads to technical difficulty in bowel preparation or at laparotomy.

However, if it is certain that the area of obstruction is in the small bowel, no such difficulties attend the oral administration of contrast medium, and frequently the site and the nature of the obstructive lesion in the small bowel can be demonstrated by this method. Barium sulfate suspensions may be administered by mouth in such patients or,

better, may be injected through a long intestinal tube of the Miller-Abbott type. In the latter instance, the progress of the tube is observed until the distention is relieved and the point of obstruction is reached. Then the introduction of the barium suspension directly through the tube is observed fluoroscopically and by appropriate filming at the time of fluoroscopy. Recently, the water-miscible contrast media long used for pyelography have been employed successfully to examine rather quickly and definitively the small intestines of people with ileus. One need not worry about giving these materials orally to patients with colonic lesions; they cannot convert a partial into a complete colonic obstruction as barium sulfate may do.

Simple stereoscopic filming of the abdomen will often permit the discovery of intestinal obstructing foreign bodies.

FOREIGN BODIES

Most foreign bodies that are ingested will pass through the gastrointestinal tract without incident. Occasionally, a large or peculiarly shaped ingested object will fail to pass, and surgical removal will be necessary. If the

TABLE 5 (*Continued*)

TEMPER-ATURE	PULSE RATE	W.B.C.	HEMATO-CRIT	SERUM AMYLASE	SERUM LACTIC DEHYDRO-GENASE	X-RAY SIGNS	OBSTIPATION
							Intermittent
Normal unless complicated by severe dehydration or infection	Normal unless complicated by severe dehydration or infection	Normal differential. Count normal unless complicated by severe dehydration or infection	Rise that is proportionate to the apparent dehydration	Normal	Normal	Intra-intestinal fluid and gas above the obstruction and very little or none below the obstruction	Often alternating diarrhea and obstipation
							Complete
						Intra-intestinal fluid and gas throughout the intestine	Variable, often incomplete
Fever	Tachycardia	Leukocytosis and shift to left (young cells)	Rise that is disproportionately greater than the apparent dehydration	Occasionally elevated	Usually much elevated	Intra-intestinal fluid and gas above the obstruction	
				Often much elevated (up to 4,000 S. U.)		Often little gas in bowel but fluid distention may be enormous (sigmoid volvulus)	Complete after evacuation of the intestine below the obstruction
		Occasionally leukopenia				Little gas or fluid in the intestine	

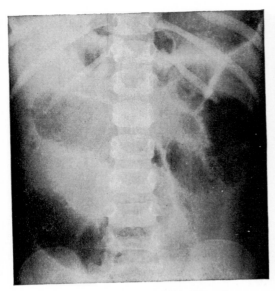

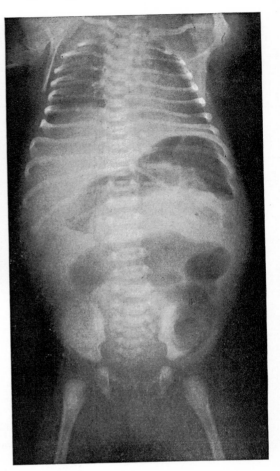

Fig. 36-6. (*Top and right*) Dilated gas-filled loops of small bowel indicate the presence of intestinal obstruction. Mechanical ileus in this case was due to a nonopaque foreign body (trichobezoar).

foreign body is opaque to x-rays, generally its location and progression can be determined. Plastic, glass and other radiolucent foreign bodies afford more difficulty, and their presence may be determined only if they produce complications. The findings of a perforated viscus may be produced by such an object, or the clinical and radiologic picture of intestinal obstruction may result (Fig. 36-6).

INTESTINAL OBSTRUCTION

The location, the level and the degree of obstruction in large or small bowel generally can be determined from radiologic examination. Except for direct inspection at laparotomy, supine abdominal x-ray examination is the most dependable means of determining the location and the degree of distention of the small bowel. If dilated gas-filled loops of small bowel are present, a diagnosis of ileus may be made with reasonable confidence.

In a typical case of low small bowel obstruction, diagnosis is usually easy. The presence of distended loops of jejunum and ileum arranged transversely in the central portion of the abdomen with little or no gas in the colon strongly suggests mechanical obstruction (Fig. 36-7). Small bowel is identified by the presence of the plicae circulares forming their characteristic pattern of circular transverse ridges in the distended lumen and by the usual central abdominal position that distended small bowel assumes. Distended colon does not have this appearance; the haustra do not cross the entire distended lumen.

In closed loop obstruction, the distended fluid-filled loop of small bowel forms an abdominal mass which displaces other abdominal viscera (Fig. 36-8). The closed loop contains fluid and no significant amount of gas. The closed loop becomes edematous and fluid-filled due largely to embarrassment of venous return. Prompt radiologic recognition of the presence of a closed loop obstruction may lead to surgical intervention prior to permanent vascular damage and gangrene.

Volvulus of the sigmoid colon is the most

FIG. 36-7. Classic roentgen appearance of mechanical ileus. Note that the "trans-lateral" view (*right*) made with the patient supine and with the radiation horizontal demonstrates the distended loops. However, it gives no useful information as to extent or the location of these loops; as a matter of fact, it fails even to make possible the differentiation of large and small bowel.

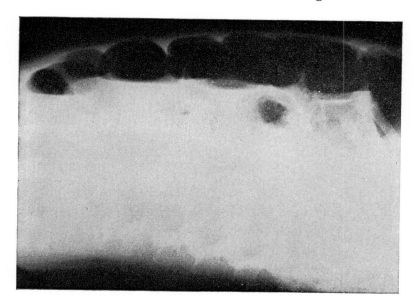

frequent form of torsion of the colon and produces a quite characteristic roentgen appearance (Fig. 36-9). There is a grossly dilated loop of bowel which has no plicae circulares (valvulae conniventes, Kerkring's folds) but it may have haustral indentations. The bowel walls lead to the two distinct points of obstruction. Barium enema demonstrates the abruptly tapering narrowing (bird-beak deformity) of the colon distal to the volvulus (Fig. 36-10). This finding is diagnostic of torsion.

The presence of distended loops of large and small bowel is said to be typical of adynamic ileus (Fig. 36-11). However, in obstructive lesions of the colon, distention of the large bowel proximal to (and occasionally even outlining) the point of obstruction is found frequently. If the ileocecal valve is incompetent, there is also small bowel distention

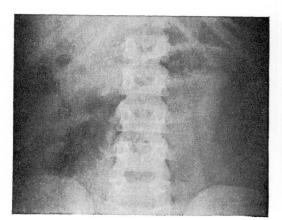

FIG. 36-8. Closed loop obstruction with large "pseudotumor" in the left lower abdominal quadrant.

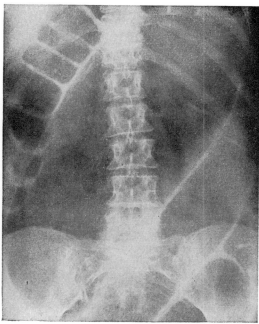

FIG. 36-9. Volvulus of the sigmoid colon.

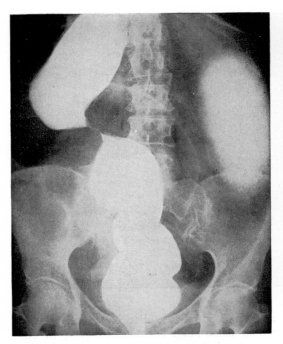

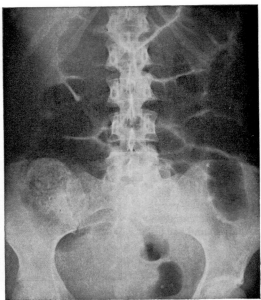

FIG. 36-11. Peritonitis with adynamic ileus.

FIG. 36-10. Typical appearance of barium enema in case of sigmoid volvulus of Figure 36-9 (bird-beak or ace of spades deformity).

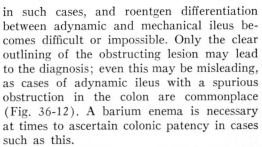

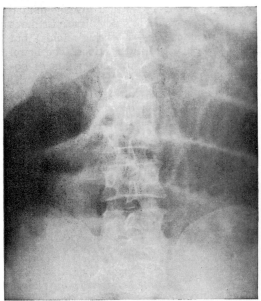

in such cases, and roentgen differentiation between adynamic and mechanical ileus becomes difficult or impossible. Only the clear outlining of the obstructing lesion may lead to the diagnosis; even this may be misleading, as cases of adynamic ileus with a spurious obstruction in the colon are commonplace (Fig. 36-12). A barium enema is necessary at times to ascertain colonic patency in cases such as this.

The most reliable method of differentiating mechanical and adynamic ileus is by auscultation of the abdomen. Fortunately, this method is accurate early. The absence of bowel sounds in functional neuromuscular disturbances is characteristic, whereas increase in borborygmi at the height of colic is a characteristic of mechanical intestinal obstruction.

Diagnosis of ileocolic or colocolic intussusceptions as the etiology of mechanical intestinal obstruction is best done by barium enema (Figs. 36-13 and 36-14).

Administration of barium sulfate suspension through a double lumen tube after it has reached the point of obstruction will demon-

FIG. 36-12. Distended small bowel and right colon leading to the erroneous conclusion that there was mechanical colon obstruction with incompetent ileocecal valve. Adynamic ileus was the true situation.

strate the point and the nature of the obstructing lesion (Fig. 36-15). The presence of normal mucosal folds in the constricted area is

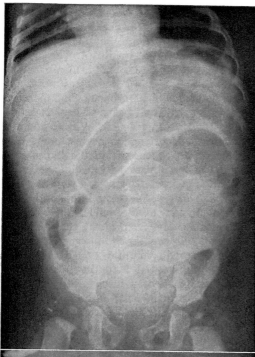

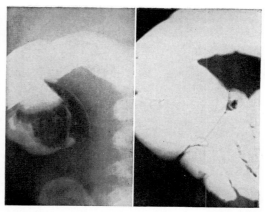

FIG. 36-14. (*Left*) The diagnosis of intussusception is made. (*Right*) The invagination is corrected during the procedure.

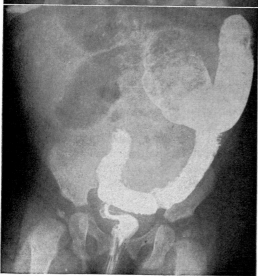

FIG. 36-13. The etiology of mechanical ileus is demonstrated by barium enema. In this case the intussusception was not reduced by this diagnostic procedure.

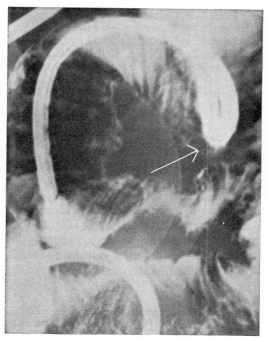

FIG. 36-15. The small bowel distention and its deflation by means of a Miller-Abbott tube may be seen. Barium administered after decompression when the tube ceased advancing demonstrates the point of obstruction that was caused by an adhesive band.

suggestive of an extrinsic obstruction, such as one caused by adhesions; occasionally, the rare small bowel tumor is demonstrated by this method.

Bowel obstruction due to the presence of a large gallstone which has perforated the gallbladder and the duodenum and entered the small bowel lumen through the resultant fis-

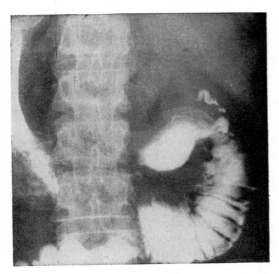

Fig. 36-16. Gallstone ileus. Air and some barium in the biliary tree are noted. A large radiolucent gallstone was found at the ligament of Treitz. The dilated duodenum is seen, and the point of obstruction is sharply outlined by orally administered barium. (Also see Fig. 36-1)

CLINICAL FEATURES

The treatment of ileus needs to fit the cause of the obstruction and the physiologic deformations that have attended it. The physiologic deformations that attend ileus are mainly hydrational, circulatory and respiratory.

The hydrational disturbance that more or less always attends all forms of ileus is extracellular fluid volume deficit. Within minutes after intestinal obstruction begins, interstitial fluid begins to collect within the lumen and the walls of the obstructed intestine; *whether this fluid is subsequently spewed out as vomitus or not does not matter;* interstitial fluid within the lumen and the walls of the intestine is as certainly lost from about the nonintestinal tissue cells and the red blood cells as if it were lost through vomiting or diarrhea. The amount of interstitial fluid that may collect within the lumen of a mechanically or adynamically obstructed small intestine within 12 hours is occasionally almost fantastically large, even constituting about one half of the entire corporal interstitial fluid. With mechanical obstructions of the terminal ileum and with toxic adynamic ileus among adults the small intestinal diameter frequently attains to 4 cm. Should such a dilated small intestine be filled only with interstitial fluid, from 7 to 9 liters would be needed to fill it.

As the intestine distends, its volume increases exponentially; it increases as the square of the radius. Within the ranges of distention that are associable with intestinal obstructions the intraluminal capacities are approximately those tabulated in Table 6.

Fortunately, the content of the distended

tula is one of the types of intestinal obstruction in which the etiology is frequently apparent on the supine abdominal film. The presence of air in the biliary tree is pathognomonic of the fistulous connection, and this finding coupled with that of bowel obstruction is sufficient to make the diagnosis (Fig. 36-16). In about one fourth of such patients, the gallstone contains sufficient calcium so that it can be identified radiographically.

TABLE 6

	Diameter of Intestine	Volume per Meter Length of Intestine		Volume in Entire Length of Uniformly Distended Bowel	
	cm.	mls.	pints	mls.	pints
Small intestine normal length —7 meters	2	300	.75	2,000	4.6
	3	700	1.5	4,900	10.9
	4	1,250	2.75	8,750	19.4
	5	2,000	4.4	13,700	30.4
	6	2,800	6.2	19,600	43.5
	7	3,850	8.5	26,950	59.5
Colon length— 1.5 meters	10	7,800	17.2	11,700	26
	11	9,500	21	14,250	31.6
	12	11,300	25.1	16,900	37.5
	13	13,200	29.3	19,800	43.9
	14	15,400	34.2	23,100	51.3

intestine is rarely only interstitial fluid; usually half or more of it consists of gas. However, interstitial fluid often constitutes practically the total amount of the content of the obstructed intestine in cases of volvulus, mesenteric vascular occlusion and strangulated closed-loop obstruction. In such cases as well as others in which fluid makes up a significant part of the distended intestine's contents, severe extracellular fluid deficit and even dehydrational shock are to be expected.

Acidosis is a rare accompaniment of ileus, except with diabetes and infancy, and usually requires for its treatment only insulin and glucose for the diabetic and glucose for the infant.

Potassium deficiency with hypokalemia is one of the primary causes of adynamic ileus and frequently complicates simple mechanical intestinal obstruction and more especially when the obstruction has been partial and accompanied by diarrhea or repetitive vomiting. Potassium deficiency very rarely complicates acute simple mechanical or strangulating intestinal obstruction.

Because of the rarity of severe acidosis or potassium deficit with acute mechanical ileus, the repair solutions best fitted to the treatment of the interstitial fluid volume deficit of mechanical ileus are glucose containing Hartmann's solution (lactated Ringer's solution), or slightly hypotonic (¾ strength) Locke's solution (bicarbonate Ringer's solution) (see Chap. 5). Occasionally, the amount of repair solution needed may be very large. Some idea of the amount needed may be gained from the assessment of the amount of the vomitus, the degree of fluid distention of the intestine measured on roentgenograms, and measurement of the volume of fluid removed from the intestine by nasogastric intubation or operative decompression. No glucose in water need be given during the restitution of the dehydration of ileus so long as the patient requires 2.5 to 3.0 liters or more of Hartmann's solution or of dilute Locke's solution containing glucose daily.

Whenever potassium deficiency occurs with or causes ileus it should be treated with appropriate solutions of potassium salts in glucose (see Chap. 5).

Occasionally, severe hypo-osmolarity (hyponatremia) complicates ileus; when it does, from 500 to 1,000 ml. of 3 per cent sodium chloride solution may be used with the other repair solutions. The hypertonic sodium chloride is especially indicated should physical signs of water intoxication exist.

The respiratory derangements that accompany intestinal obstructions are relatable to meteorism. With an adynamic ileus in which the entire small intestine is dilated to 5 cm. and the colon to 10 cm. (not unusual with toxic adynamic ileus) the intra-abdominal visceral volume has been increased by about *20 liters,* or more than 5 gallons. Such intestinal distention cannot be accommodated within the abdomen without pushing the diaphragm far up into the thoracic cavity and thereby choking the person from below. At times intestinal meteorism may so impede breathing as to threaten life immediately. The only sure way of treating acute life-threatening respiratory insufficiency related to acute meteorism of ileus is operative decompression of the intestine.

The general circulatory disturbances of ileus without organic interference with blood flow to the obstructed intestine are largely relatable to the dehydration and the meteorism, and upon proceeding far enough become manifest as peripheral circulatory failure. Adequate treatment of the dehydration and the meteorism correct these circulatory disorders. However, whenever organic obstruction of intestinal blood vessels occurs, additional circulatory disturbances take place that are relatable to the movement of bacteria and bacterial products into the peritoneal cavity and then through the peritoneum into the general circulation. Many bacterial toxins weaken heart muscle, injure capillary walls and affect vasomotion. Couple these with dehydrational oligemia and dehydrational cellular metabolic disturbances, and a very profound and often therapeutically unresponsive form of shock, called septic shock, occurs. The principles of the treatment of septic shock are: remove the bacteria-permeable intestine, treat the dehydration, use a vasopressor drug whenever there are signs of an abnormally low arteriolar peripheral resistance and give wide-spectrum antibiotics intravenously.

The treatment of the intestinal obstruction itself is individual and is outlined in Table 7.

TABLE 7. SPECIFIC TREATMENT OF MECHANICAL ILEUS

TYPES	SPECIFIC CAUSE	TREATMENT	CHAPTER REFERENCE THIS TEXT
I. Intraluminal	Bezoars, gallstones, foreign bodies	Push obstructing object back into a part of the proximal dilated intestine *that is not* inflamed and remove it through a short longitudinal antimesenteric incision that is closed transversely	This chapter
	Polyps	Local removal, or local resection of bowel	37, Part 2
	Diaphragms	Local excision, or diverting enteroenterostomy about them	46
	Atresia	Resection of proximal bulbous end and enteroenterostomy	46
	Malignant neoplasms	Small intestine and right colon—wide primary resections and anastomosis; left colon—decompressive colostomy followed by wide resection	37, Parts 1 and 2
II. Intramural and Mural	Inflammatory strictures	Resect or bypass with an appropriate enteroenterostomy	37, Part 1
	Neoplastic strictures	As for intraluminal obstructing neoplasms, or bypass enteroenterostomy if there are numerous peritoneal metastases	
	Intussusception	Reduce in infants by methods described in Chapter 46	46
		Resect without attempting to reduce in older children or adults because among older children and adults *malignant neoplasms* constitute *the lead point of the lesion* in from 30 to 50 per cent of cases	This chapter
III. Extra-intestinal and Mesenteric	Annular pancreas	Duodenojejunostomy	46
	Congenital and postinflammatory adhesions	Excise band adhesions, do not merely transect them	46
	Volvulus of sigmoid colon	Decompress through sigmoidoscope with a rectal tube if possible; otherwise surgically decompress after exteriorizing	This chapter
	Volvulus of small intestine	Reduce operatively	46
	Hernias of all types	Reduce operatively and repair	39
	Ileostomy or colostomy strictures	Excise stricture and effect a meticulous coaptation of mucous membrane to the skin with sutures	2
IV. Adynamic	*K deficit Na deficit Diabetic ketosis	Potassium salts Sodium salts Insulin	5
	*Reflex	Gastric and/or intestinal intubation	
	*Septic	Drain abscesses, remove gangrenous parts, antibiotics	3 and 4
	Vascular occlusive	Embolectomy, endarterectomy, bypass grafting, resection of dead intestine	40

* In cases of adynamic ileus of these types in which meteorism threatens life because of respiratory embarrassment, operative decompression of the intestine is the best treatment.

COMPLICATIONS OF ILEUS

Aspiration pneumonitis and disruption of the continuity of the intestine are the main complications of ileus.

Aspiration pneumonitis is to be feared with all kinds of ileus. Vomiting, while the person is weak or drugged by soporifics or analgesics, is especially prone to lead to pneumonic aspiration of the vomitus. The aspiration of a large amount asphyxiates and kills within minutes, while the aspiration of lesser amounts leads to a *gangrenous type of pneumonitis that kills within days.* To date there is *no treatment that is effective for aspirational pneumonitis.* Because of this the only thing that can be done is to prevent aspiration. Prevention rests practically in entirety upon *keeping the stomach empty!* This can be done only by the *proper placement of and attention to the continuous functioning of an inlying gastric tube.* Occasionally, a gastrostomy is needed to ensure emptiness of the stomach should the patient be comatose, very weak, or so unco-operative as to remove the nasogastric tube repeatedly.

Should the gastric tube be connected to a mechanical suction pump, the tube leading from the gastric tube to the pump should *always* be vented with a No. 20 or 22 hypodermic needle. If this is not done, the mucosa of the stomach is often sucked into the holes of the gastric tube, the stomach fills with liquid, and vomiting and aspiration occur even though the tube is properly placed. Simple straight gravity drainage of the gastric tube directly into a plastic bag that is simply fastened to the patient's gown or the mattress cover is a very simple and effective way to keep the stomach empty *provided that there are no vertical U-loops* in the tubing connecting the gastric tube with the plastic receptacle. Should there be such a loop, it acts as a hydraulic obstructive valve because the fluid part of the gastric drainage collects in the loop, and the gas part of the gastric drainage collects behind it and precedes it. *When this happens nothing will leave the stomach through the tube until the pressure in the stomach reaches a level which is higher* than the weight of the column of water in one side of the U-loop. If the vertical height of a loop, half filled with a liquid that has air in front

of and behind it, is 13 cm., the pressure in the stomach must rise above 13 cm. of water (*10 mm. Hg*) before any gas or fluid will leave the stomach through the tube. *When U-loops are kept out of the tubes, simple drainage works very satisfactorily.*

Irrigation of the gastric tube, using a syringe and a *saline solution once an hour,* is very important! It is the only way that one is able to ensure emptiness of the stomach. Saline should always be used to irrigate inlying gastric and intestinal tubes. Should water be used to flush the tubes and wash the stomach, sodium and potassium salts pass into the water from the gastric and the intestinal mucosa very rapidly and are washed out of the body.

Disruption of the continuity of the wall of an obstructed intestine is a catastrophe! The postoperative mortality rate for intestinal obstruction without peritonitis is now less than 7 per cent, while the postoperative mortality rate is about 30 per cent for intestinal obstruction when complicated by peritonitis, arising from dissolution of the continuity of the obstructed intestine.

There are a number of ways that intestinal continuity may be broken functionally: (1) localized pressure necrosis of the wall immediately under hernial rings or adhesive bands, (2) avascular necrosis from pressure occlusion or thrombo-embolic occlusions of large intestinal arteries by twisting, intussusception, hernial or adhesive bands, mesenteric arterial thrombosis or embolism, and (3) localized avascular necrosis arising from distentional occlusion of intramural intestinal arterioles, capillaries, or veins.

The first mechanism of necrosis is relatively rare but is especially important as a cause of rupture of the intestine caught in a Richter's hernia or under a fixed adhesion (see Chap. 39).

The second mechanism is the most frequent cause of intestinal disruption. The third is not rare and pertains especially to the colon.

In the past, occasional disruptions of the wall of the obstructed colon were thought to be directly attributable to simple physical rupture by the pressure built up between the ileocecal valve and the obstructing lesion. The normal small intestine of man bursts when subjected to intraluminal pressures of 120 to 230 mm. Hg, and the colon when pressured to 90 mm. Hg.[11] The ileocecal valve is forced open by intracolonic pressures of 40 to 55 mm. Hg. Obviously, the ileocecal valve will be breached before the normal colon bursts from pressure alone; if this were not true, bursting of the colon would be an important hazard of roentgenographic examination of the colon with the barium enema which, as practiced today, regularly is attended by retrograde filling of a part of the terminal ileum.

However, acute complete left-sided colonic obstruction is very dangerous because localized colonic rupture affecting usually the cecum or the ascending colon is so prone to complicate it. Van Zwalenberg[30] discovered that upon increasing the intraluminal pressure within exteriorized human appendices (exteriorized to decompress obstructed colons through appendicostomy) circulatory arrest would occur within the wall of the distended appendix. Others[8, 11, 18, 19] have demonstrated that intestinal capillary stasis occurs with intraluminal pressures of 30 to 50 mm. Hg, venular occlusion with pressures of 50 and 60, and intramural arterial occlusion with pressures higher than 90 mm. Hg.

Obviously, localized avascular necrosis of the colon may follow its being subjected to intraluminal pressures that have actually been measured in obstructed human colons, namely, 10 to 40 mm. Hg.[27]

Whatever the mechanism may be, cecal rupture does complicate complete colonic obstruction; consequently, operative decompression of the completely obstructed colon is a surgical emergency.

Peritonitis may complicate strangulated closed loop obstruction without actual physical dissolution or rupture of the intestine.[15]

Ordinarily, the intestinal wall is remarkably capable of preventing diffusion of its intraluminal contents into the peritoneal cavity and vice versa. However, when the bowel is severely distended or even distended moderately for protracted periods of time, many substances are then capable of diffusing into the peritoneal cavity. Bacteria, hemoglobin and pigments of hemoglobin may be detected in the peritoneal fluid. Colloidal dyes which normally would not diffuse into the peritoneal cavity may stain the serosal surface of the distended bowel and color the intra-abdominal fluid. Nemir *et al.* (1953)[17] and many before

them have studied the effects of the intravenous injection of peritoneal exudates obtained in the presence of strangulated obstruction. Often these exudates have been fatal to recipient animals. This type of observation has been the principal anchor for the toxic theory of mortality from intestinal obstruction.

TREATMENT

INDICATIONS FOR INTUBATIONS IN INTESTINAL OBSTRUCTION

Short Tubes. Besides being useful for the prevention of pneumonic aspiration, the short or gastric tube is employed most frequently during the early postoperative period of any operation performed upon the abdomen which is likely to produce temporary inhibition of peristaltic activity. The tube is used for 1 to 3 days, by which time peristalsis usually has returned. The short-tube intubation is often the most effective type of intubation in the prevention of further distention in paralytic ileus from peritonitis. It is also employed occasionally as a supplement to long-tube intubation to prevent accumulation of swallowed air in the stomach when the long tube lies far down the ileum.

The chief drawback to the use of short-tube or gastric suction in attempting decompression of intestinal obstruction is its failure to remove appreciable amounts of gas or fluid distal to the pylorus. This criticism is not as serious as might appear, for the usefulness of long-tube intubation in the relief of mechanical intestinal obstruction is fairly limited due to the fact that more than 80 per cent of mechanical obstruction occurs within the small bowel where short tubes are fairly effective in avoiding distention.

Long Tubes. Intestinal intubation with a tube of the Miller-Abbott type may be indicated in some patients with simple small bowel obstruction, particularly incomplete obstruction. Occasionally, the release of distention in such patients will permit the bowel to disengage itself from its point of obstruction. It may slip out from under an adhesive band, or retract from a hernial sac if not incarcerated or volvulated. However, long-tube intubation has its greatest usefulness in patients with recurring bouts of small bowel obstruction during and for a short time after acute peritonitis from any cause and in cases of multiple neo-plastic metastases to the wall of the intestine. It is also occasionally useful in the late stages of paralytic ileus from peritonitis when relief of distention occasionally hastens the return of peristaltic activity.

In most patients with intestinal mechanical obstruction, even when not associated with obstruction of blood flow to the intestine, an operation is the best treatment. Procrastination generally does not avoid necessity for operation and carries with it the threat of unrecognized bowel necrosis occurring during the interval of intubation as well as problems in fluid and electrolyte balance.

Decompression of the colon by long tubes is practically impossible; the fecal matter within an obstructed colon cannot be drawn through the tube. Consequently, the passage of a long tube in cases of colonic obstruction with the hope of decompressing the colon and preventing its disruption only wastes time. A proximal colostomy works and prevents colonic rupture.

Any sign of restricted blood flow to obstructed intestine contraindicates any attempt at passage of a long intestinal tube; one cannot afford to waste this time doing something that *cannot* take the intestine out of vascular jeopardy.

SURGICAL INTERVENTION AND PROCEDURES FOR THE RELIEF OF MECHANICAL OBSTRUCTION OF SMALL BOWEL AND COLON

Before these operations are undertaken for simple mechanical ileus, it is presumed that the deficits of fluids and electrolytes have been at least partially corrected, that blood has been administered as indicated, and that other disorders have been appropriately considered and treated insofar as possible. All of these things need to be accomplished within a matter of hours with simple mechanical intestinal obstruction. *In case of ileus with signs that the blood flow to the intestine is impaired, and with complete colon obstruction with a greatly distended cecum, there can be no time wasted.* In such cases the operating room is the place, and the period of the operation itself is the time to treat the dehydration and the shock. This can be done more readily during the operation because then the causes of the de-

hydration and the shock are removed, and the fluids given are consequently more effective than they are when given while the causes are still operative. Delay in release of an incarcerated and strangulated loop of bowel is the most important secondary factor contributing to bowel necrosis and hence to the mortality rate.

The *aims of surgical intervention* in acute mechanical obstruction are:

1. Release of obstruction
2. Re-establishment of intestinal continuity or at least of a segment sufficient in length to avoid excessive losses of water and electrolytes and to provide for adequate absorption and nutrition in the days or years ahead
3. Resection of nonviable bowel

How these aims may best be accomplished will vary from one patient to another, but the most important determining factor related to treatment is the site of obstruction. The operative procedure of choice for large bowel obstruction can be the most harmful one which may be performed on the obstructed small bowel and vice versa.

Choice of Anesthesia. The safest anesthesia for operative correction of ileus is one that permits the anesthetist to maintain full control over breathing and to keep gastric fluid out of the trachea and the lungs. A cuffed-intratracheal tube is the instrument which permits him to do both things. Whether the basal anesthetic be spinal, local, or inhalation, the intratracheal tube should be used. This can now be done by skilled anesthetists on fully conscious persons (see Chap. 12, "Anesthesia").

Relief of Simple Obstruction. Except for the performance of operative decompression for asphyxiating meteorism of adynamic ileus and for colostomy, the incision must be long enough to permit removal of the entire small intestine from the abdomen if need be. The site of the *most distal* obstruction can be located most readily by *first finding collapsed bowel* and following it upward. One should never assume that a mechanical obstruction of the intestine has been relieved *until the entire small intestine has been examined by sight and feel. Whenever the small intestine is significantly dilated with gas and fluid, it should be decompressed surgically before any attempt is made to replace it within the abdo-*

men. A person able to breathe with a meteorism before being operated upon may be readily choked by it after the operation when he is weaker and the incision hurts with each breath. Great care must be taken during the replacement of intestine into the abdomen so that the jejunum lies within the left upper abdominal quadrant, the terminal ileum in the pelvis, and that the base of the mesentery runs straight from the ligament of Treitz to the cecum to be sure that a volvulus has not been created during the replacement of the intestine.

DIVISION OF ADHESIONS. In many patients with simple obstruction of the small bowel, removal of adhesions is all that is required. Often the excision of one adhesive band is sufficient. However, the remainder of the peritoneal cavity should be inspected carefully for the presence of other adhesions likely to give rise to obstruction. Care should be taken to avoid denuding the serosal surface of bowel insofar as possible.

Reduction of Strangulated Hernia. Reduction by external pressure applied over the hernia should not be attempted with the pressure applied over the hernia if obstruction is more than 6 hours in duration, or if fever and leukocytosis are present. It is better that these patients be subjected to operation, exposing the hernial sac and opening the sac to inspect the bowel for viability before replacing it in the abdomen (see p. 917). If viable, the bowel is manipulated gently under direct vision, returned to the abdomen, and the hernia is repaired (see Chap. 39, "Hernia"). In some patients, the hernial ring may need to be enlarged by incision to allow re-entry of the bowel into the abdomen without trauma or taxis. Traction or taxis on the afferent or the efferent loops from within the abdominal cavity is to be avoided as the occluded loop may be torn with surprisingly little tension.

Occasionally, an awkward situation arises in which an incarcerated hernia with bowel obstruction of a few hours' duration cannot be reduced prior to operation but does reduce spontaneously under anesthesia in the operating room prior to operation. Then the question arises: can it be assumed that the bowel is viable and that the hernia can be repaired without inspection of the bowel to determine its viability. The answer is *no!* One must enlarge the hernial ring surgically so that the

visceral contents can be inspected adequately. Once the decision is made to operate and gentle attempts at pre-anesthetic reductions have failed, further manipulation should be avoided until the obstructed loop is exposed surgically and inspected to determine its viability while remaining *in situ.*

Removal of Foreign Bodies, Bezoars and Gallstones. Occasionally, a large gallstone obstructing the intestine may be so friable that it breaks up when a little firm pressure is applied to it. Should this happen, that is all one needs do. In general, whenever one can do so readily without risking puncture of the bowel, all obstructing intraluminal foreign bodies should be pushed up into the proximal dilated noninflamed bowel before making the intestinal incision to remove it. Making the incision through the inflamed intestine overlying the lodged body invites an intestinal fistula. The incision should be made through uninflamed bowel, linearly and antimesenterically, and closed transversely so not to obstruct the bowel by the closure.

Loop Colostomy for Relief of Distention. Decompression by colostomy of the proximal colon in simple complete colon obstruction is the safest and most satisfactory means yet devised. It affords prompt relief of distention with minimal risk of soilage or bacterial contamination.

The location of the colostomy along the course of the colon should receive special consideration. Two factors are concerned in arriving at the proper decision: (1) The colostomy must be proximal to the point of obstruction. (2) In locating and devising the type of colostomy, one needs to bear in mind the types of colostomy appliances available for subsequent usage, especially if the colostomy is to be permanent.

In general, there are 3 sites where a colostomy may be located on the anterior abdominal wall: over the descending colon (Fig. 36-17), over the transverse colon (Fig. 36-18) and over the cecum (Fig. 36-19). Each decompresses the colon proximal to the site of obstruction without leaving a long distal obstructed segment. As more than 75 per cent of obstructing lesions in the colon and the rectum are distal to the descending colon, the transverse colostomy is the one most often employed as well as the one most easily performed. Barium enema to locate the site of colon obstruction is a most helpful procedure in patients with large bowel obstruction and should be performed in all cases before the colostomy unless contraindicated by signs of perforation.

To perform a transverse colostomy, a vertical incision is made in the mid-line or, better, a right paramedian one, generally above the umbilicus. If distention is massive and its cause is established as tumor or diverticulitis without threat of strangulation, a large incision should be avoided, as it will allow distended loops of small bowel to escape to the outside and complicate wound closure. However, the incision should be large enough to permit the introduction of the hand to palpate

the site of obstruction. It is often possible to establish that the distally situated tumor is locally operable or not operable, and to establish the presence of nodules within the liver, presumably from metastatic tumor, by passing the hand over the various hepatic surfaces. If it can be satisfactorily established that the tumor is inoperable due to local extension or hepatic metastases, the patient is spared a second operation. However, it must be realized that *blind palpation is a poor substitute for palpation with inspection and biopsy,* particularly biopsy of hepatic nodules. Sclerosing hemangioma or lymphangioma, concretions or stones within the liver, hamartoma and fibroma are among the many benign lesions that may erroneously imply hepatic metas-

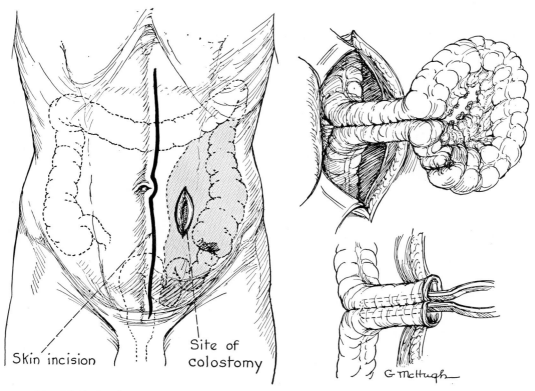

Skin incision Site of colostomy

Fig. 36-17. A colostomy of the descending colon is performed. Mikulicz type of exteriorization of the sigmoid colon for diverticulitis or necrotic bowel from volvulus of sigmoid. The mesenteric borders of afferent and efferent segments are sutured together to prevent a loop of small bowel from slipping in between and becoming obstructed. The site for colostomy is indicated. A few days later a crushing clamp is applied, necrosing the bowel between the afferent and the efferent limbs, hoping that a spontaneous fistula will develop between them and that the normal fecal current will be re-established. If successful, the colostomy often will undergo spontaneous closure. (See text pages 914 to 918)

tases, hence inoperability. Massive hepatic metastases are usually easy to recognize by palpation with a high degree of reliability, but small nodules on or just under the surface of the liver are often most deceiving.

Similar errors are common to palpation of bowel tumors. Much of the apparent fixation may represent local cellulitis secondary to infection of the bowel tumors rather than local tumor extension. Despite the drawbacks and the limitations of palpation, a fair number of inoperable cases can be established at the time of colostomy, saving the patient a useless second operation (see Carcinoma of the Colon, p. 977).

A loop colostomy of the descending colon may have several disadvantages when used as a means of decompression. It should be avoided if possible, in favor of a transverse colostomy. Colostomy at this site at times interferes seriously with a curative operative procedure planned for several weeks later, whether the obstructing lesion is inflammatory or neoplastic.

No attempt should be made to resect carcinoma of the *transverse* or *descending* or *sigmoid segments of the colon* at the time that colostomy is performed for relief of distention. The careful dissection essential to curative operations for carcinoma of the colon cannot often be carried out satisfactorily in the presence of distended loops of bowel. Moreover, even though the tumor may seem to be resectable at the time colostomy is being performed for relief of obstruction, the patient cannot be spared the need for a second operation to close the colostomy, as primary anastomosis cannot be performed safely with the colon distended.

In cases of even obstructing carcinoma of the cecum or the ascending colon without very

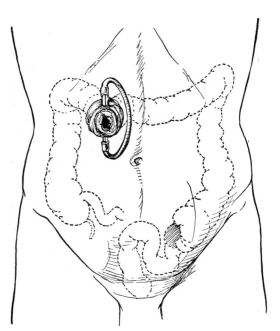

FIG. 36-18. Transverse colostomy through a right paramedian incision about 2 inches above the umbilicus. A glass rod is carried under the transverse colon and is used as a temporary support to hold the loop of colon outside the abdomen. This location of colostomy is best suited to patients whose obstructions are in the splenic flexure and distally.

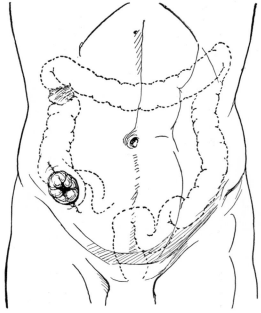

FIG. 36-19. Cecostomy drainage for decompression of the colon with lesion lying at hepatic flexure. Cecostomy here is a temporary one, and bowel resection is planned within 2 to 3 weeks. Location of the cecostomy site is too low in this illustration for a colostomy appliance, but in this instance it is purposefully placed low, as incision for the second operation will be largely above the present cecostomy.

great dilatation of the small intestine, wide and adequate resection usually can be carried out initially to advantage. In these patients the proximal bowel may be decompressed by trocar drainage at the operating table (see below). Then the necessary bowel is resected, and a careful anastomosis is performed between the terminal ileum and the transverse colon. In such patients, carcinoma of the cecum or the ascending colon may be transplanted locally by attempting cecostomy or ileostomy close to the tumor.

The location of the colostomy wound on the abdominal wall should be well away from the anterosuperior spines of the ilium, preferably about halfway along a line between the spine of the ilium and the umbilicus if a descending colostomy or cecostomy is to be performed. This precaution allows the colostomy appliance to fit snugly against skin and avoids resting upon the iliac spine, causing pressure necrosis of the skin or leakage with soiling of clothing later on. This error is illustrated in Figure 36-19.

The transverse colostomy is better suited to the majority of appliances if placed 2 to 3 inches above rather than below the umbilicus. In this location, the colostomy is cared for more easily and is less likely to be displaced, especially in patients with protuberant abdomens. Moreover, there is less chance that diastasis or colostomy hernia will occur in the upper abdomen, as the forces of gravity are less than in the lower abdomen; also the posterior rectus sheath is present in the epigastrium but not in the lower abdomen.

In most cases with loop colostomy and distention, the colostomy should be opened as soon as the abdominal incision is closed and its proximal and distal segments aspirated. A closed colostomy has no decompressing value and may distend upon the surface of the abdomen, dragging more colon to the outside.

TROCAR DECOMPRESSION of the distended small bowel is often desirable at the time of operation. This can be performed safely by carefully packing off a segment of bowel and placing a purse-string suture, encircling the site intended for the introduction of the trocar into the enteric lumen. As soon as the trocar (with its suction tube vigorously active) perforates into the intestinal lumen, the purse-string suture is immediately drawn tight about the shaft of the trocar to avoid leakage. The sharp trocar tip is then pulled back and the outer tube (sheath of the trocar) is gently directed upward, pleating the bowel onto the shaft. Then it is directed distally, and the procedure is repeated. As the metal tube is removed, the purse-string is closed, sealing the enterostomy site, which is then reinforced with 2 or 3 interrupted serosal sutures.

Trocar decompression has the following advantages: it provides better surgical exposure and avoids a large spill within the abdomen should the distended bowel wall accidentally be perforated while handling. With the bowel collapsed, wound closure is greatly facilitated. The possibility for a postoperative leak at the suture line occurring because of continual distention is hereby largely avoided. It has the physiologic advantage that the collapsed bowel affords more rapid recovery of normal bowel activity. Trocar drainage introduces no important hazards if carefully performed, and at times its usage can avoid unnecessary delay in attempting long-tube intubation as its alternative.

Should a long tube with an inflatable balloon on its tip have passed successfully beyond the ligament of Treitz, the balloon tip can be threaded down the small bowel without much difficulty. Suction applied at the head end of the tube collapses the bowel and, of course, avoids the necessity for trocar drainage. Such tubes are very difficult to manipulate distally at operation unless they have already traversed the duodenum.

Relief of Strangulated Obstruction with Bowel Necrosis.

DETERMINING BOWEL VIABILITY. This is the all-important question to be answered in strangulation obstruction. The circulation of the strangulated bowel may be impaired but recovers when obstruction is released; it may be impaired and fail to recover when released, or the bowel segment may be obviously dead when first inspected.

Although a number of valid clinical observations have been employed to determine the viability of the strangulated loop, the only practical ones are those which are decisive. There is no room for doubt. The following 3 points are likely to be valid under most circumstances in determining the viability of the segment in question.

1. Restoration of color promptly (1 to 15 minutes) when strangulation is released

2. Return of pulsation in small arterioles on the surface of the bowel

3. Return of peristaltic activity and the peristaltic contraction following stimulation (pinching, etc.)

Should doubt remain, "There is no better rule than this: . . . resect"; this statement by Wangensteen[27] summarizes all that needs to be said.

SURGICAL MANAGEMENT OF DEAD AND DISTENDED BOWEL

Colon. Exteriorization of the dead segment of colon and its excision after the abdominal wound has been closed about living colon proximal and distal to the dead part is the only safe operative procedure that can be carried out where a necrotic segment of the transverse, descending or sigmoid colon is encountered regardless of the co-existence of distention. The blood supply to the colon, being less dependable than that of the small bowel, is even less dependable when the colon is obstructed, distended or its wall edematous. Hence, primary colocolic anastomoses are to be avoided under these circumstances, because the suture line may leak a few days later. A necrotic ascending colon is treated as is necrotic small intestine. It is excised, and an ileocolic anastomosis performed.

The exteriorization of necrotic distal colon is performed as follows: mesentery at the proximal and the distal ends of the segment involved is divided, and the segment of dead bowel is lifted gently to the exterior surface of the abdomen along with about 4 or 5 cm. of the adjoining viable bowel at either end (Fig. 36-17). This technic is known as the Mikulicz exteriorization procedure or the Mikulicz-Brun-Mayo resection. Many modifications exist, but the principles embodied are the same as those described by Mikulicz. The segment of necrotic bowel is not resected or decompressed until after the abdomen is closed, thereby avoiding operative spillage or soilage within the peritoneal cavity.

The disadvantages of the Mikulicz type of resection are inconsequential when dealing with obstruction and/or a dead segment of colon. Essentially only one disadvantage exists: a second operation is required to close the colostomy that the Mikulicz procedure creates.

Small Bowel. Primary resection and anastomosis in high intestinal obstruction with a nonviable segment of the small bowel is the only practical procedure in most patients. External drainage of the mid-ileum or the jejunum nearly always creates more trouble than it solves. The volumes of fluids and electrolytes lost through most high intestinal enterostomies are no less than those of high intestinal obstruction itself. Malnutrition also continues.

Primary resection and intra-abdominal anastomosis of the obstructed dead segment of small bowel fortunately does not carry the risk entailed in similar resection of the obstructed colon. While primary resection and anastomosis of the dead distal colon is condemned, this is the only feasible and safe operation possible in small bowel obstruction with necrosis. Ordinarily, an end-to-end anastomosis of the small bowel is the operation of choice and most frequently employed after resection of an *unobstructed* segment of small bowel. However, when obstruction exists, the proximal segment may be so distended, its wall so edematous, and the diameter of its proximal lumen so large that to join it to the collapsed distal one would be unsafe.

Therefore, the proximal and the distal transected ends are carefully sutured closed, the ends enfolded and reinforced with serosal stitches, and a lateral (side-to-side) anastomosis performed to re-establish intestinal continuity. This type of anastomosis is easily carried out, and the lateral opening in the distended proximal segment can be cut to the same size as the lateral opening in the collapsed distal segment. With rubber-shod intestinal clamps applied to both the proximal and the distal segments at the proposed anastomotic site, the operative field is carefully walled-off with laparotomy pads, and a lateral anastomosis (isoperistaltic) is carried to completion without risk of spillage of intestinal contents and with only minimal surface soilage.

Trocar decompression of the small bowel prior to closure of the abdomen should be carried out whenever anastomoses of small intestine are done and the proximal intestine is distended if long-tube intubation has not been successful.

TREATMENT OF INTUSSUSCEPTION IN ADULTS

This is different than it is in infants (see Chap. 46). In infants, reduction by hydrostatic pressure or manually should be attempted if the bowel is not dead or the intussusception is not too long-standing. Intussusception in adults, excepting for very short ones with a Meckel's diverticulum as the lead point, should *not be reduced but should be resected* because, excepting the Meckel's diverticulum inversion type, malignant intestinal tumors make up a significant percentage, about 30 per cent, of the lead points of the intussusceptions in older children and adults, and one runs too much risk of breaking the tumor and spreading it if reduction of the intussusception is attempted. After all, in adult intussusception the bowel must practically always be opened to remove the lead point even if it is benign, and this is as dangerous, if not more dangerous, than a resection with anastomosis between normal bowel parts because incision through bowel that was in the intussusception and is inflamed and edematous if not ulcerated is less likely to heal well.

Mechanisms and Treatment of Primary Volvulus in Adults. The frequency with which volvulus or torsion of the small and large intestine is reported to occur varies widely. These discrepancies are in part artificial (differences in semantics) and in part true. For example, if one considers rotation of a loop of small bowel about the axis of an adhesion, an ileostomy or colostomy stoma, etc., then volvulus is a very frequent cause of acute small bowel obstruction in adults. If the term is restricted to those which are primary in origin in that torsion is due to the congenital failure of fixation of the duodenum and/or of the colon, then torsion of the intestines in the adult is indeed a rare occurrence (see chapter on Pediatric Surgery).

Using the latter definition, primary torsion or volvulus is much more frequently encountered in the cecum or sigmoid colon than in the small bowel, though still not a commonly encountered cause of acute intestinal obstruction among the populations of western Europe and the United States.

When primary volvulus occurs, obstruction is usually sudden, and always of the closed loop variety if obstruction is complete. Ischemia or total vascular occlusion is often present from the onset.

PRIMARY VOLVULUS OF THE COLON. This nearly always occurs in the cecum or the sigmoidal segments. Volvulus of the transverse colon is exceedingly rare, probably because this segment of colon is suspended posteriorly from the mesocolon and superiorly by the gastrocolic omentum (Fig. 33-1).

VOLVULUS OF THE CECUM. This is a form of torsion which nearly always involves also the terminal ileum just proximal to the cecum and the adjacent ascending colon at its distal end. This disorder accounts for about 1 per cent of all causes of acute intestinal obstruction.[1] The predisposing factor is the inadequate fixation of the ascending colon by the posterior parietes. Instead, it is generally partially or totally mobile upon a mesentery.

The severity of symptoms depends upon the extent to which torsion is possible. Minor degrees of mobility are not likely to provide the soil for a volvulus that can obstruct completely; more often partial obstruction occurs, giving rise to right lower abdominal crampy pains whose origin is not likely to be recognized unless surgical intervention is required.

Wolfer et al.[28] maintained that in addition to the unduly mobile ascending colon, the terminal ileum must be less mobile than usual if volvulus of the cecum and the ascending colon was to occur. They believed that the point of hyperfixation of the ileum is essential and that it serves as the axis about which the cecum and the ascending colon may rotate.

Other factors have been described as providing a higher degree of mobility to the ascending colon and the cecum. Among these are malrotation or incomplete rotation of the midgut embryologically, or its counterpart—too much rotation with an exaggerated degree of descension, allowing excesses of the cecum and part of the ascending colon to lie free within the right pelvis.

To some extent, dietary habits are thought to play an inciting role in volvulus of the mobile cecum and the sigmoid, too. Large amounts of diet roughage have been suggested to explain the higher frequency of volvulus of the cecum claimed for populations of the eastern European countries. In Russia, Turkey,

India and Africa, volvulus of the cecum is reported to be one of the commonest causes of acute obstruction in adults.[9] According to Donhauser and Atwell,[7] the cecum and the ascending colon are sufficiently mobile in about 20 per cent of the population to permit pathologic rotation. If this be the case, it would seem plausible that the incidence of torsion might be higher among those individuals in whom the cecum becomes heavily weighted with feces, thereby favoring rotation in response to gravity or exertion. Clinical experience possibly tends to support this thesis.

Diagnosis presents the problem of deciding upon the specific cause of acute intestinal obstruction. The nature of onset and the clinical findings are not distinctive, but the roentgenographic findings may be fairly diagnostic. Figiel and Figiel[9] describe the ectopic position of the cecum which is simulated by only a few clinical entities. Partial torsion should be suspected when the cecum is severely distended and displaced. Volvulus of the cecum without displacement is not likely to be distinguished from incomplete obstruction from other cause, such as carcinoma of the ascending colon, without the aid of contrast studies (barium enema). A large intra-abdominal abscess containing gas and lying in the right mid and lower abdomen constitutes the most difficult radiologic distinction usually encountered, but the longer history and the septic state associated with infection generally tip the scale in favor of abscess. The barium enema shows the contrast medium cut off at the hepatic flexure and having the appearance of the apex of the "ace of spades" with no alterations of mucosal pattern. The cecum tends to wander toward the left upper quadrant as distention progresses, for the cecum and the ascending colon swing mesially from their distal point of twist and fixation which is usually near the hepatic flexure.

Treatment is operative and is carried out as promptly as the diagnosis is suspected. More commonly, the nature of the distention is not discovered until the time of operative intervention for the relief of acute intestinal obstruction. This may be sufficiently late that viability of the bowel is threatened, if the bowel is not actually gangrenous.

Most surgeons believe that it is best to perform an exteriorization procedure of the Miku-licz type, resecting the cecum after the abdomen is closed, leaving the patient with a temporary ileostomy (Fig. 36-17), to be closed as a transverse ileocolostomy a few weeks later. In some patients, right hemicolectomy with a primary anastomosis may be performed safely.

When the cecum is fully viable, a cecocoloplicopexy may be performed. "Cecocoloplicopexy" (incising the lateral parietal peritoneum and suturing its cut edge to the cecum and the ascending colon) is a method devised to anchor these structures to the posterior parietes to avoid subsequent torsion. Although this technic has been employed successfully in the management of the detorsed cecum, it carries the risk of needle or suture perforation in view of the acutely distended and ischemic bowel. This hazard coupled with occasional failure to maintain anchorage of the cecum and ascending colon in position favors resection over cecocoloplicopexy; i.e., resection performed at the time of volvulus.

However, coloplicopexy for abnormal mobility of the cecum or sigmoid is at times a procedure to be elected when the conditions of abnormal mobility are discovered in the course of other abdominal operations, preferably if distention presents no problem.

VOLVULUS OF THE SIGMOID in the adult is encountered most often after the age of 50. Occasionally, it is a complication of megacolon or sigmoidal obstruction from carcinoma. In a few it is the result of adhesions suspending the sigmoid from the abdominal wall. In the latter instance, the rotational axis is about the adhesive bands; in the case of the long mesentery the volvulus is about the mesenteric axis and the sigmoidal vessels.

Usually the twist is in the counterclockwise direction with the upper loop coming to lie in front of the distal segment. This creates a very efficient check-valve at the proximal end, allowing gas and liquid feces to enter the closed loop but none to leave. Gas and feces continue to accumulate. There is no cause of bowel obstruction which produces larger coils of distended bowel loops than volvulus of the sigmoid. The heavier the loop becomes, the more tightly closed is the distal site of occlusion. The distal end, too, has a check-valve action but not when entered from below. Therefore it may be possible to introduce very gently a proctoscope or long rectal tube through the lower check-valve to enter the "omega" loop, achieving explosive decompression, often with total relief (see Figs. 36-9 and 36-10).

Clinical patterns may be those of chronic constipation associated with bouts of colicky pain, distention and obstipation. Occasionally, the condition is self-relieved by the expulsion of huge quantities of air and liquid stool. As the disease progresses, there is less likelihood of spontaneous remission. The obstructing occasion usually develops over a period of several days to a week or longer in older patients. Often by the time they present themselves, distention is pronounced; the abdomen tympanitic, and respiratory embarrassment is obvious. Bloody exudates accumulate within the bowel lumen and may lead to hypovolemic shock. Bowel necrosis is the sequela, followed by perforation.

Less commonly encountered is the sudden onset of symptoms which usually occurs in younger patients, especially those with megacolon. After the sudden onset, the course usually progresses more rapidly than that noted above for older patients. Peripheral circulatory collapse from dehydration is frequent, and necrosis of the bowel with rupture or perforation tends to occur soon.

Diagnosis of a sigmoid volvulus should be suspected in any patient with pronounced abdominal distention.

Treatment. As mentioned above, the simplest procedure to attempt is decompression by proctoscopy. If this is successful, surgery need not be performed, although peripheral collapse may occur a few hours later unless the extracellular fluid volume deficit is sufficiently treated. In order to determine the approximate amount of Hartmann's solution needed to treat the dehydration, the amount of fluid that flows out through the sigmoidoscope and the rectal tube, or that removed from the loop by trocar drainage must be measured. An amount of Hartmann's solution equal to this, plus a liter more to allow for the edema of the colon, should be given intravenously. At times this may amount to 5 to 8 liters (see Table 6). Antibiotics may be given for several days. Surprisingly, recurrence of sigmoidal volvulus after decompression in this manner is not a certainty; only about 1 out of 4 or 5 patients ever have trouble again.

Operative management is designed for detorsion. But before this can proceed safely, it is better to perform trocar decompression, being very careful to avoid splitting the colon and causing extensive fecal contamination. Once bowel distention is relieved, the volvulus may be untwisted. At this point, the decision is whether to perform a Mikulicz exteriorization of the sigmoid colon, ligating its vessels, or whether to return the bowel to the abdomen, and perform a decompressing transverse colostomy in the course of closure of the abdomen. The bowel should be left in situ only when its circulation is not impaired.

INTRAPERITONEAL ANTIBIOTICS

The intraperitoneal instillation of antibiotics after celiotomy for the relief of simple mechanical intestinal obstruction is not indicated. The "prophylactic administration" of antibiotics when overt contamination of the peritoneal cavity has *not* taken place accomplishes nothing. Should necrotic bowel have to be resected, or spillage of intestinal contents into the peritoneum have occurred, antibiotics should be given parenterally as for peritonitis (see Chap. 35) and an antibiotic may be placed in the peritoneal cavity. However, if an antibiotic is put into the peritoneal cavity, no antibiotic having a curarelike action (such as neomycin) should be used. Fatal respiratory failure may be induced. Penicillin is safe.

REFERENCES

1. Byrne, J. J., Swift, C. C., and Farrell, G. E.: Volvulus of the cecum, A.M.A. Arch. Surg. *64*:378, 1952.
2. Calman, C., Hershey, F. B., and Skaggs, J. O.: Serum lactic dehydrogenase in the diagnosis of the acute surgical abdomen, Surgery *44*:43-52, 1958.
3. Cannon, W. B.: The Mechanical Factors of Digestion, London, Longmans, 1911.
4. Cantor, M. O.: Intestinal Intubation, Springfield, Ill., Thomas, 1949.
5. Cooke, R. E., Segar, W. E., Cheek, D. B., Coville, F. E., and Darrow, D. C.: The extrarenal correction of alkalosis associated with potassium deficiency, J. Clin. Invest. *31*:798, 1952.
6. Darrow, D. C., and Pratt, E. L.: Fluid therapy, relation to tissue composition and the expenditure of water and electrolyte, J.A.M.A. *143*:365, 432, 1950.

7. Donhauser, J. L., and Atwell, S.: Volvulus of the cecum with a review of 100 cases in the literature and a report of 6 new cases, Arch. Surg. *58*:129, 1949.

8. Dragstedt, L. R., Lang, V. F., and Millet, R. F.: The relative effects of distention on different portions of the intestine, Arch. Surg. *18*:2257, 1929.

9. Figiel, L. S., and Figiel, S. J.: Volvulus of the cecum and ascending colon, Radiology *61*:495, 1953.

10. Fine, J., Banks, B. M., Sears, J. B., and Hermanson, L.: Treatment of gaseous distention of intestine by inhalation of 95 per cent oxygen: description of apparatus for clinical administration of high oxygen mixtures, Ann. Surg. *103*:375, 1936.

11. Gatch, W. D., Trusler, H. M., and Ayres, K. D.: Effects of gaseous distention on obstructed bowel: incarceration of intestine by gas traps, Arch. Surg. *14*:1215, 1927.

12. Hay, L.: Unpublished data, 1940. (Quoted by Wangensteen[24])

13. Machella, T. E., and Miller, T. G.: Treatment of idiopathic ulcerative colitis by means of a "medical ileostomy" and an orally administered protein hydrolysate-dextri-maltose mixture, Gastroenterology *10*:28, 1948.

14. McKittrick, L. S., and Sarris, S. P.: Acute mechanical obstruction of the small bowel, New England J. Med. *222*:611, 1940.

15. Medins, G., and Laufman, H.: Hypothermia in mesenteric arterial and venous occlusions, Ann. Surg. *148*:747-754, 1958.

16. Miller, T. G., and Abbott, W. S.: Intestinal intubation: a practical technique, Am. J. M. Sc. *187*:595, 1934.

17. Nemir, P., Hawthorne, H. R., Cohn, I., and Drabkin, D. L.: Cause of death in strangulation obstruction: II. Lethal action of the peritoneal fluid, Ann. Surg. *130*:874, 1949.

18. Noer, R. J., and Derr, J. W.: Effect of distention on intestinal revascularization, **Arch.** Surg. *59*:542, 1949.

19. Oppenheimer, M. J., and Mann, F. C.: Intestinal capillary circulation during distention, Surgery *13*:548, 1943.

20. Paine, J. R.: The history of the invention and development of the stomach and duodenal tubes, Ann. Int. Med. *8*:752, 1934.

21. Portis, S. A.: Diseases of the Digestive System, ed. 3, p. 176, Philadelphia, Lea & Febiger, 1953.

22. Randall, H. T.: Water and electrolyte balance in surgery, S. Clin. North America *32*:445, 1952.

23. Ravdin, I. S., and Abbott, W. O.: The use of the Miller-Abbott tube in facilitating one-stage resections of the small and large bowel, New Internat. Clin. *1*:179, 1940.

24. Schwartz, E.: Ueber Flatulenz, Med. Klin. *5*:1339, 1909.

25. Smith, G. A.: Long intestinal tubes for operative decompression and postoperative ileus, J.A.M.A. *160*:266, 1956.

26. Sperling, L., Paine, J. R., and Wangensteen, O. H.: Intra-enteric pressure in experimental and clinical obstruction, Proc. Soc. Exper. Biol. & Med. *32*:1504, 1936.

27. Wangensteen, O. H.: Intestinal Obstructions, ed. 3, Springfield, Ill., Thomas, 1955.

28. Wolfer, J. A., Beaton, L. E., and Anson, B. J.: Volvulus of the cecum: Anatomic factors in its etiology; report of a case, Surg., Gynec. & Obst. *78*:882, 1942.

29. Wright, S.: Applied Physiology, ed. 9, New York, Oxford, 1952.

30. van Zwalenburg, C.: Strangulation resulting from strangulation of hollow viscera; its bearing upon appendicitis, strangulated hernia and gallbladder disease, Ann. Surg. *46*:780, 1907.

Note: This chapter revised by Dr. Carl A. Moyer (1961).

J. GARROTT ALLEN, M.D.

—————————————— CHAPTER 37 ——————————————

Part 1

Small Bowel and Colorectum (Exclusive of Tumors of the Colorectum)

Congenital Disorders of the Intestinal Tract Afflicting Adult Patients

Traumatic Injuries to the Small Bowel and the Colorectum

Inflammatory Diseases of the Small Bowel and the Colorectum

Tumors of the Small Bowel

Preoperative Preparation of the Bowel for Intestinal Operations

Pseudomembranous Enterocolitis

The anatomy and the physiology of the small bowel, the colon and the peritoneal cavity have been discussed in the preceding 4 chapters and are not under discussion here:

Chapter 33—Peritoneum and splanchnic circulation of blood

Chapter 34—Anatomy of appendix and cecum and the differential diagnosis of the acute abdomen

Chapter 35—The peritoneum's response to peritonitis

Chapter 36—Lymphatic circulation of small bowel and colon, physiology of peristalsis, intestinal secretions and absorption, intestinal air and gases, intestinal intubation, abnormal fluid and electrolyte losses and their replacements in small and large bowel obstruction

CONGENITAL DISORDERS OF THE INTESTINAL TRACT AFFLICTING ADULT PATIENTS

Most congenital anomalies of the bowel manifest their presence shortly after birth, especially the obturator obstructions (imperforate anus, atresias of small or large bowel)

(see Chap. 46, "Pediatric Surgery"). Most others are likely to give symptoms within the first 2 years. Duplications of portions of the alimentary canal and other anomalies generally produce symptoms before the age of 10 and need only be mentioned here as they are discussed in Chapter 46, "Pediatric Surgery." The only congenital anomalies giving rise to symptoms in adults as frequently as they do in infants and children are the Meckel's diverticulum and the abnormally mobile cecum and sigmoid which may create volvulus (see Chap. 36, "Anatomy, Physiology and Treatment of Intestinal Obstruction").

MECKEL'S DIVERTICULUM

Incidence. Meckel's diverticulum is found in 1 to 2 per cent of all patients coming to autopsy, being present 3 times more often in males than in females. About half of those who become symptomatic do so before the age of 2.

Historical Considerations. This diverticulum is a developmental remnant of the vitelline duct. Normally, the duct atrophies; failure do so may leave only a residual fibrous cord which extends from the lower ileum to the umbilicus. The duct may remain patent with umbilical sinus or fecal fistula presenting, or more commonly the proximal portion remains patent on the antimesenteric margin of the ileum (95% of cases) where the ductal remnant constitutes a pouch—Meckel's diverticulum. This was named for Johann Friedrich Meckel (The Younger, 1781-1833) whose several works on comparative anatomy made Germany the center for this discipline in the early 19th century and earned him recognition as the German Cuvier.

Johann Friedrich Meckel, the elder (1724-74) of Wetzlar, was graduated at Göttingen in 1748 with a noteworthy inaugural dissertation on the 5th nerve (Meckel's ganglion) and became the first teacher of obstetrics in Berlin. His son, Philipp Friedrich Theodor Meckel (1776-1803) was graduated at Strassburg in 1777 with an important dissertation on the internal ear. He was Professor of Anatomy and Surgery in Halle in 1779 and was also a favorite obstetrician in the Russian Court. His son, in turn, Johann Friedrich Meckel (1781-1833), called the younger, was born in Halle, was an eminent pathologist and the greatest comparative anatomist in Germany before Johannes Müller. It was he who discovered Meckel's diverticulum of the intestine.

Unlike another great and almost contemporary family in anatomy, the three Monros of Edinburgh—*primus, secundus* and *tertius*—the flame of genius burned brightest with the third generation of the Meckels, rather than dimmest as with the Monros.

According to Maingot (1955), Lavater first mentioned the existence of such a diverticulum in 1671; Ruynch illustrated its presence in 1701; and Littre in 1742 described its presence in a hernial sac, but to Meckel belongs the credit for recognizing its embryologic and anatomic significance 200 years after Lavater's discovery. Zenker (1861) described the occasional presence of ectopic pancreas in its wall; Salzer (1904) reported the occasional finding of gastric mucosa lining the diverticulum; Schaetz (1925) described local peptic ulceration as accounting for the hemorrhagic complications the diverticulum occasionally presents.

Complications. A number of other complications may arise from the presence of Meckel's diverticulum. To a large extent these depend upon the structural nature of the remnant. Should a cord attachment persist between the ileum and the umbilicus, the ileum may rotate on this axis (antimesenteric), causing volvulus and closed loop obstruction. A loop of small bowel may slip innocently behind the cord, causing acute intestinal obstruction. This type of Meckel's diverticulum cannot intussuscept in the usual manner as the intussuscipiens is held in traction by the cord, tending constantly to disengage any but a retrograde type of intussusception. If the pouch only remains attached to the ileum, the diverticulum is free to intussuscept or to twist upon its own axis, producing strangulation volvulus and obstruct its own lumen, causing gangrenous Meckel's diverticulitis. If its neck is small or its lumen is obstructed by concretions or a foreign body, preventing drainage, obstruction diverticulitis, gangrenous perforation and peritonitis may follow in the same manner as acute obstructive appendicitis (see Chap. 34, "Appendicitis and the Acute Abdomen").

If its wall contains gastric mucosa, peptic ulcer may develop within the diverticulum or on the wall of the ileum, usually a little distal to the ostium of the diverticulum. Acute rectal bleeding, without pain, is the usual complaint when bleeding is from an ulcer of this sort. The ulcer may perforate, especially one lying within the diverticulum. Colonic or duodenal heterotopia may also comprise part or all of the lining of the diverticulum; each may appear singularly or in combination and are asymptomatic.

For so small an anomaly, this diverticulum has been the site of origin of a variety of tumors, benign and malignant. Among them are lipomas, fibromas, angiofibromas, fibrosarcomas, argentaffinomas, lymphosarcomas and carcinomas. However, the total number of tumors encountered is exceedingly small.

Diagnosis. The diagnosis of the diverticulum obviously is a speculative one. The physician must envisage the numerous pathologic entities which can arise from Meckel's diverticulum but realize that these are also common to many other alimentary disorders. The diagnosis may be suspected but it is difficult to prove short of operation. Usually, one or more of the following complaints are among the indications for operation:

Intestinal hemorrhage: if cramplike pain persists, one may suspect intussusception and Meckel's diverticulum with intussusception as one of many possible causes.

Hemorrhage without pain is frequently present and suggests peptic ulceration.

Intestinal obstruction from volvulus, bands, intussusception but only when the diagnosis of intestinal obstruction is tenable, Meckel's diverticulum being one of the less common causes of obstruction in adults.

Acute Meckel's diverticulitis resembles appendicitis in particular and other right lower abdominal inflammatory lesions in general.

The umbilical sinus or ileal-umbilical fecal fistula are rare conditions but are more usually recognized as due to the presence of Meckel's diverticulum.

Therefore, the indications for operation are the same as those for surgical intervention in seeking to establish the cause and to institute treatment for intestinal bleeding, acute obstruction or acute intra-abdominal inflammatory disease with or without abscess or peritonitis. About two thirds of all symptomatic Meckel's diverticula are those of intestinal obstruction or those which bleed, sharing about equally in frequency of occurrence in the adult.

The remaining third of complications caused by Meckel's diverticula are largely concerned with acute diverticulitis, perforation and tumors. In excess of 70 per cent of all patients with Meckel's diverticulum have no symptoms, its presence being established at the operating table incidentally or at autopsy.

Treatment for the complications of Meckel's diverticulum is early operation. If the diverticulum has undergone torsion or intussusception, they are relieved as described (see pp. 951 to 952). Should the bowel segment be nonviable, the segment is resected and appropriately anastomosed. If the bowel is viable and the diverticulum is necrotic, the latter is resected. A clamp is placed across its base at a 45° angle to the axis of the bowel lumen, cutting away the diverticulum and suturing with 2 layers of interrupted fine silk without infolding. Some prefer to resect a wedge of the antimesenteric edge of the ileum, which also permits closure without encroachment upon the lumen and has the advantage of resecting a segment of adjacent bowel whose blood supply may have been partially impaired.

Meckel's diverticula found incidentally in the course of another operation are usually resected unless the nature of the primary operation is one which will contraindicate any additional or elective surgery at the time, such as a long operative procedure or an operation performed for acute inflammatory disease within the abdomen. Otherwise those diverticula which are long and have a narrowed proximal lumen should be resected if they can be removed easily without risk. Similarly,

those with attachments to the umbilicus should be removed to avoid volvulus.

Other conditions exist and give rise to symptoms in the adult which may be considered "quasicongenital" in origin, as factors in addition to congenital disorders undoubtedly contribute to the onset of their complications in adult life.

These are (1) the superior mesenteric artery syndrome; (2) volvulus of the cecum; (3) volvulus of the sigmoid colon; and (4) intestinal obstruction due to internal hernia. The superior mesenteric artery syndrome results in partial obstruction of the third portion of the duodenum as the artery crosses its anterior surface, compressing and partially occluding the duodenal lumen (see Chap. 29, Stomach and Duodenum). Volvulus of the cecum or of the sigmoid colon is made possible by an unusually mobile cecum or ascending colon. Internal hernias are the result of strangulation of intestine in abnormal peritoneal folds that result from failure of normal fusion of the peritoneum. The sites at which internal intestinal incarcerations may occur are (1) diaphragmatic hernia; (2) hernia of the foramen of Winslow; (3) hernias of the paraduodenal fossae; (4) congenital hole in the mesentery; (5) hernia into the intersigmoid fossa, and (6) pericecal hernias (see Chap. 36, Anatomy, Physiology and Treatment of Intestinal Obstruction).

TRAUMATIC INJURIES TO THE SMALL BOWEL AND THE COLORECTUM

Traumatic injuries suffered by the small bowel and the colon generally are classified as nonpenetrating injuries to the abdomen, penetrating wounds from without, and perforations of the bowel arising from within the lumen.

NONPENETRATING INJURIES

The classification of injuries sustained by any part of the body necessarily is arbitrary, and a particular injury may fall into more than one category. The very nature of the trauma sustained is one of chance; so, too, is the pattern of the injury sustained.

Classification. Nonpenetrating or blunt injuries to the abdomen generally fall into 3 categories: crushing injuries where the bowel is squeezed against unyielding structures such as bone. At times it may be pinched or "exploded." Tearing injuries are usually the result of a tangential blow or one wherein the body is displaced more rapidly than the mobile intestine. Acute compression injuries may burst the bowel or shear it from its mesenteric attachment. Of course, any one of these types of trauma may produce symptoms which are characteristic of another.

Much of our knowledge on nonpenetrating abdominal wounds has been derived from military activities, although in recent decades the high-speed modes of travel provide an equally or even larger experience among the civilian population (see Chap. 23, "Military Surgery").

The pathology of traumatic lesions to the bowel produced by nonpenetrating injuries includes complete or partial tearing, rupture of the bowel, subserosal hematoma and infection following tearing of mucosa and/or the muscular coats. The bowel may be severed from its mesenteric vessels, and rents of the mesentery, the mesocolon, the gastrocolic or the greater omentum are not uncommon.

Tearing and rupture of the bowel, pathologically and clinically, can be the same entity. Only the physical forces producing them tend to differ. Tears more frequently are the result of indirect violence. For example, the individual may fall, landing on his feet or buttocks, tearing the intestine from portions of its mesenteric attachments. Intraperitoneal hemorrhage with shock occurs early. Should the bowel subsequently necrose, perforation with peritonitis is inevitable.

Delayed rupture of the bowel may occur several days later, often after the patient has been discharged from the hospital; this situation is reminiscent of delayed rupture of the spleen (see Chap. 32, "Spleen"). Such instances are rare and usually are caused by an infected subserosal hematoma which perforates or devitalizes the adjacent bowel by interference with its blood supply. Not infrequently, more than one contusion or tear in the bowel is present. At times delayed perforations are minute compared with the several centimeters of tear or the complete division of bowel that is usually seen early.

The location of the perforation may be anywhere along the 360° diameter of the bowel.

The tear may be on the retroperitoneal surface facing into the mesentery, commonly giving rise to hematoma and abscess formation which later may burst into the free peritoneal cavity. This type of injury is likely to devitalize the adjacent segment of bowel as it frequently injures the mesenteric vessels as they enter and leave the bowel.

Most tears resulting from indirect violence occur near the points of bowel fixation. Neighboring portions of bowel will move quickly, but in "rolling with the punch" a tear may occur in close proximity to a portion which is fixed. Injuries of this type are found in the upper jejunum near the ligament of Treitz or in the distal ileum. Occasionally the proximal or distal ends of the sigmoid colon are torn in a similar manner.

The mesentery of the small bowel, the transverse mesocolon, the gastrocolic omentum and the greater omentum are torn or detached in about 30 or 40 per cent of injuries sustained by the intestine. The direction of the mesenteric tear bears upon the hazard involved. Vertical tears are less likely to serve the mesenteric blood vessels.

Clinical pattern of nonpenetrating injuries sustained by the small bowel and the colon: With rare exception, the most frequent clinical finding is that associated with hypovolemic shock. The loss of blood from the torn surfaces of the bowel or one of the mesenteric vessels, the irritant action of intestinal juices and the rapid outpouring of peritoneal exudates, and the fact that other injuries also are often sustained provide adequate explanations for the pallor, the clammy and moist extremities, the thready and rapid pulse, and the hypotension commonly observed. As blood accumulates within the abdomen, pain and tenderness increase if the patient is conscious. Rigidity of the abdominal musculature with shifting dullness in the flanks and the presence of a boggy mass felt in the cul-de-sac are all indications of internal hemorrhage.

Pain and muscle spasm are usually present when the patient is first seen. Both tend to increase steadily unless the patient is treated promptly. At first pain may be localized but rapidly becomes diffuse. Occasionally, the patient complains of pain referred to the shoulder cap distribution of the phrenic nerve, due to subdiaphragmatic irritation from blood or intestinal contents.

Nausea and vomiting are frequent complaints from any acute and painful injury, whether to the abdomen or elsewhere. However, when vomiting continues an hour or 2 later, it is suggestive evidence of bowel perforation.

Muscular rigidity may be deceptive, as it can arise from associated compression fractures of the vertebrae or broken ribs and from hemorrhage into the abdominal wall.

Abdominal distention may develop very promptly or not for a day or two. Initially, the distention is in part the result of air swallowing associated with apprehension and the dyspnea caused by hemorrhage or splinting of the chest or the abdomen to avoid pain. Subsequently, distention usually results from the air which normally is swallowed but not expelled because of paralytic ileus of peritonitis or injury to the spinal cord.

Subcutaneous crepitation may occur from the escape of free intestinal air dissecting over the abdominal wall. It is found in a few patients having ruptured the bowel along its mesenteric attachments, particularly ruptures of the second and the third portions of the duodenum and the ascending and the descending colons. Intestinal emphysema can occur from air or gas dissecting under the serosa when the mucosal and the muscular layers are torn but the serosa remains intact.

X-ray examination of the abdomen is useful primarily for the detection of free air in the peritoneal cavity. Failure to do so is not acceptable evidence that rupture or perforation has not transpired.

Diagnosis of injury to the intestinal tract is not readily obvious in most patients soon after injury. However, it always should be suspected and the patient observed for more definite signs; these are early peritonitis and hypovolemic shock. It is most important that the diagnosis be made within the first few hours to avoid the hazards of generalized peritonitis or fatal hemorrhage.

One of the distressing features of a rupture of any viscus within the abdomen is that it may follow any seemingly inconsequential injury. A sneeze, a cough, or a very trivial blow to the abdomen has been at times the only history of trauma that can be elicited.

Mortality. The urgency of early diagnosis and early treatment is reflected in the mortality rates of the many reports to be found in the literature. Mortality rate increases exponentially with the duration of time after injury and perforation prior to treatment. Lockwood reported in 1934[32] mortality rates as low as 15 per cent when patients were subjected to operation within 2 to 4 hours after the injury. A year later, Counsellor and McCormack[2] reported mortality of 60 per cent among all patients injured, but Maingot in 1955[3] stated that the mortality rate from a tear of the bowel is not higher than 10 per cent if operation is carried out within the first 6 hours. Needless to say, the mortality rate is also a function of the presence or the absence of other injuries, but for the most part the high mortality rate from ruptured bowel continues attributable to delayed diagnosis, inadequate replacement of blood, and delay in surgical treatment and age of patient (Roof, Morris and DeBakey, 1960).

Treatment. Surgical intervention is indicated in any patient in whom a tear or rupture of the intestinal tract or intraperitoneal hemorrhage is suspected. Nasogastric suction is instituted immediately. Favoring early exploration are shock, intra-abdominal pain with referred pain to the shoulder cap, persistent vomiting, increasing abdominal tenderness, fever, leukocytosis and intraperitoneal air.

A matter of priority in the treatment of other injuries should be considered. For example, the co-existence of hemopericardium and/or pneumothorax must be corrected first if the patient is to survive his abdominal operation.

The correction of hypovolemic shock is mandatory. Unless the patient is bleeding actively at a brisk rate, shock can be corrected within a matter of an hour or less by the rapid infusion of blood during the period in which the operating room is being set up to receive the patient. Unless contraindicated, a general anesthetic, with supplemental oxygen, has much to recommend its use. The vasodilatation of splanchnic circulation from spinal anesthesia can be troublesome. Antibiotics, preferably penicillin, should be administered prior to operation.

A long paramedian incision is made in order to explore the entire abdominal cavity, making possible satisfactory examination of the stomach, duodenum, liver, kidneys, spleen, pancreas and rectum, as well as careful examination of the entire small bowel and colon. The exploration should be carried out expeditiously but without haste. Unless pulmonary, cardiac, or central nervous system damage has occurred, these patients withstand prolonged surgery remarkably well, provided that adequate blood replacement is continued throughout the entire period of the operation and generally for a few hours at a slower rate while the patient is in the recovery room (see Chap. 7, "Shock").

When the abdomen is opened, hemostasis should receive first attention. Continued hemorrhage not only implies continued blood loss and shock, but the dry, clean abdomen is essential if a careful search for perforations and tears is to be made. The stomach, the duodenum, the small bowel and the colon are examined thoroughly throughout for evidences of contusion, subserosal tears, or perforations. One need not fear that shock will be induced by exploring the bowel several times, provided that sufficient blood has been and is being administered. If inadequate transfusion is employed, the manipulation of any abdominal viscera, having a vagotonic action, superimposes vasodilatation upon existing hypovolemia, a bad state of affairs!

The types of lacerations and tears found within the bowel vary considerably and repair may tax the ingenuity of the surgeon. Although the perforation may be only 2 or 3 mm. in diameter, it is advisable to excise the wedge of small bowel extending 1 to 2 cm. beyond the site of perforation. This procedure removes traumatized tissue at the edges of the perforation which otherwise might subsequently become necrotic. One must bear in mind always that more than one perforation may have occurred or that the perforation can be on the mesenteric border and hidden. Consequently, the mesentery, as well as the bowel, should be explored.

When the mesentery artery or one of its branches has been severed, the segment of bowel it supplied should be inspected carefully as to viability. If any question remains, the segment should be resected.

Nonpenetrating wounds of the abdomen produce injury to the small bowel much more frequently than to the colon (Albers, Smith and Carter, 1956). When perforation of the colon is found, the loop involved should be either exteriorized (see Fig. 334 in Chap. 36, "Anatomy, Physiology and Treatment of Intestinal Obstruction") or resected with a colostomy being performed.

PENETRATING WOUNDS OF THE ABDOMEN

Penetrating wounds of the abdomen may present ever greater diagnostic problems to the surgeon in his appraisal as to whether or not the bowel has been perforated. He must recognize the well-established fact that he often may need to explore the abdomen if he is to recognize penetrating perforations early. Usually he has no other choice. Wounds with ice picks, hat pins, razors and knives in particular are difficult to evaluate. The presence of more than incisional pain and especially the presence of tenderness within the abdomen are very suggestive of bowel perforation and peritoneal soilage, demanding early surgical exploration. It is better to explore such a patient early, finding no perforation, than to delay 10 or 12 hours while a spreading peritonitis develops, when penetrating wounds are present.

Abdominal wounds inflicted by bullets and high-velocity missiles vary in extent, according to the velocity, the size and the shape of the penetrating fragment. The abdominal wound may bleed very slightly and yet several loops of bowel may have been penetrated. The introduction of a probe into such wounds to determine whether or not the probe will pass into the peritoneal cavity provides positive information only. More often than not, the probe cannot be passed freely along the path of the penetrating missile, despite the fact that the missile entered the peritoneal cavity.

A roentgenogram is valuable in 2 respects: (1) it may disclose the presence of pneumoperitoneum and be diagnostic of perforation, and (2) it may disclose the site of the missile. Except for the presence of pneumoperitoneum, the early x-ray findings are likely to be uninformative as to bowel perforation.

GUNSHOT WOUNDS

Gunshot wounds of the abdomen and the bowel encountered in the military experience during World War II and the Korean War have been discussed in Chapter 23, "Military Surgery." The best results were obtained when the simplest technical procedures were employed. For wounds of the colon, exteriorization of the injured segment was singularly the best immediate form of therapy. Wounds of the rectum were managed most effectively by closure and the performance of a proximal colostomy, supplemented with the generous use of antibiotics and blood. The average time lapse was about 11 hours from time of injury to operation, according to Chunn's experience[10] (1947), and the mortality rate was 36 per cent in his series. The cause of death was attributed to infection when death from co-existing head and thoracic wounds was excluded. 80 per cent of deaths were attributed to peritonitis.

Curiously, the mortality rate was highest for wounds of the cecum and the ascending colon and diminished when perforations were situated more distally. The lowest mortality was in injuries to the rectum. These differences have been attributed to the more liquid nature of feces in the proximal colon which allowed greater soilage of the peritoneal cavity.

Better results were achieved during the Korean campaign due to more rapid evacuation and to the more liberal usage of antibiotics, the increased availability of agents with a broader spectrum of antibacterial action, and to administration of more generous quantities of blood and, of course, to the recent experiences and lessons learned from World War II (see Chap. 23, "Military Surgery").

COMPRESSED AIR INJURIES

Pneumatic or compressed air injuries of the colon constitute a serious but rare surgical emergency occurring largely in industries employing high-pressure air guns. The usual story is that a prankster fellow worker places the nozzle of the air gun against the anus of the victim who is stooping or perched on a ladder. Occasionally, a worker falls on an air-gun nozzle or is cleaning his clothing with compressed air while wearing them, forgetting or being untutored in the hazard of the air gun. The sudden burst of air ruptures the colon completely or incompletely. Abdominal pain quickly follows. Pneumoperitoneum may or may not be present.

Rupture of the colon is believed to be due more commonly to the quick distention of the lumen more often than to the air volume introduced. However, the pressures encountered from such injuries are many times those encountered in the most severe forms of intestinal obstruction.

While numerous areas of colon may rupture from air gun injuries, there is usually only one which actually perforates (Burt, 1931). Most perforations are located in the sigmoid. The size of the rupture varies from a just discernible split, to a longitudinal laceration running the entire length of the colon (Waugh and Leonard, 1951). Swenson and Harkins (1944) and others describe the lesions as characteristically lying on the antimesenteric border. Burt (1931) found in his studies on cadavers that rupture most frequently took place longitudinally, along the teniae; however, transverse rupture was not a rare occurrence. Waugh and Leonard (1951) state that the longitudinal rupture is fundamentally a series of adjoining transverse ruptures.

Treatment is prompt surgical exploration. In some patients extreme meteorism may exist; immediate trocar decompression of the abdomen may be lifesaving and is a preliminary maneuver essential to the release of associated respiratory embarrassment prior to the administration of anesthesia.

PENETRATION OF THE BOWEL FROM WITHIN

Swallowed objects, capable of penetrating the wall of the gut, seldom succeed in doing so. Henderson and Gaston (1938) reported only 1 per cent of perforations occurring among 800 patients treated for ingested foreign bodies in the Boston City Hospital. Usually ingested small bones are completely digested within the stomach, although bones of similar size often will pass unchanged when the patient is achlorhydric (Faber, 1938). It is remarkable how many foreign bodies, open safety pins, glass and sharp metal objects pass without difficulty. Undoubtedly many pins perforate the bowel but continue to pass, and healing takes place without leakage.

Perforations more often occur from small objects entering the appendix or a Meckel's diverticulum where they become trapped and perforate (Bunch, Burnside and Brannon, 1942). Such objects may produce an abscess or peritonitis. Once the foreign body enters the peritoneal cavity, it may migrate to form an abscess some distance away.

Treatment is expectant. If the foreign body is radiopaque, its progression may be checked by serial roentgenograms or fluoroscopy. Should pain, tenderness, fever and/or leukocytosis occur, surgical exploration is advised. The feeding of a bulky diet to "coat the foreign body" is a dubious procedure. Such a program implies that the foreign body is hung up in the alimentary tract and that bread, cotton or other materials will overtake the foreign body, encase it and aid in its passage. This seldom happens; in some patients the ingested material has surrounded the foreign body and produced obturator obstruction. Catharsis is contraindicated. A regular diet seems to be best (Siddons, 1939).

Proctoscopic injuries or perforations of the bowel from the use of dilators to overcome strictures of the rectosigmoid are hazards to be borne in mind when these procedures are employed. Should such an accident occur, laparotomy should be performed with repair of the perforation and a temporary transverse loop colostomy created at the same time.

SUMMARY OF MANAGEMENT OF BOWEL TRAUMA

If the management of bowel trauma including gunshot wounds and pneumatic injuries of the abdomen and bowel can be reduced to principles in treatment, the following might be included:

1. Adequate blood replacement: preoperative, operative and postoperative.

2. Institution of gastric suction and catheter drainage of urinary bladder immediately.

3. Assume that the bowel and/or the mesentery have been injured when the bullet(s) or knives etc. have pierced the abdominal wall or are found by x-ray examination to have lodged within the abdomen; explore within 2 to 4 hours of injury if possible. It is seldom wise to wait for evidence of peritonitis before operating.

4. Secure hemostasis of mesenteric or other vessels before attempting repair of perforations.

5. Ligation of several vessels and correction of shock usually will improve the color of viable bowel and more distinctly delineate between viable and nonviable bowel. Examine carefully all other abdominal organs for perforations and lacerations, including those in the lesser peritoneal cavity.

6. Examine carefully the entire abdominal alimentary tract for contusion, subserosal hemorrhage and perforations. A missile penetration of the bowel almost always will have a point of exit as well. If none is obvious, enlarge the point of entrance with scissors and examine the mucosa. Search for the point of exit along the mesenteric attachment or the retroperitoneum, duodenum, cecum, ascending and descending segments of colon in particular.

7. Resect any segment of small bowel whose circulatory status is in question.

8. Primary, 2-layer repair of the lacerated colon if injury is not extensive. When the colon is badly damaged perform a segmental resection with 2-layer end-to-end anastomosis. Exteriorization should be used in situations where long segments of colon have been destroyed, making repair unduly hazardous or difficult. If the low sigmoid or rectum has been injured, a defunctionalizing transverse colostomy should be performed.

9. Trim back edges of perforated bowel before suturing the injured area closed, especially should subserosal hematomata exist. This avoids necrosis of the area a few days later.

10. Evacuate and drain all retroperitoneal hematomata through appropriately placed stab wounds.

11. Remove all intraperitoneal collections of intestinal contents by suction, followed by the gentle absorption of the areas involved with warm saline-moistened sponges or laparotomy pads.

12. Inspect urinary bladder.

13. Close abdomen but continue the administration of blood and plasma slowly for several hours until circulatory status is stable.

14. Dilate rectum if colostomy has not been performed.

15. Limit intravenous saline solutions in early postoperative hours.

16. Administer larger than usual dosages of antibiotics during first 4 postoperative days.

17. Continue nasogastric suction until bowel sounds are heard and flatus is expelled.

18. Observe for latent abscess formation and drain when appropriate (see Chap. 35,

"Peritoneum, Peritonitis and Intra-abdominal Abscesses").

INFLAMMATORY DISEASE OF THE SMALL BOWEL AND THE COLORECTUM

Inflammatory diseases of the intestinal tract are fairly numerous, but idiopathic diverticulitis, ulcerative colitis and regional enteritis are by far the most commonly encountered ones likely to require surgical intervention. Other diseases which on rare occasion require surgical attention are tuberculosis, amebiasis and occasionally blastomycosis or actinomycosis. The surgeon must bear in mind that bacillary dysentery, food poisoning and pseudomembranous enterocolitis are entities which may confront him in the differential diagnosis of the "acute abdomen" and which call for surgical intervention only if perforation or abscess formation develop as complications.

AMEBIASIS

Amebiasis is encountered as a surgical problem for 4 reasons: (1) the erroneous interpretation of intrahepatic or other intra-abdominal or pulmonary abscesses; uncomplicated amebic abscesses are preferably treated primarily with amebicidal drugs; (2) when the nature of such abscesses is recognized, they may require surgical drainage should they become secondarily infected with bacteria, usually one of the coliform group; they may also require surgical drainage when they fail to respond to antiamebal drugs; (3) perforation of the colon, usually the cecum; (4) obstruction from amebic granuloma, a rare complication in this disease.

Amebiasis is a systemic disease which is said to mimic as many clinical syndromes as undulant fever, syphilis and tuberculosis combined. It is world-wide in distribution; chronic carriers frequently are nearly asymptomatic. But the surgeon is usually concerned only with its consideration in his differential diagnosis of patients with hepatic or intra-abdominal abscesses of unexplained origin, and in establishing the diagnosis of idiopathic ulcerative colitis or regional enterocolitis.

Amebiasis occurs 5 to 8 times more frequently in men than in women. The pathogen is the *Endamoeba histolytica,* a protozoan

usually transmitted from person to person in contaminated food and water supplies. Once within the alimentary tract, the trophozoite resides in the cecum where it attaches itself to the mucosa and begins to invade by virtue of its mobility, aided by the cytolytic enzymes it produces (Frye, 1956). More often, only the mucosa is penetrated; the muscular coats seem better able to withstand the cytolytic action. Once beneath the mucosa, the colony tends to undermine and destroy the submucosa. The result is the small mucosal perforation with a large undermined area, the so-called "flask-shaped" abscess. These abscesses may become confluent with others nearby. For some time the mucosa between the surface perforations remains normal, and only the pinhead-sized ulcerations with their grayish-yellow exudates are seen. If the disease continues to progress, the mucosa is devitalized. It sloughs, leaving the "buffalo-hide" appearance occasionally noted upon proctoscopic examination or at autopsy. It is present more commonly in the cecum.

Lesions are found more frequently in the cecum, the rectum and in the region of haustral valves. Sawitz (1943) attributes the predilection for these regions to the assumption that the fecal current moves more slowly in these regions, affording more leisure for invasion by the protozoan.

Occasionally, the muscularis and the serosa are penetrated, giving rise to amebic peritonitis or to a perityphlic abscess. Nearly always such abscesses are also infected with bacteria of enteric origin.

The clinical pattern and complaints of intestinal amebiasis are protean, ranging from constipation to bloody diarrhea. Often malaise, fatigue, constipation and fever are the only complaints, so unless one initiates a self-stimulated search for the organism in the stool, he is not likely to make the diagnosis. In others, bloody diarrhea (occult blood is nearly always present) immediately arouses suspicion.

Representative flecks of feces or mucus are removed with an applicator and examined for the organism, using the direct film method of D'Antoni (1942) or preferably the zinc sulfate centrifugal flotation technic of Faust (1952). In the final analysis, the diagnosis is a laboratory one, depending upon the demonstration of *Endamoeba histolytica* in the stool, body fluids or tissues. As other nonpathogenic ameba may be found within the colon or the feces, e.g., *Endamoeba coli*, these are to be distinguished and not confused as pathognomonic of amebiasis. These nonpathogenic amebae often coexist with *Endamoeba histolytica*.

Occasionally, amebic granulomata, the "ameboma," occur within the small bowel, particularly in the cecum. Definite tumor formation may be observed by palpation and by roentgenogram. Ameboma is the result of massive granulomatous reaction within the cecum and occasionally is confused with carcinoma, stricture or abscess. Unless intestinal obstruction supervenes, the treatment of choice is the use of amebicidal drugs in conjunction with a low-residue diet. Operative intervention should employ only Mikulicz's exteriorization resection with ileostomy, for primary anastomoses in amebiasis of the colon are notorious for subsequent leakage.

Extra-intestinal amebic lesions occur most frequently in the liver and the lung. The amebae are transported from the primary intestinal ulcers to the liver via the portal venous system, resulting in amebic hepatitis and amebic hepatic abscesses. Amebic lesions in the lung may be embolic in origin but are usually secondary to direct extension of subcapsular liver abscesses by rupture through the diaphragm. Although free rupture into the pleural or the pericardial cavities does occur, more often the lung becomes adherent to the inflamed diaphragm, and rupture is direct into the lower lobe (Takaro and Bond, 1958).

Treatment of amebic hepatic abscesses is somewhat debated among authorities in this field. Most prefer a trial of one of the amebicidal drugs, particularly chloroquine or emetine, aspirating the abscess periodically as indicated by the clinical findings. Under this regimen the abscess may subside and disappear permanently. However, in many cases which improve markedly on drug therapy, complete recovery may be delayed until the abscesses are drained. If an amebic abscess becomes secondarily infected, extraperitoneal drainage should be employed (see Chap. 35, Peritoneum, Peritonitis, and Intra-Abdominal Abscesses). Transperitoneal or transpleural routes for drainage should be avoided.

Reports of DeBakey and Ochsner (1951) and of Ochsner and DeBakey (1943) extending over a period of 16 years clearly indicate the value of drainage of hepatic abscesses due to amebiasis. The abscess may be aspirated beforehand to determine its nature. The New Orleans group states that the "pus" is typically sterile and that in the stages of early focal necrosis, the protozoa can be demonstrated readily. Later on, however, amebae in such aspirates are difficult to detect.

DeBakey and Ochsner experienced a mortality of 42.9 per cent when amebic abscesses of the liver were present against 6.8 per cent when they were absent. Secondary infection of the amebic abscess is a grave consequence where the mortality rate of 40 per cent prevailed in contrast with 5.5 per cent when the abscess was sterile.

Should perforation of the bowel occur, nothing but bold surgical exteriorization of the involved segment will prove to be effective. Operative mortality is high, but with conservative management it approaches 100 per cent.

INTESTINAL TUBERCULOSIS

Tuberculosis of the intestinal tract is most frequently secondary to systemic tuberculosis. It may occur in the small bowel or the colon. Usually secondary intestinal tuberculosis is seen in the late stages of pulmonary tuberculosis, although it can occur when the pulmonary is healing. Most physicians consider secondary tuberculosis of the intestinal tract to be the result of the continuous swallowing of sputum containing the bacillus. Once secondary tuberculosis of the intestinal tract with ulceration of its mucosa becomes established, healing is extremely difficult to obtain unless the primary pulmonary disease can be arrested. Continued exposure of the intestinal tract to sputum containing the bacillus favors continuation of alimentary tract tuberculosis.

Primary tuberculosis of the intestinal tract rarely occurs in this country and seldom is observed in conjunction with tuberculosis of other organs. The principal form is probably bovine in origin, whereas the secondary variety is due to the human form of the tuberculous bacillus.

In a study by Rubin (1931), 30 years ago, 2 out of 3 patients dying of pulmonary tuberculosis had intestinal tuberculosis. Secondary intestinal tuberculosis is an uncommon finding today when pulmonary disease is not advanced.

Pathology. The pathologic change in secondary intestinal tuberculosis is usually one of mucosal ulceration. That of primary tuberculosis is more likely to be hypertrophic, a fact which seems to explain why many patients with regional enteritis, a hypertrophic disease of the small bowel in which non-caseating tubercules are found, formerly were considered to have an aberrant form of hypertrophic or primary intestinal tuberculosis.

In the ulcerative form, the mucosa may become necrotic and desquamate, producing an ulcer. In others, the mucosa remains intact, and the lymph nodes are the only site in which infection can be detected. Although the disease may be located from the stomach to the anus, the terminal ileum is the most frequently involved portion of the alimentary tract, possibly because of its higher content of lymphoid tissue (Peyer's patches) and the affinity of the tubercle bacillus for lymphoid tissue. Peyer's patches are gray and translucent early in the disease but later become swollen, caseous and yellow. The overlying serosa is normal or chronically inflamed. Healing usually occurs if the systemic disease can be controlled.

Clinical Course of Diagnosis. The disease when present is so frequently a complication of the terminal stages of systemic tuberculosis that secondary intestinal tuberculosis is more often diagnosed at autopsy than during life. Diarrhea with blood and pus in the stool may be observed. However, massive intestinal bleeding is unusual.

Intestinal tuberculosis in patients with pulmonary tuberculosis is to be suspected when the pulmonary disease is healing and suddenly the patient becomes febrile and his condition changes from one of improvement to one of deterioration, an unexplainable course of events on the basis of pulmonary findings. Abdominal pain is the principal symptom aside from diarrhea. If the mucosa is ulcerated and the adjacent peritoneum is irritated, tenderness is also found. Tuberculous peritonitis (the "wet" variety) may follow, but the latter is often seen in the absence of intestinal tuberculosis (Chap. 36, "Anatomy, Physiology and Treatment of Intestinal Obstruction").

The patient continues to run a downhill course with bizarre manifestations, especially his daily temperature records. Usually, his previous temperature had its maximum point of elevation in the late afternoon, but now he may exhibit his highest fever for the day before noon.

Barium studies may disclose filling defects, particularly in the lower ileum. This finding may suggest intestinal tuberculosis when the disease is known to exist elsewhere. Ileal stasis may be noted when oral barium is administered and is a finding considered suggestive of tuberculosis in this region.

The differential diagnosis centers chiefly about the distinction between other granulomatous diseases such as sarcoidosis, amebiasis, regional enteritis, lymphoma and nonspecific ulcerative ileocolitis.

The prognosis is dependent upon the ability to control pulmonary tuberculosis. If the latter can be arrested, the prognosis for secondary intestinal tuberculosis is good. On the other hand, when intestinal tuberculosis complicates advancing pulmonary tuberculosis, the prognosis is poor indeed.

The treatment is primarily medical and conservative. It consists first of all in controlling the pulmonary disease. A bland diet high in caloric value and containing supplemental vitamins usually is administered. Surgery is rarely indicated unless perforation, intestinal obstruction, abscess or fistulation occurs.

The hypertrophic form of the disease is more likely to produce partial intestinal obstruction and occasionally complete occlusion of the bowel. As this disease is seldom recognized preoperatively, most commonly the lesions are resected without suspecting its nature. This disease, like that of the secondary type, is most commonly present in the ileocecal region.

The hypertrophic form still persists fairly commonly in England and upon the continent of Europe and in other parts of the world where pasteurization of milk is seldom practiced. Its persistence in England and Europe is interesting, for despite the fact that the most effective measure for elimination of bovine tuberculosis had its origin in France, pasteurization is seldom practical in these countries.

The only patients whom the author has encountered with hypertrophic primary tuberculosis were seen on shipboard in 2 members of the British crew. Curiously, the 2 British surgeons performing the emergency operations for relief of obstruction in these patients also had been operated upon a few years previously for the same disease.

Fistula-in-ano may develop from intestinal tuberculosis, although this, too, has largely disappeared as a cause of perirectal fistulae in this country. However, all patients with fistula-in-ano should be investigated to exclude tuberculosis as its cause. A normal chest film coupled with a history of drinking pasteurized milk is generally sufficient to exclude tuberculosis as the cause of perirectal fistula in most patients in this counry, but smears of pus and tissue examination should be carried out in suspicious cases.

REGIONAL ENTERITIS

In 1932, Crohn, Ginzberg and Oppenheimer[16] resolved a group of nonspecific inflammatory tumors of the small bowel into a single pathologic entity to which they gave the name "regional ileitis." In retrospect, many granulomatous lesions of the small bowel previously attributed to hyperplastic tuberculosis and other granulomatous diseases probably were this entity instead.

For the most part, the disease is found in the terminal ileum; hence the name "terminal" ileitis was coined. As multiple diseased areas were soon described affecting different levels of the small bowel, and at times the colon, too, the names of "regional" or "segmental" enteritis seemed to be more appropriate. In other quarters, the entity is known as Crohn's disease, especially among the Europeans.

Regional enteritis and nonspecific ulcerative colitis have certain features in common, but there is no evidence that these two pathologic states are the same pathologic process. They coexist in about 2 per cent of all patients. In neither entity is the cause known. Both diseases affect more commonly the young and the middle-aged groups, and in neither disease does a predilection for predominance occur in one sex. Both have a higher attack rate in the same families than in the population at large, but the evidence of a strong familial attack rate does not exist. Regional enteritis may occur in one member of the family and ulcerative colitis in another. In both diseases personality changes occur, but the patient with ulcerative colitis suffers more. However, the pathologic findings are quite different (see pp. 934-935, 939-942, and Lockhart-Mummery and Morson, 1960, and Laipply, 1957).

Etiology of regional enteritis is unknown. No virus or bacterial agent has been recognized as causing the disease.

Pathology. The segment of small bowel involved most frequently is the terminal portion of the ileum, usually extending for a distance of a few inches to several feet. In about 15 per cent of patients, the lesions may be found elsewhere, either as single segments in continuity or as multiple segments with normal regions in between. Rarely is an isolated segment found in the colon; more often lesions in the colon are located in the region of the ileocecal valve and the cecum and are involved in continuity or by extension with that of the terminal ileum. Regional enteritis is primarily a disease of the small bowel. Ulcerative colitis is primarily a disease of the colon.

The diagnosis of regional enteritis at the operating table can be readily suspected from the gross appearance of the bowel alone, although actinomycosis, tuberculosis, sarcoidosis and intestinal lymphoma, including Hodgkin's disease, occasionally have similar gross and roentgenographic appearances. In a few instances, the diagnosis of regional enteritis is possible only when the adhesions are freed and the bowel can be inspected and microscopic examination of tissue is possible.

The involved segment of bowel is inflamed; often its color is livid. Fibrinous exudation is commonly present on the serosal surfaces of the diseased segment and its mesentery during the acute stages. The circumference of the bowel is enlarged, its wall thickened, often causing encroachment upon its lumen so that partial obstruction is a fairly frequent finding. Uninvolved proximal small bowel may be dilated or normal, depending upon the presence or the absence of obstruction. The thickened diseased portions resemble a "rubber garden hose," an analogy commonly used in the gross description of the diseased segments.

Fistulous communications between loops of adjacent small bowel and/or the colon are commonly encountered. Abscess pockets between the leaves of mesentery of nearby segments are present not infrequently. Abscesses may be located in the lateral gutters of the posterior abdomen or in the pelvis.

The mesentery is classic in its appearance. Its serosa is often slightly fibrotic so that its high gloss may be lost. More distinctive, however, is its thickness. At times, the thickness of the mesentery is equal to that of the small bowel that it sustains. The mesenteric lymph glands are always prominent and enlarged in the segment of the involved mesenteric segment concerned. These nodes may reach 2 to 4 cm. in diameter. Should operation be performed early in the stage of the disease, the lymph nodes may not be as enlarged as later on. But they may appear more prominent as the mesentery is not likely to be as edematous or as thickened as in the subacute or chronic stages of active disease.

The extent of adhesions is a matter of time and continued activity of the disease. Adhesions are usually more prominent when abscess and fistula are present. As a rule, adhesions are short and are found principally between adjacent loops of bowel and parietal peritoneum, agglutinating the gut into a mass which may be felt while palpating the abdomen. Adhesions may be scanty or absent, or they may be prolific. In some patients inspection of the gut at the time of operation discloses a large mass of adhesions, so extensive that the individual loops of bowel are not identifiable. Loops of bowel are encased in fibrous tissue. However, the diagnosis should be suspected, as there are few other pathologic conditions which produce similar pathologic states within the abdomen.

The mucosa is swollen; its transverse folds are edematous; and small ulcerations are noted fairly frequently along the mesenteric border where they may become confluent, forming linear ulcerations, oval in shape, which may be several centimeters long or run the entire length of the involved segment. Secondary infection often extends into the mesentery or into adherent adjacent loops of bowel, the bladder or the visceral peritoneum. Fistula or satellite abscesses tend to form at these sites.

Microscopically, two features dominate the picture. One is the appearance of multiple granulomatous areas which are characterized by large multinucleated giant cells not dissimilar from those seen in tuberculosis, except that caseation does not occur. Occasionally, these are centered about small foreign bodies which have the appearance of food particles, possibly cellulose, or other material which may have entered from the diseased mucosa.

The second prominent microscopic feature is sclerosing lymphangitis which appears to obstruct the lymphatics and the lacteals. Warren and Sommers (1954) describe the process as being focal with widely dilated lacteals and lymphatics in between. The end result is "elephantiasis" of the bowel segment and mesentery. Indeed, the primary disturbance may well be the obliteration of the lymph and lacteal channels of the mesentery with engorgement of the lymph nodes, lymphedema of the mesentery and finally lymphedema of the bowel itself leading to mucosal ulceration. Reichert and Mathes (1936) recognized the close relationship in the pathologic changes seen in regional enteritis and the changes following experimental chronic mesenteric lymphedema. They felt that the more extensive stenosis and mucosal ulceration found in clinical regional enteritis as compared with their experimental preparations might be due to the presence of a persistent low-grade bacterial infection in the clinical disease. This is a pathologic state resembling the lymphedema and the ulceration of the lower extremity with elephantiasis. Can regional enteritis be the end result of "mesenteric adenitis" with mesenteric lymphangitis and lactealitis? Further study will be necessary to establish its basic disturbance.

Clinical Pattern and Course. Regional enteritis is a chronic disease characterized by remissions and exacerbations and sometimes spontaneous "cures." The disease is found most frequently in young adults, the average age of onset of symptoms being about 25. However, it may have its symptomatic onset at any age, although 75 per cent of patients acquire the disease before the age of 35. The attack rate is essentially the same for both sexes.

In general the symptoms, signs and clinical course are functions of the rapidity at which the disease progresses, the segment(s) and the lengths of bowel involved, and the complications that develop.

ACUTE SYMPTOMS often simulate an attack of smoldering or subacute appendicitis and more frequently are observed in patients under 25 years of age. Nausea, vomiting, and pain in the right lower quadrant with tenderness and muscular rigidity often are observed. Fever and leukocytosis are generally parts of the total picture in all forms of the disease, although they tend to be more pronounced in the acute stages or when abscesses are present or perforation occurs. Appendicitis is the disease usually suspected, and frequently appendectomy is performed in patients of this group. The fundamental disease may not be detected at the time, as the appendix is often inflamed, and after it has been removed, the surgeon may not choose to explore for the presence of other disease. At times, acute appendicitis is coexistent but usually its inflammatory reaction is secondary to regional enteritis. Elective appendectomy is unwise when the terminal ileum is diseased, due to the high incidence of fistula formation arising from the appendiceal stump. Van Patter et al (1954) reported fistulation in about 25 per cent. If acute appendicitis coexists, resection of the diseased portion of the terminal ileum, the cecum and ascending colon with the appendix intact is preferred rather than appendectomy alone (see Treatment).

ENTERIC SYMPTOMS with chronic diarrhea, pain in the abdomen and the back, weight loss, malaise, fever, moderate leukocytosis and anemia are usually present. These are the symptoms and the symptom complexes most often observed. Gross blood in the stool may occur but is infrequent; occult blood is common. Tenderness of the abdomen is less severe than in the acute group, and a sausage-shaped mass may be felt in the abdomen, located in the right lower abdomen in about 85 per cent of patients in whom it is detected. As the disease progresses, diarrhea and pain become more troublesome. When the pain becomes crampy in nature, impending obstruction should be suspected.

OBSTRUCTIVE SYMPTOMS in this disease seldom occur in the absence of a previous history of diarrhea, mild to moderate abdominal distress or pain. Obstruction may be partial or complete. Operative intervention should not be delayed.

ABSCESS AND FISTULATION are late manifestations of the disease, although in unrelenting acute forms these complications may appear within a few months after onset of initial symptoms. They are often associated with signs of partial intestinal obstruction; less frequently they are independent of obstruction but seldom are present without a previous and fairly prolonged history of diarrhea, malaise, weight loss, increasing abdominal pain with tenderness, fever and leukocytosis. This group comprises about 30 per cent of all patients seen with regional enteritis.

Pain is the complaint most consistently given. Diarrhea is present in about 75 per cent of patients, and a palpable mass can be made out in the abdomen in about 50 per cent of patients examined.

Roentgenographic findings, when demonstrable, strongly support the diagnosis of regional enteritis but are not specific, as other granulomatous and malignant lesions of the small bowel may produce similar findings. Barium enema filling the terminal ileum may disclose the "string sign" of Kantor (1934) and can be demonstrated in many patients if the wall of terminal ileum is swollen and has encroached upon the lumen, allowing only a thin thread of barium to pass into the ileum on barium enema examination. This thin thread of the barium shadow may be several inches in length (Fig. 37-1). It is usually a late manifestation of the disease and often likely to be associated with symptoms of partial intestinal obstruction.

Other x-ray findings are "feathering" of the plica circulares with some separation of the mucosal pattern due to edema. Later the mucosal pattern is largely destroyed. These findings are helpful in detecting the presence of disease in the jejunum and the upper ileum when the diagnosis is rarely established for the terminal ileum. The lesions of the proximal small bowel are detected when the small bowel is filmed serially after the administration of oral suspensions of barium. Oral barium should not be administered when symptoms of intestinal obstruction are present.

Diagnosis and the differentiation of regional enteritis from other diseases of the small bowel is largely a presumptive one, to be con-

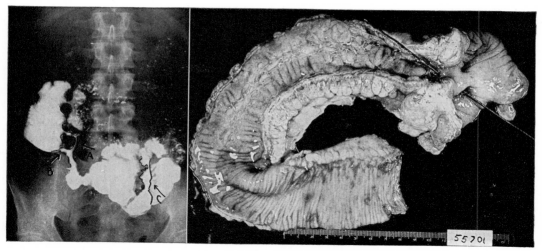

FIG. 37-1. Barium enema of a 34-year-old male with regional ileitis, showing narrowed segments of ileum at points A and C. Point A resembles a "string." Point B is a fistulous communication between the lower ileum and the cecum. Also shown is the resected specimen with the probe passing through this fistulous tract. Note the edema and the "trough" of confluent ulcerations of the mucosal folds along the mesenteric border. Thickening of the bowel wall is clearly indicated; the edematous mesentery is not shown.

firmed by microscopic examination of the resected specimen. Nonetheless, the presumptive diagnostic evidence in favor of Crohn's disease is usually strong despite the fact that at times lymphoma, tuberculosis and mycotic infections may produce local hypertrophic lesions that may simulate regional enteritis. Two of the features of regional enteritis generally are not well mimicked when the specimen is viewed at the operating table. These are the hypertrophic mesenteric lymph nodes and the thickened mesentery. The history, the physical findings and the positive x-ray findings of the bowel with negative chest films are very helpful. However, the extensive hypertrophy of the wall of the small bowel in primary intestinal tuberculosis usually is not suspected until the resected specimen is examined histologically. If in doubt at the operating table, biopsy of an enlarged lymph node usually will disclose tubercles with caseation in tuberculosis but not in regional enteritis.

Amebiasis is largely a diagnostic problem when the stools are negative for parasites in patients with amebic granuloma of the ileocecal area. In patients with amebic granuloma, "ameboma," the diagnosis may be established only when the resected specimen is examined histologically. Amebiasis much more often af-

fects the cecum and the ascending colon; regional enteritis affects primarily the small bowel. The cecum and the proximal portion of the ascending colon are usually involved in regional enteritis, secondary to this disease in the terminal ileum.

Carcinoma is exceedingly rare in the small bowel but commonly found in the cecum and the ascending colon. This seldom presents a serious diagnostic problem in regional enteritis, especially if the terminal ileum can be visualized with barium. Ulcerative colitis extending into the ileum may be very difficult to distinguish from regional enteritis extending into the cecum and the ascending colon.

Treatment of regional enteritis is primarily surgical at the present time. Symptomatic regional enteritis, all 4 clinical varieties, may improve under medical therapy, which includes corticoids and ACTH therapy. However, the treatment of choice in most patients remains surgical.

Once abscess, stricture or fistulation occurs, ·nothing short of surgical intervention affords any benefit. Crohn (1953) sums it up in the following manner:

A specific conservative or medical approach does not exist; the long, slowly downward course cannot be interfered with or changed by any method now known . . . sulfonamides occasionally produce good results. Penicillin is useless, and Aureomycin may cause diarrhea and vomiting. . . . Streptomycin, given orally or parenterally, and chloramphenicol, given orally, frequently produce strikingly favorable results, but follow-up studies are too limited to warrant definite opinions as to their ultimate value. . . . Frequently one observes a very dramatic and rapid change for the better with small doses of ACTH followed by a maintenance dose of cortisone given by mouth. The action is nonspecific, not curative. . . .

The form that surgical therapy should take is slowly becoming better defined, and there is better, though not complete, agreement as to which particular operation should be applied to the particular clinical forms of the disease.

The indications for surgical intervention are:

1. Medical failure (this should not be long continued and is best suited to patients with multiple segments involved or recurrences).

2. Abscess with or without fistula

3. Stricture with partial or complete obstruction

4. Massive hemorrhage (rare)

If resection is carried out, the enlarged lymph nodes and edematous mesentery present certain technical and pathologic considerations and problems, for which there is no very conclusive answer. The author, inclined toward the theory that primary obstruction of the mesenteric lymphatics and lacteals may be the basic disturbance responsible for the changes in the ileum or the jejunum in regional enteritis, attempts to resect the enlarged lymph nodes and edematous mesentery of the segment of bowel involved unless this procedure should entail resection of too large a bowel segment. In early cases, however, such resections along anatomic lines are readily feasible. The results are usually good.

Resection of bowel always demands the removal of 10 to 20 inches of grossly normal bowel on either side of the lesion if one is to remove all microscopic evidence of disease. This long-known fact would seem to argue in favor of the lymphostasis theory in that the lateral limits of lymphatic disease in the mesentery might be expected to extend further than the grossly diseased bowel. However, this point of view must be recognized as one of conjecture and without definite proof; its value until proved is principally one of affording a theoretic basis for a rational explanation in the extent of the surgical resection required and the desirability of excision of all of the grossly involved mesentery. This concept may be useful in the opposite direction, too, for if the amount of bowel which needs to be resected to eliminate diseased mesentery is too great, a bypass procedure may be necessary.

Ileocolostomy with exclusion is an operation which has been gaining in popularity within the past decade. It has been recommended as the primary operation when the terminal ileum is the only segment diseased. By this method, the terminal ileum is divided about 12 to 18 inches above the diseased segment. The distal portion of the divided segment is closed. The proximal end of the ileum is anastomosed to the ascending or right portion of the transverse colon. Thus all feces are diverted around the diseased terminal ileum. The chief advantage claimed for this procedure is that it carries a lower mortality rate. To date, the recurrence rate is said to remain about the same as that following resection. However, this bypass procedure is successful only if an adequate amount of normal ileum proximal to the disease is included in the distal transected portion. Subsequent exploratory laparotomy discloses in many instances regression of the disease with scarring, and in some patients evidence of gross disease disappears. However, the same course of events is noted when an ileotransverse colostomy is performed without exclusion and occurs spontaneously.

Not all accept the bypass and exclusion operation as the preferred method of surgical treatment (Colcock and Vansant, 1960). Moreover, among those who elect to perform this procedure, the indications for its use also vary considerably. In general, the bypass-exclusion procedure is preferred when more than one area of the jejuno-ileum is involved and the major disease is affecting the terminal ileum. The bypass procedure is not well suited for other diseased areas of the small bowel. Some believe it to be the procedure of choice for early disease; others prefer to restrict its use for more advanced stages.

This author prefers to limit the use of bypass procedures to patients with previous resections above the terminal ileum who now have recurrences involving the terminal ileum, or to those who have other segments of the bowel involved but in whom the dominant disease is found in the distal ileum. The results with resection are good if the mesenteric involvement also can be removed completely without resecting more than 4 or 8 feet of small bowel.

It is to be admitted that no one operation has gained universal acceptance. The diversity of procedures currently employed reflects the problems clinically encountered and the continued failures in about 15 per cent of cases regardless of which operation is performed. The most likely cause of recurrence is the inability or the failure to remove all of the disease originally present, including mesentery.

Nonspecific Ulcerative Colitis

Nonspecific ulcerative colitis may be acute and fulminant, subacute, chronic, relapsing and recurring in nature. As its cause is unknown and its course at times spontaneously remitting, methods of treatment often have been controversial. After examination of the patient and consideration of his course, appropriate treatment is often self-evident when contemplated in light of the pathologic process and the clinical facts at hand.

Etiology. As the name implies, the cause of nonspecific idiopathic ulcerative colitis is not established. There are many agents that may cause an ulcerative colitis, such as amebiasis, bacillary dysentery, tuberculosis and mercuric poisoning, but these are not of concern here.

From time to time, various suggestions have been made as to its pathogenesis. Among them are bacterial and virus infections, toxins, allergens, enzymatic disorders, collagen disturbances, and emotional or psychiatric disturbances. Some evidence can be marshalled in defense of each claim but in no instance is it sufficient to warrant the conclusion that a specific pathogen is uniformly responsible for the disease or, for that matter, solely responsible for the disease in any one patient.

A most impressive clinical feature is the emotional instability of most patients with this disorder. So striking is the psychological overlay that some have expressed the belief that such disturbances alone accounted for its pathogenesis. There is, however, no evidence to support this contention and much information to suggest that the psychological disorders are secondary. There is some evidence that pre-existing emotional disorders precipitate the *initial* attack; however, there is strong evidence that emotional or physical stress often precipitates *subsequent* ones. The precipitating role of emotional distress in acute relapse, once the disease has been established, is illustrated by the following case abstract:

A 32-year-old male salesman was admitted to the University of Chicago Clinics in March, 1939. His history was that of fairly mild ulcerative colitis of 7 months' duration. The diagnosis was arrived at by exclusion; the barium enema and the proctoscopic examination findings were compatible with mildly severe chronic ulcerative colitis. With bed rest, sedation, dietary adjustments and reassurance, symptoms remitted.

For 2 months following hospital discharge he remained symptom-free. On the 66th day, his twin brother developed acute perforative appendicitis and died 2 days later. Our patient suffered an immediate fulminant relapse from which he died 72 hours later.

Until an etiologic agent is established, the possibility exists that nonspecific ulcerative colitis is a clinical syndrome which may result from a variety of causes and that no one specific therapeutic agent may not prove to be uniformly effective.

Pathology. The systemic and local manifestations of nonspecific ulcerative colitis are sufficiently variable that it is not surprising the pathologic findings also should vary considerably.

Fulminant nonspecific ulcerative colitis with death occurring within a few days to a few weeks discloses the colon to be grossly dark and seminecrotic. Its serosal surface ranges from dusky red in color to purple or black. Fibrinous exudate is scanty. Free serosanguineous fluid is often present within the peritoneal cavity, but unless perforation has occurred, the exudate is not very purulent nor especially fibrinous. Numerous enteric bacteria often can be cultured from the fluid. The mesentery is moderately edematous, but there is remarkably little enlargement of its lymph nodes in contrast to regional enteritis.

The colon is usually shortened by one third or less of its usual length, particularly if the fulminant course is superimposed upon the chronic disease. Usually the entire colon and the rectum are involved in the fulminant form of the disease. The mucosal surface is semi-necrotic if not desquamated. The ileocecal valve and the terminal 2 to 6 inches of ileum may show similar changes.

Microscopically, there may be little or no mucosal surface remaining. That which may be found frequently contains numerous small abscesses within the crypts of the glandular epithelium. The muscular and serosal layers are infiltrated with polymorphonuclear leukocytes. Numerous thrombi are found throughout the intramural vessels of the colon. Acute vasculitis is widespread in the walls of the colon and the rectum. Focal necrosis is common and often confluent. Perforation and multiple areas with small pericolonic abscesses may be found. However, extension of thrombi beyond the marginal mesenteric vessels into the larger portal radicals is seldom observed.

Chronic nonspecific ulcerative colitis displays a less uniform pathologic appearance. It most frequently affects the rectum, least often the cecum. In order of frequency are the rectum, the rectosigmoid, the rectosigmoid-descending colon, etc. Occasionally, the disease is segmental, or at least some portions of the colon are more extensively diseased than others. In most patients with advanced disease the entire colon is involved.

Grossly, the colon is shortened considerably, often less than half of its normal length. The splenic flexure no longer rises high into the splenic fossa, the sigmoid redundancy is lost, the cecum, the ascending and the transverse colonic segments are short, all of which tend to give the x-ray appearance on barium enema examination of a "sickle-shaped" structure. The lateral portions of the colon are usually drawn to a more mesial position than its usual "picture-frame" location (Fig. 37-2). The haustral markings are lost, providing the

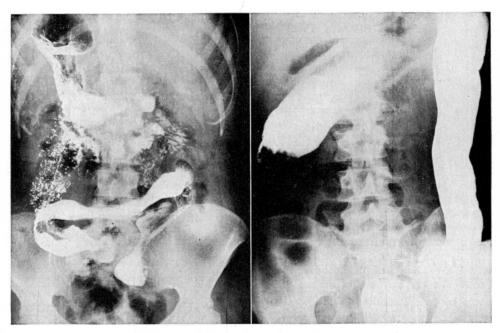

Fig. 37-2. Roentgenograms of the colons of 2 patients with chronic nonspecific ulcerative colitis. (*Left*) The shrunken colon; the ascending and the descending colon segments lie more mesially than they usually do and are contracted, drawing the transverse colon into the lower abdomen. (*Right*) Shows less shortening but not the loss of haustral markings throughout and the stricture at the hepatic flexure which proved to be inflammatory when the resected specimen was examined. Preoperative decision as to malignant or benign nature of the stricture was not possible on the basis of the barium studies alone.

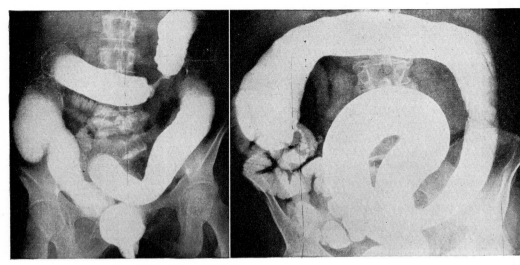

FIG. 37-3. (*Left*) Shows the "lead-pipe" appearance of the colon silhouette in nonspecific chronic ulcerative colitis. In addition, note the stricture in the left portion of the transverse colon which proved to be carcinoma. (*Right*) Also has a "lead-pipe" appearance, but this patient did not have ulcerative colitis. Instead, she suffered from chronic constipation and had taken mineral oil daily for 25 years; mineral oil, chronically administered, is known to produce this change in some patients.

"lead-pipe" characteristics seen on the barium contrast films (Fig. 37-3).

The mesentery is short and stubby, often edematous and frequently contains abscesses.

The serosal surface has lost much of its sheen; it is dull and grayish pink in color. Its surface is usually free of fibrinous exudate, save for areas of impending perforation. The wall of the colon is thickened, perhaps twice as thick as normal, but this is still an unremarkable finding compared with the thickening of the small bowel or the colonic segments in regional enteritis.

Several small perforations on the mesenteric margins with abscess formation in the mesentery are frequent findings in the advanced stages, particularly in the sigmoid-rectum where they tend to dissect downward, often forming perianal, rectovesicle or rectovaginal fistulae. Abscess formation is also a frequent finding at the sites of structure formation, the latter being a fairly common complication in the chronic state and one of the stellar indications for operation.

The mucosal surface in chronic ulcerative colitis shows a variety of changes. Ulcerations tend to run in the longitudinal axis of the colon and to be more prominent along the teniae coli with lateral cross extensions, similar to a spider web. The remaining mucosa is edematous with the ulcerated edges overhanging the denuded surfaces, often giving the appearance of multiple polyps—pseudopolyps. The strictures encountered may nearly occlude the lumen.

Carcinoma is encountered in 2 to 5 per cent of all cases with chronic ulcerative colitis and in 10 to 15 per cent of those cases which are severe enough to need surgical treatment. The longer the duration of the disease the higher the percentage of carcinoma. The threat of carcinoma does not reach such proportions that prophylactic colectomy should be considered for this reason alone.

Microscopically, the colonic mucosa is infiltrated with inflammatory cells. Its surface, where mucosa remains, is superficially ulcerated as well. Therefore, the crypts are shallow, though often plugged with detritus and leukocytes, giving rise to myriads of small, almost miliary abscesses. Submucosal layers are edematous, and fibroplasia is usually evident. Muscular hyperplasia is often described, but it is difficult to determine whether this is true hyperplasia or a functional thickening due to the longitudinal shortening of the colon.

Except where abscess or perforation is present, the seromuscular coats show surprisingly little pathologic reaction for so extensive a disease.

Clinical Course. *Fulminant or colitis gravis* form may occur as the first attack or it may be superimposed as an exacerbation upon the chronic form. Bowel movements are frequent, 15 to 30 a day, and almost always show blood with pus and mucus also. Fever, anemia and exhaustion are characteristic.

The anus and the lower rectum can be very painful; fissures often are observed. The entire colonic area of the abdomen becomes tender, and moderate distention may be present. Cramps are frequent and usually associated with an attitude of gloom, irritability and despair.

Weight loss is rapid. The hollow cheeks and the sunken eyeballs resemble those of severe shock or dehydration. These are due to excessive losses of water and salt and to loss of fat and protein. The hands, the arms and the legs show a remarkable loss of muscular substance. The bony thorax, the anterosuperior spines of the ilium, the spinous processes of the vertebrae and the bony sacrum are all prominently visible; pressure necrosis of skin and subcutaneous tissue is difficult to avoid over these weight-bearing areas when in bed.

Peristalsis is hyperactive.

Anemia is prominent, requiring frequent transfusions, often several a day, to keep ahead of blood loss and peripheral circulatory collapse. Crossmatching becomes increasingly difficult because of the frequent occurrence of "cold agglutinins" (see Chap. 8, "Blood Transfusion"). Leukocytosis is pronounced, often in excess of 25,000 cells per cu. mm. of blood.

Fever mounts higher and higher, frequently ranging between 104° and 106° F. in the fulminant state.

The patient becomes increasingly toxic and confused and lapses into coma if he fails to respond. Death then may occur from 24 to 36 hours later from irreversible shock, peritonitis, exhaustion or toxemia—singularly, in combination, or collectively.

Chronic nonspecific ulcerative colitis as well as the fulminant variety are largely diseases of the young and the middle-aged adults. The age and sex distribution of 100 illustrative

TABLE 1

DECADE	MALE	FEMALE	TOTAL
1–9	3	..	3
10–19	7	17	24
20–29	17	21	38
30–39	12	9	21
40–49	7	4	11
50–+	2	1	3
Total	48	52	100

(Kirsner, J. B., Palmer, W. L., Maimon, S. N., and Ricketts, W. E.: J.A.M.A. 137:922, 1948.)

patients studied by Kirsner and Palmer (1948) is shown in Table 1 and are fairly representative.

The duration of the disease in these patients at the time they were first seen at the University of Chicago ranged from a few months to more than 15 years. The mortality rate was highest within the first 2 years of illness and became progressively lower as the average duration of chronicity increased. The course characteristically was one of remissions and exacerbations with only 6 whom these authors were willing to consider as possible "cures."

The severity of clinical symptoms tended to parallel the degree to which the colon was involved. This relation was by no means a constant one. Nor did the severity of the roentgenographic findings correlate more than in a general way with the severity of the clinical manifestations, although the presence of stricture was more commonly associated with the more serious complications: continued hemorrhage, diarrhea, distention, cramps, abscess and fistulation.

Relapses in the Kirsner-Palmer series of patients could be associated with emotional disturbances in 34 per cent, respiratory infections in 29 per cent and physical fatigue in 14 per cent. It is to be emphasized that relapses are commonly associated with trials of everyday life, but this association is not evidence that such stresses play a fundamental etiologic role (see Etiology). As these same stimuli often cause diarrhea among the normal population, it was believed that their effects should be more pronounced among those with inflammatory disease of the colon, a postulate which, indeed, is difficult to deny.

Despite the serious pathologic changes of the bowel, many of the Kirsner-Palmer patients had little disability, and some remained in good health for longer than a decade. 14 per cent died—9 per cent while on medical management and 5 per cent after operation.

The complications were and are numerous and varied in this particular series as well as in all other similarly studied series. 19 per cent developed stricture; 17 per cent developed abscess and fistula; in 16 per cent polyps occurred; 12 per cent had severe bleeding from the bowel; 8 per cent had arthritic manifestations; perforation with peritonitis occurred in 6 per cent; and carcinoma in 2 per cent. Infections of various types were frequent, and thrombophlebitis occasionally noted. About half of the patients developed pronounced microcytic anemia; and in the more debilitated, hypoproteinemia was usually present with occasional reversal of the albumin-globulin ratio. Vitamin deficiencies occurred unless combated actively in most who were chronically ill for prolonged periods. Many patients developed more than one complication.

The initial roentgenographic findings in 24 of 89 patients were normal. The entire colon was abnormal in 30 patients; the rectosigmoid involvement alone was found in only 11. Involvement from the rectum to the splenic flexure occurred in 12 with another 8 having involvement from the rectum to the hepatic flexure (see Table 2).

This experience is rather typical for any group of carefully managed patients with this disease carried on conservative or medical therapy. Perhaps the complications of abscess, perforation, peritonitis and carcinoma are higher than this series indicates, as some patients with these complications were admitted directly to the surgical services and hence not included in the Kirsner-Palmer series.

The author has encountered 5 patients with chronic nonspecific ulcerative colitis who developed cirrhosis and portal hypertension later on. These were treated by portacaval anastomosis. It is possible that the hepatitis and the cirrhosis were secondary to ulcerative colitis, recognizing the ease with which the virus particles of hepatitis might enter the portal circulation from the ulcerative surface of the colon or that the cirrhosis could have been in part nutritional in origin or perhaps a combination of both (see Chap. 33, "Mesentery, Splanchnic Circulation, Portal Hypertension and Mesenteric Thrombosis").

The personality of the patient with nonspecific ulcerative colitis deserves special mention and understanding upon the part of the physician and the surgeon alike, if cooperation of the patient is to be elicited in the therapeutic program that they wish the patient to follow. To conclude that the personality is more than a complex combination of neuroses accumulating in the course of a most distressing illness does not seem to be warranted from the data at hand. Infantilism, dependency and emotional instability are characteristic but these are manifest expressions rather than descriptive of psychological disturbances.

Once relieved of their disease, many of the overt personality disorders disappear, although not without leaving their mark. In the meantime, persistent patience on the part of the physician is as rewarding as most other forms of conservative therapy.

Diagnosis. The diagnosis of nonspecific ulcerative colitis is one of exclusion: exclusion of amebiasis, bacillary dysentery, tuberculosis, polyposis, diverticulitis, carcinoma and specific causes of ulcerative colitis. Stool culture and repeated examinations for the presence of parasites within the bowel exclude most infections other than tuberculosis and ameboma.

Proctoscopic examination is perhaps the most direct diagnostic technic when the results of other tests are known. The diffusely granular, friable, superficially ulcerated and

TABLE 2

Extent of Roentgenographic Involvement	DURATION OF SYMPTOMS			
	Less Than 1 Yr.	1–9 Yrs.	10–20 Yrs.	Total
Normal	10	12	2	24
Rectosigmoid only	3	7	1	11
Rectum to splenic flexure	6	5	1	12
Rectum to hepatic flexure	2	6	..	8
Entire colon	10	16	4	30
Segmental	1	2	1	4
Total	32	48	9	89

(Kirsner, J. B., Palmer, W. L., Maimon, S. N., and Ricketts, W. E.: J.A.M.A. *137*:922, 1948.)

bleeding mucosa are diagnostic findings in the absence of other specific causes of inflammation.

The barium enema examination discloses the so-called "lead-pipe" character of the bowel wall with the absence of haustral markings in the involved segment. Frequently, the major or entire colon is shortened. However, the lead-pipe appearance may occur from other causes, particularly the chronic use of mineral oil (Fig. 37-3), wherein the patient's complaint is constipation rather than diarrhea. However, it is to be noted in Figure 37-3 that while the haustral markings are lost, the colon is not shortened. The loss of mucosal detail is an early finding in ulcerative colitis but not necessarily diagnostic of the disease. Roentgenographic lesions limited to the cecum and the ascending colon should raise suspicion of tumor, amebiasis or tuberculosis in addition to ulcerative colitis. The last has a predilection for the more distal portions of the colon and seldom is seen as an isolated disease entity involving only the cecum and the ascending colon alone. In about 15 to 25 per cent of the patients, the terminal ileum is also involved in ulcerative colitis and may be demonstrated by edematous folds and often with destroyed mucosal patterns in the ileum.

The repeated use of the barium enema and proctoscopic examination over the years is the best protection that can be afforded the patient against delayed detection of carcinoma in chronic ulcerative colitis. Unfortunately, carcinoma developing in the colon with ulcerative colitis carries a poor prognosis (see Part II, this Chapter). Cytology may be helpful.

The differential diagnosis, aside from amebiasis, tuberculosis, polyposis, diverticulitis, etc., should consider also nonspecific proctitis and lymphopathia venereum. Both of these latter diseases are detected proctoscopically, and the history of bubo with a strongly positive Frei test weighs heavily in favor of the diagnosis of lymphopathia venereum. Nonspecific proctitis may be a form of nonspecific ulcerative colitis and is best treated medically on a regimen similar to that used for mild ulcerative colitis.

Treatment. Divergence of opinion exists as to the best means for treating the patient with nonspecific ulcerative colitis, although the lines drawn are more rational than a decade ago. Operation after a short period of conservative management is no longer frequently practiced today. However, the persistence at medical management when the patient's condition continues to fail is equally unsound.

The chief problem centers about the indications for surgical intervention. Considerable variations exist as to the threshold levels of resistance or capitulation on the part of the physician to permit the operative management of his patient. Perhaps the one point about which there is most confusion relates to the emotional disorders of the patient. The disease in the colon may be brought under control medically, but the patient's emotional disorders may continue to be incapacitating. Freed of his colon, many of his emotional ills may disappear, but is this an indication for colectomy? Most believe not.

Patients with mild disease do well on conservative therapy about 85 per cent of the time, although recurrences are the rule. These, too, tend to be mild. About 50 per cent of those with moderately severe disease will respond to conservative management, including corticoids and ACTH, although several months are often necessary to achieve results.

Continued efforts are rewarding unless an early recurrence supervenes. Should this occur, it is well to take stock of what has been accomplished. Hospital costs and loss of gainful employment deserve serious attention, too. The treatment employed should provide not only relief of symptoms but rehabilitation and restoration to gainful employment and a useful life when possible.

Several clinical factors tend to forecast the likelihood for recovery on conservative management: the older the patient at the time of onset of the disease, the better his prognosis is likely to be. Most deaths occur within 2 years after onset and most often before the age of 30; the moderately severe disease in the younger patient may not respond well to conservative treatment. When the disease is limited to the left colon, the prognosis is a more favorable one; the longer the segment of proximal uninvolved colon, the better the outlook is likely to be. The lack of disease in the right colon, the absence of stricture, fistulation and pseudopolyposis are favorable signs, indicating that a good response to conservative treatment may be obtained.

The indications for surgical therapy are

reviewed by Dukes and Lockhart-Mummery (1957). Most physicians and surgeons would agree that surgery is indicated for:

1. Acute fulminating disease with uncontrollable hemorrhage, toxic megacolon, or a continued downhill course despite aggressive medical management

2. Complications of acute or chronic disease, such as stricture with partial or complete obstruction, perforation of the colon, peritonitis, abscess formation, fistula formation

3. Medical failure; that is, chronic invalidism or the continued presence or progression of chronic bleeding, arthritis, dermatitis, etc.

4. Carcinoma, proved or suspected. The onset of carcinoma in ulcerative colitis patients is at an average age of 42 years after an average duration of disease of 14 years.

The type of operation performed is no longer held in much dispute. *Total abdominal colectomy and ileostomy* as a 1-stage procedure is the operation of choice for the management of the above indications. Compromise and procrastination add to the complications and have been responsible for many of the poor results and much of the mortality rate. In most patients the 1-stage colectomy is feasible and safe. The rectum may be removed at the same time; this is desirable for 3 reasons: (1) it spares the patient a second operation; (2) no residual disease exists; and (3) the improvement obtained will often make difficult the persuasion of the patient that removal of the rectum is necessary at a later date.

Diversionary ileostomy performed to "place the colon at rest" seldom accomplishes anything in advanced disease. For example, in those patients with abdominal colectomy, leaving the rectum intact nearly always continues to show active disease within the rectum upon proctoscopic examination. Patients who might benefit with temporary ileostomy are those in whom the disease is mild and will improve on conservative management alone. To perform only ileostomy in fulminant nonspecific ulcerative colitis does not rid the abdomen of seminecrotic bowel, and the results are indeed poor. The author has seen no survivals among patients upon whom this was attempted as a last resort procedure. If any operation is to be performed in this moribund group of patients, it should be colectomy. The patient who will withstand ileostomy will also generally withstand at least a total abdominal colectomy.

ACUTE FULMINANT NONSPECIFIC ULCERATIVE COLITIS. Most patients with the malignant form of colitis, colitis gravis, should be subjected to total abdominal colectomy as soon as this course is evident. The clinical problem involved is largely defining when this condition exists. In another sense, the question revolves about what constitutes a medical failure in acute ulcerative colitis. There is no better answer than this: any patient whose stools continue to increase in frequency with larger quantities of blood being lost, whose fever continues to mount, whose abdomen becomes increasingly tender and whose general status continues to go down hill despite vigorous conservative management, should be subjected to colectomy. Once the decision is made to operate, the procedure should be carried out as soon as the operating room can be made ready. Tomorrow may be too late.

As these patients are critically ill, often moribund, it is difficult for the surgeon to muster sufficient courage to perform colectomy; he would rather settle for the diversionary ileostomy under local anesthesia. However, there is no disease within the abdomen other than hemorrhage and panhypersplenism where a patient so near to death will respond as promptly as these patients do once the colon is removed. Each should be given a chance, but the fair chance depends upon nothing less than complete abdominal colectomy. Diversionary ileostomy has no place here. The author has employed this approach without mortality in all fulminant cases operated upon since 1950. The abdominal rectum may be divided, closed and tucked beneath the pelvic peritoneum if desired, with extraperitoneal stab-wound drainage established, or it may be removed at the same time.

The response of a patient with the fulminant disease to 1-stage colectomy is shown in Figure 37-4. The high temperature and tachycardia promptly drop and are often near normal within 12 to 24 hours. Toxemia disappears within the same period. Within 2 to 4 days, the patient is able to eat, and complete recovery usually follows.

Corticoids are administered preoperatively if the patient is not already receiving them. If he is on corticoids or ACTH, as usually is the case, his daily dosage is doubled during the day of operation. Half of the increase is given within 2 hours prior to operation, and the remainder is distributed equally throughout the rest of the day, being added to the base-line dosage levels used prior to operation. These are administered over the next 4 doses given at 6-hour intervals. During the second 24-hour period, the increased increments of corticoids are usually cut in half so that each 6-hour dose now is only 25 per cent greater than the preoperative one. On the second postoperative day, the dosage is reduced to its preoperative level and thereafter is reduced judiciously each 2 or 3 days until discontinued between the 8th and the 10th postoperative days.

The *technical features* of ileostomy construction are important, since the future uncomplicated function of the ileostomy depends on attention to small details. We utilize the technic of Brooks (1954) as modified by Durham (1957) (see Chap. 37, Part 2).

The location of the ileostomy should be on the right side of the anterior abdominal wall at least 1½ inches away from both the umbilicus and the anterior spine of the ilium. Otherwise, a skin-tight ileostomy seal, such as that afforded by the Rutzen-type of ileostomy ap-

pliance, cannot be maintained. For this reason, the abdominal skin incision for abdominal colectomy should be in the mid-line or slightly to the left and deviating around the left of the umbilicus (Fig. 37-5). It is well to remember that the patient will wear a belt to support his ileostomy appliance so that the stoma should be placed in or near the waistline; otherwise, the belt will tend to pull the appliance out of position.

After selecting the ileostomy site, a circular excision of skin, subcutaneous fat and anterior fascia is made; the muscle fibers are separated, and the posterior fascia incised. If the fascial edges are at all tight, portions are excised so as to obviate the possibility of any stricture. Then the end of the small bowel is brought through this wound and turned back upon itself, forming a double-layered ileostomy stoma with no exposed serosal surface. This prevents the serositis, inflammation, stricture and ileostomy dysfunction which were so common with the older technics. The free edge of bowel mucosa is immediately sutured to the skin margins (see Chap. 2, Wound Healing, and Chap. 37, Part 2, Tumors of the Colon and the Rectum).

The serosal surface of the mesentery should be sutured to the parietal peritoneum about

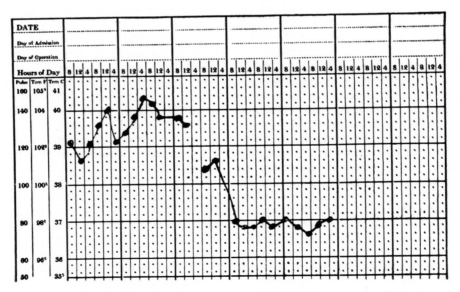

FIG. 37-4. Graphic chart shows the return of temperature to normal the day following total abdominal colectomy. The rectum was removed at the same time.

the ileostomy site internally and along the posterior and lateral surfaces of the right abdominal wall. No sutures should be placed in the bowel segment as it traverses the abdominal wall lest a fistula develop. As an alternative, the extraperitoneal tunnel technic of Goligher (1958) may be used. This internal anchoring of the mesentery to the parietes helps eliminate the possibility of three postoperative complications of ileostomy: internal hernia, rotational volvulus of the terminal ileum, and prolapse of the ileum through the ileostomy.

Early postoperative management of ileostomy. Immediate application of a temporary water-sealed ileostomy appliance or the use of catheter drainage of the terminal ileum is essential to preventing excoriation of the skin which delays the application of a permanent appliance. More important, skin excoriation promotes low-grade infection of the exteriorized ileum which contributes to stenosis of the ileostomy stoma and the partial obstruction that stenosis may cause.

A No. 26 fenestrated soft latex catheter introduced into the ileostomy for a distance of 5 to 6 inches will often drain away ileal juices for a few days, leaving the skin dry. A ligature snugging or tying the tube to the *tip* of ileal stoma to prevent leakage may be used *only* if it is realized that the distal segment will slough and may result in a skin-flush stoma if an inadequate length of ileum is exteriorized. The final stoma should protrude from ½ to 1 inch from the abdominal wall.

The catheter should be removed on or before the 5th postoperative day after which time plastic ileostomy bags are sealed to the skin and a week or two later a permanent appliance may be worn. Care must be exercised that the portion of the appliance adjacent to the ileostomy does not cause excoriation or pressure necrosis of the ileum, as this will create a small external fistula and cause leakage.

Gentle dilatation of the ileostomy should be performed with the index finger, at least 4 times a week for 5 to 6 weeks. By this time the skin and the mucosa will have united. A split skin graft applied to the ileostomy serosal surface as suggested by Dragstedt is another method of performing ileostomy so as to avoid an exposed peritoneal surface.

Before discharge, the patient should dem-

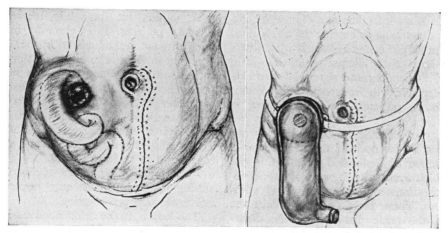

FIG. 37-5. The 2 drawings illustrate the construction of an ileostomy. Note (*left*) that the ileum adjacent to the inner aspects of the abdominal wall can twist and cause obstruction unless this portion of the ileal mesentery is sutured to the parietal peritoneum so that volvulus is prevented. (*Right*) Illustrates the application of a watertight or "skin-seal" ileostomy bag. Note that the location of the ileostomy is such that this appliance does not rest on the anterior superior iliac spine or encroach upon the umbilicus. The operative incision is placed slightly to the left of the mid-line to avoid interference with the ileostomy appliance and its seal.

onstrate to the surgeon his ability to apply the sealed bag without injury to the ileostomy and to dilate the stoma satisfactorily. His diet should be bland, avoiding fruit juices and roughages for several months, by which time the ileal contents should be semisolid, if not as formed stools.

A well-performed colectomy and ileostomy is a great satisfaction to the patient with chronic ulcerative colitis. He is free to leave his home to resume normal activity, to raise his family and to be self-supporting. Bacon (1960) has reported a personal series of 468 patients with both acute fulminant and chronic forms of ulcerative colitis who underwent colectomy. The long term survival and rehabilitation rate in this series was 98 per cent at 5 years and 90.5 per cent at 10 years postoperatively.

DIVERTICULAR DISEASE OF THE COLON

Diverticular disease includes both diverticulosis and diverticulitis. Diverticulosis eventually affects two thirds of patients who live to be 85 years of age. Diverticula are present in one fifth of all persons over 40 years of age who have barium enema examinations of the colon. Diverticulitis occurs as a complication in 15 per cent of patients who have diverticulosis (Ryan, 1958). As the name implies, this is an inflammatory disease of one or more diverticula occurring in the colon. More than 80 per cent of patients with diverticulosis have their disease situated within the distal descending and sigmoidal segments of the colon. Next in frequency is the cecum, and in some patients the entire colon is involved.

Etiology of diverticulitis is nearly always obstruction at the neck of the diverticula or the impaction of desiccated feces within the pouch which eventually is cause for stercoraceous ulcerations and inflammation of adjacent tissue. These facts do not explain the origin of the basic disturbance—the diverticula. They may be acquired, although certain anatomic features, congenital if you choose to call them, may account for their development in some individuals and not in others.

The diverticulum represents a herniation of colonic mucosa through the muscular layers. This herniation may occur between muscle coats. The muscular layers may be pushed ahead of the mucosal pouch and thinly dispersed over its surface. Diverticula rarely are found in the rectum or along the taenia coli. Generally, they are located on the mesenteric border or beneath the appendices epiploicae. However, some diverticula appear in regions of the bowel not commonly covered with appendices.

For the most part, however, diverticula appear to arise in areas penetrated by the small vessels entering and leaving the colon. Many pathologists and anatomists attribute the location of diverticula to these regions as related to etiology. It should be easier for the mucosal outcroppings or herniations to proceed along the paths made by these vessels than to make new ones.

The diverticulum tends to become larger and its wall thinned out, becoming "teardrop" in shape. The diverticulum does not perforate because of distention unless it becomes inflamed. It is surprising how frequently most or all diverticula empty readily despite the attenuation of the muscular coats. They seem to fill readily when enemas of barium sulfate suspension are administered and to empty fairly promptly soon after the enema is expelled.

Diverticulosis may be found in children and young adults but much less frequently than in older patients. It is observed more commonly in fat individuals with poor muscular tone and in those who have a history of mild or moderate constipation over a number of years. Some of these clinical features are encountered frequently in patients with hiatus hernia and cholelithiasis. In fact, the concurrence of hiatus hernia, cholelithiasis and diverticulosis is fairly common and sometimes is referred to as Saint's triad.

Pathology. Inflammation of diverticula, resulting in diverticulitis, may be acute, subacute, chronic or recurring.

The length of the colon involved is usually 4 to 10 inches. Inflammation of one diverticulum causes sufficient edema to occlude the openings of those adjacent to it. These diverticula, now closed, often become secondarily infected. The length of the segment involved may be fairly extensive if diverticula are extensive and in close approximation. Frequently, the disease may only stop its progression when there are no more diverticula

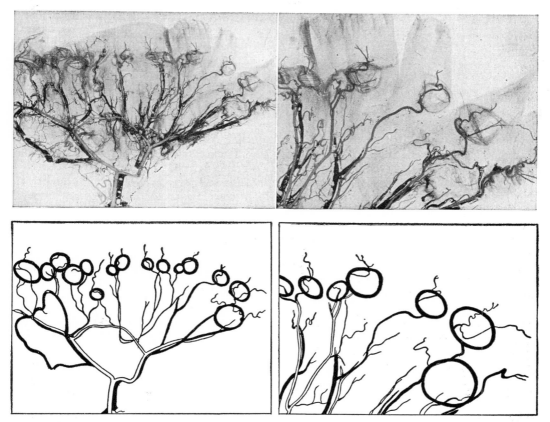

Fig. 37-6. The two photographs show the abnormal arterial blood vessels about diverticula in a resected specimen of colonic wall in which liquid latex was injected to outline the vessels. The specimens were then cleared by the Spalteholtz technic. The arteries are light and the veins are dark. The two drawings below are shown to clarify the nature of the vascular abnormalities. Each corresponds to the photograph immediately above. (Noer, R. J.: Ann. Surg. *141*:674)

above or below to be occluded by edema or the distance between them is greater than can be bridged by the inflammatory reaction. In some patients with diverticulosis of the entire colon, the disease commences in the sigmoid and extends in retrograde fashion to involve most if not all of the colon. One of the author's patients required resection from the hepatic flexure to the rectum, and in another abdominal colectomy was necessary; however, such occurrences are rare.

Slight bleeding, though often occult, is frequent, occurring in about one fourth of patients with diverticular disease. As the location of a diverticulum is usually alongside a blood vessel, it is not unexpected that ulceration caused by fecal impaction of the diverticulum may erode into blood vessels. The concept has often been expressed in past years that "if the sigmoidal lesion bleeds, it is carcinoma." This point of view is contested by Noer (1955) who believes it to be an erroneous one. Noer's studies disclosed some rather unusual features of the vessels in the regions of diverticula, which he believes to favor bleeding (Fig. 37-6). Recent studies by Ponka, Brush and Fox (1960) substantiate the opinion that bleeding is not a useful criterion in differentiating diverticulitis from carcinoma of the colon.

Although serious hemorrhage is a less frequent complication, it does occur in 12 per cent of patients with diverticular disease (Harkins, 1960). At times, hemorrhage from a diverticulum may nearly exsanguinate the patient and dictate very aggressive treatment (Ulin, Sokolic and Thompson, 1959).

The inflammatory changes in diverticulitis are often extensive locally. Whether or not perforation occurs, pericolitis is usually pronounced, the wall of the colon becomes edematous, and partial or complete obstruction not infrequently occurs. Perhaps the most impressive feature of the disease, noted at the operating table, is the extent of the edema of the mesocolon, the adjacent pelvic structures and loops of small bowel. Certainly, the extent of the gross pathology is usually greater than expected on the basis of preoperative studies. An abdominal mass may be palpated or felt on digital examination of the rectum or the vagina.

Abscess formations within the mesentery, between loops of small bowel or the adherent bladder, are not uncommon and occasionally contain several hundred milliliters of pus.

Fistulous communications between the colon and the small bowel, the bladder or the skin (usually perianal) are not as commonly encountered as in regional enteritis but are by no means rare complications. Pylephlebitis of the sigmoidal veins with miliary or larger abscesses forming in the liver is an infrequent complication. Adhesions form and are among the more common nonsurgical causes of small bowel obstruction in patients who have had no previous surgery.

Less than 1 per cent of cases have carcinoma as a co-existing feature. The major diagnostic hazard is the failure to recognize that carcinoma may be a "sleeper." There is no evidence that diverticulitis induces carcinoma; the coincidence appears to be explainable on predilection of both diseases for the sigmoid segment of colon.

Clinical Pattern and Course. The symptoms of diverticulitis and the nature of complications are dependent upon the segment of the colon involved, the length of the segment affected, the presence or the absence of intestinal obstruction, perforation, abscess formation with or without fistulation, and bleeding (see Pathology, p. 948).

Pain is the most common complaint and is located most often low in the abdomen. As the sigmoid is often redundant and may lie across the lower abdomen, bilateral lower abdominal pain is often complained of. Pain is generally constant and not very intense unless perforation or pericolitis occurs with irritation of the adjacent perietal peritoneum. The patient may state that pain is worse with defecation or if jolted when riding in an automobile. He is restless and decidedly uncomfortable in most instances.

When the lesion lies in the low sigmoid, he may complain of a sense of rectal fullness unrelieved by defecation, especially if an abscess is developing. The stools are frequently loose and may be small in caliber.

Chills and fever may be noted. A chill with high fever raises the alarming question of migratory pylephlebitis of the sigmoidal veins with possibly early intrahepatic abscess formation. On the other hand, these symptoms may be the result of abscess formation with or without cystitis and urinary tract infection, or they may imply perforation. Low-grade fever is commonly encountered in the active stages of the disease.

Bilateral lower abdominal tenderness is commonly present when the disease is active; of course, tenderness may be elsewhere if diverticulitis is in a part of the colon other than the sigmoid. Abdominal tenderness is maximum over the point of inflammation, except for perforation, abscess and pericolitis. Tenderness usually is not exquisite, although it may be pronounced.

Hemorrhage and its cause have been discussed under Pathology.

Leukocytosis is generally present, and its degree is roughly commensurate with the extent and the activity of infection.

The clinical course is one of remissions and exacerbations. Often the intervals between attacks are years rather than months apart, a point which favors conservative management. At the same time, the attacks are weeks in duration rather than days; occasionally they linger for several months. They may not clear up short of operative excision of the segment involved (see Treatment).

Proctoscopic examination is of value primarily because usually the scope will not pass readily into the narrowed sigmoid. If it does, the proctoscopist recognizes the fact that he has entered a narrowed segment whose mucosa is intact without polyps or carcinoma, and that such a finding is indirect evidence of diverticulitis. Few, if any, other inflammatory lesions of the colon mimic diverticulitis upon proctoscopic examination. Bleeding mucosa is infrequent, and ulcerations are rare. Pus may be noted upon occasion. The openings of diverticula are almost never observed in diverticulitis because edema of the mucosa generally occludes their lumina.

Barium enema should not be administered in the presence of crampy pains, as partial obstruction may be present. Iodinated oil may be used, as this will not obstruct a partially occluded lumen, but this is a technic inferior to barium sulfate examination. Pain without cramps does not contraindicate barium administration.

The features of the barium enema examination which suggest diverticulitis are: First, the mucosal pattern is normal in the narrowed segments. Second, both the proximal and the distal segments of the involved loop are funnel-shaped, indicating the more gradual narrowing of the bowel lumen in contrast to the abrupt constriction seen in carcinoma. Third and most helpful, of course, is the demonstration of diverticula of the colon adjacent to the diseased segment. As the ostia of diverticula in the inflamed narrowed segment of bowel are occluded or narrowed, they seldom visualize (Fig. 37-7).

A mass may be felt in the left lower abdomen. Aiding in the abdominal palpation is the fact that the general muscular tonus is poor in many of these patients. With gentle palpation the mass can be detected in many patients.

Digital examination of the rectum may disclose bogginess of the cul-de-sac and often a sense of a mass above the reach of the finger when the patient bears down at the time of bimanual palpation.

The diagnosis is largely one of exclusion plus the important positive findings disclosed by the barium enema. The location and the bilaterality of pain in the lower abdomen, the palpable mass, fever and leukocytosis, the absence of positive findings by proctoscopic examination, all favor the diagnosis. But it is to be remembered that carcinoma in this same segment and diverticulitis may coexist, and the tumor be obscured.

Treatment. MEDICAL OR CONSERVATIVE TREATMENT is the one most often employed unless perforation, fistulation, intestinal obstruction or serious hemorrhage prevail. Con-

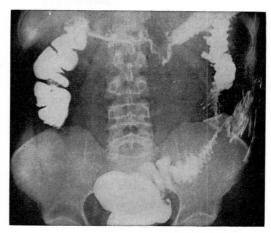

FIG. 37-7. Roentgenogram of colon in patient with diverticulosis and diverticulitis. Note the tapered narrowing of the upper and the lower ends of the constricted descending and transverse colonic segments. Diverticula are noted near the splenic flexure which were not extensively diseased, which barium could enter and leave. Absence of diverticula in diseased portions is due to closure of their ostia in the inflamed regions.

servative management consists largely of mineral oil, a bland diet, bedrest, heat to the abdomen, sulfasuxidine or sulfathalidine, streptomycin, and/or one of the tetracycline compounds administered parenterally during the acute phases. The disease subsides in most patients, although recurrences later on may be unpleasant and require a repetition of the same therapeutic program. Avoidance of constipation or diarrhea are important prophylactic measures to be carried out throughout the rest of the patient's life.

SURGICAL TREATMENT. The results of conservative management are sufficiently good and recurrences sufficiently infrequent that it is not easy for the surgeon to protest vigorously in most cases, should one wish to advocate resection instead. However, Babcock (1941); Bartlett and McDermott (1953); Judd and Mears (1955) and Rosser (1945) have expressed the view that surgical intervention has more to offer than is generally realized. This position is tenable largely because of the advent of intestinal sulfonamides and antibiotics, and a better understanding of the problems of bowel preparation with improvement in methods to accomplish this purpose. A more aggressive attitude in favor of earlier surgical intervention is desirable in many of the patients eventually referred for surgical therapy. In the past, they have been patients with difficult complications which resulted in a higher mortality rate than occurs today.

Indications for surgical intervention in diverticulitis continue to be largely those of the pre-antibiotic era of 15 years ago. They are:

1. Partial or complete obstruction
2. Abscess
3. Perforation
4. Fistulation
5. Severe hemorrhage
6. Carcinoma

Some surgeons are broadening the indications for operative treatment to include patients who fail to respond to medical management during an acute attack or have repeated attacks of diverticulitis (McCune *et al.,* 1957; Schlicke and Logan, 1959; Boyden and Neilson, 1960; Brown and Toomey, 1960, and Smithwick, 1960).

The types of operation performed depend upon the nature of the complication requiring surgical intervention.

For partial or complete intestinal obstruction, the goal of the immediate operation is decompression. One of two procedures may be employed. A transverse colostomy is all that is required in most patients in whom the disease is distal to this point. It is a very useful temporary procedure and, of course, simple to perform. The second is the Mikulicz resection wherein the involved segment of colon is freed by cutting the lateral peritoneal reflection of the colon as required. The colon segment is dissected free and reflected mesially, being careful to avoid the ureter which may be adherent to its undersurface. Then the involved segment is exteriorized, being brought to the outside through a stab-wound incision.

It is advantageous when possible to resect the area involved, for in many patients there is no significant local improvement following a diversionary colostomy, leaving the inflamed bowel in place. However, the risks entailed in freeing up the diseased bowel need to be considered for the individual case, and this usually can be assessed only at the operating table when the extent of the lesion is known.

Any abscesses encountered should be drained. Generally, such abscesses are fairly chronic, having been present for several weeks or months. For reasons not well understood, the peritoneum seems to gain some degree of immunity under these circumstances, and generalized peritonitis is not likely to follow. Pus should be thoroughly aspirated, the cavity sponged dry, a soft latex drain placed in the cavity and led to the outside, preferably through an extraperitoneal stab-wound incision. As many abscesses are situated low in the pelvis or the cul-de-sac, a drain may be inserted into the upper rectum or the vagina and led externally through the anus or the vagina, where it is sutured to the skin to avoid premature removal. Cultures are taken of the pus, and a broad-spectrum antibiotic likely to be effective in the treatment of bacteria of enteric origin is administered parenterally in large doses for several days, changing to another should the culture data so indicate.

The patient must be observed and examined for evidence of new abscesses or recurrences of old ones during his recovery period. Blood and plasma are used as indicated to prevent and combat shock. Short-tube intubation is employed to avoid distention from swallowed air until peristaltic activity returns.

Perforation requires immediate surgical intervention. The need to support the patient promptly by the administration of plasma and blood in the prevention or treatment of shock is often as essential as the operation itself (see Chap. 36, page 909). One of two operative procedures is indicated when perforation occurs. Exteriorization of the perforated segment of bowel is the procedure of choice but is not always feasible to perform; however, exteriorization should not be abandoned without serious try. Second is the closure of the perforation, resorting to a proximal colostomy. With either technic, the peritoneum and its recesses are cleared of feces and pus, extraperitoneal stab-wound drainage is instituted, and large doses of antibiotics are administered. Continued support of the patient with blood and plasma transfusions may be necessary for many hours after operation to counteract shock. Short-tube intubation is employed.

Fistulation requires exteriorization of the segment of bowel serving as a source of the fistula. Abscesses are frequently encountered along the way and are to be treated as described above.

When hemorrhage is the indication for surgical intervention in diverticulitis, the surgical problem is hemostasis. Essentially, only one method of surgical therapy exists—Mikulicz resection of that segment of bowel which is the source of bleeding.

TUMORS OF THE SMALL BOWEL

Compared with inflammatory lesions of the small bowel, tumors are remarkably rare, particularly malignant tumors. Tumors of the duodenum have been discussed elsewhere (see Chap. 29, Stomach and Duodenum). Those comprising this discussion are only those of the jejuno-ileum.

Benign Tumors. Most tumors of the small bowel are benign, as indicated in Table 3 by Shandalow (1955).

River, Silverstein and Tope (1956) have presented a most comprehensive review of benign small bowel tumors, compiling and classifying all of these tumors reported in the world literature (Table 4).

The incidence of benign tumors of the small bowel depends upon the character of reports consulted and the polysemantics of descriptive pathology. Small bowel tumors account for about 10 per cent of all benign tumors of the gastrointestinal tract. There is no striking difference in occurrence between sexes. As most of these tumors are small and asymptomatic, the numbers found at autopsy greatly exceed those encountered in surgical specimens; about 15 are incidental findings at autopsy for every one resected surgically. Even so, the occurrence at autopsy is no greater than 0.02 per cent; that of surgical specimens is about 0.002 per cent.

The association of generalized polyposis of the intestine, particularly involving the jejuno-ileum, and melanin spots of the buccal mucosa and the lips (Peutz-Jeghers syndrome) has recently been recognized (Dormandy, 1957; Staley and Schwarz, 1957; also Chap. 37, Part 2).

Despite their rare occurrence, they should be discussed briefly, as small bowel tumors are among the causes of occult abdominal pain, melena and intermittent intestinal obstruction. Failure to consider benign small bowel tumors in diagnosis accounts in part for the near 20 per cent mortality associated with operative treatment; many of these patients are seen late when intussusception,

TABLE 3. RATIO OF BENIGN AND MALIGNANT TUMORS OF THE SMALL INTESTINE

SOURCE	CASE No.	BENIGN %	BENIGN No.	MALIGNANT %	MALIGNANT No.
Morison	17	77	13	23	4
Dundon	62	77	44	29	18
Raiford	88	57.8	51	42.2	37
Eckel	19	37	7	63	12
Shandalow	25	88	22	12	3

Morison, J. E.: Tumors of the small intestine, Brit. J. Surg. 29:139, 1941.

Dundon, C. C.: Primary tumors of the small intestine, Am. J. Roentgenol. 59:492, 1948.

Raiford, T. S.: Tumors of the small intestine, Arch. Surg. 25:122, 321, 1932.

Eckel, J. H.: Primary tumors of the jejunum and ileum, Surgery 23:467, 1948.

Shandalow (this series).

Adenomas were the most frequently found, followed by myomas and leiomyomas.

(This table from Shandalow, S. L.: A.M.A. Arch. Surg. 71:761, 1955)

TABLE 4. TYPES AND NUMBERS OF TUMORS STUDIED; 20 CASES PREVIOUSLY UNREPORTED FROM COOK COUNTY HOSPITAL ARE INCLUDED

Adenomas	227
Polyps	170
Polyposis (adenomatosis) with melanin pigmentation (Peutz-Jeghers syndrome)	59
Lipomas	219
Myomas	179
Fibromas	163
Angiomas and hemangiomas	127
Neurogenic tumors	90
Fibromyomas	81
Fibromyxomas and myxofibromas	26
Lymphangiomas	18
Fibroadenomas	15
Myofibromas	12
Myxomas	8
Reticulofibromatosis	1
Teratoma	1
Hemangiopericytoma	1
Osteoma	1
Osteofibroma	1
Total	1,399

(River, L., Silverstein, J., and Tope, J. W.: Surg., Gynec. & Obst. (Internat. Abstr. Surg.) 102:1, 1956)

necrosis, perforation and hemorrhage have taken their toll.

The pathology of tumors found at operation in the survey by River *et al.* (1956) is reported as follows:

The majority of benign tumors are located in the ileum—606 of 1,399; 272 were found in the jejunum, and 198 were found in the duodenum. 323 were multiply located.

Clinical pattern and diagnosis are evident in less than 10 per cent of all benign tumors because most are asymptomatic. Obstruction was present in 877 patients, absent in 359 and unstated in 163 of the reports surveyed by River *et al.* Intussusception was the most common cause of obstruction, occurring in 627, and frequently was self-reducing. Occasionally, there is more than one clinical episode of intussusception, as many of these tumors are multiple.

Intestinal bleeding was present in 426 or 30 per cent of those included in River's review and ranged in severity from serious hemorrhage to occult blood. Adenomas, polyps, polyposis, myomas, neurogenic tumors and angiomas accounted for most of the bleeding, in the order of descending frequency.

Small bowel tumor is much more often suspected than proved preoperatively. The cramplike pain of intestinal obstruction which remits and recurs days, weeks or months later is suggestive of recurring intussusception of the small bowel due to Meckel's diverticulum or tumor. Bleeding from the rectum when the esophagus, stomach, colon, rectum and anus are negative to endoscopic and barium contrast studies leaves the small bowel the site of suspicion. Small bowel fluoroscopy is not often helpful, as many of these tumors are small, and their presence is difficult to detect. Such studies should be carried out nonetheless.

One of the most useful diagnostic technics when small bowel tumors are suspected is the use of long-tube intubation, sampling the aspirate for the presence of gross or occult blood. As soon as blood is found, barium may be introduced through the tube and the particular segment studied fluoroscopically. If this fails, the patient is explored, and the segment, a few feet on either side of the end of the tube, is thoroughly inspected and palpated. If this also fails to reveal the bleeding point, the bowel is opened 6 to 12 inches above the end of the indwelling tube, and a sterile sigmoidoscope is passed into the lumen. The mucosa is carefully explored as far as possible in both directions.

The surgeon should not be satisfied upon the finding of one tumor, as multiple ones are not infrequent. If necessary, one should not hesitate to open the bowel in 3 or 4 areas to permit inspection of the entire small bowel with the sigmoidoscope.

Treatment of benign tumors is local resection; generally a wedge resection is sufficient, although resection of a loop of small bowel may be necessary in about 20 per cent of cases. Frozen sections of such tumors are advisable and may avoid the need for a second operation.

Pneumatosis Cystoides Intestinorum. This is a rare and generally symptomless curiosity in which gas-containing cysts lined by endothelium are found in the subserosa and the submucosa, usually of the distal ileum, rarely of the duodenum, the rectum or the appendix. The origin of the gas cysts is unkown. They may spontaneously regress or slowly enlarge and ultimately project into the peritoneal cavity or into the bowel lumen. They may be mistaken for polyps.

Malignant tumors of the small bowel, excluding carcinoid tumors, account for 0.5 to 3.0 per cent of all malignancies of the gastrointestinal tract. The incidence may be slightly higher in the duodenum and the ileum than in the jejunum. Conflicting statements exist as to whether sarcoma or carcinoma is the more commonly encountered tumor.

Pathology of carcinoma discloses no outstanding differences between those of the small bowel from those of the colon. They may be polypoid, or annular and constricting. Obstruction and anemia are the usual symptoms and findings. Wide resection is indicated. The prognosis is not as favorable as for carcinoma of the large bowel, possibly because of the more extensive lymphatic and lacteal channels in the small bowel. Malignant tumors, like the benign ones of the small bowel, tend to be multiple.

The sarcomas principally encountered are leiomyosarcoma, neurofibrosarcoma, fibrosarcoma, angiosarcoma and lymphosarcoma. The prognosis of sarcoma of the small bowel, like that of carcinoma, is poor, although lympho-sarcoma is less rapidly fatal than other intestinal sarcomas.

Symptoms produced and diagnostic procedures to be employed are the same as those of benign small bowel tumors.

Carcinoids. Carcinoid tumors of the small bowel deserve special mention, as there is much confusion as to their pathologic significance and clinical consequence. As is the case with any rarely encountered tumor, the incidence varies according to the surgeon's experiences. Carcinoids may be malignant or benign. Although the author has encountered more carcinoids of the small bowel than carcinoma in this same structure, the reverse is the general experience reported.

These tumors stain with chromic acid and therefore are of argentaffin origin. When malignant, they may or may not metastasize early; of those encountered at the University of Chicago Clinics, many had metastasized at the time of operation, or metastasis became evident within a few months or a year or two later. The carcinoid syndrome occurs in about one fourth of patients with these tumors (see discussion in Chap. 37, Part 2, Tumors of the Colon and the Rectum).

These tumors are not infrequently multiple, and hemorrhage has been the complaint most commonly encountered. Some bleed with surprisingly large amounts of blood being lost within a few days, considering their small size; this seems to be explained on occasion when large dilated vessels are found within the tumor on microscopic examination. (For a discussion of carcinoids of the colorectum, see pages 975-976.)

PREOPERATIVE PREPARATION OF THE BOWEL FOR INTESTINAL OPERATIONS

A variety of technics may be employed to prepare the bowel for intestinal surgery in patients whose disease has not been complicated by obstruction, perforation, abscess formation or mesenteric thrombosis. Ulcerative colitis presents certain obstacles which impose changes in such programs; here catharsis is contraindicated, but intestinal antibiotics should still be employed. Extensive bowel preparation is not essential for surgery of the small bowel, but it is mandatory for the colon, particularly for operations on the left colon and rectum.

Two principles are involved in bowel preparation. First and probably the most important is purgation to rid the bowel of feces and gas. Second is the use of "intestinal" antibiotics and sulfonamides.

The combination of Neomycin-Sulfathalidine has been found to be most effective both clinically and in experimental animals. Pseudo-membranous enterocolitis has not been a problem when the recommended schedule of drug administration has been followed (Poth, 1960).

Cleansing the bowel can be accomplished best by catharsis. While certain routines may be set up, the surgeon must be willing to deviate from any established program as the local nature of the disease and the general health of the patient may dictate. At the same time he should be fully aware that the improperly prepared patient upon whom he plans a colonic resection and a primary anastomosis usually carries a greater operative risk than that imposed by the catharsis necessary to cleanse and deflate the bowel. In fact, should he encounter at operation a colon largely filled with feces, he should resect the bowel without primary anastomosis, using the Mikulicz exteriorization procedure. If this seems to be ill-advised, as may be the case with carcinoma, he will wisely close the abdomen, revise his method for cleansing the bowel and resect later on.

Lesions calling for resection of the right colon do not require necessarily as vigorous a catharsis schedule as those of the left colon for two reasons. First, the stool is liquid and not so highly contaminated as in the left colon. Second and more important, a lateral anastomosis can be performed with greater safety than the end-to-end procedure necessary in anastomosing the descending or sigmoid colon segments to the sigmoid rectum.

The concept of a "sterile colon" at the time of operation is a good one and is essentially accomplished within 24 hours in most patients. Sulfonamides will not achieve so extensive an inhibition of intestinal bacteria, but they do reduce the colony counts and are principally effective against the coliform group. Unfortunately, upsetting the "balance of nature" so

TABLE 5. PREOPERATIVE PREPARATION OF THE COLON*

	NO OBSTRUCTION	PARTIAL OBSTRUCTION	COMPLETE OBSTRUCTION, OR INTRA-ABDOMINAL TRAUMA, PERFORATION OR PERITONITIS
Preliminary Preparation	Liquid or low residue diet for 1-3 days.	Gastric suction, decompression until bowel movements are re-established; cleansing enemas as indicated.	None. Exploration should be performed as soon as the general condition of the patient warrants.
Purgation	Castor oil 30-60 ml. given 18-20 hours prior to operation.	Contraindicated	Contraindicated
Agent	Neomycin 1.0 Gm. and sulfathalidine 1.5 Gm. by mouth, given beginning the day before surgery at 2 P.M., 3 P.M., 4 P.M., 6 P.M., 8 P.M., 12 M., 4 A.M., and 7 A.M. Operation is scheduled for 8 A.M. If operation must be delayed, continue giving drugs every 4 hrs.	After obstruction relieved, give neomycin 1.0 Gm. and sulfathalidine 1.5 Gm. by mouth every 4 hours for a minimum of 3 days and until mechanical preparation of the bowel by suction and enemas is completed.	
Postoperative	Intestinal antisepsis maintained without further drugs throughout period of postoperative ileus. No further treatment generally needed.	Intestinal antisepsis maintained without further drugs throughout period of postoperative ileus. No further treatment generally needed.	

* After Poth (1960).

far as bacterial flora in the colon is concerned may be responsible for some of the patients who develop pseudomembranous enterocolitis (see below) (Cohn and Rives, 1956; Cohn, 1958). When antibiotics are used for prolonged periods, certain strains of the staphylococcus may proliferate, creating a serious enteritis which may terminate in death. That so simple an explanation as the upset of bacterial components of the colon accounts for this disturbance often is open to question. The disorder may occur in patients who have not received any antibiotics.

The method of preparation of the colon for surgery is outlined in Table 5.

PSEUDOMEMBRANOUS ENTEROCOLITIS

Pseudomembranous enterocolitis, a disease entity first described within recent years, occasionally occurs as a postoperative complication of bowel surgery and may be fatal. Originally, this disorder was attributed to an overgrowth of the *Micrococcus pyogenes,* one of the staphylococcal family. It was presumed

to grow excessively because of the diminished or near absence of other normal bacterial inhabitants of the colon when intestinal antibiotics were administered orally. More recently the disease has been recognized in patients receiving no antibiotics or chemotherapeutic agents; hence the initial concept as to the cause for the overgrowth by this organism may not be true.

This disturbance is characterized by gaseous distention of both the large and the small bowel, diarrhea, fever, leukocytosis, peripheral collapse and death. At autopsy, the bowel is distended, often hemorrhagic; the lumen of the colon is frequently filled with blood. The peritoneal cavity generally contains large quantities of exudate. The amount of blood and plasma lost contribute materially to peripheral vascular collapse. Most consider peripheral collapse in this disease to be the result of the enterotoxin elaborated by the Micrococcus (Prohaska, Long and Nelsen 1956).

Microscopic examination of the diseased bowel shows intense inflammatory changes involving all of its layers, with pronounced edema and partial or complete destruction of the mucosa.

Prohaska and his associates recommend combating shock vigorously, the replacement of fluids and electrolytes and the intramuscular administration of 50 mg. of ACTH 3 times a day for 2 or 3 days. He reports the response to ACTH to be rapid. After the third day, the dosage of ACTH is reduced progressively until it is discontinued by the end of a week. He believes that ACTH inhibits the action of the bacterial enterotoxin; indeed, the prompt improvement that such patients make would seem to support his contention. The *Micrococcus pyogenes* is often sensitive to Erythromycin. This drug should be administered parenterally unless contraindicated. Norepinephrine may be useful as an adjunct to blood and plasma in the treatment of shock in these patients.

REFERENCES

1. Albers, J. H., Smith, L. L., and Carter, R.: Perforation of the cecum, Ann. Surg. *143*: 251, 1956.
2. Babcock, W. W.: Diverticulitis, Rev. Gastroenterol. *8*:77, 1941.
3. Bacon, H. E., Bralow, S. P., and Berkley, J. L.: Rehabilitation and long-term survival after colectomy for ulcerative colitis, J.A.M.A. *172*:324, 1960.
4. Bartlett, M. K., and McDermott, W. V.: Surgical treatment of diverticulitis of the colon, New England J. Med. *248*:497, 1953.
5. Boyden, A. M., and Neilson, R. O.: Reappraisal of the surgical treatment of diverticulitis of the sigmoid colon, Am. J. Surg. *100*: 206, 1960.
6. Brooke, B. N.: The management of an ileostomy including its complications, Lancet *263*:102, 1952.
7. Brown, D. B., and Toomey, W. F.: Diverticular disease of the colon, Brit. J. Surg. *47*:485, 1960.
8. Bunch, G. H., Burnside, A. F., and Brannon, L. J.: Intestinal perforation from ingested fishbone, Am. J. Surg. *55*:1, 1942
9. Burt, C. A. V.: Pneumatic rupture of the intestinal canal; with experimental data showing the mechanism of perforation and the pressure required, Arch. Surg. *22*:875, 1931.
10. Chunn, C. F.: Wounds of the colon and rectum, J. Florida M.A. *34*:269, 1947.
11. Cohn, I., Jr.: Antibiotics for colon surgery, Gastroenterology *35*:583, 1958.
12. Cohn, I., Jr., and Rives, J. D.: Protection of colon anastomosis with antibiotics, Ann. Surg. *144*:738, 1956.
13. Colcock, B. P., and Vansant, J. H.: Surgical treatment of regional enteritis, New England J. Med. *262*:435, 1960.
14. Counsellor, V. S., and McCormack, C. J.: Subcutaneous perforations of the jejunum, Am. J. Surg. *102*:365, 1935.
15. Crohn, B. B.: Regional ileitis *in* Portis, S. A.: Diseases of the Digestive System, ed. 3, p. 738, Philadelphia, Lea & Febiger, 1953.
16. Crohn, B. B., Ginzberg, L., and Oppenheimer, G. D.: Regional ileitis, a pathological and clinical entity, J.A.M.A. *99*:1323, 1932.
17. D'Antoni, J. S.: Amebiasis: recent concepts of its prevalence, symptomatology, diagnosis and treatment, Internat. Clin. *1*:101, 1942.
18. Dormandy, T. L.: Gastrointestinal polyposis with mucocutaneous pigmentation (Peutz-Jeghers Syndrome), New England J. Med. *256*:1093, 1141, 1957.
19. Dukes, C. E., and Lockhart-Mummery, H. E.: Practical points in the pathology and surgical treatment of ulcerative colitis, A critical review, Brit. J. Surg. *45*:25, 1957.
20. Durham, M. W.: Simplified technique for ileostomy construction, Surgery *41*:984, 1957.
21. Faber, Knud: Quoted *in* Ingested foreign body in the intestinal tract, Arch. Surg. *36*: 66, 1938. Henderson, F. F. and Gaston, E. A.
22. Faust, E. C.: Modern criteria for the laboratory diagnosis of amebiasis, Am. J. Trop. Med. *1*:140, 1952.
23. Frye, W. W.: The pathogenesis and therapy of human amebiasis, Am. J. Gastroenterol. *25*:315, 1956.
24. Goligher, J. C.: Extraperitoneal colostomy or ileostomy, Brit. J. Surg. *46*:97, 1958.
25. Harkins, H. N.: Discussion *in* Howard, M. A.: The management of bleeding diverticula of the colon, Am. J. Surg. *100*:217, 1960.
26. Henderson, F. F., and Gaston, E. A.: Ingested foreign body in the intestinal tract, Arch. Surg. *36*:66, 1938.
27. Judd, E. S., Jr., and Mears, T. W.: Diverticulitis; progress toward wider application of single-stage resection, A.M.A. Arch. Surg. *70*:818, 1955.
28. Kantor, J. L.: Regional (terminal) ileitis: its roentgen diagnosis, J.A.M.A. *103*:2016, 1934.
29. Kirsner, J. B., Palmer, W. L., Maimon, S. N., and Ricketts, W. E.: Clinical course of chronic nonspecific ulcerative colitis, J.A.M.A. *137*:922, 1948.
30. Laipply, T. C.: Pathological anatomy of regional enteritis, J.A.M.A. *165*:2052, 1957.

31. Lockhart-Mummery, H. E., and Morson, B. C.: Crohn's disease (regional enteritis) of the large intestine and its distinction from ulcerative colitis, Gut. *1*:87, 1960.

32. Lockwood, A. L.: Traumatic lesions of the abdomen, Internat. J. Med. & Surg. *47*:35, 1934.

33. McCune, W. S., Iovine, V. M., and Miller, D.: Resection and primary anastomosis in diverticulitis of the colon, Ann. Surg. *145*:683, 1957.

34. Maingot, R.: Abdominal Operations, ed. 3, New York, Appleton, 1955.

35. Noer, R. J.: Hemorrhage as a complication of diverticulitis, Ann. Surg. *141*:674, 1955.

36. Ochsner, A., and DeBakey, M.: Amebic hepatitis and hepatic abscess, Surgery *13*:635, 1943.

36a. DeBakey, M., and Ochsner, A.: Hepatic amebiasis: a 20-year experience and analysis of 263 cases, Surg., Gynec. & Obst. (Internat. Abstr. Surg.) *92*:209, 1951.

37. van Patter, W. N.: Regional enteritis, Gastroenterology *26*:347, 1954.

38. Ponka, J. L., Brush, B. E., and Fox, J. D.: Differential diagnosis of carcinoma of the sigmoid and diverticulitis, J.A.M.A. *172*:515, 1960.

39. Poth, E. J.: The role of intestinal antisepsis in the preoperative preparation of the colon, Surgery *47*:1018, 1960.

40. Prohaska, J. V., Long, E. T., and Nelsen, T. S.: Pseudomembranous enterocolitis, A.M.A. Arch. Surg. *72*:977, 1956.

41. Reichert, F. L., and Mathes, M. E: Experimental lymphedema of the intestinal tract and its relation to regional cicatrizing enteritis, Ann. Surg. *104*:601, 1936.

42. River, L., Silverstein, J., and Tope, J. W.: Benign neoplasms of the small intestine; a critical comprehensive review with reports of 20 new cases, Surg., Gynec. & Obst. (Internat. Abstr. Surg.) *102*:1, 1956.

43. Roof, W. R., Morris, G. C., Jr., and DeBakey, M. E.: Management of perforating injuries to the colon in civilian practice, Am. J. Surg. *99*:641, 1960.

44. Rosser, C.: Diverticulitis; indications for resection, South. M.J. *38*:161, 1945.

45. Rubin, E. H.: Laryngeal intestinal tuberculosis, Am. J. M. Sc. *191*:663, 1931.

46. Ryan, P.: Emergency resection and anastomosis for perforated sigmoid diverticulitis, Brit. J. Surg. *45*:611, 1958.

47. Sawitz, W. G.: The diagnosis of amebiasis, Clinics *2*:828, 1943.

48. Schlicke, C. P., and Logan, A. H.: Surgical treatment of diverticulitis of the colon, J.A.M.A. *169*:1019, 1959.

49. Shandalow, S. L.: Benign tumors of the small intestine, A.M.A. Arch. Surg. *71*:761, 1955.

50. Siddons, A. M. H.: The fate of swallowed foreign bodies, J.A.M.A. *113*:17, 1577, 1939.

51. Smithwick, R. H.: Surgical treatment of diverticulitis of the sigmoid, Am. J. Surg. *99*:192, 1960.

52. Staley, C. J., and Schwarz, H., II: Gastrointestinal polyposis and pigmentation of the oral mucosa (Peutz-Jeghers Syndrome), Int. Abstr. Surg. *105*:1, 1957.

53. Swenson, S. A., and Harkins, H. N.: Rupture of the rectosigmoid by compressed air, Am. J. Surg. *63*:141, 1944.

54. Takaro, T. M., and Bond, W. M.: Pleuropulmonary, pericardial and cerebral complications of amebiasis, Int. Abstr. Surg. *107*:209, 1958.

55. Ulin, A. W., Sokolic, I. H., and Thompson, C.: Massive hemorrhage from diverticulitis of the colon, Ann. Int. Med. *50*:1395, 1959.

56. Warren, S., and Sommers, S. C.: Pathology of regional enteritis and ulcerative colitis, J.A.M.A. *154*:190, 1954.

57. Waugh, R. L., and Leonard, F. C.: Rupture of the colon due to compressed air, with particular reference to the character of the lesion, Mil. Surgeon *108*:294, 1951.

Henry N. Harkins, m.d.

CHAPTER 37

Part 2

Tumors of Colon and Rectum

Benign Tumors: Polyps
Benign Tumors: Rarer Lesions
Malignant Tumors: Adenocarcinoma
Malignant Tumors: Rarer Lesions

Tumors of the colon and rectum are frequent and often malignant like those in the stomach. The small bowel, on the other hand, stands in the position of a rose between two thorns because in it malignant tumors are rare. The stomach above and the colon and rectum below are like the thorns; in them malignant tumors are very common.

At the same time, unlike some other organs where tumors manifest themselves in many diverse forms, in the colon and the rectum the issue is simpler, but at the same time at least as serious. In the colon and the rectum there are essentially two important types of tumor: polyps, which often are malignant when first seen or may lead to adenocarcinoma, and adenocarcinoma itself. In the discussion which follows, main emphasis will be placed on these two lesions; rarer tumors will be considered only briefly.

Both polyps and adenocarcinoma also involve the distal 2 cm. of rectum which is designated as the upper half of the "anorectum," the anus itself forming the lower 2 cm. This region and its tumors will be considered separately in Chapter 38. The lower half of the anorectum is also the site of squamous cell carcinoma of the anus.

Since involvement of the colon and the rectum by polyps or by adenocarcinoma differs only in degree and not in kind, these two portions of the large bowel will be considered together in the discussion that follows.

BENIGN TUMORS: POLYPS

Polyps of the colon and the rectum (colorectal polyps) present certain general features. They may be pedunculated or sessile, they often present no symptoms, they tend to bleed, their presence may be associated with a mucous discharge, they may serve as the initiating point for an intussusception (but not as often as in the small bowel), they produce direct intestinal obstruction less often than do similar polyps in the small bowel (probably because of the greater diameter of the colon), they may be diagnosed with difficulty by roentgen studies or digital anal examination and with ease (in the lower 10 in., 25 cm., of the bowel) with a sigmoidoscope. Colorectal polyps may be very small, but they are extremely important.

Colorectal polyps cannot be differentiated from cancers of the colon or rectum by looking at them because small cancers are sessile tumors and many larger cancers are pedunculated. Biopsy and microscopic examination are requisite for the diagnosis of colorectal polyps.

Polyps of the colon and the rectum can be divided into 6 main clinical types: (1) polypoid adenoma, (2) villous tumor, (3) familial polyposis of the colon, (4) congenital polyposis of the entire intestinal tract, (5) pseudopolyposis and (6) juvenile polyposis. Pathologically, the polyps in cases of familial polyposis and congenital polyposis of the entire intestinal tract are examples of polypoid adenoma, and juvenile polyposis is an example of retention polyps. Villous tumor and pseudopolyposis are other discrete pathologic entities.

The 6 clinical types will be considered separately below:

POLYPOID ADENOMA

(*Synonyms:* pedunculated polyp, lobulated adenoma, adenomatous polyp)

Polypoid adenomas have until recently been considered as an important factor in the etiology of carcinoma of the colon and the rectum. More recent studies have cast doubt on this causative relationship. This type of polyp is by far the most frequent; hence, its role in leading to cancer is all the more important.

Age. Helwig (1947) reported a gradually rising incidence of polyps reaching a peak incidence in the 8th decade. Based on careful double-contrast colon studies of 3,609 patients, Andrén and Frieberg (1959) of Malmo, Sweden, found an incidence of 28 per cent in the 1st decade, dropping off markedly to only 3 per cent in the 2nd decade and *then* gradually rising to a peak incidence of 17 per cent in the 9th decade. Horrilleno, Eckert and Ackerman (1959) found the very highest incidence at ages 3 and 4 years. This increased incidence in polyps in the 1st decade is due to the occurrence of juvenile polyposis. "Polypoid adenoma is a nonentity under the age of 20 years provided the patient does not have the gene of multiple polyposis" (Moyer, 1960).

Childhood polyps (juvenile polyposis) appear to be different from the adult type, both statistically and pathologically. The juvenile ones are more inflammatory in nature with more connective tissue stroma (Mauro and Prior, 1957); they bleed more often (182 of 183 cases reported by Mallam and Thomson, 1959); and they occur mainly in the rectum. The usual sigmoidoscopic and x-ray studies are paramount for their diagnosis. For the former, except in newborn infants, Turrell and Maynard (1956) recommend an adult (usually ⅝ or ¾ in. [1.6 or 1.8 cm.] in diameter) scope rather than the often suggested "pediatric" sizes.

Sex. Helwig (1947) found that at all age levels above 30 years the condition was slightly more prevalent in males.

Symptoms may include bleeding, mucous discharge, or pain, but, as Colvert and Brown (1948) pointed out, many patients with polyps are symptomless (only 12% of their patients had symptoms).

Size. Polyps vary greatly in size. Rider, Kirsner, Moeller and Palmer (1954) reported that 68 per cent of their polyps were less than 1 cm. in diameter.

Multiple Polyps. Using the term "multiple" to mean from essentially 2 to 10 adenomatous polyps, as opposed to familial (multiple) polyposis where there may be thousands of polyps, such a condition presents special features. The occurrence of more than one polyp, in this sense, was reported by Swinton and Warren (1939) and by Van Buskirk (1955) in 35 per cent of their patients with polyps. Helwig (1947) reported a figure of 41 per cent.

Site. Figures concerning the site of polyps are influenced by the thoroughness with which sigmoidoscopic discovery is followed by x-ray examination of the upper colon. In general, the figures are weighted toward the distal end of the colorectum. (See *autopsy* series of Swinton and Doane, 1953, Table 6, in which a higher percentage of colonic polyps was found relative to rectal polyps than reported in the following *clinical* series). Both Swinton and Warren (1939) and Jackman and Mayo (1951) stated that 70 per cent of polyps are within 10 inches of the anal verge. Van Buskirk (1955) reported a similar figure of 78 per cent. As seen from Table 7, Welch, McKittrick and Behringer (1952) found 73 per cent this low; and as seen in Figure 37-8, Rider, Kirsner, Moeller, and Palmer (1954) found 88.7 per cent in the lower 10 inches, this figure again being based on clinical studies.

TABLE 6. COMPARISON OF SITES OF PREDILECTION OF COLORECTAL CARCINOMA AND POLYPS, AUTOPSY FINDING, 1935-1945

SITE	PER CENT OF PATIENTS	
	CARCINOMA (207 CASES)	POLYPS (311 CASES)
Cecum Ascending colon	13.0	20.5
Hepatic flexure Transverse colon Splenic flexure	13.5	27.3
Descending colon Sigmoid Rectum Anus	73.5	52.2
Total	100	100

(From Swinton and Doane, 1953)

TABLE 7. SITE OF COLORECTAL ADENOMATOUS
POLYPS (NON-NECROPSY DATA)

SITE OF POLYP	PER CENT OF PATIENTS
Ascending colon	2
Transverse colon	2
Descending colon	3
Middle or upper sigmoid	20
Within reach of sigmoidoscope	73
Total	100

(From Welch, McKittrick and Behringer, 1952)

Lawrence (1936), Helwig (1947) and Spratt, Ackerman and Moyer (1958) in autopsy studies found that there is a more even spread of polyps throughout the colon (Fig. 37-9) and that this distribution does not correspond to the distribution of carcinomas in the colon.

Some writers claim that the distribution of polyps is similar to that of carcinomas and use this observation as an argument for the causal relationship between these two conditions (see p. 962). Thus, Cattell and Swinton (1940) pointed out that in their series 68 per cent of colorectal adenomas were in the rectosigmoid and the rectum, while 60 per cent of the carcinomas were so located.

Incidence. The most comprehensive report is that by Rider, Kirsner, Moeller, and Palmer who collected records of 55,876 routine sigmoidoscopic examinations from the literature with 5.1 per cent incidence of rectal polyps. In 7,487 patients subjected to such an examination they found 401 with polyps (5.4%), an

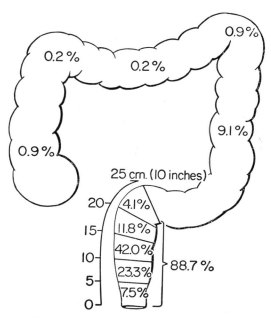

FIG. 37-8. Distribution of 583 colorectal polyps found in 401 patients (not necropsy data). (Modified from Rider, J. A., *et al.*: Am. J. Med. *16*:557)

almost identical figure. Ault (1952) analyzed 10 sources in the literature, including his own series, and found that an average of 9 per cent of otherwise normal patients over 40 years of age have rectocolonic polyps. He also reported that 7.5 per cent of these patients have no symptoms. In a later paper, Bacon, Lowell and Trimpi (1954) reported that polypoid

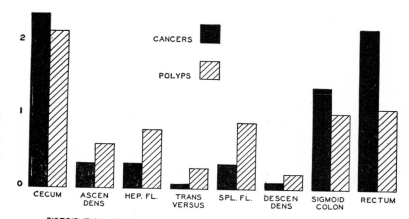

FIG. 37-9. Percentile distributions of cancers (black) versus polyps (shaded) of the colon per centimeter length of the fixed colon based on autopsy studies (Spratt, J. S., Jr., Ackerman, L. V., and Moyer, C. A.: Ann. Surg. *148*:689).

DISTRIBUTION OF 100 COLONIC CANCERS AND POLYPS PER UNIT LENGTH
OF SEGMENT

adenomas are present in 7 per cent of all adults.

Helwig (1947), on the basis of a study of the entire colon in 1,460 consecutive autopsies found 139 (9.5%) with adenomas. The elimination of 1 case of familial polyposis leaves 138 patients with 272 separate tumors. The peak incidence was reached in the 8th decade when 28 per cent of the men and 20 per cent of the women showed adenomas. In 80 (58%) of the 139 cases there were single adenomas. In 58 cases there were 2 or more tumors, and, as already stated, in 1 case there was familial polyposis.

"Sentinel Polyps." Polyps tend to be near colorectal carcinomas, and in all cases of polyps, search should be made not only for additional polyps elsewhere in the large bowel but also for an already active second carcinoma. Jackman and Mayo (1951) reported that in 18 per cent of all cases of carcinoma of the large intestine, one or more adenomas were found adjacent to the lesion. Rosenthal and Baronofsky (1960) believe that sentinel polyps are a dangerous sign, and arrest of the cancer can best be effected "by performing a subtotal or total colectomy whenever polyps are noted in the resected specimen at the time of surgery." On the other hand, Holden (1958) reported just the opposite: carcinoma with sentinel polyp, 75 per cent 6-year arrest; without, 46 per cent. Moyer (1960) has been unable to confirm Holden's observations.

Malignant Actuality and Potential of Polyps. Colvert and Brown (1948) reported that 6 per cent of their primarily removed polyps were malignant. Similar figures given by other authors are: Welch, McKittrick and Behringer (1952)—18.6 per cent in 322 polyps, this figure being high because villous adenoma is included (see Table 8); Bacon, Lowell and Trimpi (1954)—15 to 19 per cent. Of course, the percentage found to be malignant depends on the pathologic criteria used for malignancy; some of the higher percentages include cases of carcinoma-in-situ. Not only microscopic study but also gross appearance is important in this regard. Induration on palpation or ulceration suggests carcinoma (Gilchrist, 1953). Polyps in the colon (Table 8) are somewhat more apt to be malignant than in the rectum.

The intermediate pathologic subclasses of

TABLE 8. INCIDENCE OF CANCER IN COLORECTAL POLYPS

SITE	TOTAL NUMBER OF POLYPS	TOTAL POLYPS WITH CANCER
Colon	102	24 (23.6%)
Rectum	220	36 (16.6%)
Total	322	60 (18.6%)

(Welch, McKittrick and Behringer: New England J. Med. 247:959-965)

polyps have not been followed accurately enough to determine exactly which ones can be safely excised locally and which ones require radical bowel resection. As discussed on page 984, this involves an especially serious decision in the lower rectum, where the radical procedure best suited for clear-cut malignancy is an abdominoperineal resection, very radical indeed. There is little argument concerning benign polypoid nodules (thickening of folds), hyperplastic polyps, or benign adenomatous polyps at the benign end of the spectrum nor yet with carcinoma at the malignant end of the spectrum. However, as Humphreys (1956) has pointed out, there is considerable discussion regarding the intermediate grades (adenoma malignum: carcinoma-in-situ, intramucosal carcinoma, Grade I adenocarcinoma). It is quite possible that further correlative clinical and pathologic follow-up study will divide this intermediate group so that certain cases can be safely put in the benign group and others be firmly placed in the malignant category.

Many reports indicate that polyps are geographically and causally connected to carcinoma. Thus, Swinton and Warren (1939) in their series of 827 patients with colorectal carcinoma, claimed that 14 per cent could be demonstrated histologically to have arisen in benign mucosal polyps. Helwig (1947) also concluded that most carcinomas of the large intestine arise from polyps, though without any direct data supporting his claim.

The presence of evidence of malignancy in polyps also is agreed upon. However, the possibility of malignant potential in a polyp that is benign is not so definitely settled. Many surgeons claim that there is a definite potentiality of future malignant change in benign polyps, but the dissenting minority includes some authors who have studied the subject carefully. Jackman and Mayo (1951) went so far as to say that "polyps (adenomas) of the large intestine, if given sufficient time, develop into carcinomas." They admitted that the reverse may not always hold true and that not all carcinomas may arise from polyps. While it is generally believed that sessile polyps present more malignant potential than pedunculated polyps, this concept may be based partly on early studies wherein villous tumors (admittedly more potentially malignant) were included with the sessile polypoid adenomas.

Jackman and Mayo listed several factors that they considered to be in favor of the polypoid adenoma-carcinoma sequence, as follows: (1) the close parallelism between the location of polyps and the location of carcinoma in various segments of the colon (see Fig. 37-10—it is to be noted that these figures are based on clinical studies, unlike those in Fig. 37-9, which are based on autopsy studies); (2) the close parallelism in age and sex incidence; (3) the frequency with which polyps are associated with carcinoma (the "sentinel polyp"); (4) the certainty of development of cancer of the colon in familial polyposis; and (5) their claim that adenomas are replaced by carcinomas. They offered no satisfactory evidence for this 5th factor.

McKittrick and Wheelock (1954) phrase this same idea as follows: "Every so-called adenomatous polyp, sessile or pedunculated, is actually or potentially malignant."

The theory of malignant changes in these polyps is attested further by the claims of Klein and Scarborough (1952) who stated regarding lesions in the colon above reach of the sigmoidoscope that "ninety-five per cent of benign lesions are precancerous adenomatous polyps." The location of the *colonic* polyps in their series of 100 patients is as follows: ascending colon, 1 per cent; transverse colon, 5 per cent; descending colon, 13 per cent; and sigmoid colon and upper rectosigmoid, 81 per cent. A single polyp was found in 85 of the 100 patients, 2 polyps in 14, and 3 polyps in 1 patient. (Cases of familial polyposis and of frank carcinoma were excluded from the series.) Twenty-three per cent were microscopically malignant, including, of course, carcinomas-in-situ.

The contrary opinion was first advocated in part by Lawrence (1936). More recently, Colvert and Brown (1948), reported that their observations "strongly suggested that malignancy usually either develops very early in rectal polyps or is present from the start. There is no evidence available from this study that benign adenomata of the rectum became malignant with the passage of time."

In their review of 401 patients with polyps found in a series of 7,487 patients undergoing routine sigmoidoscopy, Rider, Kirsner, Moeller, and Palmer (1954) also arrived at several interesting conclusions (Table 9) that are

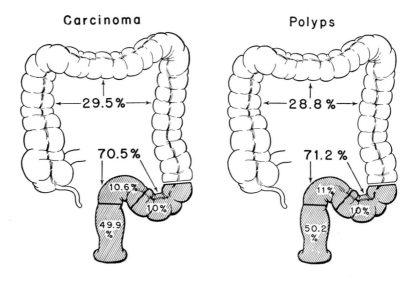

Fig. 37-10. Comparative distribution of carcinomas and polyps of the large bowel. (Jackman, R. J., and Mayo, C. W.: Surg., Gynec. & Obst. *93*: 328)

TABLE 9. SUMMARY OF DATA CONCERNING 401
PATIENTS WITH COLORECTAL POLYPS IN A
SERIES OF 7,487 ROUTINE SIGMOIDOSCOPIES

Sex: M:F:: 1.7:1
Age: Patients with polyps averaged 8 years older
than those without
Associated carcinoma:
11 per cent in 401 patients with polyps
2 per cent in 7,086 patients without polyps (see
below*)

9 per cent in patients wtih single polyps
20 per cent in patients with several polyps
*Result in 11 patients without polyp removal followed
1-5 years:*
No development of carcinoma
1 (9%) showed adenoma malignum on re-examination
Development of new polyps later:
20 per cent in patients with one original polyp
40 per cent in patients with several original polyps
5 per cent in entire series of 7,487 patients
Development of carcinoma after polyp removal:
2 per cent. (Note: this is identical with figure for
patients without polyps; see above*)

* Note that these two figures are identical, indicating a more or less irreducible minimum percentage,
or, in other words, a control figure for the incidence
of carcinoma in the absence of polyps.
(From Rider, Kirsner, Moeller and Palmer, 1954)

somewhat at variance with older reports in the literature such as those of Buie and Brust (1935) and Welch and McKittrick (1952) who attributed subsequent carcinoma to pre-existing polyps. In the group of 11 patients with biopsy-proved adenomatous polyps observed by Rider *et al.,* for from 1 to 5 years, one demonstrated adenoma malignum (equivalent to carcinoma-in-situ, intramucosal carcinoma, or Grade I adenocarcinoma according to the terminology used by their pathologist, Dr. Eleanor Humphreys), while none showed frank carcinoma. Rider and associates did not have any of their 385 removed polyps recur as frank carcinoma, and only 8 recurred as polyps. Rider *et al.* concluded that, "No conclusive direct evidence was obtained in this study to prove that benign adenomatous polyps undergo transition to carcinoma." This conclusion is comparable with that of Colvert and Brown (1948), who postulated that polyps are essentially malignant from the start or not; they rarely become malignant with the passage of time. Spratt, Ackerman and Moyer (1958) also agree, stating that ". . . the theory of origin of adenocarcinomas of the colon

within adenomatous polyps has little to support it." The data shown in Figure 37-11 uphold their concept.

In a more recent report, Kirsner, Moeller, and Renier (1956) stated that the over-all incidence of polyps in 9,669 patients examined in their clinic was 5.5 per cent. In 326 patients re-examined the incidence was 12.9 per cent, indicating a greater incidence than in the over-all gastrointestinal patient population in their clinic. Furthermore, it is of interest that of 275 patients re-examined who had had single polyps, only 10.2 per cent developed new polyps, whereas of 51 patients re-examined who had had multiple polyps, 27.4 per cent developed new polyps.

This important subject has also been discussed by Binkley, Sunderland, Miller, Stearns and Deddish (1952); Radke (1954); Bacon and Peale (1956); Enquist (1957); Turell (1957); Grinnell and Lane (1958); and by Rider, Kirsner, Moeller and Palmer (1959). The last 2 listed studies are especially comprehensive and deserve to be put on the reading list of every student, resident or practitioner. Mugrage (1959) presents an interesting summary of a questionnaire sent to 41 surgeons regarding the management of these polyps. Helwig (1959) presented a compromise view, stating, "Carcinoma *in situ* in adenomas of the colon and rectum is not capable of metastasis, but carcinoma with invasion of the core or stalk is capable of metastasis."

Treatment of polypoid adenoma can be divided under 2 headings: (1) that of polyps within reach of the sigmoidoscope (25 cm., 10 in.), and (2) that of polyps beyond reach of the sigmoidoscope.

Treatment of polypoid adenoma can be **the Sigmoidoscope.** A *biopsy* should be done. In any instance in which it is possible, this should be an *excision biopsy* with removal of the stalk and a goodly portion of the base. Humphreys (1956) pointed out that except for frank malignancy (invasive cancer in the base) the local excision is safe if the stalk and the base are *adequately* removed, and by adequately is meant at all points on its circumference and not just at the portion seen from below. Thus, treatment can be local if the polyp is still benign. Also, adequate local removal is all that is required for adenomatous polyps containing focal atypia, cancer *in situ,* and even for the adenoma malignum if the pathologist has had the opportunity to ascertain with certainty that the base of the polyp *does not contain carcinoma.* To date there has not been a reported case of metastasis from a carcinoma located entirely within the body of an adenomatous polyp (Spratt, Ackerman and Moyer, 1958). For polyps of the rectum and the rectosigmoid visible through the sigmoidoscope, the instrument is inserted to its full length (23 to 25 cm., 9 to 10 in.) and withdrawn slowly. A telescopic attachment may be helpful in visualizing small polyps. The endotherm, coagulating snare and biopsy forceps should be available for use during the examination. According to Morton (1953) the polyps can be dealt with under three headings according to type and size:

1. *Small sessile lesions, single or multiple,* are removed with biopsy forceps, knife, scissors or high-frequency current and then examined microscopically with permanent sections.

A careful 3-dimensional record of the site of each lesion is made. Fulguration of such lesions without biopsy should not be practiced, irrespective of the size of the lesion, since small carcinomas are apt to metastasize as well as large ones. After the biopsy, the base of the lesion may be cauterized for hemostatic purposes, taking especial care when the lesion is located on the anterior or lateral walls of the colon (McKittrick and Wheelock, 1954).

2. *Pedunculated polyps* are similarly removed, including the entire base. When within 12 cm. of the anal verge and if the polyps are large, two subsidiary procedures are available in indicated cases: (A) The lower edge of the internal sphincter is divided in the posterior mid-line by the method of David (1943), and the rectal mucosa is everted, and the polyp excised with its base, the resulting wound being closed transversely by catgut sutures. (B) A more conservative procedure is to use a large (3 cm. diameter) round

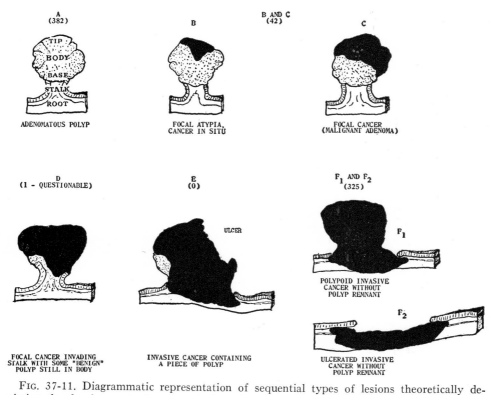

Fig. 37-11. Diagrammatic representation of sequential types of lesions theoretically depicting the development of cancer of the colon from adenomatous polyps. The actual distribution of 750 cases is shown. If polyps are a forerunner of cancer, it is reasonable to expect that types D and E would be much more frequent.

Tumors of Colon and Rectum

rectoscope after relaxation of the sphincters by local infiltration with procaine, 0.5 per cent solution. Then an instrument removal of the polyp, the stalk and a wide base (forceps and angulated scissors or knife) and transverse catgut closure of the resultant defect can be done through such a large rectoscope. If the polyp is large, it can be excised with a vertical ellipse which is then closed transversely, utilizing the Heineke-Mikulicz maneuver. All such tumors are sent for permanent microscopic examination.

With all polyps within reach of the sigmoidoscope, permanent sections are made. Three courses of action then are followed: (A) If the polyp is benign, the patient should be studied as to the rest of the colon for additional polyps by air-barium contrast roentgenogram, and also should be studied periodically every 6 to 12 months for the rest of his life; (B) if the lesion is cancer with obvious invasion of the adequately removed base, an abdominoperineal resection is required within a few days, while (C) if "carcinoma in situ" is present at the tip, and an adequate base is removed, we recommend frequent restudy, as do also McKay and McMahon (1959). Gilchrist (1959) stated that neither he nor Vernon David, his teacher, had ever ". . . seen a patient die of metastases from a carcinoma in the end of a polyp when there was a sizable pedicle" after local polypectomy. He agreed with us that the rectum should be spared in such cases.

Treatment of Polyps Beyond the Reach of the Sigmoidoscope. This involves the matter of diagnosis and then the problem of what to do about the polyps, once they are diagnosed. Diagnosis involves a preoperative suspicion based on the presence of polyps lower down or on the symptoms of bleeding, confirmed by barium and air contrast enemas. At operation, palpation is helpful, but even when the roentgenogram gives a lead as to the approximate site of the lesion, one may not be able to feel the polyp. A transverse colotomy at selected points with sterile operative coloscopy from within the abdomen (Loe, 1952; Gilchrist, 1953; Baker, Margetts and Schutt, 1955; Deddish and Hertz, 1955; McLanahan and Martin, 1957 and Shackelford and McGeehan, 1958) is a valuable procedure. Such patients should receive a complete bowel prep-

aration before such operations. If operative coloscopy is unsatisfactory, the use of extended colotomy incisions made within the antimesenteric longitudinal muscular taenia are to be considered. These should be closed after exploration with a continuous 0000 plain catgut suture for the inner row followed by 0000 interrupted silk for the outer row. If polyps are found, the required resection will decrease the length of colotomy incision that it will be necessary to close. Gants, Raymond and Pope (1956) utilized such incisions in monkeys and in 10 patients with good results. We have not adopted these long slits for operative coloscopy and believe that it is premature to advise them at this time. It is seldom necessary to make more than 3 short slits for this purpose if the two colonic flexures are adequately mobilized.

Once the polyps are found, they can be removed in two ways: (1) by colotomy with local removal (polypectomy) or (2) by segmental resection of the involved segment of colon. Judd and Carlisle (1953) based their advocacy of the second of these two on the following observations: In 264 cases of transcolonic removal, 177 (72%) developed no further polyps, 37 (15%) developed further polyps above sigmoidoscopic reach, and 32 (13%) developed further polyps requiring fulguration from below.

Welch (1951) also preferred segmental resection. He pointed out that 11 of 70 polypoid growths thought to be benign on observation through a sigmoidoscope or through a colotomy incision turned out to be carcinoma (16%). Two of these 11 already had lymph node metastases. Frozen section diagnosis is invaluable in cases such as these. It is sometimes inconclusive and when it is so, the surgeon must choose between simple polypectomy through a colotomy incision in the face of a significant chance of malignancy or elect the better cancer operation: segmental resection with deep removal of the corresponding mesenteric segment. If he elects simple polypectomy and the permanent sections show carcinoma, he is faced with the prospect of a second operation, or the worry of doing nothing. Welch concluded his argument for segmental resection of the involved bowel by pointing out that this operation in itself is little if any more dangerous than a colotomy with polypectomy. Loe (1952) was also dubious of the value of frozen sections in the average hospital.

Klein and Scarborough (1952) found frozen sections to be reliable in the diagnosis of carcinoma in colonic polyps; they preferred colotomy plus local polypectomy, as did David (1943), Morton (1953), McKittrick and Wheelock (1954), Turrell, Pomeranz, Paradny, and Vallecillo (1955), Swinton (1956) and Hellwig and Barbosa (1959). Length of stalk is of little importance. If basilar invasion exists, it is bad regardless of the length of the stalk. Moyer (1960) (Fig. 37-11) points out that actual proof that polyps become malignant is lacking. At the same time, from the practical standpoint, if a polypoid mass is demonstrated by repeated x-ray examinations, it should be removed because cancer cannot be ruled out.

In summary, it would seem to be advisable to do a wedge resection for almost all polyps above the reach of the sigmoidoscope. When the polyps are multiple or frankly malignant, an even more radical procedure may be necessary. On the other hand, Grinnell (1958) found that in 67 patients with multiple polyps of this type, only one would have benefited from subtotal or total colectomy. When resection is done, it is our opinion that the corresponding mesentery and its vessels should be removed *en bloc*. Spratt (1960) advises frequent re-examinations of simple polyps showing up on x-ray films as being less than 1.5 cm. in diameter.

Summary of treatment of adenomatous polyps below and above reach of the sigmoidoscope. This is a subject of such practical importance to the patient and of such interest to practitioners that a few general remarks are in order. If an adenomatous polyp is *below 25 cm.* from the anus (i.e., within reach of the sigmoidoscope) most surgeons would agree on removal. One feature of polypoid lesions below the peritoneal reflexion as opposed to those above this point is that below this point radical excision may require an abdominoperineal resection, while above it radical excision usually requires only wedge resection. There is a marked difference in morbidity, and even in mortality, between abdominoperineal resection and simple polypectomy in the lower lesions, while in the higher lesions there is relatively much less such difference between wedge resection and simple polypectomy. Therefore, for lower lesions a radical procedure should be approached with much more caution, particularly in cases with so-called carcinoma *in situ*.

Second, if an adenomatous polyp is removed by simple polypectomy, and the frozen section is reported benign, but the permanent sections later show carcinoma at the tip, should a second operation be performed? On the basis of the report of Spratt, Ackerman and Moyer (1958), metastases from such lesions are extremely rare and, to quote Moyer (1960), ". . . you don't need to go back." If the polyp is *above 25 cm.*, the decision is more difficult. The conventional view is to remove such polyps irrespective of size. Before making a diagnosis of the presence of a polyp, it is advisable to get at least one repeat x-ray study with barium or air contrast medium. A shadow on the roentgenogram may be a polyp, a carcinoma, or nothing (30% of cases do not prove to be positive for anatomic lesions despite repeated x-ray examinations). In certain clinics, as a part of an investigational study, apparent polyps less than 1.5 cm. in diameter are allowed to remain. This study is based on the observation that there is only 1/120 chance that the lesion will be a malignancy. This chance is less than the mortality at transabdominal polypectomy or polypectomy with wedge colectomy. For general adoption, until these newer views are more clearly established, it is to be recommended that small polyps *not* be left *in situ* and that demonstrable tumors within the bowel be removed. (It should be emphasized that the discussion in this paragraph concerns single or a few adenomatous polyps. Congenital polyposis is an entirely different subject.)

This leaves only two further decisions concerning adenomatous polyps above the reach of the sigmoidoscope. *First*, should they be removed by simple colotomy with a short diagonal slit plus polypectomy, or by polypectomy plus wedge resection? This is difficult to answer. When the "polypectomy" is done one does not know for sure whether one is dealing with a polyp or a carcinoma. This, and the fact that in some clinics wedge resection is not accompanied by a higher mortality rate, would favor wedge resection. On the other hand, in the average surgeon's hands, wedge resection cannot help being more dangerous. Hence, it is recommended that in this regard the cases be individualized. A thin patient in good condition with a suspicious lesion, had best have a wedge resection. At the other end of the spectrum of possibilities, an obese patient in poor condition with obvious polyp should be treated by simple polypectomy. Between these extremes, the decisions must be individualized.

VILLOUS TUMOR

(*Synonyms:* Villous papilloma, papillary adenoma, papilloma, true papilloma)

The malignant nature of these tumors, unlike polypoid adenoma, is so definite that they might well be classified with the malignant tumors later in this chapter, rather than here. According to Humphreys (1956), this tumor may be defined as a broad-based polyp with greatly elongated simple or branching crypts separated by delicate stroma and forming villous efflorescences at the surface. Lateral buds are absent or few; cell types vary as in benign and malignant adenomas. The tumor structure tends toward height of the epithelial elements rather than toward complexity. It may be termed "velvet carpet disease."

The soft velvetlike consistency and broad sessile arrangement of the villiform projections identify villous tumors in striking con-

trast with all other tumors of the distal bowel. This tumor should be differentiated from polypoid adenomas. It is soft, superficial, broad-based and represents an overgrowth of epithelial elements without connective tissue. Because of its softness, it is often difficult to palpate, but it is easy to see because of its whitish color and because most of such tumors are within 15 cm. of the anal verge. Thus, in Wheat and Ackerman's series of 50 cases, 79 per cent of the cases (Fig. 37-12) were in the rectosigmoid or below. In some instances the fluid discharge from such a tumor may be so extensive as to render the patient acutely ill of dehydration and sodium and potassium depletion (McKittrick and Wheelock, 1954; Goldgraber and Kirsner, 1958; and Hoffman, 1959).

With regard to the villous tumors being called papillary adenomas, this is not definitive, because, as Bacon, Lowell and Trimpi (1954) pointed out, all villous tumors are papillary, but not all adenomas are papillary. These tumors are relatively rare. In a series of 272 benign epithelial colorectal tumors, these authors found 243 polypoid adenomas (90%) and 28 villous tumors (10%). The average age of the patients with villous tumor was 55 years. They are rare in children. Bleeding occurred in 79 per cent of the 28 patients, diarrhea in 46 per cent, mucoid discharge in 31 per cent (some may pass mucus 15 to 20 times a day), and protrusion of the tumor in 21 per cent. Less frequent symptoms include constipation, weight loss, pruritis and rectal pain, while 18 per cent had no symptoms.

Size of the tumors varied from 2 × 5 cm. to 10 × 18 cm., the average being 6 × 12 cm. The levels of the tumors were as follows: 79 per cent below and 21 per cent above the peritoneal reflexion; the proximal-most tumor was in the transverse colon; 39 per cent were completely circumferential; while of the localized tumors, the majority were anterior or anterolateral. Malignant change was found in 36 per cent of the cases (36% of the 37 cases reported by Hines, Hanley and Schramel, 1955; and 32% of the 216 cases reported by Grinnell and Lane, 1958); 25 per cent were classically benign, 22 per cent revealed signs of "adenoma malignum," and 17 per cent revealed "atypism."

The malignant nature of villous tumors or

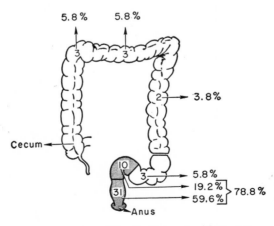

Fig. 37-12. Distribution of villous tumors of the large intestine (Wheat, M. W., Jr., and Ackerman, L. V.: Ann. Surg. *147*: 476)

their colloid propensity is attested further by the data of Sunderland and Binkley (1948) who reported the relatively large series of 48 cases of villous tumor occurring among 3,356 colorectal tumors. One of these 48 cases occurred in the rectosigmoid, and the remaining 47 in the rectum. They found that 69 per cent of the villous tumors either had carcinoma in the original tumor or developed a recurrence. It is also of interest that 40 per cent of the 48 cases developed invasive carcinoma and, furthermore, that 42 per cent of these invasive carcinomas were colloid carcinomas, while only 8 per cent of carcinomas of the rectum as a whole were colloid in their series.

Treatment should be radical. A few older publications recommended local removal if the tumor is still benign and not too large. Thus, David (1943) advocated a local procedure for certain villous tumors of the rectum. The posterior commissure was split posteriorly to the coccyx, exposing the tumor—which usually is anterior—and then the latter is excised with the cautery. The rectal defect where the tumor was is then sutured transversely and the posterior incision longitudinally in layers.

As Wheat and Ackerman (1958) stated: "Irradiation therapy of any type has no place in the treatment of villous adenomas of the large intestine." On the basis of experience with 50 cases (53 tumors), these authors divide villous tumors into 4 groups, as follows:

Group 1. Completely benign (13 cases)

Group 2. Localized areas of focal atypical change (19 cases)

Group 3. Localized areas of focal carcinoma (i.e., "carcinoma-in-situ") (13 cases)

Group 4. Invasive carcinoma (8 cases)

Thus, 76 per cent of their cases were of Groups 2 to 4. On the other hand, it is also seen that 85 per cent were of Groups 1 to 3. However, the placement of a given villous adenoma into the above categories *cannot be done with certainty from single or even multiple biopsies of the lesion.* An invasive carcinoma within a villous tumor is not readily visible, since it is usually small and situated in the depths of the tumor. Consequently, the assignation of benignancy or malignancy to one of these tumors cannot be made unless a pathologist examines the entire tumor minutely with serial sections. Since this procedure is time-consuming and invasive carcinoma is found so frequently (20-60% of cases), we recommend a proper "cancer operation" for at least all large villous adenomas, and when preoperative multiple biopsies (10 to 20 pieces) taken randomly from the body of the tumor, rather than its edge, demonstrate invasive carcinoma. Our recommendation is for *radical resection* in Group 4, in some large tumors, and in any case in which the tumor is high enough so the rectum can be spared. Except for purposes of biopsy, we deprecate "picking at" these tumors. If a villous tumor is in such a position that a proper cancer operation requires a Miles resection, we advise wide local removal if a biopsy has not shown malignancy. When the lesion is high enough so that a Miles resection is not required, we advise radical wedge resection for all villous tumors. Moyer (1960) stated: "Villous adenomas should be considered as a cancer and treated as such." Schoenberg, Fitts and Enterline (1958) and Turrell (1959) have also attested to the malignant nature of these tumors. The former authors stated that they are "frequently malignant and must be treated with special concern." The latter: "In my experience the size of (villous) adenomas is no guarantee against cancer."

In Bacon, Lowell and Trimpi's series treatment involved wide removal in 26 of the 28 patients (abdominoperineal proctosigmoidectomy, 15; abdominoperineal, 6; sigmoidectomy, 4; and resection of transverse colon, 1) while a localized Bevan-type excision of rectal mucosa was performed in only 2 cases. The results were good, and 93 per cent of the patients were still alive from 2 to 7 years after operation. Thus, these authors concluded that in cases of villous tumor, the bowel and its lymphatic drainage area should be removed radically.

Welch, McKittrick, and Behringer (1952) concluded as follows:

Radical resection with or without preservation of the sphincter, depending upon the location of the lesion, is indicated for all papillary adenomas (villous tumors).

In a later publication, McKittrick and Wheelock (1954) again advocated removal of the entire rectum for villous tumor. On the basis of their 6 cases, which were all malignant, Lee and Kay (1956) and Moran (experience with 32 cases, 18 of which, or 56%, were malignant, 1957) advocated either an anterior resection with anastomosis (for high lesions) or an abdominoperineal resection (for low lesions).

FAMILIAL POLYPOSIS OF THE COLON

(*Synonyms:* hereditary multiple polyposis, diffuse polyposis, polypoid adenomatosis, multiple adenomatosis)

This disease might also be called familial colonic carcinosity because if these individuals live long enough, all of them develop colonic carcinoma. This is what kills them.

This condition was first accurately described by Virchow (1863) in a 15-year-old boy. Cripps (1882) first recognized the familial nature of the condition, describing cases in a brother and a sister. The condition involves the appearance in childhood of innumerable small adenomatous polyps in the colon and the rectum. Cases with less than a dozen polyps usually do not represent the true condition, and in most instances the differentiation is easy because in familial polyposis the polyps are literally innumerable. The polyps may vary in size from those barely visible to the naked eye to those several centimeters in diameter, either sessile or pedunculated.

The patients with this condition are about equally distributed between the sexes, and apparently the affection can be inherited from either parent as a simple dominant Mendelian trait. In a review of 95 cases seen at the Mayo Clinic during the 15-year period ending in 1947, Mayo, DeWeerd, and Jackman (1951) reported that the majority (77%) of cases were diagnosed between the ages of 20 and 40 years. Blood in the stools or diarrhea or both were present in 90 (95%) of these cases. Physical examination, except for the rectum, was negative in all except the cases in which carcinoma had supervened. Sigmoidoscopic examination was positive in 100 per cent of 93 cases, and roentgen studies also in 100 per cent of 89 cases.

The expectation of life of a patient with familial polyposis of the colon is 41.6 years (Dukes, 1952). The rates of development of the polyps and the cancers vary from patient to patient, being somewhat similar in individual families. The earlier the disease occurs, the sooner cancer develops.

The hereditary aspect of familial polyposis of the colon, so well outlined by Lockhart-Mummery (1934) and by Dukes (1952), presents a fascinating genetic study. Brasher (1954) studied 2 families with familial polyposis of the colon. In the first family, in the 5 generations studied, there were 84 individuals, including 2 members with polyposis, 8 members with carcinoma of the large bowel, and 3 additional members with carcinoma of the large bowel and proved polyposis. The word "member" is used to describe polyposis patients, their brothers and sisters, and the direct descendants of these persons. Thus, there were 13 persons affected out of 84, an incidence of 15 per cent. The average age at death of the affected members was 41.9 years. Three patients (the 2 with polyposis, one with total colectomy, and one of the polyposis cases with carcinoma who was treated by rectosigmoidectomy) are still alive.

In the second family studied by Brasher, there were 103 individuals, including 8 members with polyposis, 3 with carcinoma of the large bowel, and 5 with polyposis plus carcinoma of the large bowel, a total of 16, or an incidence of 16 per cent.

The full key to these two family trees, as well as those of 56 other such families collected by Lockhart-Mummery, Dukes, and Bussey (1956), are filed in the Polyposis Register of St. Mark's Hospital, London, where they are available for reference. On the basis of his studies, Brasher concluded that:

. . . in accepting the responsibility of treating an affected member, the surgeon should also take the responsibility of investigating the whole family. Only if active investigations of these families are carried out will the high incidence of malignant change before treatment be lowered.

Durham (1954) reported a family with 3 generations which were studied. Eighteen of 29 members had polyposis or carcinoma of the colon, and 9 of these (50%) had carcinoma. Laberge, Sauer and Mayo (1957) described an association of soft-tissue tumors elsewhere in the body with familial polyposis. They advised that when multiple such "tumors are found on examination of a patient, proctoscopic examination and roentgenograms of the colon should be considered to exclude polyposis of the colon."

Treatment is mandatory. Mayo, DeWeerd and Jackman (1951) stated: "It is no exaggeration to say that every person with untreated, diffuse polyposis of the colon will die of carcinoma of the colon before he reaches the age of 50 years or will have an advanced malignant disease of the colon when he reaches the age of 50 years."

Treatment of familial polyposis of the colon should be radical and generally is of 2 types:

1. **Destruction of the Polyps in the Rectum Through a Sigmoidoscope, Followed by Ileorectal Anastomosis.** The stump of rectum must be observed at frequent intervals throughout the patient's life for the appearance of new polyps which are then fulgurated. While this method presents the apparent advantage of being less radical, even though the rectum is examined every 6 months in an attempt to keep it clear of polyps, this does not assure that carcinoma will not develop (Everson and Allen, 1954). Teicher and Abrahams (1956) epitomize this viewpoint by stating: "Patients with familial polyposis must be informed that preservation of normal bowel function by ileoproctostomy carries a calculated risk of carcinoma developing in the retained rectum."

This method has both opponents and adherents. Ravitch (1948) termed it "a dangerous half measure." Hoxworth and Slaughter (1948) discussed this technic and the methods discussed below but came to no definitive conclusion as to their relative merits. Mayo, DeWeerd, and Jackman (1951), Dukes (1952), Durham (1954), Everson and Allen (1954), Coller and Flotte (1955), Dukes and Lockhart-Mummery (1955) and Teicher and Abrahams (1956) favored this method. The last-named authors collected 115 cases so treated from the literature with a 5.2 per cent recurrence rate.

Lockhart-Mummery, Dukes and Bussey (1956) treated 29 of their 39 cases operated upon between 1946 and 1954 by subtotal colectomy and ileorectal anastomosis. In the entire series of 39 cases they had 2 operative deaths (5%), 5 deaths from recurrence or other disease (13%), and 1 developed a new carcinoma (3%). Thirty-one are still living. While these authors do recommend leaving the rectum in place in selected cases, they do not temporize otherwise. They advise as follows:

We now consider that once the decision to operate has been taken, removal of the whole colon is advisable, even though the polypi may still be small and scattered . . . there seem to us to be only two alternatives in most cases of polyposis, either to excise the whole large bowel and establish a permanent ileostomy or to preserve part of the rectum and join the ileum to it.

They point out an additional reason for avoiding partial colectomy, namely,

that persistent ill health and anemia may result from slight constant blood loss from polypi in even a short segment of colon.

Lockhart-Mummery, Dukes and Bussey cited 3 reasons for leaving the rectal stump—under continued close proctoscopic supervision, of course—as follows: (1) The risk of carcinoma arising under adequate supervision was small in their hands, only 1 case in 27 (4%); (2) the dislike of the patient for permanent ileostomy; (3) the special complications of ileostomy apart from its social disadvantages.

2. **Total Colectomy with Ileostomy.** This radical method eliminates all danger of recurrence, assuming that no cancer existed in the rectum at the time of colectomy. It is as good a cancer operation whether done with an *abdominal ileostomy* or an *anal ileostomy*. However, the latter procedure is more difficult for the average surgeon to perform. It is advocated by Best (1948), Ravitch (1948), Devine and Webb (1951) and by some of the same surgeons who favor its use in selected cases of nonspecific ulcerative colitis. As in cases of ulcerative colitis, when carcinoma is not present, the rectal dissection should be close to the bowel, and the anal dissection may include only mucosa. Technical details are given by Ravitch and Handelsman (1951).

Regarding the preferred age for elective operation in familial polyposis, Lockhart-Mummery, Dukes and Bussey (1956) recommend such surgery in the late teens or as soon thereafter as the condition is diagnosed. This is based on the occurrence of carcinoma in 2 of their patients with familial polyposis at the age of 20 and the report of cases in the literature at an even younger age than this.

We recommend total colectomy, because we are not sure that even if one can keep visible polyps from the rectal stumps carcinoma can be avoided. Furthermore, we believe that colectomy should be performed as soon as the diagnosis of familial multiple polyposis is confirmed.

Congenital Polyposis of the Entire Gastrointestinal Tract

This condition should be differentiated from the main one that is under consideration here, namely, familial polyposis of the colon. The generalized condition has two distinguishing features, namely, the presence of skin and oral mucosal pigmentation and the early presence in some instances of obstruction of the small bowel due to the presence of the polyps. The pigmented spots involve melanin deposits with a typical distribution on the lips, especially the lower one, in the mouth and on the face. The condition was first described by Peutz (1921) in Holland, and by Jeghers (1944) in this country. (Three of Peutz' 7 cases appeared to be malignant, and 1 of Jeghers' 12 cases appeared to be malignant.)

One of the best articles for reference is that of Jeghers, McKusick and Katz (1949). Other reviews are those of Rohrs (1957); Bartholomew and Dahlin (1958); Guillard, Laumonier, Seyer and Boulet (1958); Falkinburg and Key (1959) and Mégevand (1959). Intussusception is frequent in these cases (Bläckberg, 1960).

The condition is hereditary, involves both sexes equally and is transmitted by both males and females. The two factors, typical pigmentation and generalized polyposis, always were found together in the cases studied by Weber (1954). Sometimes the condition is referred to as Peutz-Jeghers syndrome. No special symptoms are ascribed to the syndrome other than frequently bloody stools and bouts of intestinal obstruction due to recurrent intussusception or obturative occlusion of the bowel lumen by the polyps. As Berkowitz, Pearl and Shapiro (1955) pointed out, about 10 per cent of cases of small bowel polyposis belong to the syndrome. Of the 37 cases they collected from the literature, including 3 of their own, 10 also had gastric polyps, and 10 also had colonic polyps. Apparent malignancy occurred in 9 of the 37 cases; in all but 1 of these 9, in which the location of the apparent malignancy was cited, the ileum was the site of the supposed carcinoma.

In these cases, a complete gastrointestinal study—gastroscopy from above, sigmoidoscopy from below; gastrointestinal x-ray studies from above, air contrast barium enemas from below—is mandatory. In fact, as Rubin (1956) pointed out, the examination of no case with colorectal polyps is complete without a gastroscopy.

In the first edition of this book, the section on Peutz-Jeghers syndrome concluded with the statement that "malignant change is frequent. We now believe that the polyps in this condition are benign." Bartholomew, Dahlin and Waugh (1957) stated: "There have been no reported deaths from carcinoma in this condition. . . . The so-called polyps actually are abnormal collections of normal cells in a normal location. It is clear that the evidence of muscle invasion is equivocal and in fact the findings in the [Mayo] Clinic cases suggest that actual invasion does not occur." Such polyps, even with occasional "factitious malignancy" are not at the present time an indication for extensive bowel resections. However, until these newer ideas concerning their benign nature are proved, patients with them should be examined periodically.

Pseudopolyposis

(*Synonyms:* Acquired type of polyps, secondary polyposis, post-inflammatory polyposis)

The incidence of carcinoma of the colon is definitely higher in patients with chronic ulcerative colitis than it is in the general population. The incidence of carcinoma of the colon in patients with chronic ulcerative colitis has also been shown to be much more common in cases of over 10 years' duration than in those who have had the disease less than 5 years. Such carcinomatous degeneration is more apt to occur in patients with pseudopolyposis. Such pseudopolyps are islands of normal mucosa surrounded by confluent ulcers. It is generally believed that the carcinomatous degeneration of these pseudopolyps is on a basis of repeated scarring and healing—much like Marjolin's ulcer externally—rather than on any special quality of the mucosa per se.

However, one should remember that 1 out of 3 carcinomas of the colon in ulcerative colitis arises directly as an infiltrating lesion without an intermediary phase of pseudopolyposis.

The treatment of ulcerative colitis in general is considered previously in this chapter. Suffice it to say that it is becoming more radical with more 1-stage colectomies. In most cases the colectomy is total with either an *abdominal ileostomy* (Bacon and Trimpi, 1950; Palumbo and Rugtiv, 1953; Fallis and Barron, 1955; Scarborough, 1955 and Fallis, 1956), or an *anal ileostomy* (Ravitch, 1948; Fallis and Barron, 1953, and others). Other surgeons preserve the rectum, when it is not too badly ulcerated, and perform an ileoproctostomy.

When total colectomy is done with abdominal ileostomy, we favor a "matured" ileostomy (Brooke, 1952; Crile and Turnbull, 1954; Durham, 1957; and Hamilton, Harbrecht and Lucas 1959). In such cases special care must be given to the peritoneal wound and pelvic dead space, because of the frequency of infection. Tolstedt, Bell and Harkins (1961) reported that in 27 of their 32 cases of this type, the peritoneal wound took more than 3 months to heal. These authors recommended that the posterior parietal peritoneum be left open in the pelvis so as to eliminate the dead space. The incidence of carcinoma in ulcerative colitis has been reported by other authors as varying from 2.9 per cent (Dawson and Pryse-Davis, 1959) to 6.7 per cent, a figure almost identical with that of Thorlakson, 1956 (see also: Slaney and Brooke, 1959).

The possibility of carcinomatous degeneration is one of the main reasons for surgery in ulcerative colitis, and this danger influences the selection of operation. In Thorlakson's series (1956) of 182 consecutive colectomies for ulcerative colitis, carcinoma was found in 12 (6.6%). These patients averaged 10 to 15 years younger than in the general population afflicted by colorectal carcinoma. There were from 1 to 8 carcinomas in the individual patients, a total of 23 primary malignant tumors: 1 of the 23 was in the cecum, 4 in the transverse colon, 4 at the splenic flexure or upper descending colon, 10 in the sigmoid and the rectosigmoid, and 4 in the rectum. The incidence of carcinoma in patients who had been afflicted by ulcerative colitis for 10 years or

more was much higher than in patients of the same age and sex who had not had ulcerative colitis. Malignant changes often first appeared in the quiescent stage of the disease when clinically the patient seemed to have improved. Most authors believe that carcinoma secondary to ulcerative colitis is more malignant than otherwise, but in Thorlakson's series this did not seem to be the case. (Aylett, 1959; Turnbull, 1959).

The malignant potentiality of ulcerative colitis favors the performance of at least a subtotal colectomy, contraindicates leaving the rectum in when pseudopolyposis is marked, and makes periodic proctoscopic examinations of the rectal stump mandatory in all cases where such a stump is left in place.

At the same time, unless frank carcinoma is already present, the operation can be modified from that of the classic radical colectomy plus abdominoperineal resection of the rectum. The mesentery can be cut close to the bowel. The rectal dissection should be kept close to the bowel, particularly in males, to prevent injury to the sacral nerves and possible interference with sexual function. The anal portion can be performed entirely from above, according to the method of Fallis and Barron, 1953, and others, except for the anal mucosa which can be removed from below without injuring the sphincter muscles. Technical details are well described by Ravitch and Handelsman (1951); Ravitch (1956), and by Dukes and Lockhart-Mummery (1957).

Once frank carcinoma has developed in ulcerative colitis, the prognosis is grave, although 33 per cent of Thorlakson's 12 cases are still alive after 3 years. Prophylactic excisional therapy in the stage of pseudopolyposis is thus of especial importance.

JUVENILE POLYPOSIS

(*Synonym:* Retention polyps)

Certain features of the age incidence and the pathologic nature of such polyps are discussed on page 960 under "polypoid adenoma," from which they are quite different but with which they are often confused. Juvenile polyps are more like warts than true polyps. They contain cystic space filled with mucus (Fig. 37-13). Their chief maltoward effects are hemorrhage and serving as a starting point of an intussusception. They tend to disappear

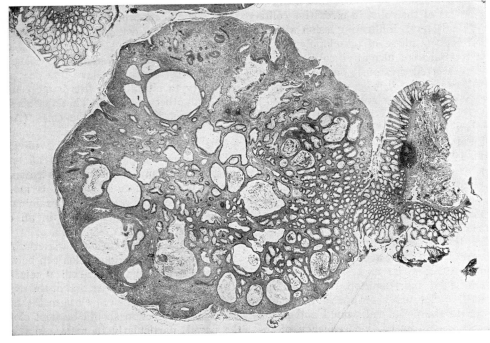

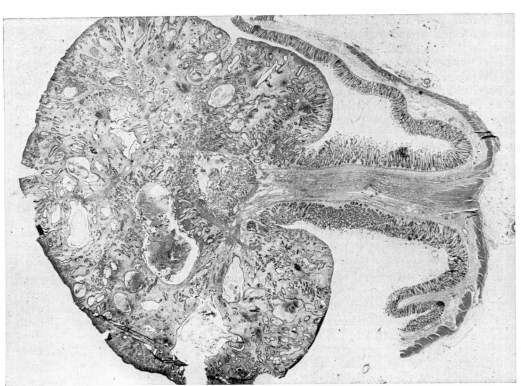

FIG. 37-13. Photomicrographs of retention polyp from a child. (*Left*) Lower power. (*Right*) Higher power shows uniformity of glandular epithelium and retention of mucus in some distended glands. (Spratt, J. S., Jr., Ackerman, L. V., and Moyer, C. A.: Ann. Surg. *148*:683)

spontaneously. Recommended management is as follows: A single polyp should be biopsied. If multiple polyps are present, in a child at least, one should be biopsied. If one is a retention polyp, all are probably retention polyps, and the rest should be observed periodically. If the biopsied polyp is adenomatous in nature, and the polyps are multiple, familial polyposis should be considered; if present, it should be managed accordingly. True juvenile retention polyposis "is universally a benign disease" (Moyer, 1960). The error of doing a colectomy in a young child for juvenile polyposis is comparable with removing a normal uterus in a young girl. Knox, Miller, Begg and Zintel (1960) also uphold the more conservative approach once the diagnosis is confirmed, on the basis of experience with 75 such juvenile polyps at St. Luke's Hospital, New York City. They stated: "Extensive operative procedures should not be employed to remove asymptomatic juvenile polyps in the proximal colon." On the basis of a study of 183 such cases at the Hospital for Sick Children in Toronto, Mallam and Thomson (1959) stated: "The risk of malignancy is remote." Turrell (1960) has recently reviewed these lesions.

BENIGN TUMORS: RARER LESIONS

The point to be emphasized here is that most, if not all, of these lesions are of such secondary importance as compared with the polyps previously discussed that any discussion of them should not detract from emphasis on polyps and their potentialities. A few rarer tumors will be listed below:

1. **Leiomyoma:** Such tumors are grossly similar to those which appear elsewhere in the intestinal tract and are essentially submucosal. Only rarely do they produce symptoms. Such tumors have recently been reviewed by Haas and Ritter (1960). Very rarely they are malignant (Sanger and Leckie, 1959).

2. **Fibroma.** Neurofibromas in patients with von Recklinghausen's disease have been reported (Grodsky, 1958).

3. **Lipoma** (Ryrberg, 1956; D'Alonzo, 1957; Kolb and Black, 1958; Henderson, Harris and Packer, 1958; Hayes, Burr and Melton, 1960, and Ochsner and Ray, 1960).

4. **Carcinoid.** About 90 per cent of the rare carcinoids of the rectum are benign, but lo-cally invasive while the other 10 per cent are quite malignant (see p. 955). This is in contrast with those in the cecum or the ileocecal valve which are almost all malignant (Stout, 1955). Carcinoids were first named by Oberndorfer (1907) to designate a benign tumorous lesion. They may represent the migration to the surface of neurocrine cells of the chromaffin system. In the rectum, unlike carcinoids of the appendix, they usually do not stain with silver salts (argentaffin reaction) (Rosser, 1951). Malignant carcinoids of the rectum are of special interest, and as in the case of the anorectum (see Chap. 38) carcinoids of the rectum are more apt to be malignant than those of the appendix. MacDonald (1956) collected 356 carcinoids from surgical and autopsy material in 7 Boston hospitals. Of the 356 cases, 207 (58%) originated in the appendix and 149 (42%) were of extra-appendiceal origin. Of the 149 extra-appendiceal cases, 67 per cent were invasive and 16 per cent had metastasized. Of the 149 cases, 26 were in the colorectum. Forty per cent of the 25 cases of carcinoid tumor of the rectum seen by Peskin and Orloff (1959) were malignant. Swinton and Freedman (1960) stated: "Rectal carcinoid potentially is highly malignant and should be managed in the same way as early adenocarcinoma."

The carcinoid syndrome (Thorson, Björck, Björkman and Waldenström, 1954; Mattingly and Sjoerdsma, 1956; MacDonald, 1956; Page, 1958; and Davies, 1959) is present in about one fourth of patients with malignant carcinoids and consists of lesions chiefly in 3 spheres: (1) cutaneous vascular, (2) gastrointestinal and (3) cardiac.

The characteristic cutaneous vascular symptom is *episodic flushing;* the flush tends to become fixed with time. A striking illustration of flushing appears in a recent article (Wilson and Storer, 1959). An additional vascular lesion is telangiectasia, particularly of the face and the neck. Cyanosis appears only after a flush; it is related to temperature (Davies, 1959), being more prominent in a cool environment, and is probably secondary to capillary stasis.

The characteristic gastrointestinal lesion is hyperactivity of the bowel, resulting in *chronic diarrhea,* frequently of disabling severity. Partial to complete bowel obstruction secondary to fibrosis around the carcinoid tumor is often the presenting complaint. Abdominal colic is a frequent symptom. Massive hepatomegaly occurs with metastases to the liver.

The characteristic cardiac lesion is *valvular disease of the right heart* secondary to endocardial fibrosis. This process results (in decreasing order of frequency) in pulmonic stenosis, tricuspid insufficiency and tricuspid stenosis. Right heart hypertrophy and congestive heart failure are natural consequences of the valvular lesions. Asthmatic symptoms and dyspnea are not uncommon and are due to serotonin induced bronchospasm rather than to congestive heart failure. Serotonin is probably removed in some way during the passage of blood through the pulmonary circulation; because of this the left heart is exposed to a lower concentration of serotonin and is usually spared the valvular lesions occurring in the right heart (Goble, Hay and Sandler, 1955).

An interesting facet of rectal carcinoids is that they differ histologically from carcinoids in other anatomic sites. The rectal carcinoid cells are more primitive, which may account for their more malignant potential, and they do not show the silver staining reaction that characterizes carcinoid (argentaffin) tissue elsewhere in the body (Davies, 1959). In some series, it is reported that a carcinoid less than 1 cm. in diameter metastasizes rarely, if at all. Before accepting this as a definitive conclusion, one must explain the case reports of massive liver metastases without a grossly discernible primary tumor elsewhere in the abdomen.

The functional cell is the argentaffin cell (first described by Heidenhain in 1870) which is ectodermal in origin. They have a characteristic silver-reducing staining reaction. The cells in rectal carcinoids are of a more primitive type than those involved in appendiceal carcinoma.

The chemical aspects of these tumors involve the following pathway: Tryptophane → 5-Hydroxytryptophane (5HTP) → 5-Hydroxytryptamine (5HT, serotonin) → 5-Hydroxyindolacetic acids (5HIAA). The first conversion to 5HTP is effected by tryptophane oxidase, the second to 5HT (serotonin) by 5HTP-oxidase, and the third conversion

by amine oxidase. Since the action of carcinoids when producing the carcinoid syndrome is believed to be due to excess 5-HT (serotonin) produced especially by the hepatic metastases, enzymatic antimetabolic methods to prevent its formation or to hasten its conversion have been tried. Isoniazid is a serotonin antagonist in high drug dosage in vitro (Horita, 1960). Its isopropyl congener, iproniazid also works only in high dosage which is toxic for man (Davies, 1959). On the other hand, blockage of the conversion of serotonin into 5-HIAA, in which form it is excreted in the urine, could theoretically exacerbate the symptoms. In this connection it is interesting to consider the recent demonstration by Sjoerdsma, Terry and Udenfriend (1957) that serotonin antagonism by phenothiazine derivatives (chlorpromazine, etc.) is spurious and an artifact of the colorimetric method for determining urinary 5-hydroxyindolacetic acid. The phenothiazines interfere with the development of the color reaction leading to falsely low readings of 5-hydroxyindolacetic acid and the assumption, also false, that serotonin blood levels were lowered.

Another point of diagnostic and prognostic interest is that if 5-HIAA is still present in the urine in abnormally large amounts after removal of a carcinoid, metastases are probably present.

As far as surgical treatment is concerned, complete removal is naturally most desirable. However, if the flushing syndrome does not develop, the patients may live for years. The condition is quantitative, and removal of as much of the tumor as possible, including hepatic lobectomy, may be helpful.

5. **Hemangioma.** Such a tumor involves the colon, or more rarely the rectum, and presents several distinguishing features, as pointed out by Bailey, Barrick, and Jenkinson (1956). Rectal bleeding is common. By roentgenographic examination, phleboliths may be seen, and the tumor usually extends over a longer segment of bowel than does carcinoma, often with no obstruction to the retrograde flow of barium. As pointed out by Scott and Brand (1957), if the tumor does not extend up into the sigmoid loop, ligation of the inferior mesenteric artery may effect improvement, but resection of large tumors may be preferable.

6. **Endometriosis.** This lesion may produce obstruction in the absence of mucosal involvement (Korn and Savage, 1957). About 40 per cent of women with endometriosis have rectosigmoid implants (Jenkinson and Brown, 1943); Colcock and Lamphier (1950) presented a somewhat lower figure in this regard, stating that in a series of 213 operated cases of endometriosis, 39 (18%) had small or large bowel involvement, and 14 of these patients had obstruction. Treatment is usually conservative.

7. **Benign Lymphoma.** Lymphoid polyps (benign lymphoma) have been reported by Keeling and Beatty (1956) in an account of 3 cases in siblings, and by Holtz and Schmidt (1958) who found 24 cases in 20 years at the University of Michigan. This condition is not rare, over 300 cases having been reported in the literature. McGraw and Bonenfant (1960) confirm the benign nature of these tumors.

8. **Granuloma.** Granulomas, amebic (Gunn and Howard, 1931) or nonspecific (D'Alonzo, 1958), are chiefly of interest because they simulate carcinoma.

9. **Congenital Cyst** (Thomson and Farmer, 1958)

10. **Xanthoma**

11. **Melanoma** (Pack and Martins, 1960)

MALIGNANT TUMORS: ADENOCARCINOMA

Squamous cell carcinoma of the anus is considered separately in Chapter 38, "Anorectum."

The importance of colorectal cancer is attested by the following facts:

First, it ranks Number 1 in mortality in the United States, accounting for 34,709 deaths in 1953, with the lung (23,502 deaths for both primary and secondary lesions) ranking second and the stomach (23,373 deaths) ranking third (see Table 10). The large intestine alone (24,015 deaths)—not including the rectum—still exceeded the mortality from any other organ. The mortality of 1,577 from poliomyelitis in the same year serves as a basis of comparison. This rating of colorectal carcinoma as the leading cancer killer may seem to disagree with that of Figure 44-1. It should be remembered that that Figure refers only to males, in which instances there is a far greater

TABLE 10. MORTALITY FROM MALIGNANT DISEASE IN THE UNITED STATES: MOST COMMON ORGANS INVOLVED 1953

MALIGNANT DISEASE OF:	DEATHS	
1. Large intestine except rectum	24,015	
2. Stomach	23,373	
3. Breast	20,566	
4. Uterus	15,547	34,709*
5. Lung, unspecified as to whether primary or secondary	12,938	
6. Prostate	12,595	23,502†
7. Rectum	10,694	
8. Lung, primary	10,564	
9. Pancreas	10,165	

* Combined figure for items 1 and 7.

† Combined figure for items 5 and 8. Even assuming that all of the lung tumors "unspecified as to whether primary or secondary" were primary, the figure of 23,502 still ranks second to that for the large intestine alone.

(From Dunn, 1955)

preponderance of carcinoma of the lung than for the colorectum. When both sexes are included, the statement given here still stands.

Second, by means of removal of colorectal polyps this mortality definitely may be reduced. An antipolyp campaign may do good directly, if one subscribes to the view that polyps may become malignant; or indirectly, by finding unexpectedly some early carcinomas, polypoid or flat. In this connection, it is of interest (see Fig. 10-1), that a colonic tumor to be visible to the naked eye (e.g., 4 mm. diameter), has already spent 70 per cent of its life span, assuming its eventual maximum size compatible with life of the patient to be 12 cm. in diameter. This assumption also implies that tumor growth proceeds exponentially. Sloughing may slow up the late phases of growth of colon carcinoma.

Third, the probability of cure following definitive operation (5-year arrest rate) is quite high (about 50%), being higher than any others of the first 9 leading organs causing death (Tables 11-11 to 11-13) with the exception of the breast and the possible exception of the stomach. Either or both the colon and the rectum respond far more favorably to definitive operation than the stomach, the lung and the pancreas.

Age. Colorectal carcinoma is usually a disease of older persons, but youth is no barrier to its occurrence. Hoerner (1958) collected reports of 262 cases in patients under 20. An unusual feature of childhood colorectal carcinoma is the high incidence of mucoid carcinoma (50%, Hoerner, 1958; 43%, Chappell, 1959). A possible relationship to juvenile polyps which often contain mucoid retention cysts is purely speculative. The results of treatment are poor, probably because of delay in diagnosis, overconservativism in treatment and because of the high percentage of intracellular mucoid carcinoma which is relatively incurable at any age (Moyer, 1960). It is true that on first reading, the paper by Wolfman, Astler and Coller (1957) would indicate otherwise, but if only the intracellular mucoid carcinomas in their paper are considered, their conclusion is "that this is a highly malignant type of tumor." As Johnson, Judd, and Dahlin (1959) pointed out, younger patients stand definitive resective procedures well, and such treatment is indicated if the diagnosis is confirmed.

Etiology. While there may be some relationship to adenomatous polyps, there most certainly is to familial polyposis, to ulcerative colitis and to villous tumor. Otherwise, the etiology is unknown. Woolf (1958) believes there is a genetic basis for carcinoma of the rectum other than that resulting from familial polyposis.

Symptoms include alteration in bowel habits: constipation, obstipation, or even continued diarrhea, small caliber of the stools, especially in low left-sided lesions, weakness, often due to anemia, and blood in or on the stools.

The subject of intestinal obstruction is dealt with separately in Chapter 36, so that only certain aspects of it will be considered here. Furthermore, the very important discussion of the blood supply to the colon and the rectum and lymphatic drainage from them, so important to the election of points of division of the colon, is elaborated upon in Chapter 33 and will only be considered here, as it applies to certain technical points. Obstruction was 7 times more frequent in the left colon carcinoma than in right colon carcinoma (Morgan, 1952). The over-all incidence of carcinoma was 1.5 times as frequent on the left.

Physical signs include only the palpation or visualization by sigmoidoscopy of a low-lying lesion in early cases. In high-lying lesions the early diagnosis usually is made only by laboratory methods, including x-ray examination. Presence of "sentinel polyps" or "sentinel hemorrhoids" may give a valuable early lead. Late physical signs include palpation of an abdominal mass, either primary in the bowel, or in the liver, or of an enlarged blown-up cecum or abdominal distention, or anemia and evidence of loss of weight. The qualitative differences between the symptoms and signs of right and left colonic lesions are listed in Table 11. This differentiation holds true only on the average, but not always in the individual patient. Thus, while more patients with right colon lesions have anemia than do those with left colon lesions, the presence of anemia does not rule out left colon carcinoma. A blown-up cecum may be the first sign of a sigmoidal carcinoma. Rupture of such a cecum is a serious complication with a 70 per cent mortality rate. Measuring the greatest diameter of the cecum as shown on a prone film, Lowman and Davis (1956) found that no case developed perforation without the diameter's having attained at least 9 cm. In 100 control patients without left colon obstruction, most could be distended by barium or air to 5 to 7 cm. Only 4 of the 100 controls exceeded 9 cm. which is thus the critical diameter.

Laboratory examination includes barium enema (best done after the sigmoidoscopic examination), biopsy in low-lying lesions, hemoglobin determination, and possibly cytologic examination of colonic washings, although this last technic is not practical in most cases at present.

Differential diagnosis includes the ruling out of diverticulitis (more apt to have fever), lymphopathia venereum (Frei test), tuberculosis (usually pulmonary tuberculosis is pres-

TABLE 11. QUALITATIVE DIFFERENCES IN
SYMPTOMS AND SIGNS OF RIGHT AND
LEFT COLORECTAL CARCINOMA

	RIGHT	LEFT
Occult blood in stools	+	−
Bright blood in stools	−	+
Anemia	+	−
Obstructive signs	−	+
Gallbladderlike symptoms	+	−
"Sentinel polyps"	+	+
"Sentinel hemorrhoids"	−	+
Small caliber of stools	−	+

ent), endometriosis (does not involve the mucosa, and the symptoms usually are made worse at the time of the menstrual periods), appendicitis (Feldman, 1958), simple ulcer of the colon (Friedman and MacKenzie, 1959), and of course, benign polyps. In all instances of low-lying lesions, biopsy is the surest and really the only way to make the diagnosis. There are many benign conditions which can be confused with carcinoma (of the cecum: Phillips, ReMine, Beahrs and Scudamore, 1960; elsewhere in the colon: Rives and Emmett, 1954).

The important differential diagnosis between diverticulitis and carcinoma of the colon was studied by Colcock and Sass (1954). These authors pointed out that the roentgenograms would differentiate most cases, but that the history is important as well. On the basis of 50 consecutive cases of each condition, nausea and vomiting, colicky pain, chills and fever, and rectal tenderness were all more common in diverticulitis. Constipation and blood per rectum were more common in carcinoma. Massive hemorrhage may occur, not only with diverticulitis but also with diverticulosis of the colon (Noer, 1955; Mobley, Dockerty and Waugh, 1957; and Knight, 1957). Abscess and fistula formation were more common in diverticulitis. However, it should be mentioned in emphasizing the difficulties of this differential diagnosis that all of these listed differential features occurred in both conditions except for rectal tenderness which, while present in only 8 cases (16%) of the patients with diverticulitis, did not occur in any of those with carcinoma.

However, the differentiation between diverticulitis and carcinoma does not solve all the problems, as Mayo and Delaney (1956) reported 50 cases in which the two conditions occurred in the same patient. Ponka, Fox and Brush (1959) pointed out that 75 (21%) of their cases of carcinoma of the colon had coexistent diverticulosis and diverticulitis.

Treatment involves preliminary decompression (colostomy, see Chap. 36) in certain acute cases followed by definitive resection at a later date. In patients without acute obstruction a definitive resective operation should be performed as soon as possible. In some cases, even in the presence of obstruction, a one-stage resection can be done (Windsberg, 1959).

Roentgen treatment is of little help, either as a palliative or a curative measure in colorectal carcinoma, although Stearns, Deddish and Quan (1959) claimed some benefit from preoperative roentgen therapy for carcinoma of the rectum in the group with lymph node metastases. In the experience of the authors, x-ray treatment is not of value except in the control of pain in the late phases of some inoperable cases.

At the present time, in patients with metastases that cannot be removed, resection with anastomosis is used more widely than is colostomy without resection. Of course, this apparently more radical procedure is accompanied by a higher mortality than is simple colostomy, but it may eliminate the colostomy and temporarily improves the general condition of the patient. Any lesion in the colon is *a priori* an infected, bleeding, fungating mass as well as a tumor. In the liver or other remote organs the metastases only sap the patients' vitality on the basis of their abnormal tumor metabolism without the added enervating influences of infection and hemorrhage. Furthermore, removal of the primary tumor prevents continued seeding of the liver.

In rare instances, removal of a single metastasis in the liver, particularly in the left lobe may be tried. Involvement of contiguous organs is also not the deterrent it used to be to definitive resection. Attachment to small bowel, requiring coincident resection of a loop of the latter, does not, in the author's experience, materially alter the ultimate prognosis. Bladder involvement is also not an absolute contraindication to definitive resection. The use of an ileal segment as a substitute bladder (Bricker, 1950) has proved to be useful in such cases. The late results with an ileal conduit in urinary diversion were analyzed recently by Baker and Graf (1956) with a generally favorable conclusion on the basis of 13 cases.

THE SECOND LOOK. Cancers of the colon offer the most favorable opportunity of utilizing this somewhat experimental technic. The second look may be either deliberate, as utilized by Wangensteen, Lewis, Arhelger, Muller, and MacLean (1954), or forced by the evidence of recurrence (Moore, 1953). In the former instance, a deliberate re-exploration of the abdomen is performed in cases which showed evidence of lymph node involvement at the time of the first operation. Such a second look usually is done within 6 to 8 months. In 103 patients with cancers of the stomach, the colon and the rectum, Wangensteen and his associates observed 6 patients who revealed carcinoma at the second operation who were found to be free of carcinoma at a subsequent operation. In cancer of the stomach (39 cases) there was one such good result, in cancer of the colon (29 cases) there were four, and in cancer of the rectum (35 cases) there was one. These authors concluded: "The second look procedure would appear to exhibit greatest promise in patients with colic cancer."

DEFINITIVE RESECTION involves a consideration of 6 factors in the spread of the tumor, as follows: (1) the local tumor and its intramural spread, (2) the lymphatic metastases, (3) the venous spread, (4) the implantation of cells from within the bowel lumen in the lines of anastomosis, (5) spread by direct extension to contiguous organs, and (6) transperitoneal spread.

1. *Intramural Spread.* Dunphy and Broderick (1951) reported that a margin of 10 cm. below the tumor is essential to remove all of the bowel involved by intramural spread of the tumor (cf. the somewhat similar situation in the stomach, Chap. 29). These authors pointed out that measurements of extent of mural spread often are based on those taken in fixed contrasted specimens in the laboratory. Such figures cannot be applied safely to the operating room where fresh, unshrunken tissues are being measured. Other studies of the extent of intramural spread of colon tumors are those of Coller, Ransom and Regan (1956), and of Lofgren, Waugh and Dockerty (1957).

2. *Lymphatic Metastases.* The lymphatic drainage of the colorectum is surgically important. It follows the blood vessels and is generally upward. Thus, Gilchrist and David (1947) found retrograde metastases, in carcinomas below the sacral promontory, to nodes 1 to 5 cm. below the tumor in only 7 of 153 cases (5%). Decision as to the uppermost point of resection is based upon the factor of stopping short of arteries that supply structures which one does not want to remove. At the same time, the arteries. the veins and the lymphatics must be removed as a unit to the uppermost point of resection. In 11 early deaths from operation in a series of colorectal carcinomas, Gilchrist and David (1947), reported that necropsy revealed retroperitoneal positive lymph nodes in 4 cases (36%). In 3 of these (27%) "complete removal of all node metastases would have been obtained if the field of resection had been 1.5 cm. wider"! Assuming that this 27 per cent would apply to those who survived operation, such an increment to the 5-year survival rate would be appreciable and welcome.

The importance of the presence of positive lymph nodes is shown in Table 12. Examples of specific instances of "going higher" to remove involved nodes are as follows: Phillips, Waugh, and Dockerty (1954) pointed out the fallacy, from the standpoint of lymph node metastases, of removing only the right branch of the middle colic artery in hepatic flexure lesions. They advocated, as we do, ligation of

TABLE 12. THE INFLUENCE OF POSITIVE LYMPH NODES IN THE OPERATIVE SPECIMEN UPON 5-YEAR SURVIVAL IN COLORECTAL CARCINOMA (FROM GILCHRIST AND DAVID, 1947)

	NUMBER OF CASES			PER CENT 5-YR. SURVIVAL		
TYPE OF TUMOR	WITH NODES	NO NODES	TOTAL	WITH NODES	NO NODES	AVERAGE
1. Right Colon	..	..	15	54	87	60
2. Left Colon	..	..	18	37	80	61
3. Intraperitoneal Rectal	35	20	55	51	90	65
4. Extraperitoneal Rectal	69	43	112	38	74	52
Total or Average			200			57

the middle colic at its source from the superior mesenteric artery.

In lesions of the left colon, Rosi and Capos (1955) showed that the 1 cm. distance between the origin of the inferior mesenteric artery from its origin from the aorta to its first branching included 8 per cent positive lymph nodes. (See Fig. 37-14 and also Fig. 33-7 in Chap. 33.)

3. *Venous Spread.* Metastases spreading by the venous route are probably more common than is popularly realized. Gilchrist and David (1947) found that the liver was the site of persistences in 10 to 16 per cent of their cases, probably on the basis of blood-borne metastases. Utilizing the injection of a radiopaque substance into the vascular tree, Madison, Dockerty, and Waugh (1954), studied 42 carcinomas of the rectum after excision. In the entire series, 43 per cent showed evidence of venous invasion, while in the 35 operations performed with a hope for cure, the incidence was 31 per cent.

Burns and Pfaff (1956) studied microscopic invasion of blood vessels. In similar studies, Swinton and Snow (1959) reported 565 cases divided into those with or without either blood vessel or lymph node involvement. The 5-year arrest rates were: with neither lymph nodes nor vessels involved, 67 per cent; with vessels only, 38 per cent; with nodes only, 27 per cent; and with both, 9 per cent. These statistics might indicate that while blood vessel involvement is important, it is not so much so as nodal involvement. Another approach to the subject is the finding of cancer cells in the venous blood, either locally, or from the antecubital vein. Roberts, Watne, McGrew, McGrath and Cole (1957) and Sandberg and Moore (1957) reported finding cancer cells in venous blood of many such patients.

Our technic (see p. 951) involves ligation of the inferior mesenteric vein at its point of confluence with the splenic vein (see Fig. 33-6, Chap. 33) in cases of abdominoperineal resection. For instances of colonic resection elsewhere, the appropriate veins are ligated near their confluence early in the operation. This step is based also on the work of Fisher and Turnbull (1955) who recovered tumor cells from the blood of the major mesenteric venous channels in 8 of 25 (32%) cases of colorectal carcinoma by a perfusion technic. Only those cells that were morphologically identical with the epithelial cells observed in direct smears from the neoplasm were considered as positive examples of tumor cells. Such cells were found in 4 instances in which histopathologic evidence of venous extension was not observed. The presence of these cells in 1 of the 5 lesions classified as "Duke's A" (the most favorable class) offers an explanation for the malignant clinical course exhibited in the patient with a lesion usually considered favorable.

4. *Implantation of Tumor Cells from Within the Bowel Lumen in the Lines of*

Fig. 37-14. Percentages of resected specimens of carcinomas of the left colon in which metastatic carcinoma was found in the lymph nodes that lay in the region of the inferior mesenteric artery (I.M.A.) and the aorta (L.C.A.-left colic artery). It is remarkable what a great difference a few centimeters make. (Rosi, P. A., and Capos, N. J.: S. Clin. North America *35*:1325)

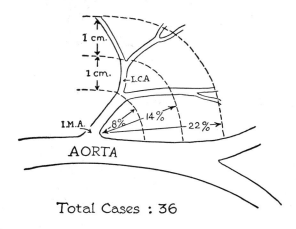

Total Cases : 36

Positive nodes:	No.	%
from aorta to bifurcation of I.M.A.	3	8 %
from aorta to 1 cm. beyond bifurcation of I.M.A.	5	14 %
from aorta to 2 cm. beyond bifurcation of I.M.A.	8	22 %

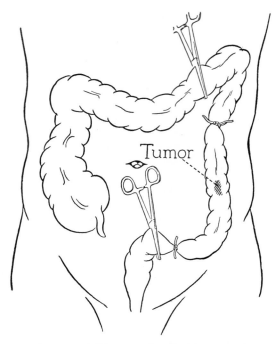

Fɪɢ. 37-15. First step in effort to prevent recurrence in colonic carcinoma from implantation of intraluminal tumor cells in suture lines: ligation of bowel on each side of tumor. (Cole, W. H.: J.A.M.A. *155*: 1549)

Anastomosis. Lloyd-Davies (1948) studied 65 rectal resections in which a rectal stump was left intact (19 with inversion of the stump, Hartmann procedure, and 46 with anastomosis) in which there were 16 local recurrences (24.6%). These local recurrences included those at the suture line, along drainage tracts and apparent second primary carcinomata. He listed 3 possible causes: (1) inadequate removal of the primary tumor, (2) implantation of cancer cells at the time of operation. In this connection he stated: "We know that this can occur as we have instances of adenocarcinomata developing at the external openings of fistulous tracks, there being no direct continuity with the primary tumour in the bowel," and (3) a traumatic factor caused by suturing since quite a number of these recurrences have occurred on the rectal rather than on the colonic side of the anastomosis. It would seen that this third explanation could be supplanted by assuming a local implanta-

tion of exuded cancer cells from the lumen along the suture tracks.

Goligher, Dukes, and Bussey (1951), on the basis of 23 recurrences following sphincter-saving operations for carcinoma of the rectum and rectosigmoid, concluded that:

there may be a danger of cancer cells, present in the lumen of the bowel below a rectal carcinoma, becoming engrafted on any raw surface with which they are allowed to come in contact . . . in possibly half the cases we think that the so-called recurrences may have been due to surgical implantation at the first operation.

Cole (1951, 1952) and Le Quesne and Thomson (1958) extended and elaborated this hypothesis. In 55 patients with local resection of the colon and the rectum, 9 or 16 per cent developed local recurrence and 6 of these (11% of all cases, 66% of the recurrences) were at the suture line. Cole pointed out that such recurrences are explained best by the downward washing of cancer cells in the lumen of the bowel, these cells becoming implanted on the raw surface at the point of anastomosis. This theory is substantiated by the fact that recurrence seldom develops at a proximal colostomy in cases of abdominoperineal resection. Colcock (1956) and Le Quesne and Thomson (1958) also advocated isolation of the tumor-bearing portion of the colon with ligatures before proceeding with the resection.

The importance of "shed cells" from bowel tumors is further substantiated by the recent studies of Le Blond (1956) who demonstrated by radioactive and other technics that the entire mucosal surface epithelium of the colon is replaced every 36 hours. This means an extensive and surprising degree of exfoliation. Millions of cells are involved, and when it is remembered that malignant cells may grow more rapidly than normal ones, the chances of such cells being in the lumen become even more understandable.

Cole advocated a technic to obviate implantation of cancer cells in the line of anastomosis following resection for carcinoma of the colon or rectosigmoid, as follows:

Step 1: Ligation of the bowel with umbilical tape several centimeters above and below the tumor before any manipulation incident to the operation is carried out (Fig. 37-15).

Step 2: Irrigation of the two ends of the bowel to be anastomosed for three to five minutes with distilled water (Fig. 37-16). (We irrigate the lower end through a previously placed enema tube from below and with aqueous Zephiran or other mild antiseptic. This obviates Step 3 so far as the lower end is concerned.)

Step 3: After the irrigation, a small segment is cut off each end before anastomosis to minimize the possibility of implanting cancer cells into these cut surfaces of the bowel.

5. *Spread by Direct Extension to Contiguous Organs.* In males spread to the prostate (Ganem, Wallwork, Jolliffe and Kay, 1957) or from the prostate to the rectum (Winter, 1957) may make the decision difficult at the time of operation as to exactly where the tumor arose. Involvement of the small bowel is a simpler matter, since the tumor has almost always arisen in the colorectum. Such spread is not a reason for defeatism, and the results of pelvic exenteration in such cases are often surprisingly good. Even in the presence of gastrocolic fistula (Clay

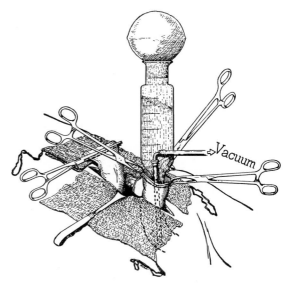

Fig. 37-16. Second step to prevent implantation of intraluminal tumor cells in suture lines: irrigation of bowel. After this irrigation, a small segment is cut off each end before anastomosis. (Cole, W. H.: A.M.A. Arch. Surg. *65*: 268)

TABLE 13. SUMMARY OF OPERATIONS SUITABLE FOR CARCINOMA IN DIFFERENT PORTIONS OF THE COLORECTUM

SITE OF TUMOR	RESECTION	ANASTOMOSIS OR COLOSTOMY
1. Cecum	Right hemicolectomy	Terminal ileum → Right transverse colon
2. Ascending colon	Right hemicolectomy	Terminal ileum → Right transverse colon
3. Hepatic flexure	Right hemicolectomy + transverse colectomy	Terminal ileum → Left transverse colon
4. Transverse colon	Right hemicolectomy + excision upper third left colon	Terminal ileum → Upper descending colon
5. Splenic flexure	Right hemicolectomy* + excision upper half left colon	Terminal ileum → Mid-descending colon
6. Descending colon	Left hemicolectomy	Left transverse colon → rectum
7. Sigmoid	Left hemicolectomy	Left transverse colon → rectum
8. Rectosigmoid	Left hemicolectomy (or left lower colectomy†)	Left transverse colon (or upper descending colon) → rectum
9. Rectum	Left lower colectomy (or left hemicolectomy†) with abdominoperineal resection	Abdominal or pull-through anal

* The lower ascending colon and cecum may be left in place (Fig. 5-C, Chap. 33). Colcock (1956) and Coller, Ransom and Regan (1956) also advocated leaving intact the cecum and the lower ascending colon in cases of resection for carcinoma of the left half of the transverse colon. Some of the Editors would remove more or less colon than advised above. Thus for sites 4, 5 and 6, one (C.M.) would have the excision go down to the sigmoid in 4 and 5 and start at the midtransverse colon in 6. In essence, this Editor performs only 3 operations for carcinoma of the colorectum: colectomy + ileosigmoidostomy, Miles, and resection with pelvic exenteration. For the same tumors, another Editor would remove only the part supplied by the middle colic artery (4), preserve the right half of the colon (5) and do as advised above (6).

† The decision as to whether to do a left hemicolectomy or a left lower colectomy (with section of the inferior mesenteric artery at its origin in either instance) is based upon the adequacy of the blood supply through the left portion of the middle colic artery at a distance from its origin and upon the relative ease with which the transverse or descending colon can be brought down for anastomosis and *not* upon the differences between these technics as a "cancer operation."

and Ravitch, 1957), the result is far from hopeless. Gilbertson (1960) found that most recurrences start locally.

Extended resection (Ault, 1953, 1958; Butcher and Spjut, 1959) is becoming recognized as a useful procedure. The facts that "after it reaches 1.5 cm. in diameter, the percentage of metastases to lymph nodes from colon carcinoma is not altered by the size of the lesion in direct contradistinction to cancer of the breast" (Moyer, 1960), and that different colon carcinomas do vary in their biologic propensities are both in favor of extended resection. At the Barnes Hospital, in cases with attachment to regional structures, if pelvic exenteration is done, removing these involved structures *en bloc*, a 5-year survival rate of 50 per cent results, as opposed to 0 per cent to 5 per cent for a Miles resection for the same sized lesion attached to contiguous organs such as the prostate, the bladder, or the uterus.

SELECTION OF OPERATION FOR TUMORS AT DIFFERENT SITES IN THE COLORECTUM. This is based on striking a proper balance between a good cancer operation, i.e., one which removes as much as possible so as to increase the percentage of 5-year arrests, and a good comfort operation, i.e., one which makes the patient's future lifespan as comfortable as possible. It is our opinion that in dealing with carcinoma of the colorectum the surgeon's first attention should be directed toward cure and *only* then should comfort be considered. In society practice, the operator may place undue stress on the avoidance of colostomy, etc. Comfort depends on lack of pain and on preservation of as many of the normal functions as possible.

Excellent plans for dealing with tumors in various parts of the left colorectum are shown in Figures 37-17 to 37-21, based on the work of Rosi (1954) and of Rosi and Capos (1955), and in Table 13. These recommendations are

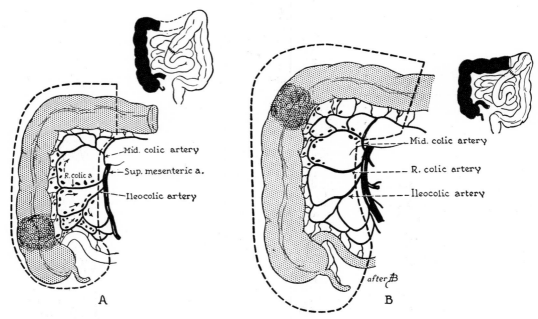

FIG. 37-17. (A) Carcinoma of the cecum. Lymphatic spread is along the ileocolic group of lymph nodes. Extent of resection, indicated by dotted line, includes tumor and potentially involved regional lymph nodes. In our opinion, the lowest branch of the superior mesenteric artery (A) should be ligated proximal to its first branching and not distally as shown. Inset shows site of ileocolic anastomosis. (B) Carcinoma of hepatic flexure. Lymphatic spread is along the right and the middle colic arteries. Line of resection includes tumor, omentum and regional lymph nodes. Inset shows the continuity of the bowel re-established by an anastomosis of the ileum to the splenic flexure. (Rosi, P. A.: S. Clin. North America *34*:225)

FIG. 37-18. Carcinoma of the splenic flexure. Lymphatic spread is to the nodes that lie on the middle colic and the left colic arterial arcade. Line of resection includes ascending (not all surgeons would remove this, since the nodes along the right colic and the ileocolic arteries are seldom involved), transverse and descending colon and all the lymph nodes along the middle colic and the left colic arteries. Inset shows anastomosis between the ileum and the sigmoid. (Rosi, P. A., and Capos, N. J.: S. Clin. North America *35*:1323)

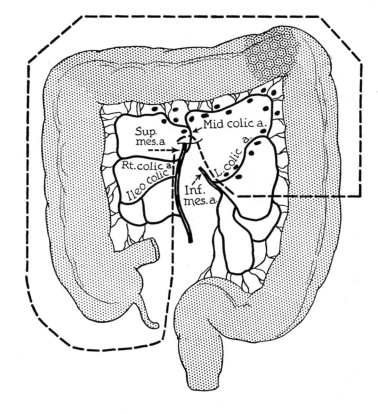

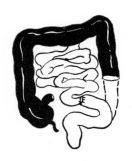

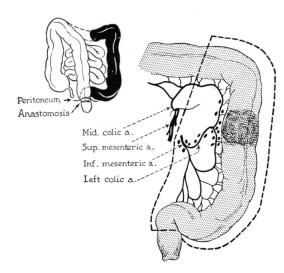

Peritoneum →
Anastomosis

Mid. colic a.
Sup. mesenteric a.
Inf. mesenteric a.
Left colic a.

quite similar to those of Hughes (1959) as portrayed in his monograph on "Surgery of the Colon," and by Abel (1957) in his Bradshaw Lecture given before the Royal College of Surgeons of England.

For lesions of the cecum and the ascending colon, ileotransverscolostomy, utilizing an anastomosis of the terminal ileum to the transverse colon but *sparing* the main trunk of the middle colic artery, is a rational procedure. For lesions of the hepatic flexure or the transverse colon, the same operation is done, *removing* the middle colic artery.

For operations to remove cancers of the

FIG. 37-19. Carcinoma of the descending colon and sigmoid. Lymphatic spread is to the regional lymph nodes and the inferior mesenteric and the periaortic group of nodes. Line of resection includes the tumor and the entire mesentery of the left colon. Inset shows continuity of the bowel reestablished by transverse colon-rectal anastomosis. (Rosi, P. A., and Capos, N. J.: S. Clin. North America *35*:1324)

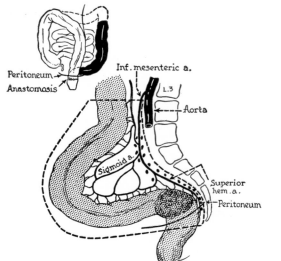

Peritoneum
Anastomosis
Inf. mesenteric a.
L.3
Aorta
Sigmoid a.
Superior hem. a.
Peritoneum

FIG. 37-20. Carcinoma of the rectosigmoid. Lymphatic spread is upward toward the inferior mesenteric group of nodes, but retrograde spread into the nodes of the mesorectum may occur. Line of resection includes the tumor, the inferior mesenteric and the periaortic nodes and from 12 to 15 cm. of bowel and mesentery below the tumor. The tumor shown in this figure is so low that only surgeons with considerable experience can safely remove it by anterior resection. Inset shows descending colon-rectal anastomosis (because of better circulation in the left transverse colon, we often anastomose it to the rectum). (Rosi, P. A., and Capos, N. J.: S. Clin. North America *35*:1326)

FIG. 37-21. Carcinoma of the lower rectum. Lymphatic spread is upward toward the inferior mesenteric group of nodes and laterally along the middle hemorrhoidal, the hypogastric and the iliac groups of nodes. Line of resection includes the tumor, the mesentery of the left colon, and nodes along the middle hemorrhoidal, the hypogastric and the iliac arteries and the perianal muscles and the skin. Inset shows completed abdominoperineal resection with colostomy in the region of the splenic flexure. Whereas the colostomy comes from the splenic flexure, in our opinion it should be placed more centrally on the abdomen. (Rosi, P. A., and Capos, N. J.: S. Clin. North America *35*: 1328)

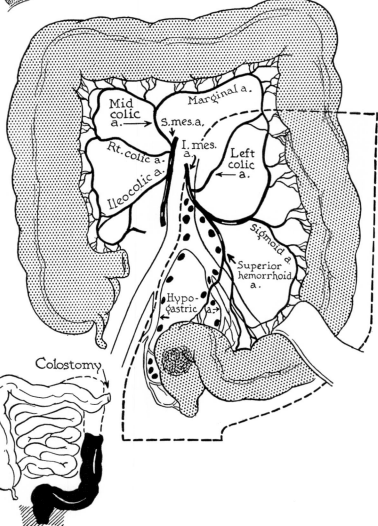

Mid colic a.
Marginal a.
S. mes. a.
I. mes. a.
Rt. colic a.
Left colic a.
Ileocolic a.
Sigmoid a.
Superior hemorrhoid. a.
Hypogastric a.
Colostomy

lower rectum that *have not infiltrated* through the rectum, the classic operation of Miles (1908) is still advocated (Beahrs and Congdon, 1957, and Black and Botham, 1957), with a higher ligation of the inferior mesenteric artery than originally described. This ligation is shown in Figure 37-21 and is based upon the lymph node spread, as shown in Figure 37-14. (See also Figure 33-7, Chapter 33, which utilizes the lower point of ligation.) Failure to ligate the artery high enough may explain in part why in the past the 5-year arrest rate has been better with right than with left colon lesions (Rosi, 1954; Morgan and Griffiths, 1959). We advise ligation of this artery at the site of its origin from the aorta, not even at Miles' point: "The inferior mesenteric artery is then ligatured below the point where it gives off its uppermost branch to the pelvic colon" (Miles, 1908) (see Fig. 37-22). Ligation of the superior hemorrhoidal artery at Sudek's critical point, just proximal to the last sigmoid branch, "was not intended to have any relationship to the Miles abdominoperineal resection or to anterior resection" (Ault, Castro and Smith, 1950, 1952). As these authors have shown, even though such a ligation is above the left colic artery, viability of the distal end of the descending colon is maintained.

However, with anterior resection, Sudek's point is applicable as demonstrated in the following anatomic review: The surgical importance of the marginal artery of the colon, formed by branches of the superior and the inferior mesenteric arteries, was first pointed out by Drummond (1913). This artery is usually adequate but may be deficient, especially in two places: at the splenic flexure (hence the need for use of the *transverse* colon for anastomosis or colostomy in cases of sigmoid or rectal carcinoma *if* the inferior mesenteric artery has been ligated at its junction with the aorta), or between the lowest sigmoid and the superior rectal arteries (hence the need for ligating *above* Sudek's point to preserve nutrition of the upper end of the rectal stump in some anterior resections of the rectum).

The *vasa recta longa* are branches of the marginal artery of Drummond. They divide at the edge of the colon in the mesocolic fat, course around the colon in the subperitoneal

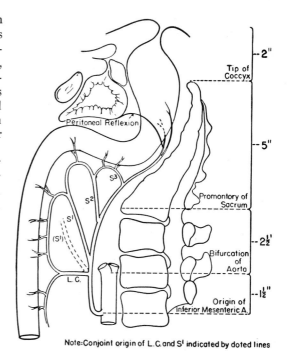

Note:Conjoint origin of L.C.and S¹ indicated by doted lines

FIG. 37-22. Diagram illustrating the most common levels at which the various branches of the inferior mesenteric artery arise. Measurements are related to the origin of the inferior mesenteric artery, the caudal edge of the aortic bifurcation, and the promontory of the sacrum. (L.C.—left colic, S—sigmoidal.) (Ault, G. W., *et al.*: Postgrad. Med. *8*:178)

coat as far as the antimesenteric taeniae, where they penetrate the circular muscular coat obliquely and lie beneath that coat all the way to their junction at the antimesenteric border (cf.: small intestine where the vasarecta penetrate the muscle coat almost immediately after division). An important surgical anatomic point is that where the vasa recta course through the subperitoneal fat just before reaching the antimesenteric teniae, they may make a U-shaped loop in the base of the appendices epiploicae which lie just on the mesenteric side of the tenia. Since this loop does not rise more than 2 mm. above the wall of the bowel, surgical removal of an appendix epiploica by ligature at its base, so long as such a ligature is not flush with the bowel wall and if traction is not applied to the appendix epiploica, can be considered a safe procedure (Brockis and Moffat, 1958), but a radical removal with a suture ligature penetrating the bowel wall may ligate the vasa recta and cause necrosis of the corresponding antimesenteric edge of the colon.

The final test of viability of any stump of rectum or colon should be the continuation of normal bowel wall color after several minutes observation period, *plus* the presence of arterial bleeding from the cut stump.

TECHNICAL POINTS IN LEFT COLON RESECTION. The technical points as outlined below are listed here, both because carcinomas in this part of the colorectum are the most frequent and because they demonstrate an application of the principles involved, particularly as regards control of spread of carcinoma, as an example. It is understood that this method is not the only way to do this type of work but serves as a basis for consideration of other technics.

OUTLINE OF PREOPERATIVE PREPARATION IN LEFT COLON SURGERY FOR CARCINOMA

1. Sterilization of bowel.
   a. Sulfasuxidine—4 Gm. t.i.d. × 5 days
   b. Mineral oil—1 oz. b.i.d. × 5 days
   c. Menadione—5 mg. b. i. d. × 5 days
2. Decompression and cleansing of bowel.
   a. Castor oil—2 oz. operative day minus 2. Repeat operative day minus 1 if poor result
   b. Clear liquid diet—operative day minus 2
   c. Nasogastric suction tube—operative day minus 1
3. Skin preparation: nipple line to below knees.

16-STEP OUTLINE OF OPERATIVE TECHNIC IN LEFT COLON SURGERY FOR CARCINOMA

1. Lithotomy position.
2. Prepare and drape one operative field: abdomen and perineum.
3. Insert Foley catheter.
4. Long mid-line incision.
5. Metastasis survey (liver, etc.).
6. Ligate proximal bowel with umbilical tape 2 inches above tumor.
7. Ligate inferior mesenteric vein near its entrance into splenic vein (Friesen, 1957).
8. Preaortic and precaval dissection, above downward (Castro, 1956).
9. Ligate inferior mesenteric artery. Such ligation, when done for surgery of the abdominal aorta in which the bowel is *not* removed, may lead to ischemic necrosis of the colon (Smith and Szilagyi, 1960).
10. Free bowel.

11. Ligate distal bowel if anterior resection is to be done.
12. Irrigate distal bowel—several liters 1:1,000 aqueous Zephiran through rectal tube.
13. Resect from 2 inches above the proximal umbilical tape to below the distal umbilical tape (or including anus, if Miles' resection or pull-through is done).
14. Anastomose for anterior resection; abdominal or anal colostomy for proctectomy procedures.
15: Drainage: pelvic
               suprapubic
               prevesical
16. If anterior resection is performed, dilate sphincter to 4 fingers.

The question as to whether to do an abdominoperineal resection with colostomy, a "pull through" operation with anal colostomy, or an anterior resection with end-to-end anastomosis in cases of upper rectal lesions arises. Both of the first two named procedures are about equally good as cancer operations. However, the anal colostomy (Babcock and Bacon, 1942) is more difficult to perform. Recent advocates of the abdominoperineal resection with preservation of the anal sphincter include Babcock (1947), Best and Rasmussen (1957), Hallenbeck (1958), and Waugh and Turner (1958). Anterior resection with anastomosis has been advocated by Fallis (1943), Wangensteen (1943), Mayo and Smith (1948), Mayo (1957), Mayo, Laberge and Hardy (1958), Muir (1958), and Wheelock, Toll and McKittrick (1959). Best and Rasmussen (1956) used the term "sphincter-preserving" operation only when the anastomosis is to a stump of rectum without peritoneum on its surface. These authors found this procedure to be as good a cancer operation as the abdominoperineal resection. In low anastomosis, particularly when done as a palliative procedure, the side-of-colon to end-of-rectal-stump method of Baker (1950) is particularly useful. Aside from the classical abdominoperineal operation, the perineoabdominal approach (Weinstein and Roberts, 1956), or the 2-team approach are to be considered. If mutiple tumors are present (McGregor and Bacon, 1958), or suspected, operative coloscopy is advised with individualization of the operation to fit the patient.

Complications. Urinary complications (Emmett, 1957; and Salvati and Kleckner (1957), and sexual malfunction (Stahlgren and Ferguson, 1958), are among those complications which follow these operations. Hughes (1959) presents a summary of fatal complications.

The complications of colorectal surgery are not inconsiderable. Nearly 100 per cent of the patients have temporary difficulties with voiding, some have serious delay in recovery in this respect, some never recover entirely. Many men have need for a later prostatectomy. Almost all patients with abdominoperineal resection for carcinoma have some postoperative sexual difficulty, either with erection or ejaculation or both, in contradistinction to a similar resection for ulcerative colitis, or congenital polyposis for which the dissection is close to the rectum. In operations for carcinoma with adequate pelvic resection there is no adequate way of preventing such a complication and younger male patients should be warned concerning it before operation. Other complications include late wound infections in the properitoneal fat, necrosis of the colostomy stump if proper attention is not paid to the blood supply of the colon loop, and leakage at the site of the anastomosis, particularly when colon is joined to colon or to rectum.

Prognosis and Results. The results vary with the location of the tumor, its extent, the presence or absence of nodes, and the operation performed. General discussions as to prognosis and results are those of Bacon (1957a, 1957b); Buckwalter (1957); Dukes and Bussey (1958); Postlethwait, Adamson and Hart (1958); Ginzburg, Freund and Dreiling (1959); and Gregg, Chamberlain and Vercillo (1959). The figures given by Rosi (1954) reveal a better result in right than in left colon lesions (right half of colon, 57 per cent 5-year survival; splenic flexure, 25

TABLE 15. FIVE- AND 10-YEAR SURVIVAL RATES FOLLOWING ABDOMINOPERINEAL RESECTION FOR CARCINOMA OF THE RECTUM AS INFLUENCED BY THE PRESENCE OF POSITIVE LYMPH NODES IN THE OPERATIVE SPECIMEN

LENGTH OF FOLLOW-UP	SURVIVAL, PER CENT		
	Nodes −	Nodes +	Total
5 years	66.8	40.0	58.8
10 years	53.0	40.0	50.0

(From Binkley and Stearns, 1951)

per cent; descending colon, 37 per cent; rectosigmoid, 47 per cent, and rectum 48 per cent. At the University of Chicago Clinics the figures are: colon, 54 per cent and rectum, 47 per cent (Allen, 1956). In general, survival figures for intraperitoneal rectum are about 10 per cent better than for the extraperitoneal rectum (Tables 12 and 14). In Table 15, the deleterious effect of the presence of positive nodes in another series is presented. On the basis of their most recent statistics, Mayo and Fly (1956) concluded that anterior resection, in lesions from 6 to 15 cm. from the dentate margin, gives as good curative results as does a nonsphincter-saving operation. Yoon (1959) reported studies indicating that the more local eosinophilic infiltration in colorectal carcinoma, the better the prognosis. On the other hand, the higher the blood eosinophil count, the worse the prognosis.

In certain unresectable tumors when cure is clearly impossible, or when the patient's general condition is too poor to stand resection, conservative treatment, especially with surgical diathermy by the method of Strauss (1935), and Strauss, Saphir, and Appel (1956) gives results which are good enough to warrant a trial. This method has also been used by Kergin (1953), Rosenthal and Turell

TABLE 14. FIVE-YEAR SURVIVAL RATES FOR CARCINOMA OF THE RECTUM DEPENDING ON THE LEVEL OF THE TUMOR

TYPE OF OPERATION	TOTAL NUMBER OF CASES	FIVE-YEAR SURVIVAL RATE		
		Nodes −	Nodes +	Total
Nonpalliative anterior resection	272	74.0	58.5	67.7
Abdominoperineal (0-4 cm. from dentate line)	51	—	—	40.7
Abdominoperineal (5-9 cm. from dentate line)	74	—	—	43.6
Abdominoperineal (10-14 cm. from dentate line)	60	—	—	57.9
Radical posterior resection with double-barreled colostomy	475	54.2	28.8	44.8

(From Dixon: Ann. Surg., 1948)

(1958), and by Wittoesch and Jackman (1958).

MALIGNANT TUMORS: RARER LESIONS

Among malignant tumors, adenocarcinoma is so preponderantly of major importance among the lesions of the colon and the rectum that other lesions will only be listed. These include: (1) fibrosarcoma, (2) leiomyosarcoma (Lewis, 1950; and Gordon and Segal, 1959), (3) lymphosarcoma, (4) malignant carcinoid metastasizing to distant organs, (5) malignant melanoma (Delaney, Scudamore and Waugh, 1954), (6) squamous cell carcinoma (Dixon, Dockerty and Powelson, 1954) and (7) hemangiopericytoma (Ault, Smith, and Castro, 1951).

BIBLIOGRAPHY

Abel, A. L.: Diagnosis and treatment of diseases of the large intestine, Ann. Roy. Coll. Surgeons England 20:329-348, 1957.

Allen, J. G.: Personal communication, June 27, 1956.

Andrén, L., and Frieberg, S.: Frequency of polyps of rectum and colon, according to age, and relation to cancer, Gastroenterology 36:631-632, 1959.

Ault, G. W.: The relationship between rectal polyps and rectal carcinoma, J. Kentucky M.A. 50:108-111, 1952.

————: Carcinoma of the rectum: factors responsible for recurrent or residual disease, Am. Surgeon 19:1035-1044, 1953.

————: A technique for cancer isolation and extended dissection for cancer of the distal colon and rectum, Surg., Gynec. & Obst. 106:467-477, 1958.

Ault, G. W., Castro, A. F., and Smith, R. S.: Carcinoma of the upper rectum and rectosigmoid, clinical report on high inferior mesenteric ligation, Postgrad. Med. 8:176-183, 1950.

————: Clinical study of ligation of the inferior mesenteric artery in left colon resections, Surg., Gynec. & Obst. 94:223-228, 1952.

Ault, G. W., Smith, R. S., and Castro, A. F.: Hemangiopericytoma of the sigmoid colon, Surgery 30:523-527, 1951.

Aylett, S.: Total colectomy and ileo-rectal anastomosis as the treatment of choice in ulcerative colitis, Acta chir. belg. 58:597-607, 1959.

Babcock, W. W.: Radical single stage extirpation for cancer of the large bowel, with retained functional anus, Surg., Gynec. & Obst. 85:1-7, 1947.

Babcock, W. W., and Bacon, H. E.: One-stage abdomino-perineal proctosigmoidectomy, S. Clin. North America 22:1631-1662, 1942.

Bacon, H. E.: Cancer of the colon, rectum and anal canal, Am. J. Surg. 94:567-572, 1957.

————: Cancer of the rectum and colon, Surgery 41:387-400, 1957.

Bacon, H. E., Lowell, E. J., Jr., and Trimpi, H. D.: Villous papillomas of the colon and rectum: a study of 28 cases with end results of treatment over a 5-year period, Surgery 35:77-87, 1954.

Bacon, H. E., and Peale, A. R.: Appraisal of adenomatous polyps of the colon, their histopathology and surgical management, Ann. Surg. 144:9-18, 1956.

Bacon, H. E., and Trimpi, H. D.: The selection of an operative procedure for patients with medically intractable ulcerative colitis, Surg., Gynec. & Obst. 91:409-420, 1950.

Bailey, J. J., Barrick, C. W., and Jenkinson, E. L.: Hemangioma of the colon, J.A.M.A. 160:658-659, 1956.

Baker, J. W.: Low end-to-side rectosigmoidal anastomosis: description of technic, Arch. Surg. 61:143-157, 1950.

Baker, J. W., Margetts, L. H., and Schutt, R. P.: Distal and proximal margin of resection in carcinoma of pelvic colon and rectum, Ann. Surg. 141:693-706, 1955.

Baker, W. J., and Graf, E. C.: Experiences with the ileal conduit in urinary diversion, J. Urol. 75:950-960, 1956.

Bartholomew, L. G., and Dahlin, D. C.: Intestinal polyposis and mucocutaneous pigmentation (Peutz-Jeghers Syndrome): further comments and report of an additional case, Minnesota Med. 41:848-852, 1958.

Bartholomew, L. G., Dahlin, D. C., and Waugh, J. M.: Intestinal polyposis associated with mucocutaneous melanin pigmentation, Gastroenterology 30:434-451, 1957 (Abstr. Proc. Staff Meet. Mayo Clin. 32:675-680, 1957).

Beahrs, O. H., and Congdon, G. H.: Morbidity and mortality following combined abdomino-perineal resection, with special reference to closure of the posterior wound, S. Clin. North America 37:999-1007, 1957.

Berkowitz, S. B., Pearl, M. J., and Shapiro, N. H.: Syndrome of intestinal polyposis with melanosis of the lips and buccal mucosa: a study of the incidence and location of malignancy, Ann. Surg. 141:129-133, 1955.

Best, R. R.: Anastomosis of the ileum to the lower part of the rectum and anus: report on experiences with ileorectostomy and ileoproctostomy, with special reference to polyposis, Arch. Surg. *57*:276-285, 1948.

Best, R. R., and Rasmussen, J. A.: Sphincter-preserving operations for cancer of the rectum, A.M.A. Arch. Surg. *72*:948-956, 1956.

————: Results of sphincter-preserving operations for carcinoma of midrectum, J.A.M.A. *164*:739-744, 1957.

Binkley, G. E., and Stearns, M. W., Jr.: Ten year surgical results of rectal cancer, Surg., Gynec. & Obst. *93*:428-430, 1951.

Binkley, G. E., Sunderland, D. A., Miller, C. J., Stearns, M., and Deddish, M. R.: Carcinoma arising in adenomas of colon and rectum, J.A.M.A. *148*:1465-1469, 1952.

Black, B. M., and Botham, R. J.: Combined abdominoendorectal resection. A critical reappraisal based on 91 cases, S. Clin. North America *37*:989-997, 1957.

Blackberg, B.: Recurrent intussusception due to gastrointestinal polyposis in Peutz-Jeghers syndrome, Acta chir. scandinav. *119*:45-54, 1960.

Brasher, P. H.: Clinical and social problems associated with familial intestinal polyposis, Arch. Surg. *69*:785-796, 1954.

Bricker, E. M.: Bladder substitution after pelvic evisceration, S. Clin. North America *30*:1511-1521, 1950.

Brockis, J. G., and Moffat, D. B.: The intrinsic blood vessels of the pelvic colon, J. Anat. *92*:52-56, 1958.

Brooke, B. N.: Management of ileostomy including its complications, Lancet *2*:102-104, 1952.

Buckwalter, J. A.: Abdominoperineal resection morbidity. Preoperative and operative factors, A.M.A. Arch. Surg. *74*:770-779, 1957.

Buie, L. A., and Brust, J. C. M.: Solitary adenomata of rectum and lower sigmoid, Tr. Am. Proct. Soc. *36*:57-67, 1935.

Burns, F. J., and Pfaff, J. P.: Vascular invasion in carcinoma of the colon and rectum, Am. J. Surg. *92*:704-709, 1956.

Buskirk, van, W. C.: Polyps of the large bowel, Ann. Surg. *141*:234-239, 1955.

Butcher, H. R., Jr., and Spjut, H. J.: An evaluation of pelvic exenteration for advanced carcinoma of the lower colon, Cancer *12*:681-687, 1959.

Castro, A. F.: Surgical technic of ligation of inferior mesenteric artery and preaortic lymphadenectomy, Surg., Gynec. & Obst. *102*:374-376, 1956.

Cattell, R. B., and Swinton, N. W.: The diagnosis and treatment of sigmoidal polyps, New England J. Med. *222*:535-540, 1940.

Chappell, F. W.: Carcinoma of the colon in young people, Am. Surgeon *25*:449-457, 1959.

Clay, R. C., and Ravitch, M. M.: Surgical treat-

ment of gastrocolic fistula due to cancer of the colon, A.M.A. Arch. Surg. *75*:793-799, 1957.

Colcock, B. P.: Surgical treatment of carcinoma of the colon, S. Clin. North America *36*:739-749, 1956.

Colcock, B. P., and Lamphier, T. A.: Endometriosis of the large bowel and small intestine, Surgery *28*:997-1004, 1950.

Colcock, B. P., and Sass, R. E.: Diverticulitis and carcinoma of the colon: differential diagnosis, Surg., Gynec. & Obst. *99*:627-633, 1954.

Cole, W. H.: Measures to combat the menace of cancer, Am. Surgeon *17*:660-663, 1951.

————: Recurrence in carcinoma of the colon and proximal rectum following resection for carcinoma, A.M.A. Arch. Surg. *65*:264-270, 1952.

Coller, F. A., and Flotte, C. T.: Multiple polyposis of the colon, J. Michigan M. Soc. *54*:1061-1063, 1955.

Coller, F. A., Ransom, H. K., and Regan, W. J., Jr.: Cancer of the Colon and Rectum, New York, American Cancer Society, 1956.

Colvert, J. R., and Brown, C. H.: Rectal polyps, diagnosis, 5 year follow-up, and relation to carcinoma of the rectum, Am. J. M. Sc. *215*:24-32, 1948.

Crile, G., Jr., and Turnbull, R. B., Jr.: The mechanism and prevention of ileostomy dysfunction, Ann. Surg. *140*:459-466, 1954.

Cripps, W. H.: Two cases of disseminated polypus of the rectum, Tr. Path. Soc., London *33*:165, 1882. Cited by Ravitch, M. M. (see reference below) 1948.

D'Alonzo, W. A.: Granuloma of the right half of the colon, J. Internat. Coll. Surgeons *29*:683-698, 1958.

————: Lipoma of sigmoid, Am. J. Surg. *94*:931-937, 1957.

David, V. C.: The management of polyps occurring in the rectum and colon, Surgery *14*:387-394, 1943.

Davies, A. J.: Carcinoid tumors (argentaffinomata), Ann. Roy. Coll. Surgeons England *25*:277-296, 1959.

Dawson, I. M. P., and Pryse-Davies, J.: The development of carcinoma of the large intestine in ulcerative colitis, Brit. J. Surg. *47*:113-128, 1959.

Deddish, M. R., and Hertz, R. E.: Symposium of early diagnosis of tumors of rectum and colon: colotomy and coloscopy in management of mucosal polyps and cancer of colon, Am. J. Surg. *90*:846-849, 1955.

Delaney, L. T., Scudamore, H. H., and Waugh, J. M.: Malignant melanoma of the rectum: report of case, Proc. Staff Meet. Mayo Clin. *29*:416-420, 1954.

Devine, J., and Webb, R.: Resection of rectal mucosa, colectomy, and anal ileostomy, with normal continence, Surg., Gynec. & Obst. 92: 437-442, 1951.

Dixon, C. F.: Anterior resection for malignant lesions of the upper part of the rectum and lower part of the sigmoid, Ann. Surg. 128:425-442, 1948.

Dixon, C. F., Dockerty, M. B., and Powelson, M. H.: Squamous cell carcinoma of the mid-rectum: report of case, Proc. Staff Meet. Mayo Clin. 29:420-423, 1954.

Dockerty, M. B.: Pathologic aspects in the control of spread of colonic carcinoma, Proc. Staff Meet. Mayo Clin. 33:157-163, 1958.

Drummond, H.: Some points relating to the surgical anatomy of the arterial supply of the large intestine, Proc. Royal Soc. Med. (Surgical Section, Subsection of Proctology) 7:185-193, 1914.

Dukes, C. E.: Familial intestinal polyposis, Ann. Roy. Coll. Surgeons England 10:293-304, 1952.

Dukes, C. E., and Bussey, H. J. R.: The spread of rectal cancer and its effects on prognosis, Brit. J. Cancer 12:309-320, 1958.

Dukes, C. E., and Lockhart-Mummery, H. E.: Familial intestinal polyposis, S. Clin. North America 35:1277-1281, 1955.

————: Practical points in the pathology and surgical treatment of ulcerative colitis, Brit. J. Surg. 45:25-36, 1957.

Dunn, H. L.: Vital Statistics of the United States, 1953, vol. 2, Washington, D. C., U. S. Government Printing Office, 1955.

Dunphy, J. E., and Broderick, E. G.: A critique of anterior resection in the treatment of cancer of the rectum and pelvic colon, Surgery 30: 106-115, 1951.

Durham, M. W.: Familial cancer of the colon, West. J. Surg. 62:26-31, 1954.

————: Simplified technique for ileostomy construction, Surgery 41:984-985, 1957.

Emmett, J. L.: Treatment of vesical dysfunction after operations on the rectum and sigmoid, S. Clin. North America 37:1009-1017, 1957.

Enquist, I. F.: The incidence and significance of polyps of the colon and rectum, Surgery 42: 681-688, 1957.

Everson, T. C., and Allen, M. J.: Subtotal colectomy with ileosigmoidostomy and fulguration of polyps in retained colon: evaluation as method of treatment of polyposis (adenomatosis) of colon, A.M.A. Arch. Surg. 69:806-817, 1954.

Falkinburg, L. W., and Key, M. N.: Intestinal polyposis with oral pigmentation (Peutz-Jeghers syndrome): report of a case with review, J. Pediat. 54:162-169, 1959.

Fallis, L. S.: Anterior resection of the rectosigmoid and upper rectum with re-establishment of continuity, Surgery 14:397-402, 1943.

————: One-stage total colectomy for ulcerative colitis, Am. J. Surg. 92:696-699, 1956.

Fallis, L. S., and Barron, J.: Modified technique for total colectomy in ulcerative colitis, A.M.A. Arch. Surg. 67:363-369, 1953.

————: Total colectomy in ulcerative colitis, West J. Surg. 63:452-455, 1955.

Feldman, M.: Unrecognized carcinoma of the cecum diagnosed preoperatively as appendicitis, Am. Surgeon 24:495-498, 1958.

Fisher, E. R., and Castro, A. F.: Diffuse papillomatous polyps (villous tumors) of the colon and rectum: pathologic and clinical observations, Am. J. Surg. 85:146-151, 1953.

Fisher, E. R., and Turnbull, R. B., Jr.: The cytologic demonstration and significance of tumor cells in the mesenteric venous blood in patients with colorectal carcinoma, Surg., Gynec. & Obst. 100:102-108, 1955.

Friedman, M. H. W., and MacKenzie, W. C.: Simple ulcer of the colon: report of four cases, Canad. J. Surg. 2:1-8, 1959.

Friesen, S. R.: Criteria for satisfactory colectomy for carcinoma of the left colon, A.M.A. Arch. Surg. 75:342-351, 1957.

Ganem, E. J., Wallwork, D. W., Jolliffe, L. S., and Kay, J.: Rectal carcinoma invading the prostate gland, A.M.A. Arch. Surg. 75:85-89, 1957.

Gants, R. T., Raymond, B. A., and Pope, J. K.: Extended colotomy incisions for intraluminal examination of the colon: a report of experimental investigation and clinical application, Ann. Surg. 144:865-871, 1956.

Gilbertsen, V. A.: Adenocarcinoma of the rectum: incidence and locations of recurrent tumor following present-day operations performed for cure, Ann. Surg. 151:340-348, 1960.

Gilchrist, R. K.: Discussion of paper by Judd and Carlisle, A.M.A. Arch. Surg. 67:362, 1953.

————: (1958): Discussion of paper by Spratt, Ackerman and Moyer (see reference below) 1958.

————: Lymphatic spread of carcinoma of the colon, Dis. Colon & Rect. 2:69-76, 1959.

Gilchrist, R. K., and David, V. C.: A consideration of pathological factors influencing five-year survival in radical resection of the large bowel and rectum for carcinoma, Ann. Surg. 126:421-438, 1947.

Ginzburg, L., Freund, S., and Dreiling, D. A.: Mortality and major complications following resection for carcinoma of the large bowel, Ann. Surg. 150:913-927, 1959.

Goble, A. J., Hay, D. R., and Sandler, M.:

5-Hydroxytryptamine metabolism in acquired heart disease associated with argentaffin carcinoma, Lancet 2:1016-1017, 1955.

Goldgraber, M. B., and Kirsner, J. B.: Papilloma of the large intestine: a clinical pathologic correlation, Gastroenterology 35:36-49, 1958.

Goligher, J. C., Dukes, C. E., and Bussey, H. J. R.: Local recurrences after sphincter-saving excision for carcinoma of the rectum and rectosigmoid, Brit. J. Surg. 39:199-211, 1951.

Gordon, E. T., and Segal, A. L.: Leiomyosarcoma of the rectum, Am. J. Surg. 98:105-106, 1959.

Gregg, R. O., Chamberlain, B. E., and Vercillo, A. A.: Carcinoma of colon and rectum; survey of surgical management in central New York State, J.A.M.A. 170:143-148, 1959.

Grinnell, R. S.: The rationale of subtotal and total colectomy in the treatment of cancer and multiple polyps of the colon, Surg., Gynec. & Obst. 106:288-292, 1958.

Grinnell, R. S., and Lane, N.: Benign and malignant adenomatous polyps and papillary adenomas of the colon and rectum. An analysis of 1856 tumors in 1335 patients, Surg., Gynec. & Obst. 106:519-538, 1958.

Grodsky, L.: Neurofibroma of the rectum in a patient with von Recklinghausen's disease, Am. J. Surg. 95:474-476, 1958.

Guillard, J., Laumonier, R., Seyer, J., and Boulet, R.: Intestinal polyposis associated with melanin spots: Peutz-Jeghers syndrome, Presse méd. 66:2076-2079, 1959; Abstr. J.A.M.A. 170:367, 1959.

Gunn, H., and Howard, N. J.: Amebic granulomas of the large bowel, J.A.M.A. 97:166-170, 1931.

Haas, A., and Ritter, S. A.: Leiomyoma of the rectum: report of a case, Dis. Colon & Rect. 3:65-66, 1960.

Hallenbeck, G. A.: Sphincter saving operations for carcinoma of the distal twenty centimeters of the rectum and colon, Gastroenterology 34:313-319, 1958.

Hamilton, J. E., Harbrecht, P. J., and Lucas, M. A.: Rehabilitation of the ulcerative colitis patient with special reference to one stage proctocolectomy and matured ileostomy, Ann. Surg. 149:822-832, 1959.

Hayes, H. T., Burr, H. B., and Melton, W. T.: Submucous lipoma of the colon: review of the literature and report of four cases, Dis. Colon & Rect. 3:145-148, 1960.

Helwig, E. B.: The evolution of adenomas of the large intestine and their relation to carcinoma, Surg., Gynec. & Obst. 84:36-49, 1947.

————: Adenomas and the pathogenesis of cancer of the colon and rectum, Dis. Colon & Rect. 2:5-17, 1959.

Hellwig, C. A., and Barbosa, E.: How reliable is biopsy of rectal polyps?, Cancer 12:620-624, 1959.

Henderson, R. P., Harris, E. J., and Packer, J. M.: Lipomas of the colon, with report of five cases, Am. J. Roentgenol. 79:843-849, 1958.

Hines, M. O., Hanley, P. H., and Schramel, R.: Villous tumors of the colon and rectum, South. M. J. 48:891-897, 1955.

Hoerner, M. T.: Carcinoma of the colon and rectum in persons under twenty years of age, Am. J. Surg. 96:47-53, 1958.

Hoffman, E.: Hyponatremia due to a villous adenoma of the rectosigmoid, Am. J. Surg. 98:99-104, 1959.

Holden, W. D.: Discussion of paper by Spratt, Ackerman and Moyer (see reference below) 1958.

Holtz, F., and Schmidt, L. A., III: Lymphoid polyps (benign lymphoma) of the rectum and anus, Surg., Gynec. & Obst. 106:639-642, 1958.

Horita, A. (Associate Professor of Pharmacology, Univ. of Washington School of Medicine): Personal communication, July, 1960.

Horrilleno, E. G., Eckert, C., and Ackerman, L. V.: Rectal and colonic polyps in children, Cancer 10:1210-1220, 1957.

Hoxworth, P. I., and Slaughter, D. P.: Polyposis (adenomatosis) of the colon, Surgery 24:188-211, 1948.

Hughes, E. S. R.: Fatal complications following colectomy, Australian & New Zealand J. Surg. 28:202-214, 1959.

————: Surgery of the Colon, Edinburgh, Livingstone, 1959.

Humphreys, E.: Personal communication, June 27, 1956.

Jackman, R. J., and Mayo, C. W.: The adenoma-carcinoma sequence in cancer of the colon, Surg., Gynec. & Obst. 93:327-330, 1951.

Jeghers, H.: Medical progress: pigmentation of the skin, New England J. Med. 231:88, 122, 181, 1944.

Jeghers, H., McKusick, V. A., and Katz, K. H.: Generalized intestinal polyposis and melanin spots of the oral mucosa, lips and digits: a syndrome of diagnostic significance, New England J. Med. 241:993-1005; 1031-1036, 1949.

Jenkinson, E. L., and Brown, W. A.: Endometriosis: A study of 117 cases with special reference to constricting lesions of the rectum and sigmoid colon, J.A.M.A. 122:349-354, 1943.

Johnson, J. W., Judd, E. S., and Dahlin, D. C.: Malignant neoplasms of the colon and rectum in young persons, Arch. Surg. 79:365-372, 1959.

Judd, E. S., Jr., and Carlisle, J. C.: Polyps of the colon: late results of transcolonic removal, A.M.A. Arch. Surg. 67:353-362, 1953.

Keeling, W. M., and Beatty, G. L.: Lymphoid

polyps of the rectum, A.M.A. Arch. Surg. *73*:753-756, 1956.

Kergin, F. G.: Diathermy fulgurization in treatment of certain cases of rectal carcinoma, Canad. M.A.J. *69*:14-17, 1953.

Kirsner, J. B., Moeller, H. C., and Renier, J.: Personal communication, June 27, 1956.

Klein, R. R., and Scarborough, R. A.: Diagnosis and treatment of adenomatous polyps of colon, A.M.A. Arch. Surg. *65*:65-71, 1952.

Knight, C. D.: Massive hemorrhage from diverticular disease of the colon, Surgery *42*:853-861, 1957.

Knox, W. G., Miller, R. E., Begg, C. F., and Zintel, H. A.: Juvenile polyps of the colon: a clinicopathologic analysis of 75 polyps in 43 patients, Surgery *48*:201-210, 1960.

Kolb, L. H., and Black, A.: Submucous lipoma of the colon, Am. J. Surg. *95*:471-473, 1958.

Korn, G. W., and Savage, P. T.: Endometrioma of the rectum, Brit. J. Surg. *44*:588-591, 1957.

Laberge, M. Y., Sauer, W. G., and Mayo, C. W.: Soft-tissue tumors associated with familial polyposis, Proc. Staff Meet. Mayo Clin. *32*: 749-752, 1957.

Lawrence, J. C.: Gastrointestinal polyps: statistical study of malignancy incidence, Am. J. Surg. *31*:499-505, 1936.

Le Blond, C. P.: Personal communication, July 5, 1956.

Lee, H. C., and Kay, S.: Papillary tumors of the rectum, Ann. Surg. *143*:780-790, 1956.

LeQuesne, L. P., and Thomson, A. D.: Implantation recurrence of carcinoma of rectum and colon, New England J. Med. *258*:587-582, 1958.

Lewis, A. E.: Leiomyosarcoma of rectum; report of a case, Northwest Med. *49*:272, 1950.

Lloyd-Davies, O. V.: Discussion on radical excision of carcinoma of the rectum with conservation of the sphincter, Proc. Roy. Soc. Med. *41*:822-827, 1948.

Lockhart-Mummery, J. P.: The causation and Bussey, H. J. R.: The surgical treatment of familial polyposis of the colon, Brit. J. Surg. *43*:476-481, 1956.

Lockhart-Mummery, J. P.: The causation and treatment of multiple adenomatosis of the colon, Ann. Surg. *99*:178-184, 1934.

Loe, R. H. (1952): Discussion of a paper by Klein and Scarborough (see reference above) 1952.

Lofgren, E. P., Waugh, J. M., and Dockerty, M. B.: Local recurrence of carcinoma after anterior resection of the rectum and the sigmoid. Relationship with the length of normal mucosa excised distal to the lesion, A.M.A. Arch. Surg. *74*:825-838, 1957.

Lowman, R. M., and Davis, L.: An evaluation of cecal size in impending perforation of the cecum, Surg., Gynec. & Obst. *103*:711-718, 1956.

MacDonald, R. A.: A study of 356 carcinoids of the gastrointestinal tract: report of four new cases of the carcinoid syndrome, Am. J. Med. *21*:867-878, 1956.

McGraw, J. Y., and Bonenfant, J. L.: Anorectal lymphomas, Canad. J. Surg. *3*:225-228, 1960.

McGregor, R. A., and Bacon, H. E.: Multiple cancers in colon surgery. Report of 162 cases, Surgery *44*:828-833, 1958.

McKay, J. L., and McMahon, W. A.: Management of adenomas of the colon and rectum showing malignant changes: report of 44 cases treated by local removal, Dis. Colon & Rect. *2*:298-302, 1959.

McKittrick, L. S., and Wheelock, F. C., Jr.: Carcinoma of the Colon, Springfield, Ill., Thomas, 1954.

McLanahan, S., Grove, G. P., and Kieffer, R. F., Jr.: Conservative surgical management for certain rectal adenomas showing malignant change, J.A.M.A. *141*:822-826, 1949.

McLanahan, S., and Martin, R. E.: Colotomy, coloscopy, and colectomy in the management of polyps of the large intestine, Ann. Surg. *145*:689-698, 1957.

Madison, M. S., Dockerty, M. B., and Waugh, J. M.: Venous invasion in carcinoma of the rectum as evidenced by venous radiography, Surg., Gynec. & Obst. *99*:170-178, 1954.

Mallam, A. S., and Thomson, S. A.: Polyps of the rectum and colon in children. A ten year review at the Hospital for Sick Children, Toronto, Canad. J. Surg. *3*:17-24, 1959.

Mattingly, T. W., and Sjoerdsma, A.: The cardiovascular manifestations of functioning carcinoid tumors, Mod. Concepts Cardiovas. Dis. *25*: 337-341, 1956.

Mauro, J., and Prior, J. T.: Gastrointestinal polypoid lesions in children, Cancer *10*:131-137, 1957.

Mayo, C. W.: Anterior resection for carcinoma of the lower portion of sigmoid, the rectosigmoid and the upper portion of rectum: present status, S. Clin. North America *37*:981-987, 1957.

Mayo, C. W., and Delaney, L. T.: Colonic diverticulitis associated with carcinoma, A.M.A. Arch. Surg. *72*:957-961, 1956.

Mayo, C. W., DeWeerd, J. H., and Jackman, R. J.: Diffuse familial polyposis of the colon, Surg., Gynec. & Obst. *93*:87-96, 1951.

Mayo, C. W., and Fly, O. A.: Analysis of five-year survival in carcinoma of the rectum and rectosigmoid, Surg., Gynec. & Obst. *103*:94-100, 1956.

Mayo, C. W., Laberge, M. Y., and Hardy, W. M.:

Five year survival after anterior resection for carcinoma of the rectum and rectosigmoid, Surg., Gynec. & Obst. *106*:695-698, 1958.

Mayo, C. W., and Smith, R. S.: Low anterior segmental resection with or without colostomy, Ann. Surg. *127*:1046-1055, 1948.

Mégevand, A.: Visceral polyposis and cutaneo-mucosal melanin pigmentation (Peutz Syndrome), Arch. franç. pédiat. *16*:353-361, 1959; Abstr. J.A.M.A. *171*:478-479, 1959.

Miles, W. Ernest: A method of performing abdominoperineal excision for carcinoma of the rectum and of the terminal portion of the pelvic colon, Lancet *2*:1812-1813, 1908.

Mobley, J. E., Dockerty, M. B., and Waugh, J. M.: Bleeding in colonic diverticulitis, Am. J. Surg. *94*:44-51, 1957.

Moore, H. G., Jr.: Repeated surgical attack on carcinoma of the sigmoid colon: a case report, Surgery *33*:761-765, 1953.

Moran, T. F.: Surgical treatment of villous tumors of the rectum, J. Internat. Coll. Surgeons *28*:227-233, 1957.

Morgan, C. N.: The management of carcinoma of the colon, Ann. Roy. Coll. Surgeons, England *10*:305-323, 1952.

Morgan, C. N., and Griffiths, J. D.: High ligation of inferior mesenteric artery for rectal and colonic carcinoma, Modern Medicine, pp. 170-173 (Sept. 15) 1959.

Morton, P. C.: Adenomas of the colon and rectum: diagnosis and treatment in relationship to cancer prevention, Ann. Surg. *138*:92-98, 1953.

Moyer, C. A.: Personal communication, July 13, 1960.

Mugrage, R. M.: The developing philosophy of surgery of cancer of the colon, Postgrad. Med. *26*:748-759, 1959.

Muir, E. G.: Carcinoma of the rectum and anterior resection, Australian & New Zealand J. Surg. *27*:174-182, 1958.

Noer, R. J.: Hemorrhage as a complication of diverticulitis, Ann. Surg. *141*:674, 1955.

Oberndorfer (1907): Cited by Rosser (see reference below) 1951.

Ochsner, S. F., and Ray, J. E.: Submucosal lipomas of the colon: experience with 12 cases, Dis. Colon & Rect. *3*:1-8, 1960.

Pack, G. T., and Martins, F. G.: Treatment of anorectal malignant melanoma, Dis. Colon & Rect. *3*:15-24, 1960.

Page, I. H.: Serotonin (5-Hydroxytryptamine): the last four years, Physiol. Rev. *38*:277-335, 1958.

Palumbo, L. T., and Rugtiv, G. M.: One-stage total colectomy including abdominoperineal resection with primary ileostomy: surgical treatment of chronic ulcerative colitis and familial polyposis, A.M.A. Arch. Surg. *67*:762-768, 1953.

Peskin, G. W., and Orloff, M. J.: A clinical study of 25 patients with carcinoid tumors of the rectum, Surg., Gynec. & Obst. *109*:673-682, 1959.

Peutz, J. L. A. (1921): Cited by Weber (see reference below) 1954.

Phillips, J. W., Waugh, J. M., and Dockerty, M. B.: The surgical significance of regional lymphatic drainage of the hepatic flexure, Surg., Gynec. & Obst. *99*:455-461, 1954.

Phillips, W. M., ReMine, W. H., Beahrs, O. H., and Scudamore, H. H.: Benign lesions of the cecum simulating carcinoma, J.A.M.A. *172*: 1465-1468, 1960.

Ponka, J. L., Fox, J. D., and Brush, B. E.: Co-existing carcinoma and diverticula of the colon, A.M.A. Arch. Surg. *79*:373-384, 1959.

Postlethwait, R. W.: Adamson, J. E., and Hart, D.: Carcinoma of the colon and rectum, Surg., Gynec. & Obst. *106*:257-270, 1958.

Radke, R. A.: Adenomatous polyps of the large intestine, Mil. Surgeon *115*:85-92, 1954.

Ravitch, M. M.: Anal ileostomy with sphincter preservation in patients requiring total colectomy for benign conditions, Surgery *24*:170-187, 1948.

————: Polypoid adenomatosis of the entire gastro-intestinal tract, Ann. Surg. *128*:283-298, 1948.

————: Total colectomy and abdominoperineal resection (pan-colectomy) in one stage, Ann. Surg. *144*:758-767, 1956.

Ravitch, M. M., and Handelsman, J. C.: One stage resection of entire colon and rectum for ulcerative colitis and polypoid adenomatosis, Bull. Johns Hopkins Hosp. *88*:59-82, 1951.

Rider, J. A., Kirsner, J. B., Moeller, H. C., and Palmer, W. L.: Polyps of the colon and rectum: their incidence and relationship to carcinoma, Am. J. Med. *16*:555-564, 1954.

————: Polyps of the colon and rectum, a four-year to nine-year follow-up study of five hundred thirty-seven patients, J.A.M.A. *170*:633-638, 1959.

Rives, J. D., and Emmett, R. O.: Melena, a survey of two hundred and six cases, Am. Surgeon *20*:458-470, 1954.

Roberts, S. S., Watne, A. L., McGrew, E. A., McGrath, R. G., and Cole, W. H.: Cancer cells in the circulating blood, Sci. Exhib., Am. Coll. Surgeons, October, 1957.

Rohrs, L. C.: Intestinal polyposis and pigmented spots of lips, J.A.M.A. *165*:208-210, 1957.

Rosenthal, I. I., and Baronofsky, I. D.: Prognostic and therapeutic implications of polyps in metachronous colic carcinoma, J.A.M.A. *172*: 37-41, 1960.

Rosenthal, I. I., and Turell, R.: Surgical diathermy (electrothermia) of cancer of the rectum, J.A.M.A. *167*:1602-1605, 1958.

Rosi, P. A.: Selection of operations for carcinomas of the colon, S. Clin. North America *34*:221-230, 1954.

Rosi, P. A., and Capos, N. J.: Selection of operations for carcinoma of the midtransverse colon to the rectum inclusive, S. Clin. North America *35*:1321-1329, 1955.

Rosser, C.: Carcinoid (neurocrine) tumors of the rectum, Surg., Gynec. & Obst. *93*:486-490, 1951.

Rubin, C. E.: Personal communication, July 2, 1956.

Ryrberg, C. H.: Lipoma of the colon: report of 4 cases and review of the literature, Acta chir. scandinav. *111*:45-53, 1956.

Salvati, E. P., and Kleckner, M. S.: Urinary retention in anorectal and colonic surgery, Am. J. Surg. *94*:114-117, 1957.

Sandberg, A. A., and Moore, G. E.: Examination of blood for tumor cells, J. Nat. Cancer Inst. *19*:1-11, 1957.

Sanger, B. J., and Leckie, B. D.: Plain muscle tumours of the rectum, Brit. J. Surg. *47*:196-198, 1959.

Scarborough, R. A.: Surgical treatment of ulcerative colitis, Am. J. Surg. *89*:1224-1229, 1955.

Schoenberg, H. W., Fitts, W. T., Jr., and Enterline, H. T.: Adenomatous polyps of the colon and rectum, Geriatrics *13*:718-724, 1958.

Scott, W. M., and Brand, N. E.: Giant haemangioma of rectum, Brit. J. Surg. *45*:294-296, 1957.

Shackelford, R. T., and McGeehan, J. S.: Improved technique of coloscopy, J.A.M.A. *167*: 280-284, 1958.

Sjoerdsma, A., Terry, L. L., and Udenfriend, S.: Malignant carcinoid, A.M.A. Arch. Int. Med. *99*:1009-1012, 1957.

Slaney, G., and Brooke, B. N.: Cancer in ulcerative colitis, Lancet *2*:694-698, 1959.

Smith, R. F., and Szilagyi, D. E.: Ischemia of the colon as a complication in the surgery of the abdominal aorta, A.M.A. Arch. Surg. *80*:806-821, 1960.

Spratt, J. S.: Cited by Moyer: Personal communication, July 25, 1960.

Spratt, J. S., Jr., Ackerman, L. V., and Moyer, C. A.: Relationship of polyps of the colon to colonic cancer, Ann. Surg. *148*:682-698, 1958.

Stahlgren, L. H., and Ferguson, L. K.: Influence on sexual function of abdominoperineal resection for ulcerative colitis, New England J. Med. *259*:873-878, 1958.

Stearns, M. W., Jr., Deddish, M. R., and Quan, S. H. Q.: Preoperative roentgen therapy for cancer of the rectum, Surg., Gynec. & Obst. *109*:225-229, 1959.

Stout, A. P.: Tumors of the colon and rectum (excluding carcinoma and adenoma), S. Clin. North America *35*:1283-1288, 1955.

Strauss, A. A., Saphir, O., and Appel, M.: The development of an absolute immunity in experimental animals and a relative immunity in human beings due to a necrosis of malignant tumors, Swiss Med. J. *86*:1-8, 1956.

Strauss, A. A., Strauss, S. F., Crawford, R. A., and Strauss, H. A.: Surgical diathermy of carcinoma of rectum: Its clinical end results, J.A.M.A. *104*:1480-1484, 1935.

Sudek, P.: Ueber die Gefässversorgung des Mastdarmes in Hinsicht auf die operative Gangrän, München. med. Wchnschr. *54*:1314-1317, 1907.

Sunderland, D. A., and Binkley, G. E.: Papillary adenomas of the large intestine: a clinical and morphological study of 48 cases, Cancer *1*:183-207, 1948.

Swinton, N. W.: The management of rectal polyps, S. Clin. North America *36*:751-760, 1956.

Swinton, N. W., and Doane, W. A.: The significance and treatment of polyps of the colon and rectum, New England J. Med. *249*:673-678, 1953.

Swinton, N. W., and Freedman, A. N.: Carcinoid tumors of the rectum: case report and review of the literature, Dis. Colon & Rect. *3*:189-193, 1960.

Swinton, N. W., and Snow, J. C.: Cancer of the colon and rectum, Lahey Clin. Bull. *2*:137-140, 1959.

Swinton, N. W., and Warren, S.: Polyps of the colon and rectum and their relation to malignancy, J.A.M.A. *113*:1927-1933, 1939.

Teicher, I., and Abrahams, J. I.: The treatment of selected cases of multiple polyps, familial polyposis, and diverticular disease of the colon by subtotal colectomy and ileoproctostomy, Surg., Gynec. & Obst. *103*:136-146, 1956.

Thomson, H. S., and Farmer, A. W.: Congenital cyst of the rectum, Canad. J. Surg. *1*:160-162, 1958.

Thorlakson, R. H.: Carcinoma of the colon and rectum associated with chronic ulcerative colitis, Surg., Gynec. & Obst. *103*:41-50, 1956.

Thorson, Å., Björck, G., Björkman, G., and Waldenström, J.: Malignant carcinoid of the small intestine, Am. Heart J. *47*:795-817, 1954.

Tolstedt, G. E., Bell, J. W., and Harkins, H. N.: Chronic perineal sinus following total colectomy for ulcerative colitis, Am. J. Surg. *101*:50-54, 1961.

Turell, R.: Adenomas of the colon and rectum, J.A.M.A. *163*:1258-1259, 1957.

————: Adenoma and cancer of the rectum and colon, advances and retreats, S. Clin. North America *39*:1291-1308, 1959.

————: Adenomas of the colon and rectum in children—A recapitulation, S. Clin. North America *40*:985-997, 1960.

Turell, R., and Maynard, A. de L.: Adenomas of the rectum and colon in juvenile patients, J.A.M.A. *161*:57-60, 1956.

Turell, R., Pomeranz, A. A., Paradny, R., and Vallecillo, L. A.: Adenomas of the colon and rectum: with special emphasis on therapy, S. Clin. North America *35*:1259-1275, 1955.

Turnbull, R. B.: Surgical management of ulcerative colitis, J.A.M.A. *169*:1025-1027, 1959.

Virchow, R.: Die Krankhaften Geschwülste, Berlin, Hirschwald, 1863. Cited by Mayo, DeWeerd, and Jackman (see reference above) 1951.

Wangensteen, O. H.: Primary resection (closed anastomosis) of the colon and rectosigmoid: including description of abdomino-anal methods for restoration of continuity accompanying excision of carcinoma of the rectal ampulla, Surgery *14*:403-432, 1943.

Wangensteen, O. H., Lewis, F. J., Arhelger, S. W., Muller, J. J., and MacLean, L. D.: An interim report upon the "second look" procedure for cancer of the stomach, colon, and rectum and for "limited intraperitoneal carcinosis," Surg., Gynec. & Obst. *99*:257-267, 1954.

Waugh, J. M., and Turner, J. C., Jr.: A study of 268 patients with carcinoma of the midrectum treated by abdominoperineal resection with sphincter preservation, Surg., Gynec. & Obst. *107*:777-783, 1958.

Weber, R. A.: The coincidence of perioral pig-
mented spots and small bowel polyps, Ann. Surg. *140*:901-905, 1954.

Weinstein, M., and Roberts, M.: The perineoabdominal operation for cancer of the rectum, A.M.A. Arch. Surg. *72*:691-708, 1956.

Welch, C. E.: Editorial: The treatment of polyps of the colon, Surg., Gynec. & Obst. *93*:368-369, 1951.

Welch, C. E., McKittrick, J. B., and Behringer, G.: Polyps of the rectum and colon and their relation to cancer, New England J. Med. *247*:959-965, 1952.

Wheat, M. W., Jr., and Ackerman, L. V.: Villous adenomas of the large intestine, Ann. Surg. *147*:476-487, 1958.

Wheelock, F. C., Jr., Toll, G., and McKittrick, L. S.: An evaluation of the anterior resection of the rectum and low sigmoid, New England J. Med. *260*:526-534, 1959.

Wilson, H., and Storer, E. H.: Malignant carcinoid syndrome, Arch. Surg. *79*:917-920, 1959.

Windsberg E.: Intestinal obstruction of the distal colon due to malignancy: single-stage decompression and resection, Surgery *46*:305-318, 1959.

Winter, C. C.: The problem of rectal involvement by prostatic cancer, Surg., Gynec. & Obst. *105*:136-140, 1957.

Wittoesch, J. H., and Jackman, R. J.: Results of conservative management of cancer of the rectum in poor risk patients, Surg., Gynec. & Obst. *107*:648-650, 1958.

Wolfman, E. F., Jr., Astler, V. B., and Coller, F. A.: Mucoid adenocarcinoma of the colon and rectum, Surgery *42*:846-852, 1957.

Woolf, C. M.: A genetic study of carcinoma of the large intestine, Am. J. Human Genet. *10*: 42-47, 1958.

Yoon, I. L.: The eosinophil and gastrointestinal carcinoma, Am. J. Surg. *97*:195-200, 1959.

HENRY N. HARKINS, M.D.

——————————————— CHAPTER 38 ———————————————

Anorectum

DEFINITION

The anorectum is the distal 1½ inches (4 cm.) of the intestinal tract. The upper ¾ inches (2 cm.) of the anorectum is the distal end of the rectum while the lower ¾ inches (2 cm.) comprise the anus itself. As seen in Figure 38-2, the rectal portion of the anorectum is bounded above by the anorectal ring and below by the pectinate line. The anal portion of the anorectum is bounded above by the pectinate margin and below by the anal verge.

The anorectum is not the anus *and* the rectum. It includes all of the anus, but only the distal ¾ inches (2 cm.) of the rectum. To avoid confusion, and yet to discuss the portion of the intestinal canal which functions as a unit, even though it is composed of 2 separate organs, we have used the term anorectum.

GENERAL CONSIDERATIONS

Even though the anorectum or distal portion of the intestinal tract is relatively short, it is, like the mouth, very important. Pathologic conditions in the anorectum are frequent, painful, sometimes dangerous (carcinoma) and often difficult to cure.

One feature of the anorectum is that an understanding of its diseases largely involves a knowledge of *anatomy*. Unlike the parathyroids or the adrenals, for example, where the problems are chiefly physiologic or chemical, in the anorectum pathologic conditions—and

their correction—have a primarily anatomic basis. The principle that different basic sciences have a different extent of application in different parts of the body is well illustrated by these contrasting conditions.

Probably the second most important feature in the anorectum is infection; it involves a knowledge of *bacteriology*. With a few exceptions involving specific infections such as syphilis (chancre and condylomata lata), tuberculosis, etc., most of the infections of the anorectum are nonspecific and have an anatomic basis of causation. Usually when an anatomic correction has been made, the nonspecific infection will be cured. Among the specific infections, lymphopathia venereum leads to stricture involving the lower rectum as well as the anus. Nonvenereal warts, condylomata acuminata, should be treated by anal hygiene, including the use of a dusting powder to keep the area dry, and 25 per cent podophyllin in tincture of benzoin applied directly to the lesions, avoiding contact of the drug with uninvolved skin. Another type of infection is that by *Schistosoma mansoni* (liver fluke). The large shift of population to the United States from Puerto Rico, where the parasite is endemic, has brought the disease to the attention of proctologists. A precise method of diagnosis (Warner, 1957) involves sigmoidoscopy with biopsy of small specimens of rectal mucosa for identification of the eggs.

The anorectum has a close relationship with surrounding structures, and particularly with the remainder of the intestinal canal above. The physician who treats the anorectum, whether he be general surgeon, proctologist, or general practitioner, must be cognizant of these relationships and must not direct his attention only at the obvious lesions at hand. An example of the danger of such a narrow approach is the report that at one large clinic over 20 per cent of the patients submitted to radical excision of the rectum for carcinoma had had a simple hemorrhoidectomy elsewhere within 3 months, invariably without a sigmoidoscopic examination.

ANATOMY

The anorectum is collapsed when empty so that it is an anteroposterior slit. Two clearly palpable landmarks are felt by the examining finger, the anorectal ring at the upper end of the anorectum and the interhemorrhoidal groove at the junction of the middle and the upper thirds of the anus proper.

The anatomy of the rectum has been worked out both by anatomists and by surgeons. Many of the surgeons who have contributed to this field were or are at St. Mark's Hospital, London, an institution devoted entirely to diseases of the anus and the rectum (see Fig. 38-1). Ernest Miles, Lockhart-Mummery, Cuthbert Dukes, Gabriel, Milligan,

Morgan, and many of the other world leaders in this field are or have been on the staff of St. Mark's Hospital. The classic anatomic studies of this region, done by Milligan and Morgan, have been accepted by proctologists throughout the world, even though in some instances they may have differed from the writings of the anatomists. Figure 38-2 presents a recent concept of the anatomy of the anorectum. Figure 38-3 depicts the classic Milligan-Morgan diagram on the left as contrasted with the recent concept based upon the observations of other surgeons, including Eisenhammer (1951, 1953), Goligher, Leacock, and Brossy (1955), also of St. Mark's, Parks (1955, 1956), Morgan and Thompson (1956), Hughes (1956), Fowler (1957), and Walls (1958). These later observations are more in accord with those of the anatomists and, it is believed, with the patient. The rest of this chapter will be based on the newer ideas of anatomy, especially those of Parks.

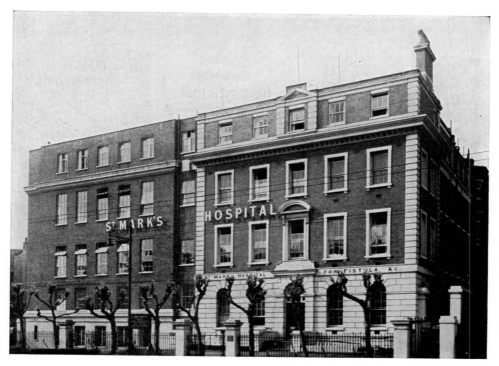

FIG. 38-1. Picture of St. Mark's Hospital For Fistula &C., London, England. This hospital has played a greater role in the development of anorectal and colorectal surgery than any other institution in the world. It was built in 1835; Charles Dickens was a subscriber. (From Mr. C. Naunton Morgan, F.R.C.S.)

MEMBRANES

The rectal mucous membrane is composed of columnar epithelium (pale pink as is the membrane above). The mucous membrane of the rectal portion of the anorectum is covered by a columnar-cuboidal epithelium (red, due to the underlying vessels of the superior hemorrhoidal plexus) according to the classical description. Goligher, Leacock, and Brossy (1955), however, found the mucous membrane between the pectinate line and the anorectal ring to be multilayered.

Going from the skin to the rectum, the epithelial lining may be divided into 4 zones. Lateral to the most median attachment of the conjoined terminating fibers of the levator ani and longitudinal muscles (Fig. 38-3) at a point which Parks (1956) terms the squamous border, there is true skin. Medial to this there are 3 additional zones, and the entire arrangement is as follows:

Zone 1. *True skin*, with sweat glands and hair follicles.

Dividing margin: squamous border (lateral hemorrhoidal groove, anal verge).

Zone 2. *Stratified squamous epithelium* with only occasional sweat glands and hair follicles (1.0-1.5 cm.).

Dividing margin: line of anal crypts (inter-hemorrhoidal groove, mucocutaneous line, point of attachment of mucosal suspensory ligament—see Fig. 38-3).

Zone 3. *Stratified columnar epithelium* (middle zone): mucus secreting and moist (0.25-1.0 cm.).

Dividing margin: pectinate or dentate line.

Zone 4. *Columnar glandular rectal epithelium*, above the pectinate line.

Zones 2 and 3, combined, are known as the pecten (Stroud, 1896). Zones 1, 2 and usually 3 are sensitive; Zone 4 is supplied by visceral nerves and is insensitive. Zone 1 has the normal color of the patient's skin elsewhere or is slightly darker. Zones 2 and 3 are slightly bluish.

The skin is adherent to the underlying structure at the squamous border. The mucous membrane is similarly adherent at the mucocutaneous line. Between these two points of attachment the subepithelial space is termed

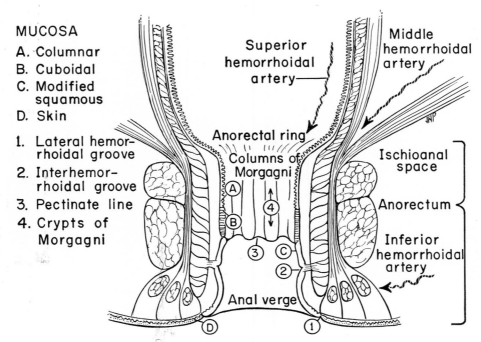

MUCOSA

A. Columnar
B. Cuboidal
C. Modified squamous
D. Skin

1. Lateral hemorrhoidal groove
2. Interhemorrhoidal groove
3. Pectinate line
4. Crypts of Morgagni

Superior hemorrhoidal artery

Middle hemorrhoidal artery

Anorectal ring

Columns of Morgagni

Ischioanal space

Anorectum

Inferior hemorrhoidal artery

Anal verge

FIG. 38-2. Master drawing of anorectum and lower rectum showing epithelium, muscles, arteries and landmarks. The anorectum itself is the portion of the intestinal canal between the anorectal ring above and the anal verge below.

the "marginal space" (in which are the external hemorrhoidal vessels); lateral to the squamous border it is the "ischiorectal space," while above the mucocutaneous line is the "submucous space" (in which are the internal hemorrhoidal vessels).

The pectinate line is made prominent by the presence of small epithelial processes, the anal papillae, on the free margins of the anal valves of Ball. These papillae represent the remnants of the proctodeal membrane which in early embryonic life separated the proctodeum from the postallantoic gut. The sinuses of Morgagni are small depressions or pockets which occur above each anal valve. These sinuses are deeper posteriorly than elsewhere and may be subject to infection through lodging of foreign material in them. The infection of the sinuses and of the anal glands at their bases is known as cryptitis and may be the starting point for other infections of the anorectum (abscess, fistula and possibly fissure). The anal glands may be several millimeters long and may extend down to the interhemorrhoidal groove or into the circular muscles. Hypertrophy of the papillae usually is associated with cryptitis and is known as papillitis.

NERVE SUPPLY

Only the external sphincter and the levator ani muscles are under voluntary control, and there is sensitivity to pain only below the pectinate line.

BLOOD SUPPLY

The superior hemorrhoidal artery sends branches which course down the rectum beneath the mucosa and are collected in 6 to 8 vertical folds or columns of Morgagni in the rectal portion of the anorectum (Fig. 38-2). The middle hemorrhoidal artery comes to the rectum at the inferior angle of the pelvirectal space. The inferior hemorrhoidal arteries approach the anus through the perianal space. These vessels anastomose freely, except at

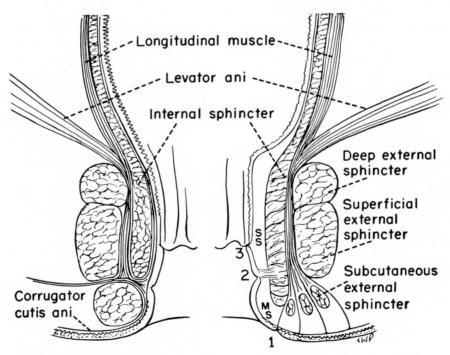

FIG. 38-3. Muscles and fascial septa of anorectum. The classical Milligan-Morgan concept is shown on the reader's left, the *newer* concept of Parks and others on the right. (1—lateral hemorrhoidal groove, 2—attachment of mucosal suspensory ligament, or interhemorrhoidal groove, 3—pectinate line, MS—marginal space, and SS—submucous space.)

the interhemorrhoidal groove, and the corresponding veins form an extensive plexus about the anorectum with many of the vessels lying just beneath the mucosa. Because of the effects of gravity upon venous congestion, the horizontal position relieves pain in most anorectal conditions.

MUSCLES (Fig. 38-3)

The external sphincter and the levator ani, being voluntary striated muscles, are red, while the internal sphincter and the longitudinal sphincter, being involuntary nonstriated muscles, are paler.

Longitudinal Sphincter. The 3 taenia coli of the colon become spread out over the wall of the rectum. The muscle is strongest and thickest on the anterior and the posterior surfaces and laterally is thinner. The longitudinal muscle, involving nonstriated fibers is continued down in this way to the rectal portion of the anorectum where it envelops the internal sphincter and ends by passing through the subcutaneous portion of the external sphincter, dividing it into many segments, and inserting in the anal skin (Wilde, 1949). The

corrugator cutis ani muscle is a continuation downward and outward from the cutaneous insertion of the longitudinal muscle. Extending upward and inside the canal from the cutaneous insertion of the longitudinal muscle (lateral hemorrhoidal groove) is the *musculus submucosae ani* (Fine and Lawes, 1940, Gorsch, 1955). These longitudinal fibers lie between the internal hemorrhoidal plexus (toward the lumen) and the circular internal sphincter (away from the lumen). They are the counterpart of the *muscularis mucosae* elsewhere in the intestinal tract. The "pecten band," so well described by Miles, is the lower portion of the internal sphincter.

External Sphincter. Santorini in 1715 first described the external sphincter as being composed of 3 parts. These 3 parts are now termed the deep, the superficial and the subcutaneous portions of the external sphincter. They are usually fused together more in the patient than the diagrams would indicate. Their respective locations are shown in Figure 38-3. The subcutaneous portion has been likened by Gabriel to an umbrella ring. It is about ¼ inch in cross section and lies immediately

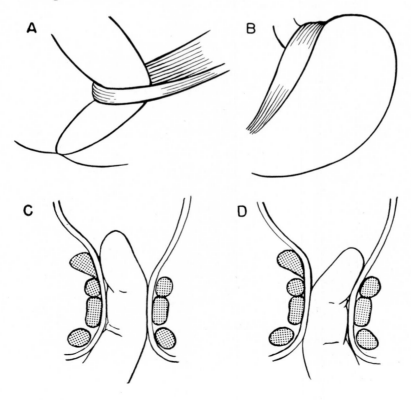

FIG. 38-4. Demonstration of the sling-like action of the puborectalis (one of the 3 components of the levator ani) muscle. (A) Lateral view of puborectalis sling (posterior to left, anterior to right). (B) Diagrammatic representation of similar situation with regard to right crus of diaphragm, forming a sling for the esophagogastric junction (Allison). (C) Lateral view shows that the finger palpating the posterior rectal wall meets resistance of puborectalis. (D) Lateral view shows that finger palpating anterior rectal wall meets no resistance at level of puborectalis.

beneath the skin lateral to the anal margin and to the lateral hemorrhoidal groove.

The muscle "seen" in the bed of a hemorrhoidectomy wound was formerly believed to be the subcutaneous portion of the external sphincter. Recent work by Eisenhammer (1951, 1953), Goligher, Leacock, and Brossy (1955), Parks (1956) and others, indicates that this is actually the lower end of the internal sphincter. Biopsy of this muscle was performed by Vetto, Harkins, McMahon and White (1956), and in 18 of 20 patients microscopic study revealed nonstriated muscle, confirming the Eisenhammer-Goligher-Parks hypothesis. The recent paper by Swinton and Mumma (1956) is the first in the American literature, to the author's knowledge, taking cognizance of these new anatomic concepts.

Associated Muscles. These include the levator ani, including the puborectalis, as well as all of the muscles of the pelvis and the perineal floor.

Anal Muscular Defects. Certain normal muscular defects are important in the surgical anatomy of the anorectum. These are as follows:

PUBORECTALIS "SLING." The puborectalis, which has been called the best-developed muscle in the pelvic diaphragm, acts like a sling around the upper portion of the anorectum, as shown in Figure 38-4. It is of interest that this slinglike action has been compared with that of the oblique muscles of the stomach around the cardia of the stomach. The result of the arrangement of the puborectalis as depicted is that the anal canal is shorter anteriorly than posteriorly, 1¼ in. (3 cm.) as opposed to 1½ in. (4 cm.).

MINOR'S TRIANGLE. Of the 3 portions of the external sphincter, 2 (the deep and the subcutaneous) are essentially circular, while the superficial is the only one of the 3 that attaches to the coccyx. The angular defect produced by this insertion is known as Minor's triangle (Fig. 38-5). It may have considerable clinical importance because of a lack of support of the anal wall at this level posteriorly. The downward passage of feces may cause

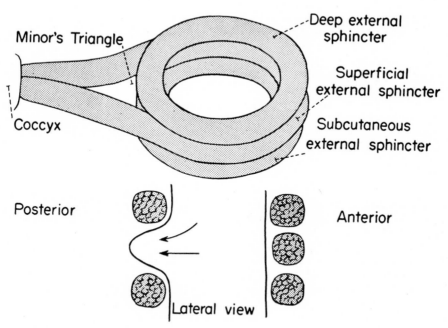

FIG. 38-5. Diagrammatic representation of Minor's triangle. The upper drawing in partially superior view shows the gap caused by the coccygeal attachment of the superficial portion of the external anal sphincter. The lower drawing is a lateral view showing the same defect as caused by the presence of Minor's triangle.

trauma because of this irregularity of the wall and may be a factor in the causation of anal fissure, which is most common in the mid-line posteriorly. The relative protuberance of the subcutaneous external sphincter below Minor's triangle is known as Blaisdell's bar. Recently, Eisenhammer (1951, 1953) has contested the importance of "Blaisdell's bar" in the genesis and the perpetuation of fistula and has stated that the only "bar" at fault is the internal sphincter.

DIAGNOSIS

In various conditions occurring in different parts of the body the diagnosis is made by the history and the physical examination, supported by laboratory studies. The inexperienced doctor is apt to fall into two errors of concept in this regard, wrongly assuming: (1) that the history is always the most important of these 3 methods and (2) that their relative importance is the same, irrespective of the lesion. Granting that the history is generally the basic diagnostic tool and that laboratory studies play in general only a supportive and corroborative role, the relative usefulness of these 3 methods varies markedly with the lesion. In cases of epilepsy or peptic ulcer the history is most important; in instances of parathyroid tumor or islet cell tumor of the pancreas laboratory studies have a special applicability; but in diseases of the anorectum, the physical examination is the *sine qua non*.

After a preliminary history, examination of the anorectum involves *inspection* of the anal orifice and the surrounding skin. Following this, a *digital examination* should be done. Since fissures usually occur in the mid-line posteriorly and since, with the exception of the thrombosed external hemorrhoids, they are the most sensitive anorectal lesion, in cases where fissure is suspected the examining finger should hug the anterior wall on introduction into the anal canal to minimize pain. The digital examination should be thorough and systematic. In postoperative cases, fecal impaction should be searched for, and a history of frequent stools may be misleading and delay disimpaction (Dresen and Kratzer, 1959).

Following the digital examination, a *proctosigmoidoscopic examination* should be performed. A sigmoidoscope is one of the first instruments that a surgeon or a general practitioner should purchase upon entering practice. The importance of the sigmoidoscope in anorectal examination is exceeded only by the palpating finger and direct inspection. An anoscope is a useful adjunct.

For a proctosigmoidoscopic examination (Jackman, 1958, and Turell, 1959, give detailed instructions), the patient should come with the rectum well cleansed and prepared. Adequate preparation includes: (1) a light or liquid supper the night before, (2) castor oil, 1½ ounces (50 cc.) the night before, (3) two enemas in the morning and (4) tea and toast for breakfast preceding the examination. Despite these measures, preparation may be incomplete, and it is advantageous to have suction available in the proctoscopy room. In old and debilitated patients it may be advisable to adopt a less rigorous preparation, and it may be preferable to avoid some of the head-down positions for examination to be listed below. The position, whether it be the knee-chest-left shoulder down position, the Sims' or left lateral position, the lithotomy position, or the prone jackknife position, is relatively immaterial so long as the surgeon is familiar with it. Any firm table is adequate for the first two positions, while special tables are necessary for the latter two. The examination should be done, if possible, to the full length (23 cm.) of the instrument, and the history sheet should have a special form, possibly a rubber stamp diagram such as is used at St. Mark's Hospital, London, for recording of the findings.

CLINICAL CONDITIONS

In the brief summary of surgery of the anorectum given in this chapter, an outline of 10 surgical conditions of this region will be given. Certain other lesions, such as lymphopathia venereum, ulcerative colitis, proctitis, viral verrucae (Young, 1957), polyps and adenocarcinoma, are considered to be more in the province of the colon or the rectum proper and are discussed in Chapter 37.

IMPERFORATE ANUS

Imperforate anus may occur in both sexes and may be classified into 4 main groups, as shown in Figure 38-6. Bill (1958) and Bill and Johnson (1958) believe that failure of migration of the rectal opening is the probable cause in the majority of cases of imperforate anus. The frequent association of fistulas with imperforate anus has been emphasized by Brayton and Norris (1958), Scott, Swenson and Fisher (1960) and by Swinton and Palmer (1960).

(For a more complete discussion of this condition, see Chap. 47, "Pediatric Surgery").

PROLAPSE

Prolapse of the rectum can be classified into 3 types as shown below:

CLASSIFICATION OF PROLAPSE OF THE RECTUM

(Modified from Altemeier, Hoxworth, and Giuseffi, 1955)

Type I. Mucosal Prolapse (Partial Protrusion of the Rectum, False Prolapse). This type occurs especially at the extremes of life and in the debilitated. Constipation, straining at stool, and reading on the toilet are etiologic factors. Treatment involves correction of these factors, but with avoidance of cathartics and diarrhea. In children the buttocks may be strapped together for a few days. The straight vertical rectal canal of children may be a factor in the etiology. This type of prolapse is seldom longer than 4 to 6 cm. and is usually shorter. Since the protrusion involves only the mucosa it is thin to palpation.

Type II. Intussuscepted Prolapse (Incomplete Prolapse). This type involves a prolapse of all layers of the rectum. It usually starts at a point above the anorectal ring, having as a point of origin one of the valves of Houston or the pelvic rectal junction. Both areas correspond to the junction of a higher, comparatively mobile portion of the rectum with a lower, more fixed portion. In early cases there may be a groove around the prolapsed bowel between it and the skin extending up to the point of invagination. If the groove is deeper than 3 cm., the lesion is more apt to be a true intussusception rather than a prolapse. In advanced cases of intussuscepted prolapse the anus becomes everted as well as the rectum, and the groove is no longer present.

Type III. Sliding Prolapse (Complete or Massive Prolapse, Pelvirectal Sliding Hernia). Such a lesion represents a herniation of the pelvic peritoneum or cul-de-sac through a defect in its underlying endo-abdominal fascia and the pelvic diaphragm. As the hernia progresses and slides downward, the cul-de-sac invaginates the anterior wall of the rectum to produce an intussusception. The anal sphincter becomes progressively relaxed with continued protrusion. Such prolapses are larger than the other types. The anterior wall is thicker than the posterior (due to contained sac and even small bowel) and may be tympanitic. As a result of this asymmetry the rectal opening faces posteriorly, while in Types I and II the opening of the bowel is centrally located. Type III is rare in children. In adults it is not restricted to the older age group as in Type I.

Treatment of Type I or Type II is relatively simple and involves sleeve excision of the mass with mucosa-to-mucosa approximation. Perisphincteric wiring (Thiersch operation) has recently been revised for Type II by Burke and Jackman (1959). The correction of true prolapse, Type III, on the other hand, is a

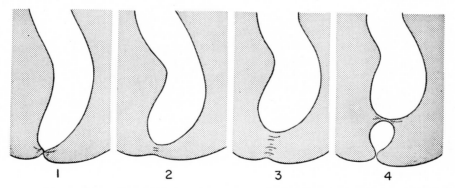

1	2	3	4

FIG. 38-6. Imperforate anus (classification of Dr. Robert Gross): Type 1: Stenosis at the anus. Type 2: Imperforate anus; obstruction only by a persistent membrane. Type 3: Imperforate anus; rectal pouch ending blindly some distance above anus. Type 4: Anus and rectal pouch normal; blind rectal pouch in hollow of sacrum.

difficult problem which has led to devising a number of operative approaches (Nigro and Walker, 1957). These involve the abdominal approach (Moschcowitz, 1912; Graham, 1942; Orr, 1947; Frykman, 1955; Tendler, 1956; Goligher, 1958; MacKenzie and Davis, 1958; Baden and Mikkelsen, 1959; Shann, 1959; Rhoads, 1960), the combined abdominal and perineal approach (Dunphy, 1948), and the perineal approach (Miles, 1954, 1933; Altemeier, Hoxworth, and Giuseffi, 1955; Inberg, 1957). The perineal approach was utilized by Altemeier and associates in 13 cases of Type III prolapse with good results in all but 1 case and presents several advantages.

This technic involves a 1-stage operation with less risk to the patient, since it utilizes the perineal approach. An incision is made about the circumference of the protruding mass 3 mm. proximal to the pectinate line. This incision is carried through the first of the 2 layers of bowel, the cut layer then being stripped distally from the underlying or inner loop. The hernial sac is located anteriorly and dissected free superiorly as far as possible. Then the sac is opened, and the peritoneal cavity is explored. The sliding character of the hernia now becomes apparent because the posterior peritoneal layer of the sac is the serosa of the rectum. The redundant loop of rectum and sigmoid with its attached mesentery is marked for the site of resection with a silk stitch. This point is selected so as to permit ready anastomosis to the anus previously cut across 3 mm. proximal to the pectinate line at the first step.

The peritoneal cavity is closed with a Y-shaped suture, the levator ani muscles are approximated in front of the rectum with interrupted sutures, the bowel is divided at the point previously marked and is anastomosed in one layer to the anus. In the event no hernial sac or levator defect is found, it can be assumed that the prolapse is Type I. If a levator defect is found without a hernial sac, the prolapse is Type II. Resection of the elongated rectum with anastomosis is performed as for Type III, with or without repair of the levators as indicated in the case at hand.

(Since Type III, or sliding prolapse, is also a type of pelvic hernia, see Chap. 39, "Hernia" in section on "Perineal Hernia.")

STRICTURE

Stricture of the anus may follow trauma, infection (Kark, Epstein and Chapman, 1959) or poorly performed hemorrhoidectomies, particularly of the Whitehead type (Anderson, Pontius and Witkowski, 1955). The best method of treatment, aside from prevention, is an S-shaped incision (S-plasty), swinging the skin flaps into the tightened anal ring (Ferguson, 1959).

INCONTINENCE

Anal incontinence is due to overenthusiastic muscle-cutting operations for anal fistula, to trauma and to neurologic conditions. Karlan, McPherson and Watman (1959), have studied factors affecting fecal incontinence in the dog. The 4 chief methods of surgical treatment in patients are as follows:

Treatment of Anal Incontinence

1. Lawson-Tait operation (like a Heineke-Mikulicz)
2. Blaisdell operation (1957)
   a. Advance muscle flaps
   b. Close as Lawson-Tait
3. Lockhart-Mummry operation (superficial external sphincter pleating)
4. Thiersch's operation (circumferential wire suture)

PRURITUS ANI

This condition is common, annoying to the patient, and difficult to treat. Possibly more than with some other anorectal lesions the patient as a whole must be considered. Psychic factors, general medical conditions, such as jaundice, spread from vaginal lesions including trichomonas, and spread of pinworms from the rectum above, are all to be considered. Furthermore, an underlying anorectal cause *per se* is often a factor, and cryptitis (with involvement of the associated anal glands), fistula, hemorrhoids, hypertrophied anal skin tags, etc., should be taken care of adequately before the diagnosis of idiopathic or primary pruritus ani is made. In secondary pruritus ani the condition is a symptom rather than a disease.

A classification of pruritus ani, modified from that of Fromer (1955) follows. The percentage figures listed after each group of patients indicate the relative frequency of such patients at the Lahey Clinic.

CLASSIFICATION OF PRURITUS ANI
(Modified from Fromer, 1955)

The percentage figures represent relative incidences of the different groups of patients as seen at the Lahey Clinic.

Type 1. Anorectal (25%). (Best treated by surgical care of the underlying condition)

a. Fissures
b. Fistulas
c. Draining sinuses
d. Ulcers
e. Mucosal prolapse

f. Papillitis
g. Cryptitis
h. Skin tags
i. Hemorrhoids
j. Neoplasms

Type 2. Dermatologic (20%). (Best treated locally by medical means)

a. Psoriasis
b. Seborrheic dermatitis
c. Bacterial dermatitis
d. Mycotic dermatitis

e. Lichen sclerosus
f. Syphilis
g. Contact dermatitis

Type 3. Medical (10%). (Best treated generally to overcome or remove the underlying condition)

a. Jaundice
b. Diabetes
c. Lymphoblastomatosis
d. Antibiotic irritation

e. Allergy (foods, deodorants, hygienic pads, etc.)
f. Parasites (especially pinworms)

Type 4. Idiopathic (45%). (Treatment difficult, see text)

Another classification, listed in Table 1, is that of Turell (1955) and, while less useful for general purposes than the Fromer classification, serves as a guide for hydrocortisone therapy.

If the pruritus continues despite a careful and thorough diagnostic study to determine causative factors with the carrying out of indicated therapeutic measures, the condition can be classified as idiopathic (essential or primary) pruritus ani. Before reaching this conclusion a dermatologic and/or a psychiatric consultation may be advisable.

In cases of idiopathic pruritus ani, as well as in some cases of secondary pruritus, 4 types of therapy should be considered. The first of these is adoption of a regimen of anal hygiene. This does no harm and may be sufficient to cure most cases of pruritus ani. Directions for anal hygiene are as follows and may be given to the patient in the form of a mimeographed schedule:

Anal Hygiene. After defecation immediately cleanse the perianal skin with wet absorbent cotton or, if possible, take a shower, or a partial bath or a partial shower, avoiding strong soaps. Basis soap or some other superfatted soap is nonirritating to most people. The lubricating action of the soap helps to reduce the hemorrhoids. Do not use toilet tissue. Dry well with cotton and powder well with cornstarch or nonaromatic powder. Cleansing with wet cotton and dusting with powder must be repeated about 4 times daily, depending on the amount of moisture and the degree of itching. Always keep the skin around

TABLE 1. GROUPING OF CASES OF PRURITUS ANI ACCORDING TO RESPONSE TO HYDROCORTISONE OINTMENT THERAPY

(Turell, 1955)

Group	No. of Cases Treated	Response
1. Intractable (with moderate lichenification), of less than 3 years' duration	36	Good
2. Intractable (with advanced lichenification), of over 3 years' duration	5	Good
3. Acute exacerbations	2	Trace
4. Refractory, without cutaneous changes	15	None
5. Secondary to diarrhea	12	Trace
6. Secondary to antibiotic therapy	14	Trace
7. Severe, accompanying fistula, fissure, or hemorrhoids	16	Trace
8. Severe, caused by pediculosis, enterobiasis or leukemia	6	None

the anus clean and dry. Carry cotton and talcum in separate envelopes on the person in a pocket or a handbag. Before retiring repeat rectal lavage and cleanse, dry and powder the anal region. Once a week, after retiring, daub a small amount of bland ointment or menthol-phenol paste into the perianal skin. The latter may cause mild burning for several minutes. Osborne and Stoll (1959) also emphasize the importance of local hygiene in the treatment of pruritus ani. In our opinion, especially as a prophylactic measure in early cases, local hygiene is the cornerstone of all treatment for this condition.

Sedatives. Phenobarbital gr. 1 $\overline{ss}$ (90 mg.) at bedtime and gr. ¼ (15 mg.) t.i.d. may be useful in quieting the nervous patient who still has to work. For patients confined to bed, larger daytime doses may be allowed. An ice bag applied to the itching area may be helpful.

Hydrocortisone Ointment. This method of treatment is very helpful for certain types of pruritus ani. Turell (1955, 1957) reported that it is particularly effective in the treatment of patients with intractable anal pruritus (Group 1, Table 1) but completely ineffective for patients of Groups 4 or 8. Hydrocortisone acetate or free alcohol in 1 per cent or 2.5 per cent ointment base is applied locally by the patient in the night and the morning, or more often in severe cases. When associated infection is present, oxytetracycline may be added to the ointment. While this treatment is almost specific in many instances, its chief danger is that it will be used indiscriminately without utilizing proper diagnostic methods. If the pruritus is due to pinworms, hydrocortisone ointment therapy, even if it helps the itching, will be of symptomatic value only; if the pruritus is due to discharges from un-diagnosed carcinoma of the rectum, the ointment, by its symptomatic benefit, may actually delay definitive treatment of the carcinoma until metastases have occurred.

Operative Management. In the most severe and intractable cases of pruritus ani when diagnostic measures have failed to reveal a causative factor and when all conservative measures (Anal Hygiene, Sedatives, and Hydrocortisone Ointment) have been tried, operative management, beyond that necessary to remove causative fistulas, etc., may be indicated. In many instances, such treatment is necessary more to heal the skin which has been damaged by incessant scratching than for the itching itself. Included in the category of treatments to be considered are tattooing with cinnabar; subcutaneous injections of procaine, long-acting anesthetics, or even alcohol; presacral neurectomy (Smith, Malkiewicz, and Massenberg, 1955); undermining of skin flaps; or even excision of skin flaps with skin grafting. Fortunately, these radical measures are becoming less and less necessary as conservative treatment is improved.

FISSURE

An anal fissure is essentially a very sensitive crack in the mucous membrane of the anal canal. Most fissures occur in the mid-line posteriorly at or above the interhemorrhoidal groove (attachment of mucosal ligament to the anal wall). The next most common site is in the mid-line anteriorly. Goodsall's fissure site rule (1900) states that anterior fissure occurs in 1 per cent of male patients with fissure and in 8 per cent of female patients with fissure; hence, there is a 1:8 ratio between the sexes for anterior fissure. The probable reason for the relatively greater incidence of anterior fissure in women is because of the associated strains and tears connected with childbirth. The probable reason for the greater incidence of posterior fissure in both sexes is that the sinuses of Morgagni and the anal glands at their bases are deeper posteriorly. Less likely reasons are the irregularity of the posterior wall caused by Minor's triangle and Blaisdell's bar (Fig. 38-5) and that when undistended the anal canal is an anteroposterior slit.

In chronic fissure one sees the circular muscle (formerly thought to be the subcutaneous portion of the external sphincter but now considered to be the lower portion of the internal sphincter). An anal fissure develops an "anal skin tag" at its lower end. This is not an anal papilla from the pectinate line but is edematous skin. It can be likened to a terminal moraine in the realm of geology, the stools corresponding to the glaciers. Tearing down of the associated anal valve may be a cause of fissure.

TREATMENT. The treatment of fissure involves 2 different types of therapy, depending on the stage of the disease:

Best in acute fissure ↑ 1. Medical treatment 2. Surgical treatment ↓ Best in chronic fissure

Medical treatment includes the avoidance of constipation and of rough foods or those containing seeds, the use of a regimen of anal hygiene, as for pruritus ani, mineral oil by mouth, soothing suppositories and externally applied ointments, and occasionally the injection of long-lasting anesthetics under the bed of the fissure. Supposedly, such injections will relax the sphincters, allow bowel movements to pass without trauma, and in turn permit healing. Because of the danger of infection and necrosis, injections are not advised.

Surgical treatment includes either dilatation or excision. Dilatation puts the sphincters at rest for several days, usually allowing a subacute fissure time to heal. Since this method requires an anesthetic, local, regional, or general, one usually excises the fissure at the same time as one performs a dilatation. In chronic fissures, Gabriel stated that, "I have come to the conclusion that cure cannot be given for certain except by operation." Recurrence does occur occasionally following surgical treatment, but the results following this type of management are generally good, despite the fact that its use is reserved for the most severe fissures.

Two features of fissurectomy are also important: (1) one should remove a triangle of skin for drainage during the healing process external to and including the anal skin tag (sentinel pile). (2) The pecten band or lower portion of the internal sphincter may be divided in the bed of the fissure (total internal sphincterotomy is advised by Eisenhammer [1951] and by Brossy [1956]), or an 0.8 mm. square section of it may be excised.

In place of this standard operation, Pope (1959) advises an anorectoplastic procedure.

ABSCESS ("THE FORERUNNER OF FISTULA")

As shown in Figure 38-7, abscesses occur with varying frequency in the different spaces near the anus. There is a 5 to 1 preponderance in males. The origin of abscesses is considered to be an infection, often originating in anal glands or crypts, which penetrates into the perirectal spaces. Perirectal abscesses are associated with malaise, fever, pain and swelling until they either rupture externally or in-

ternally into the anorectum, or are incised and drained. Because of the thickness of the skin of the buttocks, fluctuation is not felt early. Similar conditions exist around the mouth at the opposite end of the intestinal tract, or on the palm of the hand; a contrasting situation exists on the dorsum of the hand where incision seldom should be done unless definite signs of fluctuation are present. Gabriel stated in this regard: "Every anorectal abscess should be incised at the earliest possible moment. It is not desirable to procrastinate and apply palliative treatment until fluctuation has occurred. . . ."

The submucous space extends downward only as far as the interhemorrhoidal groove. It contains the internal hemorrhoidal plexus. The perianal (marginal) space is inferior and lateral to the interhemorrhoidal groove. More laterally, infections superficial to the corrugator cutis muscle usually heal spontaneously, while those beneath it generally result in low-level ana fistula.

According to Nesselrod there are 5 deep spaces:

2 ischioanal (one on each side)
2 pelvirectal (anterior and posterior)
1 retrorectal

Three papers by Eisenhammer (1953, 1958, 1959) of Johannesburg, South Africa, have emphasized a new concept in the origin, the development, the classification and consequently the treatment of anorectal abscesses. This concept is that many abscesses are of an "intermuscular" variety, lying between the internal and the external sphincters (Fig. 38-7). Such abscesses result, according to Eisenhammer, from infection of anal glands which end deep to the internal sphincter in the intermuscular space. This space may be similar to the "anal intermuscular interstice" so well described by Shropshear (1960). The classification of anorectal abscess, with etiologic factors in each instance, is given in Table 2.

The high intermuscular abscess, situated deep to the internal sphincter and occupying the intermuscular space, is universally described and diagrammatically represented as the "submucous abscess" (Fig. 38-7). A true

TABLE 2. EISENHAMMER CLASSIFICATION OF ANORECTAL ABSCESS
It is to be noted that the pelvirectal abscess, not being a primary anorectal
condition, is not included in the percentage incidences.

GROUP	TYPE	ETIOLOGY	INCIDENCE
A. Internal	1. High intermuscular	Deep cryptoglandular infection	10%
	2. Low intermuscular	Deep cryptoglandular infection	81%
	3. High submucous	Shallow cryptoglandular infection, infected hematomes, direct trauma	2%
	4. Low mucocutaneous	Shallow cryptoglandular infection, infected hematomes, direct trauma	
B. External	5. Pelvirectal	Pelviabdominal infection	..
	6. Ischiorectal	Primary lymphatic or blood borne infection	2%
	7. Subcutaneous	Local tegumentary infection	1%
C. Internoexternal	8. Intermuscular ischiorectal fistulous abscess (horseshoe type)	Secondary break-through of low intermuscular abscess into both the subcutaneous space and the outer portion of the ischiorectal fossa	4%
		TOTAL	100%

submucous abscess, a very superficial lesion, resolves spontaneously before operation is required. Eisenhammer states: "The failure to recognize the intermuscular space abscess is responsible for much of the present-day unsatisfactory treatment of the anorectal fistulous abscess." When fully developed, with a subcutaneous projection, the high intermuscular space abscess, instead of being mistaken for the simpler submucous abscess is confused with the more serious deep postanal or ischioanal abscess. This mistake results in formidable incorrect surgery, whereas the correct diagnosis requires only the simple surgical procedure of total internal sphincterotomy over the central axis of the abscess in order to bring about a cure (Eisenhammer, 1958, 1959). This author also refers to the intermuscular space as the "breeding ground of the more complicated fistulas" and "the key to the surgery of this complex subject." Table 2 also shows that the total per cent of abscesses which are of cryptoglandular origin amounts to at least 95 per cent. Similarly, at least 90 per cent of fistulas occur in the posterior quadrant because this is where the glands are.

The pelvirectal and retrorectal spaces have only visceral sensation; hence, they are not so painful and they produce only vague symptoms. The ischioanal space abscesses are painful (as well, of course, as the perianal ones). Batson's rule is also of importance in differentiating: the ischioanal space has a capacity of only 2 or 3 ounces; on the other hand, the pelvirectal space can enlarge considerably by floating up the peritoneum. Hence, if over 2 to 3 ounces is obtained by incision and drainage, the lesion is not an ischioanal abscess. Pelvirectal abscesses may be confused with true pelvic abscesses.

Eisenhammer (1960) has recently described two special varieties of the anterior anorectal intermuscular fistulous abscesses, namely the "anovulvar high" and the "anoscrotal low" varieties. Since these are so frequently misinterpreted, a separate account of each is in order.

1. **Acute Anovulvar High Intermuscular Fistulous Abscess.** In the female, the acute high anterior anorectal intermuscular fistulous abscess lies to the side of the rectovaginal septum and bulges posteriorly into the deep aspect of the lower vulva above the anorectal line. It is distinctly palpable bidigitally and is about the size of a walnut. It has the misleading features of a primary vulval abscess. There are two diagnostic features: (A) the acute pain is of distinctly anorectal distribution, and (B) there is edema at the anal verge. There are no superficial inflammatory changes of the vulva as in an acute Bartholin abscess in which the pain is vulval. This type anterior abscess is relatively rare.

2. **The Anoscrotal Low Intermuscular Fistulous Abscess.** In the male, the anterior low acute anorectal intermuscular fistulous abscess points, in the majority of cases, to the right of the median perineal raphe at the base

of the scrotum. In the ensuing recurring inflammatory attacks, the infection spreads higher up the scrotum until it is grossly involved in the chronic suppurative process and now appears to be the primary site. In the advanced scrotal involvement, the testes may be pushed up by the cicatrised scrotum. The diagnosis is made from the fact that there are no signs of epididymo-orchitis, and the testicle remains free and mobile. More important signs are telltale healed scars nearer the anal verge. The chief diagnostic sign is a well-developed cord representing the chronic granulomatous fistulous tract which is distinctly palpable from the base of the scrotum to the anal verge.

This lesion forms about 5 per cent of the lower intermuscular fistulous abscess group and is, in nearly all cases, on the right side.

Antibiotics have a limited application in the treatment of these abscesses. Their use should not delay necessary operation, as they seldom, if ever, eliminate the requirement for it. Drainage usually involves a radial or cruciate incision over the abscess, sometimes with complete unroofing of the overlying skin. Drainage is maintained for a few days with either a Penrose drain or a gauze pack. Even though abscesses are the "forerunner of fistula," there is little that one can do at the time of treating the abscess to prevent the development of a

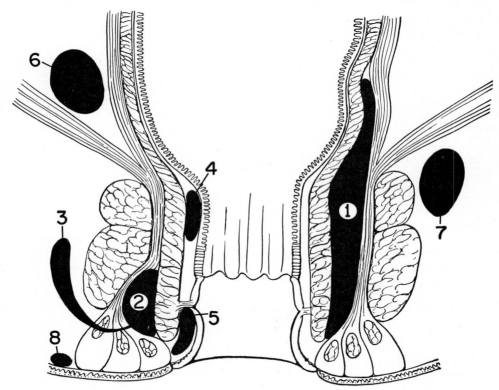

FIG. 38-7. Location of various types of anorectal abscesses. This figure incorporates the new concepts of Eisenhammer (1958). The eight types are designated by numbers in the above Figure as follows:

1. High intermuscular fistulous abscess
2. Low intermuscular fistulous abscess
3. Intermuscular ischiorectal fistulous abscess (horseshoe abscess)
4. High submucous nonfistulous abscess
5. Low mucocutaneous fistulous abscess
6. Pelvirectal abscess, nonanorectal
7. Ischiorectal fistulous abscess
8. Subcutaneous fistulous abscess

fistula although McElwain (1959) has used primary fistulotomy in the treatment of 100 consecutive anorectal abscesses of all types. The advocates of anorectoplasty also treat abscesses definitively in one stage in selected instances. The patient should be warned of this probable eventuality and be examined periodically until either the danger is over or the time for treating the fistula has come.

FISTULA

A fistula-in-ano involves the two openings of the sinus tract left behind by an abscess as shown in Figure 38-8. Because of inadequate drainage due to scarring, first one opening and then the other may clog up. If too long a period of time is allowed to elapse, both openings may close off, the abscess may become reactivated, and a new site of spontaneous rupture may occur. This process, if repeated several times, results in the so-called "pepper pot anus." Formerly, 10 per cent of fistulas were tuberculous; at present, the true percentage is undoubtedly lower (2 to 3%, Dunphy and Pikula, 1955). Martin (1957), basing his observations on experience with 29 cases, mostly at a tuberculosis sanatorium,

outlines rules for adjunctive chemotherapy. He also points out that in 112 cases with tuberculosis, viable and virulent tubercle bacilli were present in the lower portion of the rectum in 30 per cent, indicating how tuberculous fistula may originate. Differential diagnosis of fistula, tuberculous or otherwise should include furunculosis, pilonidal sinuses and perineal sinuses.

Fistulas occur mainly in adults. Males predominate 3:1 as would be expected, since antecedent abscesses are the cause ("Invariably results from abscess"—Gabriel). In truth, fistulas can lead "anywhere," and the process of tracing out their full course is often difficult but important, since unless the tract is found *in toto,* cure cannot be expected. A classification of anal fistulas is given below, with relative incidences and a diagrammatic representation of the course of these main types is shown in Figure 38-8.

The rule propounded by Goodsall (1900) is a very practical one in understanding anal fistula: Fistulas with posterior external openings have their internal opening in the midline posteriorly; fistulas with anterior external openings have their internal openings radially

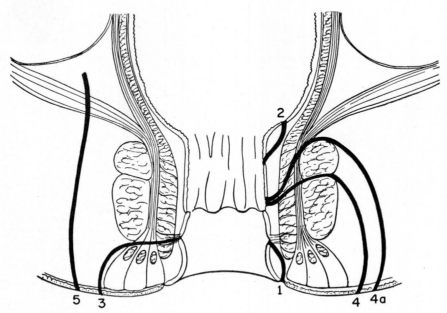

FIG. 38-8. Location of the various types of fistula-in-ano (see also table on p. 1013 for relative incidence). Gabriel classification: Type 1, subcutaneous. Type 2, submucous. Type 3, low level anal. Types 4 and 4a, high level anal. Type 5, anorectal without internal connection.

opposite therefrom (Fig. 38-9). Most fistulas, like most fissures, and possibly for the same reasons, have posterior openings.

Delineation of the course of fistulas may be made with probes, with injection of a peroxide-dye mixture (the writer uses 1% peroxide and methylene blue) and with the use of Lipiodol, bismuth paste, or other radiopaque injections followed by x-ray examination.

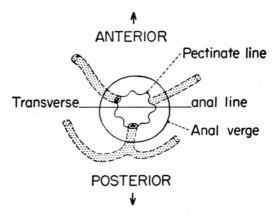

FIG. 38-9. Goodsall's rule: Fistulas with posterior external openings have their internal openings in the mid-line posteriorly; fistulas with anterior external openings have their internal openings radially opposite therefrom.

CLASSIFICATION AND RELATIVE INCIDENCE OF
ANAL FISTULAS

1. Subcutaneous	}	
2. Submucous	....	5%
3. Low level anal	....	75%
4. and 4a. High level anal	....	15%
5. Anorectal without internal connection	......	5%

Treatment is essentially surgical. The surgeon, fortified with the armor of knowledge of the exact course of the fistula, still stands between the Scylla of inadequate surgery and resultant recurrence and the Charybdis of complete excision and cure of the fistula, but with such extensive sphincter division that fecal incontinence results. Fortunately, in the subcutaneous, the submucous and the low level anal types (which comprise 80% of fistulas) this is not a problem, and the entire fistula can be laid open and excised quite safely. If a fistula is soft it should merely be laid open; if it has a hard core it should be excised. It is quite safe to cut the subcutaneous and the superficial portions of the external sphincter; it is quite unsafe to cut everything as high as the anorectal ring. (In this connection it is fortunate that some of Type 5 fistulas can be treated with thorough exposure and drainage without cutting the anorectal ring even by a 2-stage operation.) Between these extremes, the lower portion of the internal sphincter and the deep portion of the external sphincter can be cut when absolutely necessary in cases of high level anal fistulas by experienced surgeons using certain precautions. The incision should be perpendicular to the muscle and sometimes should be done in 2 stages, inserting a seton at the time of the first operation, although setons are used less often than formerly. The seton is left in place beneath the muscle to be cut at the second stage about 7 days later, the fistulous tract having been excised at the first stage. Use of the seton permits the muscle to become

fixed so that its cut ends will not separate too widely. Swerdlow (1958) advocates a 2-stage technic in most lateral fistulas.

Ischiorectal abscess and fistula in cases of ulcerative colitis present a special problem. Before a fistula is to be excised, ileostomy should be done; until the ileostomy is functioning it is only safe to drain.

Concepts concerning fistula should take cognizance of the newer ideas regarding abscess, particularly the intermuscular variety, described by Eisenhammer.

When excising the fistulous tract it is advisable to remove a generous bit of tissue from 1 to 3 mm. in thickness at the site of the internal opening so as to assure extirpation of the adjacent anal glands which so often are the origin of the fistula. Wide saucerization of the wound, especially at the external end, permits healing from the bottom upward. Thus, if the entire lesion is removed in one piece it is like a long dumbbell with the fistulous tract connecting the widely excised skin margin at one end and the less widely removed portion of mucosa at the other. Packs should be used only for hemostasis and should never be left in longer than 4 days (Stelzner, Dietl, and Hahne, 1956). Immediate split-thickness skin grafting of the fistula defect, utilizing a stent, as advocated by Hughes (1957 b, c), may save considerable time in healing. In a limited experience with this technic, the author has been impressed by how well these grafts take. Anorectoplasty, bringing down a mucosal flap to cover the internal opening, may simplify the treatment of these patients and may obviate the cutting of muscles. This has been utilized by McMahon (1956) and Rhoads (1960). The treatment of fistulas must also take cognizance of Eisenhammer's newer ideas (1958) on "Abscess" (pp. 1009-1011).

HEMORRHOIDS

A hemorrhoid is a vascular enlargement of either the internal or the external venous hemorrhoidal plexus or of both. The internal plexus is situated in the submucous space above the interhemorrhoidal groove, while the external plexus lies in the marginal space between the interhemorrhoidal groove above and the lateral hemorrhoidal groove below. The interhemorrhoidal groove is quite visible on a prolapsed combined internal-external type of hemorrhoid (Fig. 38-10). When the hemorrhoids enlarge, the whole mass tends to prolapse and to carry with it the mucosal ligament and interhemorrhoidal groove to a more superficial position, as shown on the right of Figure 38-10.

Hemorrhoids represent one of the most common ailments to afflict mankind. Fortunately, the treatment is relatively simple and safe, and the results are good when operation has been performed properly. From the anatomic standpoint it should be noted that there are 3 primary hemorrhoidal masses (piles): a left lateral and 2 right ones—anterior and posterior. These are also designated as being at 3, 7 and 11 o'clock, the mid-line anterior

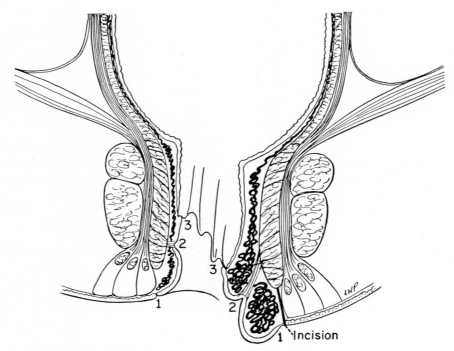

FIG. 38-10. Hemorrhoids. The portion of the drawing on the left shows the normal hemorrhoidal plexuses with the internal plexus above and the external plexus below the interhemorrhoidal groove (Point 2 on the diagram). The portion of the drawing on the right shows how advanced prolapsed internal-external hemorrhoids still maintain their relationship to the interhemorrhoidal groove. The solid black line depicts the line of first incision for either the St. Mark's Hospital operation or for submucosal hemorrhoidectomy. The surgeon should avoid cutting into the internal sphincter muscle. Point 1 is the lateral hemorrhoidal groove; Point 3 is the dentate line.

being high noon. It is interesting for the student to consider other places in the body where asymmetry exists (cerebral lobes, heart, lungs, entrance of ovarian veins into renal vein and vena cava, etc.).

Internal hemorrhoids are insensitive, except at their lower portions and when prolapsed or infected, while external ones are very sensitive. The appearance of both may be considerably altered as a result of thrombosis, infection, ulceration, sloughing, or, in their later stages, by the processes of repair.

Predisposing factors include the erect posture of all mankind, constipation, long straining at the toilet, pregnancy, and a general hereditary venous weakness or pressure factor as evidenced by the frequent concomitant presence of hemorrhoids and varicose veins. Hemorrhoids are rarely present in portal hypertension but may occur in patients with neoplasms of the rectum and the sigmoid. Hemangiomata of the anus are a rare cause of hemorrhoids, excepting in children.

Parks (1956) presented a reasonable theory of the etiology of hemorrhoids. He postulated that the descending fecal scybalous mass forces the blood in the superior hemorrhoidal vessels downward, much as an interne will "milk" a blood transfusion rubber tube. Normally the blood may escape through vascular connections penetrating the internal sphincter, but in the presence of sphincter spasm, this is interfered with. Escape of the blood below is meager, due to the mucosal ligament which separates the internal and the external hemorrhoidal plexuses. All this time, arterial blood continues to enter the venous plexus from above, until the venous pressure equals the arterial. The result is an internal hemorrhoid which bleeds easily.

Once an internal hemorrhoid occurs, partial prolapse stretches the mucosal ligament. The external plexus now begins to fill due to free communication between the two plexuses, i.e., between the submucous and the marginal spaces, and a combined internal-external pile results. At this stage when a bowel movement occurs, the pressure within the internal hemorrhoidal plexus can be dissipated by a flow of blood to the external hemorrhoidal plexus, and bleeding is less apt to result. Other factors rendering chronic prolapsed hemorrhoids less apt to bleed than some early hemorrhoids

are squamous metaplasia of the overlying rectal mucosa due to the prolapse, and recurrent minor thrombosis and resultant fibrosis.

Complications. Before considering the treatment of hemorrhoids, one point deserves special emphasis. Hemorrhoids may occur coincidentally with, be confused with (because both give rectal bleeding and possibly pain) and even may be caused by carcinoma of the rectum or the rectosigmoid. No patient ever should be operated upon for hemorrhoids (except for acute thrombosis of an external hemorrhoid and then he should be urged to return for subsequent study) without a complete anal and rectosigmoidoscopic examination. Any surgeon treating a large number of patients with carcinoma of the lower bowel has seen repeated instances in which advanced cases are admitted with a history of recent hemorrhoidectomy elsewhere.

Acute involvement of hemorrhoids may affect either the internal or the external plexuses. Prolapse of internal hemorrhoids is usually a chronic process associated with laxity of the anal musculature. In certain instances an internal hemorrhoid may be "strangulated," and reduction into the anal canal is in order. Most usually, however, advanced internal hemorrhoids become infected, ulcerated, thrombosed and permanently prolapsed. An erroneous diagnosis of strangulation is often made. In such instances reposition is not possible, the hemorrhoids being completely irreducible, and the preferred treatment is conservative, involving moist dressings, bed rest, heat and sitz baths. Operative treatment, or even attempts at forcible "replacement," in the presence of acutely infected internal hemorrhoids, may lead not only to spread of local infection but also to liver and lung abscesses due to the double (portal and systemic) venous drainage of the hemorrhoidal masses.

Acutely thrombosed *external* hemorrhoids (sometimes called "perianal hematoma"), on the other hand, if infection is not marked, may be safely treated as follows: under local infiltration anesthesia, a radial ellipse of overlying skin over the hemorrhoid (Anderson, 1959; Turell, 1960) plus a small wedge of skin lateral to it is removed. The clot is split, and the two halves are removed (Inberg, 1955). All visible clots are picked out of the vein with forceps. Because the thrombosis extends back to the nearest branches, bleeding is seldom a problem, and this operation truly is one of the most successful in all of surgical practice. However, it is usually unwise to perform simple excision of thrombosed external hemorrhoids situated in the mid-line anteriorly or posteriorly because of the danger of resultant fissure.

Treatment. The treatment of chronic internal hemorrhoids is essentially surgical. Historically, the "complete hemorrhoidectomy" of Whitehead (1882) removing a circumferential cuff of hemorrhoid-bearing mucosa is of interest. In fairness to this surgeon it should be pointed out (Starr, 1957) that not all of his hemorrhoidal operations were radical. Whitehead stated: "Whenever it is possible with strict regard to removing every evidence of hemorrhoidal growth, I invariably leave longitudinal strips of mucous membrane continuous with the skin." Injections are not recommended, because of the danger of infection, necrosis and occasional resultant stricture. The operation to be outlined here is the St. Mark's Hospital technic, a conservative one which involves the removal, after ligation, of the 3 primary internal hemorrhoids with the associated external hemorrhoid and with preservation of a bridge of mucosa of at least 8 to 10 mm. between each line of excision. In general, it is preferable to remove too little rather than too much. More radical *anorectoplastic hemorrhoidectomies* have been introduced, such as the technics of Lewis (1955), McMahon (1956) and others, which are modifications of Whitehead's second operation (1887) but utilize the principles of anorectoplasty. These radical methods have the disadvantage that they lead to a high incidence of stricture unless used by experts in this field. They are not advocated for general use.

The two other most commonly used methods of hemorrhoidectomy are the *clamp and cautery method* (which the author of this chapter was taught but does not advise; a co-editor of this book. (C. A. M.) believes that it is a relic of barbarism and should have been cast into oblivion with the rack and the iron-woman) and the *Parks submucosal hemorrhoidectomy* (which the author prefers above all other methods but will not advise until his experience with it has become greater). The

history of hemorrhoidectomy is discussed by Parks (1955).

Technical details of the St. Mark's Hospital hemorrhoidectomy are as follows:

Preoperative preparation of the lower bowel is similar to that for sigmoidoscopy. Using either general or low spinal anesthesia, the patient is placed in the lithotomy position. The anal canal and the lower rectum are cleansed with pieces of moist cotton wool introduced with the index finger.

Using a pair of nontoothed dissecting forceps, one of the anal skin tags is drawn downward and outward to expose the lower end of the internal hemorrhoid. When the dark-red mucosa covering the hemorrhoid is seen, this is grasped with an artery forceps, and the same thing is repeated with each of the 3 primary internal hemorrhoids. Morgan (1955) described the next important steps as follows:

When traction is now made on the artery forceps, pink rectal mucosa is delivered, and upon it, longitudinal ridges will be noted running downwards, one to each hemorrhoid—these are the *pedicles* of the piles. Each artery forceps is removed in turn from the pile mass and placed on each pile pedicle, which is then drawn downwards until there is a ridge of *pink* mucous membrane seen between each hemorrhoid. These ridges form a complete triangle of pink mucous membrane with a hemorrhoid at each corner. It is important to demonstrate this triangle of pink mucous membrane, which has been called, by Milligan, the *"triangle of exposure,"* since until this is produced, the hemorrhoids are not fully delivered. (Figure 38-11 A.)

The left lateral hemorrhoid is dealt with first, the right posterior one second, and the right anterior one last, so that bleeding from this anterior one will not obscure dissection of the others.

The technic of ligature of each of the hemorrhoids is essentially the same and is as follows:

A second hemostat is placed on the skin overlying the external hemorrhoid corresponding to the internal one to be removed. With a scissors the skin is cut in a V-shape up to the pectinate line on each side of the external hemorrhoid (Fig. 38-11 B). This dissection is carried upward, exposing the lower border of the pale internal sphincter (Fig. 38-11 C). Occasionally, the relaxed subcutaneous portion of the external sphincter is seen at the lateral angle of the wound and is recognized by being redder than the internal sphincter. The internal hemorrhoid is ligated with a transfixion suture of No. 1 catgut on a round needle at the level of the lower border of the internal sphincter and on the mucosal side at the level of the triangle of exposure (Fig. 38-10 and 38-11 D). The skin should not be included in the ligature.

A complete bridge of skin and mucous membrane at least 8 to 10 mm. wide should be left between each of the 3 incisions. After ligation of all 3 hemorrhoids, they are excised, leaving an adequate stump below the point of ligature. If it has been necessary to remove skin in the anterior or the posterior mid-line of the anal canal, the lower 8 mm. of the internal sphincter should be divided at this

point. Generally, except in cases with associated fissure, the hemorrhoid removal should not cross the mid-line anteriorly or posteriorly.

The skin edges are trimmed, and external hemorrhoidal masses protruding from beneath them are avulsed (Fig. 38-11 E). Ligatures are avoided here if at all possible. A proctoscope is inserted to see if the pedicles are bleeding, and after its removal a Penrose drain is inserted. No gauze is inserted into the anal canal, but saline gauze strips are placed on each side between the buttocks. The drain is removed in 24 hours, while the gauze dressings are removed by irrigation in 48 hours and changed at least daily thereafter for the first week, after which they are discontinued except for wearing a pad to protect the clothing. The second evening after the operation the patient is given 15 cc. of mineral oil and

FIG. 38-11. The St. Mark's Hospital operation for hemorrhoids. (A) The triangle of exposure. (B) Commencement of dissection with initial incisions. (C) Dissection completed with the lower end of the internal sphincter (white) and the ligamentous fibers passing to the dissected hemorrhoid exposed. (D) The left lateral hemorrhoid has already been ligated, and the right posterior hemorrhoid is in the process of being ligated. (E) The 3 flat perianal wounds with complete skin bridges in between. (Morgan, C. N.: Hemorrhoids *in* Turner, G., and Lamber, R.: Modern Operative Surgery, London, Cassell)

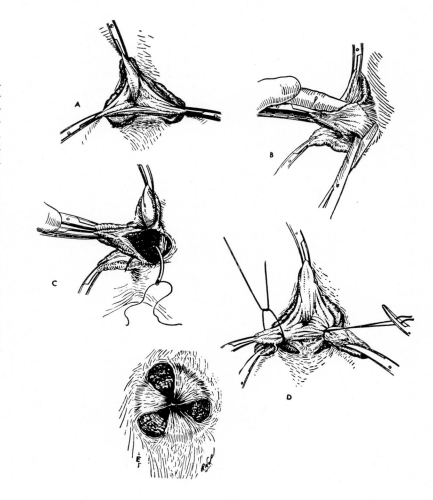

4 cc. of cascara sagrada. The next morning, 48 hours after operation, the patient is given an enema of 5 ounces (150 cc.) of olive oil.

A finger is passed very gently into the rectum on the 7th day and twice weekly thereafter until the skin wounds heal, which usually takes from 3 to 6 weeks.

A method of control of postoperative anorectal bleeding has been advocated recently by Marshall (1955). A lubricated No. 16 French urethral catheter with a 30-ml. balloon is inserted 10 cm. into the rectum, the balloon is distended, gentle traction is exerted upon the catheter, it is taped to the buttocks and usually is withdrawn in 24 to 36 hours. This method has the advantage that it does not require a second trip to the operating room or additional anesthesia.

The author has recently utilized the "submucosal hemorrhoidectomy" of Parks (1956), with good results, but it is still early to recommend this method in preference to ligature and excision, as described above, since we have used the Parks' method in only 22 cases. This method is also used by Shackelford (1958), Rainier (1959) and Silen and Brown (1960) and in modified form by Bartlett (1959). The Parks' technic involves infiltration of the skin and the mucous membrane overlying the hemorrhoids with a 1:400,000 solution of epinephrine in normal saline. The skin ellipse overlying the external hemorrhoid is excised in the usual manner, but the mucous membrane is cut longitudinally over each hemorrhoid. The artificial edema produced by the injection permits the surgeon to dissect up two mucosal flaps over each hemorrhoid and to ligate and excise each hemorrhoid without excision of any mucosa and without including any mucosa in the ligature. The method presents advantages in being radical as far as the hemorrhoidal varices are concerned but conservative as far as the mucous membrane is concerned. Thus the operation is not apt to produce pain or to lead to stricture or recurrence. It is not suitable for early hemorrhoids because of the friability of the mucosa in such instances.

The postoperative management of these cases includes the following 9 points:

1. Mineral oil—30 ml./day for 1 week
2. Dioctyl sodium sulfosuccinate (Doxinate, Colace, aerosol—O.T.), either 1 teaspoonful of liquid (1% solution) in fruit juice b.i.d. or 1 capsule (60 mg.) daily for 3 weeks
3. Ice bag over dressing for pain
4. No sulfonamides
5. No antibiotics
6. No drain or pack
7. Sitz baths beginning in 24 hours
8. Inspect wound with applicator
9. Dilatation: none except by bowel movements first week, little finger second week, and index finger third week
10. If postoperative bleeding of severe degree occurs, an attempt should be made to control it by the method of Marshall (1958), using a balloon catheter, or the technic of Blaisdell (1958), which aims at avoiding sloughing of tissue.

CARCINOMA OF THE ANUS

Such carcinomas are usually epidermoid carcinomas, although basal cell and melanotic carcinomas may occur. Basal cell carcinomas are rare, but Wittoesch, Woolner and Jackman (1957) reported 28 cases of basaloid tumors, 10 of which they called true basal cell carcinomas. Bunstock (1958) collected 47 cases from the literature, including the 10 of Wittoesch et al. Anorectal malignant melanoma is also rare (Probstein, 1957; Pack and Martins, 1960), but Hume and Marshall (1957) stated that over 100 have been reported in the literature while Quan, White and Deddish (1959) reported 21 (0.5% of all malignant tumors of the anorectal region) from the Memorial Center, New York City. Anorectal melanoma represents about 1 per cent of all malignant melanoma. Epidermoid carcinomas arise from the true anus, in other words from the portion of the anorectum external to the pectinate line. The lesion is relatively rare, and only about 3 per cent of cases of cancer of the rectosigmoid, the rectum and the anus arise from the anus. While adenocarcinoma of the rectum is twice as common in men as in women, there is little or no sex predisposition with carcinoma of the anus. Buckwalter and Jurayj (1957) believe that chronic infection plays an important etiologic role. Patients with carcinoma of the anus are usually about 4 years older than those with adenocarcinoma of the rectum (61 as opposed to 57 years). The lesion is especially apt to involve the anterior quadrant of the anorectum. In females this has a clinical application in that the posterior vaginal wall frequently has to be removed.

The routes of spread of the tumor have a relation to selection of treatment. Local extension may involve the skin, the perianal and the ischioanal spaces, and the levator ani muscles. Extension to the prostate, the vagina (except in anterior lesions, see previous paragraph), the cervix and the bladder is rare except late in the course of the disease.

Blood-borne metastases are rare when compared with those from rectosigmoid carcinomas, being respectively 4 and 11 per cent to the liver, and 0 and 8 per cent to the lungs, the spine and the brain (Grinnell, 1955). This may explain why radical surgery may give better results in the treatment of anorectal (squamous cell) carcinoma than in rectosigmoid carcinoma.

Metastases by way of the lymphatics are common. Because of the position of carcinoma of the anus it metastasizes by lymphatic spread, both to the inguinal glands and upward to the pelvic glands. Upward metastatic involvement of either the perirectal or the mesocolic lymph nodes by way of the superior hemorrhoidal artery to the inferior mesenteric vessels occurs almost as frequently as in carcinoma of the rectum (33 as opposed to 42%; Grinnell, 1955). Involvement of the inguinal nodes can occur by 2 routes: an external and an internal one. The external route is via the anal plexus through the perineal lymphatics up over the upper thigh, emptying into the superficial groin nodes. The internal route is via the middle hemorrhoidal plexus to the hypogastric and the obturator nodes, then to the external iliac nodes and finally to the inguinal nodes.

The standard treatment of carcinoma of the anus is combined abdominoperineal resection of the rectum associated with the following 7 procedures: (1) ligation of the superior hemorrhoidal vessels just below the left colic, (2) wide removal of the peritoneum, (3) wide perianal skin excision, (4) complete removal of the ischioanal fossa contents, (5) division of the levator muscles at their origin, (6) abdominopelvic node dissection which includes removal of the tissue about the aorta and its bifurcation, the vena cava, the iliacs (common, external and internal), and to obturator

and the presacral spaces, and (7) inguinal node dissection if these nodes are involved. This is essentially the method of treatment advocated by Stearns (1955, 1958) and by Grinnell (1955) and used at the Memorial and the Presbyterian Hospitals respectively, in New York.

Variations from this standard treatment should be assessed carefully before being adopted. Roentgen therapy alone is not recommended, and in combination with surgery has not been used in most big centers. Less radical surgery than a combined abdominoperineal resection should not be used for high lesions but is still used at the Memorial Hospital for small and superficial lesions very low in the anal canal. Such low lesions are sometimes treated by wide local excision.

While all surgeons agree that involved inguinal nodes are an indication for *therapeutic* groin dissection, either at the time of the posterior operation or within a few weeks thereafter, there is difference of opinions as to whether a bilateral *prophylactic* groin dissection is to be advocated. Stearns studied the 69 patients with epidermoid carcinoma of the anus treated at the Memorial Hospital during the 11-year period 1942 to 1952, inclusive. In 53 of these patients there were no recognizable inguinal metastases at the time the primary lesion was treated. Forty of these failed to develop metastases, while 13 (25%) did. Further breakdown of the 13 indicated that in only 3 could a prophylactic groin dissection have been of possible value. Thus, 53 bilateral groin dissections with their attendant morbidity, including possible leg edema, etc., would have had to be performed to salvage at the most 3 patients or 6 per cent. Further analysis of large series of patients will be necessary to settle the question as to the advisability of prophylactic groin dissection in this condition. However, one point is clear, namely, that if a prophylactic groin dissection is not done the patient should be examined periodically for the subsequent development of involved groin lymph nodes. The Memorial Hospital schedule for such check-ups is as follows: examination at monthly or bimonthly intervals the first 2 years (the time interval during which 85% of the nodes which are to become positive do so), at intervals of 3 or 4 months from then to 5 years, and at yearly intervals thereafter. Furthermore, it was found that the results following groin dissection on such delayed metastases were actually much better than in cases in which the groin nodes were involved initially, possibly because in the delayed cases the tumor is less active biologically.

The results of radical surgery for epidermoid carcinoma of the rectum are obtainable only from the few large series reported. Stearns reported an over-all 5-year survival rate of 30 per cent (50% in patients without groin metastases and 12.5% in those with groin metastases—all of the latter representing patients in whom the groin metastases occurred after removal of the primary lesion). Grinnell reported an over-all 5-year survival rate of 39 per cent, but in those with curative surgery it was 55 per cent. These figures are quite comparable with those obtained after abdominoperineal resection for carcinoma of the rectum or the rectosigmoid.

A rare but very interesting tumor of the rectum, not related to carcinoma of the anus, is *villous tumor* of the rectum. This tumor is usually sessile, occurs in adults, may cover a wide area of the rectum and extend down to but not below the pectinate line of the anorectum. Its two chief points of interest are (1) its microscopic nature—in that it is composed of numerous stalklike or frondlike thin villous processes which appear to be quite fragile—and (2) its frequent tendency to malignant change, possible in one third of cases. (For a more extensive discussion of *colorectal* villous tumors, see Chap. 37, Part 2.)

BIBLIOGRAPHY

Altemeier, W. A., Hoxworth, P. I., and Giuseffi, J.: Further experiences with the treatment of prolapse of the rectum, S. Clin. North America *35*:1437-1447, 1955.

Anderson, R. E.: The humble thrombosed hemorrhoid, Northwest Med. *58*:114-1120, 1959.

Anderson, R. E., Pontius, G. V., and Witkowski, L. J.: Complications following surgery for benign anorectal lesions, J.A.M.A. *159*:9-17, 1955.

Baden, H., and Mikkelsen, O.: The results of rectopexy in complete prolapse of the rectum in adults, Acta chir. scandinav. *116*:230-234, 1959.

Bartlett, W.: Freedom from pain after hemorrhoidectomy, A.M.A. Arch. Surg. *78*:916-922, 1959.

Bill, A. H., Jr.: Pathology and surgical treatment of "imperforate anus," J.A.M.A. *166*:1429-1432, 1958.

Bill, A. H., Jr., and Johnson, R. J.: Failure of migration of the rectal opening as the cause for most cases of imperforate anus, Surg., Gynec. & Obst. *106*:643-651, 1958.

Birnbaum, W., and Sproul, G.: The treatment of postoperative fecal incontinence, S. Clin. North America *35*:1487-1495, 1955.

Blaisdell, P. C.: Repair of the incontinent sphincter ani, Am. Surg. *94*:573-576, 1957.

————: Prevention of massive hemorrhage secondary to hemorrhoidectomy, Surg., Gynec. & Obst. *106*:485-488, 1958.

Brayton, D., and Norris, W. J.: Further experiences with the treatment of imperforate anus, Surg., Gynec. & Obst. *107*:719-726, 1958.

Brossy, J. J.: Anatomy and surgery of anal fissure, Ann. Surg. *144*:991-998, 1956.

Buckwalter, J. A., and Jurayj, M. N.: Relationship of chronic anorectal disease to carcinoma, A.M.A. Arch. Surg. *75*:352-361, 1957.

Bunstock, W. H.: Basal cell carcinoma of the anus, Am. J. Surg. *95*:822-825, 1958.

Burke, R. M., and Jackman, R. J.: A modified Thiersch operation in treatment of complete rectal prolapse, Dis. Colon & Rect. *2*:555-561, 1959.

Dresen, K-A., and Kratzer, G. L.: Fecal impaction in modern practice, J.A.M.A. *170*:644-647, 1959.

Dunphy, J. E.: A combined perineal and abdominal operation for the repair of rectal prolapse, Surg., Gynec. & Obst. *86*:493-498, 1948.

Dunphy, J. E., and Pikula, J.: Fact and fancy about fistula-in-ano, S. Clin. North America *35*:1469-1477, 1955.

Eisenhammer, S.: The internal anal sphincter: its surgical importance, South African M.J. *27*:266-270, 1953.

————: The surgical correction of chronic internal anal (sphincteric), contracture, South African M.J. *25*:486-489, 1951.

————: The internal anal sphincter and the anorectal abscess, Surg., Gynec. & Obst. *103*:501-506, 1956.

————: A new approach to the anorectal fistulous abscess based on the high intermuscular lesion, Surg., Gynec. & Obst. *106*:595-599, 1958.

————: The evaluation of the internal anal sphincterotomy operation with special reference to anal fissure, Surg. Gynec. & Obst. *109*:583-590, 1959.

————: Personal communication, August, 1960.

Ferguson, J. A.: Repair of "Whitehead deformity" of the anus, Surg., Gynec. & Obst. *108*:115-116, 1959.

Fine, J., and Lawes, C. H. Wickham: On the

muscle-fibres of the anal submucosa, with special reference to the Pecten Band, Brit. J. Surg. 27:723-727, 1940.

Fowler, R.: Landmarks and legends of the anal canal, Australian & New Zealand J. Surg. 27:2-18, 1957.

Fromer, J. L.: Dermatologic concepts and management of pruritus ani, Am. J. Surg. 90:805-815, 1955.

Frykman, H. M.: Abdominal proctopexy and primary sigmoid resection for rectal procidentia, Am. J. Surg. 90:780-789, 1955.

Gabriel, William B.: The Principles and Practice of Rectal Surgery, ed. 4, London, Lewis, 1948.

Goligher, J. C.: The treatment of complete prolapse of the rectum by the Roscoe Graham operation, Brit. J. Surg. 45:323-333, 1958.

Goligher, J. C., Leacock, A. G., and Brossy, J. J.: The surgical anatomy of the anal canal, Brit. J. Surg. 43:51-61, 1955.

Gorsch, R. V.: Proctologic Anatomy, ed. 2, Baltimore, Williams & Wilkins, 1955.

Graham, R. R.: The operative repair of massive rectal prolapse, Ann. Surg. 115:1007-1014, 1942.

Granet, Emil: Manual of Proctology, Chicago, Year Book Pub., 1954.

Grinnell, R. S.: Squamous cell carcinoma of the anus, S. Clin. North America 35:1289-1294, 1955.

Hughes, E. S. R.: Anal fissure, Brit. M.J. 2:803-804, 1953.

————: Ano-rectal Suppuration, Australian & New Zealand J. Surg. 23:41-47, 1953.

————: Fistula-in-ano, M.J. Australian 1:198-200, 1953.

————: Surgical anatomy of the anal canal, Australian & New Zealand J. Surg. 26:48-55,1956.

————: Surgery of the Anus, Anal Canal and Rectum, Edinburgh, Livingstone, 1957.

————: The classification of anorectal fistula, Australian & New Zealand J. Surg. 26:274-280, 1957.

————: Treatment of ischiorectal anal fistula, Australian & New Zealand J. Surg. 26:281-288, 1957.

Hume, A. H., and Marshall, S. F.: Anorectal malignant melanoma, Lahey Clin. Bull. 10:174-177, 1957.

Inberg, K. R.: Perianal haematoma, Acta chir. scandinav. 109:203-205, 1955.

————: Complete rectal prolapse, Acta chir. scandinav. 114:310-318, 1958.

Jackman, R. J.: Technique of proctoscopy, J.A.M.A. 166:1510-1513, 1958.

Karlan, M., McPherson, R. C., and Watman, R. N.: An experimental evaluation of fecal continence—sphincter and reservoir—in the dog, Surg., Gynec. & Obst. 108:469-475, 1959.

Kark, A. E., Epstein, A. E., and Chapman, D. S.: Nonmalignant anaorectal strictures, Surg., Gynec. & Obst. 109:333-343, 1959.

Leifer, W.: Pruritus ani, S. Clin. North America 35:1479-1482, 1955.

Lewis, A. E.: Anorectoplasty for hemorrhoidal surgery, Am. J. Surg. 90:767-772, 1955.

McElwain, J. W.: Primary fistulotomy in the treatment of anorectal abscesses, Surgery 45:945-948, 1959.

MacKenzie, R. J., and Davis, D. A.: Prolapse of the rectum in infants and children, West J. Surg. 66:323-325, 1958.

McMahon, W. A.: Personal communication, May 9, 1956.

Marshall, G. R.: A method for control of anorectal hemorrhage, J. Internat. Coll. Surgeons 24:97-99, 1955.

————: Control of anorectal hemorrhage with balloon catheter, Northwest Med. 57:334, 1958.

Martin, C. L.: Tuberculous fistula-in-ano: Diagnostic criteria and current therapy, J. Internat. Col. Surgeons 27:649-655, 1957.

Miles, W. E. (1904): Cited by Altemeier, Hoxworth, and Giuseffi (see reference above), 1955.

————: Recto-sigmoidoscopy as a method of treatment for procidentia recti, Proc. Roy. Soc. Med. 26:1445-1452, 1933.

Milligan, E. T. C.: Rectum-haemorrhoids in British Surgical Practice, vol. 7, London, Butterworth, 1948.

Milligan, E. T. C., and Morgan, C. N.: Surgical anatomy of the anal canal with special reference to anorectal fistulae, Lancet 2:1150-1156, 1213-1217, 1934.

Milligan, E. T. C., Morgan, C. N., Jones, L. E., and Officer, R.: Surgical anatomy of the anal canal, and the operative treatment of hemorrhoids, Lancet 2:1119-1124, 1937.

Milligan, E. T. C., Morgan C. N., Lloyd-Davies, O. V., and Thompson, H. R.: Fistula in ano in British Surgical Practice, vol. 4, London, Butterworth, 1948.

Morgan, C. N.: Hemorrhoids and their surgical treatment: A description of the St. Mark's Hospital operation for hemorrhoids, S. Clin. North America 35:1457-1464, 1955.

Morgan, C. N., and Hughes, E. S. R.: The anal canal and rectum, Australian & New Zealand J. Surg. 21:161-172, 1952.

Morgan, C. N., and Thompson, H. R.: Surgical anatomy of the anal canal with special reference to the surgical importance of the internal sphincter and conjoint longitudinal muscle, Ann. Roy. Coll. Surgeons England 19:88-114, 1956.

Moschowitz, A. V.: The pathogenesis, anatomy,

and cure of prolapse of the rectum, Surg., Gynec. & Obst. *15*:7-21, 1912.

Nigro, N. D., and Walker, G. L.: An evaluation of the mechanism and treatment of complete rectal prolapse, Am. J. M. Sc. *234*:213-226, 1957.

Orr, T. G.: A suspension operation for prolapse of the rectum, Ann. Surg. *126*:833-840, 1947.

Osborne, E. D., and Stoll, H. L.: Pruritis ani et vulvae, J.A.M.A. *169*:108-111, 1959.

Pack, G. T., and Martins, F. G.: Treatment of anorectal malignant melanoma, Dis. Colon & Rect. *3*:15-24, 1960.

Parks, A. G.: De haemorrhois, Guy's Hosp. Rep. *104*:135-156, 1955.

————: A note on the anatomy of the anal canal, Proc. Roy. Soc. Med. *47*:997-998, 1954.

————: The surgical treatment of hemorrhoids, Brit. J. Surg. *43*:337-351, 1956.

Pope, C. E.: An anorectal plastic operation for fissure and stenosis and its surgical principles, Surg., Gynec. & Obst. *108*:249-252, 1959.

Probstein, J. G.: Malignant melanoma of the anorectum, A.M.A. Arch. Surg. *75*:253-255, 1957.

Quan, S. H., White, J. E., and Deddish, M. R.: Malignant melanoma of the anorectum, Dis. Colon & Rect. *2*:275-283, 1959.

Ranier, W. G.: Discussion of paper by Bartlett (see reference above), 1959.

Rhoads, J. E.: Personal communication, July 16, 1960.

Scott, J. E. S., Swenson, O., and Fisher, J. H.: Some comments on the surgical treatment of imperforate anus. Long term results and postoperative management, Am. J. Surg. *99*:137-143, 1960.

Shackelford, R. T.: Personal communication, November, 1958.

Shann, H.: The complete prolapse of procidentia of the rectum, an unsolved surgical problem, Internat. Abst. Surg. *109*:521-534, 1959.

Shropshear, G.: Surgical anatomic aspects of the anorectal sphincter mechanism and its clinical significance, J. Internat. Coll. Surgeons *33*:267-287, 1960.

Silen, W., and Brown, W. B.: Submucosal hemorrhoidectomy, Am. Surgeon *26*:123-128, 1960.

Smith, C., Malkiewicz, G. M., and Massenberg, G. Y., Jr.: The autonomic nervous system in pruritus ani: perianal skin temperatures after sympathetic block in control subjects, Am. J. Surg. *90*:790-794, 1955.

Starr, K. W.: The heritage of Walter Whitehead, Surg., Gynec. & Obst. *104*:751, 1957.

Stearns, M. W., Jr.: Epidermoid carcinoma of the anal region: inguinal metastases, Am. J. Surg. *90*:727-733, 1955.

————: Epidermoid carcinoma of the anal region, Surg., Gynec. & Obst. *106*:92-96, 1958.

Stelzner, F., Dietl, H., and Hahne, H.: Results of radical operations in 143 anal fistulas (evaluation of one-step sphincteral division in one-stage and in multi-stage operations), Chirurg. *27*:158-162, 1956, Abstr. J.A.M.A. *161*:1189, 1956.

Stroud, B. B.: On the anatomy of the anus, Ann. Surg. *24*:1-15, 1896.

Swerdlow, H.: Fistulotomy and fistulectomy for fistulas about the anus and rectum, Am. J. Surg. *95*:818-821, 1958.

Swinton, N. W., and Mumma, J. F.: The treatment of hemorrhoids, S. Clin. North America *36*:761-772, 1956.

Swinton, N. W., and Palmer, T.: The management of rectal prolapse and procidentia, Am. J. Surg. *99*:144-151, 1960.

Tendler, M. S.: Massive prolapse of the rectum, A.M.A. Arch. Surg. *72*:667-672, 1956.

Turell, R.: Hydrocortisone therapy in control of anogenital pruritis, J.A.M.A. *158*:173-175, 1955.

————: Modern treatment of pruritis ani, Surg., Gynec. & Obst. *104*:233-237, 1957.

————: Colonic and anorectal function and disease, Surg., Gynec. & Obst. *107*:417-448, 1958.

————: Sigmoidoscopy and biopsy, Surgery *45*: 880-882, 1959.

————: Hemorrhoids: advances and retreats, Am. J. Surg. *99*:154-167, 1960.

Vetto, R. M., Harkins, H. N., McMahon, W. A., and White, T. T.: Unpublished data, 1956.

Walls, E. W: Observations on the microscopic anatomy of the human anal canal, Brit. J. Surg. *45*:504-512, 1958.

Warner, B. W.: Diagnosis of schistosomiasis by sigmoidoscopy and rectal mucosal biopsy, J.A.M.A. *163*:1322-1325, 1957.

Whitehead, W.: The surgical treatment of haemorrhoids, Brit. M. J. *1*:148-150, 1882.

Wilde, F. R.: The anal intermuscular septum, Brit. J. Surg. *36*:279-285, 1949.

Wittoesch, J. H., Woolner, L. B., and Jackman, R. J.: Basal cell epithelioma and basaloid lesions of the anus, Surg., Gynec. & Obst. *104*: 75-80, 1957.

Young, H. M.: Viral verrucae in the anorectum, Surgery *41*:292-305, 1957.

CHAPTER 39

Hernia

There is, perhaps, no operation which has had so much of vital interest to both physician and surgeon as herniotomy, and there is no operation which, by the profession at large, would be more appreciated than a perfectly safe and sure cure for rupture. —Halsted, 1892.

In the entire history of surgery no subject has been so controversial as the repair of groin hernias.—McVay, 1954.

INTRODUCTION

The subject of hernia is an important one in surgery today, and probably will be so for some time to come. The number of persons now alive who either have had or will develop hernia runs into the millions. Thus, hernia is a practical subject. Its repair is largely a structural one, and is based on a sound correction of the existing anatomic defects. At the same time, many of the advances in the fundamental knowledge of wound healing have and will come from a study of their almost controlled and repetitive application in the treatment of countless patients afflicted with the deformity of hernia.

One factor which is responsible today for part of the poor results following the repair of hernia is that operations for hernia are often considered to be minor or easy. On the contrary, it is difficult to learn the anatomy of the inguinofemoral region, repairs are not easy, and it is necessary to utilize great judgment in selecting the proper procedure for the particular patient being treated and to develop a facile technic in performing the operation. Only too often in training programs these operations are done by the younger and more inexperienced assistant residents. Ideas concerning the repair of hernias are passed on from one resident generation to another, often with no direct supervision by or infusion of new ideas from the chief of the service who is interested in more "major" procedures. In practice, surgeons who have learned their craft by other means than training do herniorrhaphies when they would not venture into more "major" fields. The philosophy that "anyone" can get good results with the repair of hernia makes even some trained surgeons careless. While experienced surgeons have fewer immediate complications involving such things as inadvertent division of the vas deferens, puncture of femoral vein by sutures, wound infection, etc., the matter of recurrence is the chief one at stake. For example, in good hands repair of direct hernia is followed by about a 7 per cent recurrence, while in less well-trained hands it may be 30 per cent (or higher). To the 70 out of 100 patients who may get a satisfactory result whether they go to an expert or a novice (or to the 7% who would get a recurrence anyway), the matter is not important; but to the 23 patients who do have a recurrence only because they have gone to a less capable surgeon, the matter is vitally significant.

HISTORICAL CONSIDERATIONS

The treatment of hernia has gone through an evolution similar to that in other fields of surgery. The careful anatomic repair of today had to wait for the development of anesthesia and antisepsis. Before the introduction of these two advances, operation was both hurried, because of pain, and dangerous, because of frequent sepsis permitting operation only in the larger hernias which demanded treatment and in which it was often impossible to ascertain the anatomic relationships. Mass ligatures, and even the cautery, were widely used. One clinic visitor observed even as great a surgeon as Dupuytren (1777-1835) cut into the bowel with the original skin incision during the performance of 2 consecutive herniotomies.

In the last decade of the last century there was an especially rapid advance in the knowledge of hernia, particularly in so far as surgical treatment was concerned. The stage was set for careful dissections without the previous handicaps of haste and fear of infection, and able observers in a number of countries made distinct and almost simultaneous contributions. The classic reports of Bassini (1888), Halsted (1889, 1903), Lucas-Championnière (1892), Andrews (1895), Lotheissen (1898), Ferguson (1899) and McArthur (1901) appeared during this period. Essentially, these observers devised different varieties of layer closure of the defects remaining after sac ligation, and most of today's repairs, of groin hernias at least, are based upon the technics of 60 years ago. The details of repair introduced by some of these men will be discussed in the section on groin hernia later in this chapter. The historical development of herniorrhaphy was reviewed recently by Carlson (1956), Brown and Galetti (1960) and Galletti and Brown (1960).

DEFINITION, DIAGNOSIS, INCIDENCE AND PROGNOSIS

DEFINITION

A hernia is an abnormal protrusion of an organ or a portion of it through the containing wall of its cavity, beyond its normal confines. The usual meaning of the term is restricted to the abdominal cavity, so that such things as muscle hernia of the leg are not usually considered and will not be in this chapter.

DIAGNOSIS

The diagnosis of a hernia is made primarily on the basis of the physical examination, not on the history. However, there are exceptions to this rule. If the patient, or the patient's mother in the case of a child, states that a hernia is present, the physician should not dismiss the patient with a negative diagnosis on the basis of a single examination. If repeated examination is negative, the patient should be urged to return at a time when the hernia is present. Furthermore, a patient wearing a truss may have negative findings at the first examination. In such instance he should be requested to leave the truss off for several days, or until the hernia becomes manifest, and then return for a second examination.

A dragging sensation, sometimes with pain at the onset, is the one feature in the history common to many groin hernias, but, as stated above, the diagnosis is based primarily on the physical examination. A hernia usually is most painful at the onset, while the gradual spreading of tissues in the later stages only gives a vague discomfort.

The physical examination involves 4 steps. The first 3 require that the examiner be seated on a low stool before the patient, who is standing with the area from above the groin to the knees exposed. Furthermore, the patient should be masked or should be required to hold a towel in front of his mouth when coughing to prevent the spread of germs, particularly *Mycobacterium tuberculosis*. The patient is encouraged to cough while the examiner (1) observes the groin region for appearance of a swelling; (2) palpates it to feel for an impulse and later for a swelling which gives a gurgling sensation on being reduced; and (3) palpates through the invaginated neck of the scrotum with a single examining finger for an impulse or reducible swelling. The 4th step involves repetition of the examination with the patient lying down.

The "thumb test" (Moyer, 1955) is an

added means of examination. With the hernia reduced, the flat of the thumb is held firmly over the site of the internal ring (just above a point halfway between the anterior superior iliac spine and the symphysis pubis), and the patient is encouraged to cough. If the hernia is indirect, the thumb will retain it; if the hernia is direct, the thumb cannot hold it in, and it will protrude medial to the point being pressed upon.

In infants, the "water-silk" sign (see Gross, 1953) may be helpful. The middle finger is placed over the inguinal canal and moved back and forth from below and laterally to above and medially. An increased thickness can be felt if an inguinal hernia is present, and there is a sensation of silken surfaces sliding over each other.

Zieman (1940) emphasized the importance of the second step in the physical diagnosis of hernia, as listed above. In brief, his method consists of standing behind and to the side of the erect patient and using the right hand for examination of the right side and the left hand for the left. The 1st, the 2nd and the 3rd fingers of the hand are placed over the region of Hesselbach's triangle, the external ring and the femoral region, respectively, with the fingers pointing downward and medially. When the patient coughs or strains, a peculiar gurgling, sliding or slipping motion occurs under one finger. If under the index finger, the hernia is more apt to be direct; if under the other 2, indirect or femoral hernia. If a bulge is present before coughing, it is reduced before applying the test.

Other methods also are used to decide the difficult question as to whether the hernia is indirect or direct inguinal, or femoral. An oblique impulse, a hernia which goes all the way down into the scrotum, or palpation of a rounded edge of the fascial defect medially indicates a possible indirect inguinal hernia. A more vertical or outward impulse, a hernia which protrudes diffusely anteriorly and medially and does not go all the way down into the scrotum, and a straight vertical edge of the medial fascial defect indicate a possible direct inguinal hernia. Preoperative palpation of the pulse in the superficial inferior epigastric artery through the abdominal wall and determining whether the hernial impulse is lateral

or medial to it, hence indirect or direct, is not possible in the experience of the author.

The decision as to whether the hernia is inguinal or femoral is arrived at on accurate palpation of the lower edge of the external oblique aponeurosis. If the bulge comes out above, it is inguinal; if below, it is femoral. At the same time the examiner should remember that femoral hernias first descend, then protrude, anteriorly; then they may even curl upward slightly. The common error is to overlook a femoral hernia; it is much more common to label a femoral hernia as an inguinal one than the reverse. The author's rule epitomizes this as follows: "If in doubt, it is a femoral hernia."

In the differential diagnosis from other conditions, the following must be considered: (1) inguinal adenitis (to one side of the empty inguinal canal); (2) ectopic testis (characteristic shape to mass combined with absence of testis in scrotum on that side); (3) hydrocele of the cord (usually moves when cord is tightened by scrotal traction, may be transilluminated, examining finger may get above mass with the finding of absent cough impulse); (4) psoas abscess (dull to percussion, associated with changes in the spine); (5) femoral adenitis (lacks the impulse of a femoral hernia); and (6) saphenous varix (compressible, has an impulse on percussion of saphenous vein below—Schwartz's sign—and a thrill or a transitory impulse as a result of pressure from above during coughing).

INCIDENCE AND PROGNOSIS

It is difficult to arrive at the incidence of the various types of hernia, since different hospitals treat different types of material and, furthermore, different hernias, due to diagnostic difficulties, etc., are treated in different proportions in relationship to their occurrence in the untreated population. However, for practical purposes, the following outline serves as a basis of departure. These figures are reached by combining percentages given in various texts plus personal observations, taking into special consideration the belief that direct hernia, if properly tested for and searched for at operation, is much more common than is generally realized. These figures are given in Table 1.

TABLE 1. INCIDENCE OF HERNIA

	PERCENTAGE
Indirect inguinal	56
Direct inguinal	22
Femoral	6
Ventral and incisional	10
Umbilical	3
Esophageal hiatus	1
Others	2
Total	100

As Elman (1952) pointed out in an editorial, it is a surprise to learn that in the 1948 United States mortality tables, hernia (exclusive of intestinal obstruction) is listed as responsible for 5,000 deaths, a figure which exceeded the death rate for acute appendicitis in that year. Moreover, this mortality has remained nearly constant for the past 2 decades, a period during which the mortality from acute appendicitis has been cut sharply to about one third. Elman urged more frequent practice of herniorrhaphy before the onset of the complications of strangulation and obstruction, which are responsible for the high death rate cited above.

Elman pointed out further that the hernia problem is larger than this when it is considered that the United States Public Health Service estimates that there are 800,000 individuals in this country today with unrepaired hernias, which figure correlates well with the annual sale of trusses, which is said to exceed 1 million a year. He concluded his observations by stating: "The hernia problem is a simple one which can be solved by using adequate surgery earlier and more frequently."

Hagan and Rhoads (1953) discussed the prognosis following 1,082 groin herniorrhaphies on 957 patients in 1,022 operations at the University of Pennsylvania Hospital from 1945 to 1948, inclusive. The operative mortality rate was 0.3 per cent. The distribution of these cases gives an indication of the relative incidence of the more common types of groin hernia in hospital practice, as follows: 86 per cent of the total hernias occurred in males, while 84 per cent of the femoral hernias occurred in females. It is significant that in conformity with most other reports, while femoral hernia is *relatively* more common in females, its *absolute* frequency in

females is less than indirect inguinal hernia (41% femoral, as opposed to 52% indirect inguinal, the most common among all groin hernias in women). Hagan and Rhoads reported 4.6 per cent of hernias in women as being direct or pantaloon in type. This is considerably more than has occurred on the author's service (1 in approximately 1,000, or 0.1%). However, the figure of 4.6 per cent represents only 0.4 per cent of the direct hernias in both sexes and only 0.9 per cent of the entire series of 1,082 groin hernias. For the student who may not see a large number of hernias, the rule taught the author by Andrews (1933), that "There is no such thing as a direct hernia in a woman," may be valuable as a teaching point to emphasize that such hernias are indeed very rare.

Recurrences were noted as late as 39 years after the original operation by Hagan and Rhoads: 55 per cent of the recurrences were evident within 2 years and an additional 20 per cent during the following 3 years. Thus, 25 per cent occurred after 5 years following operation. Fallis (1937) reported similar figures: 48 per cent recurrences within 2 years, an additional 20 per cent within the following 3 years and 32 per cent after 5 years following operation. Recurrence rates relative to the time since repair in various reported series are shown in Table 3 (p. 1027). The entire subject of recurrence of groin hernias has been analyzed by Ryan (1953) on the basis of his experience with 369 recurrent cases.

The recurrence rate relative to age in Hagan and Rhoads' series is of interest. The over-all recurrence rate at the end of 2 years was 5.4 per cent. There were no recurrences in children under 10 years of age. The recurrence rate rose by decades from 10 to 60 years with percentages of 2.3 rising progressively

TABLE 2. RELATIVE INCIDENCE OF
GROIN HERNIAS
(HAGAN AND RHOADS, 1953)

	PERCENTAGE
Indirect inguinal	66.1
Direct and direct-indirect	20.2
Recurrent inguinal	6.9
Femoral	6.8
Total	100.0

TABLE 3. RECURRENCE RATES IN INGUINAL HERNIA RELATIVE TO TIME
ELAPSED SINCE PRIMARY REPAIR

AUTHOR	NO. OF CASES	RECURRENCES PERCENTAGE		
		To 1 yr.	To 2 yr.	To 5 yr.
Fallis (1937)	200	37	48	68
Clear (1951)	114	17	28	62
Zawacki and Thieme (1951)	105	51	..	75
Borgström (1951)	88	55	71	87
Hagan and Rhoads (1953)	75	..	55	75

to 12.2 per cent. After 60, the recurrence rate again dropped to 3.7 per cent, probably because of less physical activity in patients over that age. The sex differences in recurrence rate also were interesting, being 6.1 per cent for males and 1.1 per cent for females.

Guy, Werelius and Bell (1955) give an over-all summary of the probable recurrence rates now occurring in the United States, as shown in Table 4.

The incidence of recurrences in different parts of the inguinal floor was studied by Zawacki and Thieme (1951), as shown in Table 5.

These authors pointed out that 75 per cent of recurrences were due to failure either to close the internal ring properly or to take a firm stitch at the pubic spine. In general, it can be said that most recurrences are direct, except when the sac has been left behind or the internal ring has not been tightened properly.

THE HERNIA PROBLEM TODAY

The hernia problem today is essentially surgical. Its major facets are two: (1) the problem of incarceration (irreducibility) and strangulation; and (2) technical factors in the repair of the 4 most common types of hernia (groin, ventral incisional, umbilical and esophageal hiatus hernias) with the prevention of recurrence.

These 2 major groups of problems, which concern the medical student, will be considered here. Then at the end of the chapter the following items which concern the specialist will be covered: (1) subsidiary general problems in the field of hernia, (2) a consideration of certain "aids" to repair which are not applicable routinely but are useful methods in the armamentarium of any surgeon, and (3) a glossary of terms, including a discussion of some of the rarer, but important, types of hernia for which a few details of therapy will be given.

THE PROBLEM OF INCARCERATION (IRREDUCIBILITY), OBSTRUCTION AND STRANGULATION

In cases of incarcerated (irreducible) hernia (see glossary at end of chapter), it is often difficult to tell whether such a hernia is strangulated or soon will be, and, from a practical viewpoint, it would seem advisable to look upon all incarcerated hernias as potentially strangulated and to treat them as emergencies along with the truly strangulated hernias. This same argument also applies to obstructed

TABLE 4. RECURRENCES AFTER
HERNIORRHAPHY

	PERCENTAGE RECURRENCE
Indirect inguinal hernia:	
Children and females	1 to 4
Adult males	5 to 10
Direct inguinal hernia	15 to 30
Recurrent inguinal hernia	15 to 40
Ventral and incisional hernias	20 to 30

TABLE 5. ANATOMIC LOCALIZATION OF 105
RECURRENCES FOLLOWING INGUINAL
HERNIORRHAPHY

TYPE OF RECURRENCE	PERCENTAGE OF TOTAL CASES	
At internal ring:		
Small at ring	18	
Above and lateral	12	
Typical indirect hernia	20	50
At pubic tubercle		22
Direct hernia		22
Miscellaneous		6
Total		100

hernias to an even greater degree. The line of differentiation between incarceration (syn.: irreducibility) and obstruction on the one hand and strangulation on the other is often tenuous and may change from hour to hour, particularly in the case of a hernia which has become incarcerated only recently. The safest procedure would be early operation for all, and emergency operation for incarceration, and always, of course, for strangulation.

Strangulation, implying obstruction of the flow of blood to the contents of a hernia, is an important catastrophe. It is one of the two most common causes of death from intestinal obstruction (the other being adhesive bands), and it kills about 5,000 persons in the United States every year. In 1946, strangulation was responsible for 3,985 deaths in England and Wales in a total population of 43 million. Smith, Moore and Perry (1955) reported that 44 per cent of all strangulating bowel obstructions at the University of Minnesota were due to external hernia with strangulation. A prophylactic means of reducing this mortality would be to treat more reducible hernias surgically. Therapeutically, 2 means are available: (1) the physician always should look at and feel the hernial rings in any patient with intestinal obstruction or abdominal symptoms which might become intestinal obstruction; (2) one should recognize the early signs of obstruction in any patient who has a hernia. These include general and abdominal symptoms (see Chap. 36) or local symptoms and signs, including pain in the region of the hernia, tenderness over an irreducible or an incarcerated hernia, recent development of irreducibility, and discoloration of the tissues over the hernia.

Certain hernias—for the most part those with small rigid rings—are more apt to become strangulated than others. Femoral hernias, umbilical hernias in adults and indirect inguinal hernias are apt to strangulate in that order, while direct inguinal hernias are less apt to do so. Hagan and Rhoads (1953) observed that of 19 strangulated hernias, 12 were indirect inguinal, 6 were femoral, 1 was recurrent inguinal and none was direct inguinal.

The treatment of a strangulated hernia involves several general principles in addition to that of anatomic repair of the hernia:

1. The operation is an urgent emergency.

2. The general condition of the patient may be precarious, and supportive measures (blood, etc.) should be given if at all indicated.

3. Infection is apt to occur, particularly if intestinal resection becomes necessary, and antibiotics may be indicated.

4. The questionable loop of bowel must not be allowed to escape into the general peritoneal cavity until the *all-important decision* as to its viability has been made. Querna (1955) pointed out that reduction of hernia en masse, even in the absence of strangulation, may be dangerous and lead to later intestinal obstruction. When strangulation is present, such reduction en masse, in which the hernia remains in its peritoneal coat—hence is not really reduced at all—is particularly hazardous. Persistent tenderness may give an indication as to the diagnosis. Such reduction usually occurs in inguinal hernias, but 1 of Querna's 3 cases was femoral. Furthermore, even when the strangulated loop of bowel is apparently viable and is not resected, late stenosis of the intestine may result. Cherney (1958) reported such a case and reviewed 82 others cited in the literature.

5. It must be recognized that the operative wound, following repair of a strangulated hernia, is especially liable to become infected. For this reason, steel-wire sutures are to be considered in the closure.

If intestinal resection proves to be necessary, it should be done with as little contamination of the wound as possible. In seriously ill or moribund patients, all the means of dealing with a complicated situation available to a thoroughly trained abdominal surgeon may be necessary. It is estimated that 20 per cent of strangulated external hernias require bowel resection. Despite all safeguards, the operation is difficult, it requires a careful decision as to viability of the bowel, the mortality is high relative to that for other hernias (about 25% or more), and, if the patient survives, the recurrence rate is higher than that for corresponding nonstrangulated hernias.

In the special instance of treatment of femoral hernia with gangrenous bowel, the method of Dennis and Varco, 1947 (elaborated upon by Enquist and Dennis, 1955), represents a distinct advance when gangrene is present and resection is required. The entire sac and contents are resected intact in order to avoid bacterial contamination of tissues to be used for repair. This is accomplished by freeing the sac and its contents above without releasing the neck. The peritoneum is opened parallel with the oblique skin incision, involved omentum is cut and ligated close to the neck, and the mesentery of the small intestine entering the sac is divided from the proximal to the distal side of the incarcerated intestinal loop. Each limb of bowel is clamped by 2 Ochsner clamps, and the intestine is divided between them with the cautery. Next, the inguinal ligament is divided near its attachment to the pubis and split laterally, enough of the heavy aponeurotic tissue being left in front of the neck of the sac to prevent it from relaxing and releasing the contaminated contents. Then the entire sac is freed by dissection down to the remains of the ring, which is cut under direct vision, and the complete contaminated mass is removed without soiling the field. A Cooper's ligament repair now is performed.

THE PROBLEM OF THE 4 MOST COMMON TYPES OF HERNIA

This problem will now be considered for each of these general types with a consideration of diagnosis, indications for operation and methods of procedure to prevent recurrence.

GROIN HERNIAS

Indirect Inguinal Hernia

This is the most common type of hernia in both sexes and at all ages. Millions of persons now alive in this country have had or will develop an indirect inguinal hernia. The operative treatment of this condition is one of the most important subjects in surgery today. This type of hernia stands in an intermediate position in its tendency to strangulate between direct hernia (rare strangulation) and femoral hernia (frequent strangulation).

Important anatomic studies within the past 10 years have clarified the structural arrangement of the fascial layers in the groin. Emphasis on ligaments which previously received scant notice, such as Cooper's ligament (ligamentum pubicum superius) and the iliopubic tract (intermediate iliopubic ligament), has altered surgical concepts. Outstanding ana-

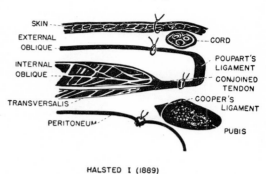

FIG. 39-1. Diagrammatic representation of groin hernia repair with cord superficial to the external oblique aponeurosis. (Harkins, H. N.: Ann. West. Med. & Surg. 6:221)

tomic studies are those of McVay and Anson (1942), Clark and Hashimoto (1946), Donald (1948), Anson, Morgan and McVay (1949), Burton (1952, 1953) and Griffith (1959).

The surgical treatment of inguinal hernia can be simplified by considering it from 3 standpoints: (1) a clarification of the exact nature of some of the historically significant operations for groin hernia; (2) a consideration of 4 grades of hernia, increasing in severity, each of which requires a different surgical operation, also increasing in complexity; and (3) a step-by-step outline of the radical operation for hernia required for the severest indirect inguinal hernia, not all of the steps being necessary in the repair of the simpler grades of hernia.

Clarification of Certain of the Historically Significant Operations for Groin Hernia. Because of the common misuse of eponymic terminology as related to certain of the classic operations, the diagrammatic representations of these are shown in Figures 39-1 to 39-5. Koontz (1949) has helped in the elucidation of the origin of these operations. It is noted that these technics are classified as to whether the cord is superficial, intermediate or deep in the first 4 diagrams, all of which portray various Poupart's ligament repairs, while the 5th shows the Cooper's ligament repair. It is of interest that just as in gastric surgery there is renewed interest in the Billroth I gastric resection, so in the

CORD INTERMEDIATE

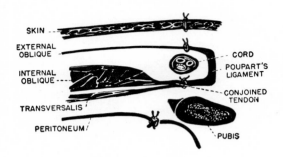

BASSINI (1888)

FIG. 39-2. Cord in intermediate position between external oblique aponeurosis and conjoined tendon. (Harkins, H. N.: Ann. West. Med. & Surg. 6:222)

CORD DEEP

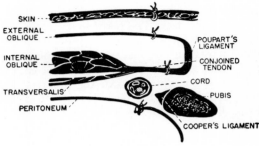

FERGUSON (1899)
HALSTED II (1903)

FIG. 39-4. Diagrammatic representation of groin hernia repair with cord deep to conjoined tendon. (Harkins, H. N.: Ann. West. Med. & Surg. 6:223)

surgery of hernia the swing is definitely toward the Halsted I herniorrhaphy among those surgeons who use a Poupart's ligament type of repair (Fig. 39-1).

Grades of Groin Hernia Repair. Groin hernias can be divided according to severity into 4 grades. The type of operation required in each grade is shown in Table 6. This grading of the severity of hernia is similar to that introduced by Ogilvie (1937) and Harkins (1952), except that the 3rd grade of these 2 previous classifications has been expanded into a 3rd and a 4th grade. Some surgeons omit the 2nd grade (McVay, 1947). It is seen that, in general, each successive grade adds an ad-

ditional step to the procedure but also keeps the steps of the lower grade. The borderline between the grades is not always sharp, and treatment in borderline cases must be individualized.

Grade 1. Infant Type of Hernia (Repair: High Ligation of Sac). Two current concepts should be emphasized: (1) in infants, as Potts, Riker and Lewis (1950) showed, there is an urgent indication for surgical repair; and (2) such a repair primarily should consist of sac ligation. When the author received his training, he was taught to avoid operation in infants under 2 years of age, except in face of the most urgent circumstances, because it

CORD INTERMEDIATE
(IMBRICATED)

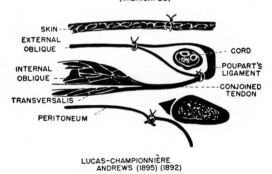

LUCAS–CHAMPIONNIÈRE
ANDREWS (1895) (1892)

FIG. 39-3. Intermediate position of cord with imbrication between layers of external oblique aponeurosis. (Harkins, H. N.: Ann. West. Med. & Surg. 6:222)

COOPER'S LIGAMENT REPAIR

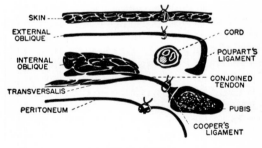

LOTHEISSEN (1898)

FIG. 39-5. Diagrammatic representation of repair with cord in intermediate position and conjoined tendon sutured to Cooper's ligament. (Harkins, H. N.: Ann. West. Med. & Surg. 6:223)

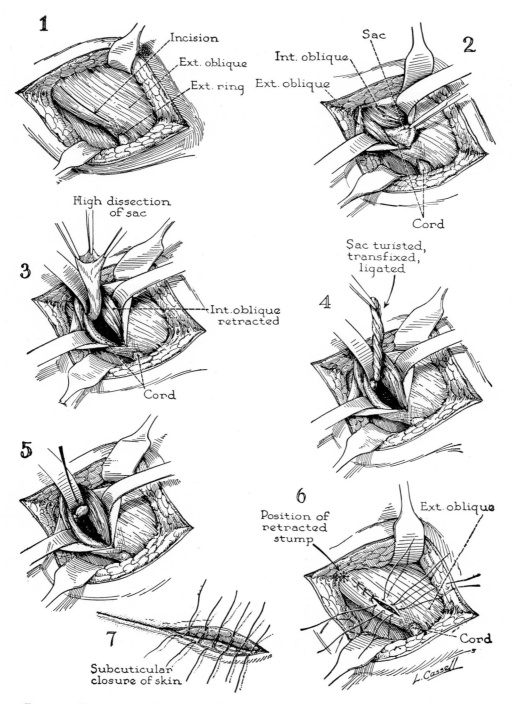

FIG. 39-6. Technic of repair of infantile hernia. (1) Opening the external oblique aponeurosis—*not* down to external ring. (2) Finding sac. (3) High dissection of sac. (4) Twisting, transfixion and ligation of sac. (5) Retraction of stump of sac. (6) Closure of external oblique aponeurosis. (7) Superficial wound closure. (Potts, W. E., Riker, W. L., & Lewis, J. E.: Ann. Surg. *132*:571)

was then believed that the repair would be easier after that age, that the danger of strangulation was slight, and that many of the hernias would be cured spontaneously. At present, less credence is given to these 3 beliefs, and early operation is urged. As Fisher (1951) pointed out, even if most infantile hernias do disappear spontaneously, many of them will reappear in later life. He stated: "Children should be operated at any age they present themselves—this, of course, providing there are no complicating conditions."

Heifetz (1953) also emphasized that inguinal sacs do not tend to obliterate themselves after birth.

The operation described by Potts (Figs. 39-6 and 39-7) embraces the following features:

1. Short transverse skin incision

2. Opening the external oblique aponeurosis in the direction of its fibers, but in the routine case *"the external ring is not opened"*

TABLE 6. GRADES OF HERNIA REPAIR

Grade 1. Infant repair. Indication: infants. Repair: high ligation of sac.

Grade 2. Simple repair. Indications: older children, young and healthy adults with indirect inguinal hernia. Repair: high ligation of sac. Tighten internal ring.

Grade 3. Intermediate repair. Indications: adults with indirect inguinal hernia plus slight weakness of Hesselbach's triangle. Repair: high ligation of sac. Tighten internal ring. Close Hesselbach's triangle, suturing transversalis fascia to iliopubic tract.

Grade 4. Radical repair. Indications: older adults with poor musculature; recurrent, direct or femoral hernias. Repair: high ligation of sac. Tighten internal ring. Close Hesselbach's triangle, suturing conjoined tendon to Cooper's ligament.

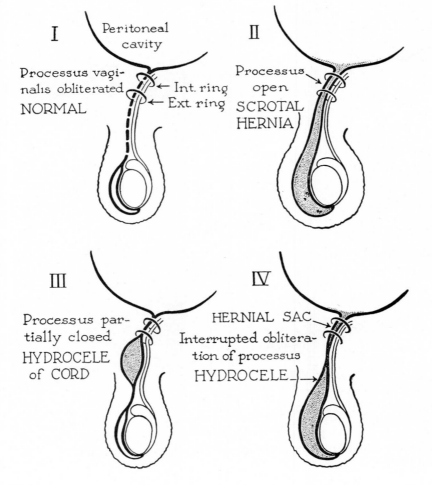

FIG. 39-7. The pathology of hernia, hydrocele of the cord and hydrocele in the male child. (Potts, W. E., Riker, W. L., & Lewis, J. E.: Ann. Surg. *132*:573)

3. Exposure, separation, division and high ligation of the sac without disturbing the cord

4. Simple closure of the external oblique aponeurosis and of the skin over the undisturbed cord

According to Potts:

The treatment of the typical inguinal hernia in infants and children is surgical removal of the sac without elevating the structures of the cord and without any plastic repair of the muscles or fascia of the inguinal region.

Packard and McLauthlin (1953) and Clatworthy and Thompson (1954) advocated essentially the same type of repair, based on an experience with 332 and 940 cases operated upon at the Denver and the Cincinnati Children's Hospitals, respectively. The Denver authors stated:

Recurrence is so rare that when it does occur, it suggests a technical error. Apparently the simple removal of the sac is as effective as any other method. Some tightening of the ring in large hernias may possibly be indicated, but it is hard to see how the approximation of the internal oblique to the inguinal ligament over the cord (Ferguson method) can be of any help; and transplantation of the cord by the Bassini method seems absolutely contraindicated.

McVay (1947), in speaking of small indirect hernias, stated this another way:

Any additional imbricating, plicating, or other sutures are not only superfluous but may damage the posterior inguinal wall so as to cause a direct or femoral recurrence.

Grade 2. Simple Type of Hernia (Repair: High Ligation of Sac Plus Plastic Closure of the Internal Ring). This grade of repair is used in older children and in young adults or in middle-aged individuals with primary indirect inguinal hernia and with good muscular and fascial structures. It is the repair most suitable for the majority of military personnel. It emphasizes the closure of the neck of the sac by high suture ligation—which may be said to be the essential foundation of the repair of all hernias—but adds a few additional steps because the structures are older and the hernia is more complex than in infants.

The surgical procedure delineates the following features:

1. Transverse skin incision

2. Opening the external oblique aponeurosis in the direction of its fibers and usually by opening the external ring

3. Exposure, separation, division and high ligation of the sac

4. Separation of the cord near the internal ring so as to delineate the margins of the latter

5. Plastic closure of the internal ring (MacGregor maneuver)

6. Closure of the external oblique aponeurosis, Scarpa's fascia, and skin over the minimally disturbed cord

Technical details of some of these steps will be given below in the discussion of the radical type of repair.

The essential added feature in the simple type of repair is the careful plastic closure of the internal ring to guard against recurrence at this point, the frequency of which has been pointed out, among others, by Levy, Wren and Friedman (1951).

Grade 3. Intermediate Type of Hernia (Repair: High Ligation of Sac Plus Plastic Closure of the Internal Ring Plus Closure of Hesselbach's Triangle, Suturing Transversalis Fascia to Iliopubic Tract). This type of hernia is that encountered in young adults with large indirect inguinal hernias, or in older persons with small hernias or especially strong inguinal floors. Most military inductees with inguinal hernias present Grade 3 (or Grade 2) indications for repair. The first 5 steps in the procedure are similar to those in Grade 2. Step 6 involves a row of interrupted fine silk sutures between the transversalis fascia above (at the upper edge of the slight bulge in the inguinal floor) and the iliopubic tract below. Step 7 then involves a closure of the external oblique aponeurosis, Scarpa's fascia, and skin over the cord.

Grade 4. Advanced Type of Hernia (Radical Repair: High Ligation of Sac Plus Plastic Closure of the Internal Ring Plus Closure of Hesselbach's Triangle, Suturing Conjoined Tendon to Cooper's Ligament) (Fig. 39-8). This grade of repair is indicated: (1) in recurrent hernias; (2) in femoral hernias; (3) in direct hernias; and (4) in indirect hernias in older individuals or in those with weak musculature or fascial structures (Harkins, 1943, 1949; McVay and Anson, 1949).

The radical repair advised involves high ligation of the sac and plastic closure of the

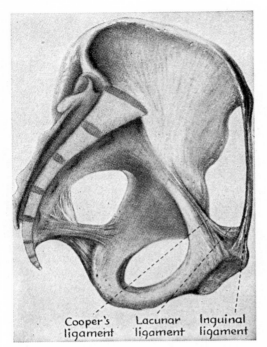

Cooper's   Lacunar   Inguinal
ligament   ligament   ligament

FIG. 39-8. Cooper's ligament. View of the left half of the pelvis with attached ligaments. The relationships between the firmly anchored Cooper's ligament and the loose inguinal ligament are clearly shown. (Harkins, H. N.: S. Clin. North America *23*: 1281)

internal ring, as discussed above in connection with the simpler grades of repair. The additional essential feature is the closure of Hesselbach's triangle by suturing the conjoined tendon to Cooper's ligament. A relaxing incision in the anterior rectus sheath facilitates this maneuver.

Within the past few years the author has adopted the "preperitoneal" approach for the majority of groin hernias (Nyhus, Condon and Harkins, 1960). While we recognize that this method has advantages, at the same time we do not feel that it is ready for recommendation for general adoption in a standard text. Through this approach, the suture of transversalis fascia to Cooper's ligament can be accomplished—and with better visualization, we believe—as is recommended below in the account of the classic Cooper's ligament repair:

Ten Steps in Radical Groin Hernia Re-

pair (**Cooper's Ligament, Lotheissen-McVay Technic**). The technical details may be divided into 10 steps, but in individual cases the available armamentarium should include use of such ancillary suture materials as steel wire and fascia lata strips and such accessory patches as tantalum mesh, cutis grafts and buried whole skin grafts. The author has utilized these adjuncts, with the exception of whole skin, in selected cases, but their use is seldom necessary.

Step 1. Exposure of the Cord and Opening the Indirect Sac. The skin incision is made in one of the skin folds, ending about 2 cm. above the pubic spine medially. The semitransverse skin incision has several advantages. It avoids part of the hairy area over the pubis and is less prone to infection. In addition, because it follows the lines of skin cleavage, the cosmetic result is better. The external oblique aponeurosis and the external ring are exposed, and the external oblique aponeurosis is split in the direction of its fibers even with the upper border of the ring to allow for an adequate lower flap. This splitting with the scalpel should be begun 3 cm. from the ring to avoid the nerves when they are adherent to the ring. Then the split is extended laterally and upward with scissors and then downward in the direction of the external ring after the iliohypogastric nerve, which is often adherent to the undersurface of the external oblique aponeurosis at this level, has been peeled away carefully. When cutting occurs accidentally, it is usually near the external ring, and it may be prevented by approaching the latter from the lateral side. The cord and the surrounding structures are separated from the lower leaf of the external oblique aponeurosis and Poupart's ligament, then from the region of the pubic spine and the conjoined tendon, so that finally the cord is freed entirely except at both ends. The cremaster muscle is split longitudinally anteriorly and posteriorly, and 2-in. segments are removed from the internal ring outward, including the internal spermatic fascia and the external spermatic vessels, which are doubly ligated. The cord is thus narrowed so that the internal ring can be closed more tightly as emphasized by Koontz (1956). The vas deferens and the internal spermatic vessels, including the veins, are carefully preserved. The indirect sac, which is

FIG. 39-9. Hoguet maneuver. The indirect sac is opened, and any femoral or direct (as shown above) sac is transposed so as to become a part of the indirect sac. In the above figure the tip of the examining finger is in a small direct sac. (Harkins, H. N.: S. Clin. North America 23:1284)

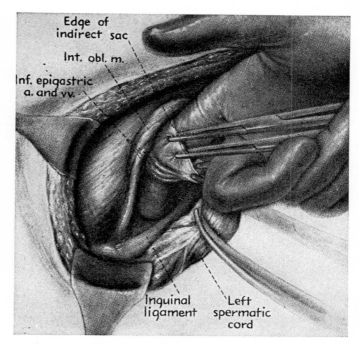

Edge of indirect sac
Int. obl. m.
Inf. epigastric a. and vv.
Inguinal ligament
Left spermatic cord

always present even in normal persons, is located upward and medially from the internal ring and is opened in all instances, whether the hernia is indirect or direct. In many instances of direct inguinal hernia or femoral hernia the indirect sac will be normal in size, but it always can be found above and medial to the cord. In cases of complete indirect inguinal hernia of the congenital type or in patients in whom the hernial sac is long, the latter is cut across near the internal ring and separated from the cord. The proximal end is closed by an internal purse-string suture, as outlined later, while the distal end is left in place.

Step 2. Exploration of Hesselbach's Triangle and of the Femoral Ring. Once the indirect sac is opened, it is a simple matter to insert the gloved finger to feel Hesselbach's triangle for a direct weakness or obvious direct hernia and to feel the femoral ring. It is indeed surprising how few surgeons will take the extra 30 seconds needed to perform this exploration, and many femoral and direct hernias that "recur" are overlooked because this maneuver was not performed. Exploration of the femoral ring and Hesselbach's triangle with the fingertip should be an essential feature of the repair of all groin hernias.

Step 3. Hoguet's Maneuver—Transposition of Direct and/or Femoral Sacs into the Indirect Sac (Fig. 39-9). If a direct sac is present, it should be transposed lateral to the inferior epigastric vessels by the technic of Hoguet (1920), which has since been popularized by Fallis (1938). Thus, the direct and the indirect sacs are converted into one. This step may be described in Hoguet's own words as follows:

By traction outward on the indirect sac, all of the peritoneum of the direct sac may be pulled external to the vessels and the two sacs converted into one. An indirect sac can always be found in these cases, although it may be very small.

The same procedure can be used to convert a femoral sac into an indirect sac, as practiced by McClure and Fallis (1939). This maneuver is extremely useful. In general, no matter how large a direct sac is, it is not opened but is merely transposed. In the case of large direct sacs the transversalis fascia can be infolded with numerous interrupted silk sutures. One advantage of not opening a direct sac is the fact that the danger of opening the bladder is largely obviated. In some instances all 3 sacs can be converted into a single indirect

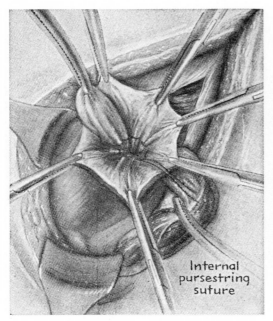

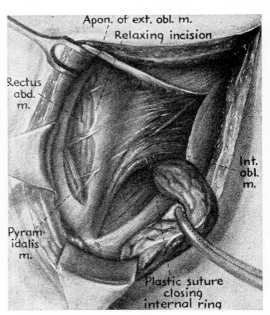

FIG. 39-10. Internal purse-string suture. The indirect sac is closed by an internal purse-string suture which obliterates all of its folds. The redundant indirect sac is usually replaced inside the internal ring, but, if large, it may be excised. The forceps in the upper left-hand portion of the figure grasp the transposed and inverted direct sac. (Harkins, H. N.: S. Clin. North America *23*:1286)

FIG. 39-11. Plastic closure of internal ring and relaxation of internal oblique muscle. The internal ring has been closed by a plastic stitch in the transversalis fascia, while the internal oblique has been relaxed close to its junction with the external oblique aponeurosis to form the linea alba. An attempt is made to spare the nerves and accompanying vessels. (Harkins, H. N.: S. Clin. North America *23*:1287)

sac, which in turn can always be dealt with as described in Step 4.

Step 4. Internal Purse-string Closure of Indirect Sac (Fig. 39-10). The indirect sac, whether it is simple or enlarged by the added conversion of direct and femoral sacs, is then closed with an internal purse-string suture of medium or heavy silk. Many stitches are taken with a round noncutting needle so as to include all crevices. Such a closure is done as high as possible to prevent indirect recurrences, although the sac is not attached beneath the abdominal wall, as is done by Collins (1942).

Step 5. Tightening of the Internal Ring—MacGregor's Maneuver (Fig. 39-11). When the free ends of the purse string are cut and the peritoneum snaps back, the defect in the transversalis fascia at the internal ring is seen to be large, and in many instances it will admit

even 3 or 4 fingers. The fascia is grasped with Allis clamps at numerous points round the internal ring above and medially as far as the inferior epigastric vessels, but not entirely around the circumference lateral to the cord, and the defect is closed vertically with interrupted silk sutures. The reason for narrowing the cord structures is now manifest, and the internal ring is narrowed so that it barely admits the tip of a little finger. This is a most important step; essentially it involves suturing the transversalis fascia, Hesselbach's ligament and the iliopubic tract to tighten the internal ring. Incomplete closure of the internal ring is a common cause of recurrence. Occasionally the conjoined tendon may be included in the sutures, but the shelving edge of Poupart's ligament should not be included, since the normal and desirable retractile sphincterlike action of the internal ring demonstrated by MacGregor (1929, 1930, 1945, 1949) would be interfered with. Occasionally the lateral sutures to close the internal ring are not placed until Step 7 is completed, so that when they are inserted there will be a continuous closure from the pubic spine to internal ring, eliminating the open space that otherwise might result. Marshall (1960) has re-emphasized recently the importance of this step.

Step 6. Relaxation of the Internal Oblique Muscle. The inner layer of the anterior rectus fascia usually is split for a distance of about 7 cm. from a point 2 cm. above the pubic spine upward and laterally, as described by Rienhoff (1940). The external oblique aponeurosis is lifted up by the assistant, and the internal oblique aponeurosis is cut just lateral to the junction of the two where they form the linea alba. The rectus and the pyramidalis muscles are exposed. The iliohypogastric nerve and the adjoining nerves and vessels which enter the rectus muscle through the internal oblique aponeurosis at this point can be avoided easily. This relaxation allows the internal oblique and the attached transversalis fascia to be pulled down for the subsequent repair without tension. This step is called the "Tanner slide" in Great Britain (Tanner, 1942) and recently has been readvocated by Doran (1955).

Step 7. Sutures into Cooper's Ligament (Fig. 39-12). The "red" muscle of the internal oblique is disregarded and elevated with a small retractor, and the conjoined tendon is located with a gauze (Küttner) dissector. If the transversalis fascia plus the transversus muscle appear strong enough, they alone are used for the upper leaf of the repair. If they are not adequate, one must go higher and include the internal oblique aponeurosis. In no instance should "red" muscle be used. The transversalis fascia plus transversus muscle, and often the conjoined tendon, therefore, form the *upper leaf* of the repair, while Cooper's ligament is the *lower leaf.* As stated previously, Cooper's ligament is an extremely tough thickening of the periosteal structures on the anterosuperior surface of the anterior ramus of the pubis. Cooper's ligament is visualized by cutting the transversalis fascia from the pubic spine lateral to and occasionally including the inferior epigastric vessels (which are doubly ligated and divided on one side). This incision in the transversalis fascia is just

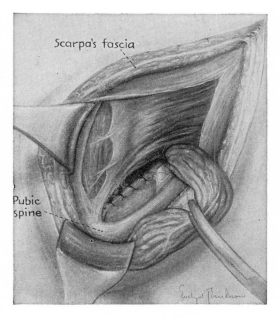

Fig. 39-12. Stitches attaching conjoined tendon and Cooper's ligament in place. (Harkins, H. N.: Arch. Surg. *55*:702)

anterior and superior to the iliopubic tract.

The left index finger now is placed on the anterior ramus of the pubis near the spine and moved laterally along the crest until the femoral vessels are reached. This is usually about 4 cm. lateral to the spine of the pubis. Since the finger is held in close contact with the bone, the vessels being kept lateral, and the 1st stitch is placed medial to the finger, there is little danger of damaging the vessels. Thus, the 1st stitch is usually from 3 to 5 cm. lateral to the pubic spine. Therefore, since the upper leaf is to be taken with the suture first, the needle goes through the transversalis fascia a corresponding distance of 3 to 5 cm. from the pubic spine and then through the thick Cooper's ligament on the upper border of the pubic ramus. Then the stitch is tied, and the intervening gap between this point and the pubic spine is closed with 3 or 4 similar sutures. The most medial sutures usually go through Gimbernat's (lacunar) ligament, as well as Cooper's. Often it is important that the most lateral suture be placed first, as otherwise it is more difficult to protect the vein. The sutures into Cooper's ligament are of double heavy 00 silk and are applied with

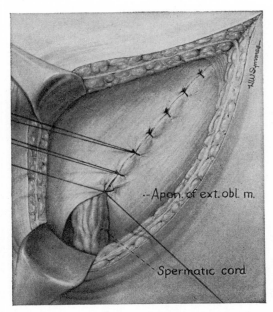

Fig. 39-13. Closure of the aponeurosis of the external oblique over the cord. Then Scarpa's fascia (well shown in this illustration) and the skin are also closed with interrupted sutures over the cord. (Harkins, H. N.: Arch. Surg. *55*:703)

a small (No. 6) round curved Mayo needle or a Davis tonsil needle, held with a Bland or a Jones needle holder. The double strands are made into a double (or triple) knot, and the individual strands are separated and tied in pairs (this is called "braiding"). The braiding technic has been found useful in other operations when one is especially anxious that a double suture should not become untied and yet the making of the knot is difficult because of the depth of the wound. The relatively large amount of silk seldom has caused trouble. In certain cases, because of the prominence of Rosenmüller's gland (a lymph gland lying over Cooper's ligament about 2 cm. medial to the femoral vessels) or because of the large size of the vein, the sutures must be placed with special care. Babcock (1927) advised one medial Cooper's ligament suture in conjunction with his operation for direct hernia.

The space between the most lateral stitch in Cooper's ligament and the plastic suture on the internal ring often seems to be a possible weak spot to those doing the operations for

the first time. Actually this is not so, because the arched internal oblique muscle will tend to close this defect on contraction. Any attempt to tighten it by suturing the internal oblique or conjoined tendon to Poupart's ligament, as is done by Baritell (1944) and others, would seem to defeat the purpose of the operation. Such a suture interferes with the sphincterlike action of the internal ring and tends to pull the transversalis fascia away from Cooper's ligament. Furthermore, the gap can be closed by an additional layer of fine interrupted silk sutures tacking down the superior edge of the lower flap of transversalis (just superior to the iliopubic tract where it was incised to expose Cooper's ligament), including the iliopubic tract and the superficial portion of the medial femoral sheath, to the outer surface of the conjoined tendon and continuing this suture line laterally to join with the line of closure of the internal ring (Griffith, 1959). The methods of McVay (1954) and of Burton (1954, 1956) to close the weak spot are also to be considered.

Step 8. Closure of the External Oblique Aponeurosis (Fig. 39-13). The external oblique aponeurosis is closed over the cord in most patients. Occasionally, in severe recurrent hernias the cord is brought out subcutaneously (Halsted I position), but in the past few years this has been done less and less. In both procedures the external oblique is closed with interrupted fine or medium silk sutures, little if any imbrication being used.

Step 9. Closure of Scarpa's Fascia. Closure of Scarpa's fascia with small bites of the suture seems more sound anatomically and leaves less silk than does suture of the fat with large bites taken at random. This closure is especially important with a Halsted I type of repair, as it gives the already superficial cord additional protection. By preference the sutures are placed so that the knot will be down.

Step 10. Closure of the Skin. Interrupted sutures of silk are advisable for this step. The proper closure of the medial fourth of the wound inside the hairline is of especial importance.

Direct Inguinal Hernia

A direct inguinal hernia is more common than is popularly believed; it is often a bulge more than a long sac; it protrudes anteriorly rather than primarily downward; it will not descend entirely into the scrotum; it affects older patients more often than does indirect inguinal hernia; for practical purposes, it never occurs in a woman; it does not strangulate as often as an indirect inguinal hernia, but more often it contains bladder (patients with bladder hernia may have to urinate twice on arising in the morning, even in the absence of prostatic obstruction); and, finally, its surgical repair is followed by a much higher recurrence rate. The results of such repair were so bad 20 years ago (about 50% recurrence in some series, and 30% even in 1947—Wangensteen) that Andrews and Bissell (Surg., Gynec. & Obst. *58*:753-761, 1934) entitled their paper: "Direct Hernia: A Record of Surgical Failure." In older patients with small direct hernias, operation is not as essential as it is in the case of inguinal and femoral hernias.

Direct inguinal hernia occurs through a weakness in Hesselbach's triangle. It represents a weakness in the inguinal floor, i.e., in the transversalis fascia. Lateral direct hernias protrude laterally to the obliterated hypogastric artery (in the lateral triangle) and medial ones medial to the artery (in the medial triangle). Medial direct hernias (Ginzburg and Freund, 1954) are more apt to be funicular in shape, whereas the lateral hernias are usually domelike.

Two technics seem to be suitable for the repair of direct inguinal hernia. These are the Halsted I procedure (especially advocated by Fallis, 1938, and by Palumbo and Mighell, 1954), and Cooper's ligament repair (McVay, 1941; Harkins, Szilagyi, Brush and Williams, 1942; and Harkins and Schug, 1947).

Since the defect in direct hernia is in Hesselbach's triangle, this area should be buttressed. The author uses only the Cooper's ligament method, but occasionally supplements it in difficult cases with imbrication of the external oblique aponeurosis beneath the cord. Such a supplemented operation could be termed a "Halsted I-McVay," or a McVay repair putting the cord in the Halsted I (superficial) position.

The technic of the Cooper's ligament repair for direct hernia is essentially as outlined in the section on indirect inguinal hernia. Usually the direct sac is not opened, but is transposed to the indirect opening by the Hoguet maneuver. Avoiding opening the sac cuts down on the incidence of trauma to the bladder.

Femoral Hernia

This type of hernia is relatively more common in the female but still is not as common in absolute figures in that sex as are indirect inguinal hernias. While femoral hernias are essentially a condition of adult life, they do occur in childhood, as Owen, Kirklin and Du Shane (1954) have pointed out. There is one important difference in the treatment of inguinal hernias as opposed to femoral hernias in early childhood; whereas the former should be treated in the simplest way possible (sac ligation only), contrariwise true radical repair of femoral hernia is indicated irrespective of age.

A rare type of femoral hernia is the "prevascular" variety, which is situated within the femoral sheath and anterior to the femoral vessels (Burton, 1950, 1953). Only when the neck of the sac extends laterally across the front of the iliac and the femoral vessels should the hernia be designated as prevascular. A hernia in which the neck traverses the femoral canal, the sac of which then deviates laterally across the femoral vessels, is a femoral hernia with lateral deviation. Turner (1953) reported a case of prevascular femoral hernia treated by means of a Cooper's ligament repair.

Femoral hernias are most important from 2 standpoints: (1) often they are overlooked, even at operation; and (2) they tend to strangulate.

As to the 1st point, the author has operated upon 3 women for femoral hernia in whom his operation was the 4th, the 5th and the 7th operation for hernia, respectively. While it is difficult to prove, it is likely that the total of 13 previous operations on these unfortunate patients was all for inguinal hernia— probably nonexistent—and that the cause of their troubles (and even of their swellings) was femoral hernia from the beginning. It is of interest that when reporting 8 cases of "ectopic recurrence" of femoral hernia after inguinal hernia repair, Easton (1933) did not even mention the possibility that they might have been overlooked at the 1st operation. The importance of exploration of the femoral region from within the peritoneal cavity with the gloved finger at the time of any operation for hernia has been emphasized in the discussion of inguinal hernia above. Whereas the differentiation between direct and indirect inguinal hernia, at least preoperatively, is somewhat academic, that between inguinal and femoral hernia is always of practical importance.

Regarding the 2nd point, Monro (1950) stated: "Strangulation of a femoral hernia is in my experience the commonest strangulation."

The subject of strangulation has been considered in the general section on strangulation above. Femoral hernias are especially liable to strangulate because of the rigid edges of the opening. The diagnosis of strangulated femoral hernia may be very easy with the patient pointing to the lesion, or very difficult. A tense, tender lump which has lost its expansile impulse on coughing should be present. Tenseness is always present, but the occasional complete absence of tenderness may throw the physician off guard. Furthermore, tenderness alone may be due to acute femoral lymphadenitis, and the corresponding foot should be examined. General signs are also late in development, particularly in the case of Richter's hernia (see below). Taxis is entirely out of place in an incarcerated or strangulated femoral hernia. In approximately 80 per cent of strangulated femoral hernia, bowel resection is not necessary, at least at the time of operation. Because the remaining 20 per cent will die without prompt surgical treatment, immediate operation is mandatory. In fact, because of the frequency of strangulation in femoral hernias (10 to 25% in *hospital* statistics, the incidence for persons with femoral hernia who do not enter hospitals is undoubtedly lower), all femoral hernias should be operated upon at once after diagnosis, irrespective of season or accompanying minor ailments. Intestinal decompression is advisable after operation in strangulated cases until bowel sounds return.

The treatment of femoral hernia per se is in a state of flux. Three methods are vying with one another for standard adoption, and all 3 have their supporters. These 3 methods are as follows:

1. The lower approach, from the thigh, below Poupart's ligament

2. The upper, or inguinal, approach

3. The abdominal extraperitoneal approach through a mid-line, or paramedian, incision

1. **The Lower Approach** (Bassini, 1893). This is the simplest and the most direct operation, and it permits one to see the sac without disturbing the inguinal region. Disadvantages of this approach include inability to treat associated inguinal hernia at the same time, inability to close the femoral weakness high up at its beginning, and, last but not least, inability to deal adequately with strangulated bowel from below. The lower approach has considerable disadvantages in cases in which resection is necessary. Monro (1950) indicated that the recurrence rate (including inguinal hernia on the same side) is about 10 per cent. Waugh and Hausfeld (1942) reported on the use of a femoral approach with sac removal without attempting to close the femoral canal (Socin-A. J. Ochsner technic). Waugh and Hausfeld used the method in 12 cases of simple femoral hernia with good results. They did not advise the technic in complicated or strangulated cases. Birt (1947) advised the femoral route for nonstrangulated hernias and the inguinal route for strangulated femoral hernias. Butters (1948) also was an advocate of the lower approach. It is of interest that Butters' experience with 120 repairs by the lower approach with 3.3 per cent recurrences plus 7 per cent inguinal recurrences (total = 10%) seemed favorable to him, yet it is the basis for Monro's critical opinion stated above.

The technic involves a low oblique incision, freeing and opening the sac, careful observation of the contents for viability, reduction of normal contents, high ligation of the sac, and closure of the femoral ring and fossa ovalis by suturing Poupart's ligament to the tenuous pectineus fascia. The saphenous vein usually is doubly ligated and divided.

Three technical points deserve comment. The first involves the fact that femoral hernias are covered with much fat, each layer of which may be confused with omentum. True omental fat appears more granular than other fat, and in addition, when the sac is opened, fluid (hernial water, the Bruchwasser of the Germans) escapes. The second is that while omentum may be ligated and amputated, one should remember that omentum descends from colon and should avoid clamping the colon. The third point is that while in 75 per cent of cases the obturator artery arises from the internal iliac, in 25 per cent it arises from the external iliac, swinging above the femoral vein to descend to the obturator foramen. A femoral hernia may push it to one side or other of the femoral ring, where it may be injured during the repair.

2. **The Inguinal Approach.** This was introduced by Annandale (1876), but modernized by Lotheissen (1898), who in a classic paper first advocated suture of the conjoined tendon to Cooper's ligament. Another type of inguinal approach involves suturing Poupart's ligament to Cooper's ligament (Ruggi, 1892; Moschcowitz, 1907), while other surgeons suture both to Cooper's ligament. The Lotheissen-McVay method seems preferable and has the advantages of treating any coincident direct inguinal weakness at the same time and of not suturing 2 such rigid structures together as Poupart's and Cooper's ligaments. The inguinal approach gives a good visualization of strangulated bowel. If the hernia is irreducible, the following means of handling the situation are available: (1) expose, and possibly open, the sac by retracting the lower skin flap; (2) cut Gimbernat's (lacunar) ligament medially; and (3) cut Poupart's ligament loose from the pubic spine (Hey Groves maneuver, 1923) to give more room in all directions. (The ligament is resutured in place at the end of the operation.) Hagan and Rhoads (1953) pointed out that the Lotheissen Mc-Vay repair of femoral hernia may not be necessary, even though adequate, since they had no femoral recurrences in 74 femoral hernias repaired as follows: 62 by the femoral route, 2 each by the Halsted I and the Bassini procedure, and only 8 by the Lotheissen-McVay repair.

Technical steps include a somewhat low inguinal incision followed by a typical Lotheissen-McVay operation, transposing the femoral sac into the indirect one by the Hoguet maneuver in simple cases. In the more difficult instances, the additional tricks mentioned above may have to be utilized. Resection may be necessary. An all-important rule is that *bowel loops in a femoral sac never should be permitted to escape into the general peritoneal cavity before first being scrutinized carefully for viability.*

3. **The Abdominal Approach.** This method gives plenty of room for bowel resection and at the same time permits a bilateral repair through a single incision. This latter factor is important, since about 20 per cent of femoral hernias are overtly bilateral. The most popular abdominal approach is extraperitoneal (Cheatle, 1920, 1921; Henry, 1936; McEvedy, 1950; Mikkelsen and Berne, 1954 and Rogers, 1959). La Roque (1919, 1922), Williams (1947) and Phetteplace (1955) have advocated an intraperitoneal approach which would seem to have the disadvantage that only the peritoneal sac is properly dealt with, even though a fascial closure is attempted. Mikkelsen and Berne reported good results using the abdominal approach (Cheatle-Henry) combined with a transversalis plus transversus to Cooper ligament repair from within in 113 cases treated in 4 years at the Los Angeles County Hospital. There were no recurrences. This operation is essentially a Lotheissen-McVay closure through a Cheatle-Henry approach. Although other types of closure (Moschcowitz, etc.) can be done through the extraperitoneal approach, the closure used by Mikkelsen and Berne would seem to be the best.

Steps in the operation include: lower midline incision, incision through the transversalis fascia, opening the sac, reduction of the hernia taking the usual precautions, closure of the peritoneum, suture of the "conjoined tendon" to Cooper's ligament, exploration of the other side, and closure of the mid-line incision.

Recurrent Groin Hernia

The subject of the prevention of recurrence has been dealt with under the headings of individual hernias (see Table 7). The present discussion emphasizes the therapeutic approach to recurrences already present. Such treatment involves a radical herniorrhaphy utilizing certain of the "Aids to Repair" considered in the section relating to them below. If the patient is old, cord division may be considered. A careful Cooper's ligament (Lotheissen-McVay) repair utilizing nonabsorbable sutures is adequate in most instances. Fascia lata sutures (Swenson and Harkins, 1943), cutis grafts (Swenson and Harkins,

TABLE 7. FACTORS LEADING TO RECURRENCE
FOLLOWING THE REPAIR OF INGUINAL HERNIA
(MACKENZIE, 1955)

Failure to:

1. Ligate the sac high enough in indirect inguinal hernia
2. Constitute the internal ring adequately
3. Close the fascial defect adequately in direct hernia
4. Rule out associated direct or femoral hernia
5. Recognize and repair sliding hernia adequately
6. Avoid tension by relaxing incisions
7. Place sutures properly and utilize adequate technic
8. Control sepsis
9. Utilize hemostasis, particularly in the cord structures

1943; Harkins, 1945) or tantalum-mesh patches, and suturing the external oblique aponeurosis beneath the cord (Halsted I position), in addition to the underlying Cooper's ligament repair, should all be considered. Thorough exploration to rule out previously overlooked femoral hernia is mandatory. Hagan and Rhoads (1953) found that in a series of 75 recurrent inguinal hernias, there were 21 per cent recurrences after secondary repair. This high figure may be significant when it is noted that in only 4 of the 75 cases was a Lotheissen-McVay repair performed. The problem is a difficult one, and a single Cooper's ligament operation for recurrent hernia may take from 90 to 120 minutes, but with care a secondary recurrence rate of less than 5 per cent can be obtained. Recurrent hernias can also be repaired by the preperitoneal approach, which has the advantage that it does not have to go through the scars of the previous operation or operations. The placing of wire-stitch markers on the edges of the layers to be approximated, as introduced by Doran and Lonsdale (1949), and extended by Olson, Kanar and Harkins (1954), enables one to determine if there is recurrence by roentgenologic means in some cases. The edges pull apart, and the markers become separated.

VENTRAL INCISIONAL HERNIAS

The occurrence of such hernias testifies to the lack of perfection in the closure of abdominal wounds. The incidence of incisional hernia varies from 0.5 to 8.0 per cent, depending on a number of factors, many of which are covered elsewhere in this book. No one incision, type of suture material, manner of closure or individual surgeon is immune from occasional wound disruption. However, careful attention to the general preoperative care of the patient, to the use of the correct incision for the particular patient, to the insertion of nonabsorbable sutures which do not "miss" the fascia and do not constrict the blood supply to the flaps being sutured, and to the maintenance of nutrition in the postoperative state—all these will help to prevent wound disruptions and ventral incisional hernias.

The surgical care of these hernias is difficult and simple at the same time. The scarred skin is removed by an elliptical incision. The fascial margins of the ring, which usually is smaller than would appear from the outside before operation, are freed, and the peritoneal cavity is opened, preferably at a point at which there are no adhesions. The sac is trimmed away, taking into consideration the fact that one does not wish to leave weak tissue behind, but at the same time does not wish to sacrifice good tissue.

A decision as to the direction of closure must now be reached. Whereas, other things being equal, one would wish to close a ventral hernia transversely (i.e., by bringing an upper flap down and a lower flap up), most herniated incisions are vertical, leaving the surgeon with no other choice than to close the gap vertically. If the closure is to be horizontal, the flaps should be tested to see if they can be imbricated. If so, fat should be cleared from the undersurface of the upper flap and from the outer surface of the lower flap for a distance equal to that to be imbricated. The surgeon should approach each incisional hernia with the aim of at least getting the edges together. With proper care usually they can be imbricated a little, even in the largest hernias.

The flaps now are sutured with a 1st row of mattress sutures at the edge of the lower flap to upper flap at the distance from the edge corresponding to the imbrication. The 2nd row of mattress sutures approximates the lower edge of the upper flap down over and to the outer surface of the lower flap. If a vertical closure is necessary, the same thing is done by overlapping one lateral flap over the other. If imbrication is not possible, the edges should be sutured together. If the edges cannot be brought together, the surgeon should consider carefully as to whether the fault is his or the anatomic situation is insurmountable. In 10 years the author did not find a ventral hernia the edges of which could not be brought together.

Next, the superficial wound is closed, often with large mattress sutures, to obliterate the dead space. A drain is inserted in the wound for 48 hours.

Additional technical points are as follows:

It is usually impossible to make a separate peritoneal closure. A common error is to mistake the anterior edge of a daughter sac for the inner fascial flap to be used for closure. The most common error is to give up too easily in trying to see if the true flap edges can be approximated. It is especially difficult to close epigastric incisional hernias because of the unyielding nature of the near-by costal margins. The surgeon will need a knowledge of all the methods listed below under "Aids to Repair" in dealing with a difficult ventral incisional hernia.

UMBILICAL HERNIAS

This type of hernia is most common in infancy and in young children. Small umbilical hernias in infants often may be treated by adhesive strapping, as many of them will close spontaneously as the patients grows. This is especially true of those umbilical hernias which are hemispheric in shape. As Gross (1953) pointed out, the two requirements are relaxation of lateral tension and the emptying of the sac. These requirements are not met by strapping a metal coin over the protruding navel or by spring trussses or rubber belts with protruding attachments. Adhesive strapping must be applied carefully if it is to be successful. Even then it is difficult to be sure if the good results are not those of a natural cure. Strapping is accomplished by cutting two pieces of 2-in. adhesive, one with a hole and the other with a tongue so that they can be interlaced. They are applied with tension after previously preparing the abdominal skin with tincture of benzoin. Such support is renewed every week or two and is maintained for several months. Strapping is of little value in the treatment of conical or "elephant-trunk" umbilical hernias. Few of this type can be controlled adequately by strapping. Strapping should be abandoned if it is unsuccessful after

6 months' trial or if the child is over 1 year of age. Surgery may be indicated more urgently in females for the same size of hernia because of the future possibility of strain upon the opening by pregnancy. On the other hand, McVay (1954) stated that in his experience the serious complication of strangulation was most common in the elderly debilitated male. After the 1st year of life, umbilical hernias larger than 8 mm. in diameter (2.0 cm. in younger infants) should be repaired surgically. The repair in children involves the following steps (Fig. 39-14):

1. A semilunar "frowning" skin incision above and sparing the umbilicus
2. Freeing the sac with transverse closure of it
3. Longitudinal closure of the fascia with interrupted fine (4-0) silk sutures. When the recti muscles are immediately adjacent to the umbilical hernia ring, the anterior and the posterior rectus sheaths can be closed longitudinally and separately in layers (Brown, 1960).
4. Interrupted subcuticular (6-0) silk closure of the wound.

In adults, an umbilical hernia with symptoms, or with incarceration, or larger than 1 cm. should be treated surgically. In the surgical repair in adults, the following steps are suggested:

1. Separate and ligate the sac.
2. Incise the anterior rectus sheath transversely on each side for about 1 cm. in small hernias and up to 3 cm. in large hernias.
3. Retract the rectus muscle and incise the posterior sheath in a similar manner.
4. Imbricate the upper flap over the lower ("vest over pants") with 2 layers of mattress sutures of nonabsorbable material.
5. If possible, preserve the umbilicus; if not, in younger patients fashion an artificial umbilicus with skin tucked down to the deeper tissues.

In any imbrication procedure, as in (4) above, it is important that the 2 layers in contact be as fat free as possible; thus, the upper flap (vest) should be fat free on its inner surface and the lower flap (pants) should be fat free on its outer surface. It is not necessary to remove fat from the surfaces which are not to be in contact, and to do so is to risk interfering with the blood supply of the flaps.

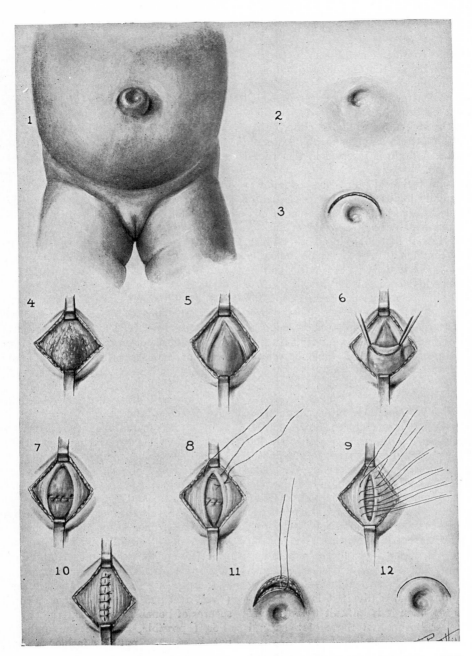

Fig. 39-14. Recommended technic for umbilical herniorraphy in a baby or a child. (1) Showing the navel swelling. (2) When relaxed under anesthesia, the navel becomes depressed. (3) Position of the curved incision in skin just above the navel. (4) Skin flaps freed from underlying tissues and retracted. (5) Rectus sheaths cleared of overlying fat. Hernial sac cleared. (6) Hernial sac cut away from undersurface of navel skin. (7) Peritoneum (hernial sac) closed. (8) Stitches (of silk) being taken in the edges of the rectus sheaths. (9) Rectus sheath stitches in place. (10) Rectus fasciae brought together in mid-line. (11) Subcuticular stitches (of 6-0 Deknatel silk) just beneath the corium. Skin edges brought together by the subcuticular stitches. (12) No cutaneous sutures are necessary. (Gross, R. E.: Surgery of Infancy and Childhood, Philadelphia, Saunders)

ESOPHAGEAL HIATAL DIAPHRAGMATIC HERNIA

General Considerations

These hernias are the most common type of herniation that occurs through the diaphragm. They are also the most common type that requires surgical treatment. Harrington (1955), whose outstanding work has helped to develop this field and whose experience based on 489 repairs of these hernias is the basis for his statements, lists a number of factors which make these hernias of general interest, as follows: their indefinite causation; their relatively frequent occurrence; the variation of the relationship between the defective esophageal hiatus and the esophagus resulting in involvement of different structures and in different types of esophageal hiatal hernias; their progressive development; their varied and complex symptoms which often simulate those of other organic disease (this, coupled with the not infrequent presence of unassociated and coincidental conditions, such as malignant disease of the esophagus or the stomach, cholecystic disease, angina pectoris, and duodenal ulcer, which may be confused with the hernia, makes appropriate its designation as the "masquerader of the upper abdomen"); the complications such as incarceration of the viscera involved in the hernia; the occurrence of incompetency of the sphincteric mechanism at the cardia which permits a retrograde flow of acid-peptic secretions into the esophagus with resultant occurrence of esophagitis, ulceration of the esophagus and the cardia, and, in some instances, stricture of the esophagus; and, finally, spasm of the esophagus which may be secondary to the herniation, or may be a primary condition causing the hernia.

Saint's triad (hiatal hernia, gallstones and diverticulosis coli) is of great interest from the diagnostic standpoint. This syndrome, first described by Muller (1948) and elaborated upon by Palmer (1951), denotes that about 10 to 15 per cent of patients with hiatal hernia will have *both* the other two conditions at the same time. Furthermore, if such patients have either of the other two conditions, they are extremely likely to have both. In most cases, symptoms which are present are attributed to the gallbladder pathology. It is significant that the symptomatic relief from the cholecystectomy is usually slight, while that from the repair of

the hiatal hernia is usually good. Saint's triad may explain the course of events in at least some of the patients with the "postcholycystectomy syndrome."

Anatomic Considerations

The esophageal hiatus permits the traversing of the diaphragm by the esophagus, both vagi and the connections between the left gastric artery and the coronary vein below and the corresponding thoracic esophageal blood vessels above. These structures actually penetrate the phreno-esophageal ligament (see below). So far as the action of the hiatus on the esophagus is concerned, in conjunction with the cardiac sphincter it maintains the flow of food in one direction, downward, and when this sphincter mechanism is impaired, the patient becomes subject to the evils of bidirectional flow with its possible complications listed above. The action of the diaphragm and the attached fascia is termed the *extrinsic mechanism* in maintaining competency; the cardiac sphincter is termed the *intrinsic mechanism*. Lendrum (1937), Allison (1951) and others believed that the extrinsic mechanism was most important, Lam (1954) favored emphasis on the intrinsic mechanism.

The oblique entry of the esophagus into the stomach acts as a valve in the opinion of Nauta (1955, 1956). This valvelike mechanism is supplemented by a rosette of stomach mucosal folds. The diaphragm plays only a passive role, except during inspiration when it compresses the rosette. Braasch and Ellis (1956) also did experimental studies which indicate that the mechanism which prevents regurgitation is primarily a sphincter mechanism rather than the action of the diaphragm.

As to the hiatus itself, Carey and Hollinshead (1955) considered the anatomy from the standpoint of 3 layers, going from outside inward: (1) muscle, (2) fascia, and (3) peritoneum.

1. **Muscular Relations of the Hiatus.** The crura of the diaphragm, right and left, arise by stout tendinous bands from the anterolateral surfaces of the first 3 or 4 lumbar vertebrae and their intervening fibrocartilages. The 2 crura are separated immediately anterior to the spine by the upper end of the abdominal aorta and its first main anterior

branches (celiac axis and superior mesenteric artery). In 25 human dissections by Carey and Hollinshead, the right crus was found to be larger than the left in 24 (Fig. 39-15). In most instances, the superficial (viewed from the abdomen, hence caudad) portion of the right crus forms the right margin of the esophageal hiatus, and the deep (craniad) portion the left margin. This confirms the observation of Low (1907), that the right crus usually sends fibers on both sides of the esophagus (Fig. 39-16). From their positions bordering the esophagus, medial fibers of the right crus continue anterior to the hiatus to complete the muscular collar, while lateral ones insert in a fan-shaped manner into the central tendon of the diaphragm. The anterior muscular collar separating the esophagus from the diaphragm is less than 1.5 cm. in almost all instances. The role of the right crus in forming a sling for the esophagogastric junction is similar to that of the puborectalis around the anorectal junction.

The left crus usually passes forward to abut against, but not to contribute to, the muscular collar of the diaphragm. The left crus then passes to the central tendon of the diaphragm.

On the basis of 204 fresh cadaver dissections, the variations in the muscular anatomy of the esophageal hiatus were divided into 11 types (Listerud and Harkins, 1958, 1959).

The most common, Type I, is that referred to in the previous paragraph (49% of total series). The next most common, Type II (31%), has a divided left crus, the right portion of which *does* contribute to the right margin of the hiatus. The important facts for the student to remember are: First, that while in the most common type, and in the rare Type VIII (0.5%), only the right crus contributes to the hiatal margins, in the other 9 types (comprising slightly over 50.5% of the series), the left crus also contributes. Second, in operating in this region, the surgeon should be aware of these anatomic variations. Allison (1951) summarizes his view of the hiatus, as follows:

Examination of the esophageal hiatus shows it to be a split in the muscle fibers of the right crus lightly reinforced by fibers from the left. In front the esophagus is supported by a sling of muscle fibers continuous on each side with the perpendicular fibers of the crus and decussating with one another to form a stoutly reinforced raphe, but behind there is less support, for it is here that the crus splits to form the hiatus. If the opening is enlarged the pressure felt in front and at the sides may cause some atrophy of muscle fibers, but it can do little more because it is acting "across the grain." The pressure at the back, however, is felt "along the grain" and splits the fibers to increase the size of the opening. This . . . forms the key to the problem of surgical repair.

2. **Fascial Relations of the Hiatus.** There are 2 fascial layers involved in the esophageal hiatus: (1) the strong diaphragmatic reflection of the endo-abdominal fascia below, and (2) the weak diaphragmatic reflection of the

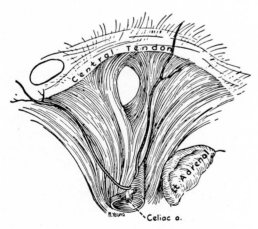

FIG. 39-15. The usual mode of formation of the esophageal hiatus as seen from below. The aorta is posterior, and the opening represents the hiatus. The right crus forms the hiatus. (Carey, J. M., & Hollinshead, W. H.: Surg., Gynec. & Obst. *100*:198)

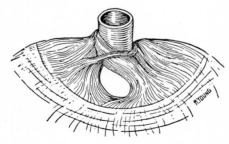

FIG. 39-16. The same as in Figure 39-15 from above and anteriorly. The accessory bundle of Low from the left crus passes forward to the right. (Carey, J. M., & Hollinshead, W. H.: Surg., Gynec. & Obst. *100*:198)

endothoracic fascia above. The fascial lining of the abdominal parietes (endo-abdominal fascia) commonly is given the local name of the muscle under which it lies (much as certain rivers used to be known locally by the name of the town through which they flowed). Thus, in the inguinal region, a portion of the endo-abdominal fascia is designated the *transversalis fascia* (see p. 1033), where it lies beneath the transversus muscle, and in the region of the esophageal hiatus a portion is designated the *diaphragmatic fascia* on the inferior surface of the diaphragm. As the diaphragmatic fascia approaches the hiatus it overlies the crura, then passing over the margins of the esophageal hiatus it ascends through the hiatus and out of the abdomen to be attached about the entire circumference of the lower end of the thoracic esophagus about 2 to 3 cm. above the cardia (Fig. 39-17). The portion involved in this attachment is known as the phreno-esophageal ligament (Laimer's ligament, 1883). It is a relatively strong fascia which normally holds the structures in their proper relationships and is stretched in cases of hernia. Another way of putting it is to state that the ligament is the normal antagonist of the longitudinal musculature of the esophagus and prevents the stomach from herniating into the chest upon esophageal contraction. Thus, while the muscular ring of the normal esophageal hiatus approximates the lower end of the esophagus, it is not directly attached to it. The phreno-esophageal ligament serves this function. Many of the hiatal hernias of elderly people result from incompetence of the hiatus due to atrophy of this protective and normally elastic membrane. This is especially true when the hiatus itself is already abnormally large and the ligament has to carry the burden of holding back increased intra-abdominal pressures from coughing, etc.

The diaphragmatic portion of the endothoracic fascia, especially where it reflects onto the esophagus is, in marked contrast with the endo-abdominal layer (true phreno-esophageal ligament), a weak and tenuous layer of loose connective tissue underlying the pleura.

3. **Peritoneal Relations of the Hiatus.** The peritoneal layer which closely invests the major portion of the stomach becomes quite loose anteriorly 2 to 3 cm. from the cardia. It becomes separated from the wall of the stomach before passing anteriorly to become firmly attached to the diaphragm by a variable amount of loose areolar tissue.

The laxity of the peritoneum at this point is the reason why the surgeon can invaginate his fingers for a short distance through the normal hiatus when doing an abdominal exploration. Surgeons are urged to do this exploratory maneuver, when the abdomen is open and when no contraindications are present, to accomplish 2 purposes: (1) to detect abnormally large hiatal openings; and (2) to acquaint themselves with the size of the normal opening—usually "2 fingers, 3 cm." (2 fingers admitted to a depth of 3 cm. The author has included this maneuver as a part of his routine abdominal exploration since 1942). Harrington (1955) stated that while there was considerable variation in the size of the hiatus, which is palpated as a part of a routine abdominal exploration,

a hiatus that will admit 1 or 2 fingers may be considered normal if there is no infolding of the peritoneum into the mediastinum but, in all cases in which the hiatus admits 3 fingers, the possibility of a hernia should be considered. Each of these patients should have a roentgenogram of the stomach. Even though hernia may not be demonstrated by a subsequent roentgenogram, it should be considered as a potentiality and the patient, if obese, should reduce and have periodic physical examinations.

There is some discussion as to whether the enlarged esophageal hiatal opening, which is usually elliptical in shape, has its long axis mainly in an anteroposterior direction (vertically) or in a transverse direction (hori-

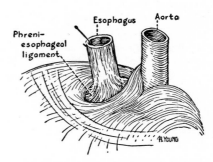

FIG. 39-17. Phrenoesophageal ligament as seen from above. (Carey, J. M., & Hollinshead, W. H.: Surg., Gynec. & Obst. *100*:198)

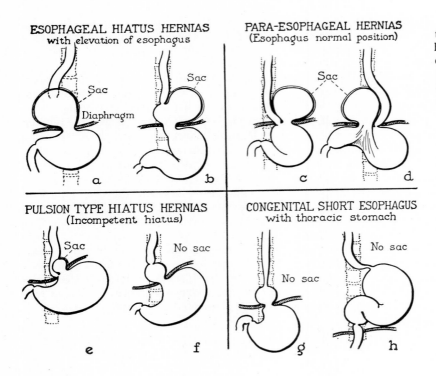

ESOPHAGEAL HIATUS HERNIAS
with elevation of esophagus

PARA-ESOPHAGEAL HERNIAS
(Esophagus normal position)

Fig. 39-18. Harrington's classification of herniation through the esophageal hiatus. (Harrington, S. W.: Surg., Gynec. & Obst. *100*:279)

PULSION TYPE HIATUS HERNIAS
(Incompetent hiatus)

CONGENITAL SHORT ESOPHAGUS
with thoracic stomach

zontally). Many published pictures of operative procedures indicate that it is transverse. The author is in accord with Lam and Kenney (1954), who stated that it is essentially vertical.

Classification

A recent classification (Harrington, 1955) of esophageal hiatal diaphragmatic hernia is as follows (Fig. 39-18). In the instance of the more common types, as seen at surgery, the percentage incidence is listed:

Esophageal Hernia with Elevation and Displacement of the Esophagus. The esophagus is of normal length but does not extend to the diaphragm (many so-called "short esophagus" cases are probably of this type). There is a true sac. This is the most common type (67%) in Harrington's series, and the incidence of recurrence was higher than with other types. Almost always the sac is anterior and incompletely embraces the portion of the stomach which has slid up posterior to the sac. Usually the herniation is of the stomach, and it may be large and into either or both sides of the thoracic cavity. (See Fig. 39-19). This type is also called a "sliding" hiatal hernia.

It almost never leads to strangulation but is a definite causative factor of esophagitis.

Para-esophageal Hernia. The esophagus is of normal length but is not displaced and remains attached to, and is not elevated above, the diaphragm. There is a true sac which lies anterior to the stomach (as shown in Fig. 39-20). This is the second most common type (15%) in Harrington's series, but, unlike Group 1, the most satisfactory results are obtained from surgical treatment in these cases, because correction of the hernia requires only repair of an abnormal and enlarged hiatus after replacement of the herniated viscera. These hernias usually are of the stomach, although other intestinal loops also may herniate, and, while they may be of any size, more often they are small or of moderate size. The herniation into the posterior mediastinum may extend into either or both sides of the thoracic cavity. This type constitutes the true "upside-down" stomach. Almost always there is a small remnant of the hiatus between the esophagus and the sac, although the main crural fibers may be found displaced by the sac.

Short Esophagus. These have no sac.

A, Sliding (Short Esophagus)

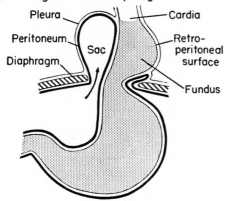

B, Parahiatal (Para-esophageal)

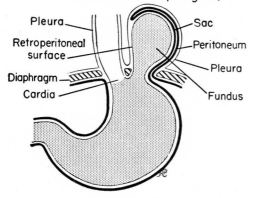

FIG. 39-19. (*Top*) Diagram illustrating the anatomic relations of the sliding type of herniation through the esophageal hiatus of the diaphragm. The drawing is made as a sagittal section through the area involved to show the relation of the herniated portion of the stomach to the hernia sac. (*Bottom*) Diagram illustrating the anatomic relations of the parahiatal type of diaphragmatic hernia. (Sweet, R. H.: Ann. Surg. *135*:2 and 5)

Congenital Type. In such instances the esophagus is not long enough to permit the stomach to reach its normal position below the diaphragm, with the result that the organ is held suspended above the diaphragm in the posterior mediastinum. This type is not a true hernia, since the stomach never has been below the diaphragm. Harrington, who reported this as being present in 5 per cent of his operative

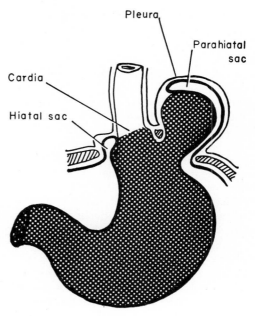

Hiatus hernia (composite type)

FIG. 39-20. Diagram illustrating the anatomic relations of the type of diaphragmatic hernia at the esophageal hiatus which consists of a combination of both sliding hiatal and parahiatal varieties. The term *composite* is suggested to designate this double arrangement. (Sweet, R. H.: Ann. Surg. *135*:5)

cases, stated: "I believe the condition could be described better as congenitally short esophagus with partially thoracic stomach than as an esophageal hiatal hernia."

Other writers put the incidence of this condition as lower than 5 per cent, while Lam (1954) stated that for practical purposes there was no such thing as a congenitally short esophagus. The editors of this textbook agree with Lam in this regard. The condition involves a mucosal factor as shown by Barrett (1950) and Morris (1955), i.e., the growth of the gastric mucosa up the esophagus. Therefore, the problem is one of esophageal surgery rather than of diaphragmatic surgery (see Chap. 28, "Esophagus"). Preoperative esophagoscopy, sometimes immediately before operation, is often helpful in cases of hiatal hernia if esophagitis is suspected. In general, it can be said that the relative roles and relationships between esophagitis and hiatal hernia are still unsettled. Moyer (1955) advocated a Finney pyloroplasty in conjunction with hernial repair when there was associated esophagitis. Peptic esophagitis, being a type of peptic ulcer, is also considered in Chapter 29, "Stomach and Duodenum."

Acquired Type. As a result of ulceration, or occasionally malignancy, of the esophagus, the cardia of the stomach may be pulled above the diaphragm. No true hernia exists, and any stricture which may be present is a result of the primary condition rather than of the elevation of the stomach. Treatment, either by dilatation or resection, is also directed toward that of the primary condition.

Pulsion Type of Hernia. Harrington adds a 4th type, which in turn is divided into (1) a small para-esophageal type of hernia with a sac and (2) incompetent hiatus without sac. The exact place which this group will occupy in the classification of hiatal hernia will be determined by future observations.

Incidence. Esophageal hiatal diaphragmatic hernia is noted most commonly in adult life, particularly in obese females over 50, but it may be found at any age, or in males, or in persons of normal weight. This type is less commonly found at birth than certain other types of congenital diaphragmatic hernia. Nelson (1953) reported 4 cases of hiatal hernia seen at the Sydney Children's Hospital. It is difficult to arrive at a figure for its overall incidence at all ages, but in the larger hospitals it may represent 1 per cent of the hernias treated surgically.

Predisposing Factors. These include: (1) age changes due to decreased elasticity of connective tissue, atony of the diaphragmatic muscles and loss of fat (or excessive fat) around the structures in the hiatus; and (2) changes due to increased subdiaphragmatic pressure caused by coughing, vomiting, constipation with flatulence, pregnancy, ascites and abdominal tumors.

Symptoms. The chief feature of the symptoms of early esophageal hiatal diaphragmatic hernia is the vagueness of their nature. Pain is substernal, precordial or epigastric. It may be exaggerated by lying down; thus, it may occur at night. It may be relieved by getting up in the morning or by sleeping in a semi-erect position at night; also by belching, swallowing and induced vomiting. Pain resulting from postural changes, particularly forward bending, is significant. Helpful diagnostic information also is supplied by a history of postural heartburn, probably due to regurgitation of acid liquid or of food, chiefly on forward bending or lying down; it may disturb sleep and is helped by assuming an erect or semierect position. Vomiting is rare, but eructation is not, and hiatal hernia should be suspected when there is aerophagia.

Additional symptoms include dysphagia, regurgitation, heartburn, hiccough, vomiting, hematemesis, anemia, palpitation, tachycardia, difficulty in breathing, and cough. Differential diagnosis should consider heart disease, especially angina pectoris, gallbladder disease, gastroduodenal ulcer, and other lesions of the esophagus, some of which may be associated with hernia, including peptic ulcer, cardiospasm, diverticula and tumors. The importance of differential diagnosis from coronary insufficiency was emphasized by Kohli and Pearson (1953).

Diagnosis. Except that most patients are over 40 years of age and are obese, physical examination is of little value. The history of symptoms referable to hiatal hernia may be of some help, but confirmation is made with roentgen examination. Such a study should be performed in a number of positions, including the prone, the supine and sometimes the head-down position. If a hiatal hernia is suspected, it is important to inform the roentgenologist about it, since the lesion may be missed easily on a routine upper gastro-intestinal examination. Pressure on the stomach region, as by bending forward during fluoroscopic examination, may force the stomach to herniate upward. Hillemand and Watteblede (1953) emphasized the importance of observation of the position of the cardia on fluoroscopic examination to determine if it was thoracic (sliding hernia) or abdominal (para-esophageal hernia). For study of the gastro-esophageal reflux, the patient swallows a few mouthfuls of water to clear the esophagus of barium. Then, in the decubitus position, retrograde flow into the esophagus is looked for. O'Connor and Ritvo (1955) pointed out that while the diagnosis of hiatal hernia by roentgen examination after the administration of opaque contrast material is a well-established procedure, it is not generally recognized that plain films of the upper abdomen may lead to a positive or a suggestive diagnosis. Observation of soft tissue densities, with or without air inclusion, is the essential feature in this method. Esophagoscopic examination also is indicated frequently.

Berry, Holbrook, Langdon and Mathewson (1955) have introduced an important new procedure in the differential diagnosis of hiatal hernias. They produced pneumoperitoneum in 15 patients with diaphragmatic hernia of the hiatal type. This caused a reduction in the hernia and concomitant cessation of certain of the symptoms which previously it had been difficult to attribute only to the hernia. They concluded that this might "be a useful technic for selecting patients who will benefit from surgical intervention."

Complications. These include ulceration, hemorrhage, incarceration and, very rarely, strangulation and rupture. Anemia frequently is present, probably because of chronic hemorrhage. Ritchey and Winsauer (1947) found anemia in 27 per cent of their series of 41 hiatal hernia patients. While as a general rule hemorrhage in cases of peptic esophagitis, with or without associated hiatal hernia, is of the chronic slow type (see Chap. 29), in exceptional instances sudden massive hemorrhage does occur (De Vito, Listerud, Nyhus, Merendino and Harkins, 1959). In the 39 cases of strangulated diaphragmatic hernia collected by Carter and Giuseffi (1948), all but 4 with the etiology stated were traumatic, and these 4 were congenital; in other words, in no instance in their collected series did strangulation occur in a hiatal hernia. The incidence of complications as reported by Stensrud (1954) in his 42 cases was 26 per cent (11 patients). These included stricture in 6, hematemesis or melena in 4, and incarceration in 1.

Treatment

When an opening which normally admits 2 fingers for 3 cm. is found on routine abdominal exploration in a patient with no symptoms attributable to the esophageal hiatus, operation is not required. A patient with a large fist-sized or larger herniation, and with symptoms most likely attributable to it, needs repair. Those cases with indications varying in intensity between these extremes pose a difficult problem. Lam (1954) pointed out that the "incidental" finding of a hiatal hernia on "routine" upper gastrointestinal examination might not be as incidental as might be thought, as otherwise why did these patients have the examination performed in the first place? Most certainly, patients with a combination of severe symptoms, complications and large hernias require operative care. Obese patients should be requested to reduce. Evarts Graham (1954) summarized his opinion concerning the operative indications in hiatal hernia by saying:

Too many roentgenologists and physicians are accustomed to think that repair is not indicated unless the symptoms are extreme. The operative risk is extremely small. Unquestionably, many more hernias should be operated on.

The author agrees that symptomatic hiatal hernias should be repaired surgically in the absence of definite contraindications. Blades (1956) recently summarized his conclusions in this regard as follows: "(1) The incidental finding of a hiatal hernia without symptoms does not justify surgical treatment at the present time. In the future this attitude may change. (2) All symptomatic hiatal hernias should be treated surgically unless the patient's condition precludes operation." Harrington (1956) stated: "At the Mayo Clinic we have operated on about 16 to 18 per cent of the hiatal hernias that have been recognized roentgenologically."

The essential decisions as to type of surgical treatment are twofold: abdominal versus thoracic approach, and placing sutures behind versus in front of the esophagus. As to the first decision, the thoracic approach now is considered preferable by most surgeons (Allison, 1951; Sweet, 1952; Lam, 1954; and others), except where a problem in intra-abdominal differential diagnosis exists, in which instance the abdominal approach is preferred. Harrington (1955) has had the most experience with the abdominal approach. As to a combined approach, Sweet (1952) stated: "It is never necessary to enlarge the incision into the abdomen or to use a thoraco-abdominal incision in order to obtain an adequate exposure of the operative field."

As to the second decision, the author believes that the sutures usually should be placed *behind* the esophagus. This technic was first reported by Merendino, Varco and Wangensteen (1949), and later by Allison (1951), Effler and Ballinger (1951), Lam and Kenney (1954) and Stensrud (1954). Tanner (1955) advocated a return to a repair of the hiatal opening in *front* of the esophagus, but with especial attention also to cleaning off all fatty tissue behind it. Madden (1956) advocated a thoracic approach, but advocated sutures between the two portions of the right crus, both in front of and behind the esophagus. In addition, he pointed out that in some instances the long axis of the enlarged hiatal ring is in the horizontal plane and that in such patients a transverse closure to the left is preferable.

The transthoracic retro-esophageal suture method is essentially a 7-step technic as follows:

1. The lower left chest is opened through the 7th interspace or the bed of the 8th rib (the latter in older patients).

2. The lower esophagus is exposed by means of a longitudinal incision through the mediastinal pleura over it, and then is mobilized, avoiding injury to the phrenic nerve, which is *not* crushed.

3. A radial incision is made in the diaphragm just in front of the spleen. This incision should be made large enough to admit either a forceps or a finger, and it should be placed so as to preserve as much as possible of the phrenic nerve terminal fibers (Merendino, Johnson, Skinner and Maguire, 1956). A second opening is made with forceps or scalpel, inserted through the first hole via the abdominal cavity, in the peritoneum and the phrenoesophageal ligament in front of and lateral to the stomach. A piece of tape is passed around the esophagus and brought through these holes in the hiatus and out through the incision in the diaphragm. This tape, grasped with a forceps, is held on tension by an assistant, moving the cardia under the diaphragm.

4. The sac is reduced, and the crura, especially the right, are cleared of areolar tissue posteriorly. Since the hernia is usually a sliding one, no useful purpose is accomplished by removing a portion of the sac.

5. The collar, consisting of the cut edges of phreno-esophageal ligament and peritoneum, then is affixed with 4 or 5 interrupted silk mattress sutures to the abdominal surface of the diaphragm in front and to the left of the cardia. If the incision in the diaphragm is large enough, these sutures can be placed through it and from below.

6. Then the esophagus is pulled forward and the 2 mobilized crural margins are joined with interrupted silk mattress sutures behind the esophagus. These sutures (usually not more than 3 or 4) are placed loosely so as not to strangulate the muscle. The orifice should admit a fingertip alongside the last stitch. The diaphragmatic portion of the endothoracic fascia usually is too weak to close over the crural sutures, but an attempt should be made to include it with the pleural closure in the region of the hiatus.

7. Next, the incision in the diaphragm is closed, followed by closure of the chest wall with water-seal drainage.

Allison (1951) summarized this technic as follows:

> The aim of surgery must be to restore those factors to normal which have already been described as being responsible for the protection of the esophagus. This is achieved by two main steps: first, by division of the extended phreno-esophageal ligament and peritoneal reflection close to the cardia, and the resuturing of these to the under aspect of the diaphragm, and second, by application of the vertical fibers of the right crus to one another behind the esophagus, and their retention thus by such light suturing as will enable them to continue to act as muscle.

The author, Tanner (1955), Beardsley (1956), Harrington and some others prefer the abdominal approach. Cooley (1956), in advocating the abdominal approach, cited as an additional advantage for it the fact that he had performed associated operative procedures within the abdomen during laparotomy for hiatal hernia in 65 per cent of the cases.

Ancillary considerations involve 2 supplemental procedures, as follows:

Phrenicotomy. Crushing the left phrenic nerve has been advised as either a concomitant or a definitive procedure in the treatment of hiatal hernia, particularly of the short esophagus type. Lam (1954) showed that in the experimental animal and in a human being, mechanical or faradic stimulation of the left phrenic nerve did not cause the left crus to contract. These studies would indicate that any beneficial effect of phrenicotomy would be indirect from elevation of the diaphragm rather than direct by relieving "spasm" of the hiatus. Amendola (1955) reported a case of late esophageal obstruction following excision of a segment of the left phrenic nerve for sliding hiatal hernia. Phrenicotomy now is seldom employed as a mode of therapy for hiatal hernia. Blades and Hall (1956) prefer procaine injection of the phrenic nerve at the end of the operation, if indicated.

Displacement of the Hiatus Anterolaterally into a New Opening. This more radical method involves an anterolateral incision in the diaphragm for about 2 to 4 cm., extending from the hiatus. The esophagus then is moved to the anterolateral end of the incision, and the diaphragm is closed behind it. This technic, first advocated by Merendino, Varco and Wangensteen in 1949, is applicable to large or difficult hiatal hernias in which the crural tissues are not satisfactory for suture.

The method of gastropexy as the only intervention for hiatus hernias is a technic now used in Europe (Nissen, 1956; Boerema, 1956) with which the author has had no experience. This method involves a suture of the anterior wall of the stomach and the lesser curvature to the anterior abdominal wall. The crura and the hiatus are not touched. This method is said to be especially suitable for elderly patients. Nissen stated that he had used the method for 10 years, while Boerema used it in 34 cases. The latter author sutures the lesser curvature to the anterior abdominal wall and the greater curvature to the under surface of the diaphragm in cases of either siding or para-esophageal hernia.

SUBSIDIARY PROBLEMS IN THE FIELD OF HERNIA

HERNIA IN INFANCY AND CHILDHOOD

This involves the following 3 factors: (1) different types of hernias; (2) indications for repair; and (3) technical differences in the type of repair. Many of the congenital hernias present in infants and children are considered in the glossary at the end of this chapter (e.g., Bochdalek hernia, paraduodenal hernia, etc.). Among the groin hernias, indirect inguinal ones are more common, and femoral, and particularly direct, hernias are much rarer in infants and children. The problem of inguinal hernia *complicated by undescended testis* also arises much more often in infants and children. Snyder and Chaffin (1955) found this combination in 7 per cent of their patients at the Los Angeles Children's Hospital and concluded that such children "may have both defects safely and simultaneously operated upon without delay."

Certain misconceptions exist concerning hernia in infants:

1. "Infants are poor surgical risks."
2. "Hernias in infants and childhood may cure spontaneously."
3. "A truss may obliterate the funicular process and cure the hernia."
4. "Hernias in infancy seldom incarcerate or strangulate."
5. "Hernias in infancy are seldom bilateral." Actually, about 25 per cent (Williams, 1959) to 60 per cent (Gilmore, 1960) are bilateral, or an inguinal hernia on the opposite side develops subsequently. McLaughlin and Coe (1960) did routine exploration of the opposite side in cases of single hernia, with a finding of previously unrecognized hernia in 55 per cent. They advised: "Routine exploration of the opposite side with single primary hernia in pediatric patients under three years of age is advised if the general condition permits." In a similar study, Kiesewetter and Parenzan (1959) found a contralateral hernia in 61 per cent of cases where it had not been suspected preoperatively. In another group of cases, these Pittsburgh authors did not explore the opposite side, and 31 per cent of these patients subsequently underwent contralateral herniorrhaphy. The evidence seems to be strong that hernias in infancy are often bilateral and that treatment should be planned accordingly.

Specific indications for treatment of 2 common hernias of infancy and childhood (indirect inguinal and umbilical) are considered under these headings. In general, the tendency is toward earlier operation. Technical differences in the type of repair likewise are treated under the discussion of these 2 last-named hernias. In infants, strangulation and particularly incarceration are recognized as being more common than was formerly thought to be the case (Potts, Riker and

Lewis, 1950; Smith, 1954; Holcomb, 1956). However, one precaution in this regard should be observed; namely, in infant females one should be alert to the possibility of the presence of an ovary in a hernia thought to be strangulated.

HERNIA IN THE AGED

Associated prostatic hypertrophy or carcinoma of the bowel must be looked for. The commonly accepted treatment in these instances is conservative. However, it must be remembered that hernias do not grow at a steady rate but may progress in size exponentially, particularly in the aged. With good anesthesia (see Chap. 12, Anesthesia), the risk of operation for hernia in the aged is quite low in the experience at the King County Hospital, Seattle, where many such patients are treated. Local infiltration anesthesia has a definite place in the surgical treatment of hernias in the aged. Operation can be made simpler in the case of groin hernias by orchiectomy in selected cases (see "Aids").

INDUSTRIAL ASPECTS OF HERNIA

The actual treatment of hernia in industry differs only in certain minor details from that in nonindustrial practice. However, there are several points that make such hernias of especial importance. Whether a hernia is congenital or has developed as a result of the occupational activities of the individual is an important consideration. The statement of a reliable industrial examiner must be given weight. Local practices in different communities may vary. Many of the industrial aspects of hernia may be subjects for litigation. If a patient with no pre-existing hernia has an "accident" during employment, after which a hernia is found, the condition usually is compensable. If a patient with a pre-existing hernia has an "accident" during employment, after which the hernia is found to be larger, the condition usually is compensable because of aggravation of the pre-existing hernia. The industrial examiner during physical examinations and the industrial surgeon at operation must pay more attention to an enlarged external ring than is the case in nonindustrial practice. (See section below on size of subcutaneous inguinal ring.) Since medical records on employed patients may be consulted

by others or may appear in court, the recorder must consider not only the medical aspects of his patient but also the legal implications of the same when writing the history and the physical examination. The last chapter of Watson's *Hernia* covers the subject of industrial aspects of hernia in detail and should be consulted by those doing industrial examinations or surgery.

TREATMENT BY NONSURGICAL MEANS

In infants, the truss treatment of indirect inguinal hernia is rapidly declining in popularity, while adhesive strapping of umbilical hernia is now restricted to infants less than 1 year old and preferably less than 6 months old. In healthy adults, the use of a truss would seem to the author to have little or no place in modern therapy. In some elderly individuals with reducible hernia (there is no place for the use of a truss in the treatment of irreducible hernia), especially those in whom operation is deemed to carry a significant risk, a carefully fitted truss may be tried. It is the responsibility of the physician who orders the truss to see that it fits and that it is applied properly. The truss should be applied in the recumbent position with the hernia reduced. These patients should be kept under careful observation because of the constant danger of strangulation.

The injection treatment of hernia involves the introduction of a sclerosing anesthetic mixture around the sac in selected cases of reducible hernia so as to produce fibrosis and eventual fixation of the sac in the reduced position. The method has suffered a progressive decline in the last 15 years. This was influenced by several factors: (1) the method never really gained a foothold in the larger surgical centers; (2) improvements in the results of the operation made a substitute procedure less necessary; (3) the unsurgical nature of the method, combined with the difficulties produced by varying positions of the sac, made little appeal to experienced surgeons; and particularly (4) the unfavorable report of the Council on Pharmacy and Chemistry of the American Medical Association on August 17, 1940, militated against it. Lawrence (1948) published a case report concerning fatal intestinal obstruction following injection treatment of hernia; he believed the method to be unreliable and hazardous. With this opinion the author is in accord. The injection treatment is mentioned only to be condemned.

BILATERAL REPAIR AT ONE OPERATION

The question has often been raised as to whether a bilateral hernia should be repaired at a single operation or whether it is best to do the second side a week later. A decision in this regard involves 3 main factors: (1) infection, (2) recurrence, and (3) mortality in poor risk patients. So far as the first factor is concerned, it seems to the author that if adequate aseptic precautions are used, and if the operation on the first side does not take over 90 minutes, the increased risk should be insignificant. In a series of over 100 bilateral repairs, infection occurred in only one instance, and then in the wound on the side *first* repaired. If bowel is entered, or an abscess is encountered on the first side, it would seem wise to do the other side later. Otherwise it may be concluded that the danger of increased risk of infection in the second side is not a frequent contraindication to bilateral operation.

The second factor of increased recurrence rate—in this instance the supposed increase applying to *either* side because of tension on the peritoneum and the endo-abdominal fascia —may be important in certain circumstances. If the hernia is very large on one side, or if the hernia is recurrent on one side, it usually is best to do a one-sided operation and then repair the smaller hernia at a later date.

In poor risk patients, the larger or otherwise more important hernia should be repaired first. If the patient is standing the procedure well, the second side may be done at the same sitting if 2 factors apply: (1) if the second hernia needs repair (which often is not so in bedridden patients with a small second side hernia); and (2) if the increased risk of a second anesthesia exceeds the risk of prolonging the first operation. Koontz (1954) was in agreement with this policy.

The additional point should be mentioned that often a bilateral hernia exists even when it is not demonstrable, except on one side, preoperatively. Rothenburg and Barnett (1955) reported that in 100 per cent of their infants under 1 year with hernia and in 66 per cent

of those from 1 to 12 years of age the lesion was bilateral. This is an additional consideration in favor of more frequent bilateral operations.

Aside from the question of *when* a bilateral hernia should be repaired at one sitting, discussed above, the problem arises as to *how* this should be done when indicated. Many surgeons advise 2 separate groin incisions. Others advise a transverse, or Pfannenstiel-type incision. And still others advise a mid-line incision with internal repair. Knott (1954) advocated a transpubic horizontal incision of the Pfannenstiel type in bilateral cases. At the same time, Knott pointed out that otherwise a "second side" hernia often is overlooked.

THE RELATIONSHIP BETWEEN INGUINAL HERNIA AND PREVIOUS APPENDECTOMY INCISIONS

While it is generally recognized that inguinal hernia is more common on the right than on the left, this increased frequency seems to be accentuated in patients with previous appendectomy incisions. Pitkänen (1948), in a study of 1,062 postappendectomy patients, found that the incidence of inguinal hernia on the right side was no greater in those patients in whom there had not been diffuse peritonitis, but was about 2 times the normal expected rate in patients who had had diffuse peritonitis at the time of the appendectomy. Hicks (1941) also stated:

We found that a considerable number of right inguinal hernias followed the McBurney incision for appendicitis. This is, no doubt, due to a blind tearing injury to nerves and muscle when this incision is used.

To obviate the difficulty, Hicks has adopted the transverse incision for appendicitis without abscess.

The different but related problem of concomitant appendectomy with herniorrhaphy is important. No hard-and-fast rule can be laid down. In general, if the appendicitis is acute and the hernia is large (hence apt to recur), the appendectomy should be done through a separate incision. On the other hand, an interval appendectomy is permissible through a herniorrhaphy incision when the hernia is small, the appendix presents itself in the wound, and the surgeon is experienced.

If these criteria are not all met, coincident interval appendectomy with herniorrhaphy should be avoided.

CHOICE OF SUTURE MATERIAL

This choice always has been a matter of debate. Since 1939 the author has used non-absorbable sutures (generally silk; although when cotton was used in a few cases at hospitals which did not regularly use silk, cotton seemed to work equally as well). During the years 1931 to 1938 he used catgut. While it is true that the catgut available in the thirties was not as good as that now on the market, it is the author's opinion that silk is preferable to catgut for the repair of hernias. At the same time, it must be admitted that an improperly performed silk repair is not as good as a properly performed catgut repair. The author is using steel wire more and more in place of silk, but has had difficulty in tying it square in the deep wound where the conjoined tendon is sutured to Cooper's ligament, so that silk is still preferred for this deep layer. Silk (and steel even more so) seems to give rise to less frequent "seroma" development, wound infection and recurrence of the hernia (see Chap. 2, Wound Healing). Even in the rare instance in which wound infection has required that the incision be laid wide open and the silk removed, recurrence has not resulted. The one objection to silk—extrusion of sutures or sinuses down to them requiring their removal ("silkosis")—rarely applies if care is taken to use aseptic technic and avoid too heavy sutures, sutures too near the skin or continuous silk sutures.

DISPOSAL OF DISTAL PORTION OF THE INDIRECT SAC

In many clinics great care is taken, after dividing a long indirect sac not only to close the proximal end but also to excise the remaining distal segment because of fear of developing a hydrocele. We believe that while high ligation of the proximal stump of the sac is the most important step in the repair of hernia, in most instances it is preferable to leave the distal portion of the sac in place. In cases of congenital hernia, generally we do not even do a bottle type of operation in the absence of a pre-existing hydrocele. The rationale behind this mode of treatment is that an almost certain danger of hematoma (from sac excision) is more to be feared than the more remote possibility of a subsequent hydrocele. Larsen (1949), speaking of hernias in infancy and in childhood, also emphasized that the distal portion of the sac should be disregarded. Griffith (1959), on the other hand, advised removal of the sac in most instances.

SIZE OF THE SUBCUTANEOUS INGUINAL RING

In physical examinations much is made of the size of the subcutaneous or external inguinal ring as an indication of both potential and actual inguinal hernia. In an excellent review, Chassin (1947) found less correlation than would be expected between these factors. A study was made of 3,199 soldiers between 18 and 36 years of age to determine the range of sizes of subcutaneous or external inguinal rings in large numbers of healthy young men. It was found that 78.1 per cent of these men had external rings sufficiently large to admit the index finger, almost half being from 1.4 to 1.9 cm. This does not agree with the previous statements of many authorities, and it indicates that normal external rings vary widely in size, and that the average is appreciably larger than was formerly believed to be the case. In 724 men with asymmetric rings, the larger occurred on the left side in 57.5 per cent, but 58.3 per cent of inguinal hernias discovered during this study occurred on the right side. There was no convincing evidence to indicate that a large subcutaneous ring was abnormal or that it predisposed to future herniation. No correlation could be demonstrated between the size of the subcutaneous ring and the weight or the height of the subject.

ERRORS AND SAFEGUARDS IN THE REPAIR OF HERNIA

Two of the chief errors are committed during the preoperative phase: (1) overlooking a strangulated hernia; and (2) delaying operation on a hernia in an older individual until both the hernia is much bigger and the patient is much older than when first seen, hence less able to withstand operation. At operation many errors can occur. One of the chief of these is a diagnostic blunder, already referred to in the section on femoral hernia, which involves the omission of finger exploration from within of Hesselbach's triangle and the femoral region for associated direct inguinal or femoral hernia when repairing an indirect inguinal hernia. In making the incision care should be taken not to cut the ilioinguinal or the iliohypogastric nerves. Similarly, in freeing the cord, the vascular supply must be preserved, and the vas (the location of which is noted by its hard feel on palpation) should not be cut. An indirect inguinal sac may not be ligated high enough, or it may be overlooked entirely. In performing a Bassini type of operation for inguinal hernia, care must be taken to see that the needle which sutures the conjoined tendon to Poupart's ligament does not penetrate the underlying femoral vein. In performing a Cooper's ligament repair the same error can be avoided more easily, but still this requires retraction of the femoral vein under direct vision during the placing of the most lateral sutures. There are many other errors and safeguards, but a final one that should not be overlooked involves the selection of operation for the particular patient at hand. Thus, even the advocates of a Bassini repair would admit that it is not adequate for a large direct hernia. On the other hand, a Cooper's ligament repair involves too much alteration of normal structures to be necessary for the repair of an indirect inguinal hernia in an infant.

AIDS TO REPAIR

The previous discussion in the main body of this chapter includes that of the procedures ordinarily used in the repair of the common types of hernia. When the hernia is unusually large or difficult, certain additional "aids" should be available in the armamentarium of the surgeon. Some of these may have frequent application; others may be needed only rarely; still others (denoted by an asterisk) are applicable so seldom that the author never has used them, even though they are popular with others. Before considering any of these individually, it should be emphasized that an aid is like a crutch; it should be used only if absolutely necessary. The aim should be always to get the fascial edges together. While certain aids may help in accomplishing this, those that consist of a type of patch (cutis, whole skin, tantalum mesh, etc., see p. 1060) generally should be reserved for reinforcement of a

suture line between fascial layers rather than for bridging a gap. Thus, Moyer (1960) states: "The use of prostheses is practically never necessary, even for the largest hernias." The aids may be classified as follows:

Preoperative and Operative Technics for Facilitation of Surgery of Massive Hernias

In certain instances a hernia may be so large that the bowel contents may be said to have lost their "right of domain" within the abdominal cavity. Aside from the general careful preparation of the patient, which in such instances may include weight reduction and studies of cardiac and pulmonary function, 3 specific methods of preparation are available:

1. **Pneumoperitoneum.** This method, used especially in large ventral hernias, was introduced by Goñi Moreno (1940), of Buenos Aires, and has been used chiefly in certain South American clinics since that time. The technic includes a series of 4 to 6 intraperitoneal air injections at intervals of from 2 to 5 days.

It is surprising how relaxed the margins of the hernial ring are at operation and how undistended the bowel appears to be. Moyer (1960) on the basis of an experience with the method in over 30 cases, most often for the secondary repair of omphalocele, agrees that the bowel actually becomes smaller in diameter and also that even if the abdominal wall stretches, the hernia usually does not increase in size. This latter point may be because the hernia is the one portion of the abdominal wall circumference that contains scar tissue. In the case of hernias, in the repair of which it would ordinarily be difficult to get the edges together, after a course of pneumoperitoneum preparation the edges often can be imbricated liberally. The author has used this technic in a few selected cases since the autumn of 1949 with uniformly good results. Among the best references to the technic in the American literature are those of Koontz and Graves (1954) and Mason (1956). These authors use a 19-gauge lumbar puncture needle, which is usually inserted in the linea semilunaris, well away from the hernia to avoid adhesions. Air is injected (in Goñi Moreno's original report he advocated the use of oxygen, but since then he has switched to the use of air) until the patient begins to have slight respiratory distress (usually after 500-1,500 cc.). Subsequent injections at 2- to 5-day intervals may be as much as several liters at 1 sitting and are continued until "the abdominal cavity has become enlarged enough to accommodate the contents of the hernial sac." An abdominal binder is worn to prevent the air simply from becoming captive in the hernial sac and not enlarging the peritoneal cavity. From 10 to 20 days should be sufficient time for preparation for operation. Koontz and Graves (and the author) have kept the patients in the hospital during this period, but this may not always be necessary. In 4 cases, Koontz and Graves injected totals of 1,700, 7,000, 5,000 and 6,700 cc. of air in series of 2, 7, 2 and 4 injections, respectively.

2. **Phrenic Crush.*** Touroff (1954) recommended a "phrenicectomy," left-sided in his case report, to be done a few days before herniorrhaphy to relax the diaphragm and better to accommodate the contents of the hernia within the abdomen. Most certainly, if such a procedure is to be done, a simple phrenic crush, which is rarely permanent, is preferable to a phrenicectomy, which almost always is permanent. A phrenic crush is something that can be done at the time of operation if necessary and takes only 5 to 10 minutes of extra operating time. It would seem that, generally, pneumoperitoneum is preferable to phrenic crush. Pneumoperitoneum is over with as soon as the operation, hence it does not impair the patient's recovery during the postoperative period. Furthermore, if respiratory embarrassment occurs, pneumoperitoneum always can be decompressed, while the effects of the phrenic crush cannot be reversed at will.

3. **Long Intestinal Tube.** Preoperative threading of the bowel on a long intestinal tube for decompression and keeping it down for 2 to 4 days after operation may not only make the operative reduction of a large hernia easier but be a lifesaving procedure during the postoperative period. A corollary of this method is the use of physostigmine to permit closure of the abdomen at the time of operation and to keep down postoperative distention. Even if a long tube is not used, in large

* See page 1057 for explanation.

hernias a regimen involving preoperative liquid diet, castor oil and enemas the day before operation and gastric aspiration for 12 hours before, is advisable.

Three other technics, which are utilizable at the time of operation rather than preoperatively, are as follows:

1. **Bowel Resection.** The temptation to do a bowel resection for mechanical reasons only to reduce the volume of bowel content to be replaced is an ever-present one, but it should be resisted, just like the temptation to do a gastroenterostomy in the presence of apparent obstruction of the duodenum after simple closure of a perforated peptic ulcer. Bowel resection is seldom necessary for the reason of reducing bowel content of the peritoneal cavity in experienced hands; it increases the chances of infection, not only of the wound, but also of the main peritoneal cavity.

2. **Relaxing Incisions.** These are of 4 types, 2 applicable to ventral hernias and 2 to groin hernias. The first 2 involve a longitudinal incision in the anterior rectus sheath either with or without turning the medial flap over medialward (Wilkie maneuver) to reinforce the suture line. It is important not to place these relaxing incisions where there is no muscle beneath them. The other 2 involve the relaxing incision already described in the Cooper's ligament repair, either with or without turning the lower flap downward.

3. **Two-Stage Wound Closure.*** Gross, of Boston, recommended 2-stage wound closure, especially for infants with large hernias of the foramen of Bochdalek, in which the intestine has lost the "right of domain" in the abdominal cavity. At the 1st stage only the skin is closed, and then 6 days later the entire wound is closed in layers as a 2nd stage. This method is not so readily applicable to adults because of poorer blood supply in the abdominal wall. Even in infants Gross has not found it necessary since 1945. In omphalocele, the 2-stage method is becoming increasingly popular (see "Rarer Hernias"). Ziffren and Womack (1950) have described a modification of this technic for use in adults with gigantic hernias, which they applied successfully to a male with a right inguinal hernia which reached to just below the knees and

* See page 1057 for explanation.

at repair was found to be irreducible because of loss of "right of domain." Therefore, a long transverse incision was made in the upper abdomen down to the peritoneum. The latter was allowed to bulge into the wound, the skin was closed, and the space thus created permitted reduction of the inguinal hernia. The upper abdominal "new hernia" was easily repaired 12 days later when the patient had adjusted himself to the newly increased abdominal contents.

METHODS TO FACILITATE CLOSURE OF THE INTERNAL RING IN A DIFFICULT INGUINAL HERNIA REPAIR

Often it has been said that the repair of inguinal hernia in males would be much simpler if one were permitted to close the internal ring entirely rather than to have to strike the delicate balance of closing it just tight enough to prevent recurrence, yet not so tight as to strangulate the cord. In large repeatedly recurrent or otherwise difficult hernias the following 2 methods are available to obviate this difficulty, generally in elderly males only:

1. **Cord Division With Orchiectomy.** This should be done only with the full understanding of the patient and his wife and with their written consent. It permits a complete closure of the internal ring. Fowler and Stephens (1959) pointed out the importance of a knowledge of testicular vascular anatomy in operations of this type. Careful hemostasis, especially in the loose tissues within the scrotum, to prevent hematoma formation and insertion of a small Penrose drain for a few days may be indicated but is not always necessary. Hagan and Rhoads (1953) noted in their series that recurrence rates in males, when concomitant orchiectomy was done, and in females were much lower than in other patients. They concluded that these observations support the "argument that adequate closure of the internal ring is of particular importance, and suggests that in difficult or recurrent hernias in older patients orchiectomy may be justified."

2. **Cord Division Without Orchiectomy.** This method, first advocated by Burdick and Higinbotham (1935), has the advantage that if the testis does not atrophy, a better cosmetic result is obtained.

These authors gave the following indications for the procedure (these would also apply to cord division *with* orchiectomy):

1. Recurrent hernias which have had one or more unsuccessful attempts at a radical cure in individuals past 50 in whom the opposite testicle apparently is normal

2. Recurrent hernias in younger subjects who are incapacitated from their usual occupation and have an apparently normal testicle on the opposite side, especially when more than one attempt at repair has been made previously

3. Large scrotal hernias in the aged, which are either irreducible or cannot be retained satisfactorily by a truss

4. Large sliding hernia

When cord division is performed in cases of scrotal hernia, the distal sac never should be removed, nor should the testicle be delivered intentionally into the wound for fear of damaging the anastomotic blood supply. Burdick and Higinbotham advocated elevating the scrotum on a bridge for a few days postoperatively. They stated that there is "always considerable swelling accompanied by redness of the skin and edema of the scrotum. . . . Gangrene did occur in four . . . . Many of the testicles atrophy, in fact some almost completely disappear, but it is surprising how many do not." 200 such cord divisions were performed, and, of 169 cases followed, there were notes as to the condition of the testicle available in 64. The testicle was normal in 42 cases (including all bilateral cord divisions), slightly atrophied in 11, and atrophied to one half or less of normal size in 11. These figures do not include the 4 cases with gangrene necessitating orchiectomy.

Heifetz and Goldfarb (1952) reported 23 cases with cord divisions with the following results: 6 without postoperative swelling or atrophy and 17 with postoperative swelling (of these 4 became atrophic, 2 slightly atrophic, 1 had to be removed because of chronic infection, and the remaining 10 were normal when last seen). In dog experiments these same workers reported no gangrene or necrosis of the testicle after division of the spermatic cord at various levels, although there was some degeneration of the tubules and the spermatic cells. Paradoxically, when the ductus deferens and its artery were preserved after division of the rest of the cord structures in the dog, the testes atrophied completely.

In patients in whom retention of the internal secretions of the testicles or a single remaining testicle is important, or in whom the psychic effect of testicular absence is important, this method should be considered in the light of its possible complications in preference to orchiectomy.

METHODS OF SUTURE REINFORCEMENT

These include the following:

1. **Attached Fascial Suture** (McArthur, 1901). These are often called living fascial sutures, and if viable they do have an advantage. Often the circulation is deficient, and they are not viable. These sutures can be obtained only from contiguous structures, usually the external oblique aponeurosis, and this practical consideration limits their length, strength and size.

2. **Free Fascial Sutures** (Gallie & Le Mesurier, 1921). Such sutures can be obtained of satisfactory size from the tensor fascia lata tendon (iliotibial tract) using a fascial stripper. The objections to them are that of necessity they make large needle holes in the tissue being sutured and also may become infected. However, they are strong and, even though inserted loosely, fill in weak spaces quite adequately.

3. **Darning and Filigree Technics.*** Such methods are especially popular in Great Britain, where faith in the classic Bassini operation is beginning to falter, and reliance has not yet been widely placed in the Cooper ligament technic. Moloney, Gill and Barclay (1948) advocated a technic using nylon darn. These authors reported on the use of this method whereby 2 layers of No. 5 nylon were used as a loose continuous suture without slack, but without tension between the lower edge of the internal oblique muscle and Poupart's ligament and *without* approximation of these structures. The suture goes back and forth and is tied at each end. From 3 to 6 lengths of 40 in. nylon are inserted. In a series of 412 inguinal darns (indirect, direct and strangulated hernia) the results were good. In the last 239 cases there were 5 wound

infections, none with extrusion of the darn, and "no inguinal case darned with nylon has yet recurred." Monro (1950) advocated a silk darn.

The filigree technic, as described by Cole (1941), involves the insertion of a prefabricated patch of laced silver wires to support the same area as is darned by the technic of Moloney *et al.* Cole reported 862 inguinal repairs (out of a total of 3,755) treated by the filigree technic at the Seamen's Hospital, Greenwich, from 1920 to 1941. He stated that there "never was an extrusion of the filigree." While these methods have the advantage of strength, they have the disadvantage, particularly when nylon or silk is used, of any *continuous* nonabsorbable suture, namely, that if one portion becomes infected the infection spreads to the remainder, in the same way that explosions will traverse a chain of firecrackers.

PATCHES

These are becoming more popular and include cutis grafts, whole skin grafts,† tantalum mesh, steel-wire mesh, Vitallium plate, Ivalon (polyvinyl alcohol sponge, used by Schofield, 1955) other plastics and cartilage (for repair of large ventral hernias, Satinsky & Kron, 1953). Of these, tantalum mesh (Koontz, 1950; Koontz and Kimberly, 1950; Smith, 1954, 1959) and cutis grafts (Cannaday, 1942; Swenson & Harkins, 1944; Harkins, 1945; Swenson, 1950; and Ali, 1954) are most popular, although Mair, in Scotland, has used whole-thickness skin-graft patches in several hundred instances of repair of hernia with reportedly good results. Theoretically, Vinyon "N" cloth could be used as a patch. It should be re-emphasized that almost always such patches should be used to *reinforce* rather than to *supplant* a layer-to-layer closure. Furthermore, it should be emphasized that these patches complicate the operation and lead to additional complications, and they do not eliminate recurrences.

Tantalum Mesh. Lam, Szilagyi and Puppendahl (1948) studied the effects of implantation of tantalum (a biologically inert metallic element) in the form of gauze as implanted in dogs with favorable results. In 24

---

* See page 1057 for explanation.

† See page 1061 for explanation.

large postoperative ventral hernias these authors also reported good results. Throckmorton (1948) in 16 cases, Koontz (1948, 1955) in several reports and a large series of 139 cases, Smith (1954) in 43 cases, and Guy, Werelius and Bell (1955) in 302 cases have all reported their experiences with the method. Smith (1954) and Erwald and Rieger (1960) pointed out that the fragmentation of the mesh may be disadvantageous in the upper abdomen. Experience by the author of this chapter would indicate that if tantalum mesh is used, tantalum sutures should be utilized to suture it in place. The large experience of Guy *et al.* is based on the use of tantalum mesh in 302 of 1,073 total hernia operations. Only 37 of the 302 were ventral hernias, the rest being groin hernias. Even though mesh was used in the more difficult hernias, so far as inguinal hernias are concerned the recurrence rate was 3.0 per cent without mesh and 1.9 per cent with mesh. The experience of Allen (1955) with tantalum mesh is less encouraging. In his clinic 7 of 10 cases had to have the tantalum removed in 2 months to 3 years. Infection was not always the dominant factor. The tantalum was fragmented and uncomfortable. In the majority of cases it was utilized above the umbilicus; hence, a warning should be voiced against its use in the upper abdomen.

Steel-wire mesh is cheaper and does not fragment as much as tantalum mesh. However, its adoption is slow despite its availability. The experimental observations of Koontz and Kimberly (1950) indicating the superiority of tantalum as compared with steel-wire mesh partly explain this reluctance to adopt the latter.

Cutis Grafts. Cutis may be defined as the deeper layers of the skin which have been stripped of their epidermal covering. Anatomically, this includes approximately the deeper three quarters of the thickness of the skin, the entire skin averaging about 1 mm., or 40/1,000 in., in depth. Histologically, cutis comprises the dermal layer with no epidermal covering, but with sebaceous and sudoriferous glands and occasional hair follicles, as well as some of the underlying subdermal fat.

Since Loewe's report, in 1913, cutis grafts have been adopted sporadically for 2 purposes: (1) in the field of plastic surgery when the cutis is utilized to fill in tissue defects; and (2) in the operative treatment of hernia when patches of cutis are applied to strengthen the repair.

Cannaday (1942) was the first writer in this country to report the use of cutis in hernial repair work; he presented 14 such cases. Two years later he had increased the size of his hernia series to 56 and reported good results. In 1945, Harkins reported experimental studies in dogs and the clinical use of cutis in 11 cases of large ventral or incisional hernias. In the animal experiments cyst formation was noted, while in the clinical cases the results seemed excellent, so that the wounds remained healed. Swenson (1950) is one of the chief workers in this field at present.

Whole Skin. This procedure is more radical than the introduction of cutis grafts. The method was introduced by Mair in 1938 (with further reports in 1945 & 1948). Mair's technic was controlled by careful animal experiments. In 2 cases in which the skin implant was examined later in human subjects, it was found to be converted into stout fibrous tissue. Mair (1948) stated:

In my own practice I have repaired 140 indirect inguinal herniae with the whole skin graft technique and with a recurrence rate of 0.71 per cent after a follow-up of 1 year. I have also repaired 40 direct inguinal herniae by the same technique without a recurrence at the end of 3 years. This is associated with a morbidity rate, both immediate and remote, which compares well with figures from both my own practice and results from other clinics for other methods. These figures embrace those repairs performed with skin only over a short period.

So far I have found no contra-indication to the routine use of the operation where sound repair is indicated, but insist on an adequate pre-operative skin preparation as being essential to elimination of sepsis as a complication.

West and Hicks (1948) have also reported favorably on the use of whole skin grafts in the repair of inguinal hernia, particularly recurrent cases, and femoral hernia. The method has been also used successfully at the University of Tennessee (Wilson, 1948), by Zavaleta and Uriburu (1950) in 211 cases and Strahan (1951) in 413 cases.

The use of plastic materials is becoming more common. Rigid plastic implants should be avoided (Fitzgerald and Mehigan, 1959); Nylon (Smith, 1959); Teflon (Adler and Firme, 1959); and Marlex meshes (Usher, Ochsner and Tuttle, 1958; Ponka, Wylie, Chäikof, Sergeant and Brush, 1959; Usher, 1959; Usher, Fries, Ochsner and Tuttle, 1959; and Usher and Gannon, 1959) have all been tried. It should be re-emphasized that while these supports are very useful when indicated, for the vast majority of hernia repairs they are entirely superfluous.

RARER HERNIAS: TREATMENT AND GLOSSARY OF TERMS

Bochdalek (Foramen of) Hernia. Hernias in posterolateral region of the diaphragm, along the old pleuroperitoneal canal (foramen of Bochdalek), are the most common among congenital hernias of the diaphragm (90% of all cases at the Boston Children's Hospital). They are 5 times as common on the left as on the right. In most instances no sac exists, and the absence of adhesions to the parietal pleura is also noteworthy. Associated malrotation of the intestine is often present. Treatment includes immediate operation, preferably during the first 48 hours of life before the intestines are distended. Most surgeons (Harrington, 1951; Gross, 1953) prefer an abdominal approach, although some use a thoracic one. On the right side it is usually preferable to replace the liver last, and on the left side to replace the stomach first. The ring is closed with interrupted silk-mattress sutures, with imbrication if possible. The abdominal wound should be closed in layers, although if the intestine truly has lost the "right of domain," skin closure with later repair of the entire wound is an available method (see section on "Aids").

Congenital Hernia. This includes any hernia which results from either abnormal persistence of a normally present opening (e.g., indirect inguinal hernia) or the presence of an abnormal opening (e.g., paraduodenal hernia, see p. 1065).

Epigastric Hernia (hernia of the linea alba above the umbilicus). Since hernia of the linea alba below the umbilicus is so rare, "epigastric" hernia is the term commonly used. The symptomatology of epigastric hernia is important; such hernias may mimic peptic ulcer, cholecystitis, acute pancreatitis, etc. The pain may be worse when the patient lies down, due to the pull on the omentum by gravity. Some of the most symptomatic epigastric hernias are so small as not to be visible. Such hernias comprise about 1 per cent of all hernias. They may occur anywhere between the xiphoid and the umbilicus, but they are most common immediately above the latter structure. The initial defect which predisposes to these hernias is most likely the aperture for a perforating blood vessel. Because of these blood vessels, in doing a repair when the herniated lobule of fat is excised, its base should be secured with a suture ligature. A closure of the fascial defect is usually done transversely, fastening the upper flap over the lower as in an umbilical hernia and utilizing relaxing incisions similar to those described under the repair of umbilical hernia.

Eventration of the Diaphragm. This is often classified as a type of diaphragmatic hernia, but actually it consists by definition merely in elevation into the thorax of one or both leaves of the diaphragm associated with defective muscular action, similar to that which follows the surgical procedure of crushing one or both phrenic nerves. Also it may occur following pneumoperitoneum, or it may be of idiopathic origin. Neuman, Ellis and Andersen (1955) advise operation more often than has been done in the past. Plication and strengthening with fascia, etc., have been used to lower the thinned-out diaphragm in cases in which symptoms of respiratory embarrassment exist.

Incarcerated Hernia (syn.: **Irreducible Hernia**). According to another definition, there is, in addition to irreducibility, obstruction to the flow of intestinal contents in any intestinal loop which may be present but in which, unlike a *strangulated hernia*, the blood flow and the lymph drainage remain intact. According to our definition, this type of hernia is an *obstructed hernia*. The term *incarceration* usually is used to denote an irreducible hernia without obstruction or strangulation.

Internal Hernia. Such hernias are of 3 main types: (1) congenital in origin, of which paraduodenal hernia (q.v.) is the most common type; (2) due to adhesive bands—congenital (e.g., attached Meckel's diverticulum), inflammatory (e.g., after appendicitis with perforation) or iatrogenic (e.g., from talcum implantation at the time of previous operation); and (3) due to volvulus around colostomies, etc. Strangulation is frequent, and careful observation with prompt laparotomy in indicated cases is mandatory. Prophylactic measures include the general abdandonment of the use of talcum on gloves about 1950 (the starch powder now used is much less noxious than talcum in this regard, see Chap. 2, "Wound Healing"), but like any foreign body, starch is not entirely innocuous. It should be washed off the gloves *carefully* before any abdominal operation and care should be taken in closing the lateral peritoneal gutter adjacent to laterally placed colostomies or ileostomies.

Interparietal Hernia. Lower and Hicken (1931) classified interparietal hernias into 3 anatomic types, as follows:

(1) Properitoneal hernia, that type in which the hernial sac lies between the peritoneum and the transversalis fascia; (2) interstitial hernia, in which the sac lies between the transversalis fascia and the transversalis, internal oblique, or external oblique muscles; and (3) superficial hernia, in which the sac is situated between the aponeurosis of the external oblique and the integument.

Of these 3 types, the interstitial is the most common and is described below:

Interstitial Hernia. A hernia which lies in one of the planes of the abdominal wall, e.g., between the internal and the external oblique aponeuroses. This type of hernia, first described by Bartholin in 1661, has many subvarieties. While most interstitial hernias are also inguinal hernias, this is not always true (Koontz & Stafford, 1955). Interstitial hernia may be very large. It is over 3 times as common in males as in females. Its treatment is essentially that of the type of hernia it represents, independent of its burrowing propensities. (See "Interparietal Hernia" above.)

Irreducible Hernia. The opposite of *reducible hernia.*

Laugier's Hernia (hernia ligamenti lacunaris gimbernati, hernie de Laugier, medical femoral hernia). This hernia was first described by Laugier in 1833. Since such hernias pass through the fibrous plate of Gimbernat's ligament, reduction may require incision into the lateral border of the ring as advocated by Priesching (1956).

Lipoma of the Cord. A soft lobulated fatty projection from the retroperitoneal space, coming out usually at the lateral margin of the internal ring. Its importance is that it may be confused with a simple indirect hernia. When seen at operation, it should always be removed to prevent a future possible misdiagnosis and unnecessary secondary operation.

Littré Hernia. A hernia of Meckel's diverticulum through a hernial opening (Littré, 1700). This type of hernia is found most frequently in adult males. Among 143 cases collected by Watson, 109 were on the right and only 34 on the left. Treatment includes that of the hernia itself plus, if possible, excision of the Meckel's diverticulum. When Meckel's diverticulitis is present—and this may have drawn the patient's attention to the hernia—resection is mandatory, possibly through a separate abdominal incision.

Lumbar Hernia (also called **Petit's Triangle Hernia**). While such hernias may occur in any part of the lumbar region, they are particularly prone to protrude through Petit's triangle (bounded by the iliac crest below, the external oblique in front, and the latissimus dorsi behind; the floor is made up by the internal oblique). Petit's triangle is also known as the inferior lumbar triangle. About 2 in. above and slightly anterior to it is the superior lumbar triangle of Grynfelt-Lesshaft. This superior triangle represents the bare space where there is neither external nor internal oblique. It has no muscular floor but has the latissimus dorsi for a roof or an outer covering. It is larger and more constant than Petit's triangle, but herniation through it is rarer. Watson collected reports of 146 lumbar hernias from the literature; of those in which the sex was stated, 103 were males and 39 were females. They occurred at all ages but were rare in young children and common in older persons. Nine per cent were strangulated. Usually there is a sac. Treatment usually is accomplished by pushing in on the sac and by overlapping muscular and aponeurotic layers over the defect. Swartz (1954) advocated free fascial sutures for the repair of these hernias, but in most instances silk or steel wire will be adequate.

While primary lumbar hernias are the third rarest of the main types of hernia according to Koontz (1955) (the 5 rare hernias being in the order of frequency, beginning with the rarest: sciatic, perineal, lumbar, obturator and internal), incisional lumbar hernias are more common. These usually follow kidney operations. Koontz described an operation used successfully in 5 cases. This involved (1) the freeing of the sac, (2) inversion and plication of the sac with interrupted mattress sutures, (3) reflection of a flap of fascia lata upward to cover the anterior portion of the defect, and (4) reflection forward of a flap of lumbar fascia to cover the posterior portion of the defect.

Mesenteric Defect Hernias. Such hernias go through a rent in the mesentery, most often that of the ileum, and represent the most common intra-abdominal hernia in the childhood period (cf. paraduodenal hernia, which is the second most common hernia of this type).

Morgagni (Foramen of) Hernia. A type of diaphragmatic hernia involving the anterior and parasternal region (space of Larrey). These hernias (which also are called subcostosternal, retrocostoxiphoid, parasternal, or retrosternal) may be congenital or acquired, and a sac is present. At the Boston Children's Hospital, hernias of the foramen of Morgagni constituted 5 per cent of congenital hernias of the diaphragm. In his thorough review of this particular type of hernia, Harrington (1940) stated that they constituted 1.5 per cent (4 cases) of his entire series of diaphragmatic hernias. Helsby and Wells (1954) collected 24 operated cases from the literature. Strangulation is more frequent than with hernias of the esophageal hiatus. The colon is present in the sac in about two thirds of the cases. Lateral roentgen examination may help in the diagnosis of these hernias, as indicated by De Nicola and Vracin (1950). As Denisart (1951) has shown, closure of the neck of the sac followed by fascial closure of the foramen is the essential feature of operative repair. Occasionally, the sac can be peeled out of the mediastinum, but such a traumatic procedure may lead to hematoma or injury to the heart of the pleura. The abdominal approach is preferable. In most cases the operation is simple, and the results are excellent.

Obturator Hernia. Such a hernia is one which passes through the obturator foramen or canal in the os inominatum. Watson collected 442 cases from the literature. In the cases in which the sex was given, females outnumbered males 5 to 1. It is of interest, as Anson, McCormack and Cleveland (1950) pointed out, that in a relatively restricted zone in the abdominopelvic wall, 4 areas of potential herniation occur. The upper 2 are inguinal (indirect and direct), the intermediate is femoral, and the lower is obturator. These follow an almost vertical line approximately 2 in. in height. Because the diagnosis of obturator hernia is difficult, treatment usually is applied only in late or complicated cases. Also, because of the unyielding nature of the internal opening of the canal, the strangulation rate in treated cases is extremely high. The combination in elderly women who have lost weight of generalized abdominal pain and rigidity, together with pain down the inner side of the thigh to the knee (Howship-Romberg sign), pain on movement of the hip and palpation of a mass on rectal examination, is characteristic of a strangulated obturator hernia.

Surgical treatment is advised and can be by several routes:

1. The abdominal route with inversion of the sac. Muraro (1959) reported a successful operation for strangulated obturator hernia in a 73-year-old woman by this approach.

2. The obturator route, using a vertical incision beginning in the femoral region with the thigh flexed and retracting the pectineus muscle outward and the adductor longus inward. After inversion or ligation of the sac, aponeurotic flaps are utilized to close the defect.

3. A combined obturator-abdominal route.

4. An inguinal approach, which is recommended only for the nonstrangulated variety because it does not give enough room to deal with gangrenous bowel.

5. The anterior preperitoneal approach. We have used this in one recent case with good exposure resulting.

The 2 chief features of obturator hernia are that diagnosis is very difficult before the onset of strangulation (and often misleading then), and that operative treatment is technically difficult.

Omphalocele (Umbilical Eventration). Such a congenital defect is a herniation of abdominal viscera into the base of the umbilical cord. The pouch is a thin translucent structure consisting only of peritoneum and amniotic membrane. Unlike its less severe counterpart, umbilical hernia, it has no skin covering. The average omphalocele is 6 to 8 cm. in diameter; the size makes considerable difference as to the prognosis. The underlying fascial opening is usually 4 to 5 cm. in diameter. The small intestine is included in the contents of almost all omphaloceles, although portions of the stomach, the spleen, the pancreas or the urinary bladder may also be included. The transverse colon participates in a third of the cases and the liver in half. Since the membrane is essentially avascular (except that the 3 umbilical vessels traverse its dome), it soon becomes infected, even if not ruptured, and prompt repair is mandatory.

The repair of omphaloceles is considered in Chapter 47, "Pediatric Surgery."

Paraduodenal (Mesentericoparietal) Hernia. Such congenital hernias have their orifices just below the ligament of Treitz. The hernia involves the space behind the mesentery, particularly the mesocolon. The sac may go to the right or the left, behind the ascending or the descending colon, respectively. In the case of left mesentericoparietal hernia, the inferior mesenteric arteries and veins course along the neck of the sac. In the case of right mesentericoparietal hernia, the superior mesenteric vessels do likewise. Hence, the neck of the sac cannot be split in either instance when reducing the hernia.

Perineal Hernia. A perineal hernia is a protrusion of abdominal viscera through the muscles and the fascia of the outlet of the pelvis. Such hernias occur most frequently between the ages of 40 and 60 years. Anterior perineal hernias protrude anterior to the transverse perinei muscles and posterior perineal hernias posterior to the same. Anterior perineal hernias start as a defect in the levator ani, they usually contain bladder, and almost always they are found in women. Posterior perineal hernias start as a defect in the levator ani or in a gap between this muscle and the coccygeus, they usually contain ileum, and, while they may occur in men, they are 5 times as common in women. A third type is complete rectal prolapse (see Chap. 39, "Anorectum." Also see Chap. 48, "Gynecology," regarding enterocele). Unlike obturator hernia, perineal

hernia is usually reducible, and strangulation is infrequent. However, the condition is progressive, and operation, usually by the abdominal route, with sac inversion and ligation, is advised.

Posterolateral Hernia. This is a foramen of Bochdalek hernia.

Reducible Hernia. One in which the sac contents can be put back into the cavity from which they originally protruded.

Richter's Hernia (partial enterocele, lateral pinching of the intestine, sometimes incorrectly called Littré's hernia). Such a hernia is a strangulated hernia in which only a part of the circumference of the intestine is caught in the constricting ring. Since the original report by Richter in 1785, Orr (1950) reported that 126 cases have been described in the literature. The vast majority are femoral in location, with right-sided involvement being more frequent than left. Of all femoral hernias, only 0.7 per cent are of the Richter type. External perforation with fistula formation may result. Butters (1948) reported an incidence of 7 out of 45 *strangulated* femoral hernias (16%) as being of the Richter type. Hagan and Rhoads (1953) observed Richter's hernia in 0.65 per cent of their entire series of groin hernias. Of these 5 were femoral and 2 indirect inguinal hernias. Their figure for the over-all incidence of Richter's hernia agrees quite closely with that of Orr. Richter's hernia is particularly dangerous because intestinal obstruction is incomplete, even though strangulation of the outpouched bowel may be complete. Thus, signs and symptoms are slow in developing. The incidence is at least 5 per cent of strangulated hernias. Treatment is similar to that of other strangulated hernias, except that even greater care than usual must be exercised in preventing escape of the involved segment of bowel into the peritoneal cavity before the extent of necrosis can be assessed. If doubt as to bowel viability exists, the involved segment should be resected. In other respects the repair is similar to that of other femoral (or inguinal) hernias.

Sacrosciatic Hernia. A sciatic hernia.

Sciatic Hernia. A sciatic hernia is one which makes its exit through the greater or the lesser sacrosciatic foramen. Watson stated that it was the rarest of all hernias, and he was able to find only 35 cases reported in the literature. Such hernias involve all ages and both sexes almost equally. The protrusion is usually posterior below the fold of the buttock. While operation can be either by the abdominal or the sciatic approach (occasionally the combined approach is used), the former is preferable with inversion and ligation of the sac.

Sliding Hernia (Hernia-en-glissade). These are inguinal hernias in which a portion of the wall is formed by a viscus that in its normal position is only partly covered by peritoneum (Walton, 1913). Moyer (1955) defines it as "an inguinal hernia containing retroperitoneal bowel." Usually the posterior wall consists of the cecum on the right, or of the sigmoid on the left. Thus, a sliding hernia involves the prolapse of a retroperitoneal or partially retroperitoneal structure (Figs. 39-21 to 39-23). Ryan (1956) divided sliding hernias into 3 types: (1) *intrasaccular*, in which the sliding component is free except for its mesentery, the peritoneum of which is continuous with that of the sac; (2) *parasaccular* (*intramural*), in

which the sliding component lies in the wall of the sac, the peritoneum of the sac being in intimate contact with it so that the two cannot be separated without danger of injury to the sliding organ; and (3) *extrasaccular*, in which the sliding element can be readily separated or may be distinctly separate from the sac, or there may be even no sac at all, the so-called sacless type. There is some doubt that Ryan's first type is a true sliding hernia, but this may be true in certain instances. In his series of 313 consecutive cases of sliding hernia, over 95 per cent were of the second (parasaccular) type, there being only one sacless sliding hernia.

Sliding hernia generally increases in incidence with advancing years. Males are more often affected, and in Ryan's series all 313 cases were in males. The incidence of sliding hernias relative to inguinal hernias is shown in Table 8.

The diagnosis of sliding hernia is difficult (large size, irreducibility, and difficulty in freeing the sac should alert one to be on the

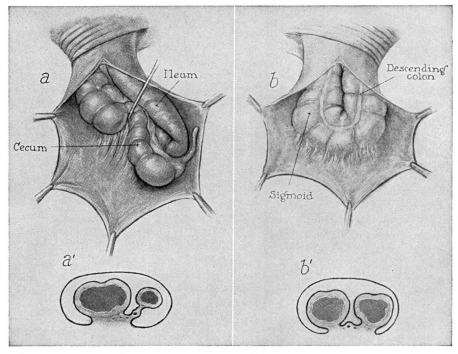

FIG. 39-21. Cross section of sliding hernia of cecum and ascending colon.
FIG. 39-22. Cross section of sliding hernia of descending colon and sigmoid.
(Bevan, A. D.: Ann. Surg. *92*:754)

lookout for this complication) so that Bevan (1930), who had a large experience with the condition, stated that he could not remember making a diagnosis of sliding hernia before operation. A true sliding hernia must be differentiated at operation from a mere adhesion, as is often present when a supposed sliding hernia involves the small bowel. A sliding hernia is usually an indirect inguinal hernia and involves an actual downward prolapse of the viscus (cecum, sigmoid or bladder) with attached mesentery and posterior parietal peritoneum. Preoperative barium enema may show sigmoid (left) or cecum (right) in an irreducible hernia, indicating the probability of sliding.

Repair is more difficult than in a hernia of similar size without true "sliding." By one simple technic (Bevan, 1930) the first step consists of cutting the peritoneum along both sides of the mesenteric attachment. The blood supply of the colon should be carefully preserved. The second step consists of longitudinal suture of the diamond-shaped defect produced (see Fig. 39-24), utilizing essentially the Heineke-Mikulicz principle of transverse closure of a longitudinal defect. With careful attention to the principles of closure of the peritoneal defect, these hernias should not be attended by the high recurrence rate that they apparently have. Since high ligation of all hernial sacs is the first step in repair, and since this is difficult to do without freeing the prolapsed cecum or sigmoid first, this incidence of high recurrence rate is probably due largely to inadequate high sac ligation. Thus, indirect sliding hernias should not be reduced en bloc.

The simple Bevan technic by an inguinal approach outlined above is applicable to smaller sliding hernias, particularly on the

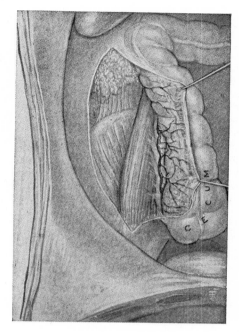

FIG. 39-23. Blood supply of sliding hernias on the right and the left with incisions necessary to mobilize safely the bowel by dividing the outer avascular layer of the mesocolon. (Bevan, A. D.: Ann. Surg. *92*:755)

right side. The Lyter method, also by an inguinal approach, of dealing with larger sliding hernias is as follows:

After opening the sac and determining that a sliding hernia is present, the cecum or mesosigmoid is separated from the vas deferens and the internal spermatic vessels to expose the iliacus (endo-abdominal) fascia covering the iliopsoas muscle. This is done through the already dilated internal ring, sometimes facilitated by a lateralward incision from the ring through the internal oblique and transversus muscles. In very difficult cases a sec-

TABLE 8. INCIDENCE OF SLIDING HERNIA

AUTHOR	PERCENTAGE INCIDENCE	TYPE OF HERNIA CONSIDERED
Zimmerman (1953)	3.0	Indirect inguinal
Ryan (1956)	6.8	Indirect inguinal
Bevan (1930)	1.0	Inguinal
Burton and Blotner (1942)	1.0–2.0	Inguinal
Sensenig and Nichols (1955)	4.9	Inguinal
Ryan (1956)	5.1	Inguinal

FIG. 39-24. Operation for sliding hernia of the large intestine. The intestinal loop and its mesentery have been freed and the sac trimmed along either side of the bowel as high as the neck of the sac. The peritoneal edges of the trimmed sac are being sutured together behind the bowel to form a new mesocolon. (Watson, L. F.: Hernia, ed. 3, St. Louis, Mosby)

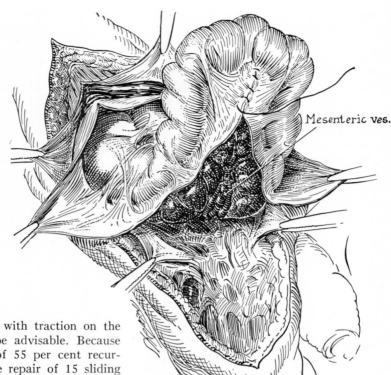

Mesenteric ves.

ond abdominal incision with traction on the prolapsed bowel may be advisable. Because of the high incidence of 55 per cent recurrence rate following the repair of 15 sliding hernias by the inguinal route alone, Hagan and Rhoads (1953) stated that they now managed all such hernias by the combined inguino-abdominal approach. Moyer (1955) also advocated a laparotomy wound in these cases. The hernia then is reduced, and the retroperitoneal aspect of the cecum or mesosigmoid (or sigmoid itself) is carefully sutured to the iliacus fascia. Next, the anteromedial edge of the sac is sutured high to the lateral edge behind the cecum or sigmoid to close the peritoneum. The internal ring, including any lateral extension incision of its margin, is closed, and the inguinal floor is repaired in the usual manner. The abdominal (La Roque) approach is also useful (Williams, 1947). The author of this chapter now advocates a preperitoneal suprapubic approach for repairing the hernia with intraperitoneal handling of the bowel through the opened sac. Sensenig and Nichols (1955) reported only 13 per cent recurrence using the inguinal approach in 53 cases of sliding hernia, and preferred this to the combined approach. Ryan (1956) also preferred the inguinal approach, reporting a 1 per cent recurrence rate.

Sliding direct, even more seldom femoral,

hernias containing the bladder are rare, but they do occur. As mentioned in the section on direct hernias, reduction of a direct hernia en bloc without opening the direct sac is considered preferable in either the simple or the sliding variety.

Spigelian Hernia (Lateral Ventral Hernia, Hernia of the Linea Semilunaris). The fold of Douglas (linea semicircularis Douglasii) is a transverse fold somewhat below the umbilicus. Above, a portion of the internal oblique and all of the transversus abdominis aponeuroses lie deep to the rectus muscle; below, all the aponeuroses lie anterior to the rectus. The transition makes the fold. More laterally, the fold turns downward from its transverse direction near the mid-line, and fibers from it descend as pillars to insert on the pubis. The fold of Douglas has considerable surgical importance aside from the connotation regarding hernia. Above the fold closure of medial abdominal incisions is different from that below the fold, because of the different arrangement of the aponeuroses.

The 2 lineae semilunaris Spigelii (named after the Flemish anatomist Adrian van der Spigelius, 1578-1625) are just lateral to the rectus. Each is vertical, but slightly convex outward, and extends from the cartilage of the 9th rib to the pubic spine. Each represents the transition of the internal oblique and the transversus abdominus muscles laterally to aponeuroses medially (Gould).

The crossing of the transverse fold of Douglas by the linea semilunaris on each side presents a weak point, the inadequacy of which may be compounded by the fact that the inferior deep epigastric vessels in their ascending course turn medially near or at this point to go behind the rectus muscle but superficial to the fold of Douglas. This crossroads of the 2 lines plus the penetration of the vessels is the site of spigelian hernias. Thus, these hernias are lateral to the rectus, medial to the muscular portion of the transversus, and below the fold of Douglas. Pull by the accessory slip of internal oblique (Chouke, 1938) may help to widen the opening.

Diagnosis should be made by palpating the area in question, which usually presents the chief complaints of tenderness and possibly a mass, with the patient supine and with the head off the pillow. In this way the abdominal wall is tense, and visceral tenderness can be excluded. Strangulation is frequent. The condition usually occurs in adults (River, 1942), but Hurwitt and Borow (1955) reported a case in an 8-year-old boy. Treatment involves inversion of the sac, aponeurotic suture and often a patch of tantalum mesh or cutis because of the weak aponeurotic structures in some patients with these hernias. There should be no hesitation about doubly ligating and dividing the deep epigastric vessels so that the hole may be sutured tightly. McVay (1954) stated that fine silk sutures were adequate, and that while the diagnosis was difficult, repair was easy and "there should be no recurrence."

Parenthetically, it should be pointed out that the medial variety of direct hernia represents a type of lateral ventral hernia, even though not spigelian in location.

Strangulated Hernia. One in which there is not only incarceration (syn.: *obstructed hernia*) but also either partial or complete occlusion of the blood supply and lymph drainage. Tardy or incorrect treatment of strangulated hernia is the major cause of death in this type of surgery. (See section on femoral hernia earlier in this chapter.)

Traumatic Hernia of the Diaphragm. Such hernias are a common result of automobile accidents (Schneider, 1956); the tear may be at any point, although usually it is on the dome or posterior part of the left half of the diaphragm (69 out of 71 cases were on the left, Harrington, 1950); associated injuries are common; and repair is difficult because of pleural adhesions (cf. lack of adhesions in foramen of Bochdalek hernia). The condition is a common one and represented 13 per cent of a total of 435 diaphragmatic hernias repaired by Harrington (1950). This high figure is all the more remarkable when it is remembered that the Mayo Clinic does not have a large emergency service. The diagnosis usually is relatively simple. The decision as to time of operation (and operative approach) often depends on the associated injury, but generally it should be as early as possible. The approach preferably is thoracic, especially on the right, thoracoabdominal if the reposition of the viscera is difficult, or possibly abdominal on the left as advocated by Harrington. The repair should be with interrupted nonabsorbable sutures.

BIBLIOGRAPHY

There are several selected classic monographs on hernia which are available to the student of the subject. Watson and Zimmerman and Anson are good reference works, while McVay presents a good brief summary of up-to-date methods in atlas form. The others are of historical interest or cover special aspects of the field. Among the monographs on hernia, the following are listed chronologically:

Richter, A. G.: Abhandlung von den Bruchen, Göttingen, Dieterich, 1785 (cited by Watson).

Marcy, Henry O.: The Anatomy and Surgical Treatment of Hernia, New York, Appleton, 1892.

Ferguson, Alexander H.: The Technic of Modern Operations for Hernia, Chicago, Cleveland Press, 1907.

Iason, Alfred H.: Hernia, Philadelphia, Blakiston, 1941.

Mair, George B.: The Surgery of Abdominal Hernia, Baltimore, Williams & Wilkins, 1948.

Watson, Leigh F.: Hernia: Anatomy, Etiology, Symptoms, Diagnosis, Differential Diagnosis, Prognosis, and Treatment, ed. 3, St. Louis, Mosby, 1948.

Iason, Alfred H.: Synopsis of Hernia, New York, Grune & Stratton, 1949.

Vogeler, Karl: Chirurgie der Hernien, Berlin, de Gruyter, 1951.

Zimmerman, Leo M., and Anson, Barry J.: Anatomy and Surgery of Hernia, Baltimore, Williams & Wilkins, 1953.

McVay, Chester B.: Hernia: The Pathologic Anatomy of the More Common Hernias and Their Anatomic Repair, Springfield, Ill., Thomas, 1954.

Ogilvie, H.: Hernia, Baltimore, Williams & Wilkins, 1959.

Nissen, R., and Rossetti, M.: Die Behandlung von Hiatushernien und Refluxosophagitis mit Gastropexie und Fundoplicatio: Indikation, Technik und Ergebnisse, Stuttgart, Thieme, 1959.

Journal references on the subject of hernia are also numerous. According to Watson, nearly 2 centuries ago, Georges Arnaud, the Parisian surgeon, published his treatise on hernia, and, in his preface, remarked that he planned a work embracing all that had been written on hernia. In the libraries of Paris alone, he transcribed 4,000 pages of writings on hernia before he abandoned his ambitious plan. The following references are selected because they represent classic contributions, in the case of some of the older ones, or are pertinent to present-day thought, in the case of some of the recent ones.

Adler, R. H., and Firme, C. N.: Use of pliable synthetic mesh in the repair of hernias and tissue defects, Surg., Gynec. & Obst. 108:199-206, 1959.

Ali, Munawar: Cutis strip and patch repair of large inguinal hernias, New England J. Med. 251:932-934, 1954.

Allen, J. G.: Personal communication, April 30, 1955.

Allison, P. R.: Reflux esophagitis, sliding hiatal hernia, and the anatomy of repair, Surg., Gynec. & Obst. 92:419-431, 1951.

Amendola, F. H.: An unusual complication of interruption of the left phrenic nerve in the management of esophageal hiatus hernia, Surg., Gynec. & Obst. 100:379-382, 1955.

Andrews, E.: Personal communication, 1933.

Andrews, E., and Bissell, A. D.: Direct hernia: a record of surgical failures, Surg., Gynec. & Obst. 58:753-761, 1934.

Andrews, E. W.: Imbrication or lap joint method: a plastic operation for hernia, Chicago M. Rec.

9:67-77, 1895. Cited by Watson (see reference below), 1948.

Annandale, T.: Case in which a reducible oblique and direct inguinal and femoral hernia existed on the same side, and were successfully treated by operation, Edinburgh M. J. 21:1087-1091, 1876.

Anson, B. J., McCormack, L. J., and Cleveland, H. C.: The anatomy of the hernial regions; III. obturator hernia and general considerations, Surg., Gynec. & Obst. 90:31-38, 1950.

Anson, B. J., Morgan, E. H., and McVay, C. B.: The anatomy of the hernial regions; I. inguinal hernia, Surg., Gynec. & Obst. 89:417-423, 1949.

Babcock, W. W.: The ideal in herniorrhaphy: a new method efficient for direct and indirect inguinal hernia, Surg., Gynec. & Obst. 45:534-540, 1927.

Baritell, A. LaM.: A review of our experience with hernioplastic procedures, Permanente Found. M. Bull. 2:114-120, 1944.

Barrett, N. R.: Chronic peptic ulcer of the oesophagus and "oesophagitis," Brit. J. Surg. 38:175-182, 1950.

Bassini, E. (1888): Cited by Watson (see reference below), 1948.

———: Nuovo metodo operativo per la cura radicale dell'ernia crurale, Padua, Draghi, 1893. Cited by Spivack, J.: The Surgical Technic of Abdominal Operations, Chicago, Debour, 1938.

Beardsley, J. M.: Esophageal hiatus hernia: repair from below, New England J. Med. 254:409-412, 1956.

Berry, W. C., Holbrook, J. P., Langdon, E. A., and Mathewson, C. W.: A study of hiatal hernias using pneumoperitoneum, U. S. Armed Forces M. J. 6:1715-1720, 1955; also A.M.A. Arch. Surg. 72:1014-1017, 1956.

Bevan, Arthur D.: Sliding hernias of the ascending colon and cecum, the descending colon and sigmoid, and of the bladder, Ann. Surg. 92:754-760, 1930.

Birt, A. B.: Some views on femoral hernia and its treatment, Practitioner 159:362-368, 1947.

Blades, B., and Hall, E. R.: The consequences of neglected hiatal hernias, Ann. Surg. 143:822-832, 1956.

Boerema, I.: Fixation of reduced esophageal hiatus hernia by suturing the lesser curvature to the anterior abdominal wall (gastropexia anterior geniculata), Abstr. J.A.M.A. 161:281-282, 1956.

Borgström, S.: Recurrence rates of lateral inguinal hernia in adults, Acta chir. scandinav. 101:429-443, 1951.

Braasch, J. W., and Ellis, F. H., Jr.: The gastroesophageal sphincter mechanism: an experimental study, Surgery 39:901-905, 1956.

Brown, R. K.: Umbilical hernia repair by layer closure of posterior and anterior rectus sheaths, Surg., Gynec. & Obst. *110*:381-382, 1960.

Brown, R. K., and Galletti, G.: Bassini's contribution to our understanding of inguinal hernia, Surgery *47*:631-635, 1960.

Burdick, C. G., and Higinbotham, N. L.: Division of the spermatic cord as an aid in operating on selected types of inguinal hernia, Ann. Surg. *102*:863-874, 1935.

Burton, C. C.: The combined Cooper's ligament and inguinal ligament hernia repair, Surg., Gynec. & Obst. *98*:153-160, 1954.

————: The critical point of Cooper's ligament hernia repair, Am. J. Surg. *91*:215-226, 1956.

————: Hernias of the supravesical, inguinal, and lateral pelvic fossae: their diagnosis, classification, and relationship, Internat. Abstr. Surg. *91*:1-16, 1950.

————: Inguinopectineal hernias—a classification and correlation, Internat. Abstr. Surg. *97*:417-431, 1953.

————: A suggested terminology for ligaments of the groin: their clinical and surgical application in repair of hernias, Surgery *31*:562-574, 1952.

Burton, C. C., and Blotner, C.: Sliding and other large bowel herniae: development, classification and operative management, Ann. Surg. *116*:394-404, 1942.

Butters, A. G.: A review of femoral herniae with special reference to the recurrence rate of the low operation, Brit. M. J. *4581*:743-745, 1948.

Cannaday, J. E.: The use of the cutis graft in the repair of certain types of incisional herniae and other conditions, Ann. Surg. *115*:775-781, 1942.

Carey, J. M., and Hollinshead, W. H.: An anatomic study of the esophageal hiatus, Surg., Gynec. & Obst. *100*:196-200, 1955.

————: Anatomy of the esophageal hiatus related to repair of hiatal hernia, Proc. Staff Meet. Mayo Clin. *30*:223-226, 1955.

Carlson, R. I.: The historical development of the surgical treatment of inguinal hernia, Surgery *39*:1031-1046, 1956.

Carter, B. N., and Giuseffi, J.: Strangulated diaphragmatic hernia, Ann. Surg. *128*:210-225, 1948.

Chassin, J. L.: The subcutaneous inguinal ring: a clinical study, Surgery *22*:540-544, 1947.

Cheatle, Sir G. L.: An operation for the radical cure of inguinal and femoral hernia, Brit. M. J. *2*:68-69, 1920.

Cheatle, G. L.: An operation for inguinal hernia, Brit. M. J. *2*:1025-1026, 1921.

Cherney, L. S.: Intestinal stenosis following strangulated hernia, Ann. Surg. *148*:991-993, 1958.

Chouke, K. S. (1938): Cited by River, L. P. (see reference below), 1942.

Clark, J. H., and Hashimoto, E. I.: Utilization of Henle's ligament, iliopubic tract, aponeurosis transversus abdominis and Cooper's ligament in inguinal herniorrhaphy: a report of 162 consecutive cases, Surg., Gynec. & Obst. *82*:480-484, 1946.

Clatworthy, H. W., Jr., and Thompson, A. G.: Incarcerated and strangulated inguinal hernia in infants: a preventable risk, J.A.M.A. *154*:123-126, 1954.

Clear, J. J.: Ten year statistical study of inguinal hernias, A.M.A. Arch. Surg. *62*:70-78, 1951.

Cole, P. P.: The filigree operation for inguinal hernia, Brit. J. Surg. *29*:168-181, 1941.

Collins, J. D.: A method of disposal of the sac in operations for oblique inguinal hernia, Ann. Surg. *115*:761-767, 1942.

Cooley, D. A.: Discussion of paper by Blades and Hall, Ann. Surg. *143*:830-831, 1956.

Council, A.M.A., Report of: Present status of injection treatment of hernia, J.A.M.A. *115*:533-534, 1940.

DeNicola, R. R., and Vracin, D. J.: Diaphragmatic hernia through the foramen of Morgagni, J. Pediat. *36*:100-104, 1950.

Denisart, P.: De la variété rétro-costo-xiphoïdienne des hernies diaphragmatiques, J. chir. *67*:407-427, 1951.

Dennis, C., and Varco, R. L.: Femoral hernia with gangrenous bowel, Surgery *22*:312-323, 1947.

DeVito, R. V., Listerud, M. B., Nyhus, L. M., Merendino, K. A., and Harkins, H. N.: Hemorrhage as a complication of reflux esophagitis, Am. J. Surg. *98*:657-663, 1959.

Donald, D. C.: The value derived from utilizing the component parts of the transversalis fascia and Cooper's ligament in the repair of large indirect and direct inguinal hernia: a group of cases, Surgery *24*:662-676, 1948.

Doran, F. S. A.: Inguinal herniorrhaphy, Lancet *2*:1307-1314, 1955.

Doran, F. S. A., and Lonsdale, W. H.: A simple experimental method of evaluation for the Bassini and allied types of herniorrhaphy, Brit. J. Surg. *36*:339-345, 1949.

Easton, E. R.: The incidence of femoral hernia following repair of inguinal hernia—ectopic recurrence: a proposed operation of external and internal herniorrhaphy, J.A.M.A. *100*:1741-1744, 1933.

Effler, D. B., and Ballinger, C. S.: Complications and surgical treatment of hiatus hernia and short esophagus, J. Thoracic Surg. *22*:235-247, 1951.

Elman, R.: Editorial: the hernia problem, A.M.A. Arch. Surg. *65*:807-808, 1952.

Enquist, I. F., and Dennis, C.: The management of strangulating external hernias, S. Clin. North America *35*:429-439, 1955.

Erwald, R., and Rieger, A.: Tantalum mesh in hernial repair, Acta chir. scandinav. *119*:55-59, 1960.

Fallis, L. S.: Direct inguinal hernia, Ann. Surg. *107*:572-581, 1938.

———: Recurrent inguinal hernia: an analysis of 200 operations, Ann. Surg. *106*:363-372, 1937.

Ferguson, A. H.: Oblique inguinal hernia: typical operation for its radical cure, J.A.M.A. *33*:6-14, 1899.

Fisher, H. C.: The surgical repair of inguinal hernia in infants and children, Rocky Mountain M. J. *48*:424-426, 1951.

Fitzgerald, P., and Mehigan, J. E.: A complication resulting from the use of a rigid inlay in the repair of an inguinal hernia, Brit. J. Surg. *46*:422, 1959.

Fowler, R., Jr., and Stephens, F. D.: The role of testicular vascular anatomy in the salvage of high undescended testes, Australia & New Zealand J. Surg. *29*:92-106, 1959.

Galletti, G., and Brown, R. K.: Halsted's operation for inguinal hernia. Exactly what is it? Surgery *47*:633-635, 1960.

Gallie, W. E., and Le Mesurier, A. B.: The use of living sutures in operative surgery, Canad. M.A.J. *11*:504-513, 1921.

Gilmore, W. E.: A technical aid in bilateral inguinal herniorrhaphy in infants and children, Surg., Gynec. & Obst. *110*:501-502, 1960.

Ginzburg, L., and Freund, S.: Hernias of supravesical fossa presenting externally through the conjoined tendon, Surg., Gynec. & Obst. *99*:295-300, 1954.

Goni Moreno, I.: XII Congreso Argentino de Cirurgia, pp. 85-87, 1940. Cited by Koontz and Graves (see reference below), 1954.

Graham, E.: Editorial comment: diaphragmatic hernia through esophageal hiatus *in* Year Book of General Surgery, 1954, Chicago, Yr. Bk. Pub., 1954.

Griffith, C. A.: Inguinal hernia: an anatomic-surgical correlation, S. Clin. North America *39*:531-556, 1959.

Gross, R. E.: The Surgery of Infancy and Childhood: Its Principles and Techniques, Philadelphia, Saunders, 1953.

Guy, C. C., Werelius, C. Y., and Bell, L. B., Jr.: Five years' experience with tantalum mesh in hernia repair, S. Clin. North America *35*:175-188, 1955.

Hagan, W. H., and Rhoads, J. E.: Inguinal and femoral hernias, Surg., Gynec. & Obst. *96*:226-232, 1953.

Halsted, W. S.: The cure of the more difficult as well as the simpler inguinal ruptures, Bull. Johns Hopkins Hosp. *14*:208-214, 1903.

———: The radical cure of hernia, Bull. Johns Hopkins Hosp. *1*:12, 1889.

———: The radical cure of inguinal hernia in the male, Bull. Johns Hopkins Hosp. *4*:17-24, 1893.

Harkins, H. N.: A Cooper's ligament herniotomy; clinical experience in 322 consecutive cases, S. Clin. North America *23*:1279-1297, 1943.

———: Cutis grafts: clinical and experimental studies on their use as a reinforcing patch in the repair of large ventral and incisional herniae, Ann. Surg. *122*:996-1015, 1945.

———: Recent advances in the treatment of hernia, Ann. West. Med. & Surg. *6*:221-225, 1952.

———: The repair of groin hernias: progress in the past decade, S. Clin. North America *29*:1457-1482, 1949.

Harkins, H. N., and Schug, R. H.: Hernial repair using Cooper's ligament: follow-up studies on 367 operations, Arch. Surg. *55*:689-708, 1947.

Harkins, H. N., Szilagyi, D. E., Brush, B. E., and Williams, R.: Clinical experiences with the McVay herniotomy, Surgery *12*:364-377, 1942.

Harrington, S. W.: Clinical manifestations and surgical treatment of congenital types of diaphragmatic hernia, Rev. Gastroenterol. *18*:243-256, 1951.

———: Diaphragmatic hernia *in* Cyclopedia of Medicine, Surgery and Specialties, Philadelphia, Davis, 1950.

———: Discussion of paper by Blades and Hall, Ann. Surg. *143*:831-832, 1956.

———: Esophageal hiatal diaphragmatic hernia, Surg., Gynec. & Obst. *100*:277-292, 1955.

———: Subcostosternal diaphragmatic hernias (foramen of Morgagni), Tr. West. S. A., pp. 332-356, 1940.

Heifetz, C. J.: Inguinal hernias: management of these hernias of infancy and childhood, M. Times *81*:238-243, 1953.

Heifetz, C. J., and Goldfarb, A.: Division of the spermatic cord as an aid in the repair of recurrent and other difficult inguinal hernias, J. Internat. Coll. Surgeons *28*:498-512, 1952.

Helsby, R., and Wells, C.: Subcostosternal hernia (hernia through the foramen of Morgagni): report of a case, Brit. J. Surg. *42*:274-275, 1954.

Henry, A. K.: Operation for femoral hernia by a midline extraperitoneal approach: with a preliminary note on the use of this route for reducible inguinal hernia, Lancet *1*:531-533, 1936.

Hey Groves, E. W.: A note on the operation for the radical cure of femoral hernia, Brit. J. Surg. *10*:529-531, 1923.

Hicks, E. S.: Inguinal hernia, Canad. M.A.J. *45*: 134-136, 1941.

Hillemand, P., and Watteblede: Une affection fréquente et trop méconnue: la hernie diaphragmatique de l'hiatus oesophagien, Presse méd. *61*:886, 1953.

Hoguet, J. P.: Direct inguinal hernia, Ann. Surg. *72*:671-674, 1920.

Holcomb, G. W.: Incarcerated inguinal hernia in infants and children: a preventable condition, J. Tennessee M.A. *49*:37, 1956.

Hurwitt, E. S., and Borow, M.: Bilateral spigelian hernias in childhood, Surgery *37*:963-968, 1955.

Kiesewetter, W. B., and Parenzan, L.: When should hernia in the infant be treated bilaterally?, J.A.M.A. *171*:287-290, 1959.

Knott, J. I.: The second side inguinal hernia and routine transpubic exposure, Am. J. Surg. *87*: 97-100, 1954.

Kohli, D. R., and Pearson, C. C.: A study of hiatus hernia, Gastroenterology *23*:294-300, 1953.

Koontz, A. R., Some common fallacies and confusions with regard to repair of inguinal hernia, J.A.M.A. *141*:366-369, 1949.

————: Failure with tantalum gauze in ventral hernia repair, A.M.A. Arch. Surg. *70*:123-127, 1955.

————: The inguinal hernia problem, Mil. Surgeon *115*:93-100, 1954.

————: An operation for massive incisional lumbar hernia, Surg., Gynec. & Obst. *101*:119-121, 1955.

————: Preliminary report on the use of tantalum mesh in the repair of ventral hernias, Ann. Surg. *127*:1079-1085, 1948.

————: Views on the choice of operation for inguinal hernia repair, Ann. Surg. *143*:868-880, 1956.

Koontz, A. R., and Graves, J. W.: Preoperative pneumoperitoneum as an aid in the handling of gigantic hernias, Ann. Surg. *140*:759-762, 1954.

Koontz, A. R., and Kimberly, R. C.: Tissue reactions to tantalum mesh and wire, Ann. Surg. *131*:666-686, 1950.

Koontz, A. R., and Stafford, E. S.: Unusual types of interparietal hernia, A.M.A. Arch. Surg. *71*: 723-726, 1955.

Lam, C. R.: Personal communication, November 16, 1954.

Lam, C. R., and Kenney, L. J.: The problem of the hiatus hernia of the diaphragm, J. Thoracic Surg. *27*:1-12, 1954.

Lam, C. R., Szilagyi, D. E., and Puppendahl, M.: Tantalum gauze in the repair of large postoperative ventral hernias, Arch. Surg. *57*:234-244, 1948.

La Roque, G. P.: The intra-abdominal operation for femoral hernia, Ann. Surg. *75*:110-112, 1922.

————: The permanent cure of inguinal and femoral hernia: a modification of the standard operative procedures, Surg., Gynec. & Obst. *29*:507-510, 1919.

Larsen, R. M.: Inguinal hernia in infancy and early childhood, Surgery *25*:307-328, 1949.

Laugier, M. (1833): Cited by Priesching (1956).

Lawrence, K. B.: Fatal intestinal obstruction following injection treatment of an inguinal hernia, New England J. Med. *238*:397-398, 1948.

Lendrum, F. C.: Anatomic features of the cardiac orifice of the stomach, with special reference to cardiospasm, Arch. Int. Med. *59*:474-511, 1937.

Levy, A. H., Wren, R. S., and Friedman, M. N.: Complications and recurrences following inguinal hernia repair, Ann. Surg. *133*:533-539, 1951.

Listerud, M. B., and Harkins, H. N.: Anatomy of the esophageal hiatus, A.M.A. Arch. Surg. *76*: 835-842, 1958.

————: Variations in the muscular anatomy of the esophageal hiatus: based on dissections of two hundred and four fresh cadavers, West. J. Surg. *67*:110-113, 1959.

Littré (1700): Cited by Watson (see reference below), 1948.

Loewe, O.: Über Hautimplantation an Stelle der Freien Faszienplastik, München. med. Wchnschr. *60*:1320-1321, 1913.

Lotheissen, G.: Zur Radikaloperation der Schenkelhernien, Zentralbl. Chir. *25*:548-550, 1898.

Low, A.: A note on the crura of the diaphragm and the muscle of Treitz, J. Anat. & Physiol. *42*:93-96, 1907.

Lower, W. E., and Hicken, N. F.: Interparietal hernias, Ann. Surg. *94*:1070-1087, 1931.

Lucas-Championnière, J. (1892): Cited by Koontz (see reference above), 1949.

Lyter, C. S.: Cited by Griffith (see reference above), 1957.

McArthur, L. L.: Autoplastic suture in hernia and other diseases; preliminary report, J.A.M.A. *37*:1162-1165, 1901.

McClure, R. D., and Fallis, L. S.: Femoral hernia; report of 90 operations, Ann. Surg. *109*: 987-1000, 1939.

McEvedy, P. G.: Femoral hernia, Ann. Roy. Coll. Surgeons England *7*:484-496, 1950.

MacGregor, W. W.: The demonstration of a true internal sphincter and its etiologic role in hernia, Surg., Gynec. & Obst. *49*:510-515, 1929.

————:The fundamental operative treatment of

inguinal hernia, Surg., Gynec. & Obst. *50*:438-440, 1930.

————: Observations on the surgical treatment of hernia, Ann. Surg. *122*:878-884, 1945.

————: Surgical repair of inguinal hernia based upon closure of internal inguinal sphincter, Grace Hosp. Bull. *117*:125, 1949.

MacKenzie, W. C.: Why do inguinal hernias recur?, Paper given before the Annual Meeting, Washington State Medical Association, Seattle, Sept. 13, 1955.

McLaughlin, C. W., Jr., and Coe, J. D.: Inguinal hernia in pediatric patients, Am. J. Surg. *99*:45-47, 1960.

McVay, C. B.: An anatomic error in current methods of inguinal herniorrhaphy, Ann. Surg. *113*:1111-1112, 1941.

————: Inguinal and femoral hernioplasty, Minnesota Med. *32*:599-607, 1949.

————: Personal communication, February 21, 1947.

McVay, C. B., and Anson, B. J.: A fundamental error in current methods of inguinal herniorrhaphy, Surg., Gynec. & Obst. *74*:746-750, 1942.

————: Inguinal and femoral hernioplasty, Surg., Gynec. & Obst. *88*:473-485, 1949.

Madden, J. L.: Anatomic and technical considerations in the treatment of esophageal hiatal hernia, Surg., Gynec. & Obst. *102*:187-194, 1956.

Mair, G. B.: The Surgery of Abdominal Hernia, London, Arnold, 1948.

————: The use of whole skin grafts as a substitute for fascial sutures in the treatment of hernias: preliminary report, Am. J. Surg. *69*:352-365, 1945.

Marshall, S. B.: Indirect inguinal hernia and the internal ring, U.S. Armed Forces M. J. *11*:191-198, 1960.

Mason, E. A.: Pneumoperitoneum in the management of giant hernia, Surgery *39*:143-151, 1956.

Merendino, K. A., Johnson, R. J., Skinner, H. H., and Maguire, R. X.: The intradiaphragmatic distribution of the phrenic nerve with particular reference to the placement of diaphragmatic incisions and controlled segmental paralysis, Surgery *39*:189-198, 1956.

Merendino, K. A., Varco, R. L., and Wangensteen, O. H.: Displacement of the esophagus into a new diaphragmatic orifice in the repair of para-esophageal and esophageal hiatus hernia, Ann. Surg. *129*:185-197, 1949.

Mikkelsen, W. P., and Berne, C. J.: Femoral hernioplasty: suprapubic extraperitoneal (Cheatle-Henry) approach, Surgery *35*:743-748, 1954.

Moloney, G. E., Gill, W. G., and Barclay, R. C.: Operations for hernia: technique of nylon darn, Lancet *2*:45-48, 1948.

Monro, A. K.: Strangulated femoral hernia *in* Maingot, Rodney: Techniques in British Surgery, Philadelphia, Saunders, 1950.

————: The treatment of inguinal hernia *in* Maingot, Rodney: Techniques in British Surgery, Philadelphia, Saunders, 1950.

Morris, K. N.: Gastric mucosa within the oesophagus, Australian & New Zealand J. Surg. *25*:24-30, 1955.

Moschcowitz, A. V.: Femoral hernia: a new operation for the radical cure, New York State J. Med. *7*:396-400, 1907.

Moyer, C.: Personal communication, January 23, 1955.

Moyer, C. A.: Personal communication, July 13, 1960.

Muller, C. J. B.: Hiatus hernia, diverticula and gall stones: Saint's triad, South African M.J. *22*:376-382, 1948.

Muraro, U.: Strangulated obturator hernia, Riforma med. *73*:332-336, 1959; Abstr. J.A.M.A. *170*:1852, 1959.

Nauta, J.: Een studie van het afsluitingsmechanisme tussen slokdarm en maag, Leiden, H. E. Stenfert Kroese N. V., 1955.

————: Movements of the lower oesophageal segment: the cardiac mechanism, Bull. Soc. Internat. de Chir. *15*:97-110, 1956.

Nelson, T. Y.: Hiatus hernia in infants and children, Australian & New Zealand J. Surg. *22*:192-197, 1953.

Neuman, H. W., Ellis, F. H., Jr., and Andersen, H. A.: Eventration of the diaphragm, Proc. Staff Meet. Mayo Clin. *30*:310-318, 1955.

Nissen, R.: Die Gastropexie als alleiniger Eingriff bei Hiatushernien, Deutsche med. Wchnschr. *81*:185, 1956.

Nyhus, L. M., Condon, R. E., and Harkins, H. N.: Clinical experiences with the preperitoneal hernia repair for all types of groin hernia: with particular reference to the importance of transversalis fascia analogues, Am. J. Surg. *100*:234-244, 1960.

O'Connor, F. J., and Ritvo, M.: Diagnosis of hiatus hernia on plain roentgenograms of thorax and abdomen, J.A.M.A. *157*:113-117, 1955.

Ogilvie, W. H.: Hernia *in* Maingot, R.: Postgraduate Surgery, vol. 3, p. 3637, New York, Appleton, 1937.

Olson, H. H., Kanar, E. A., and Harkins, H. N.: The use of wire markers in Cooper's ligament hernia repairs with roentgenologic studies; report of 72 hernioplasties, Surgery *36*:270-277, 1954.

Orr, T. G., Jr.: Richter's hernia, Surg., Gynec. & Obst. *91*:705-708, 1950.

Owen, H. W., Kirklin, J. W., and DuShane, J. W.: Femoral hernias in infants and young children, Surgery 36:283-285, 1954.

Packard, G. B., and McLauthlin, C. H.: Treatment of inguinal hernia in infancy and childhood, Surg., Gynec. & Obst. 97:603-607, 1953.

Palmer, E. D.: Saint's triad: hiatus hernia, diverticulosis coli and gall stones, Am. J. Digest. Dis. 18:240-241, 1951.

Palumbo, L. T., and Mighell, S. J.: Primary direct inguinal hernioplasty, Surgery 36:278-282, 1954.

Phetteplace, C. H.: The intra-abdominal (La Roque) approach to hernioplasty, West. J. Surg. 63:490-496, 1955.

Pitkänen, A.: The relation of incisional and inguinal herniae as well as of mechanical intestinal disturbances to previous operations for appendicitis with peritonitis, Acta chir. scandinav. (Supp. 138) 96:1-166, 1948.

Ponka, J. L., Wylie, J. H., Chaikof, L., Sergeant, C., and Brush, B. E.: Marlex mesh—a new plastic mesh for the repair of hernia, Henry Ford Hosp. M. Bull. 7:278-280, 1959.

Potts, W. J., Riker, W. L., and Lewis, J. E.: The treatment of inguinal hernia in infants and children, Ann. Surg. 132:566-576, 1950.

Priesching, A.: Laugerische Hernia, Arch. klin. Chir. 281:411-419, 1956.

Querna, M. H.: Reduction of hernia en masse: a cause of intestinal obstruction, Paper presented before Annual Meeting, North Pacific Surgical Association, Portland, Ore., Nov. 18, 1955.

Rienhoff, W. F.: The use of the rectus fascia for closure of the lower or critical angle of the wound in the repair of inguinal hernia, Surgery 8:326-339, 1940.

Ritchey, J. O., and Winsauer, H. J.: Anemia and its relation to diaphragmatic hernia, Am. J. M. Sc. 214:476-482, 1947.

River, L. P.: Spigelian hernia: spontaneous lateral ventral hernia through the semilunar line, Ann. Surg. 116:405-411, 1942.

Rogers, F. A.: Strangulated femoral hernia: a review of 170 cases, Ann. Surg. 149:9-20, 1959.

Rothenburg, R. E., and Barnett, T.: Bilateral herniotomy in infants and children, Surgery 37:947-950, 1955.

Ruggi, G. (1892): Cited by Koontz, A. R. (1956).

Ryan, E. A.: An analysis of 313 consecutive cases of indirect sliding inguinal hernias, Surg., Gynec. & Obst. 102:45-58, 1956.

————: Recurrent hernias: an analysis of 369 consecutive cases of recurrent inguinal and femoral hernias, Surg., Gynec. & Obst. 96:343-354, 1953.

Satinsky, V. P., and Kron, S. D.: Transposition

of cartilage for repair of large ventral hernia, J. Albert Einstein M. Center 1:109-113, 1953.

Schneider, C. F.: Traumatic diaphragmatic hernia, Am. J. Surg. 91:290-297, 1956.

Schofield, T. L.: Polyvinyl alcohol sponge: an inert plastic for use as a prosthesis in the repair of large hernias, Brit. J. Surg. 42:618-621, 1955.

Sensenig, D. M., and Nichols, J. B.: Sliding hernias: a follow-up study, A.M.A. Arch. Surg. 71:756-760, 1955.

Smith, G. A., Moore, J. R., and Perry, J. F., Jr.: Intestinal obstructions due to external hernia, A.M.A. Arch. Surg. 71:260-264, 1955.

Smith, I.: Irreducible inguinal herniae in children: gangrenous bowel in a 25-day-old infant, Brit. J. Surg. 42:271-274, 1954.

Smith, R. S.: The uses of tantalum mesh in hernia repair, West. J. Surg. 62:1-6, 1954.

————: Adjuncts in hernial repair, A.M.A. Arch. Surg. 78:868-877, 1959.

Snyder, W. H., Jr., and Chaffin, L.: Inguinal hernia complicated by undescended testis, Am. J. Surg. 90:325-330, 1955.

Stensrud, N.: Hiatus hernias, Acta chir. scandinav. 107:57-71, 1954.

Strahan, A. W. B.: Hernial repair by whole-skin graft with report on 413 cases, Brit. J. Surg. 38:276-284, 1951.

Swartz, W. T.: Lumbar hernias, J. Kentucky M. A. 52:673-678, 1954.

Sweet, R. H.: Esophageal hiatus hernia of the diaphragm: the anatomical characteristics, technic of repair, and results of treatment in 111 consecutive cases, Ann. Surg. 135:1-13, 1952.

Swenson, S. A., Jr.: Cutis grafts: clinical and experimental observations, Arch. Surg. 61:881-889, 1950.

Swenson, S. A., Jr., and Harkins, H. N.: Cutis grafts; application of the dermatome-flap method: its use in a case of recurrent incisional hernia, Arch. Surg. 47:564-570, 1943.

————: The surgical treatment of recurrent inguinal hernia with special reference to a Cooper's ligament herniotomy and the use of free fascial grafts, Surgery 14:807-818, 1943.

Tanner, N.: Personal communication, July, 1955.

————: A "slide" operation for inguinal and femoral hernia, Brit. J. Surg. 29:285-289, 1942.

————: Treatment of oesophageal hiatus hernia, Lancet 2:1050-1055, 1955.

Throckmorton, T. D.: Tantalum gauze in the repair of hernias complicated by tissue deficiency: a preliminary report, Surgery 23:32-46, 1948.

Touroff, A. S. W.: Phrenicectomy as aid to repair of large abdominal hernias, J.A.M.A. 154:330-332, 1954.

Turner, D. P. B.: Prevascular femoral hernia, Brit. J. Surg. *41*:77-78, 1953.

Usher, F. C.: A new plastic prosthesis for repairing tissue defects of the chest and abdominal wall, Am. J. Surg. *97*:629-633, 1959.

Usher, F. C., Fries, J. G., Ochsner, J. L., and Tuttle, L. L. D., Jr.: Marlex mesh, a new plastic mesh for replacing tissue defects. II. Clinical studies, A.M.A. Arch. Surg. *78*:138-145, 1959.

Usher, F. C., and Gannon, J. P.: Marlex mesh, a new plastic mesh for replacing tissue defects. I. Experimental studies, A.M.A. Arch. Surg. *78*:131-137, 1959.

Usher, F. C., Ochsner, J., and Tuttle, L. L. D., Jr.: Use of Marlex mesh in the repair of incisional hernias, Am. Surgeon *24*:969-974, 1958.

Walton, A. J.: Extrasaccular hernia, Ann. Surg. *57*:86-105, 1913.

Wangensteen, O. H.: Discussion of paper by McVay (see reference above), 1949.

Watson, L. F.: Hernia: Anatomy, Etiology, Symptoms, Diagnosis, Differential Diagnosis, Prognosis, and Treatment, ed. 3, St. Louis, Mosby, 1948.

Waugh, R. L., and Hausfeld, K. F.: Femoral hernia; a simple operation with report of cases, Am. J. Surg. *58*:73-78, 1942.

West, W. T., and Hicks, E. S.: Skin as a supporting graft in repair of herniae, Canad. M.A.J. *58*:178-180, 1948.

Williams, C.: Repair of sliding inguinal hernia through the abdominal (LaRoque) approach, Ann. Surg. *126*:612-623, 1947.

Williams, C., Jr.: Inguinal hernia in infants and children, Virginia M. Month. *86*:314-318, 1959.

Wilson, H.: Personal communication, January 28, 1948.

Zavaleta, D. E., and Uriburu, J. V., Jr.: Whole thickness skin grafts in the treatment of hernias; analysis of 211 cases, Surg., Gynec. & Obst. *91*:157-172, 1950.

Zawacki, S., and Thieme, E. T.: Study of the types of recurrence following inguinal herniorrhaphy, A.M.A. Arch. Surg. *63*:505-510, 1951.

Zieman, S. A.: The diagnosis of hernia, J.A.M.A. *115*:1873-1874, 1940.

Ziffren, S. E., and Womack, N. A.: An operative approach to the treatment of gigantic hernias, Surg., Gynec. & Obst. *91*:709-710, 1950.

CHAPTER 40

Peripheral Vascular Surgery

Arterial Surgery

INTRODUCTION

Much of the groundwork for the development of vascular surgery was laid when Alexis Carrel developed a simple direct method of vascular suture in 1905.[15] Surgery of the arteries, up until that time, had been confined largely to the treatment of aneurysms which had progressed from the ligation technics of Antyllus and Hunter to the endo-aneurysmorrhaphy of Matas. Interest was directed even earlier to the repair of arterial injuries by suture, and a few blood vessel grafts were used in this period successfully to restore circulation in trauma and disease. Carrel also suggested and demonstrated that vessels could be preserved by refrigeration for use as transplants.

It is remarkable that widespread application of these principles waited for 30 years. Perhaps the best reasons for the great recent impetus to the field lie in the availability of the anticoagulant, heparin, and the development of roentgen technics for arterial visualization. It was necessary for vascular surgeons of the pre-anticoagulant days to use liquid petrolatum to discourage thrombosis at every stage of surgery. Their sutures, grafts and the vessel ends under operative attack were all coated with it. As a result it is evident from their descriptions of technic that every needle hole was a site of potential bleeding, and the whole field must have been impeded seriously by this material. Roentgenograms have provided much of the information that many vascular lesions, even in diffuse arteriosclerosis, are localized and because of the more nearly normal character of the adjacent vessel, susceptible to direct repair.

Should we wish to characterize the present direction of vascular surgery, it would be to say that we are in a period of extension of the use of various types of grafts to restore circulation in the presence of obstructed arterial channels, and of surgical technics for removing the diseased inner layers of arteries to permit return of blood flow through the channel itself (thromboendarterectomy).

Fundamental knowledge of arterial pathology from the standpoint of pathogenesis of disease and etiology has had little recent impetus. Study of arterial disease from the time it chiefly concerned the anatomy and the structure of aneurysms has consisted of a gradual accumulation of data and impressions concerning arteriosclerosis, punctuated by the descriptions by Raynaud and Buerger of the conditions bearing their names. Almost everything remains to be discovered. The chemical changes which cause arteriosclerosis, the etiologies of the entities which constitute Buerger's disease, the very existence of which has been questioned by some, and the meanings of the slightly different arteridides—

periarteritis and panarteritis—are outstanding challenges.

ACUTE ARTERIAL OCCLUSION

Other than by external violence or compression, an arterial channel may become acutely occluded through 2 mechanisms—arterial embolism and arterial thrombosis. An *embolus* is a plug which has traveled through the artery to become lodged at the point at which the vessel size becomes too small to pass it. The composition of the embolus may be a mass of bacteria, a foreign body, or a thrombus which has become detached from its site of origin. Lodgment of a bacterial mass as an arterial embolus produces a very special kind of condition and is known as a *mycotic embolus*. A foreign-body embolus is, as one might suppose, a rarity. Usually it has been a bullet or other small missile, although the extremely rare tumor embolus arising in a lung tumor or a cardiac tumor might be added. A detached clot or portion of clot is the common type of arterial embolus and of particular interest.

Primary *thrombosis* of an otherwise normal artery is rare. Severe debilitating disease, such as intractable diarrhea of ulcerative colitis, has been known to lead to this complication. The increased tendency to intravascular thrombosis which accompanies polycythemia vera more frequently produces venous thrombosis but may affect an artery. The polycythemia of cyanotic congenital heart disease carries the same hazard. The more common mechanism of arterial thrombosis is an underlying arterial disease, arteriosclerosis.

Severe dehydration and periods of hypotension following surgery are factors which increase the danger of arterial thrombosis in patients with or without arteriosclerosis.

ARTERIAL EMBOLISM

Etiology. Most arterial emboli arise from thrombi which develop within the heart chambers. Two cardiac conditions are outstandingly responsible for the initial origin of the intracardiac clot. The *arrhythmia of auricular fibrillation* produces a significant degree of stasis within the 2 atria because of the failure of the chambers to empty themselves forcefully while in the abnormal rhythm. Stasis allows

for the formation and the growth of a blood clot (Fig. 40-1 A) and, although the thrombus certainly is attached to the endothelium or to trabeculae within the chamber, there is increasing likelihood of a portion being dislodged by the blood stream as it grows. Pulmonary artery emboli result when the thrombus detaches from the right atrium and peripheral arterial emboli arise when the initial thrombus is within the left side of the heart. The condition underlying the auricular fibrillation may be arteriosclerotic heart disease, hyperthyroidism, or rheumatic heart disease. If the element of mitral stenosis is added to the fibrillation in a rheumatic heart the incidence of peripheral emboli is multiplied because the stasis is increased by the stenosis. One of the common complications of long-standing mitral stenosis is peripheral or cerebral arterial embolism.

The second common cardiac condition likely to produce peripheral embolism is *myocardial infarction secondary to coronary artery occlusion*. The mechanism of development of the intracardiac thrombus in this condition is the presence of a subendocardial necrotic patch of myocardium. A thrombus, called a *mural* thrombus because of its location against the wall, develops over this area. Not all such thrombi detach to form emboli. Many undoubtedly remain securely attached and take part in the healing of the infarct. Detachment when it happens is likely to take place on the 5th to the 12th day after the original infarct (Fig. 40-1A).

In addition to their development in these two conditions, *intracardiac thrombi* may be laid down without demonstrable reason. The source of emboli has been demonstrated within the ventricle of hearts not otherwise abnormal in patients dying of the embolism. The absence of a cardiac lesion of the usual type does not rule out the heart as the source in cases of acute arterial occlusion due to embolus.

An extracardiac source of emboli to the extremities exists in patients with *advanced arteriosclerosis of the aorta*. The roughening and even ulceration which develops in the intimal lining of the diseased vessel results in the appearance of thrombi on its wall which may break loose and become emboli. (Fig. 40-1.)

When a clot detaches from any of these

sites it travels in the arterial blood stream, its final lodgment determined by chance and by its size. It may enter the carotid and cerebral circulation to lodge in the brain, enter the subclavian system and enter an arm, or proceed down the aorta to lodge in the aortic bifurcation or continue into one of the lower extremities. In either the arm or the leg it most often stops at a major bifurcation. The reason for this seems quite clearly to be that arterial caliber remains almost constant between origins of major branches to the main channel. The common sites of embolism in the upper extremity are the innominate bifurca-tion on the right and the circumflex scapular branch of either axillary artery, the profunda brachii branch of the brachial artery, and the brachial bifurcation at the elbow. In the lower extremity the common sites of lodgment are the aortic and the iliac artery bifurcations, the origin of the profunda femoris branch of the femoral and the bifurcation of the popliteal artery.

The forceful nature of lodgment of an embolus is evidenced by the expansion of the artery at the point of occlusion and the obser-vation that the clot extrudes under pressure when an incision is made over it during surgi-

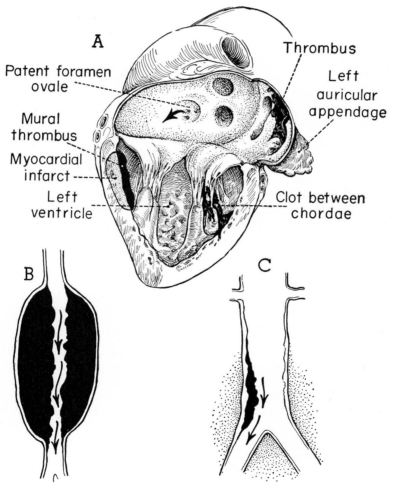

FIG. 40-1. Common sources of peripheral arterial emboli: (A) Com-posite showing sources of emboli within the heart. (B) Aneurysm with mural thrombus as source of emboli. (C) Arteriosclerotic plaques with thrombus formation.

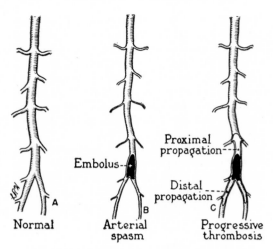

Proximal
propagation
Embolus
Distal
propagation

A
B
C
Normal   Arterial   Progressive
         spasm   thrombosis

FIG. 40-2. Mechanisms of intensification of arterial obstruction secondary to peripheral arterial embolus: (*left*) diagrammatic representation of caliber of an arterial bifurcation and the potential collateral branches; (*center*) reflex arterial spasm has constricted the collateral branches in response to lodgment of embolus; (*right*) because of stasis and the presence of a clot surface, the occluding embolus grows.

cal removal. This impact and expansion sets up a strong source of vasoconstrictor reflexes. These arise at the point of stimulus and are carried up through the sympathetic nervous system supplying the region and return to a large area of the adjacent arterial tree.

This reflex vasoconstriction multiplies the occlusive effect of the embolism, which now becomes not only a matter of mechanical block but also one of vascular constriction serving to diminish sharply the effectiveness of the collateral arterial channels which should be used to bypass the obstruction (Fig. 40-2).

Symptoms. The symptoms of an acute arterial occlusion consist of pain and loss of function. Pain is most often severe, acute and continuous. It is of a sharp constricting type. A most surprising fact is that pain may be slight or entirely absent in a considerable proportion of patients with major arterial embolism. Freedom from pain may result from a particularly severe ischemia of the peripheral nerves which renders them functionless rather acutely. Loss of function is both motor and sensory. The patient observes that he is unable to move the toes or the fingers within a

few minutes of the onset. The sensory element is interpreted as numbness by the patient and is independent of the presence or the absence of pain. Paralysis and loss of sensation are never absent in a major embolism.

Signs. The signs observed in a patient who has suffered an embolism of a major vessel of an extremity fairly soon are those of the loss of motor and sensory function. Paralysis of the small muscles of the foot or the hand is observed and, if the embolism is high enough, there will be paralysis of the muscles of the calf or the forearm. Paralysis of the thigh muscles or those of the arm is rarely observed, even with the highest acute occlusion. The loss of cutaneous sensation to touch and to pain by application of pinprick can be determined and mapped out on the extremity. The upper limit of the sensory loss is determined by the level of occlusion and the degree of reflex arterial spasm. It rarely extends above the knee and the elbow in embolism. The skin color depends on the blood present within the skin capillaries which very soon loses its oxygen and very naturally diminishes in amount. Therefore, the color changes of pallor and cyanosis are present from the distal end of the part upward for a variable distance. The appearance becomes progressively more waxy white during the early period of occlusion. The skin temperature falls rapidly after the occlusion. The extent of the zone of coldness roughly corresponds to the zone of color change.

The final characteristic signs of acute occlusion concern the changes in the pulses of the extremity as determined by palpation and by the use of the *oscillometer*. Pulses cannot be palpated at their normal locations distal to the obstruction. Immediately proximal to the embolism the arterial pulse may be slightly exaggerated in comparison with the other side because of the greater lateral pressure exerted as the blood meets the block and is thrown into eddies and cross currents. This observation is made most clearly on palpation of the common femoral artery when an embolus has lodged at the femoral bifurcation. A second kind of pulse disturbance is met with when the site of occlusion is just above a level at which pulses are normally most easily felt, such as over the common femoral artery in the groin. In this instance a weak pulse may be felt which is transmitted through the tightly lodged embolus. Finally, the pulse may be absent above the site of embolism simply because of intense arterial spasm. The oscillometer finds one of its most valuable applications in the accurate localization of the level of acute embolism. This instrument consists of a pneumatic cuff attached to an aneroid system which reacts freely and with minimum lag as the pressure changes within the cuff. When the cuff is wrapped and inflated smoothly about the extremity the aneroid needle reflects the changes in volume and therefore pressure within the cuff and the tissues included. Repeated applications of the cuff at descending points on the limb detect a level at which the swings of the needle show a marked drop. The embolus is almost always found to have lodged at the major arterial branch or bifurcation proximal to this point of change. With infrequent exceptions the lodgment will be at one of the points of common selection mentioned above.

Course. The course following the embolic occlusion is widely variable. Its severity depends on the intensity and the duration of the reflex arterial spasm, the extent of development of progressive thrombosis of the arterial lumen above and below the embolus, and upon the site of the occlusion. If spasm is unremitting and the development of progressive thrombosis rapid and extensive, the extremity will remain severely ischemic and become moribund in 8 to 10 hours. In other instances the extremity may begin to show return of motor function and sensation within a few minutes or hours of the embolism and recover without loss of tissue.

Treatment of embolism is directed to removal of the obstruction by surgery whenever possible. In the immediate stage, therapy attempts to overcome the two damaging complications: spasm and progressive thrombosis. The arterial constriction may be largely relieved by injecting with procaine the sympathetic ganglia supplying the region. In the upper extremity the 2nd and the 3rd dorsal sympathetic ganglia may be anesthetized with procaine or the stellate ganglion so treated with about equal results. In the lower extremity the 2nd and the 3rd lumbar ganglia are infiltrated.

The tendency for the intra-luminal clot to extend is combated best by the administration of heparin. As is discussed elsewhere, heparin may be given intravenously or by hypodermic injection. In arterial embolism it is given intravenously in order to obtain a rapid drop in the coagulability of the blood. This route also has the added advantage of producing an effect of short duration. If operation is done on the patient to remove the obstructing embolus, the administration of heparin into the artery at the time of surgery will not be complicated by anticoagulant remaining from an earlier dose.

These 2 steps in treatment—the administration of heparin and the blocking by procaine injection of the paravertebral ganglia —are both of real benefit and are often employed together in the same case. When both are to be used the sympathetic block must be done first, because if a needle is introduced into the loose tissue of the paravertebral region a segmental branch of the aorta or the vena cava may be perforated. Ordinarily, this is inconsequential, but in the presence of effective anticoagulant therapy a serious hemorrhage into the space may result.

SURGICAL. The final step in the treatment of an arterial embolus is its surgical removal.[33, 70, 113] In embolism of small arteries the anticoagulant and antispasmodic treatment may be sufficient to prevent any loss of tissue or troublesome symptoms after the patient is well. In larger vessels such nonsurgical treatment may succeed in preserving tissue, but the patients later suffer from symptoms of chronic arterial insufficiency. This must be prevented by doing an embolectomy whenever possible. Operation is to be undertaken as an emergency allowing as little lapse of time as possible. No all-inclusive rule can be made as to the maximum permissible delay of operation. The actual limiting factor is the viability of the part. An early sign of nonviability is development of rigidity of the muscles of the leg or the forearm. Thrombosis in superficial veins and liquefaction of subcutaneous fat also indicate nonviability. Embolectomy should be done within 8 hours of the accident, but successful long-delayed operations have been reported.[96] These have been in patients who recovered early from the vasospasm and did not develop progressive thrombosis.

This operation is performed under local

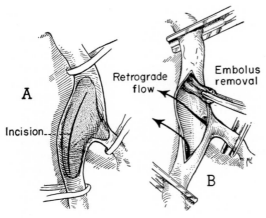

FIG. 40-3. General steps in embolectomy. (A) Control tapes are placed above and below the site of lodgment, and the incision is made directly over the embolus and slightly below its superior limits. (B) Distal aspiration is done first, and retrograde flow is assayed. Then the embolus is removed by forceps or aspiration. Distal embolectomy or retrograde flushing is done if necessary.

anesthesia in most parts of the arterial system. The aortic bifurcation is an exception, as it cannot very well be exposed surgically and operated on while the patient is awake. The anesthesia is a most important consideration, because patients suffering an embolus are frequently ill of cardiac disease and are sometimes bad risks for surgery. However, the surgical indication is greatest of all in cases of aortic bifurcation embolism, because the mortality from this accident is very high, probably 90 per cent, if the embolus is not removed. The operation virtually becomes life-saving and should be tried.

An aortic bifurcation embolus may also be approached by introduction of suction tubes through the femoral arteries from below. In this approach the patient may be spared a general anesthetic, whereas if aspiration fails the patient may be put to sleep and the embolectomy done through an abdominal incision.[116]

In any location the procedure for removing the embolus after the artery has been exposed is relatively simple and follows a definite sequence (Fig. 40-3). The exposure must be adequate for the surgeon to work comfortably on the obstructed vessel. First, the artery is exposed above the embolus, and a tape or heavy ligature is passed about it so that it may be lifted up and clamped with a suitable atraumatic arterial instrument. The same control is accomplished below the point of occlusion. Then the artery is opened over the embolus by a longitudinal incision. Clot is first aspirated from the distal part of the artery, and the clamp is applied distally when good retrograde bleeding appears. Next, the vessel is cleared proximally. Aspiration of the embolus from the vessel is usually unnecessary. The clamp above the incision is placed when good pulsatile flow has been obtained. Care should be taken during this maneuver that the blood loss is controlled and minimized, particularly when a suction tube is used, producing rapid and perhaps unrecognized loss. With the atraumatic clamps in place the vessel wall is repaired by suturing it in an over-and-over fashion with fine silk. As the artery is being closed or immediately after the distal lumen has been cleared, heparin solution should be injected peripherally into the lumen. Since very little blood flow is present, only 5 to 10 mg. in 10 cc. of saline is needed. This is the most effective method of minimizing the tendency of the artery to thrombose while being sutured.

Great persistence and thoroughness is recommended in clearing all of the intraluminal clot. This is encouraged by positioning and draping the patient in such a way that the arteries of the extremity beyond the the point of suspected primary embolism may be exposed if removal of the known embolus does not restore circulation. On occasion, removal of an embolus at the iliac or femoral bifurcation may disclose the fact that a smaller portion of the embolus has lodged at the popliteal artery bifurcation. Sometimes it is also the case that clot has formed distal to the initial obstruction and is sufficiently adherent to the vessel wall that it is difficult to aspirate from above. In these more complicated instances, the popliteal artery bifurcation may be exposed and the artery opened at this level, in order entirely to clear out the vessel within the thigh. Also, it is occasionally necessary to expose a small vessel at the ankle, such as the posterior tibial artery, and by the passage of small catheters from below, or irrigation under some pressure from below, to dislodge and wash out clots from the vessels within the calf.

Postoperatively, motion of the extremity is encouraged to avoid stasis, and the anticoagulant therapy may be continued with careful use of heparin. This last is done not only to prevent thrombosis of the operated artery but also to diminish development of more thrombi at the original source of the embolus. It may be continued for long periods after an embolus has occurred, and in this case the anticoagulant drug is changed in an orderly fashion from heparin to Dicumarol.

Treatment of the underlying condition must not be lost sight of, and careful follow-up of these patients is required to determine which might require active therapy. This would pertain particularly to patients with rheumatic heart disease who may need a mitral commissurotomy to relieve stasis in the left atrium, as well as a possible open heart procedure to evacuate clots from within the left atrium at the same time that the mitral valve was relieved of its stenosis.

ARTERIAL THROMBOSIS

Etiology. The usual underlying arterial disease leading to arterial thrombosis is arteriosclerosis. In the presence of this degenerative condition the factors leading to development of a thrombus in the lumen are the narrowing of the lumen and roughening of the lining.

Symptoms. The symptoms at the onset of an arterial thrombosis superimposed on chronic arterial disease are not necessarily very severe. The reason for this is that the pre-existing arteriosclerosis has slowly developed a certain degree of chronic obstruction. During this time collateral arterial routes have widened. When the final acute occlusion of the diseased point in the artery occurs, the resulting sudden fall in blood flow is less than is the case when a normal artery is obstructed. This mechanism may be so prominent that no acute episode is registered by the patient. This is demonstrated to be so by the fact that specimens of segments of chronic arterial occlusion removed at the operating table for replacement with vascular grafts frequently show thrombotic occlusion of the narrowed lumen in patients whose course has been gradual and without an acute episode. However, when the final thrombosis occurs in a rela-

tively wide open, diseased artery, a variable symptomatology will result.

In the acute phase there is a lesser degree of arterial spasm than accompanies arterial embolism. The pain is distinctly less than that seen in severe forms of embolism. However, since pain can be absent in either condition, this is a poor point in differentiation. On the basis of history some indication of the pre-existing arterial disease may be recognized. Intermittent claudication, the earliest symptom of chronic arterial occlusion, is most likely to be discovered as a previous complaint. The presence of a cardiac arrhythmia or disease likely to produce an embolus is helpful in differentiating arterial thrombosis from arterial embolism but is not necessarily accurate. The cardiac status of the patient can be misleading in those instances of embolism already mentioned in which the heart is not demonstrably abnormal.

The presence of a heart condition likely to cause embolism does not rule out thrombosis, particularly if a phase of the cardiac disease has been productive of a depressed blood pressure. Although arterial hypotension can develop in the course of a condition producing auricular fibrillation, the more important condition is coronary occlusion. A cardinal manifestation of myocardial infarction due to coronary occlusion is hypotension. During the period of depressed blood pressure there is the additional factor of reduced peripheral arterial flow to encourage the development of peripheral arterial thrombosis. Since coronary occlusion is usually a manifestation of degenerative arterial disease, it is frequent that the same patients have some degree of similar change in the peripheral arteries.

Therefore, a 3-fold relationship can be seen to exist between coronary occlusion and peripheral arterial obstruction of the acute type. An understanding of the problem is much more than academic in its importance. The first element is the incidence of arterial embolism in patients having myocardial infarcts. It has been mentioned that this complication occurs most often from the 5th to the 12th day. The second point is the tendency to thrombosis in arteriosclerotic vessels of the extremities during the period of hypotension, most frequently present during the initial hours of an acute myocardial infarct. The third facet, which has not been discussed so far, is the effect of hypotension of an acute coronary attack on the appearance of extremities of a patient who has chronic arterial obstruction due to arteriosclerosis but has *not* developed an arterial thrombosis. Cold skin, small pulses and a pale cyanotic color are frequently seen in this stage of the heart attack. If significant arterial disease is present the appearance can mimic very closely an acute occlusion. If the patient responds to cardiac management and heart action improves, the signs of acute peripheral arterial occlusion disappear.

In the presence of a myocardial infarct, therefore, the clinical appearance of acute peripheral arterial occlusion may denote an arterial embolus, a thrombosis of a diseased segment of peripheral artery, or a simple augmentation of a chronic arterial insufficiency due to the depressed blood pressure without additional occlusion. The treatment of arterial embolism has already been pointed out to be the removal of the obstructing embolus wherever possible and has been described in some detail. The treatment of an arterial thrombosis has the same purpose but is affected very much by the state of the patient's cardiovascular system in general and the cardiac status and blood pressure specifically.

Treatment of an arterial thrombosis offers a greater challenge to the surgeon than does treatment of arterial embolism. The fact that the obstructed segment is the site of a degenerative condition is responsible for the technical difficulties which are involved. The removal of the obstruction usually does not consist of simple removal of the clot but demands that the arteriosclerotic segment either be cleared of its atheromatous lesions or be by-passed or replaced by a graft. The elements of these procedures are discussed later in relation to treatment of chronic occlusive lesions of arteriosclerosis. However, if the best of these methods are applied in a patient who has developed the thrombosis in a period of hypotension and remains in the hypotensive state, the result will be the almost immediate recurrence of thrombosis. Therefore, the initial requirement in deciding to intervene directly in arterial thrombosis is the restoration of the patient's arterial blood pressure. The inability to do so contraindicates surgery on

the artery. This contraindication has the additional effect of preventing surgical approach to a supposed arterial occlusion when the signs are produced by the hypotensive state without arterial obstruction.

ARTERIAL TRAUMA

Improved technics and dissemination of knowledge of how to perform surgical procedures on the arteries has distinctly improved the prognosis in cases of arterial trauma. This is due in part to experience gained during World War II.[25] However, much more was learned in the postwar period because of the surgical correction of arterial damage sustained during the war but corrected months and years later.[43, 108] Application of these technics in the acute cases occurring during the Korean conflict led to a much higher proportion of immediate restoration of damaged arteries during that period than had occurred in World War II.[54, 106, 120] It has been learned that systematic handling is imperative, and the immediate surgical emergency which exists with an arterial injury has come to be appreciated more thoroughly. With proper handling correction of major arterial wounds is well within the realm of possibility.

CLASSIFICATION

A classification of the types of arterial injuries is important in order to develop a scheme of treatment which will be widely applicable. The division of arterial injuries into incision or laceration, perforation and contusion is not simply a didactic matter but is one of technical importance.

Incision or Laceration. An artery which is subjected to damage by a sharp instrument may be partially or completely transected. An incision or laceration without transection results in a gaping opening in the wall of the artery which is held open by the retraction of the vessel wall adjacent to the hole. A completely transected artery, on the other hand, is drawn back into the tissues by its elasticity. The surrounding tissues tend to close over the ends. There is also a distinct tendency for the transected ends to constrict, due to the circular coats of muscular and elastic tissue. Both of these actions aid in stopping hemorrhage, and for these reasons a partially severed artery is productive of more blood loss than is

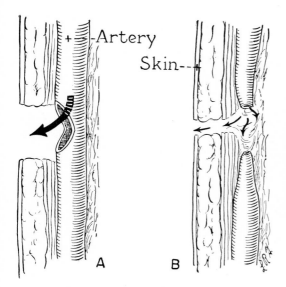

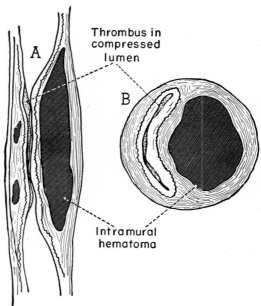

FIG. 40-4. Diagrammatic explanation of the tendency of a partial laceration of an artery (A) to bleed more profusely and longer than a complete transection (B). The retraction of the artery ends into adjacent tissue, and constriction of the cut ends minimize the bleeding in (B).

FIG. 40-5. Traumatic occlusion of an artery without blood loss occurs following a contusion. The longitudinal (A) and cross-section (B) of the artery shows compression of the lumen by the intramural hematoma plus thrombus formation in the lumen.

one which is completely divided (Fig. 40-4).

Perforations of an artery occur when a high velocity missile of small size or a small sharp instrument, such as an ice pick or a thin knife, pass through the vessel. These injuries are accompanied by a minimal amount of surrounding tissue damage and a small opening on the body surface. Usually little outside bleeding occurs. Injuries of this type may be followed by specific lesions as pulsating hematoma and arteriovenous fistulae which will be described later.

A contusion of an artery is caused by a broad, crushing or grinding force or missile.[34, 85] A large, relatively slow missile may produce this kind of lesion, as will very high velocity missiles passing through tissue near the wall of an artery. The impingement of a fractured bone against the artery, as in fractures of the lower end of the femur, can injure the vessel in this manner. It should be emphasized that contusion of an artery may be caused by a sudden blow to an extremity without there being an associated fracture or wound. This lesion has been met with most frequently in the brachial artery in patients

who have hooked their arm over some structure in order to break a fall, and in the lower thigh at about the femoral-popliteal artery junction in patients who have been struck obliquely from behind by the bumper of an automobile.

The lesion can also be described as an intramural hematoma of the artery. The crushing force produces damage within the coats of the vessel in such a way that bleeding occurs between the various layers. As the hematoma grows, it compresses the lumen of the vessel and produces obstruction (Fig. 40-5). The thoracic aorta is subject to quite a different type of damage of the general contusion type. This occurs most frequently in the portion of the descending aorta within 1 or 2 inches of the left subclavian artery. A heavy blow to the chest, either directly depressing the sternum or applied laterally in such a way as to fracture some of the ribs in the left chest, may produce a tear in the intima and the internal layers of the media of the aorta at this area. The tear is sometimes completely about the circumference of the aorta. Continuity of blood flow is maintained because of the resistance of the overlying pleura supporting the remaining layers of the vessel. This type of contusion leads to the development of a traumatic aneurysm of the descending aorta, rather than an obstruction of the intramural hematoma type.

DIAGNOSIS

The hemorrhage from arterial injury is variable. It may dissect into tissue spaces or into body cavities or viscera. The wound may coincidentally involve the adjacent vein and permit hemorrhage to occur from the artery into the vein. Finally, in cases of arterial contusion or intramural hematoma, hemorrhage may be absent. Therefore, the diagnosis of an arterial injury cannot depend primarily on the presence and the character of the bleeding. Diagnostic features other than that of hemorrhage must be sought. If bleeding is free to occur from the arterial injury to the outside, the pulsatile character of the escaping blood will make the diagnosis obvious. Hemorrhage from an arterial injury into a closed tissue space produces a pulsating swelling.

If the artery and the vein are injured simultaneously in such a way as to allow blood loss from artery into vein a permanent fistulous communication can be established immediately or develop later if the communication is at first blocked by a thrombus. The initial sign which is diagnostic of an arteriovenous communication is the continuous "machinerylike" murmur, audible with the stethoscope over the region of the injury and sometimes palpable as a thrill.

Intramural hematoma is a type of arterial injury which may escape detection with disastrous results unless other specific signs are looked for carefully. Such an injury produces an acute occlusion of the artery involved. Acute arterial occlusions tend to produce pain in the region of the body that is deprived of its blood supply. However, the injuries to other tissues may also be painful, and pain alone is not pathognomonic of arterial occlusion. If a major vessel to an extremity is bruised and closed, the distal part of the extremity may appear pale immediately because of lack of blood supply and soon thereafter becomes paralyzed and anesthetic. These

signs, together with the loss of pulses in the region in which they are normally palpable distal to the obstruction, indicates the presence of an arterial injury.

Differential Diagnosis. The presence of an intramural hematoma must be differentiated from an acute intense arterial spasm secondary to an injury not actually involving an artery at all. Such severe spasm of the vessels of an injured extremity is a common occurrence and usually attributed to a reflex which is elaborated through the sympathetic nervous system. Rarely does reflex vasospasm attain the intensity or last long enough to produce numbness and paralysis of the distal part of the involved extremity. Failure of these specific signs to appear is an aid in differentiating the two conditions. Also, spasm can make the pulses distal to the injury temporarily impalpable. Final distinction between these two conditions may depend upon interrupting the sympathetic nervous system reflex responsible for spasm by the injection of procaine into the appropriate part of the sympathetic nervous system. Sympathetic blocks, the technic of which will be described elsewhere, may be done simply and quickly.

Further accuracy of diagnosis of the traumatic arterial obstruction may be obtained by the injection of such contrast media as sodium acetrozoate (Urokon Sodium) or iodopyracet (Diodrast) into the artery proximal to the injury. These iodine-containing substances are opaque to x-rays, and if an exposure is made as the medium is being transported by the artery, an accurate picture is obtained of the vessel lumen showing obstruction if it is present. Arteriography is not often required in the diagnosis of an injury but may be of value in difficult cases (Fig. 40-6).

The differentiation of arterial hemorrhage from venous bleeding is seldom of much practical importance. The difference may be immediately obvious on the basis of the color of the blood being lost. Most venous bleeding and many instances of arterial bleeding can be controlled by moderate pressure over the region of the vascular injury. If severe bleeding which cannot be controlled by this method is present, adequate surgical exposure for the control of hemorrhage is required, and appropriate management of the vein or artery lesion accomplished.

FIG. 40-6. Arteriograms of the popliteal artery of a patient who had sustained a crushing injury to the posterior aspect of the knee. (*Left*) A preoperative arteriogram shows abrupt and near total occlusion of the artery at the level marked. It is noted that there is no dye outside the artery in the region of the injury. (*Right*) Postoperative arteriogram taken 3 weeks following resection of the damaged area of the artery and repair through the use of a short vein graft. The points of anastomosis are almost indistinguishable but are probably as marked by the two arrows.

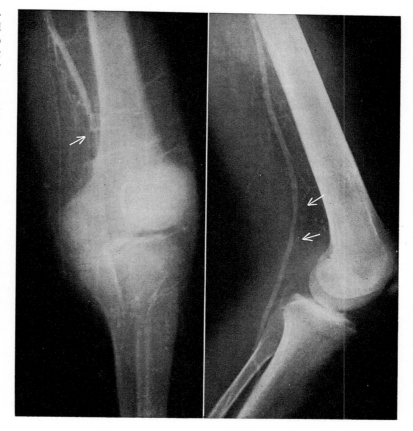

TREATMENT

Three Phases. The treatment of an arterial injury may be divided into 3 phases.

1. In the initial phase it deals with the control of hemorrhage. As is noted above, there are very few instances in which pressure or tourniquet application will fail to control bleeding from the extremities. Arterial injuries high in the groin, deep in the axillae or the base of the neck, as well as within the abdomen and the thorax, present problems which cannot always be treated adequately except in a well-equipped operating room. Injuries such as these, if they are so located and formed as to allow free hemorrhage, often will be productive of deep shock which the patient will not survive. Rapid transfusion combined with immediate surgery to control the hemorrhage is, in severe cases, the only practical means of treatment of the injury.

2. The second phase in treatment consists of restoration of the blood volume by blood transfusion until the blood pressure returns to normal and is maintained. Blood is the fluid of choice in restoring the blood volume but may be substituted in part by various solutions, such as plasma, dextran, gelatin, or in a limited degree by rapid infusion of electrolyte solution, should no other fluid be immediately available (see Chap. 7, "Shock," and Chap. 8, "Blood Transfusion").

3. The third phase involves definitive treatment of the arterial lesion. This should include, under all possible circumstances, a repair of the damaged vessel adequate to restore normal circulation to the part. Repair is undertaken as an emergency measure but should be carried out under the same optimum conditions as would accompany an elective surgical procedure on an artery.[53]

In locations where adequate facilities or personnel for arterial repair are lacking, consideration should be given to transferring the patient. This may be done if control of hemorrhage and replacement of blood loss have been accomplished and associated injuries do not contraindicate moving the patient. Time becomes a most important factor if the injury has produced ischemia of the part.

The general plan in operation upon an artery for an injury or, indeed, the general plan of operation upon any artery for any reason follows a very definite sequence. Adequate anesthesia is used without the requirement of deep muscular relaxation. Because of the specific danger of disruption of a suture line in an artery if infection results from the operation, meticulous care is taken in the preparation of the skin. Tourniquets are seldom used in operations on the vessels of the extremities.

The primary task in operating upon an artery is to expose the vessel sufficiently proximal to the lesion to be able to isolate a segment of it without disturbing the damaged area. This process is known as gaining proximal control of the artery. A length of cotton tape is passed about the artery so that it may be pulled up to be constricted against the finger or to apply suitable blood vessel clamps for stopping blood flow through the vessel. The second step of the procedure consists of gaining the same sort of control beyond the lesion. Following this, the dissection of the artery is carried out in both directions toward the actual site of operation, and finally, with the vessel constricted above and below, the repair is done.

Repair may consist of a simple *suture* of a laceration or an end-to-end anastomosis of a transected vessel. In treating high-velocity puncture wounds of large arteries, it is important to remember that the hidden damage to the inner portion of the wall is often much more extensive than the visible damage to the outer portion of the wall. This may lead to secondary blowouts if the puncture wound is merely closed by suture. Such wounds should be débrided with removal of an adequate margin of the adjacent wall or it may be best to excise the injured segment and to bring the vessel together again by end-to-end suture. Complicated lacerations which defy reconstructive suture directly along the incised edges are treated by removal of that portion of the artery which is damaged and, wherever possible, advantage is taken of the elasticity of the artery, bringing the 2 ends together for

simple anastomosis. When the amount of vessel lost is too great to bring the ends together without undue tension, the defect which is produced by its removal is replaced by the insertion of a vessel graft. In a person with normal arteries a surprising amount of lost vessel length may be compensated for by stretching.

A variety of technics of blood vessel suture are currently in use. Simple laceration of an artery is repaired with a suture of very fine silk swedged onto a fine needle, applied in an over-and-over fashion. The suture is placed 1 mm. from the edge of the vessel and the adjacent sutures are 1 mm. apart (Fig. 40-7 A and B). When carefully done, it will be almost water tight and always will be impervious to blood because of blood's greater viscosity and early fibrin deposits. An anastomosis between the ends of a severed vessel or between the vessel end and a graft may be made in this same over-and-over fashion (Fig. 40-7 C and D) or may be done so as to bring the inner lining, the intima, of the vessel ends into apposition. An everting mattress suture employs the same material, and the placement is in the same dimensions as described for an over-and-over suture (Fig. 40-7 B).

The choice of grafts in the repair of a vascular injury is dictated by availability of materials and by the diameter and the length of the arterial segment which needs replacing. Vascular tissue taken from the patient himself makes the best material, strictly on the basis of acceptance of the tissue in its new site. For this reason, a vein graft is usually selected for repair of the medium-sized vessels of the extremities. The vein often used is the patient's own long saphenous vein. It can be readily spared in any patient and is a relatively muscular vein which substitutes well for most extremity arteries. A point of great importance in the implantation of a vein graft is to remember to orient the vein graft end-to-end in such a way that the valves do not obstruct the flow of arterial blood. Arterial prostheses of woven plastic yarn are available in a wide range of sizes corresponding to the size of all vessels from the small brachial artery to the large aorta. They are reliable, and their availability without the necessity of additional surgical maneuvers, such as are necessary to obtain a vein graft, is in favor of their

Fig. 40-7. Repair of a simple linear laceration of an artery may be accomplished by anatomic suture (A and B). If the laceration is more extensive, the damaged area is removed, and closure is done by approximating the ends by traction on the atraumatic vascular clamps and reanastomosing by one of two technics. The use of a simple over-and-over suture is diagrammed (C and D).

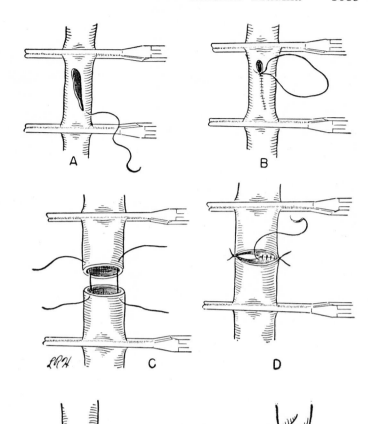

Fig. 40-7 (*Cont.*) The alternate method of performing an arterial anastomosis is an everting mattress suture. This may be done as a continuous suture, illustrated here, or as an interrupted suture. The technic is simplified by rotating the vessel with the clamps to expose the posterior aspect of the anastomosis (B).

(Continued on p. 1090)

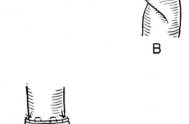

use. Arterial homografts preserved by various methods are a further type of arterial replacement. The disadvantages to their use are the difficulty attendant to obtaining them and the fact that deterioration of the graft after long periods has been observed.

Pulsating Hematoma (False Aneurysm)

Perforation of an artery by a sharp instrument or a high-speed, small-size missile often produces a pulsating hematoma or false aneurysm. If the tissues of the point of injury are sufficiently resistant, the pressure in the pool of blood lost into the area soon builds up to the mean arterial pressure. Thereafter some blood extravasates through the vessel opening into the tissue space during systole, and some

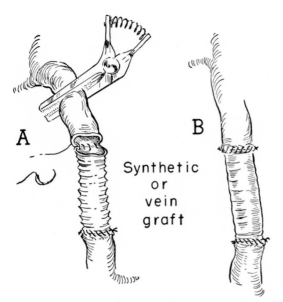

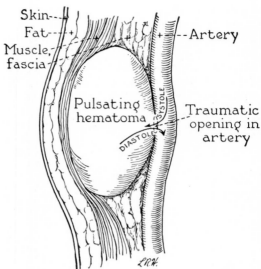

FIG. 40-7 (*Cont.*) When resection of the contused segment is necessary, the defect is bridged by a synthetic or autogenous vein graft as shown in A and B.

FIG. 40-8. Diagram of false aneurysm or pulsating hematoma. The directions of flow through the opening during diastole and systole are indicated by the arrows.

returns to the artery during diastole (Fig. 40-8). The accumulation of blood pulsates within the tissues. In many such cases the blood flow distal to the injury is maintained, and a pulsating hematoma frequently is tolerated for a long time before it is repaired. Fibrosis occurs in the wall, and in time the sac becomes endothelialized.

Indirect trauma sometimes causes a pulsating hematoma. Abrupt stretching of the femoral artery in a fall in which the thighs are abducted suddenly and forcefully, or of the popliteal artery if the knee is hyperextended, tears the vessel wall and allows this lesion to form. This is most likely to occur when the vessel is previously the site of some such disease as arteriosclerosis and therefore is weak and inelastic.

The clinical signs of a pulsating hematoma are the palpable pulsation of the mass and the sounds which are audible with the stethoscope as the blood leaves and enters the hematoma. The sound produced usually is confined to systole but may be heard also during the diastolic phase. When heard in both systole and diastole the murmur is not continuous. This is because blood flow ceases momentarily

at the end of systole and again at the end of diastole as the pressures within the sac and the artery equalize and the direction of flow through the arterial opening prepares to reverse. This interrupted character differentiates it from the murmur of arteriovenous fistula which is continuous. The location and the extent of such a lesion may be determined exactly by an arteriogram.

Treatment. Where facilities are available, surgical repair of a pulsating hematoma is indicated immediately upon making the diagnosis of the arterial injury. Formerly, it has been general practice to delay treatment of such a lesion for several months. The reason for this is that a false aneurysm to some degree produces a partial occlusion of the artery which has been damaged. This is caused by the turbulence of flow within the artery developed by the exit and the return of blood through the opening, and also by the compression of the artery resulting simply from the mass of the adjacent hematoma. Chronic occlusion stimulates the branches of the artery above and below the lesion to dilate and, by enlarging their natural communications, to form a collateral arterial bed. This may become sufficient in a moderate period of time to protect the part, usually an extremity, from gangrene if the segment of artery bearing the lesion is simply doubly ligated and removed. At the present time such ligation and excision is no longer practiced by choice but rather direct anastomosis or interposition of a vessel graft is done. In applying the principle of waiting for collateral arteries to be stimulated, operation is sometimes made necessary before the optimum period has passed because of changes which go on in the region of the pulsating hematoma. The hematoma itself may become intimately attached to the skin overlying it and by pressure and associated inflammation thin out the skin and threaten to rupture, particularly at the point of the healing skin wound which was produced by the penetrating object. Pain of compression of the adjacent nerves and other structures in the region of the pulsating hematoma may necessitate early operation. Finally, the mass of the pulsating hematoma can produce ischemia of the tissues distal to the lesion by compression of the collateral arteries and by pressure on the injured vessel itself. Such pain and ischemia make waiting the optimum period impossible. Then the operation may be required during the period of 6 to 9 days following the initial injury. At exactly this time the softening and the edema of the artery wall adjacent to the injury are at their maximum, and the least desirable condition of the vessel will be found at operation for the necessary repair. These factors, together with the relative ease with which operation can be done at the time of the injury, make immediate treatment more desirable at the present time.

The actual operation to be carried out upon the lesion, whether it is done immediately as is recommended above or as a delayed procedure after the pulsating hematoma has been present for weeks, months or years, varies, depending upon the size and the importance of the vessel concerned and the extent of damage to the vessel. A very small unimportant artery injured in such a way as to produce a pulsating hematoma is simply ligated at points above and below the traumatic opening in the vessel, and the lesion is removed. Larger vessels are preserved by excision of the segment of vessel which has been damaged, followed either by direct repair of the artery by end-to-end anastomosis or by the interposition of a graft, depending upon the

length of segment lost and the elasticity of the adjacent artery. This, of course, varies in no way from the repair of an arterial injury of any type. When the delayed method of repair has been planned, and when the symptoms of compression, ischemia or threatening rupture necessitate emergency operation, it routinely will be necessary to resect the segment of the damaged vessel because of the arterial softening.

TRAUMATIC ARTERIOVENOUS FISTULA

Etiology. An arteriovenous fistula occurs as the result of a trauma involving adjacent arteries and veins. Usually it is produced by a high-speed missile or a stab wound but also may occur because of rupture of an arteriosclerotic aneurysm into the adjacent vein to which it has gradually become adherent and into which it has finally eroded. Arteriovenous fistulae on the basis of congenital malformation are discussed elsewhere. In the traumatic type of arteriovenous fistula there is often not much external hemorrhage. The fistula which is produced by the trauma sometimes becomes active immediately after the injury. However, the actual establishment of the fistula can be delayed until there is some organization of the adjacent wounds and absorption of a thrombus which happens to occupy the opening between the 2 vessels. Sometimes fistulae are caused by surgical trauma. This occurs most frequently in thyroidectomies or in nephrectomies when the artery and the vein of the superior pole of the thyroid or of the renal pedicle are ligated together.[36] The ligature erodes through the 2 vessels in such a way as to establish a communication. Surgically produced fistulae are also known to develop when vessels not being ligated are damaged inadvertently. Fistulae have appeared between the aorta or the right common iliac artery and the inferior vena cava when these vessels have been damaged by an instrument passing between the lumbar vertebral bodies during surgery for removal of a herniated intervertebral disk.[84]

Diagnosis. The presence of an arteriovenous fistula is diagnosed on the basis of the characteristic auscultatory finding of a continuous machinerylike murmur. This continuous murmur is produced by the continuous flow of blood from the artery into the vein where

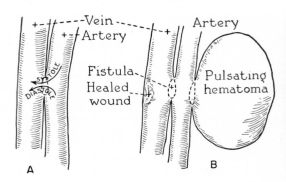

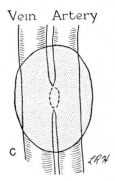

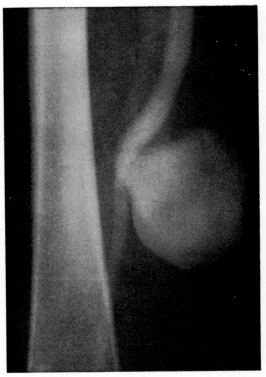

FIG. 40-9. Common forms of arteriovenous fistulae resulting from trauma. The direction of flow through the fistula during diastole and systole is indicated by the arrows (A). Combinations of pulsating hematoma with arteriovenous fistulae are diagrammed (B and C).

FIG. 40-10. Reproduction of an arteriogram in a patient who developed a superficial femoral artery-vein fistula and a pulsating hematoma after a bullet wound of the lower thigh. The artery feeding the fistula is enlarged, while the artery leaving the fistulous point is diminished in size. The superficial femoral vein proximal to the fistula is seen in the arteriogram less densely filled with dye than is the artery.

the jet produces turbulence and vibration of the vein wall. The machinerylike character of the continuous murmur is due to the fact that the velocity of this shunt and therefore the pitch of the murmur is increased during the systolic phase of the pulse. The flow of blood is not a to-and-fro action as in pulsating hematoma but is always from the artery into the vein. Such a murmur is often associated with a palpable thrill. Anatomically, an arteriovenous fistula produced by a stab wound or a missile is often a compound lesion, consisting of the fistula between the 2 vessels and a pulsating hematoma on the opposite surface of the artery. This compounding of the lesion is due to the fact that the damage to the artery, whether it be missile or stab, enters and leaves the artery, producing 2 openings. The apposed holes produce the fistula; the wound in the free surface of the artery forms the false

aneurysm. For this reason there is a pulsating mass palpable in the immediate region of an arteriovenous fistula (Fig. 40-9).

Arteriography in cases of arteriovenous fistula confirms the diagnosis and provides accurate localization to guide the surgeon in repair (Fig. 40-10).

Further points in the diagnosis depend upon a series of physiologic disturbances which are produced by the abnormality.[38, 48]

When it is established, the shunt immediately increases the venous return to the heart; velocity, pressure and minute flow into the right atrium are raised. Ventricular filling time is shortened, and the pulse rate is accelerated. An important clinical sign is made possible by this sequence of events. If the artery proximal to or directly over the fistula is compressed manually to stop flow through the fistula, the pulse rate will drop immediately. This phenomenon is called the Branham-Nicoladoni sign.[10, 94] It is almost universally present in arteriovenous fistulae so located that the maneuver can be accomplished.

The abnormal flow and pressure in the venous system in the region of the fistula causes a visible venous dilatation. There is a greater volume of blood in the tissues in the region of the fistula due to massive engorgement of the veins and increased flow. This produces a warming of the skin in the region of the fistula. For some distance beyond the lesion the skin also is warmer than on the contralateral side. When the arteriovenous fistula involves the major vessel of the thigh, the skin of the thigh will be warm, but the skin of the foot will be cooler than the opposite normal foot. This cooling distally is the result of diminished head of pressure in the artery beyond the shunt and lower arterial circulation from that point onward. Other physiologic results of the fistula are an increased cardiac output and an increase in blood volume. The arterial blood pressure is diminished by an arteriovenous fistula. Both systolic and diastolic pressures fall. Later, however, the systolic pressure rises to its former level or higher, whereas the diastolic remains lower, producing an increase in pulse pressure.

TABLE 1. PREOPERATIVE AND POSTOPERATIVE DATA AT REST OF A 32-YEAR-OLD PATIENT WITH ARTERIOVENOUS FISTULA OF 18 YEARS' DURATION*

	PRE-OPERATIVE	POST-OPERATIVE
Cardiac output (L./min. × 100)	5.36	2.16
Oxygen consumption (ml.) Stroke index (ml./beat/M²)	140	77
Heart rate (beats/min.)	61	55
Systemic pressure (mm. Hg.) Mean	69	93
Total blood volume (ml.)	6789	4835

* From Section of Cardiorespiratory Diseases, Presbyterian-St. Luke's Hospital, Chicago, Ill.

The increased cardiac output, increased blood volume, and the rapid pulse secondary to the accelerated venous return to the heart distinctly produce a strain upon the heart.

Evidence of this strain is the almost constant cardiac enlargement in those patients who have a fistula for a significant length of time. The strain is infrequently a cause of heart failure in patients with normal hearts. However, patients who have valvular heart disease, even mild, as a result of healed rheumatic fever, or have arteriosclerotic heart disease, often will go into heart failure when an arteriovenous fistula has been established.

Treatment. Treatment of an arteriovenous fistula is entirely surgical unless some degree of heart failure has occurred. In the latter case maximum competency of the myocardium should be obtained by proper treatment before surgery.

As in pulsating hematoma, arteriovenous fistulae were managed formerly by delaying the operative procedure for the purpose of development of arterial collaterals. This was for the reason that until recently the method of surgical treatment of a fistula of this type was the excision of the fistula after ligation of the 2 arterial and the 2 venous limbs. With the application of technics of vascular suture, anastomosis and grafting, the optimum treatment at the present time consists of removal of the fistula and re-establishment of the circulation. In subjects with otherwise normal vessels this procedure is sufficiently dependable that the waiting period for development of collaterals can be abandoned and surgery done as soon as the diagnosis is made. Actually, if early operation in all forms of arterial damage becomes routine, the development of arteriovenous fistula will be a rarity.

Various types of surgical procedures were done long before the 2 modern technics of quadrilateral ligation and excision and of excision with re-establishment of the circulation were developed. These technics and the changes which resulted from them are of interest from a physiologic point of view.

Proximal ligation of the artery alone produces immediate severe ischemia of the extremity distal to the fistula. This, of course, is because all the blood that enters the artery from collaterals distal to the fistula drains backward through the fistula into the vein, disastrously reducing the head of pressure in the vascular bed supplying the tissues.

Distal ligation of the artery also has a most unsatisfactory result. Ligation at this point alone immediately and sharply increases the amount of blood which is shunted into the vein. The degree of heart strain is increased, and heart failure results. Theoretically, proximal and distal ligation of both the artery and the vein would seem to result in a cure of the fistula. However, some recurrences come about through the fact that relatively small arterial branches between the ligatures are overlooked, later to re-establish arterial circulation into the occluded segment reactivating the fistula.

Simple ligation of the 4 ends was soon abandoned in favor of excising the area after ligating the vessels. This operation seldom, if ever, produces ischemic necrosis of the tissues distal to the fistula if it is delayed 3 months or more because by this time collateral arterial supply has become adequate. However, after this type of repair, the patients are limited in their ability to exercise, because the collateral bed upon which their limb depends cannot increase the blood flow to the extremity adequately to meet the needs of exercise. It has been not only the incidence of gangrene that has led to the procedures re-establishing arterial flow, but also the symptoms which result during exercise in a limb that has been treated by the ligation methods.[51]

CHRONIC OCCLUSIVE ARTERIAL DISEASE

GENERAL

The pathologic states productive of chronic arterial occlusion fall into 2 distinct groups: the degenerative arterial diseases, and a group of inflammatory arterial changes which are represented by the example of Buerger's disease.

Chronic occlusion of arteries may involve any organ or part of the body. Most by far of such occlusions are caused by degenerative arterial diseases. The symptoms produced depend on the organ or the body part involved, such as cerebral ischemia secondary to carotid artery involvement, hypertension secondary to renal artery involvement, angina caused by coronary artery obstruction, and a characteristic symptom complex caused by arterial occlusions in the extremities. The clinical picture which results from occlusive arterial disease will be considered in some detail as it involves the extremities. The effects of occlu-

sion of the arteries to the brain and the kidney will be discussed under these particular sections.

Symptomatology. INTERMITTENT CLAUDICATION. Chronic occlusion of the arterial supply to the extremities produces symptoms of essentially the same type, independent of the underlying pathology of the obstructing lesion. The earliest symptom is met with in the lower extremities during the work of the calf muscle groups in walking, running, or climbing stairs. The symptom develops initially during such exercise because, although the arterial supply may be quite adequate to meet all the needs of the part during rest, it cannot meet the increased demand of exercise. The symptom produced is a severe cramping pain in the muscle groups which are inadequately supplied with blood. Resting of the muscle by standing still or sitting down relieves the pain as soon as the metabolites are removed and an adequate ratio of work to blood supply is restored. This symptom is termed "intermittent claudication." It is not reproduced accurately by conditions other than those which restrict muscle blood supply during exercise.

Certain *characteristics of intermittent claudication* tend to distinguish it from other types of pain. One important characteristic is its independence from the general fatigue of the patient. The repeated reproducibility of the pain after the same amount of exercise and the constancy of the length of rest needed for relief in the same subject are also distinguishing characteristics of intermittent claudication. The afflicted patient has his cramping pain after walking a certain distance at a given rate of speed, and when the pain occurs he requires a definite rest period for relief. After this period of rest he is able to duplicate the exercise, and again the pain returns. The distance he can walk or the number of stairs he can climb before pain starts is the same in the morning as it is in the evening, even though the patient is tired after a day's work. No pain at all results in these patients when they walk a shorter distance than that required to produce claudication. Therefore, in walking about the home or the place of work the patient is perfectly comfortable.

Intermittent claudication particularly differs from the pain of hypertrophic arthritis in that the arthritic pain begins almost immediately at the beginning of exercise. It is worse when the patient gets up in the morning, relieved somewhat during the day as he loosens up, and increases again at night during fatigue. Much attention is paid to this symptom of intermittent claudication because it is the outstanding one, almost the hallmark, of chronic arterial occlusion.

REST PAIN. As the degree of arterial obstruction increases and intermittent claudication requires less exercise for its production and more rest for its relief, other symptoms appear. A sense of coldness in the distal part of the extremity is often the next symptom. Muscle pain of a cramping nature during rest and sleep becomes disturbing as the disease progresses. This symptom which is termed "rest pain" is, in effect, an intermittent claudication though in reverse. It is a result of the continued muscle work of normal tonus going on during the reduced circulation of repose. The patient actually finds that he may relieve the pain by stirring about or walking which increases cardiac output and local blood supply.

ISCHEMIA. The ischemia that results from chronic occlusive disease produces its most disturbing symptom by the direct effect of the lack of circulation on the peripheral nerves. The neuritic pain of ischemia differs from intermittent claudication and rest pain in that it is constant once it has become established. The pain is burning and compressing in quality and comes on relatively late in the course of the disease. It has one very distinctive characteristic. The patient so afflicted finds it difficult or impossible to elevate his legs or even to allow them to remain on a level with the rest of his body. When they are in any position other than hanging down as the patient sits, the pain is markedly exaggerated. This characteristic of the ischemic neuritis may account for some of the *edema of the feet and the ankles* which occurs in advanced arterial disease. The swelling itself is a very damaging factor in the arterial insufficiency because it renders the small vessel circulation in the part even more inefficient. The tendency to develop a *gangrenous ulcer* because of ischemic necrosis of the edematous tissue is markedly increased.

Whenever the ischemia progresses to the point at which blood supply is inadequate for tissue life, *ischemic ulcers* develop. At any time in the course of the disease ulcers may be precipitated by minor trauma or blister formation because the demand for increased metabolism of healing cannot be met. The pain of ulceration is usually severe, although the ischemic neuritis which often has preceded it may have produced enough nerve damage to reduce the pain sensation.

These common symptoms including intermittent claudication, a sense of coldness, rest pain, ischemic neuritis, and the pain of ulceration are shared by various types of chronic occlusive arterial disease, although they appear in different degrees in the various conditions.

Physical Examination. In every general physical examination, whether arterial pathology has been suggested by the history or not, the peripheral pulses in their normal locations should be sought for and compared with those of the opposite side. The pulses which are normally palpable are the femoral, the popliteal, the dorsalis pedis and the posterior tibial arteries in the lower extremities; the subclavian, the axillary, the brachial, the radial and the ulnar in the upper extremities. Not only is the loss of palpability important, but also the comparative fullness of the pulse between the two sides should be noted and recorded. At the ankle the more important pulse is the posterior tibial because of the occasional congenital absence of the dorsalis pedis artery. This infrequent anomaly is probably always bilateral. The ulnar arterial pulse may be difficult to palpate but is demonstrable by a simple maneuver described by Allen.[1]

In addition to noting the presence or the absence of pulses and comparing the fullness and the strength of the pulses on the two sides, the character of the blood vessel wall should be observed. Thickening, stiffness and calcification of the vessel wall can be palpated, particularly at the femoral, the brachial, the ankle and the wrist levels.

Auscultation over various arteries during physical examination provides very important information. Under normal circumstances, one hears only faint crisp sounds, roughly corresponding in time to the first and the second heart tones, over large vessels. In addition to characteristic abnormal sounds produced by aortic stenosis and aortic valvular insufficiency, intrinsic changes in the blood vessels proximal to the point at which auscultation is carried out may produce very characteristic abnormal sounds. Roughening of the lining of a blood vessel, or changes in its caliber, particularly in the direction of stenosis, causes the appearance of a systolic *bruit*. The character of the sound, whether it be soft or coarse or pitched high or low is determined by the character of abnormality in the vessel wall, but changes in these characters cannot be ascribed directly to different kinds of lesions. The commonest cause of a harsh bruit over a vessel is stenosis of the vessel proximal to the area. The stenosis is caused by the development of an elevated atheroma or degenerated and calcified lesion in the vessel intruding on its lumen. Much attention must be paid to the bruit and its interpretation. The bruit is absent distal to a complete occlusion of an artery, even though a small pulse may be palpable in the artery due to the fact that the collateral arterial circulation is very well developed. Therefore, if a patient exhibits pulses at both femoral levels with that on the left being stronger than that on the right, and with a bruit over the stronger left femoral pulse and none over the weaker right femoral pulse, the interpretation would be that there is a stenosis in the iliofemoral system on the left and a complete occlusion on the right with good collateral development, at least on the right side.

The objective skin temperature is an important observation rendered somewhat unreliable because of its strong vasomotor control. The finding of cold skin of the hands and the feet may indicate a physiologic response to an unfamiliar situation rather than arterial insufficiency. However, when skin temperature is diminished on one side, the finding has greater meaning.

The skin color which is observed during the examination is also of importance but is also affected by vasomotor stimuli. If the abnormal color is asymmetrical it has meaning, and its extension above the portions of the extremities which have a heavy vasomotor control also gives it importance.

Skin color changes in relation to changes in posture of the extremities can be characteristic for chronic arterial occlusion. The normal extremity blanches perceptibly during elevation. This can be demonstrated in any normal subject. Following elevation, acute dependency of the part produces a brief flushing of the skin with a quick return to normal. In arterial disease the blanching that occurs during elevation is increased, and the time required for the appearance of the heightened color following dependency is lengthened. When color does appear in the arterial-insufficient extremity, it is deeper and more intense than in the normal. It is also more lasting and in severe cases may not return to normal during the period of observation unless the extremity is brought up to the horizontal position. This phenomenon is termed *"reactive hyperemia."* It is thought to be based upon a relative ischemia and anoxia of the skin capillary walls during elevation. The vessels are then in maximum caliber as the new fill of arterial blood slowly comes into the skin when the extremity is lowered. The degree of ischemia during elevation governs the length of time it takes for the artery to regain its normal tone.

At the same time that the limb is brought into dependency after elevation to observe reactive hyperemia, one measures the length of time necessary for normal veins in the skin of the extremity to fill. In the normal subject without varicose veins or arterial insufficiency the so-called *"venous filling time"* is approximately 5 to 6 seconds. In arterial insufficiency this venous filling time is prolonged. If varicose veins are present, the retrograde flow of blood in the veins themselves renders this observation unreliable.

OSCILLOMETER AND PLETHYSMOGRAPH. Certain mechanical aids in the diagnosis of arterial insufficiency are useful. The oscillometer and the plethysmograph are respectively crude and very delicate methods of recording the changes in volume in a part coincident with the heart action. The oscillometer is a manometer attached to a blood pressure cuff and records the swing of the differences in pressure of the tissue contained within the cuff due to heart action at various pressures of inflation of the cuff. The plethysmograph records the changes in volume in a portion of the extremity, usually a portion of toe or finger, which is enclosed in a container having an air-tight seal around the tissues. Plethysmography is rarely used except in specialized examinations. The oscillometer is a valuable practical instrument to record the relative pulse volume. It is used to demonstrate the approximate level of an arterial occlusion by making readings up and down the extremity, showing the point at which the oscillometric index is diminished. The oscillometer readings are recorded as an oscillometric index of millimeters of mercury fluctuation at various pressures. The plethysmograph reading is recorded as the number of cubic millimeters change in volume per cubic centimeter of tissue that occurs during the cardiac cycle.

Angiography. Visualization of the arterial system by x-rays has been mentioned already in relation to arterial trauma. However, its essential use is in the evaluation of chronic occlusion in arterial disease.

Much of our present knowledge concerning the typical segmental distribution of arteriosclerosis, its method of progression, the production of partial occlusion of the vessel by atherosclerotic plaques, and the development of collaterals, comes from x-ray visualization of the lumens of the blood vessels. The technic of visualizing the vascular system by x-rays is known as angiography and constitutes the greatest single aid in the evaluation of chronic arterial occlusions. Typical patterns of filling defects in occlusions are demonstrated by angiography, and the extent of the disease may be mapped out accurately when this is thought to be a necessary prerequisite to surgical treatment. The trend, as experience is gained in the evaluation of a patient by physical examination, is to carry out x-ray examination less and less frequently. Fewer of these studies are done now, and surgical exploration is often done without previous angiographic studies.

In studying the arterial system several methods of angiography are available. Most commonly used is the peripheral *arteriogram*. A peripheral arteriogram is made by introducing a suitable iodine-containing solution into the artery through a needle inserted into its lumen and making one or several rapid x-ray exposures as the dye progresses through the arteries (Fig. 40-11). In the femoral and the brachial arteries the needle can be introduced under local anesthesia through the skin. However, in case of the brachial artery, the many adjacent major nerves make this

percutaneous method hazardous, and more frequently the artery is exposed through a small incision, in order that the needle may be intro-

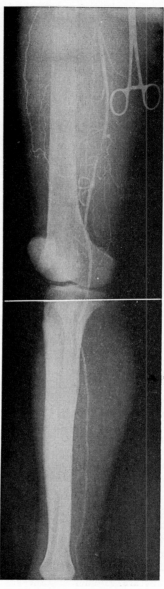

FIG. 40-11. Femoral arteriogram produced by injection of opaque iodine solution into the common femoral artery. The superficial femoral artery is shown to be completely obstructed for a small segment at the level of the adductor tendon. Many collaterals are visualized, and the artery above and below the obstruction is relatively normal.

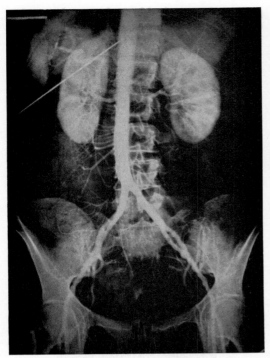

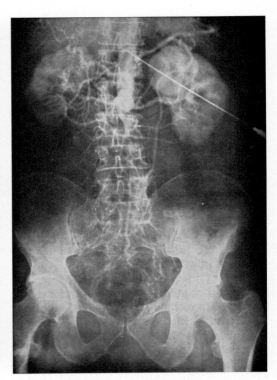

Fig. 40-12. Abdominal aortogram produced by the injection of opaque iodine solution into the aorta at the level of the 1st lumbar vertebra. The needle has been introduced through the lumbar region while the patient is under general anesthesia in the prone position. The resulting picture visualized the splenic artery, the renal arteries and several lumbar arteries as well as the aorta and the iliofemoral systems below. Mild arteriosclerotic changes in the vessels are indicated by the slight elongation of the lumbar aorta and the irregularity of the internal and the external iliac arteries.

Fig. 40-13. Abdominal aortogram demonstrating a high obstruction of the abdominal aorta just below the origins of the renal arteries; irregularities at the inferior margin of the column of the dye indicate the upper limits of the clot.

duced without endangering these other structures. In the femoral region, percutaneous introduction of the needle is routine except when the artery seems to be seriously hardened by arteriosclerosis at the site of the proposed puncture. In such instances a short incision may be made under local anesthesia so that the needle can be introduced in as atraumatic a manner as possible.

Visualization of the abdominal aorta rather than of the femoral system is indicated when absence of femoral pulses and the symptoms which are present indicate that the occlusive lesion is at iliac artery level or higher. In

order to produce an *aortogram,* a long relatively large-bore needle is introduced through the left lumbar area directly into the aorta at the level of the first lumbar vertebra with the patient in the prone position. From 5 to 8 cc. of the contrast medium is injected, and a scout film is made. This is for the purpose of determining that the tip of the needle is completely within the lumen of the aorta, rather than partially buried within its wall, or in a branch. The aortogram is made by exposing the film just at the conclusion of the rapid injection of 20 to 40 cc. of the radiopaque substance. The use of a 36-inch x-ray film cassette makes it possible to visualize not only the aorta but also a good portion of the upper part of the femoral system (Figs. 40-12 and 13).

There is a small incidence of complication with aortography which must be accepted in those cases in which the information to be obtained is important. Direct injection into the renal artery or into the superior mesenteric artery may be damaging to the tissues supplied by these vessels. An intramural injection in the wall of the aorta causes damage to the wall with some hemorrhage into the layers of the vessel. This has been known to be sufficiently extensive as to occlude an important vessel, such as a renal artery. The introduction of the needle may of itself cause dislodgment of an arteriosclerotic plaque or a clot lying against the wall of the aorta and produce an acute arterial occlusion of some smaller distal vessel.

Visualization of the thoracic aorta may be done by one of two means. A catheter introduced through one of the arteries in the arm or the leg is passed up to the arch of the aorta and the dye injected through it (Fig. 40-14). The second method of visualizing the thoracic aorta and its branches is by means of contrast medium injected very rapidly into a vein of the arm. The rapid injection causes this material to travel through the right side of the heart and the lungs, back to the left ventricle, without too much dilution. Then it travels on

into the aorta in sufficient concentration to outline it in x-ray films made at that time. If films are made as the dye passes through the cardiac chambers, an angiocardiogram results. If the exposures are made at the time the dye traverses the thoracic aorta, the visualization is termed a transvenous thoracic aortogram.

By use of the aortogram and the peripheral arteriogram, diffuse and segmental forms of arteriosclerosis obliterans and aneurysms may be studied. The dorsal aortogram produced by angiocardiography or aortogram per catheter delineates such lesions of the descending aorta as coarctation of the aorta, aneurysms of the arch or thoracic aorta wherever they may occur, and dissecting aneurysm of the dorsal aorta.

Arteriosclerosis Obliterans

Arteriosclerosis undoubtedly is the commonest pathologic condition of man. Its almost universal appearance during advancing age is evidence of the part played in its production by wear, tear and degeneration. However, the etiology of arteriosclerosis is understood only in broad terms, which include the factors of

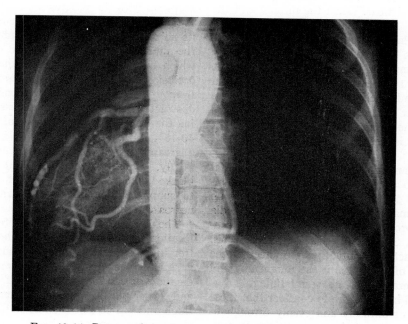

Fig. 40-14. Retrograde aortogram performed by injection through a catheter introduced by way of the left brachial artery. Aortogram shows normal aorta. It also visualizes the coronary arteries and the root of the aorta.

aging and of disturbed metabolism. Evidence of the latter is shown most strongly by the early appearance and the rapid advance of arteriosclerosis in some diabetics.

Pathology. The arterial lesion in arteriosclerosis may be described in terms of its effect on the various layers of the arterial wall. The intima, the subintimal layer, the elastic lamina, the media and the adventitia are involved to varying degrees, and on the basis of the degree to which each is involved, types of arteriosclerosis have been subdivided.

The earliest change observed in arteriosclerosis is the deposition of lipoid material in the subendothelial layer. This primary lesion is called an *atheroma*. This type of change is accelerated in diabetics, but it is often exaggerated and occurs early in certain individuals who are not diabetic. To explain this tendency in occasional individuals, apparently otherwise normal, is impossible now.

The findings in the media characteristic of arteriosclerosis include fibrosis, fragmentation of the elastic fibers, necrosis of areas of the media, hemorrhage, and later calcification of the necrotic or hemorrhagic areas. At present these changes are explained best on the basis of aging and wear. When the intimal and the subintimal layer changes are predominant, producing large plaques, yellow in color, the disease has been termed *atherosclerosis*. The medial change predominates in some patients, producing the pathologic picture of medial sclerosis and calcification. These vessels have a pipestem characteristic. They retain patency of the lumen for a surprising length of time. This is known as *Mönckeburg's medial sclerosis.*

Most commonly, the intimal and the medial changes go on together after initial preponderance of one or the other. The building up of the intima and the thickening of the media result in progressive narrowing of the vascular lumen. This finally leads to thrombosis. Another factor accentuating the effect of the narrowing of the lumen is the roughening and actual ulceration of the vessel lining.

It would be a mistake to consider that these lesions occur diffusely and evenly throughout the arterial system in any one patient. Rather, they develop to various degrees and stages and are distributed in irregular fashion. Severe degeneration in one segment of artery will be adjacent to other segments having moderate or insignificant pathology. The disease of arteriosclerosis obliterans shows a very definite tendency to be segmental and to involve primarily specific areas of the arterial tree. The commonest areas to be involved include the aortic bifurcation (producing the Leriche syndrome, described later), the iliac arteries immediately at the aortic bifurcation, and the superficial femoral artery at two points, one being just below the common femoral bifurcation, and the other at the adductor hiatus. The popliteal bifurcation, the coronary arteries, and cerebral vessels are other points at which segments of occlusion occur.

Course. The clinical characteristics of the disease and its progression are connected intimately to the tendency for segmental occurrence of the individual lesions. The early symptom of claudication becomes disturbing when a significant degree of local obstruction has developed. During the course of development of total occlusion, the progression is usually slow, allowing time for the development of the available collateral circulation. Nutrition of the involved part may not be disturbed at all if the collateral circulation keeps up with the progressing obstruction, so that the distal part of the extremity retains its normal color and resists atrophy of either the muscles or the skin. From this stage, which is usually encountered when a single occlusion has occurred, progression results from upward or downward extension of the obstructing thrombus, progressively obstructing the orifices of the collateral arteries (Fig. 40-15). As these are obstructed in sequence, a greater severity of symptoms occurs, and finally, when enough collateral has been blocked, the blood flow becomes inadequate to support tissue metabolism, and ischemic necrosis develops.

The level of the occlusion determines the location of the symptoms. In the lower extremities, superficial femoral and popliteal arterial occlusion produces intermittent claudication of the foot and the calf, while iliac and lower aortic obstruction may produce thigh and hip claudication as well. A form of claudication also occurs in the upper extremities as a result of occlusion of the subclavian or the axillary arteries. In this condition the patient suffers pain in the muscles of hand,

Fig. 40-15. Femoral arteriogram of a 58-year-old man, showing moderate ischemic changes in the foot. The needle has been introduced into the common femoral artery. The superficial femoral artery is completely occluded from the bifurcation down to the level of the adductor tendon. At this point it is seen to be patent and to contain dye which has been brought to it through collaterals from the profunda femoris branch. The most proximal collateral entering this distal segment is about to be pinched off by the advancing disease. Progressive obstruction of collateral branches above and below an occluded segment is the manner in which arteriosclerosis advances.

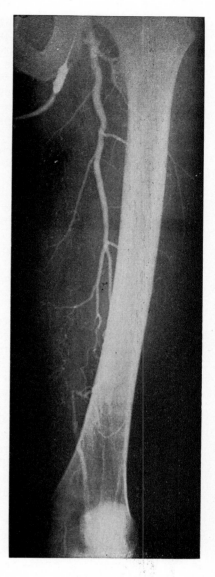

forearm and arm during prolonged activity and is particularly unable to work with the hands raised up over his head.

Attention was drawn to a clinical syndrome typically produced by chronic arteriosclerotic occlusion of the aortic bifurcation by Leriche in 1940.[76] This syndrome, which has been further clarified by others,[37, 97] consists of intermittent claudication of the lower extremities, loss of pulses everywhere in the lower extremities, impotence in male patients and the notable point that the nutrition of the feet remains good over a relatively long period of the disease.

With the exception of the impotence, which probably is due to the diminished arterial pressure within the pelvis, the same type of syndrome is produced also by unilateral or bilateral segmental arteriosclerosis of the iliac arteries or the superficial femoral arteries.

Treatment. GENERAL MANAGEMENT. Curative treatment of the arteriosclerosis is totally lacking. Any study of the histologic picture of well-established arterial lesions convinces one that the changes observed are irreversible. Perhaps at some early stage in which the initial lesion of atheromata is the only manifestations of the disease, some method of alteration of metabolism might in the future be effective. It is clear that the advance which must be sought in the general problem of arteriosclerosis is one of prevention. On the basis of information now available concerning the part played by ingested fats and lipids, some rigid regimen of a dietary nature started very early in life might succeed in producing individuals more free of arteriosclerosis than the average. For obvious reasons a major clinical work in this direction has not been done. Many patients with mild involvement require only general management, while another large group with very advanced disease is seen at a time at which only general management can be applied.

In the peripheral arteries the relief sought generally will be for symptoms of the lower extremities. The first step in treatment of a patient with symptoms in the lower extremities due to arteriosclerosis is a reduction in the work that must be done by the legs. Weight reduction to accomplish this is of prime importance in general management.

It has been amply demonstrated experimentally and clinically that smoking plays a part in the general efficiency of the peripheral arterial circulation. In relation to arteriosclerosis it does so largely through the fact that smoking increases the general vasomotor tone. When a patient with early symptoms of arteriosclerosis, such as intermittent claudication, stops smoking, improvement is frequent.

The third item of general management consists of careful instructions as to foot hygiene and protection from injury. This is important because the reduced arterial supply diminishes the ability of the tissues of the feet to heal traumatic lesions and infections. Even minor skin conditions, such as intertrigo or fungus infection, may lead to disaster and must be avoided.

DRUGS. The class of drugs which seems most likely to aid in the relief of symptoms in arteriosclerosis is the vasodilator group. A wide choice of vasodilators has been offered, and new ones are being added constantly. Their effectiveness can hardly be predicted in individual cases without trial, but most frequently they are disappointing. The principal defect in the use of vasodilator drugs is that they produce a dilatation of all the arteries in the body which are capable of dilating. They are ineffective on the diseased vessels which have become rigid, and the collateral arteries in the area of disease, although dilated, fail to benefit very much because of the general increase of the vascular bed throughout the body.

Substances which diminish the coagulability of the blood are indicated in chronic arterial insufficiency when the pathologic change in the blood vessels is arteriosclerosis. The phenomenon leading to final obstruction of an arterial lumen narrowed by arteriosclerosis is thrombosis. It is doubtful that anticoagulants prevent total occlusion, but there is good reason to believe that the rate of obstruction is slowed. When rapid and temporary alteration in coagulation is desired, heparin is used. For chronic depression of the coagulation system, one of the prothrombin depressing drugs, such as Dicumarol, is indicated.

INDIRECT SURGICAL TREATMENT. Symptomatic improvement in arteriosclerosis may be obtained by indirect surgical means in properly selected cases by removal of an appropriate portion of the sympathetic nervous system.[16, 23, 69] Other indirect means are excision of diseased portions of the artery, supposedly to reduce vasomotor reflexes,[77] and inactivation of the group of muscles most commonly involved in intermittent claudication, by cutting the Achilles tendon.[9] Achilles tenotomy and the operation of simple arteriectomy are not in wide use, and their effectiveness must be said to be in question. When properly selected patients with arteriosclerosis are subjected to sympathectomy, the majority will benefit.

SYMPATHECTOMY. On the basis of experimental evidence surgical ablation of the sympathetic nervous system in the lumbar region for arterial insufficiency of a lower extremity and in the dorsal region for an upper extremity principally improves the circulation of the skin of the part.[115] However, numerous clinical studies indicate that the operation also provides a significant degree of relief from intermittent claudication.[6, 27, 72] It is apparent that there is a very real tendency for a sympathectomy in the lumbar region to increase the rate of development of collateral arterial circulation in the lower extremity.[46] In selecting patients for lumbar sympathectomy, use is made of the fact that the sympathetic system controls the blood flow through the skin. A temporary sympathetic paralysis is produced by introducing procaine into the region directly about the lumbar sympathetic chain. Carefully measuring the changes in skin temperature which result is helpful.

Three types of skin temperature responses occur. In a patient who has a normal arterial system the elevation in skin temperature may vary between 12° and 15° C. In a patient with arterial insufficiency of an organic type which will probably benefit by doing a lumbar sympathectomy, the elevation of temperature may be between 2° and 5°. The third type of response is a fall in the skin temperature in response to sympathetic block. This is observed in advanced cases of arterial insufficiency and is usually taken to contraindicate a lumbar sympathectomy. The test is relatively unreliable unless the observations are made in a comfortable, cool room of stable temperature and humidity. Other observations, such as testing the patient's ability to walk without pain after a procaine sympathetic block has been done, are not generally considered as reliable because the procaine may diffuse to interrupt somatic sensory fibers of the adjacent nerve roots and relieve pain by this method.

DIRECT SURGICAL APPROACH. A large proportion of patients with arteriosclerosis obliterans, particularly of the lower end of the aorta and of the major vessels of the thighs, have a segmental form of the disease. This does not mean that the disease appears in one part of the vessels while the artery above and below the area is normal, but rather that certain areas are found to be in a far more advanced state than the adjacent areas at any given time. By the use of arteriography an estimate can be made of the state of the disease above and below the advanced segment. Three methods of direct surgical approach are

now available for use in these cases which provide for more definitive treatment than can be gained by the indirect technics.[60, 68]

Thrombo-endarterectomy. This type of direct surgery in arteriosclerosis consists of exposure of the segmentally obstructed portion of the artery and removal of the diseased inner coats of the vessel by one technic or another (Fig. 40-16). Thereafter, repair of the more normal muscular layers, usually consisting of about half of the media and the adventitia, is done with fine silk sutures. The opening in the artery through which the diseased portions are removed may be made longitudinally throughout the section of disease or the artery may be opened above and below the segment and the diseased tissue removed with special instruments. After the procedure, the resulting rough lining of the vessel becomes smooth, either by condensation of

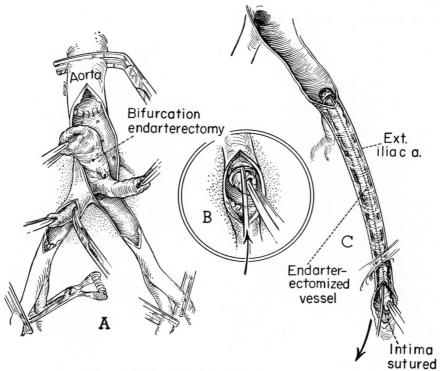

FIG. 40-16. Thrombo-endarterectomy of bifurcation of the aorta, the left iliac and the common femoral arteries. (A) Endarterectomy of bifurcation of the aorta, carried out by direct incision and dissection. Intima in the right common iliac has been sutured down. (B) Further endarterectomy of the left external iliac and the common femoral carried out by Cannon type stripper. (C) Illustrates endarterectomized vessel with core being removed.

fibrous tissue or by the direct growth of intima from each end.[4, 5, 14, 31, 62, 78, 103, 118, 119]

RESTORATION WITH VASCULAR GRAFTS. Grafts are used to restore the circulation in the presence of segmental occlusion of an artery. Sometimes they are implanted after complete excision of the segment, during which the ends of the artery above and below the area of disease are prepared for anastomosis to the grafts in an end-to-end fashion. Much more frequently, grafts are implanted as *by-pass* grafts. In this type of graft, the graft is installed simply by connecting it end-to-side to the diseased blood vessel above and below the area of obstruction.[18, 73, 83]

The by-pass method of installation of a graft has the great advantage of reducing the amount of surgical trauma, because it is not necessary to remove the obstructed segment of artery. The collateral arteries which remain open are preserved by this method (Fig. 40-17).

For either method of implantation, the grafts in common use are autogenous vein grafts, usually the saphenous vein, and prosthetic appliances woven of synthetic fiber yarns, such as Dacron or Teflon. Homologous grafts consisting of human aortic bifurcations were the type first used in treatment of abdominal aortic aneurysms and of obstructions of the bifurcation of the aorta when these lesions were initially successfully subjected to curative surgery. The convenience and the high degree of reliability of prosthetic materials has caused them virtually to replace the use of homologous arteries.[61] The autogenous vein grafts which were the first type of graft used for reconstruction of the femoral artery have continued to be a favored material, having the specific disadvantage that the saphenous vein of a certain proportion of patients is unsuitable in length or diameter for this purpose.

RENAL ARTERY DISEASE

Disturbances of the blood supply of the

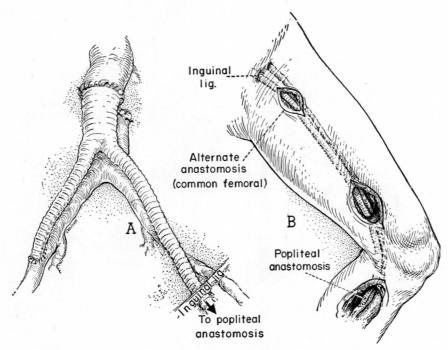

FIG. 40-17. By-pass technic of restoring flow in cases of arterial obstruction. (A) By-pass of obstruction of bifurcation of the aorta with end-to-end anastomosis to aorta above and closure of end of patient's aorta. Distal end-to-side to right external iliac. (B) By-pass on the left side carried under the inguinal ligament and down to the popliteal artery.

kidney are produced by a variety of arterial lesions, some of which have surgical importance. In the investigation of patients for the cause of hypertension or renal insufficiency it is of great practical importance to differentiate surgically correctable arterial lesions from arterial and arteriolar disease not treatable by mechanical means and from primary parenchymal lesions as well as from conditions involving the urinary tract (renal pelvis, ureters, bladder and urethra).

There is a definite relationship between renal blood flow and the systemic blood pressure.[56] The experimental background was provided by the valuable work of Goldblatt[45] in showing that arterial hypertension resulted from experimentally induced stenosis of the renal artery in dogs. The analogous relationship occurs spontaneously in man in a variety of abnormal situations.

Etiology. Disturbances of renal blood flow causing systemic arterial hypertension result from congenital narrowing of the arterial supply to the kidney. This narrowing may be as far proximal to the renal artery as the thoracic aorta where a "coarctation" produces elevated blood pressure at least in part because it changes the character of renal arterial inflow. Coarctation of the abdominal aorta above the renal arteries, also occurring as a congenital lesion, similarly causes hypertension. Parenthetically, it should be noted that complete occlusion of the aorta below the renal arteries does not per se cause hypertension. Congenital narrowing of one or both renal arteries causes hypertension and, in contrast with thoracic and abdominal aortic coarctation, the elevation of blood pressure is present in the lower extremities as well as in the upper.

The renal arteries themselves are more commonly affected by acquired lesions than by congenital ones. Two forms are presently recognized. One consists of a typical atheroma of the renal artery, usually close to the origin of the vessel but sometimes seen at other points in the renal artery or its main branches. The second lesion consists of a hypertrophy of the media of the artery which results in a localized stenosis.

Pathophysiology. These arterial lesions are found on one or both sides. In either event they rarely fail to cause a sustained systolic and diastolic hypertension probably because

the kidney is stimulated to produce abnormal amounts of vasopressor substances. Suppression of renal function need not be of such a degree as to cause nitrogen retention even in bilateral lesions. Disturbances in filtration are detected by clearance studies. This provides clear evidence when only one renal artery is involved and is more difficult to interpret when both sides are affected. In unilateral disease, the lesion tends to protect the involved kidney from arteriolar damage by the blood pressure elevation that it has produced. It does cause the involved kidney to become smaller while the contralateral kidney hypertrophies and often suffers progressive arteriolar damage because of the hypertension.

The frequency of renal artery stenosis as a cause of hypertension in comparison with parenchymal renal disease or intrarenal arterial disease is not clearly known. Its frequency in any given series of hypertensive patients is proportional to the amount of effort expended in looking for it.

Diagnosis. The finding of a bruit over the kidney area may suggest renal artery stenosis. The absolute diagnosis of renal artery stenosis depends on its demonstration by roentgenograms. Renal arteriograms may be made by injection of contrast medium into the suprarenal aorta through a needle introduced by the translumbar route or through a catheter passed upward to the renal level of the aorta from the femoral artery below (Fig. 40-18). By either route, this examination is somewhat imposing as to time, discomfort and possible dangers. Therefore, other tests are used to screen hypertensive patients before renal arteriograms are done.

None of the "screening" tests is of certain reliability, and either new methods or improvements are needed. History of onset of the hypertension, age and presence of atherosclerotic lesions elsewhere are of little value. Asymmetry of kidney size as seen in a plain roentgenogram of the abdomen suggests stenosis on the side of the smaller kidney but may also be a normal congenital variation or due to unilateral pyelonephritis.

Differential renal function studies often provide a strong lead in unilateral disease. An excretory urogram (intravenous pyelogram) in which additional x-ray exposures are

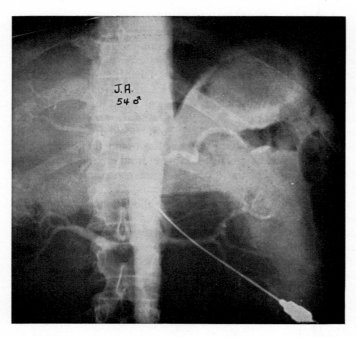

Fig. 40-18. Translumbar renal arteriogram, showing severe stenosis of the right renal artery near its origin. Obstruction was bypassed by graft from the aorta to renal artery.

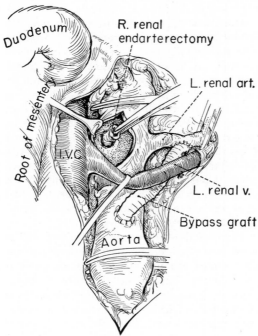

Fig. 40-19. Renal artery reconstruction. Two of the methods used to relieve obstruction to the renal arteries. Endarterectomy of the right renal artery by the transaortic route is shown. On the left a by-pass graft is used from the aorta to the left renal artery.

made ½, 1 and 2 minutes after injection of the dye is a simple form of differential renal function test.

Treatment requires reconstruction of the renal artery in order to eliminate the stenosis. A variety of technics is available; some are shown in Figure 40-19. Thromboendarterectomy, by-pass graft and reimplantation of the artery into the aorta are commonly done.[26, 87, 91, 99, 112] Anastomosis of the splenic artery to the renal artery has been carried out with success.

ARTERIAL INSUFFICIENCY AFFECTING THE BRAIN

The technics of restorative vascular surgery are applicable to obstructing lesions of the arteries supplying the brain. The principal lesion affecting the cerebral circulation is arteriosclerosis.

Blood supply of the brain is vulnerable to arteriosclerotic lesions in both the extracranial and the intracranial portions of the arteries involved. The extracranial vessels in which obstructions can be relieved by surgery are the paired internal carotid arteries and the vertebral arteries. Internal carotid blood flow can be impeded by lesions of the vessel itself between the common carotid bifurcation and the skull, or by any lesion of the common carotid artery proximal to its bifurcation.[19, 40, 52, 110] The arteries of this system are accessible to surgical repair in all parts of their extracranial course. The vertebral arterial flow can be interfered with at any point in the artery itself or by lesions of the subclavian artery proximal to the vertebral origin. The vertebral artery is accessible to surgical repair only in its proximal portion.

Surgical repair of these vessels must be done before irreversible brain damage has resulted from ischemia. In a general way, patients with cerebral ischemia can be divided into groups which are related to the selection of individuals for surgical treatment. Group I consists of patients who suffer transient episodes of cerebral ischemia. These episodes are manifested by a great variety of symptoms, common among which are dizziness or fainting, visual disturbances, aphasia and muscular weakness or lack of co-ordination. Between attacks, these patients are essentially normal. In general, the lesion responsible for attacks of this type is a partial occlusion or stenosis of one of the arteries. Group II consists of patients who show the gradual development of a neurologic deficit which does not prove to be transient. Actually, these patients are those who are seen in the early stages of an arterial occlusion which, if not relieved, will lead to a brain infarct. These patients must have relief of the obstruction early in order for surgery to be useful. In later stages, relief of the obstruction which is almost invariably a total one does not affect the irreversible brain damage. The third group of patients are those with multiple bilateral cerebral deficiencies. These patients may have multiple lesions of the carotid and the vertebral systems, some of the lesions being intracranial, and relief of partial occlusions of the extracranial vessels may be of some benefit.

Diagnosis. The diagnosis of an arteriosclerotic lesion in the carotid or vertebral artery can often be made on history and physical examination alone. The history of various symptoms related to the carotid-vertebral systems as pointed out in prior paragraphs may suggest a lesion involving one or both of these arteries. Physical examination revealing bruits over the stenosed vessel, such as the bifurcation of the carotid artery, or striking differences in amplitude of the carotid

pulse strongly supports the suspicion. This bruit may also be heard at the base of the neck in instances of stenosis of the origin of the vertebral artery. Digital compression of the uninvolved carotid artery will very quickly lead to cerebral signs in a patient who has a stenosis or an obstruction of the contralateral vessel, while the patient will withstand very well compression of the carotid artery on the side of the disease. The definitive diagnosis is provided by arteriograms which show the various portions of the carotid and vertebral systems. A single arteriogram made by the rapid intravenous injection of a bolus of dye with multiple x-ray exposures in rapid sequence of the upper dorsal and cervical region will often succeed in showing both systems in a single x-ray examination. If necessary, more complete visualization can be obtained by direct injection into either carotid artery or by retrograde injection of dye through a catheter into the arch of the aorta (Fig. 40-20).

Treatment. After a stenosing lesion has been amply localized by physical examination and arteriography, the obstruction to blood flow may be relieved by one of several different technics. The most common locations of stenosing lesions are the proximal portions of the internal carotid artery and of the vertebral artery. In partial carotid artery stenosis, endarterectomy is generally successful in restoring circulation. In the period of total occlusion of the circulation through the vessel which is being operated upon, a small plastic tube is used as a temporary shunt to avoid the possibility of damage to the brain (Fig. 40-21). The ostium of the vertebral artery is approached through a longitudinal incision in the subclavian artery, and endarterectomy is carried out up into the vessel. When long segments of obstruction are present in the carotid system, and when the carotid obstruction is at the origin of the innominate artery or the left carotid artery from the aortic arch, a by-pass graft may be used. In such a case, this graft must extend from the aorta to the common carotid artery or the internal carotid artery, by-passing all of the disease in that system.[24, 57, 79, 88, 104]

The results of such surgery are best in patients with partial obstructing lesions. In such persons, recovery is usually complete and

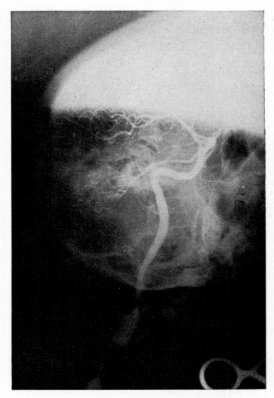

Fig. 40-20. Carotid angiogram, outlining stenosis of the internal carotid artery at its origin. The external carotid artery is not seen. This obstruction was relieved by endarterectomy.

very gratifying. These patients are not only relieved of their attacks of intermittent cerebral ischemia, but they are also relieved of the imminent day-to-day danger of complete thrombosis of the stenosed arterial segment which would be likely to cause a major stroke and a brain infarct.

Buerger's Disease—
Thromboangiitis Obliterans

Thromboangiitis obliterans is an inflammatory disease of unknown etiology of arteries and veins and of the adjacent nerves. Its inflammatory nature contrasts sharply with the degenerative, metabolic nature of arteriosclerosis. The terms "thromboangiitis obliterans" and "Buerger's disease" are used interchangeably. The condition occurs most often in young men and has its onset between the ages of 20 and 35. It involves the extremities pre-

dominantly and is more frequent in the lower extremities than in the upper. It is seen occasionally in the vessels of the viscera, such as the heart, the brain and the mesenteric vessels. It is characteristically a disease of medium-sized arteries, such as the posterior tibial, the anterior tibial, the ulnar and the radial arteries.

Leo Buerger's name (1879-1943) is applied to the condition because of his classical description of the disease in 1908.[13] This was not the first description of the condition, the first being by von Winiwarter in 1879.[117] Buerger's description was based on a study of 11 amputated limbs showing chronic arterial occlusion of this type.

Etiology. The specific etiology is not known. Secondary etiologic features which have a positive effect on the disease include age, sex, race, heredity and tobacco. Sex and age have been mentioned already. Heredity is an uncertain factor included because of the occasional occurrence of more than one case of Buerger's disease in a family. The higher incidence in Jewish people, as was assumed by Buerger, does not exist. However, the condition is rare in the colored race, but one instance of the disease has appeared in our series in a colored woman. Tobacco is the strongest secondary etiologic factor in the disease. Buerger's disease has rarely been described in nonsmokers, and all attempts at alleviating the condition fail in patients who continue to smoke. The etiologies of bacteria or virus, fungus and sensitivity to fungus have been suggested and explored, but none has been substantiated.

The suspicion must be entertained that thromboangiitis obliterans is not etiologically a single condition. It may be a common entity with many etiologies brought together by similar clinical features and pathologic appearances.

Symptoms. The symptoms in Buerger's disease are those which arise from the arterial occlusion, those which depend upon the inflammatory nature of the lesions, and those resulting from the breakdown of the tissues rendered ischemic by the arterial occlusion.

The symptoms of arterial insufficiency depend upon the area involved and the caliber of the vessels primarily attacked. Intermittent claudication occurs but is less frequent than in arteriosclerosis obliterans because, instead of attacking such major channels as the femoral artery, producing ischemia of the gastrocnemius group of muscles, the disease occurs in the smaller vessels named earlier, producing extensive tissue damage in many instances without there ever having been claudication.

The symptoms which result from the inflammatory nature of the condition are those of direct irritation of the adjacent sensory nerves producing intense pain and those resulting from the associated thrombophlebitis as the disease affects the vein. The symptoms produced by the involvement of the veins are not in any way characteristic, but the habit of the disease to affect short segments of superficial veins is a striking feature. Such superficial phlebitis occurs in short segments and in a migratory manner. Red, painful lumps appear under the skin, progressively heal and then occur in other areas over a variable

length of time. The favorite sites for these segments of segmental thrombophlebitis are over the lower extremities, although they have been seen in many areas of the body, including the upper extremity. The presence of migrating phlebitis, in the absence of obvious local cause, should raise the question of Buerger's disease.

Pathology. The lesions of superficial phlebitis may precede or accompany the acute stage of the disease and have often been biopsied. The microscopic picture found in these lesions may or may not show the histologic changes which are thought to be characteristic of the acute stage as it occurs in arteries. In the early stage the arteries show a panarteritis in which all of the layers of the artery are involved in an inflammatory reaction with a relatively sparse distribution of chronic inflammatory cells. A characteristic part of the picture is the early appearance of a diffuse sprinkling of multinucleated giant cells. Thickening of the intima progresses rapidly, and thrombosis of the lumen occurs. Organization and fibrosis of the entire artery proceeds, and

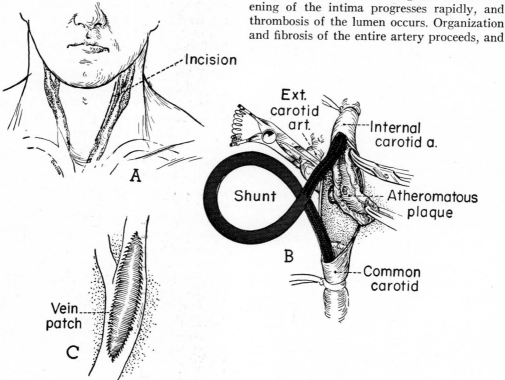

FIG. 40-21. Endarterectomy of common and the internal carotid arteries. (A) Incision over the anterior border of the sternocleidomastoid muscle. (B) Endarterectomy of the common carotid and the internal carotid, using a by-pass shunt. (C) Patch of autogenous vein or synthetic material is used to enlarge the lumen in certain cases.

in the subsided stage the vessels which have been involved are represented by fibrous cords containing a large number of small vascular channels. These vascular channels are discontinuous and do not represent an efficient recanalization of the artery. At any time in an individual active case of Buerger's disease, various stages of acute, subsiding and healed lesions are present. There are inflammation and thrombosis of the concomitant veins. This dual involvement is the basis of the name thromboangiitis obliterans rather than thromboarteritis obliterans. The accompanying perivascular inflammation involves the entire neurovascular bundle, producing a dual type of pain from involvement of sensory nerves as well as from ischemia of tissues below the vascular obstruction.

Clinical Course. The most characteristic feature of the acute stage is an appearance of pain and erythema with a co-existing coolness of the skin which is due to mechanical obstruction of the vessels and to some degree of vasospasm. A tenacity of the acute stage is often observed because new segments of the medium-sized arteries of an extremity are progressively involved with the lesion and, although healing of the initial lesions may have occurred, the new ones keep the process alive. This part of the course is completely unpredictable. Even under the best management it may be self-sustaining and be terminated only by the appearance of gangrene extensive enough to require amputation. In other instances the acute process dies out, and the patient is left with some degree of arterial insufficiency. Symptoms during the subsided stage of the disease depend upon how much arterial occlusion has occurred during the acute process.

Treatment. The relationship between superficial phlebitis of the migratory type and Buerger's disease is strong enough to suspect the disease in any patient displaying it and even to call this lesion a part of the premonitory stage of the disease. Suspicion of this disease is the signal for complete abstinence from tobacco and the institution of a variety of other supportive measures, none of which are nearly so specific. These include the eradication of areas of infection about the body, avoidance of exposure to cold, maintenance of good hydration and a regimen of sufficient rest and adequate diet, to bring the patient into the maximum possible state of health.

During the acute stage bed rest with sedation is absolutely required because of the pain. All measures should be aimed at the prevention and the reduction of swelling of the affected part. A very frequent characteristic of the pain suffered is that it becomes worse when the extremity is kept in an elevated position. Therefore, dependency is insisted upon by the patient, edema results, and the atmosphere for healing or combating of the inflammation is made less favorable by the increased intercellular fluid. Antibiotics do not seem to be indicated except in those cases in which a skin lesion goes on to the point of ulceration. Then antibiotics may be used to combat the secondary invaders. Heat is contraindicated as a direct application to the affected part but may be helpful when it is applied elsewhere to the body to produce reflex vasodilatation in the extremity. This does not appear to be too important because it is obvious from examination of the skin color that much vasodilatation is already present in response to the inflammation. During the acute stage, however, the extremity may show a tendency to become sensitive to the vasoconstrictor stimuli, such as environmental coolness and emotional upset. Then, vasodilators and heat to the abdomen particularly may be indicated. All efforts should be spent on bringing the patient through the acute stage of the disease with the minimum of tissue damage and loss. Sometimes amputation will be required in acute patients whose pain cannot be relieved otherwise.

After the acute process has subsided, the degree of arterial insufficiency with which the patient has been left is estimated. Sympathectomy and amputations are done then as they are indicated and necessary. Sympathectomy is applied when the patient is left with a cold, temperature-sensitive foot or hand. Peripheral gangrenous ulcers are indications for sympathectomy. More extensive ischemic necrosis requires amputation.

ANGIOSPASTIC CONDITIONS

The vascular system, and particularly the capillary bed, constantly fluctuates in its caliber in response to needs for blood flow, heat loss or preservation, or of secretory activity. Portions of the body principally affected by this constant change are the various mucosal surfaces and the skin of the hands and the feet. The effective stimuli other than actual physiologic need are the external application of heat and cold and emotional experience. The simplest form of derangement of this normal vasomotor mechanism is seen in persons who chronically have an increased vasomotor tonus in the hands and the feet so that these parts are always cold. This is sometimes distinctly uncomfortable but not necessarily a pathologic state.

The system is subject to pathologic states in which there is an abnormal sensitivity to the vasoconstrictor influence of exposure to cold and emotional disturbances. These responses occur largely where the density of vasomotor control is greatest, primarily in the skin of the hands and the feet. The most severe pathologic vasomotor phenomena follow a routine set of changes. In sequence, the skin color rapidly becomes white, due to arteriolar and capillary spasm, and then goes through stages of a blue cyanotic color, rubor, finally returning to normal. This progression of changes occurs as a result of a variety of underlying causes so as to suggest that the exaggerated response to a vasoconstrictor stimulus is in some way self-limited. It is not difficult to theorize a sequence of events beginning with diffuse arteriolar spasm producing the dead white appearance, which, causing an ischemic paralysis of the arteriolar muscle, leads to a stage of wide dilatation. Since the capillary-venule end of the system is most severely subject to hypoxia, it dilates first, allowing a back-filling of the gradually opening capillaries and producing a cyanotic skin color. As arterial blood is finally admitted by anoxic paralysis of the arterial end of the capillary loop, the dilated capillaries are flushed with red blood, and rubor results. In a few moments the arteriolar and capillary walls are oxygenated, and normal tonus is re-established.

The name of Raynaud's phenomenon is given to these changes on the basis of the classical description by Raynaud in 1862.[102] His thesis was entitled "On the Local Asphyxia and Symmetrical Gangrene of the Extremities." He considered the condition to be a pathologic entity. His theory based the defect on a fault in the vasomotor nerves supplying the part of the body which is affected without there being any arterial lesion per se.

The original report of Raynaud contained not only the cases which actually consisted of a functional vasomotor disturbance but also a number in which he did not recognize that arterial disease was present. We now classify patients who show this form of vasoconstrictor response into 3 groups: (1) those in whom there is apparently no primary arterial pathology; (2) those having an underlying arterial disease; and (3) a group presenting this vasomotor response because of trauma, scleroderma, certain nerve lesions and poisonings with ergot or such metals as lead. In recent years the 1st group has retained the name of Raynaud's disease. The 2nd and the 3rd groups are said to exhibit "Raynaud's phenomenon" attributable to an arterial disease or to the other etiologic agents.

Raynaud's Disease. The group remaining under the name of Raynaud's disease shows age and sex preponderance. More than three quarters of the patients presenting this complaint are women. The onset of the condition is usually between the ages of 15 and 35 years. The patients frequently are emotionally immature or inadequate. The earlier symptoms of the condition occur in the most highly innervated parts of the body in response to strong vasomotor constrictor stimuli. This results in the hands being the common primary site of the reaction and the response first occurring during local exposure to very cold water or ice or during a severe emotional upset. Later the response is noted in wider areas, that is to say, spreading from one finger to all the fingers and then to other less innervated parts, such as the feet. The reaction is caused by progressively lesser stimuli. The color changes described earlier vary in individual severity but all are present in most patients.

The disease is strongly bilateral and symmetrical. There is usually some numbness associated with the stage of pallor, particularly if it lasts very long, but pain is not present. The parts involved are quite normal between the attacks until the condition has been present for a long time. Ischemic necrosis is not observed frequently, and when it is present after years of affliction, the areas of necrosis are very small; they occur on the fingertips, heal rapidly and leave pinhead-size depressed scars. Pain occurs in Raynaud's disease while these ischemic necrotic areas are present. It is characteristic that the pulses of the extremities remain undisturbed.

Severe cases of Raynaud's disease lead to varying degrees of handicap due to the frequency of attacks and the repeated occurrence of small painful ulcers. After a long course of the disease, the skin of the fingers and the hands becomes thickened, and there is an excessive dryness. The soft tissues of the distal parts of the fingers become atrophied, and the characteristic tapered appearance of late Raynaud's disease becomes manifest.

TREATMENT. The general management which immediately suggests itself in the treatment of Raynaud's disease is the protection of the subject from the stimuli which cause the vasomotor response. Reassurance and avoidance of cold exposure are important. Therapy with drugs is relatively difficult because of the long, chronic course of the condition. Vasodilator drugs which may be taken frequently over a long period of time would be indicated. The results obtained with the best available drugs are usually disappointing.

Surgical removal of the controlling region of the sympathetic nervous system, which ought to be completely curative if the lesion were simply an abnormal vasomotor reflex, produces only comparative relief of the symptoms in reducing the frequency of the attacks and increasing the stimulus required for production. The fact that the attacks are not completely relieved by sympathectomy indicates that there is a local vascular sensitivity in effect which, in part, produces the condition. It is the opinion of most that sympathectomy should be reserved for severe cases and particularly applied in those cases showing the minute areas of necrosis characteristic of the disease.

Consistent reconsideration of the diagnosis in order to pick up an underlying organic pathologic condition is important.

Raynaud's Phenomenon. The same type of color reaction in response to cold and emotion is seen in a group of patients in whom a distinct underlying cause is present. The underlying conditions responsible are fairly diverse. This lends weight to the idea that the vasoconstrictor phenomenon which is observed is a fundamental pathologic response.

Intrinsic vascular disease, particularly in the upper extremity, of both the degenerative and the inflammatory types, is frequently a cause of Raynaud's phenomenon. The suspicion of an underlying arterial disease as a cause should be aroused when an individual patient diverges from the pattern of the condition typical to Raynaud's disease. An asymmetrical appearance of the disturbance should raise suspicion of an arterial disease. Raynaud's phenomenon developing in a patient beyond the age of 35 suggests arteriosclerosis, and the occurrence in a male indicates the possibility very strongly. Loss of pulses or more extensive gangrene than that described is further evidence of arterial disease. When pain is an important symptom in an individual case, the indication is that an underlying pathologic state exists.

Raynaud's phenomenon is also frequently associated with the early stages of *scleroderma*. Some confusion in its relation to scleroderma results from the fact that in the very late stages of Raynaud's disease the fibrosis, atrophy and stiffening of the skin resembles scleroderma. However, the sequence of events under both circumstances should be fairly clear. Raynaud's phenomenon occurs early in scleroderma, before and during the edematous stage. On the other hand, sclerodermatous change in Raynaud's disease is a late feature after a long progressive course. Furthermore, scleroderma associated with Raynaud's phenomenon may be generalized; on the other hand, sclerodermatous changes in Raynaud's disease are localized to the involved portions of the extremity.

Scalenus anticus syndrome, herniated cervical disk, chronic lead poisoning, ergotism or trauma to the extremity of a type which produces a post-traumatic sympathetic dystrophy, cervical ribs, all occasionally bring about the vasomotor discharges of Raynaud's disease.

The importance of designating a definite pathologic condition as the cause of any case of Raynaud's phenomenon leads to the constant search for new signs in patients thought to have Raynaud's disease. In every such instance the proper treatment of the patient will be directed against the underlying condition, if such therapy is available, rather than against the phenomenon.

ARTERIAL ANEURYSM

A true aneurysm is a dilatation of an artery produced when the elastic property of the vessel wall is lost because of a disease process. This loss of elasticity renders the wall unable to return to its unexpanded size following each stretching force of the systolic thrust of the blood stream. Progressive enlargement is the rule. A true arterial aneurysm is to be differentiated from the false aneurysm or pulsating hematoma resulting from trauma which has been described on page 1089 (Fig. 40-22).

CLASSIFICATION

Anatomic. The shape of the distended structure serves to classify the lesion in anatomic terms as fusiform or saccular. A *fusiform aneurysm* is one in which the dilatation is diffuse and results in the development of a spindle-shaped lesion. A diffuse change in the arterial wall and the general application of pressure from within are required for its production.

The *saccular type of aneurysm* is a bulbous expansion of a portion of the circumference of the arterial wall. This results from a more localized change in the vessel, allowing a patch of the artery to expand, or from a more localized application of pressure from within due to a jet stream of the blood impinging against a localized area of the artery wall.

Etiologic. Aneurysms are classified in terms other than anatomic on the basis of the disease which injures the wall. The causes of aneurysm are not known except for arteriosclerosis, syphilis and pyogenic infection. Other etiologies, such as trauma or congenital absence of elastic properties of an artery or a portion of an artery, are less well known. It is theoretically possible for a true aneurysm to be produced by trauma to a normal artery.

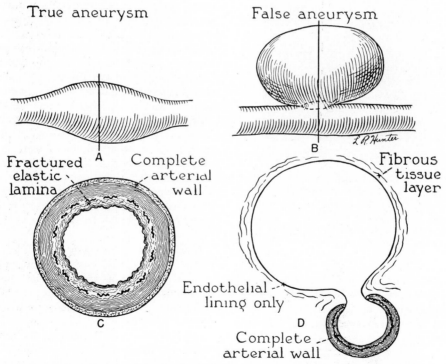

FIG. 40-22. Differentiation between true arterial aneurysm and false aneurysm. A cross section of a true aneurysm is shown (C), illustrating the presence of all vascular layers in entire circumference of lesion. (D) The only vascular layer present in the pulsating hematoma is the endothelial lining, which is present if the lesion has been in existence long enough for its growth.

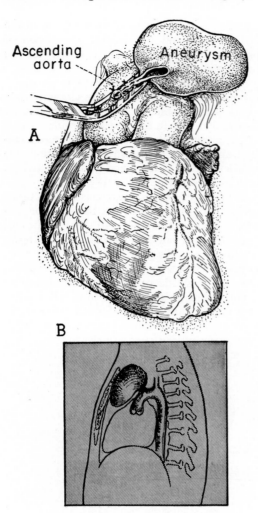

FIG. 40-23. Lateral aneurysmectomy performed for a saccular aneurysm of the aortic arch. (A) Resection of aneurysm without reduction of the aortic lumen. (B) Lateral view, showing small size of the neck of the aneurysmal sac.

This would occur if a moderate crushing injury or high-speed missile damaged the arterial wall without hemorrhage or occlusion, the blood pressure later expanding the damaged area.

SYPHILITIC ANEURYSMS

Syphilitic aneurysms are commonly saccular and occur primarily in the upper thoracic aorta, usually on the arch. Infection involves all of the vessel coats, producing an inflam-

matory infiltration of the media and the adventitia and a spotty destruction of the elastic lamina. As the condition heals the repair is by the production of inelastic scar tissue. The dilatation that produces an aneurysm is the commonest complication of syphilitic aortitis. These aneurysms grow to compress and erode the adjacent structures.

Symptoms. Their symptomatology depends entirely on the effect on their surroundings. Pain, cough, hoarseness and dysphagia are common symptoms, and dyspnea is a symptom more on the basis of an accompanying aortic regurgitation than it is of compression of the trachea. Impingement upon the superior vena cava produces the typical signs of a plethora in the arms and the head with increasing congestion and elevated venous pressure upon bending or stooping.

Diagnosis of a syphilitic aneurysm by examination occasionally is made on the basis of palpation of the pulsating mass through the intercostal spaces and in the sternal notch. Pulses in the upper extremities are usually unequal. Paralysis of one vocal cord, almost always the left, tug on the trachea, and deviation of the trachea, are important signs. A Horner's syndrome may be present because of impingement of the aneurysm on the upper dorsal sympathetic ganglia. The x-ray appearance of the lesion always must be differentiated from that of a mediastinal tumor. On fluoroscopy the pulsatile nature of an aneurysm may be observed, but inasmuch as the wall of the aneurysm is inelastic, almost by definition, the pulsation is much less than might be expected and may be entirely absent. The x-ray examination for aneurysm may be carried much further by doing an angiocardiogram.

Treatment. CONSERVATIVE. The chemotherapeutic treatment of the underlying disease, if it has not already been thoroughly accomplished, is an important primary requirement. Supportive measures directed to relief of symptoms of compression on adjacent structures are not likely to be successful. Palliative surgery has been applied, consisting of division of the sternum or excision of a portion of the sternum overlying the aneurysm in order to give more space and relieve compression of the trachea or the esophagus. The relief obtained by such treatment is temporary because the aneurysm continues to grow and fills the new space made available to it. Stimulation of the development of a thrombus within the aneurysm by threading coils of tightly wound wire was done frequently in the past with meager results in truly large symptomatic aneurysms.

Surgical. More direct surgical therapy, consisting of resection of all or part of the diseased vessel wall and re-establishing continuity, offers the most in these patients, although presently at a high expense in operative mortality. This is done in two ways. *Lateral aneurysmectomy* (Fig. 40-23) consists of removal of the lateral expanded wall of the saccular aneurysm by clamping it at its base

and oversewing the edges left by the resection.[3] *Resection and grafting* (Fig. 40-24) consists of removal of the entire length of involved aorta and replacing the defect with a graft.[3, 21, 75]

This method is also used in dissecting aneurysm of the thoracic aorta just distal to the left subclavian artery. The salvage rate is greater with this type of dissecting aneurysm than with those originating near the aortic valve. Here a decompression type of operation is done. Aneurysms involving the arch of the aorta, where it is necessary to occlude the branches of the arch during resection, require the use of a cardiopulmonary by-pass and temporary shunts to the carotid arteries

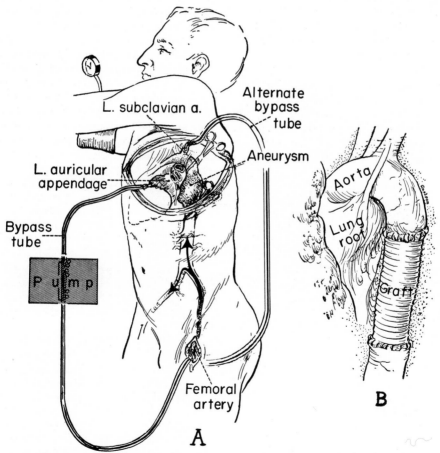

FIG. 40-24. Resection of aneurysm of descending thoracic aorta. (A) Temporary shunts are used to offset the changes resulting from crossclamping the aorta. Shunts from the left subclavian or the left auricular appendage are used. (B) Following resection of the aneurysm, a graft is inserted, and then the shunts are removed.

as well as coronary artery perfusion. Temporary by-passes alone may be used if the area involved is limited.

ARTERIOSCLEROTIC ANEURYSM

Sites. Arteriosclerotic aneurysms have been known to appear in almost all major arterial channels in the body. In the intra-abdominal viscera they develop in the mesenteric, the splenic, the renal and the hepatic arteries. More peripherally, the carotid artery, the brachial, the femoral and the popliteal arteries are sites. The most common peripheral site is the popliteal artery. The commonest location of an arteriosclerotic aneurysm is the aortic bifurcation producing a mid-line lower abdominal pulsating mass. Aneurysms of the remainder of the aorta diminish in incidence progressively upward so that the arch and the upper descending aorta are involved comparatively rarely with an arteriosclerotic aneurysm. The symptomatology produced by aneurysms is entirely dependent upon location.

Aneurysms of the commonest sites, the abdominal aorta and the popliteal artery, will be discussed to illustrate the dependence of the symptoms upon the location of the aneurysm, the diagnosis of aneurysm, and the treatment that may be applied.

Aneurysm of the Popliteal Artery. ETIOLOGY. Loss of elasticity of the popliteal segment with resulting expansion of the size of the vessel occurs in the presence of diffuse arteriosclerosis. When it reaches the clinical stature of an aneurysm, it is usually brought to the patient's attention by his discovery of a pulsating area or pulsating mass behind the knee, and he experiences some discomfort and annoyance when the affected side is crossed over the other leg. An aneurysm produces some obstruction to the flow of blood because it disturbs the smooth pattern of blood flow through a normal artery. The elongation of the vessel which accompanies the dilatation also causes obstruction (Fig. 40-25). Therefore, the patient may have some degree of intermittent claudication of the calf muscles when he walks. As the aneurysm grows it causes pain by compression of adjacent nerves and can produce swelling of the leg below the knee because it compresses the popliteal vein. The patient begins to experience difficulty in extending the knee, and a form of flexion contracture develops simply because of the mass in the popliteal space.

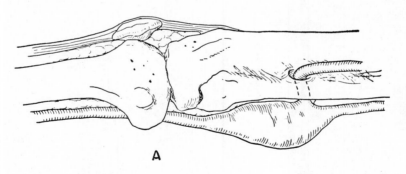

A

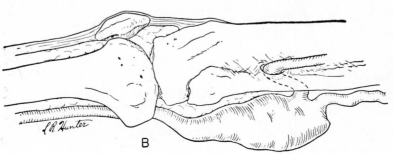

B

Fig. 40-25. Popliteal aneurysm illustrating the elongation which occurs along with the dilatation. This serves to obstruct the branches of the artery, particularly the anterior tibial as shown in (B) and is one of the mechanisms by which popliteal aneurysm causes chronic arterial obstruction.

COMPLICATIONS. Two complications of popliteal aneurysm are frequent. These are acute thrombosis of the aneurysm and rupture of the aneurysmal wall. *Acute thrombosis* causes sudden ischemia of the extremity with ensuing gangrene unless treatment is successful. *Rupture of a popliteal aneurysm* results in a massive increase in the swelling because of blood loss into the tissues. The blood loss dissects its way up through Hunter's canal to fill the fascial compartments of the thigh and downward into the calf where the limited available space usually prevents very much blood loss in this direction. Exsanguination does not occur, and the maximum effect of a ruptured popliteal aneurysm is rapidly progressive deterioration of the blood supply to the leg and gangrene.

TREATMENT. The earliest rational surgical treatment of popliteal aneurysm was the *surgical ligation of the femoral popliteal segment of artery above the lesion.* This operation has been explained best as a part of the work of Hunter in a description by one of his students, the ligation being done in the adductor canal which bears his name.[111] The ligation did not always result in gangrene of the leg, depending upon the effectiveness of the collateral circulation which had developed about the knee in response to the long-standing presence of the aneurysm.

A far better technic of taking care of popliteal aneurysm was introduced by Rudolph Matas[90] who opened directly into the aneurysm, evacuated the clots which were within it and then, without further dissection which might damage the collateral arteries, sutured the orifices of the artery entering and leaving the aneurysm from the inside of the aneurysmal sac. Much of the remaining sac was then sutured in upon the aneurysm cavity, portions of the redundant wall being resected. This operation known as *endo-aneurysmorrhaphy* results in about 10 per cent incidence of gangrene of the leg. In addition to this obliterative type of operation, Matas also used a technic which restored arterial continuity. He folded down the trimmed aneurysmal wall, suturing it in place to leave a lumen. Further improvement in the treatment consisted of *combining complete resection of the aneurysm with a lumbar sympathectomy.* The lumbar sympathectomy was depended upon to improve the efficiency of the collateral circulation and to prevent spasm of the arteries adjacent to the operative site. In the hands of surgeons who have reported on this operation the incidence of gangrene has been essentially zero.[55, 80]

The most definitive and reparative type of surgery for this lesion consists of *removal of the aneurysm followed by the implantation of a suitable vein, artery or prosthetic graft* sutured to the carefully prepared ends of the popliteal artery above and below the lesion. Although this grafting was done very early by Pringle in 1913,[100] only sporadic use has been made of this technic until recently.[63] Blakemore[8] of New York used a slightly different method of implantation, opening the aneurysm and suturing the graft ends from within to the internal proximal and distal openings. The advantage of restoring the circulation through the artery at the knee level lies in the fact that these patients are not only protected from having gangrene of any part of the extremity but, after the operation, having a normal blood supply to the calf, they are not subject to intermittent claudication or other symptoms of arterial insufficiency.

Arteriosclerotic Aneurysm of the Abdominal Aorta. Aneurysms of the abdominal aorta consistently arise just above the bifurcation and very rarely do they extend above the level of the renal artery branches of the aorta. Distally, the process of loss of elasticity and dilatation may proceed into the common iliac arteries, and it is not unusual to find 3 aneurysms—1 of the distal abdominal aorta, and 1 of each common iliac artery.

SYMPTOMS. The patient having an abdominal aortic aneurysm may remain asymptomatic even while the aneurysm grows to sizes up to 10 and 15 cm. in diameter. This is undoubtedly because of the availability of space within the abdomen among the hollow viscera. More frequently, symptoms are produced as a result of compression of the surrounding structures. Intermittent claudication is present occasionally, due to the relative obstruction to the blood flow produced by the aneurysm. Pressure on the bodies of the vertebrae, which are frequently eroded by the pulsating mass, causes back pain. When the aneurysm extends to the side of the spine, radiating pain is produced by pressure on the lumbar nerve roots. Distention of the small intestine mesentery into which the aneurysm expands may produce abdominal pain and digestive disturbances such as attacks of ileus and distention. Obstruction to the third portion of the duodenum occasionally results when the aneurysm distends upward against the duodenum held by the ligament of Treitz at the duodenal-jejunal junction. Such patients have nausea and vomiting, which may be either intermittent or progressive until the aneurysm is removed or until it ruptures.

COURSE. Occasionally, an abdominal aortic aneurysm will follow a long and benign course. Aside from the production of symptoms by compressing the spine or involving the gastro-intestinal tract, the common complication of abdominal aortic aneurysm is rupture. Reviews of collected cases by several investigators have disclosed the true, rather grave prognosis in patients with aneurysm when it is asymptomatic and the more serious prognosis when symptoms have developed.[39] Rupture is into the retroperitoneal space most commonly but also may be into any adjacent viscus of the gastro-intestinal tract or into the vena cava. When the retroperitoneal rupture occurs, free rupture into the peritoneal cavity almost always follows unless death occurs from the retroperitoneal blood loss (Fig.

40-26). Rare resolution of the retroperitoneal hematoma with temporary stabilization of the wall of the aneurysm may occur, but in the overwhelming majority of patients rupture leads progressively to a fatal outcome. Death by hemorrhage ensues rapidly when free abdominal cavity bleeding develops or when the aneurysm ruptures into the gastro-intestinal tract. The progression to death by hemorrhage is sometimes delayed for hours or days in patients with a retroperitoneal rupture. These patients show the development of a wide pulsating mass in the abdomen extending into the flanks and the lower abdomen above Poupart's ligament. Signs of hemorrhage such as increased pulse rate, falling blood pressure, and particularly a drop in the red blood count, together with such a pulsating growing mass, are diagnostic of ruptured aneurysm. Another much less common complication of abdominal aneurysm is acute thrombosis. This has been seen in 2 of 300 cases in the authors' series.

TREATMENT of abdominal aortic aneurysm has been entirely palliative until recent years when more definitive curative surgery has become well established. An early form of treatment consisted of ligation of the abdominal aorta above the aneurysm.[92] When this ligation was carried to the point of occlusion of

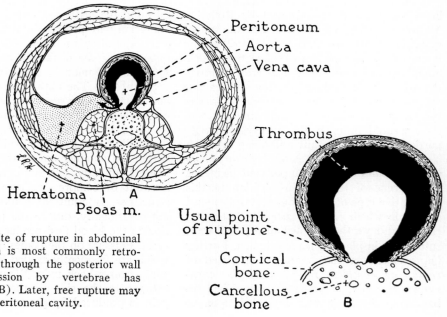

FIG. 40-26. Site of rupture in abdominal aortic aneurysm is most commonly retroperitoneal (A) through the posterior wall where compression by vertebrae has thinned it out (B). Later, free rupture may occur into the peritoneal cavity.

the aorta the pulsations within the aneurysm ceased. However, hemorrhage frequently resulted from the ligature cutting through, and there was a discouraging incidence of gangrene of both lower extremities. Stimulation of the development of a large clot within the aneurysm by the introduction of wire has been practiced similar to that used in thoracic aneurysms.[7, 81] Gradual occlusion of the aorta proximal to an aneurysm at the bifurcation can be accomplished by wrapping the vessel in this region with a cuff of polyethylene film containing a sizing compound, dicetyl phosphate.[28] This substance stimulates development of scar tissue which shrinks and gradually shuts off the blood flow. At their best,

when successful, these methods provide only a temporary cessation in growth of the aneurysm or relief of symptoms.

Real help to these patients, developed during 1952[32, 105] and used progressively more widely since,[11, 22, 66, 71] consists of the total removal of the lower abdominal aorta, its bifurcation, and a variable amount of the iliac systems with subsequent replacement of the defect with an aortic bifurcation graft (Fig. 40-27). Vein grafts are unsuitable in this region because they would certainly dilate to aneurysmal proportions. An alternative material for replacement of the aortic bifurcation is a Y-shaped tube of closely woven nylon or Dacron cloth. These surgical procedures are

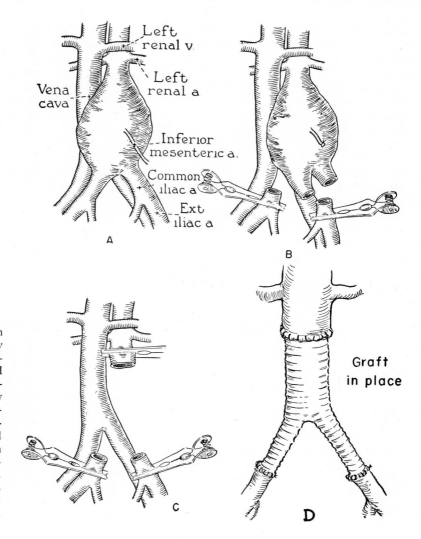

FIG. 40-27. Resection and homologous artery graft replacement of aneurysm of abdominal aorta. (A) Usual location of aneurysm below renal arteries and involving bifurcation to a varying degree. (B) Proximal and distal control with clamps is followed by removal of the aneurysm. The defect left in (C) is restored by the implantation of the graft (D).

ideally applied to patients who are found to have aneurysms of a significant size at the time of discovery, but they also may be applied in patients whose aneurysms have already undergone rupture, particularly if the rupture is retroperitoneal and a period of stabilization occurs of sufficient length to transport the patient to the hospital, give him brief preparation for surgery and take him to the operating room.[17, 58]

MYCOTIC ANEURYSMS

A rare but distinctive form of aneurysm occurs in cases of subacute bacterial endocarditis. The arterial wall at some point in the body is weakened by a bacterial infection carried to it by small emboli arising from the vegetations on the heart valve involved with the endocarditis. It is supposed that the embolus is quite small and implants itself in the vessel wall by entering one of the vaso-vasorum. It is equally likely that the embolus lodges in a small branch of the major artery and the infection involves the arterial wall by spreading along the periarterial tissues. These emboli would be the same type that produce the intensely tender fingertips by lodging in the digital vessels in patients with endocarditis. The acute episode of lodgment of the embolus is apparently entirely asymptomatic in many cases, and the first evidence of an arterial lesion is the appearance and the rather rapid development of a pulsating swelling. Mycotic aneurysms have been observed in many locations in the lower extremities. The brachial artery is the point of most frequent site in the upper extremity. They have been seen in the mesenteric arteries. The symptomatology produced by the aneurysm includes pain almost from the beginning of development. Why these aneurysms should be more painful than those of arteriosclerosis or syphilis probably depends on the acute inflammatory nature of the lesion. The inflammation causes them to attach themselves very quickly to surrounding structures or to the undersurface of the skin. Therefore, they may dissect through adjacent structures and rupture. The other frequent complication of mycotic aneurysm is early thrombosis.

In our experience the aneurysm continues to grow after subacute bacterial endocarditis and the blood stream infection which is associated with it have been arrested by chemotherapy. Therefore, though antibotics are indicated in the treatment of mycotic aneurysm they probably do not reverse the tendency for the aneurysm to enlarge because the wall already has been weakened by the inflammatory reaction.

Treatment consists of resection and restoration of the blood flow by the implantation of a vein or artery graft if a major channel is involved. This operation obviously should be deferred until the causative infection has been overcome. However, ideal timing cannot always be accomplished because the extremely painful expanding lesion may require earlier operation simply because of the pain, because of threatened rupture, or because thrombosis has led to a serious degree of ischemia in an extremity or in a viscus.

Surgery of the Venous System

INTRODUCTION

The general pathologic processes to which veins are subject are limited. They are confined largely to the changes of dilatation and elongation, intrinsic occlusion by thrombosis and inflammation, and pathologic processes not inherent to the veins which cause extrinsic venous occlusion. Additional rare processes include suppurative inflammation, intrinsic occlusion by the invasion of the vein lumen by tumor, and degenerative lesions.

Dilatation and elongation of the vein occur because of chronic increased pressure within the vein or overloading of the venous system concerned. As is the case with arteries, veins are so constructed that when they are forcibly expanded the expansion occurs both in circumference and in length. The tendency to expand is governed to some extent at least by a familial trait of generalized weakness of certain of the vein walls. This factor is in part responsible for the clinical manifestation of varicose veins of the lower extremities occurring in families. Elongation and dilatation aside from the varices of the legs is seen in varicosities of the veins of the submucosal area of the esophagus in portal vein obstruction and liver disease, anal hemorrhoids and the venous enlargement which accompanies arteriovenous fistulae in any location.

Occlusion by inflammation and thrombosis is termed *thrombophlebitis*. The clinical manifestations of the thrombophlebitis are very diverse, depending upon the severity of the acute inflammation and later on the residual vein damage. The complications of thrombophlebitis are those which reflect this damage to the veins, particularly in the lower extremities. Another complication is pulmonary artery embolism which occurs when the thrombus within the vein lumen breaks loose and travels to the lungs.

Extrinsic occlusion of a vein may be due to compression by tumor, pregnant uterus, or as a result of an adjacent chronic fibrosing inflammation. One very important clinical manifestation of this latter form of extrinsic occlusion is superior vena caval syndrome. The clinical features produced by compression of a vein by tumor are available according to region and will not be described.

VARICOSE VEINS OF THE LOWER EXTREMITY

Etiology. Varices of the lower extremities are the result of dilatation of the subcutaneous venous channels to a degree which renders the valves incompetent because they are no longer capable of coapting across the enlarged vein area (Fig. 40-28).

Certain features of the structure of the venous systems involved are important in order to understand the development of the condition and the rationale of its treatment. The veins affected are the long saphenous vein and the short saphenous vein, together with their tributaries. Both of these systems lie beneath the superficial fascia and superficial to the deep fascia throughout the major portion of their course in the thighs and the legs.

The *long saphenous vein* arises in superficial veins on the dorsum and the medial aspects of the foot. These form a channel at the level of the medial malleolus which courses directly upward along the calf medial to the tibia. At the level of the knee the course be-

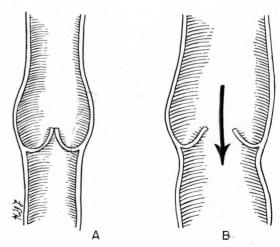

Fig. 40-28. Diagrammatic representation of vein dilatation in producing valvular incompetence.

comes somewhat more posterior, and the vein continues up the medial and then the anteromedial surface of the thigh to enter the common femoral vein high in the groin. The point of entrance into the femoral vein is approximately 2 cm. distal to Poupart's ligament. The vein gains entrance into the deep compartment of the thigh through the deep fascia by way of an oval opening, the fossa ovalis. At or near the point of entrance into the common femoral vein the saphenous vein receives tributaries which are exceedingly important from the standpoint of treatment. These tributaries are the superficial circumflex iliac, entering laterally, the superficial epigastric, entering superiorly, and the superficial pudendal entering medially. In addition the accessory saphenous veins, medial and lateral, enter the long saphenous vein a short distance below the saphenofemoral junction, right at the junction, or may even enter the femoral vein directly. Normally, only one of the accessory saphenous veins is prominent.

Throughout its course the long saphenous vein receives tributaries which drain the skin and the subcutaneous tissue of the thigh and the medial aspect of the leg and the foot. It communicates frequently with the deep veins of the extremities through branches which penetrate the deep fascia of the leg and the thigh.

The entire course of the saphenous vein is

protected by valves occurring at intervals of 4 to 8 inches which are so positioned as to permit only cephalad flow of blood. The perforating branches of the saphenous vein which communicate with the deep venous system also contain valves. These direct flow from the saphenous to the deep veins.

The *short saphenous vein* drains the posterior and the lateral aspects of the leg. It arises posterior to the lateral malleolus from superficial veins on the lateral aspect of the foot and then takes its course upward approximately in the mid-line of the calf to penetrate the deep fascia and enter the popliteal vein. The point of penetration of the fascia varies in individuals from the level of the Achilles tendon to the popliteal space. Communications with the deep system are not plentiful. The lesser saphenous vein usually communicates through a large branch with the greater saphenous vein. The position of this vessel is variable. It may leave the short saphenous vein at almost any point in the leg, entering the greater or long saphenous at the ankle level or above.

Pathology. No intrinsic pathologic change is seen as the cause of the dilatation. However, after the process has been present for a long time, fibrosis and thickening of the vein wall are present. There is also at an early stage a distinct hypertrophy of the muscularis of the vein.

Three predisposing factors seem to be active in the development of varicose veins. They are (1) a familial defect in strength of venous structure which is no doubt responsible for the appearance of the condition in families; (2) occupational influence which makes the condition common in persons who stand for long periods of time at their work; (3) increased venous pressure and collateral vein formation in an extremity following a thrombophlebitic occlusion of the deep venous system.

On the basis of these predisposing causes varicose veins are divided into two classes— primary and secondary. Primary varicose veins are those which arise because of intrinsic weakness of the vein walls, because of occupational stress, or due to pregnancy. Secondary varicose veins are those which develop as a part of the tremendous venous collateral growth which is stimulated by thrombo-

phlebitic occlusion of the deep venous system of the lower extremities.

Primary Varicose Veins. Local dilatation of a segment of the saphenous vein provides the beginning of structural failure of the entire system. The primary enlargement in circumference renders the valve or valves in the segment incompetent. This brings a longer blood column to rest on the subjacent valve. As the dilatation continues the valves of the perforating branches are rendered incompetent, allowing flow in a reverse direction in these veins from the deep to the superficial systems. The blood thus escaping into the saphenous system from the deep veins flows in a retrograde direction unhampered by the valves already incompetent. It re-enters the deep system at whatever point of leg or ankle its pressure in relation to deep vein pressure permits it to do so. It then resumes its flow upward.

SYMPTOMS. Uncomplicated varicose veins are seldom productive of severe symptoms, and frequently there may be none at all. Increased fatigue, some aching of the legs at night, and moderate pain and tenderness over the distended veins are the usual symptoms when any are present. Complaints of severe pain or disability in patients exhibiting varicose veins is a strong suggestion to search for some other cause of the symptoms, such as arthritis of the hip, the knee or the lower back, or for arterial insufficiency.

COMPLICATIONS of varicose veins of the lower extremities are productive of a more symptomatic course. The unphysiologic level of the back pressure in the local venous drainage results in a disturbance of skin nutrition causing changes in the skin and to some degree in the cutaneous nerves. Paresthesias of the skin of the leg, eczematoid dermatitis, pigmentation, fibrosis and finally ulceration may occur. The appearance of edema of the ankle or the dorsum of the foot is rare except perhaps in a very mild degree as a complication of varicose veins alone. The amount of back flow and the height of the column of blood in the superficial veins ordinarily is handled quite well by an entirely normal deep venous system. Therefore, the presence of edema is suggestive of concomitant deep vein pathology.

A second complication is acute inflammation with thrombosis of a segment of the dilated tortuous vein. This produces pain, tenderness and local heat of a magnitude which depends on the size of the varix involved.

EXAMINATION. The physical examination of the patient with varicose veins must be complete. The general portion of such an examination determines the presence of any pathologic process which might have a causal relation with the varices or might alter the treatment of the veins. The local examination determines the extent and the severity of the dilatation. It points out the presence and the location of incompetent valves in the saphenous system and in the perforating veins communicating between saphenous and deep circulation. The presence of complications of the varicose veins is sought for, and the deep venous circulation is evaluated.

The initial observation is made with the patient standing relaxed, allowing the veins time to fill to a maximum extent. This is carried out best in an oblique light, and palpation of the channels will reveal pathologically dilated veins which are invisible because of obesity. Palpation should be done by a percussing movement with the fingers, delineating veins by the ballottement of the contained blood. This percussion is done with firm, brisk strokes of one hand while the other hand is placed over the course of the vein, either above or below. The pressure wave can be felt transmitted through the column of blood. The point in local examination most frequently overlooked is an evaluation of the short saphenous vein. In its classically normal anatomic form, the short saphenous vein is subcutaneous from the popliteal space to the ankle. However, with great frequency the vessel may lie beneath the deep fascia along the posterior surface of the calf down to a point as low as the development of the Achilles tendon before it emerges as a dilated channel. When this is true the pathologic state in the short saphenous vein may be missed. Dilatation of veins under the skin of the lateral aspect of the ankle or dermatitis in this region are indicative of a varicose short saphenous vein.

The incompetence of the valves in the saphenous channels may be demonstrated by a test which allows the varicose veins to fill from above. To perform this maneuver, the *Brodie-Trendelenburg test*,[12] first the veins are emptied of blood by elevating the legs. A tourniquet is applied at thigh level, and the patient stands. With the tourniquet in place the veins tend to remain empty, filling gradually from below. If the tourniquet is removed quickly with the veins unfilled, the blood from above drops immediately into the dilated system below. This response indicates competent valves in the perforating veins and incompetent valves in the saphenous vein. If during this the veins fill rapidly with the tourniquet in place high on the thigh the test is interpreted to mean that the perforating vein valves are incompetent. The level of incompetence of valves in the perforating veins may be demonstrated by an extension of the maneuver which was described by Ochsner and Mahorner.[89] When filling from above occurs with a tourniquet in place at the midthigh level, it may be assumed that an incompetent perforating vein exists some place below the tourniquet. By repeating the test with the tourniquet at progressively lower points on the thigh and the calf, the level of the most distal incompetent perforator may be demonstrated. This actually can be done with only one change of position by putting 4 tourniquets at various levels down the thigh and the leg with the leg elevated and then, with the patient standing, removing them progressively from below until rapid filling occurs.

The ability of the deep venous system to drain off the blood collected in the varicose veins may be demonstrated by the *Perthes test*[98] which is done by occluding with a tourniquet the subcutaneous veins at the knee or thigh level. The tourniquet must be at or distal to the lowest significant incompetent perforator. The tourniquet will prevent all downward filling from above this level, and, as the patient walks, the normal pumping action of the muscles exerted on the deep veins drains the dilated varices. Failure of the veins to empty may mean that the tourniquet is above a large incompetent perforating vein which allows flow out into the varices. Also it may mean that the deep veins have been damaged by an inflammatory process so that their function is disturbed. Formerly, this latter conclusion from the test was considered as a contraindication to surgical therapy of the varicose veins. As will be discussed in the management of secondary varicose veins, the contraindication no longer is considered valid, and such veins are given definitive surgical treatment.

Secondary Varicose Veins. These are the superficial components of the general massive development of venous collaterals which results from deep vein damage due to thrombophlebitis. The differentiation between primary and secondary veins depends on the history of an attack of thrombophlebitis and the presence of other signs of deep venous insufficiency. If other complications of the past deep vein disease are present, the varicose veins must be considered only as a part of the stasis syndrome.

A rare cause of varicosities of the superficial veins is the presence of arteriovenous fistulae, usually of the congenital type. In this condition the extremity is usually the site of congenital hemangiomata of the skin and increased warmth and skin color. Sometimes a bruit is heard in the congenital fistulae and is always present in the acquired type. Finally, the abnormal filling of the veins from the arteries is manifested by increased oxygen in the venous blood which can be measured and by increased pressure in the varices. Sometimes the pressure can delay emptying of the varicose veins when the extremity is elevated.

Indications for surgery in varicose veins vary. The presence of small superficial and asymptomatic veins are not in themselves an indication for their removal. Symptoms from varicosities must be evaluated carefully, and other causes of leg discomfort should be ruled out. Large prominent and tortuous varicosities are removed on the basis of possible future phlebitis and for relief of symptoms, if any. Varicosities occurring during pregnancy present a problem. These patients with few exceptions are carried to term on conservative management. Elastic support and periods of bed rest with elevation of the extremities are used. Surgery is done after delivery with the reservation that recurrences may occur with further pregnancies. Injection therapy is seldom used as a primary treatment. It may be of value in controlling the remaining small ones following surgical removal of the major veins.

TREATMENT. The surgical treatment of varicose veins consists of removal of the long or short saphenous veins or both, together with their affected tributaries. At the same time the incompetent perforating veins must be ligated or otherwise inactivated. The ligation of the main saphenous trunk accurately at its point of entrance into the deep vein into which it would normally drain is fundamental to the surgical procedure. This is at the junction of the common femoral vein in the case of the long saphenous, and the popliteal vein in the case of the short saphenous.

The saphenous channel is then removed by withdrawing it with a long wire stripper, passed through the length of the vein from groin or popliteal space to ankle. Varicose tributaries are excised through accessory incisions if they are large or, if small, they are treated with direct injection of sclerosing solutions at a later date. Particular attention should be paid to large tributaries of the long saphenous channel because of the fact that perforator veins may communicate with these tributaries rather than with the channel itself. If they are left behind, local recurrence of the varicose condition will develop on the basis of the remaining perforating veins. (Fig. 40-29).

Emphasis has been placed in the past on an evaluation of the deep venous function as a guide to choice of therapy, particularly surgical, in secondary varicose veins. The varices were considered to be a valuable part of the collateral bed. Actually, this is rarely true. In the great majority of cases the varicose veins serve not as a collateral venous route but, because of complete loss of their valve function, lack of fascial support and their inability to be affected by muscle-pumping action, they carry blood downward. This actually increases the load to be carried by the deep venous collaterals which do serve more or less effectively. In most present-day experience complete removal of the incompetent superficial veins has been beneficial rather than detrimental to the total venous drainage of a lower extremity. Therefore, the various tests for deep vein damage are not of practical use in deciding whether extirpation of secondary varicose veins should be done. The decision as to choice of therapy depends more on the presence and the severity of the other complications of deep venous obstruction. In the absence of significant edema secondary varicose veins should be eradicated by ligation and stripping as in the case of primary varices. The presence of cutaneous ulcers and eczema reinforces the insistence on complete removal. However, if edema is present, as will be discussed in the next section, the primary therapeutic attack should be toward the control of the swelling by general management.

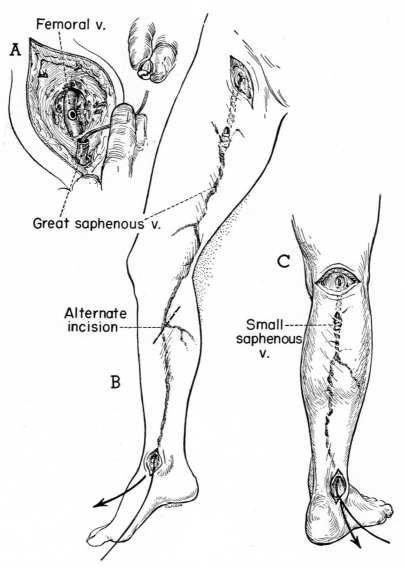

FIG. 40-29. Ligation and stripping of the great and the small saphenous veins. (A) The tributaries of the saphenous vein have been ligated, and the saphenous vein has been ligated at the saphenofemoral junction. Vein stripper has been inserted from the ankle superiorly to the groin. (B) The vein is stripped from above downward. A number of alternate incisions may be needed to remove separate varicose masses. (C) The small saphenous vein is stripped from its junction with the popliteal vein to a point posterior to the lateral malleolus.

THROMBOPHLEBITIS

Definition. Thrombophlebitis may be defined as an acute inflammatory disease of the vein wall and the surrounding tissue, including lymphatics, and usually thrombosis of the lumen of the vessel. It may involve the superficial veins (superficial phlebitis) or the deep veins (deep phlebitis). The severity of the inflammation varies widely. In some it may be very mild, producing minor febrile reaction and only slight pain. In others all features of an acute inflammation—heat, redness, tenderness and fever—are marked. This variation in the severity of the inflammatory aspect of thrombophlebitis has given rise to a purely artificial subdivision of inflammatory deep vein disease into two groups.[95]

Classification. The first group, *thrombophlebitis*, consists of those cases in which the inflammatory reaction is severe. In the second group, *phlebothrombosis*, the presence of the thrombus is the most important aspect. It is practical to use this subdivision, although fundamentally the two conditions have one identity. Morphologically, the elements are the same, merging from one to another, and both can be present in the same extremity simultaneously. Individual patients are frequently observed to enter the phase of thrombophlebitis after first exhibiting signs of the milder state for some time.

Complications. The major complications are pulmonary embolism during the early stage and stasis disease later. Pulmonary embolism results when a portion of the intraluminal clot detaches from its site of origin, travels through the venous system and the heart and lodges in a branch of the pulmonary artery. Pulmonary embolism occurs much more frequently in the milder form of the disease, namely, phlebothrombosis. Late stasis disease is the manifestation of damage to the venous drainage and to the surrounding lymphatics by the inflammation. This is more frequent after the greater destruction which occurs in the inflammation of thrombophlebitis.

Phlebothrombosis. This bland form occurs as a complication of surgery, any acute illness, unusual activity such as a long hike by an ordinarily sedentary person, or unusual inactivity such as sitting long periods in a boat while fishing. It also occurs without any determinable deviation from normal activity.

SYMPTOMS. The symptoms consist of mild pain and stiffness in the calf of the leg on active motion and a duplication of these symptoms on passive dorsiflexion of the ankle. This discomfort is accompanied by mild or moderate swelling with or without a low-grade fever and tachycardia. The course of the condition may be very benign, the fever and symptoms disappearing in a few days on bed rest. In other cases the originally bland phlebothrombosis may go on to display a picture of acute thrombophlebitis.

The clinical importance of the illness is the complication of pulmonary embolism, which sometimes occurs before the local symptoms are very manifest.

PROPHYLAXIS. Much attention has been paid to the prevention of phlebothrombosis as a complication of surgery. The factors in its production in the postoperative patient are probably 3-fold. Changes in the coagulation mechanism, hemoconcentration, and stasis resulting from bed rest and infrequent changes of position, probably all contribute. Modern fluid and electrolyte management of the surgical patient, early ambulation and the prophylactic administration of the anticoagulants Dicumarol and heparin have all been emphasized in prevention of phlebothrombosis. The incidence remains significant in spite of preventive therapy.[20]

DIAGNOSIS. Individuals developing phlebothrombosis usually have very mild symptoms. These consist of stiffness and aching of the calf and of a limp because of pain when they walk. Body temperature elevation is mild when present. The first sign of phlebothrombosis may be a pulmonary embolism, whether the patient has been well preceding the illness or it overtakes him in the hospital after surgery.

The serious nature of pulmonary embolism and its habit of occurring as a sudden unexpected complication of other disease or surgery makes the constant search for signs of phlebothrombosis in hospitalized patients mandatory. The daily inspection of the temperature chart and of the patient's lower extremities is a habit to be developed by all physicians. An early diagnosis and immediate institution of treatment will diminish the chances of embolism.

An unexplained mild simultaneous rise in pulse and temperature is one of the danger signals of phlebothrombosis.[30] Inspection of the extremities includes looking for mild edema, dilatations of the veins over the anterior tibia, congestion of the calf muscles, and a positive Homans' sign. This consists of a feeling of tightness and discomfort when the ankle is passively dorsiflexed.[49]

TREATMENT. Therapy has two purposes. One is to limit the course of the local condition, and the second is to prevent pulmonary embolism. The local treatment is not complicated. It consists of bed rest with elevation of the lower extremities. The patient is allowed good mobility in bed but massage of the legs or active exercise of the lower extremities is forbidden. Local heat is useful in increasing comfort. It should be in the form of a heat cradle at not more than 115° F. rather than hot, wet foments, which necessarily produce complete immobilization.

Good hydration must be obtained and the fluid management directed to avoid or correct dehydration. Evidences obtained through culture of the clots removed from involved veins indicate that bacterial agents probably are not responsible. Therefore, antibiotics such as penicillin or streptomycin are not required. The anticoagulant agents, heparin and Dicumarol, produce an effect which is beneficial both in the local management and in the prevention of emboli (Table 2. See also Chap. 14, p. 252, "Arterial Occlusive Edema.")

The period of local therapy is hard to determine. Ambulation may be permitted gradually when all local signs have been gone 1 or 2 days. As the patient is allowed up it is important to watch for a recurrence. The anticoagulant therapy should be kept up for longer periods. The duration of this varies in the opinions of authorities from 10 days to several months. The purpose of maintaining the depression in coagulation is to prevent upward growth in the involved vein of a nonadherent segment of thrombus which might break loose even after a week or two. Since very few emboli have occurred more than 2 weeks after subsidence of local signs, this has been taken by many surgeons as the period of

TABLE 2. ANTICOAGULANT REGIMENS

INDICATION	PURPOSE	HEPARIN	DICUMAROL
Arterial Embolism (Peripheral and Aortic)	Rapid, temporary prolongation of clotting time to limit growth of intra-arterial clot	75-100 mg. i.v. Followed by 50 mg. i.v. every 3 hours until embolectomy	None
Phlebothrombosis Therapeutic	Rapid, continued depression of clotting activity to diminish growth of thrombus in involved vein and diminish incidence of pulmonary embolism	A. Heparin Alone 30-50 mg. deep subcut. (not intramuscular) every 3 to 4 hrs. to prolong clotting time to approx. 3 times normal	None
		————————— or —————————	
Prophylactic	Depression of clotting activity effective 4-6 hrs. after surgery to diminish tendency to develop phlebothrombosis in patients thought to be likely to develop it	B. Heparin plus Dicumarol 30-50 mg. heparin subcut. every 3-4 hrs. until Dicumarol becomes effective	100 mg. by mouth every 6 hrs. for 5 doses then 25-100 mg. per day to maintain 25-40% clotting activity
Thrombophlebitis	Prolonged depression of clotting activity to: (1) diminish propagation of intraluminal venous clots to limit extent of damage to system; and (2) diminish incidence of pulmonary embolism	Either method outlined for use in phlebothrombosis	

anticoagulant therapy after subsidence of symptoms and signs.

PREVENTION of pulmonary embolism in cases of phlebothrombosis may also be obtained by *interrupting surgically the involved vein above the process*. The operation is in most cases simply a ligation of the superficial femoral vein done under local anesthesia. Almost always it is carried out bilaterally, even if the second limb is without signs of the condition. Great care must be taken to place the interruption immediately below a good-sized venous tributary such as the profunda femoris vein in order that a blind segment of vein is not left just above the ligature. Also, it is preferred to divide the vein rather than merely to ligate it. In a certain proportion of patients the thrombotic process extends so high that femoral interruption will not be central to it. In these a more extensive procedure is required to ligate the common iliac vein on the involved side (and the contralateral superficial femoral) or preferably the lower vena cava.

Thrombectomy as a primary treatment of deep venous thrombosis may be tried. The thrombus is aspirated in the early stages of the disease. The vein is closed or ligated, and anticoagulants are continued.

For several reasons *anticoagulant therapy* is preferred to vein interruption for the prevention of pulmonary embolism, except when a contraindication exists or in areas where facilities to control the anticoagulants are not available, or in patients sustaining pulmonary embolism despite good anticoagulant therapy. Statistical evaluation favors anticoagulant therapy slightly in the prevention of embolism. It is also probable that late venous stasis is intensified by mechanical block by ligation of the veins. Finally, it is quite evident that the substitution of an equally effective medical therapy for one involving an operative procedure is desirable. However, it must be remembered that vein interruption is an effective form of therapy and that the administration of anticoagulants is not without its complications. Therefore, ligation may easily be resorted to when difficulty is encountered either in the patient's response to anticoagulants or in the facilities for its management. Stasis disease may follow ligation.

ACUTE THROMBOPHLEBITIS

Although acute thrombophlebitis is considered to be less dangerous in regard to production of pulmonary embolism, it is more incapacitating than is phlebothrombosis in point of causing persistent trouble in the legs. The onset of thrombophlebitis usually is rapid, the first symptom being pain and stiffness in the foot and the calf or the thigh. There is some indication that much of the initial pain is due to reflex arterial spasm in that a procaine block of the lumbar sympathetic ganglia may afford relief at times. Further, many cases of thrombophlebitis, if observed early, will be seen to pass through a stage of arterial spasm in which pallor of arterial insufficiency precedes the plethora of venous occlusion. This so-called "white stage" can be sufficiently prolonged and intense as to produce superficial ischemic necrosis in the distal part of the extremity. This forms a subgroup of thrombophlebitis called *phlegmasia cerulea dolens*.

As the white stage, which is usually fleeting, passes the signs of inflammation and venous occlusion develop. Fever, swelling, redness and an aching pain less intense than the earlier pain of spasm develop.

A significant degree of lymphatic obstruction occurs by direct extension of the inflammation from the adjacent veins. This obstruction is manifested early by peau d' orange type of edema of the skin.

While the inflammation is present the edema persists in spite of elevation of the extremity. Complete subsidence leaves the venous and lymphatic drainage with a variable degree of obstruction. The degree is determined by the anatomic extent of the thrombophlebitis as well as its severity. Involvement may be limited to the veins of the calf or extend up through the iliac system to attack a major portion of the vena cava. Restoration of the venous drainage develops through 2 mechanisms. One is recanalization of the major vein and the second is development of collaterals. Tributaries of the major veins lying beneath the deep fascia of the limb and those in the superficial layers all are forced to dilate. The former provide relatively efficient collaterals; the latter do not. Even when a significant-sized lumen is restored in a healed vein, such as the superficial femoral vein, the channel is functionally deficient in that the valves cannot be restored. Back flow or a tendency for back flow to occur is then present. This may be demonstrated by retrograde filling of the vein with Diodrast, if this solution is injected into the common femoral vein with the patient in a nearly vertical position on the x-ray table.

The course of the patient who has healed his acute phlebitis and is not managed adequately leads to continued morbidity. The complications are development of fibrosis in the skin and the subcutaneous tissues, pigmentation and the development of hypersensitivity of the skin leading to dermatitis and finally to ulceration.

Treatment. The treatment of thrombophlebitis of the lower extremities is aimed at the limitation and the early resolution of the acute phase and at the prevention of late sequelae.

Rest and elevation of the involved extremity with local application of heat, either by fomentation or carefully controlled heat cradle, is insisted upon until all signs of inflammation have subsided. This simple treatment is often all that is required when only the superficial veins are involved. However, when the thrombus extends superiorly toward the foramen ovale, ligation of the great saphenous vein may be necessary. Heparin therapy is instituted with the aim of helping to limit the extent of vein occlusion by thrombus and possibly to limit fibrin deposition and organization of the intercellular edema fluid. Antibiotic therapy usually is applied, but the indication for its use must be questioned. The occasional bacteriologic studies which have been done on clots and tissues removed from thrombophlebitis have been negative.

The elevation of the extremity is continued after the acute process has subsided until the edema of the extremity is entirely gone. Then ambulation of the patient is conducted on a gradually increasing regimen, using elastic support with bandages and stockings. At no time should the period of ambulation be long enough to cause the development of swelling, and at the same time the increase in activity should be as rapid as possible within this limit. Such a regimen is often very time-consuming and will be tolerated by the patient only if he

understands the purpose of preventing the even more time-consuming late sequelae of his condition. Management for many months is often necessary but, in the majority, gainful occupations may be resumed early if periods of recumbency with elevation can be arranged during the working hours.

Complications of late stasis disease—dermatitis, fibrosis, pigmentation, secondary varicose veins, and ulceration—are frequently met with because the need of a careful regimen was not recognized at the beginning. The successful treatment of these complications again depends upon the complete management of the continued daily swelling.[86]

It is fundamental to the surgical treatment of late stasis disease that edema be entirely controlled before operation and that the patient's long-term postoperative regimen be directed to preventing recurrence of swelling.

The actual operative treatment consists of total removal of the varicose veins, resection of the entire fibrotic and ulcerated area, and restoration of the skin defect by a skin graft.[65, 93] When the changes in the skin and the subcutaneous tissue are less advanced, operation may consist of exposure and ligation of the incompetent perforating veins in the region. This is accomplished by raising a flap of the tissues in the stasis area, exposing these veins at the deep fascial level.[82]

SYNDROME OF SUPERIOR VENA CAVA OBSTRUCTION

An obstruction of the superior vena cava is poorly compensated for by the collateral venous system available. The collateral route is long and circuitous, carrying venous blood from head, neck, upper extremities and shoulder girdle down and around to drain into the inferior vena cava. The syndrome which develops from superior caval occlusion is usually unremitting.

The elements of the clinical picture are due to the high venous pressure in the superior caval drainage bed and to the development of collateral veins. The venous stasis produces distention of the neck veins and a plethoric appearance of the face. The distention increases markedly when the patient bends over or lies down. Edema of the face develops during recumbency at night and may be so severe that the puffed-up eyelids cannot be opened in the morning. He learns to sleep with trunk elevated to minimize this. Dizziness and even fainting may result from stooping or bending forward too long.

The collateral veins first appear beneath the skin of the upper chest and progessively become prominent downward over the trunk.

Pathology. The occluding lesion is exterior to the vein almost without exception. Benign and malignant tumors in the superior mediastinal structures, aneurysms of the aortic arch or its branches, and inflammatory lesions of the superior mediastinum are the common causes.

Of these the tumors and aneurysms are visible on roentgenograms, which also serves to some extent to differentiate between them. The inflammatory lesions produce caval obstruction by formation of contracting scar tissue and do not always produce an x-ray visible mass. In some instances healed tuberculosis is demonstrated in tissues removed at surgery. In others the fibrous tissue shows no specific causation. It is likely that the inflammation responsible was originally of a mediastinal lymph node, whether tuberculous or pyogenic. In the latter instance it seems reasonable to suggest that an upper respiratory infection of the past had involved the mediastinal node.

Treatment. In instances displaying a superior mediastinal mass by roentgenography the management is dictated by the character of the tumor. Curative resection of a malignant lesion which has occluded the cava is not likely to be possible. Roentgen therapy offers the most to the patient if the lesion is a lymphoma. Resection of a benign tumor which may occasionally compress the vessel will be curative.

The problem of relief of the venous engorgement in chronic superior vena caval syndrome has proved to be a difficult one. Most attempts to do so involve the use of grafts bridging the occluded segment. Homologous artery and prosthetic vascular grafts usually fail to remain open. An autogenous vein graft constructed from segments of the patient's femoral or jugular vein offers a better chance of continued patency. The discrepancy in caliber is overcome by incising longitudinally two segments of the selected graft and suturing them together to form one graft of double the original circumference.

The difficulties encountered in overcoming this problem illustrate the general need for methods of replacing or restoring diseased venous channels in any location.

ACUTE THROMBOSIS OF THE SUBCLAVIAN VEIN (EFFORT THROMBOSIS)

The subclavian and the axillary veins are subject to acute thrombosis probably secondary to a tear in their intima or to sustained compression by surrounding muscles. Occurrence during the prolonged or unusual use of the arms or sudden effort with the involved arm suggests the term "effort thrombosis."

The *onset* is acute and is characterized by the rapid development of edema of the extremity which often is massive. A varying degree of pain is experienced. Pallor, cyanosis, and coolness of the hand and forearm are seen in the period of onset, but very soon the extremity becomes warmer than the uninvolved one.

Distention of the veins of the extremity itself may be hidden by the edema, but the subcutaneous veins about the shoulder which dilate to act as collateral channels become visible very soon after onset. The axillary vein is palpable as a firm cord, and if the thrombosis extends peripherally the brachial vein may become similarly involved.

Prognosis. The prognosis is excellent. Venous drainage of the extremity becomes adequate in 1 to 4 weeks, either by collateral vein development or by eventual recanalization of the subclavian-axillary channel. Pulmonary emboli due to detachment of a portion of the thrombus is rare. Recurrences rarely may develop after complete recovery.

Management usually requires only bed rest with elevation of the extremity. External application of heat or cold is not useful, and a compression dressing may be harmful. The effect of anticoagulant drugs has not been evaluated, but the lack of frequent evidence of progression of the thrombus is against their use.

In the infrequent instance of recurrences, changes in the patient's occupation or method of working are useful and surgical efforts to enlarge the muscular route through which the subclavian vein passes may be required.

REFERENCES

1. Allen, E. W.: Thromboangiitis obliterans: methods of diagnosis of chronic occlusive arterial lesions distal to the wrist with illustrative cases, Am. J. M. Sc. *178*:237-244, 1929.
2. Atlas, L. N.: Lumbar sympathectomy in the treatment of selected cases of peripheral arteriosclerotic disease, Am. Heart J. *22*:75-85, 1941.
3. Bahnson, H. T.: Considerations in the excision of aortic aneurysms, Ann. Surg. *138*: 377, 1953.
4. Barker, W. F., and Cannon, J. A.: Technic of endarterectomy, Am. Surgeon *25*:912-918, 1959.
5. Bazy, L.: A propos du procès-verbal sur l'endarteriectomie désobliterante, Mém. Acad. chir. *74*:109, 1948.
6. Berry, R. E. L., Flotte, C. T., and Coller, F. A.: A critical evaluation of lumbar sympathectomy for peripheral arteriosclerotic vascular disease, Surgery *37*:115-129, 1955.
7. Blakemore, A. H.: Progressive, constrictive occlusion of the aorta with wiring and electrothermic coagulation for the treatment of arteriosclerotic aneurysms of the abdominal aorta, Ann. Surg. *137*:760, 1953.
8. ———: Restorative endoaneurysmorrhaphy by vein graft inlay, Ann. Surg. *126*:841, 1947.
9. Boyd, A. M., Ratcliffe, A. H., Jepson, R. P., and James, G. W. H.: Intermittent claudication: a clinical study, J. Bone & Joint Surg. *31-13*:325-355, 1949.
10. Branham, H. H., Aneurysmal varix of the femoral artery and vein following a gunshot wound, Internat. J. Surg. *3*:250-251, 1890.
11. Brock, R. C.: Discussion on reconstructive arterial surgery, Proc. Roy. Soc. Med. *46*: 115, 1953.
12. Brodie, B. C.: Lectures Illustrative of Various Subjects in Pathology and Surgery, London, Longmans, 1846.
13. Buerger, Leo: Thromboangiitis obliterans: a study of the vascular lesions leading to presenile spontaneous gangrene, Am. J. M. Sc. *136*:567-580, 1908.
14. Cannon, J. A., and Barker, W. F.: Successful management of obstructive femoral arteriosclerosis by endarterectomy, Surgery *38*:48-60, 1955.
15. Carrel, A.: The surgery of the blood vessels, Bull. Johns Hopkins Hosp. *17*:1907.
16. Coller, F. A., Campbell, K. N., Harris, B. M., and Berry, R. E. L.: The early results of sympathectomy in far advanced arteriosclerotic peripheral vascular disease, Surgery *26*:30-40, 1949.
17. Cooley, D. A., and DeBakey, M. E.: Ruptured aneurysms of abdominal aorta, excision and homograft replacement, Postgrad. Med. *16*:334, 1954.
18. Crawford, E. S., Creech, O., Cooley, D. A., and DeBakey, M. E.: Treatment of arteriosclerotic occlusive disease of the lower extremities by excision and graft replacement or bypass, Surgery *38*:981-992, 1955.
19. Davis, J. B., Grove, W. J., and Julian, O. C.: Thrombotic occlusion of the branches of the aortic arch, Martorell's syndrome: report of a case treated surgically, Ann. Surg. *144*:124, 1956.
20. DeBakey, M. E.: A critical evaluation of the problem of thromboembolism, Surg., Gynec. & Obst. (Internat. Abstr. Surg.) *98*:1-27, 1954.
21. DeBakey, M. E., and Cooley, D. A.: Successful resection of aneurysm of thoracic aorta and replacement by graft, J.A.M.A. *152*:673, 1953.
22. ———: Surgical treatment of aneurysm of abdominal aorta by resection and restoration of continuity with homograft, Surg., Gynec. & Obst. *97*:257, 1953.
23. DeBakey, M. E., Creech, O., and Woodhall, J. P.: Evaluation of sympathectomy in arteriosclerotic peripheral vascular disease, J.A.M.A. *144*:1227-1231, 1950.
24. DeBakey, M. E., Morris, G. C., Jr., Jordan, G. L., Jr., and Cooley, D. A.: Segmental Thromo-Obliterative Disease of Branches of Aortic Arch, J.A.M.A. *166*:998, 1958.
25. DeBakey, M. E., and Simeone, F. A.: Battle injuries of the arteries in World War II, Ann. Surg. *123*:534-579, 1946.
26. DeCamp, P. T., and Birchell, R.: Recognition and treatment of renal arterial stenosis associated with hypertension, Surgery *43*: 134, 1958.
27. de Takats, G., Fowler, E. F., Jordan, P., and Risley, T. C.: Sympathectomy in the treatment of peripheral vascular sclerosis, J.A.M.A. *144*:1227-1231, 1950.
28. de Takats, G., and Marshall, M. R.: Surgical treatment of arteriosclerotic aneurysms of the abdominal aorta, A.M.A. Arch. Surg. *64*:307, 1952.
29. Deterling, R. A., and Bhonslay, S. B.: An evaluation of synthetic materials and fabrics

suitable for blood vessel replacement, Surgery *38*:71-91, 1955.

30. Donaldson, G. A.: The therapy and prophylaxis of venous thrombosis and pulmonary embolism, S. Clin. North America *27*: 1037-1051, 1947.

31. dos Santos, J. C.: Sur la désobstruction des thromboses artérielles anciennes, Mém. Acad. chir. *73*:409-411, 1947.

32. Dubost, C., Allary, M., and Deconomas, N.: Resection of an aneurysm of the abdominal aorta, A.M.A. Arch. Surg. *64*:405, 1952.

33. Dye, W. S., Olwin, J. H., Javid, H, and Julian, O. C.: Arterial embolectomy, A.M.A. Arch. Surg. *70*:715-722, 1955.

34. Edwards, W. S., and Lyons, C.: Traumatic arterial spasm and thrombosis, Ann. Surg. *140*:319-323, 1954.

35. Edwards, W. S., and Tapp, J. S.: Chemically treated nylon tubes as arterial grafts, Surgery *38*:61-70, 1955.

36. Elkin, D. C.: Aneurysm following surgical procedure, Ann. Surg. *127*:769, 1948.

37. Elkin, D. C., and Cooper, F. W.: Surgical treatment of insidious thrombosis of aorta, Ann. Surg. *130*:417, 1949.

38. Elkin, D. C., and Warren, J. V.: Arteriovenous fistulae: their effect on the circulation, J.A.M.A. *134*:1524-1528, 1947.

39. Estes, J. E., Jr.: Abdominal aortic aneurysms; a study of 102 cases, Circulation *2*:258, 1950.

40. Fisher, M.: Occlusion of the internal carotid artery, A.M.A. Arch. Neurol. & Psychiat. *65*:346, 1951.

41. Fontaine, R.: Remarks concerning venous thrombosis and its sequelae, Surgery *41*: 6-24, 1957.

42. Fontaine, R., Buck, P., Riveaux, R., Kim, M., and Hubinot, J.: Treatment of arterial occlusion, comparative value of thrombectomy, thromboendarterectomy, arteriovenous shunt, and vascular grafts: fresh venous autografts, Lyon chir. *46*:73, 1951.

43. Freeman, N. E.: Arterial repair in the treatment of aneurysms and arteriovenous fistulae: a report of 18 successful restorations, Ann. Surg. *124*:888-919, 1946.

44. Gifford, R. W., Jr., Tarkin, T. W., and Janes, J. M.: Atherosclerotic popliteal aneurysm in a man 35 years old, Circulation *9*: 363, 1954.

45. Goldblatt, H., Lynch, J., Hanjal, R. F., and Summerville, W. W.: Studies on experimental hypertension: production of persistent elevation of systolic blood pressure by means of renal ischemia, J. Exper. Med. *59*:347, 1934.

46. Hermann, L. G., Cranley, J. J., and Prenninger, R. M.: Importance of collateral circulation in obliterative arterial disease of lower extremities, Geriatrics *9*:1-7, 1954.

47. Holden, W. D.: Reconstruction of the femoral artery for arteriosclerotic thrombosis, Surgery *27*:417-422, 1950.

48. Holman, E.: Arteriovenous Aneurysm: Abnormal Communications Between the Arterial and Venous Circulations, p. 244, New York, Macmillan, 1937.

49. Homans, J.: Thrombophlebitis of lower extremities, Ann. Surg. *87*:461, 1928.

50. Hufnagel, C. A.: The use of rigid and flexible plastic prostheses for arterial replacement, Surgery *37*:165-174, 1955.

51. Hughes, C. W., Jahnke, E. J.: Surgery of traumatic arteriovenous fistulas and aneurysms: five year follow-up study of 215 lesions, Ann. Surg. *148*:790-797, 1958.

52. Hunt, J. R.: The role of the carotid arteries in the causation of vascular lesions of the brain, with remarks on certain special features of the symptomatology, Am. J. M. Sc. *147*:704, 1914.

53. Jahnke, E. J., Jr.: Late structural and functional results of arterial injuries primarily repaired: study of 115 cases, Surgery *43*: 175-183, 1958.

54. Jahnke, E. J., and Seeley, S. F.: Acute vascular injuries in the Korean War: an analysis of 77 consecutive cases, Ann. Surg. *138*:158, 1953.

55. Janes, J. M., and Ivens, J. C.: A method of dealing with arteriosclerotic popliteal aneurysms, Surgery *29*:398, 1951.

56. Janeway, T. C.: Note on the blood pressure changes following reduction of the renal artery circulation, Proc. Soc. Exper. Biol. & Med. *6*:109, 1909.

57. Javid, H.: Surgical management of cerebral vascular insufficiency, A.M.A. Arch. Surg. *80*:883-889, 1960.

58. Javid, H., Dye, W. S., Grove, W. J., and Julian, O. C.: Resection of ruptured aneurysms of the abdominal aorta, Ann. Surg. *142*:613-623, 1955.

59. Johnson, J., Kirby, C. K., Greifenstein, F. E., and Castillo, A.: The experimental and clinical use of vein grafts to replace defects of large arteries, Surgery *26*:945-956, 1949.

60. Julian, O. C.: Chronic occlusion of the aorta and iliac arteries, S. Clin. North America *40*:139-151, 1960.

61. Julian, O. C., Deterling, R. A., Jr., Dye, W. S., Bhonslay, S., Grove, W. J., Lopez-Belio, M., and Javid, H.: Dacron tube and

bifurcation arterial prostheses produced to specification. II. Continued clinical use and the addition of microcrimping. A.M.A. Arch. Surg. *78*:260-270, 1959.

62. Julian, O. C., and Dye, W. S.: Treatment of peripheral vascular disease: modern concepts, S. Clin. North America *32*:263-285, 1952.

63. Julian, O. C., Dye, W. S., Javid, H., and Grove, W. J.: The use of vessel grafts in the treatment of popliteal aneurysms, Surgery *38*:970-980, 1955.

64. Julian, O. C., Dye, W. S., Olwin, J. H., and Jordan, P. H.: Direct surgery of arteriosclerosis, Ann. Surg. *136*:459-474, 1952.

65. Julian, O. C., Dye, W. S., and Schneewind, J.: Surgical management of ulcerative stasis disease of the lower extremities, A.M.A. Arch. Surg. *68*:757-768, 1954.

66. Julian, O. C., Grove, W. J., Dye, W. S., Javid, H., and Sadove, M. S.: New methods of surgical treatment of degenerative diseases of the abdominal aorta, Ann. Int. Med. *41*:36-49, 1954.

67. Julian, O. C., Grove, W. J., Dye, W. S., Olwin, J. H., and Sadove, M. S.: Direct surgery of arteriosclerosis: resection of abdominal aorta with homologous aortic graft replacement, Ann. Surg. *138*:387-403, 1953.

68. Julian, O. C., Javid, H., Dye, W. S., and El Issa, S.: Diagnosis and surgical approach to aorticoiliac arterial disease, Am. J. Cardiol. *4*:622-631, 1959.

69. Julian, O. C., and Shabart, E. J.: Lumbar sympathectomy in peripheral vascular disease, Arch. Surg. *61*:804-809, 1950.

70. Key, Einar: Embolectomy in the treatment of circulatory disturbances in the extremities, Surg., Gynec. & Obst. *36*:309-316, 1923.

71. Kirklin, J. W., Waugh, J. M., Grindlay, J. H., Openshaw, C. R., and Allen, E. V.: Surgical treatment of arteriosclerotic aneurysms of the abdominal aorta, A.M.A. Arch. Surg. *67*:632-644, 1953.

72. Kirtley, J. A., Jr., Garrett, S. Y., and Martin, R. S., Jr.: An evaluation of lumbar sympathectomy in 200 consecutive cases of peripheral vascular disorders, Surgery *33*:256-267, 1953.

73. Kunlin, J.: Le traitement de l'ischémie artérique par la graffe veineuse longue, Rev. chir. *70*:206, 1951.

74. ———: Venous grafts in therapy of endarteritis obliterans, Arch. mal. coeur *42*:371, 1949.

75. Lam, C. R., and Aram, H. H.: Resection of the descending thoracic aorta for aneurysm;

a report of the use of a homograft in a case and an experimental study, Ann. Surg. *134*: 743-752, 1951.

76. Leriche, R.: De la résection du carrefour aortico-iliaque avec double sympathectomie lombaire pour thrombose artéritique de l'aorte; le syndrome de l'oblitération termino-aortique pour artérite, Presse méd. *48*:601-604, 1940.

77. Leriche, R., Froment, R., and Vacton, A.: Artérectomie pour embolie de l'artére fémorale superficielle: rétrocession de tous les terribles, Lyon méd. *154*:416-422, 1934.

78. Leriche, R., and Kunlin, J.: Essais de désobstruction des artéres thromboses suivant la technique de J. Cid dos Santos, Lyon chir. *42*:675, 1947.

79. Lin, P. M., Javid, H., and Doyle, E. J.: Partial internal carotid artery occlusion treated by primary resection and vein graft: report of a case, J. Neurosurg. *13*:650, 1956.

80. Linton, R. R.: The arteriosclerotic aneurysm: a report of 14 patients treated by preliminary lumbar sympathetic ganglionectomy and aneurysmectomy, Surgery *26*:41, 1949.

81. ———: Intrasaccular wiring of abdominal arteriosclerotic aortic aneurysms by the "pack" method, Angiology *2*:458, 1951.

82. ———: A new surgical technique for the treatment of postphlebitic varicose ulcers of the lower leg, New England J. Med. *219*: 367, 1938.

83. ———: Some practical considerations in the surgery of blood vessel grafts, Surgery *38*: 817-834, 1955.

84. Linton, R. R., and White, P. D.: Arteriovenous fistula between the right common iliac artery and the inferior vena cava: report of a case of its occurrence following an operation for a ruptured intervertebral disc, with cure by operation, Arch. Surg. *50*:6-13, 1945.

85. Lord, J. W.: Traumatic lesions of arteries, S. Clin. North America *30*:377-386, 1950.

86. Luke, J. C.: The sequelae of thrombophlebitis, Angiology *4*:413, 1953.

87. Luke, J. C., and Levitan, B. A.: Revascularization of kidney in hypertension due to renal artery stenosis, Arch. Surg. *79*:269-275, 1959.

88. Lyons, C., and Galbraith, G.: Surgical treatment of atherosclerotic occlusion of internal carotid artery, Ann. Surg. *146*:487, 1957.

89. Mahorner, H. R., and Ochsner, A.: A new test for evaluating circulation in the venous system of the lower extremity affected by varicosities, Arch. Surg. *33*:479, 1938.

90. Matas, R.: Endoaneurysmorrhaphy, Surg., Gynec. & Obst. 30:456, 1920.
91. Morris, G. C., Jr., DeBakey, M. E., Cooley, D. A., and Crawford, E. S.: Surgical treatment of renal hypertension, Ann. Surg. 151: 854-66, 1960.
92. Morton, J. J., and Scott, W. J. N.: Ligation of the abdominal aorta for aneurysm, Ann. Surg. 119:457-467, 1944.
93. Moyer, C. A., and Butcher, H. R., Jr.: Stasis ulcers; an evaluation of the effectiveness of 3 methods of therapy and the implication of obliterative cutaneous lymphangitis as a credible etiologic factor, Ann. Surg. 141:577, 1955.
94. Nicoladoni, C.: Phlebarteriectasie der rechten oberen Extremität, Arch, klin. Chir. 18:252-274, 1875.
95. Ochsner, A., and DeBakey, M. E.: Thrombophlebitis and phlebothrombosis, South. Surgeon 8:269-290, 1939.
96. Olwin, J. H., Dye, W. S., and Julian, O. C.: Late peripheral arterial embolectomy, A.M.A. Arch. Surg. 66:480-487, 1953.
97. Oudot, J., and Beaconsfield, P.: Thrombosis of the aortic bifurcation treated by resection and homograft replacement: report of 5 cases, A.M.A. Arch. Surg. 66:365, 1953.
98. Perthes, G.: Ueber die Operation der Unterschenkelvaricen nach Trendelenburg, Deutsche med. Wchnschr. 1:253-357, 1895.
99. Poutasse, E. F.: Surgical treatment of renal hypertension: results in patients with occlusive disease of renal arteries, J. Urol. 82:403, 1959.
100. Pringle, J. H.: Two cases of vein grafting for the maintenance of direct arterial circulation, Lancet 1:1795-1796, 1913.
101. Rasmussen, J. A., Potter, S. E., and Best, R. R.: Management of acute massive venous occlusion, Surgery 40:387-390, 1956.
102. Raynaud, A. G. M.: De l'asphyxie locale et de la gangréne symétrique des extrémités, p. 6, Paris, Rignoux, 1862.
103. Reboul, H., and Huguier, J.: Endarteriectomic aortico-iliaque gauche datant de 16 mois, Mém. Acad. chir. 75:318, 1949.
104. Rob, C., and Wheeler, E. B.: Thrombosis of internal carotid artery treated by arterial surgery, Brit. M. J. 2:264-266, 1957.
106. Seeley, S. F., Hughes, C. W., and Jahnke, E. J.: Direct anastomosis versus ligation and excision in traumatic arteriovenous fistulae and aneurysms: experience with 150 consecutive Korean wounds, S. Forum 152:154, 1952.
107. Schafer, P. W., and Hardin, C. A.: The use of temporary polyethylene shunts to permit occlusion, resection, and frozen homologous graft replacement of vital vessel segments, Surgery 31:186, 1952.
108. Shumacker, H. B., Jr.: The problem of maintaining the continuity of the artery in the surgery of aneurysms and arteriovenous fistulae, Ann. Surg. 127:207-230, 1948.
109. Shumacker, H. B., Jr., Harris, E. J., and Siderys, H.: Pliable plastic tubes as aortic substitutes, Surgery 37:80-93, 1955.
110. Siekert, R. G., Whisnant, J. P., Baker, H. L., Jr., Bernatz, P. E., Ellis, H. F., and Millikan, C. H.: Symposium on surgical treatment of extracranial occlusive cerebrovascular disease, Proc. Staff Meet. Mayo Clin. 35:473-502, 1960.
111. Swan, H., Maaske, C., Johnson, N., and Grover, R.: Arterial homografts: II. Resection of thoracic aortic aneurysm using a stored human arterial transplant, Arch. Surg. 61:732, 1950.
112. Trippel, O. H.: Surgical management of hypertension due to renal artery occlusion, S. Clin. North America 40:177-189, 1960.
113. Veal, J. R., and Dugan, T. J.: Peripheral arterial embolism, Ann. Surg. 133:603-609, 1951.
114. Voorhees, A. B., Jaretzki, A., III, and Blakemore, A. H.: The use of tubes constructed from vinyon "N" cloth in bridging arterial defects, Ann. Surg. 135:332-336, 1952.
115. White, J. C., Smithwick, R. H., and Simeone, F. A.: The Autonomic Nervous System, p. 569, New York, Macmillan, 1952.
116. Willman, V. L., and Hanlon, C. R.: Safer operation in aortic saddle embolism: four consecutive successful embolectomies via the femoral arteries under local anesthesia, Ann. Surg. 150:568-574, 1959.
117. Winiwarter, von, Felix: Ueber eine eigenthümliche Form von Endartriitis und Endophlebitis mit Gangrän des Fusse, Arch. klin. Chir. 23:202-226, 1879.
118. Wylie, E. J.: Thromboendarterectomy for arteriosclerotic thrombosis of major arteries, Surgery 32:275-292, 1952.
119. Wylie, E. J., Kerr, E., and Davies, O.: Experimental and clinical experiences with the use of fascia lata applied as a graft about major arteries after thrombo-endarterectomy and aneurysmorrhaphy, Surg., Gynec. & Obst. 93:257, 1951.
120. Ziperman, H. H.: Acute arterial injuries in the Korean War, Ann. Surg. 139:1, 1954.

JULIAN JOHNSON, M.D.

——————————— CHAPTER 41 ———————————

Cardiac Surgery

Introduction
Congenital Heart Disease
Acquired Heart Disease
Open Cardiac Surgery Under Direct Vision
Cardiac Resuscitation

In days of old the brain was considered to be the source of the intellect; the heart, the seat of the soul. This general concept may have played some part in the fact that only relatively recently has the surgeon attempted to operate upon the heart. No doubt, the problems of the physiologic changes that occur when the thorax is opened have been important in delaying the development of cardiac surgery, as well as thoracic surgery, in general.

In recent years, thoracic surgical procedures have become commonplace, and rapid advances have been made in cardiac surgery. Initially, attention was turned to various cardiac lesions that could be corrected or improved physiologically by operations outside the heart. Later, operative procedures were carried out inside the heart by palpation without interrupting the blood flow through the heart. More recently, the heart has been opened, and intracardiac defects have been repaired under direct vision. This was first done by taking advantage of the fact that the circulation can be stopped for short periods if the patient's body temperature is lowered.

For the past several years the attention of the cardiac world has been focused on the heart-lung machine which allows the surgeon to bypass the heart and the lungs completely, so that he may open the heart and repair various defects under direct vision with deliberation. The advantage of this method was demonstrated very rapidly, and its usefulness has been conceded by all who are interested in this field. At present several varieties of heart-lung machines are being used successfully, and a major effort is being made to improve them further and perhaps simplify them. A great many advances have already been made, using this technic, and the possibilities which lie ahead seem to be almost limitless. It is evident, therefore, that much of what is recorded here may rapidly become outdated. Insofar as possible, an effort has been made to indicate the procedures that have been accepted generally at the present time and to state when the procedure is simply one for use until something better is available.

CONGENITAL CARDIAC LESIONS

THE ACYANOTIC GROUP

Patent Ductus Arteriosus

The surgical correction of a patent ductus arteriosus was first performed successfully by Gross[25] in 1938. Since that time this lesion has been operated upon all over the world with a low mortality.

The patent ductus arteriosus is a vessel connecting the pulmonary artery with the aorta, usually at a point just distal to the left subclavian artery. In normal circumstances this vessel becomes obliterated at or shortly after birth. In unusual circumstances, it remains patent.

Pathologic Physiology. In embryonal life the blood flow through the patent ductus arteriosus is from the pulmonary artery to the aorta, so that in embryo, as well as shortly after birth, the right ventricle is the predominant ventricle. At the time of birth, with the expansion of the lungs the pulmonary arterial resistance in the lungs is reduced greatly, and the blood flow through the lungs is increased greatly. With the fall in pressure in the pulmonary artery and the rise in pressure in the aorta, the direction of flow is changed in the patent ductus arteriosus and becomes a left to right shunt; that is, from the aorta to the pulmonary artery. In normal circumstances for the patent ductus arteriosus, the diastolic pressure in the aorta is higher than the systolic pressure in the pulmonary artery, so that there is a continuous flow of blood from the aorta to the pulmonary artery through the patent ductus arteriosus. In unusual circumstances secondary changes may occur in the arterioles in the lung and increase resistance to blood flow, with the consequent rise in pressure in the pulmonary artery. In such event the pulmonary artery pressure may equal the aortic pressure, except during systole, so that the flow from the aorta to the pulmonary artery is no longer continuous but is intermittent and occurs only during systole. In the presence of extreme pulmonary resistance the pulmonary artery pressure may become higher than that in the aorta, so that actually there is a right-to-left shunt through the patent ductus arteriosus; that is, from the pulmonary artery to the aorta. This produces some peripheral cyanosis with a decrease in the arterial oxygen content, particularly to the lower part of the body, since the patent ductus arteriosus usually joins the aorta distal to the left subclavian artery. It should be emphasized that this is an unusual happening, and it occurs very rarely in this disease.

Signs and Symptoms. In most instances the child with the patent ductus arteriosus will not be aware of it until the diagnosis is made at the time of a routine physical examination. The child's color is normal, since the flow, except in rare cases, is continuously from left to right, and the child may live a perfectly normal existence with little or no decrease in exercise tolerance, particularly if the patent ductus arteriosus is a small one. If, on the other hand, the patent ductus arteriosus is a large one, the child may develop dyspnea on exertion, and it is not uncommon to find such children considerably underdeveloped physically. In extreme instances, when the patent ductus arteriosus is very large, the patient may go into cardiac failure during infancy within the first few months of life.

The patient may be cyanotic in very exceptional cases, and then under only one of two conditions: either the patient is in cardiac failure and the cyanosis is caused by pulmo-nary edema and inadequate oxygenation of the blood that passes through the lungs, or there is a reversal of blood flow through the patent ductus arteriosus with blood flowing from the pulmonary artery into the aorta and bringing about the cyanosis. With few exceptions, however, the color of the patient is normal.

The characteristic *physical finding* is a continuous "machinerylike" murmur heard most readily in the second interspace to the left of the sternum anteriorly. In some patients a thrill can be felt on palpation, in addition to the continuous murmur on auscultation. Because of the large runoff from the aorta through the patent ductus arteriosus, the diastolic blood pressure is apt to be low, with a resulting widening of the pulse pressure. A roentgen examination of the patient usually will reveal a fullness in the area of the pulmonary conus with evidence of more than normal blood flow in the pulmonary vascular bed. On fluoroscopic examination there is apt to be an increased pulsation in the hilar vessels, particularly in those patients with an increased pulse pressure.

In some instances the continuous murmur may not be present, and the patient may have only a systolic murmur. This is apt to be present in those who have an increase in the pulmonary artery pressure. In those rare cases in which the aortic and pulmonary artery pressures are approximately the same throughout the cardiac cycle, no murmur will be heard. Not infrequently it is difficult to hear a continuous murmur in infants.

Diagnosis. In the vast majority of cases the diagnosis of the patent ductus arteriosus can be made on the clinical examination alone, without any special studies. The presence of the continuous murmur usually is diagnostic in itself. The two conditions in which there may be a continuous murmur not due to a patent ductus arteriosus are very uncommon: (1) an aortic window and (2) a ruptured sinus of Valsalva. In these instances the murmur is apt to be at a different location, so that the variation may be suggested. When a continuous murmur cannot be heard and only a systolic murmur is present, the diagnosis of the patent ductus arteriosus may be more difficult. This is especially important in the infant, since not infrequently the patient may be close

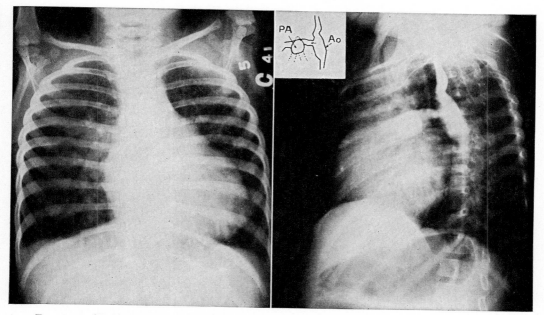

FIG. 41-1. (*Left*) Plain roentgenogram of the chest in a patient with a patent ductus arteriosus. Note the prominence of the pulmonary conus producing a convex border to the heart. Also note the prominent vascular markings especially shown in the right lung. (*Right*) Aortogram performed by injecting the contrast medium through the left subclavian artery. The contrast medium fills the aorta and passes through the patent ductus arteriosus into the pulmonary artery.

to extremis from cardiac failure, and a failure to make the diagnosis of a patent ductus arteriosus may result in a preventable death.

There are several methods by which the diagnosis of patent ductus arteriosus may be confirmed by special studies. In the infant, if a contrast medium is injected into the brachial artery quite rapidly, an aortogram may be obtained that will afford a good visualization of the aorta. If a patent ductus arteriosus is present, the contrast medium will run off through the patent ductus arteriosus into the pulmonary artery, pass through the lungs and reappear in the left auricle. In questionable cases this is perhaps the simplest method of obtaining the diagnosis of patent ductus arteriosus in the infant. It has been used less extensively in the adult by passing a catheter into the aorta through the left arm. The resistance of the catheter makes some type of power injector desirable. One is much less likely to obtain satisfactory confirmation of a patent ductus arteriosus by means of angiocardiography; that is, by the injection of the dye on the venous side of the heart. However,

angiocardiography has been used quite extensively, and not infrequently a patent ductus arteriosus can be visualized by that means. Nevertheless, in most instances the aortogram technic is far superior.

The diagnosis of patent ductus arteriosus may also be definitely confirmed by cardiac catheterization. If there is an increase in the arterial oxygen in the pulmonary artery as opposed to the right ventricle, a patent ductus arteriosus is very likely to be present. A rise in the pressure in the same area may be indicative of a patent ductus, and, in some instances, the catheter may pass directly through the patent ductus arteriosus and go down the descending aorta.

Treatment. Surgical obliteration of the patent ductus arteriosus is the treatment of choice. This treatment is advocated as a matter of election because of the poor prognosis for the patient if the lesion is not obliterated surgically. There is little, if any, chance that the patent ductus arteriosus will become obliterated spontaneously, and, according to the figures of Maud Abbott,[1] the average life

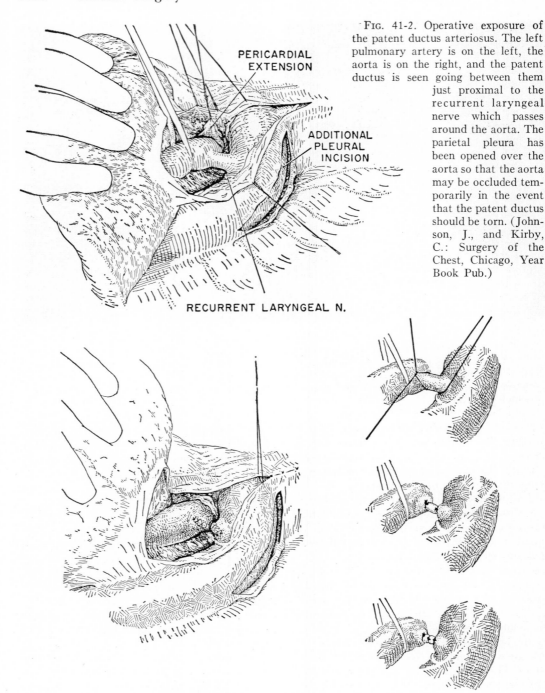

PERICARDIAL
EXTENSION

ADDITIONAL
PLEURAL
INCISION

RECURRENT LARYNGEAL N.

FIG. 41-2. Operative exposure of the patent ductus arteriosus. The left pulmonary artery is on the left, the aorta is on the right, and the patent ductus is seen going between them just proximal to the recurrent laryngeal nerve which passes around the aorta. The parietal pleura has been opened over the aorta so that the aorta may be occluded temporarily in the event that the patent ductus should be torn. (Johnson, J., and Kirby, C.: Surgery of the Chest, Chicago, Year Book Pub.)

FIG. 41-3. (*Left*) The patent ductus in this view has been divided and the 2 ends sutured with fine silk sutures. (*Right*) This view shows the obliteration of the patent ductus arteriosus by 3 ligatures. This method of closure of the patent ductus arteriosus is satisfactory when the ductus is long enough to allow the ligatures to be placed in this manner. (Johnson, J., and Kirby, C.: Surgery of the Chest, Chicago, Year Book Pub.)

expectancy in the patient with patent ductus arteriosus is about 33 years. Although these figures were collected before the advent of antibiotics, nevertheless, much of the mortality associated with patent ductus arteriosus is on the basis of vascular complications, and, furthermore, the antibiotics have not relieved us completely of the dangers and the fears of subacute bacterial endarteritis and endocarditis that are engrafted so frequently upon the patent ductus arteriosus if it is left alone.

The method of obliteration of a patent ductus arteriosus probably is not important so long as it is successful. Gross[23] and many others advocate the complete division of the ductus with closure of the two ends by suture in all cases. We, on the other hand, have felt that if the ductus is fairly long, triple ligation with silk is a satisfactory method of closure. As far as we are aware, we have had only one recurrence or persistence of a patent ductus arteriosus following this method of closure in about 300 operations. However, when the patent ductus arteriosus is short and broad, we obliterate it by division and suture as a matter of preference. This applies routinely in adults. It is our belief that in those instances in which there apparently has been a recurrence of the patent ductus arteriosus following the ligation technic, the ligature, in fact, has not been tied tightly enough, or such heavy ligature material has been used that it binds upon itself and does not allow complete obliteration of the ductus.

In the vast majority of instances when the diagnosis of a patent ductus arteriosus is made, the surgeon can proceed with its obliteration without further concern. However, there are two situations that require some comment. In an occasional patient there is some other congenital abnormality, and the patent ductus arteriosus may be acting as a compensatory factor. For example, if the patient has a tetralogy of Fallot, the patent ductus arteriosus may be keeping the patient alive. Therefore, if there is any suggestion of another congenital abnormality, particularly of the cyanotic type, the patient should be studied very carefully before a closure of the ductus is considered. The second situation in which the surgeon should go slowly is when there is reason to suspect a reversal of flow through the ductus from right to left, causing partial unsaturation of the arterial oxygen content of the peripheral blood. Now, generally, it is thought that if there is a continuous right-to-left flow, the chances are that the ductus cannot be obliterated safely. On the other hand, if the right-to-left flow is only intermittent, the secondary changes in the lung may be reversible and the patient returned to normal after obliteration of the ductus.

If the preoperative studies do not preclude completely the possibility of exploration, the surgeon may undertake to find out what happens when the ductus is occluded temporarily. If pulmonary hypertension is present, the surgeon always should be hesitant about a hasty occlusion of the ductus. If the pressure in the pulmonary artery as measured at operation or before operation is lower than that in the aorta, the chances are that the occlusion of the ductus will be successful. If it is higher than that in the aorta at all times, the chances are that it will be unsuccessful.

It is now common practice for the surgeon to measure the pressure before and after temporary occlusion of the ductus. If the pulmonary artery pressure decreases with temporary occlusion of the ductus, then permanent occlusion of the ductus would seem to be indicated. If the pulmonary artery pressure remains the same, it may also be indicated. If, however, the pulmonary artery pressure increases after a temporary occlusion of the ductus, it probably is wisest not to attempt to make the occlusion permanent for fear that the patient will die because of the inability of the right heart to force blood through the lungs satisfactorily.

Results and Prognosis. The mortality rate for the operation of patent ductus arteriosus in most of the large hospitals is in the neighborhood of 1 per cent. It is felt now that there is little reason to delay operation once the diagnosis of patent ductus arteriosus is made, and that its obliteration may be carried out at almost any age. Whereas formerly we waited electively until the child was 4 or 5 years of age, we now have abandoned that practice and are apt to operate upon the patient whenever the diagnosis is made. On the other hand, if the heart is not enlarged and the child is not having any difficulty, there is no reason why one should not wait until the age of 3 or 4 for the operative procedure.

However, if the heart is somewhat enlarged, it would seem wiser and safer to proceed with the operation without further delay, regardless of the age.

Aortic Window

The term *aortic window* is applied to a condition in which there is an opening between the aorta and the pulmonary artery just above the heart. It is apt to give the signs and symptoms of a patent ductus arteriosus, although the continuous murmur is more likely to be situated somewhat lower. Fairly frequently the opening may be quite large, and only a systolic murmur may be heard. It is a fairly uncommon lesion, and probably it cannot be differentiated from the patent ductus arteriosus on the basis of clinical grounds alone, although it may be suspected in the patient with the unusually large left-to-right shunt. A few of these patients have been operated upon successfully by obliteration of this aortic window.[44] In the future this lesion probably will be corrected only while utilizing cardiopulmonary bypass.

Coarctation of the Aorta

Coarctation of the aorta is a congenital lesion that is manifested by stenosis or complete occlusion of the aorta, usually at or about the level of the ligamentum arteriosum. Rarely, the coarctation involves some other portion of the thoracic or abdominal aorta.

When the constriction occurs at the usual level, the ductus arteriosus may or may not remain patent, but it is seldom a prominent factor in the distorted physiology. Any flow through the patent ductus arteriosus is from left to right. A marked collateral circulation develops round the site of constriction in the aorta and keeps the lower part of the body alive.

In rare instances the aortic constriction is above the ductus arteriosus, and the ductus arteriosus remains patent. In those cases the blood-flow is apt to pass from the pulmonary artery into the descending aorta, and relatively small amounts of blood-flow pass from the arch of the aorta into the descending aorta. Because of the large amount of blood-flow going from the patent ductus into the descending aorta, the usual collateral circulation has not been highly developed. This uncommon condition usually is referred to as the infantile type of coarctation of the aorta, because of the fact that these patients seldom live beyond infancy.

The physiologic response to coarctation of the aorta is an extremely interesting one. The patient develops hypertension in the upper part of the body, and the most frequent cause of death is associated with this hypertension. The hypertension certainly must be helpful in producing the collateral circulation, and the blood-flow into the descending aorta may occur by the reverse flow of blood through the large intercostal arteries distal to the constriction. The cause of the development of hypertension is not entirely certain. In some way it is related to the kidney, since it can be produced experimentally by performing a coarctation proximal to the kidney. The hypertension so produced can be relieved by transplanting the kidney to an area above the coarctation. It is not entirely a mechanical problem, as demonstrated by the fact that the blood pressure may not return to normal for several days or weeks following the correction of coarctation of the aorta. In man a few cases of coarctation of the abdominal aorta in which partial occlusion of only one renal artery exists have been reported. The hypertension in these patients has been relieved immediately by nephrectomy or a splenorenal shunt. These observations confirm the animal experiments—that the hypertension is renovascular in origin.

One other point in the physiologic response to the constriction of the aorta is the dilatation that frequently occurs distal to the constriction. This phenomenon is referred to as "poststenotic dilatation," and it has been emphasized by many writers, notably Halsted[26] and Holman.[28] The exact mechanism that brings this about is perhaps not known, but it is thought to be related to the turbulence of the blood stream distal to the constriction.

Signs and Symptoms. The patient with coarctation of the aorta may be unaware of being abnormal, and the diagnosis may be made accidentally on a routine physical examination. In many instances, however, the upper extremities and the upper part of the body are apt to be more developed than the lower. When the patient's attention is called to it, it is found that the blood-flow to the

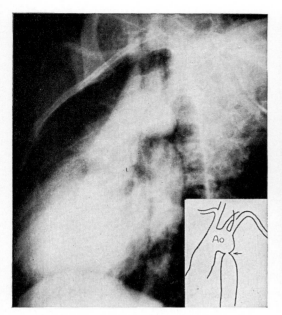

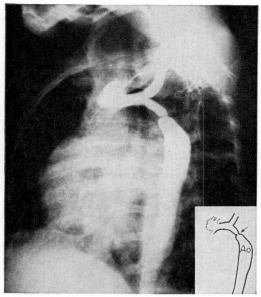

FIG. 41-4. Angiocardiogram, showing a coarctation of the aorta. While the visualization is adequate in this particular patient, this method does not always show the lesion as satisfactorily as this, particularly in an adult.

FIG. 41-5. An aortogram, showing a coarctation of the aorta in a child. The exact anatomic structure is shown much more vividly than with the angiocardiogram as seen in Figure 41-4.

lower part of his body is reduced somewhat, and that his feet are unusually cold in many circumstances. The symptoms that are most likely to direct the patient's attention to coarctation of the aorta are those associated with the hypertension.

The common causes of death are cerebral hemorrhage or rupture of an aneurysm, or factors of that type. According to Maud Abbott's survey,[1] the average life expectancy is about 35 years.

Not infrequently, a patient will be found with coarctation of the aorta who does not have hypertension to any marked degree at rest, and yet, with exercise, hypertension will be unusually severe and much beyond the usual response to such exercise. The physical findings in the patient with coarctation usually are characteristic if the diagnosis is suspected. Usually, a systolic murmur is heard not only in front but also in back on the posterior aspect of the chest. Frequently, evidence of the collateral circulation can be felt by palpating vessels between the scapulae posteriorly, and the murmur can be heard to be

transmitted in this area. With coarctations of the abdominal aorta the physical signs may be lacking except for hypertension.

A most important observation is the absence of pulses in the lower part of the body or the decrease in blood pressure in this area. In normal circumstances, as the blood pressure is taken with the sphygmomanometer the systolic blood pressure should be higher than that obtained in the upper extremities. In many instances, however, in coarctation of the aorta, a blood pressure cannot be obtained in the lower extremities, and, when it is obtained, it will be considerably lower than in the upper extremities. It should be pointed out that when the collateral circulation is very good, pulses and blood pressure may be obtained in the lower extremities, although the blood pressure will usually not be so high as that in the upper.

Frequently a diagnosis of coarctation may be suspected on the basis of the ordinary roentgen film of the chest in which the aortic arch is much less prominent than usual and evidences of collateral circulation may be seen

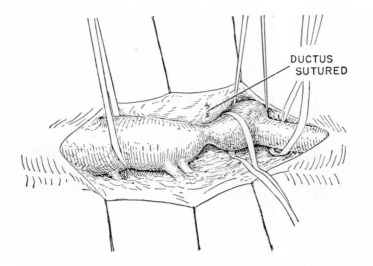

DUCTUS
SUTURED

Fig. 41-6. Operative exposure of a coarctation of the aorta. The patent ductus arteriosus has already been divided and sutured. Hernia tapes have been placed around the proximal and distal aorta and the subclavian artery. (Johnson, J., and Kirby, C.: Surgery of the Chest, Chicago, Year Book Pub).

by the notching of the inferior borders of the ribs caused by the enlarged intercostal arteries. Rib notching may be less evident early in the course of the disease in infants and in young children.

Diagnosis. As a general rule, a diagnosis of coarctation of the aorta may be made on a clinical basis, and exact information need not be obtained before the time of thoracotomy. With very few exceptions, the site of the coarctation of the aorta will be found to be just below the subclavian artery on the left, so that, for practical purposes, actual demonstration is not necessary before the time of

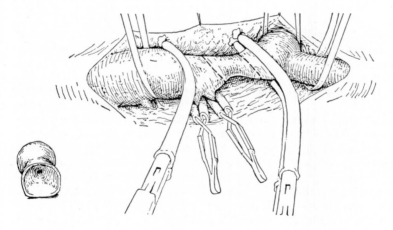

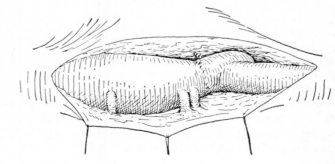

Fig. 41-7. (*Top*) Noncrushing clamps are placed across the aorta above and below the coarctation. (*Bottom*) The constricted segment is cut out and the 2 ends are sewed together with fine silk sutures. (Johnson, J., and Kirby, C.: Surgery of the Chest, Chicago, Year Book Pub.)

operation. It can be readily shown, however, particularly in infancy and childhood, by means of the angiocardiogram as administered through the right side of the heart, and, not only can the location of the coarctation of the aorta be determined, but also its configuration can be seen with considerable accuracy. In the adult, particularly the heavily built individual, the angiocardiogram is not entirely reliable, but an aortogram may outline the defect if this is desired. Actually, there seems to be very little point in carrying out this study for thoracic coarctations. However, aortography should be used when an abdominal coarctation is suspected. It is important to ascertain the exact extent of the lesion and the status of the renal arteries.

With coarctation of the thoracic aorta the clinical diagnosis of coarctation can be relied upon. Now that vascular prostheses are readily available in the event that one is necessary, it is not important to delineate the exact anatomic relationships preoperatively.

Treatment. The treatment of choice for coarctation of the aorta is excision of the constricted area with end-to-end anastomosis. This was first performed successfully by Crafoord[17] in 1944. The surgeon, naturally, is interested in the physiologic response to total occlusion of the aorta during the surgical correction of the coarctation. If the aorta has been completely occluded, obviously nothing further is done when the aorta is clamped. If the coarctation was not complete, the clamping of the aorta might add something that was not present formerly. It is common practice, however, to put noncrushing clamps across the aorta above and below the coarctation for long periods of time while the constricted area is excised and the ends are sutured, and there have been few, if any, instances of paraplegia resulting from it. The collateral blood-flow has been adequate for long periods of time. If, on the other hand, the opening in the coarctation is unusually large, and the collateral circulation appears to be small, the distal aorta may collapse appreciably when the aorta is clamped. In this situation it may be wise to reduce the patient's temperature before resecting the coarctation or utilize some type of bypass during the procedure. It is probable that paraplegia

will seldom occur with less than 20 minutes' occlusion of the normal aorta.

The ideal treatment for coarctation is an end-to-end anastomosis. In some circumstances, however, the aorta may be tapered to a degree that may not allow an opening of adequate size without cutting away an undue portion of the aorta. In the past it was common practice to turn down the subclavian artery in some of these patients. In those instances in which the subclavian artery was unusually large this gave a good result with return of the blood pressure to normal. In about half of the patients, however, the subclavian artery apparently was not sufficiently large, and a satisfactory drop in blood pressure did not occur. This procedure, therefore, has been practically abandoned in favor of aorta grafts when a satisfactory opening cannot be obtained by an end-to-end anastomosis. Aorta grafts used experimentally by Carrel[15] as early as 1906 and adapted for clinical use by Gross[24] some 40 years later were widely accepted at one time. More recently, plastic grafts have been used. Since even the aortic grafts do not grow, the grafts should be used in infancy and childhood only in dire circumstances. A satisfactory lumen can usually be obtained by some type of plastic procedure. A longitudinal strip graft enlarging the lumen of the subclavian is preferable to a circumferential graft, since the subclavian artery will continue to grow in circumference.

The time of election for operation for the patient with coarctation of the aorta has not been established. In general, it would seem that from 4 to 12 years of age would be a satisfactory period. At that time the vessels are pliable and easily brought together. Therefore, the chances of having to use a graft at this age are reduced greatly, and almost always some type of plastic procedure can be performed to give a satisfactory opening. There is probably no upper age limit for operating upon patients with coarctation of the aorta now that grafts are available and can be put into position, reducing all tension on the suture line. There may well be no age limit in the lower ages for coarctation of the aorta, for several patients have been operated upon successfully in infancy. In general, the author has preferred to attempt to carry newborn infants along, if necessary, by digitaliza-

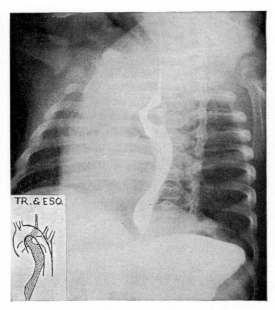

TR. & ESO.

FIG. 41-8. Esophagogram of a patient with a double aortic arch. The esophagus is displaced forward at one point by the posterior arch and constricted anteriorly by the anterior arch.

tion if cardiac failure occurs until they reach about 2 years of age.

Results and Prognosis. The results of the operation for coarctation of the aorta of the adult type have been excellent. The mortality has been in the neighborhood of 5 per cent or below. The blood-pressure response usually has returned toward normal, depending upon the surgeon's ability to obtain a sufficiently large opening at the site of the anastomosis. If the blood pressure in the lower extremities is higher than that in the upper extremities, the surgeon can be content that he has obtained a satisfactory opening, and, if hypertension persists, it is on some other basis. In the majority of instances, however, the blood pressure will return to normal or nearly normal, and it is anticipated that such patients will have a normal life expectancy. When it is necessary to use a graft, the longevity is uncertain, primarily for the lack of long-term evidence at the present time.

Only a few attempts have been made to repair the infantile type of coarctation of the aorta, and the mortality up to the present time has been high.

Vascular Rings

The congenital anomalies that occur in the aortic arch may show great variation. In themselves, they are unimportant and place no stress on the cardiocirculatory system. They are important when a vascular ring persists around the esophagus and the trachea and therefore may cause compression of these structures.

In embryo there are 2 aortic arches. Usually, the right disappears, and the left persists. Occasionally, the left disappears, and the right persists. When both vessels persist, there is a double aortic arch, one in front and one behind the trachea and the esophagus. The difficulty involved in this condition arises from the compression of these latter structures.

Similar compression from a vascular ring may occur with a right aortic arch, where the ductus arteriosus and the left subclavian artery arise from a common diverticulum on the right descending aorta to pass to the left behind the esophagus. There are many possible types of vascular rings. When the ring is incomplete, symptoms are less likely to develop, as when the right subclavian artery arises from a left descending aorta and passes to the right behind the esophagus.

The symptoms of a vascular ring usually develop in infancy and consist of a wheeze on respiration and frequent respiratory infection. Difficulty in swallowing may be noted in rather severe cases. The diagnosis should be considered in any infant with respiratory distress.

The diagnosis can be made by a careful roentgenographic examination. Compression of the trachea may be noted on a proper chest film. An esophagogram should reveal an indentation of the esophagus from behind at the level of the aortic arch.

The treatment is the division of the smaller one of the 2 vessels forming the vascular ring. When there is a double aortic arch, one is usually small, and it should be the one divided. The left thoracic approach is commonly preferred. In some instances, when the vascular ring is divided, the vessels tend to maintain their position. In such cases the pressure must be removed from the trachea and the esophagus by displacing the involved vessels by suturing them to surrounding structures.

When the constriction is caused by the ligamentum arteriosum or the subclavian behind the esophagus, these structures may be divided. In any event, great care should be taken to remove all pressure from the esophagus and the trachea.

The preoperative and postoperative care of these infants is of the greatest importance. They should be made as free as possible of respiratory infection preoperatively and watched very closely postoperatively. When diligence is exercised in providing adequate room for the trachea and the esophagus, and more than usual care is given in the postoperative period, the mortality is low and the results excellent.

Isolated Pulmonary Stenosis

The term *isolated pulmonary stenosis* refers to the congenital cardiac condition in which only the pulmonary valve is stenotic and no other congenital abnormalities are present. The stenosis usually is valvular in type. As a general rule, the valve is cone-shaped, and the small opening in the valve is at the apex of the cone, very much as a reversed megaphone. There is a great deal of variation, however, and in some instances the stenosis is infundibular in type; that is, a muscular constriction within the right ventricular outflow tract.

Since there is no communication between the 2 sides of the heart in this lesion, the patient is not cyanotic. All the blood that circulates through the heart goes through the lungs and is oxygenated, and for that reason the patient's peripheral arterial oxygen saturation is normal. The only inconvenience occasioned by the constriction of the pulmonary valve is that the right ventricle has to work harder in order to force the blood through such a small opening. For that reason, the cardiac output is apt to be reduced, even though the right ventricle may become hypertrophied and the right ventricular pressure increased greatly.

The symptoms that these patients are apt to experience are those of dyspnea and fatigue, particularly on exertion. As the heart begins to fail, the patient may have all the signs and symptoms of right heart failure. The electrocardiogram will show a right axis deviation because of the hypertrophy of the right ventricle. There is a harsh systolic murmur with

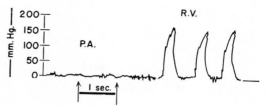

Fig. 41-9. Curves obtained on cardiac catheterization in a patient with an isolated pulmonary stenosis. First, the catheter was advanced into the pulmonary artery. The pressure curves shown were recorded as the catheter was withdrawn from the pulmonary artery into the right ventricle. The pressure in the pulmonary artery above the valve was approximately 10 mm. Hg systolic, whereas that in the right ventricle below the valve was approximately 160 mm. Hg systolic.

a thrill over the pulmonary area to the left of the sternum in the second interspace anteriorly. There is apt to be poststenotic dilatation of the pulmonary artery, frequently giving a false impression during roentgenologic studies of increased blood-flow through that vessel.

Frequently, the diagnosis of pulmonary stenosis can be made on a clinical basis by the murmur and the thrill and an apparent decrease in the amount of blood in the lungs. Cardiac catheterization, however, is essential for proper evaluation and accurate diagnosis of the condition, even though it may be suspected on the clinical examination. When the catheter is placed in the right side of the heart, there are no changes in the arterial oxygen saturation of the blood, indicating no shunts. However, the pressure in the pulmonary artery is low, and that in the right ventricle is high. If the catheter is first placed in the pulmonary artery and withdrawn slowly into the right ventricle at a time when a recording of the pressure curves is being made, a differentiation between valvular stenosis and infundibular stenosis usually is possible. In valvular stenosis there is a sudden transition from the low pulmonary artery pressure to the high right ventricular pressure. In the event of infundibular stenosis, an intermediate pressure usually is recorded as the catheter passes through the infundibular chamber.

Treatment. If the patient has a mild degree

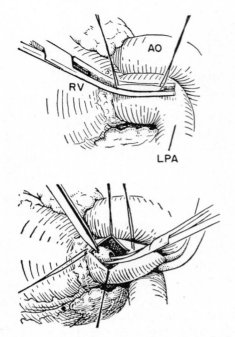

FIG. 41-10. This illustrates one method of correcting valvular pulmonary stenosis under direct vision. Utilizing moderate hypothermia, the valve may be visualized through an incision in the pulmonary artery. Cardiopulmonary bypass should be used if a right ventriculotomy is contemplated for the relief of infundibular stenosis. (Johnson, J., and Kirby, C.: Surgery of the Chest, Chicago, Year Book Pub.)

of pulmonary stenosis that does not raise the pressure in the right ventricle unduly, there probably is no indication for any surgical therapy. On the other hand, it is perfectly obvious that if these patients are to be operated upon, the operation should be carried out before the patient is in desperate condition from cardiac failure. The question arises, therefore, as to how high the right ventricular pressure should go before the operation should be done as a matter of election. The consensus at the present time is that if the pressure is as much as 100 mm. of mercury systolic in the right ventricle, operation as an elective procedure is justifiable. Some surgeons feel that 75 mm. of mercury is a proper figure to choose. Few, if any, feel that the operation should be advocated if the pressure is below 75 mm. of mercury in the right vetnricle and the patient is asymptomatic.

Several methods have been employed in the surgical treatment of pulmonary stenosis. Brock,[14] in 1947, was the first to advocate operation upon this lesion. He inserted an especially designed knife into the right ventricle that cut the valve open as it was passed out into the pulmonary artery. The same procedure has been accomplished by a cutting type instrument inserted through the wall of the pulmonary artery.

There was a fair amount of dissatisfaction with these procedures because of the feeling that the valve may be sufficiently elastic to stretch over the knife blade and not be opened completely by this maneuver. In many instances, although the patients have been improved vastly, pressures in the right ventricle have not returned to normal but perhaps only halfway to normal. If the operation is to be done blindly, the guillotine type of knife is probably the most satisfactory for opening the valve completely.

However, most surgeons are now operating upon this lesion under direct vision, using either hypothermia or cardiopulmonary bypass. If the stenosis is entirely valvular in type, hypothermia with an approach through the pulmonary artery has been successful for most surgeons. Nevertheless, many surgeons, along with the author, prefer to use cardiopulmonary bypass because of the possibility of finding some infundibular stenosis in addition to the pulmonary stenosis. Some authors feel that the infundibular stenosis may be the result of hypertrophy of the musculature of the right ventricle and will disappear in time after the relief of the valvular stenosis. However, the author prefers to relieve the pulmonary stenosis at the time of operation. In the case of infundibular stenosis, this means the excision of the muscular obstruction in the outflow tract of the right ventricle. Although this has been carried out as a blind procedure in the past,[13] it is now seldom done except under direct vision, utilizing cardiopulmonary bypass.

To date, the results of the operation on patients with pulmonary stenosis have been excellent as to mortality and morbidity, there being a very low mortality associated with the operation, particularly if it is valvular in type. In many instances in the past the stenosis has not been removed completely, and it may be that in the future some of these patients may have to be operated upon again. At the present time, however, the valvular stenosis would appear to be correctable to a nearly normal state, utilizing cardiopulmonary bypass and direct vision.

Pulmonary Stenosis with Ventricular Septal Defect

If an acyanotic patient has pulmonary stenosis plus a ventricular septal defect, the condition is often referred to as an "acyanotic tetralogy." In this condition the pulmonary stenosis is not sufficiently severe to cause a right-to-left shunt through the ventricular defect. There may be little or no shunt in either direction, or there may be a left-to-right shunt if the pulmonary stenosis is not severe.

Should the ventricular septal defect be undiagnosed and the pulmonary valvular stenosis corrected completely, the patient would suffer all the problems of a ventricular septal defect. This procedure has been carried out in the past and may be done unwittingly even now. However, if the correct diagnosis is made, all would now agree to the use of cardiopulmonary bypass for the closure of the ventricular septal defect and the relief of the pulmonary stenosis as one procedure.

The possibility of the presence of an unsuspected ventricular septal defect along with a pulmonary valvular stenosis is one reason for advocating operation upon that lesion by the right ventricular approach.

Atrial Septal Defect

An atrial septal defect should not be confused with a patent foramen ovale. In many instances there is a patent foramen ovale in which the flaplike valve over the opening is kept closed functionally by a slightly higher pressure in the left auricle. However, when a real atrial septal defect is present, there is a flow from left to right because of the higher pressures in the left atrium. The location of the atrial septal defect may be greatly varied. In general, there are two types—the so-called septum secundum, which is located high in the septum, and the septum primum, which extends low to include the area between the mitral and the tricuspid valves. In extreme cases, the defect may go on down and include the upper portion of the ventricular septum.

This is called a persistent atrioventricular canal.

Pathologic Physiology. The blood-flow is from the left to right through the atrial septal defect, so that some of the blood that has just arrived in the left atrium passes back through the defect into the right atrium, through the right ventricle, and into the lungs again. Thus, in this instance, the blood is going round and round through the lungs and the right heart in a manner somewhat similar to the patent ductus arteriosus, where the blood is going round and round through the lungs and the left heart. With the atrial septal defect the total cardiac output of the left heart will be considerably lower than that of the right heart, so that the pulmonary artery may become enormous and the aorta may be very small. It is not uncommon, for example, for the output of the right heart to be 4 or 5 times higher than that of the left heart.

As times go on, secondary obliterative vascular changes are apt to occur in the lungs, and resistance to the flow of blood is increased. Therefore, the pulmonary artery pressure will increase, and, if this process is carried to the extreme, the pressure may rise in the right ventricle and the right atrium so that the left-to-right shunt may disappear. In such circumstances, there usually is some mixing of the blood between the right and the left atria through the large defect, and the patient's systemic arterial oxygen saturation will be below normal. In such instances the right-to-left shunt and the left-to-right shunt may be approximately equal or a little bit in excess in either direction.

The symptoms of the atrial septal defect may be insignificant early in life, particularly if the defect is small. As a general rule, when the symptoms have been insignificant in early life and later develop to a significant degree, the defect is apt to be small, and surgical repair is relatively easy. If the defect has produced symptoms early, it is more likely to be a large one. The symptoms of the atrial septal defect are those of cardiac failure. When cardiac failure occurs in infancy, the lesion is apt to be a persistent atrioventricular canal.

The signs of atrial septal defect are those of an excess amount of blood-flow through the lungs and the right heart. A large pulmo-

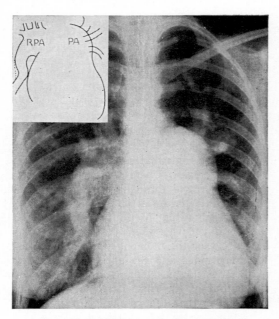

FIG. 41-11. Plain roentgenogram of the chest of a patient with an atrioseptal defect. Note the enlarged heart and the tremendously enlarged pulmonary conus, as well as the enlarged pulmonary arteries in the lung, visualized in this film, particularly in the right side.

nary artery and an excessive amount of blood in the lungs can be demonstrated readily on fluoroscopy and roentgen examination. It may be difficult to distinguish between an atrial septal defect and a ventricular septal defect on a clinical basis, but a lead in this direction is given by the nature of the murmur.

The definitive diagnosis of atrial septal defects is made by cardiac catheterization. When the catheter passes from the vena cava into the right auricle, there is an immediate increase in the arterial oxygen saturation, and in many instances the catheter may pass through the septal defect into the left auricle. After the catheter enters the right ventricle or passes into the pulmonary artery, there is no further increase in the arterial oxygen saturation. Also, the systolic pressure in the pulmonary artery and the right ventricle should be the same.

Treatment. The method first used extensively to close the atrial septal defect was that of inverting the atrial wall against the defect and suturing it in place, as suggested by

Cohn[16] and popularized by Bailey.[5] By inserting the finger into the right atrium, the size of the defect was ascertained, and some method of closure could usually be worked out in the secundum type defect. Bjork and Crafoord[12] recommend a circumferential suture around the atrial septum, and this was successful in many instances. Another method which was used successfully was that of suturing a patch over the defect by working through a rubber well attached to the wall of the right atrium.[25a]

In recent years all of the "blind" methods for the closure of these defects have given way to the use of direct vision, either under hypothermia or with cardiopulmonary bypass. The use of hypothermia has been highly successful in large series of patients.[35, 47] However, it does place a premium on speed in the closure of the defect. At a temperature of about 30° C. the circulation can be occluded safely for 4 or 5 minutes. Additional time for suture can be obtained by using 2 or 3 such periods if necessary[32] or by perfusing the coronary arteries during the inflow occlusion.[37] However, the use of cardiopulmonary bypass allows the surgeon all the time that he may need for the deliberate closure of the defect. For this reason the trend is toward the routine use of cardiopulmonary bypass for closure of atrial septal defects. At the present time the author still uses hypothermia for the closure of simple secundum type defects in children but is apt to use cardiopulmonary bypass in all complicated defects and in all adults. The use of cardiopulmonary bypass is considered essential in the septum primum type defect, since a patch is almost always necessary, and frequently a cleft mitral or tricuspid valve must be repaired.[36]

Ventricular Septal Defect

In the patient with a ventricular septal defect, the flow is from left to right because of the higher pressure in the left ventricle. The patient is not cyanotic, since oxygenated blood, which has just arrived in the left ventricle from the lungs, passes into the right ventricle, out the pulmonary artery, through the lungs and the left auricle and back into the left ventricle again. Thus, a goodly portion of the blood goes round and round through the lungs and the left heart without going to the systemic circulation in the same manner as it does in a patent ductus arteriosus.

The symptoms of a ventricular septal defect are those of heart failure when the disease is advanced. Before that time, they are apt to be few and inconsequential. The physical examination of a patient with a ventricular septal defect reveals a loud systolic murmur over the area of the base of the heart and the pulmonary artery, and fluoroscopic examination and roentgenograms show a large pulmonary artery with prominent vascular shadows in the lung fields. As a rule, the diagnosis can be made with certainty only by cardiac catheterization. As the catheter passes from the right atrium into the right ventricle, the systolic pressures increase abnormally, and the arterial oxygen saturation increases. Upon occasion, the catheter actually may pass through the septal defect.

Treatment. The surgical closure of ventricular septal defects using cardiopulmonary bypass has now been accomplished in large series of patients[34] with a low mortality. When the pulmonary artery pressure is normal or only moderately elevated, the risk should be no more than 5 per cent. As the pulmonary artery pressure rises, the risk increases. If the increased pressure is due to the increased flow, the patient is still a satisfactory risk. However, if the pressure in the pulmonary artery is roughly equivalent to that in the aorta due to abnormally high vascular resistance in the lung, and there is very little left to right shunt, the risk of operation is high.

The technical feat of obtaining a secure closure of the defect without injury to the bundle of His is the greatest problem facing the surgeon. At the same time it is advantageous to make as small a wound in the right ventricle as possible in order to reduce the efficiency of the right ventricle as little as possible during the postoperative period.

The Cyanotic Group

Tetralogy of Fallot

The congenital heart, which includes the 4 anomalies described by Fallot,[19] generally is referred to as the tetralogy of Fallot. Such a heart has a pulmonary stenosis, a ventricular septal defect, an overriding of the aorta and hypertrophy of the right ventricle. In

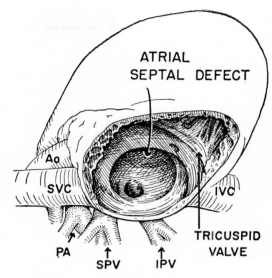

Fig. 41-12. Diagrammatic view of an atrioseptal defect of the secundum type. The opening of the right-sided pulmonary veins where they enter the left auricle can be seen through the septal defect. The opening of the coronary sinus can be seen inferior to the septal defect and superior to the opening of the inferior vena cava. Such a defect can be closed very easily under direct vision. Also it could be closed readily by various technics noted in the text.

those instances in which an atrial defect is added to this tetralogy, the term *pentalogy* sometimes has been used.

The exact pathologic anatomy present in the tetralogy of Fallot may vary tremendously. In the vast majority of instances the pulmonary stenosis is infundibular rather than valvular in type. The size of the ventricular septal defect may vary considerably from a small defect to the presence of a common ventricle. The amount of overriding of the aorta also may vary tremendously—to the extent, in fact, that the aorta apparently may arise completely from the right ventricle.

The physiologic derangement of the heart with the tetralogy of Fallot is primarily that of a right-to-left shunt; that is, the shunting of blood from the right ventricle out through the aorta rather than having it pass through the lungs. This may be accomplished because of the fact that the aorta partially overrides the right ventricle, and this shunting is in-

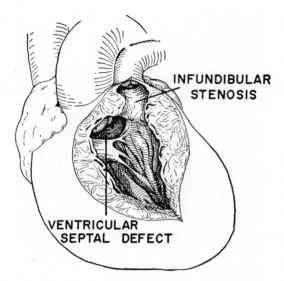

INFUNDIBULAR
STENOSIS

VENTRICULAR
SEPTAL DEFECT

Fig. 41-13. Diagrammatic sketch of the tetralogy of Fallot. Note the muscular type of infundibular stenosis in the outlet of the right ventricle proximal to the normal pulmonary valve. Also, note the ventricular septal defect through which some of the blood from the right ventricle flows into the left ventricle and out through the aorta.

creased by the stenosis that interferes with the flow of blood into the lungs through the pulmonary artery. As a result of the great right-to-left shunt, an inadequate amount of blood passes through the lungs, so that the peripheral arterial oxygen saturation may be quite low, and the patient suffers from severe oxygen deficiency and cyanosis. Incident to this tissue hypoxia, the patient may develop clubbing of the fingers and the toes and severe polycythemia.

Primarily, the symptoms of the tetralogy of Fallot are cyanosis with dyspnea on exertion. If the patient survives to childhood, he is apt to be found characteristically in the squatting position in an effort to increase his ease in breathing. If the right-to-left shunt is severe, the patient may die in infancy; if less severe, he may live into childhood. Few of these patients live past their teens without some type of surgical intervention.

Physical examination will reveal varying degrees of cyanosis, depending upon the severity of the lesion. There will be a systolic murmur over the pulmonary artery area, and

the blood count will reveal a polycythemia, although the hemoglobin may not be high if the infant is malnourished. When the polycythemia becomes severe, the danger of vascular thrombosis is increased greatly, and it is not uncommon for these patients to suffer strokes in infancy or in childhood. Fluoroscopic and roentgenographic examinations reveal characteristically a "boot-shaped" heart with a concavity at the pulmonary conus area and evidence of a decreased amount of blood in the lungs, as indicated by unusually clear lung fields.

Diagnosis. The diagnosis of the tetralogy of Fallot can be made on a clinical basis with considerable accuracy, but special studies may be necessary to make it with certainty. When the angiocardiogram is done by using a rapid cassette changer, the dye passes from the right atrium into the right ventricle and from the right ventricle into both the aorta and the pulmonary artery. This gives a positive diagnosis of an overriding aorta, or at least a ventricular septal defect, and one can feel reasonably certain of the diagnosis of the tetralogy of Fallot, although in some instances a common ventricle cannot be ruled out. If the cassette changer used is not a rapid one, there may be some fear that some of the dye may have passed from the right to the left atrium, into the left ventricle and out through the aorta, so that the aorta may be visualized at the same time as is the pulmonary artery. With a fairly rapid cassette changer, however, this mistaken diagnosis is not likely to be made.

A definitive diagnosis of the tetralogy of Fallot also may be made by cardiac catheterization. If the catheter passes from the right ventricle into the pulmonary artery and a low pressure is recorded in the pulmonary artery as compared with the right ventricle, the diagnosis of pulmonary stenosis can be made. If, then, the catheter can be passed out through the aorta, the overriding aorta, or at least a ventricular septal defect, can be assumed. This, along with the cyanosis, makes a diagnosis of tetralogy of Fallot reasonably certain.

Treatment. The first successful efforts at the surgical treatment of the tetralogy of Fallot were carried out by Blalock[10] in 1944. On the basis that methods were not available actually to correct the anatomic defects inside the heart, he and Taussig worked out a method of overcoming the physiologic inconvenience of the tetralogy of Fallot by surgical procedures outside the heart. Since the fundamental difficulty with the patient's heart in the tetralogy of Fallot is a right to left shunt, with inadequate amounts of blood going to the lungs, the Blalock operation was designed to shunt blood from the systemic circulation to the pulmonary circulation. Thus, it provides a left-to-right shunt outside the heart to compensate for the right-to-left shunt inside the heart. This is accomplished by turning down the subclavian artery and anastomosing it end to side to the pulmonary artery. There can be no doubt that this operation has been highly successful in many clinics throughout the world. The operation is usually performed on the right side, using the subclavian branch of the innominate artery, because the angle at which the subclavian artery comes off the innominate is a favorable one. However, other surgeons have preferred to use the subclavian branch of the aorta and have done so successfully. In some instances there is kinking at the angle as the subclavian is turned down from the aorta.

A side-to-side anastomosis of the descending aorta to the pulmonary artery on the left side, as suggested by Potts,[41] accomplishes the same result of a left-to-right shunt. It is preferred by many surgeons when the operation must be done during infancy, when it may be difficult to accomplish with certainty a functioning Blalock operation. Approximately 25 per cent of the patients with the tetralogy of Fallot have right-sided aortic arches. In these, except in infants, it is much more difficult to accomplish the Potts operation. The method of accomplishing the left-to-right shunt probably is not important. It can always be accomplished in some manner if a satisfactory pulmonary artery is available. If the operation is performed on the side of the aorta, a free graft from the descending aorta to the pulmonary artery is accomplished readily. By preference, the surgeon should use a section of the subclavian artery from the patient.

A direct attack upon the pulmonary stenosis in the tetralogy of Fallot was advocated by Brock.[14] In most instances this required the removal of some muscle from the outflow tract of the right ventricle, since the stenosis was

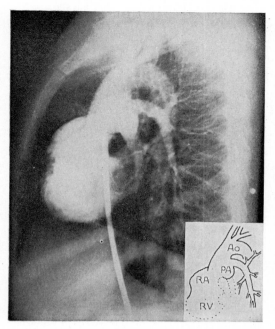

FIG. 41-14. Angiocardiogram obtained of a patient with the tetralogy of Fallot by placing a catheter up through the femoral vein into the vena cava in order to inject the contrast medium. The right side of the heart is visualized, and the aorta and the pulmonary artery are visualized simultaneously before the contrast medium has entered the left side of the heart.

usually infundibular rather than valvular. Although Brock and a few other surgeons obtained good palliative results by this procedure, it was never widely accepted.

By the use of cardiopulmonary bypass it is now possible to do corrective surgery for the tetralogy of Fallot by closing the ventricular septal defect and removing the pulmonary stenosis. Those surgeons who have had the most experience in this field now use this technic almost exclusively. The greatest difficulty has been encountered in infants and small children, especially when the patient is severely cyanotic. The author and many other surgeons are still doing shunt procedures on infants and small children and reserving the direct approach for the older children and adults. Success depends upon the ability to get an adequate outflow tract from the right ventricle without jeopardizing the efficiency of the right ventricle to too great a degree.

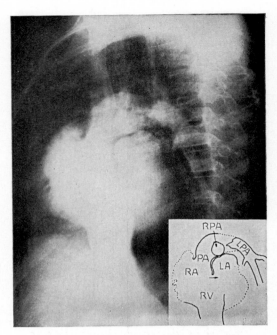

Fig. 41-15. Angiocardiogram of a patient with a valvular type of pulmonary stenosis and an atrioseptal defect. The contrast medium can be seen to have filled the right side of the heart and has passed through the atrioseptal defect into the left atrium but has not yet reached the left ventricle. The tremendously dilated pulmonary artery (poststenotic dilation) is also visualized.

Results. Patients with the tetralogy of Fallot who have been operated upon by the shunting type procedures of Blalock or Potts have been improved vastly by the procedure. By and large, the mortality has been below 15 per cent. In general, the mortality has been higher in infants and in the older age group. An ideal time for the operation, from the standpoint of low mortality, probably is from 4 to 8 years of age. However, many children will not live to this age; therefore, in such cases, the operation must be done of necessity before that time. In general, the author has tended to use the Potts operation in small infants and the Blalock operation in the children. He has had some difficulty due to unusual enlargement of the heart in the postoperative period following the Potts operation, probably due to having made the anastomosis too large. In the Blalock operation, the size of the anastomosis is limited by the size of the

subclavian artery, but, even so, some large hearts develop after this procedure. It may well be that the postoperative enlargement of the heart in some instances may be related to other phenomena rather than to too large a left-to-right shunt.

The vast majority of patients who are operated upon, either by the shunting type procedure or the Brock procedure, are much improved following the operation. Even though they do not have a normal heart again, their cyanosis will be decreased greatly and their exercise tolerance increased greatly. The polycythemia likewise will decrease. While there can be no doubt that most of the patients have been vastly improved, nevertheless these operations are palliative ones, and an increasing number of patients get into trouble as time goes on.

The results of the total correction of the tetralogy of Fallot, utilizing cardiopulmonary bypass, has improved greatly in the recent past. In the hands of those surgeons who have had the greatest experience, the immediate mortality now compares favorably with that of the shunt procedures, and it is hoped and assumed that the long-term results following a successful operation will be far superior. The execution of this procedure in infants is still hazardous in the hands of most surgeons.

Pulmonary Stenosis with Atrial Septal Defect

Frequently, this congenital defect is referred to incorrectly under the term *isolated pulmonary stenosis,* although obviously two defects are present. These patients are cyanotic because the resistance to blood-flow caused by the pulmonary stenosis increases the pressure in the right ventricle, which, in turn, increases the pressure in the right atrium, and blood flows through the atrial septal defect from right to left. Therefore, the systemic arterial oxygen saturation is decreased, and the patient is cyanotic.

The symptoms of these patients are apt to be similar to those of the tetralogy of Fallot. On physical examination the findings may be very similar, but the cardiac configuration is somewhat different, and the diagnosis usually can be suspected on a clinical basis. It is very important that this condition be differentiated from the tetralogy of Fallot, since the direct attack upon the pulmonary stenosis gives a much better result than an anastomosis type procedure in this lesion.

On physical examination the systolic thrill over the pulmonary area is present, and there is right preponderance on the electrocardiogram, as there is in the tetralogy of Fallot. On fluoroscopic and roentgenographic examinations, the lung fields are apt to be clear also, but there is likely to be poststenotic dilatation of the pulmonary artery, giving some prominence of the pulmonary conus rather than the concavity, as seen frequently in the tetralogy of Fallot. Therefore, the general cardiac configuration is helpful in making the suspected diagnosis. The diagnosis usually is confirmed, however, on the basis of the angiocardiogram, since, as a rule, the dye can be seen to pass from the right to the left atrium and into the left ventricle before appearing in the aorta. The diagnosis also can be made with reasonable certainty on cardiac catheterization if the catheter passes through the atrial septal defect, but, even so, it would be difficult to distinguish this condition from a "pentalogy" unless the catheter passed through the ventricular septal defect. The presence of a right-to-left shunt at the ventricular level may be ruled out by dye curves following a right ventricular injection of the dye.

Treatment. If the surgeon plans to make a direct attack upon the pulmonary stenosis, whether it is associated with a ventricular or an atrial septal defect, it is not important to make a differential diagnosis before operation. However, the anastomosis type procedure should not be done for this condition. If the surgeon is one who uses the anastomosis procedure for the tetralogy of Fallot, obviously it is important that a definitive diagnosis be made before operation. The treatment of the patient with pulmonary stenosis and an atrial septal defect always should be made by the direct attack. It is essentially the same as that described under isolated pulmonary stenosis above. Once the pulmonary stenosis is relieved, the atrial septal defect, which is usually a patent foramen ovale, closes and is apt to be no longer of clinical physiologic significance. However, the presence of a real atrial

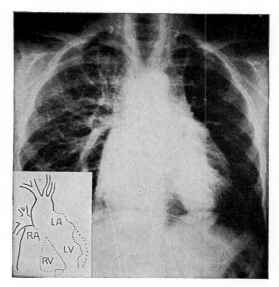

FIG. 41-16. Angiocardiogram of a patient with tricuspid atresia. The contrast medium is seen in the right atrium, in the left atrium, and partially fills the left ventricle so that the aorta and the pulmonary arteries are also shown. The contrast medium does not fill the right ventricle, a circumstance which is diagnostic of tricuspid atresia.

defect should be ruled out, and if found to be present it should be closed.

The results obtained in this lesion have been excellent, and the mortality has been low.

Tricuspid Atresia

This lesion must be associated with an atrial septal defect or it is incompatible with life. Even so, a patient with tricuspid atresia is apt to get into difficulty as a very young infant. There are various degrees of tricuspid stenosis, going on to complete atresia, but complete or almost complete atresia is the most common. Usually, the diagnosis can be made or strongly suspected clinically on the configuration of the heart on roentgenographic and fluoroscopic examinations, upon the cyanosis and the polycythemia and the left axis deviation on the electrocardiogram.

The diagnosis can be made with considerable certainty on the basis of the angiocardiogram with a rapid cassette changer. The dye passes into the right atrium, then into the left atrium, into the left ventricle and out through

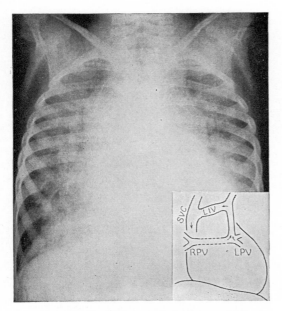

FIG. 41-17. Plain roentgenogram of the chest of a patient with abnormal venous drainage of the type illustrated in the inset. The shape of the heart on the plain roentgenogram and the tremendous engorgement of the pulmonary vessels are diagnostic in many instances. As shown in the inset, the pulmonary veins join, and the blood flows into the left innominate vein, on to the superior vena cava and back into the right atrium. The patient is kept alive by virtue of an atrioseptal defect. See text for corrective surgical procedure.

the aorta. The pulmonary artery may receive some blood from the left ventricle, but in inadequate amounts. Often the lungs may get their major blood-flow through a patent ductus arteriosus. On the angiocardiogram, the absence of dye in the right ventricle is diagnostic.

Treatment. To date, no method has been developed whereby this lesion can be totally corrected. The surgical therapy so far has been directed toward getting an increased flow of blood to the lungs. A left-to-right shunt, produced either by a Blalock or a Potts operation has been the most common method of attack. Blalock[8] has suggested making a larger atrial septal defect to avoid the possibility of partial closure of a patent foramen ovale by the increased venous return to the left atrium. Whether or not it is wise to do this routinely is an unanswered question.

In the recent past the "Glenn" operation[21] has been advocated for this condition and appears to have some advantage over the other types of anastomoses. In this procedure a side-to-end anastomosis is made between the superior vena cava and the right pulmonary artery, shunting the superior vena caval blood directly to the right lung without passing through the left heart. The work load of the left heart is thus less than it would be with either the Blalock or the Potts operation.

Abnormal Drainage of the Great Veins

The abnormal drainage of the great veins is fairly uncommon, and there may be considerable variation. Perhaps the most common type of abnormality is that of the right-sided pulmonary veins entering the right atrium in association with an atrial septal defect, as mentioned above. In that situation the cyanosis is minimal, and the defect can be corrected by closing the atrial septal defect so as to suture the septum to the right of the opening of the right-sided veins, thereby draining them into the left atrium.

The more serious type of abnormal drainage of the great veins is that in which not only the right but also the left pulmonary veins enter the right atrium. This may occur in a number of ways. In some patients (Fig. 41-17) the veins from both lungs may join on the left side to drain into a vein called the "vertical vein," from which the blood flows through the left innominate vein and on to the right atrium. In other instances, all the branches of the left pulmonary vein may join and pass inferiorly to a vein entering the inferior vena cava. In addition to the abnormal drainage of the great veins, there is an atrial septal defect, and thereby blood gets across to the left side of the heart. Therefore, these patients are cyanotic because of the mixing of the blood of the pulmonary veins and the vena cavae and its getting into the left side of the heart. Their signs and symptoms are those of tissue anoxia.

The diagnosis can be suspected on the basis of the cardiac configuration. A definitive diagnosis can be made at times by cardiac catheterization and angiocardiography, but it is difficult to be entirely certain of the complete diagnosis unless one is fortunate enough to have one of the cardiac catheters go out through the various veins and show their course with certainty.

Surgical correction of the abnormal drainage of the pulmonary veins is obviously indicated. When only the right-sided pulmonary veins enter the right atrium in association with an atrial septal defect, the correction can be carried out fairly simply by suturing the septum in front of the right-sided veins, shunting their flow into the left atrium.

When the two pulmonary veins join to drain into the right atrium by the route shown in Figure 41-17, the operation must be done utilizing cardiopulmonary bypass. A large anastomosis is made between the left atrium and the vein passing behind the heart. Then the vertical vein may be ligated and the atrial defect closed either by suture or by a patch.

Occasionally, the right pulmonary vein drains directly into the superior vena cava, usually associated with an atrial septal defect. It is usually possible to devise some means by suture or by means of a patch to have the superior vena cava blood continue to flow into the right atrium while shunting the superior pulmonary vein blood into the left atrium.

Transposition of the Great Arteries

The congenital transposition of the great arteries, so that the aorta arises from the right ventricle and the pulmonary artery arises from the left ventricle, is a very serious congenital abnormality.

The patient usually is quite cyanotic, and in most instances these patients die in early infancy. As a rule, the diagnosis is easily suspected because of the configuration of the heart, particularly when the aorta is seen to arise from the anterior position on the lateral view. If there is any doubt as to the diagnosis, it may be ascertained on angiocardiogram, which shows the dye to go from the right ventricle out through the aorta without appearing in the pulmonary artery until much later.

Patients who do not die at birth are kept alive by virtue of some communication between the right and the left circulations. This may be due to a ventricular septal defect, an atrial septal defect and/or a patent ductus arteriosus.

The problem would seem to be a simple surgical one of dividing the two vessels and

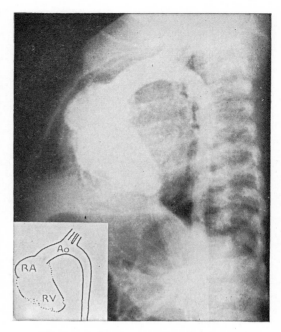

Fig. 41-18. Angiocardiogram in a patient with transposition of the great arteries. The right side of the heart is visualized with the contrast medium, and the aorta is seen to arise from the right heart and is brilliantly visualized. The contrast medium has not yet entered the left side of the heart or the pulmonary circulation.

reanastomosing in the opposite manner. However, this maneuver has not been successful as yet. It would appear that in addition to transplanting the great arteries, the coronary arteries would have to go with the aorta so as to obtain oxygenated blood from the left ventricle. This has not been carried out successfully to date, but it would appear to be feasible. In view of the failure of the efforts to transplant the great arteries, efforts have turned to transplanting the great veins. Some success has been experienced with a partitioning of the atria to reroute the blood to the opposite ventricle,[45] but to date this has appeared to be a very difficult problem. Baffes[2] has had considerable success with the palliative operation of shunting blood from the inferior vena cava to the left atrium by means of a graft, and shunting the blood from the right lung into the right atrium by direct anastomosis. Also, considerable palliation has been

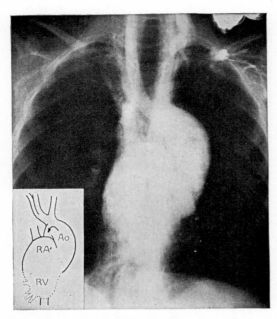

FIG. 41-19. Angiocardiogram of a patient with a truncus arteriosus. In this patient the blood flow to the lungs apparently was dependent entirely upon collateral circulation arriving from the systemic circulation.

achieved by producing a common atrium as suggested by Blalock and Hanlon.[9]

It would seem that transposition of the great vessels presents the surgeon with a purely mechanical problem. It seems unlikely that it will remain long unsolved. It may well be that the greatest problem in its solution will be the vascular changes in the lung secondary to the pulmonary hypertension.

Truncus Arteriosus

There is one variety of truncus arteriosus in which a single vessel arises from the ventricle and there is no pulmonary artery, the lung thereby receiving all the blood-flow through collateral circulation. This diagnosis can be suspected clinically on the basis of the configuration of the heart, and it can be suspected on angiocardiography because of the large single vessel and the absence of typical pulmonary arteries. The only method of surgical treatment that may be of some value to these patients is an effort to increase the collateral circulation to the lungs. In general, if the patient is doing reasonably well and the diagnosis is made preoperatively, opera-

tion is not advised. If the patient is doing poorly, however, or if the diagnosis is arrived at when the chest is opened, the parietal pleura is removed, and asbestos or talc is sprinkled over the surface of the lung in the hope of increasing the blood-flow to the lungs. This maneuver is used also in some patients with the tetralogy of Fallot when the anastomosis procedure cannot be accomplished. In the author's opinion, there is very little doubt that some of the tetralogy patients have been improved by this maneuver.

There is another type of truncus arteriosus in which a single artery coming from the heart divides very shortly into the aorta and the pulmonary artery. The cyanosis is not apt to be severe. In this situation, the pulmonary artery pressure is high, so that a continuous murmur will not be heard. In other respects, it may be difficult to differentiate between this type of truncus arteriosus and the patient with an aortic window. It is difficult to make this diagnosis with certainty except at autopsy, although it may be suspected. If the diagnosis were established, the only method of treatment at present available would be the production of pulmonary stenosis, as suggested by Muller and Dammann,[40] for the patient with a ventricular septal defect and high pulmonary artery pressure.

Eisenmenger's Complex

Eisenmenger's complex is the term applied to a congenital defect somewhat similar to the tetralogy of Fallot except that the right-to-left shunt through the ventricular septal defect is brought about by pulmonary hypertension due to vascular resistance to blood flow through the lungs rather than to a pulmonary stenosis. Sometimes this condition is present in infancy and childhood. Not infrequently, however, the child starts out with a ventricular septal defect and a left-to-right shunt, only to develop cyanosis as the years go by, due to vascular changes in the lung, increasing vascular resistance, increasing pulmonary hypertension and a reversal of the shunt to a right-to-left one. At the present time it is the objective of cardiac surgeons to repair ventricular septal defects before the above process occurs. If a considerable degree of right-to-left shunt is already present, the surgeon has little hope to offer the patient. However,

Muller and Dammann[40] have suggested that the vascular changes in the lungs may be reversed by surgically producing pulmonary stenosis as the first stage of a corrective operation. A most difficult question at the present time is how severe the pulmonary hypertension may be and how small the left-to-right shunt may be and still give hope of success in the closure of a ventricular septal defect.

Pulmonary Arteriovenous Fistula

In the presence of a pulmonary arteriovenous fistula, blood is shunted directly from the pulmonary artery to the pulmonary vein without having passed through the capillaries of the lungs to undergo oxygenation. Therefore, such a fistula would amount to the same as a right-to-left shunt inside the heart, and the patient is cyanotic. Along with the cyanosis, polycythemia develops, and in severe degrees of the condition the patient is dyspneic on exertion. In favorable circumstances a continuous murmur may be heard over a pulmonary arteriovenous fistula.

Pulmonary arteriovenous fistulas are considered to be congenital in origin, and several individuals in the same family may be afflicted with the condition. Such fistulas may be progressive, and they may not be detected until adult life. It is not uncommon to have cutaneous manifestations of telangiectasis, but this is not always present.

The patient's signs and symptoms are primarily those of cyanosis and polycythemia associated with dyspnea, particularly on exertion, when the size of the fistula is large. If the fistula is unusually large, there will be a right axis deviation on the electrocardiogram, and the right side of the heart may be larger than the left. Unlike the peripheral arteriovenous fistula, the pulmonary arteriovenous fistula is not associated commonly with cardiac enlargement.

The diagnosis of pulmonary arteriovenous fistula can be suspected on the basis of the clinical examination. Roentgenographic and fluoroscopic examinations actually may reveal the large arteriovenous communications in the lung. If these communications are large, they can be shown beautifully on an angiocardiogram.

If the pulmonary arteriovenous fistula is confined to one lobe or one lung, the resection

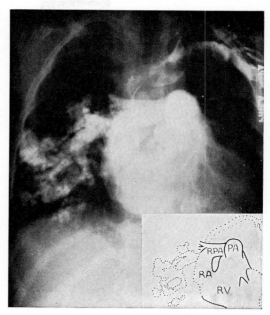

Fig. 41-20. Angiocardiogram of a 4-year-old child with a large pulmonary arteriovenous fistula. The fistula apparently was confined to the right lower lobe. It was estimated that 84 per cent of the right heart output went through this fistula. The child was severely cyanotic. Following the removal of the right lower lobe the cyanosis disappeared completely.

of the area involved will bring about a tremendous improvement in the patient. Great care should be exercised to determine the extent of the arteriovenous fistulas before operation, since it is not uncommon to have multiple small ones throughout the remaining portion of the lungs that may be overlooked. There is also some danger that after the removal of the one arteriovenous fistula, other smaller ones may increase in size as the years go on. This of course does not militate against the surgical removal of the more serious arteriovenous fistula, particularly if the patient has gone on to severe polycythemia.

ACQUIRED HEART DISEASE

SURGERY OF THE PERICARDIUM

Constrictive Pericarditis

Constrictive pericarditis is a condition in which the heart is compressed by a thickened,

TABLE 1. RIGHT HEART CATHETERIZATION

*Blood-Oxygen Saturations and Pressures in the
Heart and the Great Vessels in Cardiac Abnormalities*

Cardiac Abnormality	Vena Cava O₂ Sat.	Vena Cava Pressure	Right Auricle O₂ Sat.	Right Auricle Pressure	Right Ventricle O₂ Sat.	Right Ventricle Pressure	Pulmonary Artery O₂ Sat.	Pulmonary Artery Pressure	Systemic Artery O₂ Sat.	Systemic Artery Pressure	Remarks
Normal	75%	5/0	75%	5/0	75%	30/0	75%	30/0	96%	120/90	Approximate values
Interatrial septal defect	Normal		> V.C.	Normal or high	Same as R.A.	Normal or high	Same as R.A.	Normal or high	Normal		O₂ saturation in R.A. greater than V.C., catheter may pass into the L. A.
Ventricular septal defect	Normal or low	Normal or high	Same as V.C.	Normal or high	> R.A.	High	Same as R.V.	High	Normal		R.V. O₂ saturation is higher than R.A. or V.C., catheter may pass R.V. to L.V. and aorta.
Pulmonary stenosis	Normal	Normal or high	Same as V.C.	Normal or high	Same as V.C.	High	Same as V.C.	Low	Normal		R.V. pressures are much higher than P.A. pressures.
Tetralogy of Fallot	Low	Normal or high	Same as V.C.	Normal or high	Same as V.C.	High	Same as V.C.	Low	Low	Normal	Pulmonary stenosis with systemic arterial saturation and catheter passing through ventricular septal defect overriding aorta.
Eisenmenger's complex	Low	Normal or high	Same as V.C.	Normal or high	Same as V.C.	High	Same as V.C.	High	Low	Normal	No pulmonary stenosis, with overriding aorta. O₂ saturation of P.A. and systemic arterial blood may vary.
Patent Ductus	Normal	Normal or high	Same as V.C.	Normal or high	Same as V.C.	Normal or high	> R.V. Normal or high	Normal	Normal	Increased pulse pressure	P.A. O₂ saturation greater than R.V., R.A. and V.C. Catheter may pass into aorta.

V.C.: Vena cava   R.V.: Right ventricle   P.A.: Pulmonary artery   > : Greater than
R.A.: Right atrium   L.V.: Left ventricle   L.A.: Left atrium

diseased pericardium, so that it cannot expand to its normal size during diastole.

Frequently, the etiology cannot be ascertained. Many authors are inclined to think that it is almost always on a tuberculous basis, while others feel that rheumatic fever is the most likely etiologic factor in those instances in which the diagnosis cannot be established by microscopy.

Usually, the surgeon sees the patient with constrictive pericarditis at a time when the process appears to be a healed lesion from the pathologic standpoint. The pericardium is thick and scarred, and areas of calcification are frequently present. As a rule, the areas of calcification do not extend into the myocardium, but they may do so occasionally.

From the physiologic standpoint, constrictive pericarditis may be thought of as a constricting lesion involving the heart as a whole and preventing it from filling adequately during diastole. As a result of inadequate filling the total cardiac output is reduced, and the blood is apt to back up in the great veins. The venous pressure will be increased. As a result, enlargement of the liver with secondary ascites occurs in many instances. Passive congestion in the portal system may bring about an enlargement of the spleen with secondary hypersplenism in long-standing cases. Because of the constricting nature of the pericardium, the heart is apt to be smaller than it would be otherwise, and the effectiveness of its impulse is decreased, in respect to both palpation and auscultation.

The signs and symptoms of constrictive pericarditis on the basis of the above physiologic findings are those of cardiac failure. The diagnosis is suspected easily if the roentgenographic examination reveals calcification in the pericardium. However, when this is not the case, it may be very difficult to be certain that one is dealing with a patient with constrictive pericarditis rather than simple heart failure. The diagnostic triad suggested by Beck[6] is that of a small quiet heart, increased venous pressure and ascites. This differs from the usual patient with cardiac failure only in that the heart usually is large and more active in the latter type of patient. However, there may be many borderline situations in which it is extremely difficult to make a differential diagnosis between the two conditions. Not infrequently, the condition may be misdiagnosed as being due to primary cirrhosis of the liver.

Treatment. The treatment of constrictive pericarditis is the removal of the pericardium so as to allow the heart to expand and fill normally. In the vast majority of instances, the pericardium constricts the heart as a whole rather than any one particular area, so that, if a major portion of the pericardium is removed over a convenient area, the heart may expand, and the patient will be cured. If, for example, the pericardium can be removed from about the hilum of the lung on one side to the same area on the other side, then the heart can expand satisfactorily.

There has been some question in the surgical literature as to how decortication of the heart may be accomplished most readily. When the patient is very sick and has been allowed to reach the stage of desperation before being subjected to surgery, the greatest skill on the part of the anesthetist and the surgeon may be required to get the patient through an operative procedure.

The preoperative care is of the greatest importance. The patient should be dehydrated and made as free of excess fluid as possible before operation, and great care should be taken not to overhydrate the patient during the immediate postoperative period.

The operation itself may be performed in a number of ways. Some surgeons go through

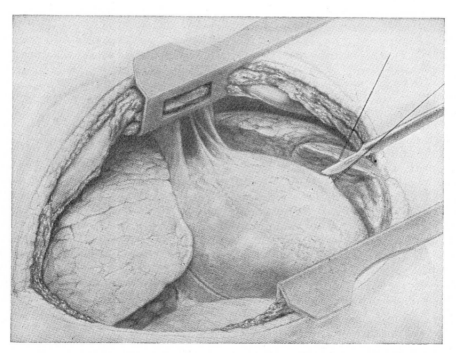

FIG. 41-21. Operative view of an operation for constrictive pericarditis. By making a transsternal incision from the anterior axillary line on one side to the anterior axillary line on the other in about the fourth interspace, it is possible to remove the pericardium from the hilum of one lung to the hilum of the other with excellent exposure. This type of exposure is also useful in a good many other procedures employing open cardiac surgery. (Johnson, J., and Kirby, C.: Surgery of the Chest, Chicago, Year Book Pub.)

the left chest and remove the major portion of the pericardium from the left side of the heart. If a large enough area of the pericardium is removed, this undoubtedly is satisfactory in most instances unless there is actual constriction of a localized area. Occasionally one encounters a patient in whom there is constriction of the venous inlet to the right auricle and one in whom there is a constriction of the venous inlet to the left atrium. However, these are the exceptions. The author has felt that a wider decortication than can be accomplished through a left pleural cavity incision probably is desirable in most patients, and he has accomplished this by a transsternal incision in the fourth or the fifth interspace, decorticating the heart from the hilum of the lung on one side to the hilum of the lung on the other. Other surgeons have accomplished essentially the same type of operation by an incision splitting the sternum from above downward. When the patient is in desperate condition, probably it is safer to do a simple left-sided thoracotomy with a decortication of the left side of the heart, with the thought of going back and doing more later if it should become necessary. In our own experience, such a secondary procedure has not been necessary if the left side of the pericardium was removed adequately.

The results of decortication of the heart in the cases of constrictive pericarditis have been excellent. When the patient goes to operation before the terminal stage, the mortality is low. Following decortication of the heart, it is the consensus at the present time that the patient should be carried along a little bit more slowly than the average patient following an operative procedure. Since the myocardium has been constricted for a long time, it may take a considerable period for it to recover from this period of constriction. It is probably wise, therefore, to advise the patient to avoid even moderate exertion for a period up to 6 months.

Recurrent Acute Pericarditis

In recent years a syndrome has been recognized[51] in which the patient may have recurrent bouts of acute pericarditis. The patient's fever and malaise may subside at rest, only to flare up again when he returns to work. The patient may have repeated attacks extending over a period of many months. Even in the absence of constriction of the pericardium, the patient may suffer considerable disability due to the recurrent nature of the disease. In recent years such patients have been subjected to pericardectomy with excellent results. The operation is technically simple, since the pericardium usually is not tightly adherent to the heart.

PERICARDIAL EFFUSION

The patient with a pericardial effusion, particularly a tuberculous one, may present a considerable problem to the surgeon. The question always arises as to whether one is dealing with a large heart or whether an effusion actually is present. The cardiologist usually can have some opinion on this subject, but in some instances it is exceedingly difficult for him to be certain.

The ultimate diagnosis of pericardial effusion is the removal of some of the fluid by needle aspiration. When the fluid is clear and obviously from the pericardial area, the diagnosis is established. After the removal of some of the fluid, a small quantity of air may be injected and roentgenographic films taken to delineate the size of the heart. Upon occasion, the fluid in the pericardial sac may be grossly bloody, and the question may arise as to whether the needle is in the cardiac cavity or in the pericardial sac. In most instances, if a hemoglobin determination is made of the fluid removed, it will be found that it is not so high as that in the blood stream. Sometimes, however, there may be some real question in the mind of the person who is doing the pericardicentesis. If air were injected into the cardiac cavity, the result might be catastrophic. An easy method of determining whether the needle is in the pericardial space with grossly bloody fluid or whether it is in the cardiac cavity is to inject some Decholin. If the patient tastes it immediately, then one can be sure that the needle is in the cardiac cavity. If the patient does not taste it, then air can be injected and a film taken to delineate the size of the heart.

The treatment of the patient with pericardial effusion depends to a considerable extent upon the etiology of the effusion. The most common variety is incident to heart failure, and the treatment depends fundamentally upon relief of that condition. In patients with either tuberculous pericarditis and effusion or with bloody pericardial effusion of uncertain etiology, a more direct attack may be worth while. If the diagnosis of tuberculosis can be established, probably the patient should be treated with antitubercular drugs for a matter of 6 months, if possible, and then undergo a resection of the pericardium. However, we have seen an occasional patient with bloody pericardial effusion in whom a diagnosis of tuberculosis could not be established and have operated without delay with resection of the pericardium. In some instances the pericardial effusion has turned out to be on the basis of metastatic malignancy, but undoubtedly there are some instances in which the etiologic agent is not determined.

In the absence of a diagnosis, we feel that operation through the left chest with removal of a large segment of the pericardium is advisable. This will prevent further accumulation of fluid in the pericardial cavity and also allow a generous biopsy for diagnostic purposes.

Acute Pyogenic Pericarditis

Acute pyogenic pericarditis was a not uncommon occurrence before the advent of antibiotics. Frequently, it was a terminal event in patients dying from various types of pneumonia. At the present time the surgeon seldom is called upon to treat a patient with acute pyogenic pericarditis. Most commonly now it is the result of trauma. However, the pericardium may be drained through the mediastinum without entering the pleural cavity should the necessity arise.

Pericarditis incident to uremia or rheumatic fever seldom is confused with pyogenic pericarditis.

SURGERY OF THE MYOCARDIUM

Stab Wounds of the Heart

The suture of stab wounds of the heart was perhaps the first operation performed upon the heart itself. It was first done successfully by Rehn in 1896.[42] The patient with a wound of the heart who survives to reach the hospital is likely to have been stabbed with a knife or an ice pick rather than to have received a gunshot wound.

The patient who dies of a stab wound of the heart is apt to do so for two reasons: one is the loss of blood from the circulation; the other—and perhaps the more frequent cause—is the filling of the pericardial sac with blood, causing tamponade of the heart. For that reason, the heart cannot fill and cannot maintain an effective cardiac output.

The diagnosis of a stab wound of the heart should be suspected in any instance in which there is a stab wound anywhere within the general neighborhood of the heart, even though the patient may not be in extremis when seen. If the patient is in shock and pulseless, the diagnosis will be suspected, of course, but, when the patient is in relatively good condition, the unwary clinician is apt to overlook the possibility of the heart wound. One of the most helpful maneuvers in the diagnosis of cardiac tamponade is fluoroscopy, the cardiac impulse being barely demonstrable. If there has been very little blood loss, the pressure in the venous side may be increased, but in most instances total blood loss has been sufficient, so that the venous pressure is not increased.

The treatment of stab wounds of the heart falls into two categories: (1) the conservative treatment in which pericardial aspiration is used; and (2) the operative treatment in which the heart is exposed and the wound in the heart sutured.

The advocates of the conservative form of treatment have come to the conclusion that in most instances the actual bleeding from the cardiac cavity will be overcome fairly early following the trauma, and that the major problem will center in the cardiac tamponade preventing effective cardiac filling. They also feel that most of the patients can be brought through satisfactorily on conservative therapy, and that only those patients who do not respond to this method of treatment should be operated upon.

The advocates of operative therapy have felt that it is better to open the pericardial sac to suture the wound in the heart and at the same time decompress the pericardium completely. The author has advocated the operative treatment in these patients largely on the theoretic basis that, if the proper operating team is available, the patient who could survive the conservative treatment would also survive the operative treatment, and that an occasional patient might be brought through by operating immediately, whereas he might have died had conservative therapy been used originally.

There can be no doubt, however, that those individuals who have had the greatest experience with stab wounds of the heart have depended more and more on conservative therapy and have had excellent results by that means. So long as the patient is watched carefully and an operating team can stand by ready to open the chest if necessary, it may well be that it is worth while to try the conservative approach. Whether treatment is operative or nonoperative, the liberal use of transfusions is most important.

Myocardial Ischemia

Undoubtedly, obliterative disease of the coronary arteries is the greatest problem facing those investigators interested in the heart. In normal circumstances, when a coronary artery becomes occluded or nearly so in one or more areas, a collateral blood-flow is apt to develop to keep the myocardium alive. If an acute area of occlusion occurs over too large an area, the patient dies. The desire of the surgeon has been to produce some means of increasing the blood-flow to the myocardium when the coronary arterial flow is inadequate.

Many procedures have been advocated in the hope of increasing the myocardial blood-flow, but, as yet, none of them has been accepted universally. The simplest of these procedures is that of putting an irritating substance into the pericardial sac, such as talcum powder, asbestos or powdered bone, with the thought that the irritating substance will cause adhesions between the myocardium and the pericardium, and that a new blood supply will grow in from the surrounding structures to supply the myocardium.

Other methods of bringing a blood supply to the myocardium have included the transplantation of muscles, skin or omentum directly to the myocardium. Transplantation of the internal mammary into the myocardium has been utilized by Vineberg.[49] Beck,[7] who has been the most persistent investigator in the field, has attempted to bring a new blood supply to the heart by an arterial graft from the aorta to the coronary sinus. None of these procedures has been widely used.

The advocates of these various procedures have felt that many patients have been improved by them. However, the greatest difficulty in evaluating these operative procedures has been the fact that many of these patients improve as they develop their own collateral circulation, and they may go on for years without any type of operative procedure. Certainly, the need in this field is tremendous. Whether or not any of the present technics will prove to be universally acceptable cannot be determined at this time.

Quite recently, endarterectomy of the coronary arteries has been used, at times with the aid of the heart-lung machine. There have been a few excellent results, but the procedure has not been widely used as yet.

Surgery of Acquired Valvular Disease

Mitral Stenosis

Almost always, mitral stenosis is incident to rheumatic heart disease, which usually occurs in childhood or the early teens. During the healing process of acute rheumatic fever with valvular involvement, the opening in the mitral valve may decrease gradually.

Pathology. At times the disease may be minimal, and mitral stenosis is produced by simple fusion of the leaflets at the commissures. In some instances, the disease is severe, causing great thickening of the leaflets with fusion, not only of the leaflets at the commissures, but there may also be shortening and fusing of the chordae tendineae and the papillary muscles. When there is necrosis of the leaflet with scarring and contraction, the edges may no longer be able to meet, and regurgitation as well as stenosis occurs. In the healing process of severe acute disease, extensive calcification may occur.

The reduced size of the opening in the mitral valve may remain relatively constant for a number of years. It is believed that, whereas the patient's heart may be able to force blood through the small opening at a satisfactory rate during the early years, following recovery from the acute disease, as time goes on the heart may fail and no longer be able to do so. The pressure in the left atrium increases gradually, and this increase

in pressure is transmitted to the vascular bed in the lungs. Over a period of time there may be hemoptysis as a result of hemorrhages into the alveoli in the lungs. With the pouring out of exudate and the organization of this exudate, there may be actual vascular constriction in the arterioles in the lungs. As a result, the pulmonary artery pressure increases in order to force the blood through the lungs. As time progresses, the patient may go into right heart failure because of the increased effort needed to push blood through the narrowed vascular bed of the lung. In many instances, the patient may do reasonably well, so long as the cardiac rhythm remains normal. However, frequently, with the onset of auricular fibrillation, which causes a loss of an effective left atrial beat, acute symptoms may develop as the result of a decreased cardiac output.

Diagnosis. The diagnosis of mitral stenosis usually is not difficult for the trained cardiologist. The presystolic rumble at the apex is fairly characteristic, and, on fluoroscopy and orthodiagram, the heart will assume a typical so-called mitral configuration with enlargement of the left atrium. The lung fields will be congested with blood in many instances, and the pulmonary artery may be increased in size. Occasionally, however, the murmur may be insignificant or absent, and the diagnosis may be a real problem. More commonly, the diagnostic problem is one of distinguishing between the relative severity of mitral stenosis and mitral regurgitation.

There are several methods by which some

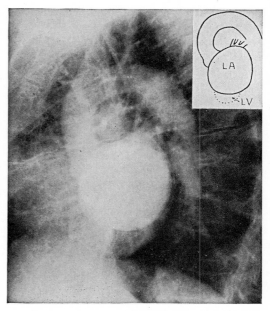

Fig. 41-22. Angiocardiogram of a patient with mitral stenosis. Note the intense opacification of the left atrium and the relatively poor visualization of the left ventricle. This represents a hang-up of the contrast medium at the level of the mitral valve.

conclusion can be reached regarding this problem. In the author's opinion, angiocardiography is a very valuable one.[50] When the mitral stenosis is severe, the contrast medium is held up in the left atrium for a considerable period of time, with the contrast medium showing poorly in the small left ventricle.

Fig. 41-23. Pressure curves obtained on left heart catheterization on two different patients, one with mitral stenosis on the right and one with mitral insufficiency on the left. In the patient with mitral stenosis note the high level of the left auricular pressure which is maintained throughout the cardiac cycle and not influenced materially by ventricular systole. In mitral insufficiency the left auricular pressure curve is similar in contour to that of the left ventricle with a peak during ventricular systole, although of course the peak does not go nearly so high.

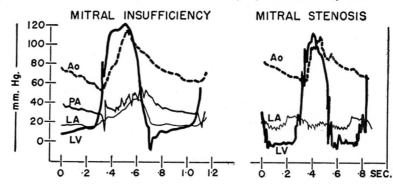

When the regurgitation (insufficiency) is the predominant factor, the medium will flow back and forth between the left atrium and the left ventricle, and the two cavities will be visualized to approximately the same extent. When mitral stenosis and regurgitation coexist, but the stenosis still is the predominant factor, the left ventricle will be visualized and may be enlarged, but the opacification will be less in the left ventricle than in the left atrium.

Another method of making this differential diagnosis is by left heart catheterization. Readings are taken simultaneously from a catheter in the left atrium and the left ventricle, so that the pressure curves may be recorded.

Whether or not significant mitral stenosis is present can be ascertained with considerable certainty by this method.

All cardiologists and surgeons in this field have been impressed in recent years by the difficulty of being certain by auscultation alone about the presence or the absence of regurgitation versus stenosis. The author has been surprised many times to find no regurgitation at the mitral valve, as judged by palpation with the finger above the valve, when he had anticipated a great deal on the basis of the auscultatory findings.

Treatment.   Mitral commissurotomy for the patient with mitral stenosis was first per-

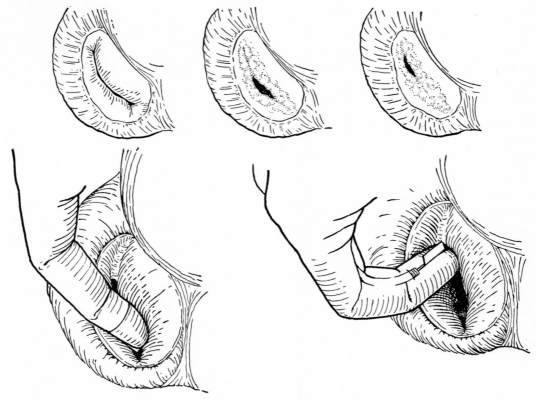

FIG. 41-24. (*Top*) The mitral valve is shown in a diagrammatic sketch. The valve on the left is a normal valve. The other two show fusion of the commissures in various locations. Both of the stenotic valves shown are relatively favorable ones for commissurotomy. (*Bottom*) Illustrating commissurotomy of a stenotic mitral valve. In many instances it is possible to open both the anterior and posterior commissures by means of finger fracture. When it is not possible to do this, some type of knife is commonly used. (*Left*) The posterior commissure is being opened by finger fracture, utilizing the fingernail to help tear open the posterior commissure. (*Right*) The knife shown in opening the anterior commissure is that designed by Brock. (Johnson, J., and Kirby, C.: Surgery of the Chest, Chicago, Year Book Pub.)

formed apparently by Souttar in 1925,[46] and more recently revived by Bailey[4] and by Harken.[27] Cutler and Beck[18] did a great deal of work on the problem of mitral stenosis in the 1920's, but abandoned the procedure because most of their work was directed toward increasing the mitral opening by cutting away a portion of the mitral valve. The amount of regurgitation obtained by this method was not tolerated by the heart. The concept of opening the fused commissures, as originally practiced by Souttar, however, was designed to obtain an increase in the size of the opening without increasing the regurgitation.

The likelihood of performing a successful mitral commissurotomy in the patient with mitral stenosis will depend to a considerable degree upon the type of valve present. In some instances, the valve leaflets are thin and pliable, and fused only at the commissures, so that they may be separated to function essentially normally again, and the patient's condition may return to normal. In other instances, however, the valve may be so severely calcified that it is difficult or impossible to obtain a reasonably functioning valve, regardless of the operative procedure employed.

The two methods of opening the mitral valve used most commonly are by finger fracture and the use of some type of knife. In recent years a few surgeons have felt that the mitral valve could be opened more satisfactorily by means of a dilator inserted through the left ventricle into the mitral valve. Most commonly, the valve is approached through the left atrium. There can be no doubt that, if the surgeon is diligent and persistent in his effort to open a stenosed mitral valve, considerable improvement can be obtained in most instances, and in a few cases a valve can be returned to a practically normal one.

In recent years some patients with mitral stenosis, especially those being operated upon for the second time, have been operated upon under direct vision, utilizing cardiopulmonary bypass.

The risk of commissurotomy in the patient with mitral stenosis centers in the possibility of some unexpected catastrophic hemorrhage, upon the possibility of a cerebral embolus (either a clot from the left atrium or some calcium from the valve), the inadvertent production of significant regurgitation, or of op-

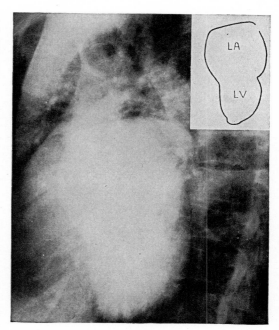

FIG. 41-25. Angiocardiogram of a patient with mitral regurgitation. The large left atrium and the large left ventricle are opacified to about the same extent by the contrast medium. This suggests that the contrast medium is going back and forth between the two cavities because of regurgitation at the mitral valve. This is shown in contrast with the angiocardiogram in a patient with pure mitral stenosis as shown in Figure 41-22.

erating upon a patient who already has reached the end stages of the disease. The operative mortality among unselected patients should not exceed 10 per cent, and in selected groups of patients it may be below 5 per cent at the present time. From 80 to 90 per cent of the surviving patients are improved—many of them startlingly so.

In patients having considerable mitral regurgitation but, at the same time, an appreciable amount of stenosis, improvement can be obtained if the stenosis can be overcome without increasing the regurgitation. We have been very much pleased with the results of this type of operation in some of these individuals, even though nothing was done to correct the regurgitation at the time of operation.

The postoperative management of the good

AORTIC STENOSIS

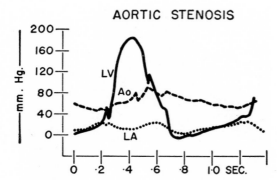

FIG. 41-26. Pressure curves obtained on left heart catheterization in a patient with aortic stenosis. Note that the peak of the pressure in the left ventricle is about 185 at a time when the peak of the pressure in the aorta is only about 90. The pressure curve in the left auricle indicates that the mitral valve is normal.

risk patient with mitral stenosis may be similar to that of any other thoracic patient. In the poor risk patient or when the valve cannot be opened satisfactorily, great care must be exercised in the patient's postoperative care. In general, the measures taken in preparing the patient for operation must be repeated, namely, low salt intake, mercurial diuretics, digitalis and careful attention to fluid balance.

Mitral Regurgitation

There can be no question that mitral regurgitation places a severe limitation on the heart as a pump. It is obviously desirable to overcome this valvular deficiency. The various methods not requiring cardiopulmonary bypass which have been used in the past have been successful occasionally, but the over-all results have left much to be desired.

At the present time there is increasing enthusiasm for what may be accomplished under direct vision, utilizing cardiopulmonary bypass. It is a little early to know whether it will be shown that this enthusiasm is justified. However, it seems evident that the results by this approach will be superior to the other methods used to date. The best results so far have been with those patients whose mitral leaflets will not meet because of a dilatation of the annulus or a shortening of the valve leaflets. Often several sutures may shorten the

annulus enough to bring the mitral leaflets together. Those leaflets which are badly calcified obviously should be replaced. Whether the efforts to replace one or both leaflets will meet with wide success is not known at this time.

Aortic Stenosis

Pathologic Physiology. In most instances, the etiology of aortic stenosis is that of rheumatic heart disease. Frequently the aortic valve is involved at the same time as the mitral valve, but aortic stenosis may occur as an isolated lesion. When the aortic valve alone is involved, it is apt to be very extensively diseased, and frequently it is severely calcified by the time the patient sees the surgeon. In some instances the aortic valve becomes stenotic by simple fusion of the commissures, in which event one still can ascertain where the commissures were located. In other instances, however, the aortic valve is completely calcified and the previous location of the commissures is not detectable by palpation alone.

As the result of aortic stenosis, the left ventricle becomes hypertrophied and the myocardium very thick in order to force the blood through the small opening. The left ventricular cavity will be small, and the patient may do quite well so long as the myocardium can overcome the obstruction at the aortic valve. However, once the patient with aortic stenosis develops heart failure, the ventricular cavity enlarges, and then his prognosis is apt to be very bad. Whereas a patient with mitral stenosis may go in and out of failure on a number of occasions and still recover, the patient with aortic stenosis is not nearly so likely to do so. The patient with aortic stenosis is not only in difficulty from the standpoint of having to overcome the obstruction due to a small opening at the aortic valve but, because of the calcification of the valves and of the adjacent aortic wall, the orifices of the coronary arteries may be cut down, and partial occlusion of the coronary arteries may be present.

Diagnosis. The diagnosis of aortic stenosis can be made readily. From the standpoint of symptoms, the patient may have periods of syncope. Anginal pain is frequently associated with it. The systolic murmur over the aortic area is often characteristic, and, as a general rule, the systolic blood pressure is low, as is the pulse pressure.

The most exact diagnostic procedure that can be used is that of left heart catheterization, so that a pressure tracing may be taken from the left ventricle at the same time that one is taken from a catheter placed in the base of the aorta. With aortic stenosis, the systolic pressure in the left ventricle will be considerably higher than that in the aorta during systole, and the pressure curves will be characteristic.

Treatment. The surgical treatment of aortic stenosis is not quite as satisfactory as that of mitral stenosis, although considerable strides are being made in that direction. Dilatation of the valve by means of an instrument inserted through the wall of the left ventricle is the method which has been used most widely in the past. Most of the complications encountered in opening the aortic valve are caused by the marked calcification of the aortic valve and by the danger of producing an arrhythmia in the large hypertrophied left ventricle. The author has obtained the best results using this method when utilizing left heart bypass. If about 2,000 ml. of blood per minute is taken from the left atrium and returned to the left common femoral artery, the work load is removed from the left ventricle. Then the dilatation of the aortic valve can be done with deliberation, and the problem of bleeding from the left ventricle is greatly reduced.

Since the left ventricle does the major work of the heart, it seemed unwise to injure it by the transventricular approach to the aortic valve. For this reason there was considerable appeal to the methods which approached the aortic valve from above. A plastic diverticulum was attached to the aorta through which the valve could be reached with the finger or instruments. The advocates of this method thought highly of it at one time.

In recent years operation upon the aortic valve under direct vision utilizing cardiopulmonary bypass has rapidly increased in popularity. Using coronary artery perfusion, the surgeon may take an hour or more to open carefully the aortic valve, removing the calcification from it when feasible. Great care in opening the valve is needed to prevent sub-

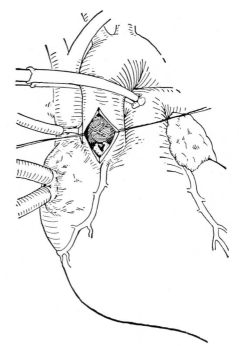

FIG. 41-27. In the past the greatest number of operations for acquired aortic stenosis were done using a dilator inserted through the left ventricle. In recent years there has been a trend toward performing the operation under direct vision utilizing cardiopulmonary bypass. The cannulae for perfusion of the coronary arteries are not shown in the diagram, but this adjunct gives the surgeon adequate time to work on the valve. (Johnson, J., and Kirby, C.: Surgery of the Chest, Chicago, Year Book Pub.)

sequent regurgitation. The approach under direct vision was first widely accepted for the congenital variety of aortic stenosis for fear of producing regurgitation by the blind methods. At present it is being increasingly widely utilized for the acquired form of the disease.

Aortic Regurgitation

The patient who suffers from severe aortic regurgitation is severely handicapped from the standpoint of his cardiac pumping mechanism. Usually, the diagnosis is established easily by the diastolic murmur extending from the base to the apex and by the wide pulse pressure. If there is any doubt about it, pressure curves taken from the aorta and, if necessary, simul-

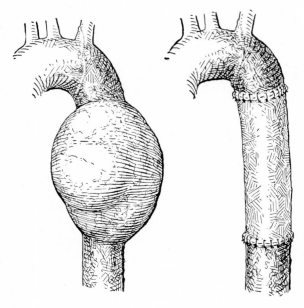

FIG. 41-28. This is a diagrammatic sketch of an aneurysm in the descending aorta distal to the left subclavian artery which has been excised and replaced by homograft. This may be carried out by utilizing partial left heart bypass. Blood is pumped from the left atrium to the left femoral artery. This method is probably safer than using hypothermia alone. Plastic grafts have now largely replaced homografts for this purpose.

Mitral and Aortic Stenosis

As a general rule the patient with mitral and aortic stenosis will have relatively mild aortic stenosis and will not have as severe calcification of the aortic valve as those patients coming to surgery with aortic stenosis alone. Likewise, the left ventricle will not have the hypertrophied musculature seen with pure aortic stenosis. As a result, these patients have done very well when subjected to mitral commissurotomy by the left-sided approach and transventricular dilatation of the aortic valve.

If the aortic valve were badly calcified but there was also some mitral stenosis, probably it would be wise to handle the patient primarily as aortic stenosis and utilize cardiopulmonary bypass.

Tricuspid Stenosis

Tricuspid stenosis is usually the result of rheumatic fever, and most often it occurs in association with involvement of the mitral and/or aortic valve. The most important problem is the danger of overlooking the diagnosis when tricuspid stenosis is present in association with other valve involvement. It is apt to occur in about 10 per cent of the patients who have involvement of both the mitral and the aortic valves, even though it may not be diagnosed preoperatively. Theoretically, the diagnosis of tricuspid stenosis should be ascertainable by right heart catheterization, by placing catheters in the right atrium and the right ventricle and taking simultaneous pressure curves. The fact that this has been done so infrequently to date is probably the result of the difficulty in suspecting the diagnosis clinically.

ANEURYSM OF THE THORACIC AORTA

Aneurysms of the thoracic aorta usually are due to weakening of the aortic wall incident to syphilis or arteriosclerosis, followed by dila-

taneously from the left ventricle can give definitive information about it.

Many different operative procedures have been attempted for the correction of aortic regurgitation. A ball-valve prosthesis was placed in the descending aorta by Hufnagel[29] with some success, even though it prevented regurgitation from only the lower half of the body. Various flap-type valves were used by various surgeons with indifferent success. In those patients with a dilated aorta, so that the valve leaflets would not meet, efforts were made to overcome this by constricting the base of the aorta proximal to the coronary ostia. None of these methods were sufficiently successful to have much appeal.

In the recent past increasing success is being achieved by utilizing cardiopulmonary bypass. With perfusion of the coronary arteries, the surgeon may take an hour or more to rebuild a functioning aortic valve or suture in new plastic cusps if need be. At times an insufficient tricuspid valve may be turned into a functioning bicuspid valve by obliterating one cusp. This is most suitable in the patients with dilatation of the base of the aorta. When a leaflet is destroyed, it may be replaced by a plastic cusp. It seems probable that an entirely new plastic valve will soon be available. At present the best results have been obtained by replacing the leaflets individually.

tation. In most instances, the symptoms produced by aortic aneurysms are due to the compression of surrounding structures. When the arch of the aorta is involved, the trachea is most commonly compressed. When the aneurysm is large, it may cause erosion of the sternum or the trachea, and death due to rupture of the aneurysm is common. Aneurysms of the descending aorta are apt to erode the spine and cause back pain.

The diagnosis of an aortic aneurysm usually is not difficult. However, it may be confused with a mediastinal tumor, since it is difficult to differentiate between the expansile pulsation of an aneurysm and the transmitted pulsation of a mediastinal tumor lying close to the heart or the aorta. When there is doubt, frequently the diagnosis can be confirmed by an angiocardiogram or an aortogram. It is possible, of course, that such studies would not be helpful if the aneurysm were filled with blood clot. In the dissecting aneurysm the double lumen of the aorta will usually be visualized.

The surgical treatment of aneurysm of the thoracic aorta is the resection of the aneurysm and repair of the defect, usually by a graft. Not very long ago it was common practice, when dealing with an aneurysm protruding from one side of the aorta, to attempt to clamp it at its neck and suture it at that point after resection of the aneurysm. That technic has been abandoned now, due to the fear of displacing old blood clots.

In aneurysms distal to the left carotid artery, the aorta may be clamped proximal and distal to the aneurysm, the aneurysm resected and replaced with a graft. Aortic homografts were used in the early experience with this technic, but at the present time plastic grafts are considered to be superior and are obtained much more easily. During the period while the aorta is clamped, partial left heart bypass is used to provide blood flow to the lower part of the body. Blood is pumped from the left atrium to the left common femoral artery at the rate of roughly half the estimated resting cardiac output. This technic is superior to the hypothermia technic formerly used. With that technic it was hoped that the oxygen requirements of the spinal cord and the kidneys would be reduced sufficiently so that the aorta could be clamped long enough to do the opera-

tion and still not injure the spinal cord or kidneys. Another objection to that technic was that with the clamping of the aorta, the cold heart might be overloaded by suddenly having to pump all of the blood against the resistance of the vascular bed supplied by the innominate and the left carotid arteries only.

When the aneurysm is located proximal to the left common carotid artery, the partial left heart bypass technic is not applicable. When the ascending aorta close to the coronary arteries is involved, total cardiopulmonary bypass is necessary during the period that the aorta is clamped. If the aneurysm is sufficiently distal to the coronary arteries, it is probably best not to use cardiopulmonary bypass since the heparinization required causes more bleeding. If enough aorta is available proximal to the aneurysm, a bypass plastic graft is first placed from the ascending aorta to the descending aorta. This serves as the new arch of the aorta. Side arms are then attached to it and then to the innominate and the left carotid arteries. Having thus established an alternate pathway for the blood to leave the heart, the arch of the aorta may be clamped on either side of the aneurysm, the innominate and the left carotid clamped proximal to the grafts, the aneurysm resected, and the free ends closed. The technical problems involved in replacing the arch of the aorta are obviously greater, and the risk is higher than when dealing with the descending aorta alone.

In a dissecting aneurysm of the aorta, the diseased intima and internal layers of the media usually have ruptured, allowing the blood from the aortic lumen to dissect out between the layers of aorta, producing a double lumen. In some instances the second lumen appears to have been due to hemorrhage from the vasa vasorum. If the second lumen extends downward, it may shut off the various branches of the aorta as the dissection proceeds, producing such phenomenon as cord paralysis, anuria, and ischemia of the legs. When the point of rupture is situated where it can be resected and a graft inserted, that should be done. If not, some palliation may be provided by dividing the descending aorta, suturing the intima to the media and the adventitia below, to prevent further downward dissection, and reuniting the aorta, leaving a point of re-entry to the main channel from the secondary lumen proximally.

OPEN CARDIAC SURGERY UNDER DIRECT VISION

The development of a technic by which intracardiac surgery could be done under direct vision was the dream of all cardiac surgeons for many years. It has now been used successfully more or less routinely in a large number of hospitals throughout the country.

Because of difficulties in the development of a satisfactory heart-lung machine, the first "open heart" operations were done with the aid of hypothermia. Swan[47] and Lewis[35] were among the first to operate on a large number of patients with atrial septal defects, utilizing this technic. The method has now been used quite widely and successfully for that lesion, as well as for operations on patients with the valvular type of pulmonary stenosis. However, most surgeons were unhappy with the limitation as to time imposed by moderate hypothermia and were desirous of a heart-lung machine which would allow the surgeon unlimited operating time.

In the development of the heart-lung machine, Gibbon[38] was perhaps the most persistent investigator over the years. It is his machine, with modifications by many other workers, which is perhaps the best one available today. It utilizes a screen-type oxygenator. However, its usefulness has been limited by the cost of its production. The bubble-type oxygenator is the least expensive to produce and has been used with real success in a few clinics. The disk-type oxygenator is probably the most widely used at the present time, since it offers a compromise as to cost and safety. It would appear that the membrane-type oxygenator would most closely simulate the action of the human lungs, but further development is necessary in this field.

Because all of the heart-lung machines require a considerable amount of effort by a fairly large team and usually a large amount of blood, there is continued interest in the field of hypothermia. By utilizing severe degrees of hypothermia with pumps to maintain the circulation during the rewarming stage, it has been possible to shut off the circulation for long periods during which time the intracardiac surgery is accomplished.[22]

Obviously, the field of open cardiac surgery is a new one in which we may expect tremendous advances within the next few years. Whether we ever shall be able to say that one method is superior to all others remains to be seen.

CARDIAC RESUSCITATION

Cardiac arrest is a term that includes ventricular asystole and ventricular fibrillation; it simply indicates that the effective pumping mechanism of the heart has stopped. It is a catastrophe that is apt to occur once or twice a year on any busy surgical service. The incidence in patients not undergoing cardiac surgery has been about 1 in 6,000 operations at the Hospital of the University of Pennsylvania.

It has been demonstrated that these patients may be revived if the diagnosis is made and treatment is instituted within about 4 minutes.[30] If the patient's pulse and blood pressure disappear suddenly and unexpectedly, the anesthetist should report it promptly to the surgeon. Unless the surgeon is in a position to deny the presence of cardiac arrest by feeling the heart or a pulsating artery, he should open the left chest promptly through an incision in the 4th left interspace from the sternum to the mid-axillary line, to re-establish the circulation by rhythmic cardiac compression, while the anesthetist maintains the respiration through an intratracheal tube. (A closed method of cardiac massage has recently been described.) A compression rate of 80 to 100 times per minute is recommended for the cardiac "massage." If it is effective, a peripheral pulse will be palpable at each compression, and the patient's color should return toward normal. If the heart has stopped due to an overdose of the anesthetic, the vagovagal reflex, or hypoxia, it should start up again after a short period of artificial circulation and respiration. If the heart is found to be in ventricular fibrillation, it can be returned to a normal rhythm most effectively by electric shock. After the tissues are well oxygenated by the artificial circulation and respiration, a shock of about 130 volts with 10 ohms resistance for 0.1 second may be applied by placing the electrodes directly on the heart. Care should be taken not to shock any of the surgical team. In cardiac surgical patients with large hearts, currents up to 280 volts have been applied for 0.1 second without apparent harm to the heart and are more effective in stopping the ventricular fibrillation in the large hearts.

Once the heart has got out of asystole or ventricular fibrillation, some drugs may be helpful in maintaining a useful heart beat. Epinephrine may speed up the heart beat and increase its effectiveness. It also increases the risk of ventricular fibrillation. Calcium chloride also has at times apparently increased the forcefulness of the heart beat. Molar sodium lactate has been helpful in certain situations by correcting the chemical disturbances brought about by metabolic changes in the myocardium. Norepinephrine has also been very helpful at times by raising the blood pressure and thereby supplying more blood to the myocardium, as well as by being a direct stimulant to the myocardium perhaps.

REFERENCES

1. Abbott, M. E.: Congenital cardiac disease *in* Nelson's Loose Leaf Medicine, New York, 1920.
2. Baffes, T. G., Lev, M., Paul, M. H., Miller, R. A., Riker, W. L., DeBoer, A., and Potts, W. J.: Surgical correction of transposition of the great vessels—a five-year survey. Read before the American Association for Thoracic Surgery, May, 1960. To be published in J. Thor. & Cardiovasc. Surg.
3. Bailey, C. P.: Surgery of the Heart, Philadelphia, Lea & Febiger, 1955.
4. Bailey, C. P.: Surgical treatment of mitral stenosis, Dis. Chest 15:377, 1949.
5. Bailey, C. P., Downing, D. F., Geckeler, G. D., Likoff, W., Goldberg, H., Scott, J. C., Jantoni, O., and Redondo-Ramirez, H. P.: Congenital interatrial communications: clinical and surgical considerations with a description of a new surgical technique: atrio-septopexy, Ann. Int. Med. 37:888, 1952.
6. Beck, C. S.: Acute and chronic compression of the heart, Am. Heart J. 14:515, 1937.
7. Beck, C. S., and Leighninger, D. S.: Scientific basis for the surgical treatment of coronary artery disease, J.A.M.A. 159:1264, 1955.
8. Blalock, A., and Hanlon, C. R.: Interatrial septal defect—its experimental production under direct vision without interruption of the circulation, Surg., Gynec. & Obst. 87:183, 1948.
9. ———: The surgical treatment of complete transposition of the aorta and the pulmonary artery, Surg., Gynec. & Obst. 90:1, 1950.
10. Blalock, A., and Taussig, H. B.: The surgical treatment of malformation of the heart in which there is pulmonary stenosis or pulmonary atresia, J.A.M.A. 128:189, 1945.
11. Bjork, V. O., Blakemore, W. S., and Malmstrom, G.: Left ventricular pressure measurements in man; a new method, Am. Heart J. 48:197, 1954.
12. Bjork, V. O., and Crafoord, C.: The surgical closure of interauricular septal defects, J. Thoracic Surg. 26:300, 1953.
13. Brock, R. C.: Infundibular resection or dilatation for infundibular stenosis, Brit. Heart J. 12:403, 1950.
14. ———: Pulmonary valvulotomy for relief of congenital pulmonary stenosis, Brit. M. J. 1:1121, 1948.
15. Carrel, A.: Results of the transplantation of blood vessels, organs and limbs, J.A.M.A. 51:1662, 1908.
16. Cohn, R.: An experimental method for the closure of interauricular septal defects in dogs, Am. Heart J. 30:453, 1947.
17. Crafoord, C., and Nylin, G.: Congenital coarctation of the aorta and its surgical treatment, J. Thoracic Surg. 14:347, 1945.
18. Cutler, E. C., Levine, S. A., and Beck, C. S.: Surgical treatment of mitral stenosis, Arch. Surg. 9:689, 1924.
19. Fallot, A.: Contribution à l'anatomic pathologique de la maladie bleue, Marseille-med. 25:77, 138, 207, 270, 341, 403, 1888.
20. Gibbon, J. H., Jr.: Artificial maintenance of the circulation during experimental occlusion of the pulmonary artery, Arch. Surg. 34:1105, 1937.
21. Glenn, W. W.: Circulatory bypass of the right side of the heart. IV. Shunt between superior vena cava and distal right pulmonary artery; report of clinical application, New England J. Med. 259:117, 1958.
22. Gordon, A. S., Meyer, B. W., and Jones, J. C.: Open heart surgery using deep hypothermia without an oxygenator. Read before the American Association for Thoracic Surgery, May 1960. To be published in J. Thor. & Cardiovasc. Surg.
23. Gross, R. E.: Patent ductus arteriosus, Am. J. Med. 12:472, 1952.
24. ———: Treatment of certain aortic coarctations by homologous grafts, Ann. Surg. 134:753, 1951.

25. Gross, R. E., and Hubbard, J. P.: Surgical ligation of patent ductus arteriosus, J.A.M.A. *112*:729, 1939.

25a. Gross, R. E., Pomeranz, A. A., Watkins, E., Jr., and Goldsmith, E. I.: Surgical closure of defects of the interauricular septum by use of the atrial wall, New England J. Med. *247*:455, 1952.

26. Halsted, W. S., and Reid, M. R.: An experimental study of circumscribed dilatation of an artery immediately distal to a partially occluding band, J. Exper. Med. *24*:271, 1916.

27. Harken, D. E., Ellis, H. B., Ware, P. F., and Norman, L. R.: Surgical treatment of mitral stenosis. 1. Valvuloplasty. New England J. Med. *239*:801, 1948.

28. Holman, E.: The obscure physiology of post-stenotic dilatation, J. Thoracic Surg. *28*:109, 1954.

29. Hufnagel, C. A., and Harvey, W. P.: The surgical correction of aortic regurgitation, Bull. Georgetown Univ. M. Center *6*:60, 1953.

30. Johnson, J., and Kirby, C. K.: Prevention and treatment of cardiac arrest, J.A.M.A. *154*:291, 1954.

31. Johnson, J., Kirby, C. K., and Blakemore, W. S.: Physiologic considerations in cardiac surgery, S. Clin. North America *35*:1729, 1955.

32. Johnson, J., Kirby, C. K., Blakemore, W. S., and Zinsser, H. F.: Intermittent inflow occlusion for the direct visual repair of atrial septal defect, J. Thor. Surg. *37*:314, 1959.

33. Johnson, J., Kirby, C. K., and Horn, R. C., Jr.: The growth of preserved aorta homografts, Surgery *31*:141, 1952.

34. Kirklin, J. W., McGoon, D. C., and DuShane, J. W.: The results of surgical treatment for ventricular septal defect. Read before the American Association for Thoracic Surgery, May 1960. To be published in J. Thor. & Cardiovasc. Surg.

35. Lewis, F. J., Taufic, M., Varco, R. L., and Niazi, S.: The surgical anatomy of atrial septal defects: experience with repair under direct vision, Ann. Surg. *142*:401, 1955.

36. Lillehei, C. W., Cohen, M., Warden, H. E., Read, R. C., Aust, J. B., DeWall, R. A., and Varco, R. L.: Direct vision intracardiac surgical correction of the tetralogy of Fallot, pentalogy of Fallot and pulmonary atresia defects, Ann. Surg. *142*:418, 1955.

37. Mahoney, E. B., Manning, J. A., DeWeese, J. A., and Schwartz, S. I.: Clinical results of correction under hypothermia of atrial septal defects and pulmonary valvular stenosis, J. Thor. & Cardiovasc. Surg. *38*:292, 1959.

38. Miller, B. J., Gibbon, J. H., Jr., and Fineberg, C.: An improved mechanical heart-lung apparatus, M. Clin. North America *37*: 1603, 1953.

39. Moffitt, G. R., Zinsser, H. F., Jr., Kuo, P. T., Johnson, J., and Schnabel, T. G., Jr.: Pulmonary stenosis with left to right intracardiac shunts, Am. J. Med. *16*:521, 1954.

40. Muller, W. H., and Dammann, F.: Results following the creation of pulmonary stenosis (personal communication).

41. Potts, W. T., Smith, S., and Gibson, S.: Anastomosis of the aorta to a pulmonary artery, J.A.M.A. *132*:627, 1946.

42. Rehn, L.: Ueber penetrierende Herzwunden und Herznaht, Arch. klin. Chir. *55*:315, 1897.

43. Scott, H. W., Jr., and Bahnson, H. T.: Evidence for a renal factor in the hypertension of experimental coarctation of the aorta, Surgery *30*:206, 1951.

44. Scott, H. W., Jr., and Sabiston, D. C., Jr.: Surgical treatment for congenital aorticopulmonary fistula, J. Thoracic Surg. *25*:26, 1953.

45. Senning, A.: Surgical correction of transposition of the great vessels, Surgery *45*:966, 1959.

46. Souttar, H. S.: Surgical treatment of mitral stenosis, Brit. M. J. *2*:603, 1925.

47. Swan, H., Virtue, R. W., Blount, S. G., Jr., and Kircher, L. T., Jr.: Hypothermia in surgery: analysis of 100 clinical cases, Ann. Surg. *142*:382, 1955.

48. Taussig, H. B.: Congenital Malformations of the Heart, New York, Commonwealth Fund, 1947.

49. Vineberg, A., Munro, D. D., Cohen, H., and Buller, W.: Four years' clinical experience with internal mammary artery implantation in human coronary insufficiency, J. Thoracic Surg. *29*:1, 1955.

50. Zinsser, H. F., Jr., and Johnson, J.: The use of angiocardiography in the selection of patients for mitral valvular surgery, Ann. Int. Med. *39*:1200, 1953.

51. Zinsser, H. F., Blakemore, W. S., Kirby, C. K., and Johnson, J.: Invalidism due to recurrent idiopathic pericarditis with recovery after pericardiectomy, J.A.M.A. *171*:274, 1959.

K. Alvin Merendino, m.d.

CHAPTER 42

Lung

ANATOMIC CONSIDERATIONS

The pulmonary arteries carry venous blood from the right ventricle to the lungs; they accompany the bronchial tubes and terminate in a dense capillary network about the alveoli. The pulmonary veins begin in the pulmonary capillaries and, coalescing with larger branches, eventually reach the hilum of the lung. Thence they convey the oxygenated blood into the left atrium for distribution to the remainder of the body.

The bronchial arteries are derived directly from the thoracic aorta or the upper intercostal arteries and are distributed to the bronchial glands, the larger bronchial tubes, the visceral pleura and the coats of the pulmonary vessels. The bronchial arteries supply oxygenated blood for the nutrition of the lung. The bronchial veins in general correspond to the branches of the arteries. On the right side they end in the azygos vein, and on the left either the highest intercostal or the accessory hemiazygos vein.

The sympathetic and the vagus nerves form anterior and posterior pulmonary plexuses which supply efferent fibers to the bronchial muscle and afferent fibers to the bronchial mucous membrane.

The lymphatic vessels of the lung originate in 2 plexuses: the superficial and the deep. The superficial plexus is immediately beneath the pleura. The deep follows the pulmonary vessels and bronchi. Little or no anastomosis occurs between these 2 sets of lymphatics except in the hilum. The superficial set empties into the hilar glands; the deep, into the tracheobronchial glands.[13]

It is recognized that the 2 lungs are composed of 5 lobes: 3 on the right and 2 on the left. Individual lobes may be subdivided into segments: on the right, a total of 10 segments, and 8 in the left lung (Fig. 42-1).[16]

The anatomic unit of pulmonary resection has been progressively reduced as shown by the shift from pneumonectomy to lobectomy and now to segmental resection. The technic of excision of an entire lung originally was performed by mass ligation of all hilar structures. Present-day technics involve the method of ligation of individual component elements. The major anatomic structures that must be ligated incident to a pneumonectomy are the pulmonary artery, the superior and the inferior pulmonary veins and the main stem bronchus. It is apparent that the performance of a lobectomy or a segmental resection requires a considerable knowledge of detailed pulmonary anatomy. Actually, until rather recently, a hiatus in precise anatomic knowledge existed. Because of the desire of the surgeon to excise only diseased tissue with the simultaneous preservation of as much normally functioning lung as possible, the need for the clarification of more detailed anatomic relationships became apparent. Through the combined efforts of anatomists and surgeons, this area of deficit has been eliminated. Consequently, the lung segments are recognized as both anatomic and surgical units which may be excised separately from the individual lobes.

While the lung segments have been considered to be bronchovascular units, they represent essentially a bronchial distribution

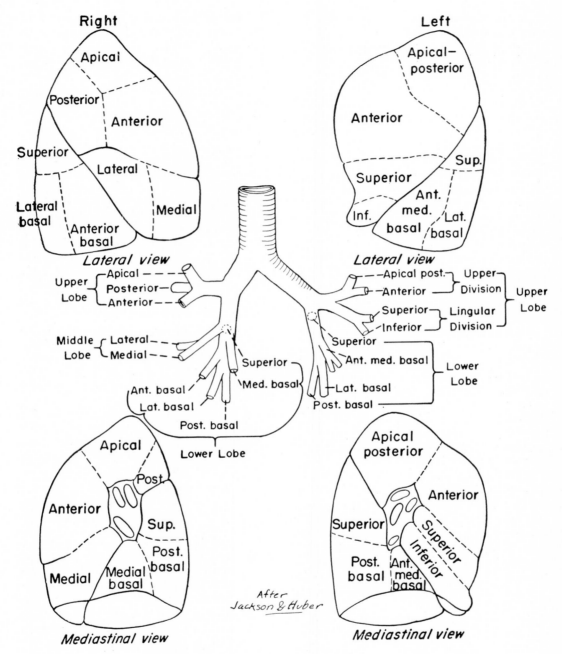

FIG. 42-1. (After Jackson, C. L., and Huber, J. F.: Dis. Chest 9:319-326)

with intersegmental planes that may be crossed by arteries from adjacent segments and contain veins draining contiguous segments. The most stable element in segmental patterns is the bronchus, next the arteries. The veins are the most variable. In general, however, the arteries follow the peripheral distribution of the bronchi, while the veins assume an intersegmental or intersubsegmental position.[3]

It has been implied that segmental resection may be carried out with facility in all instances. Of course, there are exceptions, dependent upon anatomic variations and the specific disease process present.[4, 5] However, it is not amiss to profile those areas which may be the site of the greatest number of anatomic variants.

These generalities seem to be warranted. From the standpoint of the relationship of segmental arteries to bronchi, the most variable segments appear to be the apical and the posterior segments of the right upper lobe and those of the middle lobe. Usually, in the middle lobe, the medial segmental artery tends to supply the lateral segmental bronchus. Consequently, from the practical viewpoint, the variations in the segmental anatomy of the middle lobe indicate that a clean lobectomy is preferable in situations where only the medial or the lateral segment is diseased. In the left upper lobe, it is usually advisable to resect both lingular segments together. Historically, lingulectomy constituted the first segmental resection.[9]

In each of the lower lobes, essentially 5 segments are present. Here, it is best to consider resection of the superior segment only with preservation of the 4 basal segments or excision of the basal segments with preservation of the superior segment. Because of important variations in the venous patterns of the basal segments of the lower lobes, it seems unwise to attempt to remove individual segments. There is general agreement, if more than one basal segment must be excised, that all basal segments should be sacrificed as a unit. Successes have been reported with individual basal segmental resection; nonetheless, it is difficult, if not impossible, to determine the actual venous pattern, except with deep dissection which negates any advantage in most instances. Likewise, in superior segmental resection, care must be taken to avoid the arterial supply to the middle lobe as well as the ascending artery, frequently present in this area, which supplies the posterior segment of the upper lobe. Consequently, from the surgical viewpoint, essentially 2 units of excision exist in the lower lobes. It is apparent that the segmental resection of certain areas may be gross in terms of the arterial and the venous patterns. In short, it is possible to destroy un-

knowingly the arterial supply to an area left behind, or the venous channels to an in situ element may be obstructed. While dire consequences may not result, these circumstances should be avoided if at all possible. Therefore, the properly equipped surgeon must be familiar with the usual arrangements in each segment as well as the variations that may be encountered.

As a consequence, while segmental resection is correctly considered the anatomic unit of surgical excision, the anatomic situation may preclude its use. Likewise, the extent of the disease process may indicate the need for a larger unit of resection. The disease process actually conditions the unit of resection, e.g., in general, pneumonectomy is utilized in bronchogenic carcinoma or for a totally destroyed lung for any reason; lobectomy usually is performed for lung abscess; segmental resections are used most frequently in bronchiectasis, tuberculosis and isolated solitary lesions. In addition, solitary lesions are sometimes removed by "wedge" excision, which essentially represents a wedge-shaped removal of lung between clamps without particular regard to anatomic units.

PHYSIOLOGIC CONSIDERATIONS

The control of ventilation is mainly through both central (medullary) and peripheral receptors which are affected by chemical, pressure and temperature changes. The respiratory center is rhythmically active. Stretch receptors in the lung (Hering-Breuer Reflex) may affect the rhythmicity or modify it and change the characteristics of breathing. In addition, within limits, the respiratory center is stimulated when the pCO_2 or the hydrogen ion concentration is raised. A reduced pO_2 actually depresses the center. On the other hand, peripheral receptors in the carotid and the aortic bodies are more sensitive to decreases in pO_2 than changes in pCO_2 and hydrogen ion. Receptors in the carotid bulb and the aortic arch stimulate the centers when blood pressure falls. A sneeze or a cough results from reflex stimulation of the centers; by swallowing they are inhibited.[14]

Pulmonary function per se consists of 2 components: (1) ventilatory function and (2) gas exchange. Ventilation is a term used to denote the actual mechanism of breathing in and out. Ventilatory function is dependent upon the intactness and the mobility of the thoracic cage and diaphragm, the elasticity and the distensibility of the lung, an intact pleura and a clear airway. These may be interrelated, and each facet is dependent on many other factors. Gaseous exchange is dependent upon the pressure gradient of gas between alveolar air and blood, the availability of gas and blood to the membrane surface, and the rate of the transport of blood and gas to and from the alveoli, the effective area of the membrane, and the permeability of the tissue barrier between the blood and the air.

An important function of the lung that is little emphasized is its role in the excretion of the chief acid waste product of metabolism. Daily the lungs excrete 14,000 mEq. of carbonic acid with no cation. This contrasts sharply with the relatively small daily average of 100 mEq. of free acid metabolites excreted without cations by the kidneys. Consequently, the lungs are most important organs in the regulation of acid-base balance. Any disease, acute or chronic, which interferes with the ability of the lungs to rid the body of carbonic acid, will result in respiratory acidosis.

It is apparent that any disease that affects those factors upon which ventilatory function and gaseous exchange are dependent will affect pulmonary function adversely. Many tests have been devised to study these 2 subdivisions of pulmonary function. They are utilized in reseach activities designed to further our knowledge of respiratory physiology, to evaluate alterations in function created by certain thoracic surgical procedures, and on occasion to determine whether a given patient is capable of tolerating a specific operative procedure. This latter item is of considerable importance to the surgeon. Of the many tests available, the most helpful in determining pulmonary function for the surgical needs are fluoroscopy, the timed vital capacity, maximum breathing capacity and differential bronchospirometry. As will be pointed out later, specialized tests such as these are needed only in occasional situations but are of particular value where excisional pulmonary surgery is contemplated in patients with bilateral disease, such as bronchiectasis, tuberculosis, emphysema or fibrosis.

Space does not permit a detailed description of the normal variations and the limitations in the interpretation of these tests, and the reader is referred to specialized sources of such information.[10] The normal, predicted values are based upon age, sex, etc., and in the final analysis in certain instances the results may not be conclusive in themselves. The results of such tests must be considered together with the physician's knowledge of all aspects of the patient's health status. However, it is apropos to consider briefly the fields in which these tests give valuable information.

By fluoroscopy one may ascertain the mobility of the chest wall and, particularly, the movement of the diaphragm in maximal inspiration and expiration. Lateral as well as anteroposterior views are important. This aids in determining the efficiency of the mechanics of breathing and gives insight into the volume exchange of which the lungs are capable. This in turn gives information concerning lung elasticity and mobility of the important structures. Thus, information concerning the presence of emphysema and fibrosis of the lung is gathered.

The vital capacity is the total amount of air in cubic centimeters or liters which can be expired after a maximum inspiration. This, actually, is only a measure of lung volume and does not give much information regarding function. For example, a patient with emphysema may have a large vital capacity, yet the gas exchange in his lung is poor. More important is the timed vital capacity which introduces a time factor. In short, it is important to know how rapidly one is able to expel the vital capacity. This gives information regarding the dynamics of respiration. A more reliable test of ventilatory capacity is the maximum breathing capacity. With the patient breathing as deeply and rapidly as possible over a 15-second period, one measures the maximum volume of gas breathed per minute. The ability of a patient to breathe at a sustained high velocity depends on many factors: the muscular force available, the resiliency of the lungs and the thorax, the patency of the airway, and tissue resistance.

Differential bronchospirometry is a method for obtaining separate measurements of the individual function of each lung. This is obtained by endobronchial catheterization of the patient by a double lumen tube surrounded by inflatable cuffs. This permits the collection of gas from each lung and the determination of the tidal volume, vital capacity, maximum breathing capacity and O_2 consumption of the right and the left lungs, separately. Whereas the pulmonary function of both lungs measured together may be within normal limits, conceivably one lung could be practically functionless. Thus, the advantage of differential bronchospirometry becomes apparent. This is of primary importance when a pulmonary resection is contemplated in the presence of bilateral disease.

Normally, the right lung accounts for 55 per cent of the minute ventilation and 55 per cent of the O_2 consumption, and the left lung the remainder. This congruity of ventilation and oxygen absorption is very important. For example, if by bronchospirometry the right lung was found to be responsible for 55 per cent of the ventilation and only 10 per cent of the O_2 consumption while the left was effecting 45 per cent of the ventilation and 90 per cent of the total O_2 absorbed, the conclusion is drawn that in the right lung there exists a marked impairment of diffusion of O_2 across the alveolar membrane, or a reduction in pulmonary blood flow, or both. It is apparent that if there were a reason for it, the right lung could be removed without significant loss to O_2 consumption, and with improvement of the respiratory capacity of the patient by virtue of the reduction of the dead space of the poorly absorbing right lung. As a corollary, the removal of the left lung would be contraindicated because therein resides almost the entire oxygen absorptive function of both lungs. While this gross example is clean cut, there are gradations of pulmonary insufficiency of the right and the left lungs which often make the decision more difficult.

These tests do not make a diagnosis of the disease present; they measure pulmonary function. Neither can pulmonary function tests tell the surgeon which patient will tolerate major surgery and survive. In the borderline case, the information obtained will indicate under circumstances of clean surgery without complication that the patient's function is adequate to tolerate the removal of a designated area of the lung and, if he survives, he will not be a respiratory cripple. Be mindful that pulmonary function tests must be considered as measurements of one facet of the patient's total physical assets and liabilities.

As implied earlier, special tests of pulmonary function are unnecessary except in relatively few patients. Therefore, one must be concerned with practical means of evaluating pulmonary function, using clinical methods mainly. The history and the physical examination are important, not only in assaying pulmonary function but also for selecting those patients who may require special tests. If the patient has no difficulty in meeting everyday activities without dyspnea, pulmonary function is adequate for ordinary operations. If dyspnea is present at times, this can be grossly quantitated by further questioning, e.g., how far can you walk at an average pace without shortness of breath; do hills bother you; how many stairs can you climb before becoming short of breath, etc.? If dyspnea is present, cardiac dyspnea must be differentiated from pulmonary dyspnea. A proper decision usually can be made by quantitating the patient's disability, the magnitude of the operation contemplated tempered by sound clinical judgment based on experience.

Under similar circumstances, a knowledge of the behavior of certain pulmonary diseases is essential when the removal of lung parenchyma is contemplated. Furthermore, consideration must be given to the status of the lung to be removed. If the lung is destroyed by disease and obviously nonfunctioning, and if the patient is not short of breath, it is apparent that one may remove the diseased tissue by a segmental resection, lobectomy or pneumonectomy, without reducing pulmonary function much. In short, an anatomic removal of pulmonary tissue can be accomplished without loss of pulmonary function. Actually, after the removal of a functionless lung in the absence of inflammatory pleural complications, an improvement in pulmonary function may result. By the removal of such tissue it is obligatory for all unoxygenated blood to circulate through the remaining normal lung tissue. The removal of such a lung closes a right-to-left cardiac shunt. Even if an entire lung has been destroyed, dyspnea may be improved by its removal for this reason. Removal of a destroyed lung may reduce the workload of the heart and be additionally helpful.

It has been shown that in a destroyed lung, particularly the bronchiectatic variety, the normal communications between the bronchial and the pulmonary arteries may become enlarged and constitute sizable arteriovenous shunts, increasing the workload for the left ventricle.[24]

When pulmonary resection of a normal-appearing and presumably normal-functioning lung is considered, the problem may be more complex. However, in general, an individual who exhibits normal activity without dyspnea will tolerate pneumonectomy of a functioning lung or any component thereof without much difficulty. This situation arises most frequently in bronchogenic carcinoma. On the other hand, an individual with dyspnea at rest with normal-appearing lung fields ordinarily would not be considered a candidate for pulmonary resection, because the removal of any pulmonary tissue would render him more dyspneic. Of course, one cannot always assay the function of the lung by the x-ray appearance of the lung field. However, from the x-ray appearance combined with the history, physical examination and fluoroscopy, usually a good estimate of pulmonary function can be made. In patients with dyspnea and normal-appearing lung fields the specialized pulmonary function tests find their greatest usefulness and give valuable information in this group and those patients with bilateral disease.

In the evaluation of a patient with borderline pulmonary function, it must be remembered that the most dangerous period in terms of survival is immediately postoperative, because the extensive thoracic incision of itself inactivates certain neuromuscular components of the chest wall and reduces the capacity to breathe. Postoperative pain will temporarily limit chest excursion and thereby decrease ventilation. In addition, clearing the tracheobronchial tree of secretions is hampered because coughing is painful. Consequently, consideration must be given to the patient's ability to weather these troubles as well as the eventual result in terms of pulmonary function.

THORACIC TRAUMA

A chest injury may represent the only area involved or be one aspect of a more generalized injury. One must keep in mind the structures contained within and protected by the thoracic wall. Besides the thoracic cage consisting of both hard and soft tissues, there is, in addition, the respiratory tract, the heart and the major vessels, the esophagus and the thoracic duct. Because of injuries to them a chest injury may have far-reaching and widespread general effects.

At times it is difficult to assess properly the total injury. Frequently, even in the absence of abdominal trauma, there may be abdominal signs and symptoms. This is due to the fact that the intercostal nerves also supply the abdominal wall. When they are damaged by trauma to the chest, they may give rise to severe referred abdominal spasm and pain. In addition, ileus and acute gastric dilatation may accompany "pure" thoracic injuries.

Thoracic injuries may be effected from within through the esophagus or the bronchus or from without. Esophagoscopy, gastroscopy and bronchoscopy infrequently lead to thoracic complications. With gastroscopy, rupture of the esophagus may take place. The posterior esophageal wall is thin and may be penetrated by the gastroscope, although it is a pliable instrument. For this reason, gastroscopy is contraindicated in the presence of esophageal disease, severe kyphosis and aneurysms of the thoracic aorta.

Esophagoscopy also carries a minor risk in experienced hands. The esophagoscope is a rigid instrument, and the danger of esophageal perforation is real. With partial or complete obstructions of the esophagus, the proximal esophagus may become saccularily dilated and present pouches which may be mistaken for the esophageal channel. Although the walls of such esophagi may be hypertrophied, they are usually edematous and friable. Esophageal perforations may occur posteriorly into the mediastinum or laterally into the pleural cavities. Occasional complications attend bronchoscopy. During bronchoscopic biopsy, a full thickness of the cartilaginous ring may be removed accidentally, leading to mediastinitis or pneumothorax.[1]

The wounds from without may be penetrating or contusional. Penetrating wounds are usually produced by knives or bullets. Contusional injury follows the application of a force directly to the thoracic wall. This force may be of short duration as in a fall, or prolonged as in a crush injury. Indirect injury to the contents of the chest may occur from any cause which results in increased intrapulmonic pressure such as an abdominal blow, blast or severe coughing.

All trauma to the chest, whether from within or without, may produce rupture of the thoracic duct, the esophagus, the aorta or the tracheobronchial tree. In general, thoracic duct injuries are treated by merely aspirating the chyle from the chest. Occasionally, ligation is necessary. Esophageal rupture should be treated by immediate operation and closure of the rent and closed drainage of the chest. If the tracheobronchial openings are small, they may be treated conservatively, or if severe, by surgical suture. Aortic rupture usually results in immediate death. On occasion, delayed rupture occurs. In some instances immediate operation with direct suture or the insertion of an aortic graft will be possible. Although this is feasible, the issue is often clouded by a lack of certainty in the diagnosis and the poor condition of the patient.

Most frequently, in civilian practice, one encounters hemothorax, pneumothorax, pulmonary contusion and/or laceration, rib fractures, or any combination thereof. In general, these are treated by conservative means. The major indications for exploratory thoracotomy are (1) continuing intrathoracic hemorrhage and (2) continuing air leak from the lung or the tracheobronchial tree, which cannot be controlled by the usual means, (3) large thoracic defects are an indication but rarely are seen in civilian practice.

The proper management of chest injuries is rapidly becoming more important. Chest injuries are second only to head injuries as the most common cause of death in car accidents. This section is not meant to be all-inclusive with regard to the management of chest injuries (see Chap. 24, "Military Surgery"); however, a more detailed account of 2 injuries which are not uncommonly encountered in civilian practice are included because of the severe alterations in pulmonary function which they create. If recognized and properly treated, death often can be prevented.

TENSION PNEUMOTHORAX

Tension pneumothorax exists when the pressure in the pleural cavity is atmospheric or above. Various degrees of pneumothorax may occur following spontaneous rupture of an emphysematous bleb, cyst, or in the presence of apparently normal lung. Likewise, in the presence of an intact thorax, sharp fragments of fractured ribs may lacerate the lung surface with a similar result. In order for air to enter the pleural cavity from without, a communication between the atmosphere and the pleural space must exist. Often this is secondary to penetrating wounds, e.g., knife, bullet, etc. With a penetrating wound air may reach the pleural cavity also from the lung, if injury of the latter simultaneously occurs.

Minor degrees of pneumothorax may not create much difficulty. Severe alterations occur in so-called tension pneumothorax. In order for tension pneumothorax to develop, there must exist a valvular mechanism, created usually by soft tissue adjoining the air leak, which allows air to enter the pleural cavity during inspiration more readily than it permits it to escape during expiration. Consequently, the valvular mechanism is similar to the mechanics of a one-way flutter valve.

Pathologic Physiology. Due to the presence of elastic fibers in the lung substance, the lung removed from the body tends to collapse. In its normal position, the lung is maintained in various degrees of expansion by the negative pressure in the pleural cavity. The degree of expansion is dependent upon the phases of ventilation which varies the degree of negative pressue in the pleural space. With pneumothorax, the degree of negativity is altered toward the positive side. As this occurs, the lung of the involved side begins to collapse (Fig. 42-2). The amount of collapse will be dependent upon the interplay of 2 factors, namely, the inherent elasticity of the lung in one direction and the pull created by the degree of negative pleural pressure in the opposite direction. If the lung is exposed to atmospheric pressure by means of a large communication to the outside, the pressure in the pleural cavity is atmospheric. Therefore, the position of the lung is one of maximum collapse. The degree of collapse is dependent upon the inherent elasticity of the

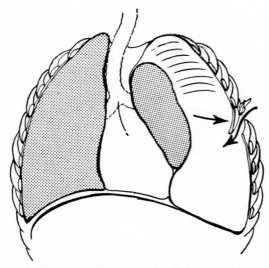

FIG. 42-2. Tension pneumothorax. Here is indicated the "flutter valve" mechanism necessary for the development of a tension pneumothorax. During inspiration, the active phase of respiration, the chest wall expands, the intercostal spaces widen, and the negativity of the pleural cavity increases. Consequently, air enters the pleural cavity. On expiration, the thorax relaxes, and the tissues surrounding the injury partially or completely prevent the escape of pleural air. It is apparent that a similar mechanism may exist in air leaks from the lung or in certain cases of bronchial or tracheal injuries with pleural communications.

lung itself. The presence of any disease which affects lung elasticity or the presence of visceroparietal pleural adhesions, etc., will affect the degree of collapse.

In tension pneumothorax, the increments of trapped air in the pleural cavity result in an increased positive pleural pressure. The adverse effects are multiple. In addition to the loss of function due to collapsed lung, as the tension increases, the mediastinum, if pliable, is displaced toward the uninvolved side. This decreases the effective expansion of the uninvolved lung. In addition to the pain due to the irritative effects of pleural air, the patient attempts to compensate for this loss by an increased respiratory rate. In addition, the circulation is affected adversely on 2 scores. Normally, the venous return via the superior and the inferior vena cavae is aided by the periodic changes in negative pressure of the

pleural cavity incident to ventilation. Not only is this action ablated, but positive pleural pressure actually may hamper venous return. Because, by location, the vena cavae are more a part of the right hemithorax, it would be expected that right pneumothorax would affect venous return more severely than one on the left side. With mediastinal shift angulation of the heart occurs. The heart may be likened to a cherry hanging by a stem. The stem consists of the major vessels by which the heart is actually suspended. When torsion of the heart occurs, the major vessels may become angulated. The aorta is thick-walled and carries a high intraluminal pressure and bends like a sapling. The cavae are thin-walled and have low intraluminal pressures and, consequently, tend to kink. When this occurs, venous return is further reduced with a resultant diminished cardiac stroke output. In order to compensate for this, tachycardia develops which may result in a further decrease of cardiac output. Thus, a vicious cycle is set up. It is apparent that tension pneumothorax may rapidly result in death unless proper therapy is instituted.

Diagnosis. Tension pneumothorax is characterized by chest pain (if due to spontaneous pneumothorax, this is of sudden onset and frequently without history of precipitating factors), rapid short respiration, tachycardia, cyanosis, anxiety and apprehension. On physical examination, in severe cases, the signs and symptoms of shock will be obvious; venous distention may or may not be present. Inspection reveals a full immobile hemithorax exhibiting little excursion with ventilation. The use of the ancillary muscles of respiration may be prominent with intercostal retraction on inspiration of the uninvolved side. Percussion reveals tympany of the involved side and on auscultation absent bronchovesicular breath sounds. X-ray examination demonstrates a collapsed lung with obvious air in the pleural cavity, a flattened diaphragm, widening of the intercostal spaces and mediastinal shift. Obviously, pulmonary disease may be apparent in the opposite lung which may give a clue to etiology in the spontaneous form, and if due to trauma, there may be additional x-ray findings. Severe abdominal pain with marked rigidity of the abdominal wall sometimes occurs and may confuse the diagnosis.

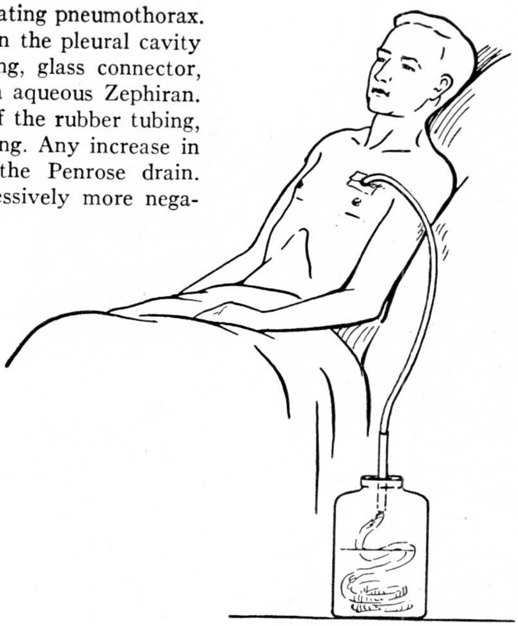

Fig. 42-3. "Water-seal" drainage. A method of treating pneumothorax. The sterilized parts consist of the plastic catheter in the pleural cavity (see text), glass adaptor, intravenous rubber tubing, glass connector, Penrose drain, and a gallon jar partially filled with aqueous Zephiran. By inserting a glass connector into the lower end of the rubber tubing, the Penrose drain can be tied firmly over the tubing. Any increase in positive pleural pressure expels pleural air out the Penrose drain. Consequently, the pleural pressure becomes progressively more negative, and the lung expands. During inspiration the Penrose drain collapses. Thus, the "flutter valve" mechanism which creates tension pneumothorax can be used in its alleviation by reversing the direction of air flow.

Treatment. Rarely, tension pneumothorax must be treated on an emergency basis outside the confines of the hospital. In the absence of any obvious penetrating injury of the chest wall, the most expedient manner of treatment is the insertion of an ordinary intravenous needle, the larger the better, into the pleural space. This is accompanied by an audible rush of air to the outside. In a desperate situation, an entry into the pleural cavity may be imperative with any instrument at hand. The wound must be maintained open by the insertion of any reasonably clean implement into the newly created wound. If a chest wound is present, it should be maintained open by any means available. By these emergency measures one creates an open communication with the atmosphere and an open pneumothorax. While the lung will not expand, the damaging effects of mediastinal shift are obviated. This situation is compatible with life and transport of the patient.

In the hospital, tension pneumothorax of the spontaneous type may be treated by multiple aspirations but preferably by a plastic catheter inserted through a No. 13 gauge needle introduced into the pleural space through the second intercostal space anteriorly. After the plastic catheter is passed into the pleural cavity a short distance, the needle is withdrawn. Then the catheter may be connected to a water seal drainage or to a negative pressure system to aid in rapid expansion (Fig. 42-3). The catheter should not be inserted low in the chest and it should have several perforations in its intrapleural portion. A small serous effusion accompanies most pneumothoraces. If the catheter is inserted into the lower chest it is apt to become plugged by

fibrin. The presence of such a catheter may give one a false sense of security. Unless it is patent it is useless; consequently, the patency of the system should be checked periodically.

If there is a penetrating wound of the chest wall, débridement should be done. Rarely, in the presence of lung injury, it may be impossible to keep abreast of the air loss into the pleural cavity. In this situation exploratory thoracotomy is indicated, in order to close the point of air loss.

FLAIL CHEST

A portion of the thoracic wall becomes "flail" when one or more ribs are fractured in at least 2 spatially separated areas. This portion of the thoracic cage becomes excessively mobile, and its direction of movements will be dependent upon the pressure relationships within the pleural cavity.

Pathologic Physiology. With inspiration the lower ribs flare outward, the sternum is elevated, and there is a descent of the diaphragm. These factors increase the volume of the thoracic cavity, which in turn creates greater negative pressure in the closed pleural space. The lung expands in response to this increased negativity of the pleural cavity. When a segment of the chest wall is flail, with in-

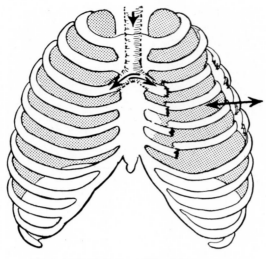

FIG. 42-4. Flail chest. The flail area moves in response to changes in intrapleural pressure. The movement of air down the trachea is mainly dependent on the degree of negative pressure created by the volume enlargement of the pleural cavity during inspiration. Because of the inward movement of the flail segment, normal expansion of the pleural cavity is reduced; consequently, the effective flow of air via the trachea to the involved lung is diminished. During expiration, as the flail segment moves outward, the expired air from the uninvolved side is not only expelled out the trachea but also into the bronchus of the involved side. With the next inspiration, the lung of the normal side receives fresh air via the trachea but also "rebreathes" air previously shunted into the opposite bronchus. Thus, the effective dead space is increased. Stabilization of the segment and tracheotomy are important measures in combating these alterations.

spiration the increased negative pleural pressure sucks in the flail portion of the chest. If the size and the mobility of this area is large, the negative pleural pressure is dissipated. Consequently, the lung does not expand completely, and the air movement down the trachea is diminished. With expiration, as pleural pressure moves toward the more positive side, the flail area is pushed outward. These movements of this mobile segment are in opposite direction of the remainder of the chest wall during both phases of ventilation. These abnormal motions of the flail portion of the

chest are referred to as paradoxical movements.

In addition, ventilation is affected adversely by the to-and-fro movement of air at the carinal level (Fig. 42-4). The limited excursion of the lung secondary to the alterations in the pleural pressure is inadequate to move air completely in and out of the tracheal dead space; and, in fact, the to-and-fro movement of air between the 2 lungs further increases the effective dead space.

It becomes apparent that with such an injury significant pain is present. Because of pain, the involved side is splinted voluntarily. In addition, involuntary splinting due to spasm occurs secondary to the localized trauma. As a consequence, aeration of the involved lung is incomplete, and coughing is inhibited. Furthermore, thoracic trauma is accompanied by increased bronchial secretion and retention. This has resulted in the term traumatic "wet lung."[7] Consequently, the stage is set for atelectasis and its sequelae. By the retention of secretions the exchange of O_2 and CO_2 may be interfered with across the alveolar membrane.

The cough is an extremely important defense mechanism, particularly in chest injuries. It is apparent that in order to clear the respiratory tract of secretions, an explosive cough is necessary. However, an explosive cough is impossible unless air is built up behind the material to be expelled. Decreased aeration of the involved side precludes this. Furthermore, with cough the closed epiglottis builds up a positive pleural pressure. However, the positive pressure build-up is dissipated because the flail segment moves outward as the remainder of chest wall actively contracts downward. Pain also is a serious deterrent to an effective cough by the patient.

Treatment. Immobilization of the flail chest is mandatory. The flail segment may be stabilized by strapping a sandbag over it or by grasping one of the involved ribs by a sterile towel clip which is connected to a weight by means of an overhead traction system; only a small incision is necessary. The former method usually suffices. Of almost equal importance is the alleviation of pain. Periodic intercostal nerve block is most effective. One should block not only the nerves of the involved ribs but 2 intercostal spaces above and below as well. By these maneuvers, immobilization of the chest wall is aided, and pain is practically abolished. As a result, paradoxical motion is obviated to a great degree, and splinting is lessened with the result that better aeration of the lung on the involved side occurs. An effective cough may now result.

If the raising of secretions becomes a problem, tracheal aspiration, bronchoscopy and tracheotomy should be resorted to in that order. Nasal oxygen may be necessary. The advantage of tracheotomy in a severe case is twofold. Not only does it serve as a readily available vent for tracheal aspiration, but it also reduces the respiratory dead space. If oxygen is required with tracheostomy, it is possible by this means to deliver O_2 under slightly positive pressure. In addition, respiratory acidosis may be avoided by washing out CO_2.

LUNG ABSCESS

Nontuberculous lung abscess occurs as a solitary unilocular or multilocular cavity. Multiple lung abscesses occur secondary to septicemia or pyemia. The latter types frequently are associated with a serious medical problem; consequently, they may fall in the province of the internist. Lung abscess is more frequent in the male than in the female; no age group is immune. The peak of incidence occurs in the 3rd, the 4th and the 5th decade. The mechanism of development is mainly aspirational; however, some abscesses are of hematogenous or embolic origin.

CLINICAL ETIOLOGY

One third of all lung abscesses occur postoperatively or postanesthetically. An equal number are of undetermined etiology. The remaining cases of lung abscess are secondary to primary respiratory infections, bronchogenic carcinoma, bronchiectasis, foreign body aspiration, pulmonary infarction, infection of congenital cysts and coma with presumed aspiration. The coma may be alcoholic, epileptic, due to trauma, brain tumor or excessive morphine sedation.

In the postoperative-anesthetic group, most abscesses follow operations on the upper respiratory tract; tonsillectomy and dental extractions are the worst offenders. Following tonsillectomy, blood in the trachea and the bronchi is a common finding after all bleeding is controlled. The Trendelenburg or Rose position during tonsillectomy offers excellent prophylaxis against this complication. Consequently, aspiration seems to be the logical explanation in the majority of cases. A similar mechanism occurs following the extraction of teeth. The unilateral dulling of the pharyngeal reflex affected by the commonly employed nerve blocks, particularly of the inferior dental and the anterior palatine nerves, allows easy access to the lower respiratory tract for the entry of infected material. Lung abscess has been known to follow anesthesia without operation and operation without anesthesia.

Of those cases classified as having an undetermined etiology, the insidious onset of symptoms defies attempts to establish the definite date of onset. Many cases in this category formerly were considered to be secondary to an atypical pneumonia. In the older literature, lung abscess frequently was diagnosed following a respiratory illness. It is probable that many cases were primary abscess with a surrounding pneumonitis. Oral sepsis is present so frequently in this group of patients that its etiologic portent cannot be overlooked.[25]

ANATOMIC LOCATION

The right lung is involved more frequently than the left in the ratio of 2:1. The right lower lobe is the most frequent site of lung abscess due to the dependent position of its bronchus, the less acute angle which the right main bronchus forms with the trachea, and its larger size. While this pertains where aspiration may have occurred in the upright position, the most dependent portion of the lung is altered by changes in position of the patient. Consequently, in the supine position the dorsal segment of the lower lobes may be involved. In the lateral recumbent position the posterior segment or the lateral (axillary) division of the anterior segment of the upper lobes become the most dependent portions of the lung.[6] Embolic abscess occurs most commonly in the lower lobes; the right lung again is involved more frequently than the left.

DIAGNOSIS AND LOCALIZATION

The history is the most important diagnostic aid and is within the reach of every physician. Cough with expectoration is the

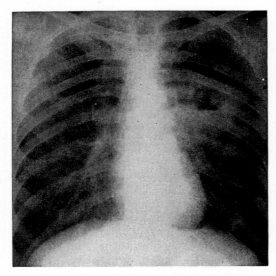

Fig. 42-5. Typical acute, thin-walled lung abscess with fluid level and surrounding pneumonitis. This lesion completely re-solved under antibiotic therapy.

most common complaint, with pleuritic chest pain, fever, malaise, headache, asthenia, hemoptysis and weight loss following in that order. The sputum is usually foul, yellow, green or dark mucopurulent material. Pleuritic chest pain is of aid in localization. The localization of pleuritic pain identifies the site of pleural adhesions. Circumscribed tenderness to pressure is often associated with pleuritic pain. Such pain is usually absent with either central or upper lobe abscesses. While hemoptyses are usually small, exsanguinating hemorrhages can occur.

On physical examination there are no pathognomonic signs of pulmonary abscess. Cavitary signs are distinctly unusual. Consolidation with or without friction rub is present in half the cases. Pneumonitis without consolidation is frequently present; 10 per cent of the patients will have a negative physical examination or reveal the presence of a complication such as pleural effusion, empyema or bronchopleural fistula. Clubbing of the fingers and the toes, when present, may be marked. This sign may be present as early as the 4th week after onset and completely disappears after cure. If there is persistence of clubbing, one should suspect an undrained focus or bronchiectasis.

LABORATORY STUDIES

In acute cases, a high leukocyte count may indicate a good prognosis. In the chronic phase, a mild normocytic anemia with slight leukocytosis is present. At this stage of the illness a high leukocyte count may indicate a complication. The bacteriologic findings are extremely complex; however, streptococcus viridans is found frequently. Anaerobic streptococcus is the most common of the strictly anaerobic micro-organisms. Pneumococci, staphylococci, fusiform bacilli and spirochetes frequently are present.

X-ray studies are important in the diagnosis and the localization of the lesion (Fig. 42-5). A cavity with a fluid level is diagnostic. Bronchograms with Lipiodol or water-soluble contrast media are sometimes essential in the differential diagnosis of lung abscess and bronchiectasis. It is difficult to fill the abscess cavity with opaque material. When filling occurs there can be no question of the diagnosis. More commonly there is an inability to fill the bronchus draining the abscess. Thus, the exact segmental localization may be made indirectly. Diagnostic bronchoscopy is indicated in all cases to establish the presence or the absence of bronchial tumor or a foreign body. A biopsy of suspected tissue is always taken, and washings are made for Papanicolaou stains. Serial roentgenograms are necessary in evaluating the progress of therapy.

TREATMENT

Medical. The use of antibiotics has reduced markedly the incidence of lung abscess. Similarly, in the subacute phase the judicious use of antibiotics, based upon the sensitivity of the organisms cultured, frequently results in cure. It is important to remember that the treatment of a lung abscess, as with abscesses anywhere in the body, entails adequate drainage. Therefore, postural drainage and, occasionally, bronchoscopy for the removal of granulation tissue remain important measures in management. In addition, supportive measures, including high protein and high vitamin diets and transfusions, are important. Significant protein loss may occur when the sputum volume is large.

Surgical. MINOR SURGICAL PROCEDURE. These include phrenic crush and pneumothorax. The success of phrenic crush is difficult to evaluate. Pneumothorax frequently results in pyopneumothorax and metastatic brain abscess. For these reasons, neither procedure warrants consideration in therapy. They are mentioned only to be condemned.

MAJOR SURGICAL PROCEDURE. If for any reason the patient shows little or no improvement in 4 to 6 weeks of adequate medical management, a major surgical procedure should be considered.

Incision and Drainage. The usefulness of external drainage of a lung abscess is determined by the relative accessibility of the cavity. A short rib resection frequently is necessary. The agglutination of visceral and parietal pleura must be adequate, otherwise a pneumothorax is produced which tends to uncap the pus pocket, resulting in pleural infection or bronchopleural fistula. If there is firm adherence between the visceral and the parietal pleura, the abscess may be drained in one stage. Otherwise, the procedure must be staged, first creating an irritation between the 2 pleural membranes by packing iodoform gauze immediately against the outside of the parietal pleura with drainage of the abscess 5 to 7 days later. External incision and drainage are utilized mainly for those patients who for any reason cannot tolerate a major thoracotomy. Some surgeons have utilized incision and drainage in the acute phase with excellent results.[19]

Excision. The excision of chronic abscess cavities has become the procedure of choice. While occasionally a wedge excision or a segmental resection may be done, the infiltrative pneumonitis surrounding the lung abscess pocket usually extends beyond the segmental confines. For this reason, frequently lobectomy must be employed in the treatment of lung abscess, except where a combination of segments (e.g., basal segments) may be removed as a unit. Because lung abscess is usually a once-in-a-lifetime occurrence, the removal of a single lobe is well tolerated. It is accomplished with low morbidity and mortality and is almost always curative.

BRONCHIECTASIS

The term implies merely a dilated bronchus. Without sputum it is considered a dry type.

However, chronic infection together with an increased secretion of mucus from the bronchial epithelium are present so frequently that the wet type must be considered as comprising the more characteristic clinical picture. The wet type is more frequently of surgical interest. Local anatomic changes in the bronchus and the bronchioles may be minimal or extensive. Cylindrical forms represent early changes, and the saccular the most severe.

ETIOLOGY

Despite considerable investigation and much speculation, the true cause of bronchial dilatation remains unknown. The main theories advanced involve the following: nutritional changes in the bronchial walls, derangement of the neuromuscular mechanism of the bronchial walls, increased fibrous tissue of the lung substance and congenital deformity of the bronchi. Whatever the fundamental causes of bronchiectasis are, the precipitating factors are not always the same. Some cases follow the aspiration of foreign bodies or infected material from the stomach and the upper respiratory tract. Others occur as a sequel to pneumonia or a lung segment which has been collapsed for any reason. Many develop as a gradual accompaniment of repeated upper respiratory infections. The association of chronic sinusitis is common and may have etiologic importance.

PATHOLOGY

Early pathologic changes are seldom confined to the ectasia of the bronchi but almost always involve the bronchial mucosa and submucosa. Chronic inflammatory changes in these layers develop and progress to a state of extensive and progressive fibrosis of the area involved. Eventually, areas of normal mucosa are destroyed and replaced by chronically infected granulation tissue. Elastic fibers and muscle bundles may become replaced partially or largely with fibrosis and occasional destruction of portions of the cartilaginous structures. Weakening of the bronchial wall is inevitable. Finally, progressive shrinkage and contraction of involved segments results. Accompanying the chronic inflammatory changes, the bronchial wall may stenose with the retention of infected secretions. Consequently, the weakened, diseased bronchi be-

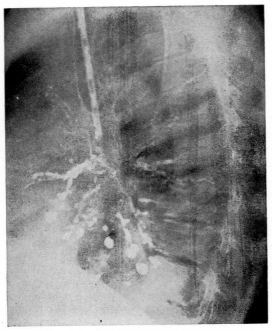

Fig. 42-6. Saccular bronchiectasis of the basal segments of the lower lobe with normal appearing superior segment.

come further dilated distal to this narrowing. These factors when combined bring about the saccular type of bronchiectasis seen as an end-stage. The bacteriologic picture is complex, and no etiologic significance can be ascribed to any single organism.

An additional change occurs in the hemodynamics of bronchial-pulmonary arterial communications (see section on Physiology).

PROGNOSIS

When the disease begins in early childhood, few survive beyond the age of 40 when untreated or treated by nonsurgical methods. Considerable impairment in the physical development begins in childhood, and chronic invalidism continues throughout life. Because of the presence of a productive cough with foul-smelling sputum, social ostracism frequently results. Eventually, many children develop psychological changes, varying in degree from mild depression to actual psychopathic personalities. Therefore, it has become apparent that untreated and medically treated bronchiectasis is attended with a high mortality, a relatively short life expectancy and

a devastating morbidity on both a physical and a psychologic basis.[8]

PATTERN OF INVOLVEMENT

Bronchiectasis may involve all lobes of the lung. However, it rarely involves all segments of the lung. There is a typical distribution in that the left lung is involved more frequently than the right. In 30 to 50 per cent of cases the disease is bilateral. The lower lobes are involved more frequently than any other lobes of the lung. More specifically, one or all of the basal segments of either lower lobe may be involved. Characteristically, the superior segments of the lower lobes are free of disease. When the left basal segments are involved, the lingula is likewise diseased in 60 to 80 per cent of cases.[9] Similarly, if the basal segments of the right lung are diseased, from 45 to 60 per cent of patients have disease in the middle lobe.

DIAGNOSIS

Dilatation of the bronchi, so-called dry bronchiectasis, gives rise to no symptoms except hemoptyses. Many patients with so-called dry bronchiectasis are converted to wet types when bronchial infection supervenes. Wet bronchiectasis gives rise to the chief symptoms of cough and purulent sputum. Hemoptyses and sputum are frequently worse in the morning, purulent secretions having accumulated during sleep. The sputum is characteristically foul. If bronchiectasis is extensive with considerable destruction of lung tissue, emphysema supervenes with dyspnea, particularly on exertion.

On physical examination, clubbing of fingers may be present, and rales may be detected over the involved lung. A roentgenogram of the chest often shows a honeycombed appearance of the affected lung fields. There may be areas of atelectasis and cavitation. The actual diagnosis of bronchiectasis rests on the demonstration of dilated bronchi on x-ray study after the intrabronchial instillation of Lipiodol or a water-soluble opaque medium (Fig. 42-6). It is of importance to map out the entire lung, both right and left, in order to determine the extent of bronchiectasis present. Particularly is this important where surgical therapy is considered, for the removal of a portion of the infected areas without removal of all bronchiectatic segments results in incomplete cure.

Pseudobronchiectasis is a term used for bronchial changes observed after atypical pneumonia (viral). These changes are reversible and should not cause any difficulty in diagnosis.[2]

COMPLICATIONS

Recurrent attacks of atypical pneumonia are common. Bronchiectasis gives rise not only to secondary lung abscess but also may develop as a complication of lung abscess. Metastatic brain abscess is an uncommon complication most frequently affecting the right frontal lobe. Empyema and pyopneumothorax do occur. Amyloid disease may follow long-standing cases with extensive involvement.

TREATMENT

Once the anatomic changes characteristic of bronchiectasis are observed, they are irreversible. Consequently, bronchiectasis is a surgical disease. Medical measures are reserved only for those cases so extensive that surgical therapy is not feasible or for patients who refuse therapy or are unable for other reasons to tolerate thoracotomy. These measures consist of rest, postural drainage and bronchoscopy. Broad-spectrum antibiotics are of value in reducing sputum, thus obtaining symptomatic relief and aborting acute respiratory infections. Intermittent usage is advocated to avoid the development of resistant strains of organisms.

Surgical therapy is directed toward the removal of all diseased tissue with the sparing of all healthy, functioning lung parenchyma. Pulmonary function studies are particularly important when there is extensive involvement or when other pulmonary changes are present which indicate borderline pulmonary function. Bronchiectasis lends itself well to segmental resection.[20]

When there is unilateral involvement, it is customary to remove all diseased segments of the entire lung on that side at one operation. If the disease is bilateral, usually the most seriously involved side is operated upon first. To avoid spill-over of secretions into the non-involved lung, endobronchial intubation and positioning of the patient with the operated side dependent are important maneuvers. Re-

cently, it has been shown that bilateral disease may be attacked simultaneously at the same operation, either by 2 separate incisions of the posterolateral type or a single anterior transsternal incision. Except for unusual indications, this approach would appear to be unwise.

When the basal segments are incompletely involved, it is considered inadvisable to leave behind less than 2 segments though they may be normal. Ordinarily, a left basal segmental resection is done with sparing of the superior segment of the lower lobe with resection of the lingula if involved; on the right side, basal segmental resection is combined with right middle-lobe lobectomy in case of its involvement.

Bronchiectasis is a surgically curable disease when all diseased segments are removed. The value of surgery in bronchiectasis has been reconfirmed in a collective review of over 800 cases. An average cure rate of 43 per cent can be anticipated, while an additional 43 per cent will be improved. Thus, 86 per cent of patients treated surgically will be benefited and capable of normal activity. Surgical treatment fails in 6 per cent of cases. This includes patients with a continued productive cough or physical limitation preventing gainful employment. While the complication rate of 23 per cent is high, the mortality rate is less than 1 per cent.[15] Recently, it has been shown that with resection of the lower lobe for bronchiectasis, the anterior segment of the upper lobe may be realigned in the chest so that it may reside in a dependent position. Subsequently, it may become involved in the bronchiectatic process. In such instances it is difficult to know whether bronchiectasis existed in the anterior segment prior to operation.

In addition to the surgical aspects of the lung itself, one must clear up any infectious disease in the upper respiratory tract with particular attention to the nasal sinuses.

EMPYEMA

Empyema, or the occurrence of pus in the pleural cavity, is usually secondary to pulmonary infections (pneumococcal, streptococcal) but may follow trauma or pulmonary surgery. With the advent of antibiotics this complication is seen less frequently. Surgical management consists of (1) closed thoracotomy drainage, (2) open thoracotomy and (3) excision or decortication of the empyema pocket.

ACUTE AND SUBACUTE EMPYEMA

Closed Thoracotomy Drainage. This term is derived from the fact that the cavity is subjected to a negative pressure in a closed system. First, an intercostal catheter is inserted into the empyema pocket and connected to a Y tube. One limb is connected to a collection bottle subjected to a constant negative pressure. The other limb is connected to an irrigation bottle. Consequently, the cavity can be irrigated periodically. At all other times, the cavity is exposed to negative pressure (Fig. 42-7).

The procedure is used primarily in acute and subacute empyema. However, a more

FIG. 42-7. Closed thoracotomy drainage. The Stedman pump generates negative pressure for the entire system. The 1st bottle is merely for the collection of aspirate; the purpose of the 3rd bottle is to protect the pump from being damaged in the event that the middle bottle is inadvertently upset. The long tube in the middle bottle is open to the atmosphere. The amount of negative pressure is dependent upon the depth of the lower end of this tube below the water level. Consequently, by adjusting the depth of the tube, the water level, or both, the degree of negative pressure can be controlled. When the negative pressure generated by the motor is greater than desired, atmospheric air is pulled in from the outside through the middle tubing. Consequently, when bubbling occurs, the negative pressure is stabilized at the desired level. This system is similar in principle to any "break-over" type manometer. This apparatus can be applied also in treating pneumothorax.

In empyema, Dakin's solution is an excellent agent for irrigation. By the application of a clamp on the tubing to the 1st bottle and release of the forceps depicted, the irrigating fluid is instilled into the cavity. This tubing is reclamped, and clamps on the tubing to the drainage bottle are reopened. At all times, except for periods of irrigation, negative pressure is maintained in the empyema cavity (see text). Usually the cavity is irrigated every 4 hours with a volume approximately half of the size of the cavity. The size of the cavity can be measured easily by allowing fluid to run in until there is no further flow or the patient complains of discomfort.

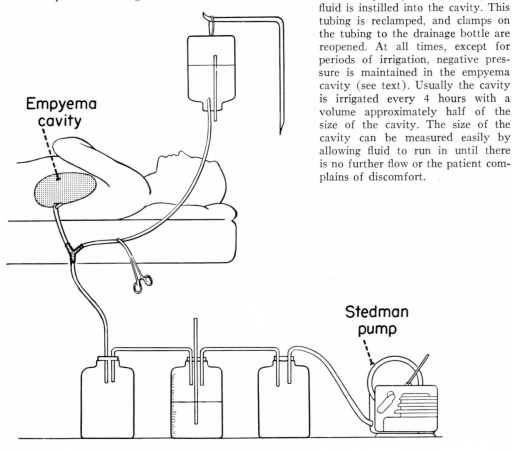

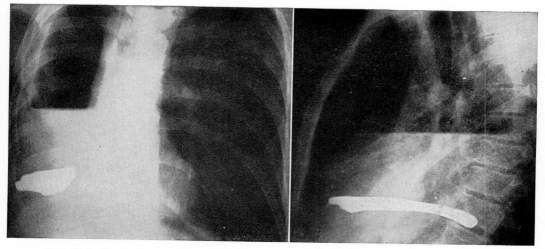

FIG. 42-8. Empyema following pneumonectomy. The instillation of Lipiodol into an empyema cavity is an excellent method to determine its lowermost level and the rib segment which should be removed for dependent drainage. First, the empyema pocket is located by the aspiration of pus, and 10 ml. of Lipiodol is instilled. The patient should remain upright for approximately 10 minutes. Since Lipiodol is heavier than the contents of the cavity, it gravitates to the bottom. Overexposed roentgenograms of the anterior and the lateral views are usually sufficient.

conservative method has partially supplanted closed thoracotomy technics. This consists of the intermittent aspiration and instillation of antibiotics combined with enzymatic débridement agents (streptokinase and streptodornase, trypsin). While this method is effective in the early stages of empyema, occasionally a sterilized empyema persists. When this occurs, it must be drained or excised, for an empyema, though sterile, still may result in a pleurocutaneous or bronchopleural fistula.

CHRONIC EMPYEMA

Open Thoracotomy Drainage. By this method the empyema cavity is opened to atmospheric pressure. A short rib segment is removed *at the most dependent portion of the empyema cavity.* A large drainage tube then is inserted into the empyema pocket (Fig. 42-8). Because the cavity is exposed to atmospheric pressure, one must be certain that the empyema is adequately sealed from the remainder of the pleural cavity. Otherwise, a pneumothorax will result with the development of a total empyema. Ordinarily, from 14 to 21 days after onset, the empyema is adequately sealed. Another empirical method for determining the safe period for open

thoracotomy is by the observation of the percentage of the aspirate which is sediment. First, the pocket is aspirated; the material is placed in a test tube and taped to the bed of the patient. In 24 hours it will be noted that a considerable cellular debris has settled in the bottom of the tube. Above it is a clear liquid. By periodic aspiration additional samples are obtained. The amount of sediment increases as the empyema matures. When the aspirate consists of approximately 80 to 85 per cent sediment, the empyema can be safely drained by open thoracotomy (Fig. 42-9).

The relationship of the etiologic organism and therapy can be credited to Dr. E. A. Graham and the U. S. Army Empyema Commission (1918) which he headed. This commission was established because of the frightening mortality of empyema treated in the military by open thoracotomy drainage during the "influenza" epidemic due to hemolytic streptococcus. It was demonstrated clearly that empyema due to streptococci accompanied the active pneumonia, and open thoracotomy was performed while the exudate was thin and watery. Thus many patients died of asphyxia resulting from an open pneumothorax. On the other hand, empyema in association with pneumococcal pneumonia (a common civilian entity) was a postpneumonic phenomenon, and drainage by open thoracotomy was done when the empyema contained frank pus and during a period when the mediastinum was stabilized by edema and adhesions. These concepts still form the basis for present-day therapy. Early in the course of empyema, regardless of the organism, periodic aspiration is carried out with the instillation of penicillin into the pleural cavity. If open thoracotomy is resorted to, frank pus must be present which ensures a localized empyema cavity and mediastinal stability.

This method is effective in curing empyema. Drainage may be prolonged, but the patient need not be hospitalized during this period. Open and closed methods require only local anesthesia.

Excision or Decortication. This procedure may be used as an alternative to open thoracotomy drainage or, in the event of a failure to cure—following open thoracotomy. Excision of all walls of the empyema is preferred by some; however, decortication of the inflammatory membrane or "peel" only over the visceral pleura allows re-expansion of the lung with ablation of the cavity. The thickening of the parietal pleura is due mainly to edema. When the empyema cavity is obliterated, the parietal pleura recedes in thickness and becomes practically normal. Unfortunately, in empyema the visceral peel is very adherent to the visceral pleura. Thus, it can be removed only piecemeal and with considerable trauma to the underlying lung. Negative pressure exerted through a chest catheter is necessary to obtain immediate and continued local pulmonary expansion. Mediastinal empyema is treated best in this fashion. Excision of the empyema pocket, if extensive, carries some risk in younger children. In the ordinary case, many prefer open thoracotomy first. A disadvantage of excision or decortication is the need for a general anesthesia and the postoperative discomfort, for considerable force may be necessary to gain exposure due to the local fixation of the chest wall involved with infection and edema. However, it is an effective and

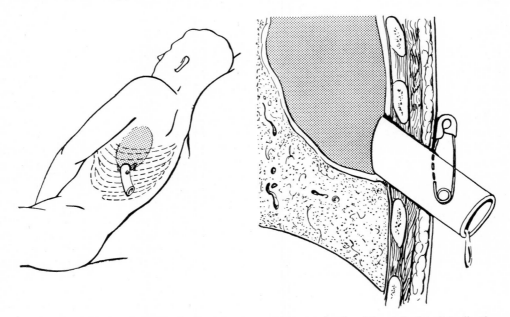

Fig. 42-9. Open thoracotomy drainage (see text). In order for this method to be effective it is essential that the thoracotomy tube be at the most dependent portion of the empyema pocket. The tube should be flush with the parietal pleura. It should be noted that the inner end of the tube has been tailored obliquely so that no lip of the tubing is above the fluid. Consequently, no puddling of undrained pus results. The safety pin is inserted through the tubing and held to the skin by adhesive tape.

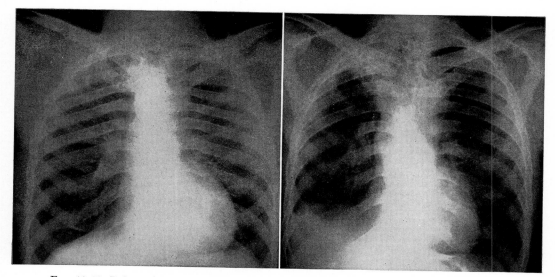

FIG. 42-10. Pulmonary coccidioidomycosis with cavity. Ordinarily, such a cavity is not considered as an indication for surgery. However, this patient had suffered 2 episodes of severe hemoptysis. (A) The cavity is present in the right upper lobe. (B) A right upper lobectomy has been performed. A lobectomy was indicated because of satellite areas of involvement.

definitive form of therapy and it reduces the duration of the illness sharply.

CERTAIN FUNGUS DISEASES

COCCIDIOIDOMYCOSIS

Coccidioidomycosis is an endemic disease peculiar to the San Joaquin valley and the Southwest portion of the United States. *Coccidioides immitis* is the causative fungus. This fungus is diphasic and thus similar to histoplasma capsulatum. In its vegetative phase it consists of long, thin mycelia which segment and form chlamydospores. These chlamydospores are highly infective. It is this form which occurs in nature and has been isolated from the soil and airborne dust in endemic areas.[21]

The inital infection is almost always respiratory and is incurred by the inhalation of fungus in contaminated dust. It is focalized in the lungs and usually subsides spontaneously and without sequela. A history of a patient having visited, traveled through, either by train or air, the endemic areas, who, in addition, exhibits a positive coccidioidin skin test, suggests the diagnosis. Hematogenous disseminated forms of the disease occur but are uncommon. In the disseminated forms, the mortality is approximately 50 per cent.

If the disease is localized or the patient survives the disseminated type of illness, lesions in the lung are found. Such lesions are seen in approximately 10 per cent of such patients. These lesions may be solid, discrete, soft granulomatous areas, or cavitation may be present. These findings are usually revealed only by roentgenogram and are unaccompanied by any constitutional symptom.

There is no specific medical therapy for coccidioidomycosis. Furthermore, surgical treatment is utilized infrequently. Cavitary lesions usually require no therapy. Some will close spontaneously. However, if hemoptyses or recurrent localized pneumonitis occur, excision is advised (Fig. 42-10). Usually, lobectomy is the procedure of choice because of the frequent presence of satellite granulomas undiagnosed by roentgenograms. Lobectomy, for what appears to be contained disease, should not be regarded as curative. One should entertain the same reservations as in the tuberculous patient. Solid discrete pulmonary granulomas are quite common. Consequently, the excision of all "coin" lesions becomes impractical in endemic areas. Such lesions must be followed periodically by roentgenograms in these areas whereas in nonendemic portions of the country usually they are excised incidental to establishing an accurate diagnosis.

HISTOPLASMOSIS

Histoplasmosis is caused by the fungus *Histoplasma capsulatum*. The fungus has 2 phases in its life cycle: the yeastlike or parasitic phase and the mycelial or saprophytic phase. Formerly, it was considered to be a disseminated disease and often fatal. This form of the disease actually is rare. Now it is recognized as a relatively benign disease which is widely prevalent. The disease is endemic in the Mississippi Valley. About 70 per cent of adults in this area are histoplasmin positive.[18] However, due to the travel characteristics of the American population and the shunting of military personnel throughout the country, histoplasmosis has been uncovered in practically all parts of the United States.

The organism is a parasite of the reticuloendothelial system and therefore is found in places where these cells are most numerous. In most fatal cases, the organism is disseminated throughout the body and can be isolated in cultures from almost every organ. The pathologic response is a granulomatous reaction which is characterized by epithelioid, giant cells and necrosis. These lesions often calcify. With pulmonary calcific deposits, a positive histoplasmin test in the presence of a negative tuberculin test would allow the diagnosis to be made. Of course, both diseases may coexist.

How man acquires an infection with histoplasma capsulatum is not clearly understood. The spores have been found in the soil in endemic areas and in the air. The inhalation of histoplasma spores is the only plausible explanation for the high incidence of positive skin tests in endemic areas. The available epidemiologic and experimental evidence strongly supports the view that the respiratory tract is the port-of-entry of the fungus, regardless of the type of illness it provokes. In the great majority of instances the inhalation of spores results in a nonfatal illness.

At present, no medications appear to be specific for histoplasma capsulatum. In view of the pathologic response to the fungus it is apparent, at some time following the sub-

acute phase of infection, that isolated pulmonary granulomas may result with or without calcifications; or cavitation may be present. Such lesions may be confused with chronic lung abscess, tuberculoma, or primary pulmonary carcinoma. Consequently, in the absence of skin testing or the fear of a more serious coexisting lesion, the surgeon occasionally removes a "coin" lesion by wedge resection, which proves to be histoplasmosis granuloma.[12] Undoubtedly, in endemic areas considerable judgment is required concerning the decision to explore patients exhibiting so-called "coin" lesions. Likewise, on occasion, a lobectomy is performed for cavitation secondary to histoplasmosis.[16] Usually, exploration is incidental to establishing an accurate histologic diagnosis of a pulmonary lesion of undetermined etiology.

ACTINOMYCOSIS

Actinomycosis is a chronic suppurative or granulomatous disease caused by a specific organism, *Actinomyces bovis*. This organism is in an intermediate position between the "higher" bacteria and fungi. From the clinical viewpoint, it may be considered as a type of pathogenic fungus.[22] The disease is characterized by multiple abscesses, draining sinuses, excess granulation tissue, dense fibrous tissue and by the appearance of mycelial masses (sulfur granules) in the discharges from involved tissue.

The thorax is involved in approximately 20 per cent of cases. Actinomycetes may reach the lung by several routes. Primary infection may occur by aspiration of saliva containing pathogenic actinomyces. Secondary infection may result from downward spread of established cervical infection or by the extension of abdominal infection through or behind the diaphragm. In the past, thoracic involvement carried a grave prognosis; however, the advent of sulfonamides and penicillin have altered the prognosis considerably.

Medical therapy is of prime importance (see Chap. 4, "Surgical Infections"). Surgery is reserved for the drainage of loculated pus and the excision of destroyed pulmonary tissue or thoracic wall.[11, 23] Surgical therapy is usually considered as an adjunct to chemotherapy and antibiotic therapy.

TRACHEA

Foreign bodies, tumors and diverticula constitute the main items of interest. The diverticula are congenital and presumably represent arrested development of supernumerary lung buds. These are rare and usually have no surgical implications. Foreign bodies occur frequently in children. When large, these may be impacted in the glottis or the trachea with acute suffocation. Sharp objects may lacerate or perforate the trachea. Most foreign bodies are held in place by the surrounding inflammatory process and seldom are coughed out spontaneously. Immediate removal by bronchoscopic methods is indicated; at times, tracheotomy is necessary for their removal. (See Chapter 43 for additional details concerning tumors of the trachea.)

REFERENCES

1. Abbott, O. A., and deOliveira, H. R.: Spontaneous pneumothoraces in patients undergoing peroral endoscopy, J. Thoracic Surg. 14:453-460, 1945.
2. Blades, B., and Dugan, D. J.: Pseudobronchiectasis, J. Thoracic Surg. 13:40-48, 1944.
3. Boyden, E. A.: The intrahilar and related segmental anatomy of the lung, Surgery 18: 706-731, 1945.
4. ———: Segmental Anatomy of the Lungs, New York, McGraw-Hill, 1955.
5. Brock, R. C.: The Anatomy of the Bronchial Tree, ed. 2, London, Oxford, 1954.
6. Brock, R. C., Hodgkiss, F., and Jones, H. O.: Bronchial embolism and posture in relation to lung abscess, Guy's Hosp. Rep. 91:131-139, 1942.
7. Burford, T. H., and Burbank, B.: Traumatic wet lung: observations on certain physiologic fundamentals of thoracic trauma, J. Thoracic Surg. 14:415-424, 1945.
8. Churchill, E. D.: Bronchiectasis: physical and psychological manifestations, New England J. Med. 218:97-101, 1938.
9. Churchill, E. D., and Belsey, R.: Segmental pneumonectomy in bronchiectasis: the lingula segment of the left upper lobe, Ann. Surg. 109:481-499, 1939.
10. Comroe, J. H., Forster, R. E., II, Dubois, A. B., Briscoe, W. A., and Carlson, E.: The Lung: Clinical Physiology and Pulmonary Function Tests, Chicago, Year Book Pub., 1955.
11. Decker, H. R.: The treatment of thoracic actinomycosis by penicillin and sulfonamide drugs, J. Thoracic Surg. 15:430-440, 1946.
12. Forsee, J. H., and Pfotenhauer, M.: Surgical management of focalized pulmonary histoplasmosis, J.A.M.A. 173:878-883, 1960.
13. Goss, C. M. (ed.): Gray's Anatomy, ed. 26, Philadelphia, Lea & Febiger, 1954.
14. Gray, J. S.: Pulmonary Ventilation and Its Physiological Regulation, Springfield, Ill., Thomas, 1950.
15. Hewlett, T. H., and Ziperman, H. H.: Bronchiectasis: results of pulmonary resection, J. Thor. & Cardiovas. Surg. 40:71-78, 1960.
16. Hodgson, C. H., Weed, L. A., and Clagett, O. T.: Pulmonary histoplasmosis: summary of data on reported cases and a report on two patients treated by lobectomy, J.A.M.A. 145:807-810, 1951.
17. Jackson, C. L., and Huber, J. F.: Correlated applied anatomy of the bronchial tree and lungs with a system of nomenclature, Dis. Chest 9:319-326, 1943.
18. Loosli, C. G.: Histoplasmosis: some clinical epidemiological and laboratory aspects, M. Clin. North America 39:171-199, 1955.
19. Neuhof, H.: The surgical treatment of acute pulmonary abscess, Dis. Chest 7:74-79, 1941.
20. Overholt, R. H., and Langer, L.: A new technique for pulmonary segmental resection; its application in the treatment of bronchiectasis, Surg., Gynec. & Obst. 84:257-268, 1947.
21. Peterson, J. C., Mapes, R., and Furcolow, M. L.: Round table discussion: systemic mycoses, coccidioidomycosis and histoplasmosis, Pediatrics 2:709-721, 1948.
22. Pittman, H. S., and Kane, L. W.: Fungus infections of the lungs, M. Clin. North America 35:1323-1331, 1951.
23. Poppe, J. K.: Treatment of pulmonary actinomycosis, with a report of severe arrested cases, J. Thoracic Surg. 15:118-126, 1946.
24. Shedd, D. P., Alley, R. D., and Lindskog, G. E.: Observations on the hemodynamics of bronchial-pulmonary vascular communications, J. Thoracic Surg. 22:537-548, 1951.
25. Stern, L.: Etiologic factors in the pathogenesis of putrid abscess of the lung, J. Thoracic Surg. 6:202-211, 1936.

CHAPTER 43

Pulmonary Tuberculosis

The surgical treatment of pulmonary tuberculosis continues to occupy an important position in surgery for diseases of the lungs. Although the future outlook for the control of this disease in the United States is quite favorable, the need for surgical therapy will continue for many years.

This area of thoracic surgery had its development at the beginning of the present century. However, progress was slow until within the past 2 decades. A number of factors have contributed to the rapid acceleration of progress in this field during recent years. Chief among these factors has been the discovery of antimicrobial agents which are effective against the tubercle bacillus. These agents include streptomycin (Schatz and Waksman, 1944),[20] para-aminosalicylic acid (P.A.S.), [12] isonicotinic acid hydrazide (Isoniazid) 1952[16] and viomycin.[8] These drugs administered alone or more often in combination, along with bed rest and other supportive measures, improve the status of the pathologic process prior to surgery, thus reducing the magnitude of the operation as well as preserving a greater percentage of pulmonary function. They also greatly reduce the risk of operative procedures and contribute materially in increasing the percentage of arrested cases following surgery. These drugs have been largely responsible for the present marked reduction in mortality following resection of the lung as compared with that of one decade ago.

A second factor of considerable significance which has contributed to the rapid acceleration of improvement during the past few years has been the development of technics for pulmonary resection and their application in the management of pulmonary tuberculosis. Although these procedures had been evolved previously and applied in the treatment of other pulmonary lesions, their application in the field of pulmonary tuberculosis was unsafe until chemotherapeutic agents became available.

Another factor of considerable importance has been the development of reliable tests for the evaluation of pulmonary function. As judged by present-day standards, tests available for this purpose were of relatively little help prior to the last decade. Although our present methods leave something to be desired and no doubt will continue to be improved, much information can now be obtained which, when correlated with roentgenologic films and other available information, aid materially in the choice of operative procedures as well as revealing the optimum time for instituting surgical therapy. The decision as to the type of surgical management of the disease process often depends mainly upon clinical evaluation of pulmonary function studies.

A fourth factor contributing to this accelerated progress has been the improvement in methods of collapse therapy. A number of technics have been developed in recent years, all based on a common principle, namely, a selective type of complete collapse of the involved lung, produced by a 1-stage operation, and with preservation of maximum pulmonary function. These procedures consist of a modified type of thoracoplasty with the removal of few or no ribs, and the use of a prosthesis for maintaining the collapse. The objectives of these newer technics have been (1) a higher percentage of arrested cases following the operation, (2) a 1-stage operative procedure, (3) avoidance of postoperative deformity and (4) preservation of maximal lung function. All 4 of these objectives have been accomplished by these procedures without increasing the risk of operation or the frequency of complications.

The rapid acceleration of progress in this field during the past decade has left the choice of surgical management of pulmonary tuberculosis in an unsettled state. There is some variance of opinion as to the best plan of therapy for different pathologic forms of the disease. There is as yet no universal agreement as to the indications and the contraindications for various surgical procedures. Furthermore, this unsettled state of thinking regarding the type of surgical therapy is due in part to the fact that many tuberculous lesions will respond equally well to two or more methods of management.

PATHOLOGY

In the surgical treatment of pulmonary tuberculosis, the time as well as the type of therapy is dictated by the pathologic status of the disease. This is determined largely by (among other things) the virulence of the organism and the resistance of the host. With the progressive nature of the disease, one or more cavities usually develop and are accompanied by some bronchogenic spread of the infection to the same or opposite side, or to both sides. The size, the location and the distribution of cavities, as well as the presence of bronchogenic dissemination, will determine if and when surgical therapy is indicated, as well as the type of management best suited for the patient.

The amount of pulmonary destruction with reduction in pulmonary reserve will have a direct bearing upon therapy. X-ray appearance of the lung may be very misleading, both as to the amount of pulmonary destruction as well as the status of pulmonary reserve. The nature of a bronchial communication with a pulmonary cavity may have considerable influence on the over-all pathologic picture presented. If the bronchus shows evidence of stenosis with partial obstruction, one of the following may develop: (1) a per-

sistent or expanding cavity, (2) atelectasis of the obstructed lung, (3) "closed cavity" with filling in of inspissated caseous material, or (4) development of tension cavity. When a tuberculous process involves a lower lobe near the hilum, a tuberculous bronchiectasis is apt to develop due to partial obstruction of the bronchial outlet. In such patients symptoms usually are due to a combination of tuberculous and nontuberculous inflammatory processes.

When the tuberculous process is near the periphery of the lung, involvement of the pleura, either in the form of a fibrous pleurisy or a pleural effusion, will result. This fluid may become contaminated with tubercle bacilli, resulting in the formation of empyema of the pleural space. If pyogenic organisms are also present, the lesion is known as a mixed tuberculous empyema. This usually occurs only when a direct communication between the lung and the pleural cavity, viz., a bronchopleural fistula, develops. The management of these various pathologic processes will be discussed under subsequent headings.

In the surgical therapy of pulmonary tuberculosis, the principal objectives may be defined as: (1) permanent arrest of the disease, (2) preservation of function of the uninvolved lung, (3) prevention of complications in surgical management and (4) early return to useful activity. Thus, as previously noted, the character and the distribution of pathologic lesions will largely determine whether these objectives may be secured. Likewise, the status and the course of the disease at the time of surgery will play a major role in this regard. A third factor of importance is the method of surgical management.

One of the most important considerations in surgical treatment of pulmonary tuberculosis is proper selection of patients for operation. In the evaluation of tuberculous patients for surgery, a number of factors concerned with the status of the disease must be taken into consideration. These factors consists of (1) the entire duration of the disease, (2) duration of the present problem presented by the patient, (3) status of the activity of the disease, (4) distribution of the lesion (unilateral or bilateral and the amount of lung involved), (5) type and status of nonsurgical therapy, (6) presence and extent of extrapulmonary disease, (7) physical factor, such as obstructed cavity and (8) consideration of the resistance.

These factors will have a direct bearing not only on the time of operative intervention but also on the type of surgical procedure indicated. In the evaluation of a patient for surgery, not only should the history, the physical findings and the laboratory examination be scrutinized carefully but, in addition, various tests to determine the status of cardiopulmonary reserve should be made in order to have a complete evaluation of the problem.

GENERAL CONSIDERATIONS

PREPARATION OF THE PATIENT FOR OPERATION

Primary consideration must be given to the proper preparation of patients for surgery in order to avoid serious complications. The nutritional condition of the individual, the status of the blood regarding hemoglobin and cell volume, as well as protein content, is of signal importance. Preparation of the patient for surgery always should be preceded by the use of chemotherapy both for pyogenic as well as acid-fast organisms, the length of time of such medication varying according to the status of the disease. The use of special x-ray examinations, such as planigrams, as well as oblique views, aids materially in accurate localization of the lesion in order to plan definitive surgery. All patients should be subjected to bronchoscopy prior to surgery, to determine the presence or the absence of tuberculous bronchitis or stenosis of the bronchus. This is particularly indicated where excisional therapy is planned but is also of value in collapse therapy. Since most patients with bilateral pulmonary tuberculosis develop some reduction in the size of the lesser circulatory bed, a careful check for evidence of cardiac strain is important prior to operation. Finally, in order to evaluate the pulmonary reserve, pulmonary function studies should be made to aid in planning the type of surgery, as well as to prognose the outcome following therapy.

ANESTHESIA

Since deep relaxation is unnecessary in thoracic surgery, a lighter type making use of simpler methods and mixtures of anesthetic agents has much to be recommended. Ether-oxygen has gained greater favor because of

its wide range of safety and the absence of depression of the respiratory center. Induction with a gas-oxygen mixture that is not depressing to respiration or circulation is advantageous. Constant adequate ventilation should be assured and oxygen administered in adequate amounts. Of the 3 principal positions of the patient for the performance of intrathoracic procedures, viz., lateral, supine and prone, the first is employed most often, except for individuals raising a considerable quantity of secretions. Because previously the tendency of infection to spread to the dependent lung had been observed when surgery was performed in the lateral position, the prone position gained favor, and at the present time some surgeons continue to consider it the position of choice.

TYPES OF SURGICAL PROCEDURES AND THEIR FUNCTION

The objective in various surgical procedures for the treatment of pulmonary tuberculosis may be divided into 4 categories: (1) local rest and relaxation of the tissues, (2) collapse of the diseased process, (3) removal of the diseased process and (4) drainage of cavities (Table 1).

The general principles governing all surgical management of pulmonary tuberculosis are: (1) preoperative determination of pulmonary reserve; (2) the use of anesthesia which assures adequate circulation and oxygenation during operation; (3) employment of a surgical approach which provides adequate exposure; (4) maintenance of normal blood

TABLE 1. OBJECTIVE OF SURGICAL PROCEDURES IN THE TREATMENT OF PULMONARY TUBERCULOSIS

1. Rest and relaxation of tissues
    A. Phrenicotomy with or without pneumothorax or pneumoperitoneum
    B. Intrapleural pneumonolysis with pneumothorax
2. Collapse of the disease process
    A. Extrapleural pneumonolysis with prosthesis
    B. Thoracoplasty
    C. Extrafascial collapse with prosthesis
3. Excisional therapy of the disease process
    A. Pneumonectomy
    B. Lobectomy
    C. Segmental resection and local excision
4. Drainage of cavity

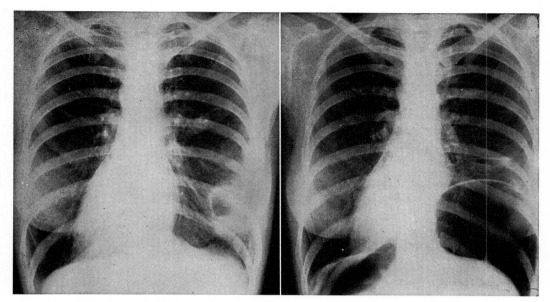

FIG. 43-1. This patient was a 37-year-old white female with a characteristic history, physical findings and laboratory findings of pulmonary tuberculosis. (*Left*) P. A. view of the chest, showing a cavitary lesion with a fluid level in the lower right lung field. Sputum examinations were strongly positive for acid-fast bacilli. Pneumoperitoneum plus temporary paralysis of the diaphragm was used in addition to antimicrobial therapy. (*Right*) P. A. view of the chest taken 3½ months following institution of therapy. Note marked change in size and shape of the cavitary lesion seen viewed at left. Complete healing of the cavitary lesion resulted following this form of therapy.

volume, normovolemia) during surgery by replacement of blood loss; and (5) postoperative care which provides for adequate oxygenation of the vital tissues and for control of infection.

OPERATIVE PROCEDURES USEFUL IN THE TREATMENT OF PULMONARY TUBERCULOSIS

PHRENIC NERVE CRUSH OR AVULSION

Paralysis of one side of the diaphragm may be temporary or permanent, according to the indications for the procedure. Crushing of the phrenic nerve in the cervical region and division of the accessory branches, if present, will lead to paralysis of the diaphragm on the same side, which will persist for 4 to 6 months. This procedure is used much more frequently than division and avulsion of the phrenic nerve, which produces a permanent paralysis. By these procedures local rest and relaxation of pulmonary tissues are obtained on the side of the operation. No actual collapse of the tissue occurs.

The indications for operation on the phrenic nerve have varied considerably since the use of this procedure in pulmonary tuberculosis was first reported by Sauerbruch in 1913.[18] They may be divided into 3 main groups, as follows: (1) to aid in pneumothorax and pneumoperitoneum treatment of tuberculosis; (2) in the preparation for more major surgery at a later date; and (3) as a definitive procedure in patients where surgical intervention of greater magnitude is contraindicated or refused. The operation is most useful: (1) for cavities not over 2.5 cm. in diameter and in the absence of marked production of scar tissue; (2) for earlier lesions with infiltration without great destruction of pulmonary tissue; and (3) in patients when pneumoperitoneum and pneumothorax are inadequate, and where operations of greater magnitude are contraindicated or refused (Fig. 43-1).

Complications following operation on the phrenic nerve are seldom seen. Hemorrhage, air embolism, pneumothorax, and injuries to the thoracic duct have been (infrequently) reported following this operation.

Intrapleural Pneumonolysis

This operation was developed and first performed by Hahns Jacobaeus in 1913.[10] It entails the severing of adhesions between the diseased lung and the chest wall, where pneumothorax has been inadequate. The procedure is accomplished through a specially devised thoracoscope, first developed by Unverricht in 1925.[23] This procedure provides severance of small stringlike adhesions which previously have prevented adequate collapse of cavities by pneumothorax. This is indicated particularly in patients where other types of surgery are refused or are contraindicated.

Complications

1. Hemorrhage. When the operation is properly performed and safeguards are taken, this complication of a serious magnitude is seldom seen. Secondary hemorrhage following surgery may occur and must be guarded against by adequate precautions at the time of surgery.

2. Empyema With or Without Bronchopleural Fistula. As in many other procedures in the treatment of pulmonary tuberculosis, if this operation is pushed beyond its limitations, empyema may result following the division of adhesions in which an active stage of the disease is present. Pleural effusion occurs to some degree in approximately 50 per cent of the patients following surgery.

However, in most cases the fluid is reabsorbed, and an empyema does not develop. Since pneumothorax therapy is used much less commonly at present than previously, this operation has lost much of its usefulness.

Extrapleural Pneumonolysis With Prosthesis

This operative procedure produces a collapse of lung tissue. Its objective is to obtain a selective and complete collapse of only the diseased portion of the lung, with preservation of as much pulmonary function as possible. The operation was first performed by Tuffier[22] in 1911 and by Baer[2] in 1913. Various materials are used as a prosthesis, the most commonly employed being paraffin, plastic materials and fiberglass. The indications for

this operation are (1) a diseased process limited to the apex of the lung in patients with low pulmonary reserve and where cavitation does not reach the surface of the lung; (2) bilateral cavitary disease of the lung; (3) apical lesions in young women; and (4) instances where for psychologic reasons other operations have been rejected (Fig. 43-2). Contraindications include: (1) large peripheral cavities; (2) marked fibrosis at the apex of the lung; (3) lung densely adherent at the periphery; and (4) cavities located below the apex of the lung.

This operative procedure offers particular advantages: (1) production of a localized and selective collapse; (2) retention of maximal functioning of normal lung tissue; (3) minimal deformity of the chest wall; and (4) necessity of only a 1-stage operation, thus assuring less discomfort, more economy and greater co-operation of the patient.

Complications. When this procedure is not pushed beyond its limitations, serious complications are seldom seen. However, when it is not used properly complications may include (1) infection of the extrapleural space by tuberculous and nontuberculous organisms; (2) bronchopleural fistula; and (3) secondary hemorrhage.

At the present time, after 8 years of experience, the author favors an extrafascial, extraperiosteal type of collapse to be described under the heading of thoracoplasty in preference to the above procedure: (1) because of the technical ease of performance; and (2) because of a much wider applicability.

Extrapleural Paravertebral Thoracoplasty

This operative procedure was one of the earliest used in the surgical treatment of pulmonary tuberculosis. It was first designed by Cerenville in 1885 and has been modified by a number of workers in this field. In order to obtain greater effectiveness and reduced surgical risk, Sauerbruch[19] developed a procedure termed extrapleural paravertebral thoracoplasty which was used for many years. The conventional present-day thoracoplasty is patterned somewhat after the Brauer[5] type of operation with the exception that it is performed in 2 or more stages in order to reduce the risk of the procedure.

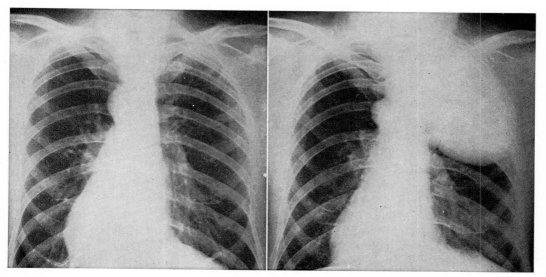

FIG. 43-2. This patient was a 47-year-old white male with a cavitary tuberculous lesion in the apex of the right lung. (*Left*) Note fibrocavernous lesion in apex of right lung. Because of the small size of the cavity and little scarring, therapy by extrapleural paraffin plombage was used. (*Right*) P. A. view of the thorax following the above operation. Note complete selective type of collapse of the upper portion of the right lung. This patient has been followed during the past 9 years and has had no further evidence of his former tuberculous lesion.

Indications. Since more prompt and effective care is now available for most patients with pulmonary tuberculosis, the indications for thoracoplasty are much less frequent than in the past. These include: (1) fibrocavernous lesions at the apex of the lung, especially in the presence of bilaterally active disease and where the organisms are no longer sensitive to antimicrobial drugs; (2) as a preliminary procedure to resection in some bilaterally cavitary lesions; (3) where pulmonary function is inadequate for safe excisional therapy; and (4) where the extent and the character of the disease or the presence of extrapulmonary lesions make resection hazardous. It is difficult to compare accurately the results of various types of surgical therapy in the treatment of pulmonary tuberculosis. However, when various advantages, disadvantages and risks are considered, it may be said that for far-advanced fibrocavitary lesions, thoracoplasty will carry less risk than resection but may produce a greater reduction in pulmonary function and in some types of lesions will not yield as high a percentage of arrested cases. For the conventional type of thoracoplasty there remain 2 real disadvantages: (1) the

necessity of performing a several-stage operation and (2) some degree of accompanying scoliosis with mild disfigurement of the body, and with reduction in pulmonary function. With the conventional type of thoracoplasty one may anticipate arrest of the disease in approximately 75 to 85 per cent of the patients, according to the nature and the extent of the disease.[11]

THORACOPLASTY WITH EXTRAFASCIAL AND EXTRAPERIOSTEAL PARAFFIN PROSTHESIS

Because of the several deficiencies in the conventional type of thoracoplasty, attempts have been made to produce a more selective type of collapse by a 1-stage procedure. The operation was developed in 1947[1] and entails the mobilization of the periosteum and the intercostal structures from the ribs and the use of an extrafascial prosthesis of paraffin placed in the collapse area. It is a 1-stage procedure which produces a selective type of collapse of the lung tissue beneath as many as 8 ribs. A short segment of approximately 2 inches of only 1 rib, usually the 3rd, is resected (Fig. 43-3 A, B).

Advantages of this procedure include: (1)

increased percentage of arrested cases (approximately 90%), (2) a single-stage operation, (3) obviation of scoliosis and resultant deformity, thus minimizing reduction in pulmonary function and (4) lessened surgical expense (Fig. 43-3, C to F). Complications observed following the use of this procedure have been minimal.[14]

RESECTION THERAPY

This type of surgical management was first suggested by Forlanini approximately 70 years ago and was attempted by Ruggi in 1884[17] and by Tuffier in 1897.[21] However, due to the delay in advancement of ancillary therapy this type of operative management did not become practical until during the past decade. Factors which contribute to the present success of resectional therapy include: (1) alteration in character and decrease in extent of the disease by the use of chemotherapy prior to surgery; (2) development of surgical technics which permit the safe excision of varying amounts of pulmonary tissue; and (3) development of tests of pulmonary function which more accurately reveal the status of cardio-pulmonary reserve prior to surgery.

Indications. Because of the increasing safety of operation, and high percentage of successful results, the value of pulmonary resection is ever increasing.

At present the principal indications for this operation are: (1) thoracoplasty failure; (2) the presence of lower lobe lesions, particularly cavities in the superior segment, or tuberculosis with secondary bronchiectasis; (3) destroyed lung; (4) closed (active) tuberculous lesions; (5) indeterminate pulmonary lesions where malignancy cannot be excluded; (6) small cavitary lesions which do not heal completely with antimicrobial therapy; and (7) very large cavities.

Excisional therapy has a number of advantages over the conventional thoracoplasty where smaller isolated lesions are present: (1) it is selective in type and is more conservative of pulmonary function; (2) only one operation is required; and (3) little or no postoperative deformity occurs (the last two advantages do not apply to extrafascial-extraperiosteal thoracoplasty with paraffin prosthesis).

Contraindication. The principal contraindication to excisional therapy is the presence of advanced bilateral fibrocavernous lesions of considerable magnitude in patients having poor host resistance, and with tubercle bacilli no longer sensitive to chemotherapy.

Mortality and morbidity following excisional therapy have been reduced markedly

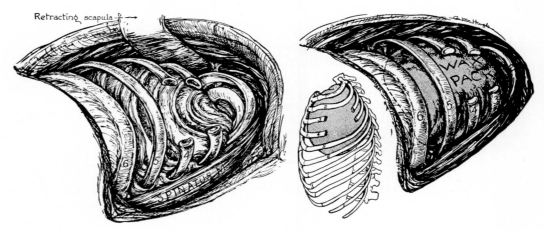

FIG. 43-3. (A, *left*) Drawing to illustrate the appearance of the collapsed area following freeing of the periosteum and the intercostal structures from the first 5 ribs in the treatment of pulmonary tuberculosis. Note that the structures are depressed from beneath these ribs and that only short segments of the 3rd and the 4th ribs were removed. (B, *right*) Appearance of chest with the wax prosthesis placed beneath the ribs from which the soft parts have been mobilized. Note the selective nature of the collapse. By resecting only short segments of 1 or 2 ribs no scoliosis results, and the wax is well maintained in position.

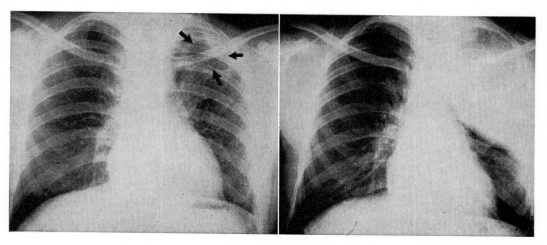

FIG. 43-3. (*Cont.*). (C, *left*) Roentgenogram of a 27-year-old East Indian student who had had pulmonary tuberculosis for several years. The patient improved temporarily and then his condition remained stationary. The tubercle bacilli became insensitive to all chemotherapeutic agents. Note large cavity in the left apex. This patient had had bilateral involvement, although at the time of surgery, the disease in the right lung was stationary. A collapse of the upper portion of the chest wall prior to resection of that portion of the lung was thought to be indicated in order to reduce the risk of resectional therapy.

(D, *right*) X-ray appearance of the chest approximately 7 weeks following a single-stage modified thoracoplasty with subscapular extrafascial paraffin prosthesis. Note the selective nature of collapse with preservation of aerated lung tissue below. The patient's sputum was converted following operation, and he was completely relieved of symptoms. In view of the size of the cavitary lesion it was concluded that complete healing was very unlikely. Therefore, a resection of the upper lobe was made a few months following the operation. The patient has made a good recovery and has had no further trouble since operation. A. P. views.

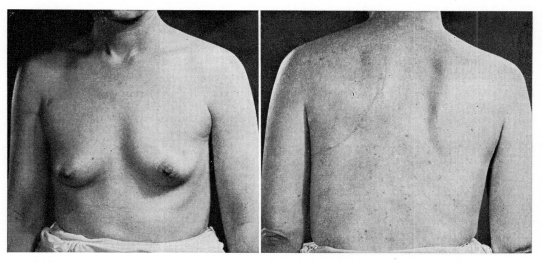

FIG. 43-3 (*Cont.*). (E, *left, and* F, *right*) Photographs of patient following extrafascial subscapular thoracoplasty with wax prosthesis in which collapse of the lung beneath the first 6 ribs was carried out. Note complete lack of deformity.

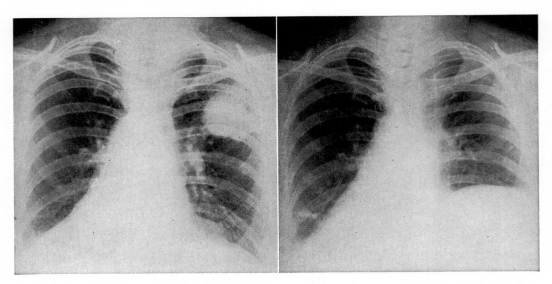

FIG. 43-4. This patient was a 62-year-old white female having had a nonproductive cough of several months' duration. She had lost no weight and was in good general condition. (*Left*) P. A. view of the thorax, showing a circumscribed opacity in the right upper lung lobe. Differential diagnosis included pulmonary tuberculosis and carcinoma of the lung. (*Right*) P. A. view of the chest following extirpation of the right upper lung lobe. The lesion was found to be a closed tuberculous abscess with evidence of activity. Note expansion of the right middle and lower lobes to fill the right thorax completely. Partial collapse of the chest wall following resection of the lung is unnecessary when the remaining portion is normal.

following the use of chemotherapy. However, when lesions of considerable magnitude are accepted for resection, complications may occur. Those most commonly observed are (1) bronchial obstruction with atelectasis of the remaining lung tissue; (2) contralateral or ipsilateral spread of the infection; (3) bronchopleural fistula with tuberculous or mixed empyema and spread of the infection; and (4) spread of the tuberculous infection to extrapulmonary tissues such as the mediastinum and the pericardium. Of these complications, the one most commonly seen is spread of the disease. However, the complication which more often contributes to the mortality of the operation is the development of a bronchopleural fistula accompanied by a tuberculous or a mixed empyema. This complication is almost always accompanied by an additional spread of infection to the contralateral or ipsilateral lung. These serious complications are observed more often following pneumonectomy or lobectomy rather than following segmental resection if this latter procedure is not pushed beyond its limitations.

Operations. Four types of procedures are employed: (1) pneumonectomy, (2) lobectomy, (3) segmental resection[4, 7] and (4) local excision. The choice of these operations is determined by the location and the extent of the lesion as well as the cardiopulmonary reserve of the patient. Temporary paralysis of the diaphragm is helpful at times in reducing the size of the pleural space following surgery (Fig. 43-4). Since tuberculous lesions are frequently considerably reduced in size with the use of antimicrobial therapy, segmental resection has become more frequently employed (Fig. 43-5, A to C).

RESULTS OF SURGERY

As stated earlier, the results of surgery for the treatment of pulmonary tuberculosis will vary considerably according to the status of the pathologic process, virulence of the organisms, host resistance, and selection of patients for operation. For this reason proper evaluation of reported statistics in this regard is quite difficult. It may be stated, however, that when various operative procedures are not pushed beyond their limitations, satisfactory results may be obtained in a high percentage of patients (80 to 90%). In the collapse type of operation the risk of surgery is somewhat less, reduction of pulmonary function may be somewhat greater, and arrestment of the disease may be anticipated in between 85 to 90 per cent of patients. Excisional therapy must be used where a collapsing operation has failed. Risk of lobectomy and pneumonectomy will average approximately 5 and 8 per cent, respectively. The risk of segmental resection is much less, being approximately 1 or 2 per cent. Arrestment of the disease may be anticipated in 80 to 85 per cent of patients where a lobectomy or a pneumonectomy is required. This figure will be somewhat higher in patients following segmental resections for smaller lesions.[6, 15]

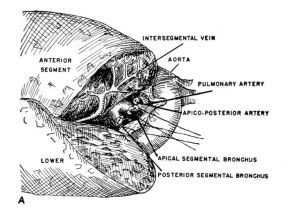

A

Fig. 43-5. (A) Drawing to show appearance of the left hilum following resection of the apical posterior segment of the left upper lung lobe. The apical posterior bronchi are closed by interrupted sutures. No attempt is made to close or pleuralize the raw surface following segmental resection. This patient was a 43-year-old female who presented a symptomless lesion in the left apex. This shadow was discovered by her physician on routine x-ray examination. Sputum examinations were positive for acid-fast bacilli. (B) P. A. view of the chest of another patient showing an ill-defined opacity at the level of the right clavicle. (C) Laminogram demonstrating multiple cavities in apical and posterior segments of right upper lobe. (D) P. A. view of the chest taken 3 months following resection of the right apical and posterior segments. Note complete filling of the right chest by the remaining pulmonary tissue. This patient has been followed for over 18 months after operation and has had no evidence of activity.

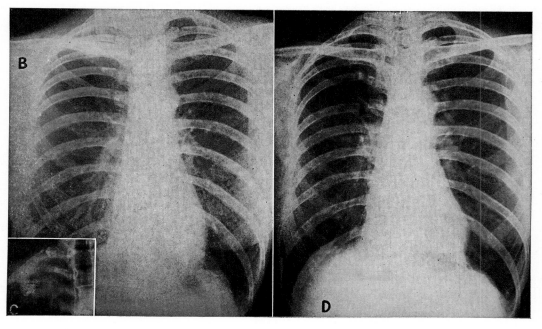

This is a far cry from statistics which were gathered not more than one decade ago before the advantages enumerated in this chapter were available. With a gradual diminution of the number of patients with severe and advanced lesions, the outlook for further improvement in these statistics is quite good.

REFERENCES

1. Adams, W. E., Lees, W. M., and Fritz, J. M.: Subcapsular paraffin pack as a supplement to thoracoplasty in the treatment of pulmonary tuberculosis, J. Thoracic Surg. 22:375, 1951.
2. Baer, G.: Ueber extrapleurale Pneumolyse mit sofortiger Plombierung bei Lungentuberkulose, Munchen. med. Wchnschr. 60:1587, 1913.
3. Björk, V. O.: Segmental resection for pulmonary tuberculosis, J. Thoracic Surg. 37:135, 1959.
4. Blades, B., and Kent, E. M.: Individual ligation technique for lower lobe lobectomy, J. Thoracic Surg. 10:84, 1940.
5. Brauer, L.: Erfahrungen und Überlegungen zur Lungenkollapstherapie: I. Die ausgedehnte extrapleurale Thorakoplastik, Beitr. Klin. Tuberk. 12:49, 1909.
6. Chamberlain, J. M., and Ryan, T. C.: Segmental resection in pulmonary diseases, J. Thoracic Surg. 19:199, 1950.
7. Churchill, E. D., and Belsey, R.: Segmental pneumonectomy in bronchiectasis; the lingual segment of the left upper lobe, Ann. Surg. 109:481, 1939.
8. Finlay, A. C., Hobby, G. L., Hochstein, F., Lees, T. M., Lenert, T. F., Means, J. A., P'an, S. Y., Regna, P. P., Routien, J. B., Sobin, B. A., Tate, K. B., and Kane, J. H.: Viomycin, a new antibiotic active against mycobacteria, Am. Rev. Tuberc. 63:1, 1951.
9. Fischer, W. W., and del Missier, P. A.: The surgical treatment of tuberculosis in children, J. Thoracic Surg. 38:501, 1959.
10. Jacobaeus, H. C.: Endopleurale Operationen unter der Leitung des Thoracoskops, Beitr. klin. Tuberk. 35:1, 1916.
11. Lees, W. M., Yang, S. C. H., Papoulakos, M., Alexander, J., and Larralde, A.: Results in 278 patients who had the modern type of thoracoplasty for tuberculosis: follow-up of living patients 5 to 15 years after operation, J. Thoracic Surg. 22:329, 1951.
12. Lehmann, J.: Para-aminosalicylic acid in the treatment of tuberculosis, Lancet 1:15, 1946.
13. Mendenhall, J. T., Cree, E., Rasmussen, H. K., Bauer, H., and Curtis, J. K.: Studies of pulmonary function before and after pulmonary resection in 450 tuberculous patients. II. Case analysis of patients with large loss of vital capacity and maximum breathing capacity, J. Thoracic Surg. 39:189, 1960.
14. Ortega, Flores, Lopez-Belio, M., Adams, W. E., Fox, R., and Lees, W. M.: La parafina como coadyuvante colapsoterapica dela toracoplastia; Estudio de 400 casos tratados por este método, presented at Decima tercera Conferencia Internacional de la Lucha contra la Tuberculosis, Madrid, Spain, September, 1954.
15. Overholt, R. H., Woods, F. M., and Ramsay, B. H.: Segmental pulmonary resection: details of technique and results, J. Thoracic Surg. 19:207, 1950.
16. Robitzek, E. H., Selikoff, I. J., and Ornstein, G. G.: Chemotherapy of human tuberculosis with hydrazine derivatives of isonicotinic acid, Quart. Bull. Sea View Hosp. 13:25, 1952.
17. Ruggi, G.: La tecnica della pneumectoma nell'uomo, Bologna, 1884.
18. Sauerbruch, F.: Die Beeinflussung von Lungenerkrankungen durch künstliche Lahmung des Zwerchfells (Phrenikotomie), München. med. Wchnschr. 60:625, 1913.
19. ————: Die chirurgie der Brustorgane, Berlin, Springer, 1920.
20. Schatz, A., and Waksman, S. A.: Effect of streptomycin and other antibiotic substances upon mycobacterium tuberculosis and related organisms, Proc. Soc. Exper. Biol. & Med. 57:244, 1944.
21. Tuffier, T.: Chirurgie du poumon, en particulier dans les cavernes tuberculeuses at la gangrene, pulmonaire, p. 31, Paris, Masson, 1897.
22. ————: Collapsthérapie par décollement pleuro-pariétal pour tuberculose limitée au sommet du poumon, greffe d'un fragment de tissu adipeux dans l'espace décollé, Bull. et mém. Soc. chirurgiens Paris 49:1249, 1923.
23. Unverricht, W.: Technik und Methodik der Thorakoskopie, Leipzig, Vogel, 1925.
24. Webb, W. R., Wofford, J. K., and Stauss, H.: Resectional therapy for residual noninfectious cavitary tuberculous lesions, Am. Rev. Res. Dis. 81:850, 1960.

JOHN H. GIBBON, JR., M.D., AND THOMAS F. NEALON, JR., M.D.

CHAPTER 44

Carcinoma of the Lung and Tumors of the Thorax

Tumors of the Lung
Tumors of the Mediastinum
Tumors of the Thoracic Wall

The widespread utilization of chest x-ray surveys in recent years has brought to light many intrathoracic tumors. These lesions have proved to be much commoner than had been realized formerly. The discovery of previously unrecognized lesions and the apparent absolute increase in cancer of the lung has made the thorax a region of great surgical significance. Thoracic tumors will be considered under 3 headings according to the site of origin: (1) tumors of the lung, (2) tumors of the mediastinum, (3) tumors of the thoracic wall.

TUMORS OF THE LUNG

Tumors of the lung are by far the largest group of thoracic tumors because of the great prevalence of cancer of the lung. They will be considered under the headings of: malignant tumors (primary and metastatic) and benign tumors (adenoma and hamartoma).

PRIMARY MALIGNANT TUMORS

Bronchogenic carcinoma is the commonest primary malignant tumor of the lung, and it is rapidly fatal if untreated. It is predominantly a disease of the male sex, about 90 per cent of all tumors occurring in men. In this sex it is the commonest cause of death from cancer (Fig. 44-1). During 1958 in the United States, 32,316 persons died of carcinoma of the lung. Approximately 95 per cent of all cases occur between the ages of 40 and 70.

Etiology. Much has been written concerning possible predisposing causes of cancer of the lung, but little is definitely known. The incidence of carcinoma has been reported to be unusually high among workers in chromate, uranium, arsenic, certain nickel and copper ores in which arsenic occurs as an impurity and in asbestos. Apparently all types of dust cannot be incriminated because the incidence is not higher in miners with anthracosilicosis.

Recently, much interest has developed regarding the relationship of smoking to cancer of the lung. Wynder and Graham[17] in this country and Doll and Hill[7] in England reported a higher incidence of cancer of the lung among heavy cigarette smokers. Shortly after this, Hammond and Horn,[11] working with large population samples, showed that both the incidence of, and the death rate from, cancer of the lung were higher among heavy cigarette smokers. Thus, there appears to be a definite relationship between cigarette smoking and cancer of the lung. The unsolved problem is whether the relationship is one of cause and effect. Investigators currently are attempting to identify some component of cigarette smoke which might be an etiologic agent of cancer of the lung.

Pathology. The 3 main histologic types of bronchogenic carcinoma in order of frequency are the epidermoid, the anaplastic and the adenocarcinomas. In any cancer of the lung, all 3 cell types usually may be found if multiple sections are taken. Nevertheless, tumors are classified according to the predominant cell type. The epidermoid, or squamous cell, carcinoma is the commonest type and accounts for about half the lesions. The epidermoid carcinoma usually originates in the segmental bronchi and extends into the lobar bronchi. It may produce a polypoid tumor projecting into the bronchus or a cicatricial narrowing of the bronchus. This cell type tends to invade the bronchial mucosa adjacent to the gross tumor mass. Cavitary carcinomas of the lung (Fig. 44-2) are most frequently squamous. This cavitation results from excavation of the cornified epithelium which forms in the center of the mass of squamous cells.

About 20 per cent of cancers of the lung are adenocarcinomas. Usually they are circumscribed peripheral lesions, although they may involve larger bronchi. This type is relatively uncommon in men but comprises approximately half of the carcinomas of the lung in women. The remaining 30 per cent are undifferentiated tumors. These tumors most frequently occur in the larger bronchi and often are characterized by massive extrabronchial involvement. Often the extrabronchial involve-

ment is so marked as to suggest a mediastinal tumor in the roentgenogram.

Finally, there is a rare type of cancer of the lung called alveolar cell carcinoma. Bronchiolar carcinoma is probably a better term, as the cells apparently arise from the epithelium of the terminal bronchioles. These tumors generally appear as ill-defined masses in the parenchyma of the lung and do not produce symptoms early.

Sarcomas may arise from the connective tissue elements in the lung but are very rare. Unless a bronchoscopic biopsy is obtained, the lesion cannot be distinguished from a carcinoma before operation. Involvement of the mediastinal lymph nodes is less common than in bronchogenic carcinoma.

Cell type affects the prognosis.[13] The epi-

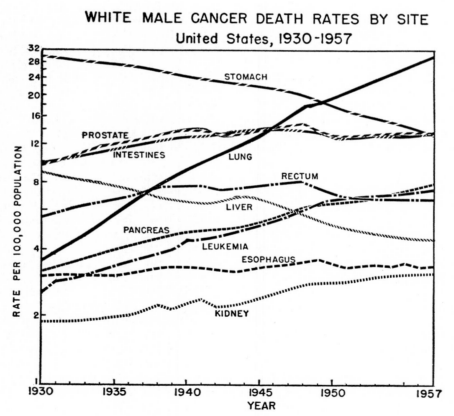

FIG. 44-1. Graph illustrating the increasing mortality from cancer of the lung. Since 1949 deaths from this cause have exceeded deaths from cancer of other organs in the male population of the United States. (Graph prepared by the American Cancer Society from data obtained from the National Office of Vital Statistics and the Bureau of the Census, U.S.)

dermoid carcinoma probably has the best prognosis. The adenocarcinomas occupy an intermediate position. The anaplastic, or undifferentiated, carcinoma is the most malignant. Regardless of cell type if metastasis to the mediastinal lymph nodes or invasion of the chest wall has occurred the prognosis is poor.

Invasion of contiguous structures is a characteristic of bronchogenic carcinomas. The trachea or the opposite bronchus, the main pulmonary artery or the pulmonary veins up to the left atrium may be invaded. Invasion of the parietal pericardium is common. Peripheral tumors may extend into the chest wall, necessitating resection of the overlying ribs and intercostal structures in continuity. The prognosis for patients with such lesions is poor. In our experience, none of these patients has lived more than 18 months after operation.

Metastasis may occur by the lymphatics or the blood stream. Hilar tumors generally metastasize by the lymphatics, while peripheral lesions are more prone to spread by the blood stream. However, cancers in either location may spread by either route. The lymphatic route is to the carinal and the paratracheal lymph nodes and then to the para-esophageal and cervical chain, particularly the supraclavicular group. The axillary nodes are less often involved by spread across the pleural space via adhesions to the chest wall or by lymphatic connections with the cervical and the mediastinal lymphatics. Hematogenous metastases appear most frequently in the liver, the adrenal glands, the brain and the bodies of the vertebrae but may occur in any part of the body. In view of the frequent finding of cancer cells in the sputum and the bronchial secretions, it is surprising that endobronchial metastasis is rare.

Symptoms. Cough is the first symptom noted by more than half the patients with cancer of the lung, and over 90 per cent have a cough by the time the diagnosis is established. In the early stages the cough is dry but later tends to become productive. The frequency and the intensity of the cough usually are out of proportion to the sputum produced. Most men who are heavy cigarette smokers have a chronic cough. When such individuals develop bronchogenic carcinoma, the cough usually becomes worse. About half the patients with cancer of the lung have expectorated

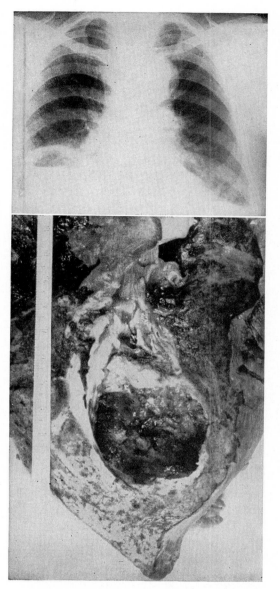

Fig. 44-2. (*Top*) Roentgenogram of a cavitary lesion with a fluid level in the right lower lobe. (*Bottom*) At operation this proved to be an epidermoid carcinoma with a large central area of cavitation.

blood-streaked sputum on one or more occasions. Severe bleeding is rare. Unfortunately, hemoptysis is rarely a first symptom. If it were, more patients undoubtedly would seek professional help earlier.

Many patients complain of vague discom-

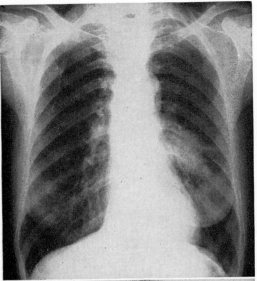

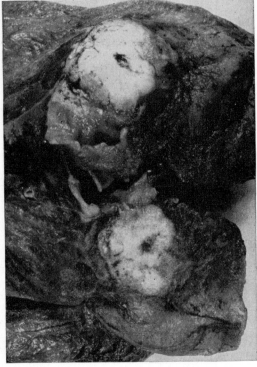

Fig. 44-3. (*Top*) Roentgenogram of a bronchogenic carcinoma of the superior segment of the left lower lobe. The x-ray density in this instance is due almost entirely to the mass of the tumor itself as shown by the photograph (*bottom*) of the lesion.

fort in the chest. Actual pain is a bad prognostic sign. It usually indicates invasion of the chest wall or the vertebrae by the tumor. More than half of the patients with resectable lesions have lost weight prior to operation. Loss of appetite and interference with normal sleep by constant cough and expectoration are probably responsible. Excessive weight loss, more than 15 lbs., is usually a bad prognostic sign. Shortness of breath, while not an early symptom, is usually present by the time a physician is consulted. The dyspnea is probably due to interference with normal aeration of all or part of the lung by the tumor.

Febrile episodes are common and are often the first indication of the cancer. The fever results from infection of the lung distal to a partial or complete obstruction of a bronchus by the tumor. Frequently, the pneumonitis is diagnosed as a viral pneumonia. Yet antibiotics usually are administered by the attending physician and often temporarily control the infection. This not infrequently results in further delay in diagnosis. The indiscriminate use of antibiotics without a definite diagnosis has deprived many patients with cancer of the lung of an opportunity to be cured.

Unilateral wheezing, due to partial obstruction of a bronchus, is an important diagnostic sign. Hoarseness may occur from involvement of the left recurrent laryngeal nerve at the level of the aortic arch by a tumor originating in the left upper lobe or left hilar region. Involvement of the right recurrent laryngeal nerve is very rare, due to its high position in the thorax as it passes around the right subclavian artery. Paralysis of a vocal cord is a generally accepted indication of inoperability. We have yet to explore a patient with a left recurrent laryngeal nerve paralysis in whom we were able to remove the cancer.

The physical signs which may be elicited depend on the size, the site and the complications of the growth. Often physical signs are lacking. Special attention should be paid in the physical examination to the common areas of metastasis. The commonest site of extrathoracic metastasis is the supraclavicular lymph nodes. The axillary lymph nodes are infrequently involved. Any enlarged supraclavicular node should be excised and examined histologically. The entire surface of the body should be examined for subcutaneous hema-

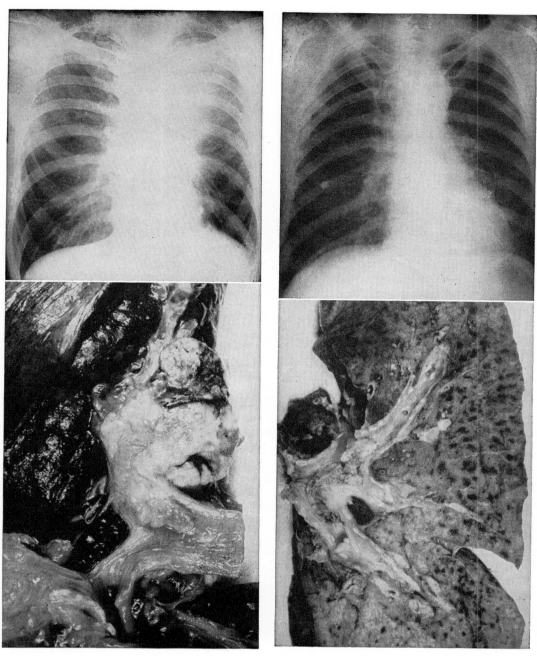

FIG. 44-4. (*Top*) Roentgenogram showing opacification of the left upper lobe. (*Bottom*) Photograph of the carcinoma completely occluding the left upper lobe bronchus with retained secretions and atelectasis distal to the tumor.

FIG. 44-5. (*Top*) Roentgenogram of the chest, revealing only a Ghon tubercle in the right lower midlung field. The patient had cough and hemoptysis. Bronchoscopic biopsy of a mass protruding from the left upper lobe revealed epidermoid carcinoma. (*Bottom*) Photograph of specimen showing tumor almost occluding the bronchus.

BRONCHO-SCOPIC BIOPSY	NEOPLASTIC CELLS NO BIOPSY	CLINICAL SYMPTOMS AND X-RAY ALONE
28 %	33 %	39 %

Fig. 44-6. Basis of the preoperative diagnosis in authors' series of 912 patients operated upon, for cancer of the lung.

togenous metastases. Neurologic symptoms may indicate metastasis to the central nervous system. Pain in the back, the pelvis or the extremities should be investigated by x-ray examination for osseous metastasis.

Diagnosis. X-ray examination of the chest is by far the most important diagnostic procedure. The radiolucency of normal pulmonary tissue provides an ideal background for the detection of densities produced by solid tumors and their complications. Thus carcinoma of the lung is the most easily detectable of all cancers of internal organs. There is some abnormality in the roentgenogram of the chest in 97 per cent of cases. In intermediate and peripheral tumors some, if not all, of the density on the film is due to the actual tumor itself (Fig. 44-3). In small cancers centrally located, the area of abnormal density may be due solely to bronchial obstruction with resultant atelectasis (Fig. 44-4). In approximately 3 per cent of cases, the usual posterior-anterior roentgenogram will not reveal any abnormality. This is due to the fact that the tumor is either within the shadow of the mediastinum or behind the heart, or is small and has not yet obstructed a bronchus (Fig. 44-5). Therefore, patients with a history and symptoms compatible with cancer of the lung should be studied completely, even though roentgenograms of the chest are normal.

Asymptomatic cancers of the lung discovered by a routine chest roentgenogram have a better prognosis than lesions which have reached the stage where they produce symptoms. Overholt[16] reported that all such cancers seen by him could be removed, and that in

over two thirds the cancer had not spread beyond the lung. Special x-ray examinations such as planography, angiography and bronchography are of only occasional value. Periodic roentgenograms to detect change in the size of a lesion never should be used because time may be lost during which an operable cancer may become inoperable. X-ray therapy as a diagnostic measure is mentioned only to be condemned.

An x-ray diagnosis of cancer of the lung is only presumptive. All patients with such a diagnosis should be examined with a bronchoscope. In approximately 25 per cent of patients with cancer of the lung, it is possible to obtain a bronchoscopic biopsy. This means that 25 per cent of cancers of the lung occur in, or project into, the main bronchus or the upper part of the lower lobe bronchus. An additional 33 per cent can be diagnosed preoperatively by finding cancer cells in the secretions, or saline washings, from the suspected bronchus. Failure to find neoplastic cells does not rule out the diagnosis of cancer. On the other hand, positive identification of cancer cells in the sputum or the bronchial secretions by an experienced cytologist is rarely erroneous. About one third of our patients have been operated upon without a positive cell, or tissue, diagnosis (Fig. 44-6). A presumptive diagnosis of cancer of the lung was made in these patients on the basis of the history and the x-ray findings.

Needle aspiration biopsy of undiagnosed pulmonary lesions should not be performed because of the danger of implantation of tumor cells in the chest wall.[1] However, needle biopsy is justified to establish a tissue diagnosis in lesions which are obviously inoperable. When pleural fluid is present, it should be aspirated and examined. If the fluid contains neoplastic cells, the lesion is inoperable. Bloody pleural fluid does not always indicate inoperable cancer of the lung or the pleura. The senior author has operated upon 2 patients with bloody pleural effusions, neither of whom had cancer.

Treatment. The proper treatment of cancer of the lung is total extirpation of the lesion together with the regional lymph nodes.[5, 9, 10] In practically all cases this requires a pneumonectomy and removal of all the mediastinal lymph nodes. Lobectomy, with removal of the adjacent mediastinal lymph nodes, should be performed when it is considered that the patient's cardiovascular status would seriously augment the risk of pneumonectomy. Patients with peripheral lesions requiring resection of the chest wall, because of direct extension, fall into this group.

X-ray therapy is helpful in alleviating the pain of chest wall invasion or the symptoms of superior caval obstruction. However, it does not appear to prolong life, with very rare exceptions. The dyspnea accompanying persistent pleural effusion may be relieved by producing pleural symphysis by talc poudrage.[4, 12] This has proved to be more effective than the injection of radioactive gold. Cytotoxic chemicals, such as Cytoxan, nitrogen mustard and 5-fluorouracil, are being evaluated in the treatment of inoperable cancer of the lung. Conclusive results are not yet available.

In reported series of patients with cancer of the lung[5, 8, 14, 15] the cancer was excised in 15 to 40 per cent. Approximately one fourth of these patients were alive without evidence of recurrence 5 years later (Fig. 44-7). The prognosis is poorer if the cancer has spread beyond the lung by either direct extension or lymph node metastasis. If the tumor is confined to the lung, approximately 40 per cent of patients will be alive after 5 years, while the figure drops to about 10 per cent if the tumor has spread beyond the lung. If the tumor cannot be removed, over 80 per cent of patients will be dead within 1 year, and less

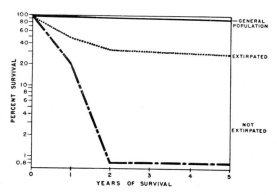

Fig. 44-8. Survival rates of patients with cancer of the lung compared with the general population (adjusted for age and sex). The patients with cancer of the lung are further subdivided with respect to whether or not the cancer was removed (Semilogarithmic scale.) (Based on 617 cases)

than 1 per cent live more than 2 years (Fig. 44-8).

Metastatic Malignant Tumors

Cancer cell emboli, with the exception of those in the portal venous system, will lodge in the lungs if the clump of cells is large enough to obstruct a pulmonary capillary. These metastatic deposits in the lungs are usually multiple and more frequently involve the lower than the upper lobes. These metastatic growths, because they rarely involve bronchi, do not produce symptoms early. A

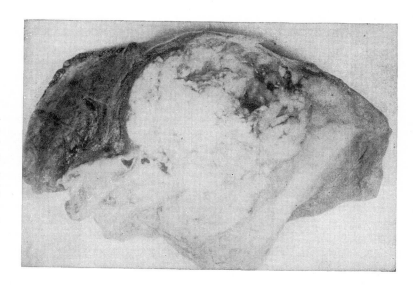

Fig. 44-7. Some cancers of the lung may grow to a considerable size and still be curable. This large epidermoid carcinoma of the lung was removed Oct. 15, 1946. Thirteen years later the patient was well and working without evidence of metastasis.

solitary pulmonary metastasis, as from a hypernephroma, an ovarian or colonic carcinoma, or a sarcoma, should be excised if there is no evidence of any other metastasis and if the primary lesion was completely eradicated at least 2 years before.

Differential Diagnosis. Tuberculosis, pneumoconiosis and lipoid pneumonitis at times may be difficult to distinguish from bronchogenic carcinoma. Sarcoidosis and histoplasmosis and the other fungus infections of the lung such as actinomycosis, nocardiosis, coccidioidomycosis, etc., are confused with bronchogenic carcinoma far less frequently. Pneumoconiosis, tuberculosis and sarcoidosis usually appear in a disseminated form which will not be confused with primary bronchogenic carcinoma. However, all 3 of these lesions occasionally produce a conglomerate mass from coalescence of adjacent nodules. If such a mass is solitary, it may be difficult or impossible to distinguish preoperatively from bronchogenic carcinoma.

Pneumoconiosis results from prolonged exposure to an irritant dust. A gradually increasing pulmonary fibrosis occurs with its attendant dyspnea. Fibrotic nodules may coalesce to produce a larger mass. Hemoptysis may occur. Such a lesion is difficult to distinguish from a bronchogenic carcinoma. Disseminated fibrosis in other portions of the lung, if present, gives a clue to the diagnosis. Tuberculosis in the healed form of a fibrous nodule may be impossible to distinguish by x-ray from a bronchogenic carcinoma. A ring of calcium in the nodule almost certainly indicates a tuberculoma, whereas small areas of density which appear to be calcium may be seen in either cancer or tuberculosis. The failure of a tuberculoma to increase in size on periodic x-ray examination in contrast with a bronchogenic carcinoma is, of course, an improper way of making the differential diagnosis, as mentioned above. It should be remembered that bronchogenic carcinoma may coexist with either tuberculosis or pneumoconiosis.

Sarcoidosis and the various fungus infections are not as likely to be confused with bronchogenic carcinoma. Nevertheless, solitary masses may appear and abscesses form which resemble a rapidly growing bronchogenic carcinoma with necrosis in its center.

The detection of eosinophilia in the circulating blood, examination of the sputum for fungi, and specific skin tests will aid in the differential diagnosis of these conditions.

Lipoid pneumonitis is usually the result of prolonged use of mineral oil for constipation, or of oily preparations to shrink the nasal mucous membranes. Some of the oil passes through the larynx and reaches the pulmonary parenchyma. A localized granulomatous reaction may occur. The resulting mass may bear a close resemblance to cancer of the lung on x-ray examination. The granuloma frequently causes hemoptysis. The demonstration of lipoid material in the sputum and the history of the use of oil may help in the differential diagnosis. In any of the diseases discussed above, if bronchogenic carcinoma cannot be ruled out, the proper procedure is an exploratory thoracotomy and a wedge excision of the suspicious lesion, with immediate histologic examination of a frozen section.

Bronchial Adenoma. Although most of these tumors may be considered as benign, some of them do metastasize after many years. Bronchial adenomas are relatively rare tumors. In our experience, they constitute from 2 to 3 per cent of all pulmonary neoplasms. These adenomas appear equally in the male and the female sexes in contrast with the strong predilection of bronchogenic carcinoma for the male sex. The tumors usually become manifest between the ages of 20 and 40 in contrast with the prevalence of bronchogenic carcinoma in the age range of 40 to 70. Eighty-five per cent of the bronchial adenomas are of the carcinoid type. The remaining 15 per cent are cylindromas. The histologic distinction between the carcinoid tumors and the cylindromas is quite clear-cut, but the symptoms and the clinical course of these pathologic types is quite similar. Bronchial adenomas generally occur in the larger bronchi and produce symptoms from obstruction and from erosion of their surface. The common symptoms are cough, hemoptysis and dyspnea. Hemoptysis is a much more frequent symptom than in carcinoma of the lung. The dyspnea is generally related to obstruction of the bronchus which, when complete, produces atelectasis.

The diagnosis is almost invariably made by bronchoscopic biopsy. The histologic appearance of the lesion is quite characteristic. Formerly, the treatment of these lesions was endoscopic removal. Recurrence was almost invariable with this treatment because of failure to excise the growth completely. The modern treatment is transthoracic excision of the tumor, together with that portion of the lung distal to the involved bronchus. A lobectomy is the usual operation. Pneumonectomy is necessary only when the adenoma involves the main bronchus. The prognosis is excellent after surgical excision.

Hamartoma. This term is applied to tumors consisting of an abnormal arrangement of normal components of an organ. Hamartomas of the lung may be made up of one or all components of pulmonary tissue. Usually, pulmonary hamartomas consist mainly of cartilage and therefore are sometimes referred to as chondromas. Hamartomas of the lung are relatively uncommon. They are apt to occur in the peripheral portion of the lungs. They rarely produce symptoms and usually are discovered on routine x-ray films of the chest. As it is generally impossible to differentiate them from a bronchogenic carcinoma, a thoracotomy with a local excision of the tumor mass should be done, and the diagnosis established by frozen section.

Tumors of the Trachea

Tumors of the trachea are rare. However, both bronchial adenomas and bronchogenic carcinomas may be primary in the trachea in any position from the bifurcation to the larynx. The symptoms are similar to those produced by tumors of the major bronchi. The treatment is local excision with plastic repair of the trachea by an autogenous graft, or a foreign material, which will prevent collapse of the tracheal wall.

TUMORS OF THE MEDIASTINUM

The mediastinum is bounded posteriorly by the vertebral bodies and anteriorly by the sternum. The lateral boundaries are the lungs; the caudad limit is the diaphragm; and the cephalad limit is at the level of the suprasternal notch. This region is occupied chiefly by the heart, the great vessels, the esophagus and the trachea. The thymus gland lies in the anterosuperior portion of the mediastinum.

The phrenic nerves and the vagus nerves and their branches traverse the mediastinum. The remainder of the space is occupied by fibrous connective tissue, fat and lymph nodes. Obviously, a wide variety of tumors can arise from these structures. Tumors of the trachea and the major bronchi have been considered already, and tumors of the esophagus are discussed in another chapter.

The symptoms produced by mediastinal tumor masses are related to their effect upon important contiguous structures. Thus, projection or growth of the tumor mass laterally compressing the lung on either side may permit the tumor to become of considerable size without producing symptoms. On the other hand, in the region of the superior mediastinum, symptoms of dyspnea, dysphagia, and congestion of the head, the neck and the upper extremities may occur from compression of trachea, esophagus or superior vena cava, respectively. If a tumor is of large size, a widening of the upper mediastinum may be noted by percussing the chest anteriorly. Usually, however, physical signs are absent, and the tumor mass is recognized by rounded projection from, or widening of, the usual mediastinal density on a posterior anterior roentgenogram of the chest. The more common types of mediastinal tumors will be discussed below, and then lesions that must be differentiated from true tumors will be considered.

Thymoma

Thymomas are relatively rare tumors. They vary considerably in their histologic characteristics. They tend to grow slowly, and it may be many years before they attain a large size. They rarely, if ever, metastasize and usually run a benign course for many years. If malignant change develops, it is apt to be of the locally invasive type rather than spread by lymphatic or hematogenous channels. Approximately three fourths of all thymomas are associated with myasthenia gravis. Removal of a thymoma usually will alleviate the symptoms of a coexisting myasthenia gravis and reduce the amount of Prostigmin required by the patient.[3] The treatment of a thymoma is surgical excision, either through a median sternotomy or through the conventional posterolateral approach for tumors presenting more predominantly on one side.

TERATOMA

The mediastinum is a common site for these interesting tumors. A teratoid tumor may be either benign or malignant. The benign teratomas are often called dermoids. These tumors are composed chiefly of ectodermal elements. Dermoid cysts are lined with squamous epithelium and contain hair and sebaceous material. However, derivatives from both endoderm and mesoderm also may be present. Teratoid tumors generally have rounded margins and project beyond the mediastinum into one or the other lung field. If a teratoid tumor ruptures into a bronchus, the diagnosis may be obvious from the expectoration of hair or sebaceous material. The x-ray finding of structures resembling bone or teeth in the tumor mass may reveal the diagnosis. When the diagnosis is established, the treatment is complete surgical excision. Preferably, these tumors should be excised before the complications of infection, fistula formation, or hemorrhage have occurred.

TUMORS OF LYMPHOID ORIGIN

The benign tumors of lymphoid origin in the mediastinum are the cystic lymphangiomas. These are cystic lymphoid structures, multilocular in character, which may communicate with a similar tumor mass presenting in the neck, especially in children. These tumor masses, presumably because of their softness, are usually asymptomatic. They are benign in character but have a tendency toward local recurrence if not completely excised.

Malignant lymphatic tumors comprise Hodgkin's disease, the lymphocytic lymphomas, the leukemias and lymphosarcoma. None of these lesions is amenable to surgical treatment in the mediastinum. Malignant lymphatic tumors are frequently associated with enlarged cervical or axillary lymph nodes. The leukemias and the malignant lymphomas may be associated with enlargement of the liver or spleen. Low-grade fever is often present. The diagnosis should be established by biopsy. Treatment of the lymphosarcomas and Hodgkin's disease by radiation therapy will often lead to palliation of symptoms arising from compression of normal structures by these bulky masses.

DIFFERENTIAL DIAGNOSIS

It is often difficult to differentiate between true tumors of the mediastinum and masses which are not neoplastic in nature. Perhaps the commonest cause of an enlarged mediastinal shadow in a posterior-anterior roentgenogram is an intrathoracic extension of the thyroid gland. This usually occurs in the anterior mediastinum, but it may present in the posterior mediastinum. Most of these intrathoracic extensions of goiters can be dealt with through the usual cervical approach, as their blood supply arises from the inferior thyroid arteries. Occasionally, it may be necessary to approach these lesions through the thorax. Adenomas of the inferior parathyroid bodies producing hyperparathyroidism also may be found occasionally in the superior mediastinum. These adenomas are too small to be recognized by physical signs or x-ray enlargement of the superior mediastinal density. The diagnosis of hyperparathyroidism is a biochemical one; once it has been made, if the adenoma cannot be found in the cervical region, then the upper mediastinum should be explored. (See Chapter 27 on the parathyroid.)

At times it may be difficult to differentiate aneurysms of the arch of the aorta from true mediastinal tumors, especially if they are filled with laminated clot and fail to show expansile pulsation on fluoroscopic examination. A history of syphilis or a positive Wassermann or Kahn test will be helpful in these cases. An angiocardiogram will succeed in making the distinction in practically all cases. Enterogenous, bronchogenic, or pericardial cysts also may at times be difficult to distinguish from true tumors arising in the mediastinum. Bronchogenic and enterogenous cysts are elements arising from the primitive foregut in the embryo and persisting as isolated cystic structures. If these structures are lined with pseudostratified ciliated epithelium, they are referred to as bronchogenic cysts. If they are lined with squamous epithelium, or gastric or intestinal epithelium, they are referred to as enterogenous cysts. The latter may be actual reduplications of portions of the gastro-intestinal tract. If they communicate with the lumen of the gut, their cystic nature will be evident from the presence of air and fluid levels. Hemorrhage or infection in these cysts is not uncommon, but malignant change is very rare. Symptoms may or may not be present, depending upon the size and the location of the cyst and the presence of complications. The treatment is always surgical excision. In the inferior mediastinum, herniation of the abdominal contents through the foramen of Morgagni may simulate a true tumor of the inferior mediastinum. (See Chap. 39, "Hernia.") The nature of the density on the x-ray examination should be suspected if a lateral roentgenogram shows the mass to be anterior. If intestines are present in the hernia, air and fluid levels may be apparent and, of course, a gastro-intestinal x-ray with barium will confirm the diagnosis.

TUMORS OF THE THORACIC WALL

PLEURAL TUMORS

Metastatic tumors of the parietal pleura are not uncommon. They usually are accompanied by a pleural effusion that is serosanguineous. As these metastatic malignant nodules grow, they may invade the contiguous ribs or the intercostal nerves and produce pain. Usually, however, the only symptom is dyspnea from the pleural effusion which will be relieved by aspiration of the fluid. The diagnosis is often apparent on posterior-anterior and oblique x-ray views of the thorax. A nodular wavy density replacing the normal straight smooth lining of the thoracic cage beneath the ribs is characteristic. Aspiration needle biopsy of such metastatic malignant tumors of the pleura is quite justifiable. The only treatment is palliative. The most effective palliation for the pleural effusion is the production of pleural symphysis by talc poudrage.[4, 12] Pain from involvement of ribs can be treated adequately by local x-ray therapy. If the pain is due to involvement of an intercostal nerve, the nerve may be sectioned proximal to the point of invasion.

MESOTHELIOMA OF THE PLEURA

In the past benign mesotheliomas of the pleura have been given the misnomer of "giant sarcoma of the pleura." However, these tumors are not malignant. Regardless of the exact origin of the cells composing these tumors, they run a characteristically slow, benign clinical course. They may arise from any portion of the pleural surface, either parietal or visceral. They grow slowly over a period of many years and adapt themselves in shape to conform to surrounding rigid structures. Generally, they produce a globular mass. They are almost invariably symptomless until they reach a considerable size; then they may produce symptoms from compression of the lung. Frequently, they are discovered on a routine x-ray film of the chest. The treatment is complete surgical excision which will be curative. These tumors do not metastasize.

Malignant mesotheliomas of the pleura are always multiple and do not attain the large size of the solitary benign lesions. These tumors are highly malignant and cause massive pleural effusion. Chest pain is often present. They are incurable.

NEUROGENIC TUMORS

Neurogenic tumors are discussed under "Tumors of the Thoracic Wall" because most of them are quite distinct and separate from the mediastinum itself. Aside from bronchogenic carcinomas and lymphoid tumors of the mediastinum, neurogenic tumors are the commonest thoracic neoplasms. The 3 main pathologic types are the ganglioneuromas which arise in the ganglia of the thoracic sympathetic chain, the neurilemmomas, and the neurofibromas which may arise in the sympathetic trunks but more commonly originate in the intercostal nerves. If a neurilemmoma or a neurofibroma arises near the origin of an intercostal nerve, it may extend through the intervertebral foramen in an hourglass fashion and produce compression of the spinal cord. Most of these tumors, when they have reached any size, may be easily recognized from their paravertebral position in the posterior-anterior and lateral roentgenograms of the chest. These neurogenic tumors are apt to be slow-growing and encapsulated, but they have the potentiality of undergoing malignant change.[2] Therefore, they should be excised surgically when first recognized. The ganglioneuromas are almost always symptomless and usually are discovered in a routine chest x-ray. The neurilemmomas and the neurofibromas are apt to produce pain from involvement of the intercostal nerves. If they are of the dumbbell-shape type growing through the intervertebral foramen, in addition they may produce symptoms of spinal cord compression. Malignant degeneration will be evident from erosion of bone and severe pain. The characteristic paravertebral position of the vast majority of these tumors makes a presumptive diagnosis easy, and surgical excision through a posterolateral thoracic incision is always indicated. Complete excision will result in cure if malignant change has not occurred. If a tumor has grown through an intervertebral foramen, a laminectomy to remove the intraspinal portion of the growth should precede thoracotomy for removal of the intrathoracic portion.

TUMORS OF RIBS AND CARTILAGES

Chondromas and chondrosarcomas are the commonest primary tumors of the ribs and the cartilages. A bony component is present not infrequently, and such tumors should be referred to as osteochondromas or osteochondrosarcomas. The benign chondromas or osteochondromas are prone to appear at the anterior ends of the ribs where they join the costal cartilages. They may involve the sternum in this region or the clavicle. Benign tumors are not apt to produce symptoms but are usually recognized first by the presence of a globular firm swelling. Malignant tumors are more common in the posterior portions of the ribs near their junction with the vertebrae. The lesions grow fairly rapidly and produce pain from involvement of the intercostal nerves and erosion of the ribs and the vertebrae. The presence of a lesion involving the ribs can be established by roentgenograms, but it is not always possible to distinguish these primary neoplasms from metastatic or other lesions of bone. The treatment is excision of the involved rib or cartilage, leaving a considerable margin of normal bone or cartilage attached to the tumor mass. The periosteum, or perichondrium, and attached intercostal muscles should be removed with the tumor.

Eosinophilic granulomas of the rib are found not uncommonly in young adults. They produce localized rarefaction of the rib which may be difficult to distinguish from a primary tumor. A solitary plasmacytoma produces an expanding lesion of the rib which gives an appearance somewhat similar to the eosinophilic granuloma. Ewing's endothelioma is also occasionally primary in a rib. The diagnosis

should be established in all these cases by complete excision of the lesion and histologic examination.

The ribs and the sternum are frequently invaded by metastatic carcinoma. Such secondary metastases to ribs, vertebra, or sternum commonly arise from primary carcinomas of the breast, the kidney, the prostate, the thyroid gland and the lungs. Pathologic fractures of ribs with metastatic carcinoma may occur on the slightest exertion, sometimes calling first attention to the lesion. If the lesion is obviously metastatic carcinoma, the proper therapy is local radiation which will relieve the pain promptly and result in healing of the pathologic fracture. If there is any question of the lesion's being a primary tumor, then complete local excision should be practiced.

REFERENCES

1. Allbritten, F. F., Jr., Nealon, T. F., Jr., Gibbon, J. H., Jr., and Templeton, J. Y., III: The diagnosis of lung cancer, S. Clin. North America 32:1657, 1952.
2. Blades, B.: Mediastinal tumors, Ann. Surg. 123:749, 1946.
3. Blalock, A.: Thymectomy in the treatment of myasthenia gravis, J. Thoracic Surg. 13: 316, 1944.
4. Chambers, J. S.: Palliative treatment of neoplastic pleural effusion with intercostal intubation and talc instillation, West. J. Surg. 66:26, 1958.
5. Churchill, E. D., Sweet, R. H., Soutter, L., and Scannell, J. S.: The surgical management of carcinoma of the lung: a study of the cases treated at the Massachusetts General Hospital from 1930 to 1950, J. Thoracic Surg. 20:349, 1950.
6. Craafoord, C.: On the Technique of Pneumonectomy in Man, Stockholm, Tryckeri Aktiebolaget Thule, 1938.
7. Doll, R., and Hill, A. B.: Smoking and carcinoma of the lung, Brit. M. J. 2:739, 1950.
8. Gibbon, J. H., Jr., Allbritten, F. F., Jr., Templeton, J. Y., III, and Nealon, T. F., Jr.: Carcinoma of the lung: an analysis of 532 consecutive cases, Ann. Surg. 138:489, 1953.
9. Gibbon, J. H., Jr., Stokes, T. L., and McKeown, J. J., Jr.: The surgical treatment of carcinoma of the lung, Am. J. Surg. 89:484, 1955.
10. Graham, E. A., and Singer, J. J.: Successful removal of an entire lung for carcinoma of the bronchus, J.A.M.A. 101:1371, 1933.

11. Hammond, E. C., and Horn, P.: The relationship between human smoking habits and death rates, J.A.M.A. *155*:1316, 1954.

12. Haupt, G. J., Camishion, R. C., Templeton, J. Y., III, and Gibbon, J. H., Jr.: Treatment of malignant pleural effusions by talc poudrage, J.A.M.A. *172*:918, 1960.

13. Kirklin, J. W., McDonald, J. R., Clagett, O. T., Moerschand, H. J., and Gage, R. P.: Bronchogenic carcinoma: cell type and other factors relating to prognosis, Surg, Gynec. & Obst. *100*:429, 1955.

14. Mason, G. A.: Cancer of the lung: review of a thousand cases, Lancet *2*:587, 1949.

15. Ochsner, A., DeCamp, P. A., DeBakey, M. E., and Ray, C. J.: Bronchogenic carcinoma; its frequency, diagnosis and early treatment, J.A.M.A. *148*:691, 1952.

16. Overholt, R. H.: Cancer detected in surveys, Am. Rev. Tuberc. *62*:491, 1950.

17. Wynder, E. L., and Graham, E. A.: Tobacco smoking as a possible etiologic factor in bronchogenic carcinoma; study of 684 proved cases, J.A.M.A. *143*:329, 1950.

JAMES BARRETT BROWN, M.D., AND MINOT P. FRYER, M.D.

—————————————— CHAPTER 45 ——————————————

Principles of General Plastic Surgery

SKIN GRAFTING AND DEEP BURNS

Treatment of the local burned areas is discussed as those due to thermal, chemical and electrical origin and irradiation effect. Depth and extent of the burns are considered because of their pertinence to the treatment and prognosis.

Fluid balance, nutrition and general care of the burned patient are covered elsewhere but are considered a part of this section and should be studied by the student with it.

The 4 phases in the care of deep, extensive burns are (1) control of shock and primary local care, (2) postmortem homograft coverage as biologic dressings when needed, (3) flat surface grafting with the patient's own skin for permanent healing and holding distortion to a minimum, (4) the repair of contractures and dysfunction and the reconstruction of features by procedures in reconstructive surgery.

CLASSIFICATION OF BURNS

Burns may be classified as to their extent, depth, or on the basis of the cause. *Estimates of extent* may be important for estimation of prognosis and usually are based on the Berkow tables of body surface, in which various areas of the body are classified as to percentage of the whole. Using this system, each thigh and leg comprise around 15 per cent; head, neck and shoulders, 15 per cent; each upper extremity, 5 to 7 per cent; and the remaining 40 per cent in the trunk. *Depth* of a burn may be reported as first, second or third degree, but since such detailed impressions may be difficult for even trained observers, more nearly accurate estimates are possible if superficially burned areas can be separated from deeply burned areas. A *superficial burn* not through the full thickness of the skin will heal because of persistent skin elements. A *deep burn* through the full thickness of the skin often requires a skin graft to heal properly. Burns can be caused by *heat, electricity, chemicals and irradiation.*

EARLY LOCAL CARE OF BURNED AREA

Dressings

Fine mesh grease gauze pressure dressing is an accepted method of local treatment for the burned area; 44-mesh gauze is recommended to make dressing change easier and not so painful, as this fine mesh will not allow the granulation tissue to grow into the bandage and in this way fine mesh gauze encourages healing. Other fine woven materials can be used. The first one was used at St. Louis Children's Hospital by us and was made from strips of old soft bed linen.

Small islands of epithelium from the deep sweat glands and the hair follicles do not become involved in the fine mesh gauze, but they do grow into a coarse mesh gauze and may be pulled off with each dressing change. A small amount of grease may be incorporated into the fine mesh gauze to make the dressings less painful. Pressure-fixation of the dressing can be secured by winding a gauze roll over clean mechanic's waste placed upon the fine mesh grease gauze. The bulk of the dressing fixes the part and promotes healing and comfort.

Dressings are changed as often as it is necessary to keep them clean and comfortable. The needs of the individually burned patient and the availability of sufficiently trained personnel regulate the schedule of burn dressings. They are done in the operating room, under anesthesia if needed.

Cleansing

Careful cleansing with soap and water and cotton sponges is done at each dressing, and loose necrotic tissue is removed with a knife or scissors without causing bleeding.

Saline baths are used, especially if the burn is first seen after a protracted time, and may hasten the cleaning up process. Allowing the dressings to soak off decreases the number of general anesthetics and lessens the pain of dressings. Normal salt solution is used for the bath rather than plain water to reduce discomfort and to prevent sodium depletion and water intoxication.

Exposure

Leaving areas open to dry heat or covered with moist loose dressings and cleaning them with saline baths has been used on this service

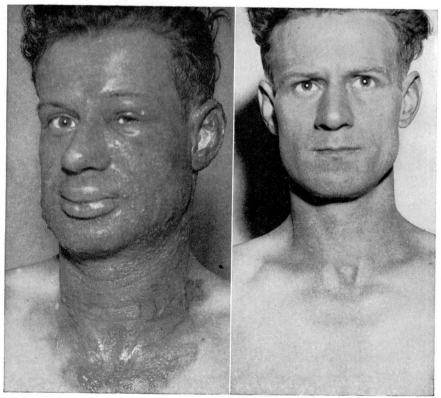

Fig. 45-1. (*Left*) Painful acute superficial burn of face and neck 24 hours following injury. Superficial blistering, weeping, generally uncomfortable. (*Right*) Immediate healing, comfort and prevention of infection promoted by pressure, fine mesh grease gauze dressing. Initial dressing left in place for 6 days. No other treatment necessary. Primary healing possible because this was a superficial burn. Comfort, promptness of healing, avoidance of infection, treatment as an outpatient made possible by dressing. (Brown, J. B., and Fryer, M. P.: J. Missouri M. A. *48*:973-981)

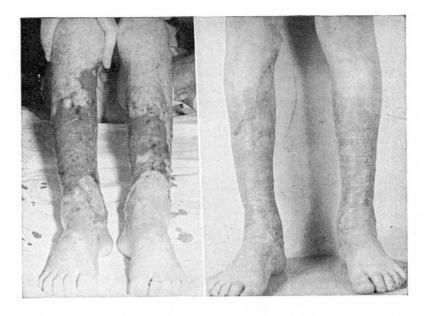

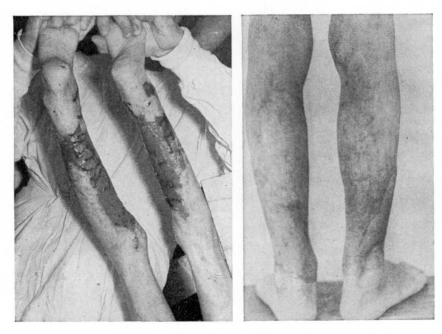

Fig. 45-2. (*Left, top and bottom*) Circular full-thickness loss of the skin of both legs resulting from deep burn when clothes caught on fire. Open areas prepared for grafting with frequent fine mesh (pressure) grease gauze dressing, done in the ward dressing room or the operating room under sterile conditions. (*Right, top and bottom*) Appearance several months following coverage of open areas with thick split-thickness grafts transferred from the back. Permanent repair in one operation. (Brown, J. B., and Fryer, M. P.: J. Missouri M. A. *48*:973-981)

for some severe burns since 1925 and still is used in some instances of severe burns difficult to handle otherwise. This is not the open coagulum treatment but one of open surgical drainage and cleanliness. The closed coagulum or so-called open treatment of burns does not have this element of cleansing of the wounds.

Leaving the burned area open and protecting the coagulum is readvocated from time to time. There is marked disadvantage if infection occurs under the coagulum and a second-degree burn is turned into a third-degree loss. This is much the same as was noted in tannic acid treatment. Another disadvantage is that hospitalization is required, whereas many could have a dressing applied and be treated as out-patients.

Healing Time

Superficial burns should be healed in 10 to 14 days and less extensive deep burns in a month.

Skin Grafting

Extensive deep burns should be ready for coverage with skin grafts in 3 weeks. Excision of the eschar and grafting in 2 weeks' time is done in some places, but usually this is not applicable to the face, the hands and the feet until the depth of the burn is known and this often takes more than 2 weeks.

Split skin grafts give the most satisfactory permanent coverage to extensive raw areas.[19] This graft contains from one third to three fourths the thickness of the skin and of course includes an appreciable pad of derma. This pad of derma is very important functionally.

Split-thickness skin grafts are cut with a long skin graft knife from areas that can be flattened by pressure or stretched into a diaphragm in the simplest way. Suction retractors aid in providing a diaphragm of skin in taking the grafts. Various mechanical, electrical or vacuum dermatomes are available and are useful in cutting split grafts from some areas.

Application of split-thickness or full-thickness grafts requires fixation and steady, even pressure for an assurance of take. Fixation may be by suture around the graft or by tying the sutures over fine mesh grease gauze and a bulk of mechanic's waste or other medium. Or the graft may be "snubbed" into place, which is accomplished by carefully rolling fine

mesh grease gauze over the graft to fix it firmly, and then firmly fixing the rest of the bulk of the dressing with soft gauze rolls, being careful not to slip the graft out of place. This is often used on extremities.

Donor site dressings aim at protection of the fresh wound from chemical, bacterial and mechanical trauma and consist of fine mesh grease gauze fixed with overlying gauze pads, held with adhesive to prevent local slipping and then gauze rolls and bandage in turn held with adhesive. Fixation of the part and the adjacent joints with steady, even pressure invites healing. Healing should be complete in 2 weeks' time. Variation in dressing technic, or no dressing to the grafted area or the donor site, can be done, but as yet these have been not proved better than the dressing described above. The healing of a donor site is comparable with a superficial burn. If the delicate exposed surface is protected, it will heal in 10 to 12 days; if not, and it is traumatized, a full-thickness loss of the remaining epidermal structures may result with subsequent scarring and distortion.

Epithelial healing of donor sites of split grafts gives one of the most interesting studies of wound healing. The deep epithelial cells in the derma, finding themselves without a normal epidermal covering, "dedifferentiate" into squamous epithelium and resurface the area in as little as 6 days' time and give solid enough healing to omit dressings after 12 days. This is considered the reverse of the formation of cancer, in which surface cells grow down and lose their differentiation.

Homografts are often important for the emergency, though temporary, coverage of extensive burns after the removal of the eschar, particularly in the very young or old.[13] Homografts are to be thought of as biologic dressings for large open wounds. They serve to prevent the excessive vaporization of water that takes place upon the cutaneously denuded surface and thereby to reduce the loss of heat from the body and the hypermetabolism characteristically associated with large burns (see Chap. 16). In addition, the number of the bacteria on the surface of the burn is very quickly reduced to the vanishing point when the wound is covered with a living homograft, just as it is when the wound is covered by a living autograft. Consequently, the living

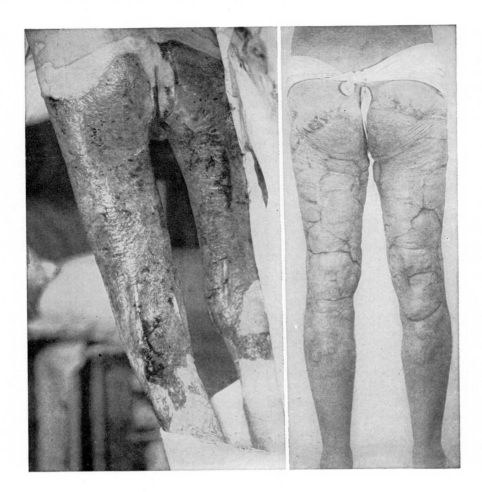

FIG. 45-3. (*Top, left*) Full-thickness loss of skin over most of both thighs and buttocks following burn with gasoline. Taken care of elsewhere for several months. Appearance after several dressings consisting of washing with soap and water, then applying fine mesh grease gauze pressure dressing. At this length of time following a burn these open areas become so painful that often a general anesthesia is necessary for adequate

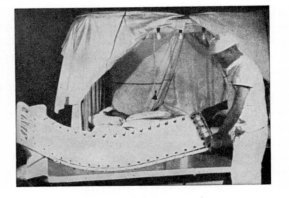

cleansing. (*Top, right*) Appearance 1 year later following resurfacing of the open areas on the thighs with long, wide, thick split-thickness grafts cut from the back with the knife and suction box. (Brown, J. B., and Fryer, M. P.: J. Missouri M. A. *48*:973-981)

(*Bottom*) Frame, tub and bed used in preparing this burn and other deep burns for rapid coverage with skin.

homograft constitutes an important means of aiding in the control of infections in burn wounds. Their use may be considered as the *second phase* in the local treatment of extensive burns. Often the extensively burned patient is deemed unable to stand the operation required for transference of his own skin to his open areas, or none of his own skin is available. Then the application of homografts stops the "leaks" of vital body fluids and may serve to carry the patient over this critical period. Covering an open wound with them also gives respite from pain and obviates the need for dressings; the patient literally walks around in another's skin. The speed with which the application of a graft abolishes the pain and the tenderness of an open wound is remarkable; all pain and tenderness disappear within a minute or two. The taking of homografts for one extensively burned patient from living donors requires a large number of them, their anesthetization, operating upon them and caring for their wounds afterward. However, *postmortem homografts* have been proved to have the same general properties as homografts taken from living donors and by using them one avoids the need of taking homografts from live donors. Postmortem grafts are removed from the clothed areas of patients who have just died. The grafts are usually taken from the cadaver in the operating room under sterile conditions by surgeons with written consent of the donor's relatives. Permission for a general postmortem examination is not necessary if proper permission for the taking of the skin is obtained. The donor should not have carcinoma, a blood dyscrasia or a transmissible disease. Using these grafts immediately obviates the need for storage. Because the skin lives for a number of hours after the heart stops, living homografts may be obtained from a cadaver for some time after death. There is no reason for not using them in place of homografts cumbersomely taken from living donors. The use of postmortem grafts has been considered for many years. We used them first in 1927 and sporadically up to 1951. Since 1951 they have been employed regularly whenever homografting was needed.[8, 15, 16, 17] It is our belief that the temporary coverage of large cutaneously denuded surfaces with homografts may have effected a reduction in the death rate from very extensive burns (larger than 50 per cent of body surface) which has remained about the same for 100 years, despite the great improvement in control of shock and general care.

However, it is important to remember that at the present time homografts do not survive indefinitely. From 3 to 12 weeks after their application they are rejected by the recipient. Much investigative work is being done in attempting to effect the permanent take of homografts.

A skin bank has been developed as an adjunct for the use of postmortem homografts because often they are needed when suitable postmortem donors are not available. Skin grafts may be stored alive in a number of ways. The simplest, most practical and suitable way is their moist storage in an ordinary household refrigerator at temperatures of $+3°$ to $+5°$ C. After removing the grafts from the body, they are rolled in fine meshed gauze and kept moist in a jar with saline in the refrigerator for as long as 3 weeks. The period of viability can be lengthened somewhat by the addition of 10 per cent serum and antibiotics to the saline. It may be prolonged further by soaking them in glycerol and then freezing and storing at $-40°$ and $-80°$ C. Recently postmortem grafts have been frozen and vacuum dried (freeze-dried). This is the easiest way to store nonviable grafts. Nonviable freeze-dried grafts serve well as temporary biologic dressings, although they are not as long lasting as fresh postmortem homografts and consequently not as good for the temporary coverage of open areas.[8, 15, 16, 17]

Homografts taken from one of *identical twins* and applied to the other survive permanently. We first effected such a transfer in 1937. Since then this demonstration has served as the basis for the transfer of organs from one identical twin to another.

Autografts. The third stage (or phase) of treatment of an extensive deep burn is that of covering the denuded areas with autografts and is carried out by using grafts from the patient as soon as he is judged capable of standing the procedure. The early coverage of flat surfaces with autografts and the securing of complete healing hold to a minimum contracture, deformity and dysfunction and in many instances are all that is needed for the complete rehabilitation of the patient.

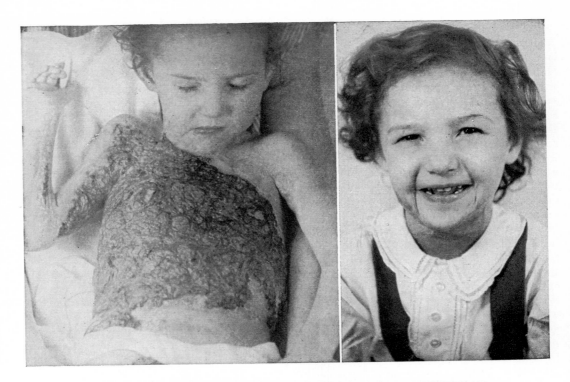

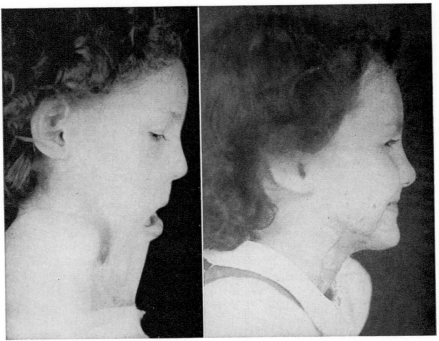

FIG. 45-4. (*Left, top*) Deep burn of abdomen, chest, neck, shoulder and arm in a child with deformity resulting from the spontaneous healing (*left, bottom*) in flexion areas. In spite of uncomfortable position of head, chief complaint was of loss of "watertight mouth." (*Right, top and bottom*) One operation has restored the "watertight mouth" and the normal neck angle. Smoothing out around the edges of the graft can be done subsequently.

Final Phase of Treatment. The final (fourth) phase in the treatment of the severely burned patient is the release and the repair of contractures, the restoration of articular function and the reconstruction of features. Frequently, the healing of raw surfaces in flexion areas is attended by contractures, requiring release of the contracture for the restoration of function and appearance. Eyelids, axilla, neck, hand or fingers are especially prone to be so affected. Excision of this contracting scar leaves a raw surface which usually can be covered best by a split-thickness graft. Local flaps and webs may be utilized when they are available, but further addition of skin grafts is almost always needed. Cumbersome distant flaps are unnecessary in most burn repairs, and this is a point that seems to be missed frequently. One patient with a burn contraction of the neck was seen on whom a large back flap was used and 100 operative procedures performed before we saw the case. Usually the whole front of the neck can be repaired in 1 to 4 operations with free skin grafts, and the functional result will be much better than with a heavy, cumbersome flap.

DISTORTION OR LOSS OF A FEATURE. This is one of the most difficult problems in repair. Loss of the alar border, the tip of the nose or the columella can best be substituted for by a free *composite graft* from the ear in one operation.[3] This graft includes both surfaces of skin and the supporting cartilaginous framework, and the resulting repair is superior to any other method.

Full-thickness skin grafts consist of the entire thickness of the skin, as the name intimates. The use of this type of graft requires antecedent closure or coverage with a split-thickness skin graft for healing before the full-thickness graft is put in place. Full-thickness skin grafts are used in small specialized areas, as about the face, the eyelids or the hands.

Full-thickness grafts from the neck give the best results in the repair of limited defects about the face because of color match and kinetic possibilities. Healing of burns of the face often is followed by eyelid contractures which leave the globe exposed, inviting irritation and ulceration, and consequently necessitate early repair in order to save the eye. The repair of eyelid contracture consists of release of the contracture, meticulous excision of the deep scar and coverage with a soft full-thickness graft from the neck. Elsewhere on the face release of contracting scars of limited size and repair with a graft from the supraclavicular region often results in a repair indistinguishable from the normal. Full-thickness grafts cannot be placed on granulating surfaces—they will not take. A bed of normal nongranulating tissue is requisite for their take.

Burns of the hands, of some degree, are usually seen accompanying burns of other areas of the body and often are the most important parts to be treated. Resurfacing of the hand is an important part of plastic surgery in general and will be outlined here for completeness. Repair of the deeper structures and treatment of infections of the hand are considered elsewhere in this text. Also a short description will be given here of the first recorded burns of the hands from atomic irradiation.

SUPERFICIAL BURNS of the hands are treated in general, as are superficial burns elsewhere in the body. Flash burns not even deep enough to cause superficial blistering are often extremely painful. Placing the hand in cold water usually will relieve the pain, but this may have to be persisted in for several hours. Following this relief of pain a light coverage with grease will give the most comfort in cases of very superficial burns of the hand. Deeper superficial burns heal in 7 to 10 days if a comfortable fine mesh grease gauze pressure dressing is applied after gentle cleansing.

DEEP BURNS of the hands should be cleansed, and the eschar excised as soon as the extent of deep burns can be recognized, and the wound covered with grafts as soon as possible to prevent deep infection and fixation of tendons and joints. It is generally agreed that dressings with open surgical drainage, fingers apart and with the hand in the position of function is the method of choice from the onset of treatment.

Early mobilization of burned hands will not be difficult if prompt healing is secured, and this is encouraged by active motion in soapy water at the time of each dressing.

Deep burns of the dorsum of the hand are usually worse than those of the palm because frequently the midportion of the extensor

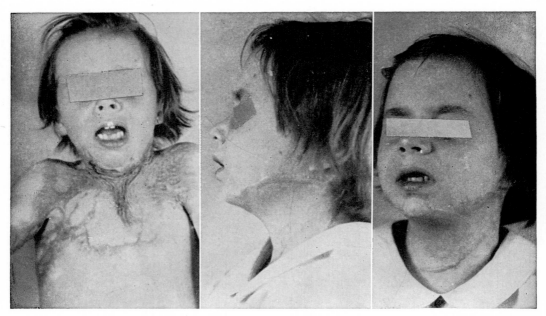

FIG. 45-5. (*Left*) Severe contracture of the neck following deep burn. (*Center and right*) Result possible by release of chin and excision of deep scar and chronically infected sinuses. Free, thick, split-thickness graft used to cover defect at same operation, which has created normal neck angle and allowed normal growth. (Brown, J. B., and Freyer, M. P.: J. Missouri M. A. *48*:973-981)

sleeve over the middle interphalangeal joints is destroyed. The lateral slips of these extensor tendons then slip volarward when extension is attempted, flexing the joint instead of extending it giving a characteristic and for the most part permanent functional loss.

Late deformities of the hand resulting from deep burns are minimized by their early coverage with free grafts. Early healing up to necrotic tendon or bone usually can be obtained by early coverage of adjacent granulating areas with free grafts. This may save function in the remainder of the hand which otherwise may be lost by waiting for complete separation of dead tissue and later total flap replacement. Contractures require careful opening, avoiding wide exposure of tendons and coverage with free grafts or flaps if the destruction is of enough depth to require the latter. The usual flap is a direct one from the inguinal region of the abdominal wall. The direct flap was developed and used hundreds of times at Valley Forge General Hospital during World War II, more for gunshot injuries than for burns.[2] Because of the change to a short, broad pedicle, from the tubed pedicle, the time element was cut from several months to days, with a tremendous saving in patient hospital days.

A DIRECT FLAP is raised and applied immediately to the recipient area with a broad, short base allowing an adequate blood supply.[2]

A DELAYED FLAP is one having a single pedicle raised in stages, progressively inducing the blood supply to enter from the attached end. The delayed flap is rarely needed because more rapid application of a flap is possible by use of a direct flap which lessens scar formation in the flap itself and saves parts that might be lost during the delay of preparation of a delayed flap graft.

TUBED PEDICLE FLAPS require even longer periods of preparation and are indicated only rarely for use on the hand.

PHYSIOTHERAPY is usually unnecessary in children, but older patients require it, depending on the depth of the burn and the rapidity of healing, and on the patient's own

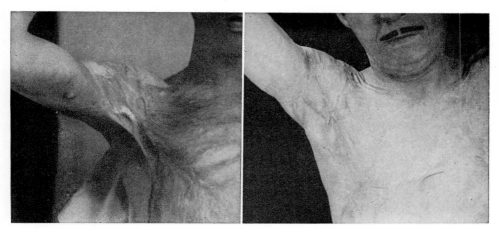

Fig. 45-6. (*Left*) Contracture of axilla resulting from spontaneous healing of a deep burn. Part of natural healing process of an open wound is contraction of the edges which, when it occurs in the neck or the axilla or any such place, pulls that part toward the heavier side or fixed part. The patient is unable to abduct the arm fully. (*Right*) Twenty years later permanent restoration of function and improvement in appearance by one operation. This consisted of the release of the contracture and excision of the deep scar, resurfacing the open area with a free graft. (Brown, J. B., and Fryer, M. P.: J. Missouri M. A. *48*:973-981)

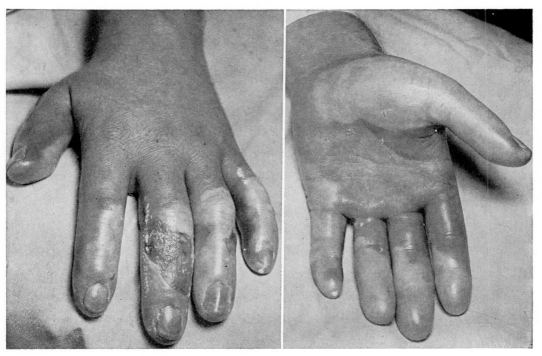

Fig. 45-7. Acute radiation burn of the hand following overexposure to fluoroscope. Blistering and deep slough. Intense pain required 3 to 5 grains of morphine a day. Received general supportive treatment and conservative management of local areas. Resection of involved skin as it definitely declared itself, with immediate coverage by free split-thickness grafts. Amputation avoided.

ideas and desires for his rehabilitation. Often in hands the setting of the joints is the most serious drawback to useful function and can occur even if the surface is restored. The sooner the surface *is* restored, however, the less joint fixation may be expected.

Irradiation burns occur frequently and often are seen in their late stages.[24, 26] They

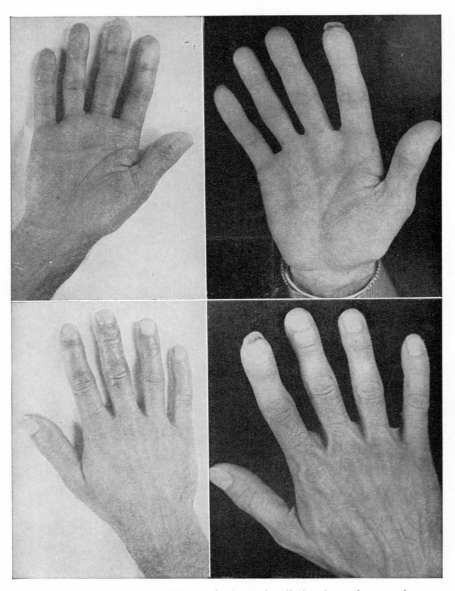

FIG. 45-8. (*Left, top and bottom*) Acute irradiation burn from cyclotron. Redness, pain and blistering following exposure to cyclotron neutron beam. Received conservative treatment to involved part with at least temporary avoidance of operation. (*Right, top and bottom*) Hand healed but result of even mild trauma to irradiated tissue seen at end of index finger. Open ulcer which looked as though it would require shortening of the finger. Again conservative care encouraged complete healing. Patient being seen at intervals with plan to excise definite, declared involvement before breakdown of the injured skin occurs.

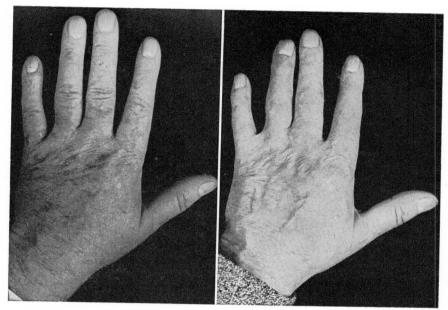

FIG. 45-9. Chronic irradiation burn of the hand. (*Left*) All the signs of chronic irradiation present with telangiectasis, "coal spots," atrophy, keratosis, ulceration and carcinoma. Due to repeated exposure to x-rays, a physician incurred these burns while taking care of others. (*Right*) Entire back of hand and the fingers was excised, and the open area was covered with split-thickness graft. One operation. Normal function. Progression to carcinoma in an irradiation burn assured if the patient lives long enough. (Brown, J. B., and Fryer, M. P.: J. Missouri M. A. *48*:973-981.

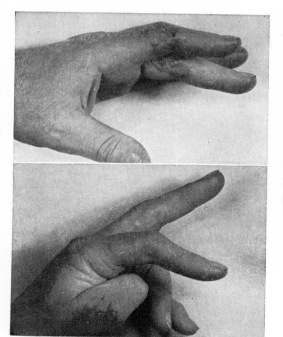

may result from recent single heavy exposure to irradiation, or from multiple smaller doses sustained years before.

THE ACUTE IRRADIATION INJURY often involves the hands, and the severe, steady, almost unbearable pain is unforgettable. Not unlike thermal burns, redness, blistering and deep slough follow the severe injuries. Resection and graft replacement of irreparably damaged skin is performed as its delimitations become clear, and the pain is relieved almost miraculously. Immediate coverage with free grafts has saved hands which appeared to be lost.

Chronic irradiation dermatitis follows a

FIG. 45-10. Chronic irradiation burn of a dentist's fingers. (*Top*) Same signs as in Figure 45-9 but had not yet proceeded to carcinoma. (*Bottom*) Involved area excised and covered immediately with free graft. One operation. Normal function. Amputation avoided.

definite predictable progression through atrophy, telangiectasis, keratosis and ulceration to ultimate carcinoma formation. Pain and itching are prominent symptoms which are relieved immediately, and carcinoma is prevented by excision of the affected areas and replacement with a free graft from other areas on the body. Usually this is done in one operation, and function is restored.

A PERMANENT PEDICLE BLOOD-CARRYING FLAP has been developed to use in the repair of some deep avascular areas resulting from irradiation.[14] Use of this type of flap actually permanently increases the vascularity of previously vascularly deficient irradiated areas which the usual pedicle flap that has to be detached from its source cannot do.

By early replacement of skin damaged by radiation, serious sequelae can be avoided, and the usefulness of irradiation therapy in general could be extended if this concept of early removal and repair were adopted.

BURNS DUE TO ATOMIC IRRADIATION are discussed because of the possible imminence of large numbers and the personal experience already obtained in the treatment of the only recorded burns of this origin.[9] In the acute phase the treatment should be the same as for any severe burn. Grease gauze pressure dressings have proved to be most satisfactory. Burns of atomic origin differ from other irradiation burns only in that local symptoms begin sooner after exposure and progress more rapidly to the chronic phase. There is local redness in a few hours, blistering begins in about a week, and the injury has either progressed to an open wound or has healed in a month. In cases of open sores early free split graft coverage is indicated. Subsequently, all injuries showing chronic irradiation effect should be resected and covered with split-thickness grafts.

It may be pointed out that at this date the only pure radiation burns of atomic origin that have been recorded have been resected and grafted without the loss of any fingers. From this first experience with such burns there is some hope offered for the control of atomic radiation damage. The only hitch is that if the whole body received such a quantity of atomic radiation as to destroy skin, life would be lost. However, when the exposure has been limited to the hand, there has

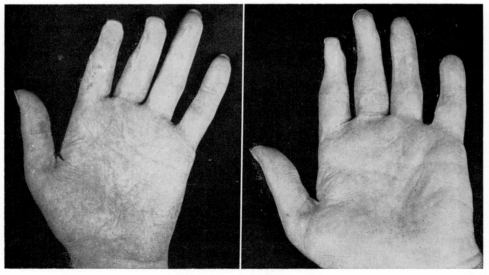

FIG. 45-11. Atomic burn of the hand. (*Left*) Rapid progression of changes to those characteristic of chronic irradiation effect, namely: atrophy, telangiectasis, "coal spots," and ulcers. (*Right*) The same hand following excision of badly damaged skin and immediate resurfacing with split-thickness grafts. The function of the hand is good. Should the excision not have been done relatively early, carcinoma would almost certainly have occurred in the damaged skin and then amputation would probably have been required.

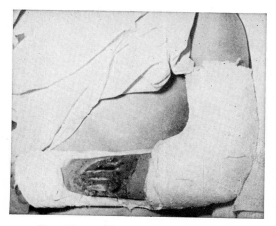
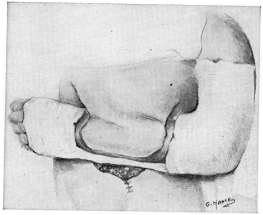

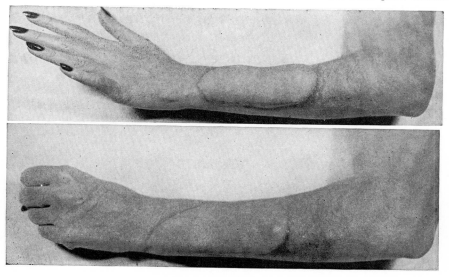

Fig. 45-12. (*Top, left*) Deep injury from gunshot wound of forearm. (*Top, right*) Drawing of application of short broad base pedicle flap from abdomen applied directly to defect in forearm. Delay of flap unnecessary. (*Bottom*) Normal function restored. Bone graft unnecessary.

been little if any systemic effect and the local repair has sufficed for good rehabilitation.

Electrical burns are considered separately because they are usually deeper but more confined than those of thermal origin. However, there may be dangerous damage to large blood vessels between the point where the electric current enters the body and its place of exit. Shock, and associated injuries, such as fractures from falling, may accompany electrical burns and require recognition and treatment. Primary or early excision and coverage of the burned areas is often possible in this type of burn. Also, a thicker type of coverage is more often necessary than that afforded by a free graft. The direct abdominal flap is of particular use in the primary repair of electrical burns to the arms and the hand and the permanent pedicle blood-carrying flaps are especially useful for the coverage of electrical burns to other parts of the body.

CLEFT LIP AND CLEFT PALATE

Cleft lip and cleft palate occur singly or in combination, at a rate of about 1 in 900 live births. The combination of cleft lip and cleft palate is slightly more common in male infants, but incomplete cleft of the palate is seen a little more often in girls. However, the ratio between sexes is almost the same, as is the side on which the cleft occurs. Double clefts of the lip and the palate are less than half as frequent as single clefts. Deformities of other parts of the body may be associated with cleft lip and palate.

Etiology of cleft lip and palate is unknown, except that it is a failure of fusion of the 3 primary segments of the face or the palate. Understanding this process, which occurs before the 2nd month of pregnancy, permits explanation for any deformity of the lip or the palate. In the face failure of fusion of the glabellar or central process with one or both lateral facial processes results in single or double cleft lip. Similarly, in the palate, when the central process does not fuse with one lateral palatine body, a single cleft of the palate results, or a double cleft of the palate follows failure on both sides.

Diagnosis of cleft lip or palate is obvious on inspection.

Deformity of the nose is usually as marked as the lip and in some instances makes acceptable repair difficult.

Scholastic standing in school by the child with a cleft lip or palate is usually above average, possibly due to greater effort or superior intelligence. Progress through life is easier now that stigma is no longer attached to this deformity. The old term of "harelip" should not be used, as it was a stigma visited on the patient because of insufficiencies of surgery and anesthesia.

Superior initial surgical repair is in a large measure responsible for the improved chance in life for these patients. Repair, when coupled with love and understanding at home, is all that is necessary to ensure a successful, happy, full life. Surgical repair is so important that some of the principles are outlined here.

CLEFT LIP REPAIR

At the initial operation prevention of deformity is sought by constructing: (1) a good alar level and direction; (2) a good nostril floor; (3) a good curve to the nostril; (4) a straight columella; (5) a full upper lip in advance of the lower lip; (6) a full vermilion; (7) if possible, a flexion crease in the lip. Widely placed sutures are avoided, as they leave "ladder" scars which are often impossible to remove without making the lip too long.[20]

Time for repair of a single cleft lip is any time after birth that it is thought safe for the child, but the sooner the better. The technical

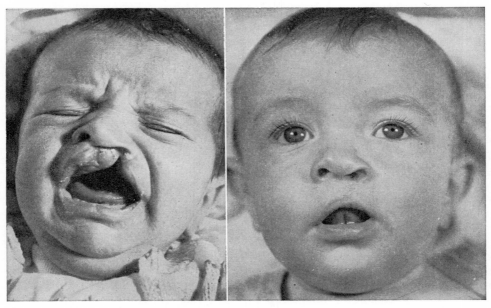

FIG. 45-13. (*Left*) Single complete cleft of lip with the usual flat nostril. (*Right*) Repaired lip and nose in one operation, using the markings illustrated in Figure 45-14. Palate to be closed later.

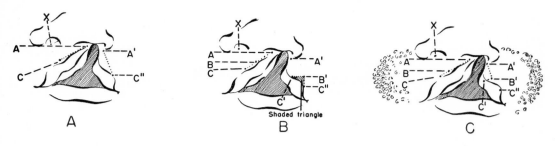

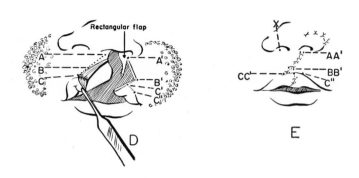

FIG. 45-14. Design for repair of single cleft lip. (A) The V-excision operation. While the columella is held over straight, A is marked at the junction of the skin and the vermilion border at the level of the base of the columella. X is in the same relation to the columella on the sound side. A′ bears the same relation to the ala on the cleft side that X bears to the ala on the normal side. C″ is on the *mucocutaneous junction* at the point where the vermilion border first begins to thin out. C is on the *mucocutaneous junction,* the same distance from A′ that C is from A. To perform the V-excision operation A′ is brought over to A, and C″ to C, after excision of the edges of the cleft.

(B) The flap operation. The V-excision operation is marked out first. C′ is on the mucocutaneous junction at the most medial point of good full vermilion border. B′ is on the line A′-C″, equidistant from C′ and C″. The incision is A′-B′-C′, saving the amount of lip indicated by the shaded isosceles triangle. B is on the mucocutaneous junction, the same distance from C that B′ is from C′.

(C) The lines A-B-C and A′-B′-C′ are incised lightly with a knife. The incision is carried upward from C′ on the mucocutaneous junction to separate the vermilion border from the skin. This is done on the other side also at A, to keep any vermilion border out of the nostril floor. The triangle (see B) is to be undermined at the next step.

(D) The lightly incised lines A-B-C and A′-B′-C′ are cut completely through the lip with a stab blade, with care to keep the knife exactly perpendicular to the lip. All angles should be opened completely. The vermilion border is inspected, and any attached skin is removed with a stab blade. The rectangular flap freed from A′-B′-C′ must be loose enough to be rotated up 180° into the nostril floor. Dotted stippling indicates areas of soft parts undermined.

(E) C and C′ are united, and the vermilion flaps are interdigitated in a zigzag fashion, fitting them so that they lie naturally together without any pull or stretching. Then suturing is continued on around the vermilion border and up the inside to the fornix. The little flap in the nostril is trimmed to fit with the one from the opposite side, and they are sutured together to form the floor. A few key mattress sutures are placed through the ala to unite the lining and the covering (which were separated during the undermining). Then the mucosa inside the lip is closed.

difficulties of repair for the surgeon should not influence this decision. It is advantageous to have the child leave the hospital with the mother, around 10 days after birth, and this is usually possible only if repair is done during the first few days of life. If the infant is jaundiced or losing weight, operation can be postponed for a few days. There is no doubt that the operation is easier to do after some weeks, and the third month has been advocated by some. Double cleft lips are not closed as soon as single clefts are. The closure is usually delayed until the infant has gained in weight or a month after birth has passed because of the longer operative time required.

The method of surgical repair of a single cleft lip summarized in Figure 45-14 is fundamentally simple and definite and permits the method of repair to fit the deformity rather than attempting the reverse. This method of marking and repair has been used for 20 years with predictably superior results.

Repair of double cleft lips is more than twice as difficult as single clefts; unfortunately, the results are usually only about half as good.[22] Notching of the vermilion is hard to avoid if full-thickness of the lip is not used in the repair, but then it is equally difficult not to make the lip too long. Repair of double cleft lips is summarized in Figure 45-16.

Secondary repair of a cleft lip or associated deformity of the nose may be necessary in spite of the best possible primary repair. When possible, tissue available in the area of the defect is readjusted. This may require flaps from the buccal fornix to advance the lip, and usually osteoplastic reconstruction of the nose, including septal resection. In extreme deformities a flap of lower lip may be set into the upper lip for proper balance between the two; "L"-shaped cartilaginous support may be added to the nose through a columellar incision; most double clefts with the usual deficient columella require elongation to get the tip of the nose up, as illustrated in the drawings in Figure 45-17. An associated "recessive ramisection" of the mandible may be necessary for proper balance between the lower jaw and the middle third of the face.

CLEFT PALATE REPAIR

Speech is a very complicated action, involving the interrelationship between thought processes and a neuro-anatomic mechanism. Children with a cleft palate may have deficiencies in any or all parts of the interacting setup. Anatomic deformities of the palate are repaired surgically as a routine procedure for perfect physiologic function. Although this does not guarantee perfect speech, because

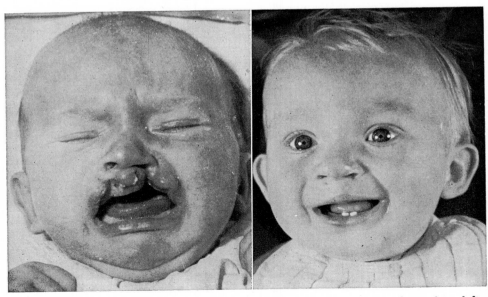

FIG. 45-15. (*Left*) Double cleft of lip with incomplete cleft on one side and complete cleft on other. (*Right*) Repaired in one operation. Palate closed later.

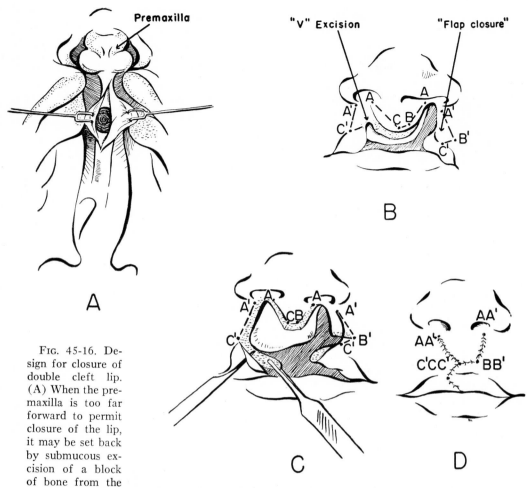

Fig. 45-16. Design for closure of double cleft lip. (A) When the premaxilla is too far forward to permit closure of the lip, it may be set back by submucous excision of a block of bone from the vomer. This removal of a block, rather than a wedge, permits the pushing of the bone directly back like closing a drawer, rather than tilting it back. This factor is of some advantage, as the finished lip should slant forward in the profile view from above downward. (B) Flap closure is done on the total side, and a V-excision operation on the partial side. (C) Both sides of the lip are opened up, going completely through the lip with a stab blade knife and using a perpendicular sawing motion. Any skin remnants are sliced off of the vermilion flaps. The vermilion border of the prolabium is cut loose from the skin and turned back all around. (D)The closure is done with many fine silk sutures, put in not more than 1 to 2 mm. from the wound edges and about as far apart. Any stay sutures are put in from the inside and are not visible. The lip is closed by interdigitating small flaps.

there may be a deficiency in other elements of this action, it should be done at as early an age as other factors will allow. *Time* for closure of a cleft palate is decided for each individual patient on the basis of growth of the maxilla which is complete enough at 4 years not to be hindered; presence of repeated attacks of otitis media, due to open communication of the middle ear with the mouth through a cleft palate, has caused deafness in some instances and has necessitated early closure of the palate. The development of faulty speech habits with an open cleft also may dictate that an earlier closure than usual be done. When necessary the palate usually can be closed in the second or the third year.

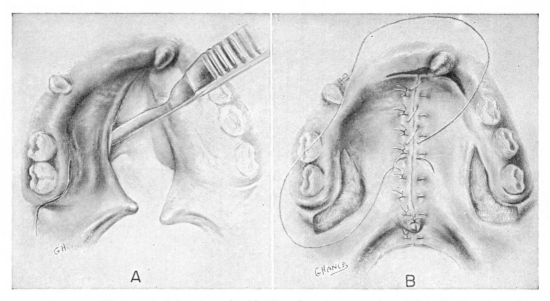

Fig. 45-17. Closure of cleft palate. (*Left*) Elevation of mucoperiosteal flaps is done through lateral incisions, including the major palatine artery, and followed by opening of medial margin. (*Right*) The medial margins of the mucoperiosteal flaps are approximated and sutured with vertical sutures. Packs in lateral incisions are removed in 48 hours.

The drawings in Figure 45-16 illustrate the method used to close a complete cleft of the palate.

CONGENITAL INSUFFICIENCY OF THE PALATE

Congenital insufficiency of the palate, wherein there is no cleft as such but a short palate with an open nasopharynx, requires elongation of the palate. Usually this can be done in one operation if there is also an incomplete cleft or if the palate actually can be split and elongated. The drawings in Figure 45-18 illustrate closure and elongation.

Careful surgical closure of a cleft palate in one operation most closely secures the approximation of the normal palatal anatomy and action. Occasionally, prosthetic appliances may be necessary to secure a degree of palatal function in swallowing and speaking if the closure has been done unsatisfactorily. These palatal prostheses are in essence a partial denture with a solid plug of plastic material attached to occlude the nasopharynx. Such an appliance cannot possibly approximate the physiologic action normally expected of a palate which has been repaired surgically in one operation.

DEFORMITIES AND INFLAMMATORY DISEASES OF THE JAWS

The common deformities of the mandible requiring surgery are micrognathia and macrognathia (mandibular, underdevelopment and overgrowth, respectively).

MICROGNATHIA

Micrognathia, which is a short underdeveloped mandible, may be associated with a short incomplete cleft of the palate. The infant with this deformity may have considerable difficulty breathing shortly after birth and requires careful nursing care to survive. Forward fixation of the tongue to the lip to pull the tongue forward so that it does not occlude the upper airway or even tracheotomy may be necessary at this time. Both of these procedures are to be avoided as long as breathing and feeding can be developed satisfactorily with meticulous nursing care.

Treatment. The surgical treatment of micrognathia is first directed toward effecting the immediate survival of the infant by securing a safely open airway by fixation of the tongue to the lip or tracheotomy. Surgical efforts to increase the rate of growth of the jaw have not been successful. Later orthodontic procedures may be very useful, especially if the jaw itself can be moved forward rather than only slanting the teeth forward. At any rate, by orthodontia the occlusion of the teeth should be achieved to the point where they will be as normal as possible. After maximal growth in the mandible has been attained, the type of treatment is decided on the basis of function and appearance. If the occlusion is relatively normal or is functional, the receding chin can be built up by adding bone or cartilage to the outer surface of the mandible beneath the periosteum without disturbing the relationship of the upper and the lower teeth. This operation is done through a small incision

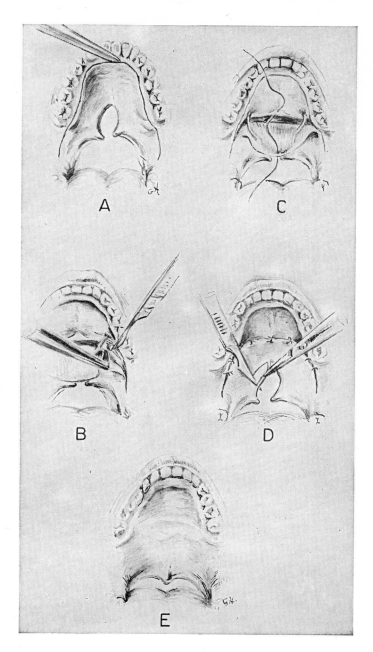

FIG. 45-18. Closure and elongation of partially cleft palate in one operation. (A) Incision is made as shown, and the entire palate is elevated as a mucoperiosteal flap. (B) Soft tissue separated and major palatine artery brought out of canal. (C) Edge of flap being sutured to band of nasal mucosa. (D) Medial margin of palatal defect opened. (E) Palate has been closed and elongated in one operation. Defect in hard palate has healed in 1 month. (Brown, J. B.: Surg., Gynec. & Obst. *63*:768)

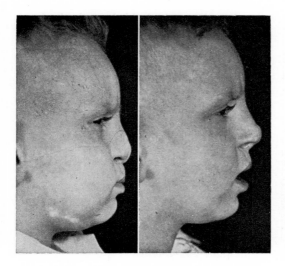

FIG. 45-19. Profile before and after elongation of columella from upper lip as illustrated in diagram Figure 45-20. (*Left*) Before and (*right*) after operation of total reconstruction of the columella from upper lip, getting tip of nose up out of lip and creating proper angle between the nose and the lip.

beneath the chin or near the angle of the jaw through which cartilage or bone is built up on the mandible by inserting it beneath the elevated periosteum in order to get the closest contact. Synthetics or bank cartilage may be employed.

If the occlusion is poor, with the upper teeth so far anterior to the lower that even

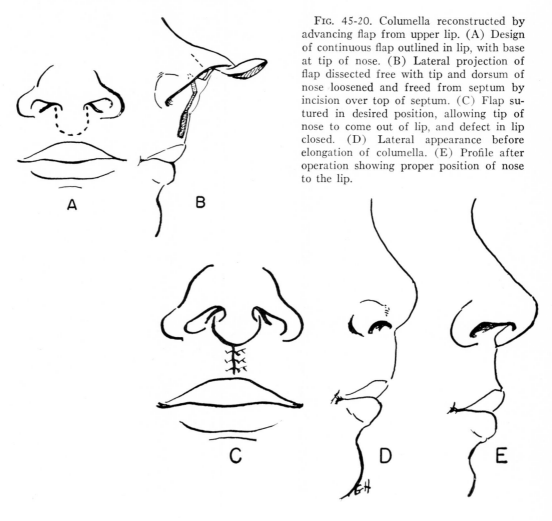

FIG. 45-20. Columella reconstructed by advancing flap from upper lip. (A) Design of continuous flap outlined in lip, with base at tip of nose. (B) Lateral projection of flap dissected free with tip and dorsum of nose loosened and freed from septum by incision over top of septum. (C) Flap sutured in desired position, allowing tip of nose to come out of lip, and defect in lip closed. (D) Lateral appearance before elongation of columella. (E) Profile after operation showing proper position of nose to the lip.

FIG. 45-21. Prognathism. Before and after views of results of recessive ramisection of lower jaw as shown in diagram Figure 45-22. (*Top, left*) Profile showing imbalance between upper and lower jaws and impossible occlusion and (*top, right*) proper balance of face and good occlusion after operation. (*Bottom, left*) Front view before operation with marked improvement (*bottom, right*) as in profile.

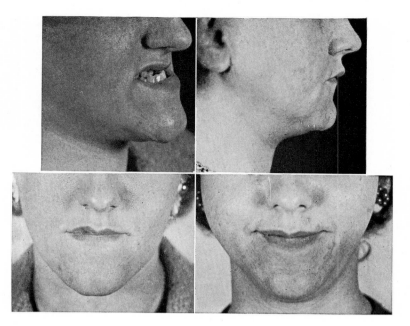

proper mastication may be impossible, they can be placed in better relationship by displacing the mandible forward after section through the rami. The technic of ramisection is illustrated in Figure 45-22 where it is used to correct macrognathia. In the case of micrognathia the jaw is moved forward instead of backward. Fixation of the jaw in its new position is maintained with interdental wires for up to 12 weeks.

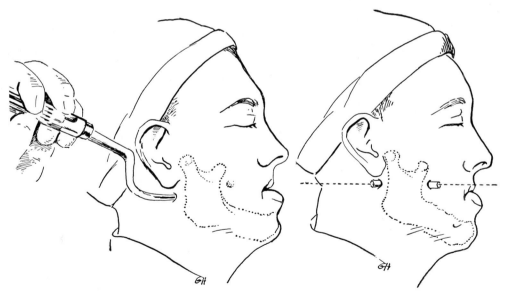

FIG. 45-22. Correction of prognathism by closed ramisection of the mandible. (*Left*) Large jaw needle passed closely behind the ascending ramus of the mandible through 1 cm. skin incisions placed at anterior and posterior borders of jaw, avoiding facial nerve and entrance into mouth. Then a Gigli saw is attached to the end of the jaw needle so that by withdrawing the needle, the saw is in position on the inside of the jaw.

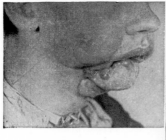
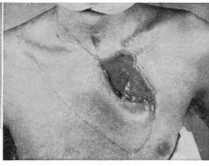
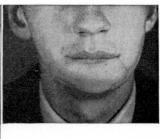

Fig. 45-23. (*Left*) Gunshot loss lower third of face with large defect in mandible. (*Center*) Delayed flat flap from chest with a side flap turned in from above to line the flap and form the lining of the inside of the mouth. Flap made mouth watertight and prevented further flow of saliva on the chest. Defect in chest covered with free graft. (*Right*) Flap has covered soft tissue defect in lower third of face and permitted bone graft to be placed between ends of the mandible. Soft tissue coverage was necessary before bone graft could be done. Jaw is solid. (Brown, J. B., and Fryer, M. P.: Am. J. Surg. *85*:401-406)

MACROGNATHIA

Macrognathia attends overgrowth of the mandible and is the opposite of micrognathia. Often the lower teeth are displaced more anteriorly relative to their upper counterparts.

Diagnosis of macrognathia is obvious on inspection alone.

Treatment depends on the position of the teeth. If the occlusion is relatively normal and does not need correction, the enlarged portion of the mandible may be removed locally by simply cutting off bone subperiosteally from the external surface. If the occlusion of the teeth is not satisfactory, the entire mandible may be set back in one operation after section through the rami has been done, as illustrated in Figure 45-22. Fixation with interdental wiring up to 12 weeks results in permanent normal relationship between the upper and the lower teeth.

In these rearrangements of the dental occlusion dental consultation is necessary, and casts of the teeth are required. In addition, cutting down of certain of the teeth is often necessary.

Other surgical methods involve resection of the body of the ramus at a high level for prognathism, and forward positioning in the body of the jaw for micrognathia.

ARTHRITIS OF THE JAW

Arthritis commonly occurs at the temporomandibular joint, and the complaint is of pain in the joint, limitation of opening, cracking, locking, with occasional progress to fixation in the joint. Roentgenograms may show erosion of the joint or narrowing.

Treatment of arthritis consists of putting the joint at rest by the patient's own efforts with foods and the gentlest uses, by bandaging from chin to vertex, or interdental wiring may be required. Reefing of the capsule has been suggested, as well as several local procedures of fixation. Resection of the joint disk should be resorted to only in very occasional instances.

INFLAMMATORY DISEASES OF THE JAWS

Osteomyelitis usually includes all inflammatory diseases of the jaw, but division can be made on the basis of etiologic agent, osteomyelitis being an inflammatory process in the bone due to staphylococcus or streptococcus, tuberculosis, actinomycosis, syphilis, metals, heat, irradiation, and trauma.[25]

The anatomy of the jaws is important, as it influences the inflammatory process, and the teeth are the most important difference between the jaws and other bones, since their normal position in the jaws establishes a path for deep infection. Where the spongiosum is thicker in the maxilla, as in the incisor, canine and tubercle regions, infection is most severe. In the mandible the thickest areas are around the angle extending forward and up, and infection here is most persistent.

Osteomyelitis usually is caused by staphylococci and streptococci, and often they are found in the smear and the culture with the other usual mouth organisms. Anaerobic culture often grows out melanogenicum. This organism may account for the foul odor of the purulent drainage. Other anaerobic organisms may also be present.

ETIOLOGY. *Affected teeth* are the commonest cause of osteomyelitis of the jaws. A periapical abscess is a localized osteomyelitis which may spread, should the tooth be extracted during the acute phase. Pericoronitis is an inflammatory process in the soft tissue pocket around a partially erupted third molar or wisdom tooth. This infection can also spread to the jaw, the mouth and the neck upon the extraction of the affected tooth during the acute phase.

Fractures of the jaw are the second most common cause of osteomyelitis because breaks of the jaw are so often associated with lacerations of the mucosa around the teeth. These mucosal breaks set up avenues for infection of the bone in the zone of fracture.

Draining cysts, blood stream infections, injuries to the mucosa around the teeth, the metastasis from osteomyelitis elsewhere are other causes of osteomyelitis but are rarely seen and then practically only in debilitated

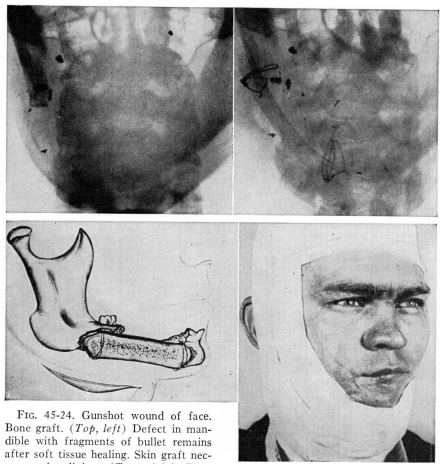

FIG. 45-24. Gunshot wound of face. Bone graft. (*Top, left*) Defect in mandible with fragments of bullet remains after soft tissue healing. Skin graft necessary for lining. (*Top, right*) Bone graft in place held with wire to ends of bone acting as its own splint. Rib graft was used in this instance. (*Bottom, left*) Diagram of bone graft held to bone with wires. (*Bottom, right*) Firm pressure dressing aids fixation of jaw and promotes healing. (Brown, J. B., and Fryer, M. P.: Postgrad. Med. 4:420-434)

patients. The nasal cavity and sinuses are additional sources of osteomyelitis in the upper jaw.

DIAGNOSIS. *Acute osteomyelitis* is diagnosed on the history of severe pain and diffuse swelling of the jaw with the general signs of infection as fever, leukocytosis and general malaise, usually starting after the extraction of an acutely infected tooth or following a fracture. Periorbital edema may be the most prominent sign of osteomyelitis in the upper jaw. Roentgenograms at this early stage usually fail to demonstrate signs of a destructive inflammatory process, but within 10 days an extension of the cavity left by the extracted tooth or dissolution of bone around the fracture may be demonstrable roentgenographically. *Chronic osteomyelitis* is diagnosed by a history of recurrent flare-ups, multiple sinus tracts and the draining of purulent material and pieces of bone. Roentgenograms show sequestra, cavities and later the formation of an involucrum.

TREATMENT of osteomyelitis is primarily prevention. This consists of postponing the extraction of the acutely inflamed tooth, and the routine drainage of the fractured jaw. Surgical drainage of acute periapical abscesses is done gently alongside the tooth over the swollen area. Large doses of antibiotics have been effective in avoiding osteomyelitis and preventing the spread if already present. Acute osteomyelitis is treated conservatively; drainage of the affected bone through soft tissues is established with the least possible operative trauma. In the chronic stage fluctuant areas are opened, but sequestra are not removed until adequate involucrum has developed to support the jaw. Tooth buds are not removed indiscriminately.

Tuberculosis. Tuberculous infection of the jaw is seen occasionally with pulmonary involvement. Diagnosis is made on the history of a slightly painful swelling over the jaw which may be fluctuant. Later a fistula may form. Roentgenograms may show spotty areas of necrosis. Final proof of diagnosis rests upon the identification of tubercle bacilli by culture methods. Treatment may be started with repeated aspiration of pus but should this,

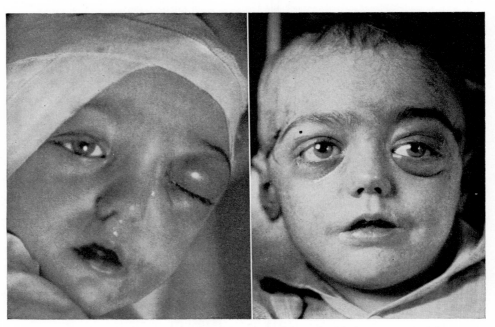

FIG. 45-25. Osteomyelitis. Typical swelling of the lids and orbital content noted in osteomyelitis of the upper jaw and the zygoma. This lesion occurred in the course of a general osteomyelitis and also occurred in the right side, as shown by the scar in the temporal region in view at right 2½ months later. (Brown, J. B., and Fryer, M. P.: The Cyclopedia of Medicine, Surgery and Specialties, vol. 7, pp. 553-562, Philadelphia, Davis)

FIG. 45-26. Actinomycosis of lower jaw. (*Left*) Brawny swelling of lower jaw treated by multiple drainage operations and sequestrectomies. (*Right*) Major portion of lower jaw saved and infection cured.

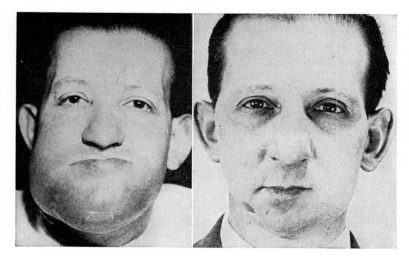

together with streptomycin, not effect a cure, excision of the affected bone is necessary. To the present, streptomycin has been the most useful antibiotic for tuberculous osteomyelitis.

Actinomycosis often follows the extraction of a tooth. Its first signs appear several days after the extraction as a slightly tender swelling over the jaw. Later the swelling extends into the neck, and still later multiple cutaneous fistulae develop. Roentgenograms may show multiple sites of decreased density in the jaw. The finding of "sulfur granules" in the drainage material and cultural identification of the organism complete the diagnosis. Treatment consists of drainage and the use of antibiotics (sulfadiazine 4 Gm. daily with penicillin 50,000 to 100,000 units daily).

Radical excision of the afflicted area may be necessary later should the treatment outlined above fail.

Irradiation necrosis is probably the most painful of the inflammatory processes involving the jaw. Usually the lesion is widespread. Radical débridement of bone and soft tissue may be necessary to relieve the pain. The reconstruction necessary is usually equally difficult because the healing of heavily irradiated tissues is slow.

Ankylosis of the jaw may follow an inflammatory process in the temporomandibular region or a gunshot wound.[28] Soft tissue scarring may require removal and replacement, along with excision of a block of bone to create a false joint. The mouth should be

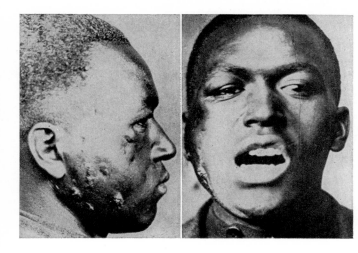

FIG. 45-27. Actinomycosis, showing multiple draining in later stages of infection than in Figure 45-25.

"blocked open" following resection. Ankylosis on both sides is extremely serious. Bilateral operation should rarely be carried out because of excessive retraction, crippling and loss of normal contour that attend it. Although arthroplasty or replacement is not uniformly successful, very careful evaluation and effort should be put forth before considering a bilateral resection of both mandibular joints.

RECONSTRUCTION OF THE JAW

Restitution of a functional arch is the aim following loss of the jaw by any means. Resection of hard, contracting scar in the mouth and on the outside and replacement with soft viable tissue may be necessary before a bone graft can be placed between the remaining ends of the jaw. Autografts of rib or ilium should be used because these defects must be bridged by living solid bone. For this reason nonviable bone from a bank is not used to repair jaw defects. However, appearance may be improved following loss of the jaw bone, by preserved cartilage placed on the remaining misshapen bone beneath its periosteum. This may have to be put upon the intact hemimandible because the intact side collapses toward the side of loss, thereby flattening out the side of the face opposite the loss and making a bulge on the damaged side.

COMPOUND FACIAL INJURIES

Compound facial injury connotes simultaneous injury to the soft parts and the bones of the face.[5] The term "compound" is outmoded for other fractures, but when the nose, the eyelids, the lacrimal duct, or other features or systems are involved, it is a compound injury by virtue of its complexity. This term emphasizes the importance of recognizing facial fractures which may be masked initially by soft tissue laceration, contusion and swelling. If bony displacement is overlooked, healing occurs, and reduction later may be impossible, though the deformity becomes obvious after the soft tissue injury has healed. Severe trauma recognizes no anatomic boundaries; separation here is only for purposes of description.

EMERGENCY CARE

Emergency care of compound facial injuries includes the provision of an airway, the control of bleeding and splinting of the injured parts. Patients with fractures of the mandible that loosen the support of the tongue or with severe intra-oral or cervical bleeding may require tracheotomy for survival. However, positioning and anchoring most mandible fractures is sufficient to secure an open airway. Bleeding from large neck muscles requires

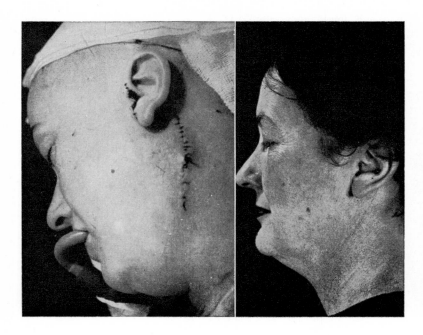

FIG. 45-28. (*Left*) Small, fine sutures placed near the edge of an incision or laceration closed the wound without adding scar. (*Right*) Wound healed. This also illustrates the author's method of approaching the parotid.

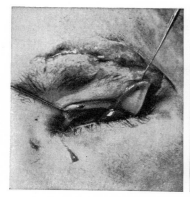
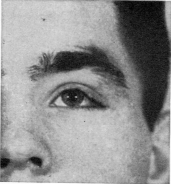
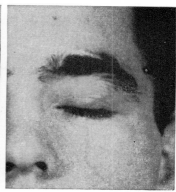

FIG. 45-29. Through-and-through laceration of upper eyelid. (*Left*) Primarily repaired in one operation, maintaining protection of eye and obviating necessity of secondary reconstruction of eyelid (*center and right*).

ligation of individual vessels near or at the point of discontinuity. Neck vessel ligation for facial or mouth hemorrhage at points distant from the site of injury is practically useless and may add further trouble. Support of a loose jaw or torn soft parts with a Barton type bandage may increase comfort and avoid the use of sedatives and analgesics which might compromise breathing.

REPAIR

The time to repair a compound facial injury is as soon as the patient's general condition permits. Shock, brain damage, dangerous cervical spine fractures, or intoxication are contraindications to early operation. However, by virtue of the fact that bony fragments become permanently fixed out of position if reduction is not done in 10 to 14 days, the reduction needs be effected within that time limit after injury.

Roentgenograms of the face, the skull and the cervical spine are important parts of the examination of all severe facial injuries, though it may be impossible to obtain all wanted views before definitive repair is undertaken.

General condition of the patient is considered after a careful physical examination and consultation with other specialists. The presence of brain or peripheral nerve damage is tested for routinely, and fractures of other bones and abdominal injury are to be suspected and sought after. It is especially important to record the function of the 2nd, the 5th and the 7th nerves before any operation upon the injured face. *Shock* is often present, and when it is it requires treatment before repairing the facial injury. However, as stated in Chapter 7, "Shock," operative intervention for the control of hemorrhage is a most important therapeutic measure in treating shock

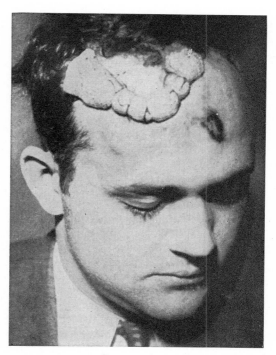

FIG. 45-30. Method of wound closure by sutures tied over roll of gauze, avoiding stay suture marks.

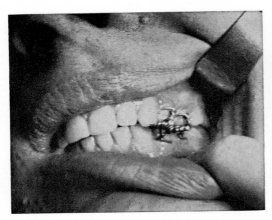

FIG. 45-31. Interdental wiring. Simple fixation of lower jaw to upper jaw by No. 24 steel wires placed around bicuspids, using upper jaw as splint for fractured mandible.

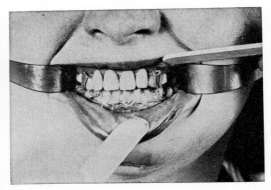

FIG. 45-32. Interdental wire and elastic fixation for fractured mandible. Elastic bands placed over twisted ends of No. 26 steel wire applied to opposing teeth in patient's normal occlusion. Continuous lower wire arch shown around lower teeth gives further fixation.

in an actively bleeding patient. Consequently, delaying the operation in order to treat shock should be practiced only in those cases in which rapid bleeding has stopped. Tetanus protection is given routinely, and antibiotics are used as indicated. (See Chap. 4, "Surgical Infections.")

The repair of facial injuries, excepting the simple superficial ones, should be done in an operating room. All facilities and assistance should be used for the best possible repair.

Anesthesia. Local block is used in small lacerations and can be used in extensive repairs, but general anesthesia is often necessary. If general anesthesia is used, an airway must be provided with an endotracheal tube.

SOFT TISSUE REPAIR

Simple Lacerations

Simple lacerations are closed carefully with adequate anesthesia secured by infiltrating the wound margins with ½ to 1 per cent procaine or lidocaine. Facial wounds never are packed open. In closing a facial laceration, known or recognizable normal coaptation points are first approximated with fine suture material placed in the subcutaneous tissue, then the remainder of the separation is closed by suturing the skin by progressively bisecting the distances between sutures until the wound is closely coapted in its entirety. Before the skin is closed bleeding points are ligated indi-

vidually, and hematomas are evacuated. Fine silk sutures placed close to the wound margins prevent slippage of the wound margins by each other. Widely placed sutures which permit slippage leave permanent "ladder type"

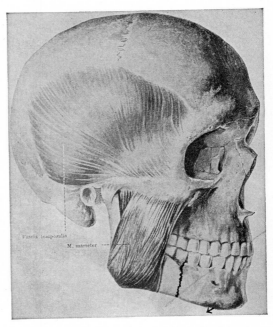

FIG. 45-33. Drawing showing attachment of muscles on angle of jaw and ascending ramus which may determine position of fragments in this area following fracture.

scars that upon the face are remarkably dis-figuring because they may never be removed by any number of secondary operations. If one cannot place stitches closely it is prefer-able to permit a facial wound to heal spon-taneously by leaving it open without packing than to leave widely placed sutures in an attempt to effect partial closure. The residual scarring is less with the wound left open than closed with widely placed sutures. If the wound must be closed under some tension, sutures may be tied over the dressing, as illus-trated in Figure 45-29.

Primary repair may require a free graft for closure, but local or distant flaps are rarely required at this stage. Innumerable secondary procedures may be avoided by a careful pains-taking initial repair. The *dressing* applied should fix the wound and apply steady, even pressure. The dressing is a most important

part of the repair. Adhesive strapping gives adequate fixation, and a gauze bandage wound around the part over fine mesh grease gauze and sterile mechanics waste secures pressure, invites healing and prevents pain. Cutaneous sutures in the face are removed after 4 or 5 days, but the fixation of the wound by adhe-sive strapping and pressure bandaging is main-tained for several more days.

FRACTURES OF THE MANDIBLE

Mandibular fractures are reduced and fixed in the simplest direct method available until union results.

Diagnosis of a fractured jaw is made by palpation which will usually elicit point

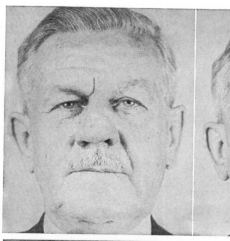
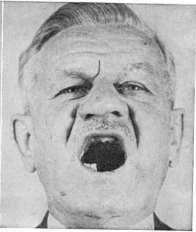
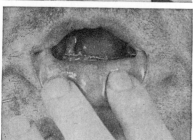
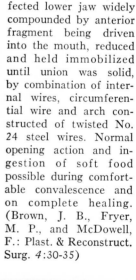
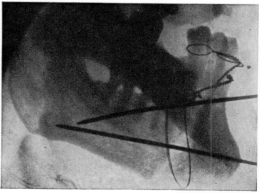

FIG. 45-34. Severe, splintered, locally in-fected lower jaw widely compounded by anterior fragment being driven into the mouth, reduced and held immobilized until union was solid, by combination of inter-nal wires, circumferen-tial wire and arch con-structed of twisted No. 24 steel wires. Normal opening action and in-gestion of soft food possible during comfort-able convalescence and on complete healing. (Brown, J. B., Fryer, M. P., and McDowell, F.: Plast. & Reconstruct. Surg. *4*:30-35)

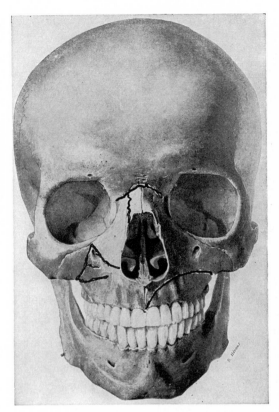

Fig. 45-35. Drawing illustrating major potential lines of separation in middle third facial fractures. One or all may be present. Comminution of smaller bones usually occurs in conjunction with displacement of larger bone elements.

tenderness, and by roentgenograms in the postero-anterior and both lateral views. Swelling is usually diffuse, but the presence of a laceration in the mouth may indicate the point of fracture.

Full reduction is judged to have been accomplished when the teeth in the maxilla and the mandible are in the patient's normal occlusion. Fractures of the edentulous mandible are palpated readily, and their reduction is determined by touch.

Drainage is established routinely from the point of mandibular fracture to the outside whenever the oral mucosa has been disrupted by placing a small incision beneath the jaw in the neck, taking care to avoid the mandibular branch of the facial nerve and vessels.

Fixation after reduction is done most simply with interdental wiring, using No. 26 or 24 steel wire, between apposing bicuspids, as illustrated in Figure 45-31. A *twisted wire arch* may give fixation in another plane by being closed around a lower molar tooth on each side and brought together in front with individual wires to other teeth as necessary. Solid union usually requires from 6 to 8 weeks of fixation.

Internal wire-pin fixation of a fractured mandible is necessary when proper teeth are not available in all fragments or the jaw is completely edentulous. They are also indicated when a prolonged period of time has elapsed before reduction and fixation; with extensive comminution; when a large soft tissue defect opening into the mouth is present; and when the fracture is in an area with a known tendency to nonunion such as the symphysis mentis.[6] Kirschner wires, .045 or .062 size, are driven across the fracture site with a power drill and may be used alone or in conjunction with interdental or direct bone wiring. The use of these wire pins often allows relatively normal eating during the period of healing. As many pins are used as the type of fracture requires.

Condylar fractures may require an open operation for reduction. However, satisfactory function usually can be obtained by fixation of the jaw in the patient's normal occlusion for 3 weeks with interdental wiring.

MIDDLE THIRD FACIAL FRACTURES

Fracture-Dislocation of the Zygoma

This is one of the commonest types of facial bone fractures. The natural position of this facial bone predisposes it to this injury—the zygoma is somewhat analogous to the bumper on an automobile. Usually the force of the trauma dislocates, rather than fractures, the bone from all of its attachments, crushing the surrounding thinner facial bones such as those of the antral walls or the orbital floor. Diplopia often follows a fracture-dislocation of the zygoma when the orbital floor is displaced. Anesthesia over the distribution of the infra-orbital nerve may be present also. Failure to bring the displaced zygoma back into normal position flattens that side of the face. *Diagnosis* usually can be made by palpation of the zygoma, even though there may be con-

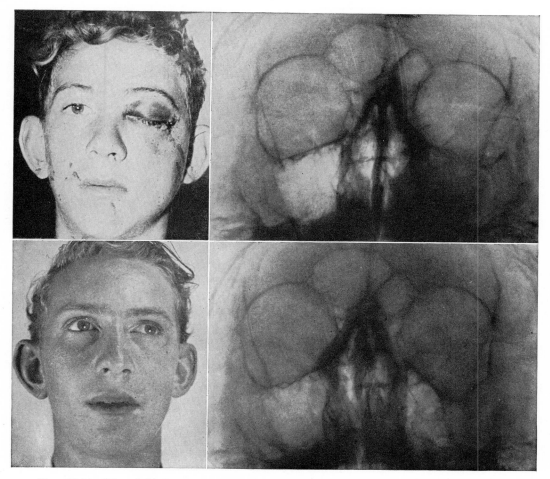

FIG. 45-36. (*Top, left*) Fracture-dislocation of the zygomatic bone with crumbling in of the antral wall and dropping of the orbital border. (*Top, right*) Appearance when first seen with contusion of eyelid, laceration and flatness of zygomatic region. (*Bottom, left*) Appearance 6 months following reduction. (*Bottom, right*) Result 6 weeks following immediate reduction by direct approach through the buccal fornix into antrum. (Brown, J. B., and Fryer, M. P.: Postgrad. Med. *6*:400-406)

siderable swelling. Roentgenograms of the facial bones in the posterior-anterior or modified Waters positions to show the orbital borders are taken routinely and are very valuable diagnostically and as means of determining adequacy of reduction in some cases.

Reduction of a fracture-dislocation of the zygoma may be done through the outside of the face with a *large jaw hook*, as shown in Figure 45-36. If the fragments become impacted during reduction, nothing further is required. However, if reduction is not maintained spontaneously, the zygoma may be sup-

ported by placing a pack in the antrum. A *wire pin* driven through the loose zygoma across the face through the opposite zygoma can give cantilever support adequate for the maintenance of reduction and the securing of solid union.[4]

Extensive comminution of the antral walls and the orbital floor by a displaced or fractured zygoma requires accurate replacement of the multiple small fragments. Entrance into the antrum is made through buccal mucosa and then through the fracture line, and after reduction of the zygoma with an elevator or a

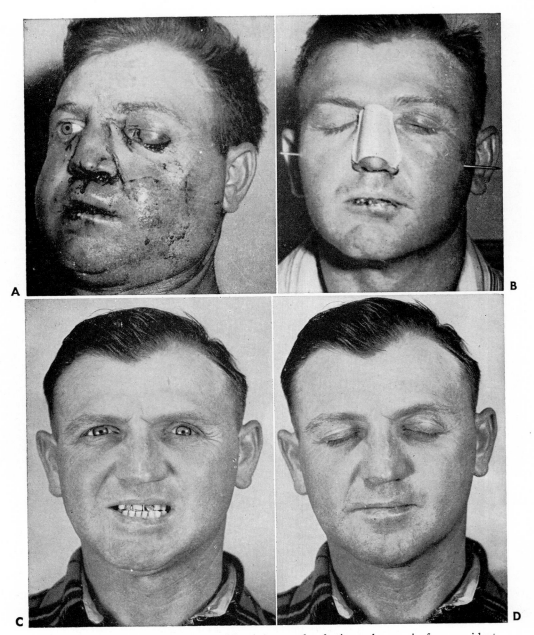

FIG. 45-37 A to D. Extensive crushing injury and soft tissue damage in farm accident. Not much stable bone was left, and practically no shape to the nose, which was torn loose and inverted into the face. Operation was performed within 12 hours under intratracheal anesthesia. The reverse of what the accident did was carried out in "unfolding" the nose and the face, elevating the left orbit and fixing the parts with cross wires and aluminum splint for the nose and with one internal wire for the shattered pyramidal fracture and the left zygomatic displacement.

Fig. 45-37 (*Cont.*) E, F. Roentgenogram shows pin in place and the zygoma restored along with the orbital border. The left eyelid is torn completely open so that the eye looks through the rent. This case is an excellent example of the necessity of early operation. To wait 10 days, as has been advised elsewhere, would result in possible eye damage and the need of multiple operations. This patient has had full restoration and rehabilitation in one operation. No further work is necessary. (Brown, J. B., Fryer, M. P., and McDowell, F.: Surg., Gynec. & Obst. *93*:676-681)

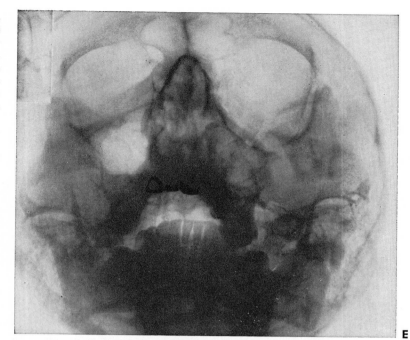

E

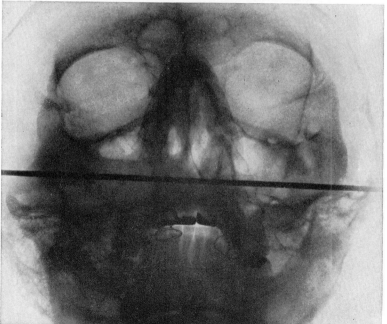

F

Kelly clamp in the antrum, the fragments are "mulched" or pressed into place and held in place with an iodoform pack into which balsam of Peru has been incorporated. The pack serves as an internal splint holding the zygoma, the antrum and the orbital floor in proper relationship until primary tissue fixation occurs. Obviously, it can be removed from 12 to 14 days after the reduction.

Transverse facial fractures may involve the alveolus above or extend up across the pyriform space into either or both zygomas. At a

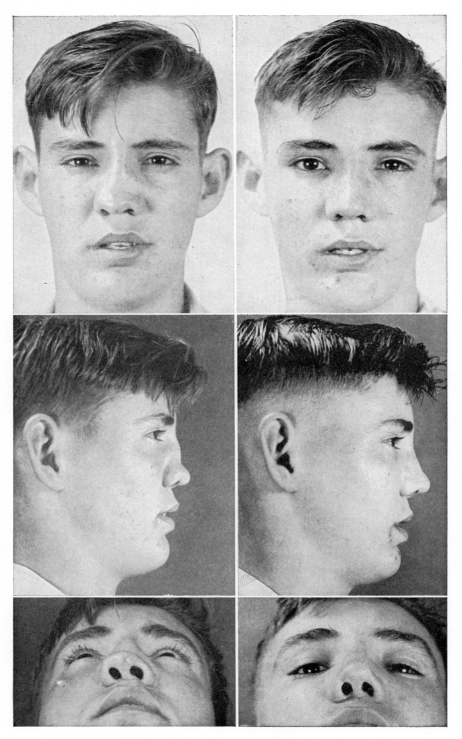

FIG. 45-38. (*Left*) Result of childhood fracture. (*Right*) Elevation and reconstruction of supports of nose done in one operation.

higher level the transverse fracture tends to extend through both orbits so as to effect a complete detachment of the entire face from the skull. A roentgenogram may show little, but an adequate examination readily shows the extent of the injury. *Alveolar fractures* after reduction may be stabilized by a wire arch with interdental wires, using the lower

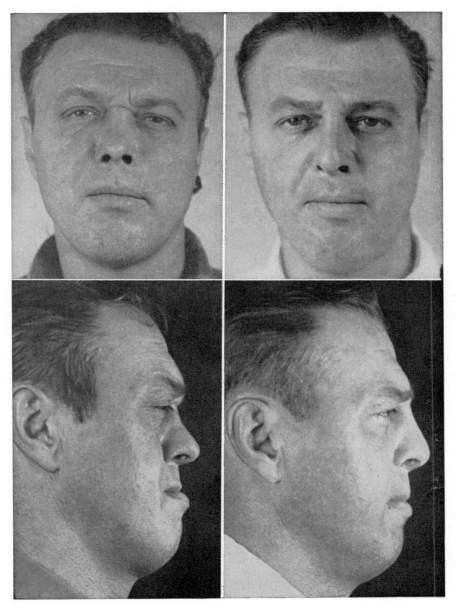

FIG. 45-39. The whole face and the nose were pushed back or caved in, from a traffic accident. The patient was seen late when bones were firm in depressed position. The whole face built forward with 4 cartilage transplants, both orbital borders, across under nose from side to side, and L-shaped transplant for dorsum of nose and columella. (Brown, J. B., and Fryer, M. P.: Postgrad. Med. 4:420-434)

jaw as a splint for the upper. However, internal wire pin fixation may be used alone or in combination with dental wiring. Other *transverse facial fractures* are reduced and then stabilized by interdental wiring in combination with internal wire pins.[13] Reduction of transverse fractures involves applying a force in the direction opposite to the force that caused the displacement. In many instances the displacing force has been applied in an upward as well as a backward direction and has pushed the upper jaw up as well as back. External traction-fixation devices actually tend to increase rather than decrease the deformity in such fractures.

Fractures of the Nose

Fractures of the nose are the most frequently seen facial fractures. They should be reduced and stabilized as in the case of any other fracture. Bleeding from the nose following trauma to the outside indicates that the lining of the nose has been lacerated by a fractured bone or cartilage.[19] Consequently, direct examination of the nasal passages and roentgenograms always should be made in order to establish the cause of the bleeding and the extent and the nature of the fracture. Nasal fractures are a particular problem in children because many remain displaced with progressive deformation of the nose until growth stops; in addition, even though the initial reduction has been good, growth deformity may occur. After reduction, fractures of the nose usually can be stabilized properly with an external aluminum splint and nasal packing. Badly depressed comminuted nasal fractures may require the passage of wires beneath the nose and their anchorage to lead plates on the sides in order to maintain proper position. In cases of residual nasal deformity in children, *secondary reconstruction* usually is done after nasal growth is complete. Marked distortion of the nose can be improved and the dorsum built up with preserved cartilage transplants after growth has been attained, as shown in Figure 45-39. Recently, plastic materials seem to have some advantage as a subcutaneous prosthesis. Dimethyl siloxanes, halogenated carbons and polyvinyl alcohol are being used as supports.[27]

Severe Facial Crushes

Severe facial crushes involving many facial bones usually require multiple means of stabilizing the multiple fragments. *Internal wire pins* can be used to hold both zygomas securely enough for union to occur, and in addition be made to serve as a base for the fixation of other fractures of the face.[6] Both antra can be held by loose packs introduced as superimposed folds through openings made in the buccal fornix. Direct bone wiring may be used wherever applicable. Alveolar and other transverse fractures can be held with internal wires driven obliquely, using the zygoma for cantilever support. External traction apparatus is expensive, cumbersome and unnecessary for the treatment of even severe facial crushes.

FACIAL PARALYSIS

The paralyzed face, whatever its cause, need not be suffered without treatment. The paralyzed face can be supported and some degree of animation secured by anchoring loops of fascia lata between the corners of the mouth and the temporalis muscle.

Etiology

Paralysis of the facial nerve may have as its origin congenital defects, infections, trauma (operative and other) and neoplastic invasion.

Congenital facial paralysis may be central or peripheral, unilateral or bilateral, complete or incomplete with involvement of any or all branches or divisions.

Infection involving the facial nerve, directly or indirectly by pressure, may induce partial paralysis when it involves a peripheral branch or complete paralysis when it affects the nerve in the parotid gland, or in the facial canal. The degree or extent of paralysis is dependent on where along the course of the nerve the inflammation, trauma or cancer impinges.

Operative paralysis of the facial nerve is usually the result of operations on the mastoid or the parotid gland. However, parotid tumors can be removed safely without damage to the facial nerve.[10]

Benign tumors in the parotid gland do not cause facial paralysis, even though very large. The facial nerve has been found flattened to a ribbon by pressure from a large benign tumor without any demonstrable evidence of distal paralysis. To the contrary, malignant tumors within the parotid gland are associated with facial nerve paralysis to a remarkably high degree, so much so that one can be fairly certain that a neoplasm within the parotid is malignant when facial paralysis and tumor coexist.

DIAGNOSIS

The diagnosis of facial paralysis is usually obvious, even with the face at rest. The face is flat and drooped, and the lid slit is widened. The degree of involvement may be judged fairly accurately by having the patient actively move all parts of the face. With acute complete paralysis, eating and talking may be very difficult.

TREATMENT

Musculofascial active support of the paralyzed face and some degree of animation can be secured by inserting loops of fascia lata beneath the skin from the corners of the mouth and anchoring them in the temporalis muscle near its tendon. By this maneuver a muscle innervated by the 5th cranial nerve is made to perform a function previously attended to by ones supplied by the 7th.

Occasionally fascial nerve anastomosis and substitution may be used to restore facial nerve function, but even if such a procedure is indicated and contemplated, overstretching of the face should be avoided by support of the face with fascial loops while nerve regeneration is awaited.

The fascial strip repair is effected by removing strips of fascia lata over 1 cm. wide and 25 to 30 cm. long with a stripper of the Masson type.[7] These strips are passed through an incision above the hairline in the temple region to the upper and the lower lips and looped back up and anchored in the temporalis muscle near the tendon. This placement near the tendon makes for the maximum

movement, as illustrated in Figure 45-40. The long fascial needle used to pass the fascia is drawn in the lower part of Figure 45-40. The smaller curved needle is used to implant the fascia in the temporalis muscle.

Support of the face by this method permits the construction of a flexion crease in the naso-labial region. The loss of this crease is the most noticeable deformity attendant upon facial paralysis, even with the face in repose.

In a somewhat similar way the drooped

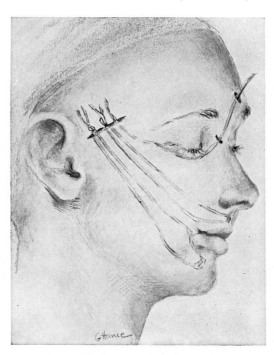

FIG. 45-40. (*Top*) Autogenous fascia lata strips looped to elevate paralyzed face, fixed in temporal muscle and tendon. Lost 7th nerve action is substituted for by 5th nerve temporal muscle action. Upper separate loop through the lower eyelid helps to hold it in contact with the globe, along with external canthoplasty. (*Bottom*) Fascia needles.

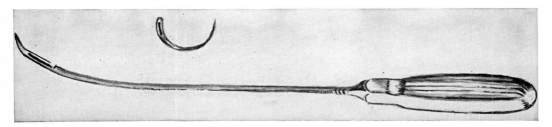

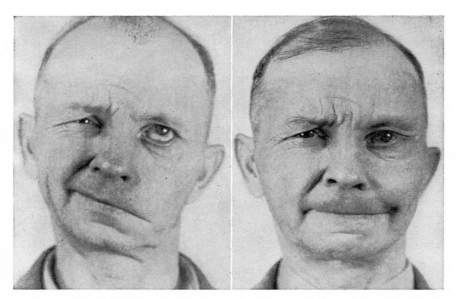

Fig. 45-41. (*Left*) Complete unilateral peripheral facial paralysis with sagged face and eyelid. (*Right*) Result of one operation one month later with face supported by loops of fascia lata anchored to temporalis tendon combined with external canthoplasty. Normal lid aperture and nasolabial fold. Comfortable and expressive movement is possible. (Brown, J. B., and Fryer, M. P.: Plastic surgery for severe facial paralysis in elderly patients, J. Am. Geriatrics Soc. 2:820-825)

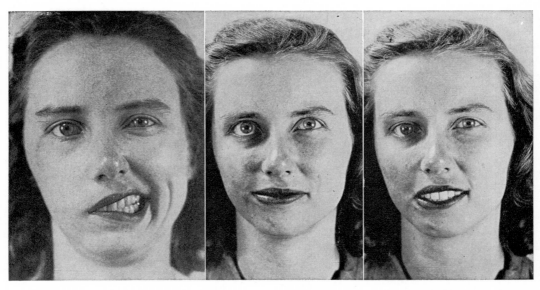

Fig. 45-42. Facial paralysis. (*Left*) From malignant parotid tumor necessitating radical operation. (*Center*) Face supported by loops of fascia lata in face anchored to temporalis muscle and fascia. (*Right*) Balanced emotional expression possible by substituting 5th cranial nerve action for lost 7th cranial nerve. No further addition of scars in the face by this operation. (Brown, J. B., McDowell, F., and Fryer, M. P.: Direct operative removal of benign mixed tumors of anlage origin in the parotid region, Surg., Gynec. & Obst. 90:257-268)

lower eyelid can be supported by a loop of fascia passed from the temporal region through the eyelid to the frontalis region. In addition, the eye can be made more comfortable and the exposure of the cornea reduced without disturbing the eyelashes with a lateral canthoplasty.

Actually, even after complete facial paralysis of long duration, eating, speaking, normal appearance, and maintenance of watertight integrity of the mouth can be practically fully restored with this fascial support method. The degree of animation is unpredictable but can be developed and improved by minor exercises.

DEFORMITIES OF THE EAR

Ear deformities may be congenital or traumatic. Congenital deformities may be of any degree and involve one or both ears. Traumatic loss of ears may follow an automobile or industrial accident but more often is the consequence of burns of the face and the ears. With burn denudation the cartilage is exposed to infection, resulting in a deformity that is more unsightly than is the actual loss of an ear.

Ears widely placed from the head or flop ears are usually of congenital origin. They can be corrected readily in one operation through

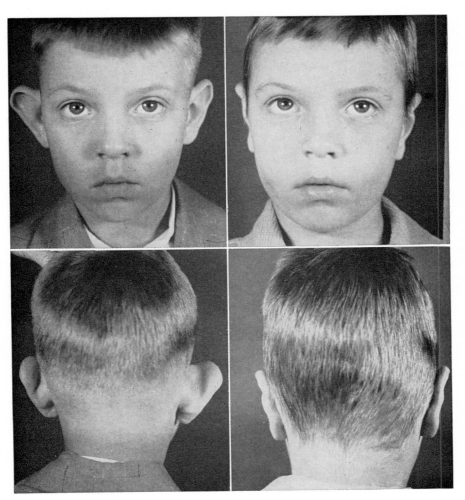

FIG. 45-43. (*Left*) Prominent ears set back in one operation through posterior incision. (*Right*) Early postoperative photograph.

an incision that is hidden behind the ear. During the operation the cartilaginous support to the ear is opened to permit permanent repositioning and the construction of normal markings.

Total construction of an absent ear can be done in 3 fundamental stages without the addition of scars in the neck or elsewhere. Vestigial remnants are smoothed out or placed in the proper direction in the first stage. The cartilaginous support for the future ear is placed in its proper position beneath the scalp in a subcutaneous pocket at the second operation. Cartilage and other materials such as dimethyl siloxanes, halogenated carbons and polyvinyl alcohol have been used to construct the support to the ear.[27] If the patient is large enough to have sufficient available cartilage, it can be used; however, fresh homografts from other members of the patient's family may be relied on; otherwise, preserved cartilage from the cartilage bank may be used. This avoids an unpleasant operation on another member of the family. At the third stage, usually done from 3 to 6 months after implantation of the support, the skin covered cartilage is raised forward from the scalp, and its posterior surface and the defect in the scalp are covered with a free split graft. Acceptable ear outlines may be made in these 3 stages and are preferred by most patients to artificial prostheses. Additional adjustments and addition of a round helix with a small tubed flap from the neck may be required after the basic procedures have been completed.

There are many suggestions as to various more laborious procedures for ear reconstruction, for which reference to specific texts is necessary if details are desired.

Traumatic loss of an ear requires essentially the same stages for reconstruction as those for the congenitally absent one.

With deep burns of the face ears are often burned off or so deformed as to require practically total reconstruction. In such cases the outer surface of the ear and the cartilage is usually so infected, wrinkled and scarred as to require total replacement.

DEFORMITIES OF THE EYELIDS

Ptosis (the inability to elevate the upper lid properly), deformities about the canthus and absence of a part of an eyelid, such as coloboma palpebrale, are the most common congenital deformities seen about the eye requiring repair. However, traumatic destruction and surgical removal constitute the most frequent causes of deformities of the eyelids.

PTOSIS

Because of the difficulty in elevating the lid above the pupil, the skin of the forehead is arched, and the head is held back so the patient may see beneath his drooped eyelids. The correction of ptosis requires elevation of the eyelid. If any levator palpebrae action remains, the tendon of this muscle may be shortened, thereby elevating the lid. However, usually there is no function remaining in this muscle, and another technic must be used. The superior tarsal plate may be shortened and brought up to the region of the frontalis muscle, or a tendon can be constructed from fascia lata and this looped down to the tarsal border and then attached to the frontalis muscle. This in effect substitutes a muscle innervated by the 7th nerve for the missing one innervated by the 3rd. Both of these technics permit the raising of the lid when the skin over the forehead is lifted. This the patient learns to do soon after operation. Postoperatively, there may be some difficulty in effecting normal closure of the eyes, especially during sleep. Should this occur, usually it can be cared for with a small piece of adhesive tape.

The operation described above is extraorbital and does not restore normal intraorbital elevation of the lid. To obtain intraorbital elevation the use of the superior rectus muscle is required in the repair. This is an ophthalmologic operation. All patients having ptosis should be examined by an ophthalmologist and the type of operation selected for a given patient on a consultative basis.

CONDITIONS REQUIRING RECONSTRUCTION OF AN EYELID

Congenital absence of an eyelid, coloboma palpebrale (a slit in the lid) or loss due to trauma or operative removal are alike in that the defect requires reconstruction of an eyelid to protect the cornea. Total eyelid reconstruction requires the formation of a mucosal lining, as well as an outer layer of skin. Protection of the exposed cornea is extremely important to the maintenance of sight; consequently, its covering may be a real emergency. Often coloboma palpebrale can be repaired in one operation by rotating the lining of the adjacent segments of the lid and utilizing local flaps for closure. This principle may be used even for the total reconstruction of lids lost from any cause. Cross-lid flaps may be used in some instances, but it is best to avoid damage to a normal lid whenever possible. However, parts of a normal companion lid must be used occasionally in order to provide a lining mucosa because skin is not tolerated by the bulbar conjunctiva.

Spontaneous reconstitution of an eyelid after its excision for carcinoma may completely obviate the necessity for secondary reconstruction, although this process may be prolonged and require the exposure of bulbar conjunctiva. However, the functional result may be more satisfactory than that which follows an attempt at primary surgical reconstruction.

Spontaneous reconstitution of the eyelid after the resection of a neoplasm of the lid is effected by the surgical coaptation of any remaining part of the resected lid to its normal partner. This may effect a spontaneous generation of mucosa and skin from the surrounding area and the adjacent lid so as to permit separation of the adherent lids later with the securance of adequate corneal coverage with but little or no addition of skin such as free full-thickness grafts from the ear or the neck, or as a small local flap.

Ectropion

Spontaneously healing deep burns of the eyelids heal with contracture and eversion of the conjunctiva of the eyelid (ectropion). This exposes the cornea with the possible result of corneal ulceration and loss of sight. The treatment consists of excising the deep scar from the eyelids while taking care to preserve all possible muscle function. This excision of scar releases the contracture and allows the lid to come in contact with the globe. The excisional defects are readily resurfaced with free full-thickness skin grafts taken from behind an ear, from the supraclavicular region or the inguinal region. Innumerable eyes of burned persons have been saved by prompt release of ectropion and immediate coverage with a skin graft.

SALIVARY GLANDS

The usual disorders of the submaxillary and the parotid glands are ductal obstruction, infection, trauma and tumors. The parotid

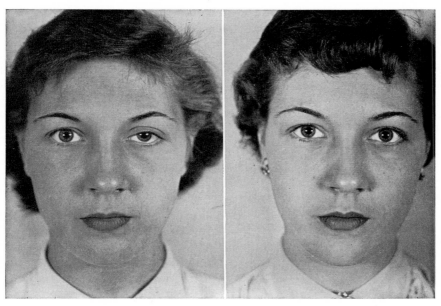

Fig. 45-44. (*Left*) Ptosis of patient's left upper eyelid repaired in one operation. (*Right*) Two weeks after repair.

glands are the most common sites of tumors, and the submaxillary gland ducts are the more frequent site of obstructions.

OBSTRUCTION

Calculi. The origin of salivary stones may be related to partial ductal obstruction and infection. The calculi usually found in the ducts may be multiple. Ductal calculi characteristically produce intermittent obstructions with swelling of the obstructed gland.

Diagnosis of salivary duct obstruction is made on the basis of acute swelling of the gland following the secretory stimulation of eating or chewing gum. Pain and swelling over the gland follows. Occasionally, fever and general malaise attend it, particularly if there is infection. When the infection occurs behind a ductal obstruction, often pus may be expressed from the duct. Simple roentgenograms may show the stones. However, sialograms may be required to demonstrate obstruction of the duct by stenosis, etc. The treatment of calculous obstruction is the removal of the calculi. Often this can be done rather easily by extracting it from the duct in the mouth, or enlarging the orifice of the duct, allowing the stone to pass spontaneously. The repeated recurrence of symptoms and calculi may require removal of the gland to cure the trouble.

Congenital narrowing of salivary ducts usually occurs at their orifices in the mouth. The signs and symptoms of congenital stenotic obstructions are the same as those caused by a calculus. Relief is afforded by enlarging the orifice in the mouth.

Infection in the salivary ducts usually is related to obstruction which, when corrected, may cure the infection. However, antibiotics are given routinely in most instances of obstruction before and for a time after its correction because some infection within the ducts is usually present by the time the patient seeks relief.

Infection in the salivary glands themselves is often secondary to obstruction or infection in the ducts. The general reaction is usually more severe than when it is confined to the ducts, but the signs of obstruction are predominant. Infection in salivary glands may occur without demonstrable obstructions of their ducts coming from infection elsewhere in the body. Surgical mumps or *parotitis* (non-

obstructive parotitis) was seen more frequently in the past in markedly debilitated patients with poor mouth care who were taking little by mouth; it was in general a symptom of some other disease process. Occasionally, all salivary glands were affected simultaneously, but the parotids alone most often. The treatment of surgical mumps is stimulation of salivary flow with chewing and mouth washes, antibiotics and care of the general debilitation. Opening of the parenchyma of the glands to the outside through multiple incisions is often necessary for the cure of parenchymal suppuration, especially when the infection is staphylococcal. Infection in a major salivary gland not apparently related to obstruction may eventually necessitate removal of the gland, but the use of light inflammatory doses of x-rays, antibiotics and salivary stimulation may avoid it.

Trauma to the salivary system is usually the result of glass cuts from automobile accidents, knife cuts or surgical exploration. Lacerations of the gland usually can be closed, and healing follows. Fistulas communicating with the intraglandular ducts usually close spontaneously. However, if a major duct has been cut, careful approximation of the two ends always should be done, or if in the mouth, the duct may be short-circuited by anastomosing the proximal end to the buccal mucosa. If neither an anastomosis nor shortening is done, persistent fistulae are prone to develop, and subsequent repair or short-circuiting is made more difficult. Secondary scarring following trauma may cause obstruction to the ducts, in which case resection of scar and reanastomosis or short-circuiting may be tried.

CONGENITAL WRYNECK

Congenital wryneck probably is seen most often by the plastic surgeon because of its related deformities of the jaw or the face.[23]

The etiology has always been indeterminate. Presumptively, it has been related to injury at birth. The microscopic appearance of the lesion is important because of its importance to the treatment. In most instances the normal structure of the sternocleidomastoid muscle is completely replaced by scar, grossly and microscopically. This scar is probably the result of fibrosis secondary to a hematoma or the tearing of the muscle. However, other theories of cause have been advanced. The mass in the muscle generally is noticed about 2 weeks after birth. It may disappear spontaneously, leaving very little deformity.

Congenital wryneck is not to be confused with spasmotic torticollis, which is an entirely different entity and cannot be relieved by removal of muscle.

Diagnosis of congenital torticollis can be made upon notation of the position of the ear and the mastoid region. They are pulled down to the shoulder of the affected side while the chin points toward the normal side. The patient cannot bend the head to the normal side. In addition, a solid mass may be felt in the sternocleidomastoid muscle during infancy. Later the mass becomes less apparent, but the mastoid process remains approximated to the clavicle by the palpably tight band of fibrous tissue representing the sternocleidomastoid muscle bundle. Roentgenograms of the cervical spine are needed to rule out congenital deformities of the cervical spine which superficially mimic congenital wryneck. Failure to correct the deformity during early childhood utimately causes deformity of the jaw and the head on the affected side.

Treatment consists of complete excision of the scarred muscle band through a low collar incision. If the lesion is of relatively long duration, the cervical fascia overlying the fibrous muscle remnant may be shortened and require opening. Casts or braces are not required after the excision if total excision of the contracting mass is done. Because spontaneous subsidence of the entire process occasionally occurs, the operation is deferred until the 6th to the 8th month of age. Should the deformity remain at this age it is looked upon as a permanent one, and operative correction should be undertaken.

INDUSTRIAL AND FARM INJURIES

Some injuries from farm and industrial machines are sufficiently peculiar to warrant their separate consideration. Tractor power take-off injuries are one of these.

TRACTOR POWER TAKE-OFF GENITAL INJURIES

These injuries attend the catching of trousers and the dragging of the leg and the lower torso over the revolving power take-off.

This tears the skin of the perineum, the penis and the scrotum and the lower abdomen and the back from the body, often completely denuding the penis and leaving the testes attached only by the cords. When the skin of the back and the abdomen are torn off, often the underlying muscles are exposed and torn.

Emergency care is directed toward the prevention and the control of shock. The prompt use of whole blood may prevent shock. However, often these patients are alone in the field when the accident occurs, and the securance of treatment is often delayed. When it is, a large volume of whole blood has been necessary to save life.

These patients should be brought to the operating room as soon as possible and individual bleeding points ligated. The poor general condition of the person may permit only cleansing with saline irrigation after controlling hemorrhage and the application of a firm comfortable fine-mesh grease gauze pressure dressing. In other words, cutaneous reconstruction is delayed. Tetanus protection with 25,000 units or more of tetanus antitoxin in cases not actively immunized with toxoid, and a booster of toxoid to those who are, and large doses of antibiotics are given.

Repair. The first steps in definitive repair of the damaged area are done when shock has been treated and the general condition permits. These steps consist of

(1) Débridement of nonviable tissue and the cleansing of open areas.

(2) Protection of the testes by implanting them beneath the skin of the thighs. A subcutaneous tunnel is made from the torn perineum into the thigh, and the testes are anchored in it. Also, temporary protection can be provided by encasing them in saline-moistened gauze packs. This will suffice for protection during immediate transportation.

After inserting the testes into the pockets, often the perineum may be closed, and this can be done safely, provided that drainage is assured. Insertion of the testes into the inner thigh tunnels may be followed by the natural withdrawal of the testes toward the mid-line, effecting the spontaneous appearance of a small bifed scrotum. During the early reconstructive period there seems to be no necessity of attempting tò construct a scrotum with local flaps. One young man who had both testes buried beneath the skin of the thighs later developed a new bifid scrotum spontaneously and begot children.

(3) Re-covering the penis usually can be accomplished with free autografts. This is done at the time of primary repair of the other damaged areas. The split-thickness graft is taken with a knife and suction retractors from the thigh and is wrapped around the penis and held in place with sutures and/or a carefully applied dressing. If a plastic surgeon is not available the penis may be temporarily buried subcutaneously with an indwelling catheter in place.

(4) Bare areas on the abdomen or the back, after cleansing and débridement, are covered by split-thickness grafts held in place by sutures and the dressing.

Subsequent care of these newly covered areas is the same as that described for any graft.

Primary definitive repair of tractor power take-off injuries is usually all that is necessary for permanent function. Rarely is complex plastic surgery necessary if the primary repair is conducted as described.

HYPOSPADIAS

Hypospadias is a congenital penile defect in which the ventral surface is foreshortened and the urethral meatus is on the ventral surface often close to the penile-scrotal junction. The ventral curvature is exaggerated by erection. Repair consists of correction of the curvature and building a tube from the opening of the short urethra to the end of the penis. This usually requires 2 or 3 operations. *Circumcision should not be done.* The repair is performed when there is sufficient tissue available, usually by the 4th or the 5th year.

Release of the curvature is the first operation. The curvature is released by dissecting the urethra free, permitting it to drop back toward the scrotum and excising the tight bands under the corpora cavernosum. The defect left by these dissections is covered by interdigitated local penile flaps, utilizing the prepuce when needed. This step may be performed before the second birthday.

Construction of the tube from the urethra to the end of the penis can be done after release of the curvature. The entire tube can

be constructed and connected to the end of the short urethra in one operation if preliminary diversion of the urinary stream is done through a perineal urethrostomy. Otherwise, the tube is constructed at one operation and connected to the urethra later. Numerous methods are available for construction of the tube, but the most satisfactory method in the author's experience has been the incision of a strip of skin on the ventral surface wide enough to circumscribe a No. 10 catheter at least and the careful approximation of the edges of this strip over a catheter with multiple sutures. The tube lined by skin but uncovered by skin is covered over by interdigitating skin flaps from the remaining normally outward-facing penile skin. The same method is used to connect the newly constructed tube to the urethra.

A firm pressure dressing encourages healing and avoids bleeding after correction of the curvature and the building of the tube.

REPAIR OF SURFACE DEFECTS OF THE FEET

Surface defects of the feet may follow removal of tumors or result from circulatory deficiency, infection or trauma. Repair may be difficult because the plantar surface, like the palm of the hand, is a specialized type of skin which cannot be reconstituted but at best can only be substituted for.

Primary closure is the simplest means of covering a defect if sufficient skin is available for closure or the resultant scar is not over a weight-bearing surface of the foot.

Coverage with a free graft can be done for larger defects if there is an adequate soft tissue pad upon which to place the graft. Skin from elsewhere on the body constitutes only a substitute type of coverage for normal plantar skin and must be protected constantly because it cannot stand the pressures of walking and standing that the original plantar skin could.

Local flaps may be necessary if the defect covers the heads of the 1st and the 5th metatarsals or the heel. The open area left by rotation of a flap from a nonweight-bearing surface of the foot to the above locations can be covered by a free graft.

Distant flaps may be necessary to cover

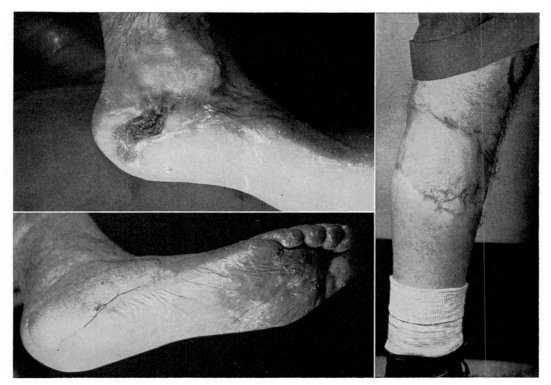

Fig. 45-45. (*Left, top*) Deep injury followed by recurrent breakdown for 20 years. (*Left, bottom*) Ulcer excised and defect covered by cross-leg flap. (*Right*) Donor site of flap.

larger deep losses of skin of the foot. Their use requires preparation in stages. The opposite thigh is used most often as a donor site. These flaps are raised in stages, training the blood supply to come in from the desired direction, and then are applied to the foot. Detachment of the flap from the thigh usually is possible within 3 weeks after its attachment to the foot. The cutaneous defect left upon the thigh is covered with a free graft.

Short, broad flaps are used whenever possible in order to avoid the delay of staging, such as in abdominal flap repair of deep injuries of the arm and the hand.

Flaps covering defects of the foot require the same permanent protection as split or free full-thickness grafts do because they, too, cannot take the pounding that the original skin could.

The preceding discussion of principles and methods in plastic surgery has been taken from the following original articles which can be consulted for detail.

REFERENCES

1. Brown, J. B.: *in* Womack, N.: On Burns, Springfield, Ill., Thomas, 1953.
1a. Brown, J. B., and Cannon, B.: Composite free grafts of skin and cartilage from the ear, Surg., Gynec. & Obst. *82*:253-255, 1946.
2. Brown, J. B., Cannon, B., Graham, W., Lischer, C., Scarborough, C., Davis, W., and Moore, A.: Direct flap repair of defects of the arm and hand: preparation of gunshot wounds for repair of nerves, bones and tendons, Ann. Surg. *122*:706-715, 1945.
3. Brown, J. B., Cannon, B., Lischer, C., and Davis, W.: Composite free grafts of skin and cartilage from the ear, J.A.M.A. *134*:1295-1296, 1947.
4. Brown, J. B., and Fryer, M. P.: Fracture-dislocation of the zygoma and orbit, Postgrad. Med. *6*:400-406, 1949.
5. ———: Management of compound facial injuries, Am. J. Surg. *76*:625-630, 1948.
6. ———: Multiple internal wire fixation of facial fractures, Am. J. Surg. *89*:814-818, 1955.
7. ———: Plastic surgery for severe facial pa-

ralysis in elderly patients, J. Am. Geriatrics Soc. *11*:820-825, 1954.

8. ———: Postmortem homografts to reduce mortality in extensive burns, J.A.M.A. *156*: 1163-1166, 1954.

9. ———: Treatment of burns: general condition, early definitive care of the local area, and repair of the sequelae; a plan for care of the survivors of an atomic attack or any mass disaster, J. Missouri M.A. *48*:973-981, 1951.

10. ———: Tumors in the parotid region: direct surgical approach and preservation of seventh nerve in benign tumors; description of radical operation for malignant tumors, Am. Surgeon *18*:880-890, 1952.

11. ———: Repair of industrial electrical burns. Plast. & Reconstruct. Surg. *18*:177-184, 1956.

12. ———: Plastic surgical principles in farm, industrial and traffic accidents, A.M.A. Arch. Surg. *72*:780-787, 1956.

13. Brown, J. B., Fryer, M. P., and McDowell, F.: Internal wire-pin stabilization for middle third facial fractures, Surg., Gynec. & Obst. *93*:676-681, 1951.

14. ———: Permanent pedicle blood-carrying flaps for repairing defects in avascular areas, Ann. Surg. *134*:486-494, 1951.

15. Brown, J. B., Fryer, M. P., Randall, P., and Lu, M.: Postmortem homografts as "biological dressings" for extensive burns and denuded areas, Ann. Surg. *138*:618-630, 1953.

16. Brown, J. B., Fryer, M. P., and Zaydon, T. J.: Establishing a skin bank; use and various methods of preservation of postmortem homografts, Plast. & Reconstruct. Surg. *16*:337-351, 1955.

17. ———: A skin bank for postmortem homografts, Surg., Gynec. & Obst. *101*:401-412, 1955.

18. Brown, J. B., and McDowell, F.: Neck Dissection (Am. Lecture Series), Springfield, Ill., Thomas, 1954.

19. ———: Plastic Surgery of the Nose, St. Louis, Mosby, 1951.

20. ———: Simplified design for repair of single cleft lips, Surg., Gynec. & Obst. *80*:12-26, 1945.

21. ———: Skin Grafting, St. Louis, Mosby, 1949; Skin Grafting, ed. 3, Philadelphia, Lippincott, 1958.

22. Brown, J. B., McDowell, F., and Byars, L. T.: Double clefts of the lip, Surg., Gynec. & Obst. *85*:20-29, 1947.

23. Brown, J. B., McDowell, F., and Fryer, M. P.: Facial distortion in wryneck prevented by early resection of the fibrosed sternomastoid muscle, Plast. & Reconstruct. Surg. *5*:301-309, 1950.

24. ———: Radiation burns, including vocational and atomic exposures; treatment and surgical prevention of chronic lesions, Ann. Surg. *130*:593-607, 1949.

25. ———: Surgery of the Face, Mouth and Jaws, St. Louis, Mosby, 1954.

26. ———: Surgical treatment of radiation burns, Surg., Gynec. & Obst. *88*:609-622, 1949.

27. Brown, J. B., Ohlwiler, D., and Fryer, M. P.: Investigation of and use of dimethyl siloxanes, halogenated carbons and polyvinyl alcohol as subcutaneous protheses, Am. Surg. *152*:534-547, 1960; Study and use of synthetic materials such as silicones and Tefton as subcutaneous prostheses, Plast. & Reconstruct. Surg. *26*:264-279, 1960.

28. Brown, J. B., Peterson, L., Cannon, B., and Lischer, C.: Ankylosis of the coronoid process of the mandible (and associated scar limitation of jaw function), Plast. & Reconstruct. Surg. *1*:277-283, 1946.

MARK M. RAVITCH, M.D.

CHAPTER 46

Pediatric Surgery

General Considerations

Head and Neck

Thorax

Gastrointestinal Tract

Sacrococcygeal Teratoma and Other Pelvic Tumors

GENERAL CONSIDERATIONS

The inclusion of a chapter on pediatric surgery in a textbook of surgery is recognition of the growth of interest in this special field and of the significance of the recent accomplishments in it. Certain subjects of pediatric surgical interest are omitted from the present discussion for considerations of space or because they are treated adequately in other chapters. The surgical problems of infancy and childhood differ from those of later life in several ways:

Newborn infants present certain conditions, the continued existence of which, uncorrected, is incompatible with life and which therefore are not seen except by those dealing with infants.

Infants and children are subject to almost all of the conditions seen in later life, but the incidence of these conditions is so different in childhood as to require a rearrangement of the clinical approach to differential diagnosis.

The physical and emotional reactions of infants and children to illness and metabolic derangements frequently differ both qualitatively and quantitatively from the response of adults to the same stimuli. This often calls for a different set of values in the evaluation of symptomatic and objective responses to illness.

In drug therapy, while infants may be more susceptible to the effects of some drugs, they have rather enormous tolerance for others when needed, such as digitalis and the barbiturates.

TIME OF OPERATION

The decision as to when an infant is to undergo an essential surgical procedure, and whether it is to be definitive or temporizing, is no longer widely discussed. It is well understood that infants and children can stand operations of any magnitude, if properly conceived and executed with appropriate preparation and after-care. There is less tendency to delay operation until the child is older or has reached some token milestone. At the same time the tendency is to make the initial operation definitively corrective rather than a means of preserving the baby until it is "large enough" to be operated upon. Tumors, benign and malignant, should be treated definitively when discovered. Malignant processes are now the leading cause of in-hospital deaths in children.[2] Far from being considered an unlikely possibility in the presence of a solid mass in an infant or a child, a malignant tumor is the most likely possibility, even at birth. Immediate, thorough, radical operations offer a rewarding percentage of cures, the opportunity for which may be lost by temporizing delays for "study" and "observation."

Congenital anomalies of every complexity, such as high anorectal atresias and esophageal atresia with tracheo-esophageal fistula, are treated definitively at birth, or soon after. At the moment, the field of cardiac surgery in which some operations are postponed, if possible for several years, constitutes a conspicuous exception. This probably is due to the newness of the field and the relative crudeness of some of the technics. In urgent situations cardiac operations are now undertaken even in the neonatal period, and the optimal age for elective procedures is being steadily revised downward.[26] In general, the tendency in pediatric surgery is for the proper operation for a given lesion to be performed whenever the necessity for it is apparent. Small size of the patient and of the structures to be dealt with tends not to be a serious limiting factor in most procedures. Scar tissue, as in intestinal and vascular anastomoses, tends to grow as the anastomosed structures grow, and little difficulty need be anticipated. In plastic reconstructive surgical procedures, as on the nose and the ear, it may be necessary to wait until the feature has attained its final shape and most of its size.

Psychologically, it is obvious that the sooner a child is like his fellows in appearance, in deglutition, defecation and urination, in vigor and general stamina, the better he is in every way.

PREPARATION FOR OPERATION

Shortly before the event, to avoid a needlessly prolonged anticipation, any child old enough to talk should know that he is coming to a hospital for an operation and that he will be put to sleep. He should be given a brief description of the anesthesia technic, or even a "dry run," and told that he will be made better and then return home. Hospitalization and operation on a well-ordered service need not be upsetting to a child. It is a "traumatic experience" chiefly to children from homes overcharged with tensions. While I am quite willing to have mothers sleep in their children's rooms, I am accustomed to point out that the most painful feature of leaving a child in the hospital is the discovery that he gets along so well. So far as possible, deceptions and misstatements should be avoided. Necessary examinations and treatments should be explained and then performed. Painful procedures should not be heralded as painless. The confidence of a child is too valuable an asset to the physician to be lost for momentary expediency, and once lost is not easily regained.

PREMEDICATION

A drowsy, sedated child is a better candidate for anesthesia than one alarmed and struggling. Children, a year of age or older, may be transported to the operating room drowsy or asleep with 3 to 4 mg. of Nembutal/ Kg. body weight given intramuscularly 1 or 1½ hours before operation, together with scopolamine or atropine.

Morphine and barbiturates should be avoided in the first 6 months of life, because of the respiratory depression induced by them. Atropine is most important to keep a dry airway, but overdosage in children should be avoided, and the drug is dangerous in hyperpyrexia, dehydration and in the presence of high ambient temperatures. If a very rapid pulse, fever, or marked flushing occur following atropine, operation should be postponed. Scopolamine is perhaps a little less likely to give such reactions. In older children, morphine sulfate is given in doses of 1 mg. for each 5 Kg. of body weight. The dosage of atropine is 0.05 mg. *total dose* in the first year of life, 0.2 to 0.3 mg. in the next 2 years, 0.2 to 0.4 mg. thereafter, increasing to the adult dose of 0.6 mg. with large adolescents. Scopolamine is given in slightly lower dosages than atropine.

ANESTHESIA

Anesthetic choices will vary with local experience and preferences. In general, local anesthesia has little place in major pediatric surgery. The struggling of an infant tied to the operating table, straining, expelling intestines through the wound, cause more harm and danger than a skillful inhalation anesthesia. Spinal anesthesia has had a vogue in some clinics but is psychologically a severe trial to older children and indefensible for infants. Intravenous barbiturates are useful but considerably more hazardous in children than in adults. Rectal supplements, of Avertin or of a barbiturate, provide excellent basal anesthesia. The choice is therefore mainly one of inhalant agents and technics. Open drip ether, by all odds the safest anesthesia for infants and children, is widely useful, frequently with cyclopropane or Vinethene induction. Fluothane is now in wide and satisfactory use. Intratracheal anesthesia, once neglected, is now abused in some clinics by too frequent use. Invaluable for intrathoracic and deep cervical procedures, it nevertheless carries its own risks. Even with smooth, flexible plastic tubes, laryngeal injury and edema may result and demand close attention after operation, in a moist atmosphere, with tracheostomy occasionally required.

Great emphasis has been placed upon conserving body heat. Yet evidence is accumulating that, at least in the presence of neonatal asphyxia, cooler temperatures are beneficial and the hot box temperatures of incubators may be harmful.[100] Potts[110] paved the way for hypothermic surgery by showing that with moderate cooling on a water mattress infants and children during cardiac surgery were protected from the dangerous and at times fatal hyperthermia which otherwise sometimes developed. In addition, he pointed out the advantages of the lowered metabolic needs of the hypothermic patient. We have been using moderate hypothermia (89° to 90° F.) for the graver operations of pediatric surgery for some time, with entire satisfaction. It would appear that the custom of swathing babies on the operating table, surrounding them with hot water bottles, has no sound physiologic basis and may be harmful.

ADMINISTRATION OF BLOOD AND PARENTERAL FLUIDS

The small amounts of parenteral fluids which a very small infant requires may be given by single subcutaneous injection between the shoulder blades or by a slow subcutaneous drip into the 2 thighs. Hyaluronidase increases the rapidity of administration of such an infusion. The intravenous route is required for continued parenteral hydration and nutrition, for patients with large fluid deficits, for administration of fluids during operation and for administration of blood. A skilled house officer with proper equipment in the form of No. 24 needles, syringes with eccentrically placed tips or scalp needles fixed to plastic tubing, and with trained assistants to hold the patient, can administer fluids regularly and easily through veins of the scalp, the hands and the feet which appear inordinately small to the physician accustomed to the gross technics of adult venoclyses. Before or after operation "stat" doses of fluids may be pumped into these small veins. Scalp needles can often be taped in place for continuous infusion. For operation, we prefer the more certain technic of the polyethylene catheter inserted in the saphenous vein through a 5-mm.

incision anterior to the internal malleolus. If the catheter is inserted in the operating room while the operative field is being prepared and draped, the surgeon will have maximal assurance that an uninterrupted flow of blood or fluids can be maintained. In adults, an unplanned-for transfusion can be given fairly readily during an operation. In the close quarters of pediatric surgery, one should not be forced into attempting the feat of entering a vein and transfusing blood into a tiny patient hidden beneath sheets and drapes.

The catheter may be left in place for as long as 2 or 3 days after operation if necessary. High fever wtih tenderness, redness or induration in the leg indicate phlebitis. The catheter is then to be removed and compresses applied to the leg. Septic thrombophlebitis is an occasional but rare complication, curable by interruption of the vein proximal to the needle or catheter site.[139]

There has been a general awareness in recent years that it is safer to carry infant surgical patients "on the dry side," that is, less than fully hydrated, although this should not be carried to excess. Infants will do well on parenteral feedings in the immediate postoperative period when receiving 75 to 100 cc. of fluid/Kg. body weight/day, apart from replacement of any special fluid losses. In the neonatal period the lower figures should be used. The sodium requirement may be taken as 1 to 2 mEq./Kg./day. Glucose, 10 per cent, in distilled water serves as the constant intravenous infusion with 0.45 per cent NaCl added as required. Five and 10 per cent glucose in water should not be given subcutaneously to sodium-depleted infants, because the subcutaneously held glucose in water abstracts sodium from the blood and the tissues, imposing an acute sodium deficit upon the infant until most of the infusion has been absorbed from the subcutaneous tissues. This abstraction of sodium into the subcutaneously given 10 per cent dextrose is occasionally sufficient to produce shock.

While potassium has great usefulness in patients who have had grave electrolyte losses from vomiting or diarrhea, it is dangerous, and in infants a miscalculation in dosage may be fatal. There is a tendency today to use potassium on almost all patients receiving intravenous therapy. Actually, it should be used only in instances of severe loss of intestinal fluids, the basic requirement being 2 to 3 mEq./Kg./day. In the case of sodium, the pendulum has swung from the old mistake of excessive dosage to the current practice of frequently inadequate dosage leading to sodium depletion. About one-quarter of the intravenous fluid may be 0.9 per cent saline, and intestinal drainage should be replaced by 0.45 per cent saline in 10 per cent glucose, volume for volume, over and above the daily requirements. The volume and the specific gravity of the urine are the practical guides to intravenous electrolyte therapy.

Blood, plasma, or human serum albumin for anemia or hypoproteinemia are given in single infusions of 10 to 20 cc./Kg. body weight. Because of the danger of acute cardiac dilatation and pulmonary edema that occasionally attend the rapid infusion of concentrated solutions of human albumin, great precautions must be taken as to the rate of the intravenous infusion of concentrated albumin solution, especially in infants with cardiac distress and any degree of dehydration. During operation blood must be administered to replace blood loss, volume for volume. In the polycythemic newborn, if blood loss is not excessive, plasma may be used instead of whole blood.

In infants requiring prolonged intravenous alimentation, protein balance becomes a serious problem. For this purpose the protein hydrolysates in 5 per cent solutions may be used in volumes up to a third of the daily fluid requirement. Human serum albumin has some limited nutritional value. On the basis of canine experiments, whole plasma can meet the entire protein requirement if supplemented with sufficient carbohydrate and fat. The small size of the younger pediatric patients makes this approach feasible in the unusual situation in which prolonged parenteral alimentation is necessary. If plasma is to be used, room temperature storage to reduce the chance of transmitting hepatitis virus is recommended (see Chap. 8, "Blood Transfusions"). Preparations of fat emulsions, suitable for intravenous use, are available and provide a high caloric intake but are still not free from undesirable effects.

ANTIBIOTICS

Penicillin remains the most widely applicable and the safest of the antibiotics. If gram-negative organisms are involved, streptomycin in dosages of 15 to 25 mg./Kg. usually is employed. The other antibiotics are reserved for special indications, based usually on the reports of sensitivity tests of the organism involved (see Chap. 3 on "Applied Surgical Bacteriology"). Chloromycetin and the successive tetracyclines have come into wide use.

DRESSINGS

For some years now, first in pediatric surgery, and then in adult surgery, we have dispensed with conventional dressings. A layer of flexible collodion, or of one of the aerosol plastic sprays, provides a neat covering, protecting the wound from saliva, urine or feces —if any such protection is required. The small patient then is examined more readily and without the necessity for removing adhesive tape and bandage. Buried subcuticular sutures spare surgeon and child the ordeal of suture removal and are employed whenever appropriate.

ACTIVITY

In general, within the restricting confines of a hospital, a child who is doing well may be permitted as much activity as he wishes.

HEAD AND NECK

Impetigo and the other troublesome pyodermas of childhood are extremely contagious because of the abundance of bacteria-laden discharge and the susceptibility of the skin of small children. Impetigo contagiosa is a staphylococcic infection of the derma. The lesions occasionally respond to gentle washing with soap and protection of the surrounding skin from constant exposure to pus. For this purpose a soap containing hexachlorophene is preferable. In stubbornly resistant cases, or in instances with sepsis, the appropriate antibiotics should be used systemically; antibiotic ointments are to be avoided, in general. As in pyogenic infections elsewhere, regional lymphadenitis usually becomes manifest while the primary lesion is still acutely inflamed.

Adenitis. Occasionally, adenitis does not appear until after the primary infection has receded, or even healed and been forgotten. In the presence of numerous small shotty nodes in the occipital area and in the posterior triangle of the neck, one should make careful search of the scalp for small crusted lesions which might escape a casual examination. Acute cervical adenitis in the anterior triangle of the neck, particularly under the angle of the mandible, is more likely to have resulted from a pharyngeal infection—not uncommonly a week or two after its subsidence. While lymphadenitis, early in its course, will yield to systemic administration of antibiotics, once suppuration has occurred, incision and drainage usually is required as in adults. There is no difficulty in determining that a superficial node, fixed to the skin, red, tender, edematous and fluctuant, is ready for incision. In a deep-lying node, fixation and a brawny elasticity are the early signs of suppuration. Superficially, there develop what ordinarily would be taken as signs of cellulitis—wide edema, induration, tenderness and a faint violaceous erythema. In general, in deep cervical adenitis, necrosis and liquefaction have occurred well before physical signs are unequivocal. If the old surgical technic of John Hilton is followed—of incising only the skin and finding the pus by blunt dissection, usually with a hemostat—injury to the nerves and the blood vessels need not be feared.

Tuberculous cervical adenitis may be difficult to distinguish from adenitis due to pyogenic bacteria. Either may present as a single node, or as a group of nodes, as a relatively indolent, nontender mass, or as an acute, red, tender, inflammatory process. Chronicity, indolence and extensiveness suggest tuberculosis, apart from the history of exposure, and a positive tuberculin test. Forty or 50 years ago, radical resection of the cervical nodes, the jugular vein and the sternocleidomastoid muscle was the standard treatment for cervical tuberculosis. Its proved inefficacy and lack of demonstrable advantage finally brought the operation into disuse in favor of rest, vitamins, ultraviolet light treatment and, for liquefied nodes, aspiration (Charcot's aspiration *à distance,* through an oblique tract commencing in healthy skin to avoid formation of a sinus tract).

The advent of streptomycin and an increasing number of other effective antituberculous drugs has altered our approach to tuberculous adenitis which is, in any case, less common than formerly. Early processes will respond to specific drug therapy. The hazard of excisional biopsy for histologic confirmation of the diagnosis has been reduced considerably; and incision and drainage of a broken-down tuberculous process under the mistaken impression that it is pyogenic is no longer so deplorable an error. Some surgeons[91, 159] protecting their patients with streptomycin and other drugs, are once more urging resection of cervical tuberculous adenitic masses. The surgeon is warned that seemingly localized masses of tuberculous lymph nodes will prove to be surrounded in all directions by other involved nodes that logically should be removed, and that an apparently movable mass may be found fixed to the jugular vein and the spinal accessory or other nerves, so that frequently a major dissection is required for what was intended as a limited resection.

B.C.G. Adenitis. Prophylaxis against tuberculosis, by inoculation with the bovine tubercle bacillus results in adenitis, axillary or cervical, in 5 per cent of infants, occasionally to an impressive degree. The disease is usually self-limited, occasionally generalized and rarely fatal.[67]

Lymphosarcoma, Hodgkin's disease and other malignant processes as well as **Letterer-Siwe's form of lipoid histiocytosis,** may produce masses of enlarged cervical lymph nodes as their first manifestation. If the remainder of the clinical picture does not make the diagnosis, local physical examination is not likely to, although in Hodgkin's disease the swelling is most likely to be unilateral and in Letterer-Siwe's, least likely. Biopsy is required to establish the diagnosis. Radical operative procedures for lymphosarcoma and Hodgkin's disease, when apparently localized, are advocated by some and have been practiced from time to time, but at present most hope is placed in the developing field of chemotherapy. Radiotherapy is often strikingly effective in temporarily reducing the size of a palpable mass.

Sternocleidomastoid tumor in newborn

babies presents as a firm tender tumor, usually in the mid-portion of the muscle. It results presumably from a tear in the taut muscle during delivery. The resultant torticollis or wryneck with the head tilted toward the shoulder of the affected side is alarming to parents who can be reassured that disappearance of the tumor and recovery of full and normal motion is the rule. The use of sandbags to hold the head straight while the baby sleeps may be of more benefit to the parents than to the baby. Excision of the tumor, counseled by some, may be postponed for 6 to 8 months, awaiting spontaneous relief. (See Chap. 45 on "Principles of General Plastic Surgery.")

Dermoid cysts about the supra-orbital ridge and the margins of the glabella are small, tense, hard, round and unattached to the skin. The frontal bone at operation will be found to be scooped out to hold the cyst, and occasionally preliminary roentgenograms will show a circular defect in the frontal bone. The cysts, even in such cases, are readily removed and have no intimate attachment to the intracranial tissues. Meningoceles in the same position are softer but become tense when the child cries.

Preauricular pits (fistula auris congenita) represent one of the curious hereditary defects associated with the embryonic branchial clefts and arches in a fashion still disputed. They occur in the tragus, in front of it or in the ascending portion of the helix and occasionally in the lobe of the ear.[151] If infected, they may require excision, a relatively simple procedure because of their superficial location and absence of ramifications. The edema of the infection may obscure a tiny external orifice, and the infection may dissect subcutaneously to the region of the angle of the mandible, making diagnosis difficult, since patients commonly are unaware of the existence of these pits.

Another and more complicated anomaly of the first branchial cleft consists of a fistula open at one end inside the external auditory canal and at the other below the angle of the mandible.[19]

The parotid gland may be the site of inflammatory processes other than the virus parotitis of mumps. In the newborn,[143] purulent parotitis occurs, with high fever, parotid swelling and pus expressible from Stensen's duct with the *Staphylococcus aureus* as the usual organism. In older children, mild, recurrent parotitis with pus in the duct and no demonstrable stones may produce a puzzling picture. Division of the sphincter of the duct and irrigation of the duct give relief. Tumors of the parotid gland in children[68] occur in all the varieties seen in adults, and some, such as hemangiomas, occur principally in children. Sarcomas, mixed salivary gland tumor, papillary cystadenoma lymphomatosum and carcinoma, both of the slower growing cylindroma type and of the more malignant muco-epidermoid type, all occur in children.[5] Once more the liability of children to malignant tumors must be borne in mind and therapy instituted appropriate to the lesion rather than some inadequate modification urged out of mistaken consideration for the tender age of the patient and the disbelief that one so young could harbor so malignant a tumor.

Oral Tumors. In the mouth, cysts of the mucous glands, on the lip, the tongue, the floor of the mouth, hemangiomas and lymphangiomas may all give smooth, rounded painless cystic tumors, inconvenient because of their location but readily excised. More diffuse hemangiomas, at times invasive, are more serious lesions but sometimes respond well to irradiation (see Chap. 18, on "Radiation Injury" for necessity of careful shielding). Diffuse lymphangiomatous tumors of tongue and lip, one cause of macroglossia[166] and macrocheilia, are deforming lesions, vexingly difficult to treat. Carefully planned repeated partial excisions may succeed in instances in which the process has not extended to invade neighboring tissues.

Epignathus. A bizarre variety of oral lesions has been reported in the newborn, epignathus, mucous cysts at the base of tongue, often causing difficulty in respiration or nursing.

Mandibular Retrusion (Pierre Robin Syndrome). Another cause of neonatal pharyngeal obstruction is mandibular retrusion.[78] With defective mandibular development and inadequate support for the tongue, the latter falls back to obstruct the pharynx, makes feeding difficult and may cause dangerous respiratory obstruction. Suture traction on tongue or the mandible is an unpleasant measure and is difficult to maintain, except as a temporary expedient. Advancing the tongue by incision and resuture in the floor of the mouth satisfactorily relieves the obstruction. Tracheostomy is an obvious first measure but can be avoided, and a tracheostomy inserted in the neonatal period is too often extraordinarily difficult to abandon. Gavage feedings may tide the infant over the first few weeks until he is able to hold his jaw forward. (See also Chap. 45.)

Choanal Atresia. Occasionally, the choanae are occluded by a bony block, covered over with unbroken mucosa so that no communication exists between the nares and the nasopharynx. Newborn infants find difficulty in breathing through the mouth and may literally suffocate before the diagnosis of choanal atresia is made, or, unable to master the technic of alternate swallowing and breathing, may starve. Associated deformities of eyes or the nasal passages, or excessive nasal discharge, and rhinorrhea of tears during crying suggest the diagnosis. Relief is afforded by transpalatine construction of an epithelium-lined nasopharyngeal passage.[96]

Ranula, a retention cyst of the sublingual and the submaxillary salivary gland ducts, presents in the floor of the mouth as a thin-walled, softly fluctuant cyst. The cause for its development, although not settled, is presumably an inflammatory obstruction. Treatment is by complete excision, or by an unroofing procedure in which the mucous membrane of the floor of the mouth and the underlying superficial wall of the cyst is removed, allowing the deep wall of the cyst to form the new oral mucosa.

Cystic hygroma (hygroma cysticum colli, cervical lymph hygroma), although occasionally seen in adults without previous history of a cervical swelling, is a characteristic lesion of infancy and childhood, usually present and recognized at birth. The swelling is rounded, extremely soft, fluctuant, usually lobulated and often transilluminates well. Characteristically, it originates in the posterior cervical triangle but may extend into the anterior triangle, the axilla or the mediastinum, or may be limited largely to one of these. The tumor is composed of a very thin-walled endothelial sac, usually multilocular.[54, 55] The several large locules, both communicating and non-communicating, generally have attached proc-

esses of tissue honeycombed by tiny cysts containing the same clear, slightly yellowish fluid, and ramifying between muscles, around vessels and nerves, often enveloping these. Hygromas occur at the time when the lymphatic system forms in the embryo from the venous system. Large hygromas cause the head to be held to the opposite side. In the anterior triangle, large hygromas, especially those suddenly increasing in size from hemorrhage within them, may cause pharyngeal compression and respiratory obstruction. Infection in the cysts, usually in association with a pharyngitis, produces severe symptoms. Antibiotic treatment should be given before decision as to incision and drainage. The uncomeliness of the swelling, the inconvenience it causes, its likelihood to infection, its tendency to growth and extension, all constitute reasons for the removal of these cysts. Irradiation, often employed, is ineffective. Operation may be undertaken as soon after birth as the patient presents himself. The delicacy of the cysts, and the difficulty of the dissection if the cysts rupture, require a painstaking dissection in the course of which the major deep structures of the neck will be exposed. Recurrence, after deliberate procedure of this type, is uncommon. About the head and the neck and elsewhere, lymphangiomas, particularly those associated with hemangiomas and classified at times as "mixed angiomas," may infiltrate tissues to such a degree as to require radical excision. In such angiomas, repeated re-recurrence is not at all uncommon.[59, 117] (See also Chap. 24.)

Lateral branchial cleft cysts, derived from the 3rd and the 4th branchial clefts,[104] appear characteristically along the anterior border of the sternocleidomastoid muscle. They are thick-walled, unilocular cysts, occasionally with open communications to the skin or the pharynx. The lining is ciliated columnar epithelium, occasionally squamous, with prominent submucosal lymphoid tissue. Diagnostic aspiration shows cholesterol crystals in the thin yellow fluid. The cysts may become infected and very rarely, late in life, may be the site of a carcinoma. Operative removal is curative and, except in those with an internal pharyngeal communication, is technically simple.

The thyroid, in the newborn, is the seat of **cellular hemangiomas, teratomata and col-**

loid goiters. These have in common the production of respiratory obstruction by laryngeal, tracheal and pharyngeal compression. Operation for relief of the obstruction by resection of the tumor or splitting of the thyroid isthmus in goiters should be undertaken at once, with tracheotomy being resorted to instead if facilities for intratracheal anesthesia and definitive surgery are lacking. In general, it may be said that whenever the advisability of tracheotomy is being considered, the procedure is already overdue. Neonatal goiters may occur in babies born of mothers treated with thiourea drugs or with cobalt during gestation.

Carcinoma of the thyroid occurs in children and forms a far higher proportion of childhood thyroid nodules than of adult thyroid nodules, so that all thyroid nodules in children should be removed with the possibility of cancer and a radical operation in mind.[6] It has been generally held that whereas malignant neoplasms in most of the body appear to grow more rapidly and kill more quickly in younger patients, thyroid cancers represent an exception and are more benign in children than in adults.[76, 87, 167] At least one publication[173] tends to cast doubt on this assertion, claiming from careful analysis of published material that cancer of the thyroid, type for type, is no more and no less malignant and no different in distribution in children than in adults. The nature, the prognosis and proper treatment of thyroid carcinoma in general is in hot dispute (cf. Chap. 26, pp. 574-575). Most clinicians have felt that any relative melioration of prognosis in childhood thyroid cancer is explained by a greater frequency of papillary carcinoma of the kind associated with the indolent metastases once thought to be lateral aberrant thyroid tissue. Diffuse goiters of the colloid type in children usually will respond to treatment with desiccated thyroid or iodides. Diffuse toxic goiter occurs in children and as a rule is usually treated nonoperatively (see Chap. 27, "Thyroid, Thymus and Parathyroids"). Thyroiditis produces the sudden appearance of a firm, tender, moderately enlarged gland. In one such we have seen regression with thyroid hormone therapy.

The thymus may falter in its embryologic descent into the thorax from the 3rd pharyngeal pouch. There may result a persistent cervical or cervicomediastinal thymus, causing pressure on the trachea and presenting as a cervical mass made more conspicuous by coughing or crying. The mass may be so soft as to suggest a hygroma. Removal of the thymus, in these uncommon instances, is curative.[4] Irradiation in this area is to be avoided because of a 1 to 2 per cent incidence of thyroid carcinoma developing later in childhood.[23]

Later cervical tumors of childhood include teratomas,[129] carotid body tumors, tumors of spinal nerves, tumors of the cranial nerves, tumors of the sympathetic nerve trunks and ganglia, and even of the ganglion nodosum of the vagus nerve.[24]

THORAX

CHEST WALL

Anomalies. A variety of deformities of the chest wall are seen in infants. In the mid-line there may be sternal defects varying from an incomplete cleft to a wide separation of the embryologically paired sternal halves. The heart, covered by thin skin or only by a transparent membranous tissue, may protrude through such a defect, in the anomaly known as *thoracic ectopia cordis*. With clefts of the upper sternum, the heart seems to be in the neck; hence the misnomer *cervical ectopia cordis*. With clefts of the lower sternum, a new syndrome has been described with a pentalogy of defects—distal sternal cleft, ventral abdominal defect, anterior diaphragmatic defect, pericardial defect and interventricular septal defect or diverticulum of the ventricle. Separation of the sternal halves is readily corrected by simple suture in the neonatal period when the chest wall is maximally flexible.[124] Later, plastic procedures are required. Major degrees of ectopia cordis seldom have been corrected successfully, in part because severe associated cardiac anomalies usually are present.[98]

Pectus Excavatum. The sternum may be either depressed or abnormally prominent. In pectus excavatum (funnel breast, trichterbrust) there is a dorsal displacement of the sternum, forming a concavity from above downward and from side to side. The costal cartilages, from the 3rd or the 4th to the costal margin, are sharply depressed toward the sunken sternum. The deformity is congenital, often familial, and usually progressive

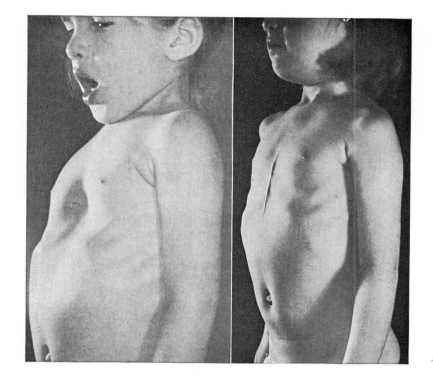

FIG. 46-1. Pectus excavatum. A 6-year-old girl with marked pectus excavatum. Before operation (*left*) note the retraction of the sternum and protrusion of the abdomen. (*Right*) 9 months after operation the chest expanded normally, with deep inspiration, and the abdomen no longer protruded.

during childhood. The children exhibit paradoxical retraction of the sternum and protrusion of the abdomen during deep inspiration. Poor posture—kyphosis, rounded shoulders, forward thrust neck—is characteristic. The heart is usually displaced to the left and rotated. Murmurs and minor degrees of electrocardiographic change indicative of rotation are common. Arrhythmias are frequent. Symptoms rarely appear before adolescence, when easy fatigability may be noticed. Mild dysphagia is not rare in infants, and in three babies we have seen severe inspiratory stridor, relieved by operation. In a few individuals, severe cardiac distress ultimately occurs. The deformity is easily corrected (Fig. 46-1) and while indications among surgeons vary, the writer of this chapter feels that the corrective operation should be performed in all infants or children with pronounced or progressive defects, in the absence of serious associated anomalies of overriding importance.[14, 89] Our preference is for subperichondrial resection of all of the deformed cartilages, division of the intercostal bundles, xiphisternal disarticulation, transverse cuneiform osteotomy of the sternum at the cephalic extrem-

ity of the defect, elevation of the sternum and maintenance in corrected position by heavy silk sutures across the sternal osteotomy. In well over 100 such procedures, symptoms have been relieved in all patients who had them; gain in weight and vigor has been extremely common, and the reconstruction has usually been excellent. Morbidity is low, and mortality almost nonexistent.[119]

In pigeon breast (pectus carinatum) the sternum buckles forward, to the accompaniment of deep lateral depression of the costal cartilages on either side. Much less common than funnel chest, this deformity is also congenital. The lateral depressions may compress the heart or significantly decrease lung volume. Operation to elevate the lateral runnels produces a gratifying result.[123]

Absence of Ribs or Costal Cartilages. One or several ribs or costal cartilages may be absent. This may occur in the upper costal cartilages in association with absence of the pectoralis major muscle—itself a common deformity. Appropriate plastic procedures with rib or fascial grafts in the chest wall fill out and bridge over these defects.[124]

Harrison's groove, a transverse groove on

either side, at the line of diaphragmatic insertion, above the costal margin which is thus made to flare, is one of the most common thoracic deformities. It may be associated with rickets. It does not appear to be surgically remediable.

Asymmetry of Thorax. The plastic, growing chest wall of a child is readily influenced by pressures from within and thoracic asymmetries must not be dismissed as idiopathic without study to be sure that the space requirements of an enormous but slow-growing dermoid or other tumor or of a hypertrophied heart or the changes associated with a congenitally absent lung are not the cause of a striking difference in the shape of one side of the chest or the other.

Tumors of the chest wall occur so early in infancy as to make it probable, despite their frequently malignant nature, that they have been present from birth. *Chondromas of ribs and sternum* occur, may reach great size and after any but radical excision tend to recur, with ultimately fatal outcome. *Sarcomas of the chest wall* occur and a wide variety of tumors of neural origin—*neurofibromas, ganglioneuromas* and *paragangliomas* of the sympathetic chain. *Ewing's tumor* may manifest itself in a rib. Whenever possible, in dealing with chest wall tumors, wide, en bloc dissection of full thickness of chest wall should be employed, except for the essentially intrathoracic nerve tumors.[126]

MEDIASTINUM

(See also Chap. 45, "Carcinoma of the Lung and Tumors of the Thorax.")

Tumors. In the anterior mediastinum, 3 principal types of tumors occur in childhood—dermoids, teratomas and lymphomas.[30] The dermoids and the teratomas are the same tumor with different manifestations. The characteristic dermoid is made up of ectodermal derivatives and shows keratinizing squamous epithelium, sweat and sebaceous glands, hair and teeth—any or all of these. Almost invariably, if sufficient care is taken, an area will be found in the wall of the cyst in which there are abnormal tissues from other germ layers. The teratomata are characteristically more obviously derived from all three germ layers, as often solid as cystic, and show vari-

ous types of abnormal appearing secretory epithelium, respiratory epithelium, glial tissue characteristically, bone and cartilage and, in fact, tissue of all types.[129] *Dermoids* rarely become malignant but may reach enormous size, compress and displace the thoracic structures, become infected and rupture into pleural cavity, pericardium or bronchus. Sudden increase in size or symptoms from an anterior mediastinal tumor, suggesting the malignant transformation of one element in a teratoma, is a frequent occurrence. Dermoids and teratomata should be removed before complications occur. The diagnosis of any mediastinal tumor is likely to be uncertain in advance of operation, and the position usually is taken that operation, when such a tumor is demonstrated by x-ray studies, is the only safe course with any mediastinal tumor. If lymphosarcoma or Hodgkin's disease is discovered, operation will have given a definitive histologic diagnosis on which to base chemotherapy and roentgenotherapy, and local extirpation itself may have some value.

The pericardium itself is, rarely, the site of a dermoid or other tumor, and occasionally a defect in the pericardium is continuous with a defect in the diaphragm so that herniation of the abdominal viscera takes place into the pericardial sac, producing a radiologic appearance suggestive of an intrapericardial tumor.[160]

Tumors of the posterior mediastinum are particularly those of the neural elements—*neurofibroma, ganglioneuroma, paraganglioma.* These are slow-growing and become malignant in an uncertain but probably high percentage of cases.[77] The roentgenographic appearance is of a dense, rounded, discrete, posteriorly placed lesion. The tumors, particularly the ganglionueuromas, are occasionally of enormous size and then may produce pressure symptoms. The neurofibromata, which always should be looked for here in patients with von Recklinghausen's neurofibromatosis, occasionally may show a dumbbell shape with extension through the vertebral foramina into the vertebral canal. Neuroblastomata, malignant and rapidly growing, may require combinations of operative therapy, irradiation and chemotherapy for maximal benefit.

The esophagus, in the posterior mediastinum, is a source of a number of lesions peculiar to infancy and childhood.

ESOPHAGEAL ATRESIA

One of the most gratifying chapters in the history of pediatric surgery deals with the development of the operation for the correction of esophageal atresia with tracheoesophageal fistula (Fig. 46-2). The condition in over 90 per cent of cases consists of a blind, proximal esophageal segment, dilated and hypertrophied as the result of obstruction to fetal deglutition and ending at the level of the 3rd to the 5th dorsal vertebra. A few strands of muscle connect it to the distal segment which communicates openly with the trachea. In the other cases, both ends may have a fistulous communication to the trachea, or neither, or solely the proximal end, or the distal esophagus may be altogether rudimentary.[84] First treated as an anatomic curiosity beyond correction and invariably fatal, atresia was then attacked in laborious multistage operations designed to establish drainage of the proximal esophagus to the exterior, close the tracheo-esophageal fistula, open the distal esophagus or stomach to the exterior, and finally to link the esophageal and gastric fistulae by a tube of skin or intestine, thus restoring deglutition and completing the operation. Leven, in 1938,[92] and Ladd, 24 hours

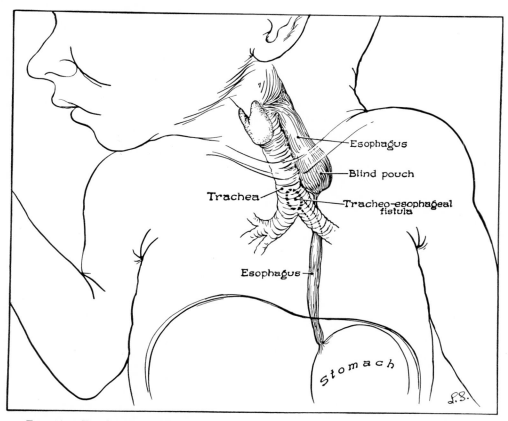

Fig. 46-2. Esophageal atresia with tracheo-esophageal fistula. In 95 per cent of the cases of esophageal atresia, the anomalies are found as pictured here. The proximal, blind esophagus is dilated and hypertrophied from the obstruction to fetal swallowing. A few strands of muscle attach it to the slender distal segment. The fistulous communication with the distal segment is to the trachea just above the carina. Aspiration of regurgitated saliva from the obstructed esophageal pouch and of gastric juice directly into the trachea through the fistula lead to atelectasis and pneumonia. The operation consists of division of the fistulous tract, closure of the tracheal opening and anastomosis of the esophageal segments. (Ravitch, M. M.: S. Clin. North America 29:1541)

later,[84] each saved the lives of the first of a series of infants operated upon by this complicated scheme. In 1941, Cameron Haight of Ann Arbor,[56] after the unsuccessful experiences of Lanman, Sampson and Shaw, performed the first successful 1-stage division and closure of a tracheo-esophageal fistula and end-to-end anastomosis of the esophageal segments. Haight's operation was performed through an extrapleural exposure of the posterior mediastinum from the left side. The right-sided extrapleural approach, which avoids the aorta, became standard soon after. At present a number of surgeons[44, 111] prefer the technically more attractive right transpleural approach, although it is not clear that the percentage of successful results has been increased thereby.

The condition is to be suspected in an infant, often premature, who bubbles spittle and chokes and becomes cyanotic when nursing. Attempted passage of a firm radiopaque rubber catheter under fluoroscopic control confirms the diagnosis. A cubic centimeter of Diontosil may be injected in the catheter which has been seen to meet an obstruction and turn back on itself. After a roentgenogram has been taken the radiopaque material is withdrawn. Pneumonia due to overflow from the blind esophageal pouch into the pharynx with reflux or aspiration into the trachea presents the greatest hazard in these infants. Gastric juice regurgitated into the trachea through the fistula is an added factor. Preoperative treatment consists of tracheal aspiration, constant-suction of the esophageal pouch, with the head of the crib elevated so that the pooled saliva is aspirated readily as it accumulates in the pouch, dehydration, and administration of antibiotics. Gastrostomy before reconstruction of the esophagus invites regurgitation of gastric feedings into the trachea through the fistula. After operation, gastrostomy may be necessary if the infant is not able to swallow fairly promptly. Postoperative strictures are not rare and may be dilated fairly readily. In the most favorable series, from 70 to 75 per cent or better of successful results have been reported.[152, 154] If the anastomosis fails or is impossible, the surgeon may resort to a swifter version of the old multistaged operations.[93] Esophageal reconstruction with a colonic loop brought up through the anterior mediastinum

is presently the simplest and most satisfactory type.[145]

ESOPHAGEAL STRICTURES

Congenital strictures of the esophagus are much more rare than atresias. At birth, the child appears to be able to swallow, but gradually the retention above the stricture leads to stasis and edema and complete occlusion of the esophagus days or weeks after birth. Immediate gastrostomy, pharyngeal suction and subsequent dilatation on a swallowed string have been regularly curative in our hands. Resection, or plastic reconstruction of the stenotic area, is feasible but rarely necessary.[142]

Acquired strictures from the ingestion of escharotics—usually lye—are better prevented than corrected. In all children thought to have swallowed lye, the immediate institution of a daily regimen of esophageal bouginage with soft-rubber catheters containing mercury or mustard seed lead shot, will usually prevent the formation of strictures.[37] If the strictures form, dilatation, with or without temporary gastrostomy, will restore deglutition in most cases.[66] In severe or neglected cases, the esophageal channel may be so tortuous that success cannot be achieved, or the lumen actually may be entirely obliterated. In such instances, some type of esophageal substitute is required. A loop of jejunum or colon is brought, preferably through the anterior mediastinum, to connect the cervical esophagus and the stomach.

Mediastinal cysts of foregut origin, the so-called duplications of the esophagus,[31, 86] like enteric cysts associated with any other part of the alimentary canal, are thick-walled, muscular structures lined by gastric, intestinal or colonic epithelium, and filled with thin mucoid secretion. Usually they are united so closely to the wall of the esophagus as to be fused to it. A communication with the esophageal lumen is rare. The cysts tend to be large, swelling out into the pleural cavity, more often the right. Symptoms are caused by compression of the esophagus, the trachea or the bronchus. In many instances, the cyst is lined by gastric mucosa, secreting acid, and eroding into the lung, the bronchus or the esophagus, with bleeding as a prominent symptom. Treatment consists of removal of the cyst or the cyst lining. Anastomosis of the cyst to the esophagus is acceptable treatment for those cysts not lined by gastric mucosa.

PLEURA

Chylothorax is seen in the neonatal period, presumably from rupture of the thoracic duct as a result of venous distention and back pressure during the birth process, and at any age from trauma or from obstruction by tumors or tuberculosis and rarely from no apparent cause. Today surgical trauma during thoracic, particularly cardiovascular, procedures is probably the most common cause. In the neonatal instances, dyspnea and signs of fluid lead to thoracentesis and discovery of a milky fluid.[169] If dyspnea is relieved by thoracentesis as needed, the accumulation of chyle will presently cease in most instances, although successful ligation of the thoracic duct on both sides of a leak usually can be achieved if aspiration therapy fails after an adequate trial. Especially in cases of traumatic chylothorax, before ligation is attempted, 3 to 4 days of intravenous alimentation with *nothing* being given orally may permit spontaneous closure. Chyle—intestinal lymph—is not formed unless food or drink is ingested.

Empyema. Once almost the only commonly treated thoracic condition in pediatric surgery, postpneumonic empyema is now almost a clinical rarity. It occurs relatively earlier in the course of the disease than in adults, and the susceptibility of the small bronchi to necrosis leads to frequent occurrence of pyopneumothorax. While persistent and continued attempts at aspiration of pus and instillation of antibiotics may result in an appreciable percentage of recoveries, early trochar thoracotomy and tube drainage will cure most childhood empyemas at the cost of the single manipulation. Delay in healing, as evidenced by persistence of fever or tachycardia or arrest in the decrease of the volume of the empyema cavity, should raise the question of rib resection and open drainage (see Chap. 43, "Surgery of the Lung").

Streptococcal and influenza pneumonia and empyema have disappeared. Pneumococcal empyema is uncommon. In the last few years staphylococcal pneumonia and empyema have become more common than any form of empyema had been for years.[125] Characteristic of staphylococcal pneumonia is the appearance of air sacs and pneumatoceles. These result from bronchial necrosis and escape of air into the parenchyma. Great enlargement of the cysts may cause dyspnea, and rupture of the cysts may cause tension pneumothorax. Earlier in the course of staphylococcal pneumonia massive effusions may cause severe dyspnea. Catheter suction drainage is required for empyema, massive effusions, pneumothorax and for rapidly expanding pneumatoceles.[140]

LUNGS

Agenesis of the lung may occur in several forms. There may be true aplasia of lung and bronchus with no trace of either, aplasia of the lung with the bronchus represented by a blind pouch or by a nodule of cartilage and fibrous tissue, or extreme hypoplasia of the lung in which the main bronchus appears to be normal but ends in a fleshy rudiment of lung. In some instances, the anomaly is little more than a physical and roentgenographic curiosity—one half of the thorax or more being occupied by the one good lung, the other containing the much-displaced heart. In other instances, in infancy, extreme respiratory difficulty and death occur.[17, 98] It is not clear why the absence of one lung should produce fatal respiratory difficulty. Maier suggests that the single pulmonary artery in its abnormal course may compress trachea or bronchus, causing a fatal respiratory obstruction.

Neonatal Atelectasis, Aspiration and Pneumothorax. In the newborn, failure of areas of the lung to expand, or obstruction by excessive aspiration of amniotic fluid or hyalin membrane disease may be suspected in the cyanotic infant with difficult respirations. Congenital pneumonia seems to be more frequent than was realized previously. Physical examination may show areas of decreased aeration and roentgenograms usually will show opaque areas in the lungs. Infants with congenital cerebral defects or brain damage may fail to breathe well enough to expand normal alveoli. In very premature infants, the pulmonary tissue may not be capable of expansion. In some infants, both term and premature, congenital alveolar dysplasia[97] interferes with aeration. Excessive aspiration of amniotic fluid leads to grave difficulties or death. Skillful bronchoscopic aspiration may produce dramatic improvement. Infants with extensive areas of unexpanded lung and making forceful (and frequently mechanically assisted) respiratory efforts may overdistend inflated segments of lung with rupture of alveoli and production of pneumothorax. Prompt aspiration of the pleural air and insertion of a catheter into the pleural cavity for under water drainage with negative pressure are lifesaving. A roentgenogram of the entire infant should be taken whenever respiratory distress or cyanosis is noted. Physical signs are not to be depended on for evidence of pneumothorax, atelectasis, diaphragmatic hernia or other lesions causing respiratory difficulty.

Congenital Cystic Disease of the Lungs. Cysts of the lungs may be single giant air-filled cysts or multiple smaller cysts containing air and/or liquid. In distribution, they may be unilobar, multilobar or, rarely, involve all lobes.[128] Air in the cysts, anthracotic pigment in their lining or entrance of contrast material on bronchography, demonstrates communication with the bronchial tree in all cases. The cysts are lined by tall, ciliated columnar epithelium and may contain cartilage in their walls. The commonest presenting clinical picture results from infection of the cysts. Such infected cysts have been mistaken for lung abscesses and for empyemas with pyopneumothorax. Single large cysts, with a flap-valve type of bronchial communication, may distend with air under tension and cause severe respiratory distress. Hemoptysis and brain abscess occasionally occur in association with lung cysts. The repeated infections result from the presence of large, ill-drained spaces connected to the bronchial tree and excision of the cyst or involved pulmonary lobes or segments is the only effective treatment. After diagnosis, early operation is indicated. Infants tolerate pulmonary resection very well, and such procedures have been performed successfully in the first weeks of life.[18]

The best analysis of the development of these cysts probably is contained in the writings of Pryce, who believes that abnormal fetal vascular supply to the lung from the aorta exerts traction on the lung and, at times, in "sequestration of the lung" and in cystic disease, "intralobar sequestration," produces resultant anomalies.[113, 114] While with cystic disease we have seen such associated systemic arteries, trilobed left lungs and other anomalies, some otherwise typical instances of congenital cystic disease of the lung seem to be innocent of such stigmata of "sequestration." Cysts are to be distinguished from bronchiectatic cavities and lung abscess, in which treatment would be similar, and in the newborn, from diaphragmatic hernia with multiple intestinal fluid levels in the chest. Infants with pneumonia, particularly that due to staphylococci, are particularly prone to develop bronchiolar necrosis and intrapulmonary pneumatoceles strongly simulating cysts with infection.[1, 13, 112, 140] Inspiratory trapping of air by mucus in the bronchi also may be responsible for such pneumatocele formation. If the true nature of pneumatoceles is appreciated, they may be watched as they slowly disappear over a course of weeks.

Pulmonary Arteriovenous Fistulae. These are single or multiple areas of communication in the pulmonary substance between pulmonary arteries and veins. They may form one or several masses, centimeters in diameter, or scores of minute almost telangiectatic communications. Cyanosis, polycythemia and clubbing of the fingers are characteristic. Violent hemoptyses may occur. The heart is normal. The lesions are demonstrable, if large enough, on ordinary roentgenograms, laminograms and by angiocardiography. Many of the reported cases are familial. Resection is the treatment of choice. Since the lesions may be multiple and the apparently uninvolved lobe or lobes may contain small communications which subsequently will enlarge, it is important to excise the vascular lesion or lesions rather than the containing lobe or segment.[148, 174] (See also Chap. 42, "Cardiac Surgery.")

Lung Tumors. Every sort of lung tumor occurring in adults occurs also in children, and treatment, as in adults, is by resection. Once more, the frequent occurrence of malignant tumors in childhood must be borne in mind. Bronchial adenoma[165] is a slowly growing malignant tumor giving early symptoms because of its intrabronchial growth and tendency to bleed or cause bronchial obstruction. If it is resected properly, the results are excellent. Carcinoma of the lung in children is rare but not unknown[22] and has been described even in infants.

GASTROINTESTINAL TRACT

ATRESIAS AND STENOSIS

Atresia (absence of an opening) and stenosis (a narrowing) may affect any portion of the intestinal tract. The standard attribution of atresia is to a failure of coalescence of vacuoles in the epithelial mass which fills the embryonic intestine. This does not explain the instances of atresia in which one or several segments of bowel are represented by little more than fibrous cord, nor the instances in which segments of the mesentery are missing, together with the segments of bowel. Cornified squamous epithelium and lanugal hairs have been found in the rectal plugs of infants with intestinal atresia, indicating the presence of a patent alimentary canal fairly late in development. Atresias have been reported in which histologic study has shown unequivocal evidence of an intra-uterine intussusception with necrosis, scarring and obliteration of the lumen.[108] It seems probable that vascular insufficiency, ischemia and necrosis by one mechanism or another, is the cause of many of the forms of atresia of the intestine. The epithelial mass mechanism may be operative, chiefly in the duodenum and the proximal jejunum, and it is here chiefly that occasionally one sees an atresia due solely to a mucosal diaphragm. An incomplete diaphragm may result in a stenosis. Other stenoses appear as narrowed areas of thickened bowel. The ileum is the commonest site of atresia and stenosis, the duodenum and the jejunum following. Atresia on the gastric side of the pylorus has been reported 2 or 3 times. Atresia of the duodenum, proximal to the ampulla of Vater, is a rarity.

The frequency with which atresias of the intestine are associated with hydramnios is recognized, although the mechanism is uncertain. Apgar has demonstrated brilliantly the utility of immediate gastric aspiration in the newborn. Accumulations of more than 25 cc. of fluid in the infant's stomach are pathologic and suggest obstruction.[144]

Vomiting, the cardinal symptom of intestinal atresia, begins within a day of birth, is unremitting and usually contains bile. Newborn babies do not normally vomit or regurgitate more than a portion of their feedings. Any excessive regurgitation, any vomiting and certainly the appearance of bile in the returned material should suggest the possibility of intestinal obstruction. In duodenal atresia, vomiting often will be effective in preventing the appearance of distention, although at times the stomach and the duodenum may be dilated tremendously and visibly.

The occurrence of duodenal obstruction by the superior mesenteric artery has long been a moot subject. Jones[73a] has adduced evidence of its occurrence, with relief by duodenojejunostomy.

A plain x-ray film of the chest and the abdomen is so extremely informative that it should be taken at the first suspicion of obstruction. Distention of stomach and duodenum with absence of air in the remainder of the abdomen indicates a duodenal atresia. Dilated loops of small bowel with no gas visible in the colon are evidence of obstruction in the ileum or jejunum (Fig. 46-3). Other causes for such obstruction must be differentiated. In meconium ileus, the opaque loops of small bowel may show a granular shadow; and in meconium peritonitis, spotty calcification may be seen in some of the opaque areas. An enema with Lipiodol will demonstrate whether the colon is in normal position or not, and in the condition known as meconium plug in which inspissated meconium simply fails to be evacuated, the enema may be curative in itself. While the meconium in infants with intestinal atresia (whose intestines, at operation, distal to the obstruction are incredibly tiny coils, relatively thick walled and empty) is generally scanty, drier and grayer than normal, it may appear surprisingly unremarkable.

Microscopic examination of the core of the rectal discharge usually will show an absence of the cornified squamous epithelial cells of the swallowed vernix caseosa normally seen in meconium (Farber's test). This is an interesting confirmatory observation but of little clinical importance since the treatment of incomplete obstructions, in the presence of which such cornified cells may be found, is often as urgent as is the treatment of complete obstructions. Much the same may be said of the test of the meconium for maternal hemoglobin which is absent in cases of atresia. In any neo-

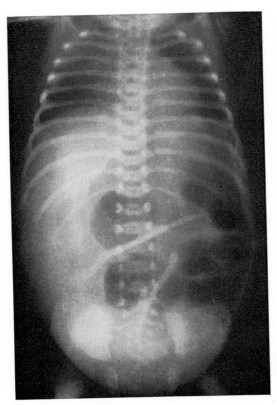

FIG. 46-3. Atresia of ileum. Roentgenogram of infant 36 hours old with great dilatation of small bowel loops and no air recognizable in the colon.

natal obstruction the patency of the bowel must be demonstrated at operation, from one end to the other.

Nothing is said about roentgenograms with ingested barium or Lipiodol, because these rarely give any more information than the plain film and even may obscure it. Barium, given to a newborn who is vomiting, may be regurgitated and aspirated. That which remains in the intestine may prove to be embarrassing. Insufflation of the stomach with air has been recommended as a safe method of obtaining contrast roentgenograms and may be useful. The water-miscible and enterally absorbable contrast media are not as objectionable as barium or Lipiodol but are not often required except in instances of suspected partial obstruction.

Treatment is directed to the establishment of a high probability of the existence of ob-

struction, and to immediate institution of gastric suction so that further swallowing of air will not increase distention. Preparation for operation includes the insertion of a polyethylene catheter in the saphenous vein, administration of glucose and electrolytes and matching of blood for transfusion. For all the causes of neonatal obstruction, the treatment is prompt operation.[9, 33, 40, 46, 74] In the newborn, a transverse incision, which rarely disrupts, made just above the umbilicus, will give access to the entire abdomen, so that no time need be lost in the intellectual exercise of pinpointing the nature and the location of the obstruction. Stenoses and mucosal diaphragm atresias are relatively more common in the duodenum than elsewhere. At operation, in duodenal obstructions, duodenojejunostomy, around the obstruction, is most satisfactory. Gastrojejunostomy lays the basis for a future anastomotic ulcer[99] although it is easier technically. Diaphragm obstructions may be excised and the longitudinal incision in the bowel closed transversely by the Heineke-Mikulicz procedure. In the jejunum and the ileum, the lateral anastomoses around the obstructions occasionally must be combined with resection of the massively distended proximal blind end. In addition, it is helpful to insert a polyethylene catheter into the dilated bowel, proximal to the anastomosis to bring it out through the abdominal wall for suction and decompression. Gastrostomy for aspiration and decompression, and subsequently for feeding, has become deservedly popular. Double-barreled ileostomies have been performed, at times successfully, but these are generally to be avoided as involving serious problems of electrolyte loss and in any case requiring a second operative procedure in the near future. Atresias may be multiple so that the few seconds required to inspect the full length of an infant's intestinal tract are well spent. Atresias of the colon, excluding rectum and anus, do occur but are very rare.

MALROTATION OF THE INTESTINE

For an understanding of the anomalies of rotation and the principles of their treatment, an outline of the embryologic development of the bowel must be borne in mind. From the 5th through the 10th week, most of the midgut—the small intestine and the proximal large intestine—lies outside the body cavity in the communicating exocoelomic space at the base of the umbilical cord. If the intestine fails to return to the abdominal cavity, the condition known as an *amniotic hernia* (exomphalos, omphalocele) results. The intestine will be found in the primitive, nonrotated position. As the intestine grows and enters the cord and then returns to the abdomen, the simple straight tube suspended on its dorsal mesentery, begins to coil. The duodenojejunal loop is bulged out and then passes behind the stalk of the superior mesenteric artery. At the same time as the cecum moves back into the abdomen, it enters on the left, moves upward and across to the right, anterior to the superior mesenteric artery, finally reaching the right lower quadrant. One more event is of clinical importance—the fusion of the duodenojejunal loop, ascending and descending colon, and the base of the mesentery of the small bowel, to the posterior parietal peritoneum. Failure of rotation usually is associated with failure of normal fusion and with abnormal peritoneal bands passing from the colon in the left upper quadrant, across the duodenum, to the posterior parietal peritoneum in the right upper quadrant. The failure of peritoneal fusion, with the entire small intestine hanging from the stalk of the superior mesenteric vessels, predisposes to volvulus of the entire small bowel on this stalk. The peritoneal bands from colon to right upper quadrant across the duodenum lead to compression of the duodenum and duodenal obstruction. It was Ladd, the father of pediatric surgery, who, in 1932,[83] pointed out the necessity for dividing these avascular peritoneal folds. In some instances, symptoms are present at birth, suggesting the volvulus existed in utero. Symptoms tend to be insidious and misleading. With a volvulus of the entire small intestine and the additional duodenal compression, vomiting begins early, and distention appears late if at all. The obstruction may be incomplete, and meconium and flatus, and later on, curds are passed intermittently. Whereas vascular obstruction and gangrene appear early in some infants, the twist in others is apparently loose enough, despite a 360° or greater anticlockwise rotation, to allow an adequate circulation in the bowel. The vomitus usually contains bile, the roentgenogram shows dilatation of stomach and the first portion of the duodenum and usually some gas in the intestines. Roentgenograms of an enema with contrast material may show an interesting picture of incompletely rotated colon.

In the newborn, then, the picture is similar to that in atresia or stenosis, and promptness in operating is even more important because of the threat of massive infarction of the intestine. Fever, leukocytosis, distention and discoloration of the abdominal wall suggest that the bowel is already gangrenous. The duodenal obstruction, without volvulus, may lead to chronic vomiting and bouts of abdominal pain for years. In some cases, malrotation of the intestine is entirely asymptomatic.

Recurrence of volvulus after operation is extremely rare. Snyder and Chaffin[150] and Gardner[35] suggest that this is due to the careful operative mobilization of the duodenojejunal loop which comes to lie in the right peritoneal gutter. Gross[48] suggests that it is due to fixation by postoperative adhesions. It seems at least as reasonable to suppose that the volvulus develops in the fetus to become symptomatic at birth or sometimes later, and that, once derotated, the free-swinging intestine will rarely develop a volvulus.

MECONIUM ILEUS AND MECONIUM PERITONITIS

Meconium ileus has come to be recognized as the neonatal manifestation of the systemic disease known as fibrocystic disease of the pancreas or mucoviscidosis. The clinical picture is that of complete intestinal obstruction from birth. Vomiting and distention attract attention to a baby who has passed no meconium or only a plug of dry, slate-gray material. Roentgenograms (Fig. 46-4) demonstrate many dilated loops of small bowel and may show granular shadows of retained meconium. At operation the distal ileum is found distended with thick, blackish, tarry, tenacious material which adheres to gloves and instruments and equally well to the mucosa of the bowel. The material can be removed only with the greatest difficulty by milking and saline washing through one or several enterostomies. Hiatt[61] published the first series of operative successes in this condition by this method. The results of Gross, with a simple resection of the "tar"-filled loop

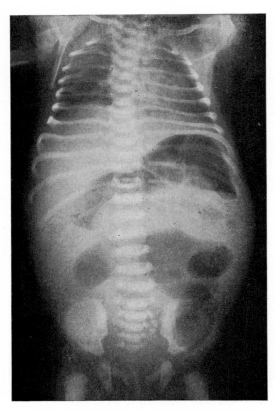

FIG. 46-4. Meconium ileus. Infant 48 hours old. Numerous loops of small bowel are dilated. Opaque, meconium-filled loops are not distinguishable in this instance, but the previous occurrence of meconium ileus in a sibling permitted the correct diagnosis to be made before operation.

and temporary double-barreled ileostomy, are spectacular—15 of the 19 treated since 1949 were relieved of their obstruction. The grim aftermath lies in the subsequent course of many of these patients. In a total group of 22 infants with meconium ileus successfully relieved by operation, 8 died of other consequences of mucoviscidosis, such as nutritional disturbances and overwhelming pulmonary infection. The condition of the survivors is said to be satisfactory. The postoperative treatment includes high caloric diet, high vitamin intake, protein hydrolysate feedings, or added pancreatic enzyme. Antibiotics are given indefinitely to ward off respiratory infections.[47]

Meconium peritonitis is the result of intra-uterine intestinal perforation with leakage of meconium into the fetal peritoneal cavity. An intense foreign body inflammatory reaction occurs, the result of which is neonatal intestinal obstruction.[94] Roentgenograms show distended loops of bowel. Spotty calcification, in the abdomen, presumably as a result of fat necrosis associated with the peritonitis, is pathognomonic (Fig. 46-5). The perforation may occur proximal to an area of atresia or stenosis, or proximal to an ileum obstructed with the glutinous meconium of meconium ileus. In almost half the cases, no cause for the perforation has been found. At operation, the adherent intestinal loops must be dissected away painstakingly and the primary condition dealt with. In most instances, the perforation itself will have healed over.

DUPLICATIONS AND ENTEROGENOUS CYSTS

At any point along the entire length of the alimentary tract there may occur intimately attached to its wall cystic structures formed of smooth muscle and lined by mucous membrane, like that of some portion of the intestinal tract. A number of embryologic explanations are offered—that embryonic diverticula are pinched off to persist as cysts or that vacuoles forming in the dissolution of the stage of epithelial plugging of the bowel fail to coalesce, hence remain as cysts. Many of these enterogenous cysts are explained inadequately by such mechanisms, particularly the instances in which an entire segment of bowel is parallel by a second and similar channel. For this reason, Ladd and Gross preferred the term duplication, implying an attempt at doubling of the bowel.[85] There is certainly a group of cases of duplication of anus, rectum and colon and external and internal genitalia which appear to be true doubling and have been interpreted as due to incomplete caudal twinning.[118] The older term of enterogenous cyst, which makes no pretense to a developmental explanation that cannot be supported strongly, probably is best retained for the more frequently occurring localized cysts. A curious feature is that the cysts may be lined by mucosa of a segment of intestine remote from that of the location of the cyst. Most of the cysts do not communicate with the lumen of the attached bowel. Symptoms are: a mass, occasionally large enough to distend the abdomen of an infant; pain from the tenseness of the mass; obstruction of the bowel to which it is attached; bleeding from necrosis of the bowel by pressure, or from erosion by the strongly acid secretion of cysts lined by gastric mucous membrane. In two instances we have seen a small enteric cyst at the ileocecal valve cause an intussusception. The treatment is operative. Because the muscular walls of the cyst and the bowel are so fused, clean excision of the cyst is not often possible. Either the adjacent bowel is resected with the cyst, or the bulk of the cyst is excised and its mucosa stripped from the common muscular wall of cyst and bowel, or the cyst is widely anastomosed to the bowel[36] in locations in which more definite treatment presents too great hazard.

Mesenteric cysts are usually lymphatic cysts, frequently chylous. They tend to be thin-walled and soft and are rarely palpable through the abdominal wall. Arising usually between the leaves of the mesentery, they may form very large sacs extending through the mesentery in dumbbell fashion and stretching the bowel over them. Intestinal obstruction, with a history of repeated attacks, and volvulus are the most common sequelae, but acute inflammation may occur in the apparent absence of obstruction.[58] Resection usually entails resection of the associated bowel. Omental cysts, lymphatic or angiomatous, are found occasionally. Torsion and infarction produce acute abdominal symptoms.[69] Very large cysts may produce vague symptoms. Mesenteric cysts and omental cysts may be so soft as to defy palpation through the intact abdominal wall.

STOMACH AND DUODENUM

Peptic Ulcer in Infancy and Childhood. Peptic ulcers associated with burns (Curling's ulcer) are well known, as are ulcers associated with manifest or occult lesions of the central nervous system (Cushing's ulcers).[141] There is now a considerable experience with peptic ulcer, largely duodenal, in infants and children without any such obvious precursor. In newborn infants, even in the first day of life, ulcers may bleed or perforate, or both.[95] Ulcers causing intractable pain or leading to stenosis are less likely to be seen in infancy than later in childhood, and the younger infants are the ones most likely to bleed. Perfora-

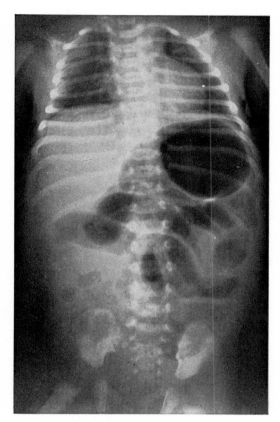

FIG. 46-5. Meconium peritonitis. Infant 48 hours old. The stomach and many loops of small bowel are distended with air. There may be some air in the colon. The generally opaque area on the right side of the abdomen contains a number of denser areas indicative of calcification and pathognomonic of meconium peritonitis. The point of perforation had sealed off and was not demonstrable at operation. A lateral anastomosis about a kink in the small bowel, probably at the site of a marked stenosis, relieved the obstruction which had been responsible for the intrauterine perforation. While there are differences in these roentgenograms (Figs. 46-3 to 46-5) which indicate the nature of the underlying lesion, all required immediate operation, and the same midabdominal transverse incision will give access to any lesion which may be found.

tion, of course, demands immediate operation, and bleeding may be massive and cause death from exsanguination. At times death has resulted from vomiting, rejection of food and cachexia without perforation or hemorrhage. A number of reports have appeared of successful treatment of these lesions by the operative procedures used in adult patients. In infants with bleeding duodenal ulcer, simple excision of the ulcer or duodenotomy and transfixion of the bleeding vessel is preferable to gastric resection.

Chronic peptic ulcer occurring in childhood and adolescence is indicative of a particularly strong ulcer diathesis, and with this in mind it is probably reasonable to apply operative therapy sooner to a child than to an adult.[11, 20, 109] In children with chronic peptic ulcers, endocrine abnormalities should be especially sought out, such as islet cell tumors of the pancreas, hyperparathyroidism, and tumors of the adrenal or the pituitary glands.

Pyloric Stenosis. Congenital hypertrophic pyloric stenosis is certainly the commonest condition requiring laparotomy in infancy. It consists of a great hypertrophy of the muscle fibers of the pyloric sphincter, such that the mass usually is large enough to be palpated through the abdominal wall and bulges inward on the lumen as well, reducing it to a thread-like channel. Males are affected more commonly than females in the proportion of 4 to 1. Classically, a vigorous and apparently normal infant begins to vomit in the 2nd or the 3rd week of life, although characteristic tumors have been found at operation in rare instances in the 1st week of life. Vomiting increases rapidly in severity until the infant empties his stomach after every feeding by a forceful emesis accurately described as projectile. As a rule, the vomitus is free of bile, but with violent effort may be blood-streaked. Immediately preceding the vomiting, the outline of the distended stomach is visible, and peristaltic waves may be seen to traverse it from left to right. The olive-shaped tumor, to the right of the right rectus muscle, can be felt in almost every instance. Its presence is pathognomic. Failure of experienced clinicians to feel the mass should lead to consideration of other conditions. Vomiting occurs in cerebral injuries but is seldom so consistent. In atresias of the intestinal tract the vomitus appears at once and usually contains bile. The radiologic picture of pyloric stenosis—delayed and incomplete emptying, threadlike pylorus with no peristalsis across it, is characteristic,[138] but

only rarely will it be necessary to resort to roentgenography for diagnosis.

In such a common disease, it is remarkable not only that the cause remains unknown but also that it is not certain whether it ever has been observed in a stillborn infant. Wallgren, in Sweden,[163] studied 1,000 male newborn infants roentgenographically. All showed pyloric canals normal in caliber and function. Five subsequently developed vomiting, typical symptoms of pyloric stenosis, and the classical roentgenographic picture. This may mean that the hypertrophy is not congenital but appears only after birth or, on the other hand, that while it may be congenital, a second factor—spasm, edema in response to gastric work—is required to produce obstruction and the roentgenographic picture. In some instances, symptoms do not develop for several months. Apparently the tumor persists indefinitely, unless a pyloromyotomy is performed.

In the United States, the Fredet-Rammstedt[34, 115] operation is generally accepted as the standard treatment. Performed electively, after deliberate rehydration and transfusion of the dry, hypochloremic, alkalotic infants (who usually show acetonuria as well) it results in cure and in discharge from the hospital in less than a week in over 99 per cent of the infants. The operation, performed preferably through a small transverse or gridiron right upper quadrant incision, consists in splitting the heavy muscular tumor from normal stomach, where it tapers off, to normal duodenum, where it ends abruptly. Glistening submucosa should bulge into the cleft in the white, gristly avascular tumor. Operative perforation of the duodenum occasionally occurs, but recovery is usual if it is recognized and repaired with fine arterial sutures. Rarely, an inadequate operation demands a second procedure. When one surgeon[29] can report 143 consecutive operations without a death, and Gross and his colleagues[45] 642 cases in 6 years (1946-1952) with 5 deaths, 2 of them in babies with serious congenital anomalies requiring operative correction, the mortality can be seen to be extremely low. Although with great effort, and much longer intensive medical care[162] many infants can be carried along nonoperatively, the risk of prolonged malnutrition, the frequent necessity for long hospitalization would appear to make the mere avoidance of an operation a questionable triumph.

BILIARY TRACT

Atresia of the Extrahepatic Bile Ducts. Newborn infants who soon become jaundiced, in whom the jaundice is intense and progressive, associated with hepatomegaly and acholic stools, may be presumed to have a mechanical obstruction of the biliary tract. Icterus neonatorum is usually milder and clears more rapidly. Hepatitis may occur in the newborn, and inclusion disease affecting the liver may cause jaundice. The icterus gravis of erythroblastosis can be anticipated in many instances before birth and diagnosed, in any event, on clinical and hematologic grounds. The commonest cause for obstruction is atresia of the extrahepatic biliary apparatus, and unfortunately in 3 to 4 cases out of 5 the atresia is total and irremediable, but in the 5th, a stubby common duct or hepatic duct can be found for anastomosis to the intestine with good recovery. In a similar number of cases, the ducts appear to be normal, apparently are plugged with thickened bile and can be induced to open up by operative or nonoperative "flushing" of the ducts.

Operation should be undertaken early before marked cirrhosis has occurred. Operative cholangiography by injection of contrast material into the gallbladder may spare the patient a detailed exploration if a patent extrahepatic biliary apparatus is demonstrated. The first successful operation was performed by Ladd in 1927.[82] Direct anastomosis of the proximal blind end of the bile duct to duodenum, over a polyethylene catheter, is the procedure of choice. Finding the proximal end may be difficult. In a number of instances a proximal end, which escaped detection at a first operation, has been found at a reoperation dilated into a structure easily anastomosed to the duodenum. When the extrabiliary ducts are entirely absent the intrahepatic architecture seems to be similarly deranged, for dilated intrahepatic ducts do not appear. When no bile duct is present, death is inevitable. Unfortunately, it is frequently delayed for 2 or 3 years and occasionally for 5 or 6.[51, 103, 133] However, almost as many children have ultimately survived to live normal lives in whom the operative report was of complete absence of extrahepatic ducts, as have been salvaged by effective anastomoses.[80, 81] Obviously, adequate ducts were present but missed in the first group so that even when no ducts are found, great care should be taken to avoid rough handling of the surrounding tissues.

Choledochal cyst is a curious anomaly in which the distal end of the common duct is dilated to form a cyst, sometimes of great size. The proximal common duct, or hepatic ducts, are not always dilated, and the thick-walled cyst is in essence a great aneurysmal dilatation of the common duct. Obstructions in the distal common duct due to valve formation or stenosis have not been reported regularly in association with choledochal cysts, and the portion of common duct beyond the cyst may be normal or in some instances dilated.[52, 131] The clinical picture is that of chronic and intermittent pain and jaundice with a palpable mass, which may vary in size and tenseness. The attacks of pain in some cases seem to have been due to bouts of acute pancreatitis.[131]

The cyst lies against and partly under the duodenum, and a direct anastomosis between cyst and duodenum provides a simple and effective treatment in the smaller cysts. With large cysts, the generally more preferable Roux-Y anastomosis with the jejunum is feasible and becomes the procedure of choice. Resection of the cyst is seldom feasible without performance of a pancreaticoduodenectomy and therefore is not attempted.

Cholelithiasis and Cholecystitis. In association, with some hemolytic diseases, the formation of bile pigment stones in the gallbladder is common in children. This is particularly true and important in congenital spherocytosis (congenital hemolytic icterus) and in sickle-cell anemia. The abdominal crises in these conditions are not unlike attacks of biliary colic or cholecystitis, and alertness is required to discover the superimposed biliary disease. Splenectomy is curative for familial hemolytic icterus, and abdominal "crises" occurring after splenectomy should be investigated for evidence of cholelithiasis. It is our practice at the time of splenectomy in patients with spherocytic familial icterus to examine the gallbladder and to remove it through a transverse extension of the subcostal incision if calculi are felt.

Acute cholecystitis may occur as a feature

of a systemic bacterial infection or apparently independently. It differs from cholecystitis in adults in the frequent occurrence of jaundice in the absence of stones. Treatment is, of course, cholecystectomy. A child with one attack of gallbladder disease can look forward to repeated distress unless cholecystectomy is performed, and even in children the complications of cholecystitis and cholelithiasis do occur.[39, 161, 168]

Liver tumors, both malignant and benign, occur in childhood. One form of neuroblastoma appears as a disseminated tumor causing enormous hepatomegaly with no evidence of a primary tumor elsewhere. Primary carcinoma of the liver is another cause of hepatic enlargement not often susceptible to treatment and manifested at first solely by the hepatomegaly. Hemangiomas of a number of varieties, cysts and other benign tumors tend to be softer and cause more localized hepatic enlargement. Resection of either lobe of the liver is feasible and has been tolerated well by children.[171]

PANCREAS

Annular and Ectopic Pancreas (see also Chap. 32, "Pancreas"). The pancreas arises from a dorsal and a ventral anlage and at times fusion of the two encircles the duodenum with a band of pancreatic tissue. Curiously enough, symptoms are characteristically produced late in life—duodenal obstruction and a more than coincidental occurrence of duodenal ulcer. Neonatal duodenal obstruction due to annular pancreas does occur. The obstruction—except in cases with associated duodenal atresia—is not complete. The roentgenogram shows a smooth, sharp obstruction in the 3rd part of the duodenum. Division of the pancreatic band is difficult in an infant and may result in pancreatitis or pancreatic fistula; duodenojejunostomy is the procedure of choice.[132]

Nodules of ectopic pancreatic tissue may occur anywhere along the gastro-intestinal tract. The most frequent locations are in a Meckel's diverticulum. The ectopic tissue may initiate an intussusception and may be the site of acute pancreatitis. It has been found also in association with intestinal bleeding, and in a prolapsing gastric polyp has caused pyloric obstruction.[25] However, most such foci

are asymptomatic and appear as incidental findings.

SPLEEN

Splenectomy in children[16] is most frequently required in association with rupture of the spleen. Other indications for this operation are discussed in Chapter 33, "Spleen."

Congenital absence of the spleen may be suspected in a child with repeated serious infections and a congenital cardiac defect. Associated may be situs inversus and other visceral anomalies, polycythemia with increased target cells, Howell-Jolly bodies, normoblastemia and decreased osmotic fragility of the red cells.[38]

UMBILICUS AND ASSOCIATED STRUCTURES

Omphalitis, a pyogenic infection, can be particularly hazardous because of transmission of inflammation along the umbilical vein to cause portal vein thrombosis. An occasional case of portal hypertension due to cavernomatous transformation of the portal vein is ascribed to a neonatal omphalitis with ascending thrombophlebitis. Happily, modern hygiene has made serious omphalitis and the tetanus that was formerly seen with it quite rare.

Umbilical granuloma, a tuft of granulation tissue on the uncicatrized umbilical stump, is a common and annoying lesion. Amputation of the granuloma with a ligature or crushing hemostat usually will permit the stump to heal over. From time to time histologic examination will discover an apparent granuloma to be a mucosal remnant of the omphalomesenteric or vitelline duct.

ANOMALIES ASSOCIATED WITH THE OMPHALOMESENTERIC DUCT

This duct represents a patent communication between midgut and yolk sac from the 3rd week of embryonic life to the 6th. Any portion of the duct, or all of it, may persist (Fig. 46-6). If all of it persists, there is found a muscular tube lined by intestinal mucosa leading from an umbilical opening to a point in the distal ileum. The tube and its external opening may be as large as the bowel so that a fecal discharge issues from the opening, or the bowel may evert itself through it. Treatment is excision of the umbilicus and the persistent duct and closure of the intestine. At the external end, cysts lined by intestinal

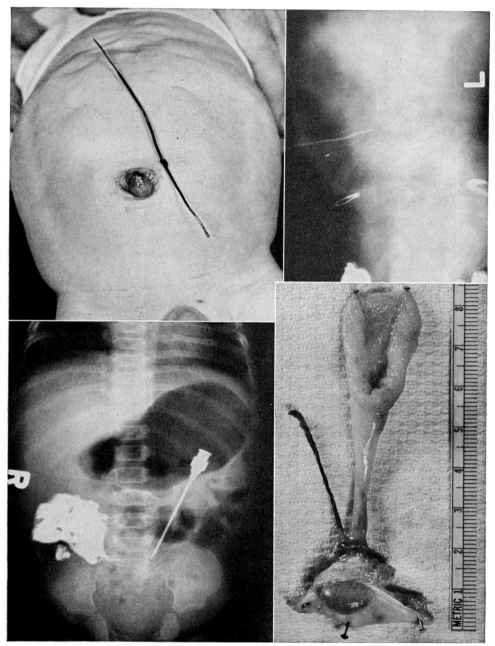

FIG. 46-6. Three-month-old male with pouting umbilical tumor obviously covered by intestinal mucosa (*top, left*). The silver probe passes deeply into the abdomen through the relatively large opening in the mucosa as seen in the lateral roentgenogram (*top, right*). Injection of Lipiodol into the sinus through a polyethylene catheter fitted to a needle shows the free communication with the intestine (*bottom, left*). The specimen (*bottom, right*) removed at operation shows the umbilicus, the tubelike patent omphalomesenteric duct, and, at its flared end, a portion of the wall of the ileum with which it connected widely. Despite the widely patent communication, only mucus discharged from the umbilicus. In some of these patients, feces or flatus may escape from the umbilical fistula.

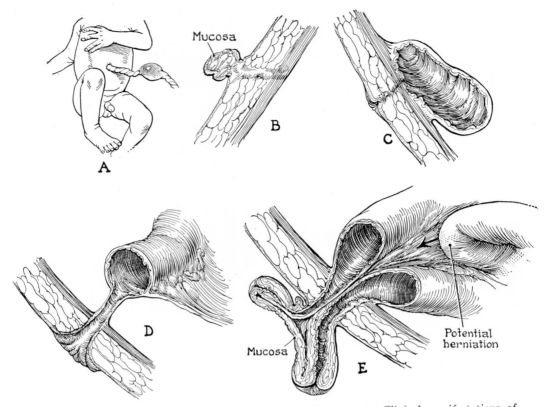

Fig. 46-7. Omphalomesenteric duct (vitelline duct) remnants. Clinical manifestations of persistence of various portions of the duct.

A. A mucosa-lined cyst exists in the umbilical cord, distant from the umbilicus. Removed when the cord is divided, it is no more than a pathologic curiosity.

B. The umbilicus is partially or completely covered with a pouting tuft of red, easily recognized intestinal mucosa, which may dip down into the abdominal wall. Sometimes small tufts are mistaken for umbilical granulomas.

C. A mucosa-lined cyst with muscular wall lies beneath the umbilicus, properitoneally, and may extend upward through the umbilicus to the skin.

D. An enteric tube forms a widely patent communication between the ileum and the umbilicus. The tube of intestine is generally much longer than shown. Gas and feces are discharged through the opening.

E. In the presence of the complete persistence of the omphalomesenteric duct, shown in D, particularly if it is short and wide, the proximal and distal loops may prolapse out through it, as when both loops prolapse in some tangential colostomies. A serosa-lined cavity, or hernial sac, is formed, into which another loop of bowel may herniate.

(Continued on facing page)

mucosa may appear in the umbilical cord at a distance from the umbilicus and may be amputated with the cord. A rosy tuft of mucosa on the umbilicus may suggest a granuloma in appearance. A cyst may persist in or under the abdominal wall, with or without communication with the skin. The obliterated omphalomesenteric vessels, persisting as a strand from ileum to umbilicus, may cause intestinal obstruction or volvulus. An intestinal cyst may persist in the middle of such a cord. Meckel's diverticulum is the result of persistence of the intestinal end of the vitelline or omphalomesenteric duct. It shows great variation in size, shape and position but usually is found within 2 or 3 feet of the ileocecal valve, occurs on the antimesenteric surface of the bowel and is marked by a

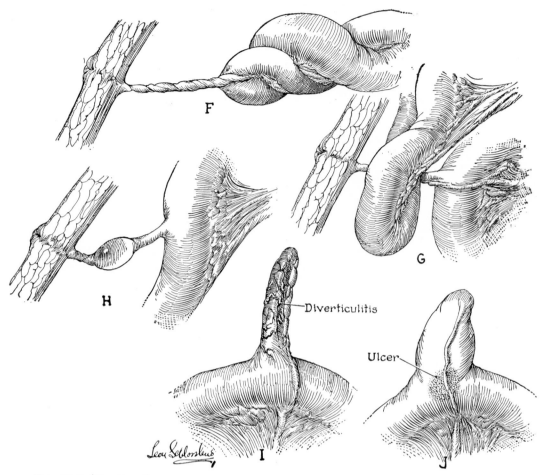

FIG. 46-7 (*Continued*)

F. The obliterated omphalomesenteric vessels persist, attaching the ileum to the abdominal wall, and creating the fixed point about which a volvulus may form.

G. A knuckle of bowel may be caught across such an obliterated omphalomesenteric artery, causing intestinal obstruction in this manner.

H. The cord of the obliterated omphalomesenteric vessels may contain in its mid-portion a mucosa-lined, smooth-muscle walled cyst, as a persistence of the mid-portion of the duct.

I & J. The intestinal end of the omphalomesenteric duct persists—the diverticulum of Meckel. If it is slender and vermiform it may be the seat of diverticulitis, indistinguishable clinically from appendicitis. Most omphalomesenteric duct remnants contain gastric mucosa. The result, in Meckel's diverticulum, is frequently a peptic ulcer of the ileum, or of the ileal mucosa in the diverticulum. Massive, painless intestinal bleeding is the only symptom in most cases. Perforation occurs occasionally.

characteristic vessel with accompanying fat running to its tip from the mesentery of the bowel. The diverticulum, if long and narrow, is subject to an acute inflammatory process clinically indistinguishable from appendicitis. In operating for appendicitis, if the appendix is normal, search always is made for a Meckel's diverticulum. Ectopic tissue—pancreatic or gastric—is commonly found in Meckel's diverticula. Peptic ulcers in the normal ileal mucosa of the diverticulum or the adjacent bowel, are not rare in association with such ectopic gastric mucosa. Like peptic ulcers elsewhere, they may bleed, or perforate, or both. The

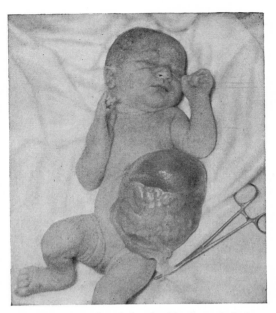

Fig. 46-8. Omphalocele. Newborn infant with massive omphalocele containing liver, spleen, stomach and intestines. The translucent sac of amniotic membrane was carefully preserved, the skin widely undermined and brought over the membrane. In this instance, the resultant ventral hernia, larger than most, posed a serious problem in repair.[57] Repeated pneumoperitoneum in massive ventral and inguinal hernias of adults, which have "lost the right of domicile" (see Chap. 39), stretches the abdominal cavity so as to permit return of the abdominal viscera without intolerable respiratory embarrassment. Pneumoperitoneum could well be used in preparation for the Stage II operation of great omphaloceles.

bleeding is characteristically painless, may be so slow as to produce dark stools and a profound chronic anemia, or so massive as to produce bright red blood and shock. Meckel's diverticulum with a peptic ulcer is an important cause of occult intestinal bleeding.[3, 79]

Anomalies Associated With the Urachus. The urachus is the fetal structure connecting allantois and bladder and derived uncertainly from either or both. At birth it persists as a mid-line cord between bladder and umbilicus. In fully a third of normal individuals, a fine probe demonstrates a connection between bladder and a short urachal sinus. In most individuals, section of the urachal cord will

show scattered epithelial persistences.[7] Like the vitelline duct, any portion of the urachus or the entire structure may persist. If the urachus persists as a patent communication between bladder and umbilicus, a urinary fistula occurs. At times a small weeping cyst or sinus at the umbilicus represents a urachal persistence in the umbilicus. The most common lesion is a cyst on the under side of the abdominal wall, in the mid-line and extraperitoneal, which causes symptoms either from its size, which may be very great, or from infection. Infected lesions are drained and subsequently, like uninfected ones, excised, care being taken to avoid injury to the bladder.

Omphalocele (amniotic hernia, exomphalos) results when the intestines fail to return to the abdomen and remain in the exocoelomic cavity of the umbilical cord, covered only by amniotic membrane. The defect in the abdominal wall may be small, 1 or 2 centimeters, or enormous, almost from flank to flank (Fig. 46-8). The contents may be only a few loops of small bowel, or liver, spleen, stomach, and almost the entire intestinal tract. The covering membrane is avascular and will ordinarily dry, crack, lead to infection and death. With care, however, in the smaller herniae it is possible to wait for spontaneous epithelialization.[42] In this country this is rarely practiced, if ever. Immediate operation is urgently required. Small omphaloceles present no problem. The contents are replaced in the abdomen, the sac excised, and the defect closed. In the presence of the very large omphaloceles, the method of Gross[43] has made the seemingly impossible repair feasible. The membrane is washed off and left undisturbed. The skin of the trunk is extensively undermined, avoiding the anterior chest wall, and is brought over the sac and sutured, producing in effect a large ventral hernia which can be repaired when the abdominal cavity has grown large enough to accept the viscera. Intestinal atresia is a frequent concomitant of omphalocele.

Gastroschisis is a condition similar to omphalocele but occurring through some point other than the umbilicus. The intestines are imbedded in a mass of gelatinous matrix uncovered by any sac. Successful outcome of surgical treatment is rare.[27, 73]

Congenital absence of the abdominal muscles is a curious condition in which the ventral musculature is represented by only a few scattered strands of abnormal muscle fibers. The skin of the mid-line frequently appears scarred as if by a burn or an operation (Fig. 46-9). The thin abdominal wall bulges in any direction, and the presence of numerous wrinkles is characteristic. The defect occurs almost exclusively in males. Unopposed pull of the diaphragm frequently results in a pigeon chest with a pronounced Harrison's groove. Of greatest importance is the almost unfailing concomitant occurrence of cryptorchidism and urinary tract anomalies—megacystica, mega-

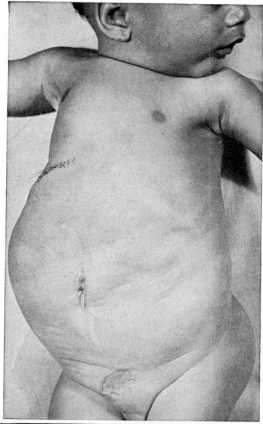

Fig. 46-9. Congenital absence of abdominal musculature. A 7-month-old male with absence of abdominal musculature. Note (A, *right*) the bulging of the contents through the flabby abdominal wall and the visible intestinal patterns. The curious midline scars are congenital stigmata. Retrograde pyelogram (B, *bottom*) shows an extensive hydronephrosis on the left. The left ureter is colossally dilated and tortuous, and there is a massively enlarged bladder. The nonfunctioning right kidney was removed, and a left nephrostomy has permitted the child to survive several years in good vigor. A convincing vesical neck obstruction was not demonstrated in this instance.

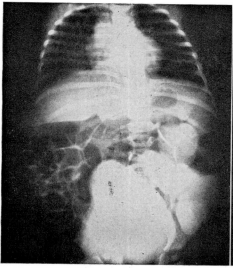
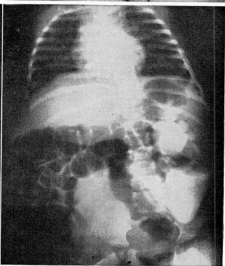

ureter and hydronephrosis. With more careful study the more recently reported cases have shown acceptable causes of lower urinary tract obstruction. Malrotations of the intestine also occur commonly in these patients. Various types of plastic procedures on the urinary tract have permitted some of these patients to survive.[146] Plastic operations upon the abdominal wall, since all the parietal muscles are not absent, achieve some success.[32]

INTESTINE AND COLON

Intussusception consists in the invagination of one portion of the intestine into another. Characteristically, it affects infants in the first 2 years of life, the peak of incidence being in the 7th, the 8th and the 9th months. Males are affected more frequently than females in the ratio of 3:2, and the victims are characteristically well nourished, breast fed, vigorous and well, up to the onset. The condition is much commoner in some areas, such as Scotland,[28] than in others. In most instances the intussusception begins at or near the ileocecal valve (Fig. 46-10). In less than 10 per cent of the cases, and in only 2.5 per cent of the patients under the age of 2 years, is a polyp, a Meckel's diverticulum or a nodule of ectopic pancreas or other local lesion such as extreme lymphoid hyperplasia in the terminal ileum seen as the obvious inciting cause. It has been pointed out that in infancy the disproportion between the caliber of the cecum and the ileum is greater than in later life, facilitating the occurrence of intussusception

and that in infancy there is great enlargement of the lymphoid patches in the bowel, perhaps arousing expulsive efforts.

Once an intussusception forms, the leading point is constant, and the increase in length occurs at the expense of the receiving loop, the intussuscipiens (Fig. 46-11). Compression of the mesenteric vessels between the 2 inner layers as well as the "U"-shaped angulation of these vessels at either end of the intussusception, leads to venous stasis, engorgement, edema, exudation, further vascular compression and ultimately gangrene. Discharge of blood is one of the first results, and the early evacuation of mucus is correlated with the appearance of great numbers of goblet cells in the mucosa of the intussusceptum. The tension of the mesentery on the intussusceptum tends to arch the bowel in a curve with its center at the mesenteric root, producing the characteristic sausage-shaped mass. Edema and compression produce intestinal obstruction, although most patients should be relieved of their intussusception before they have come to suffer from ileus. The rapidity of development of gangrene is highly variable, as Jonathan Hutchinson pointed out in 1873[70] when

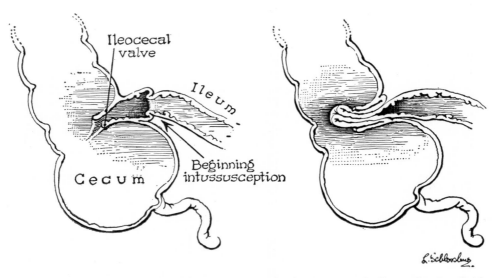

FIG. 46-10. The vast majority of intussusceptions begin at or near the ileocecal valve (*left*). In some, the ileum protrudes through the valve; in others, the valve is pushed before it. In most cases, as soon as the intussusception commences, intestinal obstruction occurs (*right*), although the condition should be recognized and the intussusception relieved before distention develops. (Ravitch *in* Holt, L., and McIntosh, R.: Holt Pediatrics, ed. 12, New York, Appleton)

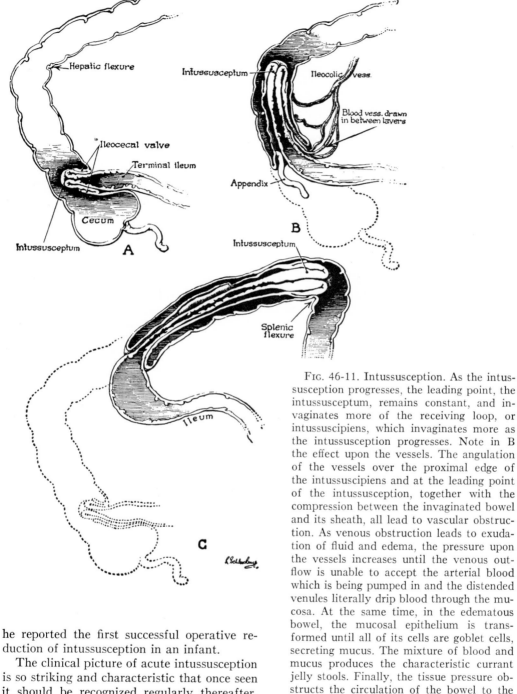

FIG. 46-11. Intussusception. As the intussusception progresses, the leading point, the intussusceptum, remains constant, and invaginates more of the receiving loop, or intussuscipiens, which invaginates more as the intussusception progresses. Note in B the effect upon the vessels. The angulation of the vessels over the proximal edge of the intussuscipiens and at the leading point of the intussusception, together with the compression between the invaginated bowel and its sheath, all lead to vascular obstruction. As venous obstruction leads to exudation of fluid and edema, the pressure upon the vessels increases until the venous outflow is unable to accept the arterial blood which is being pumped in and the distended venules literally drip blood through the mucosa. At the same time, in the edematous bowel, the mucosal epithelium is transformed until all of its cells are goblet cells, secreting mucus. The mixture of blood and mucus produces the characteristic currant jelly stools. Finally, the tissue pressure obstructs the circulation of the bowel to the point at which infarction and gangrene appear. This affects first the outer layer of the intussusception. The inner lawer of bowel becomes affected next. The outer layer of bowel remains viable. (Ravitch *in* Holt, L., and McIntosh, R.: Holt Pediatrics, ed. 12, New York, Appleton)

he reported the first successful operative reduction of intussusception in an infant.

The clinical picture of acute intussusception is so striking and characteristic that once seen it should be recognized regularly thereafter. A well-nourished infant in apparent good health suddenly cries out with obvious colic, and vomits. The attacks of colic recur regularly and with some increase in frequency. In the intervals the infant is flaccid or prostrated, although in rare instances seemingly normal and playful. There is usually one normal stool, evacuating the colonic contents. Thereafter, there is passed only thin blood or bloody mucus, the currant jelly stool of medical lore. Lassitude increases, and collapse ensues. The abdomen is relaxed, soft and nontender, except at times over the palpable intussusception. Signs of ileus—distention, vomiting, tachycardia—gradually supervene. Fever and leukocytosis are common. In almost 90 per cent of cases, a mass is palpable abdominally or rectally. Occasionally, the intussusception presents through the anus.

TREATMENT. In a few cases, without treatment the intussusception reduces spontaneously, or the gangrenous intussusceptum sloughs before the child has succumbed, leaving an intact intestinal canal behind. Reduction by enema, first practiced in antiquity, was systematized by Hirschsprung[63] and his successors.[102] Hipsley,[62] in Australia, and others accumulated a massive experience with enema reduction of intussusception. Barium enema reduction under fluoroscopic control was added by Olsson and Pallin[107] in Sweden and Retan[135] in the United States. More recently others[60, 105, 121, 122, 147] have accumulated a large experience with reduction of intussusception by barium enema (Fig. 46-12). For 70 years after Hutchinson's first operative triumph, the hydrostatic pressure method gave superior results in terms of mortality. Today there is little to choose from in mortality statistics. In hospitals accustomed to care for sick infants no child should die of intussusception regardless of the therapy employed, except for infants already moribund upon admission.[41, 49, 149] However, since in 70 to 75 per cent of infants treated primarily by barium enema, no anesthesia and no incision are required, the morbidity inevitably must be lower and the hospital stay shorter. Resection appears to be necessary much less frequently in the barium enema series. This leads to the suspicion that in some instances it is operative trauma or mistaken assumption of nonviability that necessitates bowel resection.

If operation is undertaken, it is important to prepare the infant by intravenous hydration and blood transfusion and by gastric lavage. At operation the intestine is milked back as gently as possible. Resection and anastomosis may be required for irreducible

or gangrenous bowel. White and Dennison[170] have met with success in some cases by simple anastomosis around the intussusception without resection (the old Montgomery operation). If barium enema is to be performed, the operating room should be prepared in any case, administration and intravenous fluids or blood begun and the stomach emptied by a tube. Through a securely taped balloon catheter, barium is run into the rectum from a height of 3 to 3½ feet. The flow is uninterrupted and unassisted. The abdomen is never manipulated. The intussusceptum is outlined like a cervix in the vagina. It is reduced, sometimes haltingly, sometimes swiftly. In over 70 per cent of the cases, the operating room is notified that no operation will be required. With this technic, gangrenous bowel will not be reduced, and there appears to be little or no risk of perforation. The fluoroscoping surgeon makes the diagnosis of a complete reduction by (1) complete filling of many loops of ileum, (2) disappearance of the mass, (3) passage of feces or flatus and (4) abrupt and striking improvement in the child's condition.

For further confirmation, charcoal is instilled in the stomach and recovered by enema, on the ward, in 6 hours. Operation through a simple McBurney incision is undertaken if reduction is incomplete (when the intussusception is almost always found at the cecum), or if it is not certain that it is complete.

Hirschsprung's Disease (Megacolon).[64] This is a condition in which obstinate constipation occurs from birth. In true Hirschsprung's disease if an accurate history of the period in the obstetric nursery is available the baby will invariably be found to have had neonatal difficulty in evacuation. Repeated enemata may be required, severe distention may be frequent, and in infants death may occur from respiratory insufficiency due to elevation of the diaphragm by the massively distended intestine or from intestinal obstruction due to fecal impaction, or from perforation of the cecum, or from volvulus of the redundant sigmoid, occasionally, for unexplained reasons following an enema, or in the course of repeated bouts of enteritis.[72] The colon gradually distends to an enormous size and becomes strikingly thickened and hypertrophied (Fig. 46-13). The rectum and the distal sigmoid are small. Fecal masses are felt in the abdomen. Digital rectal examination usually shows an empty ampulla. Incontinence is not a feature of this disease, and the presence of incontinence should suggest psychogenic constipation.[120] If the children survive, it is with preposterous "potbellies," flared costal margins, malnutrition and underdevelopment. In time, careful dietary habits and a regular enema regimen may effect a tolerable modus vivendi. After childhood, the symptoms tend to be less troublesome, perhaps because this is then easier to achieve. Nevertheless, we have operated upon a man of 54, gravely troubled with Hirschsprung's disease with which he had struggled from birth.

Early in infancy, before the radiologic

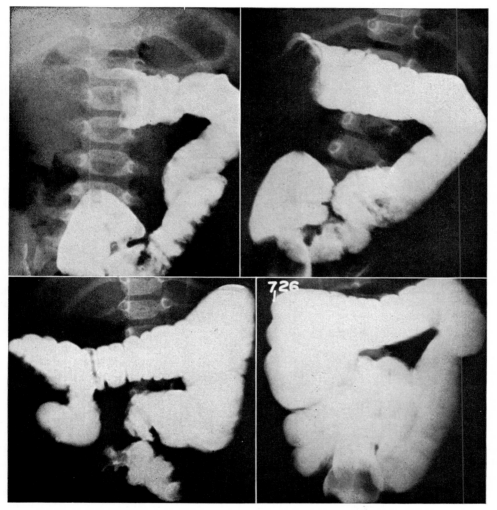

Fig. 46-12. Intussusception. Reduction by barium enema, administered under hydrostatic pressure of 3½ feet to a 9-month-old infant with characteristic history of intussusception of 29 hours' duration. (*Top, left*) Barium encounters the intussusceptum in the midtransverse colon. The concave, meniscoid appearance at the head of the barium column is typical. (*Top, right*) The intussusception is reduced by the pressure of the column of barium and has reached the hepatic flexure. (*Bottom, left*) The cecum is now filling, but no barium has yet entered the ileum. (*Bottom, right*) As the cecum distends, the intussusception is reduced through the ileocecal valve, and there is a sudden rush of barium into many loops of ileum. Free filling of these ileal loops indicates complete reduction.

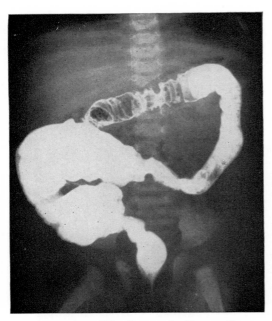

Fig. 46-13. Hirschsprung's disease. Barium enema in a 4-month-old infant with history of constipation from birth. The relatively normal-appearing distal segment is the aganglionic segment which is at fault. The grossly dilated bowel proximal to this is structurally normal. This child had severe melena, an occasional finding in infants with Hirschsprung's disease. The resected specimen showed extensive ulceration in much of the dilated, redundant sigmoid, in this infant. A low anastomosis performed by the Swenson technic, restored normal bowel evacuation and the melena gradually disappeared.

changes are marked, there may be substantial difficulty in establishing a diagnosis, and, in such cases, a transanal biopsy of the rectal musculature will show the characteristic absence of the ganglion cells of the myenteric plexus.[158]

The history of the discovery of the etiology of the disease is the history of repeated, obstinate failure to appreciate the reported observations that the ganglion cells of the myenteric plexus are lacking. This is all the more remarkable in that most pediatricians and surgeons for half a century had felt that the disease had a neurogenic basis. Even when the evidence accumulated in the reports of Kernohan[137] and of Zuelzer and Wilson,[175]

it was neglected with equanimity. Finally, Swenson,[155] demonstrating with Neuhauser that in most cases of Hirschsprung's disease the distal rectal segment is narrowed, concluded with him that it was this segment which was at fault. In a nicely devised operative procedure, he resected this narrowed distal segment, heretofore largely neglected by clinicians who had concentrated on the obvious, dilated colon above. Following Swenson's lead, Bodian,[12] in the specimens resected according to Swenson's principles by Stephens at Great Ormond Street, conclusively demonstrated that in cases of megacolon (true Hirschsprung's disease) with a narrowed distal segment of rectum or sigmoid, the ganglion cells of the myenteric plexuses were absent in the narrowed—apparently normal—distal bowel and appeared in normal numbers in the dilated and hypertrophied proximal bowel. Thus the proximal dilatation and hypertrophy were seen to be due to obstruction in the narrow, improperly functioning aganglionic distal bowel. Sympathectomy and management with parasympathomimetic drugs were abandoned, and the resections which some surgeons had long performed were now given a sound basis and direction. The Swenson procedure consists in telescoping the dissected rectum and sigmoid out through the anus, amputating close to the anus the huge prolapse thus produced and effecting an effortless 2-layer anastomosis outside the anus, then permitting the suture line to retract just inside the sphincters. The requisite upper limit of resection may be determined by frozen section identification of ganglion cells. The results in the relief of megacolon are excellent, and the mortality low. Fecal and urinary incontinence and sexual impotence in males are theoretical hazards. The latter two should not be met if pelvic dissection is held close to the bowel. The first is avoided if, in addition, resection is not too low.[153] State, Rehbein and others point out that satisfactory results may be achieved by a purely intra-abdominal resection, with a low anastomosis.[134]

In infants, Swenson prefers to delay operation until the children are 12 months old or more, performing colostomies in the more severely affected infants. Others, including this writer, operate readily on children in the first few months of life. In rare instances the entire colon is aganglionic, creating a condition extremely difficult to treat even if the diagnosis is made.[65, 156]

Atresia or stenosis of the colon is rare. Surgeons unacquainted with the appearance of the tiny, empty colon found distal to atresias of the small bowel frequently comment on microcolon and question the ability of such a colon to receive the fecal stream. In most of these cases the colon is merely collapsed because it never has been distended with meconium, but is anatomically normal.

Lymphosarcoma of the intestine is the commonest malignant intestinal tumor in childhood. Remarkable is its capacity for involving extensive segments of small bowel, the wall of which is replaced by a thick, rigid tumor mass, without any striking gastrointestinal symptoms (Fig. 46-14). In the cecum, a chronic, nonstrangulating, nonobstructing intussusception is strongly suggestive of lymphosarcoma. The mesenteric glands are almost always widely involved, and while resection of the involved intestine may be of some benefit, ultimate recovery has been rare. The newer chemotherapeutic agents may affect this picture but are not known to result in permanent cure at the present time.

Carcinoma of the colon does occur in childhood and tends to be more insidious than in adults, perhaps because little heed is given to such a possibility. The tumor is frequently inoperable by virtue of metastases, before operation is undertaken.[172]

Intestinal polyposis occurs in a wide variety of forms in infants and children. The polyps in stomach and colon may cause anemia from chronic blood loss. In the small bowel, polyps are prone to cause intussusception. In the colon, polyps may lead to or attend the development of carcinoma.

Polyps may involve the entire gastrointestinal tract,[116] may be familial or sporadic, may occur in the small bowel alone in familial form, may occur in association with the telltale melanin pigmentation of the lips, the palms and the soles known as Hutchinson's spots[71] (Peutz-Jeghers' Syndrome, see Chap. 37, Part 2) may occur in association with sexual infantilism[8] or with multiple sebaceous cysts.[106] Multiple polyposis of the colon—sporadic or familial—may cause constant bloody diarrhea, serious protein loss and malnutrition and in-

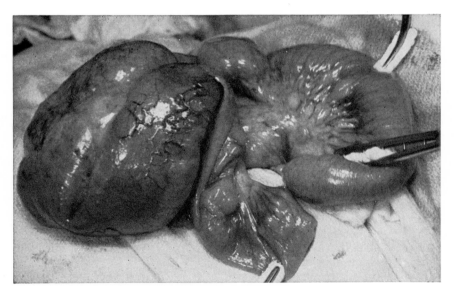

Fig. 46-14. Lymphosarcoma of intestine. The patient was a 4-year-old child with anemia and abdominal fullness. The tumor was easily palpable. The U-shaped loop at the left is diffusely replaced by tumor so that its lumen is a mere slit, and the disproportion is obvious between proximal dilated bowel, at the right, and the distal, relatively collapsed bowel, at lower center. Nevertheless, the child had no symptoms of obstruction. The mesenteric lymph nodes were widely involved.

evitably leads to death from cancer of the rectum or the colon. The only certain preventive is total colectomy.[127] Isolated rectal polyps account for many instances of blood-streaked stools and should be removed sigmoidoscopically, and the area watched thereafter by serial sigmoidoscopic examinations (see sections on polyps (Chap. 39).

Fissure in ano is common in infants and manifested by the infant's obvious reluctance to defecate, and by pain and discomfort during the act. If the little sentinel pile is clipped away, the sphincter carefully dilated with one finger and massaged daily, and measures taken to avoid costive stools, relief can be expected. In rare cases the anal ulcer is so indurated as to require excision.

Perianal abscesses and fistula in ano occur in children and are treated exactly as in adults (see Chap. 39, "Anorectum").

Rectal prolapse is commonly encountered in pediatric practice. Firm pressure will reduce the prolapse. Reduction may then be maintained for several days by the unsanitary but effective measure of strapping the buttocks together and allowing the child to defecate at will. Occasionally, a 2nd or a 3rd prolapse occurs before the measure is permanently effective. Operation is almost never required. In 2 particularly severe instances, we have performed a Mikulicz excision of the long sigmoid and the upper rectum and subsequently closed the colostomy extraperitoneally, the bowel remaining adherent to the abdominal wall.

Imperforate Anus. The formation of the anus and of the external genitalia is a sufficiently complicated process to provide opportunity for many malformations. The student should be aware that here, even more than elsewhere, there is difference of opinion both as to the embryogenesis of the organs involved and the treatment of the associated malformations. The writings of the individualistic and vastly experienced Denis Browne, of the Hospital for Sick Children at Great Ormond Street in London, are often found to be at variance with the writings of American authors, among whom in turn there is no unanimity.[15]

The anus may be closed over by no more than a translucent membrane, or there may be a pinpoint opening in the normal location or

ventral to it. Such lesions respond to instrumental and digital dilatation. The congenital median band of the anus[10] presents an anteroposteriorly directed band of tissue across a normal, or small, anal opening. The band may be excised, and the anus dilated. When, in the presence of an imperforate anus, external inspection does not reveal the location of the rectum, it may lie within reach of a perineal approach, or the distal end may be well up in the pelvis. Wangensteen and Rice[164] pointed out the usefulness of roentgenograms in demonstrating the gas-filled rectal pouch and advised the head-down position to permit air to rise. The lateral view, with the baby's head down, is the most informative. More important than the distance between the air-filled rectum and a marker at the anal dimple is the relation of the end of the rectum to the ischial tuberosities. Air will not begin to distend the rectum until toward the end of the first day of life, and roentgenograms taken too early may be misleading.

An infant can tolerate an imperforate anus for 24 to 48 hours with little hazard in most instances. If the rectal pouch is well below the ischial tuberosities, it can usually be brought down satisfactorily to the anal skin from below. Our preference is for a delicately performed operation, through the sphincteric ring, without division or wide retraction of the sphincter. A scarred perineum with divided and resutured sphincters and lacerated levatores ani is a poor basis for the development of continence. If a distal rectovaginal fistula exists, most surgeons close it by mobilizing the rectum sufficiently so that the former fistulous opening becomes the anal opening.[50]

If the rectal pouch is higher, an abdominal operation will be required. Formerly, a colostomy was often performed as a preliminary measure. If one is resorted to it must be placed in the transverse colon, well away from the sigmoid, which may have to be mobilized to permit the rectum to reach the skin. Since the publication by Rhoads, in 1948[136] in babies with imperforate anus and a high-lying rectal pouch, synchronous, combined, 1-stage abdominoperineal operation has become standard. Experienced pediatric surgeons, dealing with well-developed infants, proceed with this operation without a preliminary transverse colostomy. The freed rectal pouch is passed through a perineal opening carefully tunneled through the sphincteric ring and the pelvic floor and is sutured to the anal skin.

In all cases the urine and the vaginal vestibule should be watched for meconium or flatus. High recto-urethral fistulae are common in the males, and in the females high rectovaginal fistulae may be seen. Such fistulae are particularly well handled by the synchronous combined procedure, and it is important to be aware of their existence. Some females with fistulae low in the vagina, or at the fourchette or just between the fourchette and the normal anal site, live normal lives, with complete continence, without operation. With all repairs of imperforate anus the after-care and gentle, persistent and long-continued anal dilatation and massage of any scar tissue are important if a high percentage of satisfactory results is to be achieved.

Reoperations are difficult and unsatisfactory, and too much emphasis cannot be placed upon the importance of proper performance of a good procedure at the first operation (see Chap. 39, "Anorectum").

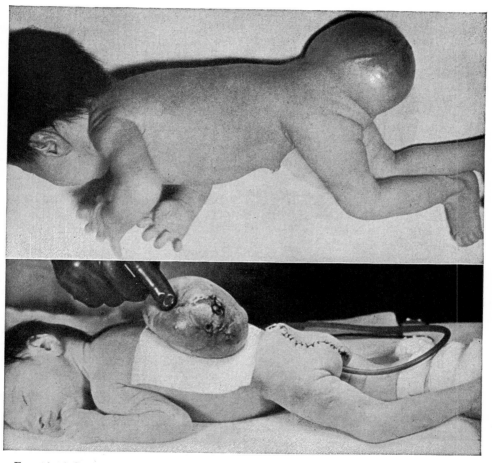

FIG. 46-15. Sacrococcygeal teratoma. (*Top*) A 10-day-old infant with a large teratoma distending the skin over it so markedly as to produce necrosis and ulceration. There was a large intrapelvic component. Such tumors may become malignant and metastasize, may ulcerate and become infected, by pressure may obstruct the rectum, the urethra or the ureters. (*Bottom*) The tumor is readily excised, with a large area of superfluous skin, leaving a posterior mid-line incision. A balloon-catheter distends the rectum and facilitates the separation of the tumor from it in the dissection.

SACROCOCCYGEAL TERATOMA AND OTHER PELVIC TUMORS

A variety of pelvic tumors occurs—neuroblastomas, sarcomas, anterior meningoceles, dermoids, chordomas, enterogenous cysts of the rectum—but perhaps the most interesting are the sacrococcygeal tumors.[53, 130] These teratomas may be entirely external (Fig. 46-15), like great coccygeal appendages, or largely internal and not visible from without, or, most commonly, both intrapelvic (occasionally intra-abdominal) and external. The tumors are often large enough to ulcerate the overlying skin with resultant infection. They may obstruct rectum, urethra, or ureters, and finally some 25 per cent of them are or become malignant. Regardless of their great size and intrapelvic and intra-abdominal extension, they can be totally removed from behind, the coccyx being excised, and the rectum dissected away. Once a malignant teratoma has invaded the surrounding tissues, cure is unlikely.

REFERENCES

1. Almklov, J. R., and Hatoff, A.: Pneumatocele during the course of pneumonia in children, Am. J. Dis. Child. *72*:521-528, 1946.
2. Ariel, I. M., and Pack, G. T.: Tumors of infancy and childhood: a general appraisal *in* Cancer and Allied Diseases of Infancy and Childhood, pp. 3-4, Boston, Little, 1960.
3. Arnheim, E. E.: Surgical complications of congenital anomalies of the umbilical region, Surg., Gynec. & Obst. *91*:71-80, 1950.
4. Arnheim, E. E., and Gemson, B. L.: Persistent cervical thymus gland: thymectomy, Surgery *27*:603-608, 1950.
5. Beahrs, O. H., Devine, K. D., and Hayles, A. B.: Tumors of the head and neck *in* Cancer and Allied Diseases of Infancy and Childhood, pp. 62-65, Boston, Little, 1960.
6. ———: Op. Cit., pp. 84-88.
7. Begg, R. C.: Urachus, its anatomy, histology, and development, J. Anat. *64*:170-183, 1930.
8. Bensaude, R., Hillemand, P., and Augier, P.: Polypose intestinale et infantilisme, Bull. et mém. Soc. méd. hôp. Paris *48*:251-257, 1932.
9. Benson, C. D., and Coury, J. J.: Congenital intrinsic obstruction of stomach and duodenum in the newborn, A.M.A. Arch. Surg. *62*:856-866, 1951.
10. Bill, A. H., Jr., and Johnson, R. S.: Congenital median band of the anus, Surg., Gynec. & Obst. *97*:307-311, 1953.
11. Bird, C. E., Limper, M. A., and Mayer, J. M.: Surgery in peptic ulceration of stomach and duodenum in infants and children, Ann. Surg. *114*:526, 1941.
12. Bodian, M., Stephens, F. D., and Ward, B. C. H.: Hirschsprung's disease and idiopathic megacolon, Lancet *1*:6-11, 1949.
13. Brock, R. C.: Lung Abscess, p. 86, Oxford, Blackwell, 1952.
14. Brown, A. L.: Pectus excavatum, J. Thoracic Surg. *9*:164, 1939.
15. Browne, D.: Some congenital deformities of the rectum, anus, vagina and urethra, Ann. Roy. Coll. Surgeons England *8*:173-192, 1951.
16. Buren, van, G., and Curtis, G. M.: Principal indications for splenectomy during childhood, Arch. Surg. *56*:125-131, 1948.
17. Burger, R. A.: Agenesis of the lung, Am. J. Dis. Child. *73*:481-488, 1947.
18. Burnett, W. E., and Caswell, H. T.: Lobectomy for pulmonary cysts in a 15 day old infant with recovery, Surgery *23*:84-91, 1948.
19. Byars, L. T., and Anderson, R.: Anomalies of the first branchial cleft, Surg., Gynec. & Obst. *93*:755-758, 1951.
20. Cameron, A. L.: Surgical aspects of chronic duodenal ulcers in childhood, A.M.A. Arch. Surg. *66*:827-842, 1953.
21. Cantrell, J. R., Haller, J. A., and Ravitch, M. M.: A syndrome of congenital defects involving the abdominal wall, sternum, diaphragm, pericardium and heart, Surg., Gynec. & Obst. *107*:602-614, 1958.
22. Cayley, C. K., Caez, H. J., and Mersheimer, W.: Primary bronchogenic carcinoma of the lung in children, A.M.A. Am. J. Dis. Child. *82*:49-60, 1951.
23. Clark, D. E.: Association of irradiation with carcinoma of the thyroid in children and adolescents, J.A.M.A. *159*:1007, 1955.
24. Clay, R. C.: Ganglioneuroma of nodose ganglion of vagus, Ann. Surg. *132*:147-152, 1950.
25. Collett, R. W.: Prepyloric polypus in stomach of child diagnosed histologically as aberrant pancreatic tissue, Am. J. Dis. Child. *72*:545-551, 1946.
26. Collins, H. A., Harberg, F. J., Soltero, L. R., McNamara, D. G., and Cooley, D. A.: Cardiac surgery in the newborn, Surgery *45*:506-519, 1959.
27. Cook, T. D.: Gastroschisis, Surgery *46*:618-623, 1959.

28. Dennison, W. M.: Acute intussusception in infancy and childhood, Glasgow M.J. *29*: 71-80, 1948.

29. Donovan, E. J.: Congenital hypertrophic pyloric stenosis in infancy, J.A.M.A. *109*: 558-561, 1937.

30. Ellis, F. H., Jr., Kirklin, J. W., Hodgson, J. R., Woolner, L. B., and Dushane, J. W.: Surgical implications of the mediastinal shadow in thoracic roentgenograms of infants and children, Surg., Gynec. & Obst. *100*:532-542, 1955.

31. Fallon, M., Gordon, A. R. G., and Lendrum, A. C.: Mediastinal cysts of foregut origin associated with vertebral anomalies, Brit. J. Surg. *41*:520-533, 1954.

32. Fitch, E. A., and Denman, F. R.: Congenital deficiencies of abdominal musculature (a syndrome): a surgical repair, Am. Surgeon *24*:371-376, 1958.

33. Fox, P. F.: Duodenal obstruction in infants and children, A.M.A. Arch. Surg. *67*:475-489, 1953.

34. Fredet, P., and Guillemot, L.: La sténose du pylore par hypertrophie musculaire chez les nourrissons, Ann. Gynec. et Obst. *7*:504-629, 1910.

35. Gardner, C. E.: The surgical significance of anomalies of intestinal rotation, Ann. Surg. *131*:879-898, 1950.

36. Gardner, C. E., and Hart, D.: Enterogenous cysts of duodenum; report of case and review of literature, J.A.M.A. *104*:1809-1812, 1935.

37. Gellis, S. S., and Holt, L. E.: The treatment of lye ingestion by the Salzer method, Ann. Otol., Rhin. & Laryng. *51*:1086-1088, 1942.

38. Gilbert, E. F., Nishimura, K., and Wedum, B. G.: Congenital malformation of the heart associated with splenic agenesis, Circulation *17*:72-86, 1958.

39. Glenn, F., and Hill, M. R.: Primary gallbladder disease in children, Ann. Surg. *139*: 302-311, 1954.

40. Glover, D. M., and Barry, F. M.: Intestinal obstruction in the newborn, Ann. Surg. *130*: 480-511, 1949.

41. Goldenberg, I. S.: Intussusception, Surgery *36*:732-739, 1954.

42. Grob, M.: Lehrbuch der Kinderchirurgie, pp. 311-315, Stuttgart, Thieme, 1957.

43. Gross, R. E.: A new method for surgical treatment of large omphaloceles, Surgery *24*:277-292, 1948.

44. ———: The Surgery of Infancy and Childhood, p. 87, Philadelphia, Saunders, 1953.

45. ———: Op. Cit., p. 143.

46. ———: Op. Cit., pp. 150-174.

47. ———: Op. Cit., pp. 185-191.

48. ———: Op. Cit., p. 202.

49. ———: Op. Cit., p. 299.

50. ———: Op. Cit., p. 359.

51. ———: Op. Cit., pp. 508-523.

52. ———: Op. Cit., p. 525.

53. Gross, R. E., Clatworthy, H. W., and Meeker, I. A.: Sacrococcygeal teratomas in infants and children, Surg., Gynec. & Obst. *92*:341-354, 1951.

54. Gross, R. E., and Goeringer, C. F.: Cystic hygroma of the neck, Surg., Gynec. & Obst. *69*:48-60, 1939.

55. Gross, R. E., and Hurwitt, E. S.: Cervicomediastinal and mediastinal cystic hygromas, Surg., Gynec. & Obst. *87*:599-610, 1948.

56. Haight, C., and Towsley, H. A.: Congenital atresia of the esophagus with tracheoesophageal fistula, Surg., Gynec. & Obst. *76*: 672-688, 1943.

57. Handelsman, J. C.: A technique for increasing abdominal capacity in the repair of massive ventral hernia, Surg., Gynec. & Obst. *108*:751-755, 1959.

58. Handelsman, J. C., and Ravitch, M. M.: Chylous cysts of the mesentery in children, Ann. Surg. *140*:185-193, 1954.

59. Harkins, G. A., and Sabiston, D. C.: Lymphangioma in infancy and childhood, Surgery *47*:811-822, 1960.

60. Hellmer, H.: Intussusception in children; diagnosis and therapy with barium enema, Acta Radiol. *65*:1-120, 1948.

61. Hiatt, R. B., and Wilson, P. E.: Celiac syndrome: VII. Therapy of meconium ileus; report of 8 cases with a review of the literature, Surg., Gynec. & Obst. *87*:317-327, 1948.

62. Hipsley, P. L.: Intussusception and its treatment by hydrostatic pressure based on analysis of 100 consecutive cases so treated, M.J. Australia *2*:201-206, 1926.

63. Hirschsprung, H.: Hundertundsieben Fälle von Darminvagination bei Kindern Behandelt im Königin Louisen-Kinderhospital in Kopenhagen Während der Jahre 1871-1904, Kurze Tabellarische Darstellung, Mitt. Grenzgeb. Med. u. Chir. *14*:555-574, 1905.

64. ———: Stuhlträgheit Neugeborener in Folge von Dilatation und Hypertrophie des Colons, Jahrb. Kinderh. *27*:1-7, 1888.

65. Hoffert, P. W., Zuber, S., Salzman, A., and Spinelli, V. A.: Aganglionosis of the entire colon, Surgery *46*:810-818, 1959.

66. Holinger, P. H., Johnston, K. C., Potts, W. J., and da Cunha, F.: The conservative and surgical management of benign stric-

tures of the esophagus, J. Thoracic Surg. 28:345-366, 1954.

67. Horwitz, O., and Meyer, J.: The safety record of BCG vaccination and untoward reactions observed after vaccination, Adv. Tuberc. Res. 8:245-271, 1957.

68. Howard, J. M., Rawson, A. J., Koop, C. E., Horn, R. C., and Royster, H. P.: Parotid tumors in children, Surg., Gynec. & Obst. 90:307-319, 1950.

69. Hurwitt, E. S.: Cystic lymphangioma of the omentum causing an acute surgical abdomen, J. Mt. Sinai Hosp. 10:294-297, 1943.

70. Hutchinson, J.: A successful case of abdominal section for intussusception; with remarks on this and other methods of treatment, Medico–Chir. Tr. 57:31-76, 1874.

71. Jeghers, H., McKusick, V. A., and Katz, K. H.: Generalized intestinal polyposis and melanin spots of the oral mucosa, lips, and digits, New England J. Med. 241:993-1036, 1949.

72. Jewett, T. C., Leahy, L. J., and Jamison, J.: Hirschsprung's disease in infants, A.M.A. Arch. Surg. 79:455-458, 1959.

73. Johns, F. S.: Congenital defect of the abdominal wall in the newborn, Ann. Surg. 123:886-899, 1946.

73a. Jones, S. A., Carter, R., Smith, L. L., and Joergenson, E. J.: Arteriomesenteric duodenal compression, Am. J. Surg. 100:262-277, 1960.

74. Jones, T. W., and Schutt, R. P.: Alimentary tract obstruction in the newborn infant, Pediatrics 20:881-895, 1957.

75. Kaye, R., Williams, M. L., and Kumagi, M.: Tolerance of infants and children to fat administered intravenously, Metabolism 6:727-734, 1957.

76. Kennedy, R. J. S.: Carcinoma of the thyroid gland in children, J. Pediat. 7:631-651, 1935.

77. Kent, E. M., Blades, B., Valle, A. R., and Graham, E. A.: Intrathoracic neurogenic tumors, J. Thoracic Surg. 13:116-161, 1944.

78. Kiskadden, W. S., and Dietrich, S. R.: Review of the treatment of micrognathia, Plast. & Reconstruct. Surg. 12:364-373, 1953.

79. Kittle, C. F., Jenkins, H. P., and Dragstedt, L. R.: Patent omphalomesenteric duct and its relation to the diverticulum of Meckel, Arch. Surg. 54:10-36, 1947.

80. Krovetz, J. L.: Congenital biliary atresia. I. Analysis of thirty cases with particular reference to diagnosis, Surgery 47:453-467, 1960.

81. ———: Congenital biliary atresia. II. Analysis of the therapeutic problem, Surgery 47:468-489, 1960.

82. Ladd, W. E.: Congenital atresia and stenosis of the bile ducts, J.A.M.A. 91:1082-1085, 1928.

83. ———: Congenital obstructions of the duodenum in children, New England J. Med. 206:277, 1932.

84. ———: The surgical treatment of esophageal atresia and tracheo-esophageal fistulas, New England J. Med. 230:625-637, 1944.

85. Ladd, W. E., and Gross, R. E.: Surgical treatment of duplications of the alimentary tract, Surg., Gynec. & Obst. 70:295-307, 1940.

86. Ladd, W. E., and Scott, H. W., Jr.: Esophageal duplications or mediastinal cysts of enteric origin, Surgery 16:815, 1944.

87. Langmann, A. C., and Bruch, H.: Carcinoma of the thyroid gland in children, Am. J. Dis. Child. 56:616-638, 1938.

88. Lattimer, J. K.: Congenital deficiencies of the abdominal musculature and associated genito-urinary anomalies: a report of 22 cases, Tr. Am. A. Genito-Urin. Surgeons 49:28-41, 1957.

89. Lester, C. W.: Deformities of the thorax of congenital or developmental origin, J. Pediat. 42:195-204, 1953.

90. ———: Pigeon breast (pectus carinatum) and other protrusion deformities of the chest of developmental origin, Ann. Surg. 137:482-489, 1953.

91. ———: Tuberculosis of the cervical lymph nodes, Surg., Gynec. & Obst. 87:719-724, 1948.

92. Leven, N. L.: Congenital atresia of esophagus with tracheoesophageal fistula, J. Thoracic Surg. 10:648, 1941.

93. Leven, N. L., and Varco, R. L.: Experiences with operative management of delayed restoration of alimentary continuity in children originally treated by multiple stage procedure for correction of congenital tracheo-esophageal defects, J. Thoracic Surg. 25:16-25, 1953.

94. Low, J. R., Cooper, G., and Cosby, L.: Meconium peritonitis, Surgery 26:223-228, 1949.

95. Lyday, J. E., Markarian, M., and Rhoads, J. E.: Perforated duodenal ulcer in a 2100 Gm. female infant with survival, Am. J. Surg. 97:346-349, 1959.

96. McKibben, B. G.: Congenital atresia of the nasal choanae, Laryngoscope 67:731-755, 1957.

97. MacMahon, H. E.: Congenital alveolar dysplasia: a developmental anomaly involv-

ing pulmonary alveoli, Pediatrics 2:43-57, 1948.

98. Maier, H. C., and Gould, W. S.: Agenesis of the lung with vascular compression of the tracheobronchial tree, J. Pediat. 43:38, 1953.

99. Marshall, J. M.: Gastrojejunal ulcers in children, A.M.A. Arch. Surg. 67:490-492, 1953.

100. Miller, J. A., Jr., and Miller, F. S.: Factors in neonatal resistance to anoxia, Surgery 36:916-932, 1954.

101. Miller, J. M., and Schumacker, H. B.: Congenital small intestinal stenosis and atresia, Surgery 46:973-981, 1959.

102. Monrad, S.: Acute invagination of the intestine in small children, Acta paediat. 6:31-52, 1926.

103. Moore, T. C.: Congenital atresia of the extrahepatic bile ducts, Surg., Gynec. & Obst. 96:215-225, 1953.

104. Neel, H. B., and Pemberton, J. de J.: Lateral cervical (branchial) cysts and fistulas, Surgery 18:267-286, 1954.

105. Nordentoft, J. M., and Hansen, H.: Treatment of intussusception in children, Surgery 38:311-320, 1955.

106. Oldfield, M. C.: The association of familial polyposis of the colon with multiple sebaceous cysts, Brit. J. Surg. 41:534, 1954.

107. Olsson, I., and Pallin, G.: Ueber das Bild der akuten Darminvagination bei Röntgenuntersuchung und über Desinvagination mit Hilfe von Kontrastlavements, Acta chir. scandinav. 61:371-383, 1927.

108. Parkkulainen, K. V.: Intrauterine intussusception as a cause of intestinal atresia, Surgery 44:1106-1111, 1958.

109. Plummer, G. W., and Stabins, S. J.: Bleeding duodenal ulcer in infancy: a surgical problem, J. Pediat. 37:899-904, 1950.

110. Potts, W. J.: Surgical treatment of congenital pulmonary stenosis, Ann. Surg. 130:342-362, 1949.

111. ——: The Surgeon and the Child, p. 51-59, Philadelphia, Saunders, 1959.

112. Potts, W. J., and Riker, W. L.: Differentiation of congenital cysts of the lung and those following staphylococcal pneumonia, Arch. Surg. 61:684-695, 1950.

113. Pryce, D. M.: Lower accessory pulmonary artery with intralobar sequestration of lung: a report of 7 cases, J. Path. & Bact. 58:457-467, 1946.

114. Pryce, D. M., Sellors, T. H., and Blair, L. G.: Intralobar sequestration of lung associated with an abnormal pulmonary artery, Brit. J. Surg. 35:18-29, 1947.

115. Rammstedt, C.: Zur Operation der Angeborenen Pylorusstenose, Med. Klin. 8:1702-1705, 1912.

116. Ravitch, M. M.: Polypoid adenomatosis of the entire gastrointestinal tract, Ann. Surg. 128:283-297, 1948.

117. ——: Radical treatment of massive mixed angiomas (hemolymphangiomas) in infants and children, Ann. Surg. 134:228-243, 1951.

118. ——: Hindgut duplication—doubling of colon and of the genital and lower urinary tracts, Ann. Surg. 137:588-601, 1953.

119. ——: Operation for correction of pectus excavatum, Surg., Gynec. & Obst. 106:618-622, 1958.

120. ——: Pseudo Hirschsprung's disease, Ann. Surg. 147:781-795, 1958.

121. ——: Intussusception in Infancy and Childhood. An analysis of 77 cases treated by barium enema, New England J. Med. 259:1058-1064, 1958.

122. ——: Intussusception in Infants and Children, Springfield, Ill., Thomas, 1959.

123. ——: The operative treatment of pectus carinatum (pigeon breast), Ann. Surg. 151:705-714, 1960.

124. ——: The operative treatment of congenital deformities of the chest, J.A.M.A. 175:1039-1044, 1961.

125. ——: The changing pattern of empyema in infants and children, J.A.M.A. in press, 1961.

126. Ravitch, M. M., and Handelsman, J. C.: Lesions of the thoracic parietes in infants and children, S. Clin. North America 32:1397-1424, 1952.

127. ——: One stage resection of the entire colon and rectum for ulcerative colitis and polypoid adenomatosis, Bull. Johns Hopkins Hosp. 88:59-82, 1951.

128. Ravitch, M. M., and Hardy, J. B.: Congenital cystic disease of the lung in infants and in children, Arch. Surg. 59:1-36, 1949.

129. Ravitch, M. M., and McGoon, D. C.: Teratoid tumors and dermoid cysts *in* Cancer and Allied Diseases of Infancy and Childhood, pp. 249-273, Boston, Little, 1960.

130. Ravitch, M. M., and Smith, E. I.: Sacrococcygeal teratoma in infants and children, Surgery 30:733-762, 1951.

131. Ravitch, M. D., and Snyder, G. B.: Congenital cystic dilatation of the common bile duct, Surgery 44:752-765, 1958.

132. Ravitch, M. M., and Woods, A. C.: Annular pancreas, Ann. Surg. 132:1116-1127, 1950.

133. Redo, S. F.: Congenital atresia of extra-

hepatic ducts, A.M.A. Arch. Surg. *69*:886-897, 1954.

134. Rehbein, F., and von Zimmerman, H.: Results with abdominal resection in Hirschsprung's disease, Arch. Dis. Childhood *35*: 29-37, 1960.

135. Retan, G. M.: Non-operative treatment of intussusception, Am. J. Dis. Child. *33*:765-770, 1927.

136. Rhoads, J. E., Pipes, R. L., and Perlingieró-Randall, J.: A simultaneous abdominal and perineal approach in operations for imperforate anus with atresia of the rectum and rectosigmoid, Ann. Surg. *127*:552-556, 1948.

137. Robertson, H. E., and Kernohan, J. W.: Myenteric plexus in congenital megacolon, Proc. Staff Meet., Mayo Clin. *13*:123-125, 1938.

138. Runström, G.: On Roentgen-anatomical appearance of congenital pyloric stenosis during and after manifest stage of disease, Acta paediat. *26*:383-433, 1939.

139. Rush, B. F., Jr., and Ravitch, M. M.: Septic thrombophlebitis due to a species of achromobacter in a four-year-old boy, J.A.M.A. *173*:254-254, 1960.

140. Sabiston, D. C., Hopkins, E. H., Cooke, R. E., and Bennett, I. L.: The surgical management of complications of staphylococcal pneumonia in infancy and childhood, J. Thor. & Cardiovas. Surg. *38*:421-434, 1959.

141. Sale, T. A.: Successful treatment of a perforated Rokitansky-Cushing ulcer, Arch. Dis. Childhood *31*:233-235, 1956.

142. Sandblom, P.: Plastic repair of congenital esophageal stenosis, Acta chir. scandinav. *97*:35-41, 1948.

143. Sanford, H. N., and Shmigelsky, I. H.: Purulent parotitis in the newborn, J. Pediat. *26*:149-154, 1954.

144. Santulli, T. V.: Management of surgical conditions of the alimentary tract in infancy, Bull. New York Acad. Med. *36*:185, 1960.

145. Sherman, C. D., and Waterston, D.: Oesophageal reconstruction in children using intrathoracic colon, Arch. Dis. Childhood *11*:11-16, 1957.

146. Silverman, F. N., and Huang, N.: Congenital absence of the abdominal muscles, Am. J. Dis. Child. *80*:91-124, 1950.

147. Sjöstrom, P. M.: Über unblutige Desinvagination von Darminvaginationsfällen mit Hilfe von Kontrasteinlauf unter Röntgendurchleuchtung, Chirurg *6*:706-714, 1934.

148. Sloan, R. D., and Cooley, R. N.: Con-

genital pulmonary arteriovenous aneurysm, Am. J. Roentgenol. *70*:183-210, 1953.

149. Snyder, N. H., Kraus, A. R., and Chaffin, L.: Intussusception in infants and children: a report of 143 consecutive cases, Ann. Surg. *130*:200-210, 1949.

150. Snyder, W. H., Jr., and Chaffin, L.: Embryology and pathology of the intestinal tract: presentation of 40 cases of malrotation, Ann. Surg. *140*:368-380, 1954.

151. Stiles, K. A.: The inheritance of pitted ear, J. Hered. *36*:53-61, 1945.

152. Swenson, O.: Diagnosis and treatment of atresia of the esophagus and tracheoesophageal fistula, Pediatrics *1*:195-203, 1948.

153. ———: Follow-up on 200 patients treated for Hirschsprung's disease during a ten year period, Ann. Surg. *146*:706-714, 1957.

154. ———: Pediatric Surgery, pp. 155-172, New York, Appleton Century Crofts, 1958.

155. Swenson, O., and Bill, A. H., Jr.: Resection of rectum and rectosigmoid with preservation of the sphincter for benign spastic lesions producing megacolon, Surgery *24*: 212-220, 1948.

156. Swenson, O., and Fisher, J. H.: Treatment of Hirschsprung's disease with entire colon involved in aganglionic defect, A.M.A. Arch. Surg. *70*:535-538, 1955.

157. ———: Small bowel atresia: Treatment by resection and primary aseptic anastomosis, Surgery *47*:823-835, 1960.

158. Swenson, O., Fisher, J. H., and Gherardi, G. J.: Rectal biopsy in the diagnosis of Hirschsprung's disease, Surgery *45*:690-695, 1959.

159. Swenson, O., and Small, W. T.: Tuberculosis of cervical lymph nodes, Pediatrics *10*:131-136, 1952.

160. Thomsen, G., Vesterdal, J., and Winkel-Smith, C. C.: Diaphragmatic hernia into the pericardium, Acta paediat. *43*:485-492, 1954.

161. Ulin, A. W., Nosal, J. L., and Martin, W. L.: Cholecystitis in childhood; associated obstructive jaundice, Surgery *31*:312, 1952.

162. Wallgren, A.: Lingual application of eumydrin in the treatment of congenital pyloric stenosis, Arch. Dis. Childhood *15*:103, 1940.

163. ———: Preclinical stage of infantile hypertrophic pyloric stenosis, Am. J. Dis. Child. *72*:371-376, 1946.

164. Wangensteen, O. H., and Rice, C. O.: Imperforate anus—a method of determining the surgical approach, Ann. Surg. *92*:77, 1930.

165. Ward, D. E., Jr., Bradshaw, H. H., and Prince, J. C.: Bronchial adenoma in children, J. Thoracic Surg. *27*:295-299, 1954.

166. Ward, G. E., and Hendrick, J. W.: Diagnosis and Treatment of Tumors of the Head and Neck, p. 232, Baltimore, Williams & Wilkins, 1950.

167. Ward, R.: Symposium on surgical lesions of the thyroid; malignant goiter, Surgery *16*:783-803, 1944.

168. Weens, H. S.: Cholelithiasis in sickle cell anemia, Ann. Int. Med. *22*:182-191, 1945.

169. Wessel, M. A.: Chylothorax in a 2 week old infant with spontaneous recovery, J. Pediat. *25*:201-210, 1944.

170. White, M., and Dennison, W. M.: Irreducible intussusception in infants, Brit. J. Surg. *40*:137-140, 1952.

171. Wilkins, L., and Ravitch, M. M.: Adreno- cortical tumor arising in liver of 3 year old boy with signs of virilism and Cushing's syndrome; report of case with cure after partial resection of right lobe of liver, Pediatrics *9*:671-680, 1952.

172. Williams, C., Jr.: Carcinoma of the colon in childhood, Ann. Surg. *139*:816-825, 1954.

173. Winship, T., and Chase, W. W.: Thyroid carcinoma in children, Surg., Gynec. & Obst. *101*:217-224, 1955.

174. Yater, W., Finnegan, S., and Griffin, H. M.: Pulmonary arteriovenous fistula; review of the literature and report of 2 cases, J.A.M.A. *141*:581-589, 1949.

175. Zuelzer, W. W., and Wilson, J. L.: Functional intestinal obstruction on a congenital neurogenic basis in infancy, Am. J. Dis. Child. *75*:40-64, 1948.

Gynecology

There are two main requirements for the surgeon who concerns himself with diseases of the female genital tract. (1) He must be thoroughly familiar with the variations in the reproductive changes which occur in women; these variations may be very wide and yet entirely normal. (2) He must be mindful that the majority of common gynecologic conditions are managed best by nonsurgical means, and that when surgery is indicated in the premenopausal woman, preservation of her reproductive function is of paramount importance.

HISTORY AND EXAMINATION

HISTORY

This includes:

1. History of the present illness.

2. Detailed menstrual history. Specifically, this includes the age of onset or cessation of menstruation, length of cycle, duration and amount of flow, date of last 2 menstrual periods. Recent menstrual changes, bleeding between the periods, pain at the time of menstruation, and amount and type of vaginal discharge should also be noted.

3. Detailed obstetric history. This includes number of children, date of last delivery, number and causes, if known, of abortions, and any complications of pregnancy, delivery or abortion.

4. Brief systemic review with special reference to the urinary and the lower intestinal tracts.

5. Past medical history, particularly with regard to gynecologic procedures.

6. Evaluation of psychological, social and environmental factors. These are of great importance in gynecology. The patient should be given an opportunity to talk about her husband, parents, children and her daily life, and the feelings that she expresses about them

should be noted. Careful listening will also give information about her attitude toward her female functions. Disgust or fear about menstruation, pregnancy, childbirth, breast feeding, motherhood or sexual intercourse are frequently related to medical problems (Newton). The fear of growing old and the fear of cancer may be very real problems to the female patient.

EXAMINATION

A brief but thorough general physical examination should be performed. It should include examination of the breasts, since these organs are frequently closely concerned with gynecologic disorders.

Pelvic and rectal examinations are disagreeable but not painful to the average woman. They should be conducted quietly, gently and without haste. The patient frequently finds it easier to relax during these examinations if she is encouraged to breathe slowly and deeply, concentrating on expiration. An attendant should be present during the examination both from the medicolegal standpoint and to give reassurance to the patient.

The examination of female infants and children often presents special problems in management. These are summarized by Schauffler.

Examination should not be postponed because a patient is apparently menstruating. Often observation of the site of the bleeding is a great help in diagnosis.

Equipment for an adequate gynecologic examination need not be elaborate. A full list is given by Greenhill. The basic requirements are: an examining table with a drop leaf at the bottom and stirrups, drapes, a small stool for the examiner, a good light either of the gooseneck or spotlight variety, a waste receptacle and a small movable table containing appropriate instruments. These instruments should include specula—medium Graves type specula are suitable for most gynecologic examinations—long forceps, malleable uterine sounds, uterine dressing forceps, tenacula, cotton swabs and lubricant. Equipment for obtaining cytologic studies should be readily available—suction pipette, Ayre spatula, clean slides and a bottle containing fixative.

It is helpful to develop a definite routine of examination so that important areas will not be missed. Sterilized gloves should always be used. Inspection and palpation of the external genitalia is followed by a speculum examination of the cervix. The use of a Pedersen speculum is helpful for the woman with a small or virginal introitus. In children, a Kelly urethroscope may be used. Next follows the vaginoabdominal examination in which the cervix, the uterine fundus, the tubes and the ovaries are palpated. The dominant hand is best used for the abdominal part of the examination and one or, preferably, two fingers of the less dominant hand for the vaginal part. Finally, a rectovaginoabdominal examination is performed, usually with the middle finger in the rectum and the index finger in the vagina and the dominant hand again on the abdomen: by this means the paracervical tissue, the cul-de-sac and the rectovaginal septum may be palpated.

CONGENITAL ABNORMALITIES

The abnormalities of congenital origin found in the female genital tract are most easily understood by reference to their embryologic development. The 3 structures concerned are the wolffian body or mesonephros, the müllerian ducts, and the urogenital sinus. The wolffian body forms the ovary; the unfused müllerian ducts, the tubes; the fused müllerian ducts, the uterus, the cervix and the upper vagina; and the urogenital sinus forms the lower vagina and the squamous epithelium of the vagina and the cervix.

Abnormalities of the ovary are rare and consist of the failure of descent of the ovary into the true pelvis or aplasia of one or both ovaries. Aplasia, atresia and duplication of the tubes are very uncommon.

Failure of one or both müllerian ducts to develop or fuse accounts for abnormalities of

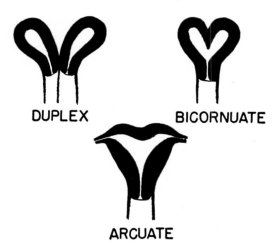

DUPLEX BICORNUATE

ARCUATE

FIG. 47-1. Congenital anomalies of the uterus. Effects of failure of fusion of müllerian ducts.

the uterus. (See Fig. 47-1.) Failure of development leads to absence of the uterus. Incomplete development with normal fusion may give rise to hypoplasia of the uterus. Failure of fusion may take various forms. The most commonly accepted classification of these anomalies is that given by Jarcho. They may range from complete duplication of uterus and cervix (uterus didelphys) down to minor septa or indentations of the top of the uterus (uterus arcuatus). These anomalies may have varying clinical significance, particularly in regard to obstetrics (Jones).

Failure of fusion of the müllerian ducts may also lead to a vagina which is completely duplicated or has a partial septum. Complete failure of development in this area may lead to partial or complete absence of the vagina.

The most important abnormality of the external genitalia is imperforate hymen (see Fig. 47-2). Double vulva or hypospadias due to failure of development of the septum between vagina and urethra may be seen.

Other congenital anomalies, especially of the urinary tract, are commonly found in association with those of the genital system.

CLINICAL FEATURES AND TREATMENT

Many of these abnormalities are not recognized until after the normal age for the onset of menstruation. Where there is obstruction to the flow of menstrual blood, symptoms usually will occur. However, the absence of normal menstruation in a girl who has reached the age of 16 or 17 should lead to a careful examination of the genital system. Many minor uterine abnormalities may not give rise to symptoms and may be discovered only incidentally during later life. There are 3 main types of clinical picture due to congenital abnormalities.

1. **Retention of Menstrual Discharge.** Imperforate hymen is the most common cause. The retained blood causes successively distention of the vagina (hematocolpos), cervix (hematotrachelos), uterine cavity (hematometra) and tubes (hematosalpinx). With each menstrual period the patient experiences increasing pain and discomfort. Distention of the lower abdomen may occur and difficulty on urination may be noted. Sometimes the symptoms may suggest an acute abdominal condition. Diagnosis in the case of imperforate hymen is easily made by examination; the bulging blue hymen is readily seen. Treatment is by cruciate incision or excision of the hymen. Infection is a not uncommon sequel of hematocolpos, and if treatment is delayed there may be permanent effects upon the reproductive capacity of the patient.

2. **Inability to Have Marital Relations.** If the absence of menstruation is not investigated, a girl may begin to consider marriage without being aware of a congenital absence of the vagina. This usually means that the whole of the lower genital tract is absent. Frequently in such instances there will be a rudi-

mentary vaginal pouch. Construction of an artificial vagina is possible in certain instances and should be attempted if the patient is anxious to have normal marital relations and is willing to co-operate fully. The most satisfactory method is by the artificial formation of a tract by dissection between the rectum and the urethra and maintenance of the tract by means of an obturator, which may be covered with a skin graft. No more than a functioning vagina can be promised to the patient. The procedure should not be undertaken until the patient is about to be married. Persistence is required on the part of both surgeon and patient to ensure adequate dilatation until the tract is completely lined by epithelium and the chance of scarring is reduced to a minimum.

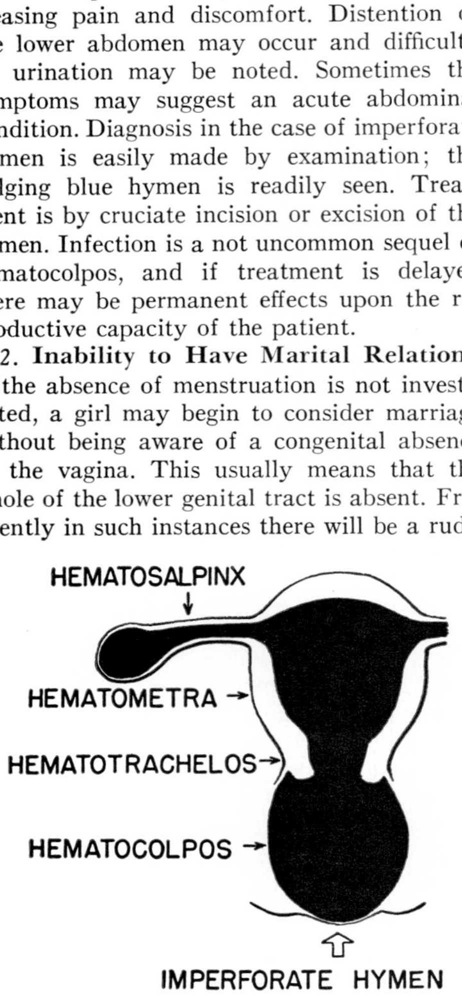

3. **Abnormalities of Pregnancy and Delivery.** Not frequently the first symptoms of an abnormality of the uterus may be discovered when the patient presents a sterility problem, has repeated abortions or has some difficulty with labor and delivery. In such cases in addition to the usual methods of examination, hysterography by means of opaque oil is valuable. Unfortunately, treatment is practical in only a few instances. For example, Strassman reports good results in selected cases by plastic unification of a double uterus.

DISPLACEMENTS OF THE UTERUS AND PELVIC RELAXATION

NORMAL POSITION AND SUPPORT OF THE PELVIC ORGANS

The uterus normally lies between the rectum and the bladder with its long axis almost in the horizontal plane so that it covers the top of the empty bladder. In this situation the cervix points almost directly backward, and the corpus bends forward slightly from the cervix. The uterus is held in this position by (1) the fascial planes of the pelvic floor (Fig. 47-3), (2) the uterine ligaments and (3) the pressure of the abdominal contents. The fascial planes of the pelvic floor consist of an area of fibromuscular thickening concentrated around the base of the broad ligament; this is variously called the cardinal or Mackenrodt's ligament. The ligaments of the uterus act as guy ropes to keep the organ in position. The broad ligaments hold it in the middle of the

HEMATOSALPINX

HEMATOMETRA →

HEMATOTRACHELOS →

HEMATOCOLPOS →

⇧
IMPERFORATE HYMEN

FIG. 47-2. Effects of retention of menstrual flow with imperforate hymen.

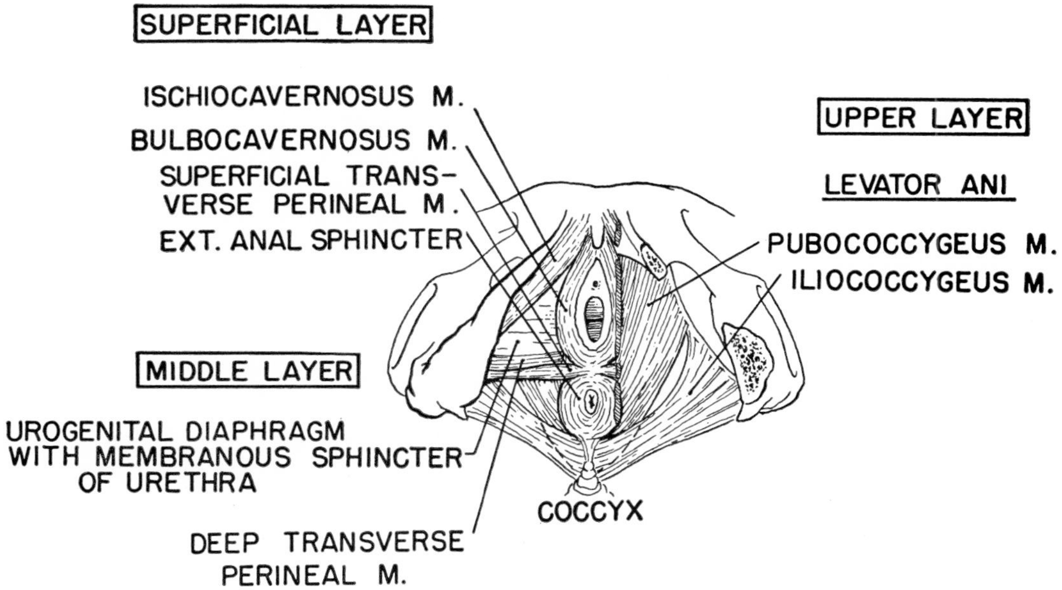

SUPERFICIAL LAYER

ISCHIOCAVERNOSUS M.

BULBOCAVERNOSUS M.

SUPERFICIAL TRANS-
VERSE PERINEAL M.

EXT. ANAL SPHINCTER

UPPER LAYER

LEVATOR ANI

PUBOCOCCYGEUS M.
ILIOCOCCYGEUS M.

MIDDLE LAYER

UROGENITAL DIAPHRAGM
WITH MEMBRANOUS SPHINCTER
OF URETHRA

COCCYX

DEEP TRANSVERSE
PERINEAL M.

FIG. 47-3. Fascia and muscles of the pelvic floor (seen from below).

pelvis and keep it up. The uterosacral ligaments pull the cervix back. The round ligaments may exert some effect on holding the fundus forward. The weight of the abdominal contents serves to keep the fundus forward.

The pelvic organs, including the bladder, the urethra and the rectum, are also supported by the muscles and the fascia of the pelvic floor. These consist of 3 layers: (1) the upper pelvic diaphragm of the levator ani muscles, (2) the triangular ligament, extending forward from the deep transverse perinei muscles at the base, (3) the superficial pelvic diaphragm, consisting of the superficial transverse perinei, the bulbocavernosus and ischiocavernosus muscles.

Childbirth and age normally result in changes in the position of the pelvic organs. Some weakening of the ligaments may be expected to follow vaginal delivery, with consequent slight descent of the uterus and increased relaxation of the walls of the vagina. After the menopause the fundus of the uterus commonly loses its forward inclination and lies in the mid-position so that it extends straight upward from the cervix.

DISPLACEMENTS OF THE UTERUS

Anterior and lateral displacements of the uterus occur occasionally, but they are usu-

ally the result of an enlarging tumor or abscess and are not of clinical importance in themselves.

Posterior displacements of the uterus are of more significance, though not as much as was thought 30 years ago. They may be divided into 3 types (Fig. 47-4): (1) retrocession, where the whole uterus is displaced toward the back of the pelvis; (2) retroversion, where the cervix is tilted forward so as to point anteriorly on vaginal examination but retains its relationship with the corpus; (3) retroflexion, where the corpus is bent backward on the cervix. The most important displacement is retroflexion but all 3 may be found together or separately and may be of varying degrees.

Cause. About 20 per cent of retrodisplacements are congenital in origin. The remainder are acquired. These may be due to: (1) childbirth, (2) age, (3) adnexal inflammation or endometriosis and (4) tumors and cysts of the uterus or the adnexa. Previously, it had been thought that trauma was a factor, but except for childbirth it is difficult to see how this could be severe enough to be important.

Clinical Features. Simple uncomplicated retrodisplacements frequently give no symptoms. However, the following may occur:

1. BACKACHE. This is characteristically of a dull aching nature and is felt in the sacral

or lumbosacral area. It is commonly worse before and during menstruation.

2. MENSTRUAL DISORDERS. Dysmenorrhea with occasional slowness in starting the flow may be noted.

3. STERILITY AND ABORTION. Relative infertility may result from the cervix being displaced anteriorly out of the apex of the vagina where the semen is pooled. Abortions may occur more frequently in patients with retrodisplacements of the uterus than in normal women. This may be due to congestion of the uterus, an unfavorable location for nidation or incarceration of the enlarging retroflexed uterus.

Diagnosis. This is made readily on pelvic examination, unless the patient is very obese or holds herself very tense. Sometimes it may be made more difficult by the presence of a myoma on the anterior surface of the uterus or by an adnexal mass which lies behind the uterus and simulates the retroflexed corpus.

Treatment. In general, if there are no symptoms, no treatment is needed. The only

possible exception to this is the retroflexion which commonly follows pregnancy; many authorities feel that this should be treated. However, many such uteri may be found later to have reverted to the anterior position without treatment.

It is important to attempt to ascertain whether the symptoms complained of are due to the retrodisplacement rather than to the associated conditions which commonly accompany acquired retrodisplacements. This is frequently difficult. In doubtful cases it may be well to treat the retrodisplacement and see if the symptoms are improved. If they are, and then return after treatment has been discontinued, one can assume that the retrodisplacement was responsible—provided that the effect of suggestion has been discounted.

If the uterus is movable, first it is replaced in the anterior position. The cervix is pushed backward toward the sacrum, and the fundus is pushed up by the fingers in the posterior fornix of the vagina. Then the fundus is grasped by the external hand and pushed

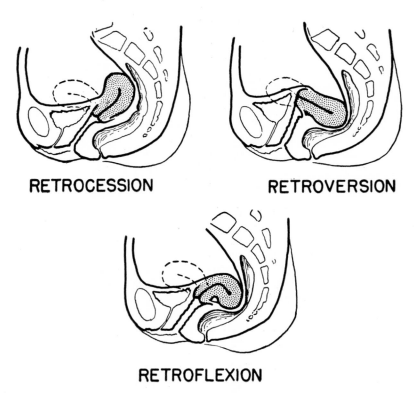

RETROCESSION   RETROVERSION

RETROFLEXION

FIG. 47-4. Retrodisplacements of the uterus.

further forward while the cervix is again pushed toward the back of the vagina. Sometimes traction on the cervix by means of a tenaculum will help the maneuver. The use of intra-uterine sounds to turn the fundus up may be successful in expert hands but is attended with the risk of perforation of the uterus.

Once the uterus is in the anterior position it may stay there of its own accord, aided by the pressure of the abdominal contents. The anterior position may be encouraged and maintained by knee-chest exercises practiced 3 or 4 times a day for 10 minutes (see Fig. 47.5).

Usually it is wise to maintain the uterus in the anterior position by means of a pessary. The best types for use in retrodisplacements are the Hodge or Smith pessaries. Insertion is relatively easy and painless. A well-fitting pessary should not cause any discomfort. The only care needed by the patient is to take a douche every day or every other day because of presence of the pessary causes a certain amount of vaginal irritation and discharge. Once a pessary has been inserted it should be removed every 6 to 8 weeks, cleaned and replaced. At this time the vaginal wall should be inspected carefully to see if any ulceration has occurred.

After the pessary has been left in place for several months and then is removed, the uterus may stay in the anterior position of its own accord. If it reverts to the posterior position, then the pessary may be replaced.

Operation should be advised for uncomplicated retrodisplacement only as a last resort. If symptoms are relieved by a pessary and return when the pessary is removed and are distressing enough so that the patient is incapacitated, then some type of operative fixation of the uterus should be considered. The principles of operative treatment are: (1) shortening of the round ligaments and changing the direction of their pull by attaching them to the back of the uterus (Baldy-Webster); (2) shortening the round ligaments by attaching them to the abdominal wall (Gilliam).

If the uterus is fixed in the posterior position, treatment is usually more difficult. However, in this case the retrodisplacement itself is less likely to be causing the patient's symptoms than the associated disease. Therefore,

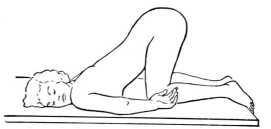

FIG. 47-5. Knee-chest position.

management may resolve itself into the treatment of the underlying condition. Manual replacement is not usually possible, though sometimes knee-chest exercises may return the uterus to the anterior position. Replacement under anesthesia may sometimes be possible under these circumstances, although if great difficulty is encountered it should not be persisted in, owing to the possibility of injury. If one is considering freeing the adhesions by laparotomy and replacing the uterus, one should be sure that there are other indications for operation than the retrodisplacement; e.g., endometriosis. Notoriously difficult to manage are the retrodisplacements associated with chronic pelvic inflammatory disease, since the mass of adhesions in the pelvis at the time of operation tends to lead to more radical surgery than would be necessary solely for the retrodisplacement.

PELVIC RELAXATION

Pelvic relaxation includes the following conditions: they may occur together or separately.

1. Prolapse of the uterus (descensus uteri)
2. Prolapse of the intestine into the pouch of Douglas (enterocele)
3. Prolapse of the bladder into the anterior vaginal wall (cystocele)
4. Prolapse of the urethra into the anterior vaginal wall (urethrocele)
5. Prolapse of the rectum into the posterior vaginal wall (rectocele)
6. Weakness of the perineum

Cause. These conditions occur most commonly, but not invariably, in parous and older women. Primarily, they are due to an exaggeration of the normal relaxation of the pelvic ligaments and support which occurs during childbirth and after the menopause. A contributing factor may be traumatic prolonged labor.

Clinical Features. Prolapse of the uterus may be divided conveniently into 3 stages (see Fig. 47-6): (1) First-degree prolapse occurs when the cervix descends below its normal position in the vaginal canal. (2) In second-degree prolapse, the cervix reaches the introitus. (3) In third-degree the whole uterus lies outside the introitus. The exact degree of prolapse of the uterus may not be realized upon examination unless the patient is asked to stand or strain down vigorously: straining may be reproduced by pulling the cervix down with a tenaculum. The descent of the cervix may be felt by the patient as a lump in the vagina, which is noticed on prolonged standing or straining. If the cervix becomes irritated or eroded as a result of its descent, vaginal discharge or bleeding may be noted.

Enterocele, in addition to accompanying other types of prolapse, may occur by itself following vaginal hysterectomy. It usually does not cause symptoms until it is felt as a protruding mass. Incarceration occurs only very rarely.

Cystocele and urethrocele are frequently associated. They may be asymptomatic, but since they predispose to the retention of urine, infection commonly occurs. In the case of urethrocele this leads to burning and frequency of urination. On occasion a urethral diverticulum may develop. In the case of cystocele, frequency and urgency of urination, together with suprapubic pain, occur. Infection is commonly recurrent and eventually may lead to upper urinary tract infection. If marked cystocele is associated with prolapse of the uterus, obstruction of the lower ureter may occur with resulting hydronephrosis and uremia.

Involuntary discharge of urine on strain-

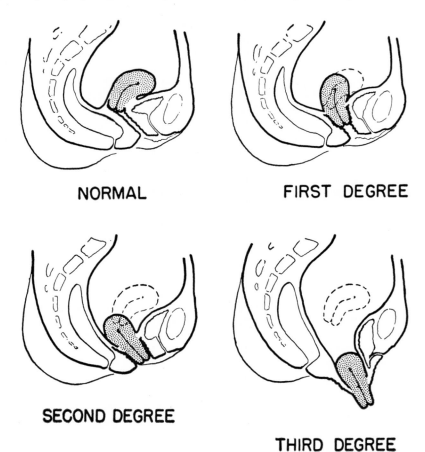

NORMAL   FIRST DEGREE

SECOND DEGREE

THIRD DEGREE

Fig. 47-6. Degrees of prolapse of the uterus.

ing, coughing, laughing or sneezing (stress incontinence) is a common concomitant of pelvic relaxation. The exact mechanism of this condition is under considerable study at present. That it is not necessarily the result of age or parity is shown by the study of Nemir and Middleton, who found that 52 per cent of 1,327 college women reported some degree of stress incontinence and that in 5 per cent this was severe.

Minor degrees of rectocele do not normally cause symptoms. If the rectocele is large, fecal material may be retained in it, and the patient may have trouble expelling it unless she manually pushes the rectocele back.

Weakness of the perineum is due to damage to the smaller muscles, such as may occur during childbirth. By itself it usually causes no symptoms, except perhaps for a sensation of gaping at the introitus. Occasionally, however, it may involve division of the fibers of the anal sphincter. This may cause incontinence of feces, especially if the bowel movements are loose.

Diagnosis. Usually the diagnosis is made readily on examination. The anterior vaginal wall may be observed by having the patient strain down while pushing the posterior wall backward. The posterior wall may be observed by having the patient strain down while pushing the anterior wall forward. Stress incontinence can be observed by having the patient strain down with a full bladder and noting the escape of urine from the urethra. The condition of the perineal body and the anal sphincter is evaluated best by rectal examination.

Treatment. Prophylaxis of pelvic relaxation by good obstetric practice is very important. During the second stage of labor the fascial supports of the uterus, the bladder and the rectum and the small muscles of the perineum are greatly stretched and may even tear. Any technic that prevents these fibers rupturing or stretching beyond their capacity to return to normal is of value. In the past 2 or 3 decades it has been felt by obstetricians in this country that shortening of the second stage of labor by performing an episiotomy and extracting the baby by forceps applied at the pelvic outlet would achieve this objective. A logical approach in most normal women would seem to be by antepartal perineal

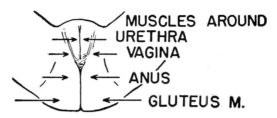

FIG. 47-7. Direction of muscle contraction in perineal exercises.

muscle exercises (Bushnell) (see Fig. 47-7). In this way adequate perineal relaxation may occur during labor, delivery of the baby is gradual and good perineal muscle tone may be promptly restored postpartally. Of course, this does not preclude the use of forceps if the second stage is abnormally prolonged or if the patient is unable to take advantage of such exercises.

In line with the prophylaxis of pelvic relaxation, the primary treatment for minor or moderate relaxation, especially in women of the child-bearing age or where stress incontinence is prominent, should be by nonoperative measures. Kegel has recommended the use of excercises to contract the perineal muscles. He finds that the strength of these muscles can be measured by a perineometer and has noted improvement in 69 per cent of patients treated in this way.

Where the anatomic changes are very marked, or where nonoperative treatment has not produced improvement, operation is indicated. Before this is done any urinary tract infection should be investigated and treated. Vaginal infection also should be treated, and in the postmenopausal woman improvement of the condition of the vaginal mucosa may be obtained by the use of estrogenic creams locally before operation.

Repair of a cystocele and urethrocele (anterior colporrhaphy) or a rectocele (posterior colporrhaphy) consists of excising the excess vaginal mucosa over the organ concerned, plicating the fascia and resuturing the vagina. Repair of a rectocele usually should be combined with repair of the perineum and narrowing of the introitus to admit 2 fingers only. Repair of the anal sphincter can be combined with a perineorrhaphy by identifying the divided ends of the muscle and suturing them together. Repair of the prolapsed uterus may be handled either by amputation of the cervix and fixation of the lower part of the parametria to the shortened cervix anteriorly (Manchester procedure) or by vaginal hysterectomy. The former is thought by many to give better support at the apex of the vagina, and, in the child-bearing age, subsequent pregnancy is possible. However, abdominal delivery by cesarean section is advisable after such a procedure. Vaginal hysterectomy may forestall the possible future development of intrauterine disease and is particularly indicated where marked prolapse is the major problem.

In the older debilitated patient who is a poor operative risk, pelvic relaxation occasionally may be treated satisfactorily by occlusion of the vagina (LeFort procedure—colpocleisis). This involves denudation and approximation of the anterior and the posterior vaginal walls, leaving lateral channels when the uterus is still present. Local anesthesia can be used, and the procedure may not be as traumatic as the other procedures described above.

When operation cannot be performed for any reason, relief of symptoms may be obtained by the use of a ring pessary. The doughnut or hard-rubber types are most useful. They act by distending the vagina and suspending the cervix at a higher level than before and work best if perineal relaxation is minimal. The care of these pessaries is the same as for the Smith or Hodge types, except that vaginal ulceration must be watched for even more carefully in the older patient.

Special problems in vaginal repair occur with enterocele or where stress incontinence is marked. As with the repair of any hernia, the sac of the enterocele must be dissected out and the peritoneum securely closed. Frequently, it is difficult to add any support to the repair from below since the uterosacral ligaments are attenuated. In the primary repair of an enterocele an attempt should be made to close these as well as possible (McCall). However, in recurrent enterocele, obliteration of the posterior cul-de-sac from the abdominal approach may be indicated (Moschcowitz procedure).

Stress incontinence occasionally presents great difficulty in treatment. Operation is indicated if conservative measures such as exercises have not succeeded, or if there is marked associated relaxation of other pelvic structures. An anterior colporrhaphy may solve the problem. In recurrent cases, however, other types of procedure may be necessary. The multitude of procedures used (Kelly urethropexy, "sling" operations, suprapubic vesicourethral suspension) indicates that no one satisfactory method has been found.

DISEASES OF THE LOWER GENITAL TRACT

Anatomically, the lower genital tract consists of the vulva and the lower two thirds of the vagina. This area is all derived embryologically from the urogenital sinus. Its arterial supply comes from the branches of the internal pudendal artery, and its lymphatics go primarily to the superficial inguinal nodes. Functionally, the upper vagina and the cervix up to the external os must also be considered as a part of the lower genital tract, since their squamous epithelium is derived from the urogenital sinus. However, this area is also developed from the lower part of the müllerian ducts, its arterial supply comes from the uterine branches of the internal iliac arteries, and its lymphatics go primarily to the nodes surrounding those vessels. Thus the cervix has to be considered as a separate entity as well as being a part of the lower genital tract.

The thickness of the vaginal epithelium and the acidity of its secretion vary with the amount of estrogen present in the woman's blood. Thus in the newborn infant, owing to the maternal estrogens which have passed through the placenta, the vaginal epithelium is thick, and the pH is low. Soon afterward it reverts to the childhood type, consisting only of a basal layer of cells and having a higher pH. Puberty brings about cyclical changes with the pH generally being in the range of 4.5 to 5.0, although it is somewhat higher just after menstruation. In the premenstrual phase it is greatly thickened, and cells become cornified. After the menopause the epithelium reverts to the childhood type.

Disorders Caused by Trauma

Direct trauma to the lower genital tract is rare. It may consist of forcible rupture of the hymen with occasional troublesome bleeding, perforation by instruments, or damage due to the retention of foreign bodies. Recognition of these injuries depends upon a careful history and thorough examination. Treatment depends upon the type of injury.

Indirect trauma is more frequent and consists chiefly of vaginal fistulae. The common ones are: (1) vesicovaginal, (2) ureterovaginal and (3) rectovaginal. They may be due to childbirth, operative injury, radiation or tumor.

Vesicovaginal Fistula. Closure of a vesicovaginal fistula by Marion Sims in 1855 marked the start of gynecology as a specialty. This condition still remains as a major problem in treatment.

CLINICAL FEATURES. There is a constant discharge of urine from the vagina with irritation and infection of the vulva and the perineal skin.

DIAGNOSIS. When the fistula is large it is usually obvious on pelvic examination. When it is small, insertion of methylene blue into the bladder and subsequent observation of it in the vagina may be conclusive.

TREATMENT. Since these fistulae do not tend to heal spontaneously, treatment is usually surgical. They may be closed from the vaginal or transvesical or from a combined approach. The primary object is to close separately the bladder mucosa, the fascia between bladder and vagina and the vaginal mucosa. Where the cervix has been removed colpocleisis of the upper vagina, as suggested by Falk and Bunkin, may succeed. When the fistula is very large and follows pelvic radiation, the shortening and the scarring of the anterior vaginal wall may be so extensive that repair is impossible. In such instances diversion of the urinary stream into an isolated loop of ileum, brought out as an ileostomy in the right lower quadrant of the abdomen, may greatly increase the patient's comfort and prolong her life (Fig. 47-8).

Ureterovaginal Fistula. This type of fistula has become more common following the more radical surgical procedures used recently in the treatment of pelvic malignancy. A certain number will close spontaneously. However, kidney function is usually lost on that side. Operative repair is discussed in the section on urology.

Rectovaginal Fistula. CLINICAL FEATURES. Discharge of feces through the vagina is the chief symptom. When the fistula is small, this may be intermittent, occurring only when the patient has diarrhea. Vaginal, vulvar and perineal infection may follow.

TREATMENT. Surgical repair is the only possible treatment. It follows the same principles as for repair of a vesicovaginal fistula: it may be performed from the vaginal approach, or if the fistula is high a combined abdominoperineal or pull-through type of procedure may be done. It is frequently advisable to divert the fecal stream by means of a loop sigmoid or transverse colostomy before proceeding to the repair.

VENEREAL INFECTIONS OF THE LOWER GENITAL TRACT

Gonorrhea is the most common veneral disease in women. It is caused by the diplococcus Neisseriae, which is identified by the fact that it is intracellular, gram-negative and oxidase-positive on culture. It is transmitted primarily by sexual intercourse, although occasional infection may occur by contact with an infected towel, toilet seat or douche nozzle.

Gonorrhea affects primarily the lower genital tract. Squamous epithelium is resistant, but the organism flourishes in the glands of the urethra (Skene's glands), the vulva (Bartholin's glands) and the cervix. Secondary invasion of the uterus and the tubes by the surface route and spread to distant parts of the body may occur, especially at the time of menstruation. These serious consequences will be considered among the diseases of the upper genital tract.

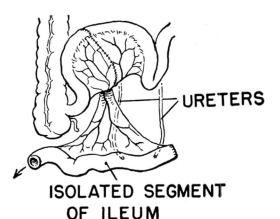

ISOLATED SEGMENT OF ILEUM

FIG. 47-8. Uretero-ileostomy.

CLINICAL FEATURES. The acute stage is relatively mild and may not be noticed by the patient. Within a few days after infection dryness and irritation of the vagina are noticed. There may be some urinary frequency and burning on urination. A small amount of discharge appears. These symptoms may become more marked or may pass away. Upon examination the vagina and the vulva appear reddened, and there may be more or less purulent discharge.

Spontaneous cure of the acute infection may occur, but it is much more likely to become subacute and chronic. In this case the organism is maintained in the cervical glands, Bartholin's glands and Skene's glands. The clinical appearance is one of continuous purulent discharge and irritation of the vagina and the vulva from the pus, associated with urethritis. From both the acute and the chronic stages infection of the upper genital tract may result, and this remains a constant hazard while the infection is untreated.

In children the organism affects primarily the vagina and the vulva. A persistent purulent vaginal discharge occurs. There is usually no spread to the upper genital tract.

DIAGNOSIS. The diagnosis can be made positively only by culture of the organism. In acute cases a smear of the discharge stained by Gram's method may be helpful (Fig. 47-9).

TREATMENT. The advent of the sulfonamide drugs and antibiotics has revolutionized the treatment of gonorrhea. Penicillin is effective, and a daily dose of 600,000 units is given for

a period of 5 days. Where the infection appears to be resistant to penicillin, other antibiotics or sulfonamide drugs may be used. Local treatment in the acute stage should be confined to rest, local washing with soap and warm water, and careful attention to avoid infecting other persons: this latter involves avoidance of intercourse as well as sterilization and disposal of infected linen, until cure is established. The tracing and the treatment of contacts is also important.

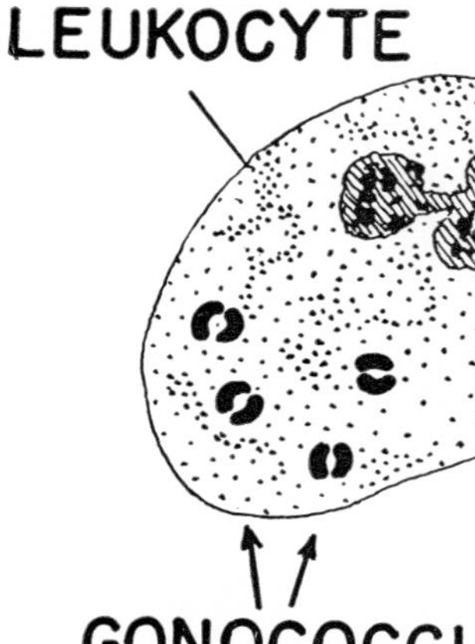

It is frequently difficult to be sure that cure of the infection has actually occurred. Ideally, at least 2 negative cultures should be obtained. It is best to take at least one of these immediately after menstruation when recrudescence of the infection commonly occurs.

In chronic cases both diagnosis and treatment are more difficult. Eradication of the foci of infection in Skene's, Bartholin's and the cervical glands is frequently necessary. Such treatment, especially in the cervix, is not without danger of infection of the upper genital tract.

In children antibiotics are the best method of treatment, but in resistant cases it may be advisable to attempt to convert the vaginal epithelium to the adult type by the administration of estrogens.

Other Venereal Infections. Syphilis, chancroid, granuloma inguinale and lymphopathia venereum may also affect the lower genital tract. These are identified by the demonstration of the specific organism involved or, in the case of lymphopathia, by the Frei test. As a rule they do not spread to involve the upper genital tract.

OTHER INFECTIONS

Trichomoniasis is caused by the flagellated protozoon, *Trichomonas vaginalis*. The organism is common and may exist for long periods in the vagina without causing symptoms. It has also been found in the upper genital tract, in urine and in the blood stream. In males it has been found in the urine, the prostatic secretion and the semen. Thus while the infection is primarily vaginal, it may also be generalized. How a quiescent is changed into an active infection is not well understood, although psychosomatic factors may be important.

CLINICAL FEATURES. The patient complains

LEUKOCYTE

GONOCOCCI

FIG. 47-9. Gonococci within a leukocyte.

of a profuse irritating vaginal discharge which frequently has a foul odor. Frequency and burning of urination are commonly noted. On examination a foamy yellow discharge is seen in the vagina. The vagina itself is reddened and may show punctate red spots. The cervix also may be involved.

DIAGNOSIS. The motile organism may be detected by microscopic examination of a small amount of discharge mixed with warm saline (Fig. 47-10). The use of lubricant for examination may destroy the motility of the organism and make diagnosis more difficult. A large number of pus cells compared with epithelial cells may indicate a more severe and resistant infection (Donald).

TREATMENT. This is by no means satisfactory as is evidenced by the large number of preparations available. The use of douches of white vinegar (3-4 tablespoonfuls to 1 quart of warm water) twice daily combined with the intravaginal application of a protozooicide probably is most effective. Treatment should be repeated through and immediately after at least 2 menstrual periods, since recrudescence is most likely to occur at this time. Careful treatment on these lines will cure from 70 to 80 per cent of cases, but relapses are not uncommon.

Moniliasis. Infection by *Candida albicans* or other fungi is relatively common especially in pregnancy.

CLINICAL FEATURES. Itching of the vulva

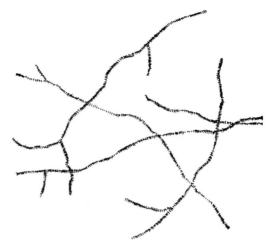

FIG. 47-11. Monilia.

usually is more prominent than discharge. The vagina and the vulva may appear inflamed on examination, and patches of white cheesy material are seen clinging to the epithelium.

DIAGNOSIS. A small amount of discharge may be mixed with 10 per cent potassium hydroxide (to obliterate the cellular elements) and examined microscopically. The fungi are seen as fine branching and budding threads (Fig. 41-11). In doubtful cases culture on Pagano-Levin medium may be helpful.

TREATMENT. The most effective remedy available is the intravaginal application of nystatin tablets twice daily for 12 days, combined with the use of nystatin ointment externally to relieve itching. If this fails (as it may do, especially in pregnancy), painting the area with 1 or 2 per cent gentian violet, or the intravaginal application of gentian violet jelly may be useful. Other preparations such as propionic acid jelly are occasionally of value.

Nonspecific Infections. Frequently no specific cause can be found for the discharge of which the patient complains, and culture reveals only a mixed group of organisms. In this connection it is well to remember that vaginal discharge is frequently a symptom of psychosomatic disturbance and attention to these factors, particularly in relation to the patient's sexual feelings, may be curative. Local treatment may consist of intravaginal application of bacteriostatic sulfa creams and attempts to restore the normal acidity of the vagina by acid jellies or by vinegar douches.

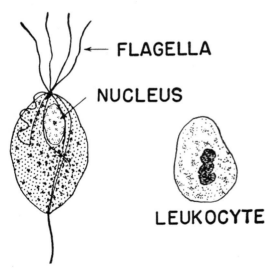

FLAGELLA

NUCLEUS

LEUKOCYTE

FIG. 47-10. *Trichomonas vaginalis.*

OTHER DISEASES OF THE LOWER GENITAL TRACT

Atrophic Vaginitis. This condition is found in postmenopausal women, and in premenopausal women who have diminished ovarian function. It is due primarily to lack of estrogens. Clinically, it is characterized by a thin irritating vaginal discharge, which at times may be bloody. On examination the vaginal mucosa is reddened and presents many petechiae. Provided that cancer of the upper and the lower genital tracts and leukoplakia have been excluded, treatment with intravaginal applications of estrogenic cream usually is helpful.

Leukoplakia. This occurs chiefly in menopausal and postmenopausal women and consists of white patches of thickened skin which appear around the introitus. The term kraurosis is used commonly for the excessive shrinkage and thinning of the skin in this area. Both conditions probably should be considered as a part of an atrophic process.

CAUSE. This is not well understood. The fact that the condition occurs at an age when ovarian function is diminishing suggests that deficiency of ovarian hormones may be a factor. Dietary deficiencies also may play a part.

PATHOLOGIC FEATURES. In the early stages areas of round cell infiltration and inflammatory changes are seen. Later atrophy and loss of the subepithelial elastic fibers become apparent. Hypertrophic changes may occur, and in the typical leukoplakic patch great thickness of the skin is seen with excessive cornification.

CLINICAL FEATURES. The patient complains of persistent itching and burning of the vulva. Increasing pain on coitus may be noted. Examination may show the skin to be thin and inelastic with white patches situated anywhere on the labia majora or minora. Cracks and inflammation in the skin may appear as a result of the scratching.

DIAGNOSIS. The important conditions to be differentiated are leukoderma in which the white areas are associated with relatively normal skin, lichen sclerosus et atrophicus and carcinoma in which induration and ulceration are prominent. Adequate biopsy is essential to differentiate between these conditions.

TREATMENT. It is important to discontinue the use of substances which may cause irritation, such as harsh soaps or detergents used in washing, contraceptives or home remedies. Tight clothing and pads should be avoided. Cotton underwear should be worn. The area should be washed only with plain water. Compresses of 1:10,000 potassium permanganate or aluminum acetate solution (diluted 1:20) and the local application of witch hazel or a simple dusting powder may help to control the itching. Analgesic ointments or creams may be helpful. Adequate diet and supplementary vitamins, especially high doses of vitamin A, have been used with success. However, in most instances early excision of the leukoplakic areas is advisable, since the chance of cancer developing eventually is considerable. On occasion this may involve a simple vulvectomy.

Pruritus Vulvae. Itching is a common concomitant of vulvitis, vaginitis and atrophic conditions of the vulva. The term pruritus has become limited conventionally to those cases where itching is the primary complaint, without clear evidence of associated disease. Frequently, it is accompanied by itching around the anus and the inner thighs. The skin in these areas eventually may become thick, fissured and inflamed. Every attempt should be made to exclude a specific cause for the itching. Many of these patients show abnormal glucose metabolism. Therefore, a glucose tolerance test should be performed routinely.

Treatment consists first in eradicating any obvious cause for the itching. Where no cause is found management may be extremely difficult. Local applications to relieve itching, dietary advice, and attention to psychological factors, which are commonly present, are important. Surgical undermining of the skin (Mering) or injection of long-acting anesthetic agents to remove sensory stimulation have been reported to be of help (Reich and Nechtow).

BENIGN CYSTS AND TUMORS OF THE LOWER GENITAL TRACT

Condylomata Acuminata. These lesions are microscopically papillomata. They are frequently multiple and are situated anywhere on the external genitalia. They may grow to a large size during pregnancy. They are due to a chronic irritating vaginal discharge of any sort. A satisfactory method of treatment is by application of 25 per cent podophyllin. Larger or resistant growths may require cauterization or surgical removal. Any infection present in the lower genital tract should also be treated vigorously.

Urethral Caruncle. Caruncle is the term given to a small red growth which develops just at or inside the external urinary meatus. Pathologically, these have the appearance of granulomata, although in some there may be evidence of papilloma formation. They are not true tumors and in general do not become malignant. Clinically, they may give no symptoms at all, or the patient may notice pain in the area, burning on urination or bleeding. They appear as small (1-2 mm. up to more than 1 cm. in diameter) red growths in the region of the urinary meatus. Care should be taken to avoid confusion in diagnosis with eversion of the mucosa of the urethra, which is common, or carcinoma of the urethra, which is very rare. Treatment, if indicated, is by excision or cauterization: for both of these adequate anesthesia, usually general, is needed.

Cysts and Abscesses of Bartholin's Glands. Obstruction of the duct of Bartholin's gland is common. This leads to retention of secretions (cyst) or pus (abscess). Abscess is a common sequel of gonorrheal infection but may be due to nonspecific causes.

CLINICAL FEATURES. A cyst may cause no symptoms except the sensation of a mass in the vulvar region. Abscess formation is accompanied by pain, redness, tenderness and fever. Tender inguinal nodes are often palpable.

DIAGNOSIS. A Bartholin's cyst lies at the posterior end of the introitus as contrasted with other labial cysts which lie more anteriorly and laterally, and with abscesses resulting from perianal infections which are felt more posteriorly.

TREATMENT. An abscess should be opened widely and antibiotics given. A permanent cure may be attempted even in the acute case by suturing the margins of the abscess to the adjacent skin. Recent work (Jacobson) has shown that this type of management by marsupialization is most satisfactory for the definitive treatment of Bartholin's cysts and is simpler than excision.

Other Cysts and Tumors. A wide variety of cysts and tumors are seen in this area. The most common are vaginal inclusion cysts, cysts of wolffian duct remnants, or tumors arising from the skin of the vulva, especially fibromata and hydroadenomata. Simple surgical excision is the treatment of choice.

MALIGNANT TUMORS OF THE LOWER GENITAL TRACT

Cancer of Vulva and Surrounding Structures. Cancer of the vulva comprises between 3 and 4 per cent of all cancers of the female genital tract. By far the greatest number (over 95%) are squamous cell carcinomata, although melanomata, adenocarcinomata of Bartholin's gland, and basal cell carcinomata are found occasionally. The lesion may start anywhere on the external genitalia. Multiple origins are not uncommon. From the initial point the disease may extend backward to the rectum, anteriorly into the urethra or upward into the vagina. Metastasis takes place to the inguinal nodes, often to the opposite side or bilaterally, and thence to the femoral and the deep pelvic nodes. Nodal spread was found by Way to have occurred in 60 of 143 operative cases (42%); in 23 of the 60 cases, the deep pelvic nodes were involved.

CLINICAL FEATURES. The symptoms of cancer of the vulva are few in the early stages. It is primarily a disease of older women, the average age being at least 60 years. Frequently, there is a history of leukoplakia. Slight itching or burning of the vulva may be noted, with bleeding only rarely being observed. Often the feeling of a hard lump in this region may be the only thing to bring the patient to a physician. Examination reveals one or more suspiciously hard nodules, parts of which may be ulcerated and may bleed easily. Inguinal nodes are frequently palpable, but this may be due to inflammation rather than metastatic tumor, unless they are very hard and fixed.

DIAGNOSIS. This usually can be suspected on examination but always should be confirmed by adequate biopsy before definitive treatment is started.

TREATMENT. Surgery provides the best treatment available at present. The most logical approach, and one which conforms to accepted standards of cancer surgery, is that originally recommended by Way. The inguinal nodes, the tissue between the inguinal region and the vulva and the vulva itself are removed en bloc in one procedure. In addition, most surgeons remove the deep pelvic nodes bilaterally at the same time (see Fig. 47-12). The success of operative treatment is indicated by reports of 5-year survival rates of 61 per cent (Green, Ulfelder and Meigs) and 54 per cent (Way). The procedure is a formidable one, since many of the patients are old, debilitated and affected by intercurrent disease. Even in the best hands these wounds do not heal well, and later postoperative swelling of the legs is common. In some poor risk patients it may be well to stage the procedure, though this sacrifices the principle of removal of the cancer and metastatic nodes in continuity. In patients who are considered to be too poor risks to stand any surgical procedure, radiation may be of palliative and possibly of curative value; it is used best in the form of

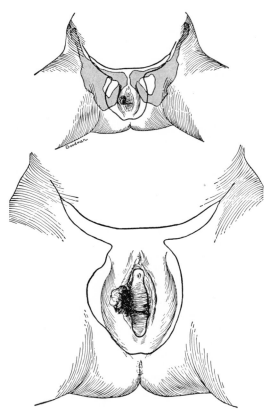

FIG. 47-12. Skin incision for radical vulvectomy and bilateral inguinal node dissection.

implantation of radium needles with or without external irradiation. It is usually unwise to use radiation first with the idea of doing surgery later, since the radiation makes the chance of healing without complications very small.

The above type of procedure is applicable to most vulvar carcinomas. In the rare instance where the anus is involved it may be necessary to perform an abdominoperineal resection of the rectum. It may be noted that it is quite practical to remove up to half of the urethra without the patient's becoming incontinent, and a large portion of the vagina also may be removed from below without difficulty.

A basal cell carcinoma of the vulva does not need extensive vulvectomy, and a wide local excision is sufficient.

Cancer of the Vagina. Primary cancer of the vagina is rare, comprising from 1 to 2 per cent of all cancers of the female genital tract. Metastatic cancer of the vagina may occur from cervix, endometrium, ovary or other organs. Primary cancer is almost always of the squamous cell type. It tends to grow in the long axis of the vagina, and because of its proximity to the rectum on the posterior wall and to the bladder on the anterior wall it may involve either of the organs at an early stage. It also spreads laterally to the paravaginal and paracervical tissues. Metastases may pass to both iliac and inguinal nodes.

CLINICAL FEATURES. Painless vaginal bleeding or discharge are usually the first symptoms, although pain and particularly dyspareunia are not uncommon. Usually it is found in the postmenopausal woman but it may occur at an earlier age. Examination reveals a hard nodule infiltrating the vaginal wall. Ulceration and a tendency to bleed easily on manipulation are common.

DIAGNOSIS. This is made on the basis of clinical examination and biopsy. All too frequently it may be delayed by lack of alertness on the part of both patient and physician.

TREATMENT. This is difficult because of the close proximity of bladder and rectum. The tumor is relatively radiosensitive, but the over-all lack of success of radiation is indicated by Murphy's figures of 24.2 per cent 5-year survivals in 124 patients. Recently, surgical treatment has been advocated. However, adequate surgery usually involves posterior, anterior or total exenteration and may include inguinal node dissection. These are formidable procedures and cannot be used in every case. It is too early to assess accurately the value of these attempts.

DISEASES OF THE CERVIX

INFECTIONS OF THE CERVIX

Acute Cervicitis. This condition is usually part of a generalized infection of the lower genital tract. Specific symptoms are not usually present. The diagnosis is made by inspection of the cervix, which appears red and inflamed; there is a profuse discharge. Treatment is primarily that of the specific infection involved and is described above. Instrumentation of the cervical canal and local applications to the cervix should be avoided for fear of spreading infection to the upper genital tract.

Chronic Cervicitis. This disease is found in at least one third of the adult female population. Frequently, it is associated with erosions, lacerations and cysts, and these 4 conditions have to be considered together. Infection itself may play a major part, such as in trichomoniasis or gonorrhea, or it may be secondary to the other disorders.

Erosions represent extension of the columnar epithelium of the endocervix outward on the external surface of the cervix. They may be congenital or acquired. The congenital type may be present in as many as one third of newborn girls. It commonly extends in a circular fashion around the external os and in the nonparous woman may not be accompanied by infection. Acquired erosions occur in association with lacerations, cysts and infections and commonly are irregular in appearance.

Lacerations result from childbirth and usually occur at 3 and 9 o'clock, giving the typical fish-mouth appearance to the parous cervix.

Cysts occur as the result of blockage of the mouth of the cervical glands by infection or trauma.

CLINICAL FEATURES. Chronic cervicitis may cause no symptoms and may be discovered only on routine pelvic examination. If symptoms are present they usually consist of mild to moderate vaginal discharge, and slight vaginal bleeding occurring following intercourse or douches. Usually pain is not noted unless inflammation involves the paracervical tissues.

Lacerations and cysts are easily visible on examination. Infection may produce a slight irregular reddening of the cervix. Erosions appear as granular and sometimes papillary red areas extending outward from the external os.

DIAGNOSIS. The most important consideration is to exclude cancer. This is frequently difficult. Available methods include cytology, colposcopy, punch biopsy and cold-knife conization. Cytology is a valuable screening technic. Material for study can be obtained by aspiration of the vaginal fornix or the cervical canal or by scraping the ectocervix with an Ayre spatula. Staining is by Papanicolaou's method or modifications thereof. Colposcopy has been used far more widely in Europe than in the United States, but interest in it is increasing in this country (Bolten). Colposcopy enables spot biopsies to be taken of suspicious areas on the cervix which cannot be seen by the naked eye. Punch biopsies can be taken from grossly suspicious lesions with little or no discomfort. Conization, with study of semiserial sections, is the most complete diagnostic tool available but requires hospitalization and anesthesia.

When all the above facilities are available, they can be used very effectively in the diagnosis of cervical conditions. When an obvious lesion is present, punch biopsy may give a definite answer. Where there is no obvious lesion, both cytology and colposcopy can be valuable and ideally should be part of the routine examination of every female patient. Spot areas can be biopsied and, in cases of continued doubt as to diagnosis, conization can be employed.

TREATMENT. Because of the likelihood, presumed though not proved, that chronic cervicitis predisposes to the development of cancer, treatment should be given to all cases where symptoms occur and to all women over 30 even if they are asymptomatic. Treatment of chronic cervicitis in the woman who is under 30 years of age and has no symptoms is usually but not always advisable.

Where nonspecific infection appears to be the main problem, restoration of the vaginal acidity by acid douches or intravaginal application of acid jelly is helpful. Sulfa creams used intravaginally are useful. Erosions may be treated in the office by radial cauterization with the electric cautery; following this the squamous epithelium usually will regenerate over the eroded area (Fig. 47-13). Cervical cysts can be punctured with a needle-point cautery. If the area of infection, erosion and laceration is very large, then more extensive cauterization may be performed as a hospital procedure. Finally, the whole area may be coned out with the electric wire and the external os reconstructed by means of a Sturmdorf or other type of inverting suture. This latter procedure should be reserved for older women, preferably those who do not plan further children, since the subsequent scarring may cause cervical dystocia.

Any procedure involving cauterization or conization should be followed by careful and regular examinations including postmenstrual sounding of the cervical canal to avoid the development of stenosis.

CERVICAL POLYPS

Cervical polyps are small pedunculated growths which arise from the endocervix or more rarely from the external surface of the cervix. They are often multiple. They are composed of a connective tissue stroma covered by columnar epithelium, which is thrown into many folds. Inflammatory changes are common, and frequently the tip is congested. They occasionally show malignant changes.

Clinical Features. There may be no symptoms, or the patient may notice slight vaginal bleeding or discharge. Examination of the cervix usually will show the lesion. Polyps are soft and sometimes may be missed on palpation.

Diagnosis. The important conditions to be distinguished from cervical polyps are endometrial polyps, pedunculated submucous myomata and cancer of the cervix.

Treatment. If irregular vaginal bleeding has occurred, particularly in the postmenopausal woman, a D. and C. should be performed to exclude intra-uterine causes. The polyp itself may be twisted off and the base cauterized to control bleeding. All polyps should be examined microscopically to rule out malignant changes.

CANCER OF THE CERVIX

Cancer of the cervix comprises more than 50 per cent of all cancers of the female genital tract (Fig. 47-14). Next to cancer of the breast it is the commonest malignant tumor in women. Thus the problem of early diagnosis and adequate treatment of this disease is of major importance.

Cause. The present-day ignorance of the exact mechanism which causes cells to become malignant applies to cancer of the cervix. Several contributory factors have been thought to be of importance. Hereditary patterns have been postulated but never proved. Early age of first coitus, early marriage and exposure to uncircumcised males may be of importance (Wynder, *et al.*). These findings are confirmed by the lower incidence of cancer of the cervix in Jewish women and in nuns. Recently there has been considerable interest in the possibility that changes in the cervical epithelium which commonly accompany chronic cervicitis may lead eventually to cancer. These changes have been given various names such as basal-cell hyperplasia, atypicalities or dyskeratosis. The possible significance of these is discussed by McKay *et al.*

Pathologic Features. 95 per cent of cervical cancers are of the squamous cell type. About 5 per cent are glandular (adenocarcinoma). The relative availability of the cervix for observation has made it possible to identify an intraepithelial and an invasive type. It seems likely that both are part of the same process, although it may be a matter of years in some instances before an intraepithelial lesion becomes frankly invasive.

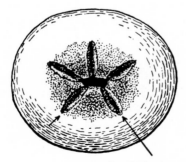

LINES OF CAUTERY

FIG. 47-13. Radial cauterization of the cervix.

The characteristics of an intraepithelial cancer are as follows: (1) lack of cellular differentiation; (2) lack of cellular polarity; (3) numerous and sometimes atypical mitotic figures throughout the whole epithelial layer; (4) pleomorphism of cells with variably enlarged hyperchromatic nuclei; (5) an intact basement membrane.

When invasive cancer is present the basement membrane is broken, and nests of tumor cells may be seen beneath it. They may have no definite arrangement, or they may show considerable differentiation with formation of epithelial pearls.

Spread. Cervical cancer spreads locally in the first instance through the cervix and into the paracervical tissues. Extension to the uterine cavity and to the vagina may occur early. Lymphatic spread occurs primarily to the hypogastric, obturator, common iliac and

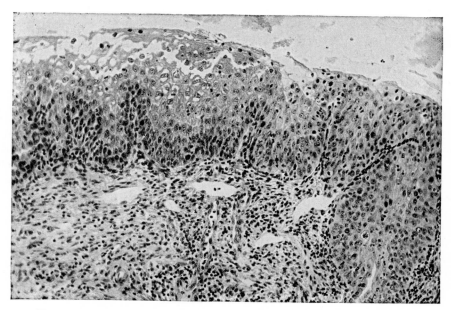

FIG. 47-14. Epithelium of the cervix, showing transition from normal stratified squamous type to intraepithelial carcinoma (A, *top*) and to invasive carcinoma (B, *bottom*). (*Continued on p. 1324*)

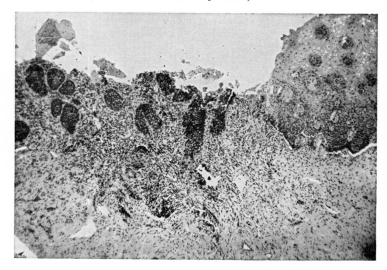

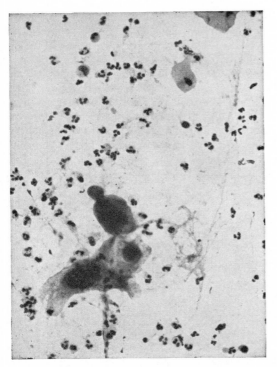

FIG. 47-14 (*Cont.*). Cervical smear showing malignant cells with large, irregular, dark-staining nuclei.

external iliac nodes. Distant metastases are found most commonly in the liver, the lungs, the bones and the intestinal tract.

Grading and Staging. Attempts to gauge the malignant potentiality of a particular tumor, based on the degree of cell differentiation seen in biopsy or excised specimens, have not been very satisfactory. The appearance of the normal vaginal cells before treatment in patients with cervical cancer has been used (Graham) as a criterion of the potentialities of the cancer. These attempts are promising but need confirmation.

Clinical staging of the disease has been of great value in prognosis and in comparing the results of treatment from different centers. The most commonly used classification is that of the Cancer Committee of the League of Nations which was first devised in 1937 and modified at the Fourth American Congress on Obstetrics and Gynecology in 1950 (International classification). This is as follows:

Stage O. Carcinoma in situ: also known as intramucosal carcinoma, preinvasive carci-noma, intraepithelial carcinoma, and similar conditions.

Stage I. The carcinoma is confined strictly to the cervix.

Stage II. The carcinoma extends beyond the cervix but has not reached the pelvic wall. The carcinoma involves the vagina but not the lower third.

Stage III. The carcinoma has reached the pelvic wall and involves the lower third of the vagina.

Stage IV. The carcinoma involves the bladder or the rectum or both or has extended beyond the limits previously described.

Other classifications have been proposed by various authors. A further modification of the International classification by Blaikley, *et al.*, may prove to be valuable.

It has been found that experienced clinicians usually will agree on the staging of a particular lesion. However, such staging depends only on examination and does not take into account the malignant potentialities of the tumor or its spread to lymph nodes, both of which greatly affect the outcome.

Clinical Features. About 75 per cent of patients with intra-epithelial and perhaps one third of those with Stage I carcinoma of the cervix have no symptoms. In fact, many far advanced lesions frequently give the unsuspicious patient little cause for concern. When symptoms occur they almost always consist of irregular bleeding which is intermenstrual in the woman of childbearing age and frequently follows coitus or other trauma such as douching. Discharge sometimes occurs. With involvement of the bladder or the rectum symptoms may be referable to these organs. If the disease extends to the pelvic wall, pain in the back or pain down the legs may be noted. It is to be noted that these symptoms are due occasionally to associated inflammatory changes in the paracervical tissues and not primarily to the cancer.

Diagnosis. The diagnosis of cervical cancer is made by the scrupulous use of all the diagnostic technics described above. A positive cytologic report (Fig. 47-14) must be confirmed by microscopic examination of a biopsy specimen. It is important to be sure whether one is dealing with an intra-epithelial or an invasive lesion. If the distinction cannot be made from a punch biopsy, then conization should be performed. Treatment should not be begun without a definite diagnosis.

The detection of early curable lesions is made more likely by regular 6-monthly or yearly pelvic examinations of women over 35 years of age. Constant awareness of the problem by both patient and physician is essential.

Treatment. INTRA-EPITHELIAL CANCER. Since it is assumed that preinvasive cancer eventually will become invasive, treatment is indicated. In the postmenopausal women or in the premenopausal woman who does not desire further children, a simple total hysterectomy with or without oophorectomy and with resection of a wide vaginal cuff is sufficient. In the woman who wants to have more children, a wide conization of the cervix, either by the knife or electrical wire, may be performed. However, such patients must be followed carefully by examinations and repeated cytologic studies of the cervix every 3 to 6 months, with further biopsies as indicated.

INVASIVE CANCER. At the present time 2 general methods of treatment are available—surgery or radiation. 50 years ago the only possible treatment was surgical, and operative technics were described by Reis, by Clark and by Wertheim, using the abdominal route. Schauta used the vaginal approach. These procedures were attended with great risk to the patient, and the results were poor, largely because of the lack of adequate supportive therapy such as antibiotics, prolonged anesthesia and blood transfusions. With the discovery of the radiosensitivity of cervical cancer and better methods of using radiation, the surgical approach fell into disuse in the United States. In the past decade interest in surgery has increased again, and large series of cases treated surgically have been reported (Liu and Meigs, Yagi, Brunschwig and Daniel). Along with this has been the recognition that radiation, while initially a safe procedure so far as the patient's life is concerned, does carry the danger of crippling complications when used in cancerocidal doses.

Adequate surgical treatment consists of a radical hysterectomy with wide excision of the parametrial and the paracervical tissues and the upper vagina with removal of the pelvic lymph nodes. Although this is a major surgical procedure, the operative mortality in good hands has been from 1 to 2.5 per cent.

The main complication to be feared is that of fistula formation. In particular, ureterovaginal fistula has been reported to occur following 2 to 9 per cent of operations.

Treatment by radiation involves the use of external radiation by means of x-rays, together with the application of radium to the cervix by means of a Manchester, Ernst or other applicator. Radium may be given in single or divided doses and may be either preceded or followed by external radiation. Whatever the technic used the amount of radiation delivered to the cervix and to the surrounding structures (rectum, bladder and ureters) should be calculated as accurately as possible in terms of roentgens. The use of fixed points in the pelvis to calculate and compare dosage has been of great advantage. Two commonly used points of reference are Point A, which lies 2 cm. above the external os and 2 cm. lateral to the center of the cervical canal, and Point B which lies 2 cm. above the external os and 5 cm. lateral to the center of the cervical canal. A suggested cancerocidal dose to point A is at least 8,000 r and to point B at least 4,000 r delivered over a period of 6 weeks. Variations in dosage may be necessary, depending on the individual lesions and on the dose delivered to neighboring organs. For patients with Stage II lesions which involve the parametria, surgery is probably contraindicated, since it may again be difficult to excise the tumor completely. The value of surgery in patients with early Stage II lesions (involving the upper vagina or the corpus uteri) is debatable.

Decision as to the best type of treatment for a particular case involves 3 considerations: (1) the stage of the patient's disease, (2) the general physical condition and age of the patient and (3) the type of treatment available in a particular center.

For patients with a Stage III or IV lesion surgical treatment would require excision of either bladder or rectum as well as the uterus and the cervix, in order to remove the lesion adequately. The high mortality of these procedures and the permanent stomata which result outweigh the possible slight improvement in survival. Even such an improvement is theoretical only.

When a patient has a Stage I lesion (and possibly an early Stage II), is relatively young and is in good general health, the choice of treatment may depend on which method is readily available. A good program of radiation will achieve better success than inadequate surgery and vice versa. Surgery may have some advantage for these patients, since the cervix can be removed with no chance of local recurrence, the lymph nodes which radiation does not easily affect can be excised, and the patient's treatment is completed at one time, rather than being continued over a 6-week period. The complications in both groups appear to be about the same, although more work on this is necessary.

Various combinations of radiation and surgical treatment have been reported. Where surgical treatment unexpectedly turns out to be inadequate, there would seem to be good reason for administering postoperative radiation. However, it is generally not advisable to give full radiation first and follow this by radical surgery. Radiation alters the tissues in the pelvis, so that dissection is made more difficult, and healing is impeded. The value of the application of less than full doses of radiation prior to surgery is questionable.

Adenocarcinoma responds to radiation in a way similar to squamous cell carcinoma, and the same considerations as to treatment apply to it.

The results of treatment of cancer of the cervix vary according to different authors. In general, provided that a patient receives adequate treatment, one may expect a 5-year survival rate of about 75 per cent for Stage I, 50 per cent for Stage II, 25 per cent for Stage III and 5 per cent or less for Stage IV lesions. In Stage I the results of radiation and radical surgery show little difference. Intra-epithelial cancer should be virtually 100 per cent curable.

Recurrent and Radioresistant Cancer of the Cervix

Close follow-up of patients is important both during and after treatment. When radiation is used, early detection of resistant lesions is important but by no means easy. Areas suspicious of recurrence should be biopsied.

Whether continued active growth of cancer is due to resistance or recurrence makes little difference. Where an adequate course of radiation has been given this type of treatment can offer little more, except perhaps in areas where

little therapy has been given (e.g., pelvic nodes), and even here palliation is all that can be hoped for. However, the development of more radical surgical procedures during the past decade has made it possible to offer selected patients among this previously doomed group a chance of survival. These procedures involve anterior exenteration (removal of uterus and bladder), posterior exenteration (removal of rectum and uterus), and complete pelvic exenteration. The immediate operative mortality is high (Brunschwig, 18%), and the patient is left with a considerable permanent disability owing to the artificial stomata. Therefore, such operations should not be performed unless actively growing cancer is present, the patient has received all possible treatment by other means, and finally unless there is a chance of cure. Furthermore, the patient must have the emotional stamina and the home circumstances to cope with the stomata involved. Under these conditions it would seem worthwhile to offer the patient what represents her only chance of survival.

THE UPPER GENITAL TRACT

INFECTIONS

Infections of the upper genital tract may affect the uterus (endometritis), tubes (salpingitis), ovaries (oophoritis), or the structures lying beside the uterus (parametritis). Frequently, all the pelvic organs are involved to a greater or less degree. The general term —pelvic inflammatory disease—is used commonly for this type of infection.

Infection usually reaches the upper genital tract from the vagina or the cervix. The following conditions may help to break down the normal barrier of the internal os of the cervix and cause the ascent of infection: (1) pregnancy and delivery, including abortion; (2) menstruation; (3) sexual intercourse; (4) instrumentation of the cervical canal. More rarely, infection may occur from the blood stream or may be spread from neighboring intra-abdominal organs.

Four common types of infection occur:

1. *Puerperal.* This usually is due to an anaerobic streptococcus and occurs following abortions or normal delivery. Spread occurs through the parametria, forming a pelvic cellulitis.

2. *Gonococcal.* This follows acute or chronic infection of the lower genital tract. Spread in this instance occurs along the surface of the uterus and along the tubes.

3. *Nonspecific.* This may be due to a variety of organisms of which the most important lie in the *E. coli* group.

4. *Tuberculous.* This is due to the *M. tuberculosis* and commonly involves the tubes first. It is usually chronic in nature and may be associated with tuberculosis elsewhere in the body.

Acute Pelvic Inflammatory Disease. CLINICAL FEATURES. A history of some exciting cause (see above) is frequently obtainable. The symptoms consist of:

1. *Abdominal pain.* This is usually in the lower abdomen and bilateral, although it may be unilateral or generalized. In gonorrhea it may be very severe.

2. *Vaginal discharge*

3. *Malaise and fever*

4. *Nausea, vomiting and abdominal distention* may occur if the infection has spread widely through the peritoneal cavity.

Examination of the abdomen may show lower abdominal tenderness, rigidity and rebound tenderness or possibly signs of peritonitis such as distention and diminished peristalsis. Pelvic examination confirms the presence of discharge. The uterus may be enlarged and soft if the patient has been pregnant. The cervix is acutely tender on motion. If adequate examination of the adnexal areas can be obtained, acute tenderness in the region of one or both tubes will be noted. In the puerperal type an area of tender brawny induration may be felt extending out from the uterus on one or both sides.

DIAGNOSIS. Culture of the cervix should be taken as soon as possible. This should include study of anaerobic organisms and Neisseria as well as the more common types. The common conditions to be considered in the differential diagnosis are:

1. *Appendicitis.* Pain is commonly localized in the right lower quadrant, the temperature is lower and intestinal symptoms are more prominent.

2. *Tubal pregnancy.* Fever is absent, and symptoms and signs of pregnancy are present. The pregnancy test may be positive. If the tubal pregnancy has ruptured, culdocentesis may be productive of nonclotting blood.

3. *Accident occurring in an ovarian cyst or uterine tumor.* Palpation of the mass may be possible.

4. *Renal tract disease,* such as pyelitis or stone. The symptoms and signs are usually unilateral, and the urine shows white or red blood cells.

TREATMENT. *Conservative.* Treatment is primarily conservative. Rest in bed is important, and adequate doses of antibiotics should be given. Penicillin is usually effective against gonococci. Broad-spectrum antibiotics are valuable in other types of infection. Supportive therapy in the form of intravenous fluids, gastric suction or blood transfusion may be indicated.

Operative treatment is not primarily indicated, and any sort of instrumentation of the uterus is to be avoided. On occasions it may be impossible to differentiate pelvic inflammation from an acute intra-abdominal condition such as appendicitis. In this case it is safer to explore the patient; but if salpingitis is found, nothing should be done. Evacuation of the uterus may be advisable in postabortal infections. In such instances it is wiser to wait until the temperature has been normal for 24 hours, unless excessive bleeding demands early intervention.

Chronic Pelvic Inflammatory Disease. This is a troublesome condition both to diagnose and to treat. It is important to avoid labeling a patient as having chronic gonorrheal pelvic inflammatory disease without sufficient proof of the cause.

PATHOLOGIC FEATURES. The following pathologic changes commonly occur in the course of the disease.

1. *Recurrent attacks of infection*—acute or subacute—in tubes, ovaries or parametria, with persistent chronic inflammation between the attacks.

2. *Development of adhesions* between the pelvic organs themselves, or between the pelvic and other intra-abdominal organs.

3. *Closure of the cornual and fimbriated ends of the tube* with formation of a serous (hydrosalpinx) or purulent (pyosalpinx) collection within the tube.

4. *Involvement of both tube and ovary in a tubo-ovarian abscess.*

5. *Rupture of a hydrosalpinx, pyosalpinx or tubo-ovarian abscess into the peritoneal cavity.*

CLINICAL FEATURES. A history of one or more attacks of acute inflammation is suggestive.

The patient with uncomplicated chronic pelvic inflammatory disease or with pelvic adhesions resulting from the disease may complain of:

1. *Chronic vaginal discharge*
2. *Pelvic pain and backache*
3. *Menstrual irregularities and secondary dysmenorrhea*
4. *Generalized weakness and tiredness*

Examination may disclose slight fever. Some lower abdominal tenderness is frequently present. Pelvic examination confirms the presence of a purulent vaginal discharge and lower genital tract infection. The cervix may be tender on motion. Thickness of the adnexal areas may be noted with a sense of adherence in the pelvis. The uterus may be fixed in retroflexion.

The presence of a hydrosalpinx, a pyosalpinx or a tubo-ovarian abscess may cause the patient to notice a tender mass in the lower abdomen, and this may be palpable on pelvic examination.

Closure of the tubes, from previous infection, may result in involuntary sterility.

Rupture of a pelvic abscess presents an acute picture of shock with low blood pressure and rapid weak pulse. The abdomen is rigid with generalized tenderness and diminished or absent peristalsis.

DIAGNOSIS. Uncomplicated chronic pelvic inflammatory disease and adhesions have to be distinguished from endometriosis, disease of the lower intestinal tract, and disease of the bladder.

Adnexal masses due to inflammatory disease may be confused with tubal pregnancy, ovarian tumors, tumors of the uterus and extragenital conditions such as tumors of the colon, diverticulitis and retroperitoneal tumors.

Rupture of a pelvic abscess may give symptoms similar to those produced by rupture of any other intra-abdominal organ, such as a tubal pregnancy, the appendix or a peptic ulcer.

TREATMENT. *Conservative.* The treatment of uncomplicated chronic pelvic inflammatory disease is primarily conservative. This is important, since many of these patients are young; and surgery, to be effective, usually involves sacrifice of childbearing function. The following measures are of value:

1. *Antibiotics.* These are of most value in acute inflammation but may be given a trial in chronic disease.

2. *Local heat* by means of hot vinegar douches, heating pads to the abdomen or short or microwave diathermy.

3. *Abstinence from intercourse or douching at the time of menstruation.*

4. *Adequate rest and emphasis on superior diet with supplemental administration of vitamins and iron.*

5. *Local treatment of disease of the lower genital tract.* It should be remembered that procedures on the cervix are likely to cause a flare-up of upper genital tract infection. They should be performed only when the disease is quiescent.

Surgical treatment is indicated in the following instances:

1. *Abscess presenting vaginally or rectally.* Drainage may be performed by opening the posterior cul-de-sac between the uterosacral ligaments, breaking up loculations with the finger and inserting a drainage tube.

2. *Rupture of a pelvic abscess.* Immediate laparotomy may be lifesaving (Lardaro). If the patient's condition permits, excision of the abscess is preferred: if not, drainage.

3. *Adnexal mass.* Any adnexal mass over 6 to 7 cms. in size requires operation and excision. It is never possible to be entirely sure on clinical examination that one is dealing with an abscess and not an ovarian tumor. If localized disease is found on one side in a young woman, local excision may be possible. However, more radical procedures are frequently necessary.

4. *Severe disability* due to recurrent disease or persistent inflammation which has not responded to conservative measures. Surgery should be resorted to only after careful deliberation since such procedures in order to be curative usually mean removal of both tubes and ovaries and the uterus.

5. *Sterility due to closed tubes* (see under sterility).

Tuberculosis. While the picture of pelvic inflammation produced by tuberculosis is frequently indistinguishable from that found with other types of infection, it does present certain particular features. For example, the infection is commonly a descending one from the tubes to the uterus and often is associated with tuberculosis elsewhere in the body. It may give no symptoms, or the patient's only complaint may be of sterility.

DIAGNOSIS is frequently impossible preoperatively. Where the diagnosis is suspected, cultures of menstrual blood or of curettings are valuable.

TREATMENT is primarily by the use of antibiotics, such as streptomycin, para-aminosalicylic acid and isoniazid, together with the commonly accepted measures for the treatment of the disease as a whole; i.e., rest and superior diet. Surgery may be indicated if the pelvic masses cause acute symptoms or if they do not respond to antibiotics. In any case the patient should be protected by antibiotics before and after operation.

TUMORS OF THE UPPER GENITAL TRACT

BENIGN TUMORS OF THE BODY OF THE UTERUS

Myoma. Myomata are the most common tumors of the female genital tract. They are present in fully 20 per cent of women over the age of 35. They are more common in nulliparous than in parous women, and in Negro than in white patients. Their etiology is unknown. Hormonal imbalance may play a part in their development, since they grow during the later years of a woman's reproductive life and decrease in size after the menopause.

PATHOLOGIC FEATURES. Various names have been applied to these tumors, such as myoma, fibromyoma, fibroid, leiomyoma. The last most accurately describes them, since they are composed of interlacing bundles of smooth muscle fibers with a varying admixture of fibrous tissue. They are frequently multiple and may grow to a very large size. They may be located underneath the peritoneal covering of the uterus (subserosal), within the uterine wall (intramural) or just beneath the endometrium (submucous) (Fig. 47-15). They may be found also in the cervix, and both the sub-

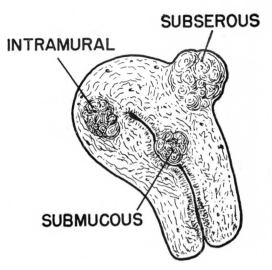

FIG. 47-15. Sites of myomata in uterus.

serosal and the submucous types may become pedunculated.

Secondary changes are common and consist of:

1. *Hyalinization.* This is very common but of little practical importance.

2. *Cyst formation.* This is common in large myomata and is due to lack of blood supply in the center.

3. *Calcification.* This is a common change in myomata of long duration.

4. *Necrosis* may occur in the center of the tumor or on the surface as in submucous myomata.

5. *Sarcomatous change* occurs in well under 1 per cent of all myomata.

CLINICAL FEATURES. Myomata may give no symptoms until they attain a large size. When symptoms occur they may be divided into the following groups.

1. *Menstrual Disturbances.* Menorrhagia, dysmenorrhea and intermenstrual bleeding may occur. The last is most common with submucous tumors.

2. *Pressure Symptoms.* These may consist of a vague sense of pressure in the lower abdomen or the back, or of bladder irritability or constipation.

3. *General Effects.* Tiredness, weakness and malaise are common.

4. *Acute Accidents.* Necrosis, or twisting of the pedicle of a pedunculated tumor may

cause acute lower abdominal pain, with fever and leukocytosis. Minor symptoms of this sort are common in myomata associated with pregnancy.

If the tumor is large, abdominal examination will reveal a hard, nodular mass arising from the pelvis. Pelvic examination will show the uterus to be enlarged irregularly and firm. Anemia is commonly present even in the absence of menorrhagia.

DIAGNOSIS. Myomata which project to the side of the uterus may be confused with adnexal masses. Acute accidents in myomata have to be distinguished from pelvic inflammatory disease, accidents in ovarian tumors, endometriosis, tubal pregnancy and other intra-abdominal disorders such as acute appendicitis or diverticulitis. The possibility of pregnancy or pregnancy associated with a myoma always must be kept in mind.

TREATMENT. Myomata can be cured only by surgical excision. No hormonal or medical treatment known at the present time will cause them to shrink or disappear. However, they are frequently small and asymptomatic: the chance of malignant change occurring is small, and spontaneous regression in size occurs after the menopause. For these reasons continued observation with examination every 6 months in the premenopausal years and every 12 months postmenopausally is advisable in the vast majority of patients with myomata. Surgery should be performed only on the following indications:

1. *Size.* Any tumor larger in size than a 3-month pregnancy generally should be removed. A sudden increase in size on repeated examinations is also an indication for operation.

2. *Pressure.* Evidence by x-rays of pressure on ureters or colon makes operation advisable.

3. *Symptoms.* It is important to be sure that the symptoms complained of really are due to myomata.

4. *Acute accidents,* such as twisting of the pedicle of a pedunculated myoma.

5. *Sterility or repeated abortions.*

The importance of doing a diagnostic curettage and cervical smear or biopsy to exclude cancer when unusual bleeding is reported cannot be overemphasized. If the curettings are suspicious of cancer, it is better to wait for a pathologic diagnosis before proceeding with definitive treatment.

Myomectomy. This procedure is of value where preservation of reproductive function is of importance. Even in the case of tumors that are of considerable size and are numerous, the persistent surgeon can restore the uterus to a remarkably normal appearance. Bleeding may be quite severe, although it can be controlled by temporary compression of the uterine arteries or by the intra-uterine injection of vasopressin. Complications in the form of adhesions are more likely than with a hysterectomy. However, the preservation of normal menstrual function and the possibility of retaining or increasing the patient's ability to have children are strong recommendations in favor of myomectomy.

Hysterectomy. This is the operation of choice in the woman who has finished having her family or where the tumor is too large or too adherent to the surrounding structures to make myomectomy practical. Both corpus and cervix should be removed (total hysterectomy) (Fig. 47-16). If the patient's condition is not good enough to permit of the extra dissection required to remove the cervix, the corpus alone may be excised (supracervical hysterectomy). When the cervix is not removed, regular postoperative examinations must be performed to watch for the possible development of cancer in the stump.

It is generally desirable to leave in both ovaries at the time of hysterectomy, provided that they appear to be normal.

Endometrial Polyps. These common growths are made up of endometrium which may undergo cyclical changes or more commonly of an unripe type of epithelium. They may occur in premenopausal and postmenopausal women and may be multiple. Sometimes they project down into the cervical canal on a pedicle. They may be associated with adenocarcinoma in another area of the uterine cavity.

The importance of endometrial polyps is that they may cause slight irregular bleeding which has to be distinguished from that due to cancer. Frequently, however, they may cause no symptoms.

Treatment is by division or avulsion of the pedicle and thorough curettage to remove the base. Sometimes polyps may be missed on routine curettage, unless the uterine cavity is explored with placental forceps in addition to the usual curette.

Malignant Tumors of the Body of the Uterus

Adenocarcinoma is by far the commonest tumor of the body of the uterus. It is the second most frequent type of cancer in the female genital tract. An interesting variant of this tumor is the adeno-acanthoma in which squamous metaplasia of the endometrial elements occurs.

Cause. The development of endometrial adenocarcinoma has long been linked to abnormal production of sex hormones and particularly of estrogens. The evidence for this connection is suggestive but not conclusive. From 10 to 27 per cent of functioning tumors of the ovary, such as granulosa cell tumors or thecomas, are reported to be associated with endometrial cancer. Again, many patients with this disease have late menopauses, indicative of prolonged estrogenic effect on the endometrium. Experimentally, hyperplasia and even adenocarcinoma have been produced in animals by the prolonged administration of estrogens. On the other hand, there is the interesting possibility, postulated by Sherman and Woolf, that abnormal hormones are produced by the hilar cells of the ovary in response to excess secretion of luteinizing hormone from the anterior pituitary. The relationship of endometrial cancer to endometrial hyperplasia is a debatable point, although there is some evidence that the two conditions are part of the same process. It seems likely that the so-called atypical hyperplasia, with excess proliferation of cells lining the glands and many mitoses, is a precancerous lesion, whereas the typical "Swiss-cheese hyperplasia" seen in premenopausal women does not predispose to cancer.

Pathologic Features. Characteristically, the microscopic picture is one of abnormal endometrial glands invading the stroma (see Fig. 47-17). These glands are of irregular shape and size and commonly appear back to back with the epithelium of one directly touching the epithelium of another. The cell nuclei are large, irregular in size and hyperchromatic. Rarely, an intra-epithelial type is seen in which the cells appear to be malignant, but no invasion is present. Attempts to gauge the degree of malignancy from the appearance of the cells may be of some value in endometrial cancer.

Adenocarcinoma of the body of the uterus spreads into the myometrium, down into the cervix and the vagina and into the parametrial tissues. Formerly, lymph node metastases were thought to be rare, but they may occur in as high as 23 per cent of cases (Liu and Meigs). Local metastases to tubes and ovaries are common, but distant metastases are rare. The average age of patients with endometrial cancer in most series is 57 to 60 years. Such patients are commonly obese, hypertensive and may be diabetic.

Clinical Features. Intermenstrual or irregular postmenopausal bleeding is the most

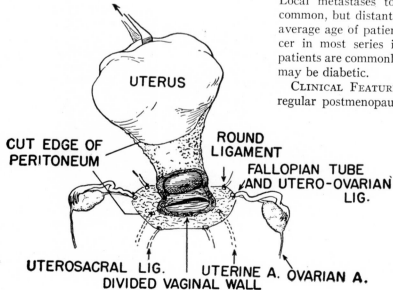

UTERUS

CUT EDGE OF PERITONEUM

ROUND LIGAMENT

FALLOPIAN TUBE AND UTERO-OVARIAN LIG.

UTEROSACRAL LIG. UTERINE A. OVARIAN A.
DIVIDED VAGINAL WALL

Fig. 47-16. Hysterectomy, showing upper vagina divided and uterus about to be removed.

common symptom. Abnormal discharge may also occur. Pain, general weakness and debility are late symptoms. Examination in the early stages may be entirely negative, or the uterus may be somewhat enlarged, soft and irregular in shape.

DIAGNOSIS. Since endometrial cancer may cause as much as 30 to 40 per cent of all postmenopausal bleeding, both gynecologist and patient must be alert to this symptom. Routine cytologic studies of material from the vagina or the cervix are not reliable, since positive smears are obtained in only about 60 per cent of patients with endometrial cancer. Endometrial biopsies, taken with a suction curette, may be useful if positive. Basically, the diagnosis rests on obtaining adequate material for study by means of a diagnostic curettage. This should be done even if there is another obvious cause for the bleeding, such as a cervical polyp.

TREATMENT. Definitive treatment should not be begun without first establishing a positive diagnosis. Sometimes gross inspection of curettings may be misleading, and frozen sections are not entirely reliable.

The most widely used method of treatment in this country is the intra-uterine application of radium (usually by the multiple source packing technic of Heiman) (Fig. 47-18), followed in 4 to 6 weeks by a total hysterectomy and bilateral salpingo-oophorectomy. From 80 to 90 per cent 5-year survivals have been reported in selected cases using this method.

Recently there has been some return to a primary surgical attack on this disease. This is due to greater operability rates and improvement in surgical and supportive technics. Furthermore, while endometrial cancer is sensitive to radiation, intra-uterine radium cannot reach a tumor which has extended far beyond the endometrial cavity, and this growth is necessarily allowed to continue unchecked until surgery is done.

At the present time it is not possible to evaluate fully the results of adequate surgical treatment. Such figures as are available indicate that the over-all survival rates of all patients treated are not greatly dissimilar from those treated by radiation and subsequent surgery (McKelvie).

Not infrequently, endometrial cancer is associated with a pyometra, or retention of pus within the uterine cavity. If such is found on preliminary curettage, a drain should be inserted through the cervical canal and the pa-

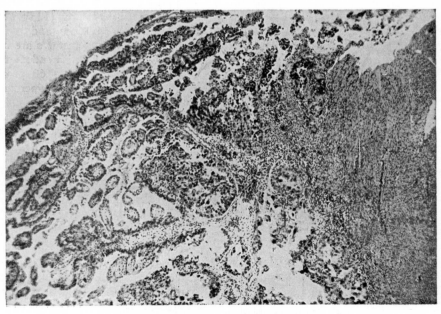

FIG. 47-17. Adenocarcinoma of the corpus uteri.

tient placed on antibiotics for several days before definitive treatment is begun.

Sarcoma of the Uterus. Sarcoma may arise in the muscle of the uterus itself or in a pre-existing myoma. The latter tends to be of a less malignant type. Sarcomata form less than 5 per cent of the total of cancers of the body of the uterus. Their incidence in myomata has been discussed above. A pedunculated submucous myoma appears to be particularly liable to develop sarcomatous change. The symptoms of sarcoma are similar to those of endometrial carcinoma in general, except that bleeding may not be so prominent. The treatment is primarily surgical by total hysterectomy and bilateral salpingo-oophorectomy, since these tumors do not respond well to radiation. Radical hysterectomy appears to offer no benefit. Chemotherapy may be helpful in palliation.

Tumors of the Fallopian Tube. Tumors of any sort in the fallopian tube are rare. The most important are the malignant ones—papillary carcinoma and sarcoma. Usually they are discovered accidentally during laparotomy. Surgical removal of the uterus and both tubes and ovaries is the best treatment.

Tumors of the Ovary

Classification. The ovary has the potentiality of developing many different kinds of cysts and tumors. The following is a classification of the more common ones.

1. NON-NEOPLASTIC CYSTS. These comprise follicle cysts and corpus luteum cysts. They are extremely common and usually of small size.

2. NEOPLASTIC CYSTS:

A. *Pseudomucinous Cysts.* These may grow to a very large size. They often are multilocular and contain a clear, viscid fluid. Microscopically, they are lined by a single layer of columnar epithelium, with basal nuclei. Goblet cells are common. (Fig. 47-19.)

B. *Serous Cysts.* These are slightly less common than the pseudomucinous cysts and usually are not so large. Microscopically, they are lined by flatter epithelium, which is frequently ciliated and bears a close resemblance to the epithelium of the tube. (Fig. 47-20.)

C. *Dermoid Cysts (Cystic Teratomata).* These tumors are derived from embryonal tissue and often show derivatives of all three germ layers. They comprise 11 per cent of all ovarian tumors and are bilateral in 12 per cent of cases. Grossly, dermoid cysts present a thick white capsule and characteristically contain a large amount of thick, yellow sebaceous material. Microscopically, they are lined by squamous epithelium; skin appendages, such as hairs, sebaceous glands and sweat glands, are usually present. Cartilage, ciliated epithelium lining small ducts and other embryonic remnants may be seen. Calcification is commonly present, and well-developed teeth may occur. This feature may enable the diagnosis to be made preoperatively by roentgenography. Malignant change, usually squamous cell carcinoma, is found in less than 1 per cent of dermoid cysts.

3. BENIGN SOLID TUMORS:

A. *Fibromata.* These are usually small asymptomatic tumors, although occasionally they may grow to a large size. Sometimes they are associated with ascites and hydro-

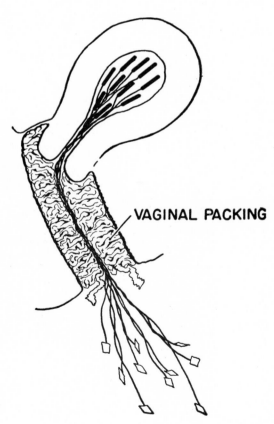

VAGINAL PACKING

Fig. 47-18. Intra-uterine application of radium.

thorax (Meigs's syndrome). The cause of this phenomenon is obscure, but the accumulation of fluid usually disappears on removal of the fibroma.

B. *Brenner Tumors.* These probably arise from the so-called Walthard cell rests which are found anywhere on the ovaries, the tubes or the surrounding ligaments. Microscopically, Brenner tumors are composed of fibrous tissue in which are situated nests of epithelial cells of a uniform type. Cyst formation is not uncommon.

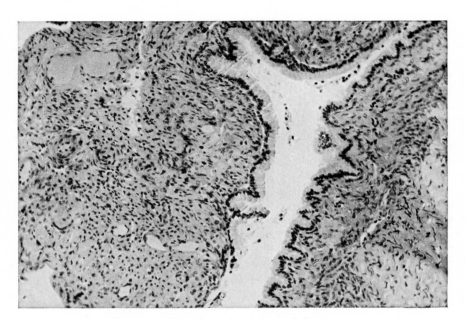

FIG. 47-19. Pseudomucinous cyst of the ovary.

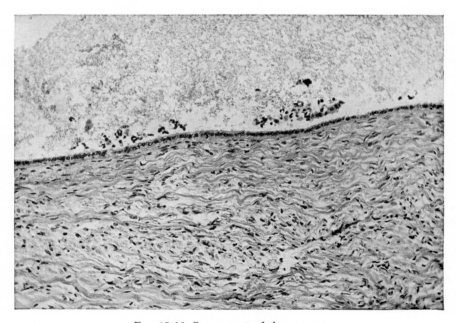

FIG. 47-20. Serous cyst of the ovary.

4. PRIMARY MALIGNANT TUMORS. These tumors of the ovary form the third largest group of malignant tumors in the female genital tract, comprising about 11 per cent of the total. They occur most commonly between the ages of 45 and 65, and more than 50 per cent are bilateral. Malignant tumors make up about 20 per cent of all ovarian tumors. Frequently, they are associated with benign lesions in the same or the other ovary.

Adenocarcinoma and papillary carcinoma are the most common pathologic types. Sarcoma forms from 2 to 5 per cent of the total and is most often of the spindle cell or round cell variety. Teratomata are not uncommon. Among these, various cell types may predominate. In this group the tumor in which thyroid tissue predominates (struma ovarii) is an example of the remarkable potentialities of ovarian tissue.

5. SEX-CELL TUMORS. These may or may not be malignant, and in any case are not common. They consist of:

A. *Functioning Tumors.* These may cause feminization—granulosa cell tumor, thecal cell tumor (thecoma), and lutein cell tumor (luteoma); or masculinization—arrhenoblastoma.

B. *Nonfunctioning Tumors.* Dysgerminoma is the main example of this group and appears to be composed of undifferentiated sex cells.

6. METASTATIC TUMORS. Metastases to the ovary can occur from tumors of the endometrium, the intestinal tract, the breast and elsewhere in the body. The most noteworthy type is the so-called Krukenberg tumor, which arises in the stomach or elsewhere in the intestinal tract. In this the ovarian metastases are frequently the most impressive part of the malignancy.

Clinical Features. Simple ovarian cysts and tumors frequently give only minor symptoms. The patient may notice a sensation of weight and pressure in the pelvis, some bladder irritability, constipation or menstrual disturbance. On examination a cystic mass may be palpable in the lower abdomen: this is confirmed on pelvic and rectal examination when a cystic mobile mass which is usually close to the lateral pelvic wall can be felt.

Diagnosis. The diagnosis of an uncomplicated cyst or tumor is often difficult to make from the history and depends on the finding of an adnexal mass on pelvic examination.

Occasionally, roentgen study of the abdomen is helpful, particularly in the case of dermoids.

Other conditions which may be confused with ovarian cysts and tumors are: myomata, especially subserous pedunculated myomata, hydrosalpinx, pyosalpinx, tubo-ovarian abscess, endometriosis and extragenital masses, such as tumors of the colon, pelvic kidney and retroperitoneal tumors.

Complications. The following complications of ovarian cysts and tumors occur frequently and are of importance because they change the clinical picture of a simple cyst and add further diagnostic problems.

1. *Size.* Ovarian cysts may grow to an enormous size and then may cause marked abdominal distention with intestinal symptoms and interference with respiration. Large cysts may be confused with a distended bladder, pregnancy, other intra-abdominal tumors and distention due to ascites.

2. *Torsion.* Many cysts and tumors are pedunculated, and the pedicle may become twisted with subsequent interference with the blood supply and necrosis and gangrene of the tumor. The patient may notice sudden or gradual onset of pain, and on examination tenderness over a cystic mass, fever and leukocytosis are commonly found. The clinical picture is very similar to that found in myomata with twisted pedicles, tubo-ovarian abscess or ectopic pregnancy.

3. *Hemorrhage* is common in cysts. Occasionally it may be so severe as to cause shock similar to that found with ruptured ectopic pregnancy.

4. *Rupture* may occur spontaneously or as a result of injury or examination. Signs of peritoneal irritation occur similar to those found with any ruptured viscus, although evidence of infection and hemorrhage is usually absent.

5. *Infection* occasionally occurs in ovarian cysts, especially dermoids, either from local ascending infection or from the blood stream.

6. *Malignant Change.* It is frequently impossible to determine whether a given ovarian cyst or tumor is malignant until after careful pathologic study. However, certain symptoms do suggest that one is dealing either with a primary malignant tumor or with a tumor that has undergone malignant change. The patient may notice sudden increase in the size of her

abdomen: she may have lost weight and give the appearance of generalized chronic disease. Examination may show ascites, a common concomitant of ovarian cancer, and on pelvic examination the ovarian mass may feel solid or may contain soft and firm areas. Bilateral masses may be present, and additional nodules may be felt in the cul-de-sac.

Treatment. At present surgery provides the only satisfactory treatment. Therefore, the problem resolves itself into when to operate. As a general rule ovarian cysts or tumors which are causing symptoms or are asymptomatic and have an estimated diameter of over 6 cm. should be removed. In a young woman of under 30 years of age observation of an asymptomatic cyst of this size for 3 months or so is justifiable, since it may disappear spontaneously. In the menopausal or postmenopausal woman the discovery of a cyst even smaller than 6 cm. in diameter, especially if it has not been noted on a previous examination, may be an indication for removal. Aspiration of ovarian cysts through the abdominal wall or the vagina is not advisable.

Frequently, it is extremely difficult to determine at the operating table whether a given ovarian cyst or tumor is benign or malignant. Evidence of ascites, peritoneal metastases, or papillary projections from the wall of the cyst are suggestive of malignancy. A frozen section may be helpful.

If the cyst is clearly benign and the patient is young, the cyst alone should be removed where possible. Sometimes the whole ovary and tube have to be removed.

Where the diagnosis is in doubt at operation, it is probably best in a younger woman to do the minimum procedure, whereas with an older woman the tumor should be treated as though it were malignant.

If the cyst or tumor is clearly malignant, a bilateral salpingo-oophorectomy and total hysterectomy should be performed. Because the lymphatic drainage of the ovary follows the ovarian vessels, pelvic node dissection is of no value. Removal of the greater omentum is indicated in some instances, since this is a common site of metastases. Care should be taken to avoid perforating a potentially malignant tumor during removal since this disseminates malignant cells through the peritoneal cavity. Even if the whole tumor mass cannot be removed, there is some advantage in excising as much as possible.

Some palliative treatment for cancer of the ovary may be hoped for by the use of x-rays postoperatively, since many tumors are radiosensitive. However, it is difficult to administer a cancerocidal dose over a large area of the abdominal cavity; therefore, the therapy is limited in usefulness. Recently, the intraperitoneal instillation of radioactive gold has been used as an adjunct to operation. Uniform distribution of the material is difficult to obtain, and its limit of penetration is only 2 to 3 mm. Its effect on any but the smallest metastases is questionable, but it does appear to retard the formation of ascitic fluid, where this is already present.

Recent advances in chemotherapy have suggested the use of these agents in ovarian carcinoma. Preliminary experience indicates the feasibility of using various drugs by the intraperitoneal, the intravenous and the oral routes. At present their effect appears to be palliative rather than curative, and further investigation is needed.

The prognosis of cancer of the ovary depends on the type of tumor, the evidence of spread beyond the ovary and upon the histologic grading of malignancy. Specific survival rates are difficult to assess because of the rarity of many ovarian tumors. In the relatively common serous cystadenocarcinoma the over-all figures indicate that from 20 to 40 per cent of patients survive more than 5 years. Long-continued observation is necessary in this disease, since late recurrences may occur.

MENSTRUAL DISORDERS

THE NORMAL MENSTRUAL CYCLE

Menstruation may be defined as the periodic discharge of bloody fluid from the uterus, occurring during the reproductive phase of a woman's life.

Menstruation normally begins between the ages of 10 and 16 and ends between the ages of 44 and 50. There is some evidence that menstruation begins earlier in the temperate climates and that women who start to menstruate earlier tend to end later in their lives.

The normal length of the menstrual cycle, as calculated from the first day of one menstruation to the first day of the next, is from 24 to 32 days, with an average of 28 days. Variations from 20 to 35 days are not uncommon and may not be abnormal.

The usual duration of the flow is from 2 to 7 days. The amount of flow varies greatly, averaging about 45 cc., of which one half to three quarters is blood. It is often difficult both for the woman and her physician to estimate accurately the actual amount of flow.

Individual variations in the cycle and in duration and amount of flow are common. These may change in the same woman at different periods of her life. They are related to certain psychological factors (Newton). Motherly women tend to menstruate more copiously and/or more frequently than less motherly women. Anxiety and elation can cause increased flow: depression may be accompanied by decreased flow. Sudden emotional shock, such as exposure to bombing or fear of pregnancy, can stop menstruation completely. Frequently, the menstrual cycle can be influenced by hypnosis, simple suggestion, administration of placebos or by superficial psychotherapy.

The events of the menstrual cycle are governed by a complex hormonal control. These can be integrated into a relatively simple schema (see Fig. 47-21). However, it must be remembered that the evidence for many of the details, such as the exact mechanism of ovulation and of the onset of bleeding, is not complete.

ABNORMAL BLEEDING

During the reproductive life any bleeding other than regular menstruation must be considered as abnormal. Occasional women do note a slight amount of vaginal bleeding at the time of ovulation: this may be due to the sudden drop of estrogens at this time and may

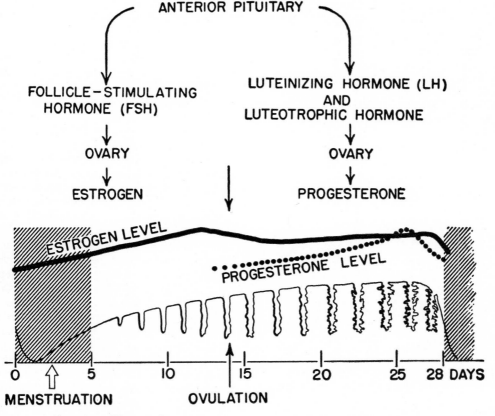

FIG. 47-21. Hormonal and endometrial changes during the menstrual cycle.

not be abnormal for that particular woman. In the prepubertal girl and in the postmenopausal woman any bleeding at all is abnormal.

Bleeding abnormalities may be divided into those which occur at the time of menstruation and those which occur between or without regular menstruation. Various symptomatic terms have been applied to the former, such as amenorrhea (absence of menstruation), oligomenorrhea (scanty menstruation), polymenorrhea (frequent menstruation), or hypermenorrhea or menorrhagia (excessive menstrual flow). The latter is known as intermenstrual bleeding, metrorrhagia (bleeding between menstruation), prepubertal bleeding or postmenopausal bleeding.

Causes. The causes of abnormal bleeding are as follows:

1. Specific causes
   A. Constitutional causes
      a. Blood dyscrasias
      b. Systemic diseases such as tuberculosis, nephritis
   B. Diseases of the vagina
      a. Trauma
      b. Foreign body
      c. Vaginitis
      d. Tumors
   C. Diseases of the cervix
      a. Infections and erosions
      b. Tumors
   D. Diseases of the uterus
      a. Infections
      b. Polyps
      c. Adenomyosis
      d. Myoma
      e. Carcinoma
   E. Diseases of the tubes and ovaries
      a. Infections
      b. Ovarian cysts
      c. Ovarian tumors
   F. Complications of pregnancy
      a. Ectopic pregnancy
      b. Abortions
      c. Hydatidiform mole and chorioepithelioma
2. General causes
   G. Endocrine causes
      a. Lack of ovulation
      b. Delayed ovulation
      c. Retention cysts of ovary
      d. Other endocrine gland disorders
   H. Emotional causes
      a. Anxiety states
      b. Emotional shock
      c. Deeper psychological disorders
   I. Nutritional causes

Diagnosis. It is of fundamental importance to discover the cause of the abnormal bleeding whenever possible before proceeding to treatment, and particularly before performing an exploratory operation which might lead to removal of any pelvic organs.

Frequently, a thorough history and physical examination as outlined on page 1306 may indicate whether or not the bleeding represents a variation of the normal menstrual pattern. It may also suggest or rule out many of the general causes of abnormal bleeding.

Additional diagnostic measures which are of value consist of:

1. *Examination under anesthesia* is helpful where the findings on pelvic examination are indeterminate because of the patient's age, resistance or obesity.

2. *Diagnostic curettage* is a relatively sim-

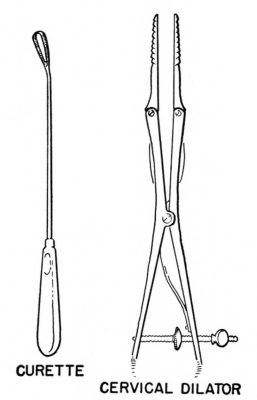

CURETTE

CERVICAL DILATOR

Fig. 47-22. Uterine curette and Goodell cervical dilator.

ple procedure, requiring dilatation of the cervix under anesthesia (Hegar or Goodell dilators) (Fig. 47-22), scraping the endometrial cavity thoroughly with a blunt or sharp curette, and careful pathologic examination of the tissue obtained. However, it does carry some risk due both to the anesthesia and also to the possibility of perforating the uterus (especially where pregnancy has occurred); it should not be considered too lightly. Curettage should generally be accompanied by appropriate studies of the cervix.

3. *More detailed psychological information,* particularly in regard to emotional shocks or problems which flared up around the time when the menstrual difficulty became manifest.

4. *Endometrial biopsy.* This office procedure can give valuable information on the state of the endometrium. However, it is not usually possible to obtain enough tissue to exclude intrauterine lesions.

5. *Additional tests of endocrine function* may include thyroid studies or assays of the excretion of gonadotrophins, estrogens or progesterone.

While all these studies are of value in certain cases, it is best not to delay curettage, especially in the woman who is over 35, since this is the best method available of excluding endometrial cancer.

Treatment should be directed to the specific cause of the irregularity if this can be determined. Attention to general nutrition and psychological problems may be of help. Diagnostic curettage itself is sometimes curative. Endocrine replacement therapy by estrogens and progesterone may be of value. Thyroid is commonly given on empirical grounds and may help.

PREMENSTRUAL TENSION

Many women suffer from this condition. In few is it severe enough to cause them to seek medical aid. The cause of it is not entirely established, but probably it is due in large part to retention of excess fluid just before menstruation. This causes a sensation of being bloated, nervous irritability and insomnia. Provided that a thorough gynecologic examination discloses no abnormalities, treatment is essentially symptomatic. It consists of attempts to remove excess water by laxatives and diuretics, dietary advice (especially vitamin B complex) and mild sedatives or tranquilizers.

DYSMENORRHEA

About 50 per cent of all women have some pain during menstruation, usually on the first day. In perhaps 15 per cent it is severe enough to cause them to go to bed. Clinically, it is convenient to divide the condition into primary dysmenorrhea, which has been present since the menarche, and secondary dysmenorrhea, which develops later in the reproductive life.

Cause. Secondary dysmenorrhea may be due to many factors, such as myomata, pelvic inflammatory disease and endometriosis among others. Primary dysmenorrhea probably is chiefly of psychological origin, although cervical stenosis and retroflexion of the uterus are sometimes responsible. Nutritional factors play a part, and the importance of hormones is shown by the fact that an anovulatory cycle usually is not accompanied by dysmenorrhea.

Diagnosis. Complete pelvic evaluation is important in every case. This should include postmenstrual sounding of the uterus to exclude cervical stenosis.

Treatment of any associated disease comes first. Cervical stenosis may be helped by dilatation of the cervix under anesthesia. A retroflexed uterus should be replaced in the anterior position and maintained with a pessary. In primary dysmenorrhea, where no organic cause can be demonstrated, simple explanation of the physiology of menstruation, psychological help and symptomatic treatment can be of great value. The last consists of advice regarding nutrition and hygiene, sedatives or tranquilizers, antispasmodics and analgesics. Frequently, patience and understanding are required to arrive at a satisfactory plan of treatment.

STERILITY

Various estimates suggest that involuntary sterility occurs in about 15 per cent of all marriages in the United States. Study of a particular problem involves a consideration of the possible factors concerned, and the application of a plan of investigation and treatment which includes both husband and wife.

CAUSES

The mechanism of fertilization in humans is still virtually unknown. Recent interest has centered around methods of transport of spermatozoa to the outer third of the tube where fertilization is presumed to take place (Hartman) and with the actual union of the spermatozoon and the ovum. Clinically, certain barriers to conception can be identified, some obvious and some more subtle.

Specific Genitourinary Tract Disorders. Any factor which may prevent the production or transport of the sperm or the ovum or prevent the meeting of the two for fertilization may be a cause of sterility. In the male this means defective spermatogenesis, obstruction of the vas deferens or urethra by trauma or infection, or inability to produce erection of the penis and entrance into the vaginal canal. In the female this involves deformities of the vagina which may prevent penetration, diseases of the cervix or the uterus, obstruction of the tubes or defective oogenesis.

General Factors. The general health of both partners is important. Debilitating disease in either husband or wife, even such mild infections as a cold, may be a barrier to pregnancy. Lack of superior nutrition may also be important.

Psychological Factors. Sterile women with no abnormality of the genital tract more frequently suffer from psychosexual disorders, such as failure to have orgasm, lack of sexual feeling or presence of pain during intercourse, as compared with fertile women (Wittkower and Wilson). In this study the sterile women frequently gave histories of ailing, timid, or unsociable childhoods, while as adults the vast majority of such sterile women showed unusual self-centeredness in their relationships with family and acquaintances. Possible psychophysiologic mechanisms are reviewed by Heiman. Impotence in the male and faulty technics of intercourse, each of which may prevent deposition of the semen near the cervix, frequently have psychological origins.

INVESTIGATION

History and Examination. This usually starts with the wife, since it is most often she who comes first to her physician for study. The usual gynecologic history should be taken, and special emphasis should be placed on her general condition, details of her marital and general relationship with her husband and possible psychological factors. This is followed by a general physical examination and a pelvic examination. The husband also should undergo a general physical examination with special attention being paid to the genitalia and to psychological factors. Additional study in both partners should include blood count, urinalysis, chest roentgenogram, serology, tests of thyroid function and nutritional evaluation. The last should include actual calculation of average daily intake of proteins and certain key vitamins and minerals, in comparison with the standards recommended by the National Research Council.

Examination of Sperm. This may be done by a semen analysis or by the Huhner (postcoital) test. Semen analysis is done best on a specimen produced by masturbation into an open-mouthed bottle. The Farris type of analysis is desirable. It includes estimation of volume (normal—2.5 to 5 cc.), motility (60-70% immediately and 25-40% after 6 to 8 hours at room temperature), cell count (more than 60 million per cc.), and morphology (80% or more of normal forms). Since masturbation is distasteful to some men on religious or other grounds, the Huhner test may be used as a substitute for this. It does not give a true picture of the sperm count. However, if the mucus taken from inside the cervical canal 4 hours after coitus contains 5 to 20 spermatozoa per high-power field with 50 per cent motility and few abnormal forms when examined microscopically, the husband is likely to be fertile. Additional information given by the postcoital test is that if active spermatozoa are seen there may be assumed to be no obvious hostility of the cervical mucus to the sperm.

Determination of Ovulation. Apart from the rather indefinite symptom of pain felt by some women at this time, ovulation can be detected only by indirect methods. These depend on the presence of a functioning corpus luteum and include: (1) absence of the "ferning" pattern when cervical mucous is spread on a slide, allowed to dry and examined microscopically; (2) decrease in the number of cornified cells seen in a cervical or vaginal smear; (3) a rise in the basal body temperature (see Fig. 47-23); and (4) the finding of secretory endometrium in an endometrial biopsy taken just before or preferably immediately after the onset of menstruation.

Tests of Tubal Patency. This may be determined by insufflation of CO_2 (Rubin test) or by hysterosalpingography. The Rubin test is performed as an office procedure, within a week after the end of menstruation. Any one of various apparatuses may be used, and the test is perfectly safe if used with care. If the Rubin test is equivocal or shows closed tubes, then hysterosalpingography should be performed. In addition to showing the site of any obstruction of the tubes, this test may also reveal any congenital abnormalities within the uterine cavity which might be acting as a barrier to fertility.

Special Endocrinologic Tests. These may be required at a later date to determine endocrine function in both partners.

TREATMENT

General Treatment. The high spontaneous cure rate in sterility has been emphasized by Bender. Of 700 sterile couples studied at Liverpool, England, from 1934 to 1949, pregnancy occurred in 46.3 per cent. In only half of these was it possible to ascribe conception to medical treatment, the remainder being due to time and chance. This emphasizes the fact that discussion of the problem and the progress

of investigation with both husband and wife is the first step in treatment. This should be combined with simple explanations about the mechanism of intercourse, conception and timing of intercourse, and detailed nutritional advice.

Specific Treatment for Husband. Oligospermia or azoospermia may be extremely difficult to treat, and the husband should be referred to a competent urologist. Even when the sperm count is very low the couple should not be discouraged. In Bender's series 33 per cent of wives whose husbands had a sperm count of under 10 million conceived.

Specific Treatment for Wife. Conditions which can be managed conservatively should be attended to first. These include infections of the lower genital tract, diseases of the cervix, and minor disorders of the upper genital tract. Major surgical procedures such as myomectomy and plastic reconstruction of the tubes should be adopted only as a last resort, if it seems that nothing else will help the couple. The best that can be expected with salpingoplasty is about 20 per cent success as measured by subsequent pregnancy. Tubal patency is obtained in a larger number of cases.

ENDOMETRIOSIS

Endometriosis is a disease produced by the growth of ectopic islands of endometrial glands and/or stroma. It may be divided into internal

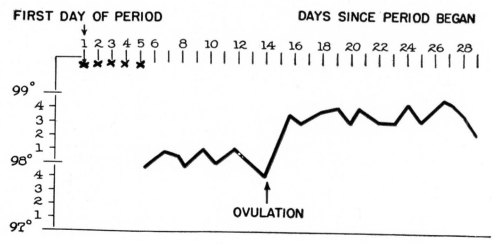

FIG. 47-23. Basal temperature chart showing postovulatory temperature rise.

and external types. In the former, which is commonly termed adenomyosis, the islands are found in the myometrium; in the latter they appear on ovaries, tubes, uterine ligaments, cervix, peritoneum and even as far away from the uterine cavity as umbilicus, appendix, intestine, vagina and vulva. Distant locations such as the skin of the arm and the thigh have been reported.

Endometriosis occurs during the reproductive life. It is seen most commonly between the ages of 30 and 50, among the higher socioeconomic groups and in white rather than Negro patients.

CAUSE

The exact cause of endometriosis has not been determined. Three main theories have been used to explain the ectopic location of the endometrial tissue: (1) transtubal regurgitation of menstrual blood and endometrial particles, (2) lymphatic dissemination and (3) metaplasia of embryonic celomic epithelium. There is little concrete evidence to support the third theory. The first, which was advanced originally by Sampson in 1921, has received recent support from the work of Scott *et al.*, and Allen *et al.* These investigators have produced experimental endometriosis in monkeys by causing the menstrual flow

to be directed into the peritoneal cavity. The idea of lymphatic dissemination has received some support from the finding of endometriosis in a considerable proportion of pelvic nodes removed during the course of radical pelvic surgery (Javert). Sampson's theory is the most attractive but does not explain all cases, and it may be that more than one mechanism is responsible. Hormonal and psychological factors have also been implicated, but it is uncertain how they act.

PATHOLOGIC FEATURES

The ectopic endometrial tissue undergoes cyclical changes, as does normal endometrium. Blood-filled (chocolate) cysts may form, or the tissue may rupture into the surrounding peritoneum or other tissues, resulting in acute symptoms or in the formation of adhesions, which may be particularly dense. (Fig. 47-24.)

CLINICAL FEATURES

Internal endometriosis usually produces secondary and increasing dysmenorrhea with menstrual irregularities. On examination the uterus may be found to be symmetrically enlarged, firm and especially tender during the premenstrual and menstrual phases of the cycle.

External endometriosis is commonly asso-

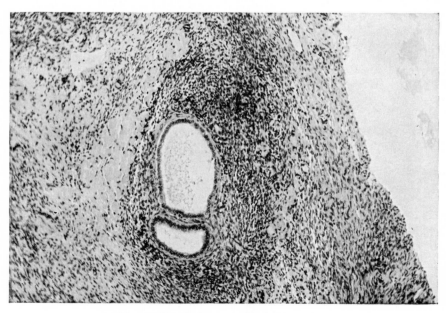

FIG. 47-24. Endometriosis of the ovary.

ciated with internal endometriosis but may exist by itself. In addition to the symptoms of internal endometriosis the patient may complain of persistent backache, especially premenstrually but also throughout the cycle. Dyspareunia is common. Sterility may result from blockage of the tubes and from pelvic adhesions. Examination will commonly show the uterus to be retroflexed and fixed. Nodules may be palpable on the uterosacral ligaments or elsewhere in the pelvis. The ovaries may be enlarged and tender. Involvement of the intestine may rarely give rise to symptoms and signs of intestinal obstruction. Thus endometriosis should be considered in the differential diagnosis of colonic and particularly rectal carcinoma in women.

DIAGNOSIS

Examination at different times of the menstrual cycle is important, since marked enlargement of the endometrial nodules usually occurs premenstrually. Chronic pelvic inflammatory disease with pelvic adhesions is the most common source of confusion in diagnosis. Ovarian cysts due to endometriosis have to be distinguished from other ovarian cysts and tumors; the latter are frequently not tender.

TREATMENT

It must be remembered that endometriosis is practically always a disease of the childbearing age. Many patients are anxious to have children; therefore, whenever possible, attempts should be made to preserve this function. Treatment may be divided into: (1) no treatment, (2) endocrine and symptomatic treatment, (3) conservative operation and (4) radical operation.

In some cases endometriosis may be discovered on routine examination and may be symptomless. No treatment is advisable in such instances, but repeated regular examinations are essential.

Where symptoms are mild, and no cysts large enough to necessitate laparotomy are found, conservative treatment should be tried. Symptomatic relief of dysmenorrhea may be offered by any one of a number of measures, such as analgesics, mild sedation, diuretics, attention to diet, and local application of heat to the abdomen. Both male and female hormones have been used with success. In part

the action of both appears to be by the suppression of ovulation, although particularly with androgens smaller doses than would be required normally for this may cause symptomatic relief. Recently, the newer progesteronelike compounds have been used with some success.

If conservative therapy does not help, or if the patient has an ovarian mass of significant size, laparotomy should be performed. In a young woman who is anxious to have children, only as little tissue as is necessary should be removed. This frequently consists of removing the cyst, or one tube and ovary, and cauterizing or excising any endometrial implants which may be found. Adhesions are freed, and suspension of a retrodisplaced uterus is advisable. Division of the pelvic nerves at the brim of the pelvis can also be performed to relieve menstrual distress and backache.

Radical operation consists of bilateral salpingo-oophorectomy and total hysterectomy. It should be reserved for older women who have had a conservative surgical procedure done or have no desire for more children, or rarely for those younger women in whom it is impossible to save any pelvic organ because of extensive involvement and adhesions.

ECTOPIC PREGNANCY

This is a most important condition, since it is potentially a major threat to the patient's life and because it can be confused with many other gynecologic disorders.

Ectopic pregnancy occurs in about 1 in 200 pregnancies. It is located most commonly in the tube but may occur on the ovary, the cervix, the uterine ligaments or in the abdominal cavity. (Fig. 47-25.)

CAUSE

Conditions which cause partial blockage of the tube may predispose to tubal pregnancy. Such are pelvic inflammatory disease, adhesions or tumors arising within or outside the tubal lumen. Patients with sterility problems due to tubal factors are more likely to have tubal pregnancies (1.7%, Bender).

PATHOLOGIC FEATURES

Tubal pregnancies may be located in the lateral part of the tube (ampullar), middle

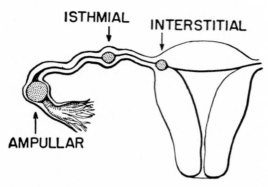

FIG. 47-25. Sites of tubal pregnancies.

(isthmial) or medial part (interstitial). Very few ectopic pregnancies reach full development, although these have been reported. They may either rupture or undergo spontaneous degeneration. Rupture may occur into the peritoneal cavity or into the uterus. Occasionally, rupture and secondary implantation on another abdominal organ may occur. Rupture occurs later with the ampullar type and is usually earlier and attended with greater hemorrhage in the interstitial type.

CLINICAL FEATURES

In a typical case the patient presents the symptoms of early pregnancy; e.g., amenorrhea, breast fullness, frequency of urination, constipation, nausea. She may also notice some slight vaginal bleeding and lower abdominal pain which is persistent and unilateral. On examination the cervix may be blue and the uterus soft and enlarged, although perhaps not to the degree expected from the length of amenorrhea. An acutely tender adnexal mass is noted.

Rupture into the uterus gives moderate to marked vaginal bleeding and intermittent lower abdominal and back pain. The picture is similar to that of abortion of an intra-uterine pregnancy.

Rupture into the peritoneal cavity causes sudden lower abdominal pain which soon becomes generalized and may spread to the shoulder. Examination may show evidence of shock with a low blood pressure and a weak and rapid pulse. The abdomen may be tender and present generalized rebound tenderness and rigidity with diminished or absent peristalsis. Pelvic examination is often difficult be-

cause of the abdominal tenderness, but an adnexal mass may be felt, and a semisolid hematoma may be palpable in the cul-de-sac.

Spontaneous degeneration may cause little except a regression of the previous symptoms and signs.

DIAGNOSIS

The typical picture of either unruptured or ruptured ectopic pregnancy is relatively clear-cut. Unfortunately, not all cases are typical. In an unruptured ectopic pregnancy, a pregnancy test may be of help, and culdoscopy, in the hands of those experienced in its use, may be of considerable value. Conditions to be considered in the differential diagnosis include:
1. Intra-uterine pregnancy with a large corpus luteum
2. Abortion
3. Pelvic inflammation with a hydrosalpinx or pyosalpinx or tubo-ovarian abscess
4. Myoma
5. Ovarian cyst or tumor
For the characteristic symptoms and signs of these conditions the reader is referred to the specific sections above.

In a ruptured ectopic pregnancy, culdocentesis is a valuable diagnostic procedure. The posterior cul-de-sac is punctured with a 15 to 18 gauge needle attached to a syringe. Aspiration of nonclotting blood indicates intraperitoneal hemorrhage and, when associated with appropriate symptoms and signs, is strongly suggestive of ruptured ectopic pregnancy. Other intra-abdominal emergencies may be confused with ruptured ectopic pregnancy. These include ruptured ovarian cyst or pelvic abscess, ruptured appendix or perforated ulcer.

TREATMENT

Since the danger of rupture is ever present, there is no place for expectant treatment. Once the diagnosis of ectopic pregnancy has been established the patient should be operated upon promptly. If shock is present, blood transfusion should be started as soon as possible, but it is not wise to wait until shock has been controlled completely before starting the operation because that time may never come, and control of the hemorrhage is vital. It is of the utmost importance to have suitable blood available for transfusion and preferably running by the time the operation is begun.

The simplest operative procedure necessary to control the bleeding and remove the pregnancy should be done. This usually involves removal of the tube, with, if possible, preservation of the ovary. A wedge of the uterine horn should be removed to prevent the chance of a subsequent pregnancy developing in the remnant of the tube. The area should be re-peritonealized as well as possible, and excess blood removed from the peritoneal cavity.

In the rare instance where an advanced abdominal pregnancy has occurred, it may be well to wait until the infant is viable before performing laparotomy, since living children have been obtained by this. At such operations the placenta is frequently found to be adherent to many organs. It should be left in situ, since castrophic bleeding may occur during attempts at removal, and if left in place, eventually it will be absorbed.

Ruptured ectopic pregnancy used to be a very serious occurrence. Now, with the aid of adequate transfusions the mortality has been decreased to 2 per cent or less. Subsequent pregnancy is quite possible by means of the other tube.

BIBLIOGRAPHY

Allen, E., Peterson, L. F., and Campbell, Z. B.: Clinical and experimental endometriosis, Am. J. Obst. & Gynec. *68*:56, 1954.

Bender, S.: End results in primary sterility, Brit. M. J. *2*:409, 1952.

Blaikley, J. B., Kottmeier, H. L., Martius, H., and Meigs, J. V.: Classification and clinical staging of carcinoma of the uterus, Am. J. Obst. & Gynec. *75*:1286, 1958.

Bolten, K. A.: Introduction to Colposcopy, New York, Grune & Stratton, 1960.

Brunschwig, A., and Daniel, W.: Total and anterior pelvic excenteration, Surg., Gynec. & Obst. *99*:324, 1954.

———: The surgical treatment of cancer of the cervix uteri, Am. J. Obst. & Gynec. *75*:875, 1958.

Bushnell, L. F.: Physiologic prevention of postpartal relaxation of genital muscles, West. J. Surg. *58*:66, 1950.

Donald, I.: Etiology and investigation of vaginal discharge, Brit. M. J. *2*:1223, 1952.

Falk, H. C., and Bunkin, I. A.: The management of vesicovaginal fistula following abdominal total hysterectomy, Surg., Gynec. & Obst. *93*:404, 1951.

Farris, E. J.: Human Fertility and Problems of the Male, White Plains, N. Y., Author's Press, 1950.

Graham, R. M.: The prognosis of cancer of the cervix by vaginal smear, Surg., Gynec. & Obst. *93*:767, 1951.

Green, T. H., Jr., Ulfelder, H., and Meigs, J. V.: Epidermoid carcinoma of the vulva: an analysis of 238 cases, Am. J. Obst. & Gynec. *75*:834, 1958.

Greenhill, J. P.: Office Gynecology, ed. 7, Chicago, Year Book Pub., 1959.

Hartman, C. G.: How do sperms get into the uterus?, Fertil. & Steril. *8*:403, 1957.

Heiman, M.: Reproduction: emotions and the hypothalamic-pituitary function, Fertil. & Steril. *10*:162, 1959.

Jacobson, P.: Marsupialization of vulvovaginal (Bartholin) cysts, Am. J. Obst. & Gynec. *79*:73, 1960.

Jarcho, J.: Malformations of the uterus, Am. J. Surg. *71*:106, 1946.

Javert, C. T.: The spread of benign and malignant endometrium in the lymphatic system with a note on coexisting vascular involvement, Am. J. Obst. & Gynec. *64*:780, 1952.

Javert, C. T., and Douglas, R. G.: Treatment of endometrial adenocarcinoma, Am. J. Roentgenol. *75*:508, 1956.

Jones, W. S.: Obstetric significance of female genital anomalies, Obst. & Gynec. *10*:113, 1957.

Kegel, A. H.: Physiologic therapy for urinary stress incontinence, J.A.M.A. *146*:915, 1951.

Lardaro, H. H.: Spontaneous rupture of tubo-ovarial abscess into the free peritoneal cavity, J.A.M.A. *156*:699, 1954.

Liu, W., and Meigs, J. V.: Radical hysterectomy and pelvic lymphadenectomy, Am. J. Obst. & Gynec. *69*:1, 1955.

McCall, M. L.: Posterior culdeplasty, Obst. & Gynec. *10*:595, 1957.

McKay, D. G., Terjanian, B., Poschyachinda, D., Younge, P. A., and Hertig, A. T.: Clinical and pathologic significance of anaplasia (atypical hyperplasia) of the cervix uteri, Obst. & Gynec. *13*:2, 1959.

Mering, J. H.: A surgical approach to intractable pruritus vulvae, Am. J. Obst. & Gynec. *64*:619, 1952.

Murphy, W. T.: Primary vaginal cancer: irradiation management and end results, Radiology *68*:157, 1957.

Nemir, A., and Middleton, R. P.: Stress incontinence in young nulliparous women, Am. J. Obst. & Gynec. *68*:1166, 1954.

Newton, M.: Maternal Emotions, New York, Hoeber, 1955.

Reich, W. J., and Nechtow, M. J.: A ten year study of treatment and its results in intractable pruritus vulvae, Am. J. Obst. & Gynec. *69*:94, 1955.

Schauffler, G. C.: Pediatric Gynecology, ed. 4, Chicago, Year Book Pub., 1958.

Scott, R. B., Te Linde, R. W., and Wharton, L. R.: Further studies on experimental endometriosis, Am. J. Obst. & Gynec. *66*:1082, 1953.

Sherman, A. I., and Woolf, R. B.: An endocrine basis for endometrial carcinoma, Am. J. Obst. & Gynec. *77*:233, 1959.

Strassman, E. O.: Plastic unification of double uterus, Am. J. Obst. & Gynec. *64*:25, 1952.

Way, S.: Carcinoma of the vulva, Am. J. Obst. & Gynec. *79*:692, 1960.

Wittkower, E., and Wilson, A. T. M.: Dysmenorrhea and sterility. Personality studies, Brit. M. J. *2*:586, 1940.

Wynder, E. L., Cornfield, J., Schroff, P. D., and Doraiswami, K. R.: A study of environmental factors in carcinoma of the cervix, Am. J. Obst. & Gynec. *68*:1016, 1954.

Yagi, H.: Extended abdominal hysterectomy with pelvic lymphadenectomy for carcinoma of the cervix, Am. J. Obst. & Gynec. *69*:33, 1955.

J. LAPIDES, M.D.

Urology

INTRODUCTION

Urology is that branch of surgery which concerns itself with the male and the female urinary tracts and the male genital organs. Therefore, the urologist deals with the following: kidney, ureter, bladder, urethra, penis, scrotum, epididymis, testis, spermatic cord, seminal vesicle and prostate, and occasionally with abnormalities of the adrenal gland.

DIAGNOSIS

Endoscopy. Urologic diagnosis is precise because methods are available for viewing the entire urinary tract directly or indirectly. The urethra, the lumen of the bladder and ureteral orifices may be viewed through instruments embodying illumination and lens systems. Through such an instrument, the cystoscope, tissue may be taken for biopsy, catheters may be passed into the ureters, and ureteral or vesicular calculi may be removed. The cystoscope cannot be used for viewing the urethra because its lens system affords only right-angle vision. However, the use of the panendoscope, which provides for seeing things ahead and to the side of it (for oblique vision) permits visualization of the urethra.

Roentgenography[2, 3, 5] is requisite to determine the condition of the ureters and the kidneys. A radiopaque material (various iodine compounds such as Urokon, Diodrast, sodium iodide and Neoiopax) is used to fill the hollow portion of the urinary tract, and then roentgenograms are taken. The ureters, the renal pelves and the calyces can be filled by injecting opaque material through ureteral catheters which have been passed up the ureters into the renal pelves. This type of urography has been designated as retrograde pyelography (Fig. 48-1). Another form, intravenous pyelography, involves the intravenous administration of radiopaque material which is cleared from the blood stream by renal excretion. If renal function is 25 per cent or more of normal, the kidneys will excrete enough radiopaque medium (e.g., Diodrast) per unit of time to outline the upper urinary tract (Fig. 48-2). This not only serves to visualize the urinary tract but also gives a gross estimation of renal function. However, extremely high concentrations of radiopaque material, such as 90 per cent Hypaque, may outline the urinary tract when renal function is less than 25 per cent of normal.

Aortography now is being used rather extensively as an aid in the diagnosis of renal hypertension[4] (Fig. 48-3). Presacral or perirenal gas insufflation (Fig. 48-4) is employed in detecting adrenal and renal neoplasms. Unlike perirenal air insufflation, which occasionally causes air embolus, carbon dioxide is safe.[1] Acute renal failure, transverse myelitis, infarction of the bowel and aortic dissection may follow aortography in rare instances.[6] Persistent renal functional impairment also may follow aortography.

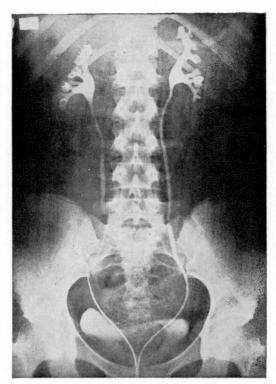

FIG. 48-1. Retrograde pyelogram, demonstrating calyces, infundibula, pelves and ureters of both kidneys. Observe the ureteral catheters through which radiopaque sodium iodide has been injected.

None of the special methods for investigation of the urinary tract is used until a medical history, a physical examination and urinalysis have been completed and evaluated.

SIGNS AND SYMPTOMS

Changes in Micturition. When eliciting symptoms and signs referable to the genitourinary tract, special attention is paid to the act of micturition, the gross characteristics of the urine, masses in the flank, the abdomen and the scrotum and pain. Normal urination is a painless function which occurs 3 to 4 times daily and occasionally once at night. The normal individual can inhibit micturition until a suitable time and place are available. On volition, a forceful urinary stream is initiable within 1 to 2 seconds; normally, the stream is continuous and uninterrupted until the bladder is emptied.

Increased frequency of urination, urgency (inability to hold urine after the sensation of bladder filling is initiated) and dysuria (painful or difficult urination) are to be observed in such conditions as inflammatory cystitis, vesical calculi, renal tuberculosis, prostatism, urethral stricture, etc. Hesitancy in starting urination, a decrease in size and force of the urinary stream, abdominal straining and an interrupted stream should lead the physician to suspect an obstruction of the urethral channel by scar tissue contraction at the vesical neck, an enlarged prostate or a stricture of the urethra, although such symptoms may be psychic in origin. Urinary incontinence is abnormal except in infancy and early childhood.[7] Incontinence associated with urgency and frequency, occurring at intervals during the day and especially at night, may be a manifestation of disease involving the central nervous system, e.g., multiple sclerosis, cerebrovascular accidents, or spinal cord tumor. In the female the involuntary loss of urine when coughing, straining or sneezing is suggestive of stretching or tearing of the ligaments holding the bladder neck in place; this condition is called stress incontinence. The continuous involuntary dribbling of urine may be associated with urinary retention of the overflow type, sometimes called paradoxical incontinence because although the patient is continually losing urine, he still has a bladder distended with urine. The continuous leaking of urine also may be associated with an empty bladder in persons who have suffered injury to the sphincter mechanisms following prostatectomy or trauma.

Hematuria is a danger signal and indicates the likely presence of cancer of the genitourinary tract. Hematuria may be associated also with renal tuberculosis, urinary tract calculi, prostatism, acute cystitis and trauma. Far too many patients with cancer of the urinary tract are seen belatedly by the urologist because the importance of hematuria is not recognized by the physician who first sees the individual. Only one episode of gross hematuria is sufficient to demand a complete investigation of the urinary tract; and this must include an endoscopic examination of the entire urethra and the bladder, as well as a roentgenographic examination of the ureters and the kidneys. From 2 to 3 red blood cells observed in the urine of a patient on more

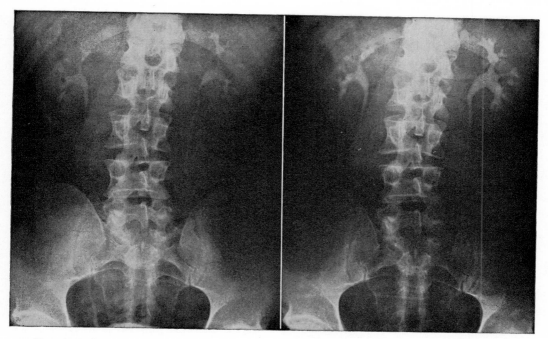

FIG. 48-2. Intravenous or excretory pyelograms made by administering radiopaque material intravenously and then obtaining roentgenograms of the kidneys, the ureters and the bladder after the material has been excreted by the nephrons into the collecting system.

than one occasion is as much of a danger signal as gross hematuria.

Pneumaturia, or air in the urine is associated with entero-urinary tract fistulae and very rarely with infections caused by *B. aerogenes, Esch. coli* and certain yeasts, the latter especially in diabetes. Fecaluria associated with pneumaturia is pathognomonic of a connection between the intestinal and the urinary systems.

Pain. Diseases of the kidney may cause characteristic pain or they may give rise solely to a discomfort or pain suggestive of disease in some other organ. Typical renal colic originates in the flank and may radiate anteriorly to the epigastrium; it is an intermittent, sharp, excruciating type of pain often associated with nausea, vomiting and hypotension. Non-obstructive calculous disease of the kidney may produce a dull boring discomfort in the epigastrium which is interpreted frequently as evidence of a peptic ulcer or cholecystic disease. Ureteral colic can be characterized as an intermittent, sharp pain radiating along the course of the ureter into the scrotum or the labium majus. This type of pain may be produced by the passage of a calculus down the ureter. On the right side it is mistaken occasionally for acute appendicitis.

The pain associated with disease of the bladder may be a vague and generalized suprapubic discomfort as in complete urinary retention and subacute cystitis, or it can be a sharp, localized suprapubic one as in interstitial cystitis. Irritation at the bladder neck is often associated with a pain at the urethral meatus.

Inflammatory swelling of the epididymis or the testis will cause severe nonradiating pain in the scrotal region. Infections involving the vas deferens may produce discomfort in the upper scrotum and along the inguinal canal.

Acute prostatitis and prostatic abscess may be associated with pain in the rectum and the perineal region.

PHYSICAL EXAMINATION

Palpation. Obviously, every patient should have a complete physical investigation. However, in this discussion the examination will be limited to the genito-urinary tract. In examining a patient for urinary tract disease one first palpates the abdomen and the flank areas. The kidneys may or may not be pal-

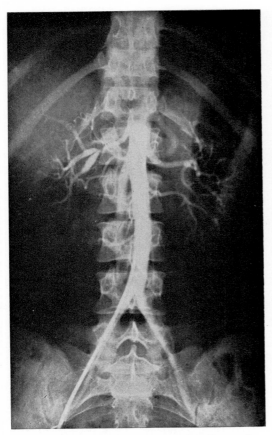

FIG. 48-3. Arteriogram depicting the renal arteries and their branches in addition to the aorta, the splenic, the hepatic, the mesenteric and the iliac vessels. Observe the stenosis of the right renal artery and the poststenotic dilatation of its two main branches.

pable, depending upon the patient's body build. The slender asthenic type of person will often have readily palpable, highly mobile normal kidneys. In examining the kidney one hand should be placed with the fingers in the costovertebral angle area and pressure applied there in order to ascertain tenderness. Renal disease may produce tenderness in this region. Should tenderness be elicited in this area, it frequently signifies renal disease. Pain produced by pressure to areas adjacent to the costovertebral angle area, e.g., sacrospinalis muscle, 12th rib, etc., does not signify renal disease.

With one hand in the costovertebral angle region and the other hand in the lower anterior abdominal quadrant, the examiner palpates for any unusual masses. The hand on the abdomen should be moved gradually up toward the lower costal margins in order to avoid missing the lower border of a large mass. The normal kidney moves with respiration and may be palpable during inspiration. Retroperitoneal structures such as the kidney may be differentiated from masses in the peritoneal cavity by the use of ballottement, i.e., pushing on the kidney with one hand in the costovertebral angle region will cause the kidney to be felt by the other hand pressing against the abdomen. A mass in the peritoneal cavity, e.g., liver, spleen, bowel neoplasm, usually cannot be balloted with one hand in the costovertebral angle region and the other on the abdomen.

Percussion and palpation are most useful procedures for ascertaining the presence of a distended bladder and other suprapubic masses. In examining the penis the foreskin is retracted first, and the urethral meatus, the glans and the coronal sulcus are inspected closely for the presence of abnormalities. Then the shaft of the penis is palpated for induration and nodules.

The scrotum and its contents are next in the order of examination. The spermatic cord is palpated, first high in the scrotum for the presence of varicocele, spermatocele, beaded vas deferens or nodules. Then the testis and the epididymis are felt carefully for unusual firmness, nodularity or large masses. If a large mass is palpated in the scrotum, then a flashlight is employed in an attempt to transilluminate the mass. If it transilluminates, it may be a spermatocele or a hydrocele. If it does not, it may be a testicular neoplasm, epididymitis, torsion of the testis or hernia. All hydroceles and spermatoceles should be aspirated because occasionally they are superimposed upon testicular cancer which cannot be felt until the overlying fluid has been withdrawn. This step may be omitted in those cases in which an operation is planned.

The rectal examination is used to determine the status of the prostate gland, the seminal vesicles and the rectum. The normal prostate is a slightly tender, elastic and firm body felt through the anterior rectal wall. Three longitudinal grooves or sulci may be

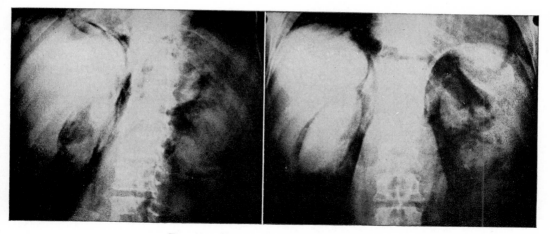

FIG. 48-4. Retroperitoneal pneumogram.

palpated on the posterior aspect of the prostate, two laterally and one centrally. The seminal vesicles lie above and lateral to the prostate and are felt as bands, beginning at the base of the prostate and running superolaterally from the prostate at an angle of about 45°. A stony hard nodular prostate suggests carcinoma, tuberculosis or calculi. A smooth hard prostate with obliteration of the sulci is indicative of infiltrating prostatic neoplasm. Early carcinoma may manifest itself as an isolated circumscribed small nodule. Marked tenderness of the prostate can be caused by acute prostatitis, while an extremely tender, bulging, tense prostate suggests abscess. A tense, exquisitely painful seminal vesicle indicates seminal vesiculitis.

Urinalysis. The examination of the urine is one of the most important aspects of the urologic investigation. In many instances it alone determines the need for detailed expensive urologic procedures entailing hospitalization. Persistent microscopic hematuria suggests the same diseases as gross hematuria and necessitates endoscopy and retrograde pyelography. A urinary tract infection which does not respond after 1 week of appropriate therapy should be investigated further with endoscopy and pyelography, since persistent pyuria may be produced by neoplasms, tuberculosis, calculous disease, hydronephrosis or pyogenic bacteria. In addition to ascertaining the presence of hematuria, pyuria and bacteriuria, the routine urinalysis may lead to the suspicion of impaired renal function.

RENAL PHYSIOLOGY[14, 15]

The purpose of the urinary tract is to aid in maintaining an optimal environment for the efficient functioning of the body cells. When the kidneys do not perform their functions in a normal fashion, either because of intrinsic disease or involvement of other components of the urinary system, illness follows. Anemia, malaise, nausea, vomiting, disorientation, coma, convulsions, weakness, paralysis and cardiac abnormalities are some of the manifestations of the general cellular dysfunction[38] at times associated with renal disease. The renal cells per se are influenced also by the results of their activities, e.g., inability of the kidneys to maintain a proper environment for all of the body means also an improper environment for the renal cells. Many of the diseases of the genito-urinary tract are of prime importance because they interfere with the homeostatic function of the kidneys.

A 70-kilo adult contains approximately 45 L. of water; 30 L. are in the cells (of which 3 are in the blood cells) and 15 L. are extracellular. Of the 15 extracellular liters of water, 11 L. are intercellular, or between the cells, and 4 L. are in the cardiovascular system as plasma.

The cells of the body carry on metabolic activities continuously and need the transport of material to them for anabolism and away from them so as to remove their catabolic products. The blood is the vehicle for the transport of these substances. The exchange of material between blood and cells is indirect in that it must pass into the intercellular fluid first. The forces accomplishing the exchange of material between blood and intercellular fluid through the capillary wall are diffusionary forces which account for 99 per cent of the movement and the intravascular protein osmotic and intravascular hydrostatic pressures. Secondary forces are tissue pressure and a small amount of protein osmotic pressure in the intercellular space.

Essentially, intravascular hydrostatic and tissue protein osmotic pressure tend to promote the movement of water and crystalloids from the blood into the intercellular space, while the intravascular protein osmotic pressure and tissue pressure tend to cause material to go from the intercellular fluid into the capillary. Thus on the arterial side of the capillary the sum (35 mm. Hg) of the intravascular hydrostatic (30 mm. Hg) and tissue protein osmotic (5 mm. Hg) pressures is greater than the sum (30 mm. Hg) of the intravascular osmotic (20 mm. Hg) and tissue hydrostatic (10 mm. Hg) pressure; therefore, material will tend here to go slightly more rapidly from the capillary into the intercellular fluid. The intravascular hydrostatic pressure drops from 30 to 15 mm. Hg on going from the arterial end of the capillary to the venous portion. Since the other pressures remain approximately constant, material here will move a little more rapidly from the intercellular space into the capillary; intravascular osmotic (20 mm. Hg) and tissue hydrostatic (10 mm. Hg) pressures now exceed intravascular hydrostatic (15 mm. Hg) and tissue protein osmotic (5 mm. Hg) pressures.

In the normal adult approximately 1,000 ml. of blood is pumped through both kidneys in 1 minute; this is about one fifth of the cardiac output. The human kidney is a tremendously vascular organ.

ANATOMY

Each kidney is composed of about 1,000,000 units, the nephrons. Each nephron consists of a glomerulus, a proximal convoluted tubule, an elongated segment (loop of Henle) and a distal convoluted tubule (Fig. 48-5). The nephron is the functional unit of the kidney; its product, urine, passes into the collecting tubule. The collecting tubule in turn empties

its contents into the calyx. The calyx propels the urine through the infundibulum into the pelvis. Then the urine is transported down the ureter into the bladder. The urine is collected in the bladder, which is emptied voluntarily at intervals through the urethra into the external environment. The nephron and the urinary collecting system are actually parts of one long conduit; therefore, an abnormality of a distal part such as the urethra may affect directly the proximal functioning unit.

The cortex of the kidney contains the glomeruli and convoluted tubules while the medulla, the portion adjacent to the pelvis, consists of elongated tubular segments (Henle's loops) and the collecting tubules. The renal artery is a short, large caliber vessel springing directly from the aorta and dividing into an anterior and a posterior branch as it enters the renal parenchyma. The branches next divide into the interlobar arteries (Fig. 48-6), which course through the medulla. At the corticomedullary junction the interlobar vessels give off the arcuate arteries which branch further to give rise to the intralobular arteries in the cortex. The afferent arteriole comes from the intralobular artery and gives off the capillaries of the glomerulus which empty into the efferent arteriole. The efferent arteriole then branches and forms the peritubular arterial capillary network which empties into the venous portion of the network. From the venous capillaries blood flows into the intralobular, arcuate, interlobar and renal veins and finally into the inferior vena cava.

The flow of blood through the glomerular capillaries is regulated, in part, by the afferent and efferent arterioles. Concomitant vasoconstriction of the afferent arteriole and vasodilation of the efferent arteriole will result in a decreased blood flow and a decreased glomerular hydrostatic pressure.

GLOMERULAR FILTRATION

As has been stated previously, 1,000 ml. of blood or about 600 ml. of plasma flows through the kidneys in 1 minute. Approximately 120 ml. of the plasma is filtered through the 2,000,000 glomeruli in 1 minute. Glomerular filtration is essentially a passive phenomenon and is very similar to the process whereby material moves from capillary into the intercellular space. In the glomerular capil-

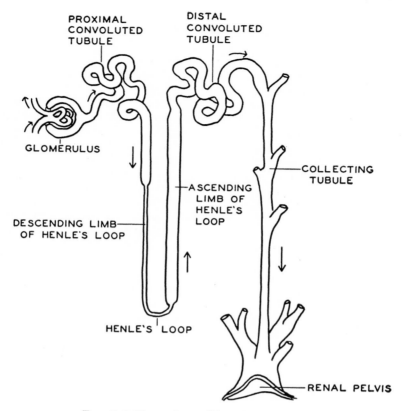

FIG. 48-5. The nephron. (From R. M. Nesbit)

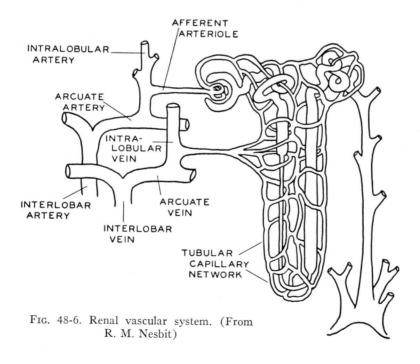

FIG. 48-6. Renal vascular system. (From
R. M. Nesbit)

lary the intravascular hydrostatic pressure is 75 mm. Hg instead of 3 mm. Hg as in capillaries elsewhere in the body. This force of 75 mm. Hg together with diffusional forces tends to promote filtration of plasma through the glomerular membrane. Opposing filtration are the intratubular hydrostatic pressure (10 mm. Hg), the interstitial pressure without tubular pressure (10 mm. Hg) and the intravascular protein osmotic pressure (20 mm. Hg)—a total opposing pressure of 40 mm. Hg. The effective glomerular filtration pressure, 35 mm. Hg, is the algebraic sum of these opposing forces. Knowing these things one need not be surprised that oliguria or anuria attend shock. Therefore, a drop in systemic blood pressure sufficient to lower the pressure in the glomerular capillary by 35 mm. of Hg may abolish glomerular filtration.

So too is the suppression of urine associated with prostatic urinary retention understandable. With acute urinary retention due to prostatism, the intravesical pressure increases as does the intra-ureteral, the intrapelvic and the *intratubular hydrostatic pressures*. Since the intratubular hydrostatic pressure opposes filtration, a rise in this pressure will decrease glomerular filtration, and urinary suppression follows. Swelling of the renal parenchyma itself can impair glomerular filtration by raising the interstitial pressure; this may attend acute pyelonephritis, which is associated with infiltration of the interstitial spaces with leukocytes. Acute inflammation of the glomerular membrane will result in impaired filtration as will vascular disease compromising the lumen of the glomerular capillary or the renal artery.

The glomerular filtrate is essentially protein-free plasma; the blood cellular elements and most of the protein are not filtered.[13] The pH of the filtrate is 7.4, specific gravity 1.010, glucose 80 mg. per 100 ml., urea nitrogen 15 mg. per 100 ml., sodium 142 mEq./L., chloride 103 mEq./L., bicarbonate 27 mEq./L. and potassium 4.5 mEq./L.

TUBULAR FUNCTION

In order to comprehend some of the functions of the tubular portion of the nephron, one need only compare the urine with the glomerular filtrate. The normal individual subsisting on the average American or Euro-

pean diet will excrete about 1,500 ml. of urine each 24 hours having a pH of 5.5, a specific gravity of 1.020, no glucose and containing urea nitrogen concentrated 70 times above its hemic concentration. The cells of the tubule perform work[25] and consume a great deal of energy in effecting these changes. In contrast, glomerular filtration is a passive process.

In 1958, Malvin, Wilde and Sullivan[24] published the "Stop Flow" method for determining the segment of renal nephron concerned with the selective reabsorption or secretion of a particular substance. As a result of work with their method, tremendous strides are being made in localizing the function of various parts of the tubule and the collecting duct.

GLUCOSE ABSORPTION

Glucose is removed from the glomerular filtrate by a tubular enzymatic carrier mechanism in the proximal convoluted tubule. The maximum amount of glucose that can be taken up by the normal mechanism is approximately 350 mg. per minute. The cells of the tubule reabsorb the glucose in as near an iso-osmotic solution as possible; thus a certain amount of water will be reabsorbed with the glucose. When there is a defect in the tubular carrier mechanism, glycosuria and polyuria result. In renal glycosuria the defect is functional and congenital, while in phlorhizin glycosuria the tubules have been damaged by a poison. The glycosuria in diabetes mellitus is a consequence of the excessive concentration of sugar in the glomerular filtrate. It is so much in excess of normal that the amount of glucose in the tubular urine exceeds the reabsorptive capacity of the tubular cells.

NaCl ABSORPTION

Other substances reabsorbed in the proximal tubule are sodium, chloride, bicarbonate, phosphates, sulfate, uric acid, and amino acids. These substances also are reabsorbed as solutes. The reabsorption of sodium chloride is in part controlled by the adrenal cortex through its hormone aldosterone.[20, 22] It is believed that the amount of aldosterone secreted is partially dependent upon the volume of the plasma or extracellular fluid; when plasma volume is low the absorption of sodium chloride and obligatory reabsorption of water are enhanced. Theoretically, in Addison's disease the patient is hypotensive and the plasma volume low, because the adrenal cortex is not secreting sufficient aldosterone to retain sufficient sodium chloride and water to maintain the plasma and interstitial fluid volumes. In secondary aldosteronism edema results because too much NaCl and water are reabsorbed.

ABSORPTION OF WATER[13, 21, 23, 27]

The reabsorption of plasma water filtered through the glomerulus occurs in many parts of the tubule and the collecting duct. Of the 120 ml. of glomerular filtrate per minute, 104 ml. is passively reabsorbed in the proximal tubule secondary to the active transport of sodium, glucose, etc. The passive diffusion of water results in osmotic equilibration, so that the fluid leaving the proximal tubule is still isosmotic with blood, i.e., it maintains a specific gravity of about 1.010.

Contrary to the previous belief that tubular water is actively reabsorbed in the distal convoluted tubule, it has been suggested that reabsorption of water is not only passive in the proximal tubule but also in the distal convoluted tubule and the collecting duct. However, the reabsorption of water in the distal portion of the nephron and the collecting duct is dependent on the hyperosmolarity or hypertonicity of the medullary tissue surrounding the distal nephron and the collecting duct. There are numerous theories[27] regarding the development of the hypertonic medullary tissue, but none has been proved.

Because the interstitial fluid surrounding the distal convoluted tubule and the collecting duct is markedly hypertonic, there is a tendency toward diffusion of hypotonic or isotonic tubular fluids across the tubular and collecting duct epithelium into the interstitial fluid. Unlike the epithelium of the proximal tubule, which is freely permeable to fluid, the cells of the distal tubule and the collecting duct require the permissive action of the antidiuretic hormone before they will allow the flow of water from the tubule into the surrounding tissue. Thus, when no ADH is being secreted, the urine will be isotonic with blood or hypotonic if sodium and other solutes continue to be reabsorbed along the distal tubule and the collecting duct. When ADH is released in large quantities, much water flows through the cells of the distal tubule and the collecting duct in response to the osmotic pressure of the peritubular fluid, and a urine with a high specific gravity or osmolarity results.

Verney[28] has presented evidence to suggest that there are osmoreceptors in the body (internal carotid, brain) which are stimulated by an increased osmolar concentration due to loss of water from or an increase in electrolytes in the plasma. Presumably, these osmoreceptors, when stimulated by hyperosmolarity, activate the hypothalamic-posterior pituitary mechanism to secrete antidiuretic hormone. ADH then acts upon the cells of the distal tubule and the collecting duct to increase their permeability to water which flows from the nephron into the peritubular fluid and thence into the plasma of the vasa recta in response to osmotic pressure. The loss of fluid from the nephron results in a low volume of concentrated urine.

When the body has taken in enough water to establish isomolarity, secretion of ADH decreases, and the cells of the distal convoluted tubule and the collecting duct become less permeable to water. Concomitantly, the urinary output will decrease, and the specific gravity or osmolarity will be lowered. Diabetes insipidus is a disease characterized by a large 24-hour output of urine with a specific gravity of 1.010 or less. It is due to a deficiency of ADH secretion by the posterior pituitary. The patient will rarely put out more than 20 liters of urine in 24 hours, even in very severe cases, because only the water absorbed in the distal tubule and the collecting duct will be lost and, at most, this amounts to 16 ml. per minute or 23 liters per 24 hours. This condition can be treated adequately with the administration of pitressin tannate in oil subcutaneously or intramuscularly, or of dried powdered posterior pituitary by nasal insufflation.

When the cells of the distal tubule are involved by disease, they may not respond to the antidiuretic hormone and thereby a urine with a fixed specific gravity of 1.010 may result. A test for tubular function is based on the ability of the kidney to absorb water under the influence of the antidiuretic hormone. The test is called the "concentration test" and consists of dehydrating the patient by withholding water for 18 to 24 hours. Tubular insufficiency is indicated whenever the urine excreted during the last 6 hours of abstinence has a specific gravity of less than 1.018. If the tubular cells are impaired by disease so that they will not respond to the antidiuretic hormone, the specific gravity of the urine will remain below 1.018.

REABSORPTION OF AVAILABLE BASE

Some of the products of oxidation of proteins and fats are the anions of organic (oxalic, citric, etc.) and inorganic acids (SO_4 and H_2PO_4). Unless neutralized by base these acids will lower the pH of the body. The kidneys when excreting the salts of these acids conserve available base by reabsorbing sodium as sodium bicarbonate and substituting within the tubular cells the hydrogen and ammonium ions for the sodium.[26] When the tubular fluid reaches the distal tubule, it has a pH of 7.4 and contains $NaCl$, Na_2HPO_4, NaH_2PO_4, Na_2SO_4, Na citrate and Na lactate among other substances. If the body is tending toward acidosis, some of the cells of the distal tubule will be stimulated to produce the ammonium and hydrogen ions. The ammonium ion is formed from glutamine and other amino acids. The hydrogen ion is formed from the ionization of carbonic acid; carbonic acid is formed from carbon dioxide and water with the aid of the enzyme carbonic anhydrase.

Interference with the base-saving mechanism by renal disease or drugs (Diamox*) will result in tubular (or hyperchloremic) acidosis. The body loses sodium that should have been reabsorbed as $NaHCO_3$. To compensate for this loss the organism presumptively attempts to keep the total body sodium and plasma volume within normal limits by increasing the reabsorption of $NaCl$. Thus in hyperchloremic acidosis serum sodium may be 142 mEq./L., serum chloride 117 mEq./L. and serum bicarbonate 13 mEq./L. The blood urea nitrogen tends to be within normal limits in disease restricted to the tubules. Tubular or hyperchloremic acidosis is seen in patients with chronic pyelonephritis, following ureterosigmoid transplantation and in the Butler-Albright syndrome.

The tubular cells excrete substances into as well as absorb them from the tubular fluid.

---

* Diamox is a sulfanilamide derivative which acts as a diuretic by inhibiting the formation of carbonic anhydrase in the distal tubule.

Renal tubular cells are capable of excreting into their lumens potassium, creatinine and a number of foreign substances such as the sulfonamides, penicillin, para-aminohippurate, phenolsulfonphthalein, Diodrast, Neoiopax and Urokon.

RENAL FUNCTION TESTS

QUALITATIVE TESTS

A gross estimation of renal function may be obtained by routine urinalysis. Albumin and casts indicate damage to the glomerulus. In the absence of diabetes mellitus, a high specific gravity of the urine indicates good tubular function. No conclusions can be drawn if the specific gravity is low and the pH neutral or alkaline, because these may be the results of dietary peculiarities and overhydration.

Intravenous or excretory pyelography is a gross test of renal function when a moderate amount (30 to 50 ml.) of 30 to 50 per cent concentration of radiopaque medium is used; under these conditions the renal collecting systems will not be visualized if more than 75 per cent of the total renal parenchyma is functionally inactive.

Determination of blood urea nitrogen, nonprotein nitrogen or creatinine will afford a gross estimate of renal function. The blood levels of these substances become elevated above normal when more than 75 per cent of total kidney tissue is damaged. With lesser damage these determinations give the physician no idea of the renal status. Other factors such as dehydration, gastrointestinal hemorrhage and excessive catabolism may cause an elevation in the blood nonprotein and urea nitrogen levels, the so-called prerenal azotemia.

QUANTITATIVE TESTS

The clearance tests provide a fairly accurate estimate of renal function. The urea and creatinine clearance[33] tests provide an estimate of glomerular filtration. The normal urea clearance[32] varies between 70 to 120 per cent of average normal, while the normal creatinine clearance value is about 140 L. per 24 hours. The onset of uremia may occur when the urea clearance drops below 25 per cent of normal or the creatinine clearance below 35 to 45 liters/24 hours.

The phenolsulfonphthalein or PSP test[31] and the concentration test estimate tubular function. The PSP determination measures the ability of the renal tubules to excrete 6 mg. of parenterally administered phenolsulfonphthalein. Normal kidneys will excrete 33 per cent of the dye in 15 minutes. The 15-minute PSP test is also a measure of glomerular status in that it has been shown[31] that the glomerular function can rarely be more impaired than tubular function. Thus, the PSP determination, in addition to giving an estimation of tubular efficiency, also provides an index of the minimal glomerular function compatible with that degree of tubular function. *The 15-minute PSP determination is the best routine clinical quantitative test of renal function.*

The concentration test can be performed in a number of ways. The urinary specific gravity obtained with it will depend on the length of the period of dehydration. The concentration test is not particularly good because: (1) it cannot follow progressive impairment of renal function after the specific gravity of the urine becomes fixed; and (2) 12 to 16 hours of dehydration may endanger the life of the patient with poor renal function.

In many situations the urologist finds it necessary to ascertain the function of each kidney separately. This knowledge is especially important in suspected cases of renal hypertension or when nephrectomy is contemplated. The performance of a nephrectomy in the presence of a contralateral poorly or nonfunctioning kidney is a catastrophe. Separate determinations of the function of each kidney (split-functions) are obtained by inserting catheters up the ureters into the renal pelves. Then, the PSP test, creatinine clearance, sodium excretion, fluid volume output or urine osmolality may be determined for each kidney.

RENAL FUNCTION IN DISEASE

Obviously, the renal tubule has many functions while the glomerulus apparently has only one. Therefore, renal abnormalities may manifest themselves in as many different ways as there are tubular functions; for example, glycosuria, cystinuria, renal rickets, etc. The more common renal diseases such as pyelonephritis,[37] hydronephrosis, glomerulotubular nephritis[35] and hypertensive renal disease tend to present the same clinical and laboratory findings when renal deterioration becomes advanced.

Impairment of glomerular filtration, whether due to increased intratubular hydrostatic pressure as in hydronephrosis, structural change in the glomerular membrane as in glomerular nephritis and intercapillary glomerular sclerosis or inflammatory involvement as in pyelonephritis, will lead to an accumulation of all metabolic end products destined to be excreted from the body primarily by the kidneys. Particularly, the products of protein metabolism, such as phosphates, sulfates, urea and uric acid, will accumulate and produce uremia when filtration is sufficiently impaired because they are excreted primarily by the kidneys. Clinically, uremia is attended by nausea, vomiting, diarrhea, malaise, dyspnea on slight exertion, hyperpnea, twitching, anemia, ease of fatigue, and occasionally by acute abdominal pain and tenderness. Blood chemical studies show elevated blood urea and nonprotein nitrogen levels, a decreased serum bicarbonate or carbon dioxide combining power, and increased phosphate and sulfate concentrations. The serum potassium level will tend to rise above 5 mEq./L. As the blood level of phosphate rises that of calcium falls. The ionized calcium may remain normal if the concomitant acidosis is sufficiently great.

ACUTE RENAL FAILURE

Etiology. Acute renal failure, for a time called the lower nephron syndrome, has been observed in patients poisoned with carbon tetrachloride, bichloride of mercury, uranium nitrate, phosphorus, bismuth, etc., and in patients in shock caused by severe dehydration, Addison's disease, hemorrhage and trauma. In other words, acute renal failure can be caused by (1) *nephrotoxins* and (2) any condition which leads to a prolonged period of *renal ischemia.*

Pathology. The kidneys of most patients dying with acute renal failure are swollen, have cortical pallor and a dark blue medulla. Microscopically, 2 types of lesions[51] are found: a generalized proximal tubular cellular (nephrotoxic) necrosis down to the basement membrane but not including it; and a randomly distributed patchy tubular necrosis, involving the basement membrane (tubulorhexic). The former is believed to be produced by toxic substances, the latter by ischemia.

Patients with acute renal insufficiency who have increased catabolism due to breakdown of traumatized tissue and fever, will deteriorate much more rapidly than the patient who is afebrile and has no tissue necrosis.

Death may occur at any time during the period of oliguria or during the first few days of recovery. Pulmonary or cerebral edema incident to the administration of too much fluid may be the cause of death during the first few days.

Diagnosis. Acute renal failure must be distinguished from acute urinary obstruction and from severe dehydration. The history will often help in differentiation. A urinary specific gravity of 1.020 or greater suggests dehydration. A specific gravity of about 1.010 suggests acute renal failure but is not absolutely diagnostic, because dehydrated patients with previous renal disease may exhibit a urinary specific gravity of 1.010. Anuria as distinguished from oliguria is seen in complete urinary obstruction but rarely in acute renal failure. Acute ureteral obstruction can be determined readily by retrograde pyelographic methods.

The therapy of oliguria depends upon the cause. Obstructive anuria or oliguria demands alleviation of the obstruction. Dehydrational oliguria requires the administration of appropriate fluids. Nephrotoxic and tubulorhexic oliguria requires the careful adjustment of diet and fluid administration. An error in diagnosis of the cause of anuria may rapidly lead to an untimely death.

Mechanism of Production of Oliguria or Anuria. An abnormal decrease in urinary output may attend a decreased blood flow[43] through the nephrons, or a complete diffusion of glomerular filtrate back through the damaged tubular wall, acting as an inert membrane.

Clinical Picture. During the early phase the 24-hour output usually will be less than 400 ml. but rarely zero. Examination of the urine may show a specific gravity between 1.010 and 1.015, a pH hovering around 7.0, albumin 1 to 2+, pigment casts, and red and white blood cells. Initially, the blood-chemistry studies may be normal.

As time passes (5 to 7 days) the blood pressure may rise to hypertensive levels, the pulse becomes rapid, the sensorium is dulled, breathing may become rapid and deeper, and vomiting may occur. As these signs of illness develop the concentrations of creatinine, urea nitrogen, polypeptide nitrogen, potassium, phosphate and sulfate increase and that of serum bicarbonate decreases. The sodium and chloride levels, although they may be increased or decreased, are frequently found to be within normal limits. Often anemia will be present. Presumably this is caused by hemolysis and depressed erythropoiesis.

After the passage of 5 to 10 days the urinary output may suddenly increase. However, usually little or no clinical or chemical improvement will attend this change for 2 to 3 days, and then improvement occurs gradually.

Therapy. Because death from acute renal failure is often attributable to hyperkalemia or the giving of excessive fluids, therapy should be directed toward alleviating processes causing hyperpotassemia, inorganic acidosis and toward maintaining proper hydration.

To decrease protein catabolism with its production of sulfate, phosphate and urea, and to decrease the formation of ketone bodies from fat, 100 Gm. of carbohydrate per day in the form of rock candy orally or 15 per cent glucose in water parenterally need be given. This amount of carbohydrate will decrease the rate of rise in nitrogen, potassium and acids. Some fatty substances may be given also to supply additional calories without nitrogen, sulfate, phosphate, or potassium. However, the giving of fat usually complicates the picture because it aggravates the nausea already present and often induces vomiting, thereby depriving the body of fluids and electrolytes. Giving much more than 100 Gm. of carbohydrate will not further decrease protein breakdown. By adhering strictly to glucose or rock candy as foodstuff, there will be no opportunity for other foods containing protein and potassium to be given to the patient inadvertently.

Unless the blood volume is below normal or the hemoglobin concentration is below 10 Gm. per 100 ml., blood transfusions should not be given during the period of oliguria because they may trigger the onset of pulmonary congestion and cardiac failure.[56] Furthermore, a mild transfusion reaction which would not endanger normal kidneys could well tip the scales against recovery in these patients. Similarly, the giving of alkaline electrolyte solutions (sodium lactate or bicarbonate) as treatment for acidosis is contraindicated unless hyperpnea due to uncompensated acidosis is present. In most cases of acute renal failure neither the anemia nor the acidosis is of sufficient severity to warrant the use of remedial measures, the side effects of which may cause death.

The daily water requirements of any patient can be calculated roughly by considering the water lost and the water gained by the body. If an individual be starved, the body will be provided approximately 300 ml. of water each day from the water of oxidation of carbohydrate, protein and fat, and from the water of solution (water holding protein and carbohydrate in solution in cells); this is water gained from within the body. The body loses water under normal conditions through the skin, the lungs, the urinary tract and the bowel. Water vapor loss through the skin and the lungs is called insensible loss and under average conditions of temperature and humidity amounts to about 600 to 800 ml. per 24 hours. Insensible loss increases with fever and hyperpnea. Unless the patient has diarrhea, water loss in the feces is negligible. Thus a patient with an oliguria of 100 ml. per 24 hours, loses 800 ml. of water by insensible loss, 100 ml. of water in the urine and gains 300 ml. of water from oxidation and water of solution. Subtracting 300 from 900 ml. leaves a 24-hour net loss of 600 ml. of water from the body. Thus fluid replacement should be 600 ml. of a 10 or 15 per cent solution of glucose in water if it is given intravenously or 600 ml. of water containing 100 Gm. of carbohydrate if it is given orally. If urinary output increases, additional water equal to urinary flow (within limits) should be added to insensible loss. Any losses through vomiting or diarrhea should be replaced *with appropriate electrolyte solutions.* (See Chap. 5, "Fluids and Electrolytes.")

It is well to start a patient on rectal ion-exchange resins as soon as the diagnosis of acute renal failure is made, for hyperkalemia is inevitable. Serum potassium levels can be kept within normal range very readily with the use of sulfonate resins. Emergency measures such as intravenous insulin and glucose or one sixth molar sodium lactate may be necessary to reduce rapidly the near-lethal serum potassium levels in patients just admitted to the hospital.

Using the therapeutic regimen just outlined, pulmonary and cardiac complications will be minimized; and as the kidneys recover, the extent of the diuresis will be limited. Some of the patients with acute renal failure will recover completely using the therapeutic regimen just outlined. However, those patients with increased catabolism due to extensive ecchymoses, massive hemorrhage into body cavities or the gastrointestinal tract, marked soft tissue trauma, high fever, active delirium and infections, will demonstrate rapidly rising levels of end products of protein metabolism associated with clouding of the sensorium. In this situation it is imperative to utilize some form of dialysis in order to save the patient's life. Intermittent irrigation of the peritoneal cavity[49] and hemodialysis[47] are the 2 methods most commonly used at the present time. We employ the Kolff coil type of artificial kidney at the University of Michigan Medical Center[48] and have found it to be extremely satisfactory from all aspects, including compactness, the time necessary to prepare the unit for use and efficiency of dialysis.

Some observers are now using a small artificial kidney to dialyze the patient daily in an effort to prevent the onset of uremia.[57]

Formerly, it was believed that persons recovering from acute renal failure pass through a phase characterized by a tremendous urinary output, up to 12 L. per day. However, evidence[56] indicates that when seen the "recovery" diuresis is usually iatrogenic, i.e., diuresis occurs mainly in those patients who have received an excessive volume of fluids during the period of oliguria or anuria. Consequently, if recovery diuresis occurs, volume for volume replacement with an electrolyte solution should not be practiced unless incontrovertible signs of dehydration attend it. The patient should be given only enough water to compensate for the insensible loss and to provide for a urinary output of about 2,000 ml.: a total of about 2,700 ml. Occasionally, an excessive urinary loss of fluid requires replacement; but in these instances replacement will be indicated by physical evidences of dehydration (see Chap. 5, "Fluid and Electrolytes"). During the recovery phase it is well to check the output of sodium and chloride in the urine, for occasionally it becomes excessive and should be replaced. A good replacement solution contains sodium, chloride and lactate or bicarbonate.

RENAL HYPERTENSION[44, 58]

During the past decade there has been a renewal of interest in hypertension caused by lesions of the renal arterial system and the parenchyma.

The increased effort to find cases of renal hypertension in the over-all group of hypertensives has led to the conclusion that renal hypertension occurs more frequently than was previously suspected.

At the present time, it is theorized that renal hypertension is caused by a disturbance in the dynamics of renal blood flow. Experimentally, the arterial vasculature may be compromised by inflammation of the renal parenchyma such as perinephritis[52] and pyelonephritis[54] or by occlusion of the renal artery.[45]

It is believed that when the renal arterial system is involved, a decrease in pulse pressure occurs,[46] and it is this phenomenon rather than ischemia which results in high blood pressure.

Diagnosis. Renal hypertension must be distinguished from elevated blood pressure produced by Cushing's syndrome, primary aldosteronism, pheochromocytoma, coarctation of the aorta, etc.

One must be particularly suspicious of renal hypertension in: (1) patients with a sudden onset of malignant hypertension; (2) patients with a history suggesting renal infarction; and (3) any patient without other demonstrable cause for the hypertension. Primary or essential hypertension is diagnosed by exclusion and simply means that the physician has been unable to find a cause.

Intravenous urography, renal angiography,[53] differential renal excretion studies[44] and radioactive renography[42] are methods used in detecting cases of renal hypertension. Intravenous pyelography and renal angiography

are the oldest and most frequently used of the diagnostic aids. The particular place and importance of the excretion test and radioactive renogram in the diagnostic armamentarium has yet to be established.

Pathology. The most frequent lesions of the renal arterial system found to be producing hypertension are fibromuscular and atherosclerotic narrowing of the renal artery (see Fig. 48-3). Other lesions include aneurysms, embolism, thrombosis, etc.

Treatment is surgical rather than medical. Nephrectomy is indicated in patients with unilateral nonfunctioning or poorly functioning kidneys and normal-functioning contralateral kidneys. Partial nephrectomy is preferred when a segmental artery is involved. In an otherwise healthy patient with a kidney worth salvaging, an attempt is made to repair the arterial defect and save the kidney. The vascular procedure may involve resection of the diseased portion of the artery and reanastomosis; resection of the arterial lesion and replacement by a homograft; bypassing the lesion with a Teflon graft extending from the aorta to the renal artery at a point distal to the lesion; or performing a splenorenal arterial anastomosis.

A high rate of cure can be expected with surgical therapy of renal hypertension if careful diagnostic studies are conducted preoperatively.

OBSTRUCTIVE URINARY TRACT DISEASE

GENERAL PHYSIOPATHOLOGY

Interference with the normal orderly propulsion of urine anywhere along the urinary tract will lead to functional and structural changes in the urinary tract proximal to the obstruction. For example, a stricture of the urethral meatus impedes urinary expulsion and after a time in a child will be attended by dilation of the urethra proximal to the stricture;* the bladder hypertrophies and becomes trabeculated. Later, outpouching cellules consisting of mucosa not covered by muscle develop; these are called diverticula. Cystoscopically, the interior of the trabeculated bladder looks like a lattice. Figure 48-7 (*Top, left*) is the cystogram of a normal blad-

* This does not occur in the adult urethra.

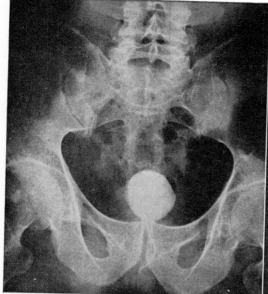
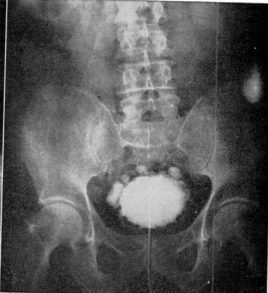
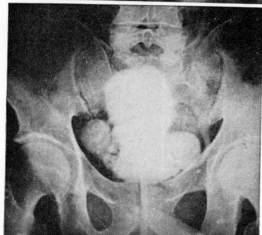

Fig. 48-7. (*Top, left*) Cystogram of a normal bladder. (*Top, right*) Cystogram of a bladder with trabeculation, cellules and small diverticula. (*Bottom*) Cystogram of a bladder with several diverticula.

der by taking a roentgenogram of the bladder filled with a solution of sodium iodide; its outline is smooth. In Figure 48-7 (*Top, right and bottom*) the irregular serrated outline indicates trabeculation, cellule and diverticulum formation.

Bladder diverticula are either acquired or congenital. A congenital diverticulum consists of muscle, mucosa and serosa, while the acquired type lacks the muscular coat. Small completely evacuable diverticula require no treatment, while large incompletely emptying ones do. Excision through a suprapubic approach is the only means of eradicating those requiring treatment. Occasionally, neoplasms arise in bladder diverticula.

Continuance of a urethral obstruction will result eventually in decompensation and atonicity of the bladder and urinary retention. Occasionally, as the bladder decompensates the valvular mechanism at the ureterovesical junction becomes incompetent and allows the reflux of urine up the ureters. This is illustrated in the cystogram shown in Figure 48-8. Ureteral reflux does not occur from normal bladders. However, even though reflux may not occur in the face of urethral obstruction, nevertheless vesical obstruction with dilatation and atonicity of the bladder is attended by hypertrophy of the ureteral musculature and later by dilatation and elongation of the ureter. A similar process occurs within the pelvis and calyces producing hydro-ureter and hydronephrosis (Fig. 48-9).

As hydro-ureter and hydronephrosis develop the hydrostatic pressure within the renal pelvis and calyces increases and impairs glomerular filtration and tubular function[60] (as discussed in Renal Physiology and Renal Function in Disease). Tubular function is

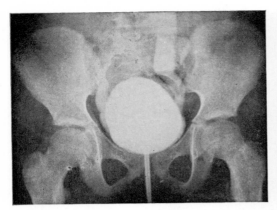

Fig. 48-8. Cystogram of a bladder with bilateral ureteral reflux.

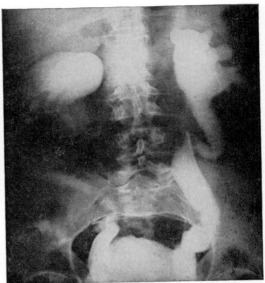

Fig. 48-9. Bilateral hydro-ureter and hydro-nephrosis.

impaired by 2 processes: by direct pressure atrophy and by compression of the peritubular capillary network. Both the direct pressure upon the renal tubules and the compression of the peritubular capillaries ultimately destroy the renal parenchyma.[59]

In brief, the effects of obstruction of the distal urinary tract are: (1) dilatation of the urethra in children (meatal obstruction); (2) hypertrophy, trabeculation, and the formation of cellules and diverticula of the bladder; (3) atonicity of the bladder; (4) ureteral reflux; (5) hydro-ureter, hydronephrosis and renal atrophy; (6) temporary or permanent loss of renal function incident to impaired glomerular filtration and tubular function.

GENERAL THERAPY

The treatment of any obstruction of a tubular organ consists of the removal or the short-circuiting of the obstruction. If the patient is very sick, a simple diversion or short-circuiting of the urinary stream is necessary. Depending upon the site of the obstruction, the diversion may be effected with an inlying urethral catheter, a perineal urethrostomy, a suprapubic cystostomy, a ureterostomy or a nephrostomy. The site of diversion needs be proximal to the obstruction. Urinary diversion permits the urinary tract and the kidneys to recover by removing back-pressure upon them. In some cases the diversion of the urine for 3 or 4 days will be attended by a fall of NPN to normal, the alleviation of the acidosis and the relief from anorexia, nausea and vomiting. In others a urinary diversion for several

months may be required to restore renal function adequately. A few patients require diversion permanently because it is not possible to restore adequate function of the urinary tract. The extent of renal impairment obtaining with an obstruction is directly related to the length of time it has existed and the completeness of the obstruction.

SPECIFIC OBSTRUCTIONAL UROGENITAL DISEASES

Congenital. URETHRA. A congenital pinpoint narrowing of the urethral meatus[69] occurs occasionally in male infants. It may manifest itself as a needlelike stream when the child voids or as a continuous wetting of the diaper with subsequent excoriation of the perineum and the lower abdomen when overflow incontinence occurs. Occasionally, the symptoms and signs of uremia may constitute the first indications of a urethral obstruction. The diagnosis is made upon physical examination and urethral calibration. The performance of a simple urethral meatotomy saves the entire urinary tract and the baby from destruction.

URETHRAL VALVES.[71] These occur only in boys and are mucosal folds extending from the veru montanum laterally toward the vesical neck so as to form a V on the floor of the prostatic urethra (Fig. 48-10). As the bladder empties, the flowing urine balloons out the mucosal folds, and these then act as valvelike structures to obstruct the urinary flow. Bed-wetting, overflow incontinence and a poor stream in males are the primary signs of this entity in childhood. Every mother, when taking the newborn male child home, should be instructed to observe the character of the urinary stream when the child urinates while lying on his back unclothed. A high stream is normal, a low stream under 1 foot in height should bring him to a urologist. Excision of the mucosal folds through the open bladder using the retropubic approach is the most effective treatment.

PENIS. Occasionally the preputial opening is so small that obstruction to urination occurs. This is called phimosis.[66] The symptoms and signs are similar to those of urethral meatal stricture. On inspection an apparent enlargement of the penis is evident, which when palpated is discovered to be a preputial sac distended with urine. The treatment is circumcision.

BLADDER. *Vesical outlet obstruction*[68, 70] may be caused by fibrosis and narrowing of the vesicourethral junction or by a large redundant mucosal fold. More often, increased resistance to urinary outflow is produced by rigidity of the urethrovesical junction. The decreased mobility can be caused by fibrosis or by muscular hypertrophy at the vesical outlet. Although the vesical outlet appears adequate on urethroscopy, it cannot be pulled open during urination as it is in the normal individual. This entity is being observed more often in young girls with histories of persistent or recurrent urinary tract infections. Appropriate diagnostic procedures, namely, cystometric examination, endoscopy, voiding cysto-urethrography, pyelography and renal function tests, will demonstrate the cause of the urinary obstruction and the extent of the damage to the upper urinary tracts. Treatment consists of (1) excision of the mucosal fold

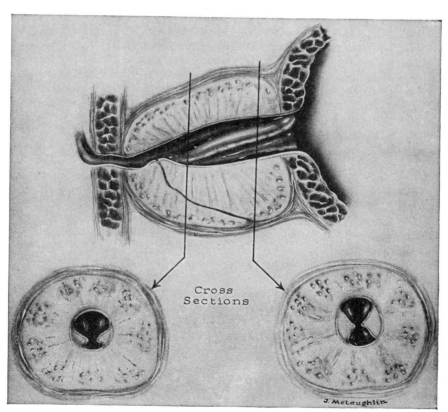

Cross
Sections

FIG. 48-10. Congenital valves of the prostatic urethra. (From R. M. Nesbit)

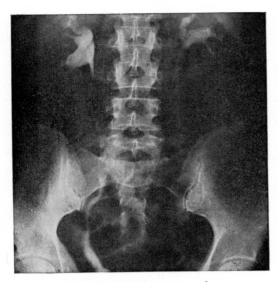

Fig. 48-11. Right ureterocele.

or (2) the plastic revision of the vesical neck to increase its mobility during micturition.

Neurogenic disturbances of the bladder are prone to occur in children suffering from myelodysplasia associated with such entities as spina bifida, myelomeningocele, etc. The signs and symptoms are those met in patients with partial or complete motor paralysis[200] of the bladder. In addition to incontinence, excoriation and increased frequency of urination, one of the characteristic signs of a congenital neurogenic bladder is the inability to void a continuous stream. Such children often void only by applying abdominal pressure. The diagnosis is made by cystometric examination and endoscopy. The treatment will vary with the ability of the patient to empty the bladder. It may involve transurethral resection or plastic revision of the vesical neck if the patient carries a large residual urine. The treatment of choice in children with neurogenic bladders due to sacral spinal cord disease is anastomosis of the ureters to an ileal conduit. Recently, the formation of a permanent vesico-cutaneous fistula to drain the bladder constantly into a collecting device appears to be superior to the ileal conduit.

URETER. *Ureterocele* (Fig. 48-11) is an abnormality of the distal end of the ureter characterized by a cystic enlargement of the ureter protruding into the bladder lumen. It is thought to be caused by a narrowing of the ureteral meatus with resultant dilatation of the intravesical portion of the ureter.[63] The ureterocele may be small, unilateral and associated with mild hydronephrosis or it may be so large that it obstructs the bladder-outlet. A ureterocele obstructing the vesical outlet causes bilateral hydro-ureter, hydronephrosis and decompensation of the bladder. The patient may be asymptomatic if the ureterocele is small. If the ureterocele obstructs micturition at the vesical neck, overflow incontinence, dysuria, increased frequency of urination and a small weak stream will attend it. Diagnosis is made by cystoscopy. The treatment consists of the transurethral enlargement of the ureteral meatus in the case of small ureteroceles or its suprapubic excision if large and obstructing.

Congenital megalo-ureter is a condition in which unilateral or bilateral dilatation of the ureters occurs without any apparent evidence of organic obstruction distal to the hydro-ureter. It is rare. To date no one has presented valid evidence to indicate that the cause of congenital megalo-ureter is a developmental defect in the neuromuscular mechanism. Most of the cases that appear to be congenital megalo-ureter, upon being examined meticulously, are found to be related to obstructions.

Persistent pyuria and ureteral reflux are the most common manifestations of the disease. Other symptoms that attend it may be due to uremia, e.g., anorexia, malaise, anemia, delayed growth, etc. The diagnosis is made by pyelography and cysto-urethrography after organic obstructive entities have been excluded by endoscopy, cystometrography and, perhaps, surgical exploration of the vesical outlet.

No completely satisfactory treatment is known for this disease.[71] Therapy may involve reimplantation of the ureters into the bladder in a manner designed to prevent ureteral reflux,[73] or conservative therapy may be employed by having the patient studiously attempt to empty the bladder and the ureters of urine with a "triple-voiding technic."[67]

Ureteropelvic obstruction may be caused by a congenital narrowing of the upper ureter, a congenital high insertion of the ureter into the renal pelvis or the compression of the ureter by anomalous renal vessels. Hydronephrosis and impaired renal function follow ureteropelvic obstruction. If the obstruction is uni-lateral, the patient may not be at all ill and carries only a ballotable mass in the flank. If infection occurs, a persistent pyuria, recur-rent episodes of chills, fever and flank pain may be the predominant manifestations. A diagnosis of obstruction at the ureteropelvic junction can be made only with pyelography which shows a hydronephrosis coupled with a normal ureter (Fig. 48-12). If the hydro-nephrosis is far-advanced and the disease is limited to one side while the other kidney is normal, a nephrectomy is the best treatment. Plastic surgical procedures[64] are requisite to correct the ureteropelvic obstruction if the kid-ney is worth saving or the disease is bilateral.

Specific Diseases

Acquired. Urethra. Strictures of the pen-dulous and bulbous portions of the urethra may follow urethral trauma or infection. The most common infection is still gonorrhea. Occa-sionally, other pyogenic organisms and the tubercle bacillus may be the cause of chronic urethritis and an inflammatory stricture.

Trauma to the urethra from straddle in-juries, auto accidents and urethral instru-mentation with sounds, catheters or resecto-scopes may, after healing, cause severe nar-rowing of the urethra.

The patient with a urethral stricture may complain of a decrease in size and force of stream, hesitancy in starting urination, dys-uria, increased frequency of urination and a feeling of incomplete emptying of the bladder. When complete urinary retention occurs, para-doxic incontinence may ensue. Often the pa-tient with a urethral stricture will present himself to the physician solely with complaints referable to uremia, i.e., fatigue, malaise, ano-rexia and weight loss, no difficulty in urination having been experienced.

In addition to the usual structural and functional abnormalities produced by obstruc-tive uropathy, a urethral stricture may cause changes peculiar to itself. Strictures are usu-ally associated with *infection and inflamma-tion* of the urethra proximal to the stricture. This, with the high intra-urethral pressure exerted in attempting to void, will frequently disrupt the urethra so that urine will escape through its wall. The escape may be slow and attended by small communicating abscesses.

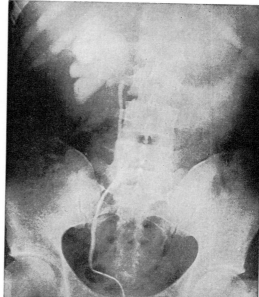

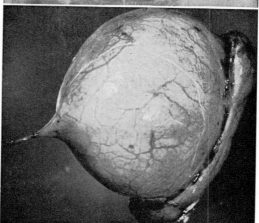

Fig. 48-12. (*Top*) Right hydronephrosis due to ureteropelvic obstruction. Ureter is normal in caliber except at UP junction. (*Bottom*) Actual specimen of a hydro-nephrotic kidney due to congenital narrow-ing of the ureter at the ureteropelvic junc-tion. The pelvis is tremendously dilated with a relatively small cap of parenchyma.

These erode the skin and perforate the skin of the penis, the scrotum or the perineum, forming urethrocutaneous *fistulae.* Numerous urethrocutaneous fistulae opening into the perineum constitute the entity of the "water-ing-pot" perineum (see Chap. 39, "Ano-rectum").

Should the escape of urine through the wall of the urethra be sudden and massive, the urine extravasates widely along fascial planes. A perforation through the urethral mucosa but within Buck's fascia produces swelling of the penis (not including the glans) and the perineum. An extravasation through Buck's fascia but still contained within Colles' fascial layer tends to give rise to swelling of the penis, the scrotum, the perineum and the anterior abdominal wall. The relationships of the pertinent structures and fascial layers are illustrated in Figure 48-13. Because Colles' fascia is limited laterally by its attachment to the fascia lata and posteriorly by its attachment to the urogenital diaphragm, the only routes for a urinary extravasation contained within this fascia to follow are the abdominoscrotal openings and along the anterior abdominal wall just beneath Camper's and Scarpa's fasciae. These fasciae are continuous with Colles' fascia.

The *diagnosis of stricture* of the urethra is made by calibration, i.e., the passage of various bougies or sounds of increasing diameters up the urethra and through the stricture to determine the diameter and the location of the urethral narrowings. Urethroscopy and urethrography may aid in the diagnosis.

The *prophylactic therapy* of urethral strictures includes (1) the prompt treatment of neisserian and nonspecific pyogenic urethral infections with appropriate antibiotics; (2)

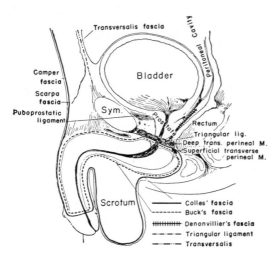

Fig. 48-13. Diagram of fascia of urogenital region concerned in urinary extravasation.

the recognition and the splinting of ruptured urethrae;[75] (3) gentleness and care in urethral instrumentation; and (4) the avoidance of prolonged urethral catheter drainage.

Until recently the only therapy available for established urethral strictures was their dilatation at intervals, frequently for the rest of the patient's life. The Johanson urethroplasty[76, 77] now may be employed to correct them.

Urethrocutaneous fistulae are treated best by excising the tracts and the elimination of the stricture. Urinary extravasation demands the immediate incision and drainage of all areas into which urine has extended and the diversion of the urinary stream by suprapubic cystostomy. After recovery from the acute phase, definitive procedures such as the Johanson urethroplasty are employed to remove the urethral stricture—the cause of all the difficulty.

PROSTATE. *Benign prostatic hypertrophy, fibrosis of the prostate* and *carcinoma of the prostate* are the 3 most common prostatic abnormalities causing prostatism. Prostatism must not be confused with prostatitis which refers to inflammation of the prostate gland. *Prostatism* is a term used to describe any or all of the pathologic and clinical manifestations of urinary obstruction caused by the prostate gland.

A knowledge of the anatomy and the physiology of the prostate is necessary to the understanding of the ways by which disease of this gland impedes the passage of urine.

Physiology. The prostate is a part of the male genital system which undergoes a remarkable pubertal development, provided that the anterior pituitary and the testes are normal. Pubertal enlargement of the prostate and the formation of the prostatic secretion are dependent upon the elaboration of a hormone from the testicular cells of Leydig. In the adult the function of the prostate is the secretion of a fluid forming a part of the ejaculate and providing a transport vehicle and a nutritional medium for the spermatozoa.

Anatomy. The relationships of the prostate to its adjacent structures are illustrated in Figure 48-14. The bladder rests upon the prostate, and the vesical outlet and the proximal urethra are surrounded by it. The ejaculatory ducts from the seminal vesicals traverse the prostate and open into the urethra on either side of the utricle. The ducts of the prostate open into the urethra on each side of the verumontanum. Figure 48-15, a cross section of the prostate, shows it to be composed of 5 lobes: 1 anterior, 2 lateral, 1 median and 1 posterior. Note how they surround the urethra! The entire gland is enclosed in a strong fibrous capsule and anteriorly is fixed to the symphysis by the puboprostatic ligaments.

Benign Prostatic Hypertrophy. After the age of 45 to 50 the submucosal glands and the smooth muscle of the prostatic urethra undergo glandular and leiomyomatous hyperplasia.[78, 79] This growth presses the normal prostatic tissue against the fibrous capsule and forms a so-called surgical capsule—the compressed normal prostatic tissue.

Primary idiopathic prostatic hypertrophy affects primarily the median and the lateral lobes; the anterior and the posterior lobes are not affected.

As the prostate enlarges, it may expand posteriorly and is readily palpated rectally. This type of enlargement may not encroach upon the vesical neck or the urethra, and consequently there may be no symptoms referable to prostatism even though the prostate may be very large. On the other hand, most or all of the hypertrophy may be toward the lumen of the urethra or upward into the bladder through the vesical outlet. In such a case great difficulty in urination occurs, while no prostatic enlargement is discernible upon rectal digital examination. Clearly, the rectal examination of the prostate gland cannot provide for any estimate of the degree of urinary obstruction that may be caused by the gland. However, the rectal examination of the prostate is very important for the determination of the presence or the absence of prostatic

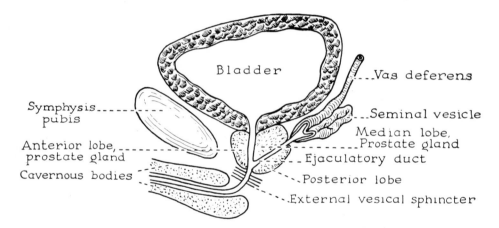

Sagittal Section of Urogenital Tract

FIG. 48-14. Relationships of prostate to its adjacent structures. (R. M. Nesbit)

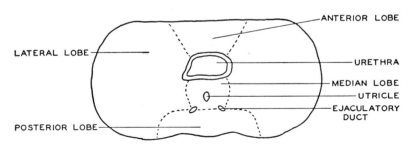

FIG. 48-15. Cross section of the prostate.

carcinoma; in the case of obstructive prostatic hypertrophy it provides the surgeon with a basis for the selection of the appropriate operative procedure.

Fibrosis of the Prostate Gland. This occurs less frequently than hypertrophy and at a younger age. Prostatitis with fibrosis and contracture of the prostatic tissue in the region of the vesical neck is its cause. Frequently, strictures of the urethra are associated with it because the inflammatory process may involve both the urethra and the prostate. Prostatic carcinomatous narrowing of the urethra and the vesical neck also cause prostatism. Carcinomas of the prostate usually originate in the posterior lobe and grow infiltratively into the other prostatic lobes, the seminal vesicles and the bladder (see section on Neoplasms for complete discussion).

Clinical Manifestations of Prostatism. The first symptoms of prostatism are those ascribable to irritation of the bladder; they consist mainly of an abnormal frequency of urination and dysuria. As the obstruction progresses there occur the complaints of difficulty in starting the urinary stream (hesitancy), a decrease in size and force of stream, an interrupted stream and abdominal straining, which may be so intense as to be associated with the passing of flatus, distention of neck veins and protrusion of the eyeballs. At last comes partial or complete urinary retention with its characteristic functional and structural change of obstructive uropathy.

Diagnosis of prostatism is based upon the history, the physical examination, cystometrography and endoscopy. All of these are necessary because urethral strictures, neurogenic bladders, bladder calculi and acute cystitis, having essentially the same signs and symptoms as prostatism, cannot be differentiated from prostatic hypertrophy, fibrosis, or cancer without them.

Treatment of prostatism varies with the cause of the obstruction, the severity of the obstruction and the condition of the patient. Prostatism with only mild symptoms of nocturia and dysuria sometimes can be treated satisfactorily with elixir of hyoscyamus, tincture of belladonna and hot sitz baths.

The patient with a weak, dribbling stream without residual urine or one carrying more than 60 ml. of residual urine requires some

form of prostatectomy, provided that he is not gravely ill from another disease.

Should the person be very ill because of uremia, cardiovascular disease, etc., and is judged incapable of recovering from a prostatectomy, urinary diversion by suprapubic cystostomy or perineal urethrostomy are performed first to permit improvement in the general health before the prostatectomy. A vasectomy is performed in such cases to reduce the incidence of epididymitis. An inlying urethral catheter is a dangerous form of urinary diversion when practiced for more than a week or two because it predisposes to urethritis, prostatitis, epididymitis, pyelonephritis, urethral strictures and urethrocutaneous fistulae.

Vesical neck contractures are sometimes remedied by transurethral resection. A more successful method of treating vesical-neck contractures involves the exposure of the vesical neck, a wedge resection of the fibrous tissue, and an alleviation of the rigidity of the vesical neck with a plastic procedure involving the insertion of a flap of mobile bladder wall into the perimeter of the vesical outlet.

The type of prostatectomy performed should be suited to the particular patient's needs. Transurethral prostatectomy[82] is well suited to the palliative treatment of advanced infiltrating prostatic carcinoma and the definitive care of the majority of patients with benign prostatic hypertrophy. The enucleative procedures such as the suprapubic, retropubic[80] or perineal prostatectomy are more suitable for the removal of very large benign hypertrophic prostates. The various enucleative procedures differ in the way the prostate is reached, but once the plane between the surgical capsule and the adenomatous tissue is found, the procedure is the same. With all types of prostatectomy the prostatic urethra is removed; it regenerates in 4 to 6 weeks. The true capsule is not removed excepting with the performance of the radical perineal or retropubic prostatectomy. This is the only known means of curing an early prostatic carcinoma. The presence of bladder calculi or diverticula in addition to an enlarged prostate may influence the surgeon to use the suprapubic or retropubic approach to the prostate. Fixation of the hip joints so that the lithotomy position, requisite for the transurethral approach, cannot be ob-

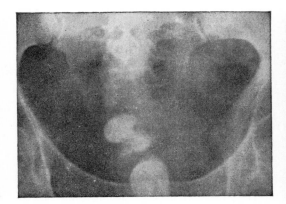

FIG. 48-16. Flat film of the pelvis showing two vesical calculi; one is dumbbell in shape; the other appears to be wedged into the prostatic urethra.

tained, necessitates the suprapubic or retropubic approach.

BLADDER. *Vesical calculi* (Fig. 48-16) occur most frequently as a complication of prostatism, though they may form about a foreign body or in conjunction with urinary tract infections or in the presence of a residual urine due to causes other than prostatism. The symptoms and signs of vesicular lithiasis may be similar to those of prostatism. However, certain symptoms are pathognomonic of a calculus in the bladder, e.g., the patient may complain of difficulty in voiding in the upright position but have no trouble in the supine position. The diagnosis can be made readily with endoscopy or roentgenography. The treatment involves their removal. This can be accomplished in several ways: (1) usually they can be crushed with a lithotrite transurethrally and the fragments evacuated (litholapaxy); (2) or when very large removed unbroken by opening the bladder suprapubically (cystolithotomy).

Vesical neoplasms may obstruct the bladder neck or the ureteral orifices.

URETER. *Ureteral stones, neoplasms and strictures* obstruct the ureter and give rise to hydro-ureter and hydronephrosis. Involvement of the ureter by an adjacent neoplasm, e.g., carcinoma of the cervix or the rectosigmoid may produce ureteral obstruction.

Pregnancy, in most cases, is associated with some degree of hydro-ureter and hydronephrosis. This dilatation of the ureters is presumed

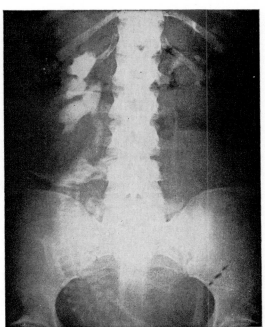

FIG. 48-17. Hydronephrosis of pregnancy.

to be due to the elaboration of progesterone.[85] An additional presumptive factor in the etiology of the hydro-ureter and hydronephrosis of pregnancy[84] is the pressure of the fetus upon the lower ureteral segments. Ureteral and renal pelvic dilatation begin about the 3rd month of pregnancy and disappear completely 6 to 8 weeks postpartum. The hydronephrosis of pregnancy is a normal physiologic phenomenon (Fig. 48-17).

Intermittent hydronephrosis and hydroureter is a syndrome characterized by recurrent episodes of obstruction with associated dilatation of the proximal ureter and renal pelvis which is at first intermittent. It is attended by recurrent attacks of pain in the costovertebral angle area which may radiate typically and be accompanied by nausea, vomiting, tachycardia, and hypotension sometimes called Dietl's crisis. Often the pain occurs while the person lies in a certain position, as upon the right side, the left side, or the back, and disappears when the position is changed, e.g., to the erect position. The entity is suspected from the history and may be confirmed by pyelography. Excretory pyelograms, taken while the patient has pain and is lying in the position inducing it, demonstrate hydroneph-

1370   Urology

rosis; while those performed after the pain has disappeared with position change may show a normal collecting system. Kinking of the ureter over an anomalous renal vessel or fascial band when the kidney shifts with change in position of the body are its causes. The treatment consists of relieving pain during the acute attack by change in position or by opiates. Occasionally, ureteral catheterization may be required for relief. Permanent relief from attacks requires the surgical excision of the causative aberrant vessel or fascial band and the plastic correction of ureteral narrowing which is frequently present.

For many years, a number of operations have been devised and used for the fixation of the highly mobile kidney—renal ptosis. All normal kidneys move downward when a person stands. Excretory pyelograms taken in both the upright and the supine positions show that normal kidneys always move downward when the person stands up. The distance of descent upon standing varies widely; it may be as little as 1 cm. or as much as 8 to 10 cm. Nevertheless, in all cases it should be considered normal, just as pulse rates varying from 60 to 90 per minute may be normal. *Renal mobility is pathologic only when it can be demonstrated objectively that it is associated with hydronephrosis*. The performance of a nephropexy for a nonhydronephrotic mobile kidney is unwarranted excepting in rare instances.

URINARY TRACT INFECTIONS

NONTUBERCULOUS INFECTIONS

Gonorrhea. ETIOLOGY. A neisserian infection[88] is a venereal disease in adults. The offending organism, the gonococcus, is a nonmotile, gram-negative, intracellular diplococcus.

PATHOLOGY. In the male the anterior urethra is invaded first by the organisms. They travel upward along the mucous membrane and in about half of the cases invade the prostatic urethra and the prostate. This in some persons ultimately produces a fibrotic contracture of the vesical neck and obstructive uropathy. In addition, the acute infection may penetrate through the mucosa of the urethra into the corpus spongiosum. The inflammatory process in the corpus spongiosum

may give rise to an urethral stricture which may not become evident until many years after the attack of gonorrhea. The most common sites of urethral strictures in gonorrhea are the bulbous and pendulous portions of the urethra.

SYMPTOMS AND SIGNS. From 3 to 5 days after exposure to the gonococcus, swelling, redness and pouting of the urethral meatus appear and are associated with the dripping of a greenish-white pus through the urethral meatus. Urination is painful, and painful nocturnal erections are frequent. These occasionally are associated with a downward curvature of the erect penis called chordee. The relative inelasticity of the inferiorly placed inflamed urethra causes the downward curvature.

As the posterior urethra becomes inflamed, the frequency of urination and the dysuria increase, and strangury, the slow painful, passage of urine, may occur.

DIAGNOSIS. The impression of urethral gonorrhea is obtained from the history and the physical examination. A positive diagnosis is made by smearing the urethral discharge and demonstrating the presence of gram-negative intracellular diplococci with stains and is further confirmed by culture.

TREATMENT. Penicillin is highly effective and inexpensive. As little as one intramuscular dose of 400,000 units may cure gonorrhea.[87] In case of an allergic sensitivity to penicillin, tetracycline and erythromycin may be used. A cure is judged to have been effected when 1 week after stopping antibiotic therapy no gonococci are grown from cultures of the urethral discharge.

Nongonorrheal Infections. Bacterial invasion of the urinary tract is a very serious matter. It causes discomfort, pain and on occasion, sepsis. It predisposes to calculus formation and strictures. Should bacterial nephritis occur, pyelonephritis may destroy the kidney, jeopardizing the person's life with renal insufficiency or renal hypertensive cardiovascular disease.

ETIOLOGY. The majority of these infections of the urinary tract are caused by members of the gram-negative bacillary group. *Escherichia coli* is the most common offender in this regard. Organisms may reach the kidney by ascending the lumen of the ureter, through the periureteral lymphatics or by way of the

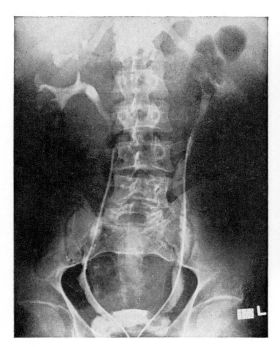

FIG. 48-18. Retrograde ureterogram, illustrating ureteritis cystica.

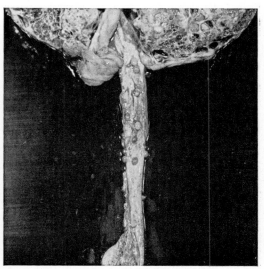

FIG. 48-19. Ureteritis cystica.

blood stream. Factors predisposing to infection of the urinary tract are urethral catheterization and instrumentation, poor vaginal hygiene, defloration, urinary stasis, calculi, diabetes mellitus, neoplasms, foreign bodies and trauma.

Occasionally, the kidney is involved by an acute staphylococcal infection. This infection is so different from the others that it will be discussed as a separate entity under perinephric abscess.

PATHOLOGY. Acute cystitis and urethritis do occur without involvement of the upper urinary tract. With these entities the bladder and the urethra are erythematous, edematous and congested. Acute pyelonephritis[91] is an inflammation of the renal pelvis, the tubules and the interstitial tissue. Acute pyelitis is a misnomer, since it is only part of the generalized process of pyelonephritis.

A chronic infection of the bladder will frequently cause hyperplastic cystitis, e.g., cystitis glandularis and cystitis cystica. If the infection is caused by an organism which splits urea with formation of ammonia, the interior of the bladder may be coated with encrusta-tions of mineral salt—the so-called ammoniacal encrustive cystitis. Cystic change (ureteritis cystica, Figs. 48-18 and 48-19) may occur in the chronically infected ureter as it does in the bladder.

Renal parenchymal suppuration may attend acute pyelonephritis. These abscesses tend to break out into the perinephritic tissue and produce perinephritis and perinephritic abscesses. Occasionally, the kidney is functionally destroyed. If the pyelonephritis is mild and subsides completely, the kidney may show no demonstrable injury. However, severe pyelonephritis always leaves residua, such as atrophy, fibrosis and cellular infiltration of the renal parenchyma and sclerosis of the renal vessels. The kidney may be smaller than normal with narrowed infundibula and hydrocalyxes (Figs. 48-20 and 48-21).

Acute pyelonephritis may clear up completely but all too often it only simmers down and smolders and becomes chronic active pyelonephritis. Chronic active pyelonephritis is an active inflammatory process of the kidney and its pelvis superimposed upon fibrosis and contracture, etc. This ultimately leads to complete destruction of the kidney and its function, an autonephrectomy.

SIGNS AND SYMPTOMS. Should the infection be limited to the lower tract, an increased frequency of urination, dysuria, urgency, pyuria and occasional hematuria are the predominant

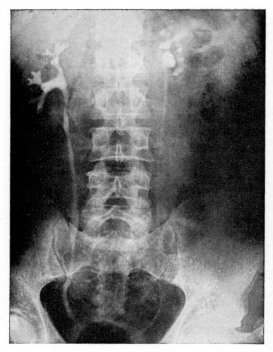

Fig. 48-20. Contracted left kidney, due to chronic pyelonephritis.

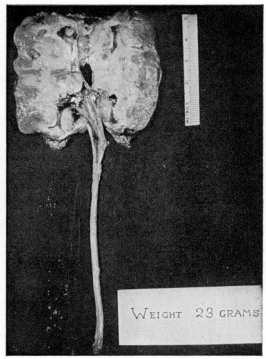

Fig. 48-21. Far-advanced chronic pyelonephritis with secondary contraction of the kidney.

signs and symptoms. Should pyelonephritis become superimposed upon cystitis, additional signs and symptoms appear: chills and fever, pain and tenderness in the costovertebral area, nausea, vomiting and prostration.

DIAGNOSIS. The presence of pathogenic bacteria and leukocytes in catheterized urine associated with the above signs and symptoms establishes the diagnosis of a urinary tract infection. Calyceal contractures and abnormalities characteristic of chronic active pyelonephritis may be demonstrated by intravenous pyelography. Retrograde ureteral catheterization may be necessary to confirm the presence and the extent of chronic active pyelonephritis.

THERAPY. Urinary tract infections must be treated in an orderly manner. The infection should be cured in the shortest time with the least cost to the patient and, most importantly, in such a way as not to permit the overlooking of serious disease of the urinary organs.

Upon finding pathogenic organisms in the urine of a person having symptoms and signs of an infection of the urinary tract cultures

should be submitted immediately for sensitivity tests (see Chap. 3, "Applied Surgical Bacteriology"). While awaiting the results of the sensitivity tests Gantrisin is prescribed for a period of 7 to 10 days in a dose of 1 Gm. Q.I.D. for urinary bacillary infections unattended with septicemia. If cocci are present in the urine, penicillin is prescribed for the same period of time. *At the end of 1 week the patient is rechecked, and if the infection is still present, a complete investigation of the urinary tract is indicated.* This must include urethroscopy, cystoscopy, retrograde pyelograms and separate urine specimens from each kidney for culture and sensitivity studies for pyogens as well as tubercle bacilli. *The practice of switching to another drug without investigating the cause of persistent pyuria is to be condemned, because the common causes of a persisting infection are neoplasms, tuberculosis, calculous disease, hydronephrosis and resistant organisms.* If the urinary tract is negative and the persistent infection is due to organisms resistant to the drugs used, culture and sensitivity studies will help in selecting the proper antibiotics.[92] If neoplasm, calculus, or obstructive uropathy is present, appropriate therapy for it is utilized first, and then the infection is treated. Obstructive uropathy is a common cause for the persistence of an infection in the urinary tract above the obstruction. In reality an infection above an obstruction is an abscess. Removal of the obstruction is requisite to the cure of the infection just as drainage of an abscess is still a definitive method of treating it wherever it exists.

If the infection clears promptly in 7 to 10 days with the use of Gantrisin, penicillin, or a combination of both, excretory pyelograms should be obtained to rule out the possibility of upper urinary tract disease.

When the urinary tract infection involves the kidney or when acute cystitis is so severe that septicemia is present, the initial medication should be a combination of potent drugs, such as streptomycin (2.0 Gm. per day) and penicillin (400,000 units per day). After a week of therapy the course of the patient will indicate the type of further studies to be done (as previously indicated).

Perinephric Abscess. Bacillary pyelonephritis, tuberculous pyelonephritis, traumatic rupture of the kidney and acute staphylococcal infections may lead to perinephric suppuration,[95] i.e., pus situated about the kidney but lying without the renal capsule.

ETIOLOGY. Infection may reach the perinephric space and tissues by direct extension from a cortical abscess, by lymphatic extension from a renal lesion or by the hematogenous route from an extra-urinary tract infection.

PATHOLOGY. Usually the perinephric infection begins within Gerota's fascia. From there it may spread downward inside the periureteral fascia and ultimately point in the floor of the bladder; it may extend through Gerota's fascia and pass superiorly to involve the diaphragm and the adjacent pleura; occasionally, it will penetrate the lung and drain into a bronchus,[97] forming a bronchoperinephric fistula; it may pass downward in the retroperitoneal space to point at Petit's triangle or to present itself in the perineum via the ischiorectal fossa.

SIGNS AND SYMPTOMS. The clinical manifestations of perinephric abscess are varied, depending upon the severity of the process and its chronicity. An acute fulminating infection is characterized by an abrupt onset with high fever to 105° F., chills, severe pain and tenderness in the costovertebral area; swelling, redness and increased warmth in the flank area; and nausea, vomiting, anorexia and prostration. The urine may contain leukocytes and bacilli if a bacillary pyelonephritis is present, or it may contain only cocci and be without leukocytes for a day or so if a staphylococcal infection is the etiologic agent. Generally, a leukocytosis exists. When the perinephric abscess is subdiaphragmatic, there may be rales, absent breath sounds and dullness to percussion in the lower lung field adjacent to the perinephric abscess.

If the perinephric abscess has been present for months, the patient may exhibit generalized debility, cachexia, anemia, low-grade fever, chronic discomfort in the flank area, infected urine and slightly elevated white count. Occasionally, these abscesses produce no signs other than fever and leukocytosis. In fact, perinephric abscesses constitute one of the important causes of "pyrexia of unknown origin."

DIAGNOSIS. In addition to the signs and symptoms, both needle aspiration of the fluctuant area through a large short-beveled needle and pyelography may aid in diagnosis. Typical x-ray findings of a perinephric abscess are: (1) absence of the psoas shadow on the involved side—this sign attends the collection of fluid in the retroperitoneal space; (2) lateral deviation of the spine with the concavity or hollow toward the abscess; and (3) fixation of the kidney on the affected side—the fibrosis and the adhesions produced by the inflammatory process immobilize the kidney. Fixation of the kidney is demonstrated by taking a pyelographic film while the patient is breathing (the renal shadow will be clear on the side of fixity and indefinite on the side of the mobile kidney) or by comparing films made in the supine and the erect positions.

TREATMENT. Prompt incision and drainage of the abscess is the treatment. Appropriate antibacterial therapy is not used unless high fever persists after the abscess is drained. If the kidney has been severely damaged or destroyed by calculus pyonephrosis, pyelonephritis, etc., and the other kidney is sufficiently functional, a nephrectomy is performed after the patient has recovered fully from the ravages of the perinephric abscess.

Staphylococcal Kidney. Staphylococcal infections of the kidney[96] are peculiar in that the organism almost invariably reaches the renal cortex by way of the blood stream. Furuncles and carbuncles of the skin and upper respiratory infections are common origins for the organism.

PATHOLOGY. Abscesses are produced in the renal cortex by the staphylococcus. The abscesses may heal spontaneously with practically no residua or they may coalesce to form large abscesses of the kidney, the so-called renal carbuncle.[93] The infection may extend to the perinephric tissue, with a resultant perinephric abscess.

SIGNS AND SYMPTOMS. Fever, chills, costovertebral tenderness, and pain are the usual manifestations of staphylococcal kidney. Early in the illness urinalysis demonstrates cocci but no leukocytes. No symptoms of cystitis occur unless there is secondary invasion of the urinary tract by the colon bacilli; this phenomenon occurs in about one half of the cases of staphylococcal kidney during the 2nd week of the disease.

THERAPY. Appropriate antibiotics administered parenterally constitute an effective form of treatment, provided that destruction of the kidney or a perinephric abscess do not exist (see Chap. 3, "Applied Surgical Bacteriology," for specific management of staphylococcal infections).

TUBERCULOUS INFECTIONS

Tuberculosis of the genitourinary system is always secondary to tuberculosis elsewhere in the body. The primary origin may be in the lung or infected lymph nodes. Many cases of urinary tract tuberculosis occur in individuals with no apparent evidence of active tuberculosis. The tubercle bacilli reach the cortex of the kidney through the blood stream; therefore, the infection tends to be bilateral. The primary renal tuberculous lesions may heal spontaneously[102] and remain unsuspected until demonstrated at autopsy.

Pathology. The initial lesion of renal tuberculosis[101] occurs in the glomerulus. From there it may break into the tubule and from the

tubule extend into the peritubular tissue, as well as down the tubule, involving the mucosa and the submucosa of the renal pelvis. Having affected the renal pelvis, then it may spread back into another portion of the kidney. It may attack the ureter and the bladder by direct mucosal or submucosal spread. Ulceration, caseating necrosis and fibrosis occur in the involved area, and these in turn give rise to strictures of the infundibula, the renal pelvis and the ureter and contraction of the bladder. In addition, the fibrosis and the stenosis may result in hydrocalysis, hydronephrosis or even complete obliteration of the ureteral lumen with resultant autonephrectomy.

Tuberculous involvement of the prostate, the seminal vesicles and the epididymides occurs in 75 per cent of males having renal tuberculosis. A small number of male patients have genital tuberculosis without apparent renal tuberculosis; the infection in these cases is believed to be hematogenous in origin.

Signs and Symptoms. The usual symptoms are those of severe bladder irritation associated with pyuria, microscopic hematuria and the absence of bacteria when the usual staining technics are used alone.

Diagnosis. A history of persistent pyuria, recurrent urinary tract infections and/or marked bladder irritability should make the clinician suspicious of tuberculosis and lead to the performance of endoscopy, retrograde pyelograms and the collection of urine specimens from each kidney and the staining and culturing of these urines for *Myobacterium tuberculosis*.

Tuberculous ulceration of the bladder mucosa may be seen through the cystoscope, and often the pyelograms will demonstrate irregular, moth-eaten-appearing calyces (Fig. 48-22 and 48-23). The ureters may be irregularly dilated and stenosed.

Positive diagnosis of tuberculosis is made after tubercle bacilli have been demonstrated in the urine by culture and guinea pig inoculation.

Treatment. The present therapy of genitourinary tuberculosis involves: (1) prolonged rest; (2) the use of antituberculous drugs; and (3) surgical procedures. Most therapeutic regimens are based on combinations of streptomycin, Isoniazid and para-aminosalicylic

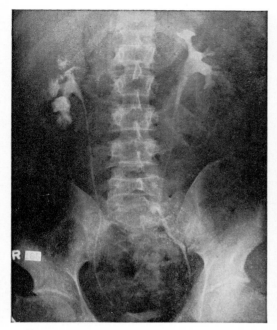

Fig. 48-22. Right renal and ureteral tuberculosis.

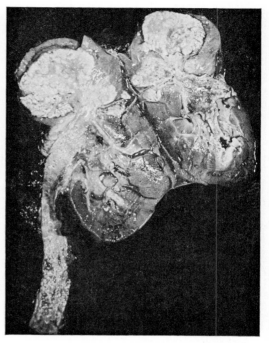

Fig. 48-23. Tuberculous involvement of the kidney and the ureter.

acid. These agents are given for periods of time varying from 1 to 2 years.[100]

Nephrectomy is indicated in cases of extensive unilateral renal tuberculosis because this type does not respond well to drug therapy. All operative procedures dealing with tuberculous organs are preceded by at least 1 week of specific drug therapy. The antituberculous drugs are continued after nephrectomy for at least 1 year.

Prognosis. The present-day antituberculous regimens have definitely improved the prognosis of genitourinary tuberculosis. Available statistics suggest an over-all arrest rate of 70 to 80 per cent for renal tuberculosis now.

NEOPLASMS OF THE GENITOURINARY TRACT

KIDNEY

Wilms's Tumor. Tumors of the kidney in children demonstrate both epithelial and connective tissue structures and have been called adenosarcoma, adenorhabdomyosarcoma, etc. The etiology is unknown.

SIGNS AND SYMPTOMS. The most common manifestation of Wilms's tumor is an abdominal mass, usually first noticed by the mother when bathing or caring for the child. Other symptoms and signs may be fever, malaise, loss of weight and anemia; these occur when the neoplasm is very large or has metastasized.

DIAGNOSIS. The suggestion of a renal neoplasm on physical examination is confirmable by pyelography.

TREATMENT. Nephrectomy combined with irradiation is a fairly effective form of therapy.[107] The x-ray therapy may be given either preoperatively or postoperatively. If the tumor is very large, preoperative irradiation will shrink the neoplasm and make it easier to remove.

PROGNOSIS. The use of irradiation in conjunction with nephrectomy has provided a 5-year survival rate varying from 50 to 60 per cent. Unfortunately, deaths from the tumor may occur after the 5th year.

Hypernephroma. The most common malignant renal tumor in the adult is the renal cell carcinoma which arises from the renal tubule.

PATHOLOGY. Grossly, the tumor is well encapsulated, vascular and composed of

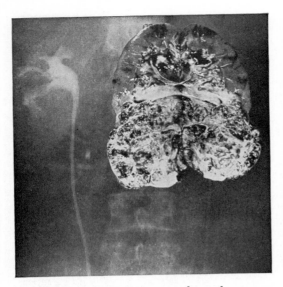

FIG. 48-24. Right retrograde pyelogram demonstrates a tumor deformity. Bivalved kidney specimen shows a hypernephroma involving the lower half of the kidney and accounting for the pyelographic abnormality.

yellowish-white lobules. Microscopically, the neoplastic cellular population contains large clear polygonal cells and small dark granular cells. The neoplasm grows into the renal venules and may block the renal veins. In the male this often gives rise to varicocele on the left side, because the left spermatic vein empties into the left renal vein. This does not happen with right renal tumors, because the right spermatic vein enters the vena cava. Consequently, these tumors metastasize frequently via the renal vein. Metastases to the lung are very common. Hypernephroma is one of the neoplasms with special predilection to bone metastases. Bilateral hypernephromas are not uncommon.

SIGNS AND SYMPTOMS. Gross hematuria is the most common sign of this primary renal parenchymal neoplasm. Some of the patients bearing it may have palpable abdominal masses as well as fever and an anemia of unknown origin.

DIAGNOSIS. Retrograde pyelography demonstrates the characteristic features of a neoplasm of the renal parenchyma, namely, distortion and elongation of the infundibula and the calyces, flattening of the collecting system

and enlargement of the renal outline (Fig. 48-24). Exfoliative cytologic smears[111] of the urine may contain neoplastic cells.

TREATMENT. A nephrectomy should be performed[110] if demonstrable metastases have not occurred and the opposite kidney is adequately functional. Irradiation may be applied to inoperable lesions, but little should be expected from it, because hypernephromas are radioresistant. Some surgeons believe that demonstrable metastasis does not contraindicate nephrectomy, because the metastases at times may grow very slowly, and removal of the primary often controls the fever and anemia.

PROGNOSIS. The 5-year survival rate is 25 per cent after nephrectomy is performed in cases without demonstrable metastases.

Neoplasms of the Collecting System. The most common cancer of the renal pelvis is the transitional cell papillary carcinoma. Other less common neoplasms are adenocarcinoma and squamous cell carcinoma. Over 50 per cent of the squamous cell carcinomata occur in association with calculi in the renal pelvis.

SIGNS AND SYMPTOMS. Compared with hypernephromas, tumors of the renal pelvis[110] give rise to episodes of gross total hematuria relatively early. The reason is obvious. The pelvic neoplasm is located in the collecting system, and any bleeding erosion thereof will be attended by the appearance of blood in the urine immediately, while before the hypernephroma causes gross hematuria it must grow extensively and break into the collecting system, and this takes time.

Other clinical evidences of renal pelvic tumors may be pain and tenderness in the costovertebral area, fever, malaise, anemia and occasional renal and ureteral colic attendant upon the passage of blood clots.

DIAGNOSIS. Pyelography will demonstrate a filling defect in the renal pelvis. Other causes for filling defects of the renal pelvis are blood clots and nonopaque calculi. Repeat pyelograms in 5 to 7 days will rule out blood clots, since clots in the pelvis tend to disappear within a week. Occasionally, cystoscopy is an aid in making the diagnosis, for one may see a papillary growth protruding through the ureteral orifice or surrounding the ureteral orifice.

TREATMENT. Nephrectomy is indicated for squamous cell carcinoma and adenocarcinoma of the renal pelvis. Nephro-ureterectomy with excision of a small cuff of bladder around the ureteral orifice is the treatment for papillary neoplasm of the renal pelvis. This extensive excision of ureter and uretervesical structure is necessary because the urothelium on the same side as the neoplasm is predisposed to formation of other papillary cancers should it not be removed.

URETER

Incidence. Primary ureteral neoplasms[115] are relatively rare. The most common type of tumor is the transitional cell papilloma and papillary carcinoma. Neoplastic growths in the ureter are more frequently metastases from carcinomas primary in the cervix, the rectum, the prostate and the bladder than they are carcinomas primary in the ureter.

Signs and Symptoms. Gross hematuria is the most common presenting symptom and sign by virtue of the erosion of the neoplasm. Neoplastic obstruction to the flow of urine through the ureter ultimately gives rise to ureteral colic, dull flank pain, costovertebral tenderness, fever and chills.

Diagnosis. A filling defect in the ureter is readily demonstrated pyelographically, and upon cystoscopy blood may be seen spurting from the ureteral orifice.

Treatment. Nephrecto-ureterectomy is indicated (provided that the opposite kidney is adequately functional).

BLADDER

Incidence. Tumors of the bladder[116, 122] are similar to those of the renal pelvis and the ureter. The most common neoplasms are the transitional cell papilloma and papillary carcinoma, while the less common tumors are the squamous cell carcinoma and the adenocarcinoma. Sarcoma is very rare, very malignant and has a poor prognosis.

Pathology. Grossly, tumors of the bladder may appear flat (sessile), polypoid or papilliferous. The neoplasms may involve only the mucosa but it ultimately extends into or through any or all of the layers of the bladder. It may be anywhere in the bladder and cover areas of all sizes. It can occlude the ureteral orifices as well as the vesical neck.

Etiology. Not all of the causes for neoplasm of the bladder epithelium are known. Chronic irritation, chronic infection and urinary steroids[120] have been suggested as possible causes, while certain aniline dyes and bilharziasis are known to contribute to the genesis of bladder carcinoma.

Signs and Symptoms. Hematuria is the most common and constant finding in patients having bladder neoplasms. Persistent and recurrent urinary tract infections are also frequent manifestations. Other symptoms of it are urgency, increased frequency of urination and dysuria.

Diagnosis. Cystoscopy and biopsy of the bladder lesion provide a positive diagnosis. The extent of the lesion can be estimated grossly by bimanual examination under anesthesia.[119] The Papanicolaou method for studying cells shed from the bladder wall is being evaluated at the present time relative to its place in diagnostic urology. It now appears that exfoliative cytology will not replace cystoscopy as the primary method for making a diagnosis. However, it may be the most important procedure for making a diagnosis in cases of sessile, infiltrating neoplasms of bladders with generalized vesical inflammation.

Prognosis. This depends somewhat upon the characteristics of the tumor. The prognosis is poorer for infiltrating than for noninfiltrating types. The growth of a tumor more than halfway through the muscularis reduces the prospect for 5 years or more of life almost to the vanishing point.

Treatment. The ideal treatment for *all bladder neoplasms* would be complete cystectomy and transplantation of the ureters into the bowel. Unfortunately, uretero-intestinal transplantation has led in the past to many troubles with ascending pyelonephritis and renal failure.[118] Therefore, cystectomy has not been adopted as the best way to treat carcinomas of the bladder. Recent experience with the implantation of the ureters into ileal segments suggests that this type of urinary diversion may obviate some of the complications seen previously with uretero-intestinal anastomoses. However, more conservative measures still are being used, e.g., transurethral resection, segmental resection of the bladder and fulguration. Without a doubt, cystectomy is indicated for multiple papillomata and superficially infiltrating lesions not amenable to less extensive procedures.

Uretero-intestinal transplantation without cystectomy is a valuable operation for patients with inoperable bladder neoplasms who have strangury and intermittent vesical obstruction by blood clots. However, transplantation does not stop hemorrhage from the vesical cancer but may reduce it.

A patient having a vesical neoplasm treated by fulguration or local irradiation must return for periodic examination of the bladder for the rest of his or her natural life, because persistent growth as well as new growths are common.

PROSTATE GLAND

Incidence. Carcinoma of the prostate occurs in 15 to 30 per cent of all males past the age of 50 years who have testes. Prostatic neoplasms do not occur in eunuchs.

Etiology is unknown.

Pathology. Adenocarcinoma usually originates in the posterior lobe of the prostate and spreads by local infiltration into the remainder of the gland, the seminal vesicles and the bladder. It may invade the lymphatics and the vertebral veins[125] and has a marked predilection for spread to the bones of the pelvis and the lumbosacral vertebrae. Terminally prostatic carcinoma may be found in practically all of the organs of the body.

Signs and Symptoms. All of the symptoms of prostatism attend the neoplastic obstruction of the prostatic urethra, osseous pain attends osseous metastases, and no symptoms are experienced so long as the lesion has neither obstructed the flow of urine nor metastasized. Rectal palpation may disclose a stony-hard, nodular prostate, or a hard, smooth prostate with obliterated lateral and median sulci.

Diagnosis. Early isolated carcinomatous nodules can be detected only by digital rectal examination of the prostate. Metastatic neoplasm often can be discovered by roentgenography of the pelvis, and the determination of serum acid phosphatase. Ultimately, carcinoma of the prostate causes metastases in most patients. When this occurs the serum acid phosphatase rises above normal in approximately 60 per cent of patients.[130] Many prostatic carcinomas are physiologically similar to normal prostatic tissue in that they produce enzymes, e.g., acid phosphatase and fibrinolysins.[132] Consequently, when they me-

tastasize into bone, lymphatics or blood vessels the concentration of fibrinolysin and acid phosphatase in the blood rises. Normally, acid phosphatase and fibrinolysin are found in the seminal fluid.

Treatment. Radical removal of the prostate and the seminal vesicles by the retropubic or perineal approach is the only method by which cure can be obtained. Radical prostatectomy is indicated only if there are no obvious signs of metastases.

Transurethral prostatectomy is utilized for the relief of obstructions due to infiltrating neoplastic glands.

Bilateral orchiectomy and stilbestrol, 1 mg. per day, are indicated for glands not amenable to radical removal, as soon as the diagnosis is made. This treatment is based on the work of Huggins and others[127] who demonstrated that the growth and the hormonal stimulation of prostatic cancer are partially dependent upon androgens elaborated by the testes and the adrenals. Suppression of the androgens by orchiectomy and stilbestrol temporarily inhibits the growth of many prostatic cancers.[129] However, the prostatic neoplasm eventually adapts itself and grows rapidly again.

Relapses after orchiectomy and stilbestrol have been treated with high doses of cortisone, hypophysectomy, stilbestrol diphosphate and radioactive phosphorus. In many cases these forms of therapy afford a further period of comfortable existence. None is curative.

Flocks[126] is using intraprostatic injections of radioactive gold to control the growth of prostatic neoplasm not confined entirely to the gland.

URETHRA

Incidence. Neoplasm of the urethra are rare in both men and women. In the male carcinoma of the urethra[133] occurs in association with stricture in 50 per cent of the cases.

Pathologically, most of the neoplasms are squamous cell in type and arise from the distal portion of the urethra which is lined by stratified squamous epithelium.

Clinical manifestations of urethral neoplasms may be bleeding from the urethra, difficulty in voiding and dysuria.

Diagnosis is made by urethroscopy and biopsy of the lesions. Condyloma accuminata and, in women, urethral caruncle may be difficult to distinguish from urethral meatal carcinoma.

Treatment of a localized urethral neoplasm is the radical excision of the urethra. However, most urethral neoplasms have infiltrated beyond the walls of the urethra when seen by the physician and are amenable only to palliative therapy. This consists of either internal or external irradiation and suprapubic urinary diversion. The prognosis of urethral carcinoma is poor.

PENIS

Incidence. Carcinoma of the penis is relatively common among uncircumcised men and rare among the circumcised.

Etiology.[138] Smegma has been demonstrated to contain material which is carcinogenic for animals. It is probable that the retention of smegma is intimately concerned with the formation of penile cancer among the uncircumcised.

Pathology. Neoplasms of the penis are squamous cell in type. Precancerous lesions are erythroplasia, leukoplakia and condylomata.[137] The penile neoplasms metastasize to the superficial and deep inguinal as well as to the external iliac lymph nodes.

Diagnosis. Carcinoma of the penis may involve the prepuce, the glans and the shaft. Inspection and palpation of the penis will suggest neoplasm which is confirmed by biopsy.

Treatment. Partial[135] or radical amputation of the penis and bilateral inguinofemoral node dissection is the therapy of choice. Radical amputation and perineal urethrotomy are done when anticipated excision of the involved penis plus 1 cm. of normal tissue will leave an inadequate stump of urethra for urination, i.e., the patient would soil his scrotum and perineum when voiding. Prophylactic treatment[134] consists of circumcision, preferably shortly after birth.

Prognosis. Cancer of the penis is relatively slow-growing and thus bears a favorable outlook if discovered early. Death in patients with far-advanced cancer of the penis may ultimately result from exsanguination caused by erosion of the iliac or the femoral blood vessels.

SCROTUM

Squamous cell carcinoma of the scrotum[140] may be caused by such skin irritants as soot and petroleum products. It is seen infrequently today. The diagnosis is made by biopsy. Therapy consists of its local excision with a wide margin of normal skin.

TESTIS

Incidence. Several of the most malignant neoplasms arise in the testicle. Although appearing at any age, they occur most commonly during the 2nd and the 3rd decades of life. Testicular cancer is insidious and metastasizes early. Statistics suggest that it is 22 times more frequent in the cryptorchid than in the normally descended testis, and this relationship pertains in both the uncorrected and the corrected cryptorchids.

Etiology. There are 2 theories[146] regarding the origin of testicular neoplasms. One theory proposes that it arises from cell rests, and the other that testicular neoplasms arise from the germinal tissue of an identical twin in the testicle.

Pathology. The types of testicular neoplasm[143] are teratoma, seminoma, embryonal carcinoma, chorio-epithelioma, teratocarcinoma and interstitial cell neoplasm. When a testicular tumor metastasizes, it usually does so by the lymphatic route and to a lesser degree through the blood vessels; chorio-epithelioma differs from the rest in that it invades and metastasizes through blood vessels early. Since the lymphatics closely follow the route of the internal spermatic vessels which supply the testes, the first lymphatic nodes to be involved usually will be the retroperitoneal nodes in the region of the renal pedicles. Spread from these nodes involves the preaortic nodes.

Signs and Symptoms. Most of the testicular neoplasms are asymptomatic and cause only slight enlargement of the testis. Occasionally, some of the neoplasms secrete estrogens, making gynecomastia an early sign. Testicular pain occurs frequently.

Fever, anemia, dyspnea and mid-line abdominal masses are late manifestations of metastatic testicular neoplasms.

Diagnosis. Since neoplasms of the testicle are so malignant, a scrotal mass should be presumed to be a cancer of the testicle until proved to be benign. A "red herring," frequently placed in the diagnostic pathway, is the history of trauma. *In the author's experience scrotal swelling due to trauma is seen less frequently than any other scrotal enlargement.* Scrotal masses may be due to acute or chronic epididymitis, hydrocele, spermatocele, hernia, torsion of the testis and testicular granulomata. Transillumination and needle aspiration (if the mass transilluminates) will establish the diagnosis of spermatocele and hydrocele. Palpation of the testis always should be done again after aspiration, because occasionally a testicular neoplasm occurs in conjunction with a hydrocele. Epididymitis is a frequent cause of scrotal swelling and is associated usually with urinary tract infections.

If there is the slightest doubt in the mind of the examiner as to the diagnosis of the scrotal swelling, the contents of the scrotum should be exposed surgically and examined without spreading tumor cells.

The Aschheim-Zondek test for chorionic gonadotropin[148] in the urine is used as an aid in diagnosis as well as prognosis. Some patients have testicular tumors which elaborate chorionic gonadotropin, and their urine will give a positive A-Z test. The A-Z test will become negative after complete excision of the tumor. Recurrence of the neoplasm is indicated by a positive A-Z test after an initial postoperative negative test.

Chest roentgenogram and intravenous pyelograms are obtained for determination of metastases. The findings on chest roentgenograms are obvious; on pyelography massive metastatic involvement of the retroperitoneal lymph nodes often will displace the upper two thirds of the ureters laterally.

Treatment. Radical orchiectomy and removal of retroperitoneal lymph nodes[145] followed by external irradiation is the modern form of therapy[144] for all malignant testicular neoplasms. If obvious metastases to the lungs or the retroperitoneal nodes are present, palliative irradiation and chemotherapy may be used.

Prognosis. The survival rate depends upon the type of testicular neoplasm. Seminomas offer the best prognosis because they are very radiosensitive. The outlook for chorio-epitheliomas is very poor. Most patients with per-

sistent testicular neoplasms die within 2 years after the diagnosis is made.

CALCULOUS DISEASE

The cause of stones in the urinary tract are unknown in at least 50 per cent of the cases.[160] Often, the normal urine is supersaturated with salts which are held in solution by chelating compounds such as amino acids, colloids, citric acid, etc. When the solute status of supersaturated urine is changed, the salts may precipitate and form calculi. Factors which may upset the solute status are: (1) a change in urinary pH, (2) a decrease in urinary chelating compounds, (3) an increase in urinary salts and (4) the presence of a nidus.

Etiology. When urine becomes highly alkaline, i.e., pH above 7.0, calcium phosphate tends to precipitate. This occurs among patients on a Sippy regimen, which not only alkalinizes the urine but tends to cause hypercalciuria. Renal tubular acidosis[149] resulting from impairment of the base-saving mechanism in the distal tubule, also gives rise to an alkaline urine and hypercalcinuria. Infections of the urine with urea-splitting ammonia-forming organisms[152] (*Pseudomonas aeruginosa, Proteus vulgaris,* etc.) alkalinizes the urine and promotes the formation of stones containing calcium, magnesium, ammonium and phosphate. It is believed that the most common cause for uric acid stones is a persistently acid urine rather than the excretion of excessive quantities of uric acid.[155]

Little is known about the role of urinary chelating compounds in the formation of urinary calculi.

Urinary salts precipitate upon foreign bodies and may even precipitate upon small areas of the renal papillae. The nidus may be a catheter, a hairpin, a piece of wire, desquamated epithelial cells (especially in vitamin A deficiency), necrotic tissue with pyelonephritis or neoplasm and clumps of bacteria. All urinary calculi are believed to have an organic matrix composed of mucoid material.[150]

The excessive excretion of urinary crystalloids is frequently the cause of urinary calculi. Patients with cystinuria[154] are notorious stone formers. Uric acid stones[157] may form in persons having gout. Any patient with hypercalciuria is prone to form stones. Hypercalciuria occurs with hyperparathyroidism, the excessive ingestion of vitamin D, acidosis, extensive bone disease, immobilization of the patient in casts, bed or frame and in idiopathic increased absorption of calcium by the gut.[151]

All patients with renal or ureteral calculi should be studied to determine the possible causes of their stones prior to any operative procedure for removal of the calculi, unless the patient's condition is so serious that immediate operative intervention is indicated. The reasoning behind this involves the possibility of recurrent stone formation during the postoperative period if the etiologic factor is not removed first. Diagnostic studies should include repeated determinations of serum calcium, phosphorus, sodium, potassium, chloride, bicarbonate, protein, uric acid, BUN and creatinine levels, urinary calcium, phosphorus and creatinine concentrations, and the pH of the urine. The serum calcium, phosphorus and creatinine, and the urinary calcium, phosphorus and creatinine levels are obtained with the patient on a normal diet and then on a low calcium phosphorus intake. With these studies one can search for hyperparathyroidism,[153] renal tubular acidosis, persistently alkaline or acid urine, etc.

Pathology. Calculi may obstruct the urinary tract anywhere and produce obstructive uropathy with renal or ureteral colic, hydro-ureter, hydronephrosis, renal atrophy and uremia. Sharp stones may lodge in the ureter and induce ulceration, erosion, perforation, urinary extravasation and stricture. Stones in the urinary tract predispose the person bearing them to urinary tract infections.

Types of Stones. In North America the most common component of the first stone is *calcium oxalate.* Calcium oxalate is radiopaque. *Calcium phosphate,* also radiopaque, is the primary constituent of recurrent calculi. Stones of *uric acid* or *cystine* are *not* radiopaque and occur less frequently than phosphate and oxalate stones.

Signs and Symptoms. Renal calculi may be silent, producing no symptoms, or, when in the renal pelvis, may be associated with constant dull flank pain or sharp, excruciating pain in the costovertebral region and flank. At times the pain of renal calculus origin may simulate closely the pain of peptic ulcer or obstruction of the biliary tract. The passage

of a calculus down the ureter is associated at times with excruciating pain, characterized by intermittency, radiation from the flank area anteriorly down the course of the ureter, ending in the scrotum or the labium majus and at times down the leg. Prostration is frequent, and hypotension may occur.

A vesical calculus usually is attended by frequency, urgency, hematuria and dysuria. Occasionally, it obstructs the vesical outlet during upright voiding but not while voiding in the supine position; this is pathognomonic of a bladder stone.

Fever and chills may accompany the pain. Anuria occurs occasionally with ureteral calculus obstruction and the more frequently in persons having only one kidney.

Diagnosis. A history characteristic of renal or ureteral colic or vesical obstruction by stone and the presence of red blood cells in the urine are suggestive of urinary calculus. Should the stone be opaque, a plain roentgenogram covering the renal, the ureteral and the vesicular areas may demonstrate an opacity. In the case of nonopaque stone, excretory pyelograms may show only the existence of a hydro-ureter, hydronephrosis or a delayed excretion of the contrast medium on the involved side. Endoscopy permits direct confirmation of the presence of bladder calculi, and retrograde catheterization that of ureteral calculus. Oblique films with the catheter in the ureter aid in differentiating ureteral calculi from extraurinary tract opacities such as phleboliths, calcified lymph nodes and gallstones.

An erroneous diagnosis of appendicitis or cholecystitis is made occasionally in cases of right ureteral calculus. All cases of suspected appendicitis should have a urinalysis, and if erythrocytes or numerous white cells are found, excretory pyelograms should be made.

Treatment. Renal and ureteral colic may be relieved by using analgesics or vasospasmolytics.[158] Morphine is an adequate analgesic, and intravenous Banthine an effective spasmolytic. Occasionally, the passage of a ureteral catheter beyond the stone is needed to relieve the pain when other methods fail.

Large vesical calculi can be removed by suprapubic cystolithotomy or transurethral crushing (litholapaxy).

Ureteral calculi smaller than 1 cm. in diameter are treated by watchful waiting. Unless the stone causes constant pain or gives rise to hydro-ureter, hydronephrosis or anuria, time is permitted for it to pass spontaneously. Stones larger than 1 cm., or smaller stones coupled with complications or renal enlargement, are removed by ureterolithotomy. If the stone is small and in the most distal portion of the ureter its transurethral removal may be attempted with the Balkus loop, the Levant basket or the Dourmashkin bag.[161]

Large calculi in the renal pelvis are removable only by pyelolithotomy or nephrolithotomy. In elderly patients it is often best to leave renal stones alone unless they cause persistent or intense pain or recurrent bouts of chills and fever.

After the removal of calculi from the urinary tract, measures should be instituted to prevent their recurrence. This may consist solely of treating a urinary tract infection; the repair of any condition leading to urinary stasis, such as a malpositioned blood vessel, positional ureteral kinking, etc.; instituting physical activity; discontinuance of the Sippy regimen, etc. Diluting the urine by the forced drinking of water is to be employed after the removal of all types of stones. The Shorr regimen is being employed[159] widely to prevent the formation of calcium phosphate calculi. This consists of a low calcium, low phosphorus diet and the ingestion of aluminum gel. In the intestine the aluminum gel forms insoluble aluminum phosphate and thereby prevents absorption of phosphorus. In this manner the urinary excretion of calcium and phosphorus is diminished. There is evidence that the Shorr regimen is effective in reducing the frequency of recurrent nephrolithiasis. Patients who have formed urinary tract stones should be investigated for possible hyperparathyroidism (see Chap. 27, "Thyroid, Thymus and Parathyroids").

If the patient shows unusual absorption of calcium by the intestine, sodium phytate[151] can be used.

Renal tubular acidosis is treated with the oral administration of a mixture of sodium citrate and citric acid, calcium gluconate, vitamin D and potassium salts.

The occurrence of uric acid, calculi and persistently acid urine is an indication for the oral administration of alkali.

TRAUMATIC LESIONS

KIDNEY

Incidence. Automobile accidents and boxing now injure the kidney more often than other forms of trauma. In the case of renal trauma sustained in automobile accidents and boxing the kidney may be crushed by the blunt force or torn from its bed by sudden deceleration of the body. Also, it is readily injured directly by penetrating objects such as knives, bullets, shell fragments, etc.[168]

Pathology. Minor renal injuries are frequent and consist solely of the rupture of small vessels, producing hematomas and hematuria. The severe renal injuries include tears or incisions through the parenchyma, the pelvis, the calyces or the renal pedicle. Hemorrhage into the collecting system and about the kidney follow such tears or cuts. It is limited by Gerota's fascia unless that too is torn or cut. Should Gerota's fascia be discontinuous, the hemorrhage extends retroperitoneally, obliterating the psoas shadow, and with it urine extravasates into the retroperitoneal space, especially after fragmentation of the kidney. Should the hematoma or the urinary extravasation become infected, a perinephric abscess may ensue.

Thrombosis and infarction without any other obvious renal injury may follow renal trauma.

Signs and Symptoms. Pain in the costovertebral area, gross or microscopic hematuria, and swelling in the flank are characteristic signs of renal injury; any or all of them may exist. Shock will follow renal injuries attended by extensive retroperitoneal hemorrhage or a fulminant infection of the hematoma or urinary extravasation. Associated injuries, including rib fracture on either side and splenic rupture on the left, are frequent.

Diagnosis. All cases with serious abdominal trauma should have a preliminary screening of a catheterized urine specimen, looking for the presence of gross or microscopic blood. Intravenous pyelography is very helpful in establishing a diagnosis of renal injury. The preliminary plain film demonstrates an enlarged renal shadow should the hemorrhage be confined within Gerota's fascia; should the hemorrhage be retroperitoneal, the psoas shadow is obscured, and a lateral deviation of the spine with the concavity toward the side of injury occurs. The injured kidney may not be visualized with excretory pyelography. In cases with visualization, distortion of the collecting system and extravasation of the dye may occur.

Treatment. Most renal injuries do not require operative intervention, and their treatment[164] consists of the treatment of hemorrhagic shock, the control of pain and rest in bed. *Special diagnostic studies should not be done while shock exists.*

Signs of continuing or life-endangering hemorrhages, such as a bulging mass in the flank and recurrent hypotension despite large blood transfusions, constitute indications for surgical intervention. The operation consists of repairing the kidney when possible, hemostasis, and evacuation of blood clots. Nephrectomy may be necessary in cases of renal avulsion or extreme fragmentation, but it should not be performed until the presence of an opposite kidney has been ascertained. Necessary treatment of associated injuries such as ruptured spleen, bowel, liver, etc., should not be overlooked (see Chap. 33, "Spleen," and Chap. 35, "Intestine," etc.).

Surgical procedures are also required in cases of injury attended by very extensive urinary extravasations or perinephric abscesses.

Prognosis. A severely traumatized kidney may live but later atrophy, and then hypertension may occur. All persons having experienced severe renal injury should be checked regularly, looking for high blood pressure. Should hypertension follow a severe renal injury, a nephrectomy should be performed, but only after ascertaining the injured kidney's function and that of its mate, employing split-function studies.

URETER

Incidence. Injuries to the ureter are practically always iatrogenic.[169] Radical surgery for cancer of the uterus and the rectosigmoid, instrumental manipulation of the ureter for calculi, and vesical diverticulectomy and segmental resection of the bladder constitute the commonest hazards to the ureter.

The most frequent type of ureteral injury is its accidental ligation. Other forms of injury include instrumental crushing, transection, tearing, excision and puncture.[170]

Pathology. Ureteral ligation is followed by hydro-ureter, hydronephrosis and eventual autonephrectomy if the ligature is nonabsorbable. A break in ureteral continuity is followed by the extravasation of urine, periureteral abscesses and entero-ureteral and cutaneous-ureteral fistula. Extensive periureteral scarring often follows transection or contusions, producing strictures with hydroureter and hydronephrosis above them.

Signs and Symptoms. Ligation of one ureter may cause no overt pain and especially so if the ligation has been performed during anesthesia. Obviously, anuria immediately follows the ligation of both ureters.

The extravasation of urine from an opening in the ureter may cause severe flank pain, abdominal distention and sepsis and at other times be attended by no symptoms. Presumptively, should the urine be of neutral pH, be nearly isotonic and not contain organisms, it should cause no more pain than saline injected beneath the skin or into the peritoneal cavity. The seeping of urine from the surgical wound or from the vagina after a ureteral injury usually requires a day or more for its appearance. It is pathognomonic of a uretero-cutaneous or ureterovaginal fistula.

Diagnosis. Retrograde pyelography with ureteral catheterization will demonstrate the obstruction if the ureter has been tied. Excretory pyelography is to be used first in cases of suspected ureteral tears or transection in order to obviate the danger associated with retrograde pyelography of introducing pathogenic organisms into the injury. If visualization is not obtained with the intravenous pyelogram, then retrograde pyelography is performed.

Treatment. Most surgical injuries to the ureter are preventable. Constant cognizance of the ease of ureteral injury during operations upon pelvic and posterior abdominal organs and the placing of catheters in the ureters through the urethra before beginning large pelvic operations will serve to prevent most of the surgical ureteral injuries. Every general surgeon or gynecologist should be prepared to repair a divided ureter on the spot when this accident is discovered. A useful method is to place a catheter upward through an incision in the ureter from below the point of division. The catheter passes through the

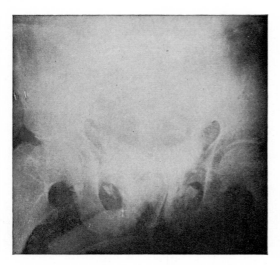

Fig. 48-25. Marked extravasation of sodium iodide beyond confines of the bladder confirms the diagnosis of ruptured bladder.

division line which in turn is resutured end-to-end with a single row of fine interrupted catgut sutures. The distal end of the catheter is then brought out through the flank. Obstructive ligatures, even though they may be absorbable, should be removed as soon as possible. Should the accident remain undetected for a long time and the patient be uremic or very ill for other reasons, nephrostomy rather than deligation is performed first. After the patient's renal function recovers, corrective procedures to restore ureteral patency and continuity are carried out.

When urinary extravasation occurs through a transected or injured ureter, incisional drainage of the urine may be indicated in addition to nephrostomy. After a suitable time interval of drainage, definitive ureteral plastic procedures to establish continuity and patency of the ureter are done. Frequently, nephrectomy must be substituted for ureteral plastic procedures, because the ureter has been so injured as to be beyond repair.

BLADDER

Rupture of the bladder occurs quite frequently with pelvic fractures. Automobile accidents and falls are the predominant causes of vesical rupture.[172] Openings through the bladder are made occasionally during transurethral resection of the prostate or of vesical neoplasms. After rupture of the bladder, urine may extravasate into the perivesical space, the peritoneal cavity, or both.

Signs and Symptoms. If the urinary extravasation is extraperitoneal, pain is suffered suprapubically, with tenderness and dullness evident suprapubically and infra-umbilically. Signs of peritonitis, such as ileus, boardlike rigidity, etc., often attend intraperitoneal urinary extravasation. Attempts to void may bring the passage of a little blood and no urine. Occasionally, the rupture of the bladder with the free flow of urine into the peritoneal cavity will be unattended by pain or signs of peritonitis. In such cases the pathognomonic signs of the accident are those of ascites, oliguria or anuria, and uremia.

When the bladder is ruptured during transurethral resection, low abdominal pain and shock attend it, and the abdomen is distended and cold—the cold irrigating fluid introduced into it having cooled the abdominal wall.

Diagnosis. In all cases of pelvic or lower abdominal trauma a catheterized urine specimen should be obtained for the detection of microscopic red cells. Unequivocal evidence of a ruptured bladder can be obtained by introducing 200 cc. of a 10 per cent solution of sodium iodide, Urokon, Diodrast, Neoiopax or Hyopaque through the urethral catheter and then taking a roentgenogram. Figure 48-25 shows the extravasation of contrast material in a case of ruptured bladder.

Treatment. Through a suprapubic incision the extravasated urine and blood are evacuated, and the rent is débrided and closed. Then a suprapubic cystostomy is done, and multiple drains are placed in the perivesical space, and the wound is closed over them. The drains and the suprapubic tube are removed after drainage through and about them has stopped and the bladder has healed.

URETHRA

Trauma to the urethra may tear it posteriorly and anteriorly. The injury may be inflicted by intra-urethral instrumentation and manipulation or by the application of external force to the para-urethral area. The common causes of intra-urethral trauma are the forceful passage of steel sounds, fiber bougies and other foreign bodies.[174] Occasionally, an irrational patient bearing a Foley catheter will pull it out while the balloon is inflated and sustain an extensive tear of the urethra. Straddle injuries caused by falling astride bars, fences, etc., crush the bulbous urethra. Sharp bony fragments from pelvic fractures may rupture the prostatic and membranous portions of the urethra.[176] Sudden arrest of the momentum of a patient with a full bladder in an automobile accident may shear the membranous urethra clear across. This is possible because the bladder and the prostatic urethra are mobile, while the membranous urethra is fixed by the urogenital diaphragm. In the female such a shear is more apt to occur at the bladder neck.

Pathology. When a break in the continuity of the urethra occurs, hemorrhage follows, and urine extravasates if the patient attempts to force urine down the ruptured urethra or if the injury is at the vesical neck.

If the rupture in the urethra is distal to the urogenital diaphragm and does not involve Buck's fascia, the urinary extravasation will be limited by Buck's fascia, and swelling will occur along the shaft of the penis and along the perineal urethra. When the injury perforates Buck's fascia, the extravasation will be limited by Colles' fascia, and the extravasated urine will swell the shaft of the penis, the scrotum, the perineum and the anterior abdominal wall. A urethral tear proximal to the urogenital diaphragm permits extraperitoneal and perivesical extravasation.

A fibrous stricture of the urethra may follow all types of traumatic lesions of the urethra.

Signs and Symptoms. The signs of an injury to the anterior urethra are pain in the region of the injury, bleeding from the urethral meatus not associated with urination, and difficulty in voiding. Straddle injury often makes a large hematoma in the perineum. If urinary extravasation occurs, swelling will take place as previously described. Posterior urethral injuries are characterized by hematuria, little urethral bleeding, suprapubic pain, tenderness and inability to void, and a hematomatous swelling in the region of the triangular ligament and displacement of the prostate discernible upon digital rectal examination.

Diagnosis. The history and the physical findings alone suffice to establish the diagnosis in many cases. A urethrocystogram readily confirms the diagnosis and aids in locating the position of the tear.

Treatment. Urinary diversion and establishment of urethral continuity are the primary therapeutic aims. If urinary extravasation has occurred, incision and drainage of the involved parts are also necessary. Urinary diversion is accomplished by suprapubic cystostomy. With prostatic and membranous urethral injuries, continuity is re-established by merely splinting the urethra over a urethral catheter passed through the site of injury into the bladder. Anterior urethral injuries are amenable to débridement and primary anastomosis of the severed parts.

POST-TRAUMATIC URETHRAL STRICTURES

Trauma as well as neisserian infections of the urethra may be followed by fibrotic narrowing[178] of the urethral lumen.

Pathology. The urethra becomes occluded by contracture of the scar about it and gives rise to obstructive uropathy. In addition, periurethral abscesses, urinary extravasations and formation of urethrocutaneous fistulae may complicate the stricture. The breaks in the continuity of the strictured urethra which give rise to these complications occur just proximal to the stricture. Through the break a small amount of urine escapes, and a localized abscess forms which may burrow its way to the skin to form a urethrocutaneous fistula. Should a large amount of bacteria laden urine escape and spread rapidly along fascial planes a life-endangering urinary phlegmon is formed.

Signs and Symptoms. The individual clinical picture varies widely, one being that of partial obstruction with hesitancy, decrease in size and force of stream and increased frequency; another that of uremia; and another that of urinary extravasation with periurethral abscesses, phlegmon, or "watering pot" perineum.

Treatment. Uncomplicated strictures generally can be managed by periodic urethral dilatations. These must be carried on from time to time for the rest of the patient's life. If the stricture is very stiff and does not respond to dilatations, internal and external urethrotomy are often performed, and these are followed by dilatations ad infinitum. Recently, a plastic procedure devised by Johanson, completely eradicates the stricture and effects reconstitution of the urethra with little scar. This may obviate the necessity of repetitive dilatation. On occasion, especially after severe trauma to the bony pelvis and the posterior urethra, impassable calcified urethral strictures may develop. Recently, the author has treated this type of case by creating an abdominal neourethra from a flap of bladder wall. The patients have been able to void voluntarily through the abdominal wall and to remain continent. The physiologic basis for this operative procedure was elucidated during experimental studies on the urinary sphincter.[173]

The complications of urinary retention, uremia and urinary extravasation are treated according to the principles previously outlined.

PENIS

Trauma to the penis may consist of denudation, amputation or transection, strangulation, or fracture.

Denudation[182] usually is effected by being caught in machinery. The early use of scrotal or free skin grafts, or in selected cases the replacement of the penile skin, is the treatment of choice. *Traumatic amputation or transection*[181] is the handiwork of psychotics or of irate wives and mistresses or husbands. In cases of such amputation or transection, the transected segment should be anastomosed to the base, even though it may have been severed for an hour or more. *Strangulation*[183] of the penis usually is a manifestation of abnormal auto-eroticism; wedding rings, washers, rubber bands and circular erection aids are the usual etiologic agents. Therapy involves the early removal of the constricting object. *Fracture* results from trauma to the organ when in the erect state. Splinting of a torn urethra, or incision and drainage of a secondary thrombosis of the corpora cavernosa may be necessary items in the treatment.

Peyronie's Disease. This condition of the penis is characterized by induration of the tunica albuginea of the corpora cavernosa and/or the intercavernous septum. The cause for the induration is not known. It occurs primarily in middle-age males.

It may produce symptoms consisting of abnormal bending of the penis on erection

associated with pain during intercourse. The curvation of the penis may be so great that sexual intercourse cannot be accomplished. On physical examination a hard plaque or cord may be palpated along the dorsal or the lateral aspects of the penile shaft; the urethra and the corpus spongiosum are not involved.

Numerous remedies have been used to treat symptomatic Peyronie's disease, but none has been completely successful. Some of the more recent therapeutic measures include cortisone,[233] vitamin E[232] and para-aminobenzoate.[185]

SCROTUM

Avulsion of scrotal skin is the most common type of scrotal trauma. The treatment[186, 187] depends upon the amount of skin lost. In any case, whenever possible, the testes should be re-covered with remaining scrotal skin, and when this is not possible skin grafts should be applied or the testis placed subcutaneously on the medial aspect of the thigh or over the anterior lower abdomen. The blood supply of the testis is independent of the scrotum; therefore, the testes usually remain viable even though all the scrotal skin is gone, and their surfaces readily accept thick split-thickness skin grafts.

BENIGN SCROTAL ENLARGEMENTS. Hydrocele, one of the most common masses occurring in the scrotum, is characterized by an accumulation of clear, straw-colored fluid within the tunica vaginalis. The hydrocele may be acute and associated with testicular tumor, epididymitis, orchitis or trauma (including herniorrhaphy, orchiopexy and varicocelectomy); most frequently the cystic enlargement of the tunica vaginalis is chronic in character and idiopathic in origin.

Acute hydroceles may be painful. The chronic hydrocele is usually asymptomatic unless it is very large, in which case the patient may complain of a heavy dragging sensation in the groin associated with difficulty in crossing the legs.

The diagnosis of hydrocele is suggested by the history of a scrotal swelling which on examination appears cystic and transilluminates. Needle aspiration of serous yellow fluid from the mass confirms the diagnosis.

Treatment includes (1) simple aspiration of

the hydrocele, (2) aspiration and injection of a sclerosing solution or (3) surgical obliteration of the sac. Hydroceles in infants should not be treated by an open operation because, in most instances, the cyst will disappear spontaneously or following simple aspiration. Excision or eversion of the hydrocele sac[236] is the treatment of choice for all chronic *symptomatic* hydroceles.

Spermatocele is a cyst within the scrotum which is attached most commonly to the epididymis or the rete testis. It is relatively rare and usually quite small in size.

It produces no symptoms unless it becomes very large and causes a heavy, dragging sensation.

The spermatocele is similar to the hydrocele in that it feels cystic and transilluminates. It differs from the hydrocele in that it usually is connected to the epididymis or the vas deferens, and its fluid, when aspirated, will be found to be white, opalescent and contain numerous spermatozoa.

No therapy except reassurance is indicated for most spermatocele. If the spermatocele is extremely large, simple excision will suffice.

Varicocele refers to venous varicosities of the vessels of the spermatic cord or the pampiniform plexus. On physical examination it feels like a mass of worms and does not transilluminate.

Varicocele may be idiopathic in origin or it may be caused by obstruction of the internal spermatic vein by retroperitoneal masses such as sarcoma, neuroblastoma or renal neoplasm. Metastases from a left renal tumor into the left renal vein will obstruct the left spermatic vein which empties into the left renal vein and cause a left varicocele.

The idiopathic varicocele is differentiated from the type caused by neoplastic obstruction in that the vein of the idiopathic type empty themselves when the patient is placed in the supine position. No change will be observed in the varicocele caused by obstruction of the internal spermatic vein when the patient is lying flat.

If the idiopathic varicocele is symptomatic, a psychotherapeutic approach is indicated. Surgical treatment is notoriously unsuccessful because most of the symptoms associated with varicocele are psychoneurotic in origin.

TESTIS

Injuries to the testis are rare. Any swelling of the testis not due to obvious inflammation (mumps orchitis) should not be attributed to injury but should be explored for the possibility of neoplasm or torsion. Torsion of the testis is a rotation of the testis and the spermatic cord. When sufficiently twisted, the blood flow to the testis stops and then is attended by testicular infarction or gangrene.

Etiology. Developmental abnormalities of the testis and the adjacent structures predispose to torsion.[188, 189] Absence of the gubernaculum and lack of attachment between epididymis and tunica vaginalis permit the testis, the epididymis and a portion of the spermatic cord to hang free in the surrounding envelope of the tunica vaginalis. Under such circumstances the cord and the testis become twisted more readily. Factors initiating torsion are not known.

Signs and Symptoms. Torsion of the testis may occur at any time but usually during physical exertion or sleep. Sudden excruciating testicular pain associated with nausea and vomiting occurs. Soon after torsion has occurred, the testis will be found high in the scrotum having been raised by the shortened twisted cord. After the passage of hours, edema, erythema and tenderness of the scrotum appear, and pain decreases. Then the scrotum and its contents become difficult to examine.

Treatment. Surgical exploration should be performed as soon as presumptive diagnosis of torsion has been made. The testis may be saved, even though much time has passed. The operation consists of untwisting the cord. If after untwisting the cord, the testis appears to be viable it is attached to the inner layers of the scrotum with several silk sutures taken through the tunica albuginea. In the case of testicular gangrene, orchiectomy is required. The other testis also should be anchored, because the developmental anomaly is usually bilateral; therefore, both testes are subject to torsion.

PHYSIOLOGY OF URINARY TRANSPORT AND MICTURITION

After urine enters the calyceal system it is propelled by co-ordinated segmented smooth muscle contractions into the infundibulum, the pelvis and down the ureter. The ureter propels the urine from the renal pelvis into the bladder where it collects for varying periods of time, depending somewhat upon the desire of the individual.

URETER

Sympathetic fibers to the ureter control its vascular elements but have no recordable effect upon ureteral peristalsis. The ureter is autonomous in that its peristalsis proceeds normally, even though the nerves to it are rendered nonconductive. The normal stimulus for ureteral peristalsis appears to be the pressure of urine high in the renal calyces.[194] The contraction of the ureter is superimposed upon a high-tensional quiescent state, the contraction is followed by relaxation and the fall of intra-ureteral pressure to a level below that existing during rest. When urine output is low, ureteral peristaltic waves are infrequent. During diuresis peristaltic waves are very frequent, and their amplitudes are so shallow as to make the ureter appear to be a rigid tube.

Ureteral contractions increase in amplitude and frequency when the intravesical or intra-ureteral pressures are raised. Traumatic irritation of the ureter by catheters or calculi can produce large irregular muscular contractions which are not related to urine volume or intravesical pressure. Portions of ureter can be excised and an anastomosis accomplished without impairing ureteral contractions, excepting for a temporary delay in conduction at the anastomotic site, provided that little fibrous tissue appears at the anastomotic site.

Human ureteral muscular tonicity and peristalsis are not affected by therapeutic doses of drugs.[193] Morphine does not cause spasm of the ureter and therefore is an effective analgesic for alleviating ureteral colic.

BLADDER

The normal individual voids 3 or 4 times during the day and occasionally once during the night. On volition the urinary stream is started within 1 to 2 seconds, and it can be stopped quickly at will. The urinary stream is continuous until terminally when efforts to evacuate the urethra interrupt the stream. Abdominal muscular contractions are not requisite for micturition.[199] However, should

they be instituted they put pressure upon the bladder and increase the force of the urinary stream once it has been started. Experimental data indicate that human bladder smooth muscle is subject to voluntary control and that micturition can be started or stopped voluntarily without the contraction or relaxation of the striated muscle of the sphincter. However, in the absence of the sphincteric striated muscle the urinary stream cannot be stopped as rapidly; instead of the normal stopping time of 1 to 2 seconds, from 6 to 10 seconds are needed.

Micturition is actually a simple process governed by the higher centers in the normal individual. The bladder consists not only of a globular portion called the fundus but also of a tubular part commonly known as the urethra. The muscular layer of the urethra is a continuation of the muscle in the wall of the bladder[204, 209] and is innervated by the same parasympathetic fibers. The smooth muscle of the bladder possesses the qualities of tonicity and accommodation which are inherent in the smooth muscle and independent of motor impulses from the central nervous system. Tonicity refers to the ability of smooth muscle to maintain continuous tension, while accommodation is that property of bladder which permits it to maintain a constant low intravesical pressure in the face of increasing volumes of fluid. Smooth muscle does not depend upon the central nervous system for its tonicity, whereas skeletal muscle does. Therefore, an atonic flaccid bladder is one that has been overdistended with urine, regardless of the cause of the retention. Bladder muscle is not weakened or rendered flaccid by cutting nerves to it.[207] A flaccid distended bladder may be rendered hypertonic and small by frequent voidings or by keeping the bladder empty through constant catheter or suprapubic cystotomy drainage, regardless of the neurologic state of the individual.

NEUROANATOMY

The fundus or globular portion of the bladder receives urine continually from the ureters and stores it at relatively low pressures until capacity is reached. The urine is prevented from flowing out of the bladder during the period of storage by the urinary sphincter

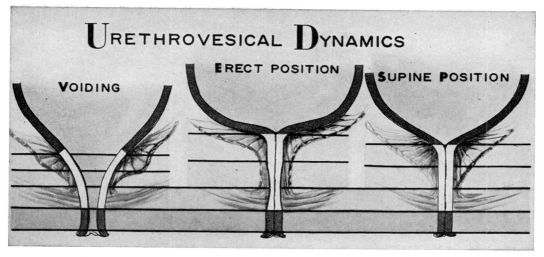

FIG. 48-26. Role of the urinary sphincter in urethrovesical dynamics.

(Fig. 48-26). The urinary sphincter has been found to be a tubular structure synonymous with the proximal three fourths of the female urethra or the prostatic and membranous portions of the male urethra; in both male and female these segments of urethra are actually the true bladder necks.[201, 202] The wall of the urethra contains much elastic tissue in addition to smooth muscle.[209] The urinary sphincter maintains continence by virtue of the resistance its apposing walls present to fluid pressure. The elastic and muscle fibers in the urethral wall keep the lumen of the urethra narrow without the aid of motor impulses from the central nervous system. Thus, the storage of urine by the bladder (fundus and neck) is a very efficient process in that it is performed in an autonomous, tireless fashion with a negligible expenditure of energy.

When intravesical pressure is markedly elevated by exertion, urethral resistance must be increased to prevent urinary incontinence. In the normal male and female human this is accomplished by the 2-fold action of the striated muscle of the urogenital diaphragm and the pelvic floor.[202] These muscles compress the urethra or urinary sphincter circumferentially as well as elongate it by pulling it cephalad toward the fundus (Fig. 48-26). The net result of the striped muscle activity is to decrease the caliber of the urethral lumen, to increase the tension of the urethral walls against its lumen and to increase the length of the urethra—all factors which increase the resistance of the urinary sphincter to the flow of fluid through it. The levator ani and muscle of the urogenital diaphragm can be contracted or relaxed voluntarily. They can contract reflexly also as in standing, coughing, sneezing, etc. These muscles are essential for the abrupt termination of urination.[197, 204]

The motor nerves to bladder muscle are quiescent when urination is not occurring. The efferent nerves conducting motor impulses to the bladder are from the craniosacral or parasympathetic nervous system and form part of the pelvic nerve. The sympathetic nervous system plays no part in the process of micturition in man. Most of the sensory nerve fibers carrying exteroceptive and proprioceptive sensations from the bladder to the central nervous system accompany the parasympathetic motor fibers in the pelvic nerve. The exteroceptive sensations include pain and temperature; the proprioceptive endings give rise to the feeling of bladder fullness and to the desire to void.

The motor neurons supplying the bladder musculature lie in the lateral horns of the sacral spinal cord at the levels of S2, S3 and S4. The motor fibers extend from the motor neuron to the wall of the bladder where ganglionic synapses and postganglionic fibers are situated (Fig. 48-27).

An intact spinal reflex arc and a normal vesical musculature are requisites for complete emptying of the bladder. As the bladder fills

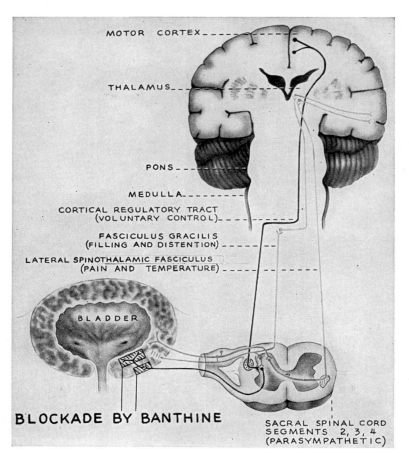

MOTOR CORTEX

THALAMUS

PONS

MEDULLA

CORTICAL REGULATORY TRACT
(VOLUNTARY CONTROL)

FASCICULUS GRACILIS
(FILLING AND DISTENTION)

LATERAL SPINOTHALAMIC FASCICULUS
(PAIN AND TEMPERATURE)

BLADDER

BLOCKADE BY BANTHINE

SACRAL SPINAL CORD
SEGMENTS 2, 3, 4
(PARASYMPATHETIC)

FIG. 48-27. Neuro-anatomy of the bladder: sites of action of Banthine.

with urine, the proprioceptive endings are stretched, and sensory impulses are carried to the spinal cord. In the spinal cord the afferent impulses bombard, and eventually cause a discharge of, the lower motor neurons. The impulses arising in the motor neurons travel over the efferent parasympathetic fibers, ganglionic synapses and neuromuscular endings to stimulate contraction of the bladder fundus and neck. The bladder fundus contracts down upon the bolus of urine and simultaneously pulls open the tubular bladder neck to expel the urine.[201, 209]

If the muscles of the pelvic floor and the urogenital diaphragm are in a state of contraction prior to urination, they must be relaxed in order for urine to transverse the urethra. These muscles are striated, and their motor neurons lie in the anterior horn of sacral spinal segments 2, 3 and 4.

The spinal reflex arc concerned with urina-tion functions without voluntary control in the infant. As the child grows, the long spinal nerve tracts linking the higher centers to the lower reflex arcs begin to operate. Pain and temperature sensations are carried to the higher centers by the lateral spinothalamic tract, and proprioceptive impulses ascend by way of the fasciculus gracilis. The lower reflex arc is brought under the control of the higher centers through the descending cortico-regulatory tracts (Fig. 48-27). The cortico-regulatory tract can initiate as well as inhibit voiding contractions of the bladder by directly influencing the lower motor neurons to the bladder—a direct cortical control over smooth muscle.[204]

Cystometry. Bladder function can be evaluated by the cystometric examination, which is conducted as follows:

1. The person is requested to void. The character of micturition is observed, noting

especially the time taken to initiate micturition, the size and the caliber of stream, the continuity of stream and the relationship of abdominal straining to micturition.

2. After voiding, a catheter is passed, and the volume of the residual urine is recorded. Through the catheter 60 ml. of cold and then 60 ml. of warm water are instilled to test exteroceptive perception.

3. The urethral catheter is then connected to a water manometric cystometer, and water is instilled into the bladder at the rate of 60 drops per minute. The person is requested to tell the examiner when he becomes conscious of the desire to micturate and again when the bladder feels full. The intravesical pressures and volumes are plotted on a cystometrographic sheet.

4. When the patient's bladder is full, the catheter is withdrawn, and the patient is requested to void. Again observations similar to those outlined in Step 1 are made. A typical normal cystometrograph is shown in Fig. 48-28.

Neurogenic Bladder. Lesions of one or

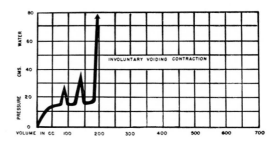

EXTEROCEPTIVE SENSATION

    HEAT - PRESENT

    COLD - PRESENT

PROPRIOCEPTIVE SENSATION

    FIRST DESIRE - PRESENT AT 75 CC. VOL.

    FULLNESS - PRESENT AT 175 CC VOL.

CAPACITY - 175 CC. VOL.

UNINHIBITED CONTRACTIONS - PRESENT

VOIDING STREAM - UNINTERRUPTED

RESIDUAL - 0 CC.

FIG. 48-29. Cystometrograph of an uninhibited neurogenic bladder.

more of the nerve tracts concerned with urination, produce dysfunction of the bladder. Bladders so affected are called neurogenic bladders and can be one of several different types or combinations thereof.

THE UNINHIBITED NEUROGENIC BLADDER.[200] This is caused by a lesion of the corticoregulatory tract and is characterized by difficulty in controlling urination. The patient complains of hesitancy, increased frequency of urination, urgency and incontinence. The sensation of filling is not disturbed, and urine is not retained in the bladder after voiding. The residual urine is within normal limits. A cystometrograph (Fig. 48-29) demonstrates uninhibited contractions of the bladder musculature. Multiple sclerosis, paresis and cerebrovascular accidents are prone to be attended by the uninhibited neurogenic bladder. Therapeutic efforts are directed toward the improvement of the control of micturition by blocking aberrant motor impulses at the terminal ganglia and nerve endings with such drugs as banthine[158] and belladonna. The dosage of these drugs is adjusted to provide

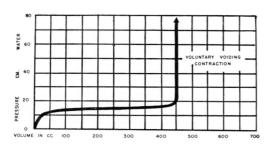

EXTEROCEPTIVE SENSATION

    HEAT - PRESENT

    COLD - PRESENT

PROPRIOCEPTIVE SENSATION

    FIRST DESIRE - PRESENT AT 175 CC. VOL.

    FULLNESS - PRESENT AT 450 CC. VOL.

CAPACITY - 500 CC. VOL.

UNINHIBITED CONTRACTIONS - NONE

VOIDING STREAM - UNINTERRUPTED

RESIDUAL - 0 CC.

FIG. 48-28. Cystometrograph of a normal bladder.

good control of micturition while maintaining the bladder's capacity to empty itself completely.

THE REFLEX NEUROGENIC BLADDER.[195, 198] This type occurs in transverse myelitis in which both the sensory and the motor tracts to and from the higher centers are interrupted above the level of sacral spinal segments 2, 3 and 4. The patient has neither exteroceptive sensation or the capacity to start or stop micturition volitionally in a normal way. The person responds as does a baby before urinary continence is acquired. The cystometrograph (Fig. 48-30) demonstrates uninhibited contractions, no sensation and frequently an abnormally high residual urine. Vesical neck contracture, a weak reflex voiding contraction or spasm of the external urethral sphincter[196] are the possible causes for the carrying of a larger urinary residual. The ultimate aim in the treatment of male patients is the complete emptying of the bladder after a voiding contraction without the use of inlying catheters. All of the male patients will need to wear the condom-type of incontinence apparatus to avoid accidental wetting. Complete emptying of the bladder can be effected by transurethral resection of vesical neck obstructions or by

pudendal neurectomy in cases of spasm of the external sphincter.

THE AUTONOMOUS NEUROGENIC BLADDER. This type characteristically attends the destruction of the sacral segment of the spinal cord and is a trouble borne by patients with myelomeningocele, spina bifida and other lesions causing destruction of the sacral spinal cord. In these patients the lower reflex arc is interrupted, and all sensations of vesical origin are absent, and no voiding contractions, voluntary or involuntary, occur (Fig. 48-31). The external urethral sphincter is flaccid, the bulbocavernous reflex is absent, and there is saddle anesthesia. The exertion of pressure upon the bladder, either manually (Credé) or by abdominal straining, is the only means of effecting interval micturition. If these maneuvers are not performed, overflow urinations keep the patients wet. Typically, micturition in these patients is characterized by inhaling deeply and then straining. Urine is expelled during the strain but stops as soon as the forced expiration against the closed glottis ceases. The residual urine may be within normal limits.

MOTOR PARALYTIC BLADDER. This is encountered most frequently in patients with

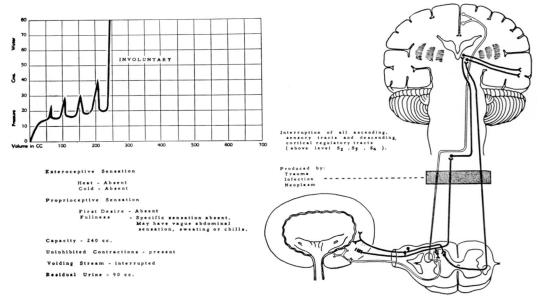

FIG. 48-30. Cystometrograph of a reflex neurogenic bladder and illustration of the involved nerve tracts.

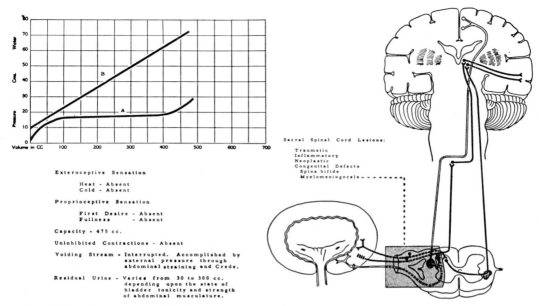

Exteroceptive Sensation

    Heat - Absent
    Cold - Absent

Proprioceptive Sensation

    First Desire - Absent
    Fullness - Absent

Capacity - 475 cc.

Uninhibited Contractions - Absent

Voiding Stream - Interrupted. Accomplished by external pressure through abdominal straining and Crede.

Residual Urine - Varies from 30 to 300 cc. depending upon the state of bladder tonicity and strength of abdominal musculature.

Sacral Spinal Cord Lesions:

    Traumatic
    Inflammatory
    Neoplastic
    Congenital Defects
    Spina bifida
    Myelomeningocele

FIG. 48-31. Cystometrograph of an autonomous neurogenic bladder and its associated nerve tract lesion.

poliomyelitis and polyradiculoneuritis (Fig. 48-32). Usually the patient suffers from complete urinary retention incident to paralysis of the lower motor neurons but has perfectly normal sensation. In the case of poliomyelitis

treatment consists of catheter drainage until the paralysis disappears. This is usually a period of seven to ten days in length. Permanent paralysis of lower motor neurons may require constant tube drainage if transurethral

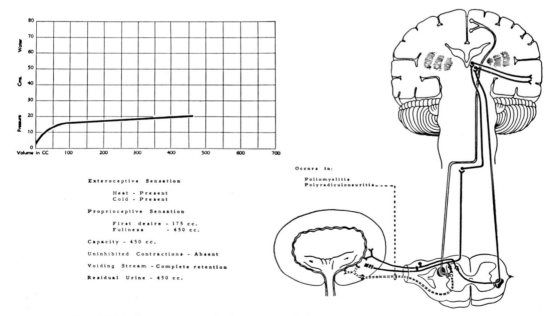

Exteroceptive Sensation

    Heat - Present
    Cold - Present

Proprioceptive Sensation

    First desire - 175 cc.
    Fullness - 450 cc.

Capacity - 450 cc.

Uninhibited Contractions - Absent

Voiding Stream - Complete retention

Residual Urine - 450 cc.

Occurs in:

    Poliomyelitis
    Polyradiculoneuritis

FIG. 48-32. Cystometrograph of motor paralytic bladder and its neuropathology.

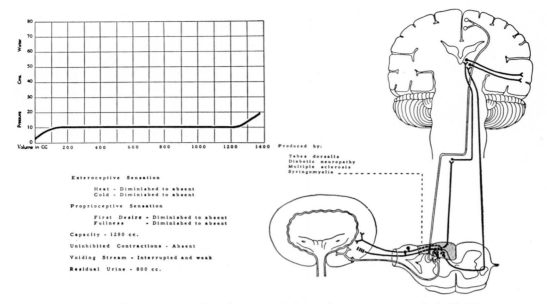

Exteroceptive Sensation

    Heat - Diminished to absent
    Cold - Diminished to absent

Proprioceptive Sensation

    First Desire - Diminished to absent
    Fullness   - Diminished to absent

Capacity - 1280 cc.

Uninhibited Contractions - Absent

Voiding Stream - Interrupted and weak

Residual Urine - 800 cc.

Produced by:

    Tabes dorsalis
    Diabetic neuropathy
    Multiple sclerosis
    Syringomyelia

Fig. 48-33. Cystometrograph and neuropathology of the sensory paralytic bladder.

resection and external pressure do not permit the expulsion of urine.

SENSORY PARALYTIC BLADDER. This type occurs with locomotor ataxia. The proprioceptive sense of fullness is lost, and consequently the musculature of the bladder becomes overdistended and as a consequence is atonic and decompensated (Fig. 48-33). Treatment is directed toward correcting the atonicity and preventing its recurrence. Continuous catheter drainage for a period of time will usually correct the atonicity, provided that the vesical musculature has not atrophied. Atonicity is prevented from recurring by having the patient void every 2 to 3 hours by the clock. In other words, the patient will depend upon a clock and vision for voiding rather than depending upon defective proprioceptive sensation.

CONGENITAL ANOMALIES

KIDNEY

Embryology. The nephrons are derived from mesodermal renal blastema, while the excretory system, including the collecting tubules, the calyces, the infundibula, the pelvis and the ureter, is derived from the entoderm of the hindgut. In the normal course of development the two systems become one when the secretory tubules of the nephrons join the collecting tubules of the excretory system.

As the embryo develops the kidneys ascend from the region of the pelvic cavity to their adult lumbar position. In the pelvic cavity the kidney lies with its medulla and pelvis facing anteriorly and the cortical and the cortical convex border facing posteriorly. As the kidney ascends, it turns through 90° so that its pelvis faces medially and the cortex laterally. While the embryonic kidney lies in the pelvis, the calyces point posteriorly and after attainment of the lumbar position they point laterally.

Renal Agenesis. During the development of some embryos, abnormalities arise in the formation of the kidneys and the ureters. Both kidneys may be absent, and the fetus consequently nonviable, or one kidney and ureter may fail to develop. This is called renal agenesis.

Duplication of the pelvis and the ureter is the most common renal anomaly. As a general rule, the ureter originating from the higher part of the kidney inserts lower into the bladder or other organ. The double ureter may be partial or complete. When 2 completely separate ureters exist unilaterally, there are 2 ureteral orifices on the same side of the ureteral ridge.

Ectopic Ureter. Occasionally, the ureter from the upper pelvis opens into the urethra, the vagina or the seminal vesicle and is called an ectopic ureter.

Ectopic Kidney. A pelvic ectopic kidney is one that fails to ascend and remains in the pelvis. This anomaly in a woman may interfere with normal pregnancy and delivery. Frequently, the kidney ascends but fails to rotate.

Horseshoe Kidney. The kidneys may join one another at their lower poles before ascending from the pelvis, forming a fused kidney. The fusion tissue may be parenchymal or fibrous. When the joined kidneys ascend into the lumbar region while each kidney attains its normal paravertebral position, the fused kidney is called a horseshoe kidney.

Crossed Renal Ectopia. If the fused kidney is located entirely to one side of the spine it is designated as crossed renal ectopia.

Aberrant Lower Pole Vessels. Abnormal blood vessels to the kidney include accessory arteries and veins to either the upper or the lower poles. The aberrant lower pole vessels may cross the ureter and compress it, giving rise to ureteral narrowing and intermittent or continuous hydronephrosis. Sometimes it may be the cause of Dietl's crises or hypertension of the Goldblatt type.

Polycystic disease of the kidney is a most interesting congenital anomaly. It is hereditary and frequently lethal, either at birth or during middle age. The polycystic kidneys of infants succumbing shortly after birth demonstrate the failure of union of the nephron tubule with the collecting tubule. Adults with polycystic disease demonstrate union between secretory and collecting tubules but show diverticula of the tubules. The adult type of polycystic kidney is thus capable of adequate functioning until the enlarging diverticula or cyst destroy most of the renal tissue by pressure atrophy.[212, 213]

The polycystic kidney is markedly enlarged and composed primarily of cysts of varying size. Polycystic kidneys are usually bilateral and palpable because of their size. They may be asymptomatic or give rise to pain, hematuria, urinary infection, hypertension and progressive renal failure. They may be associated with cystic changes in other organs, especially the liver, the pancreas and the lungs.

DIAGNOSIS can be made by pyelography which demonstrates relatively enormous collecting systems with multiple cystic deformities of the calyces and infundibula.

TREATMENT is palliative and includes measures directed toward delaying progression of renal failure.

URETER

There is a considerable variety of developmental anomalies of the ureter, but only a few are clinically important. Ureteral ectopia[214] and duplication have been mentioned before.

An ectopic ureter may be the cause of a constantly dripping incontinence when its opening enters the urogenital tract below the vesical sphincter. This happens most often in the female. The *diagnosis* is readily made by finding the ectopic ureteral orifice and this is not difficult. *Treatment* involves ureterectomy and segmental resection of the part of the kidney it drained.

Ureterocele. Congenital obstructions of the ureteral meatus lead to intravesical ureteral dilatation just proximal to the stenosis. This produces a cystlike structure inside the bladder. This ureteral cyst or ureterocele[216] may be small or be so large as to obstruct the vesical outlet and thereby lead to bilateral hydronephrosis. The *diagnosis* is made upon cystoscopy. The *treatment* consists solely of its transurethral or suprapubic excision.

Congenital megalo-ureter is a hydro-ureter having no discernibly organic obstruction as its cause. The *diagnosis* is made by exclusion. The *etiology* is unknown. Its *treatment* is still an unsolved problem.[215]

BLADDER

The most common bladder anomalies are congenital diverticula, patent urachus and exstrophy.

A congenital diverticulum[220] is an outpouching of a segment of bladder wall unassociated with obstructive uropathy. It differs from an acquired diverticulum in that it contains muscle, while the acquired type does not. When the diverticula are large they may retain urine; they predispose to cystitis, calculus formation and difficulty in micturition. The *diagnosis* is readily made upon cystoscopy and cystography. If the diverticula are large and troublesome they should be removed.

The urachus[217] is a fetal canal which connects the bladder with the allantois. After birth the urachus loses its connection with the umbilicus and becomes a cord—the middle umbilical ligament. In some people partial or complete patency of the urachus persists after birth. Complete patency is associated with leaking of urine through the umbilicus. Obliteration at the distal and the proximal ends of the urachus while the remainder is patent gives rise to cysts or abscesses beneath the anterior abdominal wall below the umbilicus. Should the umbilical end close while the vesical connection remains open, stones or neoplasms may form in it. The *diagnosis* can be made by cystoscopy and injection of the urachus with a radiopaque medium, if the urachus communicates with the bladder. Similarly, the probing or the injection of a radiopaque medium at the umbilical end of the tract, should it open there, may serve to make the diagnosis and delineate the tract. Another method of diagnosis rarely applicable is the injection of a dye into the tract and noting its appearance in the urine immediately. The *treatment* involves the complete excision of the urachus.

Exstrophy of the bladder[221] is a rather rare anomaly occurring in both the male and the female. It is said to be due to a mesodermal deficiency. It is characterized by absence of (1) the anterior wall of the bladder, (2) that portion of the anterior abdominal wall which overlies the bladder, (3) the symphysis pubis and (4) the dorsal portion of the urethra in males. Because of these defects the posterior wall of the bladder and the trigone with its ureteral orifices form the lower anterior abdominal wall, thereby exposing the mucosa of the bladder and the ureteral orifices to view. The sufferer is a social outcast because he or she constantly emanates the odor of urine and wets his pants or skirt. The abnormal development of the pelvic bones leads to a waddling gait.

TREATMENT[218, 219] until the past several years consisted primarily of excision of the bladder, supravesical urinary diversion (ileal conduit, ureterosigmoid transplantation) and

repair of the epispadias. Now many surgeons are attempting to close the bladder and the urethra so that normally functioning organs will result. Preliminary results of such reconstructive efforts seem to indicate that the motor supply to many of the reconstructed bladders is defective. If this is the case, procedures to close the bladder primarily again may have to be abandoned.

PROGNOSIS. Unless patients are treated successfully during infancy, they will soon develop hydro-ureter, hydronephrosis and ascending pyelonephritis. The exposed, infected and irritated bladder mucosa is apt to undergo malignant degeneration during the adult years, should survival be that long.

URETHRA AND PENIS

Posterior urethral valves[225] are a common cause of urinary obstruction in the male infant. They are believed to be remnants of the urogenital membrane and are found in the prostatic urethra. The valves are delicate membranes, usually extending laterally from the verumontanum toward the bladder neck. The membranes appear as folds on the floor of the urethra during endoscopy. Urinary incontinence, including bedwetting, is one of the most common manifestations of this disease. The *diagnosis* is made at the time of urethroscopy when the valves are seen. Formerly, the valves were resected transurethrally, but now their retropubic excision is the treatment of choice.

Stricture of the urethral meatus or pinpoint meatus is seen occasionally in male infants. If not treated promptly by simple incision, it will give rise to severe obstructive uropathy in early childhood.

Epispadias[223, 224] has been mentioned during the discussion of bladder exstrophy. Most cases of epispadias are associated with bladder exstrophy, but they may occur alone. The dorsal wall of the urethra is absent, and the corpora cavernosa lie ventral to the posterior wall of the urethra. The treatment consists of the plastic closure of the urethra and its transposition to the normal ventral position.

Hypospadias is a congenital abnormality of the urethra incident to failure of closure of the distal urethral groove. The urethral meatus is not found in its normal position on the glans but anywhere between the perineum and the corona. In addition, the prepuce is present only dorsally. The penis is curved ventrally (chordee) because the corpus spongiosum is absent and is replaced by fibrous tissue. The ventral curvature is exaggerated during erection. This condition should be corrected during childhood; otherwise, it may cause mental and emotional disturbances. Children having this defect frequently find it necessary to void in the sitting position because of the location of the urethral meatus. Therefore, they feel inferior to their companions who urinate while standing. In the adult phase of life the patient with untreated hypospadias cannot participate satisfactorily in sexual intercourse. The *treatment*[222] is carried out in several stages. Initially, the penis is straightened by the excision of the ventral scar tissue. At a later date a new urethra is formed from skin so that the urethral meatus comes to lie near its normal glandular position.

Phimosis is the most common congenital anomaly of the penis and is characterized by the inability to retract the prepuce over the glans. This situation predisposes to collection of smegma beneath the foreskin with resultant possibility of the formation of carcinoma of the penis in later life. Wynder recommends that all males should be circumcised during infancy and calls attention to the lower incidence of carcinoma of the cervix in wives of circumcised men. The circumcision should completely remove the prepuce, because a residual cuff of prepuce borne by an unhygienic individual predisposes the person to penile cancer.

TESTIS

Cryptorchism in the strict sense is a developmental defect in which the testes remain in the peritoneal cavity. However, it is often used as being synonymous with incomplete descent of one or both testes. In the normal male infant the testes are in the scrotum at birth. In some boys the testes are arrested in their descent. Because the testes are derived from the genital fold in the region where the kidneys come to lie eventually, undescended testes may be located anywhere from the inguinal canal up to the level of the renal pedicle.

ETIOLOGY. Bilateral undescended testes are believed to be caused by a deficiency of chorionic gonadotropin.[226] Unilateral cryptorchism is usually the result of some obstructing factor such as fascial bands, scar tissue, hernia, etc. The unilateral undescended testis must have had the same amount of hormone acting upon it as did its mate which is in its normal position.

DIAGNOSIS. In young children the testicles often ascend into the inguinal canal during play, excitement and cold. Should the physician not be aware of this, an erroneous diagnosis of cryptorchism may be readily made. Examination of the child's genitalia should be done only after the boy has been kept quiet and warm for a time.

COMPLICATIONS OF UNTREATED CRYPTORCHIDS. Moore[229] demonstrated conclusively that an undescended testis manifests aspermatogenesis because of the abnormally high temperature present in the abdomen. A testis remaining in the abdomen after puberty is aspermatogenic. Data have been accumulated regarding testicular tumors, indicating that undescended testes are 22 times as prone to develop carcinoma as are normal testes. This holds true regardless of the degree of testicular reposition attained by any means.

Treatment. The ultimate purpose of any therapy for cryptorchism is to place the testis in its normal position in the scrotum. The reason for attempting it is to avoid aspermatogenesis and the development of undetectable testicular neoplasms. The treatment may be hormonal, surgical or a combination of both. If the patient has unilateral cryptorchism, a surgical procedure should be employed to bring the testis into the scrotum no later than the age of 6 years. If both testes are undescended, hormone therapy should be instituted at the age of 6 for a short period of time. Engle[230] recommends that from 4,000 to 5,000 units of chorionic gonadotropin be given daily for 3 days and should there be no demonstrable descent of the testes within a week, operative correction is indicated.

The giving of large doses of gonadotropin for a short period of time avoids the precocious sexual development and the bone changes that occur when small doses of gonadotropin are given for a longer period of time.

Normal growth of an undescended testis is unlikely unless it is fixed in the scrotum by the age of 5 or 7 years.

REFERENCES

DIAGNOSIS

1. Blakemore, W. S., Murphy, J. J., Pendergrass, H. P., and Greening, R. R.: Carbon dioxide as contrast medium in roentgenography, J.A.M.A. *167*:310, 1958.
2. Braasch, W. F., and Emmett, J. L.: Clinical Urography, Philadelphia, Saunders, 1951.
3. Bunge, R. G.: Further observations with delayed cystograms, J. Urol. *71*:427, 1954.
4. Dustan, H. P., Page, I. H., and Poutasse, E. F.: Renal hypertension, New England J. Med. *261*:647, 1959.
5. Kerr, D. H., and Gillies, C. L.: The Urinary Tract; A Handbook of Roentgen Diagnosis, Chicago, Year Book Pub., 1944.
6. Kincaid, O. W., and Davis, G. D.: Abdominal aortography, New England J. Med. *259*:1067, 1958.
7. Lapides, J.: Urinary incontinence, M. Clin. North America *43*:1629, 1959.
8. Nesbit, R. M.: Dangers of perirenal air insufflation, Urologists' Correspondence Club Newsletter, August, 1953. (Quoted in Year Book of Urology 1953-1954, p. 32, Chicago, Year Book Pub., 1954.)

RENAL PHYSIOLOGY

10. Earle, D. P.: Introduction to the study of renal function, Am. J. Med. *9*:78, 1950.
11. Gamble, J. L.: Chemical Anatomy, Physiology and Pathology of Extracellular Fluid (A Lecture Syllabus), Cambridge, Mass., Harvard, 1947.
12. Oliver, J.: An essay toward a dynamic morphology of the mammalian nephron, Am. J. Med. *9*:88, 1950.
13. Smith, H. W.: The Kidney, New York, Oxford, 1951.
14. Symposium: Physiology and pathology of the kidney, Brit. M. Bull. *13*:1, 1957.
15. Symposium on renal physiology, Am. J. Med. *24*:659, 1958.
16. Taggart, J. V.: Mechanisms of renal tubular transport, Am. J. Med. *24*:774, 1958.

Glomerular Function

17. Bott, P. A., and Richards, A. N.: The passage of protein molecules through the glomerular membrane, J. Biol. Chem. *141*: 291, 1941.
18. Smith, H. W., Chasis, H., Goldring, W., and Ranges, H. A.: Glomerular dynamics in the normal human kidney, J. Clin. Invest. *19*:751, 1940.
19. Wearn, J. T., and Richards, A. W.: Observations on the composition of glomerular urine with particular reference to the problem of reabsorption in the tubules, Am. J. Physiol. *71*:209, 1924.

Tubular Function

20. August, J. T., Nelson, D. H., and Thorn, G. W.: Aldosterone, New England J. Med. *259*:917, 1958.
21. Berliner, R. W., Levinsky, N. G., Davidson, D. G., and Eden, M.: Dilution and concentration of the urine and the action of antidiuretic hormone, Am. J. Med. *24*:730, 1958.
22. Conn. J. W.: Presidential Address: 1. Painting background; 2. Primary aldosteronism, a new clinical syndrome, J. Lab. & Clin. Med. *45*:3, 1955.
23. Malvin, R. L.: The renal concentrating mechanism: counter-current multiplier system, Univ. Michigan M. Bull. *26*:45, 1960.
24. Malvin, R. L., Wilde, W. S., and Sullivan, L. P.: Localization of nephron transport by stop flow analysis, Am. J. Physiol. *194*: 135, 1958.
25. Newbergh, L. H.: Renal tubule work; its significance for the clinician, Bull. New York Acad. Med. *24*:137, 1948.
26. Pitts, R. F.: Some reflections on mechanisms of action of diuretics, Am. J. Med. *24*: 745, 1958.
27. Smith, H. W.: The fate of sodium and water in the renal tubule, Bull. New York Acad. Med. *35*:293, 1959.
28. Verney, E. B.: The antidiuretic hormone and the factors which determine its release, Proc. Roy. Soc., London, s. B. *135*:25, 1947.
29. Walker, A. M., and Oliver, J.: Methods for the collection of fluid from single glomeruli and tubules of the mammalian kidney, Am. J. Physiol. *134*:562, 1941.

Renal Function Tests

30. Chasis, H., Redish, J., Goldring, W., Ranges, H., and Smith, H.: The use of sodium p-aminohippurate for the functional evaluation of the human kidney, J. Clin. Invest. *24*:583, 1945.
31. Lapides, J., and Bobbitt, J. M.: Preoperative estimation of renal function, J.A.M.A. *166*:866, 1958.
32. Miller, E., McIntosh, J. F., and Van Slyke, D. D.: Studies in urea excretion, J. Clin. Invest. *6*:427, 1928.
33. Steinitz, K., and Türkand, H.: The determination of the glomerular filtration by the

endogenous creatinine clearance, J. Clin. Invest. *19*:285, 1940.

34. Weller, J. M., and Cottier, P. T.: Clinical evaluation of renal function, Univ. Michigan M. Bull. *26*:36, 1960.

Renal Function in Disease

35. Addis, T.: Glomerular Nephritis: Diagnosis and Treatment, New York, Macmillan, 1948.

36. Albright, F., Consolazio, W. V., Coombs, F. S., Sulkowitch, H. W., and Talbot, J. H.: Metabolic studies and therapy in a case of nephrocalcinosis with rickets and dwarfism, Bull. Johns Hopkins Hosp. *66*:7, 1940.

37. Boyd, W.: Changing concepts of pyelonephritis, Canad. M.A.J. *47*:128, 1942.

38. Bradley, S. E., Bradley, G. P., Tyson, C. J., Curry, J. J., and Blake, W. D.: Renal function in renal disease, Am. J. Med. *9*:766, 1951.

39. Bricker, N. S., Morrin, P. A. F., and Kime, S. W., Jr.: The pathologic physiology of chronic Bright's disease, Am. J. Med. *28*: 77, 1960.

40. Mudge, G. H.: Clinical patterns of tubular dysfunction, Am. J. Med. *24*:785, 1958.

41. Waring, A. J., Kajdi, L., and Tappan, V.: A congenital defect of water metabolism, Am. J. Dis. Child. *69*:323, 1945.

Acute Renal Failure

42. Block, J. B., and Burrows, B. A.: Diagnostic use of I^{131} Diodrast in hypertension due to unilateral renal disease, Circulation *18*: 696, 1958.

43. Bull, G. M., Joekes, A. M., and Lowe, K. G.: Renal function studies in acute tubular necrosis, Clin. Sc. *9*:379, 1950.

44. Dustan, H. P., Page, I. H., and Poutasse, E. F.: Renal hypertension. New England J. Med. *261*:647, 1959.

45. Goldblatt, H., Lynch, J., Hanzal, R. F., and Summerville, W. W.: Studies on experimental hypertension; production of persistent elevation of systolic blood pressure by means of renal ischemia, J. Exper. Med. *59*:347, 1934.

46. Kohlstaedt, K. G., and Page, I. H.: Liberation of renin by perfusion of kidneys following reduction of pulse pressure, J. Exper. Med. *72*:201, 1904.

47. Kolff, W. J., Watschinger, B., and Vertes, V.: Results in patients treated with the coil kidney (disposable dialyzing unit), J.A.M.A. *161*:1433, 1956.

48. Lakey, W. H.: The artificial kidney unit of the University of Michigan Medical Center, Univ. Michigan M. Bull. *25*:85, 1959.

49. Maxwell, M. H., Rockney, R. E., Kleeman, C. R., and Twiss, M. R.: Peritoneal dialysis, J.A.M.A. *170*:917, 1959.

50. Merrill, J. P.: The Treatment of Renal Failure: Therapeutic Principles in the Management of Acute and Chronic Uremia, New York, Grune, 1955.

51. Oliver, J., MacDowell, M., and Tracy, A.: The pathogenesis of acute renal failure associated with traumatic and toxic injury: renal ischemia, nephrotoxic damage and the ischemuric episode, J. Clin. Invest. *30*:1307, 1951.

52. Page, I. H.: Production of persistent arterial hypertension by cellophane perinephritis, J.A.M.A. *113*:2046, 1939.

53. Poutasse, E. F.: Blood pressure reduction as aid to renal angiography in hypertensive patients, Cleveland Clin. Quart. *22*:83, 1955.

54. Shapiro, A. P.: Relationships of hypertension and experimental pyelonephritis in rat, Circulation *18*:780, 1958.

55. Strauss, M. B.: Acute renal insufficiency due to lower nephron nephrosis, New England J. Med. *239*:693, 1948.

56. Swann, R. C., and Merrill, J. P.: The clinical course of acute renal failure, Medicine *32*:215, 1953.

57. Teschan, P. E., O'Brien, T. F., and Baxter, C. R.: Prophylactic daily hemodialysis in treatment of acute renal failure, Clin. Research *7*:280, 1959.

58. Yendt, E. R., Kerr, W. K., Wilson, D. R., and Jaworski, Z. F.: The diagnosis and treatment of renal hypertension, Am. J. Med. *28*:169, 1960.

OBSTRUCTIVE UROPATHY

General Physiopathology and Therapy

59. Hinman, F.: The pathogenesis of hydronephrosis, Surg., Gynec. & Obst. *58*:356, 1934.

60. Lapides, J.: Physiopathology and therapy of fluid disorders in prostatism, Geriatrics *9*:20, 1954.

61. Pilcher, F., Jr., Bollman, J. L., and Mann, F. C.: The effect of increased intra-ureteral pressure on renal function, J. Urol. *38*:202, 1937.

62. Smith, H. W., Chasis, H., Goldring, W., and Ranges, H. A.: Glomerular dynamics in the normal human kidney, J. Clin. Invest. *19*:751, 1940.

Congenital Specific Diseases

63. Campbell, M. F.: Ureterocele, Surg., Gynec. & Obst. *93*:703, 1951.
64. Gibson, T. E.: Classification and plastic re-repair of ureteropelvic obstructions, Surg., Gynec. & Obst. *80*:485, 1945.
65. Grantham, W. L., and Bunts, R. C.: Congenital obstruction of the bladder neck, South. M.J. *33*:939, 1940.
66. Jones, F. W.: The development and malformations of glans and prepuce, Brit. M.J. *1*:137, 1910.
67. Lattimer, J. K., Dean, A. L., Jr., and Furey, C. A.: The triple voiding technique in children with dilated urinary tracts, J. Urol. *76*:656, 1956.
68. Leadbetter, G. W., Jr., and Leadbetter, W. F.: Diagnosis and treatment of congenital bladder neck obstruction in children, New England J. Med. *260*:633, 1959.
69. Lloyd, E. I.: Treatment of congenital stenosis of the urinary meatus, Lancet *2*:1252, 1927.
70. Nesbit, R. M., and Baum, W. C.: Diagnosis and surgical management of obstructive uropathy in childhood, A.M.A. Am. J. Dis. Child. *88*:239, 1954.
71. Nesbit, R. M., Thirlby, R. L., and Raper, F. P.: Diagnosis and treatment of congenital urethral valves, J. Michigan M. Soc. *50*:1244, 1951.
72. Nesbit, R. M., and Withycombe, J. F.: The problem of primary megaloureter, J. Urol. *72*:162, 1954.
73. Politano, V. A., and Leadbetter, W. F.: Operative technique for correction of vesico-ureteral reflux, J. Urol. *79*:932, 1958.

Acquired Specific Diseases

Urethral Stricture

74. Harrison, J. H.: The treatment of rupture of the urethra, especially when accompanying fractures of the pelvic bones, Surg., Gynec. & Obst. *72*:622, 1941.
75. Hornaday, W. R.: Care of traumatic injuries of the male urethra, J.A.M.A. *114*:303, 1940.
76. Johanson, B.: Die Rekonstruktion der Männlichen Urethra bei Strikturen, Ztschr. Urol. *46*:361, 1953.
77. Lapides, J.: Simplified modification of Johanson urethroplasty for strictures of deep bulbous urethra, J. Urol. *82*:115, 1959.

Benign Prostatic Hypertrophy

78. Deming, C. L.: The development of prostatic hyperplasias, Surg., Gynec. & Obst. *70*:588, 1940.
79. Huggins, C.: The etiology of benign prostatic hypertrophy, Bull. New York Acad. Med. *23*:696, 1947.
80. Millin, T.: Retropubic Urinary Surgery, Edinburgh, Livingstone, 1947.
81. Moore, R. A.: Benign hypertrophy of the prostate; a morphological study, J. Urol. *50*:680, 1943.
82. Nesbit, R. M.: Transurethral Prostatectomy, Springfield, Ill., Thomas, 1943.
83. Young, H.: Some problems in surgical treatment of the prostate, J.A.M.A. *110*:280, 1938.

Hydronephrosis of Pregnancy

84. Crabtree, E. C.: Urological Disease of Pregnancy, Boston, Little, Brown & Co., 1942.
85. Wagener, van, G., and Jenkins, R. H.: Experimental examination of factors causing ureteral dilation of pregnancy, J. Urol. *42*:1010, 1939.

URINARY TRACT INFECTIONS

Nontuberculous Infections

Gonorrheal

86. Fromer, S., Cutler, J. C., and Levitan, S.: Masking of early syphilis by penicillin therapy in gonorrhea, J. Ven. Dis. Inform. *27*:174, 1946.
87. Heller, J. R., Jr.: The adequate treatment of gonorrhea, J. Ven. Dis. Inform. *27*:225, 1946.
88. Pelouze, P. S.: Gonorrhea in the Male and Female, ed. 2, Philadelphia, Saunders, 1931.

Nongonorrheal

89. Allen, A. C.: The Kidney: Medical and Surgical Diseases, New York, Grune, 1951.
90. Beer, E.: Coccal infections of the kidney, J.A.M.A. *106*:163, 1936.
91. Braasch, W. F.: Pyelonephritis and its treatment, Surg., Gynec. & Obst. *68*:534, 1939.
92. Carroll, G.: Treatment of urinary infections: choice of drug, Texas J. Med. *49*:761, 1953.
93. Graves, R. C., and Parkins, L. E.: Carbuncle of the kidney, Tr. Am. A. Genito-Urin. Surgeons *28*:41, 1935.
94. Heaney, N. S., and Kretschmer, H. L.: Pyelitis of pregnancy, J.A.M.A. *128*:407, 1945.
95. Mathe, C. P.: Diagnosis and treatment of perinephric abscess, Am. J. Surg. *37*:35, 1937.
96. Nesbit, R. M., and Dick, V. S.: Acute staphylococcal infections of the kidney, J. Urol. *43*:623, 1940.

97. ———: Pulmonary complications of acute renal and perirenal suppuration, Am. J. Roentgenol. *44*:161, 1940.

Tuberculous Infections

98. Borthwick, W. M.: Renal tuberculosis: its pathogenesis and management in patients with extraurogenital disease, Edinburgh M.J. *59*:583, 1952.

99. Hinman, F.: Tuberculosis of the kidney, Surg., Gynec. & Obst. *66*:329, 1938.

100. Lattimer, J. K., and Spirito, A. L.: The current status of the chemotherapy of renal tuberculosis, J. Urol. *75*:375, 1956.

101. Lieberthal, F.: Renal tuberculosis: the development of the renal lesion, Surg., Gynec. & Obst. *67*:26, 1938.

102. Medlar, E. M., Spain, D. M., and Holliday, R. W.: Postmortem compared with clinical diagnosis of genito-urinary tuberculosis in adult males, J. Urol. *61*:1078, 1949.

103. Nesbit, R. M., and Mackinney, C. C.: Antibiotic therapy of urinary tuberculosis: an interval report of 6 years' experience, J. Urol. *72*:296, 1954.

104. Rich, A. R.: The Pathogenesis of Tuberculosis, ed. 2, Springfield, Ill., Thomas, 1951.

NEOPLASMS OF THE GENITO-URINARY TRACT

Kidney

105. Deming, C. L.: The prognosis and problems in renal tumors, J. Urol. *55*:571, 1946.

106. Gross, R. E., and Neuhauser, E. B. D.: Treatment of mixed tumors of the kidney in children, Pediatrics *6*:843, 1950.

107. Harvey, R. M.: Wilms' tumor: evaluation of treatment methods, Radiology *54*:689, 1950.

108. Melicow, M. M.: Classification of renal tumors: a clinical and pathological study based on 199 cases, J. Urol. *51*:333, 1944.

109. Nelson, O. A., and Mousel, L. H.: Renal tumors, J.A.M.A. *148*:171, 1952.

110. O'Conor, V. J., Cannon, A. H., Laipply, T. C., Sokol, K., and Barth, E. L.: Renal tumors, Radiology *85*:830, 1952.

111. Papanicolaou, G. N.: Cytology of the urinary sediment in neoplasms of the urinary tract, Tr. Am. A. Genito-Urin. Surgeons *38*:147, 1947.

112. Smith, P. G., Rush, T. W., and Evans, A. T.: An evaluation of translumbar arteriography, J. Urol. *65*:911, 1951.

Ureter

113. Mortensen, H. J., and Murphy, L.: Primary epithelial tumors of the ureter, Brit. J. Urol. *22*:103, 1950.

114. Scott, W. W.: A review of primary carcinoma of the ureter, J. Urol. *50*:44, 1943.

115. Senger, F. L., and Furey, C. A., Jr.: Primary ureteral tumors with a review of the literature since 1943, J. Urol. *69*:243, 1953.

Bladder

116. Ash, J. E.: Epithelial tumors of the bladder, J. Urol. *44*:135, 1940.

117. Colby, F. H., and Kerr, W. S., Jr.: Carcinoma of the bladder: an evaluation of total cystectomy and other methods of treatment, New England J. Med. *244*:504, 1951.

118. Editorial: Hyperchloremic acidosis following ureterosigmoidostomy, J.A.M.A. *152*:334, 1953.

119. Jewett, H. J.: Infiltrating carcinoma of the bladder: relation of early diagnosis to 5 year survival rate after complete extirpation, J.A.M.A. *148*:187, 1952.

120. Price, J. M., Wear, J. B., Brown, R. R., Satter, E. J., and Olson, C.: Studies on etiology of carcinoma of urinary bladder, J. Urol. *83*:376, 1960.

121. Thompson, G. J.: Treatment of cancer of urinary bladder with particular reference to choice of operation, J. Missouri M.A. *49*:813, 1952.

122. Wallace, D. M.: Tumours of the Bladder, Edinburgh, Livingstone, 1959.

123. Whitmore, W. F., Jr., and Marshall, V. F.: Carcinoma of bladder, S. Clin. North America *35*:501, 1953.

Prostate

124. Baker, W. J.: Late results of bilateral adrenalectomy for advanced carcinoma of the prostate gland, J. Urol. *72*:525, 1954.

125. Batson, O. V.: The function of the vertebral veins and their role in the spread of metastases, Ann. Surg. *112*:138, 1940.

126. Flocks, R. H.: Carcinoma of the prostate, J.A.M.A. *163*:709, 1957.

127. Huggins, C. B., and Hodges, C. V.: Studies on prostatic cancer: I. The effect of castration, of estrogen and androgen injection on serum acid phosphatases in metastatic carcinoma of the prostate, Cancer Res. *1*:293, 1941; II. Effects of castration on advanced cancer of prostate gland, Arch. Surg. *43*:209, 1941.

128. Miller, G. M., and Hinman, F., Jr.: Cortisone treatment in advanced carcinoma of the prostate, J. Urol. *72*:485, 1954.

129. Nesbit, R. M., and Baum, W. C.: Endocrine control of prostatic carcinoma, J.A.M.A. *143*:1317, 1950.

130. ———: Serum phosphatase determinations

in diagnosis of prostatic cancer, J.A.M.A. *145*:1321, 1951.

131. Presti, J. C.: Carcinoma of prostate: diagnosis and treatment, California Med. *78*: 440, 1953.

132. Tagnon, H. J., Whitmore, W. F., Jr., Schulman, P., and Kravitz, S. C.: Significance of fibrinolysis occurring in patients with metastatic cancer of the prostate, Cancer *6*:63, 1953.

Urethra

133. Hotchkiss, R. S., and Amelar, R. D.: Primary carcinoma of the male urethra, J. Urol. *72*:1181, 1954.

Penis

134. Bleich, A. R.: Prophylaxis of penile carcinoma, J.A.M.A. *143*:1054, 1950.

135. Dean, A. L.: Conservative amputation of penis for carcinoma, J. Urol. *68*:374, 1952.

136. Lynch, K. M., Jr.: Carcinoma of penis, J. South Carolina M.A. *48*:298, 1952.

137. Melicow, M. M., and Ganem, E. J.: Cancerous and precancerous lesions of the penis, J. Urol. *55*:486, 1946.

138. Schrek, R., and Lenowitz, H.: Etiologic factors in carcinoma of the penis, Cancer Res. *7*:180, 1947.

Scrotum

139. Butlin, H.: Cancer of the scrotum in chimney-sweeps and others, Brit. M.J. *1*: 1341, 1892.

140. Graves, R. C., and Flo, S.: Carcinoma of the scrotum, J. Urol. *43*:309, 1940.

141. Wilson, S. R.: Cancer in cotton-mule spinners, Brit. M.J. *2*:993, 1927.

Testis

142. Beilby, J. S., Kurland, I., and Jacob, M.: Hormone excretion and bioassay of extirpated tumor in teratoma, Endocrinology *26*:965, 1940.

143. Friedman, N. B., and Moore, R. A.: Tumors of the testis, Mil. Surgeon *99*:573, 1946.

144. Kimbrough, J. C.: Tumors of the testis, Surg., Gynec. & Obst. *94*:535, 1952.

145. Lewis, L. G.: Radical orchidectomy for tumors of the testis, J.A.M.A. *137*:828, 1948.

146. Melicow, M. M.: Embryoma of testis, J. Urol. *44*:333, 1940.

147. Nesbit, R. M., and Lynn, S. M.: Malignant testicular neoplasms, Surgery *20*:273, 1946.

148. Vermooten, V., and Hettler, W. F.: The

significance of gonadotropic hormones in the urine of patients with testicular tumors, J. Urol. *61*:519, 1948.

CALCULOUS DISEASE

149. Albright, F., Burnett, C. H., Parson, W., Reifenstein, E. C., Jr., and Roos, A.: Osteomalacia and late rickets, Medicine *25*:399, 1946.

150. Boyce, W. H., and King, S. J.., Jr.: Crystal-matrix interrelation in calculi, J. Urol. *81*: 351, 1959.

151. Boyce, W. H., Garvey, F. K., and Goven, C. E.: Abnormalities of calcium metabolism in patients with "idiopathic" urinary calculi, J.A.M.A. *166*:1577, 1958.

152. Carroll, G., and Brennan, R. V.: Urea-splitting organisms in formation of urinary calculi, J. Internat. Coll. Surgeons *17*:809, 1952.

153. Chambers, E. K., Gordan, G. S., Goldman, L., and Reifenstein, E. C., Jr.: Tests for hyperparathyroidism: tubular reabsorption of phosphate, phosphate deprivation and calcium infusion, J. Clin. Endocrinol. *16*: 1507, 1956.

154. Dent, C. E., and Senior, B.: Studies on treatment of cystinuria, Brit. J. Urol. *27*: 317, 1955.

155. Henneman, P. H., Wallach, S., and Dempsey, E. F.: Metabolic defect responsible for uric acid renal stone formation, J. Clin. Invest. *37*:901, 1958.

156. Howard, J. E.: Clinical and laboratory research concerning mechanisms of formation and control of calculous disease by the kidney, J. Urol. *72*:999, 1954.

157. Kittredge, W. E., and Docons, R.: Role of gout in formation of urinary calculi, J. Urol. *67*:841, 1952.

158. Lapides, J., and Dodson, A. J., Jr.: Observations on effect of methantheline (Banthine) bromide in urological disturbances, A.M.A. Arch. Surg. *66*:1, 1953.

159. Marshall, V. F., and Green, J. L.: Aluminum gels with constant phosphorus intake for control of renal phosphatic calculi, J. Urol. *67*:611, 1952.

160. Melick, R. A., and Henneman, P. H.: Clinical and laboratory studies of 207 consecutive patients in a kidney-stone clinic, New England J. Med. *259*:307, 1958.

161. Nesbit, R. M. (Moderator): Panel discussion on urolithiasis, Urol. Survey *4*:2, 1954.

162. Nesbit, R. M., Lapides, J., and Baum, W. C.: Fundamentals of Urology, Ann Arbor, Mich., Edwards, 1953.

163. Suby, H. I.: Medical management of pa-

tients with urinary calculi, M. Clin. North America *32*:1315, 1948.

TRAUMATIC LESIONS

Kidney

164. Cheetham, J. G.: Clinical management of kidney injuries, Internat. Abstr. Surg. *72*: 573, 1941.
165. Heller, E.: War injuries of the upper urinary tract, J. Urol. *72*:149, 1954.
166. Prather, G. C.: Traumatic conditions of the kidney, J.A.M.A. *114*:207, 1940.
167. ———: War injuries of the urinary tract, J. Urol. *55*:94, 1946.
168. Sargent, J. C., and Marquardt, C. R.: Renal injuries, J. Urol. *63*:9, 1950.

Ureter

169. Aschner, P. W.: Accidental injury to ureters and bladder in pelvic surgery, J. Urol. *69*:774, 1953.
170. Rusche, C. F., and Bacon, S. K.: Injury of the ureter, J.A.M.A. *114*:201, 1940.
171. St. Martin, E. C., Trichel, B. E., Campbell, J. N., and Locke, C. M.: Ureteral injuries in gynecologic surgery, J. Urol. *70*:51, 1953.

Bladder

172. Prather, G. C.: Bladder injuries: treatment, past and present, New York J. Med. *53*: 318, 1953.

Urethra

173. Lapides, J.: Structure and function of the internal vesical sphincter, J. Urol. *80*:341, 1958.
174. Laury, R. B.: Diagnosis and treatment in traumatic injuries of bladder and urethra, New York J. Med. *52*:187, 1952.
175. O'Conor, V. J.: Repair of rupture of the male urethra, Surg., Gynec. & Obst. *63*:198, 1936.
176. Ormond, J. K., and Fairey, P. W.: Urethral rupture at apex of prostate, J.A.M.A. *149*: 15, 1952.

Urethral Strictures

177. Ainsworth-Davis, J. C.: Prevention and treatment of strictures of inflammatory origin, Brit. J. Urol. *5*:1, 1933.
178. Ballenger, E. G., and Edder, O. F.: Notes on urethral strictures, Am. J. Surg. *34*:340, 1920.
179. Dodson, A. I.: Urological Surgery, p. 554, St. Louis, Mosby, 1944.
180. Johanson, B.: Die Rekonstruktion der Männlichen Urethra bei Strikturen, Ztschr. Urol. *46*:361, 1953.

Penis

181. Adams, J. P.: Mutilations of the penis, Delaware M.J. *18*:41, 1946.
182. Douglas, P.: One-stage reconstruction for traumatic denudation of the male external genitalia, Ann. Surg. *133*:889, 1951.
183. Hoffman, H. A., and Colby, F. H.: Incarceration of the penis, J. Urol. *52*:391, 1945.
184. Kenyon, H. R., and Hyman, R. M.: Total autoemasculation, J.A.M.A. *151*:207, 1953.
185. Zarafonetis, C. J. D., and Horrax, T. M.: Treatment of Peyronie's disease with potassium para-aminobenzoate (Potaba), J. Urol. *81*:770, 1959.

Scrotum

186. Ewell, G. H., Bruskewitz, H. W., and Steeper, J. R.: Traumatic avulsion of skin of penis and scrotum, J. Internat. Coll. Surg. *19*:207, 1953.
187. Whelan, E. P.: Repair of an avulsed scrotum, Surg., Gynec. & Obst. *73*:649, 1944.

Testis

188. Ormond, J. K.: Torsion of the testicle, J.A.M.A. *111*:1910, 1938.
189. Riba, L. W., and Schmidlapp, C. J.: Torsion of the spermatic cord, Surg., Gynec. & Obst. *63*:163, 1946.

PHYSIOLOGY OF URINARY TRANSPORT
AND MICTURITION

Ureter

190. Baker, R., and Huffer, J.: Ureteral electromyography, J. Urol. *70*:974, 1953.
191. Bozler, E.: The response of smooth muscle to stretch, Am. J. Physiol. *149*:299, 1947.
192. Johnson, T. H.: Peristalsis of the upper urinary tract as demonstrated by a new x-ray technique, New York State J. Med. *52*:189, 1952.
193. Lapides, J.: Physiology of the intact human ureter, J. Urol. *59*:501, 1948.
194. Narath, P. A.: The hydromechanics of the calyx renalis, J. Urol. *43*:145, 1950.

Bladder

195. Bors, E.: Bladder disturbances and the management of patients with injury to the spinal cord, J. Internat. Coll. Surgeons *21*: 513, 1954.
196. ———: Urological aspects of rehabilitation of spinal cord injuries, J.A.M.A. *146*: 225, 1951.

197. Caine, M., and Edwards, D.: Peripheral control of micturition: a cineradiographic study, Brit. J. Urol. *30*:34, 1958.

198. Denny-Brown, D., and Robertson, E. G.. The state of the bladder and its sphincters in complete transverse lesions of the spinal cord and cauda equina, Brain *56*:397, 1933.

199. Langworthy, O. R., Kolb, L. C., and Lewis, L. G.: Physiology of Micturition, Baltimore, Williams & Wilkins, 1940.

200. Lapides, J.: Observations on normal and abnormal bladder physiology, J. Urol. *70*: 74, 1953.

201. ———: Structure and function of the internal vesical sphincter, J. Urol. *80*:341, 1958.

202. Lapides, J., Ajemian, E. P., Stewart, B. H., and Lichtwardt, J. R.: Urethrovesical dynamics in the normal human, Surg. Forum *10*:896, 1959.

203. Lapides, J., Hodgson, N. B., Boyd, R. E., Shook, E. L., and Lichtwardt, J. R.: Further observations on pharmacologic reactions of the bladder, J. Urol. *79*:707, 1958.

204. Lapides, J., Sweet, R. B., and Lewis, L. W.: Role of striated muscle in urination, J. Urol. *77*:247, 1957.

205. McClellan, F. C.: The Neurogenic Bladder, Springfield, Ill., Thomas, 1939.

206. Nesbit, R. M., Lapides, J., *et al.:* Effects of blockade of the autonomic ganglia on the urinary bladder in man, J. Urol. *57*:242, 1947.

207. Nesbit, R. M., and Lapides, J.: Tonus of the bladder during spinal shock, Arch. Surg. *56*:139, 1948.

208. Prather, G. C.: Spinal cord injuries: care of the bladder, J. Urol. *57*:15, 1947.

209. Woodburne, R. T.: Structure and function of the urinary bladder, J. Urol. *84*:79, 1960.

Congenital Anomalies

210. Arey, L. B.: Developmental Anatomy, ed. 6, Philadelphia, Saunders, 1954.

211. Patten, B. M.: Human Embryology, New York, Blakiston Div. of McGraw-Hill, 1948.

Kidney

212. Braasch, W. F., and Schacht, F. W.: Pathological and clinical data concerning polycystic kidney, Surg., Gynec. & Obst. *57*:467, 1933.

213. Lambert, P. P.: Polycystic disease of the kidney, Arch. Path. *44*:34, 1947.

Ureter

214. Moore, T.: Ectopic openings of the ureter, Brit. J. Urol. *24*:3, 1952.

215. Nesbit, R. M., and Withycombe, J. F.: The problem of primary megaloureter, J. Urol. *72*:162, 1954.

216. Thompson, G. J., and Greene, L. F.: Ureterocele, J. Urol. *47*:800, 1952.

Bladder

217. Begg, R. C.: The urachus: its anatomy, histology and development, J. Anat. *64*:170, 1930.

218. Harvard, B. M., and Thompson, G. J.: Congenital exstrophy of the urinary bladder: late results of the Coffey-Mayo method of uretero-intestinal anastomosis, J. Urol. *65*:223, 1951.

219. Higgins, C. C.: Exstrophy of the bladder, J. Urol. *63*:852, 1950.

220. Kretschmer, H. L.: Diverticula of the urinary bladder, Surg., Gynec. & Obst. *71*:491, 1940.

221. Patten, B. M.: The possible embryological mechanisms involved in the genesis of exstrophy of the bladder and epispadias, Anat. Rec. *109*:334, 1951.

Urethra and Penis

222. Burns, E., and Beckman, G. E., Jr.: Evaluation of operations for hypospadias, J. Urol. *67*:1000, 1952.

223. Campbell, M.: Epispadias, Tr. Am. A. Genito-Urin. Surgeons *43*:154, 1951.

224. Gross, R. E., and Cresson, S. L.: Treatment of epispadias, J. Urol. *68*:477, 1952.

225. Nesbit, R. M., Thirlby, R. L., and Raper, F. P.: Diagnosis and treatment of congenital urethral valves, J. Michigan M. Soc. *50*:1244, 1951.

Testis

226. Aberle, S. B. P., and Jenkins, R. H.: Undescended testes in man and Rhesus monkey; treated with the anterior pituitary-like principle from the urine of pregnancy, J.A.M.A. *103*:314, 1934.

227. Deming, C. L.: The evaluation of hormonal therapy in cryptorchidism, J. Urol. *68*:354, 1952.

228. Grove, J. S.: The cryptorchid problem, J. Urol. *71*:735, 1954.

229. Moore, C. R.: The influence of hormones on the development of the reproductive system, J. Urol. *45*:869, 1941.

230. Robinson, J. N., and Engle, E. T.: Some observations on the cryptorchid testis, J. Urol. *71*:726, 1954.

231. Torek, F.: Orchidopexy for undescended testicle, Ann. Surg. *94*:97, 1931.

Peyronie's Disease

232. Dahl, O.: Treatment of plastic induration of penis, Acta radiol. *41*:290, 1954.
233. Teasley, G. H.: Peyronie's disease: a new approach, J. Urol. *71*:611, 1954.

Interstitial Cystitis

234. Hand, J. R.: Interstitial cystitis: report of 223 cases, J. Urol. *61*:291, 1949.

235. Pool, T. L., and Crenshaw, J. L.: Treatment of interstitial cystitis with silver nitrate, Proc. Staff Meet., Mayo Clin. *16*: 718, 1941.

Hydrocele

236. Dodson, A. I.: Urological Surgery, St. Louis, Mosby, 1944.

FRED C. REYNOLDS, M.D., ARTHUR H. STEIN, JR., M.D., AND
WARREN G. STAMP, M.D.

—————————————— CHAPTER 49 ——————————————

Orthopedics (Nontraumatic)

DEVELOPMENT OF THE SKELETON

The skeleton may be looked upon as a calcified connective tissue and closely related to other tissues of mesodermal origin. In the mammalian embryo the mesenchymal cells which are to create the skeleton differentiate into two structures, a cartilaginous mold of the future skeleton and the perichondrium, a membrane which surrounds the cartilage and later becomes the periosteum. Zones of segmentation develop in this primary cartilage. These are the sites of future joints.

Once started, differentiation of the primitive mesenchymal cells into segmented cartilage with its covering perichondrium continues in an orderly way with the cells of embryologic cartilage uniformly and rapidly changing from a primitive to a relatively mature type. According to Luck,[74] a thin sheath of bone begins to form beneath the perichondrium about the 9th week of intrauterine life. At the time bone begins to form blood vessels are seen growing into the approximate center of what is eventually to be the diaphysis or shaft of the bone. The budding of capillaries beneath the perichondrium and into the area of the middle of the diaphysis of the cartilaginous mold is accompanied by calcification of the cartilage cells in this vascularized area. Subsequently, calcification of the cartilage cells spreads from the centers to the ends of the primordial osseous anlagen. Only the zones of primitive cartilage that are destined to be the epiphyseal cartilage plate escape calcification. After calcification has taken place, the cartilage is resorbed by a vascular granulationlike tissue and replaced with an immature type of cancellous bone.

Endochondral ossification is the name applied to the maturation and the calcification of the primitive cartilage, its destruction by a vascular granulation tissue, and its final replacement with cancellous bone. All the bones of the body except the skull, some face bones and the clavicle are formed in this way. In the case of the skull, the bones of the face and the clavicle the actual form of the bone develops as plates of primitive mesenchymal tissue. This tissue does not become cartilage before ossification takes place. Ossification simply involves metaplasia of the mesenchymal tissue to osseous tissue. This process is known as *intramembranous ossification.*

During endochondral ossification the primitive cartilage is not destroyed and replaced in the zones destined to be the epiphyseal plates. Here the cartilage remains as layers of primitive cartilage cells, separating the epiphyses from the metaphyses of the bones. Proliferation of cartilage within the epiphyseal plate and its subsequent conversion to bone accounts for the growth in the length of bones. Within the epiphyseal plate columns of cartilage cells grow, mature, calcify and are destroyed and replaced by bone. The calcific zone of the epiphyseal cartilage is known as the zone of provisional calcification. After having been laid down in juxtaposition to the epiphysis the osteoid trabeculae are modified so as to conform to the inherited characteristics of the bone and the stresses and strains put upon it.

Five enzymes important to carbohydrate metabolism have been measured at 4 stages of endochondral bone formation in the growing dog. Lactic dehydrogenase, phosphoglucoisomerase, malic dehydrogenase, glucose-6-phosphate dehydrogenase and alkaline phosphatase have been determined quantitatively. Enzymes mediating metabolism through aerobic pathways are more prominent in areas closest to invading blood vessels, whereas enzymes more important to anaerobic glycolysis are more active in the more avascular areas of endochondral bone formation. The enzyme content of the epiphyseal plate indicates that endochondral bone formation derives energy and synthetic intermediates from an enzymatically regulated metabolic sequence.[68]

The rate of bone growth as manifested by an increase in length can be brought about by altering the circulation to the part. The creation of an arteriovenous fistula in an extremity results in an increase in bone length and an alteration of the blood supply to the bone. The creation of an arteriovenous fistula significantly alters the normal relationship of intramedullary blood pressure in the epiphysis and the diaphysis. When the fistula is functioning the epiphyseal pressure is elevated.[62, 115]

Growth in thickness of bone occurs by the appositional formation of new bone beneath the periosteum and from the endochondral surfaces. The appositional formation and destruction of bone occurs throughout the life of the individual. In normal healthy adults the rates of bone formation and bone destruction are about equal. This causes the bones of adults to appear to be changeless structures; however, bone is not static. It is highly active metabolically; consequently the amount and the character of bone is readily altered throughout life should the individual's metabolism change. Many of the changes that take place in the life history of bone are unknown. Even the exact composition of the bone crystal is unknown. The solution of many problems in orthopedic surgery awaits the discovery of what occurs when bone is formed and what may be done to control this process.

COMPOSITION OF BONE

Although the exact organic composition of the crystal of bone is not clearly understood, it is known that bone contains approximately 25 per cent water, 30 per cent organic substances and 45 per cent inorganic substances (Luck[74]). There is evidence that the water and the organic components decrease while the inorganic salt components increase as bone ages. Bone has an important organic matrix composed of cells called osteocytes and extracellular substances. The inorganic compounds of calcium, phosphorus, magnesium and carbon are the major bone salts, and these are laid down upon and about the extracellular matrix and the cells. Besides the above salts small amounts of the salts of sodium, potassium, chloride and fluoride are found in bone. The inorganic salts, bound with protein, form a crystal structure resembling an apatite. This has been demonstrated by x-ray refraction studies, as well as by chemical analysis. Roseberry, Hastings and Morse (1931)[104] concluded that bone is a dahlite with the probable formula of $CaCa_3NCO_3(PO_4)_2$. However, others disagree with them and believe that it closely resembles a hydroxyapatite. Armstrong's[7] table of the mineral constituents of bone based upon the work of Dallemagne and Carter is as follows:

	Per Cent
Alpha tricalcium phosphate	74.6
Calcium carbonate	10.4
Calcium citrate	2.0
Trimagnesium phosphate	0.9
Magnesium carbonate	1.0
Disodium phosphate	2.4
Ca^{--} } PO_4^{++} } Protein	8.7

Employing electron microscopy, Robinson[100] showed that bone crystals are rectangular, having the dimensions 500 by 250 by 100 angstroms, and that such crystals have a surface area of about 103 square meters per gram, and that the crystals are embedded in a cement substance covering the collagen fibers, the crystals being arranged along the long axis of the collagen fiber.

COMPOSITION OF CARTILAGE

Cartilage is considered to consist of cartilage cells, known as chondrocytes, connective tissue, extracellular fluid and chondroitin sulfate.

Investigative work has begun to establish the biochemical composition of cartilage. Eichelberger[35] has studied the articular cartilage in puppies and found that in a kilogram of fresh cartilage the distribution of water and solids is as follows:

> 522 Gm. of extracellular water
> 161 Gm. of extracellular solids
> 263 Gm. of chondrocyte water
> 54 Gm. of chondrocyte solids

Mathews[80] has shown that chondroitin sulfate is present as a noncollagenous protein complex in cartilage. During the aging process, the total water content of cartilage decreases in puppies from 80 per cent to 75 per cent. The chondroitin sulfate decreases with age, but due to an increase in the connective tissues the total extracellular solids increase during the aging process.

Alterations in the chemical content of articular cartilage in various disease states is on the threshold of investigation. It has been shown that denervation of an extremity results in an alteration of chemical composition of articular cartilage. Denervation is followed by an increase in total water content, a decrease in chondroitin sulfate and a decrease in connective tissue. Chondrocyte water was found to decrease.

BONE METABOLISM

Because the exact structural composition of bone remains somewhat in doubt and knowledge of the physiology of bone is still fragmentary, the nature of the chemical processes involved in the formation and the maintenance of the skeleton cannot be described precisely.[74] However, it is known that after the dissolution of the primary mesenchymal

or calcified cartilage a collagenous substance termed osteoid is laid down by the action of the osteoblasts. This collagenous substance is either made by the osteoblasts or the osteoblasts secrete a substance that influences the deposition of the collagen from the extracellular fluids. This osteoid collagen is formed whether bone is formed by endochondral or membranous ossification. Following the laying down of this extracellular collagenous ground substance, calcium salts are precipitated upon it to form irregular, immature bony trabeculae. The chemical processes involved in precipitation of calcium salts upon the ground substances are unknown. There are a number of theories existent regarding them. Should the student be interested in them he may consult Robinson (1923),[101] Gutman and Gutman (1941),[48] Neuman et al.,[87] Albright et al.,[6] Rubin and Howard,[105] and McLean and Urist.[78]

Regardless of what exact chemical mechanisms may be involved in the formation of bone, we know that they require (1) a suitable medium for calcification and later ossification, (2) an available supply of organic and inorganic substances and (3), as Urist and McLean[120] have called them, inductor substances which start or catalyze calcification and ossification.

Duthie and Barker,[32] using radioactive sulfur and phosphorus (S^{35} and P^{32}), have studied bone growth. The S^{35} is used to tag chondroitin sulfuric acid, an important constituent of collagen. It has been shown that both epiphyseal and periosteal bone growth are accompanied by an increased utilization of chondroitin sulfuric acid and calcium phosphate complexes.

In the process of endochondral ossification it appears that maturity of the cartilage cell is the basic requirement for a suitable calcifiable medium. These mature cartilage cells, arranged in trabecular rows after calcification, are invaded by a vascular granulation tissue, and the calcified cartilage of the cells is destroyed and replaced by seams of osteoid tissue. Osteoblasts surround these immature, irregular trabeculae of cancellous bone. Then this bone is remodeled by destruction of some parts and the laying down of others. The formation and the destruction of bone goes on throughout life. Wherever bone destruction is going on mononuclear giant cells known as osteoclasts are present. These mononuclear giant cells appear to be destroying bone, since irregular indentations in the trabeculae, known as Howship's lacunae, are found about their surfaces in contact with bone. However, some believe that they have no function in bone destruction. Whatever the role played by the osteoclasts in the destruction of bone, it is possible that they are not phagocytes (McLean et al.[77]). Although osseous resorption is ordinarily a slow process, a rapid destruction of bone may occur when an increase in vascularity or change in pH to a local area of bone occurs.

RESPONSE OF BONE TO INJURY

The character of the reaction of bone to injury varies somewhat with the type and the severity of the injury received. The most common injury is a fracture.

Very soon after fracture, provided that it is not an intra-articular one, a hematoma is formed. The hematoma is later organized by the invasion of vascular connective tissue which arises from the surrounding undamaged soft tissue, periosteum, endosteum and the lining of the Haversian canals. This organized hematoma, about and interposed between the fragments, loosely glues the fragments together. The organized hematoma is called a soft callus.

Concomitant with the formation of the soft callus necrosis of the ends of the fractured bone occurs. The extent of the necrosis is directly related to the severity of trauma and the circulatory impairment attendant upon the fracture. Usually it extends only a few millimeters from the line of fracture. Because of this immutable necrosis, fractures do not unite by the direct bridging of tissue between fragments. Instead, the fragments are first loosely joined together by the connective tissue callus arising from normal tissue slightly distant from the fracture ends.

This connective tissue callus then undergoes metaplasia to cartilage and bone which results in a hard callus. The hard callus is then destroyed and reorganized by the ingrowth of bone from the edges of normal periosteum and endosteum arising some distance from the site of fracture. These new trabeculae of bone

are arranged to be parallel with the shaft of the bone and when joined from each side solidify the fracture. Rearrangement continues and after the necrotic area of the bone ends are destroyed and replaced with viable bone, complete healing of the fracture with restoration of the form of the bone including the medullary canal occurs according to Wolff's law.

The amount of cartilage found in the callus as well as the amount of callus is dependent upon (1) the blood supply, (2) the size and the character of the bone, (3) the condition of the periosteum and (4) the amount of mobility present at the fracture site during the primary stage of healing (the greater the mobility the greater the amounts of cartilage and callus). With absolute immobilization and anatomic reduction of the fracture little cartilage forms.

Duthie and Barker[33] have demonstrated that both phosphorus and chondroitin sulfate are present in high concentration during fracture healing in the rat. Chondroitin sulfate, tagged with S^{35}, is present in the greatest concentration at about 7 days and then gradually disappears by the end of the 4th week when the fracture is essentially healed.

While the trabecular construction and rearrangement is going on in the callus, the necrotic ends of the bone are being invaded and destroyed by the process called *creeping substitution*. This consists of the invasion of the necrotic bone by a highly vascular and cellular connective tissue and the progressive laying down of bony trabeculae, making the line of fracture indiscernible from the original undamaged bone on microscopic examination. Creeping substitution[91] plays a very important role in the healing of fractures where large segments of bone are deprived of circulation and thereby killed. This process is seen best in the healing of thermal, bacterial and embolic osseous injuries and also in the incorporation of osseous grafts. Creeping substitution is a slow process; consequently, the roentgen appearance of large necrotic osseous fragments may remain seemingly unchanged for long periods of time.

THE FATE OF BONE GRAFTS

Improved methods in storage of bone have stimulated a considerable interest in the use of preserved bones as grafts and also in the study of the fate of these grafts in the host. It has long been known that fixation and replacement of the graft by living bone is more rapid with cancellous grafts than with cortical grafts.[3] Likewise, much of an autogenous bone graft dies and must be replaced with living bone by action of the host tissue.[19]

There has been a question as to whether any elements of an autogenous graft survive transplantation and assist in the incorporation of the graft into the recipient part. It has now been established that some of the cells of connective tissue derivation do survive in autogenous transplants and are capable of growth. How important the presence of these viable cells of the transplant are in the process of fixation and replacement is not known. We do know that freshly taken undenatured autogenous transplants are incorporated more rapidly and more surely than any other type of graft such as fresh or preserved homografts or heterografts.

Preservation of bone by any method tends in time to kill all elements of the bone. However, Ray[96] has been able to demonstrate growth in tissue culture of bone preserved by freezing for as long as 90 days.

For the most part, the preserved graft should be considered to be dead. Utilization of the graft must be primarily the function of the host. Experimental studies comparing the effect of autogenous and various dead grafts under favorable conditions reveal few visible differences between them in the basic processes of fixation and replacement. However, replacement of the graft is more rapid with autogenous bone, and fewer are resorbed or sequestered and walled off by connective tissue. At present there is evidence that these differences may be due to unfavorable host response to the graft rather than to the state of viability of transplant. There is hope that in the future preserved bone may be so treated, that it will call forth a host response more closely allied to that of autogenous transplants. At present, however, we feel that autogenous grafts are always preferred if it is possible to obtain them. An excellent review of bone grafting is that of Chase and Herndon.[19]

DECALCIFICATION OF THE SKELETON

As stated previously, bone absorption and reconstruction go on continuously throughout life. Anything that alters the rate of absorption and reconstruction tends to lead to alteration of the skeleton. Osteoporosis is the most common consequence of altered rates of absorption and reconstruction. A rate of bone absorption more rapid than the rate of new bone formation leads to osteoporosis. Rapid destruction of bone of the type seen with hyperparathyroidism and with certain types of renal insufficiency usually leads to osteitis fibrosa cystica, while less rapid destruction results in generalized wasting and atrophy of bone without cystic changes (see Chap. 27, "Thyroid, Thymus and Parathyroids").

TABLE 1.

TYPE OF DISTURBANCE	SERUM		Alkaline Phosphatase	Serum Protein	URINE		TISSUE
	Ca	P			Ca	P	
Osteoporosis	N	N	N	N-L	N	N	Normal-appearing but slender bone trabeculae
Osteomalacia	N-L	N-L	H	N	N-L	N-L	Marked increase in osteoid formation about all trabeculae
Hyperparathyroidism	H	L	H	N	H	H	Very active bone formation and destruction-osteoblasts, osteoclasts prominent
Osteogenesis Imperfecta	N	N	N	N	N	N	Normal-appearing but slender bone trabeculae
Myeloma	N-H	N-H	N	H	Bence Jones prot.		Tumor cells
Paget's Disease	N	N	H	N	N	N	Active bone formation with mosaic pattern

When the roentgenographic picture of decalcification of the skeleton presents itself the initial problem is to differentiate between the basic physiologic disturbances—osteoporosis, osteomalacia or hyperparathyroidism. This differentiation can usually be established by means of blood chemistries and bone biopsy. In the accompanying table the usual chemical relationships are indicated. Included are the findings in osteogenesis imperfecta, myeloma and Paget's disease which at times may be confused with osteoporosis, osteomalacia and hyperparathyroidism.

OSTEOPOROSIS

When the diagnosis of osteoporosis has been made the etiologic factor must be determined in order to institute effective therapy.

Failure of formation of a proper osteoid matrix which leads to osteoporosis may attend the faulty protein metabolism seen in starvation, Cushing's syndrome and the postmenopausal period. Albright[6] differentiates between postmenopausal osteoporosis and senile osteoporosis, because in the former the skull and the extremities are somewhat less involved in the demineralization process, and the lamina dura of the teeth remain normal, while in senile osteoporosis, changes involve all of the bones, including the lamina dura.

Osteoporosis also results from disuse. This osteoporosis of disuse is to be distinguished from the localized acute bone destruction which occurs in Sudeck's atrophy in which condition the destruction of all elements of bone trabeculae occurs, presumably on the basis of increased circulation. Osteoporosis of disuse is almost always demonstrable roentgenographically in the bones of a limb long contained in a cast. With osteoporosis secondary to a deficient matrix formation, the serum calcium, phosphorus and phosphatase are within normal limits. However, disuse osteoporosis associated with immobilization in body casts and traction apparatus is associated with slight hypercalcemia and a pronounced hypercalciuria. The latter predisposes the person to renal lithiasis.

Postmenopausal osteoporosis, which occurs commonly in women between the ages of 40 and 60, may be related to disturbances in protein metabolism associated with the loss of estrogen stimulation. The picture of postmenopausal osteoporosis is one of lessening stature, rounded shoulders, a painful back with restricted motions and tenderness over the spinous processes. Compression fracture of osteoporotic vertebral bodies occurs frequently after slight injuries and lifting. The x-ray examination may show extensive deossification of the vertebral bodies. The disk spaces are widened, producing a "codfish" type of vertebrae. Prolapse of the disk material into the weakened vertebral bodies may take place. At times decalcification is so severe and the destruction so advanced that the vertebral bodies are difficult to distinguish on the roentgenogram (Fig. 49-1). The serum calcium, phosphorus and phosphatase in these individuals is usually within normal limits. However, the total serum protein is usually low. Transient hypercalcemia may occur early

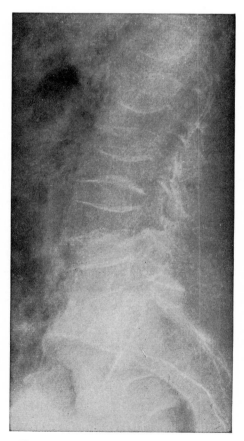

FIG. 49-1. Severe senile osteoporosis. At first glance the disk spaces may be mistaken for the vertebral bodies.

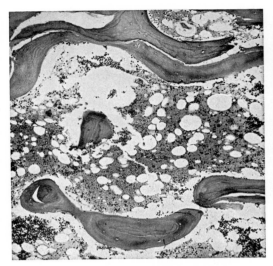

FIG. 49-2. Photomicrograph of bone from the iliac crest of a patient with osteomalacia. The symmetrical deposition of osteoid about each bone trabeculae is the characteristic histological fracture. The classical chemical findings of a high alkaline phosphatase, low serum phosphorus and normal serum calcium led to the biopsy which confirmed the diagnosis. The cause of osteomalacia in this patient (a 50-year-old woman) was faulty phosphate reabsorption.

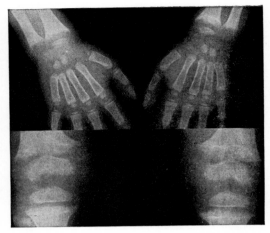

FIG. 49-3. Wrists and knees of child with rickets, showing the widened, cone-shaped epiphyseal lines. (From Shriner's Hospital, St. Louis, Mo.)

in the process. In women with severe senile decalcification the sedimentation rate is often elevated.

Treatment of the very acute phase of postmenopausal osteoporosis usually consists of bed rest and the control of pain with analgesics. However, the period of bed rest should be as short as possible and limited to the period of severe pain. The stress and strain of muscular activity conserves and improves the general condition of the patient and prevents the superimposition of disuse osteoporosis upon the postmenopausal syndrome. Androgen and/or estrogen therapy combined with adequate bracing of the spine is fairly effective. Although this form of treatment may be effective in relieving symptoms, it does not result in visible x-ray evidence of recalcification. Biopsy studies before and after hormonal therapy have been done by Levine, Gitman and Balker.[126] Bone samples were taken from the pelvis. These revealed no change in the character or amount of bone. X-ray therapy

in small doses over the painful spine may be helpful in relief of severe pain.

OSTEOMALACIA

Osteomalacia is a disturbance in the proper deposition of bone salt in the osteoid matrix. Histologically, bone trabeculae are thickened by layers of osteoid formation, but calcification of the osteoid is strikingly absent. Osteoblasts are in abundance (Fig. 49-2).

Albright[6] feels that any condition which produces this histologic change should be classified as rickets or osteomalacia, depending upon the age of the patient—rickets in children and osteomalacia in adults. An inadequate intake of vitamin D or the deficient absorption of this vitamin from the intestinal tract consequent to such diseases as sprue, celiac disease, chronic pancreatitis or steatorrhea may lead to rickets and osteomalacia. In children the pathologic process consists of a reduction of calcification at the zone of provisional calcification prefixed to the epiphyseal plate (Fig. 49-3).

As the child grows the deficient calcification within the zone of provisional calcification leads to improper calcification and ossification of the cartilaginous trabeculae, extending irregularly into the metaphyseal regions of the bone. These alterations are manifest in the x-ray picture as a widened cone-shaped epiphyseal plate with widening of the epiphysis and sclerosis of this structure along its metaphyseal margin. The epiphysis is less firmly attached to the metaphysis, permitting easier dislocation of the epiphysis among rickety children. The serum calcium is usually normal, but the inorganic phosphate of the blood is lower than normal, and the alkaline phosphatase may be increased 100 per cent or more. Calcium and phosphorus balances are less positive than normal.

Osteomalacia in the adult may be due to a variety of etiologic factors. When the diagnosis of osteomalacia has been established, the defect in calcium-phosphorus metabolism must be identified in order to institute correct therapy. Simple vitamin D lack, resistance to vitamin D, steatorrhea, renal acidosis, Fanconi syndrome, idiopathic hypercalcemia and failure of renal phosphate resorption can all produce the clinical and histologic picture of osteomalacia. However, the osseous and clinical manifestations differ somewhat from those of rickets. Decalcification of the skeleton is generalized, the epiphyseal changes are lacking because the epiphyseal plates have disappeared, the bones are softer than with rickets and deform readily, the acetabula approach one another, misshaping the pelvis. The serum calcium level is lower than normal, and hypocalcemic tetany may occur. The calcium bal-

ance is negative, and the phosphorus is near normal. The combination of a diet low in calcium and deficient in vitamin D, with an indoor life, is usually requisite to the development of osteomalacia.

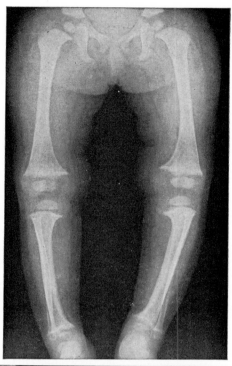

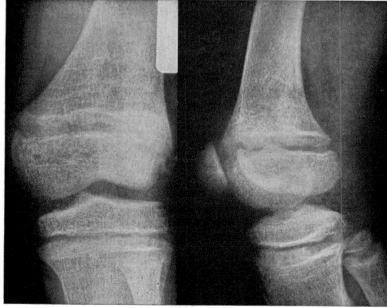

Fig. 49-4. (Top) Lower extremities of child with vitamin D resistant rickets before severe deformity has occurred. (From Dr. H. R. McCarroll, St. Louis, Mo.) (Bottom) A similar case of vitamin D resistant rickets showing healing after large doses of vitamin D. (From Shriner's Hospital, St. Louis, Mo.)

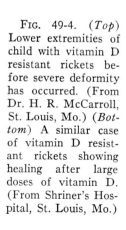

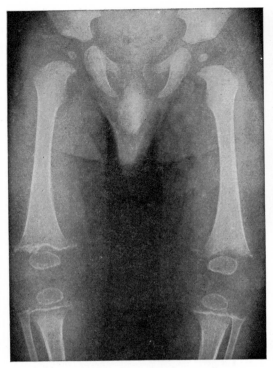

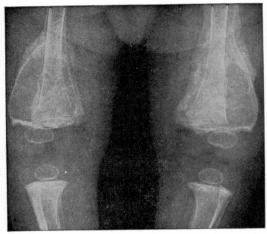

FIG. 49-5. (*Left*) Roentgenogram of childhood scurvy showing alteration of the epiphyseal lines and early subperiosteal new bone formation. The apparent increased density of the margins of the epiphyses at the knee, producing a ring appearance, is typical of this condition. (*Right*) Later stage of the disease with calcification and ossification of the large subperiosteal hematoma. The distal femoral epiphysis seems to have shifted on both sides. (From Shriner's Hospital, St. Louis, Mo.)

A predisposition to fracture and severe deformities of the pelvis which are likely to interfere seriously with childbirth constitute the clinical significance of the disease. The administration of vitamin D and a diet rich in calcium cure both rickets and osteomalacia.

There are some clinical variants of rickets and osteomalacia. Albright[6] considers the syndrome of Milkman's disease[82], characterized by symmetrical fractures starting in the cortex, to be identical with osteomalacia. Rarely, cases of rickets seem to have a familial tendency. These cases are resistant to vitamin D therapy, showing no clinical response to normal amounts of vitamin D intake. Albright,

Butler and Bloomsberg[5] described 6 cases and demonstrated that the pathologic process was exactly the same as in rickets, and that the only difference was the resistance to vitamin D therapy (Fig. 49-4). However, they found that giving very large doses of vitamin D would result eventually in healing. They termed these cases *vitamin-D-resistant rickets*. Pederson and McCarroll in 1951[90] presented a large series of such patients, pointing out that the diagnosis is commonly missed, and that these individuals were subjected to repeated surgical procedures for correction of osseous deformities, only to have the deformity recur until proper diagnosis was made and treatment was instituted. The main problem presented by these cases is that the enormous vitamin D dosage required to control the disease closely approximates the toxic level and requires very careful observation during therapy.

SCURVY

Except for the epiphyseal changes, the clinical and pathologic conditions are similar in both the child and the adult. It has been well established that a 6-month deficit of vitamin C is usually necessary before symptoms of scurvy appear. The classical pathologic changes are found in tissues of mesodermal origin. Periosteal hemorrhage, decreased osteoblastic activity in the epiphyseal regions, replacement of the myelogenous elements of the bone marrow by fibrous tissue, increased brittleness of the teeth, gingival hemorrhage, and a secondary anemia are the classic pathologic changes seen in scurvy. Severe pain in the legs is frequently the first symptom of scurvy and is the direct result of the subperiosteal hemorrhage (Fig. 49-5). Swollen, bleeding gums, loose teeth, and hemorrhagic lesions of the skin are other common findings. Epiphyseal separations and metaphyseal fractures are frequently seen in children. Due to the generalized deossification of the skeleton in late adult scurvy, pathologic fractures through the diaphyseal region of the long bones may also occur.

The classic x-ray changes are broad irregular zones in the provisional area of calcification of the growing epiphyseal plate. Ringing of the epiphysis itself, periosteal calcification and ossification, and a ground-glass translucency of the bones are also typical changes of scurvy.

If the condition remains untreated, death occurs within a few months. Pneumonia has been reported as the leading cause of death. The response to vitamin C therapy is prompt and curative. Pain and tenderness from subperiosteal hemorrhage is often relieved in 24 to 36 hours. Endochondral ossification is resumed, and frequently the ossified subperiosteal hematoma may disappear entirely.

The roentgenographic changes about the epiphysis must not be confused with the changes seen in lead poisoning. The finding of increased radiodensity of the calcified portion of the epiphyseal plate should cause a search for the other stigmata of plumbism (history of lead exposure, anemia, radial palsy, colic, increased lead level in the serum, increased urinary excretion of lead, and stippling of the red cells) (Fig. 49-6). Phosphorus and Bismuth intoxication may produce roentgenographic changes similar to those found in plumbism.

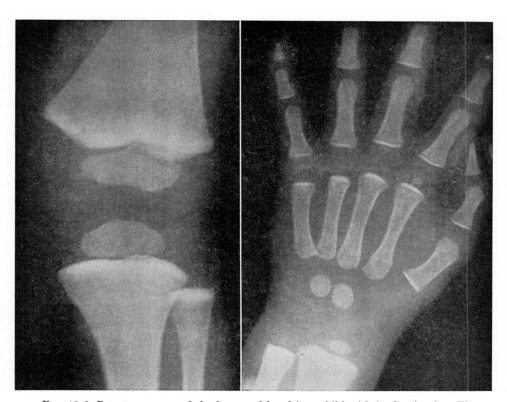

Fig. 49-6. Roentgenogram of the knee and hand in a child with lead poisoning. The increased density of metaphysis adjacent to the epiphyseal plate is characteristic. Toxic blood levels of lead and increased lead excretion in the urine confirmed the diagnosis.

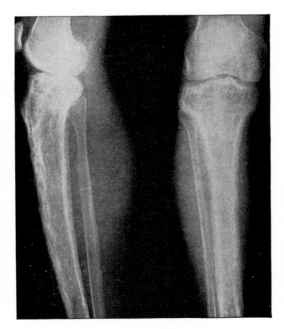

Fig. 49-7. Advanced changes in the tibia from Paget's disease. Note cortical thickening, coarse trabeculation. Transverse fissures in the anterior cortex represent pathologic fractures of a type similar to Looser's. There are no other roentgenologic evidences of Paget's disease in this patient.

OTHER METABOLIC DISEASES OF BONE

Seemingly, Paget's disease is a metabolic disease of bone. Moehlig and Abbott[85] believe it to be the result of a disturbance of carbohydrate metabolism. However, the etiology of Paget's disease remains unknown; consequently, no effective treatment has been devised. Paget's disease almost always occurs in persons past the age of 40 and in advanced stages is characterized by an increase in size of the skull (often requiring a change in hat size in men), curvature and shortening of the

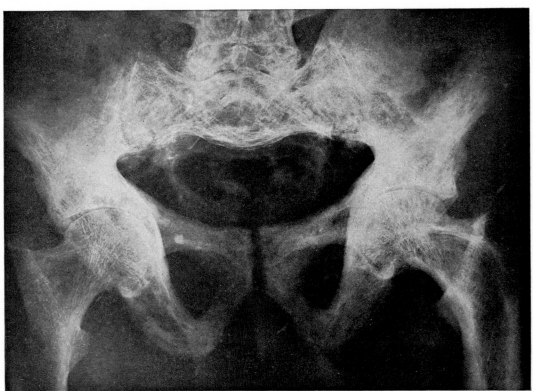

Fig. 49-8. Advanced Paget's disease, involving the lower lumbar spine, the sacrum, both innominate bones and the left femur. This patient presented himself because of painful hips, the diagnosis not having been made previously.

extremities and kyphosis. However, the disease may appear first in only one bone, all the rest of the skeleton remaining normal. When it does it is called *monostotic Paget's disease* (Fig. 49-7). Pain, thickening of the bone, increased heat and tenderness in the region of the lesion constitute the clinical signs of the monostotic form. Roentgenograms may show an irregular or fusiform lytic cavity in the bone, which may readily be confused with fibrous dysplasia.

Whether the disease is monostotic or generalized, the parts of the skeleton most commonly affected are the skull, the pelvis, the spine, the tibia and the small bones of the hands (Fig. 49-8). The feet and the ribs are rarely affected. There is an increased blood flow in the bone about the lesions in Paget's disease. The blood chemical studies may be within normal limits with the monostotic form; at times a positive diagnosis is made only from biopsy study. When the disease is more widespread, the differential diagnosis seldom offers any difficulty. With Paget's disease progressive active bone destruction or decalcification, simultaneously attended by a rapid overcompensating new bone formation, produces bones of greatly increased size. However, because of failure of proper orientation of the newly formed bone to lines of force there is decreased strength.

Fracture of the long bones is frequently found at the junction of the normal and the pathologic bone. The affected skull cap grows larger, and the progressive destruction of normal bone and the rapid overproduction results in the so-called "cottonwool" texture of the skull seen on roentgenograms. In the extremities the process results in broad irregular trabeculae lacking a definite pattern of arrangement.

The histologic examination of tissue taken from an active lesion shows active new bone formation and bone destruction going on in the same area; while broad irregular trabeculae with many cement lines produce a mosaic pattern (Fig. 49-9).

Chemical studies in Paget's disease show that the serum calcium and inorganic phosphorus content are usually within normal limits and that the calcium output in the urine is within normal limits. However, the alka-

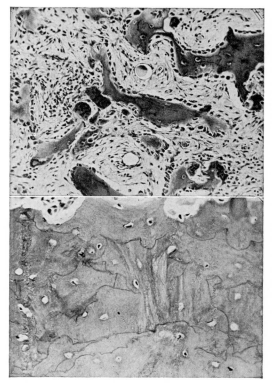

Fig. 49-9. (*Top*) Photomicrograph showing active new bone formation and bone destruction going on in a vascular fibrous stroma. (*Bottom*) Specimen from a somewhat older portion of the diseased bone showing irregular cement lines in a greatly thickened bone trabeculae resulting in a mosaic pattern.

line phosphatase is increased and may be as much as 20 or 30 times normal.

The complications of Paget's disease are: (1) pathologic fracture, (2) compression fracture of the spine, at times with spinal cord pressure, (3) deafness, (4) degenerative changes of joints secondary to incongruities and irregularities from pressure molding of the soft bone contiguous with them, and (5) the development of osteogenic sarcoma, which occurs in 5 to 10 per cent of the cases.

DISTURBANCES IN LIPID METABOLISM

The so-called lipid or lipoid granulomas of bone are Letterer-Siwe disease, Hand-Schüller-Christian disease, eosinophilic granuloma,

Gaucher's disease, Niemann-Pick disease and Hurler's disease. Letterer-Siwe disease and eosinophilic granuloma are not as a rule considered as being lipoid storage diseases. However, they appear closely related to them and therefore are discussed under this heading.

LETTERER-SIWE DISEASE

This condition is characterized by granulomatous lesions made up of collections of histiocytes (macrophages) without lipid occurring in them. These lesions occur especially in bones, spleen and other parenchymatous organs. It usually appears in children under the age of 2 or 3 years.

The clinical signs are cutaneous ecchymoses at times combined with superficial ulcerations, low-grade fever, a large liver and spleen, enlarged lymph nodes and a chronic progressive anemia. The osseous lesions destroy the bone and most commonly are found in the skull. This condition was formerly considered as being a universally fatal disease. In recent years because of its infectionlike characteristics, these patients have been treated with antibiotics, and many have recovered. Recently, Bierman et al.[11] has isolated the Arizona type of salmonella organism from a case of Letterer-Siwe disease. Antibiotic therapy was successful in arresting the lesions.

Theoretically, a patient with Letterer-Siwe disease who survives would slowly develop the clinical picture of Hand-Schüller-Christian disease. We have never seen these possibly closely related abnormalities change from one to the other.

HAND-SCHÜLLER-CHRISTIAN DISEASE

This disease is characterized by the proliferation of fibrous tissue in which are nests of histiocytes containing esters of cholesterol. Clinically, the syndrome is characterized by multiple round defects in the skull, exophthalmus, diabetes insipidus and some signs of infantilism. As no demonstrable disturbance or abnormality of cholesterol metabolism has been demonstrated, it seems likely that the collection of cholesterol in the histiocytes is not related to a generalized disturbance of cholesterol metabolism but is merely the local collection of cholesterol by the granuloma cells (Fig. 49-10).

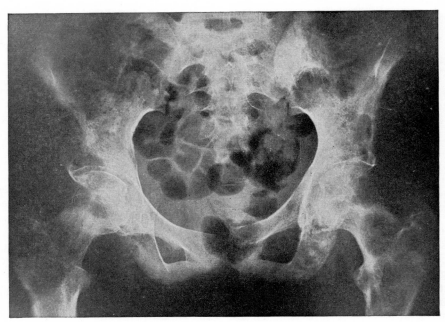

FIG. 49-10. The roentgenogram reveals multiple destruction areas in bone without new bone formation. A biopsy of one of these lesions was compatible with the diagnosis of Hand-Schüller-Christian disease.

FIG. 49-11. (*Right*) This teen-aged boy presented himself with pain and swelling of the arm of about 6-weeks' duration. Examination revealed a hard, brawny, tender enlargement of the arm with marked increase in local heat. The roentgenogram revealed a mottled, irregular area of bone destruction in the shaft of the humerus at the middle and the lower thirds with periosteal new bone formation. This, plus fever and leukocytosis suggested a clinical diagnosis of Ewing's sarcoma. However, the microscopic picture (*below*), was that of eosinophilic granuloma. Unfortunately, the eosinophils do not show without color.

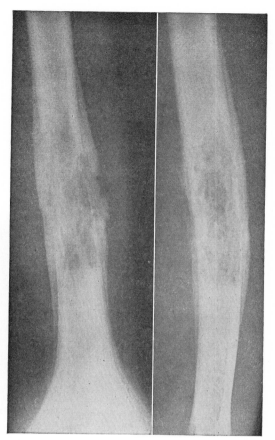

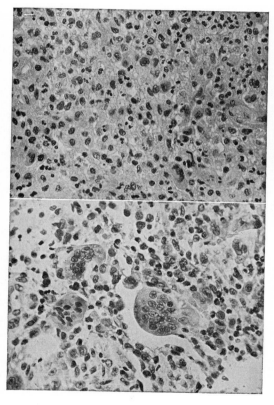

metaphyseal or epiphyseal regions (Fig. 49-11). Although the majority of the osseous eosinophilic granulomas are solitary, occasionally they are multiple. Green and Farber[46] reported that in some eosinophilic granulomas as maturity of the individual is approached deposition of lipid materials occurs, and the eosinophils tend to disappear. However, Jaffe and Lichtenstein[59] feel that the eosinophilic granuloma does not necessarily become a lipid granuloma before healing but may heal through simple resolution.

Mallory[79] tentatively expressed the relationship between these 3 conditions to be as follows: (1) Letterer-Siwe disease usually occurs in infancy and early childhood and is rapidly fatal. The histiocytic proliferations are wide scattered throughout the soft tissue, especially the lymphoid tissue and the skull. (2) Hand-Schüller-Christian's disease occurs in both children and adults and is more chronic in character. The histiocytic lesions

The eosinophilic granuloma of Jaffe and Lichtenstein[59] seems to be closely related to the preceding 2 diseases. It occurs primarily in young individuals and has not been seen in a patient over 45 years of age. Histologically, the eosinophilic granuloma is a mixture of histiocytes and eosinophils. The bone lesions are common in the skull, the pelvis, the ribs, the vertebrae, the humerus and the femur and are more common in the diaphysis than the

undergo lipidization in about one third of the patients. The prognosis is grave because of damage to heart, lungs, brain and the pituitary gland. (3) Eosinophilic granuloma occurs in children and young adults. It is comparatively benign and is largely localized in the skeleton and usually to only one bone, although rarely the lesions are multiple. As a rule it heals readily after curetting with or without x-ray therapy.

GAUCHER'S DISEASE

This is also a disease of lipid metabolism. The histiocytes and the reticular cells in the spleen, the liver and the bone marrow become filled with a gluco-galactoside kerasin. Kerasin contains nitrogen but no phosphorus. It is chemically inactive and is not stainable with the usual lipid stains. However, it can be stained with Mallory's aniline blue orange G stain. Gaucher's disease is characterized by progressive hepatic and splenic enlargement, starting early in life. Anemia, leukopenia and thrombocytopenia are frequently observed. The disease is usually familial.[111] The bone lesions may be widespread; the lower end of the femur is a common site. The roentgenogram presents a mottled moth-eaten appearance with little evidence of new bone formation. The articular cartilage is not invaded by the Gaucher cells, although aseptic necrosis and crumbling of the epiphysis or articular surface may occur. As the bone marrow contains a large number of the Gaucher cells, sternal puncture is effective in establishing a diagnosis.

NIEMANN-PICK DISEASE

This is a rather rare, strongly familial disease characterized by the collection of abnormal deposits of phospholipids and cholesterol in the reticuloendothelial tissues with a seeming predilection for the Jewish people. The predominant lipids are sphingomyelin and lecithin. It occurs most frequently in very young children and runs a short and usually fatal course. The reticulum of the bone marrow is always involved; however, a diffuse osteoporosis may be the only manifestation of bone involvement.

HURLER'S DISEASE

Hurler's disease or lipochondrodystrophy is a rare hereditary and perhaps familial disease of otherwise unknown etiology. Clinical mani-festations are a deformed head and face, dwarfism, enlarged liver and spleen, an enlarged abdomen, kyphosis and mental retardation.

DEVELOPMENTAL ABNORMALITIES

INTRODUCTION

The term "congenital abnormality" cannot be applied strictly to the broad group of pathologic changes that are manifest as aberrations of normal development of the early growing individual. Although the majority of these abnormalities are present at birth (congenital), some of them may be incipient at the time of birth and become increasingly manifest with postnatal growth and development.

The pathogenesis of developmental abnormalities is incompletely understood, although several different factors appear to be important and may be divided into 2 groups: extrinsic and intrinsic. Congenital furrows and bands as well as some congenital amputations have been thought to be due to amniotic adhesions and are examples of extrinsic influences on the developing fetus. Faulty intra-uterine position is undoubtedly important in some cases. Intrinsic factors such as primary germ plasm variation, with and without hereditary linkage, must be considered. Experimentally, various degrees and types of abnormalities may be produced by environmental alterations applied to the embryo and the fetus. These include mechanical, thermal and x-ray injury, maternal nutritional deficiencies, maternal infections and maternal metabolic and hormonal disorders. Duraiswami[30] has published an excellent review on this subject, including brilliant experimental studies. The different malformations that have been recorded are too numerous to be described here, and only those more commonly encountered and of orthopedic significance will be considered.

CONGENITAL DYSPLASIA AND DISLOCATION OF THE HIP

Etiology and Pathogenesis. The etiology and the pathogenesis of this abnormality have not been determined. At birth, one or both hips may be completely dislocated or demonstrate varying degrees of dysplasia. The terms "dysplasia" and "dislocation" are frequently used interchangeably.

A dislocated hip is either displaced out of the acetabulum posteriorly or anteriorly, or it may be dislocated upward and laterally. Subluxation implies that the head of the femur is partially but incompletely dislocated. Children with a congenital subluxation, if unrecognized, may develop an overt dislocation when they begin to walk. Congenital dysplasia of the hip consists of a retarded development of the femoral head (smaller than opposite normal femoral head) and a shallow acetabulum. A dysplastic hip may fail to develop a normal femoral head-acetabular relationship, and for this reason treatment should be instituted. It is most unusual that a dysplastic hip progresses to a frank dislocation.

Incidence. The conditions occur in females in 85 per cent of cases and is unilateral in 75 per cent of cases: they are more common in white Mediterranean racial stock and may have familial tendencies. It is extremely rare in the Negro.

As relatively few cases are completely dislocated at birth, the emphasis should be placed on the earliest possible recognition of the dysplastic hip. If adequate treatment is instituted in this stage, an essentially normal hip may be expected as the end result without the necessity of operative treatment. An outstanding monograph on this subject has been published by Vernon Hart.[53]

Signs and Symptoms of Dislocation. In children under the age of 1 (not walking) the physician must be alert to the minimal signs of dislocation. These include: (1) deepening or an increased number of the skin creases of the thigh and buttock skin secondary to shortening of the leg; (2) shortening of the involved extremity; (3) adduction contracture of the hip, best elicted by attempting to abduct the flexed hip while the child is supine. A normal infant's hip will permit an abduction of 80° to 90°; a dislocated hip will not. (4) Ortolani's sign is an audible or palpable click that occurs during abduction of the hip. This click occurs as either the dislocated or the subluxated femoral head slips over the posterior rim of the acetabulum, the so-called "click of entry"; (5) "telescoping" of the femur. This last sign is demonstrated as a pistonlike mobility of the femur that attends the pushing and the pulling of the thigh while the pelvis is fixed by a hand. This is done with the child supine, and the hip and the knee flexed to 90°.

In the child over the age of 1 (walking age), the same signs are present, but they are more obvious, and the child walks with a waddling gait.

Diagnosis of Dislocation. Presence, or suspicion of the presence, of any of these signs, should lead to a careful x-ray examination. The x-ray signs are: (1) delayed ossification of both femoral and acetabular components of the hip joint; (2) increased obliquity of the angle made by the roof of the acetabulum with the horizontal line drawn through the "Y" cartilages (Fig. 49-12); in an infant the upper limit of normal is 28° to 30°; (3) dislocation of the developing head of the femur if the epiphysis is present or of the proximal femoral shaft if the epiphysis is not present; (4) increased antiversion of the neck of the femur, demonstrated by comparing (a) an anteroposterior view of the pelvis with the hip in neutral position (knee pointing to the ceiling) and (b) with the hip held in forced internal rotation. If abnormally antiverted the hip will appear to have a valgus deformity in neutral but will appear normal when forcibly internally rotated.

Pathology of Dislocation. The characteristic abnormalities of a complete dislocation include: elongation of the joint capsule which may be associated with an hourglass constriction of the capsule located between the head of the femur and the acetabulum, a shallow acetabulum, a groove on the superior acetabular rim secondary to pressure from the head of the femur, the filling of the acetabular fossa with the inverted fibrocartilaginous rim attached to the superior rim of the acetabulum, the so-called *limbus* and the filling of the deep acetabular fossa with fibrous tissue representing a hypertrophied "haversian gland."[112] Secondary contracture of the joint capsule, muscles, nerves and vessels also occurs. The femoral neck is antiverted.

Treatment. The treatment of congenital dislocation of the hip is still a widely disputed subject. The principles advocated by Crego and Schwartzmann[27] and by McCarroll[76] are recommended. In a child less than a year old general anesthesia should be used to determine how difficult reduction is. Great force should not be used during the attempted reduction, because the epiphysis may be damaged. If it is possible to reduce the hip easily, the child is placed in a cast in a frog-leg position, and the program advocated by Ponseti and Frigerio[94] is followed. This con-sists of gradually changing the position of the leg to abduction, extension and internal rotation during a number of changes of the cast within a 6-month period. If the reduction cannot be accomplished easily, no treatment

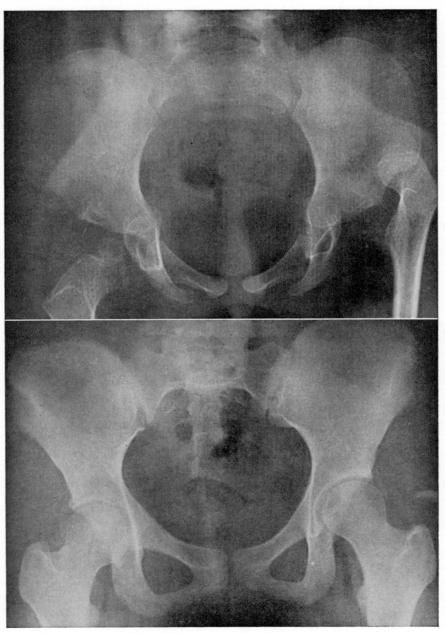

FIG. 49-12. (*Top*) Appearance of a typical congenital dislocation of the hip prior to treatment. (*Bottom*) Same patient. A very satisfactory result 14 years after adequate treatment. (From Shriner's Hospital, St. Louis, Mo.)

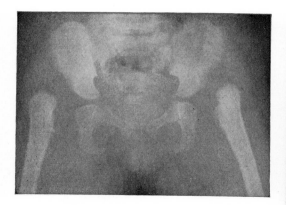

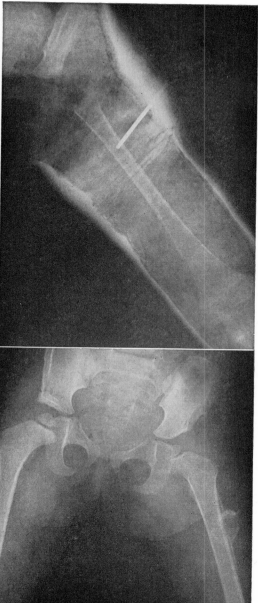

FIG. 49-13. (A, *Left, top*) Typical appearance of bilateral congenital dislocation of the hips in an infant. (B, *Left, bottom*) Same patient. Appearance of the hip during skeletal traction prior to closed reduction according to the method of Crego. (C, *Right, top*) Following closed reduction of the hip, a supracondylar derotational osteotomy has been performed to correct anteversion of the femoral neck. The position of the proximal fragment is controlled by a pin through the femoral shaft. (D, *Right, bottom*) Final appearance of the hip after removal of the cast. (From Shriner's Hospital, St. Louis, Mo.)

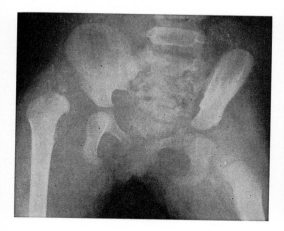

should be begun until the child is 1 year old. Then skeletal traction should be instituted. For children over 1 year old, manipulation under anesthesia is not done and traction is used first to stretch gradually the tightly contracted structures about the hip. After approximately 3 weeks of skeletal traction a closed reduction often may be done easily, and then the thigh is fully rotated internally, abducted widely and immobilized in a plaster cast. After 2 or 3 months in the cast a derotational osteotomy may be needed to correct the antiversion of the femoral neck. If the osteotomy is done, 2 more months of immobilization will be necessary (Fig. 49-13A, B, C, D). Because of gross inadequacy of the acetabulum or because of soft tissue changes, the formal head cannot be reduced in certain instances. When the dislocation cannot be easily reduced after 3 weeks of traction, an open reduction must be done. During the open reduction the fibrous tissue in the acetabulum is excised, and the poorly developed acetabular roof may be reconstructed. After an open reduction the treatment will be the same as after a closed reduction. Using these methods, excellent results may be anticipated in 80 to 90 per cent of the children if treated before the age of 4. The use of skeletal traction preliminary to reduction of the dislocation has practically eliminated the complication of a vascular necrosis of the femoral epiphysis that is not infrequent with other methods.

Signs and Symptoms of the Dysplastic Hip. This diagnosis depends a great deal on intuition. The detection of slight limitation of abduction or a little instability of the child's hip when the telescoping test is performed may be the main tips. A family history of congenital dislocation of the hip or another congenital anomaly such as club feet should make one at least suspicious that a dysplasia may exist. If a subluxation is present the Ortoloni sign may be positive, and an extra skin fold may be present. Instability of the hip will be noted on the telescoping test, but the diagnosis will be made only by an examiner who is looking for or thinking about a dislocation of the hip.

Diagnosis. The diagnosis rests upon the roentgenographic detection of (1) delayed ossification; (2) a shallow acetabulism; (3) and lateral displacement of the femoral epiphysis.

Treatment of the Dysplastic and Subluxated Hip. One may maintain constant reduction of the hip while at the same time permitting active motion of the extremity by applying a Frejka pillow splint. This consists of a firm pillow placed between the knees and holding the legs in a "frog-leg" position. The Ilfeld[58] splint is as effective, but with it excessive pressure may be placed on the epiphysis by the forcible abduction. In those children who cannot be controlled in a pillow splint, a plaster cast may be necessary. Usually, from 3 to 6 months of fixation of the thigh by one means or another will permit the acetabulum to develop and thereby cure the affliction should the apparatus be applied early in life.

DEVELOPMENTAL ABNORMALITIES OF THE FOOT

These deformities present at birth, may be unilateral or bilateral, and are somewhat more common in males; there may be familial occurrence.

Equinovarus Clubfoot. The etiology in the equinovarus "clubfoot," which occurs in all degrees of severity, is unknown. This condition has 3 separate components of deformity: adduction of the forefoot in relation to the hindfoot, varus of the entire foot, primarily of the subtalar joint, and equinus of the foot with contracture of the heel cord (Fig. 49-14). Internal torsion of the tibia is frequently associated.

PROGNOSIS. Usually at birth there is no bony deformity and if the condition is corrected properly, an essentially normal foot can be obtained. If neglected, the deformity becomes worse and more resistant to correction and actual bony deformity develops consequent to abnormal function.

DIAGNOSIS is made by inspection of the attitude of the feet and testing the range of active and passive movement.

TREATMENT. Ideally, treatment should begin as soon as the diagnosis is made. If proper management is instituted in the first few days of life, not only is correction more certain but the surgeon's task is easier.

Conservative. The method of choice in most of these cases is the use of wedging plaster casts, as described by Kite.[66] A plaster boot is used to hold, and by wedging, to correct gradually the 3 components of the deformity. It is of utmost importance to correct the adduction and the varus before starting to correct the equinus. The casts are usually wedged or changed at intervals of 1 week. Correction is obtained when the foot is in a position representing the normal extent of passive abduction, valgus and dorsiflexion. Depending on the extent and the flexibility of the deformity, correction usually can be obtained in from a few weeks to 3 or 4 months. Once full correction is obtained, a final cast is used to hold this position for 4 to 6 weeks. In the very mild cases, correction may be obtained by frequent daily passive stretching of the contracted soft parts by the mother. Such manipulation usually is done after plaster correction to restrain the tendency to recurrence. Other forms of nonoperative treatment include the Denis-Browne splint, with the various modifications and adhesive strapping, and have their advocates.

Surgical. Operative procedures should not be used as a short cut in the management of the uncomplicated club foot. If one consistently fails to obtain good correction by conservative means, the fault lies in the physician and not in the patient. However, one should be prepared to correct the resistant club foot surgically. Heyman[54] has developed an anterior capsulotomy which is done at the tarsometatarsal articulation of all 5 toes. This enables one to correct the forefoot varus. A capsulotomy of the medial tarsal joints, heel cord lengthening, and a posterior capsulotomy of the ankle and subastragalar joints are frequently required. Older children and adults will require the removal of a bone wedge, and frequently a triple arthrodesis is necessary.

Metatarsus Adductus. A more commonly encountered anomaly of the foot is a metatarsus adductus which is frequently and incorrectly called metatarsus varus. In this condition the forefoot is turned medialward in relation to the hindfoot. This deformity usually is associated with some degree of internal tibial torsion. The forefoot adduction responds well to plaster cast correction if done in the first year, and the tibial torsion will be corrected spontaneously if not too marked or may require the use of some type of splint to hold the extremity in full external rotation during the sleeping hours. A variety of satisfactory appliances which attach to shoes are available for this purpose.

Calcaneo valgus deformities are seen occasionally in which there is limitation of plantar flexion and inversion; the dorsum of the foot may be placed passively against the lower leg. The majority of these will correct with manipulative stretching of the contracted soft tissue. Rarely, the deformity is sufficiently severe to require wedging plaster correction. The deformity usually is associated with a relaxed flatfoot that will require treatment after weight-bearing is started.

Flatfoot. So-called "flatfoot" will be considered here, although many cases are in no way true developmental abnormalities. The development of longitudinal and transverse arches usually is delayed until the child has walked for a sufficient time to permit the muscles supporting these arches to develop in strength. It is quite common to see flatfeet in children who have just started to walk and to have this deformity disappear in a few weeks or months. This tendency to flatfeet may be accentuated by obesity, serious illness or malnutrition. These forms of flatfeet in

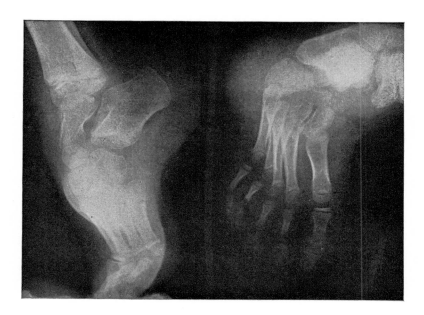

Fig. 49-14. Typical x-ray appearance of uncorrected clubfoot in an older child. (From Shriner's Hospital, St. Louis, Mo.)

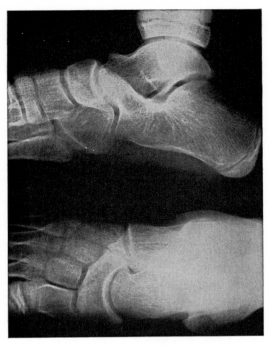

Fig. 49-15. Large calcaneonavicular horn. (From Shriner's Hospital, St. Louis, Mo.)

small children require only a good corrective shoe and time to permit attainment of a normal functioning and appearing foot.

There is a heriditary form of flatfoot that has a strong racial preponderance (Negro) that is not influenced by treatment. Fortunately, these individuals usually do not have significant disability.

There is an extreme degree of flatfoot produced by an anomaly of the astragalus in which the head of this bone is directed into the plantar aspect of the foot instead of forward toward the forefoot. This usually is disabling and can be corrected only by stabilization of the foot. This has been called a *"diving duck" astragalus* because of its x-ray appearance.

The so-called *spastic flatfoot* which we believe to be the result of altered subtalar function with or without anomalous bars is not common in children. Frequently, it may be treated adequately by manipulation and cast. Recurrent or persistent painful spastic flatfoot can be relieved only by subtalar fusion. We have not found it necessary to lengthen the peroneal tendons nor have we

seen relief with lengthening of the peroneal tendons without fusion.

A common cause of painful feet is talocalcaneal and/or calcaneonavicular bars, either bony or cartilaginous (Fig. 49-15). When only cartilaginous it may be impossible to establish the diagnosis except for restriction of motion of the involved joint, but when bony there is no difficulty in making the diagnosis, provided that oblique roentgenograms are obtained.

Treatment requires triple arthrodesis (see p. 1433 of this chapter), for resection of these bars has failed to give relief of pain or deformity, according to Harris and Beath.[51]

Developmental Abnormalities of the Hand and the Forearm

Only the more common abnormalities can be mentioned.

Syndactylism, or webbing of the fingers, is most frequent in this group (see Chap. 23, "Principles of Hand Surgery").

Congenital absence of tendons may occur in any muscle but more frequently affects the common extensors of the fingers and results in a flexion deformity. Tendon transpositions or grafts may be useful to restore function.

The so-called "thumb clutched hand" is one of the common thumb deformities of the newborn infant. The thumb is held in the acutely flexed position and may be due to either a stenosis of the flexor tendon sheath at the metacarpophalangeal joint or a congenital absence of the extensor pollicis brevis tendon. Section of the flexor tendon sheath may be necessary in the former condition, and tendon transfer in the latter situation.

Congenital absence of digits or whole finger rays is encountered and present problems of surgical closure of clefts, pollicization of fingers when the thumb is absent, and other plastic procedures (see Chap. 23).

Congenital absence (partial or total) of the radius is seen occasionally and produces a "club hand" in which the hand is fixed in radial deviation, and the thumb may be absent or deformed. The function in these extremities is sometimes surprisingly good, and the surgeon should be particularly careful not to do anything to give it a better cosmetic appearance at the expense of function.

In congenital absence of the radius or the

ulna a severe bowing of the forearm may result and require operative correction. The absent bone usually has a fibrous band in its place. The failure of the fibrous band to grow at the rate of the bone present results in severe curving. The student is referred to Riordan[97] for a discussion of the surgical management of these problems. Stretching of the soft tissue contracture by plaster casts as soon after birth as possible is indicated. Later surgical release of contracted bands, repositioning of the carpus and a bone graft to replace the missing radius are the steps necessary to improve the deformity.

Congenital fusion of carpal bones usually is nondisabling and requires no treatment.

Congenital amputation of part or all of one or more extremities is seen and presents a problem of prosthesis-fitting and stump-revision. The use of a prosthesis in the young child of 2 or 3 is worthwhile. The prosthesis is used as a helping hand surprisingly well.

Congenital Polydactylism. An additional number of partial or complete digits may be present on the hands or the feet. Such deformities are usually bilaterally symmetrical and often appear in several members of the same family. Removal of the extra digit is indicated only after the surgeon has ascertained which digit is the abnormal one.

Congenital pseudarthrosis of the tibia and the fibula with marked deformity has been a particularly difficult surgical problem for years with a high incidence of failure of bone grafting. Recent reports indicate that excision of the entire area of pseudarthrosis scar prior to bone graft and internal fixation improves the chance of success.

There are many generalized afflictions of bone that are presumed to be developmental anomalies. They are rare and usually are not amenable to surgical attack; the student is referred to Fairbank's[36] treatise for detailed description of this interesting group of afflictions.

Congenital coxa vara, although rare, appears to be due to failure of development of the neck of the femur. When treated early with fixation of the neck and the capital epiphysis and the varus deformity corrected by a subtrochanteric osteotomy of the rotational type, very satisfactory hips can be obtained. Late cases with severe deformity

and nonunion may be improved, but the end results are disappointing.

SLIPPING OF THE CAPITAL FEMORAL EPIPHYSIS

Incidence. A gradual displacement of the upper femoral epiphysis is a condition frequently encountered in adolescence. Most of the cases are seen between the ages of 12 and 14; however, the condition may be found in individuals varying from 8 to 19 years of age. It is commonly stated that this most frequently occurs in an individual who is overweight and has a body configuration similar to that which is associated with Fröhlich's syndrome. However, the condition not infrequently is seen also in the tall slender individual during a period of rapid growth. The incidence is slightly higher in males.

Etiology of the slipped capital femoral epiphysis remains unknown. Although trauma may be associated with an acute slipping of the epiphysis, more frequently the trauma that is related to the onset of symptoms is actually of a rather trivial nature. Endocrine imbalance also has been incriminated as an etiologic factor, particularly in those individuals who present the appearance of body habitus associated with Fröhlich's syndrome. More recently, it has been found that rats fed on a diet containing 50 per cent *Lathyrus odoratus* (sweet peas) seeds develop slipping of the epiphysis in the region of the knees and the shoulder (Ponseti[93]). In these animals it has been reported that there is a disintegration between the zone of proliferating cells and the calcified cartilage of the epiphysis. Slipping of the epiphysis occurred along this line of diminished resistance with the periosteum being detached at the metaphysis. The active factor of the *Lathyrus odoratus* seed has been identified chemically as an amino propionitril. With its administration the lesions appeared in areas where ground substances contained chondroitin sulfate as the only mucopolysaccharide. The fact that in man such epiphyseal slipping is seen almost solely at the upper end of the femur would lead one to believe that the obliquity of the upper femoral epiphysis or other factors may account for the displacement.

Diagnosis of a slipped femoral epiphysis must be entertained in any adolescent who complains of either pain in the hip or is walking with a limp. It must always be remembered that the pain may be referred along the path of the obturator nerve, and not infrequently the chief complaint may be pain at the inner aspect of the knee. In the early stages—the so-called preslipping stage—physical examination may be essentially normal. However, as actual slipping of the epiphysis progresses, limitation of flexion and an external rotational deformity will become increasingly apparent. In cases that have gone unrecognized there may be thigh and calf atrophy on the affected side, and limitation of abduction is a common finding in the more acute phases.

X-ray examination of both hips in the anteroposterior and lateral views will almost always confirm the diagnosis. The early changes seen on the roentgenogram are a slight roughening and widening of the epiphyseal line of the affected side. When displacement occurs, the epiphysis displaces pos-

teriorly and inferiorly. In the anteroposterior view the varus deformity is clearly evident (Fig. 49-16), but the posterior displacement is recognized most readily in the lateral view.

Treatment. In the natural course of this disease, displacement is finally stabilized by solid bony fusion of the epiphysis, and the symptoms may subside until the onset of the traumatic arthritis, which may come years after the slipping has occurred. It is generally agreed that when the diagnosis has been established, operative fixation to prevent further slipping is the best treatment provided the displacement is less than one third of the diameter of the femoral head. This fixation may be accomplished by means of the Smith-Petersen nail, the Knowles pins or the bone-pegging operation described by Howorth.[57] However, it may be impossible to drive a nail, and we prefer to use pins. In cases where the displacement has been more than one third the diameter of the neck of the femur, restoration of the anatomic relationships should be done.

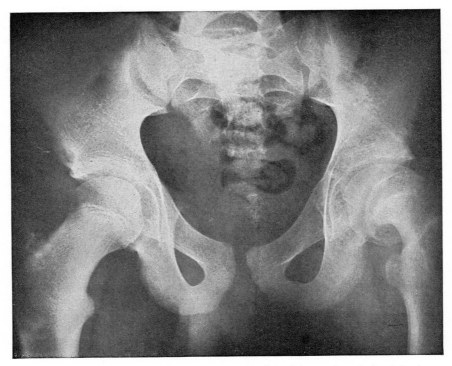

Fig. 49-16. Typical x-ray appearance of a slipped femoral capital epiphysis. Note the anterior and superior displacement of the femoral neck, the inferior bowing of the neck, and the demineralization of bone about the epiphyseal plate. The patient was a 15-year-old boy who had been limping for a year.

In such cases osteotomy of the femoral neck followed by internal fixation is often employed. However, the end results may be disappointing, for aseptic necrosis of the epiphysis or an early onset of degenerative arthritis not infrequently is a complication of this procedure. Gradual strong traction over several days or weeks occasionally has produced satisfactory reduction when the epiphyseal line is still open. Subtrochanteric osteotomy has been used successfully at times to correct the varus and rotational deformity and has the advantage of being less likely to produce an aseptic necrosis of the epiphysis. However, incongruity of the hips remains, and degenerative arthritis may be expected in later life. In the acute slipped femoral epiphysis gentle manipulative reduction followed by internal fixation may produce a satisfactory end result. Strong or overzealous manipulation is to be condemned because of its unfavorable effect upon the blood supply to the femoral head.

During the postoperative period weight-bearing of the affected side must be forbidden for 4 to 6 months or until bone has bridged the epiphysis. During the postoperative period, the opposite hip must be watched carefully, for in some series of cases it has been reported that as high as 40 per cent of individuals have developed slipping of the capital femoral epiphysis on the other side.[8, 37, 67, 113]

OSTEOCHONDRITIS

There is a group of localized bone afflictions that have been grouped together under this term because of a pathologic similarity. The common finding is an aseptic necrosis of bone that cannot be adequately explained by trauma. These cases occur almost entirely in children and adolescents, and there is accumulating evidence that disease of epiphyseal cartilage may precede the aseptic necrosis; however, the exact etiology is as yet undetermined. Aseptic necrosis is characterized by the typical x-ray finding of a relative increased density of the necrotic part in the middle stages of the disease, because atrophy of disuse of the surrounding viable bone leads to demineralization, while the dead bone does not develop demineralization because of lack of blood supply. The increased density may also result from uptake of minerals from the serum by this dead bone. As bone destruction does not occur until vascular granulation tissue reaches these necrotic areas, the increased density remains until that time. In the late stages the relative increased density of the necrotic part may be modified by patchy areas of regeneration on the one hand and of collapse and destruction of necrotic bone on the other hand.

Coxa Plana (Osteochondritis Deformans Juvenilis, Perthes' Disease). The most important of these conditions, known variously as coxa plana, osteochondritis deformans juvenilis or Perthes' disease, involves the capital femoral epiphysis. It is usually unilateral but is bilateral in approximately 10 per cent of cases. It was described independently around 1909-1910 by Calvé, Legg and Perthes, and by Waldenstrom[123] as the use of diagnostic x-rays spread. The condition is more common in boys than in girls, usually beginning between the ages of 4 and 10 years. The initial sign is a slightly painful limp which becomes worse with activity; the pain is referred to hip, thigh or knee. There is usually a history of no trauma or insignificant trauma. Physical findings are limited to slight atrophy of the musculature of the involved side, slight limitation of the hip motions, particularly extension and abduction, and discomfort at the extremes of motion. Rarely, there may be more acute pain and disability, but this will subside with rest.

The very early roentgenogram may show only slight decreased density of the upper metaphysis of the femur or only minimal changes in the epiphysis. Diagnosis at this stage may be quite difficult. Tuberculosis is the most common differential diagnostic condition. Later there is irregular sclerosis of the epiphysis leading to fragmentation (Fig. 49-17). The course of the disease may run from 2 to 4 or 5 years, which includes the time for onset of symptoms to eventual resorption of necrotic bone and replacement with new viable bone sufficient to support full, active weight-bearing.

It is felt by most authorities that some form of non-weight-bearing during the active course of the disease will protect the normally round femoral head from being flattened to the degree that would occur if unrestricted weight-bearing were permitted. The simplest way to institute non-weight-bearing in a co-

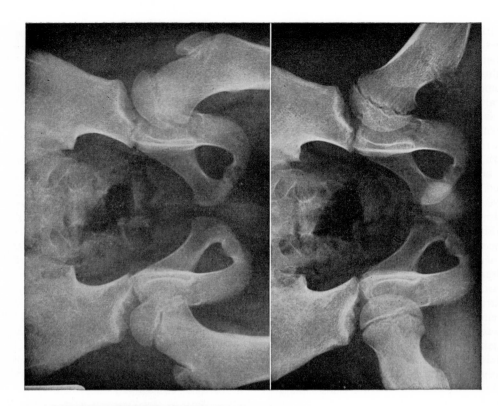

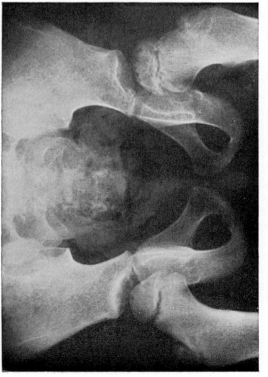

Fig. 49-17. (*Left*) Anteroposterior films of both hips of a 6-year-old child with moderately early changes in the left hip. (*Right*) Same case 18 months later, showing almost complete regeneration of the capital epiphysis.

operative child is the use of crutches with a sling-strap holding the shoe or the ankle to the belt with the knee about at 90°. An ischial weight-bearing brace may also be satisfactory at times. In the occasionally encountered bilateral case, bed rest at home with skin traction is advocated but requires intelligent and diligent parents. Operative intervention has been recommended; however, it has not been shown that a greater number of normal hips can be obtained by surgery, although the period of disability may be shortened. Neither do we subscribe to the defeatist attitude that treatment is useless and that the condition should be allowed to run its course on the chance that occasionally complete reconstruction will occur.

Osgood-Schlatter's Disease. The next most important disease in this group is Osgood-Schlatter's disease. Clinically, there is a painful enlargement of the tibial tubercle in an adolescent, usually a male, and the symptom is aggravated by physical activity and relieved by rest. A roentgenogram may show a variety of types of fragmentation of the epiphysis of the tuberosity and frequently will show some separation of the epiphysis from the shaft due apparently to the pull of the patellar tendon. The majority of cases do well with rest and protection and do not have any permanent sequelae, except for enlargement of the tibial tubercle. Surgical intervention during the early stages is absolutely unwarranted in our opinion. Occasionally, fragmentation is such that all the fragments do not solidify with healing so that a detached piece of bone remains. This may be painful on kneeling. Simple excision at this stage relieves the pain (Fig. 49-18). Rarely, the enlargement is such that it is unsightly in the female, and excision for cosmetic reasons is worthwhile.

There are several other conditions having localized bone necrosis that may or may not be etiologically similar to Perthes' and Osgood-Schlatter's disease. They are less common, less serious and usually self-limited, responding to conservative treatment. They are commonly referred to by the names of men responsible for their early description and are so listed here:

Apophysitis of os calcis—Sever and Haglund

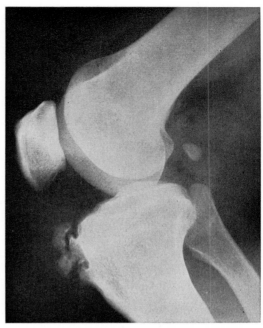

Fig. 49-18. Lateral roentgenogram of the knee in a 30-year-old white man who had Osgood-Schlatter's disease as a boy. Large fragments of the tibial tubercle failed to unite, and they remain as loose bodies. Pain eventually led to the removal of these loose pieces of bone. The pain disappeared after the loose pieces of bone were removed.

Aseptic necrosis of tarsal scaphoid—Köhler

Aseptic necrosis of carpal lunate—Kienböck

Aseptic necrosis of second metatarsal head—Freiberg's infraction

Epiphysitis of vertebrae—Scheuermann

Aseptic necrosis of patella—Sinding-Larsen, Johannson, Köhler

Aseptic necrosis of capitellum humera—Panner

Aseptic necrosis with collapse of vertebra—Vertebra plana or Calvé's disease

Some cases typical of Calvé's disease by roentgenogram have been proved to be eosinophilic granulomas (Compere et al.[21]).

ORTHOPEDIC TREATMENT OF POLIOMYELITIS

In spite of the fact that we appear to be on the threshold of control of anterior poliomyelitis, there is a tremendous reservoir of paralytic cases that will require orthopedic attention for several decades to come. Once the acute viral infection has subsided, in the paralytic cases, we are confronted with the problems of rehabilitation of all degrees of complexity. The orthopedist should begin his management during the acute illness and end only when the maximum degree of rehabilitation has been accomplished.

POSTINFECTION PERIOD

During the early weeks and months of the postinfection period the primary concern in a patient with significant paralysis is (1) control of pain, tenderness and spasm in the involved muscles and (2) prevention of deformity. This is accomplished by a variety of physical measures, including wet packs, baths, plaster splints, and passive and active exercises. As the pain and the tenderness subside, more vigorous participation in active exercise by the patient is encouraged, and resumption of activities approaching normal is allowed. Supporting and protective braces and splints are frequently necessary and helpful during this period.

Keeping in mind that recovery of muscle power after paralysis may continue for from 12 to 24 months from the time of the acute disease, final decision regarding surgical reconstructive procedures is delayed until the surgeon is satisfied that no further significant spontaneous recovery of involved muscles is likely. Hundreds of different operative procedures have been described to improve function in these patients who have an extremely variable, irregular voluntary muscle paralysis. Only those of common usage and proved value will be discussed.

APPLIANCES

Mention should be made of the use of various appliances such as braces, splints and corsets. Their use serves 2 primary purposes: (1) prevention of deformity by holding the part in the functional position and (2) permitting functional use of a part that otherwise would be useless because of paralysis and instability. For example, a child with one lower extremity having complete paralysis of the quadriceps and the peroneal muscles might be unable to bear full weight on the leg be-

cause the knee would buckle and give way and probably would develop a varus deformity of the foot. A long leg brace with a knee-lock would permit full weight-bearing, and the proper shoe attachment to the brace would tend to prevent the foot deformity.

OPERATIVE PROCEDURES

The operative procedures may be properly divided into those on the upper and the lower extremities on the basis that the aims are different in these members. In the upper extremity the primary concern is either directly to improve hand function or to improve arm function so that the hand may be better used. In the lower extremity, we are concerned with weight-bearing, stability and ambulation. With these aims in mind we can better understand the purpose of some of the procedures.

Upper Extremity. In the upper extremity any procedure must be considered in the light of whether or not it serves to improve the use of the hand. In the presence of a totally useless hand that cannot be rehabilitated in any way, obviously it is absurd to consider any reconstructive work on the remainder of the arm or the shoulder, except in rare instances in which the shoulder and the arm can be made adequate for the operation of a prosthesis. At the shoulder it is not uncommon to have a deltoid paralysis associated with good scapular musculature; in such cases with satisfactory hand function, an arthrodesis of the shoulder may be preferable to muscle transposition. Fusion may give active and stable abduction to 90°, flexion to 60° and still permit the arm to be carried at the side. Tendon transposition to replace lost deltoid power has been advocated by some, but such procedures have not gained wide acceptance. Muscle transposition may be satisfactory. Recent work suggests that this field has not been fully explored (Schottstaedt et al.[107]).

PARALYSIS OF THE TRICEPS. This condition is not badly disabling, since gravity will extend the elbow in situations not requiring force, but a paralyzed biceps and brachialis can prevent the hand from being brought to the mouth and the face. If the forearm flexor muscles are of good power, transposition of the common flexor origin from the medial epicondyle up the humerus 2 or more inches as described by Steindler[116] may produce fairly satisfactory flexion without disturbing the function of the finger and the wrist flexors.

Wristdrop due to paralysis of wrist extensors probably is treated best by arthrodesis of the wrist in a position of mild dorsiflexion. The efficiency of such an operation may be easily tested preoperatively by applying a cast or a splint to immobilize the wrist and leave the fingers free. Then the patient can tell by actual trial in exactly what manner his disability will be altered by the arthrodesis. In a few cases of wristdrop, the wrist may be stabilized by transposition of wrist flexor tendons or the pronator teres into the wrist extensors. Frequently, however, with loss of wrist extension there is also loss of finger extension, in which case the wrist flexors are needed to motivate finger extensors after the wrist is stabilized by an arthrodesis. In the severely damaged arm and hand tenodesis may give a much better functional result, as it allows motion not possible with an arthrodesis. However, function resulting from tenodesis of finger flexor tendons is completely dependent upon powerful active wrist extension.

Opposition of Thumb. One of the most common serious disabilities in the hand that can be corrected surgically is loss of opposition of the thumb. The loss of opposition is due to paralysis of the abductor pollicis brevis muscle. This may be treated by one of several tendon transpositions, using a variety of muscles for the motor power, or by putting a bone graft across the space between the first and the second metacarpals to hold the thumb in a position of opposition.[119] The choice of procedure depends upon available active muscle power and also on performance requirements and can be made only on detailed study of the individual case.

Lower Extremity. In the lower extremity with weight-bearing, stability and ambulation as the prime objectives, we desire stable joints, freedom from deformity, maximum use of remaining muscle strength and equal leg length. In order to be justified, surgical procedures should accomplish one or more of these aims.

Stabilization of the Foot. The most commonly indicated surgical procedure in the surgical reconstruction of the lower extremity involved with paralytic poliomyelitis is the stabilization of the foot, or "triple arthrode-sis." This procedure is designed to correct deformity of the foot as well as accomplish stability for weight-bearing. Regardless of the type of deformity, which may vary greatly, depending on the type of muscle imbalance around the foot, this operation can restore the position of the foot to the normal standing position by variations in technic. In essence, the procedure consists of excising the talocalcaneal, the talonavicular and the calcaneocuboid joints and allowing arthrodesis of the involved bones to occur by immobilization in a plaster cast. By taking wedges of bone with the joint excision almost any deformity may be corrected. For example, a peroneal paralysis may permit a varus or inversion deformity to occur; in stabilizing such a foot, sufficient bone is removed at the calcaneocuboid and the lateral side of the talocalcaneal joints to permit the foot to be straightened out of the varus position.

The average child does not have sufficient bone in the foot to do the stabilization until the age of 8 to 10 years; in marginal cases, a roentgenogram should be made to determine if enough bone is present. Stabilization of the foot sacrifices the motions of inversion and eversion, which has the disadvantage of making it difficult to walk on irregular surfaces. It also shortens the foot and usually increases the discrepancy of foot size. Furthermore, it may not correct a flatfoot deformity. For these reasons, plus the fact that it may be performed at an earlier age, the Grice operation (extra-articular fusion between the astragalus and the calcaneus) has a very definite place and the advantage of releasing the anterior and the posterior tibial and peroneal muscles, whichever are of significant muscle strength, for transference to aid in dorsiflexion or plantar flexion.[56] The general principal of treating the paralytic foot is to stabilize the hindfoot in order to prevent inversion and eversion. After the hindfoot has been stabilized, the tendons of the remaining and available functioning muscles may be shifted toward the mid-line to serve as dorsi and plantar flexors at the ankle. The anterior tibial and peroneal tendons work well as dorsiflexors when transposed to the midtarsus anteriorly, and the posterior tibial and peroneal tendons work well as plantar flexors when transposed to the os calcis in the mid-line posteriorly.

Anterior tibial transfer to the os calcis may work well in many instances. Thus, no remaining functioning muscle need be wasted. It must be remembered that no stabilization procedure will be successful unless muscle imbalance is also corrected.

It is not uncommon to have loss of dorsiflexors of the foot with unparalyzed dorsiflexors of the toes, so that a cockup deformity of the toes, particularly the great toe, develops as a result of the attempt to use the toe extensors to raise the foot. A very satisfactory procedure is the transposition of the great toe extensor insertion from the distal phalanx to the first metatarsal so that the muscle will dorsiflex the foot without first hyperextending the toe. This is the *Jones suspension operation*.

The stabilization procedure preserves the ankle motion, but with a completely flail leg and foot it may be necessary to do some type of bone block to prevent the foot from dropping into full plantar flexion. The *Campbell*[113] *bone block* is such a procedure and consists of elevating a flap of bone from the posterior aspect of the tuberosity of the calcaneus so that this will impinge on the posterior tibia as the foot drops down beyond a right angle. The motion of dorsiflexion is preserved by such a procedure. This operation is not always successful, but has given more satisfactory results than those obtained by a Lambrinudi type of arthrodesis.[70]

STABILIZATION OF THE KNEE. The knee joint may offer a problem of instability due to quadriceps paralysis. In some cases with good hamstring function and partial quadriceps power a very satisfactory result may accrue as a result of transposition of the tendons of the biceps femoris and the semitendinosus to the patella to aid extension. In absence of any quadriceps power or poor hamstring power, consideration must be given to an arthrodesis of the knee; some patients would prefer to wear a long leg brace with a knee lock than to have an arthrodesis. This is an example of a situation which occurs commonly in reconstructive orthopedics, in which the patient must choose between alternative plans after careful explanation of the advantages and the disadvantages of each by the surgeon. Popliteal dissection with lengthening of hamstring tendons, release of gastrocnemius origins, and posterior capsulotomy of the knee

may be necessary at times to correct flexion deformity. This is frequently associated with flexion deformity of the hip, which also may have to be corrected by surgical release of contracted soft tissue and usually is seen in neglected patients. Genu recurvatum is occasionally a disabling occurrence associated with gastrocnemius and hamstring weakness. It may be treated by constructing a check ligament or performing an osteotomy of the tibia.

STABILIZATION OF THE HIP. About the hip, the most common disability is abductor weakness; this permits a downward sag of the opposite side of the pelvis during the standing phase of the gait, called a "positive" Trendelenburg sign. The normal or "negative" Trendelenburg sign refers to the ability of the abductors to maintain the opposite side of the pelvis elevated during the standing phase of the gait. Several operative procedures have been designed to transpose muscle power to abduction; none has been sufficiently proved to gain wide usage. Instability about the hip sufficient to produce serious disability probably is best corrected by arthrodesis; such a procedure produces less disability than most people would think when done in childhood. However, in certain instances the transfer of the ileopsoas after the method of Mustard will provide functional stabilization of the hip and obviate arthrodesis.

DEFORMITIES OF LONG BONES. Osteotomy to correct deformities of long bones, particularly rotational deformities, is frequently indicated. The necessary correction is carried out under direct vision of the surgically exposed bone, and the fracture thus created is treated by immobilization in plaster.

It must be kept in mind that the indications for various of the aforementioned procedures may have to be reconsidered in light of other disabilities in the same or other extremities. That is to say, one always should consider the effect of any given surgical procedure on the whole patient.

EQUALIZATION OF LEG LENGTH. This procedure will be considered at this point because it is most frequently a problem related to poliomyelitis. The principles of its correction may be applied to other conditions that may produce a significant leg length discrepancy. As a rule, a discrepancy of leg length of 1 inch or less in an average-sized adult is usually asymptomatic and requires no treatment, other than a simple elevation of the heel of the shoe. Discrepancies of between 1¼ and 5 inches produce an ungainly limp and can and should be corrected in most cases if possible. Discrepancies of more than 5 inches usually are uncorrectable by the ordinary means and require some other management.

The group under consideration is the discrepancy of between 1¼ and 5 inches. The surgeon has a choice of: (1) operative lengthening of the shortened extremity, (2) operative shortening of the long extremity and (3) some type of epiphyseal arrest of the long extremity in childhood. The first is very seldom indicated because of technical difficulties and hazards. Suitable technics with special apparatus have been described for use in special circumstances (Abbott and Crego[1, 2]). The second is not particularly difficult or hazardous but is usually indicated only after bone growth has ceased. Epiphyseal arrest of the distal femur and/or the proximal tibia of the long extremity is the easiest method available; although applicable only in children. Permanent closure of the epiphysis by the method described by Phemister[92] or temporary closure by use of staples advocated by Blount and Clarke[12] may be carried out. With the permanent closure methods, the correct time of closing must be chosen with care so as to obtain as nearly as possible the correct amount of shortening. Several methods are available to aid the surgeon in deciding when such closures should be done. The interested student should seek further information on this subject (Green and Anderson[45]). The use of stapling to close an epiphyseal plate temporarily has the theoretical advantage that growth may be resumed by removal of the staple before closure of the plate. Either of these methods will be successful if properly employed. The most common cause of failure is to delay the operation too long, so that the anticipated amount of growth restriction does not occur.

Ideally, equalization of leg length would be accomplished best by some form of stimulation of the epiphysis or epiphyses of the short side. This problem has been and is being pursued by many investigators. So far all the published and the unpublished results have revealed failure of the various methods to produce a suitable degree of increased length. In a few instances the creation of an arteriovenous fistula between the femoral artery and vein has resulted in a significant increase in length of a shortened extremity (Janes and Musgrave[61] and Cooley et al.[23]). The possibility of severe cardiovascular changes exists in this approach to leg-length equalization, and further experience is required before the method can be employed in other than very selected cases. However, further study in experimental animals may yet result in a satisfactory method of epiphyseal stimulation (Harris and McDonald,[50] Pease[89]).

CEREBRAL PALSY

The term cerebral palsy is used to apply to a group of patients who have a variety of clinical syndromes caused by brain damage. This damage may be the result of a developmental defect, direct trauma or anoxia incident to the birth process, or even some postpartum disease affecting the central nervous system. Depending on the portion of the brain affected, an extremely wide range of clinical pictures may exist. Spasticity, rigidity and athetosis may be present alone or in combination. Monoplegia, paraplegia, hemiplegia or quadriplegia may exist. Mental deficiency may or may not exist. Potentially average or above average mentality may escape detection because of lack of opportunity of development or ability to detect it.

Numerous surgical procedures have been described to benefit victims of these conditions. Only about 25 per cent of these patients meet the criteria of suitability for surgery. It must be drawn to the attention of the families of these patients that the surgical procedure is directed at the results of the disease, e.g., flexion deformity, and not at correction of the disease itself.

A number of operations have been advocated for management of certain specific disabilities resulting from cerebral palsy, chiefly those found in spastic paralysis. Only those will be mentioned that have been well-established and accepted as beneficial. It should be pointed out that surgery may be used to improve active function of the extremity and thereby lessen physical disability, or at times is done merely to increase the ease of handling a severely crippled individual.

UPPER EXTREMITY

Contracture of the adductors and the internal rotators of the shoulder because of abnormal tonus may develop. Surgical severance of the contracted insertions of the pectoralis major and the subscapularis with immobilization for several weeks in a position of external rotation and abduction, as described by Sever,[108] is very beneficial when a good hand is present. Also, osteotomy of the humerus to correct rotational deformity has also been useful in older children.

There are several procedures to choose from for correction of pronation deformities of the forearm. A very satisfactory one is section of the pronator teres with transposition of the insertion of the flexor carpi ulnaris around the ulna dorsally into the distal radius.

Flexion deformity of the wrist is handled best by arthrodesis of this joint in a position of slight dorsiflexion. This operation must be done only in those patients who have the capacity voluntarily to release the grasp when held in the position of proposed arthrodesis. It is wise to immobilize the wrist in a cast prior to arthrodesis to be certain that hand function will be improved.

The hand is so intricate that serious spasticity or rigidity or athetosis of its muscles cannot be helped significantly by surgical procedures. Sections of adductors of the thumb to prevent premature flexion and adduction of the thumb into the palm on closure of the fist may be useful. Fusion by bone graft of the 1st and the 2nd metacarpals to hold the thumb in a position of opposition is indicated occasionally (Thompson[119]).

LOWER EXTREMITY

At the hip, spasticity produces adduction and internal rotation contractures. Adductor spasm may be handled adequately by detachment of the adductor muscles from their origin on the pubis and/or obturator nerve neurectomy. Internal rotation may be corrected by section of the anterior origin of the gluteus medius and minimus as described by Durham,[31] although this procedure may produce an undesirable abductor weakness limp. Flexion contracture of hip and knee is benefited considerably by transposition of the hamstring insertions from the tibia to the distal femur as described by Eggers.[34]

At the knee, flexion contracture is common and may be corrected by advancement of the patellar tendon insertion, as described by Chandler,[17, 18] if active but not passive full extension of the knee has been lost. Where there is fixed flexion contracture, this must be corrected by wedging casts or popliteal dissection and then a hamstring transplant done to prevent recurrence.

Equinus deformity of the foot producing a toe-to-heel gait may be corrected readily by a neurectomy of nerves supplying the gastrocnemius in mild cases without structural shortening of the heel cord or by heel cord lengthening in more severe cases. Various foot deformities occur; if significant, they usually require triple arthrodesis as described under poliomyelitis.

It should be emphasized that a child who is unable to walk with deformities will not walk without deformities. An adequate sense of balance is essential to standing and walking and it is surprising how a child with severe deformity will be able to get around if there is a good sense of balance. It is recommended that no corrective surgery be done in any child that cannot walk alone. Also, it should be noted that procedures requiring postoperative recumbency for several weeks be avoided in children who just recently have learned to walk alone, because such recumbency will "set back" the developing sense of balance so that such a child may take months relearning to walk.

One of the great challenges to the orthopedic surgeon is the management of the family of the patient with cerebral palsy so that they may have maximum legitimate hopefulness and as true an understanding as possible of the limitations of medical treatment. So many of these families go from one place to another seeking a promise of great improvement, and sometimes fall into the hands of irregular practitioners.

SCOLIOSIS

Scoliosis refers to a lateral and rotary deviation of the spine beyond normal and in most cases develops in the growing spine (Fig. 49-19). Approximately 20 per cent of

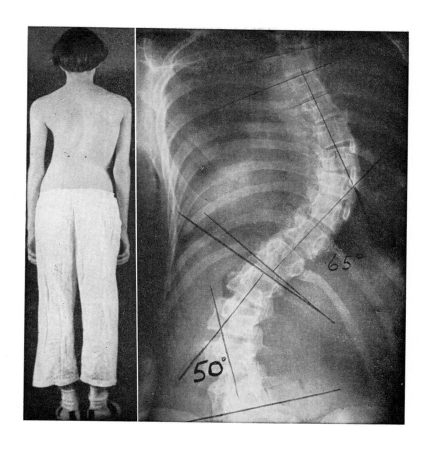

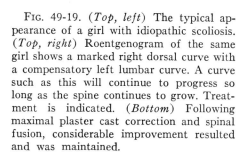

FIG. 49-19. (*Top, left*) The typical appearance of a girl with idiopathic scoliosis. (*Top, right*) Roentgenogram of the same girl shows a marked right dorsal curve with a compensatory left lumbar curve. A curve such as this will continue to progress so long as the spine continues to grow. Treatment is indicated. (*Bottom*) Following maximal plaster cast correction and spinal fusion, considerable improvement resulted and was maintained.

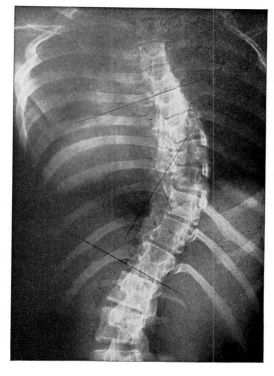

patients who are seen with this condition have some recognizable underlying etiology; this group would include cases of poliomyelitis with asymmetrical paresis of paraspinal, thoracic or abdominal musculature, patients with hemivertebrae, neurofibromatosis, muscular dystrophy, empyema and many others. The remainder of cases are referred to as idiopathic scoliosis. It is likely that the majority of these constitute a real disease entity, the cause of which may be discovered someday. Idiopathic scoliosis is seen most commonly in females between the ages of 10 and 15 years, develops insidiously, is usually asymptomatic and first noticed by someone other than the patient. Although several different types of curves are seen, the most common is right dorsal and left lumbar "S"-shaped scoliosis. As the curve develops in progressive cases there also develops associated chest cage deformity of a degree comparable with the spine deformity.

Since a wide range of severity of deformity occurs, it may be difficult to decide that a given curve is to be ultimately of such a degree of severity that expensive and rigorous surgical treatment should be instituted. In the past all too many of these adolescents have been observed over a period of years while their deformity increased to grotesque proportions. Conservative treatment consisting of exercises and braces or corsets has been of questionable value. Correction of the so-called primary curve, as contrasted with the secondary or compensatory curves, by some form of plaster cast followed by spinal fusion with the spine in the best position obtainable is the only means available at present of lessening the deformity in a lasting manner. At times a reasonably straight spine may be obtained, but even with excellent correction or even overcorrection some loss of correction can be expected as the living bone of a quite solid spinal fusion is subjected to the same stresses that produced the curves in the first place and will respond to this stress according to Wolff's Law.

As it seems likely that most cases of idiopathic scoliosis are due to a discrepancy of epiphyseal growth on one side of one or more vertebrae, retardation of growth on the more rapidly growing side should correct the deformity. So far, all procedures designed to accomplish this have been disappointing, and

further experimental study along this line appears to be necessary. It should be pointed out that considerable deformity may be compatible with good health and an essentially normal way of life. On the other hand, there is certainly an increased tendency to develop symptomatic degenerative changes in the scoliotic spine in later life.

Even though treatment by correction and spinal fusion is expensive and prolonged, frequently it is justified; an adolescent girl who develops a serious curve may have her social and physical development seriously and permanently impaired if such a curve is not improved.

When the physician sees a child with scoliosis, roentgenographic examinations of the spine and periodic observation are indicated. If the child is growing rapidly, the curvature may progress rapidly; and if such is the case, energetic therapy is indicated. The use of the Milwaukee brace, or wedging casts as advocated by Risser and Norquist[98] and Moe,[84] should be instituted promptly. Although the spine is usually not straight at the conclusion of treatment, the appearance of the patient is often greatly improved, particularly where the rotational deformity and thus the rib prominence is corrected (Fig. 49-19). Recently, internal bracing to correct the curve and hold the spine straight has been advocated; however, it is too early to know whether the method is an improvement over the older methods. For a more detailed review of the principles of scoliosis treatment the reader is referred to Schmidt.[106]

INFECTION IN BONE

OSTEOMYELITIS

Definition. Pyogenic osteomyelitis is an inflammation of any portion of the bone, produced by one of the pyogenic organisms, in contradistinction to inflammation of bone caused by such agents as tuberculosis, syphilis and fungi. The development of pyogenic inflammation of bone must be preceded by the deposition of the causative organisms, most commonly the staphylococcus and the streptococcus, in a suitable bed in the bone structure.

This may occur (1) by the organisms being carried to the bone by the circulation, (2) by the direct extension from a nearby abscess or infection and (3) by a communicating wound, such as an open fracture. There seems to be little evidence that infection of the bone can occur through the lymphatic system. Hematogenous osteomyelitis is seen most commonly in children, in which the initial area of infection is usually in the metaphyseal portion of a long bone. When hematogenous osteomyelitis occurs in adults it is said to be more common in the diaphysis. Hobo[55] and others have shown that India ink injected into the circulation of an experimental animal lodges primarily in the liver, the spleen and bone. In the bone the greatest concentration of the foreign material was in the metaphyseal area. Robertson,[99] Wilson[125] and others believe that this is due to the fact that there is a venous lake in this area in which there is a slowing of the circulation. They also believe that phagocytosis is reduced, due to the poor arterial supply. Rodet,[102] Lexer[72] and others were able to produce acute hematogenous osteomyelitis in experimental animals by the injection of bacteria into the circulation, but this has been only in young animals in which the epiphyseal line is still open. In older animals they were not able to produce osteomyelitis. Lexer[72] was perhaps the first to show that trauma can influence the localization of infection. As acute hematogenous osteomyelitis is about twice as common in boys as in girls, trauma has been cited as one of the etiologic factors. However, Key[63] reports a history of trauma in only about 25 per cent of the cases. As there must be a transient bacteremia recurring repeatedly from foci of infection in all children in whom trauma is quite prevalent, and as the incidence of acute hematogenous osteomyelitis is quite rare, it would seem that there must be many other factors in addition to those cited above to allow the successful development of this condition.

Pathogenesis. Whether the bacteria from a focus of infection in the body lodge in the bone and begin to multiply and then reseed the circulation producing a septicemia, or whether there is a septicemia with lodging of the bacteria in the bone and then the development of the picture of acute hematogenous osteomyelitis remains unsolved; in all probability both of these sequences of events may occur. Regardless of how it develops, acute hematogenous osteomyelitis should be con-

sidered a systemic disease with local manifestations.

Etiology. Key[63] reported the staphylococcus as the causative agent in about 90 per cent of the cases. Most of his strains were hemolytic *Staphylococcus aureus* (in 52 cases), and he encountered the streptococcus in 5 cases and the pneumococcus in 1, in a total of 58 cases. It is frequently stated that in infants under 2 years of age, the causative organism is more apt to be the streptococcus, and that in those over 2 years of age the staphylococcus predominates; however, in very young infants colon bacillus osteomyelitis is not uncommon. The disease produced by each of these various infectious organisms is somewhat different in that the streptococcus toxin does not seem to have the same destructive influence on bone that is present with the staphylococcus. Even in untreated cases in which recovery occurs in spite of considerable involvement of the bone, the bone lesion often heals with little, if any, sequestration. On the other hand, with the staphylococcus there is almost always a large amount of bone killed with sequestra of various sizes resulting. In addition to the necrotizing effect of the staphylococcus toxin, the amount of nonviable bone is also somewhat dependent upon the extent of the subperiosteal abscess. Such abscesses may deprive large areas of bone of circulation, either by stripping up of the periosteum or by a rapid plugging of their nutrient canals.

Treatment. SURGICAL. Because of this special ability of the staphylococcus toxins to kill bone, plus the damage to the circulation, surgeons were led to advocate early operation in these cases with the hope that if the infection could be opened and drained to the outside the amount of bone destroyed would be lessened considerably. A great effort was put forth to make a diagnosis in these cases very early in the course of the disease, long before there was x-ray evidence of bone damage, and to drain the infected area immediately as an emergency procedure. The result of this premise was to submit a critically ill child, most often dehydrated, to a surgical procedure. The mortality was rather high. Furthermore, it never was clearly shown that early operation and drainage materially limited the amount of bone destroyed; in fact, there are instances in which there was some doubt as to whether or not the early operation actually contributed to the spread of infection or caused damage to the epiphysis. Starr[114] in 1922 was one of the first to advocate delay in operation. Green[43] in 1935 and Wilson[124] in the same year also advocated delay until the acute phase had subsided and a subperiosteal abscess had formed before surgical intervention.

Orr[88] in 1927 demonstrated an entirely new principle in the treatment of osteomyelitis, namely, surgical drainage combined with rest. He reported many cases of acute hematogenous osteomyelitis which were opened early, the wound packed open with petrolatum gauze and immobilized in a plaster cast. Many of these wounds treated by this method healed without difficulty and without extensive loss of bone. This method was more generally applicable to the subacute and the chronic cases of osteomyelitis and constituted one of the greatest advances in the treatment of this condition.

CHEMOTHERAPY AND ANTIBIOTICS. With the advent of the chemotherapeutic and antibiotic drugs, not only was the treatment of acute hematogenous osteomyelitis revolutionized, but also the disease itself was practically eradicated. It is rare indeed for us now to see a case of acute hematogenous osteomyelitis, and when such a case does appear, appropriate antibiotic therapy has completely altered the course of the disease to such an extent that it is unusual for a case to come under the observation of an orthopedic surgeon. Most of the cases can be controlled by antibiotics with aspiration of the subperiosteal abscess so that open drainage is not required. However, recently acute hematogenous osteomyelitis and pyogenic joint infections are occurring more frequently, due probably to the development organisms resistant to many of the common antibiotics. Supportive therapy with blood transfusion, fluid and electrolytes is important. Sequestra, if they do occur, are sufficiently small that they will be attacked and replaced by the reparative processes of the body without surgical excision. At the present time the greatest difficulty with this form of treatment is that there is a tendency on the part of those handling these cases to fail to recognize spread of the infection to one of the adjacent joints. Although we are not called upon to see and treat many cases of extensive local abscesses with large sequestra, we do see all too often a case of osteomyelitis that is being well-managed from the bone standpoint in which the spread of infection into the adjacent joint is not recognized until irreparable damage to that joint has occurred. This is particularly true of the hip joint, in which so often the osteomyelitis is intra-articular almost from the start. Therefore, in spite of the great advances that have been made in the management of this condition (and of its almost total eradication from the general population), it still behooves those who are treating the occasional case to be on constant guard for involvement of the joints, so that early drainage of the joint may be provided. Preferably, this is accomplished by aspiration and instillation of an appropriate antibiotic agent, but if this is not immediately successful in combating the infection, the joint should be opened and drained. Otherwise, permanent damage or total loss of the joint probably will occur.

Acute flare-ups of an old hematogenous osteomyelitis may occur at any time throughout life. This is thought to be the result of lowered resistance plus local trauma. However, quite often there is no history of trauma. Often these recrudescences may be controlled by chemotherapeutic or antibiotic agents combined with rest. Occasionally, as a result of the failure of the antibiotic agent to work, either because the organisms are resistant to it or because they are so deep in an area of scar in which the blood supply is poor that the agent cannot reach them, it is necessary to carry out a saucerization procedure. Persistent pain, tenderness, fever and leukocytosis suggest the presence of an abscess. At times the roentgenogram fails to show either a localized abscess or a sequestrum because of contrast shadows or is obscured by the irregular density due to chronic infection. In these cases the laminograph may be of great aid. In these cases the area of infection is rather well sealed off, and danger of spread up and down the shaft of the medullary canal or the danger of an extensive subperiosteal abscess of the bone is not as great as in primary cases.

BRODIE'S ABSCESS

Brodie's abscess is a localized infection of bone originally described by Mr. Brodie[15] in

1832. Usually it is found in the metaphyseal area of the long bones and is characterized by a roughly spherical area of bone destruction forming a cavity which may be filled with pus, or at times if the infection is entirely burned out in an old abscess the cavity may be filled with connective tissue only. The bone surrounding this cavity is hard and eburnated and has an x-ray appearance of a sclerotic rim (Fig. 49-20). Sequestra have been reported in the cavity. The causative organism is most commonly the *Staphylococcus aureus*, and the most frequent symptom is pain, which may be more severe while resting than with activity. Local or systemic antibiotic therapy may not be sufficient to cure the condition or to relieve the pain. Surgical intervention is indicated in those cases producing symptoms. Recommended surgical procedures are of 3 types: (1) to open the abscess, unroof the abscess cavity, wash out the contents, curette the walls and close the wound. This method has been successful in a majority of cases reported by Wagner and Hanby.[122] (2) Campbell's *Operative Surgery*[113] suggests that if the abscess contains a considerable quantity of purulent material perhaps it is best to pack the wound open and close it secondarily. They recommend giving antibiotics preoperatively and postoperatively. (3) It has been suggested that in purulent cases of Brodie's abscess the wound may be closed loosely with a tube left into the cavity through which antibiotic solutions may be instilled at regular intervals.

In the majority of cases, the first of the above methods is most satisfactory. The extremity is immobilized during the period of primary wound healing. As a number of cases fail to heal by this method, it is our feeling that in those cases in which the cavity is filled with pus the second method be utilized and the wound packed open with a glycerine gauze pack. At the end of 5 to 7 days the gauze is removed in the operating room with aseptic precautions, the wound is inspected, and if it appears to be clean the cavity may be filled with cancellous bone chips and final skin closure effected at this time. However, if the cavity does not appear to be clean, the best form of treatment is to pack it with glycerin gauze, immobilize the extremity and

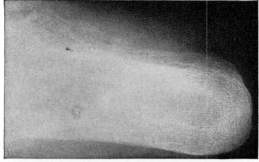
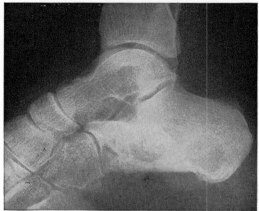

FIG. 49-20. Anteroposterior and lateral views of os calcis showing large Brodie's abscess successfully treated by curettement and closure.

let it fill in from the bottom after the method described by Orr.[88]

PYOGENIC ARTHRITIS

Pyogenic arthritis like osteomyelitis is most commonly of blood-borne origin, although of course it may result from spread of local or nearby infection or by penetrating wounds into a joint. It often occurs as a complication of osteomyelitis and, like osteomyelitis, it is not nearly so common as it was before the antibiotic age. It is more apt to occur in children; and, although any joint may be involved, the knee and the hip joints, in our experience, are involved most frequently. Any of the pyogenic organisms may be responsible, but the staphylococcus and the streptococcus are found more frequently. In infants and small children who are suffering from inflammatory diseases, the possibility of a septic joint should be kept in mind whenever the infectious process seems to flare up. There is an elevation of the pulse and the temperature with increased irritability, a limp if the child is old enough to walk, or a splinting or refusal to use the affected extremity in younger children and bed patients. Rapidly, there will be evidence of increased local heat and evidence of swelling. In the superficial joints evidence of infections of the joints almost always is recognized early, but in the hip joint infection not infrequently is overlooked until after the infection has been present for some days. It is particularly important to make the diagnosis at the earliest possible time as the articular cartilage does not withstand the toxins of the organisms and the proteolytic enzymes liberated from dead leukocytes, and the periarticular structure is damaged by the acute inflammatory process. Partial and complete ankylosis may result. In the superficial joints the physical findings are: restricted motion, pain on active or passive motion, increased local heat and evidence of effusion into the joint. Aspiration will reveal pus. At the time the joint is aspirated cultures should be taken for sensitivity tests and at the same time an instillation of penicillin may be employed. If the organisms are sensitive to penicillin, the infection may be completely overcome after a few such treatments. When the therapeutic response is not adequate following the aspiration and the instillation of penicillin, the joint should be opened and washed out thoroughly, an appropriate antibiotic instilled into it, and it should be closed, and the extremity immobilized. It is rare that continuous drainage of the joint is necessary. Such drainage is required mostly in cases of long standing, or when the chemotherapeutic or antibiotic therapy is not effective; in these cases requiring drainage, some permanent loss of function almost always results. The now rare gonococcal arthritis affects chiefly the shoulder, the elbow, the wrist, the knee and the hip; it is less acute but quite painful and usually responds to penicillin and rest.

Vertebral Osteomyelitis

Pyogenic infection involving the spinal column has not received a very great amount of attention in the literature, although it must have been very common in the preantibiotic era. Perhaps the reason for this has been the tendency of the infection to heal spontane-ously; undoubtedly, the condition has often been confused with tuberculosis. When confusion exists as to the cause of a destructive lesion of the vertebra and an associated disk, a needle biopsy of the vertebra for histologic examination and culture will usually establish a definite diagnosis. Vertebral osteomyelitis is more common at the present time in our experience than hematogenous osteomyelitis of the extremities. We see it as a complication of genitourinary and uterovaginal inflammations. Another group of cases are secondary to operations for ruptured nucleus pulposus. Ford and Key[39] presented the distinct and diagnostic x-ray findings in 3 such cases (Fig. 49-21). Kulowki[69] and more recently Sherman and Schneider[109] have reported on pyogenic osteomyelitis of the spine. In those cases not associated with the complications of surgery, Batson demonstrated a direct venous pathway to explain vertebral infection from the genitourinary tract, passing in a retrograde manner from the inferior vena cava to the veins of the vertebral system. According to Batson, vertebral veins do not have valves, so that the infection may be carried readily to the spine by the venous circulation (in much the same manner that it would be carried to any other bony site by the arteries). Rest, antibiotic therapy and drainage of the abscesses are indicated and have been satisfactory in resulting in healing of these infections. In one case of postoperative infection this regimen failed, and it was necessary to clean out the disk space and pack the wound open. It healed by second intention without drainage of the cauda equina. Spinal fusion then completed the treatment with a very satisfactory result.

Actinomycosis

This disease is caused by the ray fungus (*Actinomyces bovis*). Although the manner in which the disease is transmitted to man is not understood, it is assumed that it enters by the alimentary tract or lungs. Involvement of bone is usually secondary to an adjacent soft tissue abscess (Luck[74]), although primary bloodborne involvement of bone does occur, particularly in the spine. The pathologic picture is one of a chronic granulomatous lesion with soft tissue abscess. Those arising in the extremities are tender, the overlying skin is

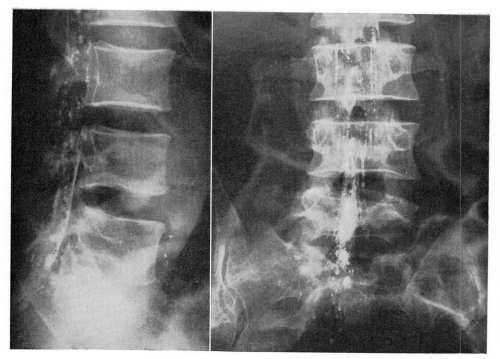

FIG. 49-21. (*Top*) Lateral and anteroposterior x-ray views of spine taken shortly after surgery for a ruptured disk. At this stage the patient had severe low back and leg pain, slight temperature elevation and leukocytosis. (*Bottom*) Anteroposterior and lateral views of same patient 2 months later. The typical changes (destruction of the vertebral plates on each side of the involved disk and early scoliosis of the vertebrae adjacent to the infection) indicating low-grade infection of the disk space are present at the L-4 space. (*Continued on following page*)

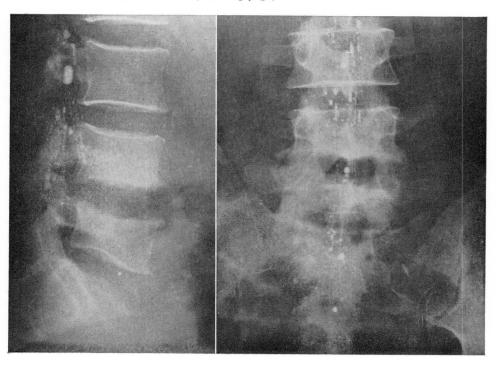

warm, and usually there is a low-grade pain. The progress is slow.

The diagnosis may be made by culture of the fungus or the finding of sulfur granules on direct smear of the pus. Many of the reported cases have responded favorably to large doses of penicillin. However, some are resistant, and the patient pursues a downhill course.

COCCIDIOIDOMYCOSIS

An infection caused by the fungus *Coccidioides immitis* is a condition firmly endemic in Southern California and Arizona, the northwestern part of Mexico and certain Central American countries. It has been called "valley fever," "desert fever" and "San Joaquin Valley fever." Bone lesions are found only in a disseminated form of the disease, which is usually in the form of multiple lesions with some predilection for cancellous bone, as the lesions occur more commonly in

the ends of long bones, the vertebral bodies and the pelvis; an occasional monarticular involvement has been reported. Primary involvement of joints is very rare, as the joints are involved through direct extension through the bone and the articular cartilage of adjacent bone lesions. There also seems to be some predilection for the bony prominences such as the tibial tubercle, the malleoli, the humeral condyles, the olecranon processes and the radial styloid. A destructive process of those particular areas should make one highly suspicious of a coccidioidal infection (see Chap. 4, "Surgical Infections").

SYPHILIS

Congenital Syphilis. Newborn infants with syphilis have a high incidence of skeletal lesions. Luck[74] reports osteochondritic changes in 97 per cent of such children. There is an extensive round cell infiltration in the metaphyseal area with a disturbance in the mecha-

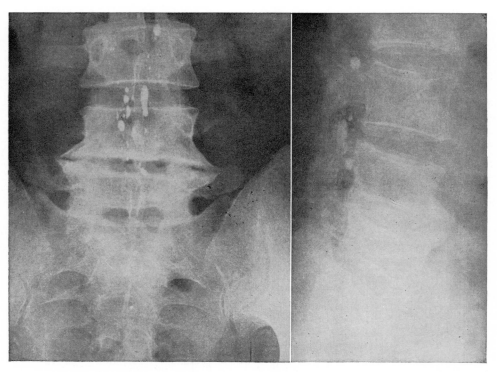

FIG. 49-21 (*Continued*). Anteroposterior and lateral views of same case after 32 months. Healing of the infection has occurred with fusion of the adjacent vertebra, and there has been complete relief of symptoms. (From Dr. Lee T. Ford, St. Louis, Mo.)

nism of destruction and resorption of mature cartilage and the formation of bone trabeculae with weakening of the epiphysio-metaphyseal junction. At the same time there is periosteal thickening and subperiosteal new-bone formation. These changes are usually bilateral.

In those syphilitics that survive, signs of latent syphilis of the bone develop, the most common lesion being the so-called "saber shin."

There may be luetic dactylitis that resembles the spina ventosa of tuberculosis, but the involvement is always bilaterally symmetrical and may be thus distinguished.

Acquired syphilis of bones and joints is primarily a periostitis. Stokes[118] reports cranium, tibia, rib cage and clavicle, in order of frequency of involvement.

TUBERCULOSIS

Bone and joint tuberculosis, like hematogenous osteomyelitis, is a blood-borne disease which of necessity must spread from infection somewhere else in the body, either from the lung or the gastro-intestinal tract. In areas where pasteurization of milk is not practiced there is a high incidence of bovine tuberculosis. At the time of the onset or the time of diagnosis of bone or joint tuberculosis, there may be no other evidence of tuberculosis, except a primary complex. On the other hand, there may be extensive systemic tuberculosis associated with the bone and joint lesions. Bone and joint tuberculosis is encountered more often in young individuals. Most commonly the spine is involved, with the hip, the knee and the ankle next most commonly involved and in that order. The small bones of the feet, the shoulder and the upper extremity joints are affected much less commonly. Still more rare is the involvement of tendon sheaths and the bursae. The involvement may be single or multiple, but more commonly only a single lesion is present. In the extremities a single lesion is more common, but in the spine multiple vertebrae are apt to be involved. Multiple joint lesions are said to occur in about 15 per cent of the cases, although in our experience it has been much less than this. The lodging of the tubercle bacilli in the bone or joint initially produces vasodilatation with the inflowing of small round cells; soon this is followed by a fibroblastic response with the formation of a

tubercle, a varying number of giant cells and thrombosis of the small vessels in the neighborhood, so that a necrotic caseous mass is formed (both by action of death of phagocytic cells and the interference with the blood supply in the area of the tubercle).

Tuberculosis of the Spine (Pott's Disease). This disease, like tuberculosis elsewhere, is usually of insidious onset, and often the patient is not brought to the doctor until the development of a "bump" is noticed on the back or even until a secondary psoas abscess first takes him to the doctor. The site of the infection is usually the anterior portion of the body of the vertebra at its inferior or superior margin. As a rule it is a destructive lesion resulting in atrophy and bone destruction without evidence of new bone formation or reaction about it. The intervertebral disk seems to be destroyed early and rapidly when the infection originates at the periphery of the vertebra (Fig. 49-22); but if the onset is within the body, there may be considerable destruction without x-ray evidence of involvement of the disk. Occasionally, the host response is such that there is increased density revealed on the roentgenogram.

In almost all cases of spinal tuberculosis a paravertebral abscess develops which is usually fusiform in nature and is helpful in establishing a diagnosis. The disease is usually more extensive than is demonstrated in the roentgenogram, as pointed out by Cleveland and Bosworth.[20] The paravertebral abscesses may form and rupture in the paravertebral area, posteriorly (rarely), or (commonly) may form a psoas abscess which presents at a point in the thigh below the inguinal ligament. Rarely, they may involve the mediastinum. The differential diagnosis is usually not difficult, although the Mantoux test may be negative early in the disease. There have been cases of proved tuberculosis of bones and joints with a negative Mantoux in children. Pyogenic secondary infection or tumor may obscure the diagnosis, and if an accurate diagnosis cannot be assured from the usual clinical method, biopsy should be undertaken. Hallock and Jones[49] found that 6.8 per cent of vertebral tuberculosis involved the posterior elements of the spine. They felt that in each instance this represented direct extension from the involved corpora. Of 192 patients with

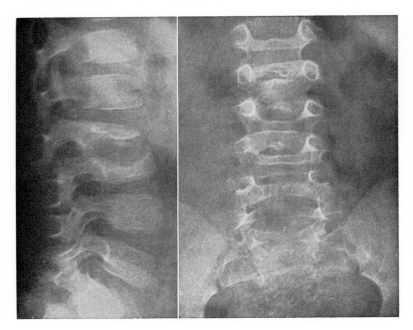

FIG. 49-22. Anteroposterior and lateral views of the lumbar spine with fairly extensive tuberculous lesion destruction of the bodies of the first and second lumbar vertebrae and involvement of the disk is present.

spinal tuberculosis reported by Hallock and Jones,[49] 23 had a paraplegia at one time or another. These were due to (1) an active granulation mass, (2) an old abscess or (3) more commonly a granuloma. Of those that developed paraplegia about one half died, most commonly from tuberculous meningitis.

Treatment of Tuberculosis of the Spine. Para-aminosalicylic acid, streptomycin, or isonicotinic acid hydrazide have not been successful in curing the bone and joint lesions without additional therapeutic measures, including surgery. Although these drugs have been very effective in contributing to the healing of sinuses, lessening the size of the abscesses, limiting the spread of the disease and perhaps making possible early intra-articular surgery, the backbone of good treatment still remains immobilization plus systemic treatment to improve the general health.

Based on the treatment of experimental bone tuberculosis with dihydrostreptomycin and isonicotinic acid hydrazide, Mora and Llamedo[86] concluded that if these drugs were administered in large quantities, there was beneficial effect in respect to the progression of experimental lesions. In all treated animals the lesions were smaller than in the controls and more sharply demarcated. They found that the drugs seemed to have the greatest in-

fluence upon the development of lymphatic lesions, but in no instance was there histologic evidence of cure of the lesions once established or did treatment prevent abscess formation. They felt that the main action of the drugs was to inhibit the spontaneous progressive course of the disease process and that it had little influence on its regression and did not in any case sterilize the wounds or lead to complete healing. Nor were they able to distinguish any beneficial effect of one drug over the other. In the chemotherapy of tuberculosis there seems to be some difference of opinion regarding the development of resistant strains. Bosworth[14] has recommended that only one drug be given at a time, as he feels that this lessens the chance of developing resistant strains of tubercle bacilli. On the other hand, Mercer[81] and others believe that the best way to lessen the development of resistant strains of tubercle bacilli is to use the drugs together because para-aminosalicylic acid apparently reduces the rate of development of a resistant strain. He has yet to find evidence of a resistant strain developing when isoniazid and streptomycin are given together. The effectiveness of the antibiotic drug may be lessened by the occlusion and the thrombosis of the vessels which may occur early in the disease. In addition, excessive connective tissue proliferation may later decrease the circulation and reduce the chance that adequate quantities of the agent will reach the bacteria.

Although the chemotherapeutic agents are very valuable, some form of immobilization for the spine remains the basis of treatment. Although bed rest and plaster-cast fixation alone may be helpful, the best method of putting the spine to rest and immobilizing it is a spinal fusion. The fusion should include at least 2 vertebrae above and below the area of disease. The operation should be done when the general condition of the patient is such as to tolerate a major operation. It must be remembered that a fusion of the spine is merely the best way to put the spine at rest; it does not cure the tuberculous process but merely affords the host a better chance to control the disease process.

Paraplegia in a patient with tuberculosis of the spine is a very serious complication. Laminectomy is usually advocated, although it does not attack the site of disease. Costotransversectomy or anterolateral decompression appears to be a more rational operation for decompression of the spinal cord in a patient with paraplegia due to tuberculous spondylitis.

Articular Tuberculosis. Joint tuberculosis may involve the periarticular soft tissues, the synovia, the cartilage, the bone, or all four. Most joint tuberculosis starts in the synovia at the point of its reflection from the articular cartilage or the epiphyseal plate.

After the involvement of the synovia, lesions may spread along the articular cartilage from the periphery by direct extension from the synovial reflection and invade and destroy the cartilage with pannus formation. In children tuberculous granulation tissue may invade the subcondylar plate or attack the epiphysis distal to the epiphyseal line, depriving a large segment of bone of its blood flow and nutrition and thus killing it. In articular tuberculosis, the weight-bearing portion of the articular cartilage tends to be preserved, while the periphery and the nonweight-bearing portions are susceptible to attack and destruction. This is in contrast with the pyogenic arthritic joint in which the weight-bearing surfaces are destroyed first. At times in tuberculous arthritis the weight-bearing surfaces are well preserved, while a large

amount of the cartilaginous bone is undermined by the fibrous granulation tissue, and as a consequence a large section of the articular surface may be deprived of support and sequestrate. Such sequestration on both sides of the joint constitutes the so-called "kissing sequestrae."

The course of the disease and treatment has changed somewhat. Before the antibiotic era, some childhood cases with the tuberculosis limited to the synovia recovered, and a useful joint was retained. The use of antibiotics has improved the outlook greatly, so that nonoperative therapy is more in favor today than it was. Green[44] and others have obtained arrest of the disease and essentially normal joints with conservative treatment without synovectomy. However, Mercer[81] and others have demonstrated that synovectomy may help in obtaining cure. It is his belief that in certain cases of synovial involvement, synovectomy is very helpful in that it allows the chemotherapeutic agent to reach the area of infection because it removes the scarred, edematous and often caseous synovial membrane. The best method of giving antibiotics for the treatment of articular tuberculosis is still unknown. The injection of streptomycin directly into the joint has been carried out by Stevenson.[117] He was able to demonstrate a level of streptomycin in the blood following this injection, suggesting that the intramuscular route might effect the establishment of an effective level of streptomycin in the joint. Jocson,[60] however, was not able to find evidence of streptomycin in the joint after intramuscular injections, implying that streptomycin moved into joints slowly. The fact that Stevenson[117] found extremely high and persistent concentrations of the drug after the intra-articular injection suggests also that the synovial membrane is not readily permeable to this chemotherapeutic agent. These observations, if supported by other evidence, may in the future constitute grounds for recommending the intra-articular administration of streptomycin in particularly obstinate or progressive cases.

Other Forms of Synovial Tuberculosis. TUBERCULOSIS OF BURSAE. This is not rare. It should be treated by radical excision in an en bloc fashion.

TENDON SHEATHS are involved not uncommonly. The process varies from a chronic relatively mild tenosynovitis to an enormous distention of the sheath with a granulomatous mass and rice bodies with matting together of neighboring tendons. The best treatment of this condition has not been clearly established. A recent survey of this problem by Key[64] from a number of orthopedic centers revealed a lack of uniformity of opinion. Our experience suggests surgical débridement of the lesion so that the sheath is completely opened, washing away of the pus and the necrotic debris, closure of the wound, immobilization and chemotherapy. This procedure offers an excellent chance of cure.

DEGENERATIVE DISEASE OF JOINTS

Degenerative Arthritis

The etiology of the degenerative changes that commonly occur in joints as individuals age is very incompletely understood. Because many patients who develop this disease early are overweight, theories suggesting endocrine or metabolic dysfunction have been formulated. Systemic infections and climatic conditions have largely been discarded as the causes. Some believe there may be hereditary developmental weakness of the articular cartilage that predisposes it to damage and early degeneration. However, these theories fail to explain the histopathologic changes that occur.

In many instances the underlying cause of degeneration is insult to the joint surfaces of a mechanical nature, i.e., (1) fractures into a joint surface with resultant irregular joint surfaces, (2) abnormal motion due to injury to ligaments and supporting structures, (3) direct damage to the articular cartilage from pyogenic arthritis or (4) atrophic arthritis, (5) impaired circulation of the subchondral bone secondary to injury and (6) developmental anomalies of the joint, resulting in incongruity of the articular surface.

Because many of the known causes of degenerative arthritis are of a mechanical nature, it seems likely that this may be the most important cause in all instances of the disease.

In studying degenerative changes of the hip joint, Harrison, Schajawiez and Trueta[52] found that without exception the initiation of the osteoarthritic process took place in the articular cartilage. There is softening, fibrillation, necrosis and frictional erosion of the cartilage. Harrison[52] et al. found that the histochemical change was a reduction of metachromasia of the cartilage and that the area of the joint in which the degenerative process started was the non-weight-bearing portion. Some of these changes were present in all the joints of persons examined who were over 14 years of age.

Hyperemia, irregular calcification of the deeper layers of cartilage, and sclerosis and thickening of the subchondral line in which both bone destruction and new bone formation is active occurs. Osteophyte and cyst formation with replacement of articular cartilage with bone occur later. Cysts filled with fluid, fibrous tissue or fibrocartilage are commonly found in juxtaposition to the articular weight-bearing area of the subchondral bone. They connect with the joint cavity and are surrounded with a rich vascular bed. The process of functional erosion of the articular cartilage is progressive, and ultimately the subchondral bone may be completely denuded of cartilage. By this time the bone has become dense and eburnated, cortical bone having replaced the lost cancellous structure of normal subchondral bone (Fig. 49-23).

Pieces of cartilage and other debris may be picked up and embedded in the synovia or may accumulate in the joint, constituting a source of loose bodies.

In some cases the synovial cells proliferate, and the synovia becomes hyperplastic, forming villi. In others the synovia and the capsule contract and become fibrotic.

Once these degenerative changes have started, continued function of the joint leads to a steady progression of the degenerative process with ultimate complete disorganization of the joint. The rate of progression varies a great deal from case to case, yet, given enough time, the end result will be about the same in all. There are no means of reversing the process, although the rate of progression may be retarded by relative immobilization of the joint.

Although marked restriction of joint motion results, bony ankylosis does not occur. The dense eburnated, relatively avascular bone surfaces opposed to each other and the absence of a vascular granulation tissue account for the failure of union at the two joint surfaces by bone. In fact, arthrodesis of the joint cannot be produced unless the avascular ends are excised to bring more vascular cancellous surfaces into contact. However, vertebral bodies may fuse by marginal osteophytic bridging. (A similar process does not occur in the major articulations of any extremities.)

Because it has not been found possible to restore the degenerative arthritic joint or even limit the progress of the disease, treatment is necessarily directed only toward relief of pain and retardation of the rate of progression. With advanced disease, treatment is directed again to the relief of pain and restoring as much function as possible. Surgery is indicated only after conservative measures have failed and then only in the severely disabled patient. Attempts at reconstruction of disorganized joints from whatever cause do not result in normal joints, and all too often the condition following surgery is not better and may be even worse than before. Therefore, it is imperative that a careful selection of both patients and procedures be made and that both the patient and the surgeon have a clear understanding of what it is hoped may be ac-

complished by operating upon degenerative arthritic joints.

ATROPHIC (RHEUMATOID) ARTHRITIS

The etiology of atrophic or rheumatoid arthritis is unknown. It is a systemic collagenous disease which is more common in young individuals but may occur at any age, although a single joint may be involved early, ultimately it becomes polyarthritic. It is a disease of temperate climates and is not often found in the tropics at or near sea level. Females are affected 3 times as often as males. Many theories of etiology have been expounded. Some of these are (1) focal infection, (2) bacterial allergy, (3) viral infection, (4) vitamin deficiencies, (5) metabolic disorders, (6) neurogenic and (7) endocrine disorders. Some believe that streptococci may be the causative agents, and most workers feel that infection may play some part in its genesis. Evidence for this are (1) fever, (2) tachycardia, (3) rapid sedimentation rate, (4) leukocytosis, (5) lymphadenopathy, (6) splenomegaly, (7) inflamed joints, (8) high titers of serum agglutinins to the *Streptococcus hemolyticus*. Comroe[22] reports, however,

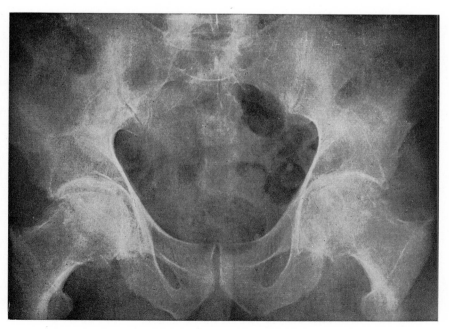

FIG. 49-23. Anteroposterior view, showing advanced degenerative changes in both hips with osteophyte formation, small subchondral cyst, sclerosis and narrowing joint line.

that a disease resembling rheumatoid arthritis can be produced by giving desoxycorticosterone acetate to adrenalectomized and thyroidectomized animals (rats), particularly if they are exposed to cold.

A peculiar form of the disease is rheumatoid spondylitis, which occurs 10 times more commonly among men than women and involves the sacro-iliac joints and the small apophyseal joints of the spine with calcification of the spinous ligaments. It does not involve the intervertebral disks. Cases of rheumatoid spondylitis do not have the high titers of agglutinins to hemolytic streptococci that are found with peripheral involvement, and pain is often relieved by small doses of deep x-ray therapy, but the course of the disease is not altered by x-ray therapy. The pathology in both conditions is essentially the same. Bennett et al.[10] found that the earliest changes in atrophic arthritis were hyperemia with lymphocyte and plasma cell infiltration of the subsynovia, showing a tendency for these cells to collect into follicles. Ghormley and Deacon[41] have pointed out the diagnostic value

of this round cell collection and demonstrated that they were not perivascular. The synovia becomes edematous and proliferative with the development of a vascular pannus which spreads over the articular cartilage, destroying and replacing the joint cartilage. There is an associated proliferation of connective tissue in the marrow spaces beneath the subchondral plate with destruction of bone and cartilage, thinning of the bone trabeculae and cortex, and effusion into the joint.

As the articular cartilage is destroyed and replaced with granulation tissue, there may be a fibrous ankylosis or a bony ankylosis. Rice bodies are frequent with rheumatoid arthritis. Orthopedic treatment of atrophic arthritis is directed at prevention of deformity by splinting in position of function and correction of the deformities that occur in spite of treatment or in latent untreated cases. Arthroplasty to restore motion almost always fails and almost always should be avoided. Considerable relief may be obtained by reconstructive procedures on the hands and the feet at times; often flexion contractures

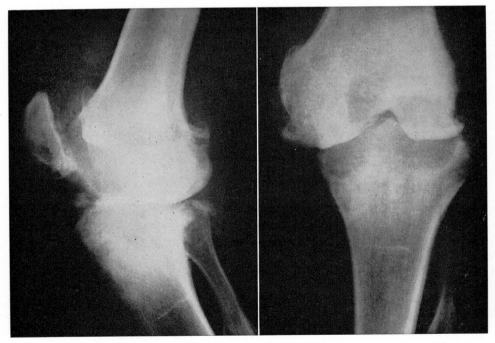

Fig. 49-24. Anteroposterior and lateral roentgenogram of a Charcot knee. The extensive disorganization of the joint is diagnostic. The neurological disorder in this case was tabes dorsalis. The patient also had a Charcot spine.

may be corrected by wedging casts and traction. Osteotomy is a useful operation in selected cases, particularly of the spine (Smith-Petersen et al.[110]). Operation must be considered carefully and undertaken only when conservative therapy has failed.

NEUROTROPHIC JOINT

When disease of the central nervous system deprives extremities of normal sensation, particularly proprioception which is important to normal joint function, destruction of the articulation may occur. Tabes dorsalis and syringomyelia are the most common central nervous system diseases to result in what is known as a Charcot joint.

The proprioceptive loss apparently allows the joint to be subjected to multiple injuries which are not painful. In the early stages the roentgenographic picture is that of degenerative arthritis; however, as the changes progress the typical Charcot joint becomes apparent. Joint surfaces are worn away—the joint fragments first; at the margins osteophytes form, and the joint becomes markedly unstable. Ultimately, complete disorganization of the joint occurs, which is characteristic of the neurotrophic joint (Fig. 49-24).

The knee is involved most often, though the ankle, the hip and the spine may be. Changes in the lower extremities are usually due to tabes dorsalis, while the neurotrophic joint in the upper extremity is more often the result of syringomyelia. Treatment consists of bracing the joint to afford some protection and stability. However, with bracing the joint changes are progressive, and ultimately the instability becomes so incapacitating as to require arthrodesis of the joint.

UPPER EXTREMITY PAIN

One of the most common conditions seen in office orthopedics is the patient with a painful neck, shoulder or arm. At times pathologic conditions responsible for these pains may make diagnosis difficult. Pain in the shoulder may be caused by (1) calcified tendinitis of a segment of the "rotator cuff," (2) so-called bursitis without calcification; (3) degenerative changes in the joint or affecting the tendon of the long head of the biceps; (4) referred pain from a lesion of the cervical spine such as ruptured disk, degenerative disk and joint changes, compression of a nerve root due to narrowing of the intervertebral foramen, by spur or degenerative changes and spinal cord tumor; referred pain from neurovascular irritation or compression at the base of the neck (scalenus anticus syndrome); pain from a tumor of the apex of the lung; (5) tumor, either primary or secondary, of any element of the scapulohumeral articulation; (6) degeneration or dislocation of the acromioclavicular joint; (7) rupture of a component of the rotator cuff; (8) atrophic or degenerative arthritis of the scapulohumeral joint; (9) referred pain from gallbladder or cardiac conditions.

CALCIFIED TENDINITIS

The etiology of this condition is unknown. Theories suggestive of repeated trauma of the tendons of the rotator cuff with subsequent degeneration of a portion allowing calcification are most popular; however, they do not answer all the questions, because (1) there is no evidence of necrotic or degenerative tendon on microscopic study, (2) the condition occurs most commonly in middle life and is rarely seen in old age while degeneration or spontaneous rupture of the rotator cuff is frequently found in the aged when calcification is seldom encountered.

Single trauma probably plays no part, as the x-ray evidence of a calcium deposit suggests its presence prior to the injury. Furthermore, the vast majority of sufferers report no injury or known cause.

Calcium and phosphorus metabolism in all studied cases has been normal. However, since calcium deposits could not be expected in normal tendon, some changes in the chemical nature of the tendon must take place to allow deposition of this material. McCarroll has shown recently that in the early "acute shoulder" without roentgenographic evidence of calcification a white liquid may be aspirated that has the appearance of a calcium suspension. However, on study it proved to have very little calcium and contained for the most part white blood cells. Later, calcification took place and reached a high degree of concentration. These findings suggest that an acute inflammatory change occurs which is followed rather rapidly with calcium deposi-

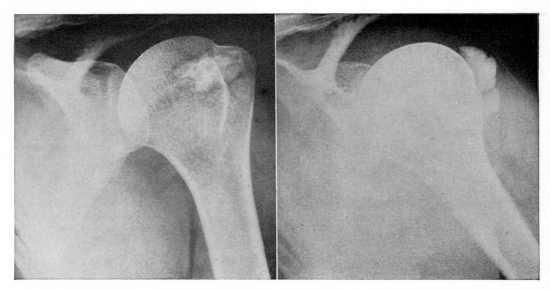

FIG. 49-25. External and internal rotational view of the upper humerus, revealing a large multilocular calcium deposit in the rotator cuff.

tion. At any rate, the picture of acute subdeltoid bursitis has its origin with calcified deposits in the tendon, the bursa being involved secondarily (Fig. 49-25).

Pain and restriction of motion may be severe and acute, or subacute or chronic. Pain is usually about the shoulder and referred to the deltoid insertion on the humerus with an ache in the arm, the forearm and the hand. Pain may radiate to the base of the neck, although neck motions are not restricted, nor does motion of the neck produce arm pain. However, there may be tenderness over the body of the muscle of the involved tendon (i.e., supraspinatus).

In most cases the roentgenogram will reveal a calcium deposit, usually a faint irregular shadow. Occasionally, there is also a dense smooth deposit in addition that represents an old calcification. In some, the calcification is so fluid that a shadow is not made out and may never show if the inflammatory process is severe enough to result in rapid absorption. We know this is true as we have been able on occasion to wash out a milky solution which we have assumed to be calcium from these shoulders presenting a picture of acute tendinitis but with a negative roentgenogram.

Treatment by irrigation with procaine by the single needle technic and instillation of

hydrocortisone has given dramatic relief of symptoms. On the other hand, even repeated injection has not been effective in some patients. In many, deep x-ray therapy is successful in relieving pain, but occasionally all measures fail to control pain, so that surgical excision of as much of the calcium deposit as possible is required. None of these measures will remove all the deposit. Often the calcification will disappear with the subsidence of symptoms. This is dependent on the inflammatory responses rather than the therapy. More often a portion remains even after complete relief of symptoms. This old deposit becomes walled off and does not produce symptoms. Recurrence of pain months or years later is usually the result of a new deposit.

Roentgenograms should be obtained of both shoulders as there often is an asymptomatic deposit in the opposite shoulder.

The complication of this condition is restriction of motion of the shoulder—the so-called frozen shoulder. After pain subsides, exercise usually will restore function. Occasionally, there is so much restriction that manipulation under anesthesia is helpful in starting recovery of function. However, the life history of the condition is such that if untreated even the severely painful and stiff shoulder may be expected to recover completely in time.

Bursitis without calcification is seldom so acute; it is more common in the female and may have a high psychogenic element. Pain and tenderness are more diffuse, and restriction of motion less marked. These are often resistant to all forms of therapy but usually can be relieved by combined psychotherapy and physical measures, such as x-ray therapy, hydrocortisone injections and appropriate psychosomatic adjustment.

A painful, swollen and often stiff hand associated with a painful shoulder which may also have considerable restriction of motion is encountered occasionally. This so-called shoulder-hand syndrome perhaps occurs more often in cardiac cases. The hand is usually warm, moist and more deeply colored than the opposite one. Frequently, sensation is increased without segmental distribution. Pain is described as a burning ache, and at times the patient will state that it feels as though a band were fixed tightly about the hand or the wrist. To complete the syndrome there is restriction of motion of the shoulder because of pain in the early stages and adhesions about the joint later on. There is diffuse pain about the shoulder with radiation down the arm, and there also may be diffuse or localized tenderness. The x-ray findings are always negative except for evidence of atrophy in long-standing cases.

As the primary condition seems to be a reflex dystrophy, treatment includes (1) sympathetic block of the stellate ganglion with procaine, (2) cortisone to control pain and (3) physiotherapy. Late cases always have some residual impairment of function of the hand.

BONE TUMORS

Primary neoplasms arising from the various elements of the skeletal system are more often benign than malignant and in either case are not common. Several lesions currently classed as tumors, i.e., osteoid osteoma, eventually may be discarded from this group. Furthermore, the most common tumor, osteochon-

TABLE 2. CLASSIFICATION OF BONE TUMORS*

TISSUE OF ORIGIN	BENIGN	MALIGNANT COUNTER-PART IF ANY	MALIGNANT
Cartilage	Osteochondroma Enchondroma Chondroblastoma	Chondrosarcoma	Chondrosarcoma
Bone	Osteoma Osteoid osteoma Ossifying fibroma		Osteosarcoma
Connective tissue	Benign giant cell tumor Metaphyseal fibrous defects	Malignant giant cell tumor	Fibrosarcoma
Mesenchymal connective tissue			Ewing's sarcoma
Hematopoietic origin			Multiple myeloma Acute and chronic leukemia Malignant lymphoma Reticular cell sarcoma Lymphosarcoma Hodgkin's disease
Nerve origin	Neurofibroma Neurilemmoma	Malignant schwannoma	
Vascular origin	Hemangioma Hemangiopericytoma	Hemangio-endothelioma Malignant hemangio-pericytoma	Hemangio-endothelioma
Fat cell			Liposarcoma
Notochordal			Chordoma

* Lichtenstein's classification slightly modified.

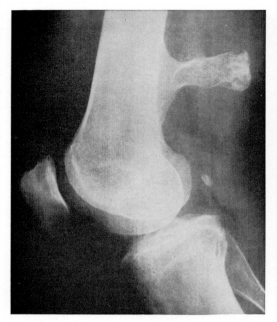

FIG. 49-26. Roentgenogram of the distal end of the femur showing a typical benign osteochondroma.

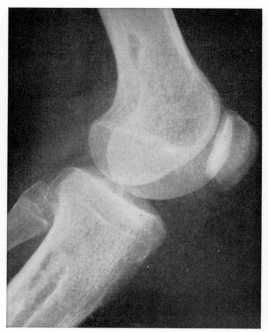

FIG. 49-27. Roentgenogram of the proximal tibia in a 15-year-old Negro boy. The eccentrically placed loculated lesions are typical of a metaphyseal fibrous defect—a benign lesion.

droma (Fig. 49-26) occurs as a result of a defect in the growth of the parent bone and is not a true neoplasm. Classification of bone tumors is often difficult and seldom worthwhile insofar as any particular lesion is concerned. However, in order to have a clear picture of the various tumors, a classification is helpful (Table 2). We prefer that given by Lichtenstein,[73] with slight modification, to those of others.

When presented with a skeletal lesion it is mandatory of course to arrive at an accurate diagnosis as early as possible. Such a diagnosis seldom can be made with any degree of certainty from roentgenologic examination alone. The possible exception to this is the osteoid osteoma and metaphyseal fibrous (Fig. 49-27) defects and even these rather characteristic lesions may have such an unusual picture as to cast doubt on the x-ray interpretation. It is imperative that a careful history, physical examination and pertinent laboratory studies be available for proper understanding of the x-ray picture. With this information an experienced radiologist or orthopedic surgeon may come reasonably close to the correct answer much of the time. Defi-

nite therapy should not be undertaken on the basis of this information alone except with regard to a few quite characteristic lesions, i.e., osteoid osteoma, metaphyseal fibrous defect and exostoses. In all other instances microscopic study of representative tissue from the lesion must be obtained before intelligently directed treatment can be instituted. There is some danger of seeding malignant cells or even spreading malignant tissue from the trauma of biopsy. The danger of tumor spread from this procedure is minor compared with the error of unnecessary amputation as a result of treatment without the knowledge gained from tissue study.

Biopsy should be done at the treatment center that is going to be responsible for the complete care of the patient. All too often we are faced with the problem of receiving a patient with a skeletal lesion who has already had a biopsy performed, in which one or all of the following circumstances exist: (1) wound infection of the biopsy site, which in some cases has profoundly influenced the course of the patient and made more difficult the proper care; (2) the slides may accompany the patient and be of such poor quality that proper interpretation is not possible; (3) the original block is lost or not available for further study; (4) the biopsy material may not be diagnostic, because the surgeon failed to get it from a representative area of the lesion; in fact, at times he has missed the lesion completely.

The biopsy material must be handled properly so that good slides are obtained. Then a pathologist experienced in the study of bone lesions usually is able to make an accurate diagnosis, but the tissue examination does not stand alone as an exact science. The pathologist must take into consideration the history, the physical findings and the laboratory studies, including the roentgenograms, and even with all information at hand it is sometimes impossible to be sure of the exact nature of the tumor.

When a complete study of the patient, together with his bone lesion, has been accomplished, then and only then should definite treatment be carried out.

Treatment will be considered here only briefly; for a more detailed study one is referred to the works of Lichtenstein,[73] Luck[74] and Ackerman.[4]

Benign tumors for the most part are not radiosensitive, with the possible exception of benign giant cell tumors. At the present not enough information is available to be sure how effective radiation in this group of tumors really is, so at present we prefer excision of benign lesions, with replacement of bone to fill surgically created defects or gaps in the involved bone where indicated because of structural weakness.

Malignant bone tumors fall into 2 groups: primary and metastatic. Operation is indicated in metastatic lesions with pathologic fractures for the purpose of relief of pain and improving function by means of internal fixation or more rarely by means of prosthetic replacement. Occasionally, amputation may be advisable to relieve the patient of a painful fungating mass. In other metastatic lesions palliative radiation should be employed (Fig. 49-28).

Primary malignant bone tumors remain an unsolved therapeutic problem. The state of

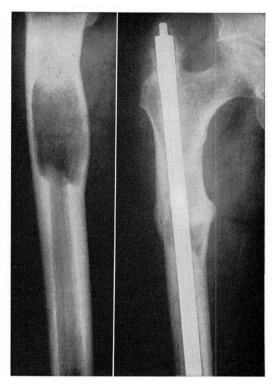

Fig. 49-28 (*Left*) This large lesion within the femur is a metastases from a carcinoma of the breast. A pathologic fracture impends. (*Right*) A femoral nail used to support the fragile femur, and x-ray therapy to the lesion has preserved a useful painless extremity for 18 months.

our present knowledge indicates that the only chance of survival is sterilization of the lesion before spreading occurs. In some very radiosensitive tumors this occasionally occurs with x-ray alone, as in Ewing's tumor. However, the author's experience is that all patients with Ewing's sarcoma and the other quite radiosensitive lesions, such as reticulum cell sarcoma, have died regardless of type of therapy. This includes: (1) radiation alone; (2) radiation followed by amputation (even when microscopic examination of the amputated extremity has failed to reveal any remaining malignant cell, nevertheless the tumor has appeared elsewhere and eventually resulted in death); and (3) cases amputated and then submitted to roentgenotherapy of regional nodes. The author feels, therefore, that radiation alone is the treatment that

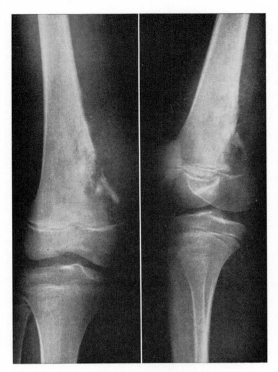

FIG. 49-29. Roentgenogram of the femur in a 9-year-old girl showing a destructive lesion of the distal metaphyseal region of the femur. It has the typical appearance of an osteosarcoma which was confirmed by biopsy. Although an amputation through the thigh was done pulmonary metastasis was apparent 9 months later.

should be employed in Ewing's and reticulum cell sarcomas but adopts this therapy in a completely defeatist attitude.

Other malignant bone tumors have a small chance of cure with early adequate surgical removal of the tumor (Fig. 49-29). So long as all the tumor cells are removed from the body it matters little what method is employed. Ideally, this would be a local resection so that some function of the extremity could be maintained. However, it is seldom possible to carry out complete eradication of the malignant growth and maintain function, so that amputation gives the best functional result at the least cost to the patient, in regard to both money and pain. Furthermore, there is a tendency for these tumors to spread up the medullary canal of the affected bone and they may even jump areas of apparently normal marrow, so

that resection may not be successful in getting around the tumor. Again, for this reason removal of the entire affected bone is advisable at the time of amputation. The author would like to suggest that chondrosarcoma has been taken too lightly (Fig. 49-30). This rather slow-growing tumor tending to metastasize late is, however, a very formidable one. One can hardly point with pride to a patient who has had a surgical resection or local excision of this tumor and remains free of trouble for a number of years only for the patient then to die of recurrence and metastases when radical removal of all the diseased tissue perhaps would have saved the patient's life. This is particularly true when these tumors involve the pelvis. In this site the first surgical procedure is often the only one that can cure the patient, and this procedure must be sufficiently radical to ensure complete eradication of all tumor cells. Often this will require hemipelvectomy.

LOW BACK PAIN

It has been estimated that from 25 to 50 per cent of all patients treated by the orthopedist have as a presenting complaint low back pain with or without sciatica. Backache, like headache, may result from a variety of abnormal conditions. It is essential, therefore, to establish an accurate pathologic diagnosis. But the desire to make such a diagnosis must be tempered with judgment so that each patient seen with low back pain is not subjected routinely to all possible diagnostic tests. The vast majority of patients can be managed satisfactorily as out patients with conservative treatment such as low back supports, rest, local heat and drugs for relief of pain and exercise. The more common causes of back pain with or without sciatica are (1) acute strain, (2) abnormality of the intervertebral disk, (3) degenerative arthritis, (4) defect of the pars interarticularis, (5) pelvic disease, (6) rheumatoid arthritis affecting the spine, (7) senile osteoporosis, (8) tumors, both primary and metastatic, (9) infection of spine, (10) psychoneurosis, (11) pathologic fracture, and others. Postural backache, although quite frequent, is seldom of such severity that the sufferer seeks medical advice.

It is apparent that a rather complete history and physical examination must be carried out for the physician to begin to grasp the patient's problem. At times the cause is quite obvious, and at other times considerable time and effort is expended before the source of trouble comes to light. These patients may be divided readily into those with a history of injury and those who cannot remember an injury.

Of those with history of injury the effort-strain type is the most common. A number of years ago the author reviewed a large series of cases with a history of this type of injury. These patients were more or less disabled and had restriction of motion, local tenderness in the low back or below, and many had radiation of pain in the legs. Of these patients, 96 per cent responded rapidly to rest and local heat and were able to return to work in less than 4 weeks. It appears that about this percentage recovers from these strains or sprains regardless of treatment. The remaining 4 per cent who did not recover in this period were found on further study to have a ruptured disk, defect of pars interarticularis, tumors or infections, with the greatest number having a ruptured disk.

Of the group having a history of back injury by a direct blow many have hematomas and muscle damage or fractures of one or more transverse processes of the lumbar vertebra. In spite of the history and the physical evidence of a direct blow, it is generally believed that the transverse processes are fractured only by muscle pull of the quadratus lumborum muscle.

The various fractures of the spine are discussed in Chapter 21, "Fractures and Dislocations of Spine, Pelvis, Sternum and Ribs."

DISEASE AND INJURY OF THE INTERVERTEBRAL DISK

Approximately 50 per cent of the patients in whom a diagnosis of a symptomatic degenerative disk condition with or without rupture of the nucleus pulposus is made give a history of trauma. A detailed description of sciatica was made by Momenico Contugno in

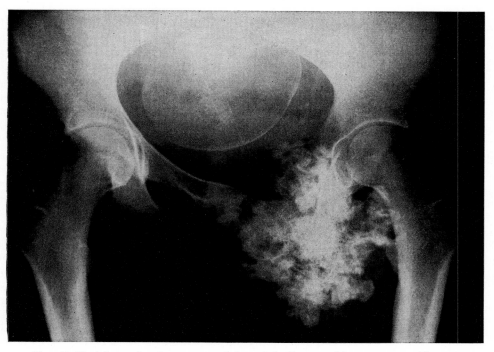

FIG. 49-30. A huge chondrosarcoma of the pelvis discovered in an 18-year-old woman seven months pregnant. The large lobulated tumor mass with areas of calcification in it is a typical chondrosarcoma. Several weeks following cesarean section, wide local resection of the tumor and all pubic rami was done.

1764; he originated the term. Further clinical description was made by Laségue (1864).[71] Virchow[121] (1857) described a fracture of the disk. Protrusion of disk material was reported by von Luschka[75] in 1858 as well as details of anatomy of the disk. Fick[38] in 1910, Brown[16] in 1921, Beadle[9] in 1939, Keyes and Compere[65] in 1932, Coventry, Ghormley and Kernohan[24, 25, 26] in 1945 have contributed to knowledge of anatomic characteristics of disks. Keyes and Compere[65] determined physiologic function of the disk and carried out experimental investigations and reviewed the literature. Virchow[121] described the nuclear cells of the disk as large cells with eccentric nuclei with clear zones. He called these physaliferous cells and thought that they were of notochordal origin. He also described cartilaginous masses of protruded disk material and called them physaliferous enchondromas. Dandy[28] in 1929 reported 2 cases of cartilaginous enchondroma compressing the cord.

Although a number of men were close to the proper understanding of the role of the disk in producing low back pain and sciatica, the placing of this in proper clinical perspective was the work of Mixter and Barr[83] who described the clinical picture in 1934, proved the existence of disk rupture with nerve root compression and demonstrated relief of symptoms by surgical removal of the protruded portion of the disk.

Puschel[95] in 1930 found that the nucleus pulposus contained 88 per cent water in newborns and that there was gradual loss of water with aging so that there was 66 per cent water at age 77. Keyes and Compere[65] substantiated these findings. DePusky[29] noted that there was increased length of the spine after resting and a decrease with standing. The extension of blood vessels into the disk substance through the cartilaginous plates has been described to about age 30. After this age none are found. Roofe[103] in 1940 found nerve fibers extending to the posterior portion of the annulus fibrosus. Also nerve fibers have been described in the anterior and the posterior longitudinal ligaments but none in the nuclear material itself.

In childhood the nucleus is well demarcated from the annulus fibrosus, while in the 2nd decade the cells become fewer and the demarcation not so clear, and in the 3rd decade cavities appear, as do also cartilage cells.

Dehydration is accompanied by a change to fibrocartilage with an associated loss of elasticity of the annulus fibrosus. All investigators have agreed that at an early age evidence of alteration of the nucleus and the annulus fibrosus of a degenerative nature are evident. These alterations reduce the elasticity of the annulus, and it appears that damage to the annulus with cracks and fissure formation is the important alteration as the elastic nature of the disk results from function of the annulus and not the nucleus pulposus.

There is evidence that low back pain or low back pain and sciatica may be caused by degeneration of the disk with alteration of the physiologic function as well as by nerve root compression when there is posterior protrusion of disk material.

Ghormley[40] has described the facet syndrome. However, there is very little evidence that alterations of the apophyseal joints are primary factors in low back pain with or without sciatica except in rheumatoid arthritis or fracture. Changes in the apophyseal joints are for the most part secondary to alterations of disk function.

Therefore, it appears that the most common cause of unexplained low back pain with or without sciatica must be due to disturbance in the disk. Whether or not the cases usually grouped under acute strains are due to slight alteration of the disk remains to be proved. So far there is no available pathologic evidence of damage to ligaments and muscles, as these cases that respond readily to treatment are not explored.

With impairment of function of the disk mechanism spine motions are altered permanently. The normal repair process is sclerosis of the adjacent vertebral borders with narrowing of the disk space, osteophyte formation and in time bony ankylosis of the involved segment or segments. Rupture of disk material with nerve root compression in the aged is quite rare. Therefore, treatment is directed to the relief of pain. Conservative measures are usually successful in all cases but those with massive posterior rupture of disk material into the spinal canal and even in these instances nonoperative treatment may successfully carry a patient through several acute episodes. Those patients with recurrent severe episodes usually can be relieved by operation and removal of the protruding disk material. However, many do well on conservative treatment with only an occasional mild recurrence.

Whether improvement is due to (1) a shift of the tissue away from the nerve, (2) desiccation or absorption of the protruded material, or (3) the nerve root becoming insensitive we do not know. However, with a large protrusion and nerve root compression the chances of relief of low back pain and sciatica are small. It is true that in time pain may be relieved, but there may be permanent nerve damage reflected in atrophy of the involved muscles, sensory loss and at times changes in the circulation.

The neurologic symptoms and signs produced by the herniated intervertebral disk are usually those of compression of a single lumbar nerve root. The history of intermittent back pain followed by sciatic radiation of pain is common. About 75 per cent of patients have the pain accentuated by coughing and sneezing. About half of them have a list or "sciatic" scoliosis which is usually away from the affected side. About 50 per cent of disk herniations occur at the L4-L5 interspace, 45 per cent at the L5-S interspace, and 5 per cent at the L3-L4 interspace. The neurologic signs depend on the level of the lesion.

Herniation of the disk at the L4-L5 interspace usually involves the 5th lumbar root. Radiation of pain is often to the great toe and the medial side of the foot, and hypesthesia in this area is frequent. Weakness of the long extensor of the great toe is also frequent, and 10 to 15 per cent will have a diminished knee jerk. Pain in the back on straight leg raising is almost always present. Local tenderness at the L4-L5 interspace is common and may be helpful in localization of the level of the lesion.

Herniation of the disk at the L5-S interspace usually compresses the first sacral root, and the radiation of pain is to the lateral side of the foot. Hypesthesia over the lateral side of the foot, a diminished or absent ankle jerk, positive straight leg raising test and tenderness at the L5-S interspace are the common signs of herniation of the lumbosacral disk.

When the signs indicate that more than a single nerve root is compressed, the possibility exists that more than one herniation has occurred, or that there is a tumor of the spinal chord or a granuloma in the spinal canal. Multiple herniations occur rather frequently. Rarely, a massive protrusion of a disk in the mid-line may result in severe neurologic abnormalities such as bilateral drop foot, quadriceps paralysis and loss of bowel and bladder control.

We feel that all patients who do not respond to conservative therapy in a reasonable period of time (1 to 4 months), depending on the severity of symptoms and the character of the physical findings, should have myelographic studies (Fig. 49-31) followed by operation if the diagnosis is confirmed. The only cases not submitted to myelography are those presenting an acute and severe picture in which the localizing neurologic signs leave little doubt as to the location of the protruding mass and in whom it is felt that because of the severity of the clinical picture further conservative treatment will be worthless. The only indications for early operation are profound

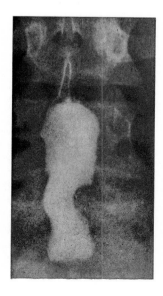

Fig. 49-31. Myelogram showing a large defect at the L4-L5 disk level. The defect is the result of a completely extruded nucleus pulposis. The myelogram is performed by injecting ethyl iodophenylundecylate (Pantopaque) into the subarachnoid space. This hyperbaric material can then be made to flow up and down the subarachnoid space by tilting the patient and clearly delineating such space-filling lesions. Spinal fluid for protein and other chemical determinations should be removed before injecting the contrast material. About half of the patients with a herniated nucleus pulposus will have a slight elevation (50-75 mgm. %) of spinal fluid protein; elevation of the spinal fluid protein greater than this are more likely due to a chord tumor than to a herniated disk.

neurologic changes when the case is first seen or a rapidly progressing neurologic deficit.

The extradural approach to the disk has greatly simplified the operative technic. Furthermore, we have used local anesthesia for further simplification.

The question still remains whether or not a spinal fusion also should be done at the time of removal of the protruded disk. As the removal of the protruded disk material only relieves nerve root compression and does not correct the altered mechanics of the spine resulting from degeneration of the disk, there remains a chance for continued low back pain and even sciatica. In our experience approximately 50 per cent of the patients with simple disk excision remain completely free of pain. There is evidence that combining disk excision with a spinal fusion will increase the over-all per cent of good results by about 10 to 15 per cent. Spinal fusion increases the operative risk and the postoperative convalescent period. It appears that local fusion is desirable, and we feel sure that when a satisfactory and simple method of obtaining fusion following disk surgery is evolved it will be employed in a larger number of cases. However, a solid spinal fusion does not ensure relief of pain; it may be that following fusion of the involved area extra stress is placed on other degenerating disks, either above or below the operated one. In spite of the theoretical and clinical evidence that the end result would be improved by the combined operation of disk removal and spinal fusion, we seldom carry out this procedure because we have felt that the results do not justify the added risk and longer period of disability entailed with our present method of spinal fusion.

At times an unstable degenerative disk without posterior protrusion may continue to cause disabling low back pain in spite of continued conservative measures, and spinal fusion may be required.

In summary, of patients with low back pain and sciatica due to degenerative disk disease with or without protrusion, only about 10 per cent require surgery. Of this group the cases without nerve root compression who fail to respond to conservative treatment may be treated by spinal fusion. Those with nerve root compression are treated by simple disk excision, and unless there is considerable instability fusion is not done.

Degenerative Arthritis of the Spine

The evidence of hypertrophic changes seen in the roentgenogram and commonly called degenerative arthritis are all probably secondary to alteration of disk function or to major trauma to the vertebra. These changes in themselves do not as a rule cause pain. However, at times a nerve root will be encroached upon in the vertebral foramen by a hypertrophic spur with resultant (and often severe) pain.

Pelvic disease of various types has been blamed for low back pain and at times neuritis of the sciatic nerve. Spread of cancer from the pelvic organs, particularly in the female, may produce low back pain and sciatica from direct involvement of the components of the sciatic nerve within the pelvis. At times the diagnosis may be difficult, but the neurologic findings usually become marked and progressive, and a negative myelogram plus the evidence of pelvic neoplasm should readily suggest the diagnosis. However, we are aware of more than one such case that had exploration for a ruptured disk. On the other hand, a considerable number of women have had pelvic operations for low back pain due to disk degeneration. It appears that tumors and chronic infections of the female pelvis may cause some back pain, but we suggest that hysterectomy not be done for back pain alone.

The roentgenogram, coupled with a good history and a physical examination, should be adequate in separating defects of the pars interarticularis, infections, tumors, senile osteoporosis and rheumatoid arthritis from cases of disk rupture. However, repeated examination and time may occasionally be required to distinguish a case of rheumatoid arthritis. Rarely, tuberculosis and slow-growing tumors present difficult diagnostic problems.

Recently, some doubt has been cast on the proper treatment of defects of the pars interarticularis. Gill et al.[42] and Bosworth et al.[13] have indicated that resection of the loose posterior element, together with complete decompression of the roots, results in relief of pain. Bosworth et al.[13] follows this with spinal fusion. We continue to believe that spinal fusion is the treatment of choice. In the presence of sciatica the involved root should be decompressed at operation, but the posterior element is not removed unless this is required to obtain adequate decompression of a root. The bone of the loose posterior element is viable, and we feel that it aids in obtaining fusion. Furthermore, Bosworth *et al.*[13] has shown that the retained posterior element helps to prevent further forward displacement of the vertebral body. For both of these reasons we see no excuse for removal of the posterior element except in the rare case where adequate exposure of the root cannot be obtained without it.

REFERENCES

1. Abbott, L. C.: The operative lengthening of the tibia and fibula, J. Bone & Joint Surg. *9*:128, 1927.
2. Abbott, L. C., and Crego, C. H.: Operative lengthening of the femur, South. M.J. *21*: 823, 1928.
3. Abbott, L. C., Schottstaedt, E. R., Saunders, J. B. de C. M., and Bost, F. C.: The evaluation of cortical and cancellous bone as grafting material: a clinical and experimental study, J. Bone & Joint Surg. *29*:381-414, 1947.
4. Ackerman, L. V.: Surgical Pathology, St. Louis, Mosby, 1953.
5. Albright, F., Butler, A. M., and Bloomsberg, F.: Rickets resistant to vitamin D therapy, Am. J. Dis. Child. *54*:629-647, 1937.
6. Albright, Fuller, and Reifenstein, E. C., Jr.: The Parathyroid Glands and Metabolic Bone Disease, Baltimore, Williams & Wilkins, 1948.
7. Armstrong, W. D.: Composition and crystal structure of the bone salt *in* Tr. Second Conf. on Metabolic Interrelations, New York, Macy, 1950.
8. Badgley, C. E., Isaacson, A. S., Walgamot, J. C., and Miller, J. W.: Operative therapy for slipped upper femoral epiphysis: an end result study, J. Bone & Joint Surg. *30*:19-28, 1948.
9. Beadle, O. A.: The intervertebral discs; observations on their normal and morbid anatomy in relation to certain spinal deformities, Rep. Med. Res. Council *161*:1-79, 1931, London, His Majesty's Stat. Off.
10. Bennett, G. A., Waine, H., and Bauer, W.: Changes in the Knee Joint at Various Ages, with Particular Reference to the Nature and Development of Degenerative Joint Disease, New York, Commonwealth Fund, 1942.
11. Bierman, H. R., Lanman, J. T., Dod, K. S., Kelly, K. H., Miller, E. R., and Shimkin, M. D.: The ameliorative effect of antibiotics on nonlipoid reticuloendotheliosis (Letterer-Siwe disease) in identical twins, J. Pediat. *40*:269-284, 1952.
12. Blount, W. P., and Clark, G. R.: Control of bone growth by epiphyseal stapling, J. Bone & Joint Surg. *31-A*:464, 1949.
13. Bosworth, D. M., Fielding, J. W., Demarest, L., and Bonaquist, M.: Spondylolisthesis; a critical review of a consecutive series of cases treated by arthrodesis, J. Bone & Joint Surg. *37-A*:767, 1955.
14. Bosworth, D. M., Wright, H. A., Fielding, J. W., and Wilson, H. J.: The use of Ipromazid in the treatment of bone and joint tuberculosis, J. Bone & Joint Surg. *35-A*: 577, 1953.
15. Brodie, B. C.: An account of some cases of chronic diseases of the tibia, Medico-Chir. Tr. *17*:239-249, 1832.
16. Brown, L. T.: Beef bone in stabilizing operations of the spine, J. Bone & Joint Surg. *20*:711, 1922.
17. Chandler, F. A.: Patellar advancement operation; a revised technique, Paper Presented at Internat. Coll. Surgeons Meeting, Chicago, Jan. 1947.
18. ———: Re-establishment of normal leverage of the patella in knee flexion deformity in spastic paralysis, Surg., Gynec. & Obst. *57*:523, 1933.
19. Chase, S. W., and Herndon, C. H.: The fate of autogenous and homogenous bone grafts: a historical review, J. Bone & Joint Surg. *37*:809-841, 1955.
20. Cleveland, M., and Bosworth, D. M.: Pathology of tuberculosis of the spine, J. Bone & Joint Surg. *24*:527-546, 1942.
21. Compere, E. L., Johnson, W. E., and Coventry, M. B.: Vertebra plana (Calvé's disease) due to eosinophilic granuloma, J. Bone & Joint Surg. *36*:969-980, 1954.
22. Comroe, B. I.: Comroe's Arthritis and Allied Conditions, ed. 5, Philadelphia, Lea & Febiger, 1953.
23. Cooley, J. C., Mussey, R. D., and Rogers, J. C. T.: Femoral arteriovenous fistula creation in the treatment of the short leg, Arch. Surg. *80*:838-842, 1960.
24. Coventry, M. B., Ghormley, R. K., and Kernohan, J. W.: The intervertebral disc: its anatomy and pathology; Part I. Anatomy, development and physiology, J. Bone & Joint Surg. *27*:105, 1947.
25. ———: The intervertebral disc: its microscopic anatomy and pathology; Part II. Changes in the intervertebral disc concomitant with age, J. Bone & Joint Surg. *27*:233, 1945.

26. ———: The intervertebral disc: its microscopic anatomy and pathology; Part III. Pathological changes in the intervertebral disc, J. Bone & Joint Surg. 27:460, 1945.

27. Crego, C. H., Jr., and Schwartzmann, J. R.: Follow-up study of the early treatment of congenital dislocation of the hip, J. Bone & Joint Surg. 30:428-442, 1948.

28. Dandy, W. E.: Loose cartilage from intervertebral disc simulating tumor of spinal cord, Arch. Surg. 19:567-770, 1929.

29. DePusky: The physiological oscillation of the length of the body, Acta orthop. scandinav. 6:338, 1935.

30. Duraiswami, P. K.: Experimental causation of congenital skeletal defects and its significance in orthopedic surgery, J. Bone & Joint Surg. 34:646-698, 1952.

31. Durham, H. A.: A procedure for the correction of internal rotation of the thigh in spastic paralysis, J. Bone & Joint Surg. 20:339, 1938.

32. Duthie, R. B., and Barker, A. N.: An autoradiographic study of mucopolysaccharide and phosphate complexes in bone growth and repair, J. Bone & Joint Surg. 37-B: 304-323, 1955.

33. ———: The histochemistry of the preosseous stage of bone repair studied by autoradiography, J. Bone & Joint Surg. 37-B: 691-710, 1955.

34. Eggers, G. W.: Transplantation of hamstring tendons to femoral condyles in order to improve hip extension and to decrease knee flexion in cerebral spastic paralysis, J. Bone & Joint Surg. 34-A:827, 1952.

35. Eichelberger, L., Akeson, W. H., and Ronia, M.: Biochemical studies of articular cartilage, J. Bone & Joint Surg. 40-A:142-162, 1958.

36. Fairbank, T. H.: Atlas of General Affections of the Skeleton, Baltimore, Williams & Wilkins, 1952.

37. Ferguson, A. B., and Howorth, M. B.: Slipping of the upper femoral epiphysis, J.A.M.A. 97:1867, 1931.

38. Fick, R.: Handb. d. Anat. und Mech. D. Gelenke, 1911.

39. Ford, L. T., and Key, J. A.: Postoperative infection of the intervertebral disc space, South. M.J. 48:1295, 1955.

40. Ghormley, R. K.: Low back pain, with special reference to the articular facets with presentation of an operative procedure, J.A.M.A. 101:1773, 1933.

41. Ghormley, R. K., and Deacon, A. E.: Synovial membranes in various types of arthritis, Am. J. Roentgenol. 35:740, 1936.

42. Gill, G. G., Manning, J. G., and White,

H. L.: Surgical treatment of spondylolisthesis without spine fusion, J. Bone & Joint Surg. 37-A:493, 1955.

43. Green, W. T.: Osteomyelitis in infancy, J.A.M.A. 105:1835, 1935.

44. ———: Personal communication.

45. Green, W. T., and Anderson, M.: Experiences with epiphyseal arrest in correcting discrepancies in length of the lower extremities in infantile paralysis; a method of predicting the effect, J. Bone & Joint Surg. 29:659, 1947.

46. Green, W. T., and Farber, S.: Eosinophilic or solitary granuloma of bone, J. Bone & Joint Surg. 30:499, 1942.

47. Griffiths, Seddon and Road: Pott's Paraplegia, New York, Oxford, 1956.

48. Gutman, A. B., and Gutman, E. B.: A phosphoranylase in calcified cartilage, Proc. Soc. Exper. Biol. & Med. 48:687-691, 1941.

49. Hallock, H., and Jones, J. B.: Tuberculosis of the spine; an end-result study of the effects of the spine-fusion operation in a large number of patients, J. Bone & Joint Surg. 36-A:219-240, 1954.

50. Harris, R. I., and McDonald, J. L.: The effect of lumbar sympathectomy upon the growth of legs paralyzed by anterior poliomyelitis, J. Bone & Joint Surg. 18:35, 1936.

51. Harris, R. T., and Beath, T.: Army Foot Survey, Ottowa, National Research Council, 1947.

52. Harrison, M. H., Schajawiez, F., and Trueta, J.: Osteoarthritis of the hip; a study of the nature and evolution of the disease, J. Bone & Joint Surg. 35-B:598, 1953.

53. Hart, V. L.: Congenital Dysplasia of the Hip Joint and Sequelae, Springfield, Ill., Thomas, 1952.

54. Heyman, C. H.: The surgical release of fibrous tissue structures resisting correction of congenital club-foot and metatarsus varus, Am. Acad. Orthop. Surgeons, Lect. 16:100-116, 1959.

55. Hobo, Teruo: Zur Pathogenese Der Akuten Haematogenen Osteomyelitis Mit Berucksichtigung Der Vtial Fabungslehe, Acta scholae med. univ. Kioto 4:1, 1921-1922.

56. Hoke, Michael: An operation for stabilizing paralytic feet, J. Orthop. Surg. 3:494-507, 1921.

57. Howorth, M. B.: Slipping of the upper femoral epiphysis in Am. Acad. Orthop. Surgeons Instructional Course Lectures, Ann Arbor, Edwards, 1951.

58. Ilfeld, F. W.: The management of congenital dislocation of the hip by means of

a special splint, J. Bone & Joint Surg. *39-A*:99-110, 1957.

59. Jaffe, H. L., and Lichtenstein, **L.**: Eosinophilic granuloma of bone, Am. J. Path. *16*:595, 1940.

60. Janes, J. M., and Musgrave, J. E.: Effect of arteriovenous fistula on the growth of bone: experimental study, S. Clin. North America *30*:1191-1200, 1950.

61. Jocson, **C. T.**: The diffusion of antibiotics through the synovial membrane, J. Bone & Joint Surg. *37*:107, 1955.

62. Kelly, P. J., Janes, J. M., and Peterson, L. F. A.: The effect of arteriovenous fistulae on the vascular pattern of the femur of immature dogs, J. Bone & Joint Surg. *41-A*: 1101-1108, 1959.

63. Key, J. A.: Osteomyelitis *in* Lewis' Practice of Surgery, vol. 2, pp. 1-95, Hagerstown, Md., Prior, 1954.

64. ——: Personal communication.

65. Keyes, D. C., and Compere, D. C.: The normal and pathological physiology of the nucleus pulposus of the intervertebral disc, J. Bone & Joint Surg. *14*:897, 1932.

66. Kite, J. H.: The treatment of congenital clubfoot, Surg., Gynec. & Obst. *61*:190, 1935.

66a. ——: Principles involved in the treatment of congenital clubfoot, J. Bone & Joint Surg. *21*:595-606, 1939.

67. Klein, A., Joplin, R. J., Reidy, J. A., and Hanelin, J.: Slipped capital femoral epiphysis, J. Bone & Joint Surg. *34*:233, 1952.

68. Kuhlman, R. E.: A microchemical study of the developing epiphyseal plate, J. Bone & Joint Surg. *42-A*:457-466, 1960.

69. Kulowski, **J.**: Pyogenic osteomyelitis of the spine, J. Bone & Joint Surg. *18*:343-364, 1936.

70. Lambrinudi, C.: A new operation on drop foot, Brit. J. Surg. *15*:193, 1927.

71. Laségue, C.: Considérations sur la sciatique Arch. gén. méd. *2*:558, 1864.

72. Lexer, E.: Über Osteomyelitis Experimente, Zentralbl. Chir. *22*:868, 1895.

73. Lichtenstein, L.: Bone Tumors, St. Louis, Mosby, 1952.

74. Luck, **J. V.**: Bone and Joint Disease, Springfield, Ill., Thomas, 1950.

75. Luschka, **H.**: Die Halbgelenke des Menschlichen Korpers, Berlin, Reimer, 1858.

76. McCarroll, H. R.: Early management of congenital dislocation of the hip *in* Lectures on Regional Orthopedic Surgery and Fundamental Orthopedic Problems, No. 2, pp. 125-156, Ann Arbor, Edwards, 1948.

77. McLean, F. C., and Bloom, W.: Calcification and ossification, Arch. Path. *32*:315, 1941.

78. McLean, F. C., and Urist, M. R.: Bone, Chicago, Univ. Chicago Press, 1955.

79. Mallory, T. B.: Diseases of bone, New England J. Med. *227*:955, 1942.

80. Mathews, M. B.: Interactions of mucopolysaccharides and some protein components of connective tissue, Circulation *14*:972, 1956.

81. Mercer, W.: The management of the tuberculous hip joint, J. Bone & Joint Surg. *36-A*:1123-1128, 1954.

82. Milkman, L. A.: Multiple spontaneous idiopathic symmetrical fracture, Am. J. Roentgenol. *32*:623-634, 1934.

83. Mixter, W., and Barr, J.: Rupture of the intervertebral disc with involvement of spinal canal, New England J. Med. *211*: 210, 1934.

84. Moe, **J. H.**: A critical analysis of methods of fusion for scoliosis, J. Bone & Joint Surg. *40-A*:529-554, 1958.

85. Moehlig, R. C., and Abbott, H. L.: Carbohydrate metabolism in osteitis deformans or Paget's disease, J.A.M.A. *134*:1521, 1947.

86. Mora, F. B., and Llamedo, L. P.: Experimental studies on the treatment of bone and joint tuberculosis with dihydrostreptomycin and isonicotinic acid hydrazide, J. Bone & Joint Surg. *37-A*:156-168, 1955.

87. Neuman, W. F., DiStefano, V., and Mulryan, B. J.: Observations and the role of phosphatase *in* Tr. Third Conf. on Metabolic Interrelations, New York, Macy, 1951.

88. Orr, H. W.: The treatment of acute osteomyelitis by drainage and rest, J. Bone & Joint Surg. *9*:733, 1927.

89. Pease, C. N.: Local stimulation of growth of long bones; a preliminary report, J. Bone & Joint Surg. *34*:1-22, 1952.

90. Pedersen, H. E., and McCarroll, H. R.: Vitamin-D resistant rickets, J. Bone & Joint Surg. *33*:203-218, 1951.

91. Phemister, D. B.: Repair of bone in presence of aseptic necrosis resulting from fractures, transplantation and vascular obstruction, J. Bone & Joint Surg. *12*:769, 1930.

92. Phemister, D. B.: Operative arrestment of longitudinal growth of bones in the treatment of deformities, J. Bone & Joint Surg. *15*:1-15, 1933.

93. Ponseti, I. V.: Lesions of the skeleton and of other mesodermal tissues in rats fed sweet peas, J. Bone & Joint Surg. *36*:1031, 1954.

94. Ponseti, I. V., and Frigerio, E. R.: Results of treatment of congenital dislocation of the

hip, J. Bone & Joint Surg. *41-A*:823-846, 1959.

95. Puschel, J.: Der Wassergehalt Normaler and Degenerierter Zwischenwirbelscheiber, Beitr. path. Anat. *84*:123, 1930.

96. Ray, R. D.: Personal communication.

97. Riordan, D. C.: Congenital absence of the radius, J. Bone & Joint Surg. *37-A*:1129-1140, 1959.

98. Risser, J. C., and Norquist, D. M.: A follow-up study of the treatment of scoliosis, J. Bone & Joint Surg. *40-A*:555-569, 1958.

99. Robertson, D. E.: Acute hematogenous osteomyelitis, J. Bone & Joint Surg. *20*: 35-47, 1938.

100. Robinson, R. A.: An electron microscopic study of the crystalline inorganic component of bone and its relationship to the organic matrix, J. Bone & Joint Surg. *34*: 389-434, 1952.

101. Robison, R.: The possible significance of hexosephosphoric esters in ossification, J. Biol. Chem. *17*:286-293, 1923.

102. Rodet, A. J.: Physiologie pathologique; étude expérimentale sur l'ostéomyelite infectieuse, Compt. rend. Acad. sc. *89*:569, 1884.

103. Roofe, P. G.: Innervation of the annulus fibrosus and the posterior longitudinal ligament, Arch. Neurol. & Psychiat. *44*:100-103, 1940.

104. Roseberry, H. H., Hastings, A. B., and Morse, J. K.: X-ray analysis of bone and teeth, J. Biol. Chem. *90*:395-407, 1931.

105. Rubin, P. S., and Howard, J. E.: Histochemical studies on the role of acid mucopolysaccharides in calcifiability and calcification *in* Tr. Second Conf. on Metabolic Interrelations, New York, Macy, 1950.

106. Schmidt, A. C.: Fundamental principles and treatment of scoliosis, Am. Acad. Orthop. Surgeons, Lect. *16*:184-212, 1959.

107. Schottstaedt, E. R., Larson, L. J., and Bost, F. C.: Complete muscle transposition, J. Bone & Joint Surg. *37*:897-919, 1955.

108. Sever, J. W.: The results of a new operation for obstetrical paralysis, Am. J. Orthop. Surg. *16*:248, 1918.

109. Sherman, M., and Schneider, G. T.: Vertebral osteomyelitis complicating postabortal and postpartum infection, South. M.J. *48*: 333-338, 1955.

110. Smith-Petersen, M. N., Larsen, C. R., and Aufranc, O. E.: Osteotomy of the spine for correction of flexion deformity in rheumatoid arthritis, J. Bone & Joint Surg. *27*:1-11, 1945.

111. Snapper, I.: Medical Clinics on Bone Diseases, ed. 2, New York, Interscience, 1949.

112. Somerville, E. W.: Development of congenital dislocation of the hip, J. Bone & Joint Surg. *35-B*:568-577, 1953.

113. Speed, J. S., and Knight, R. A. (eds.): Campbell's Operative Orthopedics, ed. 3, vols. 1 and 2, St. Louis, Mosby, 1956.

114. Starr, C. L.: Acute hematogenous osteomyelitis, Arch. Surg. *4*:567, 1922.

115. Stein, A. H., Morgan, H. C., and Porras, R.: The effect of an arteriovenous fistula on intramedullary bone pressure, Surg. Gynec. & Obst. *109*:287-290, 1959.

116. Steindler, A.: Transference of flexor muscles of forearm at elbow *in* Campbell's Operative Orthopedics, vol. 2, p. 1420, St. Louis, Mosby, 1949.

117. Stevenson, H. F.: The chemotherapy of orthopedic tuberculosis, J. Bone & Joint Surg. *36-B*:5, 1954.

118. Stokes, J. H.: Clinical Syphilology, Philadelphia, Saunders, 1934.

119. Thompson, C. F.: Fusion of the metacarpals of the thumb and index fingers to maintain functional position of the thumb, J. Bone & Joint Surg. *24*:907, 1942.

120. Urist, M. R., and McLean, F. C.: Estrogenic potency and osteogenic inductor substances of periosteum, bone marrow, bone grafts, fracture, callus and hyaline cartilage transferred to the anterior chamber of the eye *in* Tr. Third Conf. on Metabolic Interrelations, New York, Macy, 1951.

121. Virchow, R. L.: Über die Entwicklung des Schadelgrundes (cited by Waris, Berlin, 1857).

122. Wagner, L. C., and Hanby, J. E.: Brodie's abscess, pain distribution: occurrence and diagnosis, Am. J. Surg. *39*:135, 1938.

123. Waldenstrom, H.: The first stages of coxa plana, J. Bone & Joint Surg. *20*:559-656, 1936.

124. Wilson, J. C.: The delayed operative treatment of acute hematogenous osteomyelitis, Surgery *9*:666, 1941.

125. Wilson, P.: As recorded by Robertson, J. Bone & Joint Surg. *20*:35, 1938.

126. Levine, J., Gitman, L., and Balker, H.: Histological study of treated and untreated cases of osteoporosis in humans. Proceedings of Orthopedic Research Society. J. Bone & Joint Surg. *37*:624, 1955.

127. Grice, D. S.: An extra-articular arthrodesis of the subastragalar joint for the correction of paralytic flat feet in children, J. Bone & Joint Surg. *34-A*:927-940, 1952.

─────────── C H A P T E R   5 0 ───────────

Surgery of the Nervous System

Diseases Affecting the Central Nervous System
  Lesions with Surgical Implications, Intra-cranial
  Lesions with Surgical Implications, Intra-spinal
Diseases Affecting Peripheral Nervous System
Neurosurgical Operations on Normal Tissues to Relieve Disease Elsewhere
Diseases Affecting Autonomic Nervous System
Conclusion

DISEASES AFFECTING THE CENTRAL NERVOUS SYSTEM

Although the feasibility and the fruitfulness of operations on the central nervous system have been established for over 40 years, the crucial importance and the delicacy of many of the structures still limit sharply the scope of surgery here. Early recognition of disease advancing in brain or cord is especially important because of the absence of regeneration either in nerve cells or fiber tracts, as well as the vulnerability of the tissue. Hence, we shall devote our attention mainly to the symptoms, signs and simple diagnostic tests of the disorders usefully managed neurosurgically, so that the general physician or surgeon may spot them more promptly. Horsley, Krause, Cushing and Dandy, the principal pioneers, did most of their work on tumors and on relief of pain, fields which continue to present challenging problems. We begin by considering the localized intracranial lesions which the surgeon may attack profitably.

LESIONS WITH SURGICAL IMPLICATIONS, INTRACRANIAL

Symptoms and Signs

Neoplasms, infections, hematomas, trauma, aneurysms, arteriovenous malformations, congenital malformations, scars and adhesions, pseudotumor cerebri and, much more rarely, parasitic and other cysts, as well as tuberculous, syphilitic or other granulomata, comprise the lesions to be discussed. They become manifest either by (1) *generalized effects* of (A) increase in intracranial pressure, or (B) changes produced in the cerebrospinal fluid (CSF), or by (2) the *local effects* of (A) excess or (B) diminution of function.

Increased Intracranial Pressure. CHRONIC INCREASE. Chronic increase in intracranial pressure, either constant or intermittent, ensues when the lesion progresses slowly. The deleterious associated effects commonly attributed thereto may be headache, vomiting, papilledema, diplopia and enlargement of the head.

1. *Headache.* In the early stages, pain may not be severe, and its relief by aspirin or cold packs to the head may give patients and physician a false impression that the cause is inconsequential. Often the pain appears the first thing in the morning, immediately upon awakening—an unusual time for headache of less ominous etiology (if one excludes that from alcoholic imbibing the night before). Coughing, sneezing or straining raise intracranial pressure and often worsen the headache due thereto. Reference to only a portion of the head does not necessarily indicate that a mass lies just beneath, but if the pain is occipital, and especially if it is accompanied by nuchal rigidity, this is a warning that the primary lesion may be in the posterior cranial fossa or, more urgently, that the cerebellar tonsils are being crowded down into the foramen magnum against the lower medulla oblongata. Bursts of cephalic pain of agonizing intensity also warn the physician that an emergency is at hand. When there is no papilledema, the headache due to a brain tumor is referred over or near the tumor in about two thirds of these

patients. Such pain probably is due to localized rather than generalized pressure.

2. *Vomiting* is usually not so violent as to fit the term "projectile" but it may be. Virtual absence of nausea preceding the vomiting may occur, and this precipitate urge provides a clue that the cause is intracranial. In children the focal insignia of intracranial masses tend to be less conspicuous, so that headache and vomiting assume special importance, and, unless they are acted on promptly, the child may be left blind despite otherwise successful treatment. Consequently, in this age group, continuing and otherwise unexplained vomiting should lead to early investigation of a primary intracranial cause.

3. *Papilledema*—elevation of the optic disks or blurring of the disk margins, often accompanied by hemorrhages and/or exudates —is the sign of a visual impairment that can lead to blindness. The hemorrhages usually occur in or near the disks; they lie along the radially disposed fibers in the nerve fiber layer of the retina and hence tend to be thin and splinter- or flame-shaped. Even though useful vision may still be present when the mass is removed, further damage and loss of more sight may follow subsidence of a severe papilledema. The associated visual field is constricted concentrically, and the blind spot is enlarged, but central visual acuity—the function of the macula—may be preserved. In the presence of gross papilledema, the whole visual field may suddenly become dim or even black entirely for seconds to minutes with spontaneous recovery. This is another important symptom of emergency, i.e., that mechanisms compensating for the increased pressure in the head are about to fail; one must be careful not to pass it off as a hysterical symptom.

4. *Diplopia*. The 2 images are side by side and parallel, and the image seen by the abducting eye is the more lateral when an abducens paresis is present. Such weakness of the 6th cranial nerve on one or both sides may be caused by generalized increased intracranial pressure without focal lesion. This is the least frequent of the 5 manifestations of such pressure. Cushing showed this to be due to notching of the nerve from behind by any transversely directed branch of the basilar artery which shifts forward. In most instances

the diagnosis should have been made before papilledema or abducens palsy appear.

5. *Enlargement of Head.* Before the cranial sutures close at roughly 15 years of age, an expanding intracranial mass will spring the sutures apart and a "cracked-pot" note (Macewen's sign) may be heard on percussion. In infancy and early childhood, this may provoke an abnormally rapid increase in the circumference of the head with bulging fontanelles. For the range of normal sizes at various ages, see Ingraham and Matson's monograph.

ACUTE INCREASE. An acute increase in intracranial pressure, when accompanied by acute deterioration of cerebral function, evokes different responses:

1. *Headache.* This may be of extreme intensity for a few moments before the patient becomes unresponsive, as when an aneurysm at the base of the brain bursts wide open. Possibly such pain is caused partly by local stimulus to the breaking artery. Usually, however, the most important change with a less acute increase in intracranial pressure is:

2. *Increasing lethargy progressing to coma,* often without subjective complaint. This crucial sign should not be obscured by injudicious sedation in a patient initially restless.

3. Classically, the *4 vital signs alter:* (1) the systolic arterial pressure mounts while the diastolic pressure falls or stays the same; (2) the pulse becomes slower, and because of a rise in pulse pressure, fuller as well; (3) the breathing is slower, at times deeper, or irregular or of Cheyne-Stokes type; (4) the body temperature rises. However, even when increased intracranial pressure has nearly killed the patient, some or all of the vital signs may remain normal.

DECREASE IN RESPONSIVENESS OF THE PATIENT is the principal criterion of worsening in the presence of hemorrhage within the brain or into the subdural or extradural spaces, or in the later evolution of a more slowly expanding mass. An enlarging supratentorial mass soon or late pushes the ipsilateral temporal lobe's uncus and hippocampal gyrus downward and medially through the tentorial notch against the midbrain. This produces the so-called *tentorial pressure cone* (Fig. 50-1). The 3rd (oculomotor) cranial nerve is depressed, and its fibers to the constrictor pupillae muscle are usually the most affected by the external pressure. The unopposed sympathetic dilator fibers produce a widely dilated pupil ipsilaterally, which becomes fixed to light. The temporal lobe may even push the midbrain against the medial free edge of the tentorium *on the other side,* so as to indent that cerebral peduncle and thereby cause a hemiplegia on the same side as the expanding lesion. A hemiplegia of intracranial etiology usually is caused by a primary lesion on the side of the brain opposite the weakness, since the pyramidal tracts decussate in the lowermost medulla oblongata. Hence, the weakness ipsilateral to the primary lesion brought on by the tentorial pressure cone may be confusing. The intracranial mass is likely to be on the side of the dilated fixed pupil. The lateralizing value of this sign may not persist, however, because in this parlous state the opposite 3rd nerve may also shortly become compressed and the other pupil dilate. A patient whose condition is deteriorating rapidly may pass briskly through the state of anisocoria, and the one-sided dilated pupil escape careless observation. Deepening stupor and a dilating

pupil reacting sluggishly to light are then the heralds of a tentorial pressure cone; this critical state leads promptly to death unless effective surgical treatment is carried out at once.

That fibrous barrier, the tentorium cerebelli, may also cause the superior portion of the cerebellum to squeeze the midbrain in a lethal embrace if an expanding lesion in the posterior fossa pushes cerebellum upwards, a "reversed tentorial pressure cone." Finally, intracranial masses may kill by forcing the cerebellar tonsils against the medulla, in which situation the respiration at first may be more compromised than the circulation, by the *cerebellar tonsillar pressure cone* (Fig. 50-1).

In general, space-taking masses give rise to increased intracranial pressure not only by virtue of their own volume but also because they tend to impede circulation and absorption of CSF. There appears in man to be a net formation of around 100 to 150 ml. of this fluid per day in the ventricles over and above the amount reabsorbed back into the blood through the ventricular walls. As shown by Dandy, the excess fluid must be able to

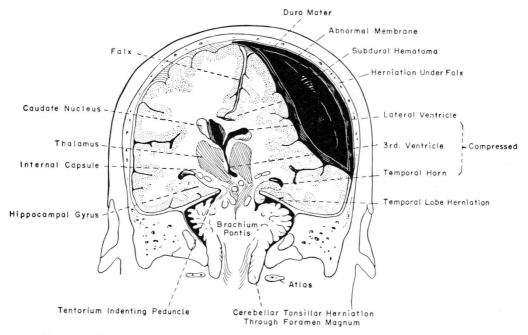

FIG. 50-1. Temporal and cerebellar tonsillar herniations—notching of cerebral peduncle. The medial herniation of the hippocampal gyrus and the downward movement of the cerebellar tonsils are also referred to respectively as tentorial and cerebellar tonsillar pressure cones.

flow from one ventricle to another, out of the lower end of the 4th ventricle, and in the subarachnoid space back up through the tentorial notch to reach the surface of the cerebral hemispheres, the locus of most of the absorbing arachnoidal villi. A mass while still small, if strategically placed near ventricular foramina, or in general in the posterior cranial fossa, may slow the flow of CSF and give ominous symptoms and signs of increased intracranial pressure. A complete obstruction can produce an acute dangerous increase in this pressure within hours. A tap into a lateral ventricle proximal to the block temporarily relieves the emergency. Slow-growing or static lesions obstructing flow of CSF may be treated merely by restoring the balance of CSF formation and absorption.

Symptoms and Signs Due to Abnormal Cerebrospinal Fluid (CSF). Bleeding into the

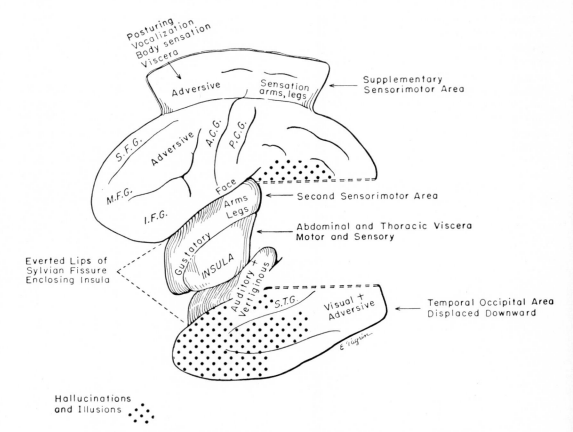

FIG. 50-2. Sites of origin of motor, sensory and psychical seizures. In this diagram, the inferior part of the brain has been displaced downward; the superior and the inferior lips of the sylvian fissure are represented as though everted with the insula between them; the central part of the medial surface of the hemisphere is drawn as though reflected upward. The main or primary sensorimotor cortex lies on either side of the rolandic fissure on the lateral surface of the hemisphere and extends slightly onto the medial surface. The second sensorimotor area, continuous with the primary area, begins on the lateral surface just above the sylvian fissure and extends onto the hidden superior lip of this fissure. A third or supplementary sensorimotor area lies on the medial surface of the hemisphere surrounding the medial end of the primary area.

S.F.G.—Superior frontal gyrus	A.C.G.—Anterior central gyrus
M.F.G.—Middle frontal gyrus	P.C.G.—Posterior central gyrus
I.F.G.—Inferior frontal gyrus	S.T.G.—Superior temporal gyrus

CSF in any quantity increases the pressure in the fluid, but even if the pressure is normal, the red cells are likely to cause nuchal pain, nuchal rigidity or even opisthotonus, along with a positive Kernig sign—meningismus, in short. A major increase in the number of white cells, which occurs in meningitis or when an abscess ruptures into the CSF, causes similar signs; an increased white cell count in the CSF may also follow as a reaction to subarachnoid hemorrhage.

Localizing Symptoms and Signs of Hyperactivity of the Brain. These arise from irritation of a particular part of the brain and cause any of the protean manifestations of a focal or generalized seizure. Following the lead of Penfield and associates, who have made the most important contributions to our knowledge in this field, we classify focal cerebral seizures as motor, sensory, autonomic and psychical. Figures 50-2 and 50-3 indicate the

portions of the brain, stimulation of which gives rise to these specific types of seizure. Reference to these figures will aid understanding of the following description.

MOTOR SEIZURES. To the casual observer, the manifestations most obviously cerebral in origin are those in which a clonic jerky or a tonic maintained contraction of muscles begins at some one part, usually in face, hand or foot because of the relatively large portion of the motor cortex representing these areas. From the starting point, there may be a progression, or, as Hughlings Jackson put it, a march, to other parts of the body on the same side, which occurs in the sequence dictated by localization of function indicated in Figure 50-3.

Vocalization, commonly a long-drawn-out cry, may start a seizure which then usually becomes rapidly generalized. The "cry" may occur upon stimulus within the face area or in the supplementary motor area.

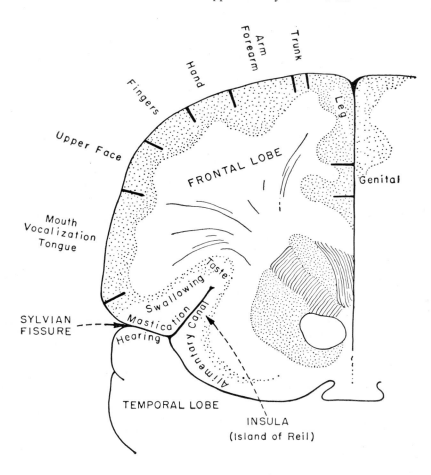

FIG. 50-3. Diagrammatic coronal section of brain through precentral gyrus. Localization of function in cerebrum.

An adversive seizure, consisting of *conjugate turning of the eyes* and often of the head, usually to the side opposite the lesion, occurs on irritation of the precentral gyrus, the posterior part of the middle frontal gyrus, the supplementary sensorimotor cortex or the occipital lobe. It is a symptom of a focal lesion which is of great importance because it usually results from discharge starting in the cortex of the prerolandic frontal or the occipital lobes —regions which are surgically resectable with minimal deficit. If the origin is anterior frontal, the patient loses consciousness before turning; if midfrontal, he may remember the turning. In the former case, only another alert observer will be able to give the crucial history of lateralizing behavior.

Mastication and *swallowing* are provoked by discharge deep in the sylvian fissure over the insula.

Aphasic arrest, i.e., an attack of inability to speak or to understand the speech of others, occurs when one of the speech areas of the dominant hemisphere is discharging.

Rhythmic movements or *adoption of a posture* involving limbs of both sides and the body as well may occur when the supplementary sensorimotor area becomes activated. For example, in one patient the first such seizure began with slow elevation and dropping of the right arm as though she were wielding an old farm pump handle. When a friend held this arm, the other arm began such movements. These were interpreted erroneously as hysterical; actually, the irritant was a small tumor.

Discharges in the midbrain produce *"decerebrate seizures"* in which all 4 limbs move into rigid extension with hyperpronation of forearms and plantar flexion of the feet. Opisthotonos—backward arching or stiffness of neck and back—may be associated. These are threatening signs of severe mesencephalic malfunction.

SENSORY SEIZURES. When a primary sensorimotor gyrus on either side of the rolandic fissure is discharging, the first experience of the patient may be of somatic sensory type, beginning in one restricted area of the opposite side of the face, torso or limbs. Tingling, numbness, a peculiar "absence of all sensation," a sense of movement of a part when none is actually occurring, or, rarely, pain,

heat or cold, are the feelings that may be evoked. Activity of the second sensorimotor area in the lowermost central gyri and adjoining upper lip of the sylvian fissure or in the supplementary sensorimotor area on the medial surface of the hemisphere (Fig. 50-2) brings on more diffuse sensations in the *opposite or in both sides* of the patient. Discharge in the second sensorimotor area often evokes sensations in the terminal portions of one or more limbs.

SEIZURES INVOLVING SPECIAL SENSES. *Visual seizures,* of positive type with the seeing of lights or of inhibitory nature with darkness or blindness, occur not only from discharges in the calcarine cortex of the occipital lobe but also in the neighboring Brodmann's areas 18 and 19 which occupy the rest of this lobe. This light or the darkness appears usually to be straight ahead but may be in the contralateral or even in the ipsilateral visual field. Likewise, in *auditory seizures* there may be a positive ringing or buzzing, or an inhibitory partial deafness. The sound usually is referred to the opposite ear but may be referred to both ears. The affected area lies in the lower lip of the sylvian fissure and the nearby superior temporal gyrus. Activity of virtually the same area may also bring on a *vertiginous seizure,* a feeling of rotation, bodily displacement or dizziness. *Olfactory seizures* occur upon stimulation of the uncus, and *gustatory attacks* probably are referable to the depths of the sylvian fissure above the insula.

Both motor and sensory seizures may be followed for hours or even a few days by impairment of function of the discharging area of cortex. The commonest form is the postictal weakness of a convulsing part, a so-called Todd's paralysis.

VISCERAL AND AUTONOMIC SEIZURES. Abdominal or thoracic sensations referred within the torso occur often as the aura of a focal seizure; a sensation in the epigastrium rising toward the head is one of the commonest of these. They suggest a discharge deep within the sylvian fissure or in the frontal lobe. Autonomic manifestations may include any or many of the following: localized or generalized flushing or sweating, lacrimation, salivation, pilo-erection, yawning, vomiting, borborygmus, abdominal cramp, defecation, urination, priapism, change in pupillary size, shivering, hiccuping, and a rise, a fall or an irregularity in rate or level of the vital signs—pulse, respiration, blood pressure or temperature. If many such features are present, the lesion probably involves thalamus or hypothalamus. Because of widespread cerebral representation of many of these functions, a few such symptoms may occur in attacks along with the cerebral somatic motor or the sensory phenomena already described.

PSYCHICAL SEIZURES AND AUTOMATISMS. Discharges in temporal lobe and inferior parietal lobule may cause attacks of altered mental or emotional attitude, classifiable as illusions, emotions or hallucinations. Thus the patient may have illusions in which objects look abnormal, e.g., too small or too large, or in which sounds seem too loud, or in which objects are abnormally placed in space. Or suddenly the environment may seem falsely familiar as though he were reliving a previous experience (the *déjà vu* phenomenon), or contrariwise it may seem absurd, strange or remote. The illusion also may have an emotional component of fear, sadness or loneliness. More complex experiences, hallucinations independent of the environment, occur and resemble dreams in which the patient e.g., sees scenes or hears conversations or songs. In all of these psychical seizures, he is able to relate the experience later.

Distinct from these are the episodes of automatism in which the patient carries out actions of greater or lesser complexity and cannot recall them later. If the movements are irrelevant or stereotyped or the patient seems confused, his associates may recognize an abnormality, but at times the patient may move for minutes or even hours in an apparently purposive fashion so that those about him are unaware of any "attack." Although automatic movements for which there is a later amnesia may occur in a variety of circumstances, lesions in the inferomedial temporal lobe are an important cause.

Paroxysmal irritative manifestations, i.e., seizures, do not occur from neuronal discharge in the cerebellum. The term "cerebellar fits" has been applied sometimes to midbrain seizures because a cerebellar mass may evoke them by irritation of the midbrain.

Any of the foregoing manifestations of localized activity of the brain may pass off within minutes, may persist for hours as an *epilepsia partialis continua,* or may extend to neighboring ipsilateral, deep, or contralateral parts. They may end as a generalized tonic-clonic seizure with any of the diffuse manifestations thereof, such as unconsciousness, tongue biting, salivation, urinary or fecal incontinence and stertorous breathing with cyanosis. Should the point of irritation lie in a "silent" area of the brain whose activity evokes no apparent change in behavior, the cerebral excitation spreading from this region may reach the whole sensorimotor areas of both hemispheres or deeper motor structures at about the same time, producing a seizure generalized at onset and indistinguishable clinically from those often seen with epilepsy of unknown cause. *It is especially important that such patients with generalized seizures be studied carefully,* because even gliomatous tumor in a silent area may be removable in toto along with a safe margin of normal brain and yet leave a functionally normal individual. Unfortunately, such patients are often treated with anticonvulsant drugs without full and repeated special diagnostic studies. The initial seizure caused by a space-taking mass may not be followed by another for weeks or even years.

ENDOCRINE HYPERFUNCTION. The overactivity of endocrine glands may arise by overstimulation from the controlling neural centers or from pituitary neoplasms producing an excess of hormone. In the former category are the rare lesions, including neoplasm, in the region of the 3rd ventricle which produce sexual precocity in male children. In the latter are the eosinophilic tumors of the anterior pituitary gland producing an excess of growth hormone, leading to gigantism in the young and to acromegaly in the adult. More rarely, functioning chromophobe adenomas provoke galactorrhea, and, after adrenalectomy for Cushing's disease, chromophobe adenomas which produce ACTH may develop.

Localizing Symptoms and Signs of Intracranial Hypoactivity. Proceeding as we did with the irritative features, we may consider the motor, sensory, autonomic, psychical and endocrine phenomena encountered.

MOTOR. In the initial phases of a juxta-rolandic cerebral mass, and in cerebellar tumors also, clumsiness, slight weakness, terminal tremor on precise movement, and slowing of rapid alternating movement occur— contralateral to a cerebral mass, ipsilaterally in the case of the cerebellum. As a cerebral lesion progresses, the weakness dominates the disability, and abnormal resistance to passive movement appears. The increased tonus is often of lead pipe or cogwheel type in deep lesions involving the basal ganglia or the diencephalon. It is usually of a spastic or clasp-knife type in more superficial lesions of the hemisphere. Often the tendon jerks are increased in the contralateral limbs, along with forced grasping, and such superficial reflex changes as the positive Hoffmann, Babinski, and Rossolimo signs, with absence of abdominal and cremasteric reflexes on the affected side. Any facial weakness affects the contralateral *lower* facial muscles much more than those in the forehead and usually is incomplete because of bilateral representation in each hemisphere. This *upper motor neuronal paresis* is thus distinguished from the *lower motor neuronal involvement* of the facial nucleus in the brain stem or the emergent facial nerve. Here the weakness affects about equally and usually severely all the facial muscles on the ipsilateral side.

When a cerebellar hemisphere is involved, there may be past pointing and deviation of gait toward the side of the lesion, with hypotonia, the rebound phenomenon, overshooting on precise motion, slight weakness and pendular tendon jerks in the ipsilateral limbs. The arm is usually worse than the leg. Horizontal nystagmus on lateral gaze to either side occurs; the quick component of the eye movement is in the direction of gaze with a slower return toward the central point; the movements are slower and coarser when the patient looks toward the side of the lesion. When the cerebellar vermis only is injured, a symmetrical unsteadiness of gait is likely without nystagmus or specific motor signs on testing an individual limb. As the lesion advances in the cerebellum, compensatory assumption of its function by other areas occurs; hence, the signs of a huge slow-growing mass in the cerebellum may be slight, and removal of cortex and subcortical white matter of an entire cerebellar hemisphere happily leaves a minimal permanent deficit. The in-co-ordination, lateral deviation and hypotonia become severe

only when the lesion invades or compresses a cerebellar peduncle or the brain stem.

SOMATIC SENSORY. Involvement of the cerebral pathways leading to the somatic sensory areas in one parietal lobe produces a contralateral defect in discriminative capacities. Tests likely to show impairment are those for stereognosis, for determining the distance of separation of two points on the skin requisite for perception as a dual stimulus, for recognition of numbers written on the skin, for localizing the spot touched, for distinguishing textures of cloth or weights, and for proprioception. Any major decrease in acuity of appreciation of the basic modalities of touch, pain, heat or cold points to a lesion encroaching on thalamus, posterior limb of internal capsule or some lower level.

SPECIAL SENSES. Hyposmia or anosmia is a symptom which the patient usually ignores; when the examiner finds it and can exclude disease in the upper air passages as the cause, it points to affection of the olfactory bulb or tract, an inferomedial frontal lesion. Impairment in the sense of taste is rarely observed clinically and only when the primary afferent pathway in the entering 7th nerve or brain stem is involved. The same applies to the sense of hearing and the 8th nerve; auditory pathways in the brain are so diffuse that lesions therein are rarely extensive enough to cause deafness, although this does occur if both inferior colliculi of the midbrain are afflicted. Tumor in the cerebellopontine angle, the commonest type being the 8th nerve's acoustic neuroma, produces ipsilateral deafness usually preceded by tinnitus. This involvement of the cochlear division of the nerve often appears years before any other sign. The clinical insignia of malfunction of the vestibular component of the 8th nerve consist of whirling vertigo or of less definite giddiness. A tendency to fall on abrupt turning of the head without subjective warning of unsteadiness also occurs. Audiometric measurements quantitate the hearing loss at each frequency tested; caloric testing yields a semiquantitative measure of equilibratory dysfunction. The audiometric test for loudness recruitment is of special value to distinguish between pressure on the cochlear nerve by a tumor (no recruitment) and disorder of the organ of Corti as in Ménière's syndrome in which recruitment is present. With the aid of this test, a mass in the cerebellopontine angle may be diagnosed and removed while only 8th nerve signs are present and before it becomes embedded in the site of the brain stem or produces an elevation of intracranial pressure.

Painstaking examination of the visual functions is one of the most important means for detecting and localizing intracranial lesions at an early, or indeed, any stage. The intracranial visual pathways extend anteriorly from the optic foramina back to the cells of the lateral geniculate bodies; fibers from these nuclei pass into the optic radiations, expanding widely in the temporal and inferior parietal region to reach cortical visual areas as far back as the tip of the occipital lobe. So, many intracranial masses may encroach on this sensitive apparatus at some point. Focal pressure directly on the optic nerve causes primary atrophy of the disk on that side. Painstaking charting of the visual fields permits quantitative assessments, and serial studies may enable one to establish the slight worsening of a lesion so suggestive of tumor. Superior or inferior altitudinal defects point respectively to pressure from below or from above against the optic nerve. Bitemporal defects indicate a chiasmal lesion; homonymous defects go with unilateral encroachment on optic tract, optic radiations or calcarine cortex. An upper quadrantic homonymous defect usually implicates the inferior or temporal portion of the optic radiations, whereas the superior or parietal radiations are correlated with the lower quadrants of the fields. Hughes' *The Visual Fields* documents beautifully the great scope of the deductions feasible from such studies.

AUTONOMIC AND METABOLIC EFFECTS. Recognizable autonomic effects are confined largely to the irritative sphere, already discussed, or to lesions in the descending pathway in the medulla. A striking example of this is the vasodilatation, Horner's sign and reduction in sweating often seen on the side of a thrombosis of the posterior-inferior cerebellar artery. Medial lesions in the posterior part of either frontal lobe may bring on involuntary micturition, perhaps by impairing inhibitory mechanisms. One metabolic effect of a disturbance in the hypothalamus is obesity. Other metabolic features of involvement of the hypothalamic-pituitary mechanism are considered below. Associated with many of the autonomic centers in the hypothalamus are those concerned with arousal. Depression of these causes drowsiness, stupor or excessive requirement of sleep.

PSYCHICAL CHANGES. Subtle changes in personality may be the first clue to disease in the so-called "silent areas" of the cerebrum. Thus a patient of Cushing with a bilateral inferior frontal meningioma made such an obviously unsuitable marriage that her friends were dumbfounded. After Cushing had removed her tumor, her mental recovery was accompanied by mystification equalling that of her friends at her choice of a husband, and she terminated the marriage. Decreases in energy and ambition, impaired memory, inattention to the courtesies of conversational intercourse, carelessness in personal habits, poor business judgment, or deviations in sexual mores may be the first symptoms of a brain tumor but are rarely recognized as such. An astute examiner usually must acquire data from an observant close associate of the patient before such symptoms lead to intensive diagnostic study.

With more serious involvement, defects in memory, especially for recent events, disorientation, indifference, apathy and drowsiness become obvious. There may be a stage of euphoria with a tendency to make silly jokes. Lesions in the frontal lobes or the corpus callosum or those causing high intracranial pressure are among the commonest to produce this picture.

Disturbances in the sphere of understanding and expressing language, called *aphasias*, have specific localizing value—in a right-handed person to some portion of the left cerebral hemisphere. In a left-handed person the language dominance of one hemisphere is not likely to be so pronounced. The related *apraxia* is an inability to carry out acts with a specific purpose, despite adequate strength and co-ordination in the necessary part, and *agnosia* refers to the inability to appreciate the significance of stimuli that are perceived. An aphasia may be largely *expressive* or *motor* in type in that the patient may know what he wishes to say, to repeat, or to read aloud but is unable to do so. This oral expressive aphasia is likely to be associated with a lesion in the posterior part of the inferior frontal gyrus of the dominant hemisphere. A lesion just above this in the posterior part of the middle frontal gyrus may produce inability to write or print words despite adequate strength in the hand and the fingers, an *agraphia.*

The lesions causing the *receptive* or *sensory* aphasias lie in general posteriorly in the dominant hemisphere. There may be loss of ability to read (a visual agnosia for words, word-blindness or *alexia*) seen especially in lesions of the dominant angular gyrus, which surrounds the upturned posterior end of the superior temporal sulcus (Fig. 50-2). If the lesion involves much of the occipital lobe behind this but spares the striate or calcarine cortex, the visual agnosia may be more severe, with inability to identify many sorts of objects which, however, the patient sees clearly enough. Lesions in the posterior half of the dominant superior temporal gyrus cause an auditory receptive aphasia or word deafness. Although the patient can hear, he cannot understand the words and may even be unable to repeat what he hears. Inability of the patient to understand his own spoken words may result in senseless speech or even gibberish—paraphasia or jargon aphasia. A more extensive lesion in this area produces a more severe auditory agnosia with incomprehension of the cause of such simple sounds as the rattling of coins. *Amnesic aphasia, nominal aphasia* and *anomia* are the terms applied to the inability to think of nouns even though the patient understands the concept embodied in a noun or name. Thus, when shown a pencil he may not be able to think of the word "pencil," describes the object as "something you write with" but usually can select the proper word from a series presented for his choice. Lesions in the dominant posterior temporal region and those around the posterior part of the sylvian fissure may produce this picture, or it may occur with diffuse lesions of the subcortical association pathways between the various language areas already described.

In most aphasic patients there is a mixture of a number of the above features, because the lesion involves either a correspondingly extensive area of cortex or the subcortical connecting fibers between them. Especially likely to be implicated are those deep to the insula and the inferior parietal lobule. There may be even a total loss of the appreciation and the expression of language, a global aphasia. Perseveration, i.e., inappropriate repetition of a syllable, a word or a phrase is common in many types of aphasia.

ENDOCRINE HYPOFUNCTION. The thyroid, the adrenal cortex, the gonads and possibly the breasts are all under control of specific trophic hormones secreted by the anterior pituitary gland. In addition, there is the anterior pituitary growth hormone which does not act via another gland. The antidiuretic hormone is secreted by certain hypothalamic nuclei and then passes down within the fibers of the hypophyseal stalk to the posterior lobe of the pituitary gland for storage and appropriate release into the blood stream.

Tumors which encroach on the sellar area before puberty tend to produce dwarfism plus incomplete or absent sexual development and a varying degree of polyuria and polydipsia (diabetes insipidus). Decrease in gonadotrophic hormone is nearly always the first evidence of hypofunction in the adult. Cessation of menses is the common early sign in women, and both men and women may be sterile. Libido as well as other primary and secondary sexual characteristics deteriorate. Next comes decreased production of thyrotrophic and finally of adrenocorticotrophic hormones (TSH and ACTH) to produce symptoms similar to those of myxedema and Addison's disease, respectively. Other manifestations of hypopituitarism are an easy fatigability, progressing to apathy associated with anorexia and weight loss. The skin is pale from loss of its melanin as well as from a mild normocytic anemia which develops. In addition, the skin is likely to be delicate, finely wrinkled and hairless. Vascular hypotension, a fasting hypoglycemia, a flat oral glucose tolerance curve and a lowered basal metabolic rate, a low protein-bound iodine in the blood and decreased radioiodine uptake are all likely to be found in study of more advanced patients with compression of the normal pituitary gland.

Accessory Diagnostic Tests

Lumbar Puncture. With the patient recumbent and fully relaxed, any initial pressure greater than 200 mm. of CSF is abnormally high. If papilledema, lethargy or agonizing headache already point to marked elevation of this pressure, and especially if there is a mass in the temporal lobe or the posterior cranial fossa, the withdrawal of lumbar fluid may provoke a dangerous temporal (tentorial) or cerebellar tonsillar movement against the brain stem. Deaths from this cause remain unfortunately frequent. Hence, in the above circumstances lumbar puncture should be carried out cautiously with a fine-bore needle, if at all, and when gross elevation of pressure is found, usually it is good judgment to remove only the contents of the manometer (enough for a cell count). When an intracranial mass is strongly suspected, but a sample of CSF is needed to aid diagnosis, often it is better judgment to have a neurosurgeon secure this via ventricular tap. An atraumatic lumbar tap which yields more than a few hundred red cells/cu. mm. indicates a spontaneous subarachnoid hemorrhage. The commonest causes, roughly in order of frequency, are a rupture of an aneurysm, an arteriovenous malformation, a vessel in a tumor, or a spread from an intracerebral hematoma into the CSF.

Extra white blood cells, usually lymphocytes, in the lumbar CSF, and especially an elevation of the total protein may occur if a mass lies next to a ventricle or a subarachnoid space. Meningiomas and in particular acoustic neuromas commonly are accompanied by a lumbar CSF total protein greater than 100 mg. %. Polymorphonuclear leukocytes, even a few, suggest the presence of an abscess or a granuloma. Cells that resemble lymphocytes, but are actually tumor cells, may be found when the tumor invades the meninges.

Plain Roentgenograms of the Skull. The following roentgenographic signs of *generalized increased intracranial pressure* occur: (1) in adults, decalcification or thinning of the dorsum sellae; (2) in children, separation of the unclosed cranial sutures or increased prominence of convolutional markings in the inner table of the skull, the "beaten silver" appearance.

These are some of the roentgenologic signs of *focal intracranial disease:* The sella turcica may be symmetrically expanded beyond its maximal normal roentgenographic measurements of 15 mm. length and 8 mm. depth by an intrasellar, i.e., pituitary, tumor. However, a similar picture can also be given by any obstructive lesion which raises intraventricular pressure, dilating the lateral and the third ventricles. Tumors or aneurysms contiguous to the sella can sometimes give the same appearance, but more often they produce an asymmetrical or parasellar erosion at the point of most direct pressure. Any other part of the skull may be eroded by neoplasm, by a benign eosinophilic granuloma or by lipoid storage disease. There is enough calcification in the pineal gland to permit its roentgenographic identification in about 60 per cent of adults, and a lateral shift of greater than 2 mm. from the mid-sagittal plane is seen frequently— away from a space-taking mass, or toward an atrophic cerebral hemisphere. The pineal gland may also be displaced in the lateral projection of the skull. Normally it lies in the zone from 55 to 59 per cent of the anteroposterior distance and from 51 to 57 per cent of the supero-inferior distance, as measured from the farthest point on the inner table in each of the four quadrants to the center of the pineal shadow. Figure 50-4 illustrates the tactic to be used. Abnormal intracranial calcification may occur in the slower growing gliomas, meningiomas, tumors arising from congenital rests, such as craniopharyngiomas, and in the walls of old hematomas and aneurysms. Such deposits may be so delicate that stereoscopic views, an essential in cranial work, are required for their identification. Abnormal thickening of the cranial bone adjoining a meningioma occurs either in the floor or the vault of the skull in the so-called hyperostosing types. A similar roentgenogram is given by the benign slowly growing osteoma composed only of bone cells. Extensive new bone formation, usually around the orbit, is also provoked in fibrous dysplasia, a benign disorder in which the overgrowth may require operative decompression of the optic nerve and of the orbit. Asymmetrically broad and numerous vascular markings in one area of the skull suggest the presence of an underlying vascular meningioma. Special views of the foramina for passage of the cranial nerves out of the skull may reveal enlargement on one side indicative of tumor of that nerve, most frequently of the optic or the acoustic nerves.

Electro-encephalography, the EEG. Fol-

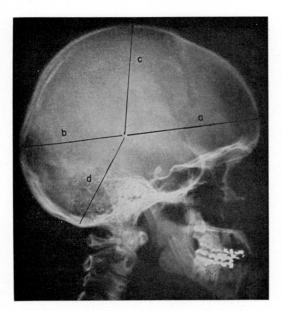

Fig. 50-4. The calcified pineal gland—
normal position. Measurements are made
from the center of the pineal shadow to the
far point of the inner table anteriorly (a);
posteriorly (b); superiorly (c) and inferiorly (d). In this patient a = 11.3 cm.,
b = 8.3 cm. so that $\dfrac{a}{a+b}$ = .58, or 58%
of the anteroposterior distance. c = 8.7 cm.,
d = 7.8 cm., and $\dfrac{c}{c+d}$ = .53, or 53%
of the superoinferior distance. Both param-
eters fall within the range of normal.

lowing Grey Walter's pioneer studies, this
innocuous procedure has been developed into
a great aid in distinguishing focal organic from
other forms of cerebral disease. Painstaking
technics that blanket the scalp with numerous
electrodes and include simultaneous recording
from many channels are likely to disclose
localizable abnormal potentials. These include
single or multiple waves or irregular deflections at 1 to 4 per second, called delta waves,
and waves at 4 to 7 per second, classed as
theta waves. The abnormal waves, present
over large and varied extents of the patient's
brain, may reach a maximum voltage and be
the slowest in the vicinity of the tumor. One
seeks to find the point or points at which
these waves show reversal of phase—since this
provides the most accurate localization of the
origin of the abnormal potential (Fig. 50-5).

A small amount of theta rhythm may be present symmetrically in the normal record; it
becomes pathologic when its amplitude exceeds by > 50 per cent that of the normal
9-11/second alpha rhythm. In general, the
main criterion of focal abnormality is any
asymmetry of electrical activity. An exception is that the voltage and the amount of the
posterior alpha rhythm (8-13/second) may
normally be mildly asymmetrical. Episodic
sharp waves or spikes lasting 1/10 to 1/50 of
a second are also found infrequently in the
neighborhood of most focal lesions, but are
commoner as the electrical insignia of such
lesions when they are epileptogenic. All of
the focal electrographic changes may occur
with localized trauma, atrophy, inflammation
or vascular accident as well as with a space-
taking mass. The method may give only a
rough clue as to the precise location of the
lesion since (1) it is the brain itself and not
the mass that is giving rise to the abnormal
discharges; (2) the most striking abnormal
potentials may arise at some distance from
the main lesion, e.g., in edematous brain or
because of neuronal conduction; (3) the abnormal features may occur at irregular intervals and may be missed in the sample obtained
on the tracing; (4) tactics for judging the
depth of the lesion are inadequate. However,
a roughly correct localization is achieved in
about 75 per cent of supratentorial space-
taking masses; accuracy is less in posterior
fossa neoplasms, dropping to about 40 per cent.

Radioactive Isotopes. There is a formidable
barrier phenomenon between blood and normal brain, by virtue of which many substances
in the blood stream gain delayed or meager
access to the brain. This barrier is much less
effective between blood and the tissue comprising the great majority of tumors, abscesses
and granulomata. Hence, radioactively tagged,
gamma-emitting isotopes, which concentrate
differentially in these lesions as compared with
the normal brain, may be injected intravenously and the zone of increased isotopic
uptake plotted with appropriate apparatus
to detect the gamma ray photons emerging
through the skull. Since gamma rays scatter
markedly as they traverse solid matter, the
image outside the head of an intracranial area
with moderate increase in isotopic uptake
tends to blur into the background and may

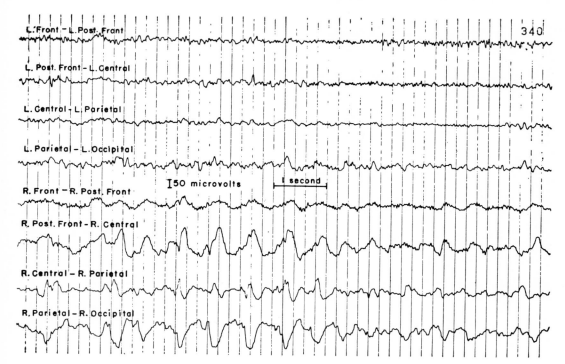

FIG. 50-5. Electro-encephalogram—right parietal hemorrhage. This 10-second sample of a 1-hour tracing shows a burst of high voltage delta waves in the right-sided leads. These deflections are in opposite directions—i.e., show a reversal of phase—between the 2 posterior tracings. The electrode common to these is in the parietal region, which places the origin of the abnormal waves nearest to this electrode. (Interpretation of Dr. John Abbott)

escape detection. Rejection of the scattered gamma rays from the recorded image is achieved in one of two ways. So-called pulse height spectroscopy may be applied to the individual rays. When the original gamma ray photon is scattered, i.e., deflected from its original course by collision with a subnuclear particle, it loses some of its original energy. The electronic detector can be designed to ignore these weaker, "degraded" gamma rays, and this tactic is usefully combined with a focusing collimator consisting of a number of tapered apertures in a metal shield coming to a focus at the detector. Radio-iodinated human serum albumin is the commonest gamma source used with this system.

Rejection of the scattered gamma rays is also possible if one uses positron-emitting isotopes coupled with coincidence counting. A positron, once it is given off, undergoes within a tiny fraction of a second an "annihilation" collision with an electron. The mass of the two particles appears as the energy of a pair of gamma rays which leave the site of the collision back to back, i.e., they move in precisely opposite directions. A pair of detectors —one on either side of the head—is connected to circuits which tally a count only when each member of the pair of annihilation gamma rays reaches its detector. If one or both of these rays scatter, no count ensues. The detectors move continuously, and their coincidence counts are recorded automatically as marks on paper, so that a slow motion televisionlike scan of the head appears. This picture, called a *positrocephalogram* or *PCG* (Fig. 50-6, *top*), shows the precise projection in the lateral view of the area of increased uptake of isotope but does not indicate its side or its depth. The nearer the mass is to one detector, i.e., the farther it is from the mid-line, the higher the total gamma count

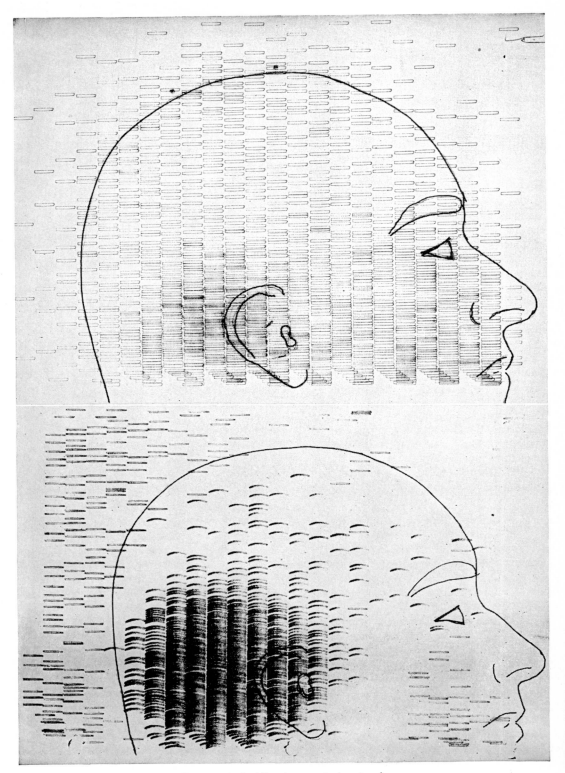

FIGURE 50-6. (*Caption on facing page*)

at the nearer detector, because of the inverse square effect of increasing distance. Therefore, one can usefully obtain simultaneously with the PCG another record of the degree of side-to-side asymmetry of the total gamma counts. This *asymmetrogammagram* or *AGG* (Fig. 50-6, *bottom*), indicates the side and the depth of the lesion.

When one uses the positron emitting isotopes arsenic[72] and arsenic[74], injected as a mixture of arsenate and arsenite, one can see in the radioactive scan an abnormal concentration corresponding well with the locus of the neoplasm or abscess in about 80 per cent of such verified lesions. An abnormal uptake of arsenic occurs in only about 60 per cent of patients with a major cerebral hemorrhage or infarct. When an increased uptake does occur it guides the surgeon's aspirating needle to the right spot and helps him with this supplementary maneuver to distinguish a clot requiring surgical removal from an area of softening. The radioactive scans, like the EEG, are painless, harmless and repeatable at will. They are at their best in spotting neoplasm or abscess in a cerebral hemisphere, the sites of most frequent failure with pneumography or angiography. The scans achieve a high percentage of accuracy in the mengioma—a benign tumor which is often difficult to diagnose at an early stage and is revealed early by the scans. Glioblastoma multiforme and carcinomatous metastases also scan well, but slow-growing gliomas such as the astrocytomas are more likely to be missed.

Pneumography. *Pneumo-encephalography* (roentgenography of the head after injection of air or other gas into the lumbar or cisternal CSF) and *ventriculography* (similar films after the air is introduced directly into one or both lateral ventricles) have played a major role in the final diagnosis and the definitive location of intracranial masses ever since the tactic was introduced by Dandy in 1918. Subsequent refinements from many quarters enable one to spot over 90 per cent of intracranial tumors by this method. In most clinics the air is introduced into the subarachnoid space only when the intracranial pressure is normal. Even then, if the films demonstrate a space-taking mass, operation the same day is advisable because abrupt severe worsening in the patient's condition may occur following the dynamic upset involved in the instillation of air whether it is added to or exchanged for CSF. When the intracranial pressure is elevated, it is advisable to do a ventriculogram and follow it with a craniotomy as soon as the locus of the mass is clear. By displacement of, enlargement of, or filling defects in ventricles, basal cisternae or cerebral sulci, the position of the mass is inferred. In Figure 50-7 one sees how a sheet of adhesions blocking outflow from the 4th ventricle led to enlargement of all 4 ventricles. The photograph permits one to pinpoint precisely the tiny lesion. Figures 50-8 and 50-9 demonstrate the clarity with which tumors may be shown. Infrequently, the ventricular needle encounters a cyst, or the wall thereof may rupture

Fig. 50-6. Radioactive scanning with positron-emitting arsenic. (*Top*) PCG—positrocephalogram. (*Bottom*) ACG—Asymmetrogammagram. *Case Summary:* 39-year-old female. For 4 years before entry, brief attacks of suboccipital pressure sensation, L > R. Three years before entry, an episode of severe headache, vomiting, dizziness and unsteady gait, apathy and disorientation with spontaneous recovery after several weeks in hospital. For 2 years unsteady gait, progressively worse with tendency to deviate to right; for 1 year progressive clumsiness in right hand and deafness in right ear; for 6 months dysphagia; recently blurring of vision on right lateral gaze. Abnormal findings confirmed symptoms plus slightly diminished sensation right cornea, face and soft palate. Loudness recruitment test: no recruitment in the nearly deaf right ear. Lumbar puncture: pressure 210 mm. CSF; total protein 23 mg. %. Roentgenograms of skull normal. Radioarsenic scan: PCG—area of marked increase in isotopic uptake just behind right ear; ACG—extreme right-sided asymmetry in this zone indicated by dense concentration of ⌢ marks; unequivocal diagnosis of tumor. Suboccipital craniectomy with total removal of large meningioma arising from right sigmoid sinus. Discharged 12th postoperative day free of symptoms and signs except for deafness, a lucky result because the severe temporary neurologic illness 3 years before entry with full recovery led to erroneous diagnosis of multiple sclerosis or vascular lesion, and growth of a huge tumor.

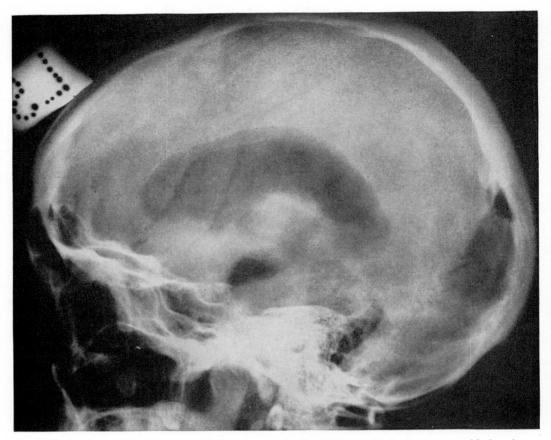

FIG. 50-7 A. Ventriculogram. Enlargement of all ventricles. Patient: 22-year-old female. History: frontal and occipital headache for 5 weeks. Vomiting, 2 weeks. Unsteady gait, nystagmus on lateral gaze, 1 week. Findings: drowsiness; tendency to veer equally to each side in walking, coarse horizontal nystagmus, in-co-ordination on heel-shin and finger-nose tests. No papilledema. Ventriculogram: symmetrical enlargement of all ventricles to over 2 times normal size; extremely marked in 4th ventricle. Absence of air in basal cisternae and sulci points to block at outlets of 4th ventricle. Operation: suboccipital craniectomy; fibrous veil obliterating foramen of Magendie was removed with complete permanent recovery.

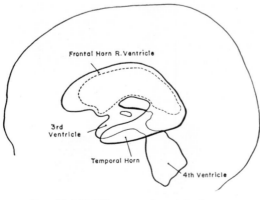

FIG. 50-7 B. Diagram of ventriculogram.

into the CSF pathways, so that the cyst itself fills and is displayed directly.

Angiography, introduced a decade later by Moniz, has steadily gained favor. Injection of the carotid in the neck on each side and of one vertebral artery is usually necessary if nearly all of the vascular supply to the head is to be shown. Puncture of the desired artery through the intact skin is nearly always successful, and open exposure is rarely required. In Figure 50-10 one sees an extraordinarily complete filling following injection of one carotid artery. Rapid serial films following a single injection show arterial, capillary and venous phases of the circulation and reveal not only displacement of the normal vessels but also may demonstrate a total absence of vessels in the zone occupied by an avascular mass (Fig. 50-11).

This technic may also depict the abnormal vessels in a highly vascularized tumor or an arteriovenous malformation, i.e., a positive demonstration of the lesion. Moreover, following the demonstration of a tumor, there is no dynamic change which makes immediate craniotomy mandatory. Precise delineation of the feeding arteries and the draining veins in a

highly vascular lesion may be especially helpful to guide the surgeon's attack. The paucity of clinical localizing features of arteriovenous malformations and aneurysms, the usual absence of displacement of CSF channels or even normal arteries by these lesions, and the normal EEG's and radioactive scans accompanying them, make angiography indispensable in their detailed diagnosis and management (Fig. 50-14).

Continuing improvements in injection media and injection technic have reduced the risk to almost insignificant proportions in competent

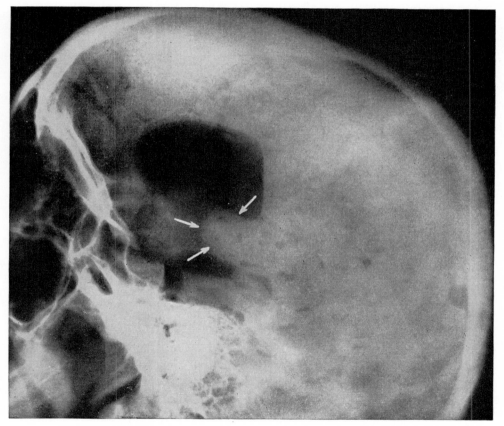

FIG. 50-8. Ventriculogram—colloid cyst, third ventricle. *Case Summary:* 41-year-old-female. Brief attacks of frontal headache and vomiting when she became "carsick." For 6 months infrequent and transient in-co-ordination left limbs; for 3 weeks right fronto-temporal headaches with screaming and vomiting for which she was amnesic—duration only 2 to 3 minutes, suggesting lesion with ball-valve action on flow of CSF. Neurologic examination, roentgenograms of skull, radioarsenic scans—all normal. Ventricular puncture: initial pressure, 180 mm. CSF; total protein, 10 mg.%. Ventriculogram: arrows indicate a cherry-sized filling defect in anterior part of third ventricle with dilated lateral ventricles—a striking picture even though lesion producing it is small. Operation: removal of colloid cyst. Slow but satisfactory recovery.

hands. The diatrizoates of sodium or methyl glucamine are currently the least irritant agents available and also are unlikely to induce arterial constriction so that even intracranial arterial occlusive disease may be studied with relative safety.

Neoplasms

The majority of the primary intracranial tumors arise either from the glial connective tissue or from the meninges, i.e., are either gliomas or meningiomas. We owe our basic knowledge regarding the behavior within these two groups mainly to Bailey and Cushing.

Gliomas. All gliomas infiltrate the brain. Those with the most differentiated type of cell may be composed mainly of slow-growing astrocytes or of oligodendroglia, and patients with astrocytomas or oligodendrogliomas have average survival times of over 5 years. The most favorable of all of the gliomas for a cure is the astrocytoma which occurs typically in childhood in a cerebellar hemisphere and is often predominantly cystic. Extirpation of cyst wall, as well as of the neoplastic mural nodule and a safe margin of cerebellum, is usually possible without permanent neurologic deficit and with a postoperative mortality of around 5 per cent. In general, the presence of a largely cystic content improves the prognosis in such tumors as gliomas, hemangioblastomas or acoustic neuromas. More rapidly growing gliomas are the astroblastoma, the polar spongioblastoma and the ependymoma,

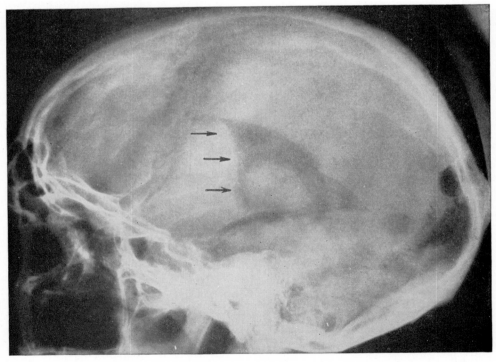

Fig. 50-9. Ventriculogram—right frontal tumor. *Case Summary:* 47-year-old male. Intermittent bilateral frontal headache and poor memory for 1 month—progressively worse. Vomiting for 1 week. Abnormal findings: unable to give consistent history, apathetic, long delays in replies to questions; diminished left abdominal reflexes. Roentgenograms of skull: normal with no pineal shift. Lumbar puncture: initial pressure 160 mm. CSF. Total protein 276 mg.%. EEG: bilateral frontal 1½/second, high voltage waves. Radioarsenic scan: PCG—inferior frontal concentration; AGG—slight right-sided asymmetry. Ventriculogram: irregular cutoff of anterior part of body right lateral ventricle (indicated by arrows). Operation: right frontal lobectomy with only partial removal of glioblastoma invading basal ganglia and other hemisphere via corpus callosum. Death 11th postoperative day.

Fig. 50-10. Normal arteriogram. (A) Injection of a single carotid usually fills carotid branches on one side only. Occlusion in neck of opposite carotid during the injection often permits simultaneous filling of the opposite anterior and middle cerebral arteries. Filling as well of the basilar artery and its posterior cerebral and superior cerebellar branches as occurred here is rare.

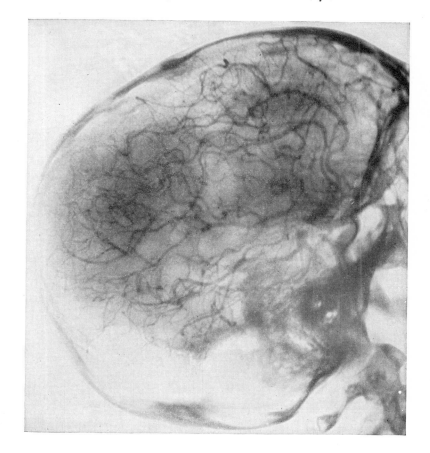

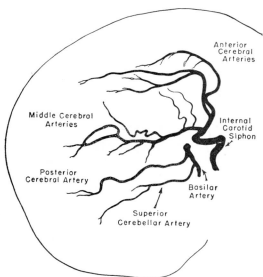

Fig. 50-10 B. Diagram of lateral view.
(*Continued on p. 1484*)

with average survival times of 2 to 3 years. The polar spongioblastoma is one of the commoner tumors of the brain stem. Despite the proximity to aqueduct and 4th ventricle, oddly enough, neoplasms here do not cause increased intracranial pressure until late in their evolution; instead, both lower cranial nerve and long tract signs predominate. Ependymomas arise from the ependyma of any of the ventricles, those in the 4th ventricle occurring much more commonly in children. The highly malignant gliomas, unfortunately the commonest, are the glioblastoma multiforme, seen mainly in the cerebral hemispheres of adults, and the medulloblastomas, which usually arise in the posterior cranial fossa and are about 4 times as common in children as in adults. There are almost no recorded cures of either of these 2 vicious lesions.

Meningiomas. The meningiomas, on the other hand, present an encouraging challenge to the surgeon; these encapsulated tumors are

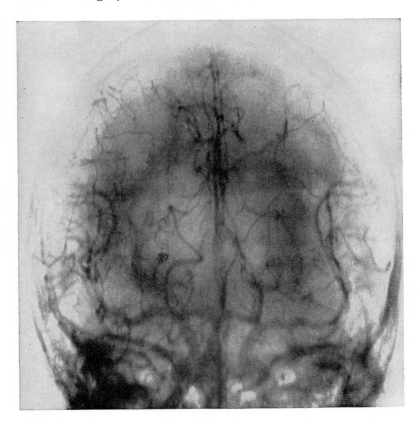

Fig. 50-10 (*Cont.*).
(C) Normal arterio-
gram. Sagittal view.

usually benign, grow slowly and may even attain large size before any symptoms appear. Then intracranial compensatory mechanisms may fail rapidly, leading to the erroneous impression of a rapidly growing tumor. Meningiomas usually lie on the surface of the brain, but so do the arteries nourishing the cerebral cortex; hence, early operation gives the best chance of saving the nutrient vessels of the brain. The vasculartiy of these tumors may be formidable and require the surgeon to employ not only multiple transfusions but also ganglionic blocking agents to lower the blood pressure during the operation. In patients with normal cerebral blood vessels the systolic pressure may be carried safely at 70 to 90 mm. Hg while the tumor is being extirpated in order to reduce the blood loss. Under these circumstances it is especially important that blood replacement keep pace with the actual loss which occurs. The total removal of the dural origin of the tumor required for cure can be achieved in the majority, but even if this is not attainable, subtotal extirpation

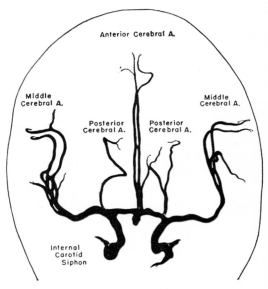

Fig. 50-10 D. Diagram of Sagittal view.

often results in remission of symptoms for many years. Dr. Cushing's practice of having these and other patients report annually follow-

Fig. 50-11. Sagittal and lateral right carotid arteriograms: sphenoidal wing meningioma. *Case Summary*: 37-year-old male. In previous 6 months, a few attacks of right temporal pounding headache, each lasting "a few minutes," relieved promptly by aspirin. Five weeks previously, awoke in middle of night, smelling peculiar odor of "rotten damp dirt" for few seconds only. Two weeks previously, a seizure beginning with illusion that a lamp in front of him was whirling clockwise in horizontal plane; shortly, the same olfactory aura recurred, followed by violent shaking of both upper limbs, whereupon he pitched forward and remembers no more. A generalized seizure ensued. On entry, general physical and neurologic examinations were normal. Lumbar puncture: initial pressure only 75 mm. CSF: total protein, 265 mg.%. EEG: spike focus, right temporal. Arsenic scan: PCG gross increase in isotopic concentration temporal and posterior inferior frontal area, suggesting meningioma; AGG marked right-sided asymmetry in same area. Right carotid arteriogram: extreme upward and medial displacement right middle cerebral artery and slight displacement to left of anterior cerebral artery, indicated by arrows. Operation: total removal of massive meningioma arising from right sphenoidal wing. Discharged 13 days later with no abnormal signs.

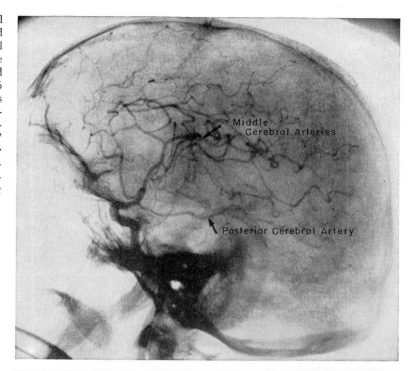

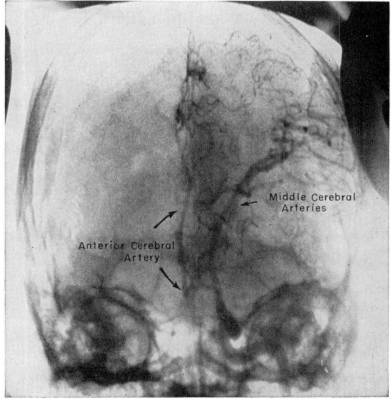

ing tumor operations is an important routine to aid in the early detection of a recurrence.

Metastatic Tumors. Metastatic intracranial tumors are not necessarily hopeless problems. Solitary metastases to cerebellum or a resectable portion of cerebrum occur so often that a previous history of malignant tumor elsewhere should not lead to incomplete study when the next symptoms of a mass lesion point to the brain. Those individuals with carcinomas which are usually slower growing, such as the ones of renal origin, or those amenable to some control by hormones, e.g., the cancers of the breast, may be particularly propitious candidates for surgery. This may consist of removal of the metastases, usually technically easy, or in extensive cranial decompression to control headache. A bronchogenic carcinoma is often clinically silent until its cerebral metastasis speaks. Hence, such a lesion should always be sought in roentgenograms of the chest of any patient at or beyond middle age whose clinical picture intimates a rapidly growing intracranial mass.

Tumors from Congenital Rests. The tumors arising from congenital rests occur mainly in regions where there is complex folding of ectoderm for skin and nerve along with mesodermal elements, principally in the mid-line in the neighborhood of the 3rd and the 4th ventricles. The commonest, the *craniopharyngioma,* arises from squamous epithelial remnants of the craniopharyngeal duct, from which the anterior lobe of the hypophysis forms. It lies above and/or within the sella turcica and usually contains one or more cysts. Its symptoms usually begin in childhood. When it is so adherent to the hypothalamus that its total removal is not feasible, the varieties of surgical treatment then to be tried are representative of the management of irremovable intracranial masses in general. The cyst may be aspirated and the content partially replaced with fluid containing a β-emitting isotope in order to retard growth and reaccumulation of cystic fluid. Larger cysts encroach from below on the floor of one or both lateral ventricles, and opening of the cystic cavity widely into a lateral ventricle may permit continuous drainage of the cystic fluid into the CSF. If the tumor has a large intrasellar extension, transsphenoidal removal of the anterior bony wall and floor of the sella will enable one to drain the cyst via sphenoid sinus into nasopharynx. If the tumor is largely solid and blocks outflow of CSF from the lateral ventricles, the short-circuiting ventriculocisternostomy operation of Torkildsen may help. In this procedure a plastic or rubber catheter is placed to connect one or both lateral ventricles with the subarachnoid space at the cisterna magna, which is just below the cerebellum. Any inoperable obstruction in the 3rd ventricle, the aqueduct or the 4th ventricle is effectively by-passed, and that considerable portion of the symptoms due to accumulation of ventricular CSF is controlled. In order of increasing complexity in their tissue content are *epidermoid, dermoid, teratoid and teratomatous* tumors. The epidermoids are usually filled with a white, scaly, totally avascular debris, which is readily ladled out of otherwise inoperable loci. Remnants of the notochord in sellar and prepontine regions may give rise to a *chordoma.*

Glandular Tumors. Those of the anterior lobe of the hypophysis are usually *chromophobe adenomas,* rarely develop before the 3rd decade, and give signs of endocrine deficiency along with the visual field defects of lesions pressing on optic nerve or chiasm. Rotational x-ray therapy centered on the sella turcica, transsphenoidal decompression of the sella and transfrontal craniotomy with partial removal are the 3 common methods vying with one another at present in the management of these lesions.

The *eosinophile adenomas* producing acromegaly, rarely starting early enough to cause gigantism, are ordinarily held well in check by x-ray treatment but may burgeon upward against the optic nerves and chiasm with sufficient insistence to require operation in order to prevent loss of vision.

Pinealomas, which press downward on the superior colliculi and thereby cause paresis of upward gaze as their most striking localizing sign, are the commonest cause of a ventriculographic filling defect in the posterior part of the 3rd ventricle. The preferred treatment of ventriculocisternostomy or ventriculovascular shunt combined with x-ray therapy often gives long remissions; direct removal has a discouragingly high mortality.

Acoustic Neuromas. Tumors of nerve sheaths within the cranial cavity rarely occur on any but the 8th nerve. The acoustic neuromas give the syndrome of a mass in the cerebellopontine angle. This includes, initially, (1) disturbance of hearing and equilibrium; then a progressive involvement of (2) the trigeminal nerve with ipsilateral reduction of corneal reflex, facial paresthesias and later numbness, (3) the facial nerve with ipsilateral facial weakness and loss of taste, (4) the cerebellar hemisphere with signs as mentioned earlier, (5) the lower 4 cranial nerves with dysphagia, dysarthria and hoarseness, and (6) the abducens nerve with external rectus paresis. With the aid of the sitting position, often these benign encapsulated tumors can be totally removed by a skillful surgeon, especially if diagnosis is made early. It may be necessary to sacrifice the lateral half of the cerebellar hemisphere in order to gain adequate exposure; maximal skill and patience are required to avoid injury to the side of the brain stem and the vessels running in its pia.

Miscellaneous Tumors of Mesodermal Origin. A variety of intracranial neoplasms arise from other connective tissue. These include the *hemangioblastoma,* a cystic tumor with a mural nodule of compact blood vessels, found nearly always in the cerebellum of adults. An as yet mysterious association with polycythemia vera often occurs. The lesion may be a part of the complex known as Lindau's disease. In this hereditary disorder, multiple tumors are present, of which the easiest to see is a capillary hemangioma of the retina (von Hippel's disease). Multiple cysts in pancreas or kidney, or tumors in kidney or epididymis also occur. Regardless of the presence or the absence of other features of Lindau's disease, the total or subtotal removal of the cerebellar hemangioblastoma is usually a fruitful procedure. Sarcomas, melanomas and even lipomas occur in the intracranial cavity.

Papillomas arising from the choroid plexus in any ventricle and *colloid cysts* in the anterior end of the 3rd ventricle are other benign tumors whose critical locus calls for special judgment and care in removal. Adherence to vital portions of ventricular walls may dictate leaving a remnant of the tumor or the cyst in order to leave a functional patient.

Orbital Tumors and Exophthalmos. Retrobulbar tumors and some other lesions provoking protrusion of the eyeball, such as the ill-understood proptosis accompanying thyrotoxicosis, are approached best surgically by a transfrontal or temporal exposure. When CSF is evacuated via a lumbar puncture needle, the frontal lobe with its dura literally falls away from the orbit. Removal of its bony roof and if necessary of the lateral and posterior wall gives easy access to the area behind the eyeball and the best chance to preserve that structure and vision if the type of lesion does not make mandatory an exenteration of the orbit. Proptosis, at times with displacement of the eyeball out of its central axis, loss of visual acuity, a field defect, weakness of extraocular muscles with diplopia and strabismus, impaired pupillary reactions, and papilledema or optic atrophy may all occur. Over a score of different types of space-taking pathologic processes—no one of them common—may be responsible for this clinical picture.

Infections

This type of lesion has become less common and presents a less stereotyped clinical picture since the antibiotics have come into use. Intensive use of the agent or agents to which the patient's organism is sensitive remains a major part of the treatment when the bacteria settle in the skull or the brain. Local application at the site of the pus after its removal permits a high concentration at the right spot and properly supplements high parenteral dosage. The principal available avenue of attack may be local when one uses such drugs as bacitracin, with which systemic levels effective against staphylococci threaten renal function. Those agents which do not enter CSF readily from the blood should be injected directly into ventricle or lumbar region if there is any suspicion of meningitis, but penicillin may not be so used in high concentration because of its convulsant effect.

Brain Abscess. Focal infection almost never begins in the brain in the absence of direct open trauma or operation. The primary source may be infections of the accessory nasal or mastoid air sinuses, which may lead by direct extension or by infected venous emboli to abscess within the brain. Usually bacteria in the nasal sinuses spread to the frontal lobe, while those from the mastoid go to the temporal lobe or the cerebellar hemisphere, but such relations are not always found. Bacteria starting from any part of the body and reaching the arterial blood may lodge in any part of the brain. Children with congenital cardiac lesions involving a right-left shunt and patients of any age with pulmonary infection are especially likely to develop a brain abscess. The systemic reactions to infection of fever, chills and leukocytosis are usually completely absent in the brain abscesses; despite this, they may evolve in devastating fashion with extensive edema or "cerebritis." *Development of any intracranial symptoms or signs in the presence either of infection elsewhere or in patients with congenital heart disease producing cyanosis should lead to an emergency analysis and full study,* even though the primary lesion may be smoldering or subsiding. The surgical portion of the treatment may consist of aspiration, or open drainage of the pus via a small bony opening, of a total excision of abscess plus capsule at a craniotomy, or a combination of these maneuvers. Aspiration, especially of a deep abscess, is properly followed by Kahn's tactic of injecting a small amount of Thorotrast which is phagocytized by the capsule and enables serial roentgenograms to show the locus and the course of the lesion as a guide to therapy. In cerebral lesions, convulsions during treatment should be forestalled with anticonvulsant therapy. Convulsions as a sequel to the disease from the residual scar in the brain are less likely to occur if the entire abscess capsule is removed. Late seizures are not a problem when the abscess is in the cerebellum.

Subdural Abscess. When pus spreads in the subdural space, the source is usually a severe nasal sinusitis, and the clinical picture is often fulminant with coma succeeding rapidly upon focal neurologic signs such as adversive seizures and hemiparesis. Pus spreads along the medial and inferior as well as the superolateral surfaces of one or both cerebral hemispheres. Catheter irrigation and drainage via multiple burr holes at all of these sites are necessary.

Cranial Osteomyelitis. Cranial osteomyelitis now occurs rarely. Antibiotic therapy, en block excision of the infected sector of the cranial vault, and cranioplastic repair after many months represent the therapeutic sequence.

Hematoma, Intracerebral

This may arise from (1) trauma (see below), (2) rupture of diseased vessels as seen in arteriosclerosis and hypertension, vascular malformations, aneurysms and tumors, and (3) systemic hemorrhagic diathesis. In the absence of trauma, abrupt evolution of focal symptoms and signs, especially with the finding of blood in the CSF, should lead to suspicion of this diagnosis. The fact that in many patients the hemorrhage does not lie in a deep-seated inoperable area makes it incumbent to study each of them critically and urgently. Often the patient's parlous clinical condition precludes his giving the examiner much assistance in diagnosis, and there may be time only to place a burr opening in the skull over the most likely site of hemorrhage and to tap into the brain with a blunt ventricular needle in the hope of striking clot which can be aspirated. This may relieve acute embarrassment of vital functions enough to permit a full exposure via craniotomy with evacuation of all the clot and management of the causative lesion under direct vision.

Craniocerebral Trauma

The rising number of traffic accidents in which head injuries present acute problems makes a basic knowledge of this subject a must for most physicians. Whenever there is any question of cerebral injury, *opiates such as morphine or methadone should be avoided,* even though they effectively control pain and restlessness. These drugs tend to aggravate a rising intracranial pressure, to depress already impaired respiratory functions to a lethal low and, by causing pupillary constriction, to obscure the important lateralizing sign of unilateral pupillary dilation. The profuse bleeding from a scalp laceration may be controlled by digital compression along the scalp margins until hemostats can be applied to the galea and reflected backward to evert this layer, which closes the vessels and makes direct ligation of most of the bleeders unnecessary. If a depressed fracture can be seen, either directly or in roentgenograms, or can be palpated with a gloved finger, the wound should be repaired as soon as traumatic shock has been treated. It is important to remove indriven bone fragments lest they form a nidus for later development of a brain abscess. A thorough, gentle débridement, including discreet removal of necrotic brain, is needed not only to promote primary healing but also to minimize post-traumatic convulsive seizures, which occur in a high percentage of penetrating cerebral wounds. The dura should be closed tightly, if necessary, with a fascial or pericranial graft, in order to prevent a progressive outward herniation or cerebral fungus of edematous, injured brain. This must be done even in the presence of probable bacterial contamination. Otherwise, cerebral veins on the surface of and draining the herniating gyri are compressed by the dural edge, whereas the arteries continue to pour in blood, and a vicious circle of steadily increasing herniation develops.

Signs of Focal Hemorrhage. A major initial task in assaying an acute head injury is the detection of intracranial hemorrhage or pulpified hemorrhagic brain. In Figure 50-12 are shown the sites of predilection for the occurrence of extradural, subdural and intracerebral hematomas. The most important indication of such a lesion is progressive decrease in responsiveness. This may follow a period of normal behavior after the injury, the so-called lucid interval. Alternatively, the patient may decline steadily from a state of decreased responsiveness to a deep coma. In such a patient a surgically removable lesion is so likely that the search for a focal clot or area of pulpification should be pursued exhaustively by every diagnostic means available. The faster the deterioration, the more urgent the indication for surgery. Increasing intracranial pressure is also likely to produce an elevation in systolic and pulse pressures, a rising temperature, bradycardia, and slow, irregular breathing. However, these warning signs may all be absent, and the lumbar CSF pressure even be normal or subnormal in the presence of a huge intracranial clot.

The side of supratentorial bleeding is shown most reliably, but not with certainty by an ipsilateral dilating pupil unresponsive to light. In patients with even minor head injuries, the size of the pupils should be checked regularly for at least 24 hours, as anisocoria may warn of an impending tentorial pressure cone before lethargy becomes severe. Its presence should lead to efforts to rouse an apparently

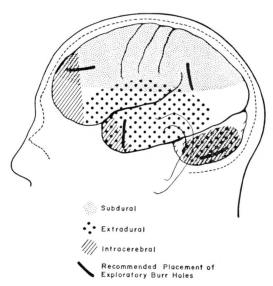

Subdural

Extradural

Intracerebral

Recommended Placement of Exploratory Burr Holes

FIG. 50-12. Traumatic intracranial hematoma. Sites of predilection for the occurrence of various types.

sleeping patient; the sleep may prove to be a coma! Decerebrate rigidity, even bilaterally, may be evoked by a unilateral supratentorial hematoma in the temporal region; the primary causative lesion need not necessarily lie within the midbrain; if removed promptly, recovery may follow. A stiff neck, cerebellar or bulbar signs, or a fracture entering the foramen magnum suggest the possibility of bleeding in the posterior cranial fossa.

Extradural Hematoma. In general, a fracture line which crosses one of the grooves for the middle meningeal vessels or the venous sinuses should lead to suspicion of an extradural hematoma underlying the crossing—X marks the spot. When the clinical signs are in agreement, this is the first place to look. If the patient's downhill course is extremely rapid, extradural arterial bleeding from a main middle meningeal vessel is a likely and the most remediable cause. To check for this, an opening may be made (even through unshaved scalp with any unsterile drill in a grave emergency) just above and in front of the ear. Provision of space for the blood clot to spout out or be aspirated through a hole in the skull, thereby relieving acute high pressure against the brain, is even more important than securing the bleeding point, which is of course the next order of business. If an experienced surgeon is not at hand, an inexperienced doctor may find himself obligated to carry out these dramatic, lifesaving gestures.

Subdural Hematoma. This lesion often presents a picture of subacute or chronic illness because it usually arises from a tiny tear in a vein from the cerebrum bridging this space to enter a venous sinus—most commonly the superior sagittal sinus. A minimal blow in the long axis of the head, so minor as to appear negligible, may provoke such bleeding, especially in an older person or an alcoholic. In the subdural space a striking semipermeable membrane forms around the clot which not only precludes its absorption after the bleeding stops but actually results in a slow increase in the size of the mass. This "growth" is attributed to increasing osmolar concentration from splitting of protein molecules and consequent net entry of more water into the sac. Symptoms may be indistinguishable from those of neoplasm; headache and mental changes are prominent; fluctuation in symptoms, especially in the level of responsiveness, is often seen. This disorder is treated so simply and effectively, frequently requiring only drainage of the brownish fluid content of the sac through one or two burr holes, that often it should be sought even when the chance of finding it seems to be small.

Subdural Hematoma in Infancy. This presents a special picture in which one may note at first only irritability, failure to gain weight and vomiting. Later, the head and the facies suggest the development of hydrocephalus, and convulsions and retinal hemorrhages may be present. Puncture at the lateral aspect of one or both sides of the anterior fontanelle yields yellow fluid. Repeated aspirations or drainage may eliminate the abnormal fluid or it may prove necessary to turn down a bone flap and remove the abnormal membranes.

Intracerebral Hematoma. Recognition of the peculiar torsion movements often undergone by the brain within the skull when the head is struck has led to realization that one or both temporal or frontal poles may become contused and hemorrhagic, even when the blow is delivered elsewhere (Fig. 50-12). Especially since one or more of these areas may be sacrificed without permanent deficit,

the internal decompression of the remainder of the brain purchased by removal of such destroyed zones is beneficial at small cost. Much less often, occipital poles or cerebellar hemisphere become contused and hemorrhagic. If a hematoma is found in the occipital lobe above the transverse sinus, it is often advisable to seek one below it in the cerebellum and vice versa.

As indicated in Figure 50-12, exploration by as many as 4 burr holes on each side may be advisable in searching for a removable hemorrhage. If none is found and the brain continues to bulge at the openings, ventriculography or angiography may be necessary.

Cerebrospinal Rhinorrhea and Otorrhea. Leakage of CSF from nose or ear occurs in about 2 per cent of patients following a closed head injury. A fistulous pathway for the fluid is created by a fracture plus dural and mucosal tears. Such a communication permits infection from the upper respiratory passages to gain direct access to the subarachnoid space and the brain, at times with a rapidly fatal result. The hazard of such infection is much less in otorrhea than in rhinorrhea because a fracture in the petrous bone tends to close promptly and effectively. The blood from nose or ear at the time of the original injury should be collected; if it does not clot, probably it is mixed with some CSF. Usually the fistula is not suspected until water-clear fluid drips from the nose later on. A collected sample of nasal fluid does indeed contain CSF if its glucose or chloride concentrations approach those in the patient's lumbar CSF and differ thereby from blood samples obtained at the same time. If the sample is water-clear, the presence of even a few milligrams per cent of glucose establishes it as CSF and not the secretion of vasomotor rhinitis. Even if the leak stops spontaneously, as it usually does, the possibility of direct infection into the intracranial cavity persists. One or more attacks of meningitis with such a mechanism may appear even as late as a decade after the injury. Formerly, the rhinorrhea was treated merely by urging the patient not to blow his nose or sniff up; operative repair was advised only if the leak did not stop in a week or two. However, long-term follow-up of patients with a CSF rhinorrhea reveals that about one fourth of them develop a later meningitis which is of a fulminant fatal type in about half of those affected. Consequently, we now advise prophylactic administration of antibiotics and, early after recovery from the original injury, a transfrontal craniotomy with repair of the dural tear. This relatively minor operation has a mortality of less than 2 per cent when done electively.

Aneurysms

These are usually saccular out-pouchings on any of the larger intracranial arteries and are principally of congenital or arteriosclerotic origin. They may rarely have a traumatic, mycotic or syphilitic cause. In another type, a fusiform dilation and tortuosity of one of the major arterial trunks at the base of the brain occurs. These lesions may give rise initially to focal signs whose nature depends on their locus; oculomotor, trigeminal or optic nerves are those most frequently indented by the expanded vessel. But a spontaneous subarachnoid hemorrhage commonly provokes the first symptoms; the converse of this, that an aneurysm is the commonest cause of such hemorrhage, is also true. The rupture of the aneurysm is signalized by the abrupt onset of severe pain in the head, often occipital, but occurring anywhere. This is followed by pain and rigidity in the nuchal region and on down the spine—promptly in major bleeding, but not for some hours if the hemorrhage is smaller. Unconsciousness may come on almost at once if bleeding is severe; in other patients recurrent bouts of leakage of blood may lead to such mistaken diagnoses as "sinusitis," especially if intense pain is preceded by duller headache. Careful questioning may elicit a history of brief focal motor or sensory symptoms at the onset or later. Retinal and/or more massive subhyaloid hemorrhages appear shortly in about 10 per cent of the patients; papilledema may come on later. The diagnosis of a spontaneous subarachnoid hemorrhage is confirmed by lumbar puncture. Persistent neurologic deficit suggests that a hematoma remains around the affected cranial nerve or within the brain.

About 60 per cent of the patients who survive the initial hemorrhagic ictus will bleed again within a month. On the conservative management of bed rest, roughly half of all the patients will survive the initial and any subsequent hemorrhages without crippling neurologic deficit. Neurosurgeons are improving on this figure and are treating many unruptured lesions as well. Since over 80 per cent of the intracranial aneurysms are on one or both carotid portions of the arterial tree, carotid angiography, simpler and safer than that of the vertebral artery, will demonstrate the great majority of the lesions. Recurrent hemorrhage and death, a great risk at first, become less likely with the passage of each successive week after the initial episode. The sooner one operates the less the likelihood of a fatal recurrent hemorrhage; but the more serious the original ictus, the greater the arterial spasm and cerebral damage, and the more dangerous is early surgery. Appraisal of the results of early and later operation has not yet reached a point at which even tentative rules of surgical conduct can be suggested. It is clear though that angiography is virtually indispensable to proper management; this is performed percutaneously in the carotids— on both sides because the aneurysms are multiple in 10 to 20 per cent of cases. Figure 50-13 indicates how striking the lesion may be.

Surgical treatment may consist of (1) carotid occlusion in the neck, or of intracranial approach with (2) proximal occlusion of the vessel bearing the aneurysm, (3) "trapping" of the lesion between proximal and distal clips on the parent vessel, (4) occlusion of the neck of the aneurysm, (5) packing of muscle or other supportive substance around the lesion, or (6) removal of the aneurysm and repair of the parent vessel. The least dangerous of these is occlusion of the cervical carotid. The intra-arterial systolic pressure in the neck distal to occlusion of the internal carotid falls to an average of about one half and the pulse pressure to about one third of that with the flow free. This degree of residual pressure usually suffices to prevent dangerous cerebral ischemia. However, the collateral inflow varies tremendously in different patients, and it is advisable to carry out a measurement in each. The percentage drop in pressure found in the cervical internal carotid is the same in all parts of that carotid's larger arterial branches, so that the location of the aneurysm on the tree would appear by this criterion to be immaterial in determining the value of carotid closure. If the drop in pressure is small or, contrariwise, is excessive, a direct intracranial approach may be advisable. However, in the case of marked drop in pressure or the development of signs of cerebral ischemia during a period of trial occlusion under local anesthesia, a fractional staged closure, leading finally to full shutoff, may be tolerated. By the use of such precautionary measures, the eventual mortality and major morbidity following cervical carotid operation have been brought below 10 per cent, a figure not strictly comparable with that for conservative treatment, since some patients die before surgery is feasible.

The intracranial operations at present carry a higher immediate mortality but are receiving a thorough trial because they permit a curative attack on the lesion, whereas later fatal hemorrhages still occur in a few patients after arterial ligations proximal to the aneurysm. Cerebral metabolism drops to $\frac{1}{4}$ to $\frac{1}{3}$

normal levels when the patient is deliberately cooled to 25° C., and at this hypothermic level a temporary clamping of both carotid and both vertebral vessels can be maintained for a succession of 10- to 15-minute periods without permanent ischemic damage. Shorter periods of occlusion and somewhat higher body temperature usually suffice when hypothermia is used in intracranial operations. The lower the body temperature the greater the danger of ventricular fibrillation. The virtually dry field obtainable by closure of the feeding arteries permits a definitive repair of the lesion with minimal trauma to contiguous brain and nerves. A ganglionic blocking agent such as Arfonad to produce hypotension may also be used here, as one does in vascular tumors, to reduce hemorrhage, and such use may be combined with hypothermia.

We doubt that aneurysms of the vertebral arterial tree may be treated effectively by

FIG. 50-13. Aneurysm of right internal carotid artery. Carotid arteriogram. *Case summary:* 44-year-old male. Abrupt onset of "terrible" knifelike pain above right eye radiating to vertex; 1 hour later lost consciousness. Lumbar puncture: bloody CSF. Roentgenograms showed

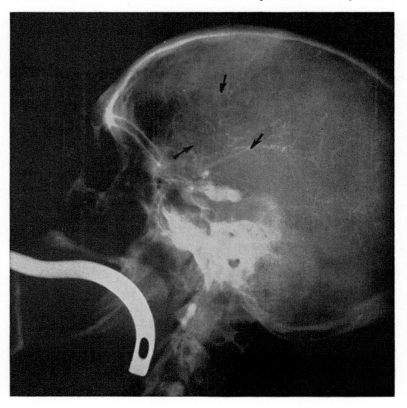

normal skull. Discharged from hospital after 5 weeks of bed rest. One week later same pain recurred followed shortly by right ptosis; CSF freshly bloody. Arteriogram: massive trilobed aneurysm projecting backward from the internal carotid at its bifurcation. The 2 anterior arrows point to anterior cerebral vessels; the posterior arrow, to the middle cerebral artery; all are in normal position. Occlusion of right common and external carotid arteries caused pressure in right internal carotid to drop from 132/100 to 66/55. Ten years later the patient was still symptom-free.

proximal ligation of one vertebral artery, since no distal fall in pressure occurs if the other vertebral artery is of roughly normal size.

Arteriovenous Fistulas and Malformations

Rupture of the intracranial carotid artery in its subclinoid, intracavernous portion permits the blood to pass directly into the cavernous sinus, thereby creating a carotid cavernous fistula. This may occur spontaneously but usually cephalic trauma is its cause. A striking picture develops within hours to weeks, characterized by pulsating exophthalmos on the side of the lesion with chemosis and redness of the conjunctiva, impaired vision, weakness of the extra-ocular muscles and a loud bruit often heard by the patient himself or even by a person standing near him. Cervical carotid ligation may control the symptoms; if not, one must occlude as well the intracranial internal carotid distal to the lesion and possibly also the ophthalmic artery.

Small or massive remnants of the embryonic vascular networks in the brain may persist and enlarge to form arteriovenous malformations. The 3 commonest manifestations of this disorder are: (1) focal convulsive seizures, (2) spontaneous subarachnoid and/or intracerebral hemorrhage and (3) headaches, often migrainous in type. A bruit occurs in a minority of the patients. The fistulous shunts are rarely large enough to provoke cardiac hypertrophy. A pneumogram may show focal or generalized cerebral atrophy, which perhaps occurs because of significant diversion of the brain's blood directly to the veins. The sovereign aid to diagnosis and planning of treatment is angiography (Fig. 50-14). These lesions usually have so little normal brain between their tangle of vessels that their total extirpation will not increase neurologic deficit, if trauma during control of bleeding can be avoided. The problem of knowing where to seek the feeding arteries is solved by the angiogram, and many of these lesions in the cerebral hemispheres are now removed readily, provided that one divides the feeding arteries *before* the draining veins. If total removal is not feasible, occlusion of as many feeding arteries as possible and evacuation of any intracerebral hematoma may still be rewarding.

Congenital Malformations

Hydrocephalus. Overproduction of the CSF by a papilloma of the choroid plexus, overwhelming normal absorptive mechanism and producing dilated cerebral ventricles, has been recorded but is an extreme rarity. Some CSF is absorbed throughout the chambers containing it, but the excess must attain the subarachnoid space over the cerebral hemispheres for final absorption. The usual cause of hydrocephalus is a lesion interfering with the essential flow or absorption of that excess. When this occurs in infancy without other major cerebral hypogenesis, the baby usually looks relatively normal at birth. However, within a few months, a frankly hydrocephalic infant with enlarged head, prominent cranial bosses, bulging fontanelles and apathetic expression is readily recognized. When this diagnosis is suspected, in order to confirm it before the stage of excessive pressure atrophy of the brain has been reached, the physician should measure the occipitofrontal circumference of the head several times a week in order to establish that an abnormal rate of increase is present. When the lesion prevents dye injected into the lateral ventricles from reaching a needle in the lumbar spinal canal, one speaks of obstructive hydrocephalus. When the lesion does not prevent such flow of the dye, the hydrocephalus is of the "communicating" type. Although tumors are the commonest cause of an obstruction to the outflow of CSF from the ventricles, congenital stenosis of the aqueduct of Sylvius or at the outflow foramina of Magendie and Luschka in the 4th ventricle may cause dilation of all ventricles rostral to the obstruction and evidence of increased intracranial pressure. The block is by-passed by a shunting tube from lateral ventricle to upper cervical spinal canal rather than cisterna magna, because the latter structure is too tiny in infancy.

The site of obstruction in congenital communicating hydrocephalus may be at the foramen magnum and be produced by the Arnold-Chiari malformation or may lie in closure of or failure of development of the subarachnoid channels. Myelomeningoceles are nearly always associated with the Arnold-Chiari deformity, which consists of a downward displacement and often a folding of the medulla through the foramen magnum along with crowding of the cerebellar tonsils into this small space. Because of this caudal position of the medulla, CSF may flow from the 4th ventricle directly into the spinal canal and be unable to pass up through the foramen magnum into the cerebral subarachnoid space. Hence hydrocephalus often develops in association with a myelomeningocele, and a decompressive enlargement of the foramen mag-

num with upper cervical laminectomy may aid in the treatment. However, for the vast majority of children with communicating hydrocephalus, no direct therapy of the lesion is feasible. Then one may attack the problem of excess CSF by decreasing its rate of formation. Electrocoagulation of the choroid plexuses of the lateral ventricles has achieved this with some success, but drainage of the excess CSF into some other area of the body

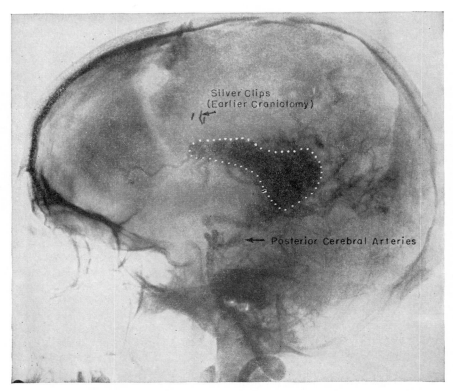

Fig. 50-14. Arteriovenous malformation. Vertebral angiograms. *Case summary:* 17-year-old male. Bouts of spontaneous subarachnoid hemorrhage from malformation filling from both carotid and both vertebral arteries. In illustrations dotted lines enclose the main mass of lesion below corpus callosum, above midbrain and between thalami. Arrow points to metal clips applied at earlier operation to both anterior cerebral arteries feeding the lesion. Neither this operation nor clipping of right posterior cerebral and posterior communicating arteries stopped the hemorrhages. Under hypothermia at 25° C. the lesion itself was exposed, and the immediate feeding arteries were occluded. To aid this, both carotid and both vertebral arteries were closed for a total of 47 min. over a 2-hr. period; longest single period of closure was 14½ min., the first such deliberate procedure in man. Probable maximal tolerable period of such closure *at normal temperature* is 3 to 5 min. Good postoperative recovery, but death 5 days later from thrombosis of right vertebral artery, propagating from site of temporary occlusions in neck. We now carry out these occlusions so as to minimize local injury.

is simpler. Catheters placed with one end in the subarachnoid space and the other in the distal ureter after nephrectomy, or in some part of the peritoneal cavity, the pleural cavity, a fallopian tube or a vein have all been tried. This predominantly mechanical problem probably is solved best by placement in a lateral ventricle of a plastic catheter which leads to a pair of one-way valves lying subcutaneously behind the ear or in the uppermost neck. Caudally, a silicone tube passes into the internal jugular, thence into the innominate vein, the superior vena cava or the uppermost right atrium. The subcutaneous position of crucial portions of the system makes them readily available for checking. The placement of the caudal tip of the shunting tube in a turbulent portion of the circulation, along with occasional digital pressure on the tube between

the 2 valves, has solved the problem of occlusion of the lower end of the tube by clot. Since the fluid is taken from the lateral ventricle, the method applies to both communicating and obstructive types of hydrocephalus.

Cranium Bifidum and Encephalocele. Failure of tissues overlying the brain to develop properly usually occurs somewhere along the mid-line from the bridge of the nose back to the nuchal region. The outward herniation of brain at this site may be accompanied by other more serious intracranial anomalies. In only about one third of the patients does surgical repair yield a relatively normal child.

Craniosynostosis. The reverse type of defect occurs in which one or more of the cranial sutures closes prematurely. If the coronal suture is involved, the head is too short and wide; if the sagittal suture is affected, the

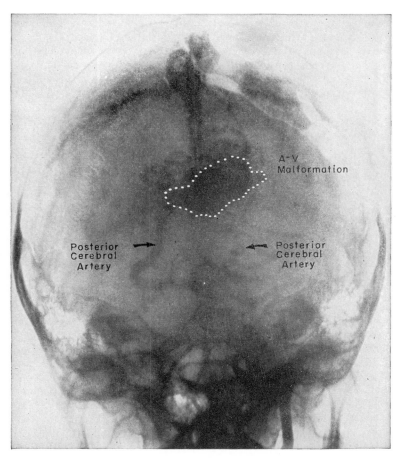

FIGURE 50-14. (*Continued*)

head is too long and narrow. If all of the sutures are involved the brain bulges up at the fontanelles and down into the orbits. Mental retardation will follow unless the brain is given enough room for growth. The successful treatment consists of removal of bone along the closed suture, and then lining the bone edges with strips of a plastic such as polyethylene to prevent bony regrowth and closure, which is a very active process in infants.

Anomalies at the Craniovertebral Junction. A variety of skeletal lesions in this region may produce neurologic malfunction or be accompanied by neurologic malformation. The commonest of the bony disorders has been called *platybasia* or, perhaps better, *basilar impression*. The latter term describes the nature of the lesion in which the anterior part of the cervical spine becomes invaginated or impressed upward into the base of the occiput, encroaching on the foramen magnum from in front. Compression of the ventral aspect of the pons, the medulla and the emergent lower cranial nerves with crowding of the cerebellum occurs. An enormous variety of clinical pictures ensues, depending upon which of these regions bears the brunt of the pressure. Long tracts moving into the cord, local bulbar nuclei, cranial nerves from V to XII, sensory pain fibers to the occiput and the neck, the cerebellum, or pathways for CSF flow may be involved singly or in combination. Symptoms rarely appear before adolescent or adult life, usually progress slowly, perhaps with remissions. An erroneous diagnosis of some intrinsic disease of the nervous system such as syringomyelia or multiple sclerosis is often made. Roentgenograms may reveal: (1) an elevation of the tip of the odontoid process more than 6 mm. above "Chamberlain's line" (drawn on a lateral view of the skull to join the dorsal surface of the hard palate and the dorsal lip of the foramen magnum). Or (2) the films may show an angle of 13° or more between the plane of the hard palate and the plane of the atlas vertebra. Normally, these two planes are nearly parallel. Although such abnormal findings may occur in some asymptomatic people, their presence in company with advancing local neurologic signs suggests that decompressive craniectomy and laminectomy will provide more space for the cramped nervous structures and may permit them to

perform properly. Basilar impression may also occur as an acquired disorder in any condition which produces softening of the base of the skull; the commonest such cause is Paget's disease.

Scars and Adhesions

The residual scar in the cerebrum following trauma, infection, vascular lesions or operation may give rise to convulsive seizures which in turn may provoke some mental deterioration. If the seizures are not controlled by nontoxic doses of anticonvulsant agents, operative removal of the abnormal tissue and of the nearby abnormally discharging cerebral cortex is advisable. Recognition that small scars and other lesions in the temporal lobe are a frequent cause of paroxysmal behavior disorders or seizures has come recently. Ischemic or other damage to the medial aspect of the temporal lobe at birth appears to occur and to cause seizures at a much later date. The seizures of temporal lobe origin, the automatisms or "psychomotor" seizures, have been especially refractory to medication and are among the commonest to require surgical treatment.

Adhesions in the subarachnoid space following upon meningitis or severe subarachnoid hemorrhages may interfere with the absorption of CSF. The communicating hydrocephalus which ensues is to be treated as indicated in the discussion of the congenital form of this disorder. Localized adhesions may develop around the optic nerves or chiasm, producing progressive visual impairment which requires operative lysis of the contracting bands of tissue.

Pseudotumor Cerebri
(Benign Intracranial Hypertension)

A benign, self-limited disorder occurs in which increased intracranial pressure with the appropriate symptoms and signs thereof is caused by a disturbance in intracranial fluid balance. No space-taking mass or block of flow in the CSF pathways proper is demonstrable by pneumoventriculography or encephalography. The disease may come on in patients with extensive thrombosis or occlusion of (1) cerebral veins, (2) a dural venous sinus, or (3) cervical veins. The probable mechanism of the rise in CSF pressure in this group seems to be impaired absorption of CSF. However, in most of the patients, who are often obese, middle-aged women, evidence of venous obstruction is lacking, and the mechanism is obscure. Although the patient ordinarily seems to be unusually well for the degree of papilledema that he shows, this may cause blindness so rapidly that the conservative treatment of repeated drainage of CSF by lumbar puncture may not suffice to protect vision. In this situation, unilateral or bilateral subtemporal decompression is likely to effect prompt improvement.

Granulomatous and Parasitic Cysts

In the United States, tuberculomas and syphilitic gummas are now rarely seen in the brain because of the effectiveness with which these infections are controlled by prophylactic measures and at their primary sites. Parasitic invasions by echinococcus and cysticercus are also rare in the United States. One sees them most often in patients who come from other quarters of the world where the dog is infested with the echinococcus tapeworm and where food is contaminated with excreta of human carriers of the *Taenia solium*. The first 3 types of lesion present clinically and are treated surgically as one would a neoplasm, with special care to avoid contamination of the brain by the infection or the cystic fluid. Cysticerci usually invade diffusely, and the need for surgical treatment is most likely to arise when the cysts block the CSF flow out of the ventricles or along the subarachnoid channels, precluding absorption. If the cysts themselves cannot be removed, one resorts to the tactics for treating obstructive or communicating hydrocephalus.

Supportive Aspects of Treatment After Intracranial Injuries, Hemorrhages or Operations

The airway requires special attention in the unconscious patient with a lesion in the brain who tends to have excessive secretions in the respiratory tract and inadequate expulsion thereof by coughing. Careful positioning *on the side* with the head low encourages postural drainage. But if cephalic venous congestion or possible intracranial bleeding are problems, these dictate elevation of the head. The lateral position is still needed to keep the tongue from falling back and obstructing the oral pharynx. A plastic oral airway may be required. The use of oxygen by nasal catheter may permit adequate exchange in the lungs. But if tracheobronchial secretions are profuse, neither drugs nor oral suction will suffice, and a tracheotomy should be done promptly. Gentle sterile suctioning via the tracheotomy tube, not exceeding a vacuum of 4 lb./sq. in., along with input of a proper mixture of humidified air or oxygen, may play a major role in the patient's recovery. Swelling of the brain is increased by even mild hypoxia, so that every effort to avoid this is rewarding. Suction with a greater vacuum, or even a bronchoscopy, may become mandatory to remove tenacious bronchial plugs of mucus.

Hyperthermia as a consequence of impaired central regulation of temperature, formerly a major threat to patients with severe cerebral lesions, is now avoided by prompt administration of aspirin, alcohol sponging or the exposure of the unclothed patient to a cool atmosphere, such as that conveniently provided by a refrigerated oxygen tent. The more drastic measures used to produce deep hypothermia should be invoked without delay if necessary. External cooling by plastic bags filled with ice cubes should be used if special cooling units are not available. Chlorpromazine, Demerol and/or anesthesia may be required to prevent shivering as well as to make the intense cold tolerable to the patient.

Convulsive seizures increase cerebral edema or bleeding; one seeks to prevent their initial appearance by prophylactic use of Dilantin, 100 mg., or phenobarbital, 100 mg., 3 or 4 times per day—intramuscularly in the unconscious patient. If seizures do occur, one must use parenteral anticonvulsants intensively, changing to another drug promptly if the first is ineffective. One need not hesitate to use intravenous Pentothal Sodium.

Restlessness. Moderate restlessness to wild thrashing about may be a problem, especially in young men. Barbiturates may make the patient even less controllable; morphine and related alkaloids are contraindicated; paraldehyde is perhaps the most satisfactory sedative and Demerol the best analgesic agent in conjunction with such tranquilizers as chlorpromazine. Straining at stool may be dangerous, and easy bowel movements must be assured by cathartics or enemas.

Cerebral edema is the unsolved problem in many of these patients. We know that over-hydration, especially if NaCl is given, will worsen this and kill them, but do not know exactly how much we should dehydrate the whole patient to try to keep his brain from becoming waterlogged. It is standard practice to give a daily intake to adults of 1,500 ml. of fluid for the first several days with frequent measurements of hemoglobin, hematocrit and urinary output to guide daily intake. If coma continues beyond 2 or 3 days, fluids, drugs and high caloric mixtures should be given via a long tube extending from the nose to the stomach. For the differential abstraction of water from edematous brain, intravenous injection of hypertonic urea 10 to 30 per cent (introduced by Javid and associates) has replaced all previous agents. Urea in the blood exchanges rapidly with nearly all extracellular areas but that of the brain. Hence, the increased osmolarity of the blood stream dehydrates only the brain. Provided that the edema or the injury is not too severe, the urea does not enter the brain in sufficient amounts to cause a later reversal of the net flow of water with exacerbation of the original process. Sucrose in 50 per cent concentration behaves similar to urea in this respect, but the large amounts injected are excreted less easily by the kidneys. When the ventricles are large, increased intracranial pressure is relieved effectively by tapping these cavities, and if necessary by maintaining continuous catheter drainage to a sterile reservoir at a level that will maintain roughly normal pressure.

Metabolic disturbances of varying types, all leading to coma, may occur. In one of these there is excessive protein catabolism, with a high level of NPN and urea in blood and an enormous output of these in urine. In this situation a large volume of urinary water must accompany these molecules, and the body, by excreting no sodium chloride and hence no water to go with it, conserves water as best it can, permitting extreme rises in sodium and chloride in the blood. Major occult gastrointestinal bleeding may appear, and the absorption back into the blood of the digested fragments of the blood proteins produces a

similar picture. The proper treatment of these malfunctions is obscure. Conversely, in other types of cerebral lesion, there may be salt wasting, with an insidious but excessive urinary output of these 2 ions and a resultant hyponatremia and hypochloremia; increased salt intake is required and may need to be supplemented by cortisone. Even a mild diabetic may slip into acidosis under the stress of serious cerebral disease, but parasellar disorders, with or without diabetes, may provoke a hypoglycemic coma.

The blood volume appears also to be subject to cerebral regulation, and the patient may slip into hypovolemic shock in the absence of occult bleeding. For these reasons we must keep a vigilant watch over the blood volume and the content in it of urea or NPN, sodium, chloride, carbon dioxide and glucose. We are only at the threshold of our efforts to understand how to help the injured brain regulate metabolism of the body as a whole and of the local lesion—a challenging task, since we know that much of the damage in edematous brain is reversible.

Cranioplasty to repair major skull defects is a much later step in the management of these patients. Plates utilizing tantalum or acrylic resins or the patient's own ribs or ilium are the favored materials.

Lesions with Surgical Implications, Intraspinal

Symptoms and Signs

Protrusions of intervertebral disks, neoplasms, abscesses, traumatic disorders, vascular malformations and congenital malformations are the main lesions encountered. Although CSF circulates around the spinal cord, neither increased pressure in nor block to the outflow of this fluid is a significant cause of disturbed function of the cord. So the symptoms arise from local effects of the lesion producing (1) *stimulation* or (2) *diminution* of function.

Stimulation of Function. The spectacular variety of responses of the brain upon irritation is absent in the cord. Pain and paresthesias, muscle spasm and excessive autonomic discharge are the main clinical manifestations of excessive neural activity seen with disease in the spinal canal.

PAIN OR PARESTHESIAS. Three different types of pain or paresthesias occur: (1) local pain in the back at the level of the lesion comes from stimuli to small neighboring nerves and nerve endings; (2) segmental pain or paresthesia lies in the distribution of one or more posterior nerve roots affected by the lesion. This is referred along a limb when the affected roots enter the brachial or lumbosacral plexuses, and often in a girdle fashion in the case of the thoracic roots. But at other times when pain arising from the thoracic posterior roots is referred to various local areas in the torso, one tends to think first of some commoner disease affecting that thoracic or abdominal viscus nearest the site of reference of the pain. (3) Pain is also produced by irritation of the specific pain pathways in the cord itself. Because of the compactness of this bundle of fibers, a small lesion on one side may cause pain referred over wide areas of the opposite side.

The following features are characteristic of an intraspinal origin of pain: (1) exacerbation upon maneuvers which raise CSF pressure, such as coughing, sneezing or straining. Such activities also raise pressure within the chest or the abdomen, but if one compresses both internal jugular veins, the subsequent rise in pressure will be confined to the head and the spinal canal. If this provokes the patient's pain in torso or limbs, the hyperirritable focus almost certainly lies in the spinal canal. (2) Worsening during motions of the spine, or relieved only in certain positions of the spine or the legs. (3) Tendency to waken the patient out of sleep. Tonic muscular activity splinting the diseased area probably is decreased in sleep, and when the patient then turns, his nerves are more likely to be pinched.

Spasms of localized muscle groups occur— ordinary cramps—and intraspinal lesions are a cause to be thought of, especially if the cramps are frequent and waken the patient from sleep. Major lesions of the cord, causing severe weakness or paralysis of one or both legs, may be accompanied by bursts of painful contraction of the muscles in the affected limb, throwing it into involuntary flexion at all joints. Extensor spasms in this situation may also be seen.

Hyperactivity of autonomic fibers is seen most often in the severe chronic lesions of the cord producing muscle spasm. The patient may have episodes of high blood pressure or of excessive sweating, with chilliness and faintness spontaneously or on other autonomic activity such as urinating or defecating. Priapism may occur in acute high lesions of the cord.

Diminution of Function. Somatic motor, sensory and autonomic deficits occur, and, as in the case of intracranial lesions, when their evolution is rapid, operations for a removable cause must be carried out as an emergency measure if they are to have their best chance of success.

Lesions affecting the *lower motor neuron,* i.e., anterior horn cells or anterior rootlets, produce a weakness that is associated with (1) atrophy, (2) flaccidity, (3) diminished or absent tendon jerks, (4) normal abdominal and cremasteric reflexes and (5) no sign of Babinski. When the lesion is in the cauda equina, the motor involvement is of this type. Inasmuch as the lower end of the spinal cord lies at the first lumbar vertebra when adult stature is attained, lumbar and sacral lesions usually involve only the rootlets of the cauda equina. Visible twitching of small or larger segments of muscle, called fasciculation, occurs spontaneously or may be brought out by tapping the weak muscle when the anterior horn cell is deteriorating. In contrast, the weakness produced by involvement of the *upper motor neuron* within the white matter of the cord proper is associated with (1) little or no atrophy, (2) increased resistance to passive movement, (3) increased tendon jerks, (4) absent abdominal and cremasteric reflexes and (5) positive Babinski and Hoffmann signs.

Somatic sensory loss includes impairment of ipsilateral proprioceptive and vibratory sense when a posterior white column is affected, and of contralateral pain and temperature sense when an anterolateral white column is involved. For complete loss of touch to be present, both anterior and posterior white matter must be nonfunctional.

Insignia of autonomic hypofunction are sudomotor and vasoconstrictor inactivity with hot, dry limbs and, if the lesion is in the cervical or upper thoracic cord, vascular hypotension. These changes are pronounced in the early stage of spinal injury but tend to fade out in the later stages when, as noted above,

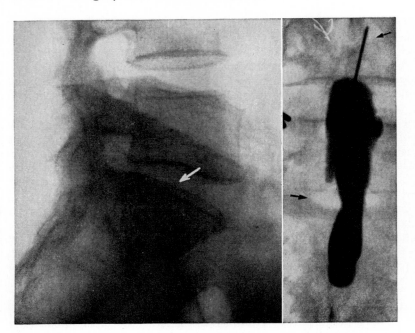

FIG. 50-15. Ruptured intervertebral disk. (A, *Left*) Plain film, lumbosacral junction. Arrow indicates the abnormally narrow interspace at L5-S1 level associated with massive posterior protrusion of the disk. (B, *Right*) Myelogram (*Upper arrow*) Lumbar puncture needle in situ during fluoroscopy. (*Lower arrow*) Filling defect caused by medial part of huge extruded fragment.

autonomic hyperactivity may appear. A lesion of these pathways in the cord down to the T1 level also produces an ipsilateral Horner's sign. One sees bladder dysfunction (1) with an atonic detrusor and urinary retention or (2) with better detrusor activity but impaired synergism between this and the sphincters giving irregular retention and overflow incontinence. Constipation or obstipation and in males impotence or sterility also occur.

Accessory Diagnostic Measures

Spinal Puncture. Following measurement of the resting initial pressure, one checks the patency of the spinal CSF pathway whenever a spinal (not an intracranial) lesion is suspected. A high-grade block will be shown by the Queckenstedt test of bilateral jugular compression, carried out digitally or by means of a blood pressure cuff around the neck inflated to 30 mm. Hg. The increased intracranial pressure should produce a rise in the pressure at the lumbar needle. An absent or a delayed rise or a delayed fall on release indicates an almost complete block in the CSF sleeve around the cord or in the cauda equina above the needle. The CSF below the block is often yellow and contains an elevated total protein.

Plain Roentgenography of Spine. A nar-

rowing of the interspace between the vertebral bodies (Fig. 50-15 A), often with a bony spur formation at the margins of the bodies (Fig. 50-20 A), indicates degeneration and/or extrusion of the intervertebral disk, the commonest lesion in the spinal canal. Destruction of bone, proliferation of bone or calcification occurs in a variety of tumors. Sites vulnerable to pressure are the vertebral pedicles, which may show a widening of the interpediculate distance at one or more vertebrae or an erosion of their medial surfaces. Examination of the lateral film may show a similar widening of the canal by erosion of the lamina and the vertebral body. The foramina of emergence of the spinal nerves revealed in oblique views may show enlargement by tumor or constriction by collapse of disk.

Myelography. Intrathecal introduction of 3 to 12 ml. of a radiopaque oil, Pantopaque, followed by fluoroscopy and spot films of the spinal canal, enables one to confirm the clinical suspicion of a significant space-taking intraspinal lesion in the great majority of instances, with the exception of ruptured disks placed far laterally. Not only the site but also the type of the lesion often can be foretold by the character of the filling defects. The fact that one can aspirate the opaque oil back out of the spinal canal makes the pro-

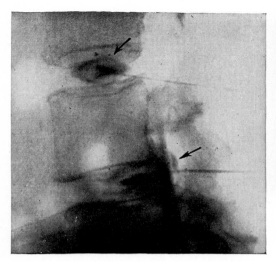

FIG. 50-16. Ruptured intervertebral disk. Diskogram. (*Upper arrow*) Ellipsoidal shadow of Diodrast in normal nucleus pulposus at lumbar 3-4 interspace. (*Lower arrow*) Diodrast shadow in ventral aspect of spinal canal; flow thence through hole in posterior annulus after injection into lumbar 4-5 disk.

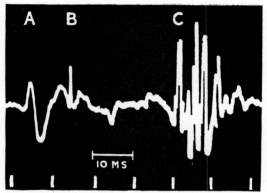

FIG. 50-17. Electromyographic recording from biceps muscle (partial denervation with recovery). (A) Normal motor unit potential. (B) Fibrillation potential. (C) Polyphasic motor unit potential (regeneration). (Richardson, A. T.: Proc. Roy. Soc. Med. *44*:992-994)

cedure almost innocuous. Cisternal puncture and introduction of contrast medium may be used to demonstrate the upper level of a complete block in the spinal canal.

Diskography. Direct injection of the intervertebral disk itself with an absorbable radiopaque agent such as Diodrast is a more recent innovation. Normally, one is able to inject less than 1 cc. of fluid into the substance of the disk inside its confining annulus fibrosus. If more can be injected, the annulus must have ruptured, and roentgenograms will show the site of the tear. The lowest 3 lumbar and the lowest 3 cervical disks are those most commonly studied (Fig. 50-16).

Electromyography. The action potentials in muscles give objective evidence of the functional state of the *lower motor neurons:* (1) for normality in the form of normal motor-unit action potentials (Fig. 50-17 A), (2) for neuronal *degeneration* with excitable tissue present in the form of fibrillation potentials (Fig. 50-17 B), and (3) one of the earliest signs of neuronal *regeneration* in the form of spike and polyphasic motor-unit potentials (Fig. 50-17 C). Thorough exploration by

needle electrodes is required to find the fibrillation potentials in a slightly denervated muscle.

Protrusion of Intervertebral Disks

Most of these lesions occur at one or both of the lowest 2 intervertebral spaces in the spinal column—below the 4th or the 5th lumbar vertebra. Protrusions below lumbar 3, or below the 5th, the 6th or the 7th cervical vertebrae are the next most likely to appear. The syndromes earlier called sciatic and brachial neuritis are now known to have as their commonest cause a posterior protrusion of the intervertebral fibrocartilage into the lateral part of the spinal canal so as to press on the emergent nerve root (Fig. 50-18). Minor or major strain or injury may play a causative role but is often absent from the history.

When one or more lumbar disks are involved, attacks of low back pain with or without relation to acute or chronic strain usually usher in the syndrome. Often bed rest, a tight corset or a back brace relieve the symptoms promptly. In later attacks the pain may start in or spread to the buttock, the posterior thigh and the calf or the foot. Paresthesias and objective hypalgesia or hypesthesia in the anterolateral leg, the medial foot and the great toe, along with a diminished or normal ankle jerk, suggest that the protrusion is at the lumbar 4-5 space, whereas such sensory findings in the posterolateral leg, the lateral foot and the small toes, along with a diminished or absent ankle jerk, point to a protrusion at the L5-S1 level (Fig. 50-15 B). Careful examination may reveal weakness of the dorsiflexors of the toes and of the peronei everting the foot in lesions at either of the 2 lowest disks. Sensory findings in the anterior thigh and the medial leg and a diminished knee jerk may occur in the much less common lesions at L3-4. In lesions at the lower 2 levels, sciatic pain is provoked upon stretching that nerve by straight leg raising from the supine position; the pain is often referred only to the side of protrusion, whichever leg is raised. In lesions at lumbar disks above L4-5, pain in the anterior thigh may be started upon stretching the femoral nerve by extension of the thigh at the hip. Tenderness over or to one side of the spinous processes at the level of the lesion and decreased mobility of the lumbar spine with loss of the lordosis in this region are typical findings.

In the cervical region, an extruding disk causes pain in the back of the neck, radiating into the lateral aspect of an upper limb. Either sudden movements of head and neck or maintenance of a fixed position of these parts may worsen the pain. In the hand and the fingers, numbness and paresthesia occur more often than actual pain. Pressure on the 6th cervical root as it emerges between the 5th and the 6th cervical vertebrae is likely to cause these sensations in the thumb and the 1st meta-

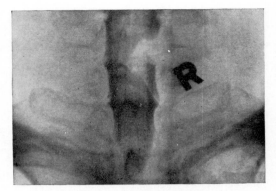

FIG. 50-19. Ruptured intervertebral disk. Cervical myelogram. Protrusion of intervertebral disk at C 6-7 interspace, right side.

carpal area, whereas pressure on the 7th cervical root tends to cause the reference of abnormal sensation mainly to the index and the middle fingers and, to a lesser degree, to the thumb. Objective sensory changes are usually slight, but demonstrable weakness of the biceps or the triceps and decrease in the corresponding tendon reflex occur, respectively, with 6th or 7th root compression (Fig. 50-19). Pressure at the level of the lesion in the back of the neck and just to the painful side of the mid-line may produce local tenderness and radicular pain or paresthesias. The same response may be evoked by the *foraminal compression test,* which consists of tilting the head and the neck to the painful side and pounding the top of the head. Tilting head and neck to the side opposite the lesion may give relief. Multiple disk protrusions, especially in the lumbar region, occur in perhaps 5 to 10 per cent of the patients. Myelography is especially valuable in the dual diagnosis.

Conservative management by bed rest on a firm mattress or with boards beneath the mattress may stop the pain. Appropriate traction may also be used. The wearing of a back or neck brace, depending on the site of the lesion, may permit resumption of full activity. When this is not successful, and particularly when significant weakness is present, surgical removal of the offending disk is advisable. In the lumbar region, one takes away most of the disk inside the lateral and ventral margins of the annulus fibrosus in order to avoid a later recurrent protrusion; in the cervical re-

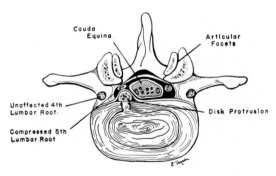

FIG. 50-18. Anatomic relations in protruded intervertebral disk. Superior view of 5th lumbar vertebra. Lesion at lumbar 4-5 interspace. Note that it usually compresses the root emerging one vertebra lower, rather than the one at the same interspace.

gion, excision of the tissue between the vertebral bodies is less necessary. In the presence of a frank posterior protrusion or rupture, the yield of such surgery is a grateful patient after 80 to 95 per cent of the procedures, which have become by far the commonest of neurosurgery. However, the proliferation of surgeons in this country interested in performing this operation has exceeded the supply of patients requiring such treatment—to the detriment both of the patients and the profession. In certain patients a "fusion" or insertion of bone grafts between the lumbar vertebral bodies or behind the laminae is required to strengthen the spine.

In the neck, the protruding disk may lie more medially as well and press against the spinal cord, giving far more serious long tract symptoms and signs resembling those of cord tumors. A similar syndrome may result from multiple osteoarthritic bars at the level of several cervical disks, a cervical spondylosis, which typically yields the picture of slow degeneration of the upper motor neurons with little or no sensory loss. This is often mistaken for degenerative disease such as amyotrophic lateral sclerosis. A decompressive laminectomy and division of the dentate ligaments which anchor the cord to the inner surface of the dura may suffice to control the symptoms, or the more hazardous curetting away of the bars from ventral to the cord may be necessary. In some patients, centrally placed bars may combine with lateral protrusions to produce weak, stiff legs along with pain and paresthesias in one or both arms (Fig. 50-20 A, B and C). The rare thoracic disk protrusions usually are not diagnosed until the cord is compressed.

Neoplasms

New growths in the spinal canal may arise primarily from any of the neural or mesodermal tissues in the neighborhood or may present secondarily after origin elsewhere. The metastatic or multiple tumors are almost always extradural, and, as would be expected, the symptoms they provoke progress rapidly. Despite their poor eventual prognosis, useful palliation is often achieved by prompt removal of laminae and the readily excisable tumor. The disconcerting speed with which a slight weakness becomes a paralysis means that

many of these patients, including those with curable maladies, often must receive emergency operations if they are not to end their days with paralyzed legs, bowels and bladder. Of the remaining intradural tumors, about two thirds are happily benign and lie outside the cord, i.e., are extramedullary. The overwhelming majority grow either from a nerve rootlet as neurofibromas or from the meninges as meningiomas. Even when their slow compression has greatly deformed the cord before they are completely removed, gradual full recovery is still a probability. The intramedullary tumors, on the other hand, are only rarely susceptible of total removal. They are, though, often cystic and slow growing; drainage of the cyst or a longitudinal incision in the cord over the tumor permitting it to extrude or grow outside the cord may purchase a surprisingly protracted relief of symptoms. The same is true of that cystic disease in the spinal cord called syringomyelia.

In children the commonest cord tumors are those arising from congenital rests and range in histologic complexity from dermoids to teratomas. Congenital bony malformations or extensive erosions often accompany them. Although they may be so attached to the cord that only subtotal removal is feasible, again a prolonged satisfactory result may be obtained. In general, in childhood the difficulty in eliciting symptoms and signs of intraspinal disease makes advisable a prompt resort to lumbar puncture as well as plain and myelographic roentgenograms of the whole spine whenever a space-taking mass is faintly suspected. Many children incubate their spinal tumors to massive proportions while being treated for their "infantile paralysis."

Abscesses

Infection in the spinal canal is usually secondary to a source elsewhere in the body and is usually in the epidural space, a locus favorable for drainage. Exceedingly prompt institution of such drainage via extensive laminectomy is vital to success, and any patient with infection elsewhere who develops severe pain plus local tenderness and rigidity in the back should be operated on at the slightest confirmatory sign on neurologic examination, lumbar puncture or myelography. A flaccid paraplegia may develop in less than

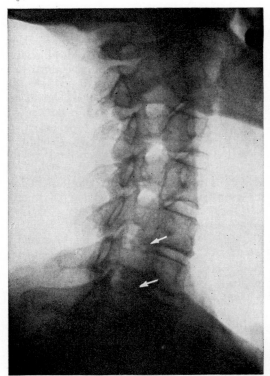

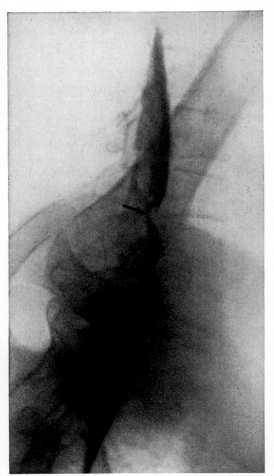

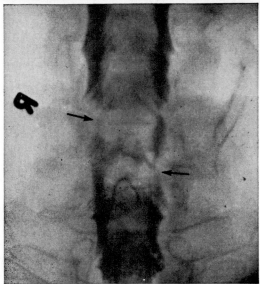

and to right at C 5-6, in mid-line and to left at C 6-7. (C, *Right*) Cervical myelogram, lateral view. Patient's arm alongside head. Arrows point to transverse bars encroaching on spinal canal at C 5-6 and C 6-7, confirming impression from plain films. Patient: 67-year-old male with severe pain in left arm and forearm; paresthesias in left index finger; moderately weak, stiff legs.

FIG. 50-20. (A, *Left, top*) Cervical spondylosis. Lateral roentgenogram, cervical spine. Arrows point to enostoses into ventral aspect of spinal canal at narrowed interspaces C 5-6 and C 6-7. (B, *Left, bottom*) Cervical myelogram, sagittal view. Arrows point to filling defects in mid-line

24 hours and once present will shortly prove to be irreversible.

Traumatic Disorders

The cervical spine and cord are particularly likely to be impaired in diving accidents and in the whiplash movements of the head and the neck that occur in many automobile accidents. A fracture or a fracture-dislocation may take place, at times with spontaneous return of the cervical vertebrae to normal position after delivery of a blow to the cord. When weakness or sensory loss abruptly follows an injury to the neck, the patient should be transported with maximal caution, utilizing traction applied to the long axis of the neck by pulling manually or via a halter applied to chin and occiput.

As soon as thorough roentgenograms have indicated the site of the lesion, it may be reduced or maintained in reduction by the amazingly comfortable maneuver of skeletal traction. This consists of placing a pair of metal tongs in the skull on each side just above and in front of the ears and applying a weight of 2 to 15 Kg. to these. The larger thoracic and lumbar vertebrae tend to hold their post-traumatic positions, and these patients may be transported with a pillow under the lumbar spine or in the prone position. In order to avoid further injury, it is vital to avoid flexion of the lumbar vertebrae.

The following are the unequivocal indications for surgical exploration: (1) worsening of the neurologic deficit after injury; (2) a partial or complete block of CSF indicated by the Queckenstedt test of bilateral jugular compression or seen at myelography; (3) a penetrating wound of the spine; (4) bony or foreign fragments within the spinal canal; (5) persistent gross dislocation of bone despite skull or other traction or hyperextension. Other indications are less clear-cut. A peculiarly dangerous injury is a fracture at the base of the odontoid process, often demonstrable only by roentgenograms through the open mouth. The only complaint may be of pain, tenderness and stiffness in the back of the neck, but a later sharp movement of the head may permit vertebral movements with fatal crushing of the upper cervical cord. Immediate skull traction and operative posterior bony fusion at this level are necessary to forestall this catastrophe.

Even when a total transverse lesion of the spinal cord persists despite early treatment, remarkable rehabilitation of the patient is still feasible. Vigilant medical and nursing care is required to avoid bedsores and to keep infection of the urinary tract at a minimum. Involuntary muscle spasms may be such a problem that extensive anterior rhizotomy, e.g.,

T11 through S1 roots on both sides, may be needed before the patient can even sit in a chair. Tenotomies, peripheral neurectomies or more limited rhizotomies may suffice when spasm is less extensive. Incredible though it may seem, a person with paralyzed legs can learn to walk with crutches and braces which keep the legs straight and permit them to bear weight. Development of mighty muscles in the shoulder girdle is prerequisite to this achievement.

Vascular Malformations

A fascinating variety of such anomalies occurs within the spinal canal. When a spontaneous subarachnoid hemorrhage is superimposed on the clinical picture of a cord lesion or when the myelogram reveals large tortuous vessels, this diagnosis may be ventured preoperatively. Decompression of such lesions, clipping of the feeding arteries or, rarely, total removal may be utilized in treatment.

Congenital Malformations

Spina Bifida. Failure of the posterior vertebral bony arch to close may have no other abnormal accompaniment and occurs at the first sacral vertebra in about 25 per cent of otherwise normal people. But if signs or symptoms in legs, bowel or bladder coming on in childhood are accompanied by a *spina bifida occulta,* shown in the x-ray film, operation may disclose a lipoma or a stalk of tissue whose removal will help the patient. If the defect is larger, a dural sac may protrude back through it, reaching the surface as a flat membrane or, more commonly, blossoming out as a posterior mass called a *meningocoele.*

If the sac contains spinal cord or nerves, i.e., is a *myelomeningocoele,* there will be weakness, sensory loss and sphincteric disturbance, whose degree will depend on the extent of malformation. Three fourths of these lesions are in the lumbar and/or the sacral areas; the remainder are more rostral. Most neurosurgeons feel that a baby born with such a lesion and with paralyzed legs should not be operated upon. When the dismal spectacle of termination of cord and nerve roots in the wall of the sac is seen, surgical repair can accomplish nothing.

In less severe lesions, after such surgical

repair as may be done one must follow the baby carefully for signs of hydrocephalus. If this develops, the Arnold-Chiari malformation is almost certainly the cause and should be treated promptly by suboccipital craniectomy and upper cervical laminectomy, followed by a shunting operation should the decompression be ineffective in controlling the hydrocephalus.

Congenital Dermal Sinuses. A tract of persisting stratified squamous epithelium may project inward from the skin along the midline anywhere from sacrum to skull. At the skin one may see only a tiny dimple, or there may be dermal thickening, pigmentation or red coloration, and hairs may protrude from the opening. These tracts often extend to the brain or the cord and may be accompanied by small dermoid tumors beneath the skin and/or at their neural end. Roentgenographs may or may not reveal a bifid spine or the tiny hole in the occipital bone by which the tracts reach the interior. Their special importance arises from the fact that they may conduct infection from the surface to the meninges, and a fulminant meningitis may ensue, destroying a significant part of the patient's nervous system. These tracts should be recognized and removed completely along with any associated tumors, if possible before meningitis develops —and certainly after meningitis has helped draw attention to their presence.

Diastematomyelia. This lesion, whose embryologic basis is obscure, consists of a bony spike projecting backward from a vertebral body into the middle of the spinal canal and dividing the spinal cord or the cauda equina into halves. Cutaneous accompaniments in the mid-line of the back at the level of the lesion are similar to those seen with congenital dermal sinuses. Major neurologic deficits may be arrested or improved by removing the offending spicule. This may be seen in roentgenographs anywhere in the thoracic or the lumbar region.

DISEASES AFFECTING THE PERIPHERAL NERVOUS SYSTEM

The principal intrinsic lesions of the peripheral nerves arise as a consequence of trauma or as neoplasms. Extrinsic pressure against the nerves also produces local disease.

INTRINSIC DISEASE

A vast number of peripheral nerve injuries occurs in wartime, largely from wounds by missiles; it is from the study of collected experiences of the two World Wars that we base our management of these lesions. From such studies has come the realization that the primary task in restoring an injured limb to action devolves around providing optimal conditions for regeneration of the nerve. Adequate repair of other soft tissues, vascular injury and the shattered bones usually is carried out at a preliminary operation, and the nerve is sutured a month later when swelling and infection have subsided.

The rarity with which peripheral nerve injuries occur in peace time, the ease with which such injury can be recognized by a decent examination, the variation from person to person in distribution of any normal nerve, and a lack of grave urgency about definitive repair make it unnecessary to treat the subject in detail in a general text. Even in a clean cut or a stab wound of a nerve in which a prompt end-to-end suture may be feasible and advisable, there is ample time for the operator to consult detailed anatomic and surgical texts regarding the nerve in question before performing the operation. Such a practice would result in fewer sutures of a severed median or ulnar nerve to a tendon, for instance, in the course of repairing a wrist laceration by capable surgeons of broad general experience.

Birth or other traumata, in which the brachial plexus is stretched unduly, may result in actual avulsion of the nerve roots from the spinal cord, often demonstrable by myelography, the contrast medium showing an abnormal configuration. The complex possibilities in any injury of the brachial plexus make it essential to study each case in detail. As knowledge in the domain of medicine increases, it becomes progressively more imperative to select fields of information in which the student need keep very few facts constantly in mind. Peripheral nerve injuries belong in this category.

Many tumors in peripheral nerves are benign neurofibromas, which may cause local pain and tenderness. The pain radiates into the distribution of the nerve on local pressure or may be confined to the site of the pressure. Later a sensory or motor loss may develop. Even when no tumor is palpable through the skin, local exploration may reveal a neurofibroma whose removal may well be possible without division of the fibers of the nerve trunk. Occasionally, some of the many neurofibromata seen in von Recklinghausen's disease may become painful and require removal. Malignant tumors of peripheral nerves are happily an extreme rarity.

EXTRINSIC DISEASE

Only 2 examples will be given of conditions in which extrinsic pressure against peripheral nerves occurs. The *syndrome of the scalenus anterior* arises as a consequence of pinching of the lower trunk of the brachial plexus and/or the subclavian artery as they cross above the first rib between the anterior scalene muscle in front and some firm structure behind. This latter may be a bony cervical rib or other osseous anomaly visible in a roentgenograph or may be a tendinous structure or cartilaginous rib which cannot thus be visualized. Symptoms tend to come on in early adult years because of the descent at puberty of the shoulder girdle with respect to the thorax. This occurs more markedly in women, who develop the disorder more frequently. Local tenderness may be present lateral to the sternocleidomastoid just above the clavicle. Pain, paresthesias, numbness and objective sensory loss to pin, touch or temperature develop along the ulnar aspect of arm, forearm, hand or fingers, the distribution of much of the medial cord of the brachial plexus arising from the anterior primary divisions of the 8th cervical and the 1st thoracic nerves. Symptoms may be exacerbated upon stretching the plexus by forcibly snapping the head away from the shoulder while pulling downward on the arm. Atrophy and weakness may appear, especially in the intrinsic muscles of the hand supplied by the ulnar nerve. Compression of the subclavian artery by the lesion may cause generalized weakness of the limb, blanching of fingers, and a low brachial blood pressure, worsened by elevation of the arm. Progression of symptoms may necessitate thorough operative exploration and removal of the offending structures

Late ulnar neuritis may occur months or years following a severe injury at the elbow or upon repeated minor traumata to the ulnar nerve at the olecranon groove, particularly when the nerve slips over the epicondyle each time the elbow is flexed. Symptoms are similar to those in the preceding syndrome, but the zone of focal tenderness is at the olecranon groove. There is no sensory loss above the hypothenar eminence, no worsening of the symptoms on elevation of the arm and no evidence of arterial compression. Transplantation of the ulnar nerve to a position anterior to the medial condyle of the humerus but deep to the muscles arising therefrom is the treatment of choice.

NEUROSURGICAL OPERATIONS ON NORMAL TISSUES TO RELIEVE DISEASE ELSEWHERE

Tissues which are presumed to be normal may be sacrificed in order to improve symptoms in an increasing variety of situations. These include the relief of (1) pain, (2) psychiatric symptoms, (3) involuntary movements, (4) Ménière's syndrome, (5) malignant disease, and (6) diabetic retinopathy. Such a sacrifice of tissue in some of the procedures to treat hydrocephalus has been discussed already.

PAIN

The earliest operations of this sort were those for the treatment of pain of unknown or incurable etiology. Often the full extent of the pain pathways involved in any particular case is unclear, and in such a situation it is good practice to utilize for diagnosis or even treatment procaine or, in selected sites, alcohol block of the nervous pathways under suspicion.

Peripheral Neurotomy. Denervation of the area of reference of pain was first tried by *interruption of impulses in the peripheral nerves thereto.* Since most peripheral nerves have a major motor component and are capable of sensory regeneration, division of such nerves has practical value in only 2 common problems: (1) In the treatment of pain confined to the foot or a finger, such as one sees in some vascular occlusive disorders. Crushing of digital nerves to a finger or of the superficial and the deep peroneal and tibial nerves a few inches above the ankle knocks out no consequential motor fibers. By the time the sensation has returned, peripheral collateral circulation may be adequate to preclude pain. (2) In the treatment of trigeminal neuralgia. In the peripheral divisions of this nerve, the sensory branches take a course different from the masticator branch, and avul-

sion or alcohol injection of them is a simple and at times desirable maneuver.

Cranial Posterior Rhizotomy. This was historically the next operation tried and remains the sovereign tactic in the treatment of idiopathic *trigeminal, nervus intermedius, glossopharyngeal and upper vagal neuralgias* (Fig. 50-21, Nos. 2 and 3). In these disorders,

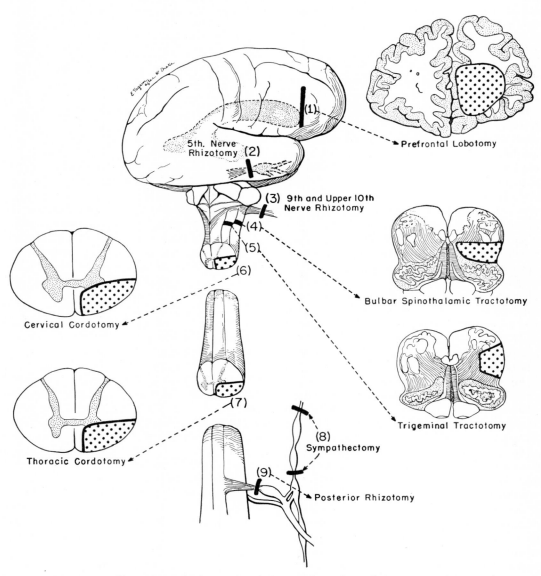

FIG. 50-21. Sites of standard neurosurgical procedures for relief of pain. The 9th, the 10th, and the 11th nerves leave the brain stem along a line dorsal to which lies the descending trigeminal tract (incision 5) and ventral to which lies the crossed pain pathway from the limbs and the torso (incision 4).

the patient has pain with most or all of the following characteristics: (1) it is *paroxysmal*, lasting seconds to a few minutes; (2) it is *provoked by obvious stimuli* to the face, the ear or the pharynx; (3) it is confined to the zone of the affected nerve; (4) in any one paroxysm it is unilateral; (5) it is accompanied by no objective sensory loss on routine clinical testing. The paroxysms tend to come in cycles, each lasting several weeks or months. When the trigeminal zone is afflicted, the reference of pain is to some part of the face or the mouth; when nervus intermedius, gossopharyngeal or upper vagal fibers are concerned, the paroxysms start in the throat or deep in the ear. After a cutting of all posterior root fibers, which provokes anesthesia to touch and temperature as well as pain, the denervated zone after trigeminal rhizotomy exhibits a major degree of constant peculiar unpleasant sensation in about 4 per cent of patients. With the exception of this group and the < 2 per cent who die after operation, the procedure nearly always affords gratifying and permanent relief of pain which often had previously attained such agonizing intensity that the patient lived in terror of the next attack. Idiopathic facial pains without the above-described features, "atypical facial neuralgias," especially when there are continuous pains unaffected by external stimuli, are unlikely to be relieved by section of trigeminal rootlets, and if this is done the postoperative paresthesias tend to be more exasperating to the sufferer.

For the control of pain associated with cephalic or facial tumors, single or multiple cranial posterior rhizotomies may be needed, at times in combination with the operation to be discussed next.

Spinal Posterior Rhizotomy. Cutting of the upper cervical posterior roots (Fig. 50-21, No. 9) often stops pain in the neck or the occiput caused by malignant tumors or trauma to the roots emerging from the spinal canal. It may be efficacious in a few other situations in which one or only a few roots are specifically involved in the disorder. In general, however, spinal posterior rhizotomy has been disappointingly inadequate, partly because of the remarkable overlap in the innervation of any zone by nerves from several somatic segments and partly because other pain fibers travel with the sympathetic nerves and enter the spinal cord many segments away from those which enter the cord directly.

Intrathecal Injection of Destructive Chemicals. Injection of alcohol into the subarachnoid space has proved to be so poorly controllable that it is now used only in patients with malignant tumors to stop pain in the saddle area and the upper sacral dermatomes when rectal and vesical sphincters have already lost their function. Then the simple maneuver of injection into the most caudal part of the subarachnoid space with the patient prone and his buttocks elevated will result in a rise of the absolute alcohol to the top of the CSF column around the sacral rootlets, usually with immediate relief of pain here for the remaining months of the patient's life.

Recently, a method has been found to combine the use of intrathecal injection with the control afforded by fluoroscopy. Phenol, which dissolves in the radiopaque oil, Pantopaque, is injected in such solution under fluoroscopic observation and the patient promptly tilted so that the fluid is placed in a layer over those thoracic, lumbar, or sacral rootlets likely to be conducting the undesired pain impulses. The phenol moves briskly from its Pantopaque and becomes fixed within a few minutes in the nerves it is bathing. Half an hour later some or all of the Pantopaque can be removed. Useful relief is afforded in perhaps half of the patients.

Sympathectomy. This (Fig. 50-21, No. 8) is usually effective when denervation is needed in the control of pain arising exclusively from certain abdominal viscera, from the heart, and from the limbs in the conditions called causalgia and sympathetic dystrophy. A small number of painful disorders associated with *disease confined to the biliary tree, the small intestine, the kidney and the pancreas* are managed most satisfactorily by splanchnicectomy. As shown by White, there is also a small fraction of the patients with *angina pectoris* in whom an alcohol block or surgical excision of the upper 3 or 4 thoracic sympathetic ganglia on one or both sides may be needed to stop otherwise intractable attacks of such pain. *Causalgia* may develop after a penetrating wound or other trauma which produces a partial injury of a peripheral nerve. A peculiar burning pain spreads to involve much of the whole affected limb, rather than being limited to the area of any one nerve; the patient tends to immobilize the whole extremity. A thin, shiny, smooth skin and long, uncut nails develop; there may be excessive sweating along with abnormal coolness and whiteness or heat and redness of the part. The touch of clothing, winter's cold and summer's heat, any emotional upset, even casual activity of others nearby, may provoke unbearable pain, and the patient may become a motionless recluse. A similar but less spectacular picture infrequently ensues after trauma, infection or arthritis in any portion of a limb. Sudomotor, vasomotor and trophic changes may be accompanied by a patchy osteoporosis which is most striking in roentgenographs of the affected hand or foot (Sudeck's atrophy). This picture, often called a "sympathetic dystrophy," is, like causalgia, dramatically amenable to change for the better upon repeated paravertebral chemical blocks of the sympathetic ganglia supplying the affected limb. Sympathectomy is often required to achieve a permanent cure.

Bulbar Trigeminal Tractotomy. After *the primary afferent neurons* enter the central neuraxis, those for pain and temperature split away from those for other sensory modalities. The pain and temperature fibers entering with the trigeminal, nervus intermedius, glossopharyngeal and upper vagal rootlets all move caudally in a bundle which becomes superficial in the lower medulla, the so-called descending trigeminal tract (Fig. 50-21, No. 5). This conveniently contains the pain fibers from the whole head on the ipsilateral side, and its division does not destroy the sense of touch. Hence, such an operation is of particular value when one must denervate the 1st trigeminal division in neuralgia, yet wishes to leave the protective afferent component of the corneal reflex arc intact. Preservation of the sense of touch to the cornea accomplishes this. Touch must also be left intact over at least some of the lower face when bilateral trigeminal neuralgia occurs in order to permit the patient to know the position of food in his mouth; otherwise he cannot eat effectively. The agonizing pain associated with inoperable malignant tumors of the face or the head may also be treated by a bulbar tractotomy of this sort, or one may divide the rootlets of

all the nerves concerned with faciocephalic pain as they enter the pons and the medulla.

Cordotomy. One of the most satisfactory of all of the procedures for relief of pain is a cordotomy, in which one incises the cord so as to divide the pain and temperature fibers of *the secondary afferent neuron* on their way to the brain. These fibers arise in the posterior horn of spinal gray matter, usually cross within 1 to 6 segments to the opposite side, where they ascend in the anterolateral and the anterior white matter. The pain fibers traveling with the sympathetic and those with the somatic nerves both converge into this area. This happy dispensation permits a single simple incision into the cord on one side to provide relief of nearly all types of pain referred to the opposite side of the body anywhere up to 5 or 6 segments below the level of the incision. If the pain is bilateral or is soon likely to be so because of a malignant midline tumor, one may make the incisions bilaterally, usually separating them by a few centimeters.

Upper thoracic incisions (Fig. 50-21, No. 7) are commonly used for pain below the costal margin; upper cervical incisions, just caudal to the decussation of the pyramids (Fig. 50-21, No. 6), are required if pain is in the chest or arm. Bilateral thoracic incisions are followed occasionally by persisting urinary retention or incontinence or by weakness in a leg. Even when such annoying sequelae appear, the patient may consider them a small price to pay for relief from the relentless misery provoked by an advancing cancer.

Incurable neoplasms are the usual cause of pain sufficiently diffuse and severe to require cordotomy; recourse to this operation is advisable as soon as direct attack on the lesion by surgical, radiation or chemical therapy can no longer control the pain, and before addiction to Demerol or other habit-forming analgesics depletes still further the patient's reserves.

Other disorders in which pain in limbs or torso may lead to cordotomy, often followed by success, are: (1) neuralgias seen with amputation stumps, phantom limbs, after peripheral nerve injuries, other trauma or surgery and after herpes zoster; (2) intraspinal lesions such as tabes dorsalis (causing tabetic crises), chronic arachnoiditis or trauma to cauda equina. Lesions of the cord itself are less likely to be relieved by cordotomy at a higher level.

Tractotomy in Medulla or Mesencephalon. The crossed pathway for pain and temperature may also be conveniently cut in the medulla (Fig. 50-21, No. 4) or in the upper midbrain. An electrode transmitting power at radiofrequencies may be inserted into the exposed brain stem to achieve the same objective. The bulbar operation has fewer disadvantages than the one in the mesencephalon and finds its chief use in patients whose extensive cancer is causing pain which extends into middle or upper cervical segments.

Thalamotomy. Stereotactic methods discussed below under "Involuntary Movements" are being used to guide the placement of electrical lesions in the terminal nuclei of afferent pathways lying in the posterior and the ventral portions of the thalamus, or in the fibers converging thereon as they lie in the midbrain, or in the dorsomedial thalamic nuclei. Although a number of patients have been relieved of pain, the tactic is still experimental.

Frontal Lobotomy. The foregoing procedures have as their objective the blocking of impulses for pain before they reach the sentient areas in the brain. Another procedure, frontal lobotomy, also may eliminate suffering, not only that due to activity of specific pain fibers but also that on a psychological basis. Division of some of the frontal cerebral white matter in the coronal plane at the anterior tip of the lateral ventricles (Fig. 50-21, No. 1) produces a state in which the individual is aware of his pain but disregards it, no longer complains about it or requests medication. Cutting too many of the frontal white fibers produces an undesirable state of mental apathy; cutting too few gives inadequate relief of pain. A pair of small lesions in each frontal lobe or a complete division of white fibers on one side may be made initially. If this is inadequate, or its originally satisfactory effect wears off, the area of destruction may be enlarged. The simplest way to achieve and later to increase a fractional lobotomy is by means of the radiofrequency electrode technic. After the initial making of small openings in the frontal skull and the meninges, the next and any necessary later stages are carried out in the radiologic suite, involving only free-

hand placement of the small electrodes with radiologic control of their positions. Not only widespread organic pain referred to any part of the patient but also mental anguish as a consequence of other symptoms and signs such as disfiguring malignant ulcers or fear of imminent death may be effectively assuaged thereby.

PSYCHIATRIC SYMPTOMS

Akin to the relief of the psychological suffering in organic disease is the relief of tension in some functional psychiatric disorders afforded by frontal lobotomy (Fig. 50-21, No. 1). Although originally proposed for this purpose and used effectively for disorders ranging in severity from obsessive compulsive neuroses to schizophrenia, frontal lobotomy's useful effects are usually reproduced, at least in the major psychoses, by the drugs chlorpromazine or reserpine. At present the operation is less often used in the management of psychiatric patients. More extensive or more posterior incisions, detaching more of the frontal tips from association with the brain, are required for the more severe psychoses.

INVOLUNTARY MOVEMENTS

In a variety of neurologic disorders characterized by nearly constant undesired movements in the waking state, destruction of various portions of the brain has been carried out in an effort to stop the distressing tremor or other less rhythmic activity while preserving voluntary power and co-ordination. These efforts have culminated in the demonstration that relatively small lesions of volume 1.0 to 1.5 cc. in the neighborhood of the medial globus pallidus or of a lesser size in the lateral thalamus are likely to produce gratifying relief in a number of these disorders. Lesions in some of the adjoining fibers of the internal capsule may play an as yet undetermined role in the beneficial effects which ensue. However, in nearly all the successful cases there is no weakness, spasticity, or abnormality of reflexes in the limbs. More recently, surgical lesions in the substantia nigra have also proved to be efficacious. In the commonest of these disorders, parkinsonism, major incapacitating features are the cogwheel or lead-pipe type of rigidity and a tremor, usually worst at rest. Both of these manifestations disappear or revert markedly toward normal on one side in over three fourths of patients following the placement of one of the above-mentioned lesions in the opposite side of the brain. The severely handicapped individual welcomes the effective use of half his limbs, and the patient with unilateral affliction resumes normal mobility. Other phenomena seen in some patients with the disorder such as extreme paucity of movement when rigidity is small or absent, a feeble speaking voice, and autonomic hyperactivity are not affected favorably. If mental deterioration is present, it may be worsened following operation. Those with cerebral atrophy or of advanced years are poor candidates; hence, careful preoperative study and selection of patients are important. After a substantial interval, presently many months rather than weeks, the opposite side of the brain is being attacked in the common bilaterally affected patient.

Other less frequent types of involuntary movement in which surgery has a high degree of success are the intention tremors seen in such disorders as multiple sclerosis and cerebellar degenerative disease. The utterly incapacitating twisting movements of body and trunk in dystonia musculorum deformans and the violent, exhausting movements of hemiballismus have signally subsided with this type of surgery, and such patients have enjoyed some of the most spectacular returns from bed-ridden incapacitation to almost unfettered productivity. The tremor of Huntington's chorea and the disability of spasmodic torticollis have yielded to this therapy in some cases; the place of surgery here is still undecided. On the other hand, the choreoathetotic movements of cerebral palsy have tended to persist.

Technics for finding the precise site at which to make the lesion as well as the tactic for producing and controlling the destruction are still evolving but have attained great safety. In fact, the lack of more postmortem confirmation of the site of effective and inefficient lesions is holding up progress in the field, even though several thousand such operations have now been performed in the active centers concerned. New "stereotactic" methods have been developed for placing the device producing the lesion at the desired point in the depth of the brain. Most of the pioneers —Myers, Speigel and Wycis, Leksell, Riechert, Talairach and others—have used precision placement almost to the desired cubic millimeter in relation to specific points in the wall of the third ventricle, such as the anterior and the posterior commissures. The definitive lesion is made via electrodes usually passing a radiofrequency current. Cooper with great originality has sought to make a trial lesion by brisk but less precise placement of a balloon cannula which he inflates with $\frac{1}{4}$ to $\frac{1}{2}$ ml. of sodium diatrizoate. If the desired degree of improvement is not achieved, he deflates the balloon and tries it in a new position. His permanent lesion is made by instillation of alcohol in cellulose into the cavity left by deflation of the balloon.

Knowledge of the neurophysiologic basis of normal movement in man, not to mention that of the neuropathologic basis of abnormal movements, is still fragmentary. The study of these deeper-seated mechanisms during therapeutic procedures in man is in its infancy.

Ménière's Syndrome

In this disorder, abrupt attacks of severe nausea, vomiting and vertigo are superimposed upon a continuous and progressive deafness and tinnitus in one ear. The second ear becomes affected in 10 to 20 per cent of the patients. The pathologic lesion includes a dilation of the endolymphatic system of the inner ear with a hydrops of the vestibular and cochlear labyrinth. Loudness recruitment is demonstrable when hearing is tested, and caloric stimulation of the affected ear yields diminished responses of vertigo, nystagmus and past pointing. When the vertiginous attacks are incapacitating and uncontrolled by medical treatment, cutting of the auditory nerve will permanently stop them in over 90 per cent of the patients. Oddly enough, division of the whole nerve, including the cochlear fibers, relieves the tinnitus of only one third of the group. When the vestibular fibers alone are sectioned, the same likelihood of relief of vertigo continues, and usable hearing is preserved in 40 per cent of the patients, at the price of an operative mortality of 1 per cent and a permanent facial paralysis in 2 per cent. In view of the chance that bilateral disease will develop, the differential neurotomy to preserve the hearing is often considered preferable to total section of the nerve or to destruction of the labyrinth.

MALIGNANT DISEASE

Total hypophysectomy is one of the procedures used to deprive the body of its normal hormones in an effort to arrest a cancer. The only tumors thus far favorably affected are cancers of the breast and possibly of the prostate. Using transfrontal operations for direct surgical removal of the gland Olivecrona and Ray in two independent series have achieved objective evidence of remission in about 50 per cent of their patients. Destruction of the pituitary gland by transphenoidal instillation of a beta-emitting isotope has in two centers yielded a less complete destruction of the gland and a lower rate of remission. In a third series of Forrest, in which a more precise placement of the beta-emitting yttrium has destroyed the gland, the results have been marred by a CSF rhinorrhea and consequent meningitis with some fatalities. Lawrence and Tobias have perfected use of a high-energy proton beam to concentrate 25,000 to 30,000 rad in the sella turcica, producing gradual destruction of the gland over several months with inconsequential side-effects and no mortality.

All of these forms of hypophysectomy are both less hazardous and less annoying to the patient than bilateral adrenalectomy. Patients whose cancers have been affected favorably by hormonal treatment or ovariectomy are particularly likely to have another remission after hypophysectomy.

This operation or section of the pituitary stalk will also by an unknown mechanism stop the hemorrhages which destroy vision in diabetic retinopathy.

DISEASES AFFECTING THE AUTONOMIC NERVOUS SYSTEM

Neurosurgical procedures on this portion of the nervous system might well have been discussed fully under the previous heading of operations on normal structures, since there is essentially no evidence that the parasympathetic or sympathetic nerves divided are themselves abnormal. We have already considered the place of sympathectomy in the treatment of pain. In the disorders next to be discussed, as in the problems connected with pain, preliminary anesthetic blocking of the sympathetic fibers is often a valuable diagnostic procedure. A favorable response makes both the surgeon and his patient more confident of the effectiveness of the proposed denervation.

PARASYMPATHETIC SYSTEM

Cranial Parasympathectomy. The only operation of established value in this area to be discussed is *denervation of the carotid sinus* in certain patients with a hypersensitive reflex arising from this structure. Such individuals on even minor movements of the head or the neck or mild pressure over the region of the bifurcation of the common carotid artery may have one of the following: (1) bradycardia or asystole, (2) arterial hypotension, (3) cerebrally induced syncope or seizures, or (4) any combination of the foregoing. No treatment except surgical denervation is effective in eliminating epileptic seizures of sinus origin. Atropine may prevent slowing of the heart rate, and vasoconstrictor agents may preclude a fall in blood pressure, but when medical management is ineffective, denervation of the afferent pathway of the hyperactive reflex arc is likely to stop the symptoms. To assure removal of the sinus nerve of Hering, the sensory portion of the reflex arc, one decorticates the common, external and internal carotid arteries for 2 cm. above and below the carotid sinus at the arterial bifurcation.

For the results of vagal denervation in the treatment of peptic ulcer see Chapter 29.

Sacral Parasympathectomy. In lesions of the spinal cord producing paraplegia, the spasm of the bladder neck which produces urinary retention may require relief by division of parasympathetic fibers to the bladder as they travel in the 2nd, the 3rd and/or the 4th pairs of sacral nerves. Thorough but unsuccessful conservative efforts to restore an "automatic bladder" and demonstration of ability to void after sacral foraminal nerve block are indispensable prerequisites to this operation.

SYMPATHETIC SYSTEM

The dividing of sudomotor and vasoconstrictor fibers which occurs in sympathectomy may control the symptoms of a number of disorders.

Hyperhidrosis. A rare individual has such an extreme tendency to sweat in the palms and the fingers or in the feet that he soon soaks whatever he touches or wears and finds himself under a major social or professional handicap. Effective denervation is provided by removal of the 2nd and the 3rd thoracic sympathetic ganglia for the upper limb and of the 3rd and the 4th lumbar sympathetic ganglia for the lower limb. The long-term results are excellent, since the regeneration of sudomotor fibers does not reach a troublesome degree.

Raynaud's Disease. In this peripheral vascular disorder, there occur episodes of tonic contraction of the smaller arteries in the limbs. Exposure to cold and emotional stimuli are the main precipitants that evoke coldness, cyanosis and at times pain in fingers or toes, often in symmetrical areas on the 2 sides. A white asphyxia of the parts supervenes when the vasoconstriction is maximal and is succeeded by redness and painful tingling on rewarming. In between these episodes of phasic color change, the hands may be constantly cold and clammy with sweat. When the disorder is severe and chronic, the tips of the phalanges may develop dry ulcers, the skin of the digits may become shiny, hard and smooth, and the bone of the terminal phalanges be decalcified. Peripheral pulses in the main arteries of the limbs remain excellent because the abnormal constriction is distal to them. When, as is usual, vasodilator drugs fail to control the symptoms, sympathetic denervation is likely to provide excellent relief if the feet are affected. When the hands are involved, the early result is usually good, but a late return of the trouble has plagued most of the patients despite a variety of maneuvers to secure complete sympathetic denervation and prevent regeneration.

In *acrocyanosis* the peripheral vasoconstriction tends to be present constantly. Otherwise, the disorder resembles Raynaud's disease in signs and treatment.

Occlusive Disease of Major Peripheral Vessels. The ischemia caused by thromboangiitis obliterans, arteriosclerosis, laceration, embolic occlusion or ligation of the main arteries has been partially relieved in past years by appropriate sympathectomy which opens the collateral channels. Direct arterial grafting has now replaced the simpler operation of

denervation in all but the poorest risk patients.

Paralysis of Legs with Ischemia. Both in anterior poliomyelitis involving the lower motor neuron and in other lesions of the cord involving the upper motor neuron a paralysis of one or both legs may be accompanied by gross impairment of circulation in the involved limb. Sympathectomy not only relieves the circulatory insufficiency but in children is followed by an accelerated growth rate in the abnormally short, cyanotic limb. In order to secure a maximal effect, the 3 upper lumbar ganglia must be removed, which brings the vasoconstrictor paralysis up to midthigh.

Vascular Hypertension. Although neurogenic vasoconstriction does not appear to be the cause of the elevated systolic and diastolic blood pressure in "essential" hypertension, often these pressures will be lowered by extensive bilateral sympathectomy. Decreased vasoconstrictor tonus at rest and a reduction in neurovascular constrictor reflexes upon psychologic and physiologic stimuli may be responsible for dropping the pressure, and denervation of adrenals and kidneys may eliminate humoral vasoconstrictor agents. In the decade of the forties before adequate nontoxic vasodilator drugs became available, extensive sympathectomy, including splanchnicectomy, was given a thorough trial in patients with the mildest to the severest forms of the disease. The patients may be grouped according to the severity of changes in the optic fundi, those with hemorrhages and/or exudates in addition to visible retinal arterial disease falling in Group 3 and those with measurable papilledema as well being placed in Group 4. On the pre-1940 medical treatment, about 80 per cent of those in Group 3 and 99 per cent of those in Group 4 were dead within 5 years. The comparable mortality 5 years after extensive sympathectomy was around 40 per cent and 55 per cent, respectively, in these 2 groups, so that the life-saving effect of operation was unequivocally shown. Symptomatic improvement occurred in the vast majority, 85 per cent of patients having relief of headache. In the operation devised by Smithwick, the sympathetic chains from the 8th thoracic to the 1st lumbar ganglia inclusive are removed bilaterally along with the splanchnic nerves arising from this segment of the chain. In Poppen's operation, the 4th thoracic through the 2nd lumbar ganglia and the splanchnic nerves are excised. The principal contraindications to operation have been poor cardiac or renal function. Candidates for operation are individuals up to the middle fifties in age in whom the objective signs of the disease are severe or are advancing rapidly and in whom the symptoms are not responding to a nonsurgical regimen. However, the medical armamentarium of vasodilator agents and diet now has sufficient therapeutic potency to permit the overwhelming majority of hypertensives to retain their sympathetic nerves.

Paroxysmal Auricular Tachycardia or Fibrillation. When medical treatment is ineffective in controlling bouts of such ectopic cardiac activity, a bilateral removal of the upper 4 thoracic sympathetic ganglia is advisable. This surgical elimination of the cardio-accelerator impulses converts the patient's life from one of frequent, incapacitating attacks of arrhythmia to a status in which the attacks are infrequent, mild and readily controlled by quinidine.

CONCLUSION

Many of the operations used routinely or undergoing trial by neurosurgeons depend upon detailed critical knowledge of normal neuro-anatomy and neurophysiology or of the functional pathology of a specific disease. Such information about the nervous system of man, in contrast with that of experimental animals, is still in an early phase of evolution. More and more we are coming to realize that the operative effort at therapy of a patient presents a favorable opportunity to increase our general knowedge and that such increase is likely to aid that particular patient. For example, information regarding localization of function gained from the statements of the epileptic consequent upon stimulation of his cerebral cortex may be essential to treatment of his seizures; and knowledge of variations in site of pain pathways which may be inferred from the patient's description of pain upon stimulus within his cord or brain is of course necessary in making a lesion to stop the pain. Moreover, the explorations incident to gaining these data have yielded unexpected dividends in other new basic knowledge. The mechanisms of disease of the nervous system and the treatment are not of comparatively simple nature, and the cream of major dis-

coveries has not yet been skimmed from this field. Its wide-open character and its complexity present a generous challenge to the finest minds.

BIBLIOGRAPHY

Bailey, P.: Intracranial Tumors, ed. 2, p. 478, Springfield, Ill., Thomas, 1948.

Bradford, K. F., and Spurling, G. R.: The Intervertebral Disc, ed. 2, p. 192, Springfield, Ill., Thomas, 1947.

Brock, S. (ed.): Injuries of the Brain and Spinal Cord and Their Coverings, ed. 4, p. 739, New York, Springer Publishing Co., 1960.

Cushing, H., and Eisenhardt, L.: Meningiomas: Their Classification, Regional Behaviour, Life History, and Surgical End Results, p. 785, Springfield, Ill., Thomas, 1938.

Dandy, W. E.: Intracranial Arterial Aneurysms, p. 147, Ithaca, N. Y., Comstock, 1944.

Davidoff, L. M., and Epstein, B. S.: The Abnormal Pneumoencephalogram, p. 506, Philadelphia, Lea & Febiger, 1950.

Ecker, A., and Riemenschneider, P. A.: Angiographic Localization of Intracranial Masses, p. 433, Springfield, Ill., Thomas, 1955.

Freeman, W., and Watts, J. W.: Psychosurgery in the Treatment of Mental Disorders and Intractable Pain, ed. 2, p. 598, Springfield, Ill., Thomas, 1950.

Hamby, W. B.: Intracranial Aneurysms, p. 564, Springfield, Ill., Thomas, 1952.

Hughes, B.: The Visual Fields: A Study of the Applications of Quantitative Perimetry to the Anatomy and Pathology of the Visual Pathways, p. 174, Oxford, Blackwell, 1954.

Ingraham, F. D., and Matson, D. D.: Neurosurgery of Infancy and Childhood, p. 456, Springfield, Ill., Thomas, 1954.

Kahn, E., Bassett, R. C., Schneider, R. C., and Crosby, E. C.: Correlative Neurosurgery, p. 413, Springfield, Ill., Thomas, 1955.

Krayenbühl, H., and Richter, H. R.: Die zerebrale Angiographie, p. 217, Stuttgart, Thieme, 1952.

Penfield, W., and Jasper, H.: Epilepsy and the Functional Anatomy of the Human Brain, ed. 1, p. 896, Boston, Little, Brown, 1954.

Seddon, H. J. (ed.): Peripheral Nerve Injuries (Med. Res. Council Special Rep. Ser. No. 282), p. 451, London, Her Majesty's Stat. Off., 1954.

White, J. C., Smithwick, R. H., and Simeone, F.: The Autonomic Nervous System: Anatomy, Physiology and Surgical Application, ed. 3, p. 569, New York, Macmillan, 1952.

White, J. C., and Sweet, W. H.: Pain: Its Mechanism and Neurosurgical Control, p. 736, Springfield, Ill., Thomas, 1955.

PETER D. OLCH, M.D. AND HENRY N. HARKINS, M.D., PH.D.

—————————————— CHAPTER 51 ——————————————

A History of Surgery

In the continual remembrance of a glorious past individuals and nations find their noblest inspiration—Sir William Osler

INTRODUCTION

In this modern age of specialization in all fields of medicine, one is very apt to lose sight of the forest because of one's intense pre-occupation with the trees. Specialization within the field of surgery has about reached the limits set by the anatomic and physiologic structure of the human body. As the accumulated knowledge in each of these divisions and subdivisions grows, it is only practical, if not essential, that a single individual limit the scope of his active participation if he intends to gain more than a superficial knowledge of the subject. However, it is very important that one does not lose sight of the common foundation shared by all surgeons. Therefore, it is perhaps quite fitting that a comprehensive textbook on the principles and the practice of surgery should include a chapter tracing the origin and the development of the surgical art. Of necessity, a history of surgery must mention the development of ancillary factors that lowered those barriers interfering with progress. In a brief review of the development of surgery, one can only hope to scrape the surface. Therefore, the reader is referred to the texts noted in the bibliography for a more comprehensive coverage of this subject. The authors at this point wish to apologize for any sins of omission or elements of personal bias in the selection of material and representative individuals to illustrate the development of surgery.

SURGERY IN THE PREHISTORIC PERIOD

The earliest evidence of surgery is perhaps found in the Paleolithic caverns in Spain where silhouettes depicting amputation of the fingers as a superstitious rite are found (25,000-20,000 B.C.). Decompressive trephining was also performed during this period, and Neolithic man 10,000 years ago performed trephining for headache and possibly for epilepsy and blindness. Primitive man dressed his wounds with moss, fresh leaves, ashes and natural balsams. When poisoned he treated with sucking and cauterization. The earliest surgical instruments were sharp fragments of rock or bone, and later iron. It was not until the Roman period that jointed or articulated surgical instruments were developed with which cutting was done by indirect action. Among the diseases known to have occurred in the prehistoric period are the arthritides, rickets, acromegaly, Pott's disease and osteomyelitis.

SURGERY OF ANCIENT CIVILIZATIONS

We are indebted to the ancient Egyptians for the earliest written records of surgery. The Edwin Smith Papyrus (1600 B.C.) contains a discussion of 48 cases in clinical surgery, covering head, chest and spine injuries with a methodical arrangement of data including provisional diagnosis, physical examination, diagnosis, prognosis and treatment. The Papyrus Ebers (1552 B.C.) makes reference to circumcision, trephining, and removal of superficial tumors. Medicine was intimately associated with religion in Egypt, being administered by the priesthood.

The ancient Jews likewise did not practice medicine as a separate profession. Their outstanding merit in medicine was their social hygiene; indeed, they contributed little to the evolution of surgery until the advent of the Alexandrian School centuries later. According to the Talmud (written during the Jewish captivity in Babylon) prior to A.D. 500, the priests were familiar with sutures, freshening wound edges, employment of the uterine sound to determine the site of bleeding, anesthetic substances, operation for imperforate anus, venesection, cesarean section, splenectomy, amputations, trephining, fractures and dislocations, crutches, artificial limbs and teeth.

The ancient Hindus on the other hand excelled all other nations of their time in operative surgery. *Susruta* (A.D. 5th Century) described approximately 121 different surgical instruments, including scalpels, saws, scissors, needles, probes, sounds, trocars, catheters, syringes, bougies and a rectal speculum. He was familiar with many materials for suturing, including plaited horsehair, cotton, strips of leather, fibers of tree bark, and animal sinews. The Hindus amputated limbs, checking hemorrhage with boiling oil, cauterization, or pressure. They treated fractures and dislocations with bamboo splints. They performed cesarean section, lithotomy, and excision of tumors. They were especially competent in plastic surgery, using skin grafts and performing rhinoplasty. The Hindus were excellent surgical teachers, using models, plants and dead animals to instruct the student in venepuncture, incision, bandaging, etc.

The first mention of surgery in ancient Greece appears in the poems of Homer (1000 B.C.). He writes of *Aesculapius* and his two sons, Machaon and Podalirius, the latter two being military surgeons as well as gallant warriors. Legend relates that Aesculapius was destroyed by a thunderbolt of Zeus because he was so proficient in the healing arts that Pluto accused him of diminishing the number of shades in Hades. Thereafter he became an object of worship, and his followers made up an organized guild of physicians, the Aesclepiads. The most famous temples of this cult were at Cos and Cnidus. Medicine in ancient Greece was practiced not only by the priest-physicians of the temples of Aesculapius but also by lay-physicians trained at their temples. Medicine was also studied by the philosophers and practiced in some detail by the gymnasts.

European medicine actually begins in the Age of Pericles, and its scientific advancement

centers around *Hippocrates* (460-370 B.C.). The eminence of Hippocrates is 3-fold, according to Garrison. He dissociated medicine from theology and philosophy, crystallized the loose knowledge of the Coan and the Cnidian Schools in a systematic science and gave physicians the highest moral inspiration. His surgical contributions are found in his treatises on "Fractures, Dislocations, and Wounds of the Head." He favored decompressive trephining but advised expectant treatment in an open depressed fracture. He noted that a wound of the left temporal region will cause right-sided convulsions and vice versa. Numerous fractures and dislocations and their treatment were described by him. He first noted the association of Pott's disease and a pulmonary tubercle. Hippocrates also recognized the importance of rest and immobilization in the healing process, gave the first description of healing by first and second intention, used boiled water or wine for wound irrigation, and stressed the cleanliness of the nails of the operator.

After Hippocrates there was a void in Greek contributions to surgery. *Aristotle* (384-322 B.C.) gave strong impetus to the study of anatomy, and his pupils founded the school at Alexandria (331 B.C.). The names of *Herophilus* and *Erasistratus* (300 B.C.) are associated with this school. Though it is believed that their knowledge of human anatomy was obtained in part through the practice of vivisection on prisoners, they made substantial contributions. Herophilus was the first to differentiate the cerebrum and the cerebellum, to describe the meninges, the choroid, the retina, the parotid and the submaxillary glands, the pulmonary artery, the duodenum, the ovary and the prostate. The first description of the aortic and the pulmonary valves and the chordae tendineae of the heart is credited to Erasistratus.

Greek medicine migrated to Rome about 146 B.C. The best record of surgery in this period is found in the seventh of eight books (*De re Medicina*) compiled by *Celsus*, the Roman encyclopediast who, though not a physician, compiled a vast amount of current medical knowledge. One of the first accounts of the use of ligature appears in this book. In this Roman period, surgery reached a peak it was not to see again until the time of Ambroise Paré. Numerous specialized surgical instruments were developed. Herniotomy, plastic surgery and cesarean section were practiced. Examples of surgeons of this period are *Heliodorus*, who first described ligation and torsion of blood vessels, and *Antyllus*, whose name is associated with the method of treating aneurysms that was in vogue until the time of John Hunter.

Soranus of Ephesus (A.D. 79-138) wrote a treatise on gynecology, obstetrics and pediatrics. It was the authority on obstetrics for the next 1500 years.

Galen (A.D. 131-201), a true disciple of Hippocrates, was the first to practice and teach laboratory methods through animal experimentation (and the last for many centuries) and may be listed as one of the earliest and the first great physiologist. He was the first to recognize that arteries transmit blood rather than air and observed that arterial and venous blood differed. He observed that arteries and veins anastamosed through minute passages. He was aware of the use of the ligature in arteries but did not apply it to amputations. He recognized a relationship between brain, spinal cord and peripheral nerves and taught that the nerves conveyed impressions of sensation and motion. Unfortunately, his genius delighted in speculation, and it was this rather than the depth of his science and methodical experimentation that imposed upon and was furthered by the Middle Ages.

Following Galen, medical progress all but came to a standstill, and the Byzantine Period (A.D. 476-732) is noted mainly for the compilers *Oribasius* (A.D. 325-403), *Alexander of Tralles* (A.D. 525-605) and *Paul of Ægina* (A.D. 625-690) who preserved and recorded the medicine of the ancients for the Arabians and then Western Europeans to draw upon.

With the rise of Mohammedan power and their capture of Alexandria (A.D. 640), the Arabians became the inheritors and the preservers of the science of the Greeks. The Oriental philosophy that it is sinful to touch the dead body with the hands did little to advance surgery or anatomy. Furthermore, the most famous of the Arabian writers, *Avicenna* (A.D. 980-1036), whose "Canon" was an unwieldy storehouse of learning that was very popular in the Middle Ages, set back the progress of surgery by spreading the doctrine that the surgical art is an inferior and separate branch of medicine. The most celebrated Arabian writer on surgery, *Albucasis* (1013-1106), composed a surgical work of three books, including the use of the cautery, descriptions of numerous surgical procedures and the treatment of wounds, and a treatise on fractures and dislocations.

SURGERY IN THE MIDDLE AGES

The fundamental error of medieval medical science was the separation of medicine from surgery. Beginning with Avicenna, Galen's dictum that "surgery is only a mode of treatment" was advanced to the degree of treating the surgeon as a lackey and inferior to the internist. Further damage was done by the Arabian obsession that it was unclean or unholy to touch the human body. Scholastic and monastic minds gradually became penetrated with the conviction that surgery was a most undesirable, lowly art. This feeling culminated in the edicts of the Council of Rheims (1125) and of Lateran (1139) that restricted the surgery of the clerical or educated class and finally the famous but infamous edict of the Council of Tours (1163), "Ecclesia abhorret a sanguine" (the Church shuns blood).

The period of Monastic medicine (5th-10th century) was only of note because of the translating and the compiling of ancient medical works by such as the Benedictine order in the cloisters of Monte Cassino and Benevente. Surgery at this time can best be termed barbaric. In the 11th century medicine was greatly elevated by the School of Salerno, a secular school of obscure origin on the best of relations with the Benedictine monks. The teachings of this first independent medical school were most invigorating for the times. In 1060 *Constantinus Africanus* arrived in Salerno, having traveled extensively and carried back the works of the Greeks and the Arabs. Arabic medical doctrine was thereby introduced at Salerno and incorporated in Western European culture until the 17th century. Constantinus, shortly after his arrival at Salerno, retired to the cloisters of Monte Cassino where he spent the remainder of his life translating and annotating the medical works he had collected. The principal outcome of the School of Salerno was the work of two surgeons, *Roger of Palermo* and his pupil

Roland of Parma in the early 13th century. Roger's *Practica,* re-edited by Roland, became a standard text at Salerno. He knew of cancer, treated goiter with ashes of sponge, introduced the seton and suture of the intestine over a hollow tube, and taught the use of styptics, sutures and ligatures in hemorrhage.

Roger and Roland were succeeded by *Hugh of Lucca* (died 1252) and his disciple *Theodoric* (1205-96), both of the School of Bologna. These two surgeons are notable as advocates of aseptic wound treatment and for contradicting the dogma of laudable pus or healing by second intention. Hugh and Theodoric, followed later by Mondeville and Paracelsus, were the only surgeons who upheld these principles prior to Lister. Hugh and Theodoric are also associated with medieval substitutes for anesthesia.

The most celebrated surgeon of the 13th century was *William of Salicet* (1210-77) of Bologna. He kept an excellent record of his case histories, wrote the first known treatise on surgical anatomy and sutured divided nerves. His pupil *Lanfranc* (died 1315) of Milan carried on his sound surgical principles and, having been driven from his native surroundings because of political strife, settled in Lyons and then Paris where he became associated with the College de Saint Come (1295). With his style of lecturing and his bedside teaching he became the virtual founder of French surgery. To his credit, he valiantly stood against the schism between surgery and medicine. He was the first to describe concussion of the brain. He differentiated between cancer and hypertrophy of the female breast. According to Garrison the work of William of Salicet and Lanfranc, coincident with the development of the great medieval universities of Paris (1110), Bologna (1113), Oxford (1167), Montpellier (1181), Padua (1222) and Naples (1224), and the false dawn of culture and liberalism in the 13th century, did much to further the growth of surgery in France, England and Flanders.

Henri de Mondeville (1260-1320), a loyal follower of Lanfranc, stressed the importance of avoiding suppuration by simple cleanliness as originally taught by Hippocrates. His surgical treatise contains such statements as these: "God did not exhaust all His creative power in making Galen," and "Many more surgeons know how to cause suppuration than to heal a wound."

The Flemish surgeon *Jean Yperman* (1295-1351) was a pupil of Lanfranc and became the great authority on surgery in the Low Countries in the 14th century. The pre-Renaissance period (14th century) also was the time of *Guy de Chauliac* (1300-68), the most eminent authority on surgery for the next 200 years. Thoroughly educated at Paris, Montpellier and Bologna, he was well qualified to write his *Chirurgia Magna.* Included in this text was the first account of medical history since the time of Celsus. He stressed the importance of human anatomy in surgery, apparently was the first to employ extension in the treatment of fractures, and attempted to excise early cancer by the knife while cauterizing the later fungating stages.

In this same period, the first English surgeon of whom there is record was in practice. *John of Arderne* (1306-90), educated at Montpellier, practiced in Newark and then London; he is noted for his graphic description of carcinoma of the rectum and his operation for fistula in ano. It should be stated that in this pre-Renaissance period with some development of surgery there was necessarily some effort to improve upon the status of human anatomy. The name *Mundinus* of Bologna is associated with the revival of human dissection (1275).

It is important to digress for a moment in order to stress the fact that the contributions and the progress in surgery in the 13th and the 14th centuries as exemplified by the foregoing individuals were the exceptions rather than the rule. For after the edict of the Council of Tours in 1163, books on surgery and midwifery were removed from the libraries, some universities excluded all those who worked with their hands, and medicine and surgery became totally divorced. To quote T. Clifford Allbutt, "But by the expulsion of surgery from the liberal arts, Medicine herself was eviscerated; the pernicious bisection of Medicine was made which has not yet spent its evil: the very foundation of the art was gone, . . ." Therefore in the 13th and the 14th centuries, surgery began to grow from the roots in the hands of lowly and unlettered men, while (internal) medicine became progressively more withdrawn into its shell and did not begin to emerge again until the 17th century.

The surgeons in base apprenticeships, not only illiterate but forbidden the means of learning, began making slow progress by practical experience, eventually reinforced by the new and urgent problems attendant upon the wounds of firearms. In England and France a caste system among the surgeons complicated matters further. In France the lower echelon was composed of the ordinary or lay barbers called barber-surgeons or surgeons of the short robe. These individuals owed their surgical background to the custom that the person who shaved the monks also gave the monks their required periodic bleeding. In some instances the barber was often a bath keeper who, in addition to bleeding and leeching, gave enemas and extracted teeth. The upper echelon consisted of individuals (few in number) who performed surgery but were not ordinary barbers. These were the surgeons of the long robe. As early as 1268 the surgeons of the long robe attempted to limit the surgical practice of the barber-surgeons with little success. In this manner barber-surgery became wound-surgery. The surgeons of the long robe became further and further removed from the practice of surgery and eventually more closely resembled the Faculty of Medicine. Therefore, it remained for the progress to be made by the surgeons of the short robe, the provencial surgeons as opposed to the Paris surgeon. A similar split occurred in England between master surgeons and barber-surgeons.

SURGERY IN THE RENAISSANCE

With the freedom of thought and escape from dialectic authority in the 15th century, surgery made important strides. The invention of printing had an obvious effect. The most important fundamental factor in the progress of surgery was the restoration of human dissection and the development of accurate anatomic studies. *Leonardo da Vinci* (1452-1519), the greatest artist and scientist of the Italian Renaissance, was the founder of physiologic anatomy and the originator of cross-sectional anatomy. *Andreas Vesalius* (1514-64) even surpassed Leonardo in making anatomy a living science. After 5 years as public prosector at Padua where he taught, he composed the *De Fabrica Humani Corporis* (1543), a work that broke with the past and

threw aside Galenical tradition. Another great individualist of this period, *Paracelsus* (1493-1541), felt by many to be the most original medical thinker of the 16th century, is not primarily remembered for his surgical contributions. However, he was about the only physician between Mondeville and Lister to stress asepsis and to teach that wounds are healed by nature and not by the surgeon. He also stressed the unity of medicine and surgery. Further anatomic contributions by *Fallopius* (1523-62), a pupil of Vesalius, included the discovery and the description of the chorda tympani, the semicircular canal, the sphenoid sinus and the fallopian tubes. His pupil, *Fabricius ab Aquapendente* (1537-1619), was Harvey's teacher at Padua and the discoverer of the valves of the veins. *Eustachius* (1524-74) discovered the adrenal glands, the abducens nerve and the eustachian tube, to name but a few.

Without question the high point of Renaissance surgery is seen in *Ambroise Paré* (1510-90) (Fig. 51-1), a provencial barber's apprentice when he arrived in Paris. He became a dresser at the Hotel Dieu, then an Army surgeon in 1537. Here by his courage, ability and common sense, he developed into the greatest surgeon of his time. He was snubbed and ridiculed by the surgeons of the long robe because he wrote in his native tongue. Among his contributions were the demonstration that the application of boiling oil to gunshot wounds was a great hindrance to healing and not necessary to rid the wound of poisons as suggested by di Vigo and Brunschwig; the reintroduction of the use of the ligature in amputations; the popularization of the truss in the treatment of hernia; and the reintroduction of artificial limbs and eyes.

A discussion of Renaissance surgery would not be complete without mention of such men as *Tagliacozzi* (1546-99), an Italian surgeon who wrote a treatise on plastic surgery and revived the operation of rhinoplasty; *Pierre Franco* (1500), an example of the itinerant provencial surgeon trained in hernias and lithotomy who did much to put the operations on a dignified basis; *Felix Wurtz* (1518-75), a follower of Paracelsus in the simple treatment of wounds; *William Clowes* (1540-1604), the greatest of English surgeons during the Elizabethan period; and *Peter Lowe*

(1550-1612), founder of the Faculty of Physicians and Surgeons of Glasgow (1599).

In closing the narrative of the Renaissance surgery, it should be noted that the status of the barber-surgeon was improved in both France and England through legislative means.

SURGERY IN THE 17th CENTURY

This 100-year period was not one of great surgical progress when compared with other branches of medicine. Beyond question the greatest name in medicine in the 17th century was *William Harvey* (1578-1657). His discovery of the circulation of the blood, and more importantly his quantitative and mathematical demonstration of the same as appears in *De Motu Cordis,* was the beginning of dynamic physiology. The 17th century was also an age of specialized anatomic research and was notable for a long list of individual discoveries, among which were the following: *Aselli* (1622) discovered the lacteals; *Pecquet* (1651) discovered the thoracic duct; *Wirsung* (1642) discovered the pancreatic duct; *Brunner* (1682) discovered the duodenal glands; *de Graaf* (1672) described the graafian follicles of the ovary; *Malpighi* (1661) discovered the capillary anastomoses in the lungs.

In the mid-17th century Holland and the schools of Amsterdam and Leyden became the centers of anatomy. The names of Swammerdam, Ruysch and Nuck are associated with these institutions.

As we have stated, in comparison with the development of anatomy in the 17th century, surgical progress was rather meager. In Germany there were two surgeons of note. *Fabricius Hildanus* (1560-1624), who has been referred to as the father of German surgery, stressed the necessity of anatomic study by surgeons; he was a bold and skillful operator and invented many new instruments. *Scultetus* (1595-1645), whose name is still familiar on the surgical ward (Scultetus binder), is remembered chiefly for his *Armamentarium Chirurgicum*, a collection of illustrations of surgical instruments and operations of the time. In England the outstanding surgeon of the century was *Richard Wiseman* (1622-76).

The strife and the rivalry between physicians, surgeons of the long robe and barber-

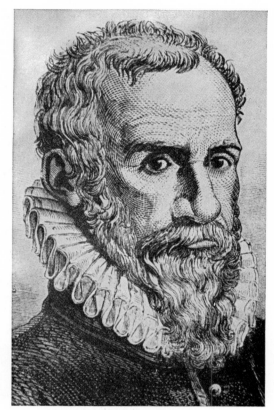

FIG. 51-1. Ambroise Paré (1510-1590). (Bettman Archive)

surgeons continued unabated in the 17th century.

SURGERY IN THE 18th CENTURY

At the beginning of the 18th century, Paris was the center of surgical study. *Jean-Louis Petit* (1674-1750) was the most distinguished surgeon of the first half of the 18th century. He invented the screw and the tourniquet for amputation and was the first to recognize the role of blood clot in stopping arterial hemorrhage. *Pierre Joseph Desault* (1744-95) was supposedly the first teacher of surgical anatomy and contributed much to the perfection of surgical technic. In Germany, *Lorenz Heister* (1683-1758) was the first surgeon of importance in this century. Perhaps the most outstanding name connected with surgery in Germany in this era was *Albrecht von Haller* (1708-1777), who never performed a surgical operation upon a human. His *Bibliotheca Chirurgica* in two volumes "is the most valuable work on the history and literature of surgery that has ever been published," according to J. S. Billings. He placed the experimental method on firm foundations in dealing with surgical problems. In the latter 18th century the leading German surgeon was *August Gottlieb Richter* (1742-1812), who wrote a treatise on hernia that is still a classic. In England the leading surgeon of the first half of the 18th century was *William Cheselden* (1688-1752), surgeon to St. Thomas' and St. George's Hospitals. In the mid-18th century *Percivall Pott* (1714-1788), surgeon to St. Bartholomew's Hospital, made significant contributions to the treatment of hernia, head injuries, hydrocele, and diseases of the spine, among others.

Because of *John Hunter* (1728-93) Fig. 51-2), surgery began to develop as a branch of scientific medicine from its former state as a mere mode of treatment. It is not possible in a short review of surgery to do justice to the multiple contributions of this rugged Scotch individualist. He is considered to be the founder of experimental and surgical pathology and a pioneer in comparative physiology and experimental morphology. He was the teacher of Jenner, Astley Cooper, Abernethy, Parkinson, Blizard, Home, Wright Post and Physick. He made outstanding contributions in the fields of surgery, anatomy, pathology and dentistry and is understandably considered one of the greatest biologists and surgeons of all time. Hunter's immediate successor in London was his pupil *John Abernethy* (1764-1831), a forceful and vigorous teacher who first ligated the external iliac artery for aneurysm (1796).

Generally speaking, the status of surgery was quite low during the greater part of the 18th century, except in France. The foundation of the Academy of Surgery in 1731 through the efforts of *de la Peyronie* (1678-1747) and *Mareschal* (1658-1736) did much

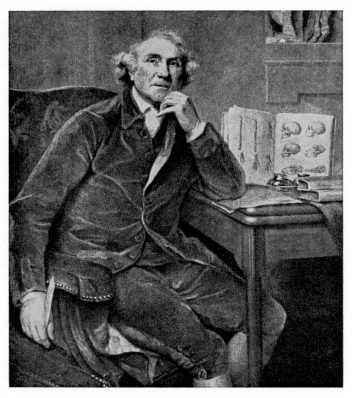

Fig. 51-2. John Hunter (1728-1793). (Sigerist, H.: The Great Doctors, New York, Norton)

to elevate surgery to an educated profession. This advancement was temporarily halted by the French Revolution. In 18th century England there were no great surgeons before the time of Pott, Cheselden, Hunter and Abernethy. In 1745 the English surgeons became formally separated from the barbers, and in 1800 the Corporation of Surgeons was rechartered as the Royal College of Surgeons of London (in 1843 this group became the Royal College of Surgeons of England). Surgical teaching was sporadic, and generally, it was conducted privately. However, in this century the hospital medical school with clinical instruction attained a definite status at such institutions as Guy's Hospital (1723), the Edinburgh Hospital (1736) and St. Bartholomew's Hospital (1790).

SURGERY IN THE 19th CENTURY

John Shaw Billings lists a number of factors as salient points in the history of surgery in the 19th century. Among these are:

1. The discovery of anesthetics
2. The establishment of aseptic and antiseptic surgery upon the scientific foundation of the new science of bacteriology
3. The development of conservative surgery in the treatment of diseases and injuries of the extremities with the development of orthopedic and plastic surgery into specialties
4. The rise and progress of abdominal and intracranial surgery
5. The entrance of two new nations, the United States and Russia, into the field of surgical discovery, literature and teaching
6. The change in the methods of educating surgeons
7. The formation of surgical societies and associations
8. The removal of restrictions on the study of anatomy
9. The great advances made in pathologic anatomy and experimental pathology
10. The development of further specialties such as gynecology.

Early 19th century surgery shifted its center of progress and teaching from Paris to London because of the impact of Hunter's teaching and the French Revolution. Many bold operative feats were performed, plastic surgery became revived, and most of the larger

arteries were ligated successfully. However, the abdomen, the cranium and the joints were still generally "off limits" until well after 1867, the year of Lister's publications on antisepsis.

The leading surgeons of the 19th century in the pre-Listerian period were the following: in Great Britain, one must include the brothers *John* (1763-1820) and *Charles Bell* (1774-1842); *Sir Astley Paston Cooper* (1768-1841), pupil of Hunter and surgeon to Guy's Hospital in 1800, renowned for his writings on hernia and diseases of the testes and his knowledge of anatomy and bedside teaching; *Abraham Colles* (1773-1843) of Dublin, remembered for his original description of the fracture of the carpal end of the radius; *Sir Benjamin Collins Brodie* (1783-1862), who devoted himself to the scientific side of surgery rather than the operative and whose work *On the Pathology and Surgery of Diseases of the Joints* remains a classic; *Robert Liston* (1794-1847), a great promoter of clinical hospital teaching; *James Syme* (1799-1870) of Edinburgh, father-in-law of Joseph Lister and a cousin of Liston's; and *Sir William Fergusson* (1808-77), considered the founder of conservative surgery in cases of bone and joint disease; his name is associated with operations for harelip and cleft palate.

In France there were *Dominique-Jean Larray* (1766-1842), a great military surgeon of the Napoleonic wars who introduced the use of the ambulance to remove the wounded from the battlefield, whose ideas of wound care and handling were amazingly ahead of his time; *Guillaume Dupuytren* (1777-1835), the ablest and best French surgeon of his time, a shrewd diagnostician, excellent clinical teacher, unrivaled operator and a competent physiologist and pathologist, chief surgeon to the Hotel Dieu (1814), whose personality was described as contemptuous, unscrupulous and overbearing; *A. A. Louis-Marie Velpeau* (1795-1867), who contributed to our knowledge of surgical anatomy, the diagnosis of tumors, and diseases of the breast; *J. M. Delpech* (1777-1832), a pioneer of orthopedic surgery in France; *J. F. Malgaigne* (1806-65), perhaps best remembered as a great surgical historian and critic; *Auguste Nélaton* (1807-73), who made many improvements in surgical technic; and *Paul*

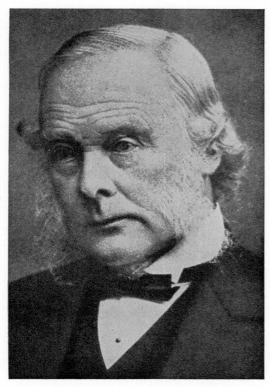

FIG. 51-3. Joseph Lister (1827-1912). (Sigerist, H.: The Great Doctors, New York, Norton)

Broca (1824-80), pioneer of modern neurosurgery with his research on cerebral localization.

Among the pre-Listerian surgeons of note in this century in Germany were *Conrad Johann Martin Langenbeck* (1776-1851), professor of anatomy and surgery at Göttingen; *Carl Ferdinand von Graefe* (1787-1840), the first professor of surgery at the University of Berlin and the founder of modern plastic surgery; *Johann Friedrich Dieffenbach* (1792-1847), successor to von Graefe at Berlin, who devoted himself largely to orthopedic and plastic surgery; *George Friedrich Louis Stromeyer* (1804-76), who greatly extended the field of conservative joint surgery; *Bernhard von Langenbeck* (1810-87), the nephew of Conrad, succeeded Dieffenbach at Berlin and started with his pupils Billroth and Gurlt the *"Archiv für klinische Chirurgie"* and founded the German Society for Surgery, both of which exerted a profound influence. His greatest contribution to surgery was his excellence as a

teacher as exemplified by his pupils Billroth, von Esmarch, Lücke, Kocher, Krönlein and Pirogoff.

The first great Russian surgeon about whom there is information belongs to this period. *Nikolai Ivanovitch Pirogoff* (1810-81) introduced the teaching of applied topographic anatomy in Russia, made many contributions of note to the treatment of gunshot wounds, amputations and bone surgery as a military surgeon, was using ether anesthesia in 1847 and composed an anatomic atlas using frozen sections.

The pre-Listerian period in American surgery was distinguished by bold operating on the vascular and the osseous systems, the foundation of modern operative gynecology and the permanent introduction of surgical anesthesia. Among the outstanding individuals in this period were *Philip Syng Physick* (1768-1837) of Philadelphia, a pupil of Hunter's referred to as the Father of American Surgery; *John Warren* (1753-1815), founder and first professor of surgery of the Harvard Medical School; his son, *John Collins Warren* (1778-1856), a pupil of Astley Cooper and Dupuytren, who succeeded his father at Harvard and practically introduced ether anesthesia in surgery. *Wright Post* (1776-1822) and *Valentine Mott* (1785-1865) of New York are examples of bold vascular surgeons of the day with many firsts in the ligations of major vessels. The early history of the introduction of anesthesia in America is still a matter of controversy in regard to credit. Suffice it to say that the following men had important roles in the development and the popularization of ether anesthesia: *Crawford W. Long* (1815-78) of Danielsville, Ga.; *William T. G. Morton* (1819-68) of Charlton, Mass.; *John C. Warren* of Boston Mass.; *Henry J. Bigelow* (1816-90) of Boston, Mass.; and *Charles T. Jackson* of Massachusetts. Those individuals in this period associated with the development of gynecology will be covered in the discussion of specialties.

With the advent of *Joseph Lister* (1827-1912) (Fig. 51-3), surgery was truly revolutionized. With surgical anesthesia, Lister's contributions to surgical antisepsis composed the greatest wedge in opening the door to the modern period in surgery. Lister was graduated from the University of London and acquired his surgical training at Edinburgh under Syme. In 1860 he became professor of surgery at Glasgow, where he began his studies in surgical antisepsis. Stimulated by Pasteur's work, he set out to prevent the development of microorganisms in wounds. In 1865 he employed a chemical antiseptic (carbolic acid) in a case of compound fracture with complete success, and in 1867 he published the results of 2 years' work in 2 papers. In 1869 Lister succeeded Syme at Edinburgh, and in 1877 he accepted the chair of surgery at Kings College, retiring from practice in 1896. He was the first medical man to be raised to the peerage (1897). Lister initially had little support from his English colleagues; in fact, he was criticized and ridiculed by such as Lawson Tait of Liverpool. It remained for the German School of Surgery in the form of such men as von Bergmann, Mikulicz, von Volkmann and Thiersch, and Lucas-Championniére in France to achieve the first advance of the Listerian doctrine.

Prominent surgeons of the early post-Listerian period include Billroth, Mikulicz, Wölfler, Czerny, Thiersch, von Volkmann, von Esmarch, von Bergmann and Gurlt in Germany; Paget, Hutchinson, Horsley and Thomas in Great Britain; S. D. Gross and S. W. Gross, Keen, Agnew and McBurney in America. Many of these individuals were influential in the development of specialized fields of surgery and will be mentioned again in the appropriate sections.

THE DEVELOPMENT OF THE SURGICAL SPECIALTIES (LATE 19th CENTURY)

Before discussing *briefly* the development of some of the major surgical specialties and the personalities involved, it is important to note the ancillary factors of importance in this development and progress.

First and foremost is the tremendous impetus given at the onset of this era by the development of surgical anesthesia and antisepsis. By the end of the 19th century, ether, nitrous oxide and chloroform were in use. Lister's concept of antisepsis (1867) was followed by Koch's concept of asepsis and the introduction of steam sterilization by *von Bergmann* in 1886. By 1895 dry heat and steam were the accepted methods of steriliza-

tion. *Mikulicz* operated in sterile linen gloves, which he changed several times during surgery, and used a face mask as early as 1896. Halsted introduced the use of rubber gloves in America in 1891.

The development of blood transfusion had an obvious effect upon surgery. First practiced by Denys of Paris in 1867, the modern period begins in 1901 when Landsteiner and later Moss (1910) described the 4 blood groups. The introduction of citrate as an anticoagulant by Hustin (1911) (diluted citrated blood for transfusion) and Agote and Lewisohn separately in 1915 (citrated whole blood for transfusion) enabled the development of blood banks. Equally important were the studies of Blalock and Parsons, and Phemister in 1930 that brought about a better understanding of the pathogenesis of surgical shock.

The field of fluid replacement therapy was founded on the concept of *le milieu interieur* of Claude Bernard (1878). In recent time Coller, Marriott, Gamble, Hartmann, Moore and others have advanced the knowledge of this subject. Closely allied with this field are the contributions of Wangensteen (1932), Miller and Abbott (1934) and Cantor on the importance of gastrointestinal suction.

The development of diagnostic radiology following Röntgen's discovery of the x-ray in 1895 was a tremendous addition to the surgeon's armamentarium. It was applied immediately for the diagnosis of fractures, dislocations and foreign bodies, and the eventual use of contrast media to aid in determining the morphology and the function of the internal organs led to such innovations as ventriculography (Dandy, 1918), cholecystography (Graham and Cole, 1923-24), cerebral angiography (Moniz, 1931) and more recently aortography in the study of peripheral vascular disease and contrast studies in the diagnosis of cardiac lesions.

Needless to say, the refinement and progress in the fields of general inhalation, local and conductive infiltration, spinal, intratracheal, and intravenous anesthesia have opened new fields to the surgeon.

The last ancillary factor to be discussed before taking up specific specialties is the important role of the new mode of surgical training that developed in the late 19th and early 20th centuries. As we have noted, surgical training through the ages was chiefly through the apprentice system. It was often haphazard, extremely variable as to quality, and seldom, if ever, a program of progressive responsibility that would produce a well-rounded capable surgeon. In the late 18th century, hospital teaching became more prevalent, but a formal competitive program with responsibility was lacking. In the 19th century the German universities became centers of the scientific spirit and method. The basic sciences and clinical medicine were under one roof. It was the natural setting for great strides and advancement in clinical medicine. It was in this setting that the origin of our present-day surgical training programs was developed. The house surgeon or chief resident (called first assistant in Germany) was selected after years of service (8 to 12) from a number of well-trained assistant residents. There was no regular advancement from the bottom to the top of the staff of assistant residents, and only a small proportion of these entertained the hope of becoming a first assistant. First assistants occasionally were brought in from other universities over the heads of those who had served for many years. The first assistant, if all went well, eventually was offered the chair of surgery in another university. However, there were many more first assistants than available chairs of surgery, and often after 8 or 9 years of service he was compelled to resign himself to an instructorship (Privat-Docent).

William S. Halsted (1852-1922) Fig. 51-4), professor of surgery at the Johns Hopkins University (1889-1922), has made innumerable monumental contributions to the art and the science of surgery. One of the greatest was his appreciation and subsequent modification and application of the German residency system to surgical training in the United States at a time when surgical training consisted of an internship of 12 to 16 months, with 4 to 6 months of operative work. In 1889 he appointed residents from qualified surgical interns, who served from 4 to 6 years before becoming chief resident for 2 years. However, this concept of surgical training was not generally accepted until the 1920's. This establishment of residency training in the university surgical clinics in the United States is con-

sidered by many to be the greatest advance in surgical training in the history of surgery.

The following are brief statements regarding the development of some of the major surgical specialties.

GENERAL SURGERY (ABDOMINAL)

Lister's principles of antisepsis opened the door to abdominal surgery, and the "wedge" in that door was the treatment of acute appendicitis. Associated with this break-through are the names of Fitz (the classic pathologic identification of the disease in 1886), Krönlein (1884), Hall (1886) and Morton. The latter 3 individuals were among the first to perform appendectomy. The leaders in abdominal surgery at the end of the 19th century were the Germans, headed by *Theodor Billroth* (1829-94) (Fig. 51-5) and his pupils von Eiselsberg, Mikulicz, Czerny, Wölfler, Gersuny, von Hacker and Gussenbauer. These were truly the pioneers of visceral surgery (See Fig. 51-6). Important events in the development of surgery for gastric and duodenal ulcer were the following:

1881   Billroth performed the first success-

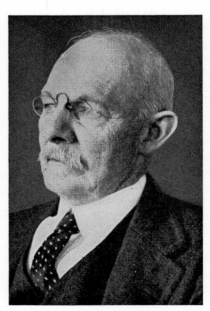

FIG. 51-4. William Stewart Halsted (1852-1922). (The Johns Hopkins University School of Medicine, 1893-1943, Baltimore, Johns Hopkins Press)

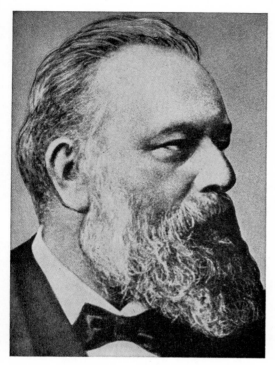

Fig. 51-5. Theodor Billroth (1829-1894). (Hurwitz, A., and Degenshein, G.: Milestones in Modern Surgery, New York, Hoeber)

ful resection of the pyloric portion of the stomach for neoplasm.

1881 Wölfler introduced gastroenterostomy.

1882 Loreta performed the first pyloroplasty.

1884 Ransohoff performed the first gastroenterostomy in America.

1885 von Hacker described the posterior gastroenterostomy.

1892 Heusner successfully sutured a perforated gastric ulcer.

1897 Schlatter performed the first successful total gastrectomy.

Generally speaking, in the first half of the 20th century, gastroenterostomy was the accepted treatment for peptic ulceration. From 1925 partial gastrectomy of the Polya type began to supplant gastroenterostomy, due to the work of such men as Balfour, Finsterer and Hofmeister. More recently, peptic ulceration has been treated by partial gastrectomy with gastrojejunostomy or gastroduode-

nostomy, gastroenterostomy combined with vagotomy (Dragstedt, 1944) or partial gastrectomy with gastrojejunostomy or gastroduodenostomy plus vagotomy.

In the field of intestinal resection and anastomosis, great progress was made by such men as Payr, Mikulicz, Kocher, Halsted, Murphy and the Mayos in the late 19th and early 20th centuries. Associated with the development of colon surgery are Paul (1895), Block (1892) and Mikulicz (1903) who described extraperitoneal resection of the colon for carcinoma. Von Volkmann first excised a rectal carcinoma (1878), Maunsell performed the first planned abdominoperineal resection of the rectum (1894), and Miles first performed a one-stage abdominoperineal resection for carcinoma of the rectum (1908). In 1948 Swenson described the treatment of Hirschsprung's disease by rectosigmoidectomy.

In 1890 Bassini of Padua and Halsted described their operations for the radical cure of hernia. Since that time there have been numerous modifications with the use of fascial strips, steel wire, tantalum mesh, etc., in more recent years.

The surgery of cancer was advanced by the popularization of the concept of complete local removal "en bloc" with the regional lymph nodes. Examples of this are seen in Mikulicz's commentary on the metastatic pathways of gastric carcinoma (1898) and the operations of radical mastectomy described by Halsted (1890) and Willy Meyer (1894). In more recent years tremendous strides have been made in the surgical treatment of head and neck cancer by Hayes Martin and others and in pelvic cancer by such men as Brunschwig and Bricker. Endocrine ablative surgery (oophorectomy, adrenalectomy and hypophysectomy) has been shown to have a definite role in specific instances.

Before closing this brief commentary on general surgery, one must acknowledge the outstanding contributions to surgery of the thyroid gland made by Kocher (1872) and Halsted (1918).

THORACIC SURGERY

Progress in esophageal surgery was made by such men as Billroth (first esophagectomy, 1872), Torek (removed a carcinoma of the esophagus and bridged the defect with a rubber prosthesis, 1913), Turner (employed an antethoracic skin tube following esophageal resection), and Yudin (employed an antethoracic segment of jejunum). However, results were rather disheartening until 1933 when Ohsawa reported 8 recoveries in 18 resections for tumors of the lower esophagus

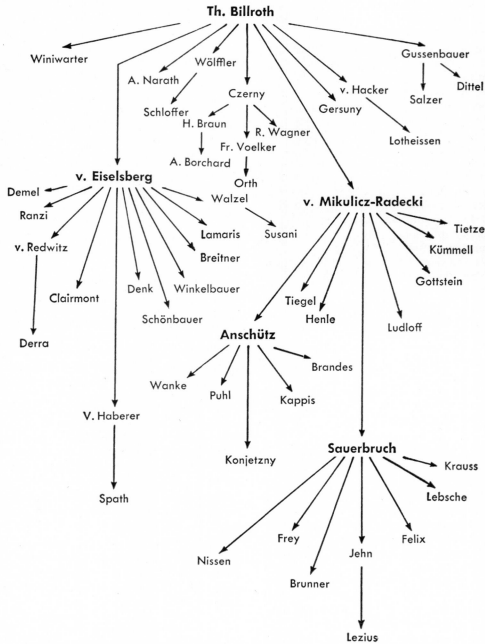

Fig. 51-6. The Billroth Tree. The surgical genealogy of Billroth's pupils and of their pupils in turn. (Killian and Krämer: Meister der Chirurgie und die Chirurgenschulen im Deutschen Raum, Stuttgart, Thieme)

and the cardia. Renewed interest was also stimulated by the report of Adams and Phemister in 1938 on successful transthoracic-abdominal resection of the lower esophagus and esophagogastrostomy. In 1944 Garlock and Sweet individually described methods of stomach mobilization to permit anastomosis of the upper esophagus and the stomach.

Progress in thoracic surgery was not possible until methods of more accurate localization of pulmonary disease were obtained with the use of x-rays (1895) and the development of bronchoscopy (1898). The other major obstruction was anesthesia administration in the face of an open pneumothorax. In 1908 Sauerbruch developed a negative pressure cabinet to permit chest surgery. In 1909 Metzler and Auer perfected positive pressure intratracheal insufflation and the problem was solved. Milestones in thoracic surgery include Evarts Graham's fundamental investigations of cardiorespiratory physiology with the Empyema Commission (1918), the report of Brunner (1929) and Shenstone and Jones (1932) emphasizing the feasibility and the value of lobectomy in bronchiectasis, the successful one-stage pneumonectomy for bronchiectasis by Nissen (1931) and Haight (1932), and the first one-stage pneumonectomy for carcinoma of the lung by Graham (1933). Perhaps the most important milestone of recent years was the consideration by Churchill and Belsey (1939) of the bronchopulmonary segment rather than the lobe as the fundamental surgical unit of the lung.

GYNECOLOGY

Operative gynecology had no special existence before the beginning of the 19th century; it was largely the creation of certain American surgeons and had its origin mainly in attempts to repair the errors and the omissions of backwoods obstetrics. The founder of operative gynecology was *Ephraim McDowell* (1771-1830), who performed his first ovariotomy in 1809, and *James Marion Sims* (1813-83) whose greatest contribution to the field was the first successful repair of a vesicovaginal fistula (1852). In England, the field was advanced by *Sir Thomas Spencer Wells* (1818-97) and *Robert Lawson Tait* (1845-99). The latter, truly a pioneer in all phases

of operative gynecology, was one of Lister's more violent critics. *Howard Atwood Kelly* (1858-1943) of Philadelphia and Baltimore is credited with important contributions to general surgery, gynecology, female urology and medical history. Ernest Wertheim's radical operation for cancer of the cervix (1906) was another bold advance in this field. Innumerable advances have been made in the understanding of ovarian function, the menstrual cycle and gynecologic pathology within the past 75 years, but they cannot be dealt with here.

UROLOGY

Prior to the turn of the century, urology was closely allied with general medicine or surgery, and the urologist chiefly treated venereal disease. It was easily recognized that progress in treatment of bladder and kidney disease depended upon adequate visualization. Various primitive methods of viewing the bladder were developed, but in 1877 Nitze produced the first cystoscope, employing the principles still used today. The history of the development of specialized instruments for handling problems of obstruction of the bladder neck is quite interesting. Suffice it to say that from 1875 when Bottini introduced his galvanocautery, which was used without visualization to destroy an obstructing prostatic lobe, to the precise instruments of today, there is a long list of contributions by such men as Young, Braasch, Bumpus and Stern.

Contributions to suprapubic prostatectomy were made by Belfield, McGill, Fuller (1895), Young and Guiteras (1900). Perineal prostatectomy was propagated and advanced by Watson (1888), Goodfellow (1891), Sims (1902) and Young (1904). The first radical prostatectomy for a carcinoma of the prostate was performed by Young in 1904. With the founding of the Brady Urological Institute under the directorship of *Hugh H. Young* in 1915, a new era in the training of competent urologists began with the establishment of the new residency system as initiated by Halsted. As the system became adopted throughout the country, institutions such as the Mayo Clinic, the Lahey Clinic and the Brady Clinic of the New York Hospital exerted great influence in stabilizing urologic practice.

ORTHOPEDICS

The specialty of orthopedic surgery was born in Paris, with the publication of the first orthopedic textbook entitled *L'Orthopédie* (Greek derivation meaning "straight child") in 1741. However, during the subsequent 100 years there were few physicians who limited their practice to the bone-and-joint field. However, in the second quarter of the 19th century, orthopedics as a specialty began to achieve minor recognition in France, Great Britain and the United States. As in other specialties, the development of anesthesia, antisepsis and then asepsis stimulated the development of surgical procedures and technics. A great contribution was made by Mathijsen in 1852 with the development of plaster-of-Paris impregnated bandages. *Hugh Owen Thomas* (1834-91) advocated uninterrupted immobilization in the treatment of fractures, and the Thomas splint which he developed is still in active use. *Sir Robert Jones* and *John Ridon* were great disciples of Thomas and are especially noted as excellent teachers. The discovery of the x-ray in 1895 was another stimulus to progress in orthopedics. Many new operative technics were developed; Lane of England and Lambotte of Belgium described open operations for reduction and internal fixation of fractures.

It was not until World War I that orthopedics gained recognition as a major specialty. Associated with the magnificent job of handling the battle casualties were such men as Jones, Osgood, Allison, Wilson, Goldthwait and Orr. The value of early and adequate surgical care with proper immobilization was established. Until World War I there were two definite schools of orthopedics—one school adhering closely to the principles of brace, manipulation and exercise treatment, and the other leaning toward surgical treatment of orthopedic diseases and deformity. Following the war, these two schools were fairly well co-ordinated.

Although the surgical technic of metal internal fixation of fractures was adequately described at the turn of the century, the complications of such a procedure were too great for general acceptance until the valuable contribution by Venable and Stuck in 1938, establishing the importance of using an inert metal which was nonelectrolytic in the host tissue. Intramedullary nails for internal fixation of long bones were first described in 1937 and since World War II have been adopted for use in most of the long bones.

NEUROSURGERY

This specialty had its inception in the latter part of the 19th century, building upon the basic contributions in neuroanatomy and neurophysiology accumulated over the preceding many years. The contributors are too numerous to mention but include such men as Magendie, Brown-Séquard, Fritsch and Hitzig, Flourens, Broca and Betz. Also of great importance were the great schools of neurology in the preneurosurgical era including the French school (Charcot *et al.*), the German school (Romberg *et al.*), the English school (Jackson *et al.*), and the American school (Mitchell *et al.*).

Early pioneers in neurosurgery include William Macewen, Sir Rickman Godlee, Sir Victor Horsley, Ernst von Bergmann, Fedor Krause, W. W. Keen and Robert Weir. However, the true founder of neurosurgery as a specialty was *Harvey Cushing* (1869-1939). Trained in the surgical technics of Halsted, Cushing was admirably suited to handle problems dealing with the tissues of the nervous system. On his return to Johns Hopkins in 1901, after a tour of Europe during which he visited Horsley, Sherrington, Kocher and many others, he had decided upon a career in neurologic surgery. In the ensuing 11 years at Johns Hopkins, he taught, adopted new surgical technics to the nervous system and experimented or reported upon increased intracranial pressure, visual fields, pituitary disorders, trigeminal neuralgia, tumors of the 8th cranial nerve and many other problems. Throughout his subsequent career at Harvard and Yale until his death in 1939, he did more than any other man to advance neurosurgery. Another great in neurosurgery followed close on the heels of Cushing in the person of *Walter E. Dandy* (1886-1946). Also Halsted trained, his contributions include classic studies on hydrocephalus and the circulation of the cerebrospinal fluid, the development of ventriculography (1918—while a surgical resident), classic monographs on tumors of the third and lateral ventricles, the treatment of intracranial aneurysm by isolation of the lesion with a silver clip. Other men in the early part of the 20th century who advanced the specialty were Elsberg of New York, Frazier in Philadelphia, and de Martel and Vincent in France. A dramatic advance in the field of diagnosis was made by Egas Moniz of Portugal in 1931 when he reported successful cerebral arteriography. More recently individuals such as Wilder Penfield, A. E. Walker and Donald Matson exemplify the continuing progress in this field.

PLASTIC SURGERY

The term "plastic surgery" was first used by Zeis as the title of his book, *Handbuch der Plastichen Chirurgie* in 1838. Although sporadic individuals throughout the history of medicine are remembered for their interest in and contributions to the field of corrective surgery of deformities, it was not until the first quarter of the 20th century that the field of plastic surgery as we know it today was developed. The principal founders were Vilray P. Blair of St. Louis and John Staige Davis of Baltimore, Harold Gillies of England, Erich Lexer of Germany and Hippolyte Morestin of France. The important role of plastic surgery became recognized in World War I.

Closely allied with plastic surgery is the development of skin grafting. Associated with the development of split-thickness grafts are Reverdin (1869), Ollier (1872), Thiersch (1886) and Blair. Full-thickness grafts were developed by Wolfe (1875) and Krause. Staige Davis described the use of "pinch grafts" in 1941. Skin flaps, though in use from early times for rhinoplasty, were first tubed by Harold Gillies in 1918.

CARDIOVASCULAR SURGERY

The history of vascular surgery dates back to antiquity with the ancient Antyllus operation for aneurysm in the first century A.D. However, the groundwork for the developments in the last few decades dates back only to the late 19th century. Eck and Heidenhain among others had done blood vessel suture and anastomoses, but their methods were not satisfactory. In 1896 Jaboulay and Brian performed vessel anastomoses and grafts in the dog, using through-and-through, intima-to-intima interrupted sutures. In the same year,

J. B. Murphy performed the first planned resection and anastomosis of an artery in the human. Alexis Carrel in 1908 with his method of triangulating the cut ends of the vessel before anastomosing, contributed significantly to the advancement of this field. In 1903 Rudolph Matas of New Orleans described his technic of endoaneurysmorrhaphy. In 1948 Gross successfully resected a coarctation of the aorta and bridged the defect with a homologous graft. In 1951 Dubost resected an abdominal aortic aneurysm and employed a homologous graft to bridge the defect. In more recent years plastic materials such as nylon, Orlon, Vinyon N, Dacron and Teflon have been employed in bridging the ends of arteries. In the past decade the advances in this field have been phenomenal due to Gross and Hufnagel, Blakemore, DeBakey, Cooley, Julian and Bahnson as well as many others.

The surgery of the venous system and the portal bed in particular was advanced by Eck, Blakemore, Whipple, Rousselot, Linton and others.

Experimental cardiac surgery was born in the laboratory of M. H. Block who in 1883 successfully sutured experimental cardiac wounds in rabbits. In 1896 Rehn of Frankfurt performed the first successful repair of a cardiac laceration in a human. Direct attack upon intrinsic lesions of the heart began with the finger dilatation of a stenotic aortic valve through the invaginated aortic wall by Tuffier in 1913. In the same year Doyen unsuccessfully attempted finger dilatation of a stenotic pulmonary valve. In 1925 Henry Souttar first successfully dilated digitally a stenotic mitral valve. Shortly thereafter the procedure was dropped because of the high mortality rate until 1945 when Bailey, Harken, Brock, Smithy and others began operating on the stenotic mitral valve with success. After Tuffier, the names of Smithy, Bailey and Merendino are associated with the surgery of aortic stenosis. Aortic insufficiency was attacked by Hufnagel in 1950 when he devised a plastic ball valve. The surgery of mitral insufficiency, in similar fashion is an epic of courageous trial, increasing experience and progressively more success.

Definitive surgery directed toward congenital heart lesions include the following: 1938, Gross successfully ligated a patent ductus arteriosus; 1944, Blalock and Taussig developed and performed the first subclavian to pulmonary artery anastomosis for tetralogy of Fallot; 1944, Crafoord first successfully resected a coarctation of the aorta; 1946, Pott performed an aorta-to-pulmonary-artery anastomosis for tetralogy of Fallot; 1948, Brock performed a pulmonary valvulotomy for pulmonic stenosis. Individuals associated with the development of closed repair of inter-atrial septal defects, utilizing a variety of ingenious methods, include Cohn (1947), Murray (1948), Swan (1950), Bailey (1952) and Gross (1952). Repair under direct vision, utilizing venous inflow occlusion and hypothermia was first performed by Bailey (1952) and Lewis (1952).

The most recent advance in cardiac surgery is the development of total cardiopulmonary bypass. Gibbon began experimenting with a pump oxygenator in 1937 in an attempt to develop a method to decrease the tremendous mortality associated with the Trendelenburg operation (extraction of a pulmonary embolus). The problems encountered were staggering. However, these difficulties were overcome, and he first used the complex apparatus to repair successfully an atrial septal defect in 1953. Andreason and Watson (1953) and Lillehei (1954) made a significant advance in this field with their new concept of cardiopulmonary bypass (azygos flow principle). In the past 5 years pump oxygenators have been developed and modified at various medical centers and are being used with success on many congenital lesions and with progressively more success on acquired valvular lesions.

BIBLIOGRAPHY

1. Allbutt, T. C.: The Historical Relations of Medicine and Surgery, New York, Macmillan, 1905.
2. Bauer, L. H. (ed.): Seventy-five Years of Medical Progress (1878-1953), Philadelphia, Lea & Febiger, 1954.
3. Billings, J. S.: History and Literature of Surgery in Dennis' System of Surgery, vol. 1, New York, Appleton, 1895.
4. Garrison, F. H.: An Introduction to the History of Medicine, ed. 4, Philadelphia, Saunders, 1929.
5. Hurwitz, A., and Degenshein, G. A.: Milestones in Modern Surgery, New York, Hoeber, 1958.
6. Killian, H., and Krämer, G.: Meister der Chirurgie und die Chirurgenschulen im Deutschen Raum; Stuttgart, Thieme, 1951.

Bibliographic Index

1533

Index